Drug	midazolam HCl	morphine sulfate	nalbuphine HCl	pentazocine lactate	pentobarbital Na	perphenazine	phenobarbital Na	prochlorperazine edisylate	promazine HCl	promethazine HCl	ranitidine HCl	scopolamine HBr	secobarbital Na	sodium bicarbonate	thiethylperazine maleate	thiopental Na
atropine sulfate	Y	P	Y	P	P	Y		P	P	P	Y	P				
butorphanol tartrate	Y	Y		Y	N	Y		Y		Y		Y			Y	
chlorpromazine HCl	Y	P		P	N	Y		P	P	P	N*	P				N
cimetidine HCl	Y	Y	Y	Y	N	Y		Y	Y	Y		Y	N			
codeine phosphate																
dexamethasone sodium phosphate											Y					
dimenhydrinate	N	P		P	N	Y		N	N	N	Y	P				N
diphenhydramine HCl	Y	P	Y	P	N	Y		P	P	P	Y	P				N
droperidol	Y	P	Y	P	N	Y		P	P	P		P				
fentanyl citrate	Y	P		P	N	Y		P	P	P	Y	P				
glycopyrrolate	Y	Y	Y	N	N			Y	Y	Y	Y	Y	N	N		N
heparin Na		N*		N			P(5)		N							
hydromorphone HCl	Y			Y	Y			N*		Y	Y	Y			Y	
hydroxyzine HCl	Y	P	Y	P	N	Y		P	P	P	N	P				
meperidine HCl	Y	N		P	N	Y		P	P	P	Y	P				N
metoclopramide HCl	Y	P		P		P*		P	P	P*	Y	P		N		
midazolam HCl		Y	Y		N	N		N	Y	Y	N	Y			Y	
morphine sulfate	Y			P	N*	Y		P*	P	P*	Y	P				N
nalbuphine HCl	Y			N				Y		N*	Y	Y			Y	
pentazocine lactate		P			N	Y		P	P*	P*	Y	P				
pentobarbital Na	N	N*	N	N		N		N	N	N	N	P		Y		Y
perphenazine	N	Y		Y	N			Y		Y	Y	Y			N	
phenobarbital Na											N					
prochlorperazine edisylate	N	P*	Y	P	N	Y			P	P	Y	P				N
promazine HCl	Y	P		P*	N			P		P		P				
promethazine HCl	Y	P*	N*	P*	N	Y		P	P		Y	P				N
ranitidine HCl	N	Y	Y	Y	N	Y	N	Y		Y		Y			Y	
scopolamine HBr	Y	P	Y	P	P	Y		P	P	P	Y					Y
secobarbital Na																
sodium bicarbonate				Y												N
thiethylperazine maleate	Y		Y			N				Y						
thiopental Na		N			Y			N		N		Y		N		

23rd Edition

Nursing2003

DRUG HANDBOOK®

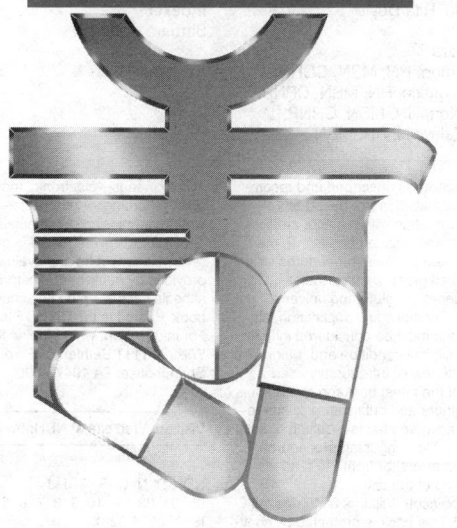

LIPPINCOTT WILLIAMS & WILKINS
A **Wolters Kluwer** Company

Philadelphia • Baltimore • New York • London
Buenos Aires • Hong Kong • Sydney • Tokyo

Staff

Publisher
Judith A. Schilling McCann, RN, MSN

Editorial Director
William J. Kelly

Clinical Director
Marguerite S. Ambrose, RN, MSN, CS

Art Director
Elaine Kasmer

Clinical Manager
Eileen Cassin Gallen, RN, BSN

Senior Associate Editor
Ann E. Houska

Drug Information Editor
Melissa M.Devlin, PharmD

Editors
Michael Anello, Rita Doyle

Clinical Editors
Shari A. Cammon, RN, MSN, CCRN;
Christine M. Damico, RN, MSN, CPNP;
Lori Mustoff Neri, RN, MSN, CRNP;
Kimberly A. Zalewski, RN, MSN

Copy Editors
Leslie Dworkin, Caryl Knutsen, Dolores
Connors Matthews, Leanne Sullivan,
Jenifer F. Walker

Designers
Arlene Putterman (senior art director),
Doug Smock (art director), Risa J. Clow,
Donald G. Knauss

Electronic Production Services
Diane Paluba (manager),
Joyce Rossi Biletz (technician)

Manufacturing
Patricia K. Dorshaw (manager), Beth
Janae Orr (book production manager)

Editorial Assistants
Danielle J. Barsky, Carol A. Caputo,
Arlene P. Claffee

Indexer
Barbara Hodgson

Visit our Web site at NDHnow.com

NDH-D N O S A J J
05 04 03 02 10 9 8 7 6 5 4 3 2
ISSN 0273-320X
ISBN 1-58255-170-7

Contents

iii

Autonomic Nervous System Drugs

Respiratory Tract Drugs

Gastrointestinal Tract Drugs

Hormonal Drugs

Drugs for Fluid and Electrolyte Balance

Hematologic Drugs

Antineoplastics

Immunomodulation Drugs

Ophthalmic, Otic, and Nasal Drugs

Topical Drugs

Contributors and consultants

At the time of publication, the contributors and consultants held the following positions.

Steven R. Abel, PharmD
Professor
Head, Department of Pharmacy
  Practice
Purdue University
West Lafayette, Ind.

Tricia M. Berry, PharmD, BCPS
Assistant Professor of Pharmacy
  Practice
St. Louis College of Pharmacy
St. Louis, Mo.

James Caldwell, PharmD
Clinical Pharmacy Professor
Anne Arundel Medical Center
Annapolis, Md.

Lawrence Carey, PharmD
Senior Medical Information
  Specialist
CoMed Communications
Philadelphia, Pa.

**Michele A. Danish, RPh, PharmD,
  BCPS**
Pharmacy Clinical Manager
St. Joseph Health Services
N. Providence, R.I.

Jennifer L. Defilippi, PharmD, BCPP
Clinical Pharmcy Specialist,
  Psychiatry
Central Texas Veterans Health Care
  System
Temple, Tex.

**Christopher A. Fausel, PharmD,
  BCPS, BCOP**
Clinical Pharmacist, Adult
  Hematology, Oncology, Bone
  Marrow Transplant
Indiana University Hospital
Indianapolis, Ind.

Tatyana Gurvich, PharmD
Clinical Pharmacologist
Glendale Adventist Family Practice
  Residency Program
Glendale, Calif.

AnhThu Hoang, PharmD
Medical Director
IntraMed Educational Group
New York, N.Y.

Mary Kate Kelly, PharmD
Owner
Health Content Consultants
Sanatoga, Pa.

Maureen Ketz, PharmD
Independent Consultant
North Royalton, Ohio

Michelle Kosich, PharmD
Clinical Pharmacist
Mercy Community Hospital
Havertown, Pa.

Kristy L. Lenz, PharmD
Associate Professor of Pharmacy
Medical University of South
  Carolina
Charleston, S.C.

Kristy H. Lucas, PharmD
Clinical Assistant Professor
West Virginia University
Charleston, W.Va.

Randall A. Lynch, RPh, PharmD
Assistant Director, Pharmacy
  Services
Presbyterian Medical Center
Philadelphia, Pa.

John S. Markowitz, PharmD, BCPP
Associate Professor
Department of Pharmaceutical
  Sciences
Medical University of South
  Carolina
Charleston, S.C.

George Melko, PharmD
Independent Consultant
West Chester, Pa.

William O'Hara, BS, PharmD
Clinical Coordinator
Thomas Jefferson University
  Hospital
Philadelphia, Pa.

Christine K. O'Neil, PharmD, BCPS
Associate Professor
Duquesne University
Pittsburgh, Pa.

Robert Lee Page II, PharmD, BCPS
Assistant Professor
University of Colorado Health
  Sciences Center
School of Pharmacy
Denver, Colo.

Christine Price, PharmD
Clinical Coordinator
Department of Pharmacy
Morton Plant Meare Health Care
Dunedin, Fla.

Barbara S. Wiggins, PharmD
Clinical Pharmacist, Cardiology,
  Clinical Instructor
University of Washington Medical
  Center
Seattle, Wash.

How to use *Nursing2003 Drug Handbook*

Nursing2003 Drug Handbook was created by pharmacists and nurses to provide the nursing profession with drug information that zeroes in on precisely what nurses need to know. With that goal clearly in mind, *Nursing2003 Drug Handbook* emphasizes clinical aspects of drugs without attempting to replace detailed pharmacology texts. In addition, the book is designed to make the content readily accessible and applicable in any clinical setting.

Features in this edition
The 2003 edition contains several features to enhance nursing knowledge and skills:
• New monographs on 39 new FDA-approved drugs.
• An "I.V. administration" section that provides step-by-step guidance on preparing and administering I.V. drugs.
• "Adjust-a-dose" logos that draw attention to dosage adjustments that may be needed in specific patient populations.
• Tables that show the route, onset, peak, and duration of each drug.
• An "Alert" logo that signals cautionary tips to help you avoid common medication errors, such as confusing one drug for another with a similar name.
• An "Effects on lab test results" section in every monograph.
• An "Interactions" section that includes interactions with other drugs, herbs, foods, and lifestyle behaviors.
• A guide to abbreviations in the front of the book that lists common abbreviations used throughout.
• An appendix on herbal medicines.
• Free NDH2003*Plus!* CD-ROM (inside the back cover) that lets you take 10 continuing education tests (and earn 40 contact hours), view and print complete drug monographs and customizable patient-teaching instructions for 200 commonly used drugs, and learn about potentially dangerous drug interactions.
• A link from NDH2003*Plus!* to NDHnow.com, the *Nursing2003 Drug Handbook* Web site that provides monthly drug updates, important drug news, patient teaching aids, and more.

Introductory chapters
Chapter 1 explains, in a general way, how drugs work. It also discusses adverse reactions and gives general guidelines about drug use in pregnancy and the presence of drugs in breast milk. Chapters 2 and 3 address the unique problems of administering drugs to children and elderly patients, respectively, and offer guidelines to minimize problems in these areas.

Therapeutic class chapters
Chapters 4 to 96 classify all drugs according to their approved therapeutic uses. Drugs with multiple therapeutic uses are classified according to their most common use; they are also listed (with a cross-reference to the major drug entry) in drug groups that share their secondary applications. For example, nadolol, a beta blocker, is described in the chapter that covers antianginals because its major therapeutic application is the management of angina pectoris. Because the drug is less commonly used to treat hypertension, it's also listed among the generic drugs grouped as antihypertensives, with a cross-reference to Chapter 20, Antianginals.

Such classification by therapeutic use offers several advantages. It helps you identify an unknown drug by its clinical application alone. It also identifies all other drugs that share the same use and provides easy comparison of their dosages and effects. In this way, it quickly identifies potential pharmacotherapeutic alternatives for patients who can't tolerate or who fail to respond to a particular drug.

Each chapter, representing a major therapeutic use, begins with an alphabetical list of the generic drugs described in the chapter. This is followed by a list of selected combination products in which these drugs are found. Specific information on each drug is arranged under the following headings: *Pregnancy risk category, Controlled substance schedule* (where applicable), *Available forms, Indications & dosages, I.V. administration*

Controlled substance schedules

Drugs regulated under the jurisdiction of the Controlled Substances Act of 1970 are divided into the following groups, or schedules:

● Schedule I (C-I): High abuse potential and no accepted medical use. Examples include heroin, marijuana, and LSD.

● Schedule II (C-II): High abuse potential with severe dependence liability. Examples include narcotics, amphetamines, and some barbiturates.

● Schedule III (C-III): Less abuse potential than schedule II drugs and moderate dependence liability. Examples include nonbarbiturate sedatives, nonamphetamine stimulants, anabolic steroids, and limited amounts of certain narcotics.

● Schedule IV (C-IV): Less abuse potential than schedule III drugs and limited dependence liability. Examples include some sedatives, anxiolytics, and nonnarcotic analgesics.

● Schedule V (C-V): Limited abuse potential. This category includes mainly small amounts of narcotics, such as codeine, used as antitussives or antidiarrheals. Under federal law, limited quantities of certain C-V drugs may be purchased without a prescription directly from a pharmacist if allowed under specific state statutes. The purchaser must be at least age 18 and must furnish suitable identification. All such transactions must be recorded by the dispensing pharmacist.

(where applicable), *Action, Adverse reactions, Interactions, Effects on lab test results, Contraindications, Nursing considerations,* and *Patient teaching.* (See *Controlled substance schedules* and *Pregnancy risk categories.*)

In each drug entry, the generic name is followed by an alphabetized list of its brand names. A brand name followed by an open diamond (◊) indicates an OTC drug. Canadian brands are designated with a dagger (†); Australian brands are followed by a double dagger (‡); and British brands are followed by a section mark (§). A brand name with no symbol is available in the United States, Canada, and possibly Australia and the United Kingdom (U.K.). The mention of a brand name in no way implies endorsement of that product or guarantees its legality.

Alcohol and tartrazine content
Many liquid drug preparations for oral use contain alcohol. Although the slight sedative effect that alcohol produces isn't harmful in most patients—and can sometimes be beneficial—alcohol ingestion can be undesirable and even dangerous. Oral drugs that contain alcohol should be given cautiously, if at all, to certain patients:

● those who concurrently take potent CNS depressants such as barbiturates

● those who take drugs that may produce a disulfiram-type reaction (such as chlorpropamide or metronidazole)

● those who take disulfiram as part of a treatment program for their alcoholism. Such patients, upon ingestion of alcohol, will develop a severe reaction that may include blurred vision, confusion, dyspnea, flushing, sweating, and tachycardia.

To help prevent inadvertent exposure to alcohol, the text signals alcohol content with a single asterisk (*) after each brand name of a liquid preparation that may contain it. In many of the preparations so marked, the alcohol content is small. Nevertheless, these drugs should be avoided by patients susceptible to adverse effects after exposure to alcohol.

Tartrazine dye, also known as FD&C Yellow No. 5, is a common coloring product in some foods and drugs. Usually harmless, it can provoke a severe reaction in susceptible persons. Because of this, most drug manufacturers have started to eliminate tartrazine from their products, but many drugs still contain it.

Tartrazine sensitivity occurs in about 1 in 10,000 people in the general population, somewhat more in people with asthma or aspirin sensitivity. The reason for this is unknown. The most common signs and symptoms of tartrazine sensitivity are urticaria, rhinorrhea, asthma, and angioedema. Acutely sensitive persons may develop allergic vascular purpura, tachycardia, dyspnea, and chest pain. These allergic reactions typically subside spontaneously with discontinuation of the drug but may require treatment with antihistamines or epinephrine.

Tartrazine may be present in yellow-colored drugs and those of many other colors, including turquoise, green, and maroon. This text signals tartrazine content with a double asterisk (**) after each brand name that may contain it. If you suspect tartrazine sensitivity in a patient receiving such a drug, inform the prescriber and contact the manufacturer to determine which dosage forms contain tartrazine.

Available forms

This section lists the preparations available for each drug (for example, tablets, capsules, solutions for injection) and specifies available dosage forms and strengths. Dosage strengths specifically available in Canada are designated with a dagger (†), those available in Australia with a double dagger (‡), and those in the U.K. with a section mark (§). Preparations that don't require a prescription are marked with an open diamond (◊).

Indications & dosages

This section lists general dosage information for adults, children, and elderly patients, as applicable. Dosage instructions reflect current clinical trends in therapeutics and can't be considered absolute or universal recommendations. For individual application, dosage instructions must be considered in light of the patient's clinical condition. The logo for "Adjust-a-dose" appears in this section.

I.V. administration

This section provides guidelines for reconstituting and mixing I.V. drugs, administering them safely, and storing them properly.

Action

This section succinctly describes the mechanism of action—that is, how the drug provides its therapeutic effect. For example, although all antihypertensives lower blood pressure, they don't all do so by the same pharmacologic process.

Also included, in table form, are the onset, peak (described in terms of effect or peak blood level), and duration of drug ac-

---

Pregnancy risk categories

The Food and Drug Administration has assigned a pregnancy risk category to each systemically absorbed drug based on available clinical and preclinical information. The five categories (A, B, C, D, and X) reflect a drug's potential to cause birth defects. Although drugs are best avoided during pregnancy, this rating system permits rapid assessment of the risk-benefit ratio should drug administration to a pregnant woman become necessary. Drugs in category A are generally considered safe to use in pregnancy; drugs in category X are generally contraindicated.

● A: Adequate studies in pregnant women have failed to show a risk to the fetus.

● B: Animal studies haven't shown a risk to fetus, but controlled studies haven't been conducted in pregnant women; or animal studies have shown an adverse effect on fetus, but adequate studies in pregnant women haven't shown a risk to fetus.

● C: Animal studies have shown an adverse effect on fetus, but adequate studies haven't been conducted in humans. The benefits from use in pregnant women may be acceptable despite potential risks.

● D: The drug may cause risk to human fetus, but the potential benefits of use in pregnant women may be acceptable despite the risks (such as in a life-threatening situation or a serious disease for which safer drugs can't be used or are ineffective).

● X: Studies in animals or humans show fetal abnormalities, or adverse reaction reports indicate evidence of fetal risk. The risks involved clearly outweigh potential benefits.

● NR: Not rated.

---

tion for each route of administration, if data are available or applicable. Values listed are for patients with normal renal function, unless specified otherwise.

Adverse reactions

This section lists adverse reactions to each drug by body system. The most common adverse reactions (those experienced by at least 10% of people taking the drug in clinical trials) appear in *italic* type; less common reactions are in roman type; life-threatening reactions are in ***bold italic*** type; and reactions that are common *and* life-threatening are in BOLD CAPITAL LETTERS.

Interactions

This section lists each drug's confirmed, *clinically significant* interactions with other drugs (additive effects, potentiated effects, and antagonistic effects); herbs; foods, with specific suggestions for avoiding dangerous drug or food interactions (for example, by reducing doses or monitoring food intake); and lifestyle (such as alcohol use or smoking). Drug interactions are listed under the drug that is adversely affected. For example, magnesium trisilicate, an ingredient in antacids, interacts with tetracycline to cause decreased absorption of tetracycline. Therefore, this interaction is listed under tetracycline. To check on the possible effects of using two or more drugs simultaneously, refer to the interaction entry for each of the drugs in question.

Effects on lab test results

This section lists increased and decreased levels, counts, and other values in laboratory test results, which may be caused by the drug's systemic effects.

Contraindications

This section lists any conditions, especially diseases, in which the use of the drug is undesirable.

Nursing considerations

This section lists recommendations for cautious use, followed by other useful information, such as monitoring techniques and suggestions for prevention and treatment of adverse reactions. Also included are suggestions for patient comfort and for preparing, administering, and storing each drug.

    An "Alert" logo provides cautionary tips to avoid medication errors, such as drug names that sound alike or are commonly confused.

Patient teaching

This section focuses on explaining the drug's purpose, promoting compliance, and ensuring proper use and storage of the drug. It also includes instructions for preventing or minimizing adverse reactions.

Photoguide to tablets and capsules

To make drug identification easier and to enhance patient safety, *Nursing2003 Drug Handbook* offers a 32-page full-color photoguide to the most commonly prescribed tablets and capsules. Shown in actual size, the drugs are arranged alphabetically for quick reference, along with their most common dosage strengths. Below the name of each drug, you'll find a cross-reference to information on the drug. Page references to the drug photos appear in boldface type in the index.

Guide to abbreviations

ACE	angiotensin-converting enzyme	GU	genitourinary
ADH	antidiuretic hormone	G6PD	glucose-6-phosphate dehydrogenase
AIDS	acquired immunodeficiency syndrome	H_1	histamine$_1$
ALT	alanine transaminase	H_2	histamine$_2$
AST	aspartate transaminase	HDL	high-density lipoprotein
AV	atrioventricular	HIV	human immunodeficiency virus
b.i.d.	twice daily	h.s.	at bedtime
BPH	benign prostatic hypertrophy	I.D.	intradermal
BSA	body surface area	I.M.	intramuscular
BUN	blood urea nitrogen	INR	International Normalized Ratio
cAMP	cyclic 3', 5' adenosine monophosphate	IPPB	intermittent positive-pressure breathing
CBC	complete blood count	IU	international unit
CK	creatine kinase	I.V.	intravenous
CMV	cytomegalovirus	kg	kilogram
CNS	central nervous system	L	liter
COPD	chronic obstructive pulmonary disease	LDH	lactate dehydrogenase
CSF	cerebrospinal fluid	LDL	low-density lipoprotein
CV	cardiovascular	M	molar
CVA	cerebrovascular accident	m^2	square meter
D_5W	dextrose 5% in water	MAO	monoamine oxidase
dl	deciliter	mcg	microgram
DNA	deoxyribonucleic acid	mEq	milliequivalent
ECG	electrocardiogram	mg	milligram
EEG	electroencephalogram	MI	myocardial infarction
EENT	eyes, ears, nose, throat	ml	milliliter
FDA	Food and Drug Administration	mm^3	cubic millimeter
		Na	sodium
g	gram	NaCl	sodium chloride
G	gauge	NSAID	nonsteroidal anti-inflammatory drug
GFR	glomerular filtration rate	OTC	over-the-counter
GGT	gamma-glutamyltransferase	PABA	para-aminobenzoic acid
GI	gastrointestinal	PCA	patient-controlled analgesia
gtt	drops		

P.O.	by mouth
P.R.	by rectum
p.r.n.	as needed
PT	prothrombin time
PTT	partial thromboplastin time
PVC	premature ventricular contraction
q	every
q.i.d.	four times daily
RBC	red blood cell
RDA	recommended daily allowance
REM	rapid eye movement
RNA	ribonucleic acid
RSV	respiratory syncytial virus
SA	sinoatrial
S.C.	subcutaneous
SIADH	syndrome of inappropriate antidiuretic hormone
S.L.	sublingual
T_3	triiodothyronine
T_4	thyroxine
TCA	tricyclic antidepressant
t.i.d.	three times daily
tsp	teaspoon
USP	United States Pharmacopeia
WBC	white blood cell

1

Drug actions, interactions, and reactions

Whenever you give any drug to a patient, it provokes a series of physicochemical events within the patient's body. The first event, when a drug combines with cellular drug receptors, is known as the drug action. What follows as a result of this action is the drug effect. Depending on the type of cellular drug receptors affected by a given drug, an effect can be local, systemic, or both. Usually, application to the skin produces a local effect. However, transdermal absorption can also produce systemic effects. Moreover, local effects can follow systemic absorption. For example, the antipeptic ulcer drug cimetidine acts solely by blocking histamine receptors in the parietal cells of the stomach. This is known as a local drug effect because the drug action is restricted to one area and doesn't spread to other parts of the body. However, diphenhydramine produces a systemic effect that blocks histamine receptors in widespread areas of the body. In short, local drug effects are specific to a limited number of organ systems, whereas systemic drug effects are generalized and affect different and diverse organ systems.

Drug properties
Drug absorption, distribution, metabolism, and excretion make up a drug's pharmacokinetic profile. This branch of pharmacology also describes a drug's onset of action, peak level, duration of action, and bioavailability.

Absorption
Before a drug can act in the body, it must be absorbed into the bloodstream—usually after oral administration, the most commonly used route. Before a drug contained in a tablet or capsule can be absorbed, the dosage form must disintegrate, resulting in smaller particles that can dissolve in gastric juices. Only after dissolving can a drug be absorbed. Most absorption of orally given drugs occurs in the small intestine, where the mucosal villi provide extensive surface area. Once absorbed and circulated in the bloodstream, the drug is bioavailable, or ready to produce a drug effect. Whether absorption is complete or partial depends on several factors: the drug's physicochemical effects, its dosage form, its route of administration, its interactions with other substances in the GI tract, and various patient characteristics. These same factors also determine the speed of absorption. Consequently, oral solutions and elixirs, which bypass the need for disintegration and dissolution, are usually absorbed more rapidly. Some tablets have enteric coatings that prevent disintegration in the acidic environment of the stomach; others may have coatings of varying thickness that delay release of the drug.

Drugs given I.M. must first be absorbed through the muscle into the bloodstream. Rectal suppositories must dissolve to be absorbed through the rectal mucosa. Drugs given I.V., which are injected directly into the bloodstream, are completely and immediately bioavailable.

Distribution
After absorption, a drug moves from the bloodstream into various fluids and tissues in the body—this is distribution. Individual patient variations can change the amount of drug distributed throughout the body. For example, in an edematous patient, a given dose must be distributed to a larger volume than in a nonedematous patient. Occasionally, a dose must be increased to account for this difference. Remember, the dose should be decreased when the edema is corrected. Conversely, in an extremely dehydrated patient, the drug will be distributed to a much smaller volume, so the dose must then be decreased. The total area to which a drug is distributed is known as volume of distribution. Patients who are particularly obese may present another problem when considering drug distribution. Some drugs—such as digoxin, gentamicin, and tobramycin—aren't well distributed to fatty tissue. Sometimes, dosing based on actual

body weight may lead to overdose and serious toxicity. In these cases, dosing must be based on lean body weight, or adjusted body weight, which may be estimated from actuarial tables that give average weight range for height.

Metabolism

Most drugs are metabolized in the liver. Hepatic diseases may affect one or more of the metabolic functions of the liver and may cause the normal metabolism of a drug to be increased or decreased. Closely monitor all patients with hepatic disease for drug effect and toxicity.

The rate at which a drug is metabolized varies with the individual. In some patients, drugs are metabolized so quickly that their blood and tissue levels prove therapeutically inadequate. In others, the rate of metabolism is so slow that ordinary doses can produce toxic results.

Excretion

The body eliminates drugs by metabolism (usually hepatic) and excretion (usually renal). Drug excretion refers to the movement of a drug or its metabolites from the tissues back into circulation and from the circulation into the organs of excretion, where they are removed from the body. Although most drugs are excreted by the kidneys, some drugs can be eliminated via the lungs, exocrine glands (sweat, salivary, or mammary), liver, skin, and intestinal tract. Drugs may also be removed artificially by direct intervention, such as peritoneal dialysis or hemodialysis.

Other modifying factors

An important factor that influences a drug's action and effect is its binding to plasma proteins, especially albumin, and other tissue components. Because only a free, unbound drug can act in the body, such binding greatly influences effectiveness and duration of effect. Protein-binding can be influenced by malnutrition, renal failure, and other protein-bound drugs. When protein-binding is altered, drug dosing may need to be modified.

The patient's age is another important factor. Elderly patients usually have decreased hepatic function, less muscle mass, diminished renal function, and decreased serum albumin. These patients need lower doses and sometimes longer dosage intervals to avoid toxicity. Neonates have underdeveloped metabolic enzyme systems and inadequate renal function. They need highly individualized dosages and careful monitoring.

Underlying disease can also markedly affect drug action and effect. For example, acidosis may cause insulin resistance. Genetic diseases, such as G6PD deficiency and hepatic porphyria, may turn drugs into toxins with serious consequences. Patients with G6PD deficiency may develop hemolytic anemia when given sulfonamides or a number of other drugs. A genetically susceptible patient can develop an acute porphyria attack if given a barbiturate. Also, patients with a highly active hepatic enzyme system, such as rapid acetylators, can develop hepatitis when treated with isoniazid from the rapid intrahepatic buildup of a toxic metabolite.

Drug administration issues

Factors related to the administration of a drug can also influence a drug's action in the body. The dosage form of a drug is important. Some tablets and capsules are too large to be easily swallowed by ill patients. Although an oral solution may be substituted, it produces higher drug blood levels than a tablet because the liquid is more easily and completely absorbed. When a potentially toxic drug (such as digoxin) is given, the increased amount absorbed could cause toxicity. Sometimes a change in dosage form requires a change in dosage itself.

Routes of administration aren't therapeutically interchangeable. For example, diazepam is readily absorbed orally but is slowly and erratically absorbed I.M. On the other hand, gentamicin must be given parenterally because oral administration yields blood levels inadequate to treat systemic infections.

Improper storage can alter a drug's potency. Most drugs should be stored in tight containers protected from direct sunlight and extremes in temperature and humidity that can cause them to deteriorate. Some may require special storage conditions, such as refrigeration. Caution patients not to store drugs in a bathroom because of the constantly changing environment.

The timing of drug administration can be important. Sometimes, giving an oral drug during or shortly after mealtime decreases the amount of drug absorbed. This isn't clinically significant with most drugs and may be desirable with irritating drugs such as aspirin. But penicillins and tetracyclines shouldn't be scheduled for administration at mealtimes because certain foods can inactivate them. If in doubt about the effect of food on a certain drug, check with a pharmacist.

Consider the patient's age, height, and weight. The prescriber will need this information when calculating the dosage for many drugs. It should be accurately recorded on the patient's chart. This chart should also include current laboratory data, especially renal and liver function studies, so the prescriber can adjust the dosage, as needed.

Watch for metabolic changes. Monitor the patient for physiologic changes (depressed respiratory function, acidosis, or alkalosis) that might alter drug effect.

Know the patient's medical history. Whenever possible, obtain a comprehensive family history from the patient or his family. Ask about past reactions to drugs, possible genetic traits that might alter drug response, and the current use of other drugs. Multiple drug therapy can cause drug interactions and dramatically change many drug effects.

Drug interactions
A drug interaction occurs when one drug given with or shortly after another drug alters the effect of one or both drugs. Usually the effect of one drug is increased or decreased. For instance, one drug may inhibit or stimulate the metabolism or excretion of the other, or free it for further action by releasing the drug from plasma protein-binding sites.

Combination therapy is based on drug interaction. For example, one drug may be given to potentiate the effects of another. Probenecid, which blocks the excretion of penicillin, is sometimes given with penicillin to maintain adequate blood levels of penicillin for a longer period. In many cases, two drugs with similar actions are given together precisely because of the additive effect that results. For instance, aspirin and codeine, both analgesics, are commonly given in combination because together they provide greater pain relief than either alone.

Drug interactions are sometimes used to prevent or antagonize certain adverse reactions. Hydrochlorothiazide and spironolactone, both diuretics, are commonly given in combination because the former is potassium-depleting, whereas the latter is potassium-sparing.

Not all drug interactions are beneficial. Multiple drugs can interact to produce effects that are undesirable and sometimes hazardous. Harmful drug interactions decrease efficacy or increase toxicity. For example, in a patient taking both diuretics and lithium, the diuretics may cause an increase in serum levels of lithium, resulting in lithium toxicity. This drug effect is known as antagonism. Drug combinations that produce these effects should be avoided, if possible. Another kind of inhibiting effect occurs when a tetracycline is given with calcium- or magnesium-containing drugs or foods (such as antacids or milk). These bind with tetracycline in the GI tract and cause inadequate absorption of tetracycline.

Adverse reactions
Any drug effect other than what is therapeutically intended can be called an adverse reaction. It may be expected and benign, or unexpected and harmful. Expected adverse reactions are sometimes called adverse effects. Drowsiness caused by antihistamines is an example of this. During hay fever season, a patient may have to contend with this drowsiness to get relief from hay fever symptoms. In such a case, the dosage may be adjusted up or down to balance therapeutic effects with adverse effects.

An adverse reaction may be tolerated to obtain a necessary therapeutic effect, or it may be hazardous and unacceptable and require discontinuation of the drug. Some adverse reactions subside with continued use. For example, the drowsiness caused by paroxetine and the orthostatic hypotension caused by prazosin usually subside after several days as the patient develops a tolerance to these effects. But many adverse reactions are dosage-related and lessen or disappear only if the dosage is reduced. Although most adverse reactions aren't therapeutically desirable, a few can be put to clinical use. An outstanding example of this is the drowsiness caused by diphenhydramine, which makes it clinically useful as a mild sedative.

Hypersensitivity, a term sometimes used interchangeably with drug allergy, is the result of an antigen-antibody immune reaction that occurs in the body when a drug is given to a susceptible patient. One of the most dangerous of all drug hypersensitivities is penicillin allergy. In its most severe form, penicillin anaphylaxis can rapidly become fatal.

Rarely, idiosyncratic reactions occur. These are highly unpredictable, individual, and unusual. One of the best known idiosyncratic drug reactions is aplastic anemia caused by the antibiotic chloramphenicol. This reaction appears in only 1 of 40,000 patients, but when it does occur it can be fatal. A more common idiosyncratic reaction is extreme sensitivity to very low doses of a drug, or insensitivity to higher-than-normal doses.

To deal with adverse reactions correctly, you need to be alert to even minor changes in the patient's clinical status. Such minor changes may be an early warning of pending toxicity. Listen to the patient's complaints about his reactions to a drug, and consider each objectively. You may be able to reduce adverse reactions in several ways. Obviously, dosage reduction can help. But, in many cases, so does a simple rescheduling of the same dose. For example, pseudoephedrine may produce stimulation that will be no problem if it's given early in the day. Similarly, the drowsiness that occurs with antihistamines or tranquilizers can be harmless if given at bedtime. Most important, your patient needs to be told what adverse reactions to expect, so that he won't become worried or even stop taking the drug on his own. Always advise the patient to report adverse reactions to the prescriber immediately.

Recognizing drug allergies or serious idiosyncratic reactions can sometimes be lifesaving. Ask each patient about the drugs he is taking or has taken in the past and what, if any, unusual reactions he experienced from taking them. If a patient claims to be allergic to a drug, ask him to tell you exactly what happens when he takes it. He may be calling a harmless adverse effect such as upset stomach an allergic reaction, or he may have a true tendency toward anaphylaxis. In either case, you and the prescriber need to know this. Of course, you must record and report clinical changes throughout the patient's hospital stay. If you suspect a severe adverse reaction, withhold the drug until you can check with the pharmacist and the prescriber.

Toxic reactions

Chronic drug toxicities are usually caused by the cumulative effect and resulting buildup of the drug in the body. These effects may be extensions of the desired therapeutic effect. For example, glyburide will normalize blood sugar when given in usual doses but can produce undesired hypoglycemia when given in higher doses.

Drug toxicities typically occur when drug blood levels rise as a result of impaired metabolism or excretion. For example, blood levels of theophylline rise when hepatic dysfunction impairs metabolism of the drug. Similarly, impaired renal function may cause digoxin toxicity because digoxin is eliminated from the body almost exclusively by the kidneys. Of course, excessive dosage can cause toxic blood levels. For instance, tinnitus is usually a sign that the safe dose of aspirin has been exceeded.

Most drug toxicities are predictable and dosage-related and are reversible once the dosage is adjusted. So, be sure to monitor patients carefully for physiologic changes that might alter drug effect. Watch especially for impaired hepatic and renal function. Warn the patient about signs of pending toxicity, and tell him what to do if a toxic reaction occurs. Also, be sure to emphasize the importance of taking a drug exactly as prescribed. Warn the patient about serious problems that could arise if he changes the dose or the schedule for taking it.

Drugs and pregnancy

Drug administration during pregnancy has been a source of serious medical concern and controversy since the thalidomide tragedy of the late 1950s when thousands of malformed infants were born after their mothers were prescribed this mild sedative-hypnotic while pregnant. To identify drugs that may cause such teratogenic effects, preclinical drug studies always include tests on pregnant laboratory animals. While these tests reveal gross teratogenicity, they don't establish absolute safety. This is because different animal species react to drugs in different ways. Consequently, animal studies can't reveal all possible teratogenic effects in humans. For example, the preliminary studies on thalidomide gave no warning of teratogenic effects, and it was subsequently released for general use in Europe.

What about the placental barrier? Once thought to protect the fetus from drug effects, the placenta isn't much of a barrier at all. Almost every drug a pregnant woman takes crosses the placenta and enters the fetal circulation, except for drugs with exceptionally large molecular structure, such as heparin, the injectable anticoagulant. By this standard, heparin could be used in a pregnant woman without fear of harming the fetus. However, even heparin carries a warning for cautious use during pregnancy. Conversely, just because a drug crosses the placenta doesn't necessarily mean it's harmful to the fetus.

Actually, only one factor—stage of fetal development—seems clearly related to exaggerated risk during pregnancy. During the first and the third trimesters of pregnancy the fetus is especially vulnerable to damage from maternal use of drugs. During these times, *all* drugs should be given with extreme caution.

The most sensitive period for drug-induced fetal malformation is the first trimester, when fetal organs are differentiating (organogenesis). During this time, all drugs except those labeled category A or B should be withheld unless this would jeopardize the mother's health. Even aspirin could harm the fetus at this sensitive time. So, strongly advise your patient to avoid *all* self-prescribed drugs during early pregnancy.

Fetal sensitivity to drugs is also of special concern during the last trimester. At birth, when separated from his mother, the neonate must rely on his own metabolism to eliminate any remaining drug. Because his detoxifying systems aren't fully developed, any residual drug may take a long time to be metabolized—and thus may induce prolonged toxic reactions. For this reason, drugs should be used only when absolutely necessary during the last 3 months of pregnancy.

Of course, in many circumstances, pregnant women must continue to take certain drugs. For example, a woman with a seizure disorder that is well controlled with an anticonvulsant should continue to take the drug during pregnancy. Similarly, a pregnant woman with a bacterial infection must receive antibiotics. In such cases, the potential risk to the fetus is outweighed by the mother's medical needs. The relative risk to the fetus is expressed by the drug's pregnancy risk category (see *Pregnancy risk categories,* page xi).

Following these general guidelines can prevent indiscriminate and harmful use of drugs in pregnancy:
● Before a drug is prescribed for a woman of childbearing age, ask the date of her last menstrual period and whether she may be pregnant. If a drug is a known teratogen (for example, isotretinoin), some manufacturers may recommend special precautions to ensure that the drug not be given to a woman of childbearing age until pregnancy is ruled out and that contraceptives are used throughout the course of therapy.
● Caution the pregnant patient to avoid all drugs except those essential to maintain the pregnancy or maternal health—especially during the first and the third trimesters.
● Topical drugs are equally subject to the same warning against their use during pregnancy. Many topically applied drugs can be absorbed in large enough amounts to be harmful to the fetus.
● When a pregnant patient needs a drug, the prescriber should order the safest possible drug in the lowest possible dose to minimize any harmful effect to the fetus.
● Instruct pregnant patients to check with their prescribers before taking any drug.

Drugs and lactation

Most drugs a breast-feeding mother takes appear in breast milk. Drug levels in breast milk tend to be high when drug levels in the blood are high—especially, right after taking each dose. Therefore, advise the mother to breast-feed *before* taking medication, not *after*.

Nevertheless, with few exceptions, a mother who wishes to breast-feed may continue to do so with her prescriber's permission. However, breast-feeding should be temporarily interrupted and replaced with bottle-feeding when the mother must take tetracyclines, chloramphenicol, sulfonamides (during the first 2 weeks postpartum), oral anticoagulants, drugs that contain iodine, or antineoplastics.

Caution the breast-feeding mother to protect her infant by not taking drugs indiscriminately. Instruct the mother to first check with her prescriber to be sure of taking the safest drug at the lowest dose.

Patient teaching

The following general guidelines will help to ensure that the patient receives the maximum therapeutic benefit and avoids adverse reactions, accidental overdose, and harmful changes in effectiveness.

● Tell the patient to store each drug in its original container, at room temperature (unless directed otherwise), and in places that aren't accessible to children or exposed to sunlight. Avoid storage in the bathroom medicine cabinet, in the kitchen close to heat, or in the glove compartment or trunk of an automobile, where extremes of temperature and humidity will cause deterioration.

● Instruct the patient to learn the brand and generic names of all drugs he is taking and to inform his regular prescriber about their use. Before a patient receives a drug, ask him to report unusual reactions experienced in the past, allergies to foods and other substances, special medical problems, and drugs taken over the last few weeks, including OTC medications or herbs.

● Advise the patient to always read the label before taking a drug, to take it exactly as prescribed, and never to share prescription drugs.

● Instruct the patient to check the expiration date before taking a drug.

● Warn the patient not to change brands of a drug without prescriber approval to avoid harmful changes in effectiveness. Certain generic preparations aren't equivalent in effect to brand-name preparations of the same drug.

● Caution the patient never to mix different drugs in a single container, remove a drug from its original container, or remove the label. Relying on memory to identify a drug and specific directions for its use is hazardous.

● Instruct the patient to safely discard drugs that are outdated or no longer needed and to keep discarded drugs out of the reach of children and pets.

● Advise the patient to inform medical personnel about use of drugs before undergoing surgery (including dental surgery).

● Stress the importance of informing the prescriber about adverse reactions experienced during drug therapy.

● Instruct the patient to call the prescriber, poison control center, or pharmacist immediately if he or someone else has taken an overdose. Tell the patient to keep these telephone numbers and other emergency numbers handy at all times. The patient should have syrup of ipecac available at home to induce vomiting but should use it only if instructed to do so by these professionals.

● Advise the patient to have all prescriptions filled at the same pharmacy so that the pharmacist can identify and warn against potentially harmful drug interactions. Also, tell the patient to inform the pharmacist and prescriber about any OTC medications or herbal medicines being taken.

● Tell the patient to have a sufficient supply of drugs when traveling. He should carry them with him and not stow them in his luggage.

2
Drug therapy in children

Providing drug therapy to children and adolescents is challenging. Physiologic differences between children and adults, including those in vital organ maturity and body composition, can significantly influence a drug's effectiveness.

Physiologic changes affecting drug action

A child's absorption, distribution, metabolism, and excretion processes undergo profound changes that affect drug dosage. To ensure optimal drug effect and minimal toxicity, consider these factors when giving drugs to a child.

Absorption

Drug absorption in children depends on the form of the drug, its physical properties, other drugs or substances such as food taken simultaneously, physiologic changes, and concurrent disease.

The pH of neonatal gastric fluid is neutral or slightly acidic and becomes more acidic as the infant matures, affecting drug absorption. For example, nafcillin and penicillin G are better absorbed in an infant than in an adult because of low gastric acidity.

Various infant formulas or milk products may increase gastric pH and impede absorption of acidic drugs. If possible, give a child oral drugs on an empty stomach.

Gastric emptying time and transit time through the small intestine—which is longer in children than in adults—can affect absorption. Also, intestinal hypermotility, as occurs in diarrhea, can diminish the drug's absorption.

A child's comparatively thin epidermis allows increased absorption of topical drugs.

Distribution

As with absorption, changes in body weight and physiology during childhood can significantly influence a drug's distribution and effects. In a premature infant, body fluid makes up about 85% of total body weight; in a full-term infant, 55% to 70%; in an adult, 50% to 55%. Extracellular fluid (mostly blood) constitutes 40% of a neonate's body weight, compared with 20% in an adult. Intracellular fluid remains fairly constant throughout life and has little effect on drug dosage.

Extracellular fluid volume influences a water-soluble drug's concentration and effect because most drugs travel through extracellular fluid to reach their receptors. Children have a larger proportion of fluid to solid body weight, so their distribution area is proportionately greater.

Because the proportion of fat to lean body mass increases with age, the distribution of fat-soluble drugs is more limited in children than adults. As a result, a drug's lipid or water solubility affects the dosage for a child.

Binding to plasma proteins

A decrease in albumin concentration or in intermolecular attraction between drug and plasma protein causes many drugs to be less bound to plasma proteins in infants than in adults.

Drugs that strongly bind plasma proteins may displace endogenous compounds, such as bilirubin or free fatty acids. Conversely, an endogenous compound may displace a weakly bound drug. For example, displacement of bound bilirubin can increase unbound bilirubin, which can lead to increased risk of kernicterus at normal bilirubin levels.

Because only an unbound, or free, drug has a pharmacologic effect, a change in ratio of a protein-bound to an unbound active drug can greatly influence its effect.

Several diseases and disorders, such as nephrotic syndrome and malnutrition, can decrease plasma protein and increase the concentration of an unbound drug, intensifying the drug's effect or producing toxicity.

Metabolism

A neonate's ability to metabolize a drug depends on the integrity of the hepatic enzyme system, intrauterine exposure to the drug, and the nature of the drug itself.

Certain metabolic mechanisms are underdeveloped in neonates. Glucuronidation is a metabolic process that renders most drugs more water soluble, facilitating renal excretion. This process isn't fully developed enough to permit full pediatric doses until the infant is 1 month old. For example, the use of chloramphenicol in a neonate may cause gray baby syndrome because the infant can't metabolize the drug. When using chloramphenicol, give neonates a decreased dosage (25 mg/kg/day) and periodically monitor blood levels of the drug.

Conversely, intrauterine exposure to drugs may induce precocious development of hepatic enzyme mechanisms, increasing the infant's capacity to metabolize potentially harmful substances.

Older children can metabolize some drugs (theophylline, for example) more rapidly than adults can. This ability may come from their increased hepatic metabolic activity. Doses larger than those recommended for adults may be required.

Also, preparations given concurrently to a child may alter hepatic metabolism and induce production of hepatic enzymes. Phenobarbital, for example, causes hepatic enzyme production and accelerates the metabolism of drugs taken with it.

Excretion
Renal excretion of a drug is the net effect of glomerular filtration, active tubular secretion, and passive tubular reabsorption. Because so many drugs are excreted in the urine, the degree of renal development or presence of renal disease can profoundly affect a child's dosage requirements. If a child can't excrete a drug renally, drug accumulation and toxicity may result unless the dosage is reduced.

Physiologically, an infant's kidneys differ from an adult's because they have a high resistance to blood flow and receive a smaller proportion of cardiac output. Infants have incomplete glomerular and tubular development and short, incomplete loops of Henle (a child's GFR reaches adult values between ages 2½ and 5 months; his tubular secretion rate may reach adult values between 7 and 12

months). Besides their low GFR, infants are also less able to concentrate urine or reabsorb certain filtered compounds. The proximal tubules in infants are less able to secrete organic acids, as well.

Both children and adults have diurnal variations in urine pH that correlate with sleep-awake patterns.

Special administration considerations

Biochemically, a drug displays the same mechanisms of action in all people. However, the response to a drug can be affected by a child's age and size as well as the maturity of the target organ. To ensure optimal drug effect and minimal toxicity, consider the following factors when giving drugs to children.

Adjusting dosages for children
When calculating children's dosages, don't use formulas that just modify adult dosages. Pediatric dosages should be based on either body weight (mg/kg) or body surface area (mg/m²). A child isn't a scaled-down version of an adult.

Reevaluate dosages at regular intervals to ensure necessary adjustments as the child develops. Although body surface area provides a useful standard for adults and older children, use the body weight method instead in premature or full-term infants. Don't exceed the maximum adult dosage when calculating amounts per kilogram of body weight (except with certain drugs such as theophylline, if indicated).

Obtain an accurate maternal drug history—prescription and nonprescription drugs, vitamins, and herbs or other health foods taken during pregnancy. Drugs passed into breast milk can also have adverse effects on the breast-feeding infant. Before a drug is prescribed for a breast-feeding mother, the potential effects on the infant should be investigated.

For example, sulfonamides given to a breast-feeding mother for a urinary tract infection appear in breast milk and may cause kernicterus in an infant with low levels of unconjugated bilirubin. Also, high levels of isoniazid appear in the breast milk of a mother who is taking this drug. Because this drug is metabolized by the liver, the infant's immature hepatic enzyme mechanisms can't metabolize the drug, and he may develop CNS toxicity.

Administering oral drugs

Consider the following when giving oral drugs to a child.

If the patient is an infant, give drug in liquid form, if possible. For accuracy, measure and give the preparation by oral syringe. Be sure to remove the cap of the syringe to prevent the infant from aspirating it. Never use a vial or cup. Lift the patient's head to prevent aspiration of the drug, and press down on his chin to prevent choking. You may also place the drug in a nipple and allow the infant to suck the contents.

If the patient is a toddler, explain how you're going to give him the drug. If possible, have the parents enlist the child's cooperation. Don't mix the drug with food or call it "candy," even if it has a pleasant taste. Let the child drink liquid drug from a calibrated medication cup rather than a spoon. It's easier and more accurate. If the preparation is available only in tablet form, crush and mix it with syrup. (Check with the pharmacist to verify that the tablet can be crushed without compromising its effectiveness.)

If the patient is an older child who can swallow a tablet or capsule by himself, have him place the drug on the back of his tongue and swallow it with water or fruit juice, as milk or milk products may interfere with drug absorption.

Administering I.V. infusions

In infants, use a peripheral vein or a scalp vein in the temporal region for I.V. infusions. The scalp vein is safe because the needle isn't likely to dislodge; however, the head must be shaved around the site. Temporary disfigurement may also result from the needle and infiltrated fluids. For these reasons, the scalp veins aren't used as commonly today as they were in the past.

The limbs are the most accessible insertion sites; however, because patients tend to move about, take these precautions:

● Protect the insertion site to prevent catheter or needle dislodgment.

● Use a padded arm board to reduce the risk of dislodgment. Remove the arm board during range-of-motion exercises.

● Place the clamp out of the child's reach. If extension tubing is used to allow the child greater mobility, securely tape the connection.

● Explain in simple terms to the child why he must be restrained while asleep, to allay anxiety and maintain trust.

During an I.V. infusion, monitor flow rates and check the child's condition and insertion site hourly, or more frequently if indicated.

Titrate the flow rate only while the patient is composed; crying and emotional upset can constrict blood vessels. Flow rate may vary if a pump isn't used. Flow should be adequate because some drugs (calcium, for example) can be irritating at low flow rates. Infants, small children, and children with compromised cardiopulmonary status are particularly vulnerable to fluid overload with I.V. drug administration. To prevent this problem and help ensure that a limited amount of fluid is infused in a controlled manner, use a volume-control device in the I.V. tubing and an infusion pump or a syringe. Don't place more than 2 hours of I.V. fluid at a time in the volume-control set.

Administering I.M. injections

I.M. injections are preferred when a drug can't be given by other parenteral routes and rapid absorption is necessary.

The vastus lateralis muscle is the preferred injection site in children younger than age 2. The ventrogluteal area or gluteus medius muscle can be used in older children. To select the correct needle size, consider the patient's age, muscle mass, nutritional status, and drug viscosity. Record and rotate injection sites. Explain to the patient that the injection will hurt but that the medication will help him. Restrain him during the injection, if needed, and comfort him afterward.

Administering topical drugs and inhalants

Consider the following when giving topical drugs or inhalants.

Use eardrops warmed to room temperature. Cold drops can cause considerable pain and possibly vertigo. To give drops, turn the patient on his side, with the affected ear up. If he is younger than age 3, pull the pinna down and back. If he is age 3 or older, pull the pinna up and back.

Avoid using inhalants in young children, because it's difficult to get them to cooperate. Before attempting to give a drug through a metered-dose nebulizer to an older child, explain the inhaler to him. Then have him hold the nebulizer upside down and close his lips around the mouthpiece. Have him exhale and pinch his nostrils shut. When he starts to inhale, release one dose of the drug into his mouth. Tell the patient to continue inhaling until his lungs feel full. Most inhaled drugs aren't useful if taken orally—if you doubt the patient's ability to use the inhalant correctly, don't use it. Such devices as spacers or assist devices may help; check with a pharmacist or the prescriber.

Use topical corticosteroids with caution because prolonged use in children may delay growth. When topical corticosteroids are used on the diaper area of infants, avoid covering this area with plastic or rubber pants, which act as an occlusive dressing and enhance systemic absorption.

Administering parenteral nutrition

Give I.V. nutrition to patients who can't or won't take adequate food orally and to patients with hypermetabolic conditions who need supplementation. The latter group includes premature infants and children who have burns or other major trauma, intractable diarrhea, malabsorption syndromes, GI abnormalities, emotional disorders (such as anorexia nervosa), and congenital abnormalities.

Before giving fat emulsions to infants and children, weigh the potential benefits against any possible risks. Fats—supplied as 10% or 20% emulsions—are given both peripherally and centrally. Their use is limited by the child's ability to metabolize them. For example, an infant or child with a diseased liver can't efficiently metabolize fats.

Some fats, however, must be supplied both to prevent essential fatty acid deficiency and to permit normal growth and development. A minimum of calories (2% to 4%) must be supplied as linoleic acid—an essential fatty acid found in lipids. In infants, fats are essential for normal neurologic development.

Nevertheless, fat solutions may decrease oxygen perfusion and may adversely affect children with pulmonary disease. This risk can be minimized by supplying only the minimum fat needed for essential fatty acid requirements and not the usual intake of 40% to 50% of the child's total calories.

Fatty acids can also displace bilirubin bound to serum albumin, causing a rise in free, unconjugated bilirubin and an increased risk of kernicterus. However, fat solutions may interfere with some bilirubin assays and cause falsely elevated levels. To avoid this complication, a blood sample should be drawn 4 hours after infusion of the lipid emulsion; or if the emulsion is introduced over 24 hours, the blood sample should be centrifuged before the assay is performed.

3

Drug therapy in elderly patients

If you're administering drugs to elderly patients, you'll want to understand the physiologic and pharmacokinetic changes that may alter appropriate drug dosage, cause common adverse reactions, or create compliance problems.

Physiologic changes affecting drug action

As a person ages, gradual physiologic changes occur. Some of these age-related changes may alter the therapeutic and toxic effects of drugs.

Body composition

Proportions of fat, lean tissue, and water in the body change with age. Total body mass and lean body mass tend to decrease, while the proportion of body fat tends to increase.

Body composition varies from person to person, and these changes in body composition affect the relationship between a drug's concentration and distribution in the body.

For example, a water-soluble drug such as gentamicin isn't distributed to fat. Because there's relatively less lean tissue in an elderly person, more drug remains in the blood.

GI function

In elderly patients, decreases in gastric acid secretion and GI motility slow the emptying of stomach contents and movement through the entire intestinal tract. Also, research suggests that elderly patients may have more difficulty absorbing drugs than younger patients. This is a particularly significant problem with drugs that have a narrow therapeutic range, such as digoxin, in which any change in absorption can be crucial.

Hepatic function

The liver's ability to metabolize certain drugs decreases with age. This decrease is caused by diminished blood flow to the liver—which results from an age-related decrease in cardiac output—and from the diminished activity of certain liver enzymes. When an elderly patient takes sleep medications such as flurazepam, the liver's reduced ability to metabolize the drug can produce a hangover effect the next morning.

Decreased hepatic function may cause more intense drug effects caused by higher blood levels, longer-lasting drug effects caused by prolonged blood levels, and a greater risk of drug toxicity.

Renal function

Although an elderly person's renal function is usually sufficient to eliminate excess body fluid and waste, the ability to eliminate some drugs may be reduced by 50% or more.

Many drugs commonly used by elderly patients, such as digoxin, are excreted primarily through the kidneys. If the kidneys' ability to excrete the drug is decreased, high blood levels may result. Digoxin toxicity can be relatively common in elderly patients who don't receive a reduced digoxin dosage to accommodate decreased renal function.

Drug dosages can be modified to compensate for age-related decreases in renal function. Aided by laboratory tests such as BUN and serum creatinine, prescribers may adjust drug dosages so the patient receives therapeutic benefits without the risk of toxicity. Observe the patient for evidence of toxicity. A patient taking digoxin, for example, may experience anorexia, nausea, vomiting, or confusion.

Special administration considerations

Aging is usually accompanied by a decline in organ function that can profoundly affect drug distribution and clearance. This physiologic decline is likely to be exacerbated by a disease or chronic disorder. Together, these factors can significantly increase the risk of adverse reactions and drug toxicity, as well as noncompliance. Be aware of these changes when giving a drug to an elderly patient.

Adverse reactions

Compared with younger people, elderly patients experience twice as many adverse drug reactions relating to greater drug consumption, poor compliance, and physiologic changes.

Signs and symptoms of adverse drug reactions—confusion, weakness, and lethargy—are often mistakenly attributed to senility or disease. If the adverse reaction isn't identified, the patient may continue to receive the drug. Furthermore, he may receive unnecessary additional drugs to treat complications caused by the original drug. This regimen can sometimes result in a pattern of inappropriate and excessive drug use.

Although any drug can cause adverse reactions, most of the serious reactions in the elderly are caused by relatively few drugs. Be particularly alert for toxicities resulting from diuretics, antihypertensives, digoxin, corticosteroids, anticoagulants, sleeping aids, and OTC drugs.

Diuretic toxicity

Because total body water content decreases with age, normal dosages of potassium-wasting diuretics, such as hydrochlorothiazide and furosemide, may result in fluid loss and even dehydration in an elderly patient.

These diuretics may deplete serum potassium, causing weakness in the patient, and they may raise blood uric acid and glucose levels, complicating gout and diabetes mellitus.

Antihypertensive toxicity

Many elderly people experience lightheadedness or fainting when taking antihypertensives, partly in response to atherosclerosis and decreased elasticity of the blood vessels. Antihypertensives can lower blood pressure too rapidly, resulting in insufficient blood flow to the brain, which can cause dizziness, fainting, or even a CVA.

Consequently, dosages of antihypertensives must be carefully individualized. In elderly patients, aggressive treatment of high blood pressure may be harmful. Treatment goals should be reasonable. Bringing blood pressure down to 135/90 mm Hg is appropriate, but it needs to be done more slowly in elderly patients than in younger patients.

Digoxin toxicity

As the body's renal function and rate of excretion decline, digoxin levels in the blood may build to toxic levels, causing nausea, vomiting, diarrhea, and—most seriously—cardiac arrhythmias. Try to prevent severe toxicity by monitoring serum levels and observing the patient for early signs and symptoms, such as appetite loss, confusion, or depression.

Corticosteroid toxicity

Elderly patients taking corticosteroids may experience short-term effects, including fluid retention and psychological effects ranging from mild euphoria to acute psychotic reactions. Long-term toxic effects such as osteoporosis can be especially severe in elderly patients who have been taking prednisone or related steroidal compounds for months or even years. To prevent serious toxicity, carefully monitor patients on long-term regimens. Observe them for subtle changes in appearance, mood, mobility, impaired healing, and fluid and electrolyte disturbances.

Anticoagulant effects

Elderly patients taking anticoagulants have an increased risk of bleeding, especially when they take NSAIDs at the same time, which is common. Observe the patient's INR carefully, and monitor him for bruising and other signs of bleeding.

Sleeping aid toxicity

Sedatives and sleeping aids such as flurazepam may cause excessive sedation or residual drowsiness. Keep in mind that ingestion of alcohol may exaggerate depressant effects, even if the sleeping aid was taken the previous evening. These drugs should be used sparingly in elderly patients.

OTC drug toxicity

When aspirin, aspirin-containing analgesics, and other OTC NSAIDs (such as ibuprofen, ketoprofen, and naproxen) are used in moderation, toxicity is minimal. However, prolonged ingestion may cause GI irritation—even ulcers—and gradual blood loss resulting in severe anemia. Prescription NSAIDs may cause similar problems. Although anemia from prolonged aspirin consumption can affect all age groups, elderly patients may be less able to compensate because of their already reduced iron stores.

Laxatives may cause diarrhea in elderly patients who are extremely sensitive to drugs such as bisacodyl. Long-term oral use of mineral oil as a lubricating laxative may result in lipid pneumonia from aspiration of small residual oil droplets in the patient's mouth.

Noncompliance

Poor compliance can be a problem with patients of any age. A significant number of hospitalizations result from noncompliance with a medical regimen. In elderly patients, factors linked to aging—such as diminished visual acuity, hearing loss, forgetfulness, the common need for multiple drug therapy, and socioeconomic factors—can combine to make compliance a special problem. About one-third of elderly patients fail to comply with their prescribed drug therapy. They may fail to take prescribed doses or to follow the correct schedule. They may take drugs prescribed for previous disorders, discontinue drugs prematurely, or indiscriminately use drugs that are to be taken as needed. Elderly patients may also have multiple prescriptions for the same drug and inadvertently take an overdose.

Review the patient's drug regimen with him. Make sure he understands the dose amount, the time and frequency of doses, and why he is taking the drug. Also, explain in detail if a drug is to be taken with food, water, or without any other drugs.

Help the patient avoid drug therapy problems by suggesting that he use drug calendars, pill sorters, or other aids to help him comply. Refer him to the prescriber or pharmacist if he needs further information.

4

Amebicides and antiprotozoals

atovaquone
chloroquine hydrochloride
(See Chapter 7, ANTIMALARIALS.)
chloroquine phosphate
(See Chapter 7, ANTIMALARIALS.)
metronidazole
metronidazole hydrochloride
pentamidine isethionate

COMBINATION PRODUCTS
HELIDAC: metrodiazole 250 mg (with povidone), tetracycline 500 mg, bismuth subsalicylate 262.4 mg (with povidone)

---

atovaquone
Mepron, Wellvone§

Pregnancy risk category C

AVAILABLE FORMS
Suspension: 750 mg/5 ml

INDICATIONS & DOSAGES
➤ **Acute, mild to moderate** *Pneumocystis carinii* **pneumonia in patients who can't tolerate co-trimoxazole—**
Adults: 750 mg P.O. b.i.d. with food for 21 days.
➤ **Prevention of** *P. carinii* **pneumonia in patients who can't tolerate co-trimoxazole—**
Adults and adolescents ages 13 to 16: 1,500 mg (10 ml) P.O. daily with food.

ACTION
Unknown. Appears to interfere with electron transport in protozoal mitochondria, inhibiting enzymes needed for the synthesis of nucleic acids and adenosine triphosphate.

Route	Onset	Peak	Duration
P.O.	Unknown	Unknown	Unknown

ADVERSE REACTIONS
CNS: *headache, insomnia,* asthenia, anxiety, dizziness.
CV: hypotension.

EENT: sinusitis, rhinitis.
GI: *nausea, diarrhea, vomiting,* constipation, *abdominal pain,* anorexia, dyspepsia, *oral candidiasis,* taste perversion.
Hematologic: anemia, *neutropenia.*
Metabolic: hypoglycemia, hyponatremia.
Respiratory: *cough.*
Skin: *rash,* pruritus, *diaphoresis.*
Other: *fever, pain.*

INTERACTIONS
Drug-drug. *Rifabutin, rifampin:* Decreases atovaquone's steady-state level. Avoid using together.

EFFECTS ON LAB TEST RESULTS
● May increase alkaline phosphatase, ALT, and AST levels. May decrease sodium and glucose levels.
● May decrease hemoglobin and neutrophil count.

CONTRAINDICATIONS
Contraindicated in patients hypersensitive to drug.

NURSING CONSIDERATIONS
● Drug has appeared in breast milk. Use cautiously in breast-feeding patients.
● Because drug is bound to plasma protein, use cautiously with other highly protein-bound drugs, and assess patient for toxicity when used together.
● *Alert:* Because of risk of concurrent pulmonary infections, monitor patient closely during therapy.

PATIENT TEACHING
● Instruct patient to take drug with meals because food significantly enhances absorption.

Reactions may be *common*, uncommon, *life-threatening*, or COMMON AND LIFE-THREATENING.

metronidazole
Apo-Metronidazole†, Flagyl,
Flagyl 375, Flagyl ER, Metric 21,
Metrogyl‡, Novonidazol†,
Protostat, Trikacide†

metronidazole hydrochloride
Flagyl IV RTU, Novonidazol†

Pregnancy risk category B

AVAILABLE FORMS
Capsules: 375 mg
Injection: 500 mg/100 ml ready to use
Oral suspension (benzoyl metronidazole):
200 mg/5 ml‡
Powder for injection: 500-mg single-dose
vials
Tablets: 200 mg‡, 250 mg, 400 mg‡,
500 mg
Tablets (extended-release): 750 mg

INDICATIONS & DOSAGES
➤ **Amebic liver abscess**—
Adults: 500 to 750 mg P.O. t.i.d. for 5 to
10 days.
Children: 30 to 50 mg/kg daily in three
divided doses for 10 days.
➤ **Intestinal amebiasis**—
Adults: 750 mg P.O. t.i.d. for 5 to 10 days;
then therapy with a luminal amebicide,
such as iodoquinol, paromyomycin, or
diloxanide.
Children: 30 to 50 mg/kg daily in three
divided doses for 10 days; then therapy
with a luminal amebicide, such as iodo-
quinol, paromyomycin, or diloxanide.
➤ **Trichomoniasis**—
Adults: 250 mg P.O. t.i.d. for 7 days or 2 g
P.O. in single dose. May give the 2-g dose
in two 1-g doses, each on the same day; 4
to 6 weeks should elapse between courses
of therapy.
Children: 5 mg/kg P.O. t.i.d. for 7 days.
➤ **Refractory trichomoniasis**—
Adults: 250 mg P.O. b.i.d. for 10 days. Or,
500 mg P.O. b.i.d. for 7 days.
➤ **Bacterial infections caused by anaerobic microorganisms**—
Adults: Loading dose is 15 mg/kg I.V. infused over 1 hour. Maintenance dose is
7.5 mg/kg I.V. or P.O. q 6 hours. First
maintenance dose should be given 6 hours

after loading dose. Maximum dose not to
exceed 4 g daily.
➤ **Prevention of postoperative infection
in contaminated or potentially contaminated colorectal surgery**—
Adults: 15 mg/kg I.V. infused over 30 to
60 minutes and completed about 1 hour
before surgery. Then, 7.5 mg/kg I.V. infused over 30 to 60 minutes at 6 and 12
hours after initial dose.
➤ **Bacterial vaginosis**—
Adults: 500 mg P.O. b.i.d. for 7 days.

I.V. ADMINISTRATION
● No preparation is needed for Flagyl IV
RTU.
● To prepare lyophilized vials of metronidazole, add 4.4 ml of sterile water for
injection, bacteriostatic water for injection, sterile normal saline solution for injection, or bacteriostatic normal saline solution for injection. Reconstituted drug
contains 100 mg/ml.
● Add contents of vial to 100 ml of D_5W,
lactated Ringer's injection, or normal saline solution for a final concentration of
5 mg/ml. The resulting highly acidic solution must be neutralized before administering.
● Carefully add 5 mEq sodium bicarbonate
for each 500 mg metronidazole; carbon
dioxide gas will form and may need to be
vented.
● Don't use equipment containing aluminum (needles, hubs) to reconstitute the
drug or to transfer reconstituted medication. Equipment that contains aluminum
will turn the solution orange; the potency
isn't affected.
● *Alert:* Infuse drug over at least 1 hour.
Don't give by I.V. push.
● Don't refrigerate the neutralized diluted
solution; precipitation may occur. If
Flagyl IV RTU is refrigerated, crystals
may form. These disappear after the solution warms to room temperature.

ACTION
A direct-acting trichomonacide and amebicide that works at both intestinal and extraintestinal sites. It's thought to enter the
cells of microorganisms that contain ni-
troreductase. Unstable compounds are

then formed that bind to DNA and inhibit synthesis, causing cell death.

Route	Onset	Peak	Duration
I.V.	Immediate	1 hr	Unknown
P.O.	Unknown	2 hr	Unknown

ADVERSE REACTIONS

CNS: vertigo, *headache,* ataxia, dizziness, syncope, incoordination, confusion, irritability, depression, weakness, insomnia, *seizures,* peripheral neuropathy.
CV: flattened T wave, edema, flushing, thrombophlebitis after I.V. infusion.
EENT: rhinitis, sinusitis, pharyngitis.
GI: abdominal cramping or pain, stomatitis, epigastric distress, *nausea,* vomiting, anorexia, diarrhea, constipation, proctitis, dry mouth, metallic taste.
GU: darkened urine, polyuria, dysuria, cystitis, dyspareunia, dryness of vagina and vulva, vaginal candidiasis, *vaginitis,* genital pruritus.
Hematologic: *transient leukopenia, neutropenia.*
Musculoskeletal: fleeting joint pains.
Respiratory: upper respiratory tract infection.
Skin: rash.
Other: fever, decreased libido, overgrowth of nonsusceptible organisms, especially *Candida.*

INTERACTIONS

Drug-drug. *Cimetidine:* Increased risk of metronidazole toxicity because of inhibited hepatic metabolism. Monitor patient closely.
Disulfiram: Acute psychoses and confusional states. Don't use within 2 weeks of last disulfiram dose.
Lithium: Increased lithium levels, resulting in possible toxicity. Monitor serum lithium levels closely.
Oral anticoagulants: Increased anticoagulant effects. Monitor PT and INR periodically.
Phenobarbital, phenytoin: Decreased metronidazole effectiveness; may reduce total phenytoin clearance. Monitor patient closely.
Drug-lifestyle. *Alcohol use:* Disulfiramlike reaction, including nausea, vomiting, headache, cramps, and flushing. Warn patient not to use together or for 3 days after completion of drug therapy.

EFFECTS ON LAB TEST RESULTS
● May decrease WBC and neutrophil counts.

CONTRAINDICATIONS
Contraindicated in patients hypersensitive to drug or other nitroimidazole derivatives and in patients in first trimester of pregnancy.

NURSING CONSIDERATIONS
● Metronidazole may interfere with the chemical analyses of aminotransferases and triglycerides, leading to falsely decreased values.
● Use cautiously in patients with history of blood dyscrasia or CNS disorder and in those with retinal or visual field changes. Also use cautiously in patients with hepatic disease or alcoholism and in those who take hepatotoxic drugs.
● Monitor liver function tests carefully in elderly patients.
● Drug is contraindicated in the first trimester of pregnancy. However, if pregnant patient must take drug for trichomoniasis, the 7-day regimen is preferred over the 2-g, single-dose regimen because the 2-g dose produces a high serum level that's more likely to reach the fetal circulation.
● Give oral form with meals.
● Observe patient for edema, especially if receiving corticosteroids; Flagyl IV RTU (ready to use) may cause sodium retention.
● Record number and character of stools when drug is used to treat amebiasis. Metronidazole should be used only after *Trichomonas vaginalis* infection has been confirmed by wet smear or culture, or *Entamoeba histolytica* has been identified. Asymptomatic sexual partners of patients being treated for *T. vaginalis* infection should be treated simultaneously to avoid reinfection.

PATIENT TEACHING
● Instruct patient to take oral form with food to minimize GI upset, although extended-release tablets should be taken at least 1 hour before or 2 hours after meals.

Reactions may be *common*, uncommon, *life-threatening*, or COMMON AND LIFE-THREATENING.

● Inform patient that sexual partners should be treated simultaneously to avoid reinfection.

● Instruct patient in proper hygiene.

● Tell patient to avoid alcohol or alcohol-containing drugs during therapy and for at least 3 days after therapy is completed.

● Tell patient that metallic taste and dark or red-brown urine may occur.

● Tell patient to report symptoms of candidal overgrowth.

---

pentamidine isethionate
NebuPent, Pentam 300

Pregnancy risk category C

AVAILABLE FORMS
Aerosol, injection: 300-mg vial

INDICATIONS & DOSAGES
➤ **Pneumocystis carinii pneumonia**—
Adults and children: 3 to 4 mg/kg I.V. or I.M. once daily for 14 to 21 days.
➤ **Prevention of P. carinii pneumonia in high-risk patients**—
Adults: 300 mg by inhalation using a Respirgard II nebulizer once q 4 weeks.

I.V. ADMINISTRATION
● Reconstitute drug with 3 ml sterile water for injection; then dilute in 50 to 250 ml D₅W. Infuse over at least 60 minutes.
● *Alert:* To minimize risk of hypotension, infuse drug slowly with patient lying down. Closely monitor blood pressure.

ACTION
Unknown. Believed to interfere with biosynthesis of DNA, RNA, phospholipids, and proteins in susceptible organisms.

Route	Onset	Peak	Duration
I.M., inhalation	Unknown	0.5 hr	Unknown
I.V.	Unknown	1 hr	Unknown

ADVERSE REACTIONS
CNS: confusion, hallucinations, *fatigue, dizziness,* headache.
CV: *hypotension, ventricular tachycardia, chest pain,* edema.

EENT: burning in throat (with inhaled form), *pharyngitis.*
GI: *nausea, metallic taste, decreased appetite, vomiting,* diarrhea, abdominal pain, anorexia, *pancreatitis.*
GU: *acute renal failure.*
Hematologic: *leukopenia, thrombocytopenia,* anemia.
Metabolic: *hypoglycemia,* hyperglycemia, hypocalcemia.
Musculoskeletal: myalgia.
Respiratory: *cough, bronchospasm, shortness of breath,* pneumothorax, *congestion.*
Skin: rash, *Stevens-Johnson syndrome.*
Other: *night sweats, chills, sterile abscess, pain, induration at injection site.*

INTERACTIONS
Drug-drug. *Aminoglycosides, amphotericin B, capreomycin, cisplatin, methoxyflurane, polymyxin B, vancomycin:* Increased risk of nephrotoxicity. Monitor patient closely.
Antineoplastics: Additive bone marrow suppression. Use together cautiously.

EFFECTS ON LAB TEST RESULTS
● May increase BUN, creatinine, and potassium levels. May increase or decrease glucose levels.
● May decrease WBC and platelet counts, hemoglobin, and hematocrit.

CONTRAINDICATIONS
Contraindicated in patients with history of anaphylactic reaction to drug.

NURSING CONSIDERATIONS
● Use cautiously in patients with hypertension, hypotension, hypoglycemia, hypocalcemia, leukopenia, thrombocytopenia, anemia, diabetes, pancreatitis, Stevens-Johnson syndrome, or hepatic or renal dysfunction.
● Use cautiously in breast-feeding patients.
● Give aerosol form only by Respirgard II nebulizer. Dosage recommendations are based on particle size and delivery rate of this device. To give aerosol, mix contents of one vial in 6 ml sterile water for injection. Don't use normal saline solution. Don't mix with other drugs.

● Don't use low-pressure (less than 20 pounds per square inch [psi]) compressors. The flow rate should be 5 to 7 L/minute from a 40- to 50-psi air or oxygen source.

● For I.M. injection, reconstitute drug with 3 ml sterile water for a solution containing 100 mg/ml; administer deeply. Expect patient to report pain and induration at injection site. Rotate injection sites.

● *Alert:* Monitor glucose, calcium, creatinine, and BUN levels daily. After parenteral administration, glucose level may decrease initially; hypoglycemia may be severe in 5% to 10% of patients. After several months of therapy, this may be followed by hyperglycemia and type 1 diabetes mellitus, which may be permanent because of pancreatic cell damage.

● In patients with AIDS, pentamidine may produce less severe adverse reactions than co-trimoxazole.

PATIENT TEACHING

● Instruct patient to use the aerosol device until the chamber is empty, which may take up to 45 minutes.

● Warn patient that I.M. injection is painful.

● Instruct patient to complete the full course of pentamidine therapy, even if feeling better.

Reactions may be *common*, uncommon, *life-threatening*, or **COMMON AND LIFE-THREATENING.**

5
Anthelmintics

mebendazole
pyrantel pamoate

COMBINATION PRODUCTS
None.

---

mebendazole
Vermox

Pregnancy risk category C

AVAILABLE FORMS
Tablets (chewable): 100 mg

INDICATIONS & DOSAGES
➤ **Pinworm—**
Adults and children older than age 2:
100 mg P.O. as a single dose; repeated if
infestation persists 2 to 3 weeks later.
➤ **Roundworm, whipworm, and hook-worm—**
Adults and children older than age 2:
100 mg P.O. b.i.d. for 3 days; repeated if
infestation persists 3 weeks later.

ACTION
Selectively and irreversibly inhibits uptake
of glucose and other nutrients in susceptible helminths.

Route	Onset	Peak	Duration
P.O.	Unknown	2-4 hr	Variable

ADVERSE REACTIONS
CNS: *seizures.*
GI: occasional, transient abdominal pain
and diarrhea in massive infestation and
during expulsion of worms.
Skin: urticaria.
Other: fever.

INTERACTIONS
Drug-drug. *Carbamazepine, hydantoins:*
Reduced plasma mebendazole levels,
which may decrease drug's effect. Monitor
patient closely.
Cimetidine: Increased plasma mebendazole levels. Monitor patient closely.

EFFECTS ON LAB TEST RESULTS
None reported.

CONTRAINDICATIONS
Contraindicated in patients hypersensitive
to drug.

NURSING CONSIDERATIONS
● Tablets may be chewed, swallowed
whole, or crushed and mixed with food.
● Administer drug to all family members,
as prescribed, to decrease risk of spread-
ing the infestation.
● Dietary restrictions, laxatives, or enemas
aren't necessary.
● Safe use in children younger than age 2
hasn't been established.

PATIENT TEACHING
● Teach patient about personal hygiene,
especially good hand-washing technique.
Advise him to refrain from preparing food
for others.
● To avoid reinfestation, teach patient to
wash perianal area daily, change undergarments and bedclothes daily, and wash
hands and clean fingernails before meals
and after bowel movements.

---

pyrantel pamoate
Antiminth, Combantrin†,
Pin-Rid◇, Pin-X◇, Reese's
Pinworm◇

Pregnancy risk category C

AVAILABLE FORMS
Liquid: 50 mg pyrantel (as pamoate)/ml
Oral suspension: 50 mg/ml
Tablets: 62.5 mg

INDICATIONS & DOSAGES
➤ **Roundworm and pinworm—**
Adults and children age 2 and older:
11 mg/kg P.O. as a single dose. Maximum
dose is 1 g. For pinworm, repeat dose in 2
weeks.

---

*Liquid contains alcohol. **May contain tartrazine. †Canada ‡Australia §U.K. ◇OTC

ACTION
Blocks neuromuscular action, paralyzing the worm and causing its expulsion by normal peristalsis.

Route	Onset	Peak	Duration
P.O.	Variable	1-3 hr	Variable

ADVERSE REACTIONS
CNS: headache, dizziness, drowsiness, insomnia, weakness.
GI: anorexia, nausea, vomiting, gastralgia, abdominal cramps, diarrhea, tenesmus.
Skin: rash.
Other: fever.

INTERACTIONS
Drug-drug. *Piperazine salts:* May antagonize drug effects. Don't give together.

EFFECTS ON LAB TEST RESULTS
• May increase AST level.

CONTRAINDICATIONS
Contraindicated in patients hypersensitive to drug.

NURSING CONSIDERATIONS
• Use cautiously in patients with severe malnutrition or anemia and in patients with hepatic dysfunction.
• Dietary restrictions, laxatives, or enemas aren't needed.
• Drug should be given to all family members.

PATIENT TEACHING
• Inform patient that pyrantel may be taken with food, milk, or fruit juices. Tell him to shake suspension well.
• Teach patient about personal hygiene, especially good hand-washing technique. To avoid reinfestation, teach patient to wash perianal area daily, to change undergarments and bedclothes daily, and to wash hands and clean fingernails before meals and after bowel movements.
• Advise patient to refrain from preparing food for others.
• Tell patient to take entire dosage as prescribed.

Reactions may be *common*, uncommon, *life-threatening*, or COMMON AND LIFE-THREATENING.

6

Antifungals

amphotericin B
amphotericin B cholesteryl
   sulfate complex
amphotericin B lipid complex
amphotericin B liposomal
caspofungin acetate
fluconazole
flucytosine
griseofulvin microsize
griseofulvin ultramicrosize
itraconazole
ketoconazole
nystatin
terbinafine hydrochloride

COMBINATION PRODUCTS
None.

---

amphotericin B
Amphocin, Amphotericin B for
Injection, Fungilin‡, Fungizone
Intravenous

Pregnancy risk category B

AVAILABLE FORMS
Lozenges: 10 mg‡
Oral suspension: 100 mg/ml‡
Powder for injection: 50 mg
Tablets: 100 mg‡

INDICATIONS & DOSAGES
➤ **Systemic fungal infections (histoplasmosis, coccidioidomycosis, blastomycosis, cryptococcosis, disseminated candidiasis, aspergillosis, phycomycosis, zygomycosis), meningitis—**
Adults: Initially, test dose of 1 mg in 20 ml of D₅W infused I.V. over 20 to 30 minutes. If tolerated, daily dose is then initiated as 0.25 to 0.3 mg/kg daily by slow I.V. infusion (0.1 mg/ml) over 2 to 6 hours. Dose is gradually increased to maximum of 1.5 mg/kg daily in potentially fatal infections. If drug is discontinued for 1 week or longer, it's resumed with initial dose and increased gradually.

➤ **Infections of the GI tract caused by** *Candida albicans—*
Adults: 100 mg P.O. q.i.d. for 2 weeks.
➤ **Oral and perioral candidal infections—**
Adults: 1 lozenge q.i.d. for 7 to 14 days.
Lozenge should dissolve slowly.

I.V. ADMINISTRATION
● After you give initial test dose, monitor patient's pulse, respiratory rate, temperature, and blood pressure for at least 4 hours.
● Use an infusion pump and in-line filter with mean pore diameter larger than 1 micron. Rapid infusion may cause CV collapse.
● Choose I.V. sites in distal veins. If veins become thrombosed, alternate administration sites.
● Monitor vital signs every 30 minutes; fever, shaking chills, and hypotension may appear 1 to 2 hours after start of I.V. infusion and should subside within 4 hours of stopping drug.
● Give antibiotics separately; don't mix or piggyback them with amphotericin B.
● Amphotericin B appears to be compatible with limited amounts of heparin sodium, hydrocortisone sodium succinate, and methylprednisolone sodium succinate.
● Store the dry form at 36° to 46° F (2° to 8° C). Protect from light. Reconstitute amphotericin B with 10 ml of sterile water. To avoid precipitation, don't mix with solutions containing sodium chloride, other electrolytes, or bacteriostatic products such as benzyl alcohol. Don't use if solution contains precipitate or foreign matter.
● Reconstituted solution is stable for 1 week under refrigeration or 24 hours at room temperature. It has 8-hour stability in room light.

ACTION
Binds to sterol in the fungal cell membrane, altering cell permeability and allowing leakage of intracellular compo-

---

nents. Fungal cell death occurs in part as a result of membrane permeability changes.

Route	Onset	Peak	Duration
I.V.	Immediate	Unknown	Unknown
P.O.	Unknown	Unknown	Unknown

ADVERSE REACTIONS
CNS: *headache,* peripheral neuropathy, transient vertigo, *malaise,* **seizures.**
CV: hypotension, **arrhythmias, asystole,** hypertension, tachycardia, flushing, *phlebitis, thrombophlebitis.*
EENT: hearing loss, tinnitus, blurred vision, diplopia.
GI: *anorexia, nausea, vomiting, dyspepsia, diarrhea, epigastric pain, cramping,* melena, steatorrhea, **hemorrhagic gastroenteritis.**
GU: *abnormal renal function with hypokalemia, azotemia, hyposthenuria, renal tubular acidosis, nephrocalcinosis;* **permanent renal impairment;** anuria; oliguria.
Hematologic: *normochromic anemia, normocytic anemia,* **thrombocytopenia, leukopenia, agranulocytosis,** eosinophilia, leukocytosis.
Hepatic: *hepatitis,* jaundice, **acute liver failure.**
Metabolic: *weight loss,* hypokalemia, hypoglycemia, hyperglycemia, hyperuricemia, hypomagnesemia.
Musculoskeletal: arthralgia, myalgia.
Respiratory: dyspnea, tachypnea, **bronchospasm,** wheezing.
Skin: **maculopapular rash,** pruritus.
Other: tissue damage with extravasation, *fever, chills, generalized pain,* **anaphylactoid reaction,** pain at injection site.

INTERACTIONS
Drug-drug. *Antineoplastics such as mechlorethamine:* May cause renal toxicity, bronchospasm, and hypotension. Use together cautiously.
Cardiac glycosides: Increased risk of digitalis toxicity in potassium-depleted patients. Monitor patient closely.
Corticosteroids: Enhanced potassium depletion. Monitor potassium levels.
Flucytosine: Synergistic effect; may cause increased toxicity of flucytosine. Monitor patient closely.

Leukocyte transfusions: Risk of pulmonary reactions, such as acute dyspnea, tachypnea, hypoxemia, hemoptysis, and interstitial infiltrates. Use together cautiously; separate administration times as much as possible and monitor pulmonary function if drugs are used together.
Nephrotoxic drugs such as antibiotics, pentamidine: May cause additive renal toxicity. Use together cautiously.
Thiazides: May intensify electrolyte depletion, especially potassium. Monitor patient for hypokalemia.
Drug-herb. *Gossypol:* Enhanced or increased risk of renal toxicity when given together. Discourage use together.

EFFECTS ON LAB TEST RESULTS
• May increase nitrogenous compounds (urea), uric acid, BUN, creatinine, alkaline phosphatase, ALT, AST, GGT, LDH, and bilirubin levels. May decrease potassium and magnesium levels. May increase or decrease glucose levels.
• May decrease hemoglobin and platelet and granulocyte counts. May increase or decrease WBC and eosinophil counts.

CONTRAINDICATIONS
Contraindicated in patients hypersensitive to drug.

NURSING CONSIDERATIONS
• Use cautiously in patients with impaired renal function.
• Because of drug's dangerous adverse effects, it's used primarily for treatment of patients with progressive and potentially fatal fungal infections.
• Infusion-related reactions, including fever, shaking chills, hypotension, anorexia, nausea, vomiting, headache, dyspnea, and tachypnea, may occur 1 to 3 hours after starting infusion.
•*Alert:* Different amphotericin B preparations aren't interchangeable and dosages will vary.
•*Alert:* To reduce severe adverse effects, patient may receive premedication with antipyretics, antihistamines, antiemetics, or small doses of corticosteroids and be given an alternate-day schedule. For severe reactions, discontinue drug and notify prescriber.

Reactions may be *common,* uncommon, *life-threatening,* or COMMON AND LIFE-THREATENING.

• Infusion-related reactions occur most frequently with initial doses and usually lessen with subsequent doses.

• Monitor fluid intake and output; report change in urine appearance or volume. Monitor BUN and creatinine levels or creatinine clearance at least weekly. Kidney damage may be reversible if drug is stopped at first sign of dysfunction.

• Hydration before infusion may reduce risk of neprotoxicity.

• Obtain liver and renal function studies weekly, if ordered. Drug may be stopped if alkaline phosphatase or bilirubin levels increase. If BUN level exceeds 40 mg/100 ml or if creatinine level exceeds 3 mg/100 ml, prescriber may reduce or stop drug until renal function improves. Monitor CBC weekly.

• Monitor potassium levels closely, and report signs of hypokalemia. Hypokalemia occurs commonly and can be life-threatening. Potassium supplementation may be needed.

• Check calcium and magnesium levels twice weekly.

• Drug is potentially ototoxic. Report evidence of hearing loss, tinnitus, vertigo, or unsteady gait.

PATIENT TEACHING
• Warn patient of possible discomfort at I.V. site and of other potential adverse reactions. Instruct patient to report signs and symptoms of hypersensitivity immediately.

• Inform patient that therapy may take several months. Stress importance of compliance and recommended follow-up.

amphotericin B cholesteryl sulfate complex
Amphocil§, Amphotec

Pregnancy risk category B

AVAILABLE FORMS
Injection: 50 mg/20 ml, 100 mg/50 ml

INDICATIONS & DOSAGES
➤ **Invasive aspergillosis in patients for whom renal impairment or unacceptable toxicity precludes use of amphotericin B deoxycholate in effective doses and in those with invasive aspergillosis for whom prior amphotericin B deoxycholate therapy has failed—**
Adults and children: 3 to 4 mg/kg/day I.V. Dilute in D_5W and administer by continuous infusion at 1 mg/kg/hour. Perform a test dose before beginning new course of treatment; infuse 10 ml of final preparation containing 1.6 to 8.3 mg of drug over 15 to 30 minutes and monitor patient for next 30 minutes. Can shorten infusion time to 2 hours or lengthen infusion time based on patient tolerance.

I.V. ADMINISTRATION
• Reconstitute 50-mg vial with rapid addition of 10 ml of sterile water for injection, and 100-mg vial with rapid addition of 20 ml sterile water. Shake vial gently. Don't use diluent other than sterile water for injection.

• Reconstituted drug is clear or opalescent liquid and is stable for 24 hours when refrigerated. Discard partially used vials. Don't administer undiluted drug.

• For infusion, add to bag of D_5W to final concentration of about 0.6 mg/ml. Don't reconstitute lyophilized powder with saline or dextrose solutions, or mix reconstituted liquid with saline or electrolytes. The presence of a bacteriostatic product in the solution may cause precipitation of drug. Don't use a filter, including an in-line filter, and don't freeze.

• Infuse drug over at least 2 hours. Don't mix with other drugs. If administered through an existing I.V. line, flush line with D_5W before infusion or use a separate line.

• Store unopened vials at room temperature.

ACTION
Binds to sterols in cell membranes of sensitive fungi, resulting in leakage of intracellular contents and causing cell death from changes in membrane permeability. The spectrum of activity includes *Aspergillus fumigatus, Candida albicans, Coccidioides immitis,* and *Cryptococcus neoformans.*

Route	Onset	Peak	Duration
I.V.	Unknown	3 hr	Unknown

ADVERSE REACTIONS
CNS: abnormal thinking, anxiety, agitation, confusion, depression, dizziness, hallucinations, headache, hypertonia, neuropathy, nervousness, paresthesia, psychosis, *seizures,* somnolence, speech disorder, stupor, asthenia.
CV: *arrhythmias, atrial fibrillation, bradycardia, cardiac arrest, heart failure, hemorrhage,* hypertension, *hypotension,* phlebitis, chest pain, orthostatic hypotension, *shock, supraventricular tachycardia,* syncope, *tachycardia,* vasodilation, *ventricular extrasystoles,* edema.
EENT: amblyopia, deafness, epistaxis, eye hemorrhage, pharyngitis, tinnitus, rhinitis, sinusitis.
GI: anorexia, diarrhea, dry mouth, *GI hemorrhage,* gingivitis, glossitis, hematemesis, melena, mouth ulceration, *nausea,* oral candidiasis, stomatitis, *vomiting,* abdominal pain.
GU: albuminuria, dysuria, glycosuria, hematuria, oliguria, urinary incontinence or urine retention, *renal failure.*
Hematologic: anemia, coagulation disorders, ecchymosis, hypochromic anemia, leukocytosis, *leukopenia,* petechiae, *thrombocytopenia.*
Hepatic: *hyperbilirubinemia,* jaundice, *abnormal liver function test results, hepatic failure.*
Metabolic: weight changes, acidosis, dehydration, *hypokalemia,* hypocalcemia, hypoglycemia, hypoproteinemia, hyperglycemia, hypervolemia, hypophosphatemia, hyponatremia, hyperkalemia, hyperlipemia, hypernatremia, hypomagnesemia.
Musculoskeletal: arthralgia, myalgia, neck or back pain.
Respiratory: *apnea,* asthma, dyspnea, hemoptysis, hyperventilation, hypoxia, increased cough, lung or respiratory disorders, pleural effusion, *pulmonary edema.*
Skin: acne, alopecia, pruritus, rash, sweating, skin discoloration, nodules, ulcers, urticaria.
Other: allergic reaction, *anaphylaxis, chills, fever,* peripheral or facial edema, infection, mucous membrane disorder, pain or reaction at injection site, *sepsis.*

INTERACTIONS
Drug-drug. *Antineoplastics:* May enhance renal toxicity, bronchospasm, and hypotension. Use together cautiously.
Cardiac glycosides: May enhance potassium excretion and increase digitalis toxicity. Monitor potassium level closely.
Corticosteroids: Enhanced potassium depletion, which could predispose patient to cardiac dysfunction. Monitor electrolyte levels.
Cyclosporine, tacrolimus: May increase creatinine levels. Monitor renal function.
Flucytosine: May increase toxicity by amphotericin. Use together cautiously.
Imidazoles (clotrimazole, fluconazole, ketoconazole, miconazole): May antagonize effects of amphotericin, although significance hasn't been determined. Monitor patient closely.
Leukocyte transfusions: Increased risk of pulmonary reactions, such as acute dyspnea, tachypnea, hypoxemia, hemoptysis, and interstitial infiltrates. Use together cautiously; separate administration times as much as possible and monitor pulmonary function if drugs are used together.
Nephrotoxic drugs (such as aminoglycosides, pentamidine): May enhance renal toxicity. Monitor renal function closely.
Skeletal muscle relaxants: Amphotericin B–induced hypokalemia may enhance effects of skeletal muscle relaxants. Monitor potassium level closely.

EFFECTS ON LAB TEST RESULTS
• May increase BUN, creatinine, alkaline phosphatase, ALT, AST, bilirubin, GGT, and LDH levels. May decrease calcium, phosphate, magnesium, and protein levels. May increase or decrease glucose, sodium, and potassium levels.
• May decrease hemoglobin, platelet count, and INR. May increase or decrease WBC count and PT.

CONTRAINDICATIONS
Contraindicated in patients hypersensitive to drug or its components unless the benefits outweigh risks.

NURSING CONSIDERATIONS
• It's unknown if drug appears in breast milk. Because of the potential for serious adverse reactions in breast-fed infants, a

---

Reactions may be *common,* uncommon, ***life-threatening,*** or **COMMON AND LIFE-THREATENING.**

decision should be made to either discontinue breast-feeding or stop treatment, taking into account importance of drug to the mother.

• **Alert:** Different amphotericin B preparations aren't interchangeable and dosages will vary.

• **Alert:** Monitor vital signs every 30 minutes during initial therapy. Acute infusion-related reactions, including fever, chills, hypotension, nausea, and tachycardia, usually occur 1 to 3 hours after starting I.V. infusion. These reactions are usually more severe after initial doses and usually diminish with subsequent doses. If severe respiratory distress occurs, stop infusion immediately and don't treat further with drug.

• Pretreating with antihistamines, antipyretics, and corticosteroids; reducing infusion rate; or maintaining sodium balance may reduce acute infusion-related reactions.

• Hydration before infusion may reduce risk of nephrotoxicity.

• Monitor intake and output; report changes in urine appearance or volume.

• Monitor renal and hepatic function test results, electrolyte levels (especially potassium, magnesium, and calcium), CBC, and PT.

PATIENT TEACHING

• Instruct patient to immediately report symptoms of hypersensitivity.

• Warn patient of possible discomfort at I.V. site.

• Advise patient of potential adverse effects, such as fever, chills, nausea, and vomiting. Tell patient that these can be severe with initial treatment but usually subside with repeated doses.

amphotericin B lipid complex
Abelcet

Pregnancy risk category B

AVAILABLE FORMS
Suspension for injection: 50 mg/10-ml vial, 100 mg/20-ml vial

INDICATIONS & DOSAGES
➤ **Invasive fungal infections, including *Aspergillus* and *Candida* species, in patients who are refractory to or intolerant of conventional amphotericin B therapy—**
Adults and children: 5 mg/kg daily I.V. as a single infusion administered at rate of 2.5 mg/kg/hour.

I.V. ADMINISTRATION
• To prepare, shake vial gently until there is no yellow sediment. Using aseptic technique, withdraw calculated dose into one or more 20-ml syringes, using an 18-gauge needle. More than one vial will be needed. Attach a 5-micron filter needle to syringe and inject dose into I.V. bag of D_5W. One filter needle can be used for up to four vials of amphotericin B lipid complex. Volume of D_5W should be sufficient to yield a final concentration of 1 mg/ml.

• For children and patients with CV disease, recommended final concentration is 2 mg/ml.

• Don't mix with saline solution or infuse in same I.V. line as other drugs. Don't use an in-line filter.

• Discard any unused drug because drug doesn't contain a preservative.

• Use an infusion pump and administer by continuous infusion at rate of 2.5 mg/kg/hour. If infusion time exceeds 2 hours, mix contents by shaking infusion bag every 2 hours.

• If infusing through an existing I.V. line, flush first with D_5W.

• If severe respiratory distress occurs, stop infusion, provide supportive therapy for anaphylaxis, and notify prescriber. Don't reinstitute drug.

• Monitor vital signs closely. Fever, shaking chills, and hypotension may appear within 2 hours of starting infusion. Slowing infusion rate may decrease risk of infusion-related reactions.

• Infusions are stable for up to 48 hours if refrigerated (36° to 46° F [2° to 8° C]) and up to 6 hours at room temperature.

ACTION
Binds to sterols of fungal cell membranes. Fungal cell damage or death results from

---

increased membrane permeability and leakage of intracellular contents.

Route	Onset	Peak	Duration
I.V.	Unknown	Unknown	Unknown

ADVERSE REACTIONS
CNS: headache, pain.
CV: chest pain, *cardiac arrest,* hypertension, hypotension.
GI: abdominal pain, diarrhea, *GI hemorrhage,* nausea, vomiting.
GU: *renal failure.*
Hematologic: anemia, *leukopenia, thrombocytopenia.*
Hepatic: bilirubinemia.
Metabolic: hypokalemia.
Respiratory: dyspnea, respiratory disorder, *respiratory failure.*
Skin: rash.
Other: *chills, fever,* infection, MULTIPLE ORGAN FAILURE, *sepsis.*

INTERACTIONS
Drug-drug. *Antineoplastics:* Increased risk of renal toxicity, bronchospasm, and hypotension. Use together cautiously.
Cardiac glycosides: Increased risk of digitalis toxicity from amphotericin B–induced hypokalemia. Monitor potassium level closely.
Clotrimazole, fluconazole, itraconazole, ketoconazole, miconazole: May antagonize amphotericin B. Monitor patient closely.
Corticosteroids, corticotropin: Enhanced hypokalemia, which may lead to cardiac toxicity. Monitor electrolyte levels and cardiac function.
Cyclosporine: Increased renal toxicity. Monitor patient closely.
Flucytosine: Increased risk of flucytosine toxicity from increased cellular uptake or impaired renal excretion. Use together cautiously.
Leukocyte transfusions: Risk of pulmonary reactions such as acute dyspnea, tachypnea, hypoxemia, hemoptysis, and interstitial infiltrates. Use together cautiously, separate administration times as much as possible, and monitor pulmonary function if drugs are used together.
Nephrotoxic drugs (such as aminoglycosides, pentamidine): Increased risk of renal toxicity. Use together cautiously and monitor renal function closely.
Skeletal muscle relaxants: Enhanced effects of skeletal muscle relaxants resulting from amphotericin B–induced hypokalemia. Monitor potassium level closely.
Zidovudine: Increased myelotoxicity and nephrotoxicity. Monitor renal and hematologic function.

EFFECTS ON LAB TEST RESULTS
• May increase BUN, creatinine, alkaline phosphatase, ALT, AST, bilirubin, GGT, and LDH levels. May decrease potassium levels.
• May decrease hemoglobin and WBC and platelet counts.

CONTRAINDICATIONS
Contraindicated in patients hypersensitive to amphotericin B or its components.

NURSING CONSIDERATIONS
• Use cautiously in patients with renal impairment. The need for dosage adjustment should be based on overall clinical status of patient. Renal toxicity is more common at higher dosages.
• *Alert:* Different amphotericin B preparations aren't interchangeable and dosages will vary.
• Premedicate patient with acetaminophen, antihistamines, or corticosteroids to prevent or lessen severity of infusion-related reactions such as fever, chills, nausea, and vomiting, which occur 1 to 2 hours after start of infusion.
• Hydration before infusion may reduce risk of nephrotoxicity.
• Monitor creatinine and electrolyte levels (especially magnesium and potassium), liver function, and CBC during therapy.
• It's unknown if drug appears in breast milk. A decision should be made to either discontinue drug or stop breast-feeding.

PATIENT TEACHING
• Inform patient that fever, chills, nausea, and vomiting may occur during infusion and that these reactions usually subside with subsequent doses.
• Instruct patient to report any redness or pain at infusion site.

• Teach patient to recognize and report signs or symptoms of acute hypersensitivity such as respiratory distress.
• Warn patient that therapy may take several months.
• Tell patient to expect frequent laboratory testing to monitor kidney and liver function.

amphotericin B liposomal
AmBisome

Pregnancy risk category B

AVAILABLE FORMS
Injection: 50-mg vial

INDICATIONS & DOSAGES
➤ **Empirical therapy for presumed fungal infection in febrile, neutropenic patients—**
Adults and children: 3 mg/kg I.V. infusion over 2 hours daily.
➤ **Systemic fungal infections caused by *Aspergillus* species, *Candida* species, or *Cryptococcus* species refractory to amphotericin B deoxycholate or in patients for whom renal impairment or unacceptable toxicity precludes use of amphotericin B deoxycholate—**
Adults and children: 3 to 5 mg/kg I.V. infusion over 2 hours daily.
➤ **Visceral leishmaniasis in immunocompetent patients—**
Adults and children: 3 mg/kg I.V. infusion over 2 hours daily on days 1 to 5, 14, and 21. A repeat course of therapy may be beneficial if initial treatment fails to clear parasites.
➤ **Visceral leishmaniasis in immunocompromised patients—**
Adults and children: 4 mg/kg I.V. infusion over 2 hours daily on days 1 to 5, 10, 17, 24, 31, and 38. Expert advice regarding further treatment is recommended if initial therapy fails or patient experiences relapse.
✱ *NEW INDICATION:* **Cryptococcal meningitis in HIV-infected patients—**
Adults and children: 6 mg/kg/day I.V. infusion over 2 hours. Infusion time may be reduced to 1 hour if well tolerated. Infusion time may be increased if discomfort occurs.

I.V. ADMINISTRATION
• Reconstitute each 50-mg vial of amphotericin B liposomal with 12 ml of sterile water for injection to yield a solution of 4 mg amphotericin B per ml.
• *Alert:* Don't reconstitute with bacteriostatic water for injection and don't allow bacteriostatic product in solution. Don't reconstitute with saline solution, add saline solution to reconstituted concentration, or mix with other drugs.
• After reconstitution, shake vial vigorously for 30 seconds or until particulate matter is dispersed.
• Withdraw calculated amount of reconstituted solution into a sterile syringe and inject through a 5-micron filter into appropriate amount of D_5W to further dilute to final concentration of 1 to 2 mg/ml. Lower concentrations (0.2 to 0.5 mg/ml) may be appropriate for children to provide sufficient volume of infusion.
• An existing I.V. line must be flushed with D_5W before infusion of drug. If this isn't feasible, give drug through separate line.

ACTION
Antifungal activity is derived from amphotericin B, which binds to the sterol component of a fungal cell membrane, leading to alterations in cell permeability and cell death.

Route	Onset	Peak	Duration
I.V.	Unknown	Unknown	Unknown

ADVERSE REACTIONS
CNS: *anxiety, confusion, headache, insomnia, asthenia.*
CV: *chest pain, hypotension, tachycardia, hypertension, edema, flushing.*
EENT: *epistaxis, rhinitis.*
GI: *nausea, vomiting, abdominal pain, diarrhea,* **GI hemorrhage.**
GU: *hematuria.*
Hepatic: *bilirubinemia.*
Metabolic: *hyperglycemia,* hypernatremia, *hypocalcemia, hypokalemia, hypomagnesemia.*
Musculoskeletal: *back pain.*
Respiratory: *increased cough, dyspnea,* hypoxia, *pleural effusion, lung disorder,* hyperventilation.
Skin: *pruritus, rash, sweating.*

---

*Liquid contains alcohol. **May contain tartrazine. †Canada ‡Australia §U.K. ◇OTC

Other: *chills, infection,* **anaphylaxis,** *pain,* **sepsis,** *fever, blood product infusion reaction.*

INTERACTIONS
Drug-drug. *Antineoplastics:* May enhance potential for renal toxicity, bronchospasm, and hypotension. Use together cautiously.

Cardiac glycosides: Increased risk of digitalis toxicity caused by amphotericin B–induced hypokalemia. Monitor potassium level closely.

Clotrimazole, fluconazole, ketoconazole, miconazole: May induce fungal resistance to amphotericin B. Use cautiously.

Corticosteroids, corticotropin: May increase potassium depletion, which could result in cardiac dysfunction. Monitor electrolyte levels and cardiac function.

Flucytosine: May increase flucytosine toxicity by increasing cellular reuptake or impairing renal excretion of flucytosine. Use together cautiously.

Leukocyte transfusions: Risk of pulmonary reactions, such as acute dyspnea, tachypnea, hypoxemia, hemoptysis, and interstitial infiltrates. Use together cautiously, separating administration times as much as possible and monitoring pulmonary function if drugs used together.

Other nephrotoxic drugs, such as antibiotics, antineoplastics: May cause additive nephrotoxicity. Use together cautiously; monitor renal function closely.

Skeletal muscle relaxants: Enhanced effects of skeletal muscle relaxants resulting from amphotericin B–induced hypokalemia. Monitor potassium levels.

EFFECTS ON LAB TEST RESULTS
• May increase BUN, creatinine, glucose, sodium, alkaline phosphatase, ALT, AST, bilirubin, GGT, and LDH levels. May decrease potassium, calcium, and magnesium levels.

CONTRAINDICATIONS
Contraindicated in patients hypersensitive to drug or its components.

NURSING CONSIDERATIONS
• Use cautiously in patients with impaired renal function, in elderly patients, and in pregnant women.

• Patients also receiving chemotherapy or bone marrow transplantation are at greater risk for additional adverse reactions, including seizures, arrhythmias, and thrombocytopenia.

• *Alert:* Different amphotericin B preparations aren't interchangeable and dosages will vary.

• Premedicate patient with antipyretics, antihistamines, antiemetics, or corticosteroids.

• Hydration before infusion may reduce the risk of nephrotoxicity.

• Monitor BUN and creatinine and electrolyte levels (particularly magnesium and potassium), liver function, and CBC.

• Watch for signs and symptoms of hypokalemia (ECG changes, muscle weakness, cramping, drowsiness).

• Patients treated with amphotericin B liposomal have a lower risk of chills, elevated BUN level, hypokalemia, hypertension, and vomiting than patients treated with conventional amphotericin B.

• Therapy may take several weeks to months.

• It's unknown if drug appears in breast milk. Because of potential for serious adverse reactions in breast-fed infants, a decision should be made to either discontinue breast-feeding or stop treatment, taking into account importance of drug to mother.

• Use a controlled infusion device and an in-line filter with a mean pore diameter less than 1 micron. Initially, infuse drug over at least 2 hours. Infusion time may be reduced to 1 hour if treatment is well tolerated. If patient experiences discomfort during infusion, increase duration of infusion.

• Observe patient closely for adverse reactions during infusion. If anaphylaxis occurs, stop infusion immediately, provide supportive therapy, and notify prescriber.

• Store unopened vial at 36° to 46° F (2° to 8° C). Once reconstituted, store concentrate for up to 24 hours at 36° to 46° F. Don't freeze.

PATIENT TEACHING
• Teach patient signs and symptoms of hypersensitivity, and stress importance of reporting them immediately.

• Warn patient that therapy may take several months; teach personal hygiene and

---

other measures to prevent spread and recurrence of lesions.
- Instruct patient to report any adverse reactions that occur while receiving drug.
- Tell patient to watch for and report signs and symptoms of hypokalemia (muscle weakness, cramping, drowsiness).
- Advise patient that frequent laboratory testing will be needed.

✳ **NEW DRUG**

caspofungin acetate
Cancidas

Pregnancy risk category C

AVAILABLE FORMS
Lyophilized powder for injection: 50-mg, 70-mg single-use vials

INDICATIONS & DOSAGES
➤ **Invasive aspergillosis in patients who are refractory to or intolerant of other therapies (amphotericin B, lipid formulations of amphotericin B, or itraconazole)—**
Adults: Single 70-mg I.V. loading dose on day 1, followed by 50 mg daily thereafter. Administer by slow I.V. infusion of about 1 hour. Duration of treatment is based on severity of patient's underlying disease, recovery from immunosuppression, and clinical response.
Adjust-a-dose: Patients with mild hepatic insufficiency (Child-Pugh score 5 to 6) don't need dosage adjustment. For patients with moderate hepatic insufficiency (Child-Pugh score 7 to 9), after initial 70-mg loading dose, give 35 mg daily. No clinical experience exists in patients with severe hepatic insufficiency (Child-Pugh score > 9).

I.V. ADMINISTRATION
- Allow refrigerated vial to warm to room temperature.
- Drug is usually diluted in 250 ml normal saline solution for all (70-mg, 50-mg, 35-mg) doses. For patients on fluid restriction, the 50-mg and 35-mg doses may be diluted in 100 ml normal saline solution.
- Don't use diluents containing dextrose.
- Use reconstituted vials within 1 hour or discard.

- Administer drug by slow I.V. infusion over about 1 hour.

ACTION
An intravenously administered antifungal that inhibits synthesis of beta (1,3)-D-glucan in susceptible *Aspergillus* species. Drug is extensively distributed and has a prolonged plasma half-life.

Route	Onset	Peak	Duration
I.V.	Unknown	Unknown	Unknown

ADVERSE REACTIONS
CNS: headache, *paresthesia.*
CV: *tachycardia,* phlebitis, infused vein complications.
GI: nausea, vomiting, diarrhea, abdominal pain, *anorexia.*
GU: proteinuria, hematuria.
Hematologic: eosinophilia, *anemia.*
Metabolic: hypokalemia.
Musculoskeletal: *pain, myalgia.*
Respiratory: *tachypnea.*
Skin: histamine-mediated symptoms including rash, facial swelling, pruritus, sensation of warmth.
Other: fever, *chills, sweating.*

INTERACTIONS
Drug-drug. *Cyclosporine:* May significantly increase levels of caspofungin. Because of increased risk of elevated alanine transaminase levels, don't use together unless potential benefit outweighs potential risk.
Inducers of drug clearance or mixed inducer-inhibitors (carbamazepine, dexamethasone, efavirenz, nelfinavir, nevirapine, phenytoin, rifampin): May reduce caspofungin levels. May need to adjust dosage.
Tacrolimus: May reduce levels of tacrolimus. Monitor levels of tacrolimus. May need to adjust dosage.

EFFECTS ON LAB TEST RESULTS
- May increase alkaline phosphatase level. May decrease potassium level.
- May increase eosinophil count. May decrease hemoglobin.

CONTRAINDICATIONS
Contraindicated in patients hypersensitive to drug or its components.

---

*Liquid contains alcohol.   **May contain tartrazine.   †Canada   ‡Australia   §U.K.   ◊OTC

NURSING CONSIDERATIONS

• The efficacy of a 70-mg dose regimen in patients who aren't clinically responding to the 50-mg daily dose isn't known. Limited safety data suggest that an increase in dosage to 70 mg daily is well tolerated. Safety and efficacy of doses above 70 mg haven't been adequately studied.

• The safety information on treatment durations longer than 2 weeks is limited; however, available data suggest that drug continues to be well tolerated with longer courses of therapy.

• Monitor I.V. site carefully for phlebitis.

• Observe patients for histamine-mediated reactions, including rash, facial swelling, pruritus, and a sensation of warmth.

• *Alert:* Never mix drug in or dilute with dextrose solution.

• Don't mix or infuse with other drugs.

• Safety and efficacy in patients younger than age 18 isn't known.

• It's unknown if drug appears in breast milk. Use cautiously in breast-feeding women.

PATIENT TEACHING

• Instruct patient to report signs and symptoms of phlebitis.

---

fluconazole
Diflucan

Pregnancy risk category C

AVAILABLE FORMS

Injection: 200 mg/100 ml, 400 mg/200 ml
Powder for oral suspension: 10 mg/ml, 40 mg/ml
Tablets: 50 mg, 100 mg, 150 mg, 200 mg

INDICATIONS & DOSAGES

➤ **Oropharyngeal candidiasis—**
Adults: 200 mg P.O. or I.V. on first day, then 100 mg once daily. Therapy should last at least 2 weeks.
Children: 6 mg/kg P.O. or I.V. on first day, then 3 mg/kg daily for 2 weeks.

➤ **Esophageal candidiasis—**
Adults: 200 mg P.O. or I.V. on first day, then 100 mg once daily. Up to 400 mg daily has been used, depending on patient's condition and tolerance of treatment. Patients should receive drug for at least 3 weeks and for 2 weeks after symptoms resolve.
Children: 6 mg/kg P.O. or I.V. on first day, then 3 mg/kg daily for at least 3 weeks, and for at least 2 weeks after symptoms resolve. Doses up to 12 mg/kg may be used based on clinical judgment.

➤ **Vulvovaginal candidiasis—**
Adults: 150 mg P.O. for one dose only or 50 mg P.O. daily for 3 days.

➤ **Systemic candidiasis—**
Adults: 400 mg P.O. or I.V. on first day, then 200 mg, once daily. Doses up to 400 mg/day have been used. Some prescribers recommend that treatment continue for at least 4 weeks and for 2 weeks after symptoms resolve.
Children: 6 to 12 mg/kg/day P.O. or I.V.

➤ **Cryptococcal meningitis—**
Adults: 400 mg P.O. or I.V. on first day, then 200 mg once daily. Higher doses, up to 400 mg daily, may be used. Treatment should continue for 10 to 12 weeks after CSF culture is negative.
Children: 12 mg/kg/day P.O. or I.V. on first day, then 6 mg/kg daily for 10 to 12 weeks after CSF culture is negative.

➤ **Prevention of candidiasis in bone marrow transplant—**
Adults: 400 mg P.O. or I.V. once daily. Start prophylaxis several days before anticipated agranulocytosis. Continue therapy for 7 days after neutrophil count rises above 1,000 cells/mm^3.

➤ **Suppression of relapse of cryptococcal meningitis in patients with AIDS—**
Adults: 200 mg P.O. or I.V. daily.
Children: 3 to 6 mg/kg/day P.O. or I.V.
Adjust-a-dose: For renally impaired patients, if creatinine clearance is 11 to 50 ml/minute, dosage is reduced by 50%. Patients receiving regular hemodialysis treatment should receive usual dose after each dialysis session.

I.V. ADMINISTRATION

• Don't remove protective overwrap from I.V. bags until just before use to ensure product sterility. The plastic container may show some opacity from moisture absorbed during sterilization. This doesn't affect drug and diminishes over time. Don't add other drugs to I.V. bag.

• *Alert:* Administer by continuous infusion at rate not exceeding 200 mg/hour. Use an

---

infusion pump. To prevent air embolism, don't connect in series with other infusions.

ACTION
Inhibits fungal cytochrome P-450 (responsible for fungal sterol synthesis) and weakens fungal cell walls.

Route	Onset	Peak	Duration
I.V.	Immediate	Immediate	Unknown
P.O.	Unknown	1-2 hr	30 hr

ADVERSE REACTIONS
CNS: headache, dizziness.
GI: *nausea,* vomiting, abdominal pain, diarrhea, dyspepsia, taste perversion.
Hematologic: *leukopenia, thrombocytopenia.*
Skin: rash.
Other: *anaphylaxis.*

INTERACTIONS
Drug-drug. *Cyclosporine, phenytoin, theophylline:* May increase plasma levels of these drugs. Monitor cyclosporine and phenytoin levels.
Isoniazid, oral sulfonylureas, phenytoin, rifampin, valproic acid: Increased risk of elevated hepatic transaminase levels. Monitor patient closely.
Oral antidiabetics (such as glipizide, glyburide, tolbutamide): May increase plasma levels of these drugs. Monitor patient for enhanced hypoglycemic effect.
Rifampin: Enhanced metabolism of fluconazole. Monitor patient for lack of response.
Warfarin: Increased risk of bleeding. Monitor PT and INR.
Zidovudine: May increase zidovudine activity. Monitor patient closely.

EFFECTS ON LAB TEST RESULTS
● May increase alkaline phosphatase, ALT, AST, bilirubin, and GGT levels.
● May decrease WBC and platelet counts.

CONTRAINDICATIONS
Contraindicated in patients hypersensitive to drug. Don't use in breast-feeding patients.

NURSING CONSIDERATIONS
● Use cautiously in patients hypersensitive to other antifungal azole compounds; no data exist regarding cross-sensitivity.
● Serious hepatotoxicity has occurred in patients with underlying medical conditions.
● Periodically monitor liver function during prolonged therapy.
● If patient develops mild rash, monitor him closely. Discontinue drug if lesions progress, and notify prescriber.
● Risk of adverse reactions appears to be greater in HIV-infected patients.

PATIENT TEACHING
● Tell patient to take drug as directed, even after he feels better.
● Instruct patient to report adverse reactions promptly.

flucytosine (5-FC, 5-fluorocytosine)
Ancobon, Ancotil‡

Pregnancy risk category C

AVAILABLE FORMS
Capsules: 250 mg, 500 mg

INDICATIONS & DOSAGES
➤ **Severe fungal infections caused by susceptible strains of *Candida* species, including septicemia, endocarditis, urinary tract, and pulmonary infections, and of *Cryptococcus* species, including meningitis, pulmonary infection, and urinary tract infection—**
Adults: 50 to 150 mg/kg daily P.O. in four equally divided doses q 6 hours.

ACTION
Unknown. Appears to penetrate fungal cells and cause defective protein synthesis.

Route	Onset	Peak	Duration
P.O.	Unknown	1-2 hr	Unknown

ADVERSE REACTIONS
CNS: headache, vertigo, sedation, fatigue, weakness, confusion, hallucinations, psychosis, ataxia, hearing loss, paresthesia, parkinsonism, peripheral neuropathy.

CV: *cardiac arrest,* chest pain.
GI: nausea, vomiting, diarrhea, abdominal pain, dry mouth, duodenal ulcer, *hemorrhage,* ulcerative colitis, anorexia.
GU: azoturia, crystalluria, *renal failure.*
Hematologic: anemia, *leukopenia, bone marrow suppression, thrombocytopenia,* eosinophilia, *agranulocytosis, aplastic anemia.*
Hepatic: jaundice.
Metabolic: hypoglycemia, hypokalemia.
Respiratory: *respiratory arrest,* dyspnea.
Skin: occasional rash, pruritus, urticaria, photosensitivity.

INTERACTIONS
Drug-drug. *Amphotericin B:* May cause synergistic effects and may enhance toxicity. Monitor patient closely.

EFFECTS ON LAB TEST RESULTS
● May increase alkaline phosphatase, ALT, AST, bilirubin, creatinine, and BUN levels. May decrease glucose and potassium levels.
● May increase eosinophil count and nitrogenous compounds (urea). May decrease hemoglobin and WBC, platelet, and granulocyte counts.

CONTRAINDICATIONS
Contraindicated in patients hypersensitive to drug.

NURSING CONSIDERATIONS
● Use with extreme caution in patients with impaired hepatic or renal function or bone marrow suppression.
● Administer capsules over 15 minutes to reduce adverse GI reactions.
● Monitor blood, liver, and renal function studies frequently during therapy; obtain susceptibility tests weekly to monitor drug resistance.
● If possible, regularly perform blood level assays of drug, to maintain flucytosine at therapeutic level of 40 to 60 mcg/ml. Blood levels above 100 mcg/ml may be toxic.
● Monitor fluid intake and output; report marked changes.

PATIENT TEACHING
● Tell patient that therapeutic response may take weeks or months.

● Advise patient to report adverse reactions promptly.
● Instruct patient to take capsules over 15 minutes to reduce adverse GI reactions.

---

griseofulvin microsize
Fulcin‡, Fulvicin-U/F, Grifulvin V, Grisactin 500, Grisovin‡, Grisovin, Grisovin FP†

griseofulvin ultramicrosize
Fulvicin P/G, Grisactin Ultra, Griseostatin‡, Gris-PEG

Pregnancy risk category C

AVAILABLE FORMS
griseofulvin microsize
Capsules: 125 mg, 250 mg
Oral suspension: 125 mg/5 ml
Tablets: 250 mg, 500 mg
griseofulvin ultramicrosize
Tablets: 125 mg, 165 mg, 250 mg, 330 mg

INDICATIONS & DOSAGES
➤ **Ringworm infections of skin, hair, or nails caused by** *Trichophyton,* *Microsporum,* **or** *Epidermophyton*—
Adults: 500 mg of microsize P.O. daily in single or divided doses. Severe infections may need up to 1 g daily. Or, 330 to 375 mg ultramicrosize P.O. daily in single or divided doses. Duration of therapy is 2 to 8 weeks depending on site of infection.
➤ **Tinea pedis, tinea unguium**—
Adults: 0.75 to 1 g of microsize P.O. daily. Or, 660 to 750 mg of ultramicrosize P.O. daily in divided doses. Duration of therapy is individualized and may range from 4 to 8 weeks for tinea pedis and from 4 months to 1 year or more for tinea unguium.
Children: 11 mg/kg/day of microsize P.O. Or, 7.3 mg/kg/day of ultramicrosize P.O.

ACTION
Arrests fungal cell activity by disrupting mitotic spindle structure.

Route	Onset	Peak	Duration
P.O.	Unknown	4-8 hr	Unknown

ADVERSE REACTIONS
CNS: headache in early stages of treatment, fatigue with large doses, occasional

---

mental confusion, impaired performance of routine activities, psychotic symptoms, dizziness, insomnia, paresthesia of hands and feet after extended therapy.
EENT: transient decrease in hearing.
GI: nausea, vomiting, flatulence, diarrhea, epigastric distress, *bleeding,* oral thrush.
GU: proteinuria, menstrual irregularities.
Hematologic: *leukopenia, agranulocytosis,* porphyria.
Hepatic: *hepatic toxicity.*
Skin: *rash, urticaria,* photosensitivity.
Other: hypersensitivity reactions, lupus erythematosus, *angioedema.*

INTERACTIONS
Drug-drug. *Coumarin anticoagulants:* Decreased effectiveness. Monitor PT and INR when used together.
Cyclosporine: Decreased cyclosporine levels. Monitor patient closely.
Oral contraceptives: Decreased effectiveness. Suggest alternative methods of contraception.
Phenobarbital: Decreased griseofulvin levels from decreased absorption or increased metabolism. Avoid using together or give griseofulvin t.i.d.
Drug-food. *High-fat meals:* Increased absorption. Give together.
Drug-lifestyle. *Alcohol use:* May cause tachycardia, diaphoresis, and flushing. Tell patient to avoid alcohol consumption.
Sun exposure: May increase risk of photosensitivity reaction. Tell patient to avoid unprotected sun exposure.

EFFECTS ON LAB TEST RESULTS
● May decrease WBC and granulocyte counts.

CONTRAINDICATIONS
Contraindicated in patients hypersensitive to drug and in those with porphyria or hepatocellular failure. Also contraindicated in pregnant patients and in women who intend to become pregnant during therapy.

NURSING CONSIDERATIONS
● Use cautiously in penicillin-sensitive patients because griseofulvin is derived from *Penicillium* species and cross-sensitivity may occur.
● *Alert:* Because of potential toxicity, drug is used only when topical treatment fails.

● Obtain laboratory tests to confirm diagnosis. Continue drug until clinical and laboratory examinations confirm eradication.
● *Alert:* Because griseofulvin ultramicrosize is dispersed in polyethylene glycol, it's absorbed more rapidly and completely than microsize preparations and is effective at one-half to two-thirds the usual griseofulvin dose. Don't interchange preparations.
● Give drug after a high-fat meal to enhance absorption and minimize GI distress.
● Assess hematologic, renal, and hepatic function periodically during prolonged therapy.
● Discontinue drug in patients who experience agranulocytosis.
● Effective treatment of tinea pedis may require concomitant use of a topical drug.
● Safety in children younger than age 2 hasn't been established.

PATIENT TEACHING
● Tell patient to take drug after a high-fat meal to enhance absorption and minimize GI distress.
● Advise patient that prolonged treatment may be needed to control infection and prevent relapse, even if symptoms abate in first few days of therapy.
● Tell patient to keep skin clean and dry and to maintain good hygiene.
● Instruct patient to avoid intense sunlight. Unprotected sun exposure may cause photosensitivity reactions.

itraconazole
Sporanox

Pregnancy risk category C

AVAILABLE FORMS
Capsules: 100 mg
Injection: 10 mg/ml
Oral solution: 10 mg/ml

INDICATIONS & DOSAGES
➤ **Pulmonary and extrapulmonary blastomycosis, nonmeningeal histoplasmosis—**
Adults: 200 mg P.O. daily. Increase as needed and tolerated in 100-mg incre-

ments to maximum of 400 mg daily. Dosages that exceed 200 mg daily should be given in two divided doses. Or, give 200 mg I.V. b.i.d. over 1 hour for four doses, followed by 200 mg I.V. daily for up to 14 days; then change to P.O. form. Treatment should continue for a minimum of 3 months. In life-threatening illness, give a loading dose of 200 mg P.O. t.i.d. for 3 days.

➤ **Aspergillosis—**
Adults: 200 to 400 mg P.O. daily, or 200 mg I.V. b.i.d. over 1 hour for four doses followed by 200 mg I.V. daily for up to 14 days; then change to P.O. form.

➤ **Onychomycosis of the toenail—**
Adults: 200 mg P.O. once daily for 12 consecutive weeks.

➤ **Onychomycosis of the fingernail—**
Adults: Initially, 200 mg P.O. b.i.d. for 1 week; after 3 weeks without itraconazole, repeat dosage.

➤ **Oropharyngeal candidiasis—**
Adults: 200 mg oral solution swished in mouth vigorously and swallowed daily, for 1 to 2 weeks.

➤ **Oropharyngeal candidiasis in patients unresponsive to fluconazole tablets—**
Adults: 100 mg oral solution swished in mouth vigorously and swallowed b.i.d., for 2 to 4 weeks.

➤ **Esophageal candidiasis—**
Adults: 100 to 200 mg oral solution swished in mouth vigorously and swallowed daily, for a minimum treatment of 3 weeks. Treatment should continue for 2 weeks after symptoms resolve.

I.V. ADMINISTRATION
● Use only components provided in the kit. Don't substitute.
● Dilute contents of 250-mg ampule in 50-ml bag of normal saline solution to provide 75 ml of a solution containing 3.33 mg itraconazole per ml.
● Diluted injection may be stored at 36° to 46° F (2° to 8° C) or at room temperature for up to 48 hours when protected from light.
● Give by I.V. infusion over 60 minutes, using infusion set provided and a controlled infusion device.

● Don't mix with other drugs or administer through same I.V. line as other drugs.
● Flush infusion set via the 2-way stopcock with 15 to 20 ml of normal saline solution injection over 30 seconds to 15 minutes, then discard I.V. line.

ACTION
Interferes with fungal cell-wall synthesis by inhibiting formation of ergosterol and increasing cell-wall permeability that makes the fungus susceptible to osmotic instability.

Route	Onset	Peak	Duration
I.V.	Unknown	Unknown	Unknown
P.O.	Unknown	3-4 hr	Unknown

ADVERSE REACTIONS
CNS: headache, dizziness, somnolence, fatigue, malaise.
CV: hypertension, edema.
GI: *nausea,* vomiting, diarrhea, abdominal pain, anorexia.
GU: albuminuria, impotence.
Hepatic: impaired hepatic function.
Metabolic: hypokalemia.
Skin: rash, pruritus.
Other: fever, decreased libido.

INTERACTIONS
Drug-drug. *Antacids, H_2-receptor antagonists, phenytoin, rifampin:* May lower itraconazole plasma levels. Avoid using together.
Cyclosporine, digoxin, tacrolimus: May increase plasma levels of these drugs. Monitor plasma levels.
Dofetilide, pimozide, quinidine: May increase the plasma concentration of these drugs by CYP3A4 metabolism, causing serious CV events, including torsades de pointes, QT prolongation, ventricular tachycardia, cardiac arrest, and sudden death. Avoid using together.
Isoniazid: May decrease plasma levels of itraconazole. Monitor patient.
Oral anticoagulants: May enhance anticoagulant effects. Monitor PT and INR.
Oral antidiabetics: Similar antifungals have caused hypoglycemia. Monitor glucose levels.
Drug-food. *Grapefruit juice:* May decrease plasma levels and therapeutic effect

---

of itraconazole. Take with liquid other than grapefruit juice.

EFFECTS ON LAB TEST RESULTS
● May increase alkaline phosphatase, ALT, AST, bilirubin, and GGT levels. May decrease potassium levels.

CONTRAINDICATIONS
Contraindicated in patients hypersensitive to drug or receiving oral triazolam or midazolam, in those with ventricular dysfunction or a history of heart failure, and in those who are breast-feeding.

NURSING CONSIDERATIONS
● Use cautiously in patients with hypochlorhydria; they may not absorb drug readily.
● Because hypochlorhydria can accompany HIV infection, use cautiously in HIV-infected patients.
● Use cautiously in patients receiving other highly bound drugs because drug and its metabolites are bound to plasma proteins.
● Confirm the diagnosis of onychomycosis before starting therapy by having nail specimens undergo appropriate laboratory testing.
● Perform baseline liver function tests and monitor results periodically.

PATIENT TEACHING
● Teach patient to recognize and report signs and symptoms of liver disease (anorexia, dark urine, pale stools, unusual fatigue, and jaundice).
● Tell patient to take capsule with food to ensure maximal absorption.
● Instruct patient not to use oral solution interchangeably with itraconazole capsules.
● Tell patient that oral solution should be used 10 ml at a time.
● Advise patient to take solution without food and to take capsules with a full meal.
● Urge patient to tell prescriber about all drugs he is taking to avoid potential drug interactions.

ketoconazole
Nizoral

Pregnancy risk category C

AVAILABLE FORMS
Oral suspension: 100 mg/5 ml†
Tablets: 200 mg

INDICATIONS & DOSAGES
➤ **Systemic candidiasis, chronic mucocandidiasis, oral candidiasis, candiduria, coccidioidomycosis, blastomycosis, histoplasmosis, chromomycosis, and paracoccidioidomycosis; severe cutaneous dermatophyte infections resistant to therapy with topical or oral griseofulvin—**
Adults and children weighing more than 40 kg (88 lb): Initially, 200 mg P.O. daily in a single dose. Dosage may be increased to 400 mg once daily in patients who don't respond.
Children age 2 and older: 3.3 to 6.6 mg/kg P.O. daily in a single dose.

ACTION
Interferes with fungal cell-wall synthesis by inhibiting formation of ergosterol and increasing cell-wall permeability that makes the fungus susceptible to osmotic instability.

Route	Onset	Peak	Duration
P.O.	Unknown	1-2 hr	Unknown

ADVERSE REACTIONS
CNS: headache, nervousness, dizziness, somnolence, *suicidal tendencies,* severe depression.
EENT: photophobia.
GI: *nausea, vomiting,* abdominal pain, diarrhea.
GU: impotence.
Hematologic: *thrombocytopenia,* hemolytic anemia, *leukopenia.*
Hepatic: *fatal hepatotoxicity.*
Metabolic: hyperlipidemia.
Skin: pruritus.
Other: fever, gynecomastia with tenderness, chills.

INTERACTIONS
Drug-drug. *Antacids, anticholinergics, H_2-receptor antagonists:* Decreased absorption of ketoconazole. Wait at least 2 hours after ketoconazole dose before administering these drugs.
Anticoagulants: May enhance effects. Monitor INR, PT, and PTT and adjust dosage, as needed.
Cyclosporine: May increase cyclosporine plasma levels. Monitor serum levels.
Isoniazid, rifampin: Increased ketoconazole metabolism. Monitor patient for decreased antifungal effect.
Paclitaxel: Inhibited metabolism. Use together cautiously.
Theophylline: May decrease theophylline plasma levels. Monitor serum levels.
Drug-herb. *Yew:* Inhibited ketoconazole metabolism. Discourage use together.

EFFECTS ON LAB TEST RESULTS
• May increase lipid, alkaline phosphatase, ALT, and AST levels.
• May decrease hemoglobin and platelet and WBC counts.

CONTRAINDICATIONS
Contraindicated in patients hypersensitive to drug.

NURSING CONSIDERATIONS
• Use cautiously in patients with hepatic disease and in those who are taking other hepatotoxic drugs.
• Because of potential for serious hepatotoxicity, don't use ketoconazole for less serious conditions, such as fungal infections of skin or nails.
• Monitor patient for signs and symptoms of hepatotoxicity, including elevated liver enzyme levels, nausea that doesn't subside, and unusual fatigue, jaundice, dark urine, or pale stool.
• Doses up to 800 mg/day can be used to treat fungal meningitis and intracerebral fungal lesions.

PATIENT TEACHING
• Instruct patient with achlorhydria to dissolve each tablet in 4 ml aqueous solution of 0.2 N hydrochloric acid, sip mixture through a glass or plastic straw, and then drink a glass of water because ketoconazole needs gastric acidity for dissolution and absorption.
• Instruct patient to wait at least 2 hours after dose before taking antacids.
• Make sure patient understands that treatment should be continued until all tests indicate that active fungal infection has subsided. If drug is stopped too soon, infection will recur. Minimum treatment for candidiasis is 7 to 14 days; for other systemic fungal infections, 6 months; for resistant dermatophyte infections, at least 4 weeks.
• Reassure patient that nausea, which is common early in therapy, will subside. To minimize nausea, instruct patient to divide daily amount into two doses or take drug with meals.

---

nystatin
Mycostatin*, Nadostine†, Nilstat, Nystex*

Pregnancy risk category C

AVAILABLE FORMS
Lozenges: 200,000 units
Oral suspension: 100,000 units/ml
Powder: 50, 150, or 500 million units; 1, 2, or 5 billion units
Tablets: 500,000 units
Vaginal suppositories: 100,000 units

INDICATIONS & DOSAGES
➤ **Intestinal candidiasis—**
Adults: 500,000 to 1 million units as oral tablets t.i.d.
➤ **Oral candidiasis (thrush)—**
Adults and children: 400,000 to 600,000 units oral suspension q.i.d. or 200,000 to 400,000 units lozenges 4 to 5 times daily for up to 14 days.
Infants: 200,000 units oral suspension q.i.d.
Neonates and premature infants: 100,000 units oral suspension q.i.d.
➤ **Vaginal candidiasis—**
Adults: 100,000 units, as vaginal tablets, inserted high into vagina, daily at h.s. or b.i.d. for 14 days.

ACTION
Unknown. Probably binds to sterols in fungal cell membrane, altering cell perme-

---

ability and allowing leakage of intracellular components.

Route	Onset	Peak	Duration
P.O., topical	Unknown	Unknown	Unknown

ADVERSE REACTIONS
GI: transient nausea, vomiting, diarrhea.

INTERACTIONS
None significant.

EFFECTS ON LAB TEST RESULTS
None reported.

CONTRAINDICATIONS
Contraindicated in patients hypersensitive to drug.

NURSING CONSIDERATIONS
• Nystatin isn't effective against systemic infections.
• Vaginal tablets can be used by pregnant patients up to 6 weeks before term to treat maternal infection that may cause oral candidiasis in neonates.
• For treatment of oral candidiasis: After the mouth is clean of food debris, have patient hold suspension in mouth for several minutes before swallowing. When treating infants, swab medication on oral mucosa. Prescriber may instruct immunosuppressed patients to suck on vaginal tablets (100,000 units) because this provides prolonged contact with oral mucosa.

PATIENT TEACHING
• Instruct patient not to chew or swallow lozenge, but to allow it to dissolve slowly in mouth.
• Advise patient to continue taking drug for at least 2 days after signs and symptoms disappear. Consult prescriber for exact length of therapy.
• Instruct patient to continue therapy during menstruation.
• Explain that factors predisposing patient to vaginal infection include use of antibiotics, oral contraceptives, and corticosteroids; diabetes; reinfection by sexual partner; and tight-fitting pantyhose. Encourage patient to use cotton underwear.

• Instruct women in careful hygiene for affected areas, including cleaning perineal area from front to back.
• Advise patient to report redness, swelling, or irritation.
• Tell patient that overusing mouthwash or wearing poorly fitting dentures, especially in elderly patients, may promote infection.

terbinafine hydrochloride
Lamisil

Pregnancy risk category B

AVAILABLE FORMS
Tablets: 250 mg

INDICATIONS & DOSAGES
➤ **Fingernail onychomycosis caused by dermatophytes (tinea unguium)—**
Adults: 250 mg P.O. once daily for 6 weeks.
➤ **Toenail onychomycosis caused by dermatophytes (tinea unguium)—**
Adults: 250 mg P.O. once daily for 12 weeks.

ACTION
Inhibits squalene epoxidase, a key enzyme in sterol biosynthesis of fungi. This enzyme inhibition results in a deficiency of ergosterol and a corresponding accumulation of sterol within the fungal cell.

Route	Onset	Peak	Duration
P.O.	Unknown	2 hr	Unknown

ADVERSE REACTIONS
CNS: *headache.*
EENT: visual disturbances.
GI: taste disturbances, diarrhea, dyspepsia, abdominal pain, nausea, flatulence.
Hepatic: hepatobiliary dysfunction, including cholestatic jaundice.
Hematologic: *neutropenia.*
Skin: rash, pruritus, urticaria, *Stevens-Johnson syndrome, toxic epidermal necrolysis.*
Other: hypersensitivity reactions, *anaphylaxis.*

INTERACTIONS
Drug-drug. *Caffeine:* Decreased I.V. caffeine clearance. Use cautiously together.

Cimetidine: Decreased clearance of terbinafine by one-third. Don't use together.

Cyclosporine: Increased cyclosporine clearance. Monitor cyclosporine levels.

Rifampin: Increased terbinafine clearance by 100%. Monitor response to therapy.

EFFECTS ON LAB TEST RESULTS
● May decrease neutrophil and lymphocyte counts.

CONTRAINDICATIONS
Contraindicated in patients hypersensitive to drug. Drug isn't recommended for pregnant or breast-feeding patients and those with liver disease or renal impairment who have creatinine clearance below 50 ml/minute.

NURSING CONSIDERATIONS
●*Alert:* Rare cases of liver failure, some leading to death or liver transplant, have occurred in patients with and without pre-existing liver disease.

● Monitor CBC and hepatic enzyme levels in patients receiving drug for longer than 6 weeks. Drug should be discontinued if hepatobiliary dysfunction or cholestatic hepatitis develops.

● Tablets not recommended for patients with acute or chronic liver disease. Obtain ALT and AST levels before starting therapy.

● Safety in children hasn't been established.

●*Alert:* Don't confuse terbinafine with terbutaline or Lamictal with lamisal.

PATIENT TEACHING
● Inform patient that successful treatment may take 10 weeks for toenail infections and 4 weeks for fingernail infections.

● Tell patient to report visual disturbances immediately; changes in the ocular lens and retina have occurred. Patient should also immediately report persistent nausea, anorexia, fatigue, vomiting, right upper quadrant pain, jaundice, dark urine, or pale stools.

7
Antimalarials

**atovaquone and proguanil
  hydrochloride**
chloroquine hydrochloride
chloroquine phosphate
doxycycline
  (See Chapter 12, TETRACYCLINES.)
hydroxychloroquine sulfate
mefloquine hydrochloride
primaquine phosphate
pyrimethamine
pyrimethamine with sulfadoxine

COMBINATION PRODUCTS
None.

✱ *NEW DRUG*

atovaquone and proguanil hydrochloride
Malarone, Malarone Pediatric

Pregnancy risk category C

AVAILABLE FORMS
Tablets: 62.5 mg atovaquone and 25 mg proguanil hydrochloride; 250 mg atovaquone and 100 mg proguanil hydrochloride

INDICATIONS & DOSAGES
➤ **Prevention of *Plasmodium falciparum* malaria, including where chloroquine resistance has been reported—**
Adults and children weighing more than 40 kg (88 lb): 1 adult-strength (250 mg atovaquone and 100 mg proguanil hydrochloride) tablet P.O. once daily with food or milk, beginning 1 or 2 days before entering a malaria-endemic area. Continue prophylactic treatment during stay and for 7 days after return.
Children weighing 31 to 40 kg (68 to 88 lb): 3 pediatric-strength (62.5 mg atovaquone and 25 mg proguanil hydrochloride) tablets P.O. once daily with food or milk, beginning 1 or 2 days before entering endemic area. Total daily dose is 187.5 mg atovaquone and 75 mg proguanil hydrochloride. Continue during stay and for 7 days after return.

Children weighing 21 to 31 kg (46 to 68 lb): 2 pediatric-strength tablets P.O. once daily with food or milk, beginning 1 or 2 days before entering endemic area. Total daily dose is 125 mg atovaquone and 50 mg proguanil hydrochloride. Continue during stay and for 7 days after return.
Children weighing 11 to 20 kg (24 to 45 lb): 1 pediatric-strength tablet P.O. daily with food or milk, beginning 1 or 2 days before entering endemic area. Continue during stay and for 7 days after return.
➤ **Treatment of acute, uncomplicated *P. falciparum* malaria—**
Adults and children weighing more than 40 kg (88 lb): 4 adult-strength tablets (total daily dose 1 g atovaquone and 400 mg proguanil hydrochloride) P.O. once daily, with food or milk, for 3 consecutive days.
Children weighing 31 to 40 kg (68 to 88 lb): 3 adult-strength tablets P.O. once daily, with food or milk, for 3 consecutive days. Total daily dose is 750 mg atovaquone and 300 mg proguanil hydrochloride.
Children weighing 21 to 31 kg (46 to 68 lb): 2 adult-strength tablets P.O. once daily, with food or milk, for 3 consecutive days. Total daily dose is 500 mg atovaquone and 200 mg proguanil hydrochloride.
Children weighing 11 to 20 kg (24 to 45 lb): 1 adult-strength tablet P.O. once daily, with food or milk, for 3 consecutive days.

ACTION
Thought to interfere with nucleic acid replication in the malarial parasite by inhibiting the biosynthesis of pyrimidine compounds. Atovaquone selectively inhibits mitochondrial electron transport in the parasite. Cycloguanil, an active metabolite of proguanil hydrochloride, disrupts deoxythymidilate synthesis through inhibition of dihydrofolate reductase. Atovaquone and cycloguanil are

active against the erythrocytic and exo-erythrocytic stages of *Plasmodium* species.

Route	Onset	Peak	Duration
P.O.	Unknown	Unknown	Unknown

ADVERSE REACTIONS
CNS: asthenia, dizziness, *headache.*
GI: *abdominal pain*, diarrhea, anorexia, dyspepsia, gastritis, *nausea, vomiting.*
Musculoskeletal: back pain, *myalgia.*
Respiratory: cough, upper respiratory tract infection.
Skin: pruritus.
Other: fever, flulike syndrome.

INTERACTIONS
Drug-drug. *Metoclopramide:* May decrease atovaquone bioavailability. Consider alternative antiemetics.
Rifampin: Reduces atovaquone levels by about 50%. Avoid using together.
Tetracycline: Reduces atovaquone levels by about 40%. Monitor patient with parasitemia closely.

EFFECTS ON LAB TEST RESULTS
• May increase alkaline phosphatase, ALT, and AST levels. May decrease sodium and glucose levels.
• May decrease hemoglobin and neutrophil count.

CONTRAINDICATIONS
Contraindicated in patients hypersensitive to atovaquone, proguanil hydrochloride, or any component of the formulation.

NURSING CONSIDERATIONS
• Use cautiously in patients with severe renal failure because proguanil hydrochloride is renally eliminated.
• Use cautiously in vomiting patients.
• Atovaquone absorption may be decreased by persistent diarrhea or vomiting. Patients with persistent diarrhea or vomiting may need alternative antimalarial therapy.
• Atovaquone and proguanil hydrochloride haven't been studied in the treatment of cerebral malaria or other forms of complicated malaria.

• In the event of a treatment or prophylaxis failure, an alternative antimalarial is indicated.
• Give atovaquone and proguanil hydrochloride at the same time each day with food or milk.
• Store tablets at controlled room temperature 59° to 86° F (15° to 30° C).
• It isn't known if atovaquone appears in breast milk. However, proguanil does appear in breast milk in small amounts, so use caution when giving to breast-feeding patients.
• Safety and efficacy haven't been established in children weighing less than 11 kg.
• It isn't known whether elderly patients respond differently than younger patients. Use cautiously in elderly patients because they have a greater frequency of decreased renal, hepatic, and cardiac function.

PATIENT TEACHING
• Tell patient to take dose at the same time each day.
• Advise patient to take his medication with food or milk.
• If patient vomits within 1 hour after taking a dose, tell him to repeat dose.
• Advise patient to contact his prescriber if he is unable to complete his course of therapy, as prescribed.
• Instruct patient that, in addition to drug therapy, malaria prophylaxis should include the use of protective clothing, bed nets, and insect repellents.

---

chloroquine hydrochloride
Aralen HCl, Chlorquin‡

chloroquine phosphate
Aralen Phosphate, Avloclor§, Chlorquin‡

Pregnancy risk category C

AVAILABLE FORMS
chloroquine hydrochloride
Injection: 40 mg/ml base
chloroquine phosphate
Tablets: 150 mg base, 300 mg base

INDICATIONS & DOSAGES

➤ **Acute malarial attacks caused by** *Plasmodium vivax, P. malariae, P. ovale,* **and susceptible strains of** *P. falciparum*—

Adults: Initially, 600 mg base P.O.; then 300 mg at 6, 24, and 48 hours. Or, 160 to 200 mg base I.M. initially, repeated in 6 hours, p.r.n. Switch patient to oral therapy as soon as possible.

Children: Initially, 10 mg/kg base P.O.; then 5 mg/kg base at 6, 24, and 48 hours. Don't exceed adult dose. Or, 5 mg/kg base I.M. initially, repeated in 6 hours, p.r.n. Don't exceed 10 mg/kg base in 24 hours. Switch patient to oral therapy as soon as possible.

➤ **Malaria prophylaxis**—

Adults: 300 mg base P.O. once weekly on the same day each week, for 1 to 2 weeks before entering a malaria-endemic area and continued for 4 weeks after leaving the area. If treatment begins after exposure, initial dose is 600 mg P.O. in two divided doses 6 hours apart, followed by the usual dosing regimen.

Children: 5 mg/kg base P.O. once weekly on the same day each week, for 1 to 2 weeks before entering a malaria-endemic area and continued for 4 weeks after leaving the area. Don't exceed 300 mg. If treatment begins after exposure, initial dose is 10 mg/kg base P.O. in two divided doses 6 hours apart, then the usual dosing regimen.

➤ **Extraintestinal amebiasis**—

Adults: 600 mg base P.O. once daily for 2 days; then 300 mg base daily for 2 to 3 weeks. Treatment is usually combined with an intestinal amebicide. When oral therapy isn't feasible, give 160- to 200-mg base I.M. daily for 10 to 12 days. Resume oral therapy as soon as possible.

Children: 10 mg/kg base P.O. once daily for 2 to 3 weeks. Maximum dose is 300 mg base daily.

ACTION

Unknown. May bind to and alter the properties of DNA in susceptible parasites.

Route	Onset	Peak	Duration
I.M.	Unknown	0.5 hr	Unknown
P.O.	Unknown	1-3 hr	Unknown

ADVERSE REACTIONS

CNS: mild and transient headache, psychic stimulation, *seizures,* dizziness, neuropathy.

CV: hypotension, ECG changes.

EENT: blurred vision; difficulty in focusing; reversible corneal changes; typically irreversible, sometimes progressive or delayed retinal changes such as narrowing of arterioles, macular lesions, pallor of optic disk, optic atrophy, patchy retinal pigmentation, typically leading to blindness; ototoxicity; nerve deafness; vertigo; tinnitus.

GI: anorexia, abdominal cramps, diarrhea, nausea, vomiting, stomatitis.

Hematologic: *agranulocytosis, aplastic anemia,* hemolytic anemia, *thrombocytopenia.*

Skin: pruritus, lichen planus eruptions, skin and mucosal pigmentary changes, pleomorphic skin eruptions.

INTERACTIONS

Drug-drug. *Cimetidine:* Decreased hepatic metabolism of chloroquine. Monitor patient for toxicity.

Kaolin, magnesium, and aluminum salts: Decreased GI absorption. Separate administration times.

Drug-lifestyle. *Sun exposure:* May exacerbate drug-induced dermatoses. Advise patient to avoid excessive sun exposure.

EFFECTS ON LAB TEST RESULTS

● May decrease hemoglobin and granulocyte and platelet counts.

CONTRAINDICATIONS

Contraindicated in patients hypersensitive to drug and in those with retinal or visual field changes or porphyria.

NURSING CONSIDERATIONS

● Use with extreme caution in patients with severe GI, neurologic, or blood disorders.

● Use cautiously in patients with hepatic disease or alcoholism because drug concentrates in the liver. Also use cautiously in those with G6PD deficiency or psoriasis because drug may exacerbate these conditions.

● *Alert:* Drug dosage may be discussed in mg or mg base; be aware of the difference.

• Ensure that baseline and periodic ophthalmic examinations are performed. Check periodically for ocular muscle weakness after long-term use.

• Assist patient with obtaining audiometric examinations before, during, and after therapy, especially if therapy is long-term.

• Monitor CBC and liver function studies periodically during long-term therapy. If a severe blood disorder not attributable to the disease develops, drug may need to be discontinued.

• *Alert:* Monitor patient for possible overdose, which can quickly lead to toxic symptoms: headache, drowsiness, visual disturbances, CV collapse, and seizures, then cardiopulmonary arrest. Children are extremely susceptible to toxicity; avoid long-term treatment.

PATIENT TEACHING

• To enhance compliance for prophylaxis, advise patient to take drug immediately before or after meals on same day each week.

• Instruct patient to avoid excessive sun exposure to prevent exacerbation of drug-induced dermatoses.

• Tell patient to report adverse reactions promptly, especially blurred vision, increased sensitivity to light, tinnitus, hearing loss, or muscle weakness.

• Instruct patient to keep drug out of reach of children. Overdose may be fatal.

---

hydroxychloroquine sulfate
Plaquenil Sulfate

Pregnancy risk category C

AVAILABLE FORMS
Tablets: 155 mg base

INDICATIONS & DOSAGES
➤ **Suppressive prophylaxis of malaria attacks caused by** *Plasmodium vivax, P. malariae, P. ovale,* **and susceptible strains of** *P. falciparum*—
Adults: 310 mg base P.O. weekly on same day of week, beginning 1 to 2 weeks before entering malaria-endemic area and continuing for 4 weeks after leaving area. If not started before exposure, double initial dose to 620 mg base in two divided doses 6 hours apart.
Children: 5 mg/kg base P.O. weekly on same day of week, beginning 1 to 2 weeks before entering malaria-endemic area and continuing for 4 weeks after leaving area. Don't exceed adult dose. If not started before exposure, double initial dose to 10 mg/kg base in two divided doses, 6 hours apart.
➤ **Acute malarial attacks**—
Adults: Initially, 620 mg base P.O.; then 310 mg base 6 to 8 hours after initial dose; then 310 mg base daily for 2 days.
Children: Initially, 10 mg/kg base P.O.; then 5 mg/kg base at 6, 24, and 48 hours after the initial dose.
➤ **Lupus erythematosus**—
Adults: 310 mg base P.O. daily or b.i.d., continued for several weeks or months, depending on response. For prolonged maintenance dose, 155 to 310 mg base daily.
➤ **Rheumatoid arthritis**—
Adults: Initially, 310 to 465 mg base P.O. daily. When good response occurs, usually in 4 to 12 weeks, cut dosage in half.

ACTION
Unknown. May bind to and alter the properties of DNA in susceptible organisms.

Route	Onset	Peak	Duration
P.O.	Unknown	2-4.5 hr	Unknown

ADVERSE REACTIONS
CNS: irritability, nightmares, ataxia, *seizures,* psychosis, vertigo, dizziness, hypoactive deep tendon reflexes, lassitude, headache.
CV: T-wave inversion or depression, widening of QRS complex.
EENT: blurred vision; difficulty in focusing; reversible corneal changes; nystagmus; typically irreversible, sometimes progressive or delayed retinal changes such as narrowing of arterioles, macular lesions, pallor of optic disk, optic atrophy, visual field defects, patchy retinal pigmentation, commonly leading to blindness; ototoxicity.
GI: anorexia, abdominal cramps, diarrhea, nausea, vomiting.
Hematologic: *agranulocytosis, leukopenia, thrombocytopenia, hemolysis in pa-*

---

tients with G6PD deficiency, aplastic anemia.
Metabolic: weight loss.
Musculoskeletal: skeletal muscle weakness.
Skin: pruritus, lichen planus eruptions, skin and mucosal pigmentary changes, pleomorphic skin eruptions, worsened psoriasis, alopecia, bleaching of hair.

INTERACTIONS
Drug-drug. *Cimetidine:* Decreased hepatic metabolism of hydroxychloroquine. Monitor patient for toxicity.
Kaolin, magnesium and aluminum salts: Decreased GI absorption. Separate administration times.

EFFECTS ON LAB TEST RESULTS
• May decrease hemoglobin and granulocyte, WBC, and platelet counts.

CONTRAINDICATIONS
Contraindicated in patients hypersensitive to drug and in those with retinal or visual field changes or porphyria; also contraindicated as long-term therapy for children.

NURSING CONSIDERATIONS
• Use with extreme caution in patients with severe GI, neurologic, or blood disorders.
• Use cautiously in patients with hepatic disease or alcoholism because drug concentrates in liver. Also use cautiously in those with G6PD deficiency or psoriasis because drug may worsen these conditions.
• *Alert:* Drug dosage may be discussed in mg or mg base; be aware of the difference.
• Ensure that baseline and periodic ophthalmic examinations are performed. Check periodically for ocular muscle weakness after long-term use.
• Assist patient with obtaining audiometric examinations before, during, and after therapy, especially if therapy is long-term.
• Monitor CBC and liver function studies periodically during long-term therapy; if severe blood disorder not attributable to disease develops, drug may need to be discontinued.
• *Alert:* Monitor patient for possible overdose, which can quickly lead to toxic signs

or symptoms: headache, drowsiness, visual disturbances, CV collapse, and seizures, then cardiopulmonary arrest. Children are extremely susceptible to toxicity; avoid long-term treatment.

PATIENT TEACHING
• To enhance compliance for prophylaxis, advise patient to take hydroxychloroquine immediately before or after meals on same day each week.
• Instruct patient to report adverse reactions promptly.

---

mefloquine hydrochloride
Lariam

Pregnancy risk category C

AVAILABLE FORMS
Tablets: 250 mg

INDICATIONS & DOSAGES
➤ **Acute malaria infections caused by mefloquine-sensitive strains of *Plasmodium falciparum* or *P. vivax*—**
Adults and children: 15 mg/kg P.O. as a single dose, then a second dose of 10 mg/kg P.O. 6 to 8 hours later. Maximum total dose is 1,250 mg. Patients with *P. vivax* infections should receive subsequent therapy with primaquine or other 8-aminoquinolines to avoid relapse after treatment of the initial infection.
➤ **Malaria prophylaxis—**
Adults and children weighing more than 45 kg (99 lb): 250 mg P.O. once weekly. Prophylaxis should be initiated 1 week before entering endemic area and continued for 4 weeks after returning. If patient returns to an area without malaria after a prolonged stay in an endemic area, prophylaxis should end after three doses.
Children weighing 31 to 45 kg (67 to 99 lb): 187.5 mg P.O. once weekly.
Children weighing 20 to 30 kg (44 to 66 lb): 125 mg P.O. once weekly.
Children weighing 15 to 19 kg (33 to 43 lb): 62.5 mg P.O. once weekly.
Children weighing less than 15 kg (33 lb): 5 mg/kg P.O. once weekly.

ACTION
Unknown. Antimalarial action may be related to drug's ability to form complexes with hemin; may also act by raising intravesicular pH in parasite acid vesicles.

Route	Onset	Peak	Duration
P.O.	Unknown	7-24 hr	Unknown

ADVERSE REACTIONS
CNS: dizziness, syncope, headache, psychotic changes, hallucinations, confusion, anxiety, fatigue, vertigo, depression, *seizures.*
EENT: tinnitus, visual disturbances.
GI: anorexia, vomiting, *nausea,* loose stools, diarrhea, abdominal discomfort or pain.
Hematologic: decreased hematocrit, *leukopenia, thrombocytopenia.*
Musculoskeletal: myalgia.
Skin: rash.
Other: fever, chills.

INTERACTIONS
Drug-drug. *Beta blockers, quinidine, quinine:* May cause ECG abnormalities and cardiac arrest. Avoid using together.
Chloroquine, quinine: Increased risk of seizures. Avoid using together.
Valproic acid: Decreased valproic acid blood levels and loss of seizure control at start of mefloquine therapy. Monitor anticonvulsant blood levels.

EFFECTS ON LAB TEST RESULTS
• May increase transaminase levels.
• May decrease hematocrit and WBC and platelet counts.

CONTRAINDICATIONS
Contraindicated in patients hypersensitive to mefloquine or related compounds.

NURSING CONSIDERATIONS
• Use cautiously in patients with cardiac disease or seizure disorders.
• Because administering quinine and mefloquine together poses a health risk, mefloquine therapy shouldn't begin sooner than 12 hours after the last dose of quinine or quinidine.
• Patients with *P. vivax* infections are at high risk for relapse because drug doesn't eliminate the hepatic-phase exoerythrocytic parasites. Follow-up therapy with primaquine is advisable.
• Monitor liver function test results periodically.
• If overdose is suspected, induce vomiting or perform gastric lavage as appropriate because of potential for cardiotoxicity. Mefloquine has produced cardiac actions similar to quinidine and quinine.

PATIENT TEACHING
• Advise patient to take drug on the same day of the week when using it for prophylaxis.
• Tell patient not to take drug on an empty stomach and always to take it with at least 8 ounces of water.
• Advise patient to use caution when performing activities that require alertness and coordination because dizziness, disturbed sense of balance, and neuropsychiatric reactions may occur.
• Instruct patient taking mefloquine prophylactically to stop drug and to notify prescriber if signs or symptoms of impending toxicity, such as unexplained anxiety, depression, confusion, or restlessness, occur.
• Advise patient undergoing long-term therapy to have periodic ophthalmic examinations because drug may cause ocular lesions.
• Advise women of childbearing age to use reliable contraception during treatment.

primaquine phosphate

Pregnancy risk category C

AVAILABLE FORMS
Tablets: 15 mg base

INDICATIONS & DOSAGES
➤ **Radical cure of relapsing vivax malaria, eliminating symptoms and infection completely; prevention of relapse—**
Adults: 15 mg base P.O. daily for 14 days. Begin therapy during the last 2 weeks of, or after, a course of suppression with chloroquine or comparable drug.
Children: 0.3 mg/kg/day base P.O. for 14 days. Maximum 15 mg base/dose. Begin

therapy during the last 2 weeks of, or after, a course of suppression with chloroquine or comparable drug.

ACTION
Unknown. May bind to and alter the properties of DNA in susceptible parasites.

Route	Onset	Peak	Duration
P.O.	Unknown	1-3 hr	Unknown

ADVERSE REACTIONS
GI: nausea, vomiting, epigastric distress, abdominal cramps.
Hematologic: *hemolytic anemia* in G6PD deficiency, methemoglobinemia in NADH methemoglobin reductase deficiency.

INTERACTIONS
Drug-drug. *Magnesium and aluminum salts:* Decreased GI absorption. Separate administration times.
Quinacrine: Enhanced toxicity of primaquine. Avoid using together.

EFFECTS ON LAB TEST RESULTS
• May increase or decrease WBC count. May decrease RBC count and hemoglobin.

CONTRAINDICATIONS
Contraindicated in patients with systemic diseases in which agranulocytosis may develop, such as lupus erythematosus or rheumatoid arthritis, and in those taking bone marrow suppressants and potentially hemolytic drugs. Administration with quinacrine is also contraindicated.

NURSING CONSIDERATIONS
• Use cautiously in patients with previous idiosyncratic reaction, involving hemolytic anemia, methemoglobinemia, or leukopenia; in those with a family or personal history of favism; and in those with erythrocytic G6PD or NADH methemoglobin reductase deficiency.
• **Alert:** Drug dosage may be discussed in mg or mg base; be aware of the difference.
• Give drug with meals.
• Drug is used along with a fast-acting antimalarial such as chloroquine, to reduce possibility of drug-resistant strains.
• Obtain frequent blood studies and urinalysis, in light-skinned patients taking more than 30 mg base daily, dark-skinned patients taking more than 15 mg base daily, and patients with severe anemia or suspected sensitivity.
• Monitor patient for marked darkening of the urine and for sudden reduction in hemoglobin level or erythrocyte or leukocyte count, which suggest impending hemolytic reactions. Stop drug immediately and notify prescriber.

PATIENT TEACHING
• Instruct patient to take drug with meals to minimize stomach upset. If nausea, vomiting, or stomach pain persists, tell patient to notify prescriber.
• Tell patient to report chills, fever, chest pain, and cyanosis; these signs and symptoms may suggest a hemolytic reaction.
• Tell patient to stop drug and notify prescriber immediately if marked darkening of urine occurs.
• Stress importance of completing full course of therapy.

---

pyrimethamine
Daraprim

pyrimethamine with sulfadoxine
Fansidar

Pregnancy risk category C

AVAILABLE FORMS
pyrimethamine
Tablets: 25 mg
pyrimethamine with sulfadoxine
Tablets: pyrimethamine 25 mg, sulfadoxine 500 mg

INDICATIONS & DOSAGES
➤ **Malaria prophylaxis and transmission control—**
pyrimethamine
Adults and children age 10 and older: 25 mg P.O. weekly for 6 to 10 weeks or longer after leaving malaria-endemic areas.
Children ages 4 to 10: 12.5 mg P.O. weekly continued for 6 to 10 weeks or longer after leaving malaria-endemic areas.

Children younger than age 4: 6.25 mg P.O. weekly continued for 6 to 10 weeks or longer after leaving endemic areas.

pyrimethamine with sulfadoxine

Adults and children age 14 and older: 1 tablet weekly, or 2 tablets q 2 weeks during exposure and for 4 to 6 weeks after exposure.

Children ages 9 to 14: ¾ tablet weekly, or 1½ tablets q 2 weeks during exposure and for 4 to 6 weeks after exposure.

Children ages 4 to 8: ½ tablet weekly, or 1 tablet q 2 weeks during exposure and for 4 to 6 weeks after exposure.

Children younger than age 4: ¼ tablet weekly, or ½ tablet q 2 weeks during exposure and for 4 to 6 weeks after exposure.

➤ **Acute attacks of malaria—pyrimethamine**

Adults: 50 mg P.O. daily for 2 days, then 25 mg once weekly for at least 10 weeks.

Children ages 4 to 10: 25 mg P.O. once daily for 2 days, then 12.5 mg once weekly for at least 10 weeks.

pyrimethamine with sulfadoxine

Adults and children age 14 and older: 3 tablets as a single dose, given on the last day of quinine therapy.

Children ages 9 to 14: 2 tablets as a single dose, given on the last day of quinine therapy.

Children ages 4 to 8: 1 tablet as a single dose, given on the last day of quinine therapy.

Children ages 1 to 3: ½ tablet as a single dose, given on the last day of quinine therapy.

Children ages 2 to 11 months: ¼ tablet as a single dose, given on the last day of quinine therapy.

➤ **Toxoplasmosis—pyrimethamine**

Adults: Initially, 50 to 75 mg P.O. with 1 to 4 g sulfadiazine; continue for 1 to 3 weeks. After 3 weeks, reduce dosage by half and continue for 4 to 5 weeks.

Children: Initially, 1 mg/kg/day P.O. in two equally divided doses for 2 to 4 days; then 0.5 mg/kg daily for 4 weeks, along with 100 mg sulfadiazine/kg P.O. daily, divided q 6 hours. Don't exceed 100 mg.

ACTION

Inhibits the enzyme dihydrofolate reductase, thereby impeding reduction of dihydrofolic acid to tetrahydrofolic acid. Sulfadoxine competitively inhibits use of PABA.

Route	Onset	Peak	Duration
P.O.	Unknown	1.5-8 hr	2 wk

ADVERSE REACTIONS

CNS: headache, peripheral neuritis, mental depression, *seizures,* ataxia, hallucinations, fatigue.
CV: *arrhythmias,* allergic myocarditis.
EENT: scleral irritation, periorbital edema.
GI: anorexia, vomiting, atrophic glossitis.
Hematologic: *agranulocytosis, aplastic anemia,* megaloblastic anemia, *leukopenia, thrombocytopenia, pancytopenia.*
Skin: *Stevens-Johnson syndrome,* generalized skin eruptions, urticaria, pruritus, photosensitivity.

INTERACTIONS

Drug-drug. *Co-trimoxazole, methotrexate, sulfonamides:* Increased risk of bone marrow suppression. Avoid using together.
Lorazepam: Increased risk of hepatotoxicity. Avoid using together.
PABA: Decreased antitoxoplasmic effects. May need to adjust dosage.

EFFECTS ON LAB TEST RESULTS

● May decrease hemoglobin and granulocyte, WBC, platelet, and RBC counts.

CONTRAINDICATIONS

Pyrimethamine is contraindicated in patients hypersensitive to drug and in those with megaloblastic anemia from folic acid deficiency. Pyrimethamine with sulfadoxine is contraindicated in patients with porphyria.

Repeated use of pyrimethamine with sulfadoxine is contraindicated in patients with severe renal insufficiency, marked parenchymal damage to the liver, blood dyscrasias, known hypersensitivity to pyrimethamine or sulfonamides, or documented megaloblastic anemia from folate deficiency. Also contraindicated in infants younger than 2 months old and in pregnant (at term) and breast-feeding women.

NURSING CONSIDERATIONS
• Use cautiously after treatment with chloroquine and in patients with impaired hepatic or renal function, severe allergy or bronchial asthma, G6PD deficiency, or seizure disorders (smaller doses may be needed).

• Pyrimethamine alone isn't recommended for treatment of malaria in nonimmune patients. Drug should be used with faster-acting antimalarials such as chloroquine for 2 days to initiate transmission control and suppressive cure.

• Obtain twice-weekly blood counts, including platelets for the patient with toxoplasmosis because dosages used approach toxic levels. If signs of folic acid or folinic acid deficiency develop, dosage should be reduced or discontinued while patient receives parenteral folinic acid (leucovorin) until blood counts become normal.

• Adverse drug reactions related to sulfadiazine are similar to sulfonamides.

• When used to treat toxoplasmosis in patients with AIDS, therapy may be lifelong.

• Pyrimethamine with sulfadoxine should be used only in areas where chloroquine-resistant malaria is prevalent and only if the traveler plans to stay longer than 3 weeks.

PATIENT TEACHING
• Instruct patient to take drug with meals.
• Inform patient with toxoplasmosis of importance of frequent laboratory studies and compliance with therapy. Tell patient he may need long-term therapy.
• Warn patient taking pyrimethamine with sulfadoxine to stop drug and notify prescriber at first sign of rash, sore throat, or glossitis.
• Tell patient to take first prophylactic dose 1 to 2 days before traveling.

8

Antituberculotics and antileprotics

clofazimine
cycloserine
dapsone
ethambutol hydrochloride
isoniazid
pyrazinamide
rifabutin
rifampin
rifapentine
streptomycin sulfate
(See Chapter 9, AMINOGLYCOSIDES.)

COMBINATION PRODUCTS
RIFAMATE: isoniazid 150 mg and rifampin 300 mg
RIFATER: isoniazid 50 mg, rifampin 120 mg, and pyrazinamide 300 mg

---

clofazimine
Lamprene

Pregnancy risk category C

AVAILABLE FORMS
Capsules: 50 mg

INDICATIONS & DOSAGES
➤ **Dapsone-resistant leprosy (Hansen's disease)—**
Adults: 100 mg P.O. daily with other antileprotics for 3 years. Then, clofazimine alone, 100 mg daily.
➤ **Erythema nodosum leprosum—**
Adults: 100 to 200 mg P.O. daily for up to 3 months; when prolonged, must use with corticosteroid therapy. Dose is tapered to 100 mg daily as soon as possible. Maximum dose is 200 mg daily.

ACTION
Unknown. Thought to inhibit mycobacterial growth by binding preferentially to mycobacterial DNA. Also has anti-inflammatory effects that suppress skin reactions of erythema nodosum leprosum.

Route	Onset	Peak	Duration
P.O.	Unknown	1-6 hr	Unknown

ADVERSE REACTIONS
EENT: *conjunctival and corneal pigmentation, dryness, burning, itching, and irritation.*
GI: *epigastric pain, diarrhea, nausea, vomiting, GI intolerance,* **bowel obstruction, bleeding.**
Hematologic: eosinophilia.
Metabolic: hypokalemia, hyperglycemia.
Skin: *pink to brownish black pigmentation, ichthyosis and dryness,* rash, pruritus.
Other: *splenic infarction,* discolored body fluids and excrement.

INTERACTIONS
Drug-drug. *Dapsone:* May inhibit antiinflammatory effects of clofazimine. No intervention is needed.
Isoniazid: May decrease level of drug in skin and increase serum and urine levels of clofazimine. Monitor patient for decreased effectiveness.
Rifampin: Decreased rifampin bioavailability. Monitor patient for decreased effectiveness.

EFFECTS ON LAB TEST RESULTS
● May increase albumin, bilirubin, and AST levels. May decrease potassium and glucose levels.
● May increase eosinophil count.

CONTRAINDICATIONS
No known contraindications.

NURSING CONSIDERATIONS
● Use cautiously in patients with GI dysfunction, such as abdominal pain and diarrhea.
● Give doses exceeding 100 mg daily for as short a period as possible and only under close medical supervision.
● If patient complains of colic, burning abdominal pain, or other GI symptoms, notify prescriber, who may reduce dose or increase interval between doses.

PATIENT TEACHING
● Advise patient to take drug with meals or milk.

Reactions may be *common*, uncommon, *life-threatening*, or COMMON AND LIFE-THREATENING.

• Warn patient that clofazimine may discolor skin, body fluids, and excrement. The color ranges from pink to brownish black. Reassure patient that the unsightly skin discoloration is reversible but may not disappear until several months or years after drug treatment ends.
• Tell patient to apply skin oil or cream to help reverse skin dryness or ichthyosis.

---

cycloserine
Seromycin

Pregnancy risk category C

AVAILABLE FORMS
Capsules: 250 mg

INDICATIONS & DOSAGES
➤ **Adjunctive treatment in pulmonary or extrapulmonary tuberculosis—**
Adults: Initially, 250 mg P.O. q 12 hours for 2 weeks; then, if blood levels are below 25 to 30 mcg/ml and no toxicity has developed, increase dosage to 250 mg q 8 hours for 2 weeks. If optimum blood levels still aren't achieved and no toxicity has developed, then increase dosage to 250 mg q 6 hours. Maximum dose is 1 g/day. If CNS toxicity occurs, stop drug for 1 week, then resume at 250 mg daily for 2 weeks. If no serious toxic effects occur, increase dosage by 250-mg increments q 10 days until blood level of 25 to 30 mcg/ml is obtained.
Children: 10 to 20 mg/kg/day P.O. in two divided doses. Maximum dose is 0.75 to 1 g.
➤ **Acute urinary tract infections—**
Adults: 250 mg P.O. q 12 hours for 2 weeks.

ACTION
Inhibits cell-wall biosynthesis by interfering with the bacterial use of amino acids. Action may be bacteriostatic or bactericidal, depending on the concentration of drug attained at the site of infection and the susceptibility of the infecting organism.

Route	Onset	Peak	Duration
P.O.	Unknown	4-8 hr	Unknown

ADVERSE REACTIONS
CNS: *seizures,* drowsiness, somnolence, headache, tremor, dysarthria, vertigo, confusion, loss of memory, *possible suicidal tendencies,* psychosis, hyperirritability, paresthesia, paresis, hyperreflexia, *coma.*
CV: *sudden heart failure.*
Other: hypersensitivity reactions.

INTERACTIONS
Drug-drug. *Ethionamide:* May potentiate neurotoxic adverse reactions. Monitor patient closely.
Isoniazid: Increased risk of CNS toxicity, including dizziness or drowsiness. Monitor patient closely.
Drug-lifestyle. *Alcohol use:* Increased risk of CNS toxicity, including seizures. Advise patient to avoid alcohol.

EFFECTS ON LAB TEST RESULTS
• May increase transaminase level.

CONTRAINDICATIONS
Contraindicated in patients hypersensitive to drug and in those with seizure disorders, depression, severe anxiety, psychosis, or severe renal insufficiency. Also contraindicated in patients who use alcohol excessively.

NURSING CONSIDERATIONS
• Use cautiously in patients with impaired renal function; these patients need reduced dosage.
• Obtain specimen for culture and sensitivity tests before therapy begins and then periodically to detect possible resistance.
• Cycloserine is considered a second-line drug in tuberculosis treatment and should always be administered with other antituberculotics to prevent the development of resistant organisms.
• Cycloserine should be used to treat urinary tract infections only when better alternatives are contraindicated and susceptibility to cycloserine is confirmed.
• Monitor serum cycloserine levels periodically, especially in patients receiving high doses (over 500 mg daily) because toxic reactions may occur with blood levels above 30 mcg/ml.
• Observe patient receiving doses of more than 500 mg daily for signs and symptoms

---

of CNS toxicity, such as seizures, anxiety, and tremor.

• Monitor results of hematologic tests and renal and liver function studies.

• Observe patient for psychotic symptoms, hallucinations, and possible suicidal tendencies.

• Monitor patient for hypersensitivity reactions, such as allergic dermatitis.

• Give pyridoxine, anticonvulsant, tranquilizer, or sedative to relieve adverse reactions.

PATIENT TEACHING

• Warn patient to avoid alcohol, which may cause serious neurologic reactions.

• Advise patient not to perform hazardous activities if drowsiness occurs.

• Tell patient to report adverse reactions promptly; dosage may need to be adjusted or other drugs prescribed to relieve adverse reactions.

---

dapsone
Avlosulfon†, Dapsone 100‡

Pregnancy risk category C

AVAILABLE FORMS
Tablets: 25 mg, 100 mg

INDICATIONS & DOSAGES
➤ **Multibacillary leprosy—**
Adults and children older than age 14:
100 mg P.O. daily for 12 months, given with one or more antileprotics.
Children ages 10 to 14: 50 mg P.O. daily for 12 months, given with one or more antileprotics.
Children younger than age 10: 25 mg P.O. daily for 12 months, given with one or more antileprotics.
➤ **Paucibacillary leprosy—**
Adults and children older than age 14:
100 mg P.O. daily with rifampin 600 mg once monthly for 6 months.
Children ages 10 to 14: 50 mg P.O. daily with rifampin 450 mg once monthly for 6 months.
Children younger than age 10: 25 mg P.O. daily with rifampin 300 mg once monthly for 6 months.

➤ **Dermatitis herpetiformis—**
Adults: Initially, 50 mg P.O. daily; usual maintenance dose in adults ranges from 25 to 400 mg daily.

ACTION
Unknown. May inhibit folic acid biosynthesis in susceptible organisms.

Route	Onset	Peak	Duration
P.O.	Unknown	4-8 hr	Unknown

ADVERSE REACTIONS
CNS: insomnia, psychosis, paresthesia, peripheral neuropathy, headache, vertigo.
CV: tachycardia.
EENT: tinnitus, blurred vision.
GI: anorexia, abdominal pain, nausea, vomiting, *pancreatitis.*
GU: albuminuria, nephrotic syndrome, renal papillary necrosis, male infertility.
Hematologic: *hemolytic anemia, agranulocytosis, aplastic anemia.*
Respiratory: pulmonary eosinophilia.
Skin: lupus erythematosus, phototoxicity, exfoliative dermatitis, *toxic erythema, erythema multiforme, toxic epidermal necrolysis,* morbilliform and scarlatiniform reactions, urticaria, *erythema nodosum.*
Other: fever, infectious mononucleosis-like syndrome, *sulfone syndrome.*

INTERACTIONS
Drug-drug. *Activated charcoal:* May decrease dapsone's GI absorption and enterohepatic recycling. Monitor patient.
Didanosine: May cause therapeutic failure of dapsone, leading to increased infection. Avoid using together.
Folic acid antagonists such as methotrexate: Increased risk of adverse hematologic reactions. Avoid using together.
PABA: May antagonize effect of dapsone by interfering with primary mechanism of action. Monitor patient for lack of efficacy.
Probenecid: Reduced urinary excretion of dapsone metabolites, increasing plasma levels. Monitor patient.
Rifampin: Increased hepatic metabolism of dapsone. Monitor patient for lack of efficacy.
Trimethoprim: May increase serum levels of both drugs, possibly increasing phar-

---

macologic and toxic effects of each drug. Monitor patient.

Drug-lifestyle. *Sun exposure:* May cause photosensitivity. Tell patient to avoid prolonged exposure to sunlight or sunlamps.

EFFECTS ON LAB TEST RESULTS
• May decrease hemoglobin and granulocyte count.

CONTRAINDICATIONS
Contraindicated in patients hypersensitive to drug. Also contraindicated in breast-feeding women because of risk of tumorigenicity.

NURSING CONSIDERATIONS
• Use cautiously in patients with chronic renal, hepatic, or CV disease; refractory types of anemia; and G6PD deficiency.
• Obtain baseline CBC. Monitor CBC weekly for first month, monthly for 6 months, and then semiannually.
• Reduce or temporarily discontinue dapsone if hemoglobin falls below 9 g/dl, WBC count falls below 5,000/mm³, or RBC count falls below 2.5 million/mm³ or remains low.
• If generalized diffuse dermatitis occurs, notify prescriber and prepare to interrupt therapy.
• Give antihistamines to combat allergic dermatitis.
• Watch for signs and symptoms of erythema nodosum reaction, such as malaise, fever, painful inflammatory induration in skin and mucosa, iritis, and neuritis, which may occur during therapy as a result of *Mycobacterium leprae* bacilli. In severe cases, stop therapy and give glucocorticoids cautiously.
• Watch for and report signs and symptoms of sulfone syndrome, including fever, malaise, jaundice with hepatic necrosis, lymphadenopathy, methemoglobinemia, and hemolytic anemia.

PATIENT TEACHING
• *Alert:* Instruct breast-feeding patient to immediately notify prescriber if cyanosis occurs in infant.
• Inform patient of need for long-term therapy. Stress importance of compliance with drug therapy.

• Advise patient to avoid unprotected exposure to sunlight or sunlamps.

---

ethambutol hydrochloride
Etibi†, Myambutol

Pregnancy risk category B

AVAILABLE FORMS
Tablets: 100 mg, 400 mg

INDICATIONS & DOSAGES
➤ **Adjunctive treatment in pulmonary tuberculosis—**
Adults and children older than age 13: In patients who haven't received previous antitubercular therapy, 15 mg/kg P.O. as a single daily dose.

Retreatment: 25 mg/kg P.O. daily as a single dose for 60 days (or until bacteriologic smears and cultures become negative) with at least one other antituberculotic; then decreased to 15 mg/kg/day as a single dose.

ACTION
Unknown. Appears to interfere with the synthesis of one or more metabolites of susceptible bacteria, altering cellular metabolism during cell division (bacteriostatic).

Route	Onset	Peak	Duration
P.O.	Unknown	2-4 hr	Unknown

ADVERSE REACTIONS
CNS: headache, dizziness, mental confusion, hallucinations, malaise, peripheral neuritis.
EENT: optic neuritis.
GI: anorexia, nausea, vomiting, abdominal pain, GI upset.
Hematologic: *thrombocytopenia.*
Metabolic: hyperuricemia.
Musculoskeletal: joint pain.
Respiratory: bloody sputum.
Skin: dermatitis, pruritus, *toxic epidermal necrolysis.*
Other: *anaphylactoid reactions,* fever, precipitation of acute gout.

INTERACTIONS
Drug-drug. *Aluminum salts:* May delay and reduce absorption of ethambutol. Sep-

---

arate administration times by several hours.

EFFECTS ON LAB TEST RESULTS
• May increase ALT, AST, bilirubin, and uric acid levels. May decrease glucose level.

CONTRAINDICATIONS
Contraindicated in children younger than age 13, patients hypersensitive to drug, and patients with optic neuritis.

NURSING CONSIDERATIONS
• Use cautiously in patients with impaired renal function, cataracts, recurrent eye inflammation, gout, or diabetic retinopathy.
• Perform visual acuity and color discrimination tests before and during therapy.
• Ensure that any changes in vision don't result from an underlying condition.
• Obtain AST and ALT levels before therapy, and monitor these levels every 3 to 4 weeks.
• Anticipate dosage reduction in patients with impaired renal function.
• Always give ethambutol with other antituberculotics to prevent development of resistant organisms.
• Monitor serum uric acid level; observe patient for signs and symptoms of gout.

PATIENT TEACHING
• Reassure patient that visual disturbances usually disappear several weeks to months after drug is stopped. Optic neuritis is related to dose and duration of treatment.
• Inform patient that drug is given with other antituberculotics.
• Stress importance of compliance with drug therapy.

isoniazid (INH, isonicotinic acid hydrazide)
Isotamine†, Nydrazid**, PMS-Isoniazid†

Pregnancy risk category C

AVAILABLE FORMS
Injection: 100 mg/ml
Oral solution: 50 mg/5 ml
Tablets: 50 mg, 100 mg, 300 mg

INDICATIONS & DOSAGES
➤ **Actively growing tubercle bacilli—**
Adults: 5 mg/kg P.O. or I.M. daily in a single dose, up to 300 mg/day, with other drugs, continued for 6 months to 2 years.
Infants and children: 10 to 20 mg/kg P.O. or I.M. daily in a single dose, up to 300 mg/day, continued long enough to prevent relapse. Drug should be used with at least one other antituberculotic.
➤ **Prevention of tubercle bacilli in those exposed to tuberculosis or those with positive skin test results whose chest X-rays and bacteriologic studies are consistent with nonprogressive tuberculosis—**
Adults: 300 mg P.O. daily in a single dose, continued for 6 months to 1 year.
Infants and children: 10 mg/kg P.O. daily in a single dose, up to 300 mg/day, continued for up to 1 year.

ACTION
Unknown. Appears to inhibit cell-wall biosynthesis by interfering with lipid and DNA synthesis (bactericidal).

Route	Onset	Peak	Duration
I.M., P.O.	Unknown	1-2 hr	Unknown

ADVERSE REACTIONS
CNS: *peripheral neuropathy, seizures,* toxic encephalopathy, memory impairment, toxic psychosis.
EENT: optic neuritis and atrophy.
GI: nausea, vomiting, epigastric distress.
Hematologic: *agranulocytosis,* hemolytic anemia, *aplastic anemia,* eosinophilia, *thrombocytopenia,* sideroblastic anemia.
Hepatic: *hepatitis,* jaundice, bilirubinemia.
Metabolic: hyperglycemia, metabolic acidosis, hypocalcemia, hypophosphatemia.
Skin: irritation at I.M. injection site.
Other: rheumatic and lupuslike syndromes, hypersensitivity reactions, pyridoxine deficiency, gynecomastia.

INTERACTIONS
Drug-drug. *Antacids and laxatives containing aluminum:* May decrease isoniazid absorption. Give isoniazid at least 1 hour before antacid or laxative.
Benzodiazepines such as diazepam, triazolam: Isoniazid may inhibit metabolic

clearance of benzodiazepines that undergo oxidative metabolism, possibly increasing benzodiazepine activity. Monitor patient.

Carbamazepine, phenytoin: Increased plasma levels of these drugs. Monitor plasma levels closely.

Cycloserine: May increase CNS adverse reactions. Institute safety precautions.

Disulfiram: May cause neurologic symptoms, including changes in behavior and coordination. Avoid using together.

Enflurane: In rapid acetylators of isoniazid, may cause high-output renal failure because of nephrotoxic levels of inorganic fluoride. Monitor renal function.

Ketoconazole: May decrease serum levels of ketoconazole. Monitor patient for lack of efficacy.

Meperidine: May increase CNS adverse reactions and hypotension. Institute safety precautions.

Oral anticoagulants: May enhance anticoagulant activity. Monitor patient.

Phenytoin: Inhibited phenytoin metabolism and increased phenytoin levels. Monitor patient for phenytoin toxicity.

Drug-food. *Foods containing tyramine:* May cause hypertensive crisis. Tell patient to avoid such foods or eat in small quantities.

Drug-lifestyle. *Alcohol use:* May increase risk of isoniazid-related hepatitis. Discourage using together.

EFFECTS ON LAB TEST RESULTS
• May increase transaminase, glucose, and bilirubin levels. May decrease calcium and phosphate levels.
• May increase eosinophil count. May decrease hemoglobin and granulocyte and platelet counts.

CONTRAINDICATIONS
Contraindicated in patients with acute hepatic disease or isoniazid-related liver damage.

NURSING CONSIDERATIONS
• Use cautiously in elderly patients and in those with chronic non–isoniazid-related liver disease, and seizure disorders (especially those taking phenytoin). Also use cautiously in patients with severe renal impairment or chronic alcoholism.

• Always give isoniazid with other antituberculotics to prevent development of resistant organisms.

• Isoniazid pharmacokinetics may vary among patients because drug is metabolized in the liver by genetically controlled acetylation. Fast acetylators metabolize drug up to five times as fast as slow acetylators. About 50% of blacks and whites are slow acetylators; more than 80% of Chinese, Japanese, and Inuits are fast acetylators.

• Peripheral neuropathy is more common in patients who are slow acetylators or who are malnourished, alcoholic, or diabetic.

• Isoniazid alters results of urine glucose tests that use cupric sulfate method such as Benedict's reagent or Diastix.

• Monitor hepatic function closely for changes. Elevated liver function study results occur in about 15% of patients; most abnormalities are mild and transient, but some may persist throughout treatment.

• **Alert:** Severe and sometimes fatal hepatitis may develop, even after many months of treatment. Risk increases with age. Monitor liver studies closely.

• Give pyridoxine to prevent peripheral neuropathy, especially in malnourished patients.

PATIENT TEACHING
• Instruct patient to take drug exactly as prescribed; warn against stopping drug without prescriber's consent.

• Advise patient to take drug 1 hour before or 2 hours after meals.

• Tell patient to notify prescriber immediately if signs and symptoms of liver impairment occur, such as anorexia, fatigue, malaise, jaundice, and dark urine.

• Advise patient to avoid alcoholic beverages while taking drug. Also tell him to avoid certain foods (fish such as skipjack and tuna and products containing tyramine, such as aged cheese, beer, and chocolate) because drug has some MAO inhibitor activity.

• Encourage patient to comply fully with treatment, which may take months or years.

---

pyrazinamide
PMS-Pyrazinamide†, Tebrazid†, Zinamide‡

Pregnancy risk category C

AVAILABLE FORMS
Tablets: 500 mg

INDICATIONS & DOSAGES
➤ **Adjunctive treatment of tuberculosis when primary and secondary antituberculotics can't be used or have failed—**
Adults: 15 to 30 mg/kg P.O. once daily. Maximum dose is 3 g daily. Or, when compliance is a problem, 50 to 70 mg/kg based on lean body mass P.O. twice weekly.

ACTION
Unknown.

Route	Onset	Peak	Duration
P.O.	Unknown	1-2 hr	Unknown

ADVERSE REACTIONS
CNS: malaise.
GI: anorexia, nausea, vomiting.
GU: dysuria, interstitial nephritis.
Hematologic: sideroblastic anemia, *thrombocytopenia.*
Hepatic: *hepatotoxicity, hepatitis.*
Metabolic: hyperuricemia.
Musculoskeletal: *arthralgia, myalgia.*
Skin: rash, urticaria, pruritus, photosensitivity.
Other: fever, gout, porphyria.

INTERACTIONS
None significant.

EFFECTS ON LAB TEST RESULTS
● May increase uric acid level.
● May decrease platelet count and hemoglobin.

CONTRAINDICATIONS
Contraindicated in patients hypersensitive to drug and in those with severe hepatic disease or acute gout.

NURSING CONSIDERATIONS
● Use cautiously in patients with diabetes mellitus, renal failure, or gout.

● Always give pyrazinamide with other antituberculotics to prevent the development of resistant organisms.
● Drug is administered for the initial 2 months of a 6-month or longer treatment regimen for drug-susceptible patients. Patients with HIV infection may need longer courses of therapy.
● Doses that exceed 35 mg/kg may cause liver damage.
● Perform baseline serum uric acid and liver function tests before treatment.
● Monitor hematopoietic studies and serum uric acid levels.
● Monitor liver function studies; assess patient for jaundice and liver tenderness or enlargement before and frequently during therapy.
● Pyrazinamide may interfere with urine ketone determinations. Drug's systemic effects may temporarily decrease 17-ketosteroid levels. Drug may increase protein-bound iodine and urate levels.
● *Alert:* Immediately report signs and symptoms of gout and liver impairment, such as anorexia, fatigue, malaise, jaundice, dark urine, and liver tenderness.
● When used with surgical management of tuberculosis, start pyrazinamide 1 to 2 weeks before surgery and continue for 4 to 6 weeks postoperatively.

PATIENT TEACHING
● Inform patient that he must take drug together with other antituberculotics.
● Tell patient to report adverse reactions promptly, especially fever, malaise, loss of appetite, nausea, vomiting, dark urine, yellow skin or eye discoloration, and pain or swelling of the joints.
● Stress importance of compliance with drug therapy. If daily therapy poses a problem, tell patient to ask prescriber about twice-weekly dosing.

rifabutin
Mycobutin

Pregnancy risk category B

AVAILABLE FORMS
Capsules: 150 mg

INDICATIONS & DOSAGES
➤ **Prevention of disseminated** *Mycobacterium avium* **complex in patients with advanced HIV infection—**
Adults: 300 mg P.O. daily as a single dose or divided b.i.d.

ACTION
Inhibits DNA-dependent RNA polymerase in susceptible bacteria, blocking bacterial protein synthesis.

Route	Onset	Peak	Duration
P.O.	Unknown	2-4 hr	Unknown

ADVERSE REACTIONS
CNS: headache.
GI: dyspepsia, eructation, flatulence, diarrhea, nausea, vomiting, abdominal pain, anorexia, taste perversion.
GU: discolored urine.
Hematologic: *neutropenia, leukopenia, thrombocytopenia,* eosinophilia.
Musculoskeletal: myalgia.
Skin: *rash.*
Other: fever.

INTERACTIONS
Drug-drug. *Drugs metabolized by the liver; zidovudine:* May alter serum levels of these drugs. May need to adjust dosage.
Oral contraceptives: Decreased effectiveness. Tell patient to use alternate form of birth control.
Drug-food. *High-fat foods:* Reduced rate but not extent of absorption. Advise patient to avoid using together.

EFFECTS ON LAB TEST RESULTS
• May increase aminotransferase levels.
• May decrease neutrophil, WBC, and platelet counts.

CONTRAINDICATIONS
Contraindicated in patients hypersensitive to drug or other rifamycin derivatives such as rifampin. Also contraindicated in patients with active tuberculosis because single-drug therapy with rifabutin increases risk of inducing bacterial resistance to both rifabutin and rifampin.

NURSING CONSIDERATIONS
• Use cautiously in patients with neutropenia and thrombocytopenia. Obtain baseline hematologic studies and repeat periodically.
• Mix drug with soft foods such as applesauce for patients who have difficulty swallowing.
• Dosage may be divided to take twice daily to decrease GI adverse effects.
• *Alert:* Don't confuse rifabutin with rifampin or rifapentine.

PATIENT TEACHING
• Instruct patient to take drug for as long as prescribed, exactly as directed, even after feeling better.
• Tell patient that drug or its metabolites may color urine, feces, sputum, saliva, tears, and skin brownish orange. Tell him to avoid wearing soft contact lenses because they may be permanently stained.
• Instruct patient to report photophobia, excessive lacrimation, or eye pain immediately; drug may rarely cause uveitis.
• Advise patient to report paresthesia and joint stiffness, swelling, or tenderness; these symptoms indicate arthralgias or myositis.

---

rifampin (rifampicin)
Rifadin, Rimactane, Rimycin‡, Rofact†

Pregnancy risk category C

AVAILABLE FORMS
Capsules: 150 mg, 300 mg
Injection: 600 mg

INDICATIONS & DOSAGES
➤ **Pulmonary tuberculosis—**
Adults: 600 mg P.O. or I.V. daily in single dose 1 hour before or 2 hours after meals.
Children older than age 5: 10 to 20 mg/kg P.O. or I.V. daily in single dose 1 hour before or 2 hours after meals. Maximum daily dose is 600 mg. Administration with other antituberculotics is recommended.
➤ **Meningococcal carriers—**
Adults: 600 mg P.O. or I.V. q 12 hours for 2 days; or 600 mg P.O. or I.V. once daily for 4 days.
Children ages 1 month to 12 years: 10 mg/kg P.O. or I.V. q 12 hours for 2 days, not to exceed 600 mg/day; or 20 mg/kg once daily for 4 days.

Neonates: 5 mg/kg P.O. or I.V. q 12 hours for 2 days.

I.V. ADMINISTRATION
● Reconstitute drug with 10 ml of sterile water for injection to make a solution containing 60 mg/ml.
● Add to 100 ml of D₅W and infuse over 30 minutes, or add to 500 ml of D₅W and infuse over 3 hours.
● When dextrose is contraindicated, drug may be diluted with normal saline solution for injection. Don't use other I.V. solutions.
● Prepare and use solution within a 4-hour period.

ACTION
Inhibits DNA-dependent RNA polymerase, thus impairing RNA synthesis (bactericidal).

Route	Onset	Peak	Duration
I.V.	Unknown	Unknown	Unknown
P.O.	Unknown	2-4 hr	Unknown

ADVERSE REACTIONS
CNS: headache, fatigue, drowsiness, behavioral changes, dizziness, mental confusion, generalized numbness, ataxia.
CV: *shock.*
EENT: visual disturbances, exudative conjunctivitis.
GI: epigastric distress, anorexia, nausea, vomiting, abdominal pain, diarrhea, flatulence, sore mouth and tongue, pseudomembranous colitis, *pancreatitis.*
GU: hemoglobinuria, hematuria, *acute renal failure,* menstrual disturbances.
Hematologic: eosinophilia, *thrombocytopenia, transient leukopenia,* hemolytic anemia.
Hepatic: *hepatotoxicity.*
Metabolic: hyperuricemia.
Musculoskeletal: osteomalacia.
Respiratory: shortness of breath, wheezing.
Skin: pruritus, urticaria, rash.
Other: flu syndrome, discoloration of body fluids, porphyria exacerbation.

INTERACTIONS
Drug-drug. *Acetaminophen, analgesics, anticonvulsants, barbiturates, beta blockers, cardiac glycosides, clofibrate, chlor-amphenicol, corticosteroids, cyclosporine, dapsone, diazepam, disopyramide, methadone, mexiletine, narcotics, oral contraceptives, progestins, quinidine, sulfonylureas, theophylline, verapamil:* Reduced effectiveness of these drugs. Monitor patient.
Anticoagulants: Increased requirements for these drugs. Monitor PT and INR closely and adjust dosage of anticoagulant as needed.
Halothane: May increase risk of hepatotoxicity of both drugs. Monitor liver function closely.
Isoniazid: Increased risk of hepatotoxicity. Monitor patient closely.
Ketoconazole, para-aminosalicylate sodium: May interfere with absorption of rifampin. Give these drugs 8 to 12 hours apart.
Probenecid: May increase rifampin levels. Use together cautiously.
Drug-lifestyle. *Alcohol use:* May increase risk of hepatotoxicity. Tell patient to avoid alcohol during therapy.

EFFECTS ON LAB TEST RESULTS
● May increase ALT, AST, alkaline phosphatase, bilirubin, and uric acid levels.
● May increase eosiniphil counts. May decrease hemoglobin and platelet and WBC counts.

CONTRAINDICATIONS
Contraindicated in patients hypersensitive to rifampin or related drugs.

NURSING CONSIDERATIONS
● Use cautiously in patients with liver disease.
● Treatment with at least one other antituberculotic is recommended.
● Give 1 hour before or 2 hours after meals for optimal absorption; however, if GI irritation occurs, patient may take rifampin with meals.
● Monitor hepatic function, hematopoietic studies, and serum uric acid levels. Drug's systemic effects may cause asymptomatic elevation of liver function test results and serum uric acid level.
● Watch for and report to prescriber signs and symptoms of hepatic impairment.
● Drug may cause hemorrhage in neonates of rifampin-treated mothers.

Reactions may be *common,* uncommon, ***life-threatening***, or **COMMON AND LIFE-THREATENING.**

• Rifampin alters standard serum folate and vitamin B_{12} assays. Rifampin may cause temporary retention of sulfobromophthalein in the liver excretion test. It may also interfere with contrast material in gallbladder studies and urinalysis based on spectrophotometry.

• **Alert:** Don't confuse rifampin with rifabutin or rifapentine.

PATIENT TEACHING
• Instruct patient who develops drug-induced GI upset to take drug with meals.
• Warn patient about drowsiness and possible red-orange discoloration of urine, feces, saliva, sweat, sputum, and tears. Soft contact lenses may be permanently stained.
• Advise patient to avoid alcohol during drug therapy.

rifapentine
Priftin

Pregnancy risk category C

AVAILABLE FORMS
Tablets (film-coated): 150 mg

INDICATIONS & DOSAGES
➤ **Pulmonary tuberculosis, with at least one other antituberculotic to which the isolate is susceptible—**
Adults: During intensive phase of short-course therapy, 600 mg P.O. twice weekly for 2 months, with an interval between doses of not less than 3 days (72 hours).

During continuation phase of short-course therapy, 600 mg P.O. once weekly for 4 months with isoniazid or another drug to which the isolate is susceptible.

ACTION
Inhibits DNA-dependent RNA polymerase in susceptible strains of *Mycobacterium tuberculosis.* Demonstrates bactericidal activity against the organism both intracellularly and extracellularly.

Route	Onset	Peak	Duration
P.O.	Unknown	5-6 hr	Unknown

ADVERSE REACTIONS
CNS: headache, dizziness, pain.
CV: hypertension.

GI: anorexia, nausea, vomiting, dyspepsia, diarrhea.
GU: pyuria, proteinuria, hematuria, urinary casts.
Hematologic: *neutropenia,* lymphopenia, anemia, *leukopenia,* thrombocytosis.
Metabolic: *hyperuricemia.*
Musculoskeletal: arthralgia.
Respiratory: hemoptysis.
Skin: rash, pruritus, acne, maculopapular rash.

INTERACTIONS
Drug-drug. *Antiarrhythmics (disopyramide, mexiletine, quinidine, tocainide), antibiotics (chloramphenicol, clarithromycin, dapsone, doxycycline, fluoroquinolones), anticonvulsants (phenytoin), antifungals (fluconazole, itraconazole, ketoconazole), barbiturates, benzodiazepines (diazepam), beta blockers, calcium channel blockers (diltiazem, nifedipine, verapamil), cardiac glycosides, clofibrate, corticosteroids, haloperidol, HIV protease inhibitors (indinavir, nelfinavir, ritonavir, saquinavir), immunosuppressants (cyclosporine, tacrolimus), levothyroxine, narcotic analgesics (methadone), oral anticoagulants (warfarin), oral hypoglycemics (sulfonylureas), oral or other systemic hormonal contraceptives, progestins, quinine, reverse transcriptase inhibitors (delavirdine, zidovudine), sildenafil, theophylline, tricyclic antidepressants (amitriptyline, nortriptyline):* Rifapentine induces metabolism of the hepatic cytochrome P-450 enzyme system, decreasing activity of these drugs. May need to adjust dosage.

EFFECTS ON LAB TEST RESULTS
• May increase uric acid, ALT, and AST levels.
• May increase platelet count. May decrease hemoglobin and neutrophil and WBC counts.

CONTRAINDICATIONS
Contraindicated in patients hypersensitive to a rifamycin (rifapentine, rifampin, or rifabutin).

NURSING CONSIDERATIONS
• Use drug cautiously and with frequent monitoring in patients with liver disease.

• Rifamycin antibiotics have been linked to hepatotoxicity. Monitor liver function test results before beginning drug therapy.

• Giving with pyridoxine (vitamin B$_6$) is recommended in malnourished patients; in those predisposed to neuropathy, such as alcoholics and diabetics; and in adolescents.

• May alter serum assays for folate and vitamin B$_{12}$.

• *Alert:* Give drug with appropriate daily companion drugs. Compliance with all drug regimens, especially with daily companion drugs on the days when rifapentine isn't given, is crucial for early sputum conversion and protection from relapse of tuberculosis.

• Taken during the last 2 weeks of pregnancy, drug may lead to postnatal hemorrhage in mother or infant. Monitor clotting parameters closely if drug is given.

• Notify prescriber of persistent or severe diarrhea.

• *Alert:* Don't confuse rifapentine with rifabutin or rifampin.

PATIENT TEACHING

• Stress importance of strict compliance with this drug regimen and that of daily companion drugs, as well as necessary follow-up visits and laboratory tests.

• Advise a woman to use nonhormonal methods of birth control.

• Tell patient to take drug with food if nausea, vomiting, or GI upset occurs.

• Instruct patient to report fever, loss of appetite, malaise, nausea, vomiting, darkened urine, yellowish discoloration of skin and eyes, pain or swelling of the joints, or excessive loose stools or diarrhea.

• Instruct patient to protect pills from excessive heat.

• Tell patient that rifapentine can turn body fluids red-orange and permanently stain contact lenses.

Reactions may be *common*, uncommon, *life-threatening*, or COMMON AND LIFE-THREATENING.

9

Aminoglycosides

amikacin sulfate
gentamicin sulfate
neomycin sulfate
streptomycin sulfate
tobramycin sulfate

COMBINATION PRODUCTS
NEOSPORIN G.U. IRRIGANT: 40 mg neomycin sulfate and 200,000 units polymyxin B sulfate/ml.

---

amikacin sulfate
Amikin

Pregnancy risk category D

AVAILABLE FORMS
Injection: 50 mg/ml, 250 mg/ml

INDICATIONS & DOSAGES
➤ **Serious infections caused by sensitive strains of *Pseudomonas aeruginosa*, *Escherichia coli*, *Proteus*, *Klebsiella*, *Serratia*, *Enterobacter*, *Acinetobacter*, *Providencia*, *Citrobacter*, or *Staphylococcus*—**
Adults and children: 15 mg/kg/day divided q 8 to 12 hours I.M. or I.V. infusion.
Neonates: Initially, loading dose of 10 mg/kg I.V.; then 7.5 mg/kg q 12 hours.
➤ **Uncomplicated urinary tract infection caused by organisms not susceptible to less toxic drugs—**
Adults: 250 mg I.M. or I.V. b.i.d.
Adjust-a-dose: For adult patients with impaired renal function, initially, 7.5 mg/kg. Subsequent doses and frequency determined by amikacin levels and renal function studies. For adults undergoing hemodialysis, give supplemental doses of 50% to 75% of initial loading dose at end of each dialysis session. Monitor drug levels and adjust dosage accordingly.

I.V. ADMINISTRATION
● Dilute I.V. drug in 100 to 200 ml of D₅W or normal saline solution and infuse over 30 to 60 minutes.

● After I.V. infusion, flush line with normal saline solution or D₅W.

ACTION
Inhibits protein synthesis by binding directly to the 30S ribosomal subunit. Generally bactericidal.

Route	Onset	Peak	Duration
I.M.	Unknown	1 hr	8-12 hr
I.V.	Immediate	30 min	8-12 hr

ADVERSE REACTIONS
CNS: *neuromuscular blockade.*
EENT: *ototoxicity.*
GU: *azotemia;* **nephrotoxicity;** possible increase in urinary excretion of casts.
Musculoskeletal: arthralgia.
Respiratory: *apnea.*

INTERACTIONS
Drug-drug. *Acyclovir, amphotericin B, cephalosporins, cisplatin, methoxyflurane, vancomycin, other aminoglycosides:* Increased nephrotoxicity. Use together cautiously.
Dimenhydrinate: May mask symptoms of ototoxicity. Use together cautiously.
General anesthetics, neuromuscular blockers: May increase neuromuscular blockade. Monitor patient.
Indomethacin: May increase trough and peak levels of amikacin. Monitor amikacin level.
I.V. loop diuretics (such as furosemide): Increased ototoxicity. Use together cautiously.
Parenteral penicillins (such as ticarcillin): Amikacin inactivation in vitro. Don't mix.

EFFECTS ON LAB TEST RESULTS
● May increase BUN, creatinine, nonprotein nitrogen, and nitrogenous compound (urea) levels.

CONTRAINDICATIONS
Contraindicated in patients hypersensitive to drug or other aminoglycosides.

NURSING CONSIDERATIONS
• Use cautiously in patients with impaired renal function or neuromuscular disorders, in neonates and infants, and in elderly patients.
• Obtain specimen for culture and sensitivity tests before giving first dose. Therapy may begin pending results.
• Evaluate patient's hearing before and during therapy if patient will be receiving drug for longer than 2 weeks. Notify prescriber if patient complains of tinnitus, vertigo, or hearing loss.
• Weigh patient and review renal function studies before therapy begins.
• Correct dehydration before therapy because dehydration increases risk of toxicity.
• Obtain blood for peak amikacin level 1 hour after I.M. injection and 30 minutes to 1 hour after I.V. infusion ends; for trough levels, draw blood just before next dose. Don't collect blood in a heparinized tube; heparin is incompatible with aminoglycosides.
• Peak drug levels more than 35 mcg/ml and trough levels more than 10 mcg/ml may be linked to a higher risk of toxicity.
• Monitor renal function: output, specific gravity, urinalysis, BUN and creatinine levels, and creatinine clearance. Report to prescriber any declining renal function.
• Watch for superinfection: continued fever and other signs and symptoms of new infection, especially of upper respiratory tract.
• Therapy is usually continued for 7 to 10 days. If no response occurs after 3 to 5 days, therapy may be stopped and new specimens obtained for culture and sensitivity testing.
• *Alert:* Don't confuse Amikin with Amicar.

PATIENT TEACHING
• Instruct patient to report adverse reactions promptly.
• Encourage patient to maintain adequate fluid intake.

gentamicin sulfate
Cidomycin†, Garamycin, Genticin§

Pregnancy risk category D

AVAILABLE FORMS
Injection: 40 mg/ml (adult), 10 mg/ml (pediatric)
I.V. infusion (premixed): 40 mg, 60 mg, 70 mg, 80 mg, 90 mg, 100 mg, 120 mg, in normal saline solution

INDICATIONS & DOSAGES
➤ **Serious infections caused by sensitive strains of** *Pseudomonas aeruginosa,* *Escherichia coli, Proteus, Klebsiella, Serratia, Enterobacter, Citrobacter,* **or** *Staphylococcus*—
Adults: 3 mg/kg daily in three divided doses I.M. or I.V. infusion q 8 hours. For life-threatening infections, patient may receive up to 5 mg/kg daily in three to four divided doses; dose should be reduced to 3 mg/kg daily as soon as clinically indicated.
Children: 2 to 2.5 mg/kg q 8 hours I.M. or by I.V. infusion.
Neonates older than 1 week and infants: 2.5 mg/kg q 8 hours I.M. or by I.V. infusion.
Neonates younger than 1 week and preterm infants: 2.5 mg/kg q 12 hours I.M. or by I.V. infusion.
➤ **Endocarditis prophylaxis for GI or GU procedure or surgery**—
Adults: 1.5 mg/kg I.M. or I.V. 30 minutes before procedure or surgery. Maximum dose is 80 mg. Given with ampicillin (vancomycin in penicillin-allergic patients).
Children: 2 mg/kg I.M. or I.V. 30 minutes before procedure or surgery. Maximum dose is 80 mg. Given with ampicillin (vancomycin in penicillin-allergic patients).
Adjust-a-dose: For adult patients with impaired renal function, doses and frequency are determined by gentamicin levels and renal function. After hemodialysis to maintain therapeutic blood levels, adults should receive 1 to 1.7 mg/kg I.M. or by I.V. infusion after each dialysis, and children should receive 2 to 2.5 mg/kg I.M. or by I.V. infusion after each dialysis.

I.V. ADMINISTRATION
• When giving by intermittent I.V. infusion, dilute with 50 to 200 ml of D_5W or normal saline solution for injection and infuse over 30 minutes to 2 hours.
• After completing I.V. infusion, flush the line with normal saline solution or D_5W.

ACTION
Inhibits protein synthesis by binding directly to the 30S ribosomal subunit. Usually bactericidal.

Route	Onset	Peak	Duration
I.M.	Unknown	30-90 min	Unknown
I.V.	Immediate	30-90 min	Unknown

ADVERSE REACTIONS
CNS: headache, lethargy, encephalopathy, confusion, dizziness, *seizures,* numbness, peripheral neuropathy, vertigo, ataxia, tingling.
CV: hypotension.
EENT: *ototoxicity,* blurred vision, tinnitus.
GI: vomiting, nausea.
GU: *nephrotoxicity,* possible increase in urinary excretion of casts.
Hematologic: anemia, eosinophilia, *leukopenia, thrombocytopenia, agranulocytosis.*
Musculoskeletal: muscle twitching, myasthenia gravis–like syndrome.
Respiratory: *apnea.*
Skin: rash, urticaria, pruritus.
Other: fever, *anaphylaxis,* injection site pain.

INTERACTIONS
Drug-drug. *Acyclovir, amphotericin B, cephalosporins, cisplatin, methoxyflurane, vancomycin, other aminoglycosides:* Increased ototoxicity and nephrotoxicity. Use together cautiously.
Dimenhydrinate: May mask symptoms of ototoxicity. Use together cautiously.
General anesthetics, neuromuscular blockers: May increase neuromuscular blockade. Monitor patient closely.
Indomethacin: May increase peak and trough levels of gentamicin. Monitor gentamicin levels.
I.V. loop diuretics (such as furosemide): Increased ototoxicity. Use together cautiously.

Parenteral penicillins (such as ampicillin and ticarcillin): Inactivates gentamicin in vitro. Don't mix.

EFFECTS ON LAB TEST RESULTS
• May increase BUN, creatinine, nonprotein nitrogen, ALT, AST, bilirubin, and LDH levels.
• May increase eosinophil count. May decrease hemoglobin and WBC, platelet, and granulocyte counts.

CONTRAINDICATIONS
Contraindicated in patients hypersensitive to drug or other aminoglycosides.

NURSING CONSIDERATIONS
• Use cautiously in neonates, infants, elderly patients, and patients with impaired renal function or neuromuscular disorders.
• Obtain specimen for culture and sensitivity tests before giving first dose.
• Evaluate patient's hearing before and during therapy. Notify prescriber if patient complains of tinnitus, vertigo, or hearing loss.
• Weigh patient and review renal function studies before therapy begins.
• *Alert:* Use preservative-free formulations of gentamicin when intrathecal route is ordered.
• Obtain blood for peak gentamicin level 1 hour after I.M. injection or 30 minutes after I.V. infusion finishes; for trough levels, draw blood just before next dose. Don't collect blood in a heparinized tube; heparin is incompatible with aminoglycosides.
• Maintain peak levels at 4 to 12 mcg/ml and trough levels at 1 to 2 mcg/ml. Increased risk of toxicity may occur with prolonged peak levels at 10 to 12 mcg/ml or prolonged trough levels greater than 2 mcg/ml.
• Monitor urine output, specific gravity, urinalysis, BUN and creatinine levels, and creatinine clearance. Notify prescriber of signs of decreasing renal function.
• Hemodialysis for 8 hours may remove up to 50% of drug from blood.
• Watch for superinfection: continued fever and other signs and symptoms of new infection (especially of upper respiratory tract).

---

*Liquid contains alcohol. **May contain tartrazine. †Canada ‡Australia §U.K. ◇OTC

● Therapy usually continues for 7 to 10 days. If no response occurs in 3 to 5 days, therapy may be stopped and new specimens obtained for culture and sensitivity testing.

PATIENT TEACHING
● Instruct patient to promptly report adverse reactions, such as dizziness, vertigo, ataxia, tinnitus, hearing loss, numbness, tingling, or muscle twitching.
● Encourage patient to maintain adequate fluid intake.
● Warn patient to avoid hazardous activities if adverse CNS reactions occur.

---

neomycin sulfate
Mycifradin†, Neo-fradin, Neosulf‡, Nivemycin§

Pregnancy risk category D

AVAILABLE FORMS
Oral solution: 125 mg/5 ml
Tablets: 500 mg

INDICATIONS & DOSAGES
➤ **Infectious diarrhea caused by enteropathogenic *Escherichia coli*—**
Adults: 50 mg/kg daily P.O. in four divided doses for 2 to 3 days; maximum of 3 g daily is usually adequate.
Children: 50 to 100 mg/kg daily P.O. divided q 4 to 6 hours for 2 to 3 days.
➤ **Suppression of intestinal bacteria preoperatively—**
Adults: 1 g P.O. q hour for four doses; then 1 g q 4 hours for the balance of the 24 hours. A saline cathartic should precede therapy. Or, 88 mg/kg in six equally divided doses at 4-hour intervals. Or, 1 g neomycin with 1 g erythromycin base at 1 p.m., 2 p.m., and 11 p.m. on day preceding 8 a.m. surgery.
Children: 40 to 100 mg/kg daily P.O. divided q 4 to 6 hours. First dose should follow saline cathartic. Or, 88 mg/kg in six equally divided doses at 4-hour intervals.
➤ **Adjunct treatment in hepatic coma—**
Adults: 1 to 3 g P.O. q.i.d. for 5 to 6 days; or 200 ml of 1% solution or 100 ml of 2% solution as enema retained for 20 to 60 minutes q 6 hours. For patients with chronic hepatic insufficiency, 4 g/day indefinitely may be needed.
Children: 50 to 100 mg/kg/day P.O. in divided doses for 5 to 6 days.

ACTION
Inhibits protein synthesis by binding directly to the 30S ribosomal subunit. Generally bactericidal.

Route	Onset	Peak	Duration
P.O.	Unknown	1-4 hr	8 hr

ADVERSE REACTIONS
EENT: *ototoxicity.*
GI: nausea, vomiting, diarrhea, malabsorption syndrome, *Clostridium difficile*–related colitis.
GU: *nephrotoxicity,* possible increase in urinary excretion of casts.

INTERACTIONS
Drug-drug. *Acyclovir, amphotericin B, cephalosporins, cisplatin, methoxyflurane, vancomycin, other aminoglycosides:* Increased nephrotoxicity. Use together cautiously.
Digoxin: Decreased digoxin absorption. Monitor patient closely.
I.V. loop diuretics (such as furosemide): Increased ototoxicity. Use together cautiously.
Oral anticoagulants: Inhibited vitamin K–producing bacteria; may increase anticoagulant effect. Monitor PT and INR.

EFFECTS ON LAB TEST RESULTS
● Increased BUN, creatinine, and nonprotein nitrogen levels.

CONTRAINDICATIONS
Contraindicated in patients hypersensitive to other aminoglycosides and in those with intestinal obstruction.

NURSING CONSIDERATIONS
● Use cautiously in patients with impaired renal function, neuromuscular disorders, or ulcerative bowel lesions and in elderly patients. Never administer drug parenterally.
● Monitor renal function: output, specific gravity, urinalysis, BUN and creatinine levels, and creatinine clearance. Notify

prescriber about signs and symptoms of declining renal function.
• Evaluate patient's hearing before and during prolonged therapy. Notify prescriber if patient complains of tinnitus, vertigo, or hearing loss. Onset of deafness may occur several weeks after drug is stopped.
• Watch for signs and symptoms of superinfection, such as fever or other evidence of new infection.
• In adjunctive treatment of hepatic coma, decrease patient's dietary protein and assess neurologic status frequently during therapy.
• For preoperative disinfection, provide a low-residue diet and a cathartic immediately before oral administration of neomycin.
• The ototoxic and nephrotoxic properties of neomycin limit its usefulness.
• Neomycin is nonabsorbable at recommended dosage, but more than 4 g/day may be systemically absorbed and lead to nephrotoxicity.
• Drug is available with polymyxin B as a bladder irrigant.

PATIENT TEACHING
• Instruct patient to promptly report adverse reactions.
• Encourage patient to maintain adequate fluid intake.

streptomycin sulfate

Pregnancy risk category D

AVAILABLE FORMS
Injection: 1 g/2.5-ml ampules

INDICATIONS & DOSAGES
➤ Streptococcal endocarditis—
Adults: 1 g q 12 hours I.M. for 1 week; then 500 mg I.M. q 12 hours for 1 week, given with penicillin.
Elderly patients: 500 mg I.M. q 12 hours for entire 2 weeks, given with penicillin.
➤ Primary and adjunctive treatment in tuberculosis—
Adults: 15 mg/kg (maximum of 1 g) I.M. daily for 2 to 3 months; then 1 g I.M. two or three times weekly.

Children: 20 to 40 mg/kg (maximum of 1 g) I.M. daily in divided doses injected deeply into large muscle mass. Given with other antituberculotics, but not with capreomycin; continued until sputum specimen becomes negative.
Elderly patients: 10 mg/kg I.M. daily.
➤ Enterococcal endocarditis—
Adults: 1 g I.M. q 12 hours for 2 weeks; then 500 mg I.M. q 12 hours for 4 weeks, given with penicillin.
➤ Tularemia—
Adults: 1 to 2 g I.M. daily in divided doses injected deeply into upper outer quadrant of buttocks; continued for 7 to 14 days or until patient is afebrile for 5 to 7 days.

ACTION
Inhibits protein synthesis by binding directly to the 30S ribosomal subunit. Generally bactericidal.

Route	Onset	Peak	Duration
I.M.	Unknown	1-2 hr	Unknown

ADVERSE REACTIONS
CNS: *neuromuscular blockade,* vertigo, paresthesia of the face.
EENT: *ototoxicity.*
GI: vomiting, nausea.
GU: *nephrotoxicity,* possible increase in urinary excretion of casts.
Hematologic: eosinophilia, *leukopenia, thrombocytopenia, hemolytic anemia.*
Respiratory: *apnea.*
Skin: exfoliative dermatitis.
Other: hypersensitivity reactions, *anaphylaxis.*

INTERACTIONS
Drug-drug. *Acyclovir, amphotericin B, cephalosporins, cisplatin, methoxyflurane, vancomycin, other aminoglycosides:* Increased nephrotoxicity. Use together cautiously.
General anesthetics, neuromuscular blockers: May increase neuromuscular blockade. Monitor patient closely.
I.V. loop diuretics (such as furosemide): Increased ototoxicity. Use together cautiously.

EFFECTS ON LAB TEST RESULTS
• May increase BUN, creatinine, and nonprotein nitrogen levels.

• May increase eosinophil count. May decrease WBC and platelet counts and hemoglobin.

CONTRAINDICATIONS
Contraindicated in patients hypersensitive to drug or other aminoglycosides.

NURSING CONSIDERATIONS
• Use cautiously in elderly patients and in patients with impaired renal function or neuromuscular disorders.
• Obtain specimen for culture and sensitivity tests before giving first dose except when treating tuberculosis. Therapy may begin pending results.
• Evaluate patient's hearing before therapy and for 6 months afterward. Notify prescriber if patient complains of hearing loss, roaring noises, or fullness in ears.
• Protect hands when preparing because drug is irritating.
• For I.M. administration, inject deeply into upper outer quadrant of buttocks or midlateral thigh. Rotate injection sites.
• In children, give I.M. injection in midlateral thigh if possible to minimize possibility of damaging sciatic nerve.
• Obtain blood for peak streptomycin level 1 to 2 hours after I.M. injection; for trough levels, draw blood just before next dose. Don't use a heparinized tube; heparin is incompatible with aminoglycosides.
• Drug has been given as I.V. infusion over 30 to 60 minutes without unusual adverse effects in patients unable to tolerate I.M. injections.
• Watch for signs and symptoms of superinfection, such as continued fever and other signs of new infection.
• Nephrotoxicity occurs less frequently with streptomycin than with other aminoglycosides.
• In primary treatment of tuberculosis, streptomycin is stopped when sputum becomes negative.
• Streptomycin may cause a false-positive reaction in copper sulfate tests for urine glucose such as Benedict's reagent or Diastix.

PATIENT TEACHING
• Instruct patient to report adverse reactions promptly.

• Encourage patient to maintain adequate fluid intake.
• Emphasize need for blood tests to monitor streptomycin levels and determine effectiveness of therapy.

tobramycin sulfate
Nebcin, TOBI

Pregnancy risk category D

AVAILABLE FORMS
Multidose vials: 80 mg/2 ml, 20 mg/2 ml (pediatric)
Nebulizer solution (for inhalation): 300 mg/5 ml
Powder for injection: 40 mg/ml
Premixed parenteral injection for I.V. infusion: 60 mg or 80 mg in normal saline solution

INDICATIONS & DOSAGES
➤ **Serious infections caused by sensitive strains of** *Escherichia coli, Proteus, Klebsiella, Enterobacter, Serratia, Morganella morganii, Staphylococcus aureus, Citrobacter, Pseudomonas,* **or** *Providencia*—
Adults: 3 mg/kg I.M. or I.V. daily in divided doses. Up to 5 mg/kg daily divided q 6 to 8 hours for life-threatening infections; dosage should be reduced to 3 mg/kg daily as soon as clinically indicated.
Children: 6 to 7.5 mg/kg I.M. or I.V. daily in three or four divided doses.
Neonates younger than age 1 week or premature infants: Up to 4 mg/kg/day I.V. or I.M. in two equal doses q 12 hours.
Adjust-a-dose: For patients with renal impairment, loading dose is 1 mg/kg; then decreased doses at 8-hour intervals or same dose at prolonged intervals. For patients with severe cystic fibrosis, initial dose is 10 mg/kg/day I.V. or I.M. in 4 divided doses.
➤ **Management of cystic fibrosis patients with** *Pseudomonas aeruginosa*—
Adults and children age 6 and older: 300 mg via nebulizer q 12 hours for 28 days. Continue cycle of 28 days on drug and 28 days off.

I.V. ADMINISTRATION
- For adults, dilute in 50 to 100 ml of normal saline solution or D_5W; use a smaller volume for children.
- Infuse over 20 to 60 minutes.
- After I.V. infusion, flush line with normal saline solution or D_5W.

ACTION
Inhibits protein synthesis by binding directly to the 30S ribosomal subunit. Generally bactericidal.

Route	Onset	Peak	Duration
I.M.	Unknown	30-60 min	8 hr
Inhalation	Unknown	Unknown	Unknown
I.V.	Immediate	30 min	8 hr

ADVERSE REACTIONS
CNS: headache, lethargy, confusion, disorientation, *seizures.*
EENT: *ototoxicity, hoarseness, pharyngitis.*
GI: vomiting, nausea, diarrhea.
GU: *nephrotoxicity,* possible increase in urinary excretion of casts.
Hematologic: anemia, eosinophilia, *leukopenia, thrombocytopenia, agranulocytosis.*
Metabolic: electrolyte imbalances.
Musculoskeletal: muscle twitching.
Respiratory: *bronchospasm.*
Skin: rash, urticaria, pruritus.
Other: fever.

INTERACTIONS
Drug-drug. *Acyclovir, amphotericin B, cephalosporins, cisplatin, methoxyflurane, other aminoglycosides, vancomycin:* Increased nephrotoxicity. Use together cautiously.
Dimenhydrinate: May mask symptoms of ototoxicity. Use together cautiously.
General anesthetics, neuromuscular blockers: May increase neuromuscular blockade. Monitor patient.
I.V. loop diuretics (such as furosemide): Increased ototoxicity. Use together cautiously.
Parenteral penicillins (such as ticarcillin): Inactivates tobramycin in vitro. Don't mix.

EFFECTS ON LAB TEST RESULTS
- May increase BUN, creatinine, and nonprotein nitrogen and nitrogenous compound levels. May decrease calcium, magnesium, and potassium levels.
- May increase eosinophil count. May decrease WBC, platelet, and granulocyte counts.

CONTRAINDICATIONS
Contraindicated in patients hypersensitive to drug or other aminoglycosides.

NURSING CONSIDERATIONS
- Use cautiously in patients with impaired renal function or neuromuscular disorders and in elderly patients.
- Obtain specimen for culture and sensitivity tests before giving first dose. Therapy may begin pending results.
- Weigh patient and review renal function studies before therapy.
- Evaluate patient's hearing before and during therapy. Notify prescriber if patient complains of tinnitus, vertigo, or hearing loss.
- Don't dilute or mix TOBI with dornase alpha in the nebulizer.
- Unrefrigerated TOBI, which is normally slightly yellow, may darken with age. This change doesn't indicate a change in product quality.
- Avoid exposing TOBI ampules to intense light.
- Administer nebulizer solution over 10 to 15 minutes using handheld Pari LC Plus reusable nebulizer with DeVilbiss Pulmo-Aide compressor.
- Obtain blood for peak level 1 hour after I.M. injection or ½ hour after infusion stops; draw blood for trough level just before next dose. Don't collect blood in a heparinized tube; heparin is incompatible with aminoglycosides.
- *Alert:* Peak blood levels over 12 mcg/ml and trough levels over 2 mcg/ml may increase the risk of toxicity.
- Monitor renal function: output, specific gravity, urinalysis, creatinine clearance, and BUN and creatinine levels. Notify prescriber about signs and symptoms of decreasing renal function.
- Watch for evidence of superinfection, such as continued fever and other signs of new infection.
- If no response occurs in 3 to 5 days, therapy may be stopped and new speci-

mens obtained for culture and sensitivity testing.
● *Alert:* Don't confuse tobramycin with Trobicin.

PATIENT TEACHING

● Instruct patient to report adverse reactions promptly.
● Caution patient not to perform hazardous activities if adverse CNS reactions occur.
● Encourage patient to maintain adequate fluid intake.
● Teach patient how to use and maintain nebulizer.
● Tell patient using multiple inhaled therapies to use TOBI last.
● Instruct patient not to use TOBI if it's cloudy, if there are particles in the solution, or if it has been stored at room temperature for longer than 28 days.

amoxicillin/clavulanate potassium
amoxicillin trihydrate
ampicillin
ampicillin sodium
ampicillin sodium/sulbactam
 sodium
ampicillin trihydrate
cloxacillin sodium
dicloxacillin sodium
mezlocillin sodium
nafcillin sodium
oxacillin sodium
penicillin G benzathine
penicillin G potassium
penicillin G procaine
penicillin G sodium
penicillin V potassium
piperacillin sodium
piperacillin sodium/tazobactam
 sodium
ticarcillin disodium
ticarcillin disodium/clavulanate
 potassium

COMBINATION PRODUCTS
None.

---

amoxicillin/clavulanate potassium (amoxycillin/ clavulanate potassium)
Augmentin, Augmentin ES-600,
Clavulin†

Pregnancy risk category B

AVAILABLE FORMS
Tablets (chewable): 125 mg amoxicillin trihydrate, 31.25 mg clavulanic acid; 200 mg amoxicillin trihydrate, 28.5 mg clavulanic acid; 250 mg amoxicillin trihydrate, 62.5 mg clavulanic acid, 400 mg amoxicillin trihydrate, 57 mg clavulanic acid
Tablets (film-coated): 250 mg amoxicillin trihydrate, 125 mg clavulanic acid; 500 mg amoxicillin trihydrate, 125 mg clavulanic acid; 875 mg amoxicillin trihydrate, 125 mg clavulanic acid

Oral suspension: 125 mg amoxicillin trihydrate and 31.25 mg clavulanic acid/5 ml (after reconstitution); 200 mg amoxicillin trihydrate and 28.5 mg clavulanic acid/ 5 ml (after reconstitution); 250 mg amoxicillin trihydrate and 62.5 mg clavulanic acid/5 ml (after reconstitution); 400 mg amoxicillin trihydrate and 57 mg clavulanic acid/5 ml (after reconstitution); 600 mg amoxicillin trihydrate and 42.9 mg clavulanic acid/5 ml after reconstitution

INDICATIONS & DOSAGES
➤ **Recurrent or persistent acute otitis media caused by *S. pneumoniae*, *Haemophilus influenzae*, or *Moraxella catarrhalis* in patients 2 years old or younger or in day care facilities, exposed to antibiotics within the last 3 months. Use Augmentin ES-600 only—**
Children ages 3 months to 12 years:
90 mg/kg/day Augmentin ES-600, based on amoxicillin component, P.O. q 12 hours for 10 days.
➤ **Lower respiratory infections, otitis media, sinusitis, skin and skin-structure infections, and urinary tract infections caused by susceptible strains of gram-positive and gram-negative organisms—**
Adults and children weighing 40 kg (88 lb) or more: 250 mg, based on amoxicillin component, P.O. q 8 hours; or 500 mg q 12 hours. For more severe infections, 500 mg P.O. q 8 hours or 875 mg P.O. q 12 hours.
Children age 3 months and older and weighing less than 40 kg: 20 to 90 mg/kg, based on amoxicillin component and severity of infection, P.O. daily in divided doses q 8 to 12 hours.
Children younger than age 3 months: 30 mg/kg/day P.O. divided q 12 hours, based on amoxicillin component. The 125 mg/5-ml oral suspension is recommended.
Adjust-a-dose: Don't give the 875-mg tablet to patients with renal impairment and creatinine clearance less than 30 ml/ minute. If clearance is 10 to 30 ml/minute, dosage is 250 to 500 mg P.O. q 12 hours.

If clearance is less than 10 ml/minute, dosage is 250 to 500 mg P.O. q 24 hours. Give hemodialysis patients 250 to 500 mg P.O. q 24 hours with an additional dose both during and at the end of dialysis.

ACTION
An aminopenicillin that prevents bacterial cell-wall synthesis during replication. Clavulanic acid increases amoxicillin effectiveness by inactivating beta-lactamases, which destroy amoxicillin.

Route	Onset	Peak	Duration
P.O.	Unknown	1-2.5 hr	6-8 hr
P.O. (extended)	Unknown	1-4 hr	Unknown

ADVERSE REACTIONS
CNS: agitation, anxiety, insomnia, confusion, behavioral changes, dizziness.
GI: *nausea,* vomiting, *diarrhea,* indigestion, gastritis, stomatitis, glossitis, black hairy tongue, enterocolitis, pseudomembranous colitis.
GU: vaginitis.
Hematologic: anemia, *thrombocytopenia, thrombocytopenic purpura,* eosinophilia, *leukopenia, agranulocytosis.*
Other: hypersensitivity reactions, *anaphylaxis,* overgrowth of nonsusceptible organisms.

INTERACTIONS
Drug-drug. *Allopurinol:* Increased risk of rash. Monitor patient.
Oral contraceptives: May decrease efficacy of oral contraceptives. Recommend additional form of contraception during penicillin therapy.
Probenecid: Increased blood levels of amoxicillin and other penicillins. Probenecid may be used for this purpose.
Drug-herb. *Khat:* May decrease antimicrobial effect of certain penicillins. Discourage khat chewing, or tell patient to take amoxicillin 2 hours after khat chewing.

EFFECTS ON LAB TEST RESULTS
• May increase eosinophil count.

CONTRAINDICATIONS
Contraindicated in patients hypersensitive to drug or other penicillins and in those with a history of amoxicillin-related cholestatic jaundice or hepatic dysfunction.

NURSING CONSIDERATIONS
• Use cautiously in patients with other drug allergies (especially to cephalosporins) because of possible cross-sensitivity and in those with mononucleosis because of high risk of maculopapular rash.
• Use cautiously in breast-feeding women; drug appears in breast milk.
• Before giving drug, ask patient about allergic reactions to penicillin. However, a negative history of penicillin allergy is no guarantee against an allergic reaction.
• Obtain specimen for culture and sensitivity tests before giving first dose. Therapy may begin pending results.
• Give drug at least 1 hour before a bacteriostatic antibiotic.
• If large doses are given or if therapy is prolonged, bacterial or fungal superinfection may occur, especially in elderly, debilitated, or immunosuppressed patients.
• *Alert:* Don't interchange the oral suspensions because of varying clavulanic acid contents.
• Augmentin ES-600 is intended for pediatric patients only.
• Drug alters results of urine glucose tests that use cupric sulfate such as Benedict's reagent or Clinitest. Make urine glucose determinations with glucose oxidase methods such as Diastix or Chemstrip uG. Ampicillin may falsely decrease aminoglycoside levels.
• Avoid use of 250-mg tablet in children weighing less than 40 kg (88 lb). Use chewable form instead.
• *Alert:* Both 250- and 500-mg film-coated tablets contain the same amount of clavulanic acid (125 mg). Therefore, two 250-mg tablets aren't equivalent to one 500-mg tablet.
• This drug combination is particularly useful in clinical settings with a high prevalence of amoxicillin-resistant organisms.
• After reconstitution, refrigerate the oral suspension; discard after 10 days.
• *Alert:* Don't confuse amoxicillin with amoxapine.

Reactions may be *common,* uncommon, *life-threatening,* or COMMON AND LIFE-THREATENING.

PATIENT TEACHING
• Tell patient to take entire quantity of drug exactly as prescribed, even after feeling better.
• Instruct patient to take drug with food to prevent GI upset. If he's taking the oral suspension, tell him to keep drug refrigerated, to shake it well before administration, and to discard remaining drug after 10 days.
• Tell patient to call prescriber if a rash occurs because rash is a sign of an allergic reaction.

---

amoxicillin trihydrate
(amoxycillin trihydrate)
Alphamox‡, Amoxil, Apo-Amoxi†, Cilamox‡, Moxacin‡, Novamoxin†, Nu-Amoxi†, Trimox, Wymox

Pregnancy risk category B

AVAILABLE FORMS
Capsules: 250 mg, 500 mg
Oral suspension: 50 mg/ml (pediatric drops), 125 mg/5 ml, 250 mg/5 ml (after reconstitution)
Tablets: 500 mg, 875 mg
Tablets (chewable): 125 mg, 250 mg

INDICATIONS & DOSAGES
➤ **Systemic infections, acute and chronic urinary tract infections caused by susceptible strains of gram-positive and gram-negative organisms—**
Adults and children weighing 20 kg (44 lb) or more: 250 to 500 mg P.O. q 8 hours.
Children weighing less than 20 kg: 20 mg/kg P.O. daily in divided doses q 8 hours; in severe infection, 40 mg/kg P.O. daily in divided doses q 8 hours or 500 mg to 1 g/m² P.O. in divided doses q 8 hours.
➤ **Uncomplicated gonorrhea—**
Adults and children weighing more than 45 kg (99 lb): 3 g P.O. with 1 g probenecid given as a single dose.
Children age 2 and older weighing less than 45 kg: 50 mg/kg to a maximum of 3 g P.O. with 25 mg/kg to a maximum of 1 g of probenecid as a single dose. Don't give probenecid to children younger than age 2.

➤ **Endocarditis prophylaxis for dental, GI, and GU procedures—**
Adults: 2 g P.O. 1 hour before procedure.
Children: 50 mg/kg P.O. 1 hour before procedure.

ACTION
An aminopenicillin that inhibits cell-wall synthesis during bacterial multiplication. Bacteria resist amoxicillin by producing penicillinases—enzymes that hydrolyze amoxicillin.

Route	Onset	Peak	Duration
P.O.	Unknown	1-2 hr	6-8 hr

ADVERSE REACTIONS
CNS: lethargy, hallucinations, *seizures,* anxiety, confusion, agitation, depression, dizziness, fatigue.
GI: *nausea,* vomiting, *diarrhea,* glossitis, stomatitis, gastritis, enterocolitis, abdominal pain, pseudomembranous colitis, black hairy tongue.
GU: interstitial nephritis, nephropathy, vaginitis.
Hematologic: anemia, *thrombocytopenia, thrombocytopenic purpura,* eosinophilia, *leukopenia,* hemolytic anemia, *agranulocytosis.*
Other: hypersensitivity reactions, *anaphylaxis,* overgrowth of nonsusceptible organisms.

INTERACTIONS
Drug-drug. *Allopurinol:* Increased risk of rash. Monitor patient.
Oral contraceptives: May decrease efficacy of oral contraceptives. Recommend additional form of contraception during penicillin therapy.
Probenecid: Increased blood levels of amoxicillin and other penicillins. Probenecid may be used for this purpose.
Drug-herb. *Khat:* May decrease antimicrobial effect of certain penicillins. Discourage khat chewing, or tell patient to take amoxicillin 2 hours after khat chewing.

EFFECTS ON LAB TEST RESULTS
• May increase eosinophil count. May decrease hemoglobin and granulocyte, platelet, and WBC counts.

CONTRAINDICATIONS
Contraindicated in patients hypersensitive to drug or other penicillins.

NURSING CONSIDERATIONS
• Use cautiously in patients with other drug allergies (especially to cephalosporins) because of possible cross-sensitivity and in those with mononucleosis because of high risk of maculopapular rash.
• Obtain specimen for culture and sensitivity tests before giving first dose. Therapy may begin pending results.
• Before giving, ask patient about allergic reactions to penicillin. A negative history of penicillin allergy is no guarantee against allergic reaction.
• If large doses are given or if therapy is prolonged, bacterial or fungal superinfection may occur, especially in elderly, debilitated, or immunosuppressed patients.
• Drug alters results of urine glucose tests that use cupric sulfate such as Benedict's reagent or Clinitest. Make urine glucose determinations with glucose oxidase methods such as Diastix or Chemstrip uG. Ampicillin may falsely decrease aminoglycoside levels.
• Store Trimox oral suspension in refrigerator, if possible. It also may be stored at room temperature for up to 2 weeks. Be sure to check individual product labels for storage information.
• Amoxicillin usually causes fewer cases of diarrhea than does ampicillin.
• *Alert:* Don't confuse amoxicillin with amoxapine.

PATIENT TEACHING
• Tell patient to take entire quantity of drug exactly as prescribed, even after he feels better.
• Instruct patient to take drug with food.
• Tell patient to notify prescriber if rash, fever, or chills develop. A rash is the most common allergic reaction, especially if allopurinol is also being taken.
• Tell parent to place pediatric drops directly on child's tongue for swallowing or add to formula, milk, fruit juice, water, ginger ale, or a cold drink; patient should take immediately and consume entirely.

ampicillin
Apo-Ampi†, Novo Ampicillin†, Nu-Ampi†, Omnipen-N

ampicillin sodium
Ampicin†, Ampicyn‡, Omnipen-N, Penbritin†, Totacillin-N

ampicillin trihydrate
Omnipen, Penbritin†, Principen, Totacillin

Pregnancy risk category B

AVAILABLE FORMS
Capsules: 250 mg, 500 mg
Injection: 125 mg, 250 mg, 500 mg, 1 g, 2 g
Oral suspension: 125 mg/5 ml, 250 mg/5 ml

INDICATIONS & DOSAGES
➤ **Respiratory tract or skin and skin-structure infections—**
Adults and children weighing 40 kg (88 lb) or more: 250 to 500 mg P.O. q 6 hours.
Children weighing less than 40 kg: 25 to 50 mg/kg/day P.O. in equally divided doses q 6 hours. Pediatric dosages shouldn't exceed recommended adult dosages.
➤ **GI or urinary tract infections—**
Adults and children weighing 40 kg (88 lb) or more: 500 mg P.O. every 6 hours. For severe infections, larger doses may be needed.
Children weighing less than 40 kg: 50 to 100 mg/kg/day P.O. in equally divided doses every 6 hours.
➤ **Bacterial meningitis or septicemia—**
Adults: 150 to 200 mg/kg/day I.V. in divided doses q 3 to 4 hours. May be given I.M. after 3 days of I.V. therapy. Maximum recommended daily dose is 14 g.
Children: 100 to 200 mg/kg I.V. daily in divided doses q 3 to 4 hours. Give I.V. for 3 days; then give I.M.
➤ **Uncomplicated gonorrhea—**
Adults and children weighing more than 45 kg (99 lb): 3.5 g P.O. with 1 g probenecid given as a single dose.
➤ **Endocarditis prophylaxis for dental, GI, and GU procedures—**
Adults: 2 g I.M. or I.V. within 30 minutes before procedure.

Reactions may be *common*, uncommon, *life-threatening*, or COMMON AND LIFE-THREATENING.

Children: 50 mg/kg I.M. or I.V. within 30 minutes before procedure.
Adjust-a-dose: In patients who have severe renal impairment, increase drug interval to 12 hours. Use same dose.

I.V. ADMINISTRATION
● For I.V. injection, reconstitute with bacteriostatic water for injection. Use 5 ml for the 125-mg, 250-mg, or 500-mg vials; 7.4 ml for the 1-g vials; or 14.8 ml for the 2-g vials. Give direct I.V. injections over 10 to 15 minutes to avoid the possibility of seizures. Don't exceed 100 mg/minute.
● For intermittent infusion, dilute in 50 to 100 ml of normal saline solution for injection and give over 15 to 30 minutes.
● *Alert:* Don't mix with solutions containing dextrose or fructose; these substances promote rapid breakdown of ampicillin.
● Use initial dilution within 1 hour. Follow manufacturer's directions for stability data when ampicillin is further diluted for I.V. infusion.
● Give I.V. intermittently to prevent vein irritation. Change site every 48 hours.

ACTION
An aminopenicillin that inhibits cell-wall synthesis during microorganism multiplication.

Route	Onset	Peak	Duration
I.M.	Unknown	1 hr	Unknown
I.V.	Immediate	Immediate	Unknown
P.O.	Unknown	2 hr	6-8 hr

ADVERSE REACTIONS
CNS: lethargy, hallucinations, *seizures,* anxiety, confusion, agitation, depression, dizziness, fatigue.
CV: vein irritation, thrombophlebitis.
GI: *nausea,* vomiting, *diarrhea,* glossitis, stomatitis, gastritis, abdominal pain, enterocolitis, pseudomembranous colitis, black hairy tongue.
GU: interstitial nephritis, nephropathy, vaginitis.
Hematologic: anemia, *thrombocytopenia, thrombocytopenic purpura,* eosinophilia, *leukopenia,* hemolytic anemia, *agranulocytosis.*

Other: hypersensitivity reactions, overgrowth of nonsusceptible organisms, pain at injection site.

INTERACTIONS
Drug-drug. *Allopurinol:* Increased risk of rash. Monitor patient.
Oral contraceptives: May decrease efficacy of oral contraceptives. Recommend additional form of contraception during penicillin therapy.
Probenecid: Increased levels of ampicillin and other penicillins. Probenecid may be used for this purpose.

EFFECTS ON LAB TEST RESULTS
● May increase eosinophil count. May decrease hemoglobin and platelet, WBC, and granulocyte counts.

CONTRAINDICATIONS
Contraindicated in patients hypersensitive to drug or other penicillins.

NURSING CONSIDERATIONS
● Use cautiously in patients with other drug allergies (especially to cephalosporins) because of possible cross-sensitivity and in those with mononucleosis because of high risk of maculopapular rash.
● Before giving drug, ask patient about allergic reactions to penicillin. A negative history of penicillin allergy is no guarantee against a future allergic reaction.
● Obtain specimen for culture and sensitivity tests before giving first dose. Therapy may begin pending results.
● Give drug I.M. or I.V. only if prescribed and the infection is severe or if patient can't take oral dose.
● Give drug 1 to 2 hours before or 2 to 3 hours after meals. When given orally, drug may cause GI disturbances. Food may interfere with absorption.
● Drug alters results of urine glucose tests that use cupric sulfate such as Benedict's reagent or Clinitest. Make urine glucose determinations with glucose oxidase methods such as Diastix or Chemstrip uG. Ampicillin may falsely decrease aminoglycoside levels.
● Monitor sodium level because each gram of ampicillin contains 2.9 mEq of sodium.

---

*Liquid contains alcohol.   **May contain tartrazine.   †Canada   ‡Australia   §U.K.   ◊OTC

• If large doses are given or if therapy is prolonged, bacterial or fungal superinfection may occur, especially in elderly, debilitated, or immunosuppressed patients.
• Watch for signs and symptoms of hypersensitivity, such as erythematous maculopapular rash, urticaria, and anaphylaxis.
• Dosage should be decreased in patients with impaired renal function.
• In pediatric meningitis, ampicillin may be given with parenteral chloramphenicol for 24 hours pending cultures.
• For prophylaxis of bacterial endocarditis in patients at high risk, give drug with gentamicin.

PATIENT TEACHING
• Tell patient to take entire quantity of drug exactly as prescribed, even after he feels better.
• Instruct patient to take oral form on an empty stomach 1 hour before or 2 hours after meals.
• Inform patient to notify prescriber if rash, fever, or chills develop. A rash is the most common allergic reaction, especially if allopurinol is also being taken.
• Advise patient to report discomfort at I.V. injection site.

---

ampicillin sodium/sulbactam sodium
Unasyn

Pregnancy risk category B

AVAILABLE FORMS
Injection: Vials and piggyback vials containing 1.5 g (1 g ampicillin sodium with 0.5 g sulbactam sodium), 3 g (2 g ampicillin sodium with 1 g sulbactam sodium), and 15 g (10 g ampicillin sodium with 5 g sulbactam sodium)

INDICATIONS & DOSAGES
➤ **Intra-abdominal, gynecologic, and skin-structure infections caused by susceptible strains—**
Adults and children weighing more than 40 kg (88 lb): 1.5 to 3 g I.M. or I.V. q 6 hours. Maximum daily dose is 12 g.
Children age 1 and older, weighing less than 40 kg: 300 mg/kg/day I.V. in divided doses q 6 hours. Don't exceed 4 g daily.

Adjust-a-dose: For renally impaired patients with creatinine clearance of 15 to 29 ml/minute, give 1.5 to 3 g q 12 hours; if clearance is 5 to 14 ml/minute, give 1.5 to 3 g q 24 hours.

I.V. ADMINISTRATION
• When preparing I.V. injection, reconstitute powder with one of the following diluents: normal saline solution, sterile water for injection, D_5W, lactated Ringer's injection, 1/6 M sodium lactate, dextrose 5% in half-normal saline solution for injection, and 10% invert sugar. Stability varies with diluent, temperature, and concentration of solution.
• After reconstitution, let vials stand for a few minutes to allow foam to dissipate. This will permit visual inspection of contents for particles.
• When giving I.V., don't add or mix with other drugs because they might be incompatible.
• Give drug at least 1 hour before a bacteriostatic antibiotic.
• *Alert:* Give I.V. dose by slow injection over 10 to 15 minutes or dilute in 50 to 100 ml of a compatible diluent, and infuse over 15 to 30 minutes. If permitted, give intermittently to prevent vein irritation. Change site every 48 hours.

ACTION
An aminopenicillin that inhibits cell-wall synthesis during microorganism multiplication. Sulbactam inactivates bacterial beta-lactamase, which inactivates ampicillin, causing bacterial resistance to it.

Route	Onset	Peak	Duration
I.M.	Unknown	Unknown	Unknown
I.V.	Immediate	15 min	Unknown

ADVERSE REACTIONS
CV: thrombophlebitis.
GI: *nausea,* vomiting, *diarrhea,* glossitis, stomatitis, gastritis, black hairy tongue, enterocolitis, pseudomembranous colitis.
Hematologic: anemia, *thrombocytopenia, thrombocytopenic purpura,* eosinophilia, *leukopenia, agranulocytosis.*
Other: hypersensitivity reactions, *anaphylaxis,* overgrowth of nonsusceptible organisms, *pain at injection site,* vein irritation.

Reactions may be *common*, uncommon, *life-threatening*, or COMMON AND LIFE-THREATENING.

INTERACTIONS
Drug-drug. *Allopurinol:* Increased risk of rash. Monitor patient.

Oral contraceptives: May decrease efficacy of oral contraceptives. Recommend additional form of contraception during penicillin therapy.

Probenecid: Increased levels of ampicillin. Probenecid may be used for this purpose.

EFFECTS ON LAB TEST RESULTS
● May increase BUN, creatinine, ALT, AST, alkaline phosphatase, bilirubin, LDH, CK, and GGT levels.
● May increase eosinophil count. May decrease hemoglobin and platelet, WBC, and granulocyte counts.

CONTRAINDICATIONS
Contraindicated in patients hypersensitive to drug or other penicillins.

NURSING CONSIDERATIONS
● Use cautiously in patients with other drug allergies (especially to cephalosporins) because of possible cross-sensitivity and in those with mononucleosis because of high risk of maculopapular rash.
● Before giving drug, ask patient about allergic reactions to penicillin. However, a negative history of penicillin allergy is no guarantee against future allergic reaction.
● Obtain specimen for culture and sensitivity tests before giving first dose. Therapy may begin pending results.
● Dosage is expressed as total drug. Each 1.5-g vial contains 1 g ampicillin sodium and 0.5 g sulbactam sodium.
● Decrease dosage in patients with impaired renal function.
● For I.M. injection, reconstitute with sterile water for injection or 0.5% or 2% lidocaine hydrochloride injection. Add 3.2 ml to a 1.5-g vial (or 6.4 ml to a 3-g vial) to yield a concentration of 375 mg/ml. Give deeply.
● Don't use I.M. route in children.
● Ampicillin alters results of urine glucose tests that use cupric sulfate such as Benedict's reagent or Clinitest. Make urine glucose determinations with glucose oxidase methods such as Diastix. In pregnant women, transient decreases in estradiol,

conjugated estrone, conjugated estriol, and estriol glucuronide levels may occur.
● Monitor liver function test results during therapy, especially in patients with impaired liver function.
● If large doses are given or if therapy is prolonged, bacterial or fungal superinfection may occur, especially in elderly, debilitated, or immunosuppressed patients.

PATIENT TEACHING
● Tell patient to report rash, fever, or chills. A rash is the most common allergic reaction.
● Advise patient to report discomfort at I.V. insertion site.
● Warn patient that I.M. injection may cause pain at injection site.

cloxacillin sodium
Apo-Cloxi†, Cloxapen, Novo-Cloxin†, Nu-Cloxi†, Orbenin†

Pregnancy risk category B

AVAILABLE FORMS
Capsules: 250 mg, 500 mg
Oral solution: 125 mg/5 ml (after reconstitution)

INDICATIONS & DOSAGES
➤ **Systemic infections caused by penicillinase-producing staphylococci—**
Adults and children weighing more than 20 kg (44 lb): 250 to 500 mg P.O. q 6 hours.
Children weighing 20 kg or less: 50 to 100 mg/kg P.O. daily, in divided doses q 6 hours. Maximum of 4 g daily.

ACTION
A penicillinase-resistant penicillin that inhibits cell-wall synthesis during microorganism multiplication. Bacteria resist penicillins by producing penicillinases—enzymes that convert penicillins to inactive penicillic acid. Cloxacillin resists these enzymes.

Route	Onset	Peak	Duration
P.O.	Unknown	0.5-2 hr	6 hr

ADVERSE REACTIONS
CNS: lethargy, hallucinations, *seizures,* anxiety, confusion, agitation, depression, dizziness, fatigue.
GI: *nausea,* vomiting, *epigastric distress, diarrhea,* enterocolitis, pseudomembranous colitis, black hairy tongue, abdominal pain.
GU: interstitial nephritis, nephropathy.
Hematologic: eosinophilia, anemia, *thrombocytopenia, leukopenia,* hemolytic anemia, *agranulocytosis.*
Other: hypersensitivity reactions, *anaphylaxis,* overgrowth of nonsusceptible organisms.

INTERACTIONS
Drug-drug. *Oral contraceptives:* May decrease efficacy of oral contraceptives. Recommend additional form of contraception during penicillin therapy.
Probenecid: Increased blood levels of cloxacillin and other penicillins. Probenecid may be used for this purpose.
Drug-food. *Any food:* May interfere with absorption. Give 1 to 2 hours before or 2 to 3 hours after meals.

EFFECTS ON LAB TEST RESULTS
● Increased ALT, AST, alkaline phosphatase, and LDH levels.
● May increase eosinophil count. May decrease hemoglobin and platelet, WBC, RBC, and granulocyte counts.

CONTRAINDICATIONS
Contraindicated in patients hypersensitive to drug or other penicillins.

NURSING CONSIDERATIONS
● Use cautiously in patients with other drug allergies (especially to cephalosporins) because of possible cross-sensitivity and in those with mononucleosis because of high risk of maculopapular rash.
● Before giving drug, ask patient about allergic reactions to penicillin. However, a negative history of penicillin allergy is no guarantee against a future allergic reaction.
● Obtain specimen for culture and sensitivity tests before giving first dose. Therapy may begin pending results.
● Give drug 1 to 2 hours before or 2 to 3 hours after meals. Drug may cause GI disturbances. Food may interfere with its absorption.
● Periodically assess renal, hepatic, and hematopoietic function in patients receiving long-term therapy.
● Elevated liver function test results may indicate drug-induced cholestasis or hepatitis.
● If large doses are given or if therapy is prolonged, bacterial or fungal superinfection may occur, especially in elderly, debilitated, or immunosuppressed patients.
● Drug alters test results for urine and serum proteins; it produces false-positive or elevated results in turbidimetric urine and serum protein tests using sulfosalicylic acid or trichloroacetic acid; it also may cause false results on the Bradshaw screening test for Bence Jones protein.

PATIENT TEACHING
● Tell patient to take entire quantity of drug exactly as prescribed, even after he feels better.
● Instruct patient to take drug on an empty stomach.
● *Alert:* Instruct patient to take each dose with a full glass of water and not with fruit juice or carbonated beverage because their acid will inactivate drug.
● Advise patient to notify prescriber if rash, fever, or chills develop. A rash is the most common allergic reaction.

dicloxacillin sodium
Diclocil‡, Dycill, Dynapen, Pathocil

Pregnancy risk category B

AVAILABLE FORMS
Capsules: 125 mg, 250 mg, 500 mg
Oral suspension: 62.5 mg/5 ml (after reconstitution)

INDICATIONS & DOSAGES
➤ **Systemic infections caused by penicillinase-producing staphylococci—**
Adults and children weighing more than 40 kg (88 lb): 125 to 250 mg P.O. q 6 hours.
Children weighing 40 kg or less: 12.5 to 25 mg/kg P.O. daily in divided doses q 6 hours depending on severity.

ACTION

A penicillinase-resistant penicillin that inhibits cell-wall synthesis during microorganism multiplication. Bacteria resist penicillins by producing penicillinases—enzymes that convert penicillins to inactive penicillic acid. Dicloxacillin resists these enzymes.

Route	Onset	Peak	Duration
P.O.	Unknown	2 hr	6 hr

ADVERSE REACTIONS

CNS: neuromuscular irritability, *seizures,* lethargy, hallucinations, anxiety, confusion, agitation, depression, dizziness, fatigue.
GI: *nausea,* vomiting, *epigastric distress,* flatulence, *diarrhea,* enterocolitis, pseudomembranous colitis, black hairy tongue, abdominal pain.
GU: interstitial nephritis, nephropathy.
Hematologic: anemia, *thrombocytopenia,* eosinophilia, *leukopenia,* hemolytic anemia, *agranulocytosis.*
Other: hypersensitivity reactions, overgrowth of nonsusceptible organisms.

INTERACTIONS

Drug-drug. *Oral contraceptives:* May decrease efficacy of oral contraceptives. Recommend additional form of contraception during penicillin therapy.
Probenecid: Increased blood levels of dicloxacillin and other penicillins. Probenecid may be used for this purpose.

EFFECTS ON LAB TEST RESULTS

• May increase ALT, AST, alkaline phosphatase, and LDH levels.
• May increase eosinophil count. May decrease hemoglobin and platelet, WBC, and granulocyte counts.

CONTRAINDICATIONS

Contraindicated in patients hypersensitive to drug or other penicillins. It isn't recommended for use in newborns.

NURSING CONSIDERATIONS

• Use cautiously in patients with other drug allergies (especially to cephalosporins) because of possible cross-sensitivity and in those with mononucleosis because of high risk of maculopapular rash.

• Before giving drug, ask patient about allergic reactions to penicillin. However, a negative history of penicillin allergy is no guarantee against a future allergic reaction.
• Obtain specimen for culture and sensitivity tests before giving first dose. Therapy may begin pending results.
• Give drug 1 to 2 hours before or 2 to 3 hours after meals. Drug may cause GI disturbances. Food may interfere with absorption.
• Drug produces false-positive or elevated results in turbidimetric urine and serum protein tests using sulfosalicylic acid or trichloroacetic acid; it also may produce false results on the Bradshaw screening test for Bence Jones protein.
• Watch for hypersensitivity reactions, such as pruritus, urticaria, rash, and anaphylaxis.
• As ordered, periodically assess renal, hepatic, and hematopoietic function in patients receiving long-term therapy.
• Elevated liver function test results may indicate drug-induced cholestasis or hepatitis.
• If large doses are given or if therapy is prolonged, bacterial or fungal superinfection may occur, especially in elderly, debilitated, or immunosuppressed patients.

PATIENT TEACHING

• Tell patient to take entire quantity of drug exactly as prescribed, even after he feels better.
• Instruct patient to take drug on an empty stomach.
• Advise patient to notify prescriber if rash, fever, or chills develop. A rash is the most common allergic reaction.

mezlocillin sodium
Mezlin

Pregnancy risk category B

AVAILABLE FORMS
Injection: 1 g, 2 g, 3 g, 4 g, 20 g

INDICATIONS & DOSAGES
➤ **Systemic infections caused by susceptible strains of gram-positive and especially gram-negative organisms**

including *Proteus species* and
Pseudomonas aeruginosa—
Adults: 100 to 300 mg/kg daily I.V. or
I.M. in four to six divided doses. Usual
dose is 3 g q 4 hours or 4 g q 6 hours. For
serious infections, up to 24 g daily may be
given.
Children ages 1 month to 12 years:
50 mg/kg q 4 hours I.V. or I.M.
➤ **Acute, uncomplicated gonococcal
urethritis caused by susceptible strains
of *Neisseria gonorrhoeae*—**
Adults: 1 to 2 g I.M. or I.V. with 1 g P.O.
probenecid.
Adjust-a-dose: For renally impaired patients with creatinine clearance of 10 to
30 ml/minute, 1.5 g q 6 hours for urinary
tract infection or 3 g q 8 hours for serious
infection; for clearance less than 10 ml/
minute, 1.5 g q 8 hours for urinary tract
infection or 2 g q 8 hours for serious infection.

I.V. ADMINISTRATION
● Reconstitute drug with at least 10 ml/g
of drug using sterile water for injection,
D_5W, or normal saline solution for injection. Solutions with a concentration not
exceeding 10% may be given by direct injection over 3 to 5 minutes.
● For intermittent infusion, dilute in about
50 to 100 ml of suitable I.V. solution, and
give over 30 minutes.
● Give I.V. intermittently to prevent vein
irritation. Change site every 48 hours.

ACTION
An extended-spectrum penicillin that inhibits cell-wall synthesis during microorganism multiplication. Bacteria resist
mezlocillin by producing penicillinases—
enzymes that hydrolyze mezlocillin.

Route	Onset	Peak	Duration
I.M.	Unknown	45-90 min	Unknown
I.V.	Immediate	Immediate	Unknown

ADVERSE REACTIONS
CNS: neuromuscular irritability, *seizures.*
CV: vein irritation, phlebitis.
GI: nausea, diarrhea, vomiting, abnormal
taste, pseudomembranous colitis.
GU: interstitial nephritis.

Hematologic: *bleeding, neutropenia,
thrombocytopenia,* eosinophilia, *leukopenia, hemolytic anemia.*
Metabolic: *hypokalemia.*
Other: hypersensitivity reactions, *anaphylaxis,* overgrowth of nonsusceptible
organisms, pain at injection site.

INTERACTIONS
Drug-drug. *Aminoglycoside antibiotics
(such as amikacin, gentamicin, tobramycin):* Chemically incompatible; don't
combine in I.V. solution. Give 1 hour
apart, especially in patients with renal
impairment.
Oral contraceptives: May decrease efficacy of oral contraceptives. Recommend
additional form of contraception during
penicillin therapy.
Probenecid: Increased levels of mezlocillin. Probenecid may be used for this
purpose.
Vecuronium: Prolonged neuromuscular
blockade. Use together cautiously.

EFFECTS ON LAB TEST RESULTS
● May increase ALT, AST, alkaline phosphatase, and LDH levels. May decrease
potassium level.
● May increase eosinophil count. May decrease neutrophil, WBC, and platelet
counts, and hemoglobin.

CONTRAINDICATIONS
Contraindicated in patients hypersensitive
to drug or other penicillins.

NURSING CONSIDERATIONS
● Use cautiously in patients with other
drug allergies, especially to cephalosporins, because of possible cross-sensitivity,
and in those with bleeding tendencies,
uremia, or hypokalemia.
● Before giving drug, ask patient about
allergic reactions to penicillin. A negative
history of penicillin allergy, however, is no
guarantee against future allergic reaction.
● Obtain specimen for culture and sensitivity tests before giving first dose. Therapy may begin pending results.
● When giving I.M., don't give more than
2 g per injection. Inject deeply and slowly
over 12 to 15 seconds into the body of a
large muscle.

Reactions may be *common,* uncommon, *life-threatening,* or COMMON AND LIFE-THREATENING.

• Check CBC and platelet counts often. Drug may cause thrombocytopenia.
• Monitor potassium level.
• Drug alters tests for urine or serum proteins; it interferes with turbidimetric methods that use sulfosalicylic acid, trichloroacetic acid, acetic acid, or nitric acid. Mezlocillin doesn't interfere with tests using bromphenol blue (Albustix, Albutest, Multistix). Positive Coombs' tests have been reported in patients taking mezlocillin.
• If large doses are given or if therapy is prolonged, bacterial or fungal superinfection may occur, especially in elderly, debilitated, or immunosuppressed patients.
• *Alert:* Don't confuse methicillin with mezlocillin.

PATIENT TEACHING
• Instruct patient to report adverse reactions promptly.
• Tell patient to report discomfort at I.V. site.
• Caution patient to limit salt intake during mezlocillin therapy because of drug's high sodium content.

nafcillin sodium
Unipen

Pregnancy risk category B

AVAILABLE FORMS
Capsules: 250 mg
Injection: 500 mg, 1 g, 2 g, 10 g
I.V. infusion piggyback: 1 g, 2 g

INDICATIONS & DOSAGES
➤ **Systemic infections caused by penicillinase-producing staphylococci—**
Adults: 250 to 500 mg P.O. q 4 to 6 hours. More severe infections may be treated with 1 g P.O. q 4 to 6 hours; or 500 mg I.M. q 4 to 6 hours or I.V. q 4 hours. Or, for more severe infections, 1 g I.M. or I.V. q 4 hours. Maximum recommended daily dose is 6 g.
Children older than age 1 month and weighing less than 40 kg (88 lb): 25 to 50 mg/kg P.O. daily in divided doses q 6 hours; or 25 mg/kg I.M. b.i.d. or 100 to 200 mg/kg I.M. or I.V. daily in divided doses q 4 to 6 hours.

Neonates: 10 mg/kg I.M. b.i.d. or 10 mg/kg P.O. t.i.d. or q.i.d.

I.V. ADMINISTRATION
• For direct injection, reconstitute piggyback containers according to manufacturer's instructions. Reconstitute 500-mg, 1-g, or 2-g vials with sterile water for injection, D_5W, or normal saline solution for injection. Add 1.7 ml for each 500 mg of drug.
• Reconstituted drug may be given I.M. Or, dilute with 15 to 30 ml of sterile water for injection or half-normal or normal saline solution for injection, and give by direct injection into a vein or into the tubing of a free-flowing I.V. solution over 5 to 10 minutes.
• For intermittent infusion, dilute drug to a concentration of 2 to 40 mg/ml and give by over 30 to 60 minutes.
• Avoid continuous I.V. infusions to prevent vein irritation. Change site every 48 hours.

ACTION
A penicillinase-resistant penicillin that inhibits cell-wall synthesis during microorganism multiplication. Bacteria resist penicillins by producing penicillinases—enzymes that hydrolyze penicillins. Nafcillin resists these enzymes.

Route	Onset	Peak	Duration
I.M.	Unknown	0.5-1 hr	Unknown
I.V.	Immediate	Immediate	Unknown
P.O.	Unknown	0.5-2 hr	Unknown

ADVERSE REACTIONS
CV: thrombophlebitis.
GI: *nausea,* vomiting, diarrhea.
Hematologic: *neutropenia, agranulocytosis, thrombocytopenia.*
Other: hypersensitivity reactions, *anaphylaxis,* vein irritation.

INTERACTIONS
Drug-drug. *Aminoglycosides:* Synergistic effect; chemically and physically incompatible. Don't combine in same I.V. solution.
Oral contraceptives: May decrease efficacy of oral contraceptives. Recommend additional form of contraception during penicillin therapy.

---

*Liquid contains alcohol.   **May contain tartrazine.   †Canada   ‡Australia   §U.K.   ◊OTC

Probenecid: Increased blood levels of nafcillin. Probenecid may be used for this purpose.
Rifampin: Dose-dependent antagonism. Monitor patient closely.
Warfarin: Increased risk of bleeding when used with I.V. nafcillin. Monitor PT and INR closely.

EFFECTS ON LAB TEST RESULTS
● May decrease neutrophil, granulocyte, and platelet counts.

CONTRAINDICATIONS
Contraindicated in patients hypersensitive to drug or other penicillins.

NURSING CONSIDERATIONS
● Use cautiously in patients with GI distress and in those with other drug allergies, especially to cephalosporins, because of possible cross-sensitivity.
● Before giving drug, ask patient about allergic reactions to penicillin. However, a negative history of penicillin allergy is no guarantee against a future allergic reaction.
● Obtain specimen for culture and sensitivity tests before giving first dose. Therapy may begin pending results.
● Give drug 1 to 2 hours before or 2 to 3 hours after meals. When given orally, drug may cause GI disturbances. Food may interfere with absorption.
● If large doses are given or if therapy is prolonged, bacterial or fungal superinfection may occur, especially in elderly, debilitated, or immunosuppressed patients.
● Monitor sodium level because each gram of nafcillin contains 2.9 mEq of sodium.
● Monitor WBC counts twice weekly in patients receiving I.V. nafcillin for longer than 2 weeks. Neutropenia commonly occurs in the third week.
● Turbidimetric urine and serum proteins are falsely positive or elevated in tests using sulfosalicylic acid or trichloroacetic acid.
● In children, give I.M. in the midlateral or anterolateral thigh. Rotate injection sites.
● An abnormal urinalysis result may indicate drug-induced interstitial nephritis.

PATIENT TEACHING
● Tell patient to take entire quantity of drug exactly as prescribed, even after he feels better.
● Instruct patient to take oral form of drug on an empty stomach.
● Advise patient to notify prescriber if rash, fever, or chills develop. A rash is the most common allergic reaction.

---

oxacillin sodium
Bactocill

Pregnancy risk category B

AVAILABLE FORMS
Capsules: 250 mg, 500 mg
Injection: 250 mg, 500 mg, 1 g, 2 g, 4 g
I.V. infusion: 1 g, 2 g
Oral solution: 250 mg/5 ml (after reconstitution)

INDICATIONS & DOSAGES
➤ **Systemic infections caused by penicillinase-producing staphylococci—**
Adults and children weighing more than 40 kg (88 lb): 500 mg to 1 g P.O. q 4 to 6 hours; or 250 mg to 1 g I.M. or I.V. q 4 to 6 hours.
Children older than age 1 month weighing 40 kg or less: 50 to 100 mg/kg P.O. daily in divided doses q 6 hours; or 50 to 100 mg/kg I.M. or I.V. daily in divided doses q 4 to 6 hours, depending on severity.
Premature infants and neonates: 25 mg/kg/day I.M. or I.V. in equally divided doses q 6 to 12 hours.

I.V. ADMINISTRATION
● For direct I.V. injection, reconstitute drug with sterile water for injection or normal saline solution for injection.
● Use 5 ml of diluent for a 250- or 500-mg vial, 10 ml of diluent for a 1-g vial, 20 ml of diluent for a 2-g vial, or 40 ml of diluent for a 4-g vial. When the solution is clear, withdraw the ordered dose and inject over 10 minutes.
● When giving by piggyback injection, reconstitute 1-g piggyback vial with 20 to 100 ml of diluent; reconstitute 2-g vial with 19 to 99 ml of diluent. For intermit-

---

Reactions may be *common*, uncommon, *life-threatening*, or COMMON AND LIFE-THREATENING.

tent infusion, further dilute drug to a concentration of 5 to 40 mg/ml.
● To prevent vein irritation, avoid continuous infusions. Change site every 48 hours.

ACTION
A penicillinase-resistant penicillin that inhibits cell-wall synthesis during microorganism multiplication. Bacteria resist penicillins by producing penicillinases—enzymes that convert penicillins to inactive penicillic acid. Oxacillin resists these enzymes.

Route	Onset	Peak	Duration
I.M.	Unknown	0.5 hr	Unknown
I.V.	Immediate	Immediate	Unknown
P.O.	Unknown	0.5-2 hr	Unknown

ADVERSE REACTIONS
CNS: neuropathy, neuromuscular irritability, *seizures,* lethargy, hallucinations, anxiety, confusion, agitation, depression, dizziness, fatigue.
CV: *thrombophlebitis.*
GI: oral lesions, nausea, vomiting, diarrhea, enterocolitis, pseudomembranous colitis.
GU: interstitial nephritis, nephropathy.
Hematologic: *thrombocytopenia,* eosinophilia, *hemolytic anemia, neutropenia,* anemia, *agranulocytosis.*
Other: hypersensitivity reactions, *anaphylaxis,* overgrowth of nonsusceptible organisms.

INTERACTIONS
Drug-drug. *Aminoglycosides:* May cause synergistic effect; chemically and physically incompatible. Don't combine in same I.V. solution.
Oral contraceptives: May decrease efficacy of oral contraceptives. Recommend additional form of contraception during penicillin therapy.
Probenecid: Increased blood levels of oxacillin and other penicillins. Probenecid may be used for this purpose.
Rifampin: May cause antagonism. Monitor patient closely.

EFFECTS ON LAB TEST RESULTS
● May increase ALT, AST, alkaline phosphatase, and LDH levels.

● May increased eosinophil count. May decrease hemoglobin and platelet, neutrophil, and granulocyte counts.

CONTRAINDICATIONS
Contraindicated in patients hypersensitive to drug or other penicillins.

NURSING CONSIDERATIONS
● Use cautiously in neonates, infants, and patients with other drug allergies, especially to cephalosporins, because of possible cross-sensitivity.
● Before giving drug, ask patient about allergic reactions to penicillin. However, a negative history of penicillin allergy is no guarantee against a future allergic reaction.
● Obtain specimen for culture and sensitivity tests before giving first dose. Therapy may begin pending results.
● Give drug I.M. or I.V. only if ordered and the infection is severe or if the patient can't take oral dose.
● Give drug 1 to 2 hours before or 2 to 3 hours after meals. When given orally, drug may cause GI disturbances. Food may interfere with absorption.
● Monitor sodium level; each gram of oxicillin contains 2.5 to 3.1 mEq of sodium.
● Monitor periodic liver function test results; watch for elevated AST and ALT levels. Elevations in these test results may indicate drug-induced hepatitis or cholestasis.
● Abnormal urinalysis results may indicate drug-induced interstitial nephritis.
● If large doses are given or if therapy is prolonged, bacterial or fungal superinfection may occur, especially in elderly, debilitated, or immunosuppressed patients.
● Turbidimetric urine and serum proteins are falsely positive or elevated in tests using sulfosalicylic acid or trichloroacetic acid.

PATIENT TEACHING
● Tell patient to take entire quantity of drug exactly as prescribed, even after he feels better.
● Instruct patient to take drug on an empty stomach.

---

*Liquid contains alcohol.   **May contain tartrazine.   †Canada   ‡Australia   §U.K.   ◊OTC

• Advise patient to notify prescriber if rash, fever, or chills develop. A rash is the most common allergic reaction.
• Tell patient to report signs and symptoms of hepatic dysfunction, such as abdominal discomfort, nausea, vomiting, malaise, or jaundice.

---

penicillin G benzathine (benzylpenicillin benzathine)
Bicillin L-A, Permapen

Pregnancy risk category B

AVAILABLE FORMS
Injection: 300,000 units/ml, 600,000 units/ml, 1,200,000 units/2 ml, 2,400,000 units/4 ml

INDICATIONS & DOSAGES
➤ **Congenital syphilis—**
Children younger than age 2: 50,000 units/kg I.M. as a single dose.
➤ **Group A streptococcal upper respiratory tract infections—**
Adults: 1.2 million units I.M. as a single injection.
Children weighing 27 kg (60 lb) or more: 900,000 units I.M. as a single injection.
Children weighing less than 27 kg: 300,000 to 600,000 units I.M. as a single injection.
➤ **Prophylaxis of poststreptococcal rheumatic fever—**
Adults and children: 1.2 million units I.M. once monthly or 600,000 units I.M. every 2 weeks.
➤ **Syphilis of less than 1 year's duration—**
Adults: 2.4 million units I.M. as a single dose.
Children: 50,000 units/kg I.M. as a single dose. Don't exceed adult dosage.
➤ **Syphilis of more than 1 year's duration—**
Adults: 2.4 million units I.M. weekly for 3 weeks.
Children: 50,000 units/kg I.M. weekly for 3 weeks.

ACTION
A natural penicillin that inhibits cell-wall synthesis during microorganism multiplication. Bacteria resist penicillins by producing penicillinases—enzymes that convert penicillins to inactive penicillic acid.

Route	Onset	Peak	Duration
I.M.	Unknown	13-24 hr	1-4 wk

ADVERSE REACTIONS
CNS: neuropathy, **seizures,** lethargy, hallucinations, anxiety, confusion, agitation, depression, dizziness, fatigue.
GI: nausea, vomiting, enterocolitis, pseudomembranous colitis.
GU: interstitial nephritis, nephropathy.
Hematologic: eosinophilia, hemolytic anemia, ***thrombocytopenia, leukopenia,*** anemia, ***agranulocytosis.***
Skin: maculopapular rash, exfoliative dermatitis.
Other: hypersensitivity reactions, ***anaphylaxis,*** pain, sterile abscess at injection site.

INTERACTIONS
Drug-drug. *Aminoglycosides:* Physical and chemical incompatibility. Give separately.
Colestipol: Decreased concentrations of penicillin G benzathine. Give penicillin G benzathine 1 hour before or 4 hours after colestipol.
Oral contraceptives: May decrease efficacy of oral contraceptives. Recommend additional form of contraception during penicillin therapy.
Probenecid: Increased blood levels of penicillin. Probenecid may be used for this purpose.
Tetracycline: May antagonize the effects of penicillin G benzathine. Avoid using together.

EFFECTS ON LAB TEST RESULTS
• May increase eosinophil count. May decrease hemoglobin and platelet, WBC, and granulocyte counts.

CONTRAINDICATIONS
Contraindicated in patients hypersensitive to drug or other penicillins.

NURSING CONSIDERATIONS
• Use cautiously in patients with other drug allergies, especially to cephalosporins, because of possible cross-sensitivity.

• Before giving drug, ask patient about allergic reactions to penicillin. However, a negative history of penicillin allergy is no guarantee against a future allergic reaction.
• Obtain specimen for culture and sensitivity tests before giving first dose. Therapy may begin pending results.
• Shake well before injection.
• Penicillin G interferes with turbidimetric methods using sulfosalicylic acid, trichloroacetic acid, acetic acid, and nitric acid. It doesn't interfere with tests using bromphenol blue (Albustix, Albutest, Multistix). Drug alters urine glucose testing using cupric sulfate (Benedict's reagent); use Diastix or Chemstrip uG instead. Penicillin G may falsely elevate results of urine specific gravity tests in patients with low urine output and dehydration and falsely elevate Norymberski and Zimmerman test results for 17-ketogenic steroids. It causes false-positive CSF protein test results (Folin-Ciocalteau method) and may cause positive Coombs' test results. Drug may falsely decrease aminoglycoside levels. Adding beta-lactamase to the sample inactivates the penicillin, rendering the assay more accurate. Or, the sample can be spun down and frozen immediately after collection.
• **Alert:** Never give by I.V. route. Inadvertent I.V. administration has caused cardiac arrest and death.
• Inject deeply into upper outer quadrant of buttocks in adults and in midlateral thigh in infants and small children. Rotate injection sites. Avoid injection into or near major nerves or blood vessels to prevent permanent neurovascular damage.
• Give drug at least 1 hour before a bacteriostatic antibiotic.
• Drug's extremely slow absorption time makes allergic reactions difficult to treat.
• If large doses are given or if therapy is prolonged, bacterial or fungal superinfection may occur, especially in elderly, debilitated, or immunosuppressed patients.
• **Alert:** Don't confuse drug with Polycillin, penicillamine, or the various types of penicillin.

PATIENT TEACHING
• Tell patient to report adverse reactions promptly.
• Inform patient that fever and eosinophilia are the most common reactions.
• Warn patient that I.M. injection may be painful but that ice applied to the site may ease discomfort.

penicillin G potassium (benzylpenicillin potassium)
Megacillin†, Pfizerpen

Pregnancy risk category B

AVAILABLE FORMS
Injection: 1 million units, 5 million units, 10 million units, 20 million units
Oral suspension: 250,000 units†, 500,000 units†
Premixed injection: 1 million units/50 ml, 2 million units/50 ml, 3 million units/50 ml
Tablets: 500,000 units†

INDICATIONS & DOSAGES
➤ **Moderate to severe systemic infection—**
Adults and children age 12 and older:
Highly individualized; 1.6 to 3.2 million units P.O. daily in divided doses q 6 hours; 1.2 to 24 million units I.M. or I.V. daily in divided doses q 4 to 6 hours.
Children younger than age 12: 25,000 to 100,000 units/kg P.O. daily in divided doses q 6 hours; or 25,000 to 400,000 units/kg I.M. or I.V. daily in divided doses q 4 to 6 hours.

I.V. ADMINISTRATION
• Reconstitute drug with sterile water for injection, D_5W, or normal saline solution for injection. Volume of diluent varies with manufacturer.
• For intermittent I.V. infusion, give drug over 1 to 2 hours.
• For continuous I.V. infusion, add reconstituted solution of drug to 1 to 2 liters of compatible I.V. solution. Determine the volume of fluid and rate of administration required by the patient in a 24-hour period, and add the ordered drug dose to this fluid.

ACTION
A natural penicillin that inhibits cell-wall synthesis during microorganism multiplication. Bacteria resist penicillins by producing penicillinases—enzymes that convert penicillins to inactive penicillic acid.

Route	Onset	Peak	Duration
I.M.	Unknown	15-30 min	Unknown
I.V.	Immediate	Immediate	Unknown
P.O.	Unknown	30-60 min	Unknown

ADVERSE REACTIONS
CNS: neuropathy, *seizures*, lethargy, hallucinations, anxiety, confusion, agitation, depression, dizziness, fatigue.
CV: thrombophlebitis.
GI: nausea, vomiting, enterocolitis, pseudomembranous colitis.
GU: interstitial nephritis, nephropathy.
Hematologic: hemolytic anemia, *leukopenia, thrombocytopenia,* anemia, eosinophilia, *agranulocytosis.*
Metabolic: *possible severe potassium poisoning.*
Skin: maculopapular eruptions, exfoliative dermatitis.
Other: hypersensitivity reactions, *anaphylaxis,* overgrowth of nonsusceptible organisms, pain at injection site.

INTERACTIONS
Drug-drug. *Aminoglycosides:* Physical and chemical incompatibility. Give separately.
Colestipol: Decreased levels of penicillin G potassium. Give penicillin G potassium 1 hour before or 4 hours after colestipol.
Oral contraceptives: May decrease efficacy of oral contraceptives. Recommend additional form of contraception during penicillin therapy.
Potassium-sparing diuretics: May increase risk of hyperkalemia. Don't use together.
Probenecid: Increased blood levels of penicillin. Probenecid may be used for this purpose.

EFFECTS ON LAB TEST RESULTS
• May increase potassium level.
• May increase eosinophil count. May decrease hemoglobin and platelet, WBC, and granulocyte counts.

CONTRAINDICATIONS
Contraindicated in patients hypersensitive to drug or other penicillins.

NURSING CONSIDERATIONS
• Use cautiously in patients with other drug allergies, especially to cephalosporins, because of possible cross-sensitivity.
• Before giving drug, ask patient about allergic reactions to penicillin. However, a negative history of penicillin allergy is no guarantee against a future allergic reaction.
• Obtain specimen for culture and sensitivity tests before giving first dose. Therapy may begin pending results.
• For I.M. injection, give deeply into large muscle; may be extremely painful.
• Give drug 1 to 2 hours before or 2 to 3 hours after meals. When given orally, drug may cause GI disturbances. Food may interfere with absorption.
• Penicillin G interferes with turbidimetric methods using sulfosalicylic acid, trichloroacetic acid, acetic acid, and nitric acid. It doesn't interfere with tests using bromphenol blue (Albustix, Albutest, Multistix). Drug alters urine glucose testing using cupric sulfate (Benedict's reagent); use Diastix or Chemstrip uG instead. Penicillin G may falsely elevate results of urine specific gravity tests in patients with low urine output and dehydration and falsely elevate Norymberski and Zimmerman test results for 17-ketogenic steroids. It causes false-positive CSF protein test results (Folin-Ciocalteu method) and may cause positive Coombs' test results. Drug may falsely decrease aminoglycoside levels. Adding beta-lactamase to the sample inactivates the penicillin, rendering the assay more accurate. Or, the sample can be spun down and frozen immediately after collection.
• Monitor renal function closely. Patients with poor renal function are predisposed to high blood levels of drug.
• Monitor potassium and sodium levels closely in patients receiving more than 10 million units I.V. daily.
• Observe patient closely. With large doses and prolonged therapy, bacterial or fungal superinfection may occur, especially in elderly, debilitated, or immunosuppressed patients.

Reactions may be *common*, uncommon, *life-threatening*, or COMMON AND LIFE-THREATENING.

• *Alert:* Don't confuse drug with Polycillin, penicillamine, or the various types of penicillin.

PATIENT TEACHING
• Tell patient taking oral form to take entire amount exactly as prescribed, even after he feels better.
• Instruct patient to take oral drug on empty stomach.
• Tell patient to notify prescriber if rash, fever, or chills develop. A rash is the most common allergic reaction.
• Warn patient that I.M. injection may be painful but that ice applied to the site may help alleviate discomfort.

**penicillin G procaine
(benzylpenicillin procaine)**
Ayercillin†, Wycillin

Pregnancy risk category B

AVAILABLE FORMS
Injection: 600,000 units/ml, 1,200,000 units/ml, 2,400,000 units/ml

INDICATIONS & DOSAGES
➤ **Moderate to severe systemic infection—**
Adults: 600,000 to 1.2 million units I.M. daily for a minimum of 10 days.
Children older than age 1 month: 25,000 to 50,000 units/kg I.M. daily in a single dose.
➤ **Uncomplicated gonorrhea—**
Adults: 1 g probenecid P.O.; after 30 minutes, 4.8 million units of penicillin G procaine I.M. divided between two injection sites as a single dose.
➤ **Anthrax caused by *Bacillus anthracis*, including inhalation anthrax (postexposure)—**
Adults: 1,200,000 units I.M. q 12 hours.
Children: 25,000 units/kg I.M.; not to exceed 1,200,000 units q 12 hours.
➤ **Cutaneous anthrax—**
Adults: 600,000 to 1,000,000 units I.M. daily.

ACTION
A natural penicillin that inhibits cell-wall synthesis during microorganism multiplication. Bacteria resist penicillins by producing penicillinases—enzymes that convert penicillins to inactive penicillic acid.

Route	Onset	Peak	Duration
I.M.	Unknown	1-4 hr	1-5 days

ADVERSE REACTIONS
CNS: *seizures,* lethargy, hallucinations, anxiety, confusion, agitation, depression, dizziness, fatigue.
GI: nausea, vomiting, enterocolitis, pseudomembranous colitis.
GU: interstitial nephritis, nephropathy.
Hematologic: *thrombocytopenia, hemolytic anemia, leukopenia,* anemia, eosinophilia, *agranulocytosis.*
Musculoskeletal: arthralgia.
Other: hypersensitivity reactions, *anaphylaxis,* overgrowth of nonsusceptible organisms.

INTERACTIONS
Drug-drug. *Aminoglycosides:* Physical and chemical incompatibility. Give separately.
Colestipol: Decreased concentrations of penicillin G procaine. Give penicillin G procaine 1 hour before or 4 hours after colestipol.
Oral contraceptives: May decrease efficacy of oral contraceptives. Recommend additional form of contraception during penicillin therapy.
Probenecid: Increased blood levels of penicillin. Probenecid may be used for this purpose.

EFFECTS ON LAB TEST RESULTS
• May increase eosinophil count. May decrease hemoglobin and platelet, WBC, and granulocyte counts.

CONTRAINDICATIONS
Contraindicated in patients hypersensitive to drug or other penicillins.

NURSING CONSIDERATIONS
• Use cautiously in patients with other drug allergies, especially to cephalosporins, because of possible cross-sensitivity. Some formulations contain sulfites, which may cause allergic reactions in sensitive persons.

---

*Liquid contains alcohol.   **May contain tartrazine.   †Canada   ‡Australia   §U.K.   ◇OTC

• Before giving drug, ask patient about allergic reactions to penicillin. However, a negative history of penicillin allergy is no guarantee against a future allergic reaction.

• Obtain specimen for culture and sensitivity tests before giving first dose. Therapy may begin pending results.

• Give deep I.M. in upper outer quadrant of buttocks in adults; in midlateral thigh in small children. Rotate injection sites. Don't give S.C. Don't massage injection site. Avoid injection near major nerves or blood vessels to prevent permanent neurovascular damage.

• Penicillin G interferes with turbidimetric methods using sulfosalicylic acid, trichloroacetic acid, acetic acid, and nitric acid. It doesn't interfere with tests using bromphenol blue (Albustix, Albutest, Multistix). Drug alters urine glucose testing using cupric sulfate (Benedict's reagent); use Diastix or Chemstrip uG instead. Penicillin G may falsely elevate results of urine specific gravity tests in patients with low urine output and dehydration and falsely elevate Norymberski and Zimmerman test results for 17-ketogenic steroids. It causes false-positive CSF protein test results (Folin-Ciocalteau method) and may cause positive Coombs' test results. Drug may falsely decrease aminoglycoside levels. Adding beta-lactamase to the sample inactivates the penicillin, rendering the assay more accurate. Or, the sample can be spun down and frozen immediately after collection.

• **Alert:** Treatment for inhalation anthrax (postexposure) must be continued for a total of 60 days. Prescriber should consider the risk-benefit ratio of continuing penicillin longer than 2 weeks, compared to switching to an effective alternate drug.

• **Alert:** Never give by I.V. route. Inadvertent I.V. administration has resulted in death from CNS toxicity.

• Allergic reactions are hard to treat because of drug's slow absorption rate.

• Monitor renal and hematopoietic function periodically.

• If large doses are given or if therapy is prolonged, bacterial or fungal superinfection may occur, especially in elderly, debilitated, or immunosuppressed patients.

• Treatment duration depends on site and cause of infection.

• **Alert:** Don't confuse drug with Polycillin, penicillamine, or the various types of penicillin.

PATIENT TEACHING
• Tell patient to report adverse reactions promptly. A rash is the most common allergic reaction.

• Warn patient that I.M. injection may be painful but that ice applied to the site may help alleviate discomfort.

penicillin G sodium (benzylpenicillin sodium)
Crystapen†

Pregnancy risk category B

AVAILABLE FORMS
Injection: 5 million-unit vial

INDICATIONS & DOSAGES
➤ **Moderate to severe systemic infection—**
Adults and children age 12 and older: 1.2 to 24 million units daily I.M. or I.V. in divided doses q 4 to 6 hours.
Children younger than age 12: 25,000 to 400,000 units/kg daily I.M. or I.V. in divided doses q 4 to 6 hours.
➤ **Neurosyphilis—**
Adults: 18 to 24 million units I.V. daily in divided doses every 4 hours for 10 to 14 days.

I.V. ADMINISTRATION
• Reconstitute drug with sterile water for injection, normal saline solution for injection, or D_5W. Check manufacturer's instructions for volume of diluent necessary to produce desired drug level.

• Give by intermittent I.V. infusion: Dilute drug in 50 to 100 ml, and give over 30 minutes to 2 hours q 4 to 6 hours.

• In neonates and children, give divided doses over 15 to 30 minutes.

ACTION
A natural penicillin that inhibits cell-wall synthesis during active multiplication. Bacteria resist penicillins by producing

penicillinases—enzymes that convert
penicillins to inactive penicillic acid.

Route	Onset	Peak	Duration
I.M.	Unknown	15-30 min	Unknown
I.V.	Immediate	Immediate	Unknown

ADVERSE REACTIONS
CNS: neuropathy, *seizures,* lethargy, hallucinations, anxiety, confusion, agitation, depression, dizziness, fatigue.
CV: *heart failure,* thrombophlebitis.
GI: nausea, vomiting, enterocolitis, pseudomembranous colitis.
GU: interstitial colitis, nephropathy.
Hematologic: hemolytic anemia, *leukopenia, thrombocytopenia, agranulocytosis,* anemia, eosinophilia.
Musculoskeletal: arthralgia.
Other: hypersensitivity reactions, *anaphylaxis,* overgrowth of nonsusceptible organisms, pain at injection site, vein irritation.

INTERACTIONS
Drug-drug. *Aminoglycosides:* Physical and chemical incompatibility. Give separately.
Colestipol: Decreased levels of penicillin G sodium. Give penicillin G sodium 1 hour before or 4 hours after colestipol.
Oral contraceptives: May decrease efficacy of oral contraceptives. Recommend additional form of contraception during penicillin therapy.
Probenecid: Increased blood levels of penicillin. Probenecid may be used for this purpose.

EFFECTS ON LAB TEST RESULTS
• May increase eosinophil count. May decrease hemoglobin and platelet, WBC, and granulocyte counts.

CONTRAINDICATIONS
Contraindicated in patients hypersensitive to drug or other penicillins and in those on sodium-restricted diets.

NURSING CONSIDERATIONS
• Use cautiously in patients with other drug allergies, especially to cephalosporins, because of possible cross-allergenicity.

• Before giving drug, ask patient about allergic reactions to penicillin. However, a negative history of penicillin allergy is no guarantee against a future allergic reaction.
• Obtain specimen for culture and sensitivity tests before giving first dose. Therapy may begin pending results.
• Penicillin G interferes with turbidimetric methods using sulfosalicylic acid, trichloroacetic acid, acetic acid, and nitric acid. It doesn't interfere with tests using bromphenol blue (Albustix, Albutest, Multistix). Drug alters urine glucose testing using cupric sulfate (Benedict's reagent); use Diastix or Chemstrip uG instead. Penicillin G may falsely elevate results of urine specific gravity tests in patients with low urine output and dehydration and falsely elevate Norymberski and Zimmerman test results for 17-ketogenic steroids. It causes false-positive CSF protein test results (Folin-Ciocalteau method) and may cause positive Coombs' test results. Drug may falsely decrease aminoglycoside levels. Adding beta-lactamase to the sample inactivates the penicillin, rendering the assay more accurate. Or, the sample can be spun down and frozen immediately after collection.
• Observe patient closely. With large doses and prolonged therapy, bacterial or fungal superinfection may occur, especially in elderly, debilitated, or immunosuppressed patients.
• *Alert:* Don't confuse drug with Polycillin, penicillamine, or the various types of penicillin.

PATIENT TEACHING
• Tell patient to report adverse reactions promptly.
• Instruct patient to report discomfort at I.V. site.
• Warn patient receiving I.M. injection that the injection may be painful but that ice applied to site may help alleviate discomfort.

---

*Liquid contains alcohol. **May contain tartrazine. †Canada ‡Australia §U.K. ◊OTC

penicillin V potassium (phenoxymethylpenicillin potassium)
Abbocillin VK‡, Apo-Pen-VK†, Beepen-VK, Cilicaine VK‡, Nadopen-V 200†, Nadopen-V 400†, Novo-Pen-VK†, Nu-Pen-VK†, Pen Vee†, Pen Vee K, PVF K†, PVK‡, V-Cillin K, Veetids**

Pregnancy risk category B

AVAILABLE FORMS
Capsules: 250 mg‡
Oral suspension: 125 mg/5 ml, 250 mg/5 ml (after reconstitution)
Tablets: 250 mg, 500 mg
Tablets (film-coated): 250 mg, 500 mg

INDICATIONS & DOSAGES
➤ **Mild to moderate systemic infections—**
Adults and children age 12 and older: 125 to 500 mg or 200,000 to 800,000 units P.O. q 6 hours.
Children younger than age 12: 15 to 62.5 mg/kg or 25,000 to 100,000 units/kg P.O. daily in divided doses q 6 to 8 hours.
➤ **Prevention of recurrent rheumatic fever—**
Adults and children: 250 mg P.O. b.i.d.

ACTION
A natural penicillin that inhibits cell-wall synthesis during microorganism multiplication. Bacteria resist penicillins by producing penicillinases—enzymes that convert penicillins to inactive penicillic acid.

Route	Onset	Peak	Duration
P.O.	Unknown	0.5-1 hr	Unknown

ADVERSE REACTIONS
CNS: neuropathy.
GI: *epigastric distress,* vomiting, diarrhea, *nausea,* black hairy tongue.
GU: nephropathy.
Hematologic: eosinophilia, hemolytic anemia, *leukopenia, thrombocytopenia.*
Other: hypersensitivity reactions, *anaphylaxis,* overgrowth of nonsusceptible organisms.

INTERACTIONS
Drug-drug. *Oral contraceptives:* May decrease efficacy of oral contraceptives. Recommend additional form of contraception during penicillin therapy.
Probenecid: Increased blood levels of penicillin. Probenecid may be used for this purpose.

EFFECTS ON LAB TEST RESULTS
● May increase eosinophil count. May decrease hemoglobin and platelet, WBC, and granulocyte counts.

CONTRAINDICATIONS
Contraindicated in patients hypersensitive to drug or other penicillins.

NURSING CONSIDERATIONS
● Use cautiously in patients with GI disturbances and in those with other drug allergies, especially to cephalosporins, because of possible cross-sensitivity.
● Before giving drug, ask patient about allergic reactions to penicillins. However, a negative history of penicillin allergy is no guarantee against a future allergic reaction.
● Obtain specimen for culture and sensitivity tests before giving first dose. Therapy may begin pending results.
● Periodically assess renal and hematopoietic function in patients receiving long-term therapy.
● If large doses are given or if therapy is prolonged, bacterial or fungal superinfection may occur, especially in elderly, debilitated, or immunosuppressed patients.
● Drug interferes with turbidimetric methods using sulfosalicylic acid, acetic acid, trichloroacetic acid, and nitric acid. It doesn't interfere with tests that use bromphenol blue (Albustix, Albutest, Multistix).
● The American Heart Association considers amoxicillin the preferred drug for endocarditis prophylaxis because GI absorption is better and serum levels are sustained longer. Penicillin V is considered an alternative drug.
● *Alert:* Don't confuse drug with Polycillin, penicillamine, or the various types of penicillin.

Reactions may be *common*, uncommon, *life-threatening*, or COMMON AND LIFE-THREATENING.

PATIENT TEACHING
• Instruct patient to take entire quantity of drug exactly as prescribed, even after he feels better.
• Tell patient to take drug with food if stomach upset occurs.
• Advise patient to notify prescriber if rash, fever, or chills develop. A rash is the most common allergic reaction.

---

piperacillin sodium
Pipracil, Pipril‡

Pregnancy risk category B

AVAILABLE FORMS
Injection: 2 g, 3 g, 4 g, 40 g

INDICATIONS & DOSAGES
➤ **Systemic infections from susceptible strains of gram-positive and especially gram-negative organisms including *Proteus species* and *Pseudomonas aeruginosa*—**
Adults and children older than age 12: 100 to 300 mg/kg I.V. or I.M. daily in divided doses q 4 to 6 hours, not to exceed 24 g daily. Patients with cystic fibrosis may receive up to 600 mg/kg/day.
➤ **Prophylaxis of surgical infections—**
Adults: 2 g I.V., given 30 to 60 minutes before surgery. Dose may be repeated during surgery and once or twice more after surgery.
Adjust-a-dose: For patients with creatinine clearance of 20 to 40 ml/minute, 3 to 4 g I.V. q 8 hours; if creatinine is less than 20 ml/minute, 3 to 4 g I.V. q 12 hours, depending on severity of infection.

I.V. ADMINISTRATION
• For injection, reconstitute each gram of drug with 5 ml of diluent, such as sterile or bacteriostatic water for injection, normal saline solution for injection (with or without preservative), D₅W, or dextrose 5% in normal saline solution for injection. Shake until dissolved. Inject reconstituted solution directly into a vein or into the tubing of a free-flowing I.V. solution over 3 to 5 minutes.
• For intermittent infusion, dilute with at least 50 ml of a compatible I.V. solution,

and give by intermittent infusion over 30 minutes.
• Avoid continuous infusions to prevent vein irritation. Change site every 48 hours.
• Aminoglycoside antibiotics, such as gentamicin and tobramycin, are chemically incompatible with piperacillin. Don't mix in the same I.V. container.

ACTION
Extended-spectrum penicillin that inhibits cell-wall synthesis during microorganism multiplication. Bacteria resist penicillins by producing penicillinases—enzymes that convert penicillins to inactive penicillic acid.

Route	Onset	Peak	Duration
I.M.	Unknown	30-50 min	Unknown
I.V.	Immediate	Immediate	Unknown

ADVERSE REACTIONS
CNS: *seizures,* headache, dizziness, fatigue.
CV: phlebitis.
GI: nausea, diarrhea, pseudomembranous colitis, vomiting.
GU: interstitial nephritis.
Hematologic: *neutropenia,* eosinophilia, *leukopenia, thrombocytopenia, bleeding.*
Metabolic: *hypokalemia,* hypernatremia.
Musculoskeletal: prolonged muscle relaxation.
Other: hypersensitivity reactions, *anaphylaxis,* overgrowth of nonsusceptible organisms, pain at injection site, vein irritation.

INTERACTIONS
Drug-drug. *Oral contraceptives:* May decrease efficacy of oral contraceptives. Recommend additional form of contraception during penicillin therapy.
Probenecid: Increased blood levels of piperacillin. Probenecid may be used for this purpose.
Vecuronium: Prolonged neuromuscular blockade. Don't use together.

EFFECTS ON LAB TEST RESULTS
• May increase ALT, AST, alkaline phosphatase, LDH, and sodium levels. May decrease potassium level.
• May increase eosinophil count. May decrease hemoglobin and platelet, WBC, and granulocyte counts.

CONTRAINDICATIONS
Contraindicated in patients hypersensitive to drug or other penicillins.

NURSING CONSIDERATIONS
• Use cautiously in patients with bleeding tendencies, uremia, hypokalemia, and other drug allergies, especially to cephalosporins, because of possible cross-sensitivity.
• Before giving drug, ask patient about allergic reactions to penicillin. However, a negative history of penicillin allergy is no guarantee against a future allergic reaction.
• Drug may falsely decrease aminoglycoside levels and may cause positive Coombs' tests.
• Obtain specimen for culture and sensitivity tests before giving first dose. Therapy may begin pending results.
• For I.M. injection, reconstitute with sterile or bacteriostatic water for injection, normal saline solution for injection (with or without preservative), or 0.5% to 1% lidocaine hydrochloride. Add 2 ml of diluent for each gram of drug. Final solution will contain 1 g/2.5 ml.
• Check CBC and platelet counts frequently. Drug may cause thrombocytopenia.
• Monitor potassium and sodium levels.
• Monitor INR in patients receiving warfarin therapy because drug may prolong PT.
• If large doses are given or if therapy is prolonged, bacterial or fungal superinfection may occur, especially in elderly, debilitated, or immunosuppressed patients.
• Patients with cystic fibrosis tend to be most susceptible to fever or rash.
• Drug may be better suited for patients on sodium-free diets than ticarcillin (piperacillin contains 1.85 mEq of sodium/g).
• Piperacillin is typically used with another antibiotic such as gentamicin.

PATIENT TEACHING
• Tell patient to report adverse reactions promptly.
• Instruct patient receiving drug I.V. to report discomfort at I.V. site.
• Advise patient to limit salt intake during therapy because drug contains 1.85 mEq of sodium/g.

piperacillin sodium/ tazobactam sodium
Zosyn

Pregnancy risk category B

AVAILABLE FORMS
Powder for injection: 2 g piperacillin and 0.25 g tazobactam per vial, 3 g piperacillin and 0.375 g tazobactam per vial, 4 g piperacillin and 0.5 g tazobactam per vial

INDICATIONS & DOSAGES
➤ **Appendicitis complicated by rupture or abscess and peritonitis caused** *by Escherichia coli, Bacteroides fragilis, B. ovatus, B. thetaiotaomicron,* **or** *B. vulgatus;* **skin and skin-structure infections caused by** *Staphylococcus aureus;* **postpartum endometritis or pelvic inflammatory disease caused by** *E. coli;* **moderately severe community-acquired pneumonia caused by** *Haemophilus influenzae—*
Adults: 3 g piperacillin and 0.375 g tazobactam I.V. q 6 hours.
Adjust-a-dose: For renally impaired adults with creatinine clearance of 20 to 40 ml/minute, dosage is 2 g piperacillin and 0.25 g tazobactam I.V. q 6 hours; if it's below 20 ml/minute, 2 g piperacillin and 0.25 g tazobactam I.V. q 8 hours.
➤ **Moderate to severe nosocomial pneumonia caused by piperacillin-resistant, beta-lactamase–producing strains of** *S. aureus—*
Adults: Initially, 3.375 g I.V. over 30 minutes q 4 hours. Give with an aminoglycoside.

I.V. ADMINISTRATION
• Reconstitute each gram of piperacillin with 5 ml of diluent, such as sterile or bacteriostatic water for injection, normal saline solution for injection, bacteriostatic normal saline solution for injection, D_5W, dextrose 5% in normal saline solution for injection, or dextran 6% in normal saline solution for injection.
• Don't use lactated Ringer's injection. Shake until dissolved. Further dilute to a final volume of 50 ml before infusion.
• Infuse over at least 30 minutes. Discontinue any primary infusion during admin-

---

istration, if possible. Don't mix with other drugs. Aminoglycoside antibiotics, such as amikacin, gentamicin, and tobramycin, are chemically incompatible with this drug. Don't mix in the same I.V. container.

• Use drug immediately after reconstitution. Discard unused drug after 24 hours if stored at room temperature or 48 hours if refrigerated. Once diluted, drug is stable in I.V. bags for 24 hours at room temperature or 1 week if refrigerated.

• Change I.V. site every 48 hours.

ACTION
Piperacillin is an extended-spectrum penicillin that inhibits cell-wall synthesis during microorganism multiplication. Tazobactam increases piperacillin's effectiveness by inactivating beta-lactamases, which destroy penicillins.

Route	Onset	Peak	Duration
I.V.	Immediate	Immediate	Unknown

ADVERSE REACTIONS
CNS: *headache, insomnia,* agitation, dizziness, anxiety, *seizures.*
CV: hypertension, tachycardia, chest pain, edema.
EENT: rhinitis.
GI: *diarrhea, nausea, constipation,* vomiting, dyspepsia, stool changes, abdominal pain.
GU: interstitial nephritis, candidiasis.
Hematologic: *leukopenia,* anemia, eosinophilia, *thrombocytopenia.*
Respiratory: dyspnea.
Skin: rash, pruritus.
Other: fever, pain, *anaphylaxis,* inflammation, phlebitis at I.V. site, hypersensitivity reactions.

INTERACTIONS
Drug-drug. *Oral anticoagulants:* Prolonged effectiveness. Monitor PT and INR closely.
Oral contraceptives: May decrease efficacy of oral contraceptives. Recommend additional form of contraception during penicillin therapy.
Probenecid: Increased levels of piperacillin. Probenecid may be used for this purpose.
Vecuronium: Prolonged neuromuscular blockade. Monitor patient closely.

EFFECTS ON LAB TEST RESULTS
• May increase eosinophil count. May decrease hemoglobin and WBC and platelet counts.

CONTRAINDICATIONS
Contraindicated in patients hypersensitive to drug or other penicillins.

NURSING CONSIDERATIONS
• Use cautiously in patients with bleeding tendencies, uremia, hypokalemia, and other drug allergies, especially to cephalosporins, because of possible cross-sensitivity.
• Obtain specimen for culture and sensitivity tests before giving first dose. Therapy may begin pending results.
• Because hemodialysis removes 6% of the piperacillin dose and 21% of the tazobactam dose, supplemental doses may be needed after hemodialysis.
• As with other penicillins, piperacillin and tazobactam may result in a false-positive reaction for urine glucose using a copper reduction method (such as Clinitest). Glucose tests based on enzymatic glucose oxidase reactions (such as Diastix) are recommended.
• If large doses are given or if therapy is prolonged, bacterial or fungal superinfection may occur, especially in elderly, debilitated, or immunosuppressed patients.
• Drug contains 2.35 mEq sodium/g; monitor patient's sodium intake.
• Patients with cystic fibrosis may have a higher rate of fever and rash. Monitor these patients closely.

PATIENT TEACHING
• Tell patient to report adverse reactions promptly.
• Advise patient to alert nurse if discomfort occurs at I.V. site.

---

ticarcillin disodium
Ticar

Pregnancy risk category B

AVAILABLE FORMS
Injection: 1 g, 3 g, 6 g
I.V. infusion: 3 g

INDICATIONS & DOSAGES

➤ **Severe systemic infections caused by susceptible strains of gram-positive and especially gram-negative organisms, including *Pseudomonas* and *Proteus* species—**
Adults and children older than 1 month: 200 to 300 mg/kg I.V. daily in divided doses q 4 to 6 hours.

➤ **Urinary tract infections—**
Adults and children weighing 40 kg (88 lb) or more: 1 g I.M. or I.V. every 6 hours. For complicated infections, 150 to 200 mg/kg I.V. infusion daily in divided doses every 4 to 6 hours.
Children older than age 1 month weighing less than 40 kg: 50 to 100 mg/kg I.M. or I.V. daily in divided doses every 6 to 8 hours. For complicated infections, 150 to 200 mg/kg I.V. infusion daily in divided doses every 4 to 6 hours.
Adjust-a-dose: For patients with renal failure, if creatinine clearance is 30 to 60 ml/minute, dosage is 2 g I.V. q 4 hours; if clearance is 10 to 29 ml/minute, 2 g I.V. q 8 hours; and if below 10 ml/minute, 2 g I.V. q 12 hours or 1 g I.M. q 6 hours.

I.V. ADMINISTRATION

● For injection, reconstitute drug using D_5W, normal saline solution for injection, sterile water for injection, or other compatible solution. Add 4 ml of diluent for each gram of drug.
● Further dilute to a maximum concentration of 50 mg/ml, and inject slowly directly into a vein or into the tubing of a free-flowing I.V. solution.
● For intermittent infusion, dilute to a concentration of 10 to 100 mg/ml, and give over 30 to 120 minutes in adults or 10 to 20 minutes in neonates.
● Aminoglycoside antibiotics, such as amikacin, gentamicin, and tobramycin, are chemically incompatible with this drug. Don't mix in the same I.V. container.
● Avoid continuous infusion to prevent vein irritation. Change site every 48 hours.

ACTION

An extended-spectrum penicillin that inhibits cell-wall synthesis during microorganism multiplication. Bacteria resist penicillins by producing penicillinases—enzymes that convert penicillins to inactive penicillic acid.

Route	Onset	Peak	Duration
I.M.	Unknown	30-75 min	Unknown
I.V.	Immediate	Immediate	Unknown

ADVERSE REACTIONS

CNS: neuromuscular excitability, *seizures.*
CV: phlebitis.
GI: nausea, diarrhea, vomiting, pseudomembranous colitis.
Hematologic: *leukopenia, neutropenia,* eosinophilia, *thrombocytopenia,* hemolytic anemia.
Metabolic: hypokalemia, hypernatremia.
Other: hypersensitivity reactions, *anaphylaxis,* overgrowth of nonsusceptible organisms, pain at injection site, vein irritation.

INTERACTIONS

Drug-drug. *Lithium:* Altered renal elimination of lithium. Monitor lithium levels closely.
Oral contraceptives: May decrease efficacy of oral contraceptives. Recommend additional form of contraception during penicillin therapy.
Probenecid: Increased blood levels of ticarcillin and other penicillins. Probenecid may be used for this purpose.

EFFECTS ON LAB TEST RESULTS

● May increase ALT, AST, alkaline phosphatase, LDH, and sodium levels. May decrease potassium level.
● May increase eosinophil count. May decrease hemoglobin and platelet, WBC, and granulocyte counts.

CONTRAINDICATIONS

Contraindicated in patients hypersensitive to drug or other penicillins.

NURSING CONSIDERATIONS

● Use cautiously in patients with other drug allergies, especially to cephalosporins, because of possible cross-sensitivity, and in those with impaired renal function, hemorrhagic conditions, hypokalemia, or sodium restrictions. Drug contains 5.2 to 6.5 mEq sodium/g.

Reactions may be *common,* uncommon, *life-threatening,* or COMMON AND LIFE-THREATENING.

• Before giving drug, ask patient about allergic reactions to penicillin. However, a negative history of penicillin allergy is no guarantee against a future allergic reaction.
• Ticarcillin interferes with turbidimetric methods that use sulfosalicylic acid, trichloroacetic acid, acetic acid, or nitric acid. Ticarcillin doesn't interfere with tests using bromphenol blue (Albustix, Albutest, Multistix). Ticarcillin may falsely decrease aminoglycoside concentrations. Systemic effects of ticarcillin may cause positive Coombs' test.
• Obtain specimen for culture and sensitivity tests before giving first dose. Therapy may begin pending results.
• Give ticarcillin at least 1 hour before a bacteriostatic antibiotic.
• For I.M. injection, reconstitute drug using sterile water for injection, normal saline solution for injection, or lidocaine 1% (without epinephrine). Use 2 ml diluent for each gram of drug. Only the 1-g vial should be used for I.M. administration. Give deeply I.M. into large muscle. Don't exceed 2 g per injection.
• Monitor potassium and sodium levels.
• Check CBC and platelet counts frequently. Drug may cause thrombocytopenia.
• Ticarcillin is typically used with another antibiotic such as gentamicin.
• If large doses are given or if therapy is prolonged, bacterial or fungal superinfection may occur, especially in elderly, debilitated, or immunosuppressed patients.
• Monitor INR in patients receiving warfarin therapy because drug may prolong PT.

PATIENT TEACHING
• Tell patient to report adverse reactions promptly.
• Advise patient to report discomfort at I.V. insertion site.

---

ticarcillin disodium/ clavulanate potassium
Timentin

Pregnancy risk category B

AVAILABLE FORMS
Injection: 3 g ticarcillin and 100 mg clavulanic acid in 3.1-g vials
Premixed: 3.1 g/100 ml

INDICATIONS & DOSAGES
➤ **Lower respiratory tract, urinary tract, bone and joint, intra-abdominal, gynecologic, and skin and skin-structure infections and septicemia caused by beta-lactamase–producing strains of bacteria or by ticarcillin-susceptible organisms—**
Adults and children weighing more than 60 kg (132 lb): 3 g ticarcillin and 100 mg clavulanic acid, given by I.V. infusion q 4 to 6 hours.
Children ages 3 months to 16 years weighing less than 60 kg: 200 mg ticarcillin/kg I.V. daily in divided doses q 6 hours. For severe infections, 300 mg ticarcillin/kg I.V. daily in divided doses q 4 hours.
Adjust-a-dose: For renally impaired patients, if creatinine clearance is 30 to 60 ml/minute, dosage is 2 g I.V. q 4 hours; if clearance is 10 to 29 ml/minute, 2 g I.V. q 8 hours; and if clearance is less than 10 ml/minute, 2 g I.V. q 12 hours.

I.V. ADMINISTRATION
• Reconstitute drug with 13 ml of sterile water for injection or normal saline solution for injection. Further dilute to a maximum of 10 to 100 mg/ml (based on ticarcillin component), and give by I.V. infusion over 30 minutes. In fluid-restricted patients, dilute to a maximum of 48 mg/ml if using D_5W, 43 mg/ml if using normal saline solution for injection, or 86 mg/ml if using sterile water for injection.
• Drug is chemically incompatible with aminoglycoside antibiotics (amikacin, gentamicin, tobramycin). Don't mix in the same I.V. container.

ACTION
Ticarcillin is an extended-spectrum penicillin that inhibits cell-wall synthesis during microorganism replication. Clavulanic acid increases ticarcillin's effectiveness by inactivating beta-lactamases, which destroy ticarcillin.

Route	Onset	Peak	Duration
I.V.	Immediate	Immediate	Unknown

ADVERSE REACTIONS
CNS: neuromuscular excitability, headache, *seizures,* giddiness.

CV: phlebitis.
EENT: taste and smell disturbances.
GI: nausea, diarrhea, stomatitis, vomiting, epigastric pain, flatulence, pseudomembranous colitis.
Hematologic: *leukopenia, neutropenia,* eosinophilia, *thrombocytopenia,* hemolytic anemia, anemia.
Metabolic: hypokalemia, hypernatremia.
Other: hypersensitivity reactions, *anaphylaxis,* overgrowth of nonsusceptible organisms, pain at injection site, vein irritation.

EFFECTS ON LAB TEST RESULTS
● May increase ALT, AST, alkaline phosphatase, LDH, and sodium levels. May decrease potassium level.
● May increase eosinophil count. May decrease hemoglobin, and platelet, WBC, and granulocyte counts.

INTERACTIONS
Drug-drug. *Oral contraceptives:* May decrease efficacy of oral contraceptives. Recommend additional form of contraception during penicillin therapy.
Probenecid: Increased blood levels of ticarcillin. Probenecid may be used for this purpose.

CONTRAINDICATIONS
Contraindicated in patients hypersensitive to drug or other penicillins.

NURSING CONSIDERATIONS
● Use cautiously in patients with other drug allergies, especially to cephalosporins, because of possible cross-sensitivity, and in those with impaired renal function, hemorrhagic conditions, hypokalemia, or sodium restrictions. Drug contains 4.5 mEq sodium/g.
● Before giving drug, ask patient about allergic reactions to penicillin. However, a negative history of penicillin allergy is no guarantee against a future allergic reaction.
● Drug interferes with turbidimetric methods that use sulfosalicylic acid, trichloroacetic acid, acetic acid, or nitric acid. Drug doesn't interfere with tests using bromphenol blue (Albustix, Albutest, Multistix). Systemic effects of drug may cause positive Coombs' test.

● Obtain specimen for culture and sensitivity tests before giving first dose. Therapy may begin pending results.
● Give drug at least 1 hour before a bacteriostatic antibiotic.
● Check CBC and platelet counts frequently. Drug may cause thrombocytopenia.
● Monitor potassium and sodium levels.
● If large doses are given or if therapy is prolonged, bacterial or fungal superinfection may occur, especially in elderly, debilitated, or immunosuppressed patients.

PATIENT TEACHING
● Tell patient to report adverse reactions promptly.
● Instruct patient to report discomfort at I.V. site.
● Advise patient to limit salt intake during drug therapy because of high sodium content.

Reactions may be *common,* uncommon, *life-threatening,* or COMMON AND LIFE-THREATENING.

11
Cephalosporins

cefaclor
cefadroxil
cefazolin sodium
cefdinir
cefditoren pivoxil
cefepime hydrochloride
cefixime
cefmetazole sodium
cefonicid sodium
cefoperazone sodium
cefotaxime sodium
cefotetan disodium
cefoxitin sodium
cefpodoxime proxetil
cefprozil
ceftazidime
ceftizoxime sodium
ceftriaxone sodium
cefuroxime axetil
cefuroxime sodium
cephalexin hydrochloride
cephalexin monohydrate
cephradine
loracarbef

COMBINATION PRODUCTS
None.

---

cefaclor
Ceclor, Distaclor§,
Distaclor MR§

Pregnancy risk category B

AVAILABLE FORMS
Capsules: 250 mg, 500 mg
Oral suspension: 125 mg/5 ml, 187 mg/5 ml, 250 mg/5 ml, 375 mg/5 ml
Tablets (extended-release): 375 mg, 500 mg

INDICATIONS & DOSAGES
➤ **Respiratory or urinary tract infections, skin and soft-tissue infections, and otitis media caused** *by Haemophilus influenzae, Streptococcus pneumoniae, S. pyogenes, Escherichia coli, Proteus*

mirabilis, Klebsiella species, **and staphylococci—**
Adults: 250 to 500 mg P.O. q 8 hours. For pharyngitis or otitis media, daily dose may be given in two equally divided doses q 12 hours. For extended-release forms, 500 mg P.O. q 12 hours for 7 days for bronchitis; for pharyngitis or skin and skin-structure infections, 375 mg P.O. q 12 hours for 10 days and 7 to 10 days, respectively.
Children: 20 mg/kg daily P.O. in divided doses q 8 hours. For pharyngitis or otitis media, daily dose may be given in two equally divided doses q 12 hours. In more serious infections, 40 mg/kg daily are recommended, not to exceed 1 g daily.

ACTION
A second-generation cephalosporin that inhibits cell-wall synthesis, promoting osmotic instability; usually bactericidal.

Route	Onset	Peak	Duration
P.O.	Unknown	0.5-1 hr	Unknown
P.O. (extended)	Unknown	1.5-2.5 hr	Unknown

ADVERSE REACTIONS
CNS: dizziness, headache, somnolence, malaise.
GI: *nausea,* vomiting, *diarrhea,* anorexia, dyspepsia, abdominal cramps, pseudomembranous colitis, oral candidiasis.
GU: vaginal candidiasis, vaginitis.
Hematologic: *transient leukopenia,* anemia, eosinophilia, *thrombocytopenia,* lymphocytosis.
Skin: *maculopapular rash,* dermatitis, pruritus.
Other: hypersensitivity reactions, *serum sickness, anaphylaxis,* fever.

INTERACTIONS
Drug-drug. *Aminoglycosides:* Increased risk of nephrotoxicity. Avoid using together.
Antacids: Decreased absorption of extended-release cefaclor if taken with-

---

in 1 hour. Separate administration by 1 hour.

Chloramphenicol: Causes antagonistic effect. Avoid using together.

Probenecid: May inhibit excretion and increase blood levels of cefaclor. Monitor patient.

EFFECTS ON LAB TEST RESULTS
● May increase ALT, AST, alkaline phosphatase, bilirubin, GGT, and LDH levels.
● May decrease eosinophil count. May decrease hemoglobin and WBC and platelet counts.

CONTRAINDICATIONS
Contraindicated in patients hypersensitive to drug or other cephalosporins.

NURSING CONSIDERATIONS
● Use cautiously in patients hypersensitive to penicillin because of the possibility of cross-sensitivity with other beta-lactam antibiotics. Also use cautiously in breast-feeding women and in patients with a history of colitis and renal insufficiency.
● Obtain specimen for culture and sensitivity tests before giving first dose. Therapy may begin pending results.
● If large doses are given, therapy is prolonged, or patient is at high-risk, monitor patient for signs and symptoms of superinfection.
● Cephalosporins may cause false-positive Coombs' test results and false-positive results in urine glucose tests using cupric sulfate (Benedict's reagent or Clinitest); use glucose oxidase tests (Diastix or Chemstrip uG) instead. Drug also falsely elevates serum or urine creatinine levels in tests using Jaffe reaction.
● Store reconstituted suspension in refrigerator. Suspension is stable for 14 days if refrigerated. Shake well before use.
● *Alert:* Don't confuse drug with other cephalosporins that sound alike.

PATIENT TEACHING
● Tell patient to take entire amount of drug exactly as prescribed, even after he feels better.
● Tell patient that drug may be taken with meals. If suspension is used, instruct him to shake container well before measuring dose and to keep the drug refrigerated.

● Advise patient to notify prescriber if rash develops or signs and symptoms of superinfection appear.
● Inform patient not to crush, cut, or chew extended-release tablets.

---

cefadroxil
Duricef

Pregnancy risk category B

AVAILABLE FORMS
Capsules: 500 mg
Oral suspension: 125 mg/5 ml, 250 mg/5 ml, 500 mg/5 ml
Tablets: 1 g

INDICATIONS & DOSAGES
➤ **Urinary tract infections caused by** *Escherichia coli*, *Proteus mirabilis*, **and** *Klebsiella species*; **skin and soft-tissue infections caused by staphylococci and streptococci; pharyngitis or tonsillitis caused by group A beta-hemolytic streptococci—**
Adults: 1 to 2 g P.O. daily, depending on infection being treated. Usually given once daily or b.i.d.
Children: 30 mg/kg P.O. daily in two divided doses q 12 hours.
Adjust-a-dose: For renally impaired patients with creatinine clearance of 25 to 50 ml/minute, 1 g P.O. then 500 mg q 12 hours. If clearance is between 10 and 24 ml/minute, give 500 mg q 24 hours; if clearance is less than 10 ml/minute, give 500 mg q 36 hours.

ACTION
A first-generation cephalosporin that inhibits cell-wall synthesis, promoting osmotic instability; usually bactericidal.

Route	Onset	Peak	Duration
P.O.	Unknown	1-2 hr	Unknown

ADVERSE REACTIONS
CNS: *seizures,* dizziness, headache.
GI: pseudomembranous colitis, *nausea,* vomiting, *diarrhea,* glossitis, abdominal cramps, oral candidiasis.
GU: genital pruritus, candidiasis, vaginitis, renal dysfunction.

Reactions may be *common*, uncommon, *life-threatening*, or COMMON AND LIFE-THREATENING.

Hematologic: *transient neutropenia,* eosinophilia, *leukopenia,* anemia, *agranulocytosis, thrombocytopenia.*
Respiratory: dyspnea.
Skin: *maculopapular and erythematous rashes,* urticaria.
Other: hypersensitivity reactions, *anaphylaxis, angioedema,* fever.

INTERACTIONS
Drug-drug. *Aminoglycosides:* Increased risk of nephrotoxicity. Avoid using together.
Probenecid: May inhibit excretion and increase blood levels of cefadroxil. Use together cautiously.

EFFECTS ON LAB TEST RESULTS
● May increase ALT, AST, alkaline phosphatase, bilirubin, GGT, and LDH levels.
● May increase eosinophil count. May decrease hemoglobin and neutrophil, WBC, granulocyte, and platelet counts.

CONTRAINDICATIONS
Contraindicated in patients hypersensitive to drug or other cephalosporins.

NURSING CONSIDERATIONS
● Use cautiously in patients with a history of sensitivity to penicillin and in breast-feeding women. Also use cautiously in patients with impaired renal function; dosage adjustments may be necessary.
● Obtain specimen for culture and sensitivity tests before giving first dose. Therapy may begin pending results.
● If creatinine clearance is below 50 ml/minute, dosage interval should be lengthened so drug doesn't accumulate. Monitor renal function in patients with renal dysfunction.
● Cephalosporins may cause false-positive Coombs' test results and false-positive results in urine glucose tests using cupric sulfate (Benedict's reagent or Clinitest); use glucose oxidase tests (Diastix or Chemstrip uG) instead. Drug also falsely elevates serum or urine creatinine levels in tests using Jaffe reaction.
● If large doses are given, therapy is prolonged, or patient is high-risk, monitor patient for superinfection.
● **Alert:** Don't confuse drug with other cephalosporins that sound alike.

PATIENT TEACHING
● Instruct patient to take drug with food or milk to lessen GI discomfort.
● Tell patient to take entire amount of drug exactly as prescribed, even after he feels better.
● Advise patient to notify prescriber if rash develops or if signs and symptoms of superinfection, such as recurring fever, chills, and malaise, appear.

---

cefazolin sodium
Ancef, Kefzol, Zolicef

Pregnancy risk category B

AVAILABLE FORMS
Infusion: 500 mg/50-ml vial, 1 g/50-ml vial
Injection (parenteral): 250 mg, 500 mg, 1 g, 5 g, 10 g, 20 g

INDICATIONS & DOSAGES
➤ **Perioperative prophylaxis in contaminated surgery—**
Adults: 1 g I.M. or I.V. 30 to 60 minutes before surgery; then 0.5 to 1 g I.M. or I.V. q 6 to 8 hours for 24 hours. In operations lasting longer than 2 hours, another 0.5- to 1-g dose I.M. or I.V. may be given intraoperatively. Prophylaxis may be continued for 3 to 5 days if life-threatening infection is likely.
➤ **Serious infections of respiratory, biliary, and GU tracts; skin, soft-tissue, bone, and joint infections; septicemia; endocarditis caused by** *Escherichia coli,* **Enterobacteriaceae, gonococci,** *Haemophilus influenzae,* **Klebsiella species,** *Proteus mirabilis,* **Staphylococcus aureus,** *Streptococcus pneumoniae,* **and group A beta-hemolytic streptococci—**
Adults: 250 mg I.M. or I.V. q 8 hours to 1.5 g I.M. or I.V. q 6 hours. Maximum 12 g/day in life-threatening situations.
Children older than age 1 month: 25 to 50 mg/kg/day I.M. or I.V. in three or four divided doses. In severe infections, dose may be increased to 100 mg/kg/day.
Adjust-a-dose: For patients with renal failure whose creatinine clearance is 35 to 54 ml/minute, give full dose q 8 hours; if clearance is 11 to 34 ml/minute, give 50% usual dose q 12 hours; if clearance is be-

low 10 ml/minute, give 50% of usual dose q 18 to 24 hours.

I.V. ADMINISTRATION

● Reconstitute drug with sterile water, bacteriostatic water, or normal saline solution as follows: 2 ml to 500-mg vial or 2.5 ml to 1-g vial. Shake well until dissolved. Resulting concentration: 225 mg/ml or 330 mg/ml, respectively.

● Reconstituted cefazolin is stable for 24 hours at room temperature or 96 hours under refrigeration.

● For direct injection, further dilute Ancef with 5 ml, or Kefzol with 10 ml, of sterile water for injection. Inject into a large vein or into the tubing of a free-flowing I.V. solution over 3 to 5 minutes. For intermittent infusion, add reconstituted drug to 50 to 100 ml of compatible solution or use premixed solution. Commercially available frozen solutions of cefazolin in D_5W should be given only by intermittent or continuous I.V. infusion.

● Alternate injection sites if I.V. therapy lasts longer than 3 days. Use of small I.V. needles in larger available veins may be preferable.

ACTION

A first-generation cephalosporin that inhibits cell-wall synthesis, promoting osmotic instability; usually bactericidal.

Route	Onset	Peak	Duration
I.M.	Unknown	1-2 hr	Unknown
I.V.	Immediate	Immediate	Unknown

ADVERSE REACTIONS

CNS: confusion, *seizures.*
CV: *phlebitis, thrombophlebitis with I.V. injection.*
GI: pseudomembranous colitis, nausea, anorexia, vomiting, *diarrhea,* glossitis, dyspepsia, abdominal cramps, anal pruritus, oral candidiasis.
GU: genital pruritus, candidiasis, vaginitis.
Hematologic: *neutropenia, leukopenia,* eosinophilia, *thrombocytopenia.*
Skin: *maculopapular and erythematous rashes, urticaria, pruritus, pain, induration, sterile abscesses, tissue sloughing at injection site,* **Stevens-Johnson syndrome.**

Other: hypersensitivity reactions, *serum sickness, anaphylaxis,* drug fever.

INTERACTIONS

Drug-drug. *Aminoglycosides:* Increased risk of nephrotoxicity. Avoid using together.
Probenecid: May inhibit excretion and increase blood levels of cefazolin. Use together cautiously.

EFFECTS ON LAB TEST RESULTS

● May increase ALT, AST, alkaline phosphatase, bilirubin, GGT, and LDH levels.
● May increase eosinophil count. May decrease neutrophil, WBC, and platelet counts.

CONTRAINDICATIONS

Contraindicated in patients hypersensitive to drug or other cephalosporins.

NURSING CONSIDERATIONS

● Use cautiously in patients hypersensitive to penicillin because of the possibility of cross-sensitivity with other beta-lactam antibiotics. Also use cautiously in breast-feeding women and in patients with a history of colitis and renal insufficiency.

● Obtain specimen for culture and sensitivity tests before giving first dose. Therapy may begin pending results.

● Dose and dosing interval will be adjusted if creatinine clearance is below 55 ml/minute.

● After reconstitution, inject drug I.M. without further dilution. This drug isn't as painful as other cephalosporins. Give injection deeply into a large muscle, such as the gluteus maximus or lateral aspect of the thigh.

● If large doses are given, therapy is prolonged, or patient is at high risk, monitor patient for signs and symptoms of superinfection.

● Cephalosporins may cause false-positive Coombs' test results and false-positive results in urine glucose tests using cupric sulfate (Benedict's reagent or Clinitest); use glucose oxidase tests (Diastix or Chemstrip uG) instead. Drug also falsely elevates serum or urine creatinine levels in tests using Jaffe reaction.

Reactions may be *common,* uncommon, *life-threatening,* or **COMMON AND LIFE-THREATENING.**

• *Alert:* Don't confuse drug with other cephalosporins that sound alike.

PATIENT TEACHING
• Instruct patient to report adverse reactions promptly.
• Tell patient to report discomfort at I.V. injection site.

cefdinir
Omnicef

Pregnancy risk category B

AVAILABLE FORMS
Capsules: 300 mg
Suspension: 125 mg/5 ml

INDICATIONS & DOSAGES
➤ **Mild to moderate infections caused by susceptible strains of microorganisms for conditions of community-acquired pneumonia, acute exacerbations of chronic bronchitis, acute maxillary sinusitis, acute bacterial otitis media, and uncomplicated skin and skin-structure infections—**
Adults and children age 13 and older: 300 mg P.O. q 12 hours for 5 to 10 days; or 600 mg P.O. q 24 hours, for 10 days. Give q 12 hours for pneumonia and skin infections.
Children ages 6 months to 12 years: 7 mg/kg P.O. q 12 hours or 14 mg/kg P.O. q 24 hours, for 10 days, up to maximum dose of 600 mg daily. Give q 12 hours for skin infections.
➤ **Pharyngitis, tonsillitis—**
Adults and children age 13 and older: 300 mg P.O. q 12 hours for 5 to 10 days; or 600 mg P.O. q 24 hours, for 10 days.
Children ages 6 months to 12 years: 7 mg/kg P.O. q 12 hours for 5 to 10 days; or 14 mg/kg P.O. q 24 hours, for 10 days.
Adjust-a-dose: If creatinine clearance is below 30 ml/minute, reduce dosage to 300 mg P.O. once daily for adults and 7 mg/kg up to 300 mg P.O. once daily for children. In patients receiving long-term hemodialysis, dosage is 300 mg or 7 mg/kg P.O. at end of each dialysis session and subsequently every other day.

ACTION
A third-generation cephalosporin whose bactericidal activity results from inhibition of cell-wall synthesis. Drug is stable in the presence of some beta-lactamase enzymes, causing some microorganisms resistant to penicillins and cephalosporins to be susceptible to cefdinir. Excluding *Pseudomonas, Enterobacter, Enterococcus,* and methicillin-resistant *Staphylococcus* species, cefdinir's spectrum of activity includes a broad range of gram-positive and gram-negative aerobic microorganisms.

Route	Onset	Peak	Duration
P.O.	Unknown	2-4 hr	Unknown

ADVERSE REACTIONS
CNS: headache.
GI: abdominal pain, *diarrhea,* nausea, vomiting, pseudomembranous colitis.
GU: vaginal candidiasis, vaginitis, increased urine proteins and RBCs.
Skin: rash, cutaneous candidiasis.

INTERACTIONS
Drug-drug. *Aminoglycosides:* Increased risk of nephrotoxicity. Avoid using together.
Antacids containing aluminum and magnesium, iron supplements, multivitamins containing iron: Decreased cefdinir rate of absorption and bioavailability. Give such preparations 2 hours before or after cefdinir.
Probenecid: Inhibited renal excretion of cefdinir. Monitor patient.

EFFECTS ON LAB TEST RESULTS
• May increase GGT and alkaline phosphatase levels.

CONTRAINDICATIONS
Contraindicated in patients hypersensitive to drug or other cephalosporins.

NURSING CONSIDERATIONS
• Use cautiously in patients hypersensitive to penicillin because of the possibility of cross-sensitivity with other beta-lactam antibiotics. Also use with caution in patients with history of colitis and renal insufficiency.

• Prolonged drug treatment may result in emergence and overgrowth of resistant organisms. Monitor patient for signs and symptoms of superinfection.

• Pseudomembranous colitis has been reported with cefdinir and should be considered in patients with diarrhea after antibiotic therapy and in those with history of colitis.

• Cephalosporins may cause false-positive Coombs' test results and false-positive results in urine glucose tests using cupric sulfate (Benedict's reagent or Clinitest); use glucose oxidase tests (Diastix or Chemstrip uG) instead. Drug also falsely elevates serum or urine creatinine levels in tests using Jaffe reaction.

• **Alert:** Don't confuse drug with other cephalosporins that sound alike.

PATIENT TEACHING

• Instruct patient to take antacids and iron supplements 2 hours before or after a dose of cefdinir.

• Inform diabetic patient that each teaspoon of suspension contains 2.86 g of sucrose.

• Tell patient that drug may be taken without regard to meals.

• Advise patient to report severe diarrhea or diarrhea accompanied by abdominal pain.

• Tell patient to report adverse reactions or signs and symptoms of superinfection promptly.

✳ *NEW DRUG*

---

cefditoren pivoxil
Spectracef

Pregnancy risk category B

AVAILABLE FORMS
Tablets: 200 mg

INDICATIONS & DOSAGES

➤ **Acute bacterial exacerbation of chronic bronchitis caused by *Haemophilus influenzae, H. parainfluenzae, Streptococcus pneumoniae, Moraxella catarrhalis*—**
Adults and adolescents age 12 and older: 400 mg P.O. b.i.d. with meals for 10 days.

➤ **Pharyngitis or tonsillitis caused by *S. pyogenes*—**
Adults and adolescents age 12 and older: 200 mg P.O. b.i.d. with meals for 10 days.

➤ **Uncomplicated skin and skin structure infections caused by *S. pyogenes*—**
Adults and adolescents age 12 and older: 200 mg P.O. b.i.d. with meals for 10 days.
Adjust-a-dose: For patients with moderate renal impairment (creatinine clearance 30 to 49 ml/min), don't give more than 200 mg b.i.d. For patients with severe renal impairment (clearance less than 30 ml/min), give 200 mg daily.

ACTION

Bactericidal antibiotic that acts by adhering to bacterial penicillin-binding proteins, thereby inhibiting cell-wall synthesis. Cefditoren is active against many gram-positive and gram-negative organisms, including *Staphylococcus aureus* (methicillin-susceptible strains, including beta-lactamase–producing strains), *S. pneumoniae* (penicillin-susceptible strains only), *S. pyogenes, H. influenzae* (including beta-lactamase–producing strains), *H. parainfluenzae* (including beta-lactamase–producing strains), and *M. catarrhalis* (including beta-lactamase–producing strains).

Route	Onset	Peak	Duration
P.O.	Unknown	1.5-3 hr	Unknown

ADVERSE REACTIONS
CNS: headache.
GI: abdominal pain, dyspepsia, *diarrhea*, nausea, vomiting.
GU: vaginal candidiasis, hematuria, increased WBC count in urine.
Metabolic: hyperglycemia.

INTERACTIONS
Drug-drug. *H₂-receptor antagonists, magnesium and aluminum antacids:* Reduced cefditoren absorption. Avoid using together.
Probenecid: Increased cefditoren levels. Avoid using together.
Drug-food. *Moderate- or high-fat meal:* Increased cefditoren bioavailability. Advise patient to take drug with meals.

EFFECTS ON LAB TEST RESULTS
- May decrease glucose level.
- May decrease hematocrit.

CONTRAINDICATIONS
Contraindicated in patients hypersensitive to drug or other cephalosporins. Also contraindicated in patients with carnitine deficiency or inborn errors of metabolism that may result in clinically significant carnitine deficiency. Because cefditoren tablets contain sodium caseinate, a milk protein, they shouldn't be given to patients hypersensitive to milk protein (as distinct from those with lactose intolerance).

NURSING CONSIDERATIONS
- Cephalosporins appear in breast milk and should be used cautiously in breast-feeding women. Safe use hasn't been established.
- Use cautiously in patients with impaired renal function or penicillin allergy.
- Give drug with a fatty meal to increase its bioavailability.
- If patient develops diarrhea after receiving cefditoren, keep in mind that this drug may cause pseudomembranous colitis.
- Don't use this drug if patient needs prolonged treatment.
- Monitor patient for overgrowth of resistant organisms.
- Cefditoren may cause a false-positive direct Coombs' test result. It also produces a false-positive reaction for glucose in the urine in copper reduction tests (using Benedict's or Fehling's solution or Clinitest tablets).
- Patients with renal or hepatic impairment, in poor nutritional state, receiving a protracted course of antibiotics, or previously stabilized on anticoagulants may be at risk for decreased prothrombin activity. Monitor PT in these patients.

PATIENT TEACHING
- Instruct patient to take medication exactly as prescribed.
- Tell patient to take drug with food to increase its absorption.
- Caution patient not to take drug with an H_2 antagonist or an antacid because they may reduce cefditoren absorption.
- Instruct patient not to stop drug before completing treatment and to immediately

call prescriber if he experiences any unpleasant adverse reactions.
- Instruct patient to contact prescriber if signs and symptoms of infection don't improve after several days of therapy.
- Inform patient of potential adverse reactions.
- Urge patient not to miss any doses. However, if he does, tell him to take the missed dose as soon as possible unless it's within 4 hours of the next scheduled dose. In that case, tell him to skip the missed dose and go back to the regular dosing schedule. Tell him not to double the dose.

---

cefepime hydrochloride
Maxipime

Pregnancy risk category B

AVAILABLE FORMS
Injection: 500 mg/vial, 1 g/100-ml piggyback bottle, 1 g/ADD-Vantage vial, 1 g/15-ml vial, 2 g/100-ml piggyback bottle, 2 g/vial

INDICATIONS & DOSAGES
➤ **Mild to moderate urinary tract infections caused by** *Escherichia coli,* *Klebsiella pneumoniae,* **or** *Proteus mirabilis,* **including concurrent bacteremia with these microorganisms—**
Adults and children age 12 and older: 0.5 to 1 g I.M. or I.V. infused over 30 minutes q 12 hours for 7 to 10 days. I.M. route used only for *E. coli* infections.
➤ **Severe urinary tract infections, including pyelonephritis, caused by** *E. coli* **or** *K. pneumoniae—*
Adults and children age 12 and older: 2 g I.V. infused over 30 minutes q 12 hours for 10 days.
➤ **Moderate to severe pneumonia caused by** *Streptococcus pneumoniae,* *Pseudomonas aeruginosa,* *K. pneumoniae,* **or** *Enterobacter* **species—**
Adults and children age 12 and older: 1 to 2 g I.V. infused over 30 minutes q 12 hours for 10 days.
➤ **Moderate to severe skin infections, uncomplicated skin infections, and skin-structure infections caused by**

S. pyogenes or methicillin-susceptible strains of *Staphylococcus aureus*—
Adults and children age 12 and older: 2 g I.V. infused over 30 minutes q 12 hours for 10 days.

➤ **Complicated intra-abdominal infections caused by *E. coli*, viridans group *streptococci*, P. aeruginosa, *K. pneumoniae*, Enterobacter species, or B. fragilis**—
Adults: 2 g I.V. infused over 30 minutes q 12 hours for 7 to 10 days. Use with metronidazole.

➤ **Empiric therapy for febrile neutropenia**—
Adults: 2 g I.V. q 8 hours for 7 days or until neutropenia resolves.

➤ **Uncomplicated and complicated urinary tract infections (including pyelonephritis), uncomplicated skin and skin-structure infections, pneumonia; as empiric therapy for febrile neutropenic children**—
Children ages 2 months to 16 years, weighing up to 40 kg (88 lb): 50 mg/kg/dose I.V. infused over 30 minutes q 12 hours, or q 8 hours for febrile neutropenia, for 7 to 10 days. Don't exceed 2 g/dose.

Adjust-a-dose: For renally impaired patients with creatinine clearance of 30 to 60 ml/minute, give full dose q 24 hours; if clearance is 11 to 29 ml/minute, give 50% usual dose q 24 hours; and if clearance is less than 11 ml/minute, give 25% of usual dose q 24 hours.

I.V. ADMINISTRATION
● Follow manufacturer's guidelines closely when reconstituting drug. Variations occur in reconstituting drug for administration, depending on concentration of drug ordered and how drug is packaged (piggyback vial, ADD-Vantage vial, or regular vial).
● The type of diluent used for reconstitution varies, depending on the product used. Use only solutions recommended by the manufacturer. The resulting solution should be given over about 30 minutes.
● Intermittent I.V. infusion with a Y-type administration set can be accomplished with compatible solutions. However, during infusion of a solution containing cefepime, discontinuing the other solution is recommended.

ACTION
A fourth-generation cephalosporin that inhibits bacterial cell-wall synthesis, promotes osmotic instability, and destroys bacteria.

Route	Onset	Peak	Duration
I.M., I.V.	0.5 hr	1-2 hr	Unknown

ADVERSE REACTIONS
CNS: headache.
CV: phlebitis.
GI: colitis, diarrhea, nausea, vomiting, oral candidiasis.
GU: vaginitis.
Skin: rash, pruritus, urticaria.
Other: pain, inflammation, fever, hypersensitivity reactions, *anaphylaxis.*

INTERACTIONS
Drug-drug. *Aminoglycosides:* May increase risk of nephrotoxicity. Monitor renal function closely.
Potent diuretics: May increase risk of nephrotoxicity. Monitor renal function closely.
Probenecid: Inhibited renal excretion of cefepime. Monitor patient.

EFFECTS ON LAB TEST RESULTS
None reported.

CONTRAINDICATIONS
Contraindicated in patients hypersensitive to drug, cephalosporins, beta-lactam antibiotics, or penicillins.

NURSING CONSIDERATIONS
● Use cautiously in patients hypersensitive to penicillin because of possibility of cross-sensitivity with other beta-lactam antibiotics. Also use cautiously in breast-feeding women and in patients with history of colitis and renal insufficiency.
● Safety of drug in children younger than age 12 hasn't been established.
● Obtain culture and sensitivity tests before giving first dose, if appropriate. Therapy may begin pending results.
● Dosage adjustment is necessary in patients with impaired renal function. Monitor renal function.
● For I.M. administration, reconstitute drug using sterile water for injection, nor-

mal saline solution for injection, D₅W injection, 0.5% or 1% lidocaine hydrochloride, or bacteriostatic water for injection with parabens or benzyl alcohol. Follow manufacturer's guidelines for quantity of diluent to use.

• Inspect solution for particulate matter before use. The powder and its solutions tend to darken, depending on storage conditions. Product potency isn't adversely affected when stored as recommended.

• Monitor patient for superinfection. Drug may cause overgrowth of nonsusceptible bacteria or fungi.

• Drug may reduce PT activity. Patients at risk include those with renal or hepatic impairment or poor nutrition and those receiving prolonged cefepime therapy. Monitor PT and INR in these patients, as ordered. Give exogenous vitamin K, as indicated.

• Cephalosporins may cause false-positive Coombs' test results and false-positive results in urine glucose tests using cupric sulfate (Benedict's reagent or Clinitest); use glucose oxidase tests (Diastix or Chemstrip uG) instead. Drug also falsely elevates serum or urine creatinine levels in tests using Jaffe reaction.

• *Alert:* Don't confuse drug with other cephalosporins that sound alike.

PATIENT TEACHING
• Warn patient receiving drug I.M. that pain may occur at injection site.
• Instruct patient to report signs and symptoms of superinfection or GI disturbance.

---

cefixime
Suprax

Pregnancy risk category B

AVAILABLE FORMS
Oral suspension: 100 mg/5 ml (after reconstitution)
Tablets: 200 mg, 400 mg

INDICATIONS & DOSAGES
➤ **Uncomplicated urinary tract infections caused by** *Escherichia coli* **and** *Proteus mirabilis*; **otitis media caused by** *Haemophilus influenzae* **(beta-**

lactamase–positive and –negative strains), *Moraxella catarrhalis,* **and** *Streptococcus pyogenes*; **pharyngitis and tonsillitis caused by** *S. pyogenes*; **acute bronchitis and acute exacerbations of chronic bronchitis caused by** *S. pneumoniae* **and** *H. influenzae,* **beta-lactamase–positive and –negative strains—**
Adults and children older than age 12, or weighing more than 50 kg (110 lb):
400 mg/day P.O. as a single 400-mg tablet or 200 mg q 12 hours.
Children age 12 and younger, or weighing 50 kg or less: 8 mg/kg/day suspension P.O. as a single daily dose or 4 mg/kg q 12 hours.
➤ **Uncomplicated gonorrhea caused by** *Neisseria gonorrhoeae*—
Adults: 400 mg P.O. as a single dose.
Adjust-a-dose: For patients with renal failure, if creatinine clearance is 20 to 60 ml/minute or patient undergoes hemodialysis, give 75% of dose at usual intervals; if clearance is less than 20 ml/minute, give 50% of usual dose at usual intervals.

ACTION
A third-generation cephalosporin that inhibits cell-wall synthesis, promoting osmotic instability; usually bactericidal.

Route	Onset	Peak	Duration
P.O.	Unknown	3.1-4.4 hr	Unknown

ADVERSE REACTIONS
CNS: headache, dizziness.
GI: *diarrhea,* loose stools, abdominal pain, nausea, vomiting, dyspepsia, flatulence, pseudomembranous colitis.
GU: genital pruritus, vaginitis, genital candidiasis.
Hematologic: *thrombocytopenia, leukopenia,* eosinophilia.
Skin: pruritus, rash, urticaria, *erythema multiforme, Stevens-Johnson syndrome.*
Other: drug fever, hypersensitivity reactions, *serum sickness, anaphylaxis.*

INTERACTIONS
Drug-drug. *Aminoglycosides:* Increased risk of nephrotoxicity. Avoid using together.

Carbamazepine: Elevated carbamazepine levels. Avoid using together.
Probenecid: May inhibit excretion and increase blood levels of cefixime. Use together cautiously.

EFFECTS ON LAB TEST RESULTS
• May increase BUN, creatinine, ALT, AST, alkaline phosphatase, bilirubin, GGT, and LDH levels.
• May increase eosinophil count. May decrease platelet and WBC counts.

CONTRAINDICATIONS
Contraindicated in patients hypersensitive to drug or other cephalosporins.

NURSING CONSIDERATIONS
• *Alert:* Use cautiously and reduce dosage in patients with renal dysfunction. Monitor renal function.
• Use cautiously in patients hypersensitive to penicillin because of possibility of cross-sensitivity with other beta-lactam antibiotics. Also use with caution in patients with history of colitis and in breast-feeding women.
• Obtain specimen for culture and sensitivity testing before giving first dose. Therapy may begin pending results.
• To prepare oral suspension, add required amount of water to powder in two portions. Shake well after each addition. After mixing, suspension is stable for 14 days. No need to refrigerate, but keep tightly closed. Shake well before use.
• If large doses are given, therapy is prolonged, or patient is high-risk, monitor patient for superinfection.
• Cephalosporins may cause false-positive Coombs' test results and false-positive results in urine glucose tests using cupric sulfate (Benedict's reagent or Clinitest); use glucose oxidase tests (Diastix or Chemstrip uG) instead. Drug also falsely elevates serum or urine creatinine levels in tests using Jaffe reaction.
• *Alert:* Don't confuse drug with other cephalosporins that sound alike.

PATIENT TEACHING
• Tell patient to take all of the drug prescribed, even after he feels better.
• Instruct patient using oral suspension to shake container before measuring dose.

Tell him that suspension doesn't need to be refrigerated.
• Advise patient to notify prescriber if rash or signs and symptoms of superinfection develop.

---

cefmetazole sodium
Zefazone

Pregnancy risk category B

AVAILABLE FORMS
Injection: 1-g vial, 2-g vial, 1 g/50 ml, 2 g/50 ml premixed solution

INDICATIONS & DOSAGES
➤ **Lower respiratory tract infections caused by *Streptococcus pneumoniae*, *Staphylococcus aureus* (penicillinase- and non–penicillinase-producing strains), *Escherichia coli*, and *Haemophilus influenzae* (non–penicillinase-producing strains); intra-abdominal infections caused by *E. coli* or *Bacteroides fragilis*; skin and skin-structure infections caused by *S. aureus* (penicillinase- and non–penicillinase-producing strains), *S. epidermidis*, *Streptococcus pyogenes*, *S. agalactiae*, *E. coli*, *Proteus mirabilis*, *Klebsiella pneumoniae*, and *B. fragilis*; urinary tract infections caused by *E. coli*—**
Adults: 2 g I.V. q 6 to 12 hours for 5 to 14 days.
➤ **Prophylaxis in patients undergoing vaginal hysterectomy—**
Adults: 2 g I.V. 30 to 90 minutes before surgery as a single dose; or 1 g I.V. 30 to 90 minutes before surgery, repeated in 8 and 16 hours.
➤ **Prophylaxis in patients undergoing abdominal hysterectomy—**
Adults: 1 g I.V. 30 to 90 minutes before surgery, repeated in 8 and 16 hours.
➤ **Prophylaxis in patients undergoing cesarean section—**
Adults: 2 g I.V. as a single dose after clamping cord; or 1 g I.V. after clamping cord, repeated in 8 and 16 hours.
➤ **Prophylaxis in patients undergoing colorectal surgery—**
Adults: 2 g I.V. as a single dose 30 to 90 minutes before surgery. May follow with additional 2-g doses in 8 and 16 hours.

Reactions may be *common*, uncommon, *life-threatening*, or COMMON AND LIFE-THREATENING.

➤ **Prophylaxis in high-risk patients undergoing cholecystectomy—**
Adults: 1 g I.V. 30 to 90 minutes before surgery, repeated in 8 and 16 hours.
Adjust-a-dose: For renally impaired patients, if creatinine clearance is 50 to 90 ml/minute, give 1 to 2 g q 12 hours; if clearance is 30 to 49 ml/minute, give 1 to 2 g q 16 hours; if clearance is 10 to 29 ml/minute, give 1 to 2 g q 24 hours; if clearance is less than 10 ml/minute, give 1 to 2 g q 48 hours given after hemodialysis.

I.V. ADMINISTRATION
● Reconstitute drug with bacteriostatic water for injection, sterile water for injection, or normal saline solution for injection.
● After reconstitution, drug may be further diluted to concentrations ranging from 1 to 20 mg/ml by adding it to normal saline solution for injection, D_5W, or lactated Ringer's injection.
● Reconstituted or dilute solutions are stable for 24 hours at room temperature (77° F [25° C]) or 1 week if refrigerated at 46° F (8° C).

ACTION
A semisynthetic cephamycin antibiotic pharmacologically similar to second-generation cephalosporins that inhibit cell-wall synthesis, promoting osmotic instability; usually bactericidal.

Route	Onset	Peak	Duration
I.V.	Unknown	Immediate	Unknown

ADVERSE REACTIONS
CNS: headache, dizziness.
CV: *shock,* hypotension, phlebitis, thrombophlebitis.
EENT: epistaxis, altered color perception.
GI: nausea, vomiting, *diarrhea,* epigastric pain, pseudomembranous colitis, candidiasis, bleeding.
GU: vaginitis, hot flashes.
Musculoskeletal: joint pain and inflammation.
Respiratory: pleural effusion, dyspnea, respiratory distress.
Skin: rash, pruritus, generalized erythema.
Other: fever, bacterial or fungal superinfection, hypersensitivity reactions, *serum sickness, anaphylaxis,* pain at injection site.

INTERACTIONS
Drug-drug. *Aminoglycosides:* Increased risk of nephrotoxicity. Avoid using together.
Probenecid: May inhibit excretion and increase blood levels of cefmetazole. May use together for this effect.
Drug-lifestyle. *Alcohol use:* May cause disulfiram-like reaction. Tell patient to avoid alcohol for 24 hours before and after administration of cefmetazole.

EFFECTS ON LAB TEST RESULTS
● May increase ALT, AST, alkaline phosphatase, bilirubin, GGT, and LDH levels.

CONTRAINDICATIONS
Contraindicated in patients hypersensitive to drug or other cephalosporins.

NURSING CONSIDERATIONS
● Use cautiously in patients hypersensitive to penicillin because of possibility of cross-sensitivity with other beta-lactam antibiotics. Also use cautiously in breast-feeding women and in patients with history of colitis and renal insufficiency.
● Obtain specimen for culture and sensitivity tests before giving first dose. Therapy may begin pending results.
● Monitor patient for signs or symptoms of bacterial and fungal superinfections. Prolonged use may result in overgrowth of nonsusceptible organisms.
● Monitor INR in patients at risk from renal or hepatic impairment, malnutrition, or prolonged therapy. Although the drug's chemical structure has the methylthiotetrazole side chain that may cause bleeding disorders, such bleeding hasn't been reported with this drug.
● Monitor renal function.
● Cephalosporins may cause false-positive Coombs' test results and false-positive results in urine glucose tests using cupric sulfate (Benedict's reagent or Clinitest); use glucose oxidase tests (Diastix or Chemstrip uG) instead. Drug also falsely elevates serum or urine creatinine levels in tests using Jaffe reaction.
● *Alert:* Don't confuse drug with other cephalosporins that sound alike.

---

*Liquid contains alcohol.   **May contain tartrazine.   †Canada   ‡Australia   §U.K.   ◇OTC

PATIENT TEACHING
● Tell patient to report adverse reactions promptly.
● Instruct patient to report any discomfort at I.V. insertion site.

---

cefonicid sodium
Monocid

Pregnancy risk category B

AVAILABLE FORMS
Infusion: 1 g/100 ml
Injection: 1 g

INDICATIONS & DOSAGES
➤ **Perioperative prophylaxis in contaminated surgery—**
Adults: 1 g I.M. or I.V. 30 to 60 minutes before surgery; then 1 g I.M. or I.V. daily for 2 days after surgery. If used for prophylaxis in cesarean section, 1 g I.M. or I.V. after umbilical cord is clamped.
➤ **Serious infections of the lower respiratory and urinary tracts; skin and skin-structure infections; septicemia; bone and joint infections; preoperative prophylaxis. Susceptible microorganisms include *Streptococcus pneumoniae, Klebsiella pneumoniae, Escherichia coli, Haemophilus influenzae, Proteus mirabilis, Staphylococcus aureus, S. epidermidis,* and *Streptococcus pyogenes*—**
Adults: Usual dosage is 1 g I.V. or I.M. q 24 hours; in life-threatening infections, 2 g q 24 hours.
Adjust-a-dose: For renally impaired patients, if creatinine clearance is 60 to 79 ml/minute, give 10 to 25 mg/kg q 24 hours; if clearance is 40 to 59 ml/minute, give 8 to 20 mg/kg q 24 hours; if clearance is 20 to 39 ml/minute, give 4 to 15 mg/kg q 24 hours; if clearance is 10 to 19 ml/minute, give 4 to 15 mg/kg q 48 hours; if clearance is 5 to 9 ml/minute, give 4 to 15 mg/kg q 3 to 5 days; if clearance is below 5 ml/minute, give 3 to 4 mg/kg q 3 to 5 days.

I.V. ADMINISTRATION
● Reconstitute drug in 1-g vial with 2.5 ml of sterile water for injection (yields a concentration of 325 mg/ml). Shake well. Reconstitute drug in piggyback vials with 50 to 100 ml of sterile water for injection, bacteriostatic water for injection, or normal saline solution.
● Infuse over 20 to 30 minutes.

ACTION
A second-generation cephalosporin that inhibits cell-wall synthesis, promoting osmotic instability; usually bactericidal.

Route	Onset	Peak	Duration
I.M.	Unknown	1-2 hr	Unknown
I.V.	Immediate	Immediate	Unknown

ADVERSE REACTIONS
CNS: dizziness, headache, malaise, paresthesia.
CV: *phlebitis, thrombophlebitis.*
GI: pseudomembranous colitis, diarrhea.
GU: *acute renal failure,* interstitial nephritis.
Hematologic: *neutropenia, leukopenia,* eosinophilia, anemia, thrombocytosis, *thrombocytopenia,* prolonged PT and INR.
Musculoskeletal: myalgia.
Skin: *maculopapular and erythematous rashes, urticaria, pain, induration, sterile abscesses, tissue sloughing at injection site.*
Other: hypersensitivity reactions, *serum sickness, anaphylaxis,* fever.

INTERACTIONS
Drug-drug. *Aminoglycosides:* Increased risk of nephrotoxicity. Avoid using together.
Probenecid: May inhibit excretion and increase blood levels of cefonicid. Use together cautiously.

EFFECTS ON LAB TEST RESULTS
● May increase ALT, AST, alkaline phosphatase, bilirubin, GGT, and LDH levels.
● May increase PT and INR and eosinophil counts. May decrease neutrophil and WBC counts and hemoglobin. May increase or decrease platelet count.

CONTRAINDICATIONS
Contraindicated in patients hypersensitive to drug or other cephalosporins.

Reactions may be *common*, uncommon, **life-threatening**, or COMMON AND LIFE-THREATENING.

NURSING CONSIDERATIONS
• Use cautiously in patients hypersensitive to penicillin because of possibility of cross-sensitivity with other beta-lactam antibiotics. Also use cautiously in breast-feeding women and in patients with history of colitis and renal insufficiency.
• Obtain specimen for culture and sensitivity tests before giving first dose. Therapy may begin pending results.
• Dosing interval will be adjusted for patients with renal impairment.
• When giving 2-g I.M. doses once daily, divide the dose equally and inject deeply into large muscle, such as the gluteus maximus or the lateral aspect of the thigh. Rotate injection sites.
• If large doses are given or if therapy is prolonged, monitor patient for superinfection, especially in high-risk patients.
• Although the drug's chemical structure has the methylthiotetrazole side chain that may cause bleeding disorders, such bleeding hasn't been reported with this drug. Monitor PT and INR and watch for signs of bleeding.
• Cephalosporins may cause false-positive Coombs' test results and false-positive results in urine glucose tests using cupric sulfate (Benedict's reagent or Clinitest); use glucose oxidase tests (Diastix or Chemstrip uG) instead. Drug also falsely elevates serum or urine creatinine levels in tests using Jaffe reaction.
• *Alert:* Don't confuse drug with other cephalosporins that sound alike.

PATIENT TEACHING
• Tell patient to report adverse reactions or signs and symptoms of superinfection promptly.
• Instruct patient to report discomfort at I.V. insertion site.

---

cefoperazone sodium
Cefobid

Pregnancy risk category B

AVAILABLE FORMS
Infusion: 1 g, 2 g piggyback
Parenteral: 1-g, 2-g vials; 1 g, 2 g premixed

INDICATIONS & DOSAGES
➤ Serious infections of the respiratory tract; intra-abdominal, gynecologic, and skin infections; bacteremia; septicemia caused by susceptible microorganisms (*Streptococcus pneumoniae* and *S. pyogenes*; *Staphylococcus aureus* [penicillinase- and non–penicillinase-producing] and *S. epidermidis*; enterococci; *Escherichia coli*; *Haemophilus influenzae*; *Enterobacter, Citrobacter, Klebsiella,* and *Proteus* species; some *Pseudomonas species,* including *P. aeruginosa*; and *Bacteroides fragilis*)—
Adults: Usual dosage is 1 to 2 g q 12 hours I.M. or I.V. In severe infections or in infections caused by less sensitive organisms, total daily dose or frequency may be increased to 16 g/day.
Adjust-a-dose: For patients with hepatic or biliary obstruction, total daily dose shouldn't exceed 4 g/day. For patients with hepatic and substantial renal impairment, total daily dose shouldn't exceed 2 g/day.

I.V. ADMINISTRATION
• Reconstitute drug in 1- or 2-g vial with a minimum of 2.8 ml of compatible I.V. solution; manufacturer recommends using 5 ml/g.
• Give by direct injection into a large vein or into tubing of a free-flowing I.V. solution over 3 to 5 minutes.
• When giving by intermittent infusion, add reconstituted drug to 20 to 40 ml of a compatible I.V. solution and infuse over 15 to 30 minutes.

ACTION
A third-generation cephalosporin that inhibits cell-wall synthesis, promoting osmotic instability; usually bactericidal.

Route	Onset	Peak	Duration
I.M.	Unknown	1-2 hr	Unknown
I.V.	Immediate	Immediate	Unknown

ADVERSE REACTIONS
CV: *phlebitis, thrombophlebitis.*
GI: pseudomembranous colitis, nausea, vomiting, *diarrhea.*
Hematologic: *transient neutropenia, eosinophilia,* anemia, hypoprothrombinemia, bleeding.

---

*Liquid contains alcohol. **May contain tartrazine. †Canada ‡Australia §U.K. ◇OTC

Skin: *maculopapular and erythematous rashes, urticaria, pain, induration, sterile abscesses, temperature elevation, tissue sloughing at I.M. injection site.*
Other: hypersensitivity reactions, ***serum sickness, anaphylaxis,*** fever.

INTERACTIONS
Drug-drug. *Aminoglycosides:* Increased risk of nephrotoxicity. Monitor renal function.
Probenecid: May inhibit excretion and increase blood levels of cefoperazone. Use together cautiously.
Drug-lifestyle. *Alcohol use:* May cause disulfiram-like reaction. Warn patient not to drink alcohol for several days after discontinuing cefoperazone.

EFFECTS ON LAB TEST RESULTS
• May increase ALT, AST, alkaline phosphatase, bilirubin, GGT, and LDH levels.
• May increase INR and eosinophil count. May decrease hemoglobin and neutrophil count. May increase or decrease PT.

CONTRAINDICATIONS
Contraindicated in patients hypersensitive to drug or other cephalosporins.

NURSING CONSIDERATIONS
• Use cautiously in patients hypersensitive to penicillin because of possibility of cross-sensitivity with other beta-lactam antibiotics. Also use cautiously in breastfeeding women and in patients with history of colitis and renal insufficiency.
• Give doses of 4 g/day cautiously to patients with hepatic disease or biliary obstruction. Higher dosages require monitoring of serum levels.
• Periodically monitor liver and renal function and compare to baseline.
• Obtain specimen for culture and sensitivity tests before giving first dose. Therapy may begin pending results.
• To prepare drug for I.M. injection, follow these steps: Using the 1-g vial, dissolve drug with 2 ml of sterile water for injection; then add 0.6 ml of 2% lidocaine hydrochloride for a final concentration of 333 mg/ml. Or, dissolve drug with 2.8 ml of sterile water for injection; then add 1 ml of 2% lidocaine hydrochloride for a final concentration of 250 mg/ml. When

using the 2-g vial, dissolve drug with 3.8 ml of sterile water for injection; then add 1.2 ml of 2% lidocaine hydrochloride for final concentration of 333 mg/ml. Or, dissolve drug with 5.4 ml of sterile water for injection; then add 1.8 ml of 2% lidocaine hydrochloride for a final concentration of 250 mg/ml.
• For I.M. administration, inject deeply into a large muscle, such as the gluteus maximus or the lateral aspect of the thigh.
• If large doses are given, therapy is prolonged, or patient is at high risk, monitor patient for signs or symptoms of superinfection.
• Monitor PT and INR regularly. The drug's chemical structure has the methylthiotetrazole side chain that may cause bleeding disorders. Vitamin K promptly reverses bleeding if it occurs.
• Cephalosporins may cause false-positive Coombs' test results and false-positive results in urine glucose tests using cupric sulfate (Benedict's reagent or Clinitest); use glucose oxidase tests (Diastix or Chemstrip uG) instead. Drug also falsely elevates serum or urine creatinine levels in tests using Jaffe reaction.
• *Alert:* Don't confuse drug with other cephalosporins that sound alike.

PATIENT TEACHING
• Tell patient to report adverse reactions and signs and symptoms of superinfection promptly.
• Instruct patient to report discomfort at I.V. insertion site.

---

cefotaxime sodium
Claforan

Pregnancy risk category B

AVAILABLE FORMS
Infusion: 1-g, 2-g premixed package
Injection: 500-mg, 1-g, 2-g vials, 10-g bottle

INDICATIONS & DOSAGES
➤ **Perioperative prophylaxis in contaminated surgery—**
Adults: 1 g I.M. or I.V. 30 to 60 minutes before surgery. Patients undergoing bowel surgery should receive preoperative me-

chanical bowel cleansing and a nonabsorbable anti-infective drug such as neomycin. Patients undergoing cesarean section should receive 1 g I.M. or I.V. as soon as the umbilical cord is clamped; then 1 g I.M. or I.V. 6 and 12 hours later.

➤ **Uncomplicated gonorrhea caused by penicillinase-producing strains of *Neisseria gonorrhoeae* or non–penicillinase-producing strains of the organism—**
Adults and adolescents: 500 mg I.M. as a single dose.

➤ **Serious infections of the lower respiratory and urinary tracts, CNS, skin, bone, and joints; gynecologic and intra-abdominal infections; bacteremia; septicemia caused by susceptible microorganisms, such as *streptococci* (including *Streptococcus pneumoniae* and *S. pyogenes*), *Staphylococcus aureus* (penicillinase- and non–penicillinase-producing) and S. epidermidis, *Escherichia coli*, *Klebsiella*, *Haemophilus influenzae*, *Serratia marcescens*, and species of *Pseudomonas* (including P. aeruginosa), *Enterobacter*, *Proteus*, and *Peptostreptococcus*—**
Adults and children weighing 50 kg (110 lb) or more: Usual dose is 1 g I.V. or I.M. q 6 to 8 hours. Up to 12 g daily can be given in life-threatening infections.
Children ages 1 month to 12 years weighing less than 50 kg: 50 to 180 mg/kg/day I.M. or I.V. in four to six divided doses.
Neonates ages 1 to 4 weeks: 50 mg/kg I.V. q 8 hours.
Neonates to age 1 week: 50 mg/kg I.V. q 12 hours.
Adjust-a-dose: For patients with renal failure, if creatinine clearance is below 20 ml/minute, give half usual dose at usual interval.

I.V. ADMINISTRATION
● For direct injection, reconstitute drug in 500-mg, 1-g, or 2-g vials with 10 ml of sterile water for injection. Solutions containing 1 g/14 ml are isotonic. Inject drug into a large vein or into the tubing of a free-flowing I.V. solution over 3 to 5 minutes.
● For I.V. infusion, reconstitute drug in infusion vials with 50 to 100 ml of D_5W or normal saline solution. Infuse drug over

20 to 30 minutes. Interrupt flow of primary I.V. solution during infusion.

ACTION
A third-generation cephalosporin that inhibits cell-wall synthesis, promoting osmotic instability; usually bactericidal.

Route	Onset	Peak	Duration
I.M.	Unknown	30 min	Unknown
I.V.	Immediate	Immediate	Unknown

ADVERSE REACTIONS
CNS: headache, dizziness.
CV: *phlebitis, thrombophlebitis.*
GI: pseudomembranous colitis, nausea, vomiting, *diarrhea.*
GU: vaginitis, candidiasis, interstitial nephritis.
Hematologic: *transient neutropenia,* eosinophilia, hemolytic anemia, *thrombocytopenia, agranulocytosis.*
Skin: maculopapular and erythematous rashes, urticaria, pain, induration, sterile abscesses, temperature elevation, tissue sloughing at I.M. injection site.
Other: hypersensitivity reactions, *serum sickness, anaphylaxis,* fever.

INTERACTIONS
Drug-drug. *Aminoglycosides:* May increase risk of nephrotoxicity. Monitor patient closely.
Probenecid: May inhibit excretion and increase blood levels of cefotaxime. Use together cautiously.

EFFECTS ON LAB TEST RESULTS
● May increase ALT, AST, alkaline phosphatase, bilirubin, GGT, and LDH levels.
● May increase eosinophil count. May decrease hemoglobin and neutrophil, platelet, and granulocyte counts.

CONTRAINDICATIONS
Contraindicated in patients hypersensitive to drug or other cephalosporins.

NURSING CONSIDERATIONS
● Use cautiously in patients hypersensitive to penicillin because of possibility of cross-sensitivity with other beta-lactam antibiotics. Also use cautiously in breast-feeding women and in patients with history of colitis and renal insufficiency.

---

*Liquid contains alcohol.   **May contain tartrazine.   †Canada   ‡Australia   §U.K.   ◇OTC

• Obtain specimen for culture and sensitivity tests before giving first dose. Therapy may begin pending results.
• For I.M. administration, inject deeply into a large muscle, such as the gluteus maximus or the lateral aspect of the thigh.
• For I.M. doses of 2 g, divide the dose and give at different sites.
• Cefotaxime may cause positive Coombs' test results.
• If large doses are given, therapy is prolonged, or patient is at high risk, monitor patient for superinfection.
• **Alert:** Don't confuse drug with other cephalosporins that sound alike.

PATIENT TEACHING
• Tell patient to report adverse reactions and signs and symptoms of superinfection promptly.
• Instruct patient to report discomfort at I.V. insertion site.

cefotetan disodium
Cefotan

Pregnancy risk category B

AVAILABLE FORMS
Infusion: 1 g, 2 g piggyback and premixed
Injection: 1 g, 2 g, 10 g

INDICATIONS & DOSAGES
➤ Serious urinary tract and lower respiratory tract infections and gynecologic, skin and skin-structure, intra-abdominal, and bone and joint infections caused by susceptible streptococci, *Staphylococcus aureus* (penicillinase- and non–penicillinase-producing) and *S. epidermidis, Escherichia coli, Haemophilus influenzae, Neisseria gonorrhoeae,* and species of *Proteus, Klebsiella, Enterobacter,* and *Bacteroides,* including *B. fragilis*—
Adults: 1 to 2 g I.V. or I.M. q 12 hours for 5 to 10 days. Up to 6 g daily in life-threatening infections.
➤ Perioperative prophylaxis—
Adults: 1 to 2 g I.V. given once 30 to 60 minutes before surgery. In cesarean section, dose should be given as soon as umbilical cord is clamped.

Adjust-a-dose: For patients with renal failure, if creatinine clearance is 10 to 30 ml/minute, give usual dose q 24 hours; if clearance is less than 10 ml/minute, give usual dose q 48 hours.

I.V. ADMINISTRATION
• Reconstitute drug with sterile water for injection. Drug may then be mixed with 50 to 100 ml of D$_5$W or normal saline solution. Interrupt flow of primary I.V. solution during cefotetan infusion.
• Infuse over 20 to 60 minutes.

ACTION
A second-generation cephalosporin that inhibits cell-wall synthesis, promoting osmotic instability; usually bactericidal.

Route	Onset	Peak	Duration
I.M.	Unknown	1.5-3 hr	Unknown
I.V.	Immediate	Immediate	Unknown

ADVERSE REACTIONS
CV: *phlebitis, thrombophlebitis.*
GI: pseudomembranous colitis, nausea, *diarrhea.*
GU: *nephrotoxicity.*
Hematologic: *transient neutropenia,* eosinophilia, hemolytic anemia, hypoprothrombinemia, bleeding, thrombocytosis, *agranulocytosis, thrombocytopenia.*
Skin: *maculopapular and erythematous rashes, urticaria, pain, induration, sterile abscesses, tissue sloughing at injection site.*
Other: hypersensitivity reactions, *serum sickness, anaphylaxis,* fever.

INTERACTIONS
Drug-drug. *Aminoglycosides:* May cause synergistic effect and increased risk of nephrotoxicity. Use together cautiously.
Probenecid: May inhibit excretion and increase blood levels of cefotetan. May use together for this effect.
Drug-lifestyle. *Alcohol use:* May cause disulfiram-like reaction. Tell patient to avoid alcohol for several days after discontinuing cefotetan.

EFFECTS ON LAB TEST RESULTS
• May increase ALT, AST, alkaline phosphatase, bilirubin, and LDH levels.

Reactions may be *common,* uncommon, *life-threatening,* or COMMON AND LIFE-THREATENING.

• May increase PT and INR and eosin-ophil count. May decrease hemoglobin and neutrophil and granulocyte counts. May increase or decrease platelet count.

CONTRAINDICATIONS
Contraindicated in patients hypersensi-tive to drug or other cephalosporins.

NURSING CONSIDERATIONS
• Use cautiously in patients hypersensitive to penicillin because of possibility of cross-sensitivity with other beta-lactam antibiotics. Also use cautiously in breast-feeding women and in patients with history of colitis and renal insufficiency.
• Obtain specimen for culture and sensitivity tests before giving first dose. Therapy may begin pending results.
• Reconstitute for I.M. injection with sterile water or bacteriostatic water for injection, normal saline solution for injection, or 0.5% or 1% lidocaine hydrochloride. Shake to dissolve and let stand until clear.
• Give I.M. injection deep into the body of a large muscle.
• Reconstituted solution is stable for 24 hours at room temperature or 96 hours refrigerated.
• If large doses are given, therapy is prolonged, or patient is at high risk, monitor patient for signs and symptoms of super-infection.
• Although the drug's chemical structure has the methylthiotetrazole side chain that may cause bleeding disorders, such bleeding hasn't been reported with this drug. Monitor PT and INR.
• Cephalosporins may cause false-positive Coombs' test results and false-positive results in urine glucose tests using cupric sulfate (Benedict's reagent or Clinitest); use glucose oxidase tests (Diastix or Chemstrip uG) instead. Drug also falsely elevates serum or urine creatinine levels in tests using Jaffe reaction.
• *Alert:* Don't confuse drug with other cephalosporins that sound alike.

PATIENT TEACHING
• Tell patient to report adverse reactions and signs and symptoms of superinfection promptly.
• Instruct patient to report discomfort at I.V. site.

• Tell patient to notify prescriber about loose stools or diarrhea.

cefoxitin sodium
Mefoxin

Pregnancy risk category B

AVAILABLE FORMS
Infusion: 1 g, 2 g in 50-ml or 100-ml container
Injection: 1 g, 2 g, 10 g

INDICATIONS & DOSAGES
➤ **Serious infections of respiratory and GU tracts; skin, soft-tissue, bone, and joint infections; bloodstream and intra-abdominal infections caused by suscep-tible organisms (such as *Escherichia coli* and other coliform bacteria, *Staphy-lococcus aureus* [penicillinase- and non–penicillinase-producing] and S. epidermidis, *streptococci*, *Klebsiella*, *Haemophilus influenzae*, and Bac-teroides, including *B. fragilis*); perioper-ative prophylaxis—**
Adults: 1 to 2 g I.V. or I.M. q 6 to 8 hours for uncomplicated infections. Up to 12 g daily in life-threatening infections.
Children older than age 3 months: 80 to 160 mg/kg daily I.V. or I.M., given in four to six equally divided doses. Maximum daily dose is 12 g.
➤ **Uncomplicated gonorrhea—**
Adults: 2 g I.M. with 1 g probenecid P.O. as a single dose.
➤ **Prophylaxis in surgery—**
Adults: 2 g I.M. or I.V. 30 to 60 minutes before surgery, then 2 g I.M. or I.V. q 6 hours for up to 24 hours.
Children age 3 months and older: 30 to 40 mg/kg I.M. or I.V. 30 to 60 minutes before surgery, then 30 to 40 mg/kg q 6 hours for up to 24 hours.
Adjust-a-dose: For patients with renal failure, if creatinine clearance is 30 to 50 ml/minute, give 1 to 2 g q 8 to 12 hours; if clearance is 10 to 29 ml/minute, give 1 to 2 g q 12 to 24 hours; and if clearance is less than 10 ml/minute, give 500 mg q 24 to 48 hours.

I.V. ADMINISTRATION
● Reconstitute 1 g with at least 10 ml of sterile water for injection and 2 g with 10 to 20 ml of sterile water for injection. Solutions of D_5W and normal saline solution for injection can also be used.
● For direct injection, inject drug into a large vein or into the tubing of a free-flowing I.V. solution over 3 to 5 minutes. For intermittent infusion, add reconstituted drug to 50 or 100 ml of D_5W or dextrose 10% in water or normal saline solution for injection. Interrupt flow of primary I.V. solution during infusion.
● Assess I.V. site frequently. Such use has been linked to development of thrombophlebitis.

ACTION
A second-generation cephalosporin that inhibits cell-wall synthesis, promoting osmotic instability; usually bactericidal.

Route	Onset	Peak	Duration
I.M.	Unknown	20-30 min	Unknown
I.V.	Immediate	Immediate	Unknown

ADVERSE REACTIONS
CV: hypotension, *phlebitis, thrombophlebitis.*
GI: pseudomembranous colitis, nausea, vomiting, *diarrhea.*
GU: *acute renal failure.*
Hematologic: *transient neutropenia,* eosinophilia, hemolytic anemia, anemia, *thrombocytopenia.*
Respiratory: dyspnea.
Skin: *maculopapular and erythematous rashes, urticaria,* exfoliative dermatitis, *pain, induration, sterile abscesses, tissue sloughing at injection site.*
Other: hypersensitivity reactions, *serum sickness, anaphylaxis,* fever.

INTERACTIONS
Drug-drug. *Aminoglycosides:* May increase risk of nephrotoxicity. Monitor patient closely.
Probenecid: May inhibit excretion and increase blood levels of cefoxitin. Sometimes used for this effect.

EFFECTS ON LAB TEST RESULTS
● May increase ALT, AST, alkaline phosphatase, bilirubin, and LDH levels.

● May increase eosinophil count. May decrease hemoglobin and neutrophil and platelet counts.

CONTRAINDICATIONS
Contraindicated in patients hypersensitive to drug or other cephalosporins.

NURSING CONSIDERATIONS
● Use cautiously in patients hypersensitive to penicillin because of possibility of cross-sensitivity with other beta-lactam antibiotics. Also use cautiously in breast-feeding women and in patients with history of colitis and renal insufficiency.
● Obtain specimen for culture and sensitivity tests before giving first dose. Therapy may begin pending results.
● *Alert:* Mefoxin in Galaxy containers is for I.V. use only.
● For I.M. use, reconstitute each 1 g of drug with 2 ml of sterile water for injection or 0.5% or 1% lidocaine hydrochloride (without epinephrine) to minimize pain. Inject deeply into a large muscle, such as the gluteus maximus or the lateral aspect of the thigh.
● Cephalosporins may cause false-positive Coombs' test results and false-positive results in urine glucose tests using cupric sulfate (Benedict's reagent or Clinitest); use glucose oxidase tests (Diastix or Chemstrip uG) instead. Drug also falsely elevates serum or urine creatinine levels in tests using Jaffe reaction.
● After reconstitution, store for 24 hours at room temperature or 1 week under refrigeration.
● If large doses are given, therapy is prolonged, or patient is at high risk, monitor patient for signs and symptoms of superinfection.
● *Alert:* Don't confuse drug with other cephalosporins that sound alike.

PATIENT TEACHING
● Tell patient to report adverse reactions and signs and symptoms of superinfection promptly.
● Instruct patient to report discomfort at I.V. site.
● Advise patient to notify prescriber about loose stools or diarrhea.

Reactions may be *common,* uncommon, ***life-threatening,*** or COMMON AND LIFE-THREATENING.

cefpodoxime proxetil
Vantin

Pregnancy risk category B

AVAILABLE FORMS
Oral suspension: 50 mg/5 ml, 100 mg/ 5 ml in 100-ml bottles
Tablets (film-coated): 100 mg, 200 mg

INDICATIONS & DOSAGES
➤ **Acute, community-acquired pneumonia caused by strains of *Haemophilus influenzae* or *Streptococcus pneumoniae* that don't produce beta-lactamase—**
Adults and children age 13 and older: 200 mg P.O. q 12 hours for 14 days.
➤ **Acute bacterial exacerbation of chronic bronchitis caused by *S. pneumoniae* or *H. influenzae* (strains that don't produce beta-lactamase only), or *Moraxella catarrhalis*—**
Adults and children age 13 and older: 200 mg P.O. q 12 hours for 10 days.
➤ **Uncomplicated gonorrhea in men and women; rectal gonococcal infections in women—**
Adults and children age 13 and older: 200 mg P.O. as a single dose. Follow with doxycycline 100 mg P.O. b.i.d. for 7 days.
➤ **Uncomplicated skin and skin-structure infections caused by *Staphylococcus aureus* or *S. pyogenes*—**
Adults and children age 13 and older: 400 mg P.O. q 12 hours for 7 to 14 days.
➤ **Acute otitis media caused by *S. pneumoniae*, *H. influenzae*, or *M. catarrhalis*—**
Children age 6 months and older: 5 mg/kg P.O. q 12 hours or 10 mg/kg P.O. daily for 10 days. Don't exceed 200 mg/ dose.
➤ **Pharyngitis or tonsillitis caused by *S. pyogenes*—**
Adults: 100 mg P.O. q 12 hours for 5 to 10 days.
Children age 6 months and older: 5 mg/kg P.O. q 12 hours for 10 days. Don't exceed 100 mg/dose.
➤ **Uncomplicated urinary tract infections caused by *Escherichia coli*, *Kleb-*** *siella pneumoniae*, *Proteus mirabilis*, or *S. saprophyticus*—
Adults: 100 mg P.O. q 12 hours for 7 days.
➤ **Mild to moderate acute maxillary sinusitis caused by *H. influenzae*, *S. pneumoniae*, or *M. catarrhalis*—**
Adults and adolescents age 12 and older: 200 mg P.O. q 12 hours for 10 days.
Children ages 2 months to 11 years: 5 mg/ kg P.O. q 12 hours for 10 days; maximum is 200 mg/dose.
Adjust-a-dose: For patients with renal failure, if creatinine clearance is below 30 ml/minute, dosage interval should be increased to q 24 hours. Dialysis patients should receive drug three times weekly after dialysis.

ACTION
A third-generation cephalosporin that inhibits cell-wall synthesis, promoting osmotic instability; usually bactericidal.

Route	Onset	Peak	Duration
P.O.	Unknown	2-3 hr	Unknown

ADVERSE REACTIONS
CNS: headache.
GI: *diarrhea*, nausea, vomiting, abdominal pain, pseudomembranous colitis.
GU: vaginal fungal infections.
Skin: rash.
Other: hypersensitivity reactions, *anaphylaxis*.

INTERACTIONS
Drug-drug. *Aminoglycosides:* Increased risk of nephrotoxicity. Monitor patient closely.
Antacids, H_2-receptor antagonists: Decreased absorption of cefpodoxime. Avoid using together.
Probenecid: Decreased excretion of cefpodoxime. Monitor patient for toxicity.
Drug-food. *Any food:* Increased absorption. Give drug with food.

EFFECTS ON LAB TEST RESULTS
None reported.

CONTRAINDICATIONS
Contraindicated in patients hypersensitive to drug or other cephalosporins.

---

*Liquid contains alcohol.   **May contain tartrazine.   †Canada   ‡Australia   §U.K.   ◇OTC

NURSING CONSIDERATIONS
• Use cautiously in patients with a history of penicillin hypersensitivity because of risk of cross-sensitivity and in patients receiving nephrotoxic drugs because other cephalosporins have been shown to have nephrotoxic potential. Because drug appears in breast milk, use cautiously in breast-feeding women.
• Monitor renal function and compare with baseline.
• Obtain specimen for culture and sensitivity tests before giving first dose. Therapy may begin pending results.
• Give drug with food to enhance absorption. Shake suspension well before using.
• Store suspension in the refrigerator (36° to 46° F [2° to 8° C]). Discard unused portion after 14 days.
• Monitor patient for superinfection. Drug may cause overgrowth of nonsusceptible bacteria or fungi.
• Cephalosporins may cause false-positive Coombs' test results and false-positive results in urine glucose tests using cupric sulfate (Benedict's reagent or Clinitest); use glucose oxidase tests (Diastix or Chemstrip uG) instead. Drug also falsely elevates serum or urine creatinine levels in tests using Jaffe reaction.
• **Alert:** Don't confuse drug with other cephalosporins that sound alike.

PATIENT TEACHING
• Tell patient to take all of the drug as prescribed, even after he feels better.
• Instruct patient to take drug with food. If patient is using suspension, tell him to shake container before measuring dose and to keep container refrigerated.
• Tell patient to call prescriber if rash or signs and symptoms of superinfection occur.
• Instruct patient to notify prescriber about loose stools or diarrhea.

---

cefprozil
Cefzil

Pregnancy risk category B

AVAILABLE FORMS
Oral suspension: 125 mg/5 ml, 250 mg/5 ml
Tablets: 250 mg, 500 mg

INDICATIONS & DOSAGES
➤ **Pharyngitis or tonsillitis caused by** *Streptococcus pyogenes*—
Adults and children age 13 and older: 500 mg P.O. daily for at least 10 days.
➤ **Otitis media caused by** *S. pneumoniae, Haemophilus influenzae,* **and** *Moraxella catarrhalis*—
Infants and children ages 6 months to 12 years: 15 mg/kg P.O. q 12 hours for 10 days.
➤ **Secondary bacterial infections of acute bronchitis and acute bacterial exacerbation of chronic bronchitis caused by** *S. pneumoniae, H. influenzae,* **and** *M. catarrhalis*—
Adults and children age 13 and older: 500 mg P.O. q 12 hours for 10 days.
➤ **Uncomplicated skin and skin-structure infections caused by** *Staphylococcus aureus* **and** *S. pyogenes*—
Adults and children age 13 and older: 250 or 500 mg P.O. q 12 hours or 500 mg daily for 10 days.
➤ **Acute sinusitis caused by** *S. pneumoniae, H. influenzae* **(beta-lactamase–positive and –negative strains), and** *M. catarrhalis* **(including beta-lactamase–producing strains)**—
Adults and children age 13 and older: 250 mg P.O. q 12 hours for 10 days; for moderate to severe infection, 500 mg P.O. q 12 hours for 10 days.
Children ages 6 months to 12 years: 7.5 mg/kg P.O. q 12 hours for 10 days; for moderate to severe infections, 15 mg/kg P.O. q 12 hours for 10 days.
Adjust-a-dose: For renally impaired patients, if creatinine clearance is less than 30 ml/minute, give 50% of usual dose. Give after hemodialysis treatment is completed; drug is removed by hemodialysis.

ACTION
A second-generation cephalosporin that interferes with cell-wall synthesis during microorganism replication, leading to osmotic instability and cell lysis (bactericidal).

Route	Onset	Peak	Duration
P.O.	Unknown	1.5 hr	Unknown

ADVERSE REACTIONS
CNS: dizziness, hyperactivity, headache, nervousness, insomnia, confusion, somnolence.
GI: diarrhea, nausea, vomiting, abdominal pain.
GU: genital pruritus, vaginitis.
Hematologic: eosinophilia.
Skin: rash, urticaria, diaper rash.
Other: superinfection, hypersensitivity reactions, *serum sickness, anaphylaxis.*

INTERACTIONS
Drug-drug. *Aminoglycosides:* May increase risk of nephrotoxicity. Monitor patient closely.
Probenecid: May inhibit excretion and increase blood levels of cefprozil. Use together cautiously.

EFFECTS ON LAB TEST RESULTS
● May increase BUN, creatinine, ALT, AST, alkaline phosphatase, bilirubin, and LDH levels.
● May increase eosinophil count. May decrease WBC, leukocyte, and platelet counts.

CONTRAINDICATIONS
Contraindicated in patients hypersensitive to drug or other cephalosporins.

NURSING CONSIDERATIONS
● Use cautiously in patients hypersensitive to penicillin because of possibility of cross-sensitivity with other beta-lactam antibiotics. Also use cautiously in breast-feeding women and in patients with history of colitis and renal insufficiency.
● Monitor renal function and liver function test results.
● Obtain specimen for culture and sensitivity tests before giving first dose. Therapy may begin pending results.
● Monitor patient for superinfection. May cause overgrowth of nonsusceptible bacteria or fungi.
● Cephalosporins may cause false-positive Coombs' test results and false-positive results in urine glucose tests using cupric sulfate (Benedict's reagent or Clinitest); use glucose oxidase tests (Diastix or Chemstrip uG) instead. Drug also falsely elevates serum or urine creatinine levels in tests using Jaffe reaction.

● *Alert:* Don't confuse drug with other cephalosporins that sound alike.

PATIENT TEACHING
● Advise patient to take drug as prescribed, even after he feels better.
● Tell patient to shake suspension well before measuring dose.
● Inform patient or parent that oral suspensions contain the drug in a bubble gum–flavored form to improve palatability and promote compliance in children. Tell him to refrigerate reconstituted suspension and to discard unused drug after 14 days.
● Instruct patient to notify prescriber if rash or signs and symptoms of superinfection occur.

ceftazidime
Ceptaz, Fortaz, Fortum§, Kefadim§, Tazicef, Tazidime

Pregnancy risk category B

AVAILABLE FORMS
Infusion: 1 g, 2 g in 50-ml and 100-ml vials (premixed)
Injection (with arginine): 1 g, 2 g, 6 g
Injection (with sodium carbonate): 500 mg, 1 g, 2 g

INDICATIONS & DOSAGES
➤ **Serious infections of the lower respiratory and urinary tracts; gynecologic, intra-abdominal, CNS, and skin infections; bacteremia; and septicemia caused by susceptible microorganisms, such as** *streptococci* **(including** *Streptococcus pneumoniae* **and** *S. pyogenes***),** *Staphylococcus aureus* **(penicillinase- and non–penicillinase-producing),** *Escherichia coli, Klebsiella,* **Proteus,** *Enterobacter, Haemophilus influenzae,* *Pseudomonas,* **and some strains of** *Bacteroides*—
Adults and children age 12 and older: 1 to 2 g I.V. or I.M. q 8 to 12 hours; up to 6 g daily in life-threatening infections.
Children ages 1 month to 11 years: 25 to 50 mg/kg I.V. q 8 hours. Maximum dose is 6 g/day. Use sodium carbonate formulation.

Neonates up to age 4 weeks: 30 mg/kg I.V. q 12 hours. Use sodium carbonate formulation.

➤ **Uncomplicated urinary tract infections**—
Adults: 250 mg I.V. or I.M. q 12 hours.

➤ **Complicated urinary tract infections**—
Adults and children age 12 and older: 500 mg to 1 g I.V. or I.M. q 8 to 12 hours.

Adjust-a-dose: For renally impaired patients, if creatinine clearance is 31 to 50 ml/minute, give 1 g q 12 hours; if clearance is 16 to 30 ml/minute, give 1 g q 24 hours; if clearance is 6 to 15 ml/minute, give 500 mg q 24 hours; if clearance is less than 5 ml/minute, give 500 mg q 48 hours. Ceftazidime is removed by hemodialysis; give a supplemental dose of drug after each dialysis treatment.

I.V. ADMINISTRATION
● Reconstitute solutions containing sodium carbonate with sterile water for injection. Add 5 ml to a 500-mg vial, or add 10 ml to a 1-g or 2-g vial. Shake well to dissolve drug.
● Carbon dioxide is released during dissolution, and positive pressure will develop in vial.
● Reconstitute solutions containing arginine with 10 ml of sterile water for injection. This formulation won't release gas bubbles.
● Each brand of ceftazidime includes specific instructions for reconstitution. Read and follow them carefully.
● Infuse drug over 15 to 30 minutes.

ACTION
A third-generation cephalosporin that inhibits cell-wall synthesis, promoting osmotic instability; usually bactericidal.

Route	Onset	Peak	Duration
I.M.	Unknown	1 hr	Unknown
I.V.	Immediate	Immediate	Unknown

ADVERSE REACTIONS
CNS: headache, dizziness, paresthesia, *seizures.*
CV: *phlebitis, thrombophlebitis.*
GI: pseudomembranous colitis, nausea, vomiting, diarrhea, abdominal cramps.
GU: vaginitis, candidiasis.

Hematologic: eosinophilia; thrombocytosis, *leukopenia,* hemolytic anemia, *agranulocytosis, thrombocytopenia.*
Skin: *maculopapular and erythematous rashes, urticaria, pain, induration, sterile abscesses, tissue sloughing at injection site.*
Other: hypersensitivity reactions, *serum sickness, anaphylaxis.*

INTERACTIONS
Drug-drug. *Aminoglycosides:* Causes additive or synergistic effect against some strains of *Pseudomonas aeruginosa* and Enterobacteriaceae; increased risk of nephrotoxicity. Monitor patient for effects and monitor renal function.
Chloramphenicol: Causes antagonistic effect. Avoid using together.

EFFECTS ON LAB TEST RESULTS
● May increase ALT, AST, alkaline phosphatase, bilirubin, and LDH levels.
● May increase eosinophil count. May decrease hemoglobin and WBC and granulocyte counts. May increase or decrease platelet count.

CONTRAINDICATIONS
Contraindicated in patients hypersensitive to drug or other cephalosporins.

NURSING CONSIDERATIONS
● Use cautiously in patients hypersensitive to penicillin because of possibility of cross-sensitivity with other beta-lactam antibiotics. Also use cautiously in breast-feeding women and in patients with history of colitis and renal insufficiency.
● Obtain specimen for culture and sensitivity tests before giving first dose. Therapy may begin pending results.
● For I.M. administration, inject deeply into a large muscle, such as the gluteus maximus or the lateral aspect of the thigh.
● If large doses are given, therapy is prolonged, or patient is at high risk, monitor patient for signs and symptoms of superinfection.
● Cephalosporins may cause false-positive Coombs' test results and false-positive results in urine glucose tests using cupric sulfate (Benedict's reagent or Clinitest); use glucose oxidase tests (Diastix or Chemstrip uG) instead. Drug also falsely

---

Reactions may be *common,* uncommon, *life-threatening,* or COMMON AND LIFE-THREATENING.

elevates serum or urine creatinine levels in tests using Jaffe reaction.

• *Alert:* Commercially available preparations contain either sodium carbonate (Fortaz, Tazicef, Tazidime) or arginine (Ceptaz) to facilitate dissolution of drug. Safety and efficacy of solutions containing arginine in children younger than age 12 haven't been established.

• *Alert:* Don't confuse drug with other cephalosporins that sound alike.

PATIENT TEACHING

• Tell patient to report adverse reactions or signs and symptoms of superinfection promptly.

• Instruct patient to report discomfort at I.V. insertion site.

• Advise patient to notify prescriber about loose stools or diarrhea.

---

ceftizoxime sodium
Cefizox

Pregnancy risk category B

AVAILABLE FORMS
Infusion: 1 g, 2 g in 100-ml vials or in 50 ml of D$_5$W
Injection: 500 mg, 1 g, 2 g, 10 g

INDICATIONS & DOSAGES
➤ Serious infections of the lower respiratory and urinary tracts, gynecologic infections, bacteremia, septicemia, meningitis, intra-abdominal infections, bone and joint infections, and skin infections caused by susceptible microorganisms, such as *streptococci* (including *Streptococcus pneumoniae* and *S. pyogenes*), *Staphylococcus aureus*, *S. epidermidis*, *Escherichia coli*, *Haemophilus influenzae*, and *Klebsiella, Enterobacter, Proteus, Peptostreptococcus*, and some *Pseudomonas species*—
Adults: Usual dosage is 1 to 2 g I.V. or I.M. q 8 to 12 hours. In life-threatening infections, give up to 2 g q 4 hours.
Children older than age 6 months: 50 mg/kg I.V. q 6 to 8 hours. For serious infections, up to 200 mg/kg/day in divided doses may be used. Don't exceed 12 g/day.
➤ Uncomplicated gonorrhea—
Adults: 1 g I.M. as a single dose.

Adjust-a-dose: For renally impaired patients, if creatinine clearance is 50 to 79 ml/minute, give 500 mg to 1.5 g q 8 hours; if clearance is 5 to 49 ml/minute, give 250 mg to 1 g q 12 hours; if clearance is below 5 ml/minute or patient undergoes hemodialysis, give 500 mg to 1 g q 48 hours, or 250 to 500 mg q 24 hours.

I.V. ADMINISTRATION
• To reconstitute powder, add 5 ml of sterile water to a 500-mg vial, 10 ml to a 1-g vial, or 20 ml to a 2-g vial.
• Inject directly into vein over 3 to 5 minutes or slowly into I.V. tubing with free-flowing compatible solution.
• Reconstitute drug in piggyback vials with 50 to 100 ml of normal saline solution or D$_5$W. Shake well.
• Infuse drug over 15 to 30 minutes.

ACTION
A third-generation cephalosporin that inhibits cell-wall synthesis, promoting osmotic instability; usually bactericidal.

Route	Onset	Peak	Duration
I.M.	Unknown	0.5-1.5 hr	Unknown
I.V.	Immediate	Immediate	Unknown

ADVERSE REACTIONS
CV: *phlebitis, thrombophlebitis.*
GI: pseudomembranous colitis, nausea, anorexia, vomiting, *diarrhea.*
GU: vaginitis.
Hematologic: *transient neutropenia,* eosinophilia, hemolytic anemia, thrombocytosis, anemia, *thrombocytopenia.*
Respiratory: dyspnea.
Skin: *maculopapular and erythematous rashes, urticaria, pain, induration, sterile abscesses, tissue sloughing at injection site.*
Other: hypersensitivity reactions, *serum sickness, anaphylaxis,* fever.

INTERACTIONS
Drug-drug. *Aminoglycosides:* May increase nephrotoxicity. Monitor renal function.
Probenecid: May inhibit excretion and increase blood levels of ceftizoxime. May be used for this effect.

EFFECTS ON LAB TEST RESULTS
• May increase BUN, creatinine, ALT, AST, alkaline phosphatase, bilirubin, GGT, and LDH levels. May decrease albumin and protein levels.
• May decrease hemoglobin and PT and RBC, WBC, platelet, granulocyte, and neutrophil counts.

CONTRAINDICATIONS
Contraindicated in patients hypersensitive to drug or other cephalosporins.

NURSING CONSIDERATIONS
• Use cautiously in patients hypersensitive to penicillin because of possibility of cross-sensitivity with other beta-lactam antibiotics. Also use cautiously in breast-feeding women and in patients with history of colitis and renal insufficiency.
• Obtain specimen for culture and sensitivity tests before giving first dose. Therapy may begin pending results.
• To prepare I.M. injection, mix 1.5 ml of diluent per 500 mg of drug. For I.M. administration, inject deeply into a large muscle, such as the gluteus maximus or the lateral aspect of the thigh. Larger doses (2 g) should be divided and given at two separate sites.
• Cephalosporins may cause false-positive Coombs' test results and false-positive results in urine glucose tests using cupric sulfate (Benedict's reagent or Clinitest); use glucose oxidase tests (Diastix or Chemstrip uG) instead. Drug also falsely elevates serum or urine creatinine levels in tests using Jaffe reaction.
• If large doses are given, therapy is prolonged, or patient is at high risk, monitor patient for signs or symptoms of superinfection.
• *Alert:* Don't confuse drug with other cephalosporins that sound alike.

PATIENT TEACHING
• Tell patient to report adverse reactions and signs and symptoms of superinfection promptly.
• Instruct patient to report discomfort at I.V. site.
• Tell patient to notify prescriber about loose stools or diarrhea.

ceftriaxone sodium
Rocephin

Pregnancy risk category B

AVAILABLE FORMS
Infusion: 1 g, 2 g piggyback; 1 g, 2 g/ 50 ml premixed
Injection: 250 mg, 500 mg, 1 g, 2 g, 10 g

INDICATIONS & DOSAGES
➤ **Uncomplicated gonococcal vulvovaginitis—**
Adults: 125 mg I.M. as a single dose, plus azithromycin 1 g P.O. as a single dose or doxycycline 100 mg P.O. b.i.d. for 7 days.
➤ **Most infections caused by susceptible organisms; serious infections of the lower respiratory and urinary tracts; gynecologic, bone and joint, intraabdominal, and skin infections; bacteremia; septicemia; and Lyme disease caused by such susceptible microorganisms as** *streptococci* **(including** *Streptococcus pneumoniae* **and** *S. pyogenes***);** *Staphylococcus aureus* **(penicillinase- and non–penicillinase-producing) and** *S. epidermidis, Escherichia coli, Haemophilus influenzae, Neisseria meningitidis, N. gonorrhoeae, Serratia marcescens,* **and** *Enterobacter, Klebsiella, Proteus, Peptostreptococcus,* **and** *Pseudomonas* **species—**
Adults and children older than age 12: 1 to 2 g I.M. or I.V. daily or in equally divided doses q 12 hours. Total daily dose shouldn't exceed 4 g.
Children age 12 and younger: 50 to 75 mg/kg I.M. or I.V., not to exceed 2 g/ day, given in divided doses q 12 hours.
➤ **Meningitis—**
Adults and children: Initially, 100 mg/kg I.M. or I.V. Don't exceed 4 g; then 100 mg/kg I.M. or I.V., given once daily or in divided doses q 12 hours, not to exceed 4 g, for 7 to 14 days.
➤ **Perioperative prophylaxis—**
Adults: 1 g I.V. as a single dose 30 minutes to 2 hours before surgery.
➤ **Acute bacterial otitis media—**
Children: 50 mg/kg I.M. as a single dose. Don't exceed 1 g.

I.V. ADMINISTRATION
• Reconstitute drug with sterile water for injection, normal saline solution for injection, D_5W or dextrose 10% in water injection, or a combination of normal saline solution and dextrose injection and other compatible solutions.
• Reconstitute by adding 2.4 ml of diluent to the 250-mg vial, 4.8 ml to the 500-mg vial, 9.6 ml to the 1-g vial, and 19.2 ml to the 2-g vial. All reconstituted solutions yield a concentration that averages 100 mg/ml.
• After reconstitution, dilute further for intermittent infusion to desired concentration. I.V. dilutions are stable for 24 hours at room temperature.

ACTION
A third-generation cephalosporin that inhibits cell-wall synthesis, promoting osmotic instability; usually bactericidal.

Route	Onset	Peak	Duration
I.M.	Unknown	1.5-4 hr	Unknown
I.V.	Immediate	Immediate	Unknown

ADVERSE REACTIONS
CNS: headache, dizziness.
CV: phlebitis.
GI: pseudomembranous colitis, nausea, vomiting, diarrhea.
GU: genital pruritus, candidiasis.
Hematologic: eosinophilia, thrombocytosis, *leukopenia.*
Skin: pain, induration, tenderness at injection site, *rash,* pruritus.
Other: hypersensitivity reactions, *serum sickness, anaphylaxis,* fever, chills.

INTERACTIONS
Drug-drug. *Aminoglycosides:* Causes synergistic effect against some strains of *P. aeruginosa* and *Enterobacteriaceae* species. Monitor patient.
Probenecid: High doses (1 or 2 g/day) may enhance hepatic clearance of ceftriaxone and shorten its half-life. Avoid using together.

EFFECTS ON LAB TEST RESULTS
• May increase BUN, ALT, AST, alkaline phosphatase, bilirubin, and LDH levels.
• May increase eosinophil and platelet counts. May decrease WBC count.

CONTRAINDICATIONS
Contraindicated in patients hypersensitive to drug or other cephalosporins.

NURSING CONSIDERATIONS
• Use cautiously in patients hypersensitive to penicillin because of possibility of cross-sensitivity with other beta-lactam antibiotics. Also use cautiously in breast-feeding women and in patients with history of colitis and renal insufficiency.
• Obtain specimen for culture and sensitivity tests before giving first dose. Therapy may begin pending results.
• A commercially available I.M. kit containing 1% lidocaine as a diluent is available from the manufacturer.
• For I.M. administration, inject deeply into a large muscle, such as the gluteus maximus or the lateral aspect of the thigh.
• If large doses are given, therapy is prolonged, or patient is at high risk, monitor patient for signs and symptoms of superinfection.
• Monitor PT and INR in patients with impaired vitamin K synthesis or low vitamin K stores. Vitamin K therapy may be needed.
• Cephalosporins may cause false-positive Coombs' test results and false-positive results in urine glucose tests using cupric sulfate (Benedict's reagent or Clinitest); use glucose oxidase tests (Diastix or Chemstrip uG). Drug also falsely elevates serum or urine creatinine levels in tests using Jaffe reaction.
• Drug is commonly used in home antibiotic programs for outpatient treatment of serious infections such as osteomyelitis and community-acquired pneumonia.
• *Alert:* Don't confuse drug with other cephalosporins that sound alike.

PATIENT TEACHING
• Tell patient to report adverse reactions promptly.
• Instruct patient to report discomfort at I.V. insertion site.
• Teach patient and family receiving home care how to prepare and give drug.
• If home care patient is a diabetic who is testing his urine for glucose, tell him drug may affect results of cupric sulfate tests; he should use an enzymatic test instead.

• Tell patient to notify prescriber about loose stools or diarrhea.

---

cefuroxime axetil
Ceftin, Zinnat§

cefuroxime sodium
Kefurox, Zinacef

Pregnancy risk category B

AVAILABLE FORMS
cefuroxime axetil
Suspension: 125 mg/5 ml, 250 mg/5 ml
Tablets: 125 mg, 250 mg, 500 mg
cefuroxime sodium
Infusion: 750 mg, 1.5-g premixed, frozen solution
Injection: 750 mg, 1.5 g, 7.5 g

INDICATIONS & DOSAGES
➤ *Cefuroxime sodium.* **Serious infections of the lower respiratory and urinary tracts, skin and skin-structure infections, bone and joint infections, septicemia, meningitis, gonorrhea, and perioperative prophylaxis**
Cefuroxime axetil. **Otitis media, pharyngitis, tonsillitis, infections of the urinary and lower respiratory tracts, and skin and skin-structure infections caused by *Streptococcus pneumoniae* and *S. pyogenes, Haemophilus influenzae, Staphylococcus aureus, Escherichia coli, Moraxella catarrhalis* (including beta-lactamase–producing strains), *Neisseria gonorrhoeae,* and *Klebsiella* and *Enterobacter species*—**
Adults and children age 12 and older:
Usual dosage of cefuroxime sodium is 750 mg to 1.5 g I.M. or I.V. q 8 hours for 5 to 10 days. For life-threatening infections and infections caused by less susceptible organisms, 1.5 g I.M. or I.V. q 6 hours; for bacterial meningitis, up to 3 g I.V. q 8 hours.

Or, give 250 mg of cefuroxime axetil P.O. q 12 hours. For severe infections, dosage may be increased to 500 mg q 12 hours.
Children and infants older than age 3 months: 50 to 100 mg/kg/day of cefuroxime sodium I.M. or I.V. in equally divided doses q 6 to 8 hours. Higher dosage of 100 mg/kg/day, not to exceed maximum adult dosage, should be used for more severe or serious infections. For bacterial meningitis, 200 to 240 mg/kg I.V. in divided doses q 6 to 8 hours. For other infections, 125 to 250 mg of cefuroxime axetil P.O. q 12 hours for a child who can swallow pills.
➤ **Uncomplicated urinary tract infections—**
Adults: 125 to 250 mg P.O. q 12 hours.
➤ **Otitis media—**
Children ages 3 months to 12 years:
250 mg P.O. q 12 hours for 10 days for children who can swallow tablets whole. Or, 30 mg/kg/day of oral suspension P.O. in 2 divided doses for 10 days for children who can't swallow tablets.
➤ **Perioperative prophylaxis—**
Adults: 1.5 g I.V. 30 to 60 minutes before surgery; in lengthy operations, 750 mg I.V. or I.M. q 8 hours. For open-heart surgery, 1.5 g I.V. at induction of anesthesia and then q 12 hours for a total dose of 6 g.
➤ **Early Lyme disease (erythema migrans) caused by *Borrelia burgdorferi*—**
Adults and children age 13 and older:
500 mg P.O. b.i.d. for 20 days.
➤ **Secondary bacterial infection of acute bronchitis—**
Adults: 250 to 500 mg tablets P.O. b.i.d. for 5 to 10 days.
➤ **Uncomplicated gonorrhea—**
Adults: 1.5 g I.M. with 1 g probenecid P.O. for one dose.
➤ **Acute bacterial maxillary sinusitis caused by *Streptococcus pneumoniae* or *Haemophilus influenzae* (only strains that don't produce beta-lactamase)—**
Adults and children age 13 and older:
250-mg tablet P.O. b.i.d. for 10 days.
Children ages 3 months to 12 years:
30 mg/kg/day oral suspension P.O. in two divided doses for 10 days.
Adjust-a-dose: For parenteral administration in patients with renal failure, if creatinine clearance is 10 to 20 ml/minute, give 750 mg I.M. or I.V. q 12 hours; if clearance is less than 10 ml/minute, give 750 mg I.M. or I.V. q 24 hours.

I.V. ADMINISTRATION
• For each 750-mg vial of Kefurox, reconstitute with 7 ml of sterile water for injection. For each 1.5-g vial of Kefurox, re-

---

Reactions may be common, uncommon, *life-threatening*, or COMMON AND LIFE-THREATENING.

constitute with 14 ml of sterile water for injection; withdraw entire contents of vial for a dose. For each 750-mg vial of Zinacef, reconstitute with 8 ml of sterile water for injection; for each 1.5-g vial, reconstitute with 16 ml. In each case, withdraw entire contents of vial for a dose.
• To give by direct injection, inject into a large vein or into the tubing of a free-flowing I.V. solution over 3 to 5 minutes.
• For intermittent infusion, add reconstituted drug to 100 ml D_5W, normal saline solution for injection, or other compatible I.V. solution. Infuse over 15 to 60 minutes.

ACTION
A second-generation cephalosporin that inhibits cell-wall synthesis, promoting osmotic instability; usually bactericidal.

Route	Onset	Peak	Duration
I.M.	Unknown	2 hr	Unknown
I.V.	Immediate	Immediate	Unknown
P.O.	Unknown	15-60 min	Unknown

ADVERSE REACTIONS
CV: *phlebitis, thrombophlebitis.*
GI: pseudomembranous colitis, nausea, anorexia, vomiting, *diarrhea.*
Hematologic: *transient neutropenia,* eosinophilia, *hemolytic anemia,* ***thrombocytopenia.***
Skin: *maculopapular and erythematous rashes, urticaria, pain, induration, sterile abscesses, temperature elevation, tissue sloughing at I.M. injection site.*
Other: hypersensitivity reactions, ***serum sickness, anaphylaxis.***

INTERACTIONS
Drug-drug. *Aminoglycosides:* Causes synergistic activity against some organisms; may increase nephrotoxicity. Monitor patient closely.
Loop diuretics: Increased risk of adverse renal reactions. Monitor patient closely.
Probenecid: May inhibit excretion and increase blood levels of cefuroxime. Sometimes used for this effect.
Drug-food. *Any food:* Increased absorption. Give drug with food.

EFFECTS ON LAB TEST RESULTS
• May increase ALT, AST, alkaline phosphatase, bilirubin, and LDH levels.

• May increase PT and INR and eosinophil count. May decrease hemoglobin and hematocrit and neutrophil and platelet counts.

CONTRAINDICATIONS
Contraindicated in patients hypersensitive to drug or other cephalosporins.

NURSING CONSIDERATIONS
• Use cautiously in patients hypersensitive to penicillin because of possibility of cross-sensitivity with other beta-lactam antibiotics. Also use cautiously in breast-feeding women and in patients with history of colitis and renal insufficiency.
• Obtain specimen for culture and sensitivity tests before giving first dose. Therapy may begin pending results.
• For I.M. administration, inject deeply into a large muscle mass, such as the gluteus maximus or the lateral aspect of the thigh.
• Absorption of cefuroxime axetil is enhanced by food.
• Cefuroxime axetil tablets may be crushed for patients who can't swallow tablets. Tablets may be dissolved in small amounts of apple, orange, or grape juice or chocolate milk. However, the drug has a bitter taste that is difficult to mask, even with food.
• Cephalosporins may cause false-positive Coombs' test results and false-positive results in urine glucose tests using cupric sulfate (Benedict's reagent or Clinitest); use glucose oxidase tests (Diastix or Chemstrip uG) instead. Drug also falsely elevates serum or urine creatinine levels in tests using Jaffe reaction.
• **Alert:** Cefuroxime axetil film-coated tablet and oral suspension aren't bioequivalent. Don't substitute on a mg/mg basis.
• If large doses are given, therapy is prolonged, or patient is at high risk, monitor patient for signs and symptoms of superinfection.
• **Alert:** Don't confuse drug with other cephalosporins that sound alike.

PATIENT TEACHING
• Tell patient to take all of the drug as prescribed, even after he feels better.

---

*Liquid contains alcohol.   **May contain tartrazine.   †Canada   ‡Australia   §U.K.   ◊OTC

• Instruct patient to take oral form with food. If patient has difficulty swallowing tablets, show him how to dissolve or crush tablets but warn him that the bitter taste is hard to mask, even with food. If suspension is being used, tell patient to shake container well before measuring dose.
• Instruct patient to notify prescriber about rash or evidence of superinfection.
• Advise patient receiving drug I.V. to report discomfort at I.V. insertion site.
• Tell patient to notify prescriber about loose stools or diarrhea.

---

cephalexin hydrochloride
Keftab

cephalexin monohydrate
Apo-Cephalex†, Biocef, Keflex, Novo-Lexin†, Nu-Cephalex†

Pregnancy risk category B

AVAILABLE FORMS
cephalexin hydrochloride
Tablets: 500 mg
cephalexin monohydrate
Capsules: 250 mg, 500 mg
Oral suspension: 125 mg/5 ml, 250 mg/5 ml
Tablets: 250 mg, 500 mg, 1 g

INDICATIONS & DOSAGES
➤ **Respiratory tract, GI tract, skin, soft-tissue, bone, and joint infections and otitis media caused by *Escherichia coli* and other coliform bacteria, group A beta-hemolytic streptococci, *Klebsiella species*, *Proteus mirabilis*, *Streptococcus pneumoniae*, and staphylococci—**
Adults: 250 mg to 1 g P.O. q 6 hours or 500 mg q 12 hours. Maximum 4 g daily.
Children: 25 to 50 mg/kg/day P.O. in two to four equally divided doses. In severe infections, dose can be doubled.
Adjust-a-dose: For adults with impaired renal function, initial dose is the same. Recommended subsequent dosing for creatinine clearance less than 5 ml/minute, 250 mg P.O. q 12 to 24 hours; for clearance of 5 to 10 ml/minute, 250 mg P.O. q 12 hours; and for clearance of 11 to 40 ml/minute, 500 mg P.O. q 8 to 12 hours.

ACTION
A first-generation cephalosporin that inhibits cell-wall synthesis, promoting osmotic instability; usually bactericidal.

Route	Onset	Peak	Duration
P.O.	Unknown	1 hr	Unknown

ADVERSE REACTIONS
CNS: dizziness, headache, fatigue, agitation, confusion, hallucinations.
GI: pseudomembranous colitis, *nausea, anorexia,* vomiting, *diarrhea,* gastritis, glossitis, dyspepsia, abdominal pain, anal pruritus, tenesmus, oral candidiasis.
GU: genital pruritus, candidiasis, vaginitis, interstitial nephritis.
Hematologic: *neutropenia,* eosinophilia, anemia, *thrombocytopenia.*
Musculoskeletal: arthritis, arthralgia, joint pain.
Skin: *maculopapular and erythematous rashes, urticaria.*
Other: hypersensitivity reactions, *serum sickness, anaphylaxis.*

INTERACTIONS
Drug-drug. *Aminoglycosides:* Increased risk of nephrotoxicity. Avoid using together.
Probenecid: May increase blood levels of cephalosporins. May be used for this effect.

EFFECTS ON LAB TEST RESULTS
• May increase ALT, AST, alkaline phosphatase, bilirubin, and LDH levels.
• May increase eosinophil count. May decrease hemoglobin and neutrophil and platelet counts.

CONTRAINDICATIONS
Contraindicated in patients hypersensitive to cephalosporins.

NURSING CONSIDERATIONS
• Use cautiously in patients hypersensitive to penicillin because of possibility of cross-sensitivity with other beta-lactam antibiotics. Also use cautiously in breast-feeding women and in patients with history of colitis and renal insufficiency.
• Ask patient about past reaction to cephalosporin or penicillin therapy before giving first dose.

Reactions may be *common,* uncommon, **life-threatening**, or COMMON AND LIFE-THREATENING.

● Obtain specimen for culture and sensitivity tests before giving first dose. Therapy may begin pending results.
● To prepare oral suspension: Add required amount of water to powder in two portions. Shake well after each addition. After mixing, store in refrigerator. Mixture will remain stable for 14 days. Keep tightly closed and shake well before using.
● If large doses are given or if therapy is prolonged, monitor patient for superinfection, especially in high-risk patients.
● Group A beta-hemolytic streptococcal infections should be treated for a minimum of 10 days.
● Cephalosporins may cause false-positive Coombs' test results and false-positive results in urine glucose tests using cupric sulfate (Benedict's reagent or Clinitest); use glucose oxidase tests (Diastix or Chemstrip uG) instead. Drug also falsely elevates serum or urine creatinine levels in tests using Jaffe reaction.
● *Alert:* Don't confuse drug with other cephalosporins that sound alike.

PATIENT TEACHING
● Tell patient to take all of the drug exactly as prescribed, even after he feels better.
● Instruct patient to take drug with food or milk to lessen GI discomfort. If patient is taking suspension form, instruct him to shake container well before measuring dose and to store in refrigerator.
● Tell patient to notify prescriber if rash or signs and symptoms of superinfection develop.

cephradine
Velosef**

Pregnancy risk category B

AVAILABLE FORMS
Capsules: 250 mg, 500 mg
Oral suspension: 125 mg/5 ml, 250 mg/ 5 ml

INDICATIONS & DOSAGES
➤ **Serious infections of respiratory, GU, or GI tract; skin and soft-tissue infections; bone and joint infections; septicemia; endocarditis; and otitis media**

caused by such susceptible organisms as *Escherichia coli* **and other coliform bacteria, group A beta-hemolytic streptococci,** *Klebsiella, Proteus mirabilis, Staphylococcus aureus, Streptococcus pneumoniae, S. viridans,* **and staphylococci; perioperative prophylaxis—**
Adults: 250 to 500 mg P.O. q 6 hours or 500 mg to 1 g P.O. q 12 hours. For severe or chronic infections, doses up to 1 g every 6 hours may be given.
Children older than age 9 months: 25 to 50 mg/kg P.O. daily in divided doses q 6 to 12 hours. For severe or chronic infections, doses up to 1 g every 6 hours may be given.
➤ **Otitis media—**
Children: 75 to 100 mg/kg P.O. daily in equally divided doses q 6 to 12 hours. Don't exceed 4 g daily.
Adjust-a-dose: For patients with creatinine clearance of 20 ml/minute or more, give 500 mg q 6 hours; for clearance of 5 to 20 ml/minute, give 250 mg q 6 hours; for clearance of less than 5 ml/minute, give 250 mg q 12 hours. In hemodialysis patients, initially 250 mg at the start of dialysis, then 250 mg 12 hours later and 250 mg 36 to 48 hours later.

ACTION
First-generation cephalosporin that inhibits cell-wall synthesis, promoting osmotic instability; usually bactericidal.

Route	Onset	Peak	Duration
P.O.	Unknown	1 hr	Unknown

ADVERSE REACTIONS
CNS: dizziness, headache, malaise, paresthesia.
GI: pseudomembranous colitis, *nausea, anorexia,* vomiting, heartburn, abdominal cramps, *diarrhea,* oral candidiasis.
GU: genital pruritus, candidiasis, vaginitis.
Hematologic: *transient neutropenia,* eosinophilia, *thrombocytopenia.*
Skin: *maculopapular and erythematous rashes, urticaria.*
Other: hypersensitivity reactions, *serum sickness, anaphylaxis.*

INTERACTIONS
Drug-drug. *Aminoglycosides:* Increased risk of nephrotoxicity. Avoid using together.
Probenecid: May increase blood levels of cephalosporins. Sometimes used for this effect.

EFFECTS ON LAB TEST RESULTS
• May increase ALT, AST, alkaline phosphatase, bilirubin, and LDH levels.
• May increase eosinophil count. May decrease neutrophil and platelet counts.

CONTRAINDICATIONS
Contraindicated in patients hypersensitive to drug and to other cephalosporins.

NURSING CONSIDERATIONS
• Use cautiously in patients hypersensitive to penicillin because of possibility of cross-sensitivity with other beta-lactam antibiotics. Also use cautiously in breast-feeding women and in patients with history of colitis and renal insufficiency.
• Monitor renal function.
• Obtain specimen for culture and sensitivity tests before giving first dose. Therapy may begin pending results.
• Group A beta-hemolytic streptococcal infections should be treated for a minimum of 10 days.
• Cephalosporins may cause false-positive Coombs' test results and false-positive results in urine glucose tests using cupric sulfate (Benedict's reagent or Clinitest); use glucose oxidase tests (Diastix or Chemstrip uG) instead. Drug also falsely elevates serum or urine creatinine levels in tests using Jaffe reaction.
• If large doses are given, therapy is prolonged, or patient is at high risk, monitor patient for signs and symptoms of superinfection.
• *Alert:* Don't confuse drug with other cephalosporins that sound alike.

PATIENT TEACHING
• Instruct patient to take all of the drug as prescribed, even after he feels better.
• Advise patient to take drug with food or milk to lessen GI discomfort. If patient is taking suspension form, tell him to shake it well before measuring dose.

• Tell patient to notify prescriber if rash or signs and symptoms of superinfection occur.
• Instruct patient to notify prescriber about loose stools or diarrhea.

---

loracarbef
Lorabid

Pregnancy risk category B

AVAILABLE FORMS
Powder for oral suspension: 100 mg/5 ml, 200 mg/5 ml in 50-ml, 75-ml, and 100-ml bottles
Pulvules: 200 mg, 400 mg

INDICATIONS & DOSAGES
➤ **Secondary bacterial infections of acute bronchitis—**
Adults: 200 to 400 mg P.O. q 12 hours for 7 days.
➤ **Acute bacterial exacerbations of chronic bronchitis—**
Adults: 400 mg P.O. q 12 hours for 7 days.
➤ **Pneumonia—**
Adults: 400 mg P.O. q 12 hours for 14 days.
➤ **Pharyngitis, sinusitis, tonsillitis—**
Adults: 200 to 400 mg P.O. q 12 hours for 10 days.
Children ages 6 months to 12 years: 15 mg/kg P.O. daily in divided doses q 12 hours for 10 days.
➤ **Acute otitis media—**
Children ages 6 months to 12 years: 30 mg/kg oral suspension P.O. daily in divided doses q 12 hours for 10 days.
➤ **Uncomplicated skin and skin-structure infections—**
Adults: 200 mg P.O. q 12 hours for 7 days.
➤ **Impetigo—**
Children ages 6 months to 12 years: 15 mg/kg P.O. daily in divided doses q 12 hours for 7 days.
➤ **Uncomplicated cystitis—**
Adults: 200 mg P.O. daily for 7 days.
➤ **Uncomplicated pyelonephritis—**
Adults: 400 mg P.O. q 12 hours for 14 days.
Adjust-a-dose: Patients with creatinine clearance of 50 ml/minute or more don't

---

need dosage adjustments. If clearance is 10 to 49 ml/minute, give half usual dose at same interval; if clearance is less than 10 ml/minute, give usual dose q 3 to 5 days. Hemodialysis patients require an additional dose after dialysis.

ACTION

A synthetic beta-lactam antibiotic of the carbacephem class with actions similar to second-generation cephalosporins. Inhibits cell-wall synthesis, promoting osmotic instability; usually bactericidal.

Route	Onset	Peak	Duration
P.O.	Unknown	0.5-1 hr	Unknown

ADVERSE REACTIONS

CNS: headache, somnolence, nervousness, insomnia, dizziness.
CV: vasodilation.
GI: diarrhea, nausea, vomiting, abdominal pain, anorexia, pseudomembranous colitis.
GU: vaginal candidiasis.
Hematologic: *transient thrombocytopenia, leukopenia,* eosinophilia, *pancytopenia, neutropenia.*
Skin: rash, urticaria, pruritus, *erythema multiforme.*
Other: hypersensitivity reactions, *anaphylaxis.*

INTERACTIONS

Drug-drug. *Probenecid:* Decreased excretion of loracarbef, causing increased plasma levels. Monitor patient for toxicity.
Drug-food. *Any food:* Decreased absorption. Have patient take drug on empty stomach at least 1 hour before or 2 hours after a meal.

EFFECTS ON LAB TEST RESULTS

• May increase BUN, creatinine, ALT, AST, and alkaline phosphatase levels.
• May increase PT and INR, and eosinophil count. May decrease platelet, WBC, RBC, and neutrophil counts.

CONTRAINDICATIONS

Contraindicated in patients hypersensitive to drug or other cephalosporins.

NURSING CONSIDERATIONS

• Use cautiously in patients hypersensitive to penicillin because of possibility of cross-sensitivity with other beta-lactam antibiotics. Also use cautiously in breast-feeding women and in patients with history of colitis and renal insufficiency.
• Safety and efficacy of drug haven't been established in infants younger than age 6 months.
• Obtain specimen for culture and sensitivity tests before giving first dose. Therapy may begin pending results.
• To reconstitute powder for oral suspension, add 30 ml of water in two portions to the 50-ml bottle or 60 ml of water in two portions to the 100-ml bottle; shake after each addition.
• After reconstitution, store oral suspension for 14 days at 59° to 86° F (15° to 30° C).
• Monitor patient for superinfection. May cause overgrowth of nonsusceptible bacteria or fungi.
• Monitor renal function.
• For otitis media, the more rapidly absorbed oral suspension produces higher peak plasma levels than do capsules.
• *Alert:* Don't confuse Lorabid with Lortab.

PATIENT TEACHING

• Instruct patient to take all of the drug prescribed, even after he feels better.
• Tell patient to take drug on an empty stomach, at least 1 hour before or 2 hours after meals. Tell him to shake container of suspension well before measuring dose.
• Advise patient to discard unused portion after 14 days.
• Instruct patient to notify prescriber if rash or signs and symptoms of superinfection appear.
• Instruct patient to notify prescriber if loose stools or diarrhea occurs.

---

doxycycline calcium
doxycycline hyclate
doxycycline hydrochloride
doxycycline monohydrate
minocycline hydrochloride
tetracycline hydrochloride

COMBINATION PRODUCTS
HELIDAC: tetracycline 500 mg, bismuth salicylate 262.4 mg, and metronidazole 250 mg
UROBIOTIC: oxytetracycline hydrochloride 250 mg, sulfamethizole 250 mg, and phenazopyridine hydrochloride 50 mg

---

doxycycline calcium
Vibramycin

doxycycline hyclate
Apo-Doxy†, Doryx, Doxy Caps, Doxy 100, Doxy 200, Doxychel Hyclate, Doxycin†, Novo-Doxylin†, Periostat, Vibramycin, Vibra-Tabs

doxycycline hydrochloride
Doryx‡, Doxylin‡, Vibramycin‡

doxycycline monohydrate
Monodox, Vibramycin

Pregnancy risk category D

AVAILABLE FORMS
doxycycline calcium
Oral suspension: 50 mg/5 ml
doxycycline hyclate
Capsules: 20 mg, 50 mg, 100 mg
Capsules (enteric-coated pellets): 100 mg
Injection: 100 mg, 200 mg
Tablets (film-coated): 50 mg, 100 mg
doxycycline hydrochloride
Capsules: 50 mg‡, 100 mg‡
Tablets: 50 mg‡, 100 mg‡
doxycycline monohydrate
Capsules: 50 mg, 100 mg
Oral suspension: 25 mg/5 ml

INDICATIONS & DOSAGES
➤ **Infections caused by susceptible gram-positive and gram-negative organisms (including *Haemophilus ducreyi*, *Yersinia pestis*, and *Campylobacter fetus*), *Rickettsiae species*, *Mycoplasma pneumoniae*, *Chlamydia trachomatis*, and *Borrelia burgdorferi* (Lyme disease); psittacosis; granuloma inguinale—**
Adults and children older than age 8, weighing at least 45 kg (99 lb): 100 mg P.O. q 12 hours on first day; then 100 mg P.O. daily. Or, 200 mg I.V. on first day in one or two infusions; then 100 to 200 mg I.V. daily.
Children older than age 8, weighing less than 45 kg: 4.4 mg/kg P.O. or I.V. daily, in divided doses q 12 hours on first day; then 2.2 to 4.4 mg/kg daily in one or two divided doses.

Give I.V. infusion slowly (minimum 1 hour). Infusion must be completed within 12 hours (within 6 hours in lactated Ringer's solution or dextrose 5% in lactated Ringer's solution).
➤ **Inhalation, GI, and oropharyngeal anthrax in conjunction with one or two additional antimicrobials—**
Adults: Initially, 100 mg I.V. q 12 hours until susceptibility tests are known; then 100 mg P.O. b.i.d. for 60 days.
Children older than age 8, weighing more than 45 kg (99 lb): Initially, 100 mg I.V. q 12 hours; then 100 mg P.O. b.i.d. for 60 days.
Children older than age 8, weighing 45 kg or less: Initially, 2.2 mg/kg I.V. q 12 hours; then 2.2 mg/kg P.O. b.i.d. for 60 days.
Children age 8 and younger: Initially, 2.2 mg/kg I.V. q 12 hours; then 2.2 mg/kg P.O. b.i.d.
➤ **Gonorrhea in patients allergic to penicillin—**
Adults: 100 mg P.O. b.i.d. for 7 days. Use for 10 days for epididymitis.
➤ **Primary or secondary syphilis in patients allergic to penicillin—**
Adults: 300 mg P.O. daily in divided doses for at least 10 days.

Reactions may be *common*, uncommon, *life-threatening*, or COMMON AND LIFE-THREATENING.

➤ **Uncomplicated urethral, endocervical, or rectal infections caused by *C. trachomatis* or *Ureaplasma urealyticum*—**
Adults: 100 mg P.O. b.i.d. for at least 7 days. Use for 10 days for epididymitis.

➤ **Prevention of malaria—**
Adults: 100 mg P.O. daily beginning 1 to 2 days before travel to endemic area and continued for 4 weeks after travel.
Children older than age 8: 2 mg/kg P.O. once daily beginning 1 to 2 days before travel to endemic area and continued until 4 weeks after travel. Dosage shouldn't exceed 100 mg daily.

➤ **Pelvic inflammatory disease—**
Adults: 100 mg I.V. q 12 hours with cefoxitin or cefotetan and continued for at least 2 days after symptomatic improvement; then 100 mg P.O. q 12 hours for a total course of 14 days.

I.V. ADMINISTRATION
• Reconstitute powder for injection with sterile water for injection. Use 10 ml in 100-mg vial and 20 ml in 200-mg vial. Dilute solution to 100 to 1,000 ml for I.V. infusion.
• Don't infuse solutions that are more concentrated than 1 mg/ml.
• Infusion time varies with dose but usually ranges from 1 to 4 hours. Infusion must be completed within 12 hours.
• Monitor I.V. infusion site for signs and symptoms of thrombophlebitis, which may occur with I.V. administration.
• Don't expose drug to light or heat. Protect it from sunlight during infusion.

ACTION
Unknown. Thought to exert bacteriostatic effect by binding to the 30S and possibly 50S ribosomal subunits of microorganisms, thus inhibiting protein synthesis. May also alter the cytoplasmic membrane of susceptible microorganisms.

Route	Onset	Peak	Duration
I.V.	Immediate	Unknown	Unknown
P.O.	Unknown	1.5-4 hr	Unknown

ADVERSE REACTIONS
CNS: *intracranial hypertension.*
CV: pericarditis, thrombophlebitis.
GI: anorexia, glossitis, dysphagia, *epigastric distress, nausea,* vomiting, *diarrhea,*

oral candidiasis, enterocolitis, anogenital inflammation.
Hematologic: *neutropenia,* eosinophilia, *thrombocytopenia,* hemolytic anemia.
Musculoskeletal: bone growth retardation in children younger than age 8.
Skin: *maculopapular and erythematous rashes, photosensitivity, increased pigmentation, urticaria.*
Other: hypersensitivity reactions, *anaphylaxis,* superinfection; permanent discoloration of teeth, enamel defects.

INTERACTIONS
Drug-drug. *Antacids (including sodium bicarbonate) and laxatives containing aluminum, magnesium, or calcium; antidiarrheals:* Decreased antibiotic absorption. Give antibiotic 1 hour before or 2 hours after any of these drugs.
Carbamazepine, phenobarbital: Decreased antibiotic effect. Avoid using together.
Ferrous sulfate and other iron products, zinc: Decreased antibiotic absorption. Give drug 2 hours before or 3 hours after iron administration.
Methoxyflurane: May cause nephrotoxicity with tetracyclines. Avoid using together.
Oral anticoagulants: Increased anticoagulant effect. Monitor PT and INR, and adjust dosage.
Oral contraceptives: Decreased contraceptive effectiveness and increased risk of breakthrough bleeding. Advise use of a nonhormonal contraceptive.
Penicillins: May interfere with bactericidal action of penicillins. Avoid using together.
Drug-lifestyle. *Alcohol use:* Decreased antibiotic effect. Discourage use together.
Sun exposure: May cause photosensitivity reactions. Advise patient to avoid excessive sunlight exposure.

EFFECTS ON LAB TEST RESULTS
• May increase BUN and liver enzyme levels.
• May increase eosinophil count. May decrease hemoglobin and platelet, neutrophil, and WBC counts.

---

*Liquid contains alcohol.   **May contain tartrazine.   †Canada   ‡Australia   §U.K.   ◇OTC

CONTRAINDICATIONS

Contraindicated in patients hypersensitive to drug or other tetracyclines.

NURSING CONSIDERATIONS

• Use cautiously in patients with impaired renal or hepatic function. Use of these drugs during last half of pregnancy and in children younger than age 8 may cause permanent discoloration of teeth, enamel defects, and bone growth retardation.

• Obtain specimen for culture and sensitivity tests before giving first dose. Therapy may begin pending test results.

• *Alert:* Check expiration date. Outdated or deteriorated tetracyclines have been linked to reversible nephrotoxicity (Fanconi's syndrome).

• Give drug with milk or food if adverse GI reactions occur.

• Reconstituted injectable solution is stable for 72 hours if refrigerated and protected from light.

• If large doses are given, therapy is prolonged, or patient is at high risk, monitor patient for signs and symptoms of superinfection.

• Check patient's tongue for signs of fungal infection. Stress good oral hygiene.

• Drug isn't indicated for treatment of neurosyphilis.

• Photosensitivity reactions may occur within a few minutes to several hours after exposure. Photosensitivity lasts for some time after therapy ends.

• Drug causes false-negative results in urine glucose tests using glucose oxidase reagent (Diastix or Chemstrip uG). Parenteral dosage form may cause false-positive Clinitest results. Drug also falsely elevates fluorometric tests for urine catecholamines.

• *Alert:* Don't confuse doxycycline, doxylamine, and dicyclomine.

PATIENT TEACHING

• Tell patient to take entire amount of drug exactly as prescribed, even after he feels better.

• Instruct patient to report adverse reactions promptly. If drug is being given I.V., tell him to report discomfort at I.V site.

• Advise patient to take oral form of drug with food or milk if stomach upset occurs. Also advise patient to increase fluid intake and not to take oral tablets or capsules within 1 hour of bedtime because of possible esophageal irritation or ulceration.

• Warn patient to avoid direct sunlight and ultraviolet light, wear protective clothing, and use sunscreen.

• Tell patient to report signs and symptoms of superinfection to prescriber.

---

minocycline hydrochloride

Apo-Minocycline†, Dynacin, Minocin*, Minomycin‡, Vectrin

Pregnancy risk category D

AVAILABLE FORMS

Capsules (pellet-filled): 50 mg, 75 mg, 100 mg
Injection: 100 mg
Oral suspension: 50 mg/5 ml*
Tablets (film-coated): 50 mg, 100 mg

INDICATIONS & DOSAGES

➤ **Infections caused by susceptible gram-negative and gram-positive organisms (including *Haemophilus ducreyi*, *Yersinia pestis*, and *Campylobacter fetus*), *Rickettsiae species*, *Mycoplasma pneumoniae*, and *Chlamydia trachomatis*; psittacosis; granuloma inguinale—**
Adults: Initially, 200 mg I.V.; then 100 mg I.V. q 12 hours. Don't exceed 400 mg/day. Or, 200 mg P.O. initially; then 100 mg P.O. q 12 hours. May use 100 or 200 mg initially; then 50 mg q.i.d.
Children older than age 8: Initially, 4 mg/kg P.O. or I.V.; then 2 mg/kg q 12 hours.
Give I.V. in 500-ml to 1,000-ml solution without calcium and give over 6 hours.

➤ **Gonorrhea in patients allergic to penicillin—**
Adults: Initially, 200 mg P.O.; then 100 mg q 12 hours for at least 4 days.

➤ **Syphilis in patients allergic to penicillin—**
Adults: Initially, 200 mg P.O.; then 100 mg q 12 hours for 10 to 15 days.

➤ **Meningococcal carrier state—**
Adults: 100 mg P.O. q 12 hours for 5 days.

➤ **Uncomplicated urethral, endocervi-cal, or rectal infection caused by *C. tra-chomatis* or *Ureaplasma urealyticum*—**
Adults: 100 mg P.O. b.i.d. for at least 7 days.
➤ **Uncomplicated gonococcal urethritis in men—**
Adults: 100 mg P.O. b.i.d. for 5 days.

I.V. ADMINISTRATION
• Reconstitute 100 mg of powder with 5 ml of sterile water for injection, with further dilution to 500 to 1,000 ml for I.V. infusion. Although reconstituted solution is stable for 24 hours at room temperature, use as soon as possible.
• Infusions are usually given over 6 hours.
• Patient may develop thrombophlebitis with I.V. administration. Switch to oral therapy as soon as possible.

ACTION
Unknown. Thought to exert bacteriostatic effect by binding to the 30S and possibly 50S ribosomal subunits of microorgan-isms, thus inhibiting protein synthesis. May also alter the cytoplasmic membrane of susceptible microorganisms.

Route	Onset	Peak	Duration
I.V.	Immediate	Immediate	Unknown
P.O.	Unknown	1-4 hr	Unknown

ADVERSE REACTIONS
CNS: headache, ***intracranial hyperten-sion,*** light-headedness, dizziness, vertigo.
CV: pericarditis, *thrombophlebitis.*
GI: *anorexia,* dysphagia, glossitis, epigas-tric distress, oral candidiasis, *nausea,* vomiting, *diarrhea,* enterocolitis, inflam-matory lesions in anogenital region.
Hematologic: *neutropenia,* eosinophilia, ***thrombocytopenia,*** hemolytic anemia.
Musculoskeletal: bone growth retardation in children younger than age 8.
Skin: *maculopapular and erythematous rashes, photosensitivity, increased pig-mentation, urticaria.*
Other: hypersensitivity reactions, ***ana-phylaxis,*** superinfection; permanent dis-coloration of teeth, enamel defects.

INTERACTIONS
Drug-drug. *Antacids (including sodium bicarbonate) and laxatives containing aluminum, magnesium, or calcium; anti-diarrheals:* Decreased antibiotic absorp-tion. Give antibiotic 1 hour before or 2 hours after any of these drugs.
Ferrous sulfate and other iron products, zinc: Decreased antibiotic absorption. Give drug 2 hours before or 3 hours after iron administration.
Methoxyflurane: May cause nephrotoxici-ty when given with tetracyclines. Avoid using together.
Oral anticoagulants: Increased anticoagu-lant effect. Monitor PT and INR, and ad-just dosage.
Oral contraceptives: Decreased contra-ceptive effectiveness and increased risk of breakthrough bleeding. Advise patient to use nonhormonal contraceptive.
Penicillins: May disrupt bactericidal ac-tion of penicillins. Avoid using together.
Drug-lifestyle. *Sun exposure:* May cause photosensitivity reactions. Advise patient to avoid excessive sunlight exposure.

EFFECTS ON LAB TEST RESULTS
• May increase BUN and liver enzyme levels.
• May increase eosinophil count. May de-crease hemoglobin and platelet and neu-trophil counts.

CONTRAINDICATIONS
Contraindicated in patients hypersensitive to drug or other tetracyclines.

NURSING CONSIDERATIONS
• Use cautiously in patients with impaired renal or hepatic function. Use of these drugs during last half of pregnancy and in children younger than age 8 may cause permanent discoloration of teeth, enamel defects, and bone growth retardation.
• Monitor renal and liver function test re-sults.
• Minocycline causes false-negative re-sults in urine glucose tests using glucose oxidase reagent (Diastix or Chemstrip uG). Drug also falsely elevates fluoromet-ric tests for urine catecholamines. Par-enteral form may cause false-positive reading of copper sulfate tests (Clinitest).
• Obtain specimen for culture and sensi-tivity tests before first dose. Therapy may begin pending test results.

• *Alert:* Check expiration date. Outdated or deteriorated tetracyclines may cause reversible nephrotoxicity (Fanconi's syndrome).

• Don't expose drug to light or heat. Keep cap tightly closed.

• If large doses are given, therapy is prolonged, or patient is at high risk, monitor patient for signs and symptoms of superinfection.

• Check patient's tongue for signs of candidal infection. Stress good oral hygiene.

• Drug may cause tooth discoloration in young adults. Watch for brown pigmentation, and notify prescriber if it occurs.

• Drug isn't indicated for treatment of neurosyphilis.

• Photosensitivity reactions may occur within a few minutes to several hours after exposure. Photosensitivity lasts for some time after therapy ends.

• *Alert:* Don't confuse Minocin, niacin, and Mithracin.

PATIENT TEACHING

• Tell patient to take entire amount of drug exactly as prescribed, even after he feels better.

• Instruct patient to take oral form of drug with a full glass of water. Drug may be taken with food. Tell patient not to take within 1 hour of bedtime, to avoid esophageal irritation or ulceration.

• Warn patient to avoid driving or other hazardous tasks because of possible adverse CNS effects.

• Caution patient to avoid direct sunlight and ultraviolet light, wear protective clothing, and use sunscreen.

---

tetracycline hydrochloride
Apo-Tetra†, Novo-Tetra†,
Nu-Tetra†, Panmycin**, Sumycin,
Sustamycin§, Tetrachel§

Pregnancy risk category D

AVAILABLE FORMS
Capsules: 100 mg, 250 mg, 500 mg
Oral suspension: 125 mg/5 ml
Tablets: 250 mg, 500 mg

INDICATIONS & DOSAGES
➤ **Infections caused by susceptible gram-negative and -positive organisms (including *Haemophilus ducreyi, Yersinia pestis*, and *Campylobacter fetus*), *Rickettsiae* species, *Mycoplasma pneumoniae*, and *Chlamydia trachomatis*; psittacosis; granuloma inguinale—**
Adults: 250 to 500 mg P.O. q 6 hours.
Children older than age 8: 25 to 50 mg/kg P.O. daily, in divided doses q 6 hours.
➤ **Uncomplicated urethral, endocervical, or rectal infections caused by *C. trachomatis*—**
Adults: 500 mg P.O. q.i.d. for at least 7 days, 10 days for epididymitis, and 21 days for lymphogranuloma venereum.
➤ **Brucellosis—**
Adults: 500 mg P.O. q 6 hours for 3 weeks with 1 g of streptomycin I.M. q 12 hours for first week; once daily for second week.
➤ **Gonorrhea in patients allergic to penicillin—**
Adults: Initially, 1.5 g P.O.; then 500 mg q 6 hours for total dose of 9 g; for epididymitis, 500 mg P.O. q 6 hours for 7 days.
➤ **Syphilis in patients allergic to penicillin—**
Adults and adolescents: 500 mg P.O. q.i.d. for 2 weeks. Patients whose infection has lasted 1 year or longer may receive dose for 4 weeks.
➤ **Acne—**
Adults and adolescents: Initially, 250 mg P.O. q 6 hours; then 125 to 500 mg daily or every other day.
➤ ***Helicobacter pylori* infection—**
Adults: 500 mg P.O. q 6 hours for 10 to 14 days with other drugs, such as metronidazole, bismuth subsalicylate, amoxicillin, or omeprazole.
➤ **Cholera—**
Adults: 500 mg P.O. q 6 hours for 48 to 72 hours.
➤ **Malaria caused by *Plasmodium falciparum*—**
Adults: 250 to 500 mg P.O. daily for 7 days with quinine sulfate 650 mg P.O. q 8 hours for 3 to 7 days.

ACTION
Unknown. Thought to exert bacteriostatic effect by binding to the 30S and possibly 50S ribosomal subunits of microorgan-

---

isms, thus inhibiting protein synthesis. May also alter the cytoplasmic membrane of susceptible microorganisms.

Route	Onset	Peak	Duration
P.O.	Unknown	1-4 hr	Unknown

ADVERSE REACTIONS
CNS: dizziness, headache, *intracranial hypertension.*
CV: pericarditis.
EENT: sore throat.
GI: anorexia, dysphagia, glossitis, *epigastric distress, nausea,* vomiting, *diarrhea,* esophagitis, stomatitis, enterocolitis, oral candidiasis.
GU: inflammatory lesions in anogenital region.
Hematologic: *neutropenia,* eosinophilia, *thrombocytopenia.*
Musculoskeletal: *bone growth retardation in children younger than age 8.*
Skin: *candidal superinfection, maculopapular and erythematous rash, urticaria, photosensitivity, increased pigmentation.*
Other: hypersensitivity reactions, permanent discoloration of teeth, enamel defects.

INTERACTIONS
Drug-drug. *Antacids (including sodium bicarbonate) and laxatives containing aluminum, magnesium, or calcium; antidiarrheals containing kaolin, pectin, or bismuth subsalicylate:* Decreased antibiotic absorption. Give antibiotic 1 hour before or 2 hours after these drugs.
Ferrous sulfate and other iron products, zinc: Decreased antibiotic absorption. Give tetracyclines 2 hours before or 3 hours after these products.
Methoxyflurane: May cause severe nephrotoxicity with tetracyclines. Avoid using together.
Oral anticoagulants: Increased anticoagulant effects. Monitor PT and INR, and adjust anticoagulant dosage.
Oral contraceptives: Decreased contraceptive effectiveness and increased risk of breakthrough bleeding. Advise patient to use nonhormonal contraceptive.
Penicillins: May interfere with bactericidal action of penicillins. Avoid using together.

Drug-food. *Dairy products, other foods:* Decreased antibiotic absorption. Give antibiotic 1 hour before or 2 hours after any of these products.
Drug-lifestyle. *Sun exposure:* May cause photosensitivity reactions. Advise patient to avoid excessive sunlight exposure.

EFFECTS ON LAB TEST RESULTS
• May increase BUN and liver enzyme levels.
• May increase eosinophil counts. May decrease platelet and neutrophil counts.

CONTRAINDICATIONS
Contraindicated in patients hypersensitive to drug or other tetracyclines.

NURSING CONSIDERATIONS
• Use with extreme caution in patients with impaired renal or hepatic function. Monitor renal and liver function test results. Also use with extreme caution (if at all) during last half of pregnancy and in children younger than age 8 because drug may cause permanent discoloration of teeth, enamel defects, and bone growth retardation.
• Obtain specimen for culture and sensitivity tests before giving first dose. Therapy may begin pending test results.
• *Alert:* Check expiration date. Outdated or deteriorated tetracyclines have been linked to reversible nephrotoxicity (Fanconi's syndrome).
• Don't expose drug to light or heat.
• If large doses are given, therapy is prolonged, or patient is at high risk, monitor patient for signs and symptoms of superinfection.
• Check patient's tongue for signs of candidal infection. Stress good oral hygiene.
• Drug isn't indicated for treatment of neurosyphilis.
• Photosensitivity reactions may occur within a few minutes to several hours after sun exposure. Photosensitivity lasts for some time after therapy ends.
• Tetracycline causes false-negative results in urine glucose tests using glucose oxidase reagent (Diastix or Chemstrip uG) and falsely elevates fluorometric tests for urine catecholamines.

---

*Liquid contains alcohol.   **May contain tartrazine.   †Canada   ‡Australia   §U.K.   ◊OTC

PATIENT TEACHING

● Tell patient to take drug exactly as prescribed, even after he feels better, and to take entire amount prescribed.

● Explain that effectiveness is reduced when drug is taken with milk or other dairy products, food, antacids, or iron products. Tell patient to take each dose with a full glass of water on an empty stomach, at least 1 hour before or 2 hours after meals. Also tell him to take it at least 1 hour before bedtime to prevent esophageal irritation or ulceration.

● Warn patient to avoid direct sunlight and ultraviolet light, wear protective clothing, and use sunscreen.

13

Sulfonamides

co-trimoxazole
sulfadiazine
sulfamethoxazole
sulfisoxazole
sulfisoxazole acetyl

COMBINATION PRODUCTS

AZO GANTANOL, AZO-SULFAMETHOXA-
ZOLE† tablets (film-coated): sulfamethoxazole 500 mg and phenazopyridine hydrochloride 100 mg
AZO GANTRISIN, AZO-SULFISOXAZOLE
tablets (film-coated): sulfisoxazole
500 mg and phenazopyridine hydrochloride 50 mg
ERYZOLE, PEDIAZOLE, SULFIMYCIN suspension: sulfisoxazole 600 mg and erythromycin ethylsuccinate 200 mg/5 ml

---

co-trimoxazole
(sulfamethoxazole-
trimethoprim)

Apo-Sulfatrim†, Apo-Sulfatrim
DS†, Bactrim*, Bactrim DS,
Bactrim IV, Cotrim, Cotrim D.S.,
Cotrim Pediatric*, Novo-Trimel†,
Novo-Trimel D.S.†, Nu-Cotrimox†,
Resprim‡, Roubac†, Septra*,
Septra DS, Septra IV, Septrin‡,
SMZ-TMP, Sulfatrim

Pregnancy risk category C

AVAILABLE FORMS

Injection: trimethoprim 16 mg/ml and sulfamethoxazole 80 mg/ml in 5-ml, 10-ml,
20-ml, and 30-ml vials
Oral suspension: trimethoprim 40 mg and
sulfamethoxazole 200 mg/5 ml*
Tablets (double-strength): trimethoprim
160 mg and sulfamethoxazole 800 mg
Tablets (single-strength): trimethoprim
80 mg and sulfamethoxazole 400 mg

INDICATIONS & DOSAGES

➤ **Shigellosis or urinary tract infections
(UTIs) caused by susceptible strains of
Escherichia coli, *Proteus* (indole positive
or negative), *Klebsiella*, or *Enterobacter
species*—**
Adults: 160 mg trimethoprim/800 mg sulfamethoxazole, one double-strength tablet,
P.O. q 12 hours for 10 to 14 days in UTIs
and for 5 days in shigellosis. If indicated,
I.V. infusion is given: 8 to 10 mg/kg/day
based on trimethoprim component in two
to four divided doses q 6, 8, or 12 hours
for 5 days for shigellosis or up to 14 days
for severe UTIs. Maximum daily dose is
960 mg trimethoprim (as co-trimoxazole).
Children age 2 months and older: 8 mg/
kg/day based on trimethoprim component
P.O., in two divided doses q 12 hours for
10 days for UTIs and 5 days for shigellosis. If indicated, I.V. infusion is given: 8
to 10 mg/kg/day based on trimethoprim
component, in two to four divided doses q
6, 8, or 12 hours. Don't exceed adult dose.
➤ **Otitis media in patients with penicillin allergy or penicillin-resistant
infections—**
Children age 2 months and older: 8 mg/
kg/day based on trimethoprim component
P.O., in two divided doses q 12 hours for
10 to 14 days.
➤ **Chronic bronchitis, upper respiratory tract infections—**
Adults: 160 mg trimethoprim and 800 mg
sulfamethoxazole P.O. q 12 hours for 10 to
14 days.
➤ **Traveler's diarrhea—**
Adults: 160 mg trimethoprim and 800 mg
sulfamethoxazole P.O. b.i.d. for 3 to 5
days. Some patients may only need up to
2 days of therapy.
➤ **Prophylaxis for *Pneumocystis carinii*
pneumonia—**
Adults: 160 mg of trimethoprim and
800 mg sulfamethoxazole P.O. daily; or
80 mg trimethoprim/400 mg sulfamethoxazole P.O. three times weekly.
Children age 2 months and older:
150 mg/m² trimethoprim/750 mg/m² sulfamethoxazole P.O. daily in two divided
doses on 3 consecutive days each week.
➤ **P. carinii pneumonia—**
*Adults and children older than age 2
months:* 15 to 20 mg/kg/day based on

---

*Liquid contains alcohol.   **May contain tartrazine.   †Canada   ‡Australia   §U.K.   ◇OTC

trimethoprim I.V. or P.O. in three or four divided doses for 14 to 21 days.

Adjust-a-dose: For patients with renal failure whose creatinine clearance is 15 to 30 ml/minute, daily dose should be reduced by 50%. Drug isn't recommended for patients with creatinine clearance below 15 ml/minute.

I.V. ADMINISTRATION
• Dilute each 5 ml of concentrate for I.V. infusion in 75 to 125 ml of D₅W before administration. Don't mix with other drugs or solutions.
• Infuse slowly over 60 to 90 minutes. Don't give by rapid infusion or bolus injection.
• Don't refrigerate; use within 6 hours if diluted in 125 ml and within 2 hours if diluted in 75 ml. Discard solution if cloudiness or evidence of crystallization is noted after mixing.

ACTION
Sulfamethoxazole inhibits formation of dihydrofolic acid from PABA; trimethoprim inhibits dihydrofolate reductase formation. Both decrease bacterial folic acid synthesis; bactericidal.

Route	Onset	Peak	Duration
I.V.	Immediate	1-1.5 hr	Unknown
P.O.	Unknown	1-4 hr	Unknown

ADVERSE REACTIONS
CNS: headache, mental depression, aseptic meningitis, tinnitus, apathy, *seizures,* hallucinations, ataxia, nervousness, fatigue, vertigo, insomnia.
CV: thrombophlebitis.
GI: *nausea, vomiting, diarrhea,* abdominal pain, anorexia, stomatitis, *pancreatitis,* pseudomembranous colitis.
GU: *toxic nephrosis with oliguria and anuria,* crystalluria, hematuria, interstitial nephritis.
Hematologic: *agranulocytosis, aplastic anemia,* megaloblastic anemia, *thrombocytopenia, leukopenia, hemolytic anemia.*
Hepatic: jaundice, *hepatic necrosis.*
Musculoskeletal: arthralgia, myalgia, muscle weakness.
Respiratory: pulmonary infiltrates.
Skin: *erythema multiforme, Stevens-Johnson syndrome, generalized skin*

eruption, **epidermal necrolysis, exfoliative dermatitis,** photosensitivity, urticaria, pruritus.
Other: hypersensitivity reactions, *serum sickness, drug fever, anaphylaxis.*

INTERACTIONS
Drug-drug. *Cyclosporine:* May decrease cyclosporine levels and increase nephrotoxicity risk. Avoid using together.
Dofetilide: May increase dofetilide levels and effects. Increased risk of prolonged QT syndrome and fatal ventricular arrhythmias. Avoid using together.
Methotrexate: May increase methotrexate levels. Use together cautiously.
Oral anticoagulants: Increased anticoagulant effect. Monitor patient for bleeding.
Oral antidiabetics: Increased hypoglycemic effect. Monitor glucose levels.
Oral contraceptives: Decreased contraceptive effectiveness and increased risk of breakthrough bleeding. Advise patient to use a nonhormonal contraceptive.
Phenytoin: May inhibit hepatic metabolism of phenytoin. Monitor patient closely.
Drug-herb. *Dong quai, St. John's wort:* Increased photosensitivity risk. Advise patient to avoid excessive sunlight exposure.
Drug-lifestyle. *Sun exposure:* May cause photosensitivity reactions. Advise patient to avoid excessive sunlight exposure.

EFFECTS ON LAB TEST RESULTS
• May increase BUN, creatinine, aminotransferase, and bilirubin levels.
• May decrease hemoglobin and granulocyte, platelet, and WBC counts.

CONTRAINDICATIONS
Contraindicated in patients hypersensitive to trimethoprim or sulfonamides and in those with severe renal impairment (creatinine clearance less than 15 ml/minute), porphyria, or megaloblastic anemia from folate deficiency. Also contraindicated in pregnant women at term, in breast-feeding women, and in infants younger than age 2 months.

NURSING CONSIDERATIONS
• Use cautiously and in reduced dosages in patients with impaired hepatic or renal function (creatinine clearance 15 to 30 ml/

minute), severe allergy or bronchial asthma, G6PD deficiency, and blood dyscrasia.

• Obtain specimen for culture and sensitivity tests before first dose. Therapy may begin pending results.

• *Alert:* Double-check dosage, which may be written as trimethoprim component.

• *Alert:* "DS" product means "double strength."

• Never administer drug I.M.

• Monitor renal and liver function test results.

• Trimethoprim can interfere with serum methotrexate assay as determined by the competitive binding protein technique. No interference occurs if radioimmunoassay is used.

• Promptly report rash, sore throat, fever, cough, mouth sores, or iris lesions—early signs and symptoms of erythema multiforme, which may progress to the sometimes-fatal Stevens-Johnson syndrome. These symptoms may also represent early signs of blood dyscrasias.

• Watch for superinfection: fever or other signs or symptoms of new infection.

• *Alert:* Adverse reactions, especially hypersensitivity reactions, rash, and fever, occur much more frequently in patients with AIDS.

PATIENT TEACHING
• Tell patient to take drug as prescribed, even if he feels better.

• Encourage patient to maintain adequate fluid intake.

• Tell patient to report adverse reactions promptly.

• Instruct patient receiving drug I.V. to report discomfort at I.V. insertion site.

• Advise patient to avoid prolonged sun exposure, wear protective clothing, and use sunscreen.

• Instruct patient to take oral form with 8 ounces (240 ml) of water on an empty stomach.

---

sulfadiazine
Coptin†

Pregnancy risk category C

AVAILABLE FORMS
Tablets: 500 mg

INDICATIONS & DOSAGES
➤ **Asymptomatic meningococcal carriers—**
Adults: 1 g P.O. q 12 hours for 2 days.
Children ages 1 to 12: 500 mg P.O. q 12 hours for 2 days.
Children ages 2 to 12 months: 500 mg P.O. daily for 2 days.
➤ **Rheumatic fever prophylaxis, as an alternative to penicillin—**
Children weighing more than 30 kg (66 lb): 1 g P.O. daily.
Children weighing less than 30 kg: 500 mg P.O. daily.
➤ **Adjunct treatment in toxoplasmosis—**
Adults: 4 to 6 g P.O. daily divided q 6 hours for 6 to 8 weeks or until improvement occurs. Usually given with pyrimethamine.
Children: 100 to 200 mg/kg P.O. daily divided q 6 hours for 6 to 8 weeks or until improvement occurs. Maximum 6 g daily. Usually given with pyrimethamine.
➤ **Malaria, chloroquine-resistant *Plasmodium falciparum*—**
Adults: 500 mg P.O. q.i.d. for 5 days with quinine sulfate and pyrimethamine.
Children: 25 to 50 mg/kg P.O. q.i.d. for 5 days with quinine sulfate and pyrimethamine. Maximum 2 g daily.
➤ **Nocardiosis—**
Adults: 4 to 8 g P.O. daily given in divided doses for a minimum of 6 weeks.

ACTION
Inhibits formation of dihydrofolic acid from PABA, decreasing bacterial folic acid synthesis; bacteriostatic.

Route	Onset	Peak	Duration
P.O.	Unknown	4-6 hr	Unknown

ADVERSE REACTIONS
CNS: headache, mental depression, *seizures,* hallucinations.
GI: *nausea, vomiting, diarrhea,* abdominal pain, anorexia, stomatitis.
GU: *toxic nephrosis with oliguria and anuria,* crystalluria, hematuria.
Hematologic: *agranulocytosis, aplastic anemia,* megaloblastic anemia, *thrombocytopenia, leukopenia, hemolytic anemia.*
Hepatic: jaundice.

Skin: *erythema multiforme, Stevens-Johnson syndrome, generalized skin eruption, epidermal necrolysis, exfoliative dermatitis,* photosensitivity, urticaria, pruritus.
Other: hypersensitivity reactions, *serum sickness, drug fever, anaphylaxis,* local irritation, extravasation.

INTERACTIONS
Drug-drug. *Methotrexate:* May increase methotrexate levels. Use together cautiously.
Oral anticoagulants: Increased anticoagulant effect. Monitor patient for bleeding.
Oral antidiabetics: Increased hypoglycemic effect. Monitor glucose levels.
Oral contraceptives: Decreased contraceptive effectiveness and increased risk of breakthrough bleeding. Advise patient to use a nonhormonal contraceptive.
PABA-containing drugs: Inhibited antibacterial action. Avoid using together.
Drug-herb. *Dong quai, St. John's wort:* Increased photosensivity risk. Advise patient to avoid excessive sunlight exposure.
Drug-lifestyle. *Sun exposure:* May cause photosensitivity reaction. Advise patient to avoid excessive sunlight exposure.

EFFECTS ON LAB TEST RESULTS
● May increase BUN, creatinine, transaminase, and bilirubin levels.
● May increase eosinophil count. May decrease hemoglobin and PT and fibrinogen, granulocyte, platelet, and WBC counts.

CONTRAINDICATIONS
Contraindicated in patients hypersensitive to sulfonamides, in those with porphyria, in infants younger than age 2 months (except in congenital toxoplasmosis), in pregnant women at term, and in breast-feeding women.

NURSING CONSIDERATIONS
● Use cautiously and in reduced doses in patients with impaired hepatic or renal function, bronchial asthma, history of multiple allergies, G6PD deficiency, and blood dyscrasia.
● Give drug on schedule to maintain constant blood level.
● Monitor patient for signs and symptoms of blood dyscrasia (purpura, ecchymoses,

sore throat, fever, and pallor). Report these immediately.
● Promptly report rash, sore throat, fever, cough, mouth sores, or iris lesions— early signs and symptoms of erythema multiforme, which may progress to the sometimes-fatal Stevens-Johnson syndrome.
● Monitor urine cultures, CBCs, and urinalyses before and during therapy.
● Monitor renal and liver function test results.
● Watch for superinfection: fever or other signs or symptoms of new infection.
● Folic or folinic acid may be used during rest periods in toxoplasmosis therapy to reverse hematopoietic depression or anemia associated with pyrimethamine and sulfadiazine.
● Monitor fluid intake and output. Maintain intake between 3,000 and 4,000 ml daily for adults to produce output of 1,500 ml daily. If fluid intake isn't adequate to prevent crystalluria, sodium bicarbonate may be given to alkalinize urine. Monitor urine pH daily.
● Drug alters urine glucose tests using cupric sulfate (Benedict's reagent or Chemstrip uG).
● **Alert:** Don't confuse sulfadiazine with sulfasalazine. Don't confuse sulfonamide drugs.

PATIENT TEACHING
● Tell patient to take drug as prescribed, even if he feels better.
● Urge patient to drink a glass of water with each dose, plus plenty of water each day to prevent crystalluria.
● Instruct patient to report adverse reactions promptly.
● Warn patient to avoid prolonged exposure to sunlight, wear protective clothing, and use sunscreen.

sulfamethoxazole (sulphamethoxazole)
Apo-Sulfamethoxazole†, Gantanol

Pregnancy risk category C

AVAILABLE FORMS
Tablets: 500 mg

Reactions may be *common*, uncommon, *life-threatening*, or COMMON AND LIFE-THREATENING.

INDICATIONS & DOSAGES
➤ **Urinary tract and systemic infections—**
Adults: Initially, 2 g P.O.; then 1 g P.O. b.i.d. up to t.i.d. for severe infections.
Children and infants older than age 2 months: Initially, 50 to 60 mg/kg P.O.; then 25 to 30 mg/kg b.i.d. Maximum daily dose shouldn't exceed 75 mg/kg.

ACTION
Inhibits formation of dihydrofolic acid from PABA, decreasing bacterial folic acid synthesis; bacteriostatic.

Route	Onset	Peak	Duration
P.O.	Unknown	2 hr	Unknown

ADVERSE REACTIONS
CNS: headache, mental depression, *seizures,* hallucinations, aseptic meningitis, apathy, dizziness.
EENT: tinnitus.
GI: *nausea, vomiting, diarrhea,* abdominal pain, anorexia, stomatitis, *pancreatitis,* pseudomembranous colitis.
GU: *toxic nephrosis with oliguria and anuria,* crystalluria, hematuria, interstitial nephritis.
Hematologic: *agranulocytosis, aplastic anemia,* megaloblastic anemia, *thrombocytopenia, leukopenia, hemolytic anemia.*
Hepatic: jaundice.
Skin: *erythema multiforme, Stevens-Johnson syndrome,* generalized skin eruption, *epidermal necrolysis, exfoliative dermatitis,* photosensitivity, urticaria, pruritus.
Other: hypersensitivity reactions, *serum sickness, drug fever, anaphylaxis.*

INTERACTIONS
Drug-drug. *Methotrexate:* May increase methotrexate levels. Use together cautiously.
Oral anticoagulants: Increased anticoagulant effect. Monitor patient for bleeding.
Oral antidiabetics: Increased hypoglycemic effect. Monitor glucose levels.
Oral contraceptives: Decreased contraceptive effectiveness and increased risk of breakthrough bleeding. Advise patient to use a nonhormonal contraceptive.
Phenytoin: May increase phenytoin effect. Monitor patient closely.

Drug-herb. *Dong quai, St. John's wort:* Increased photosensivity. Advise patient to avoid excessive sunlight exposure.
Drug-lifestyle. *Sun exposure:* May cause photosensitivity reactions. Advise patient to avoid excessive sunlight exposure.

EFFECTS ON LAB TEST RESULTS
• May increase BUN, creatinine, aminotransferase, and bilirubin levels.
• May increase eosinophil count. May decrease PT and hemoglobin and fibrinogen, granulocyte, platelet, and WBC counts.

CONTRAINDICATIONS
Contraindicated in patients hypersensitive to sulfonamides, in those with porphyria, in infants younger than age 2 months (except in congenital toxoplasmosis), in pregnant women at term, and in breast-feeding women.

NURSING CONSIDERATIONS
• Use cautiously and in reduced dosages in patients with impaired hepatic or renal function, severe allergy or bronchial asthma, G6PD deficiency, and blood dyscrasia.
• Obtain specimen for culture and sensitivity tests before first dose. Therapy may begin pending results.
• Monitor urine cultures, CBCs, and urinalyses before and during therapy.
• Watch for superinfection: fever or other signs or symptoms of new infection.
• Monitor fluid intake and output. Maintain intake between 3,000 and 4,000 ml daily for adults to produce output of 1,500 ml daily. If fluid intake isn't adequate to prevent crystalluria, sodium bicarbonate may be given to alkalinize urine. Monitor urine pH daily.
• Monitor renal and liver function test results.
• Drug alters results of urine glucose tests using cupric sulfate (Benedict's reagent or Clinitest).
• **Alert:** Don't confuse sulfamethoxazole with sulfamethizole. Don't confuse the combination products with sulfamethoxazole alone.

PATIENT TEACHING
• Tell patient to take drug as prescribed, even if he feels better.

---

*Liquid contains alcohol.   **May contain tartrazine.   †Canada   ‡Australia   §U.K.   ◇OTC

• Instruct patient to drink a glass of water with each dose, plus plenty of water each day to prevent crystalluria.

• *Alert:* Tell patient to notify prescriber of sore throat, fever, and pallor (early signs and symptoms of blood dyscrasia). Also tell patient to be alert for flulike symptoms, cough, and lesions of the iris, skin, and mucous membranes.

• Warn patient to avoid prolonged exposure to sunlight, to wear protective clothing, and to use sunscreen.

---

sulfisoxazole (sulfafurazole, sulphafurazole)
Novo-Soxazole†

sulfisoxazole acetyl
Gantrisin Pediatric

Pregnancy risk category C

AVAILABLE FORMS
sulfisoxazole
Tablets: 500 mg
sulfisoxazole acetyl
Liquid: 500 mg/5 ml*

INDICATIONS & DOSAGES
➤ **Urinary tract and systemic infections—**
Adults: Initially, 2 to 4 g P.O.; then 4 to 8 g daily divided in four to six doses.
Children older than age 2 months: Initially, 75 mg/kg P.O. daily or 2 g/m² P.O.; then 150 mg/kg or 4 g/m² P.O. daily in divided doses q 6 hours. Total daily dose shouldn't exceed 6 g.
➤ **Chlamydia trachomatis (lymphogranuloma venereum)—**
Adults: 500 mg to 1 g P.O. q.i.d. for 21 days.
➤ **Uncomplicated urethral, endocervical, or rectal infections with *C. trachomatis*—**
Adults: 500 mg P.O. q.i.d. for 10 days.
Adjust-a-dose: For patients with renal failure, use normal dose at longer intervals. If creatinine clearance is 10 to 50 ml/minute, give q 8 to 12 hours; if clearance is less than 10 ml/minute, give q 12 to 24 hours.

ACTION
Inhibits formation of dihydrofolic acid from PABA, decreasing bacterial folic acid synthesis; bacteriostatic.

Route	Onset	Peak	Duration
P.O.	Unknown	1-4 hr	Unknown

ADVERSE REACTIONS
CNS: headache, mental depression, *seizures,* hallucinations, dizziness.
CV: tachycardia, palpitations, syncope, cyanosis.
GI: *nausea, vomiting, diarrhea,* abdominal pain, anorexia, stomatitis, pseudomembranous colitis.
GU: *toxic nephrosis with oliguria and anuria,* crystalluria, hematuria, *acute renal failure.*
Hematologic: *agranulocytosis, aplastic anemia,* megaloblastic anemia, *thrombocytopenia, leukopenia, hemolytic anemia.*
Hepatic: jaundice, *hepatitis.*
Skin: *erythema multiforme, generalized skin eruption, epidermal necrolysis,* exfoliative dermatitis, photosensitivity, urticaria, pruritus.
Other: hypersensitivity reactions, *serum sickness, drug fever, anaphylaxis.*

INTERACTIONS
Drug-drug. *Methotrexate:* May increase methotrexate levels. Use together cautiously.
Oral anticoagulants: Increased anticoagulant effect. Monitor patient for bleeding.
Oral antidiabetics: Increased hypoglycemic effect. Monitor glucose levels.
Oral contraceptives: Decreased contraceptive effectiveness and increased risk of breakthrough bleeding. Advise patient to use a nonhormonal contraceptive.
Drug-herb. *Dong quai, St. John's wort:* Increased photosensivity. Advise patient to avoid excessive sunlight exposure.
Drug-lifestyle. *Sun exposure:* May cause photosensitivity reactions. Advise patient to avoid excessive sunlight exposure.

EFFECTS ON LAB TEST RESULTS
• May increase BUN, creatinine, aminotransferase, and bilirubin levels.
• May increase eosinophil count. May decrease hemoglobin and PT and fibrinogen, granulocyte, platelet, and WBC counts.

Reactions may be *common,* uncommon, *life-threatening,* or **COMMON AND LIFE-THREATENING.**

CONTRAINDICATIONS

Contraindicated in patients hypersensitive to sulfonamides, in infants younger than age 2 months (except in congenital toxoplasmosis), in pregnant women at term, and in breast-feeding women.

NURSING CONSIDERATIONS

• Use cautiously in patients with impaired hepatic or renal function, severe allergy or bronchial asthma, and G6PD deficiency.
• Obtain specimen for culture and sensitivity tests before giving first dose. Therapy may begin pending results.
• Monitor urine cultures, CBC, PT, INR, and urinalyses before and during therapy.
• Monitor renal and liver function test results.
• Report moderate to severe diarrhea to prescriber.
• Watch for superinfection: fever or other signs or symptoms of new infection.
• Monitor fluid intake and output. Maintain intake between 3,000 and 4,000 ml daily for adults to produce output of 1,500 ml daily. If fluid intake isn't adequate to prevent crystalluria, sodium bicarbonate may be given to alkalinize urine. Monitor urine pH daily.
• Drug alters results of urine glucose tests using cupric sulfate (Benedict's reagent or Chemstrip uG).
• *Alert:* Don't confuse sulfisoxazole with sulfasalazine. Don't confuse the combination products with sulfisoxazole alone.

PATIENT TEACHING

• Tell patient to take drug as prescribed, even if he feels better.
• Instruct patient to drink a glass of water with each dose, plus plenty of water each day to prevent crystalluria.
• Advise patient to report rash, sore throat, fever, pallor, or jaundice immediately.

---

*Liquid contains alcohol. **May contain tartrazine. †Canada ‡Australia §U.K. ◊OTC

14

Fluoroquinolones

ciprofloxacin
enoxacin
gatifloxacin
levofloxacin
moxifloxacin hydrochloride
nalidixic acid
norfloxacin
sparfloxacin
trovafloxacin mesylate,
   alatrofloxacin mesylate

COMBINATION PRODUCTS
None.

---

ciprofloxacin
Cipro, Cipro I.V., Ciproxin‡

Pregnancy risk category C

AVAILABLE FORMS
Infusion (premixed): 200 mg in 100 ml
D_5W, 400 mg in 200 ml D_5W
Injection: 200 mg, 400 mg
Suspension (oral): 5 g/100 ml (5%), 10 g/
100 ml (10%)
Tablets (film-coated): 100 mg, 250 mg,
500 mg, 750 mg

INDICATIONS & DOSAGES
➤ **Mild to moderate urinary tract infections (UTIs) caused by** *Escherichia coli, Klebsiella pneumoniae, Enterobacter cloacae, Serratia marcescens, Proteus mirabilis, Providencia rettgeri, Morganella morganii, Citrobacter diversus, C. freundii, Pseudomonas aeruginosa, Staphylococcus epidermidis,* **and** *Enterococcus faecalis*—
Adults: 250 mg P.O. or 200 mg I.V. q 12
hours.
➤ **Severe or complicated UTIs; mild to moderate bone and joint infections caused by** *E. cloacae, P. aeruginosa,* **and** *S. marcescens;* **mild to moderate respiratory infections caused by** *E. coli, K. pneumoniae, E. cloacae, P. mirabilis, P. aeruginosa, Haemophilus influenzae,* **and** *H. parainfluenzae;* **mild to moder-**
ate skin and skin-structure infections caused by *E. coli, K. pneumoniae, E. cloacae, P. mirabilis, P. vulgaris, Providencia stuartii, M. morganii, C. freundii, Streptococcus pyogenes, P. aeruginosa, Staphylococcus aureus,* **and** *S. epidermidis;* **infectious diarrhea caused by** *E. coli, Campylobacter jejuni, Shigella flexneri,* **and** *S. sonnei;* **typhoid fever**—
Adults: 500 mg P.O. or 400 mg I.V. q 12
hours.
➤ **Severe or complicated bone or joint infections, severe respiratory tract infections, severe skin and skin-structure infections**—
Adults: 750 mg P.O. q 12 hours or 400 mg
I.V. q 8 to 12 hours.
➤ **Chronic bacterial prostatitis caused by** *E. coli* **or** *P. mirabilis*—
Adults: 500 mg P.O. q 12 hours or 400 mg
I.V. q 12 hours for 28 days.
➤ **Complicated intra-abdominal infections caused by** *E. coli, P. aeruginosa, P. mirabilis, K. pneumoniae,* **or** *Bacteroides fragilis*—
Adults: 500 mg P.O. or 400 mg I.V. q 12
hours for 7 to 14 days. Give with metronidazole.
➤ **Acute uncomplicated cystitis**—
Adults: 100 mg P.O. q 12 hours for 3 days.
➤ **Mild to moderate acute sinusitis**—
Adults: 500 mg P.O. or 400 mg I.V. q 12
hours for 10 days.
➤ **Mild to moderate acute sinusitis caused by** *H. influenzae, Streptococcus pneumoniae,* **or** *Moraxella catarrhalis;* **mild to moderate chronic bacterial prostatitis caused by** *E. coli* **or** *P. mirabilis*—
Adults: 400 mg I.V. infusion given over
60 minutes q 12 hours or 500 mg P.O. q
12 hours.
➤ **Empirical therapy in febrile neutropenic patients**—
Adults: 400 mg I.V. q 8 hours used with
pipercillin 50 mg/kg I.V. q 4 hours (not to
exceed 24 g/day maximum).

Reactions may be *common*, uncommon, *life-threatening*, or COMMON AND LIFE-THREATENING.

➤ **To reduce the incidence of progression of disease following exposure to aerosolized *Bacillus anthracis* (anthrax)—**
Adults: 500 mg P.O. every 12 hours for 60 days, beginning as soon as possible after suspected or confirmed exposure.
Children: 15 mg/kg/dose P.O. every 12 hours for 60 days, beginning as soon as possible after suspected or confirmed exposure. Maximum dose 500 mg.
Adjust-a-dose: For patients with renal failure, if creatinine clearance is 30 to 50 ml/minute, give 250 to 500 mg P.O. q 12 hours or the usual I.V. dose; if clearance is 5 to 29 ml/minute, give 250 to 500 mg P.O. q 18 hours or 200 to 400 mg I.V. q 18 to 24 hours. If patient is on hemodialysis, give 250 to 500 mg P.O. q 24 hours after dialysis.

I.V. ADMINISTRATION
● Dilute drug using D₅W or normal saline solution for injection to a final concentration of 1 to 2 mg/ml before use. Infuse slowly (over 1 hour) into a large vein to minimize discomfort and reduce the risk of venous irritation.
● If administering drug through a Y-type set, discontinue the other I.V. solution during ciprofloxacin infusion.

ACTION
Inhibits bacterial DNA synthesis, mainly by blocking DNA gyrase; bactericidal.

Route	Onset	Peak	Duration
I.V.	Unknown	Immediate	Unknown
P.O.	Unknown	0.5-2.3 hr	Unknown

ADVERSE REACTIONS
CNS: headache, restlessness, tremor, dizziness, fatigue, drowsiness, insomnia, depression, light-headedness, confusion, hallucinations, *seizures,* paresthesia.
CV: thrombophlebitis, edema, chest pain.
GI: *nausea, diarrhea,* vomiting, abdominal pain or discomfort, oral candidiasis, pseudomembranous colitis, dyspepsia, flatulence, constipation.
GU: crystalluria, interstitial nephritis.
Hematologic: eosinophilia, *leukopenia, neutropenia, thrombocytopenia.*
Musculoskeletal: arthralgia, arthropathy, joint or back pain, joint inflammation,

joint stiffness, tendon rupture, aching, neck pain.
Skin: *rash,* photosensitivity, ***Stevens-Johnson syndrome, toxic epidermal necrolysis,*** exfoliative dermatitis, burning, pruritus, erythema.
Other: hypersensitivity reactions.

INTERACTIONS
Drug-drug. *Antacids containing aluminum hydroxide or magnesium hydroxide, iron supplements, multivitamins containing iron or zinc, sucralfate:* Decreased ciprofloxacin absorption. Don't give ciprofloxacin 2 hours before or 6 hours after antacid.
NSAIDs: May increase risk of CNS stimulation. Monitor patient closely.
Probenecid: May elevate serum level of ciprofloxacin. Monitor patient for toxicity.
Theophylline: Increased plasma theophylline levels and prolonged theophylline half-life. Monitor blood levels of theophylline and observe for adverse effects.
Drug-herb. *Dong quai, St. John's wort:* May cause photosensitivity. Advise patient to avoid excessive sunlight exposure.
Yerba maté: May decrease clearance of yerba maté's methylxanthines and cause toxicity. Discourage use together.
Drug-food. *Caffeine:* Increased effect of caffeine. Monitor patient closely.
Dairy products, other foods: Delayed peak serum levels. Advise patient to take drug on an empty stomach.
Drug-lifestyle. *Sun exposure:* May cause photosensitivity. Advise patient to avoid excessive sunlight exposure.

EFFECTS ON LAB TEST RESULTS
● May increase BUN, creatinine, ALT, AST, alkaline phosphatase, bilirubin, LDH, and GGT levels.
● May increase eosinophil count. May decrease WBC, neutrophil, and platelet counts.

CONTRAINDICATIONS
Contraindicated in patients sensitive to fluoroquinolones.

NURSING CONSIDERATIONS
● Use cautiously in patients with CNS disorders, such as severe cerebral arteriescle-

---

*Liquid contains alcohol.   **May contain tartrazine.   †Canada   ‡Australia   §U.K.   ◊OTC

rosis or seizure disorders, and in those at risk for seizures. Drug may cause CNS stimulation.

• Obtain specimen for culture and sensitivity tests before giving first dose. Therapy may begin pending results.

• Give oral form 2 hours after a meal or 2 hours before or after taking antacids, sucralfate, or products that contain iron (such as vitamins with mineral supplements). Food doesn't affect absorption but may delay peak serum levels.

• Monitor patient's intake and output and observe for signs of crystalluria.

• Tendon rupture has been reported in patients receiving quinolones. Discontinue if pain, inflammation, or tendon rupture occurs.

• Long-term therapy may result in overgrowth of organisms resistant to ciprofloxacin.

• Safety in children younger than age 18 hasn't been established. Drug may cause cartilage erosion.

PATIENT TEACHING

• Tell patient to take drug as prescribed, even after he feels better.

• Advise patient to drink plenty of fluids to reduce risk of crystalluria.

• Tell patient to take drug on an empty stomach, 2 hours after a meal.

• Warn patient to avoid hazardous tasks that require alertness, such as driving, until CNS effects of drug are known.

• Instruct patient to avoid caffeine while taking drug because of potential for increased caffeine effects.

• Advise patient that hypersensitivity reactions may occur even after first dose. If a rash or other allergic reaction occurs, tell him to stop drug immediately and notify prescriber.

• Tell patient to report pain, inflammation, or tendon rupture immediately.

• Tell patient to avoid excessive sunlight or artificial ultraviolet light during therapy and to stop drug and call prescriber if phototoxicity occurs.

• Because drug appears in breast milk, advise woman to discontinue breast-feeding during treatment or to consider treatment with another drug.

enoxacin
Penetrex

Pregnancy risk category C

AVAILABLE FORMS
Tablets (film-coated): 200 mg, 400 mg

INDICATIONS & DOSAGES
➤ **Uncomplicated urinary tract infections (UTIs) caused by susceptible strains of *Escherichia coli, Staphylococcus epidermidis,* and *S. saprophyticus*—**
Adults age 18 and older: 200 mg P.O. q 12 hours for 7 days.
➤ **Severe or complicated UTIs caused by susceptible strains of *E. coli, Proteus mirabilis, Pseudomonas aeruginosa, S. epidermidis,* and *Enterobacter cloacae*—**
Adults age 18 and older: 400 mg P.O. q 12 hours for 14 days.
➤ **Uncomplicated urethral or endocervical gonorrhea—**
Adults: 400 mg P.O. as a single dose.

Doxycycline therapy may follow to treat coexisting chlamydial infection.
Adjust-a-dose: For patients with renal failure, if creatinine clearance is 30 ml/minute or less, therapy starts with usual initial dose. Subsequent doses are decreased by 50%.

ACTION
Inhibits bacterial DNA synthesis, mainly by blocking DNA gyrase; bactericidal.

Route	Onset	Peak	Duration
P.O.	Unknown	1-3 hr	Unknown

ADVERSE REACTIONS
CNS: headache, restlessness, tremor, light-headedness, confusion, hallucinations, *seizures.*
GI: *nausea, diarrhea,* vomiting, abdominal pain or discomfort, oral candidiasis, pseudomembranous colitis.
GU: crystalluria.
Hematologic: eosinophilia.
Respiratory: dyspnea, cough.
Skin: *rash,* photosensitivity, pruritus.
Other: hypersensitivity reactions.

INTERACTIONS
Drug-drug. *Aminophylline, cyclosporine, theophylline:* Increased levels of these drugs because of decreased metabolism. Use together cautiously.
Antacids containing aluminum hydroxide or magnesium hydroxide, oral iron supplements, sucralfate: Decreased enoxacin absorption. Don't give enoxacin 2 hours before or 6 hours after antacid.
Bismuth subsalicylate: Decreased bioavailability of enoxacin when given within 60 minutes of bismuth subsalicylate. Avoid using together.
Digoxin: May increase digoxin serum levels. Monitor patient closely for toxicity.
NSAIDs: Increased risk of seizures. Use together cautiously.
Oral anticoagulants: Increased anticoagulant effect. Use together cautiously.
Drug-herb. *Dong quai, St. John's wort:* May cause photosensitivity. Advise patient to avoid excessive sunlight exposure.
Drug-food. *Any food:* Decreases absorption. Give drug on empty stomach.
Caffeine: Increased effect of caffeine. Monitor patient closely.

EFFECTS ON LAB TEST RESULTS
● May increase BUN, creatinine, ALT, AST, alkaline phosphatase, bilirubin, LDH, and GGT levels.
● May increase eosinophil count.

CONTRAINDICATIONS
Contraindicated in patients hypersensitive to drug or other fluoroquinolones.

NURSING CONSIDERATIONS
● Use cautiously in patients with CNS disorders, such as severe cerebral arteriosclerosis or seizure disorders, and in those at risk for seizures. Drug may cause CNS stimulation.
● Use cautiously and with dosage adjustments in patients with impaired renal or hepatic function. Monitor renal function and liver function tests.
● Obtain specimen for culture and sensitivity tests before giving first dose. Therapy may begin pending results.
● *Alert:* Before treatment for gonorrhea begins, patient should have an initial serologic test for syphilis. Drug hasn't been effective in treating syphilis and may mask

signs and symptoms of infection. Repeat serologic test in 1 to 3 months.
● Administer 2 hours after a meal or 2 hours before or after giving antacids containing magnesium hydroxide or aluminum hydroxide, sucralfate, or products that contain iron (such as vitamins with mineral supplements).
● Monitor patient closely for signs and symptoms of superinfection.
● Safety in children younger than age 18 hasn't been established. Drug has caused cartilage erosion.
● Tendon rupture has been reported in patients receiving quinolones. Discontinue if pain, inflammation, or rupture of a tendon occurs.

PATIENT TEACHING
● Tell patient to take drug as prescribed, even after he feels better.
● Instruct patient to take drug on an empty stomach.
● Advise patient to drink plenty of fluids to reduce risk of crystalluria.
● Warn patient to avoid hazardous tasks until adverse CNS effects of drug are known.
● Warn patient not to drink beverages containing caffeine. Enoxacin inhibits the metabolism of caffeine and can result in toxicity.
● Advise patient to avoid overexposure to direct sunlight, use a sunblock, and wear protective clothing while outdoors.
● Caution patient to discontinue drug and report pain, inflammation, or tendon rupture and to rest and refrain from exercise until diagnosis of tendonitis or rupture is excluded.
● Instruct patient to stop taking drug at first signs of an allergic reaction and to notify prescriber.

gatifloxacin
Tequin

Pregnancy risk category C

AVAILABLE FORMS
Injection: 200 mg/20-ml vial, 400 mg/40-ml vial; 200 mg in 100 ml D_5W, 400 mg in 200 ml D_5W
Tablets: 200 mg, 400 mg

INDICATIONS & DOSAGES

➤ **Acute bacterial exacerbation of chronic bronchitis** caused by *Streptococcus pneumoniae, Haemophilus influenzae, H. parainfluenzae, Moraxella catarrhalis,* or *Staphylococcus aureus*; **complicated urinary tract infection (UTI)** caused by *Escherichia coli, Klebsiella pneumoniae,* or *Proteus mirabilis*; **acute pyelonephritis** caused by *E. coli*—

Adults: 400 mg I.V. or P.O. daily for 7 to 10 days for acute pyelonephritis and complicated UTIs and 5 days for chronic bronchitis.

➤ **Acute sinusitis** caused by *S. pneumoniae* or *H. influenzae*—

Adults: 400 mg I.V. or P.O. daily for 10 days.

➤ **Community-acquired pneumonia** caused by *S. pneumoniae, H. influenzae, H. parainfluenzae, M. catarrhalis, S. aureus, Mycoplasma pneumoniae, Chlamydia pneumoniae,* or *Legionella pneumophila*—

Adults: 400 mg I.V. or P.O. daily for 7 to 14 days.

Adjust-a-dose: For patients with creatinine clearance less than 40 ml/minute, those on hemodialysis, and those on continuous peritoneal dialysis, initial dose is 400 mg I.V. or P.O. daily, and subsequent doses are 200 mg I.V. or P.O. daily. For patients on hemodialysis, administer after hemodialysis session is complete.

➤ **Uncomplicated urethral gonorrhea in men and cervical gonorrhea or acute uncomplicated rectal infections in women** caused by *Neisseria gonorrhoeae*—

Adults: 400 mg P.O. as single dose.

➤ **Uncomplicated UTIs** caused by *E. coli, K. pneumoniae,* or *P. mirabilis*—

Adults: 400 mg I.V. or P.O. as single dose, or 200 mg I.V. or P.O. daily for 3 days.

I.V. ADMINISTRATION

● Dilute drug in single-use vials with D_5W or normal saline solution to a final concentration of 2 mg/ml before administration. Diluted solutions are stable for 14 days at room temperature or refrigerated. Frozen solutions are stable for up to 6 months except for 5% sodium bicarbonate solutions. Thaw at room temperature. Thawed solutions are stable for 14 days after being removed from the freezer when stored at room temperature or under refrigeration. Don't mix with other drugs.

● Infuse over 60 minutes.

● Discard any unused portion of the single-dose vials.

ACTION

Inhibits DNA gyrase and topoisomerase, preventing cell replication and division.

Route	Onset	Peak	Duration
I.V.	Unknown	Unknown	Unknown
P.O.	Unknown	1-2 hr	Unknown

ADVERSE REACTIONS

CNS: headache, dizziness, abnormal dreams, insomnia, paresthesia, tremor, vertigo.
CV: palpitations, chest pain.
EENT: tinnitus, abnormal vision, pharyngitis.
GI: nausea, diarrhea, abdominal pain, constipation, dyspepsia, oral candidiasis, glossitis, stomatitis, mouth ulcer, vomiting, taste perversion.
GU: dysuria, hematuria, vaginitis.
Musculoskeletal: arthralgia, myalgia, back pain.
Respiratory: dyspnea.
Skin: rash, sweating.
Other: *anaphylaxis,* redness at injection site, chills, fever, peripheral edema.

INTERACTIONS

Drug-drug. *Antacids containing aluminum or magnesium, didanosine buffered solution tablets or buffered powder, products containing zinc, magnesium, or iron:* Decreased absorption of gatifloxacin. Give gatifloxacin 4 hours before these products.
Antidiabetics (glyburide, insulin): May cause symptomatic hypoglycemia or hyperglycemia. Monitor glucose level.
Antipsychotics, erythromycin, TCAs: May prolong QTc interval. Use together cautiously.
Class IA antiarrhythmics (procainamide, quinidine), class III antiarrhythmics (amiodarone, dofetilide, sotalol): May prolong QTc interval. Avoid using together.
Digoxin: May increase digoxin levels. Watch for signs of digoxin toxicity.

Reactions may be *common,* uncommon, *life-threatening,* or COMMON AND LIFE-THREATENING.

NSAIDs: May increase risk of CNS stimulation and seizures. Use together cautiously.

Probenecid: Increased gatifloxacin levels and prolongation of its half-life. Monitor patient closely.

Warfarin: May enhance effects of warfarin. Monitor PT and INR.

Drug-herb. *Dong quai, St. John's wort:* May cause photosensitivity. Advise patient to avoid excessive sunlight exposure.

Drug-lifestyle. *Sun exposure:* May cause photosensitivity. Advise patient to avoid excessive sunlight exposure.

EFFECTS ON LAB TEST RESULTS
None reported.

CONTRAINDICATIONS
Contraindicated in patients hypersensitive to fluoroquinolones. Don't use in patients with prolonged QTc interval or uncorrected hypokalemia.

NURSING CONSIDERATIONS
● Use cautiously in patients with clinically significant bradycardia, acute myocardial ischemia, known or suspected CNS disorders, or renal insufficiency.
● Monitor glucose level in patients with diabetes.
● Monitor patients also receiving digoxin for signs and symptoms of digoxin toxicity.
● Monitor kidney function in patients with renal insufficiency.
● Stop drug if patient experiences seizures, increased intracranial pressure, psychosis, or CNS stimulation leading to tremors, restlessness, light-headedness, confusion, hallucinations, paranoia, depression, nightmares, and insomnia.
● Stop drug if rash or other sign of hypersensitivity occurs.
● Stop drug if patient experiences pain, inflammation, or rupture of a tendon.
● In patients being treated for gonorrhea, test for syphilis at time of diagnosis.

PATIENT TEACHING
● Tell patient to take drug as prescribed and to finish all of it even if symptoms disappear.

● Advise patient to take drug 4 hours before taking products containing aluminum, magnesium, zinc, or iron.
● Advise patient to use sunblock and protective clothing when exposed to excessive sunlight.
● Warn patient to avoid hazardous tasks until adverse CNS effects of drug are known.
● Advise diabetic patient to monitor glucose levels and notify prescriber if hypoglycemia occurs.
● Advise patient to immediately report palpitations, fainting spells, rash, hives, difficulty swallowing or breathing, tightness in throat, hoarseness, swelling of lips, tongue, or face or other symptoms of allergic reaction.
● Advise patient to stop drug, refrain from exercise, and notify prescriber if pain, inflammation, or rupture of a tendon occurs.

levofloxacin
Levaquin

Pregnancy risk category C

AVAILABLE FORMS
Infusion (premixed): 250 mg in 50 ml D_5W, 500 mg in 100 ml D_5W
Single-use vials: 500 mg
Tablets: 250 mg, 500 mg

INDICATIONS & DOSAGES
➤ **Acute maxillary sinusitis caused by susceptible strains of** *Streptococcus pneumoniae, Moraxella catarrhalis,* **or** *Haemophilus influenzae*—
Adults: 500 mg P.O. or I.V. daily for 10 to 14 days.
➤ **Acute bacterial exacerbation of chronic bronchitis caused by** *Staphylococcus aureus, S. pneumoniae, M. catarrhalis, H. influenzae,* **or** *H. parainfluenzae*—
Adults: 500 mg P.O. or I.V. daily for 7 days.
➤ **Community-acquired pneumonia caused by** *S. aureus, S. pneumoniae, M. catarrhalis, H. influenzae, H. parainfluenzae, Klebsiella pneumoniae, Chlamydia pneumoniae, Legionella*

pneumophila, or *Mycoplasma pneumoniae*—
Adjust-a-dose: If creatinine clearance is 20 to 49 ml/min, give initial dose of 500 mg, then 250 mg daily. If clearance is 10 to 19 ml/min, give initial dose of 500 mg, then 250 mg q 48 hours. For patients on dialysis or chronic ambulatory peritoneal dialysis, give initial dose of 500 mg, then 250 mg q 48 hours.
Adults: 500 mg P.O. or I.V. daily for 7 to 14 days.
➤ **Mild to moderate skin and skin-structure infections caused by** *S. aureus* **or** *S. pyogenes*—
Adults: 500 mg P.O. or I.V. daily for 7 to 10 days.
➤ **Mild to moderate uncomplicated urinary tract infection caused by** *Escherichia coli,* *K. pneumoniae,* **or** *S. saprophyticus*—
Adults: 250 mg P.O. daily for 3 days.
✳ *NEW INDICATION:* **Complicated skin and skin-structure infections caused by methicillin-sensitive** *Staphylococcus aureus, Enterococcus faecalis, Streptococcus pyogenes,* **or** *Proteus mirabilis*—
Adults: 750 mg P.O. or I.V. infusion over 90 minutes q 24 hours for 7 to 14 days.
Adjust-a-dose: If creatinine clearance is 20 to 49 ml/minute, give 750 mg initially, then 750 mg q 48 hours; if clearance is 10 to 19 ml/min, or patient is receiving hemodialysis or chronic ambulatory peritoneal dialysis, give 750 mg initially, then 500 mg q 48 hours.
Adjust-a-dose: If creatinine clearance is 20 to 49 ml/minute, give subsequent doses at half the initial dose. If clearance is 10 to 19 ml/minute, give subsequent doses at half the initial dose and increase the interval to q 48 hours.
➤ **Urinary tract infections (mild to moderate) caused by** *Enterococcus faecalis, Enterobacter cloacae, E. coli, K. pneumoniae, Proteus mirabilis,* **or** *Pseudomonas aeruginosa*—
Adults: 250 mg P.O. or I.V. daily for 10 days.
➤ **Acute pyelonephritis (mild to moderate) caused by** *E. coli*—
Adults: 250 mg P.O. or I.V. daily for 10 days.

Adjust-a-dose: If creatinine clearance is 10 to 19 ml/minute, increase dosage interval to q 48 hours.
➤ **Community-acquired pneumonia caused by penicillin-resistant** *S. pneumoniae*—
Adults: 500 mg P.O. or I.V. infusion over 60 minutes once daily for 7 to 14 days.
Adjust-a-dose: If creatinine clearance is 20 to 49 ml/minute, give initial dose of 500 mg, then 250 mg once daily; if clearance is 10 to 19 ml/minute, give initial dose of 500 mg, then 250 mg q 48 hours. For patients on hemodialysis or chronic ambulatory peritoneal dialysis, give initial dose of 500 mg, then 250 mg q 48 hours.

I.V. ADMINISTRATION

● Levofloxacin injection should be given only by I.V. infusion.
● Dilute drug in single-use vials, according to manufacturer's instructions, with D_5W or normal saline solution for injection to a final concentration of 5 mg/ml.
● Reconstituted solution should be clear, slightly yellow, and free of particulate matter.
● Reconstituted drug is stable for 72 hours at room temperature, for 14 days when refrigerated in plastic containers, and for 6 months when frozen. Thaw at room temperature or in refrigerator. Don't mix with other drugs. Infuse over 60 minutes.

ACTION
Inhibits bacterial DNA gyrase and prevents DNA replication, transcription, repair, and recombination in susceptible bacteria.

Route	Onset	Peak	Duration
I.V., P.O.	Unknown	1-2 hr	Unknown

ADVERSE REACTIONS
CNS: headache, insomnia, dizziness, encephalopathy, paresthesia, *seizures.*
CV: chest pain, palpitations, vasodilation.
GI: nausea, diarrhea, constipation, vomiting, abdominal pain, dyspepsia, flatulence, *pseudomembranous colitis.*
GU: vaginitis.
Hematologic: eosinophilia, hemolytic anemia, lymphopenia.
Metabolic: hypoglycemia.
Musculoskeletal: back pain, tendon rupture.

Reactions may be *common,* uncommon, *life-threatening,* or COMMON AND LIFE-THREATENING.

Respiratory: allergic pneumonitis.
Skin: rash, photosensitivity, pruritus, *erythema multiforme, Stevens-Johnson syndrome.*
Other: pain, hypersensitivity reactions, *anaphylaxis, multisystem organ failure.*

INTERACTIONS

Drug-drug. *Antacids containing aluminum or magnesium, iron salts, products containing zinc, sucralfate:* May interfere with GI absorption of levofloxacin. Don't take levofloxacin 2 hours before or 6 hours after antacid.
Antidiabetics: May alter glucose levels. Monitor glucose levels closely.
NSAIDs: May increase CNS stimulation. Monitor patient for seizure activity.
Theophylline: May decrease clearance of theophylline. Monitor theophylline levels.
Warfarin and derivatives: May increase effect of oral anticoagulant. Monitor PT and INR.
Drug-herb. *Dong quai, St. John's wort:* May cause photosensitivity. Advise patient to avoid excessive sunlight exposure.
Drug-lifestyle. *Sun exposure:* May cause photosensitivity. Advise patient to avoid excessive sunlight exposure.

EFFECTS ON LAB TEST RESULTS

• May decrease glucose level.
• May increase eosinophil count. May decrease hemoglobin and WBC count.

CONTRAINDICATIONS

Contraindicated in patients hypersensitive to drug, its components, or other fluoroquinolones.

NURSING CONSIDERATIONS

• Safety and efficacy of drug in children younger than age 18 and in pregnant and breast-feeding women haven't been established.
• Use cautiously in patients with history of seizure disorders or other CNS diseases, such as cerebral arteriosclerosis. If patient experiences symptoms of excessive CNS stimulation (restlessness, tremor, confusion, hallucinations), stop drug and notify prescriber. Institute seizure precautions.
• Use cautiously and with dosage adjustment in patients with renal impairment.

• Patients with acute hypersensitivity reactions may need treatment with epinephrine, oxygen, I.V. fluids, antihistamines, corticosteroids, pressor amines, and airway management.
• Most antibacterial drugs can cause pseudomembranous colitis. Notify prescriber if diarrhea occurs. Drug may be stopped.
• Drug may cause an abnormal ECG.
• Obtain specimen for culture and sensitivity tests before starting therapy and as needed to determine if bacterial resistance has occurred.
• Monitor glucose and renal, hepatic, and hematopoietic blood studies.

PATIENT TEACHING

• Tell patient to take drug as prescribed, even if signs and symptoms disappear.
• Advise patient to take drug with plenty of fluids and to avoid antacids, sucralfate, and products containing iron or zinc for at least 2 hours before and after each dose.
• Warn patient to avoid hazardous tasks until adverse CNS effects of drug are known.
• Advise patient to avoid excessive sunlight, use sunblock, and wear protective clothing when outdoors.
• Instruct patient to stop drug and notify prescriber if rash or other signs or symptoms of hypersensitivity develop.
• Tell patient to notify prescriber if he experiences pain or inflammation; tendon rupture can occur with drug.
• Instruct diabetic patient to monitor glucose levels and notify prescriber if a hypoglycemic reaction occurs.
• Instruct patient to notify prescriber if loose stools or diarrhea occurs.

---

moxifloxacin hydrochloride
Avelox, Avelox I.V.

Pregnancy risk category C

AVAILABLE FORMS

Injection: 400 mg/250 ml
Tablets (film-coated): 400 mg

INDICATIONS & DOSAGES

➤ **Acute bacterial sinusitis caused by** *Streptococcus pneumoniae, Haemoph-*

ilus influenzae, or *Moraxella catarrhalis*—
Adults: 400 mg P.O. or I.V. once daily for 10 days.
➤ **Mild to moderate community-acquired pneumonia caused by** *S. pneumoniae, H. influenzae, Mycoplasma pneumoniae, Chlamydia pneumoniae,* or *M. catarrhalis*—
Adults: 400 mg P.O. or I.V. once daily for 7 to 14 days.
➤ **Acute bacterial exacerbation of chronic bronchitis caused by** *S. pneumoniae, H. influenzae, H. parainfluenzae, Klebsiella pneumoniae, Staphylococcus aureus,* or *M. catarrhalis*—
Adults: 400 mg P.O. or I.V. once daily for 5 days.
❋ *NEW INDICATION:* **Uncomplicated skin and skin-structure infections caused by** *Staphylococcus aureus* or *S. pyogenes*—
Adults: 400 mg P.O. or I.V. once daily for 7 days.

I.V. ADMINISTRATION
• Give only by I.V. infusion over 1 hour.
• Avoid rapid or bolus infusion.
• Don't mix with other drugs.
• Flush I.V. line with a compatible solution such as D_5W, normal saline, or Ringer's lactate solution before and after use.
• Don't use if particulate matter is visible.

ACTION
Interferes with action of enzymes necessary for bacterial replication. Inhibits topoisomerases I (DNA gyrase) and IV, thereby impairing processes of bacterial DNA replication, transcription, repair, and recombination.

Route	Onset	Peak	Duration
I.V., P.O.	Unknown	1-3 hr	Unknown

ADVERSE REACTIONS
CNS: dizziness, headache.
GI: taste perversion, abdominal pain, diarrhea, dyspepsia, nausea, vomiting.

INTERACTIONS
Drug-drug. *Antacids, didanosine, metal cations (such as aluminum, iron, magnesium, zinc), multivitamins, sucralfate:* Metal cations chelate with moxifloxacin, resulting in decreased absorption and lower serum levels. Administer drug at least 8 hours before or 6 hours after drugs containing metal cations.
Class IA antiarrhythmics (such as procainamide, quinidine), class III antiarrhythmics (such as amiodarone, sotalol): Lack of clinical experience with drug. Avoid using together.
Drugs known to prolong QT interval, such as antipsychotics, erythromycin, TCAs: May have an additive effect. Avoid using together.
NSAIDs: May increase risk of CNS stimulation and seizures. Avoid using together.
Drug-lifestyle. *Sun exposure:* Photosensitivity hasn't occurred with moxifloxacin but has been reported with other fluoroquinolones. Advise patient to avoid excessive sunlight exposure.

EFFECTS ON LAB TEST RESULTS
• May increase ALT, AST, alkaline phosphatase, and bilirubin levels.

CONTRAINDICATIONS
Contraindicated in patients hypersensitive to drug or other fluoroquinolones and in those with prolonged QT interval or uncorrected hypokalemia.

NURSING CONSIDERATIONS
• Use cautiously in patients with ongoing proarrhythmic conditions, such as clinically significant bradycardia or acute myocardial ischemia. Also use cautiously in patients with known or suspected CNS disorders and in the presence of other risk factors that may predispose to seizures or lower the seizure threshold.
• Safety and efficacy in children, adolescents younger than age 18, and pregnant or breast-feeding women haven't been established.
• Drug may be given without regard to meals. Give at same time each day.
• *Alert:* Monitor patient for adverse CNS effects, including seizures, dizziness, confusion, tremors, hallucinations, depression, and suicidal thoughts or acts. If these reactions occur, stop drug and institute appropriate measures.
• Serious hypersensitivity reactions, including anaphylaxis, have occurred in patients receiving fluoroquinolones. Stop drug and institute supportive measures, as indicated.

- Consider the diagnosis of pseudomembranous colitis if diarrhea develops after therapy begins.
- Rupture of the Achilles and other tendons has been linked to fluoroquinolones. If pain, inflammation, or rupture of a tendon occurs, stop moxifloxacin.
- Store drug at controlled room temperature.

PATIENT TEACHING
- Instruct patient to take drug once daily, at the same time each day, without regard to meals.
- Tell patient to finish entire course of therapy, even if symptoms are relieved.
- Advise patient to drink plenty of fluids.
- Tell patient to take drug 4 hours before or 8 hours after antacids, sucralfate, and products containing iron and zinc.
- Instruct patient to contact prescriber and stop drug if he experiences allergic reaction, rash, heart palpitations, fainting, or persistent diarrhea.
- Direct patient to contact prescriber, stop drug, rest, and refrain from exercise if he experiences pain, inflammation, or rupture of a tendon.
- Warn patient that drug may cause dizziness and light-headedness. Tell patient to avoid hazardous activities, such as driving or operating machinery, until CNS effects of drug are known.
- Instruct patient to take sun precautions, avoid ultraviolet light, and report photosensitivity reactions to prescriber.

---

nalidixic acid
NegGram

Pregnancy risk category C

AVAILABLE FORMS
Caplets: 250 mg, 500 mg, 1 g
Oral suspension: 250 mg/5 ml

INDICATIONS & DOSAGES
➤ **Acute and chronic urinary tract infections caused by susceptible gram-negative organisms *(Proteus, Klebsiella, Enterobacter,* and *Escherichia coli)*—**
Adults: 1 g P.O. q.i.d. for 7 to 14 days; 2 g daily for long-term use.

Children older than age 3 months:
55 mg/kg P.O. daily divided q.i.d. for 7 to 14 days; 33 mg/kg daily divided q.i.d. for long-term use.

ACTION
A quinolone antibiotic that inhibits microbial DNA synthesis.

Route	Onset	Peak	Duration
P.O.	Unknown	1-2 hr	Unknown

ADVERSE REACTIONS
CNS: drowsiness, weakness, headache, dizziness, vertigo, *seizures,* malaise, confusion, hallucinations, psychosis, *increased intracranial pressure and bulging fontanelles in infants and children.*
EENT: sensitivity to light, change in color perception, diplopia, blurred vision.
GI: *abdominal pain, nausea, vomiting,* diarrhea.
Hematologic: eosinophilia, *leukopenia, thrombocytopenia,* hemolytic anemia.
Musculoskeletal: arthralgia, joint stiffness.
Skin: pruritus, photosensitivity, urticaria, rash.
Other: *angioedema, anaphylactoid reaction.*

INTERACTIONS
Drug-drug. *Antacids containing aluminum, calcium, or magnesium; iron salts; products containing zinc; sucralfate:* May interfere with GI absorption of levofloxacin. Give nalidixic acid at least 2 hours before or 6 hours after antacid.
Cyclosporine: Increased cyclosporine levels. Monitor serum cyclosporine levels.
Nitrofurantoin: Antagonizes effects of nalidixic acid. Monitor patient closely.
Oral anticoagulants: Increased anticoagulant effect. Monitor patient for bleeding.
Theophylline: Decreased clearance of theophylline with some quinolones. Monitor theophylline levels and watch for signs and symptoms of toxicity.
Drug-herb. *Dong quai, St. John's wort:* May cause photosensitivity. Advise patient to avoid excessive sunlight exposure.
Drug-food. *Caffeine:* Increased effect of caffeine. Monitor patient closely.

Drug-lifestyle. *Sun exposure:* May cause photosensitivity reactions. Advise patient to avoid excessive sunlight exposure.

EFFECTS ON LAB TEST RESULTS
• May increase AST, BUN, and creatinine levels.
• May increase eosinophil count. May decrease hemoglobin and platelet and WBC counts.

CONTRAINDICATIONS
Contraindicated in patients hypersensitive to drug, in those with seizure disorders, and in infants younger than age 3 months.

NURSING CONSIDERATIONS
• Use with extreme caution in prepubertal children; drug has caused cartilage erosion.
• Use cautiously in patients with impaired hepatic or renal function or with severe cerebral arteriosclerosis. Monitor renal and liver function test results.
• Obtain specimen for culture and sensitivity tests before starting therapy and repeat, p.r.n. Therapy may begin pending results.
• Monitor CBC and renal and liver function studies during long-term therapy.
• Resistant bacteria may emerge in the first 48 hours of therapy.
• Drug may cause false-positive results in urine glucose tests using cupric sulfate (such as Benedict's reagent, Fehling's solution, and Chemstrip uG). Urine 17-ketosteroid and urine 17-ketogenic steroid levels may be falsely elevated because nalidixic acid interacts with *M*-dinitrobenzene, used to measure these urine metabolites. Urine vanillylmandelic acid levels also may be falsely elevated.

PATIENT TEACHING
• Tell patient to take drug as prescribed, even after he feels better.
• Instruct patient to take drug with food to prevent GI upset.
• Tell patient to drink plenty of fluids while taking drug.
• Advise patient to limit caffeine intake while taking drug.
• Tell patient to avoid exposure to sunlight, wear protective clothing, and use sunscreen.

• Tell patient to report visual disturbances or CNS symptoms immediately.

---

norfloxacin
Noroxin, Utinor§

Pregnancy risk category C

AVAILABLE FORMS
Tablets (film-coated): 400 mg

INDICATIONS & DOSAGES
➤ **Complicated or uncomplicated urinary tract infections caused by susceptible strains of** *Enterococcus faecalis,* *Escherichia coli, Klebsiella pneumoniae, Enterobacter aerogenes, E. cloacae, Proteus mirabilis, P. vulgaris, Pseudomonas aeruginosa, Citrobacter freundii, Staphylococcus agalactiae, S. aureus, S. epidermidis, S. saprophyticus,* **or** *Serratia marcescens*—
Adults: For uncomplicated infections, 400 mg P.O. q 12 hours for 7 to 10 days. For complicated infections, 400 mg P.O. q 12 hours for 10 to 21 days.
➤ **Prostatitis**—
Adults: 400 mg P.O. q 12 hours for 28 days.
➤ **Cystitis caused by** *E. coli, K. pneumoniae,* **or** *P. mirabilis*—
Adults: 400 mg P.O. q 12 hours for 3 days.
Adjust-a-dose: For adult patients with creatinine clearance of 30 ml/minute or less, 400 mg once daily for above indications.
➤ **Acute, uncomplicated urethral and cervical gonorrhea**—
Adults: 800 mg P.O. as a single dose, then doxycycline therapy to treat any coexisting chlamydial infection.

ACTION
Inhibits bacterial DNA synthesis, mainly by blocking DNA gyrase; bactericidal.

Route	Onset	Peak	Duration
P.O.	Unknown	0.5-2 hr	Unknown

ADVERSE REACTIONS
CNS: fatigue, somnolence, headache, dizziness, *seizures,* depression, insomnia.

Reactions may be *common,* uncommon, *life-threatening,* or COMMON AND LIFE-THREATENING.

GI: nausea, constipation, flatulence, heartburn, dry mouth, abdominal pain, diarrhea, vomiting, anorexia.
GU: crystalluria.
Hematologic: eosinophilia, *neutropenia.*
Musculoskeletal: back pain.
Skin: rash, photosensitivity, hyperhidrosis.
Other: hypersensitivity reactions, *anaphylaxis,* fever.

INTERACTIONS
Drug-drug. *Iron products, sucralfate:*
May hinder absorption. Separate administration times by 2 hours.
Antacids: Decreased antibiotic absorption: Don't give drug 2 hours before or 6 hours after antacid.
Cyclosporine: Increased serum levels of cyclosporine. Monitor serum levels.
Nitrofurantoin: Antagonized effects of norfloxacin. Monitor patient closely.
Oral anticoagulants: Increased anticoagulant effect. Monitor patient closely.
Probenecid: May increase serum levels of norfloxacin by decreasing its excretion. Monitor patient for toxicity.
Theophylline: May impair theophylline metabolism, resulting in increased plasma levels and risk of toxicity. Monitor patient closely.
Drug-herb. *Dong quai, St. John's wort:*
May cause photosensitivity reactions. Advise patient to avoid excessive sunlight exposure.

EFFECTS ON LAB TEST RESULTS
• May increase BUN, creatinine, ALT, AST, and alkaline phosphatase levels.
• May increase eosinophil count. May decrease hematocrit and neutrophil count.

CONTRAINDICATIONS
Contraindicated in patients hypersensitive to drug or other fluoroquinolones.

NURSING CONSIDERATIONS
• Use cautiously in patients with conditions such as cerebral arteriosclerosis that may predispose them to seizure disorders. Also use cautiously in those with renal impairment. Monitor renal function.
• Obtain specimen for culture and sensitivity testing before starting therapy.

• Tendon rupture has been reported in patients receiving quinolones. Discontinue if pain, inflammation, or rupture of a tendon occurs.
• Safety in children younger than age 18 hasn't been established. Drug has caused cartilage erosion.

PATIENT TEACHING
• Tell patient to take drug as prescribed, even after he feels better.
• Advise patient to take drug 1 hour before or 2 hours after meals because food, antacids, iron products, and sucralfate may hinder absorption.
• Warn patient not to exceed the recommended dosages and to drink several glasses of water throughout the day to maintain hydration and adequate urine output.
• Warn patient to avoid hazardous tasks that require alertness until CNS effects of drug are known.
• Instruct patient to avoid exposure to sunlight, wear protective clothing, and use sunscreen while outdoors.
• Tell patient to report pain, inflammation or tendon rupture, and to refrain from exercise until diagnosis of rupture or tendonitis is excluded.

sparfloxacin
Zagam

Pregnancy risk category C

AVAILABLE FORMS
Tablets: 200 mg

INDICATIONS & DOSAGES
➤ **Acute bacterial exacerbation of chronic bronchitis caused by** *Staphylococcus aureus, Streptococcus pneumoniae, Chlamydia pneumoniae, Enterobacter cloacae, Klebsiella pneumoniae, Moraxella catarrhalis, Haemophilus influenzae,* **or** *H. parainfluenzae—*
Adults older than age 18: 400 mg P.O. on first day as a loading dose; then 200 mg daily for total of 10 days of therapy.
➤ **Community-acquired pneumonia caused by** *S. pneumoniae, M. catarrhalis, H. influenzae, H. parainfluenzae,*

C. pneumoniae, or *Mycoplasma pneumoniae*—
Adults older than age 18: 400 mg P.O. on first day as a loading dose; then 200 mg daily for total of 10 days of therapy.
Adjust-a-dose: For renally impaired patients with creatinine clearance below 50 ml/minute, give a loading dose of 400 mg P.O.; then, 200 mg P.O. q 48 hours for total of 9 days of therapy.

ACTION
Inhibits bacterial DNA gyrase and prevents DNA replication, transcription, repair, and deactivation in susceptible bacteria.

Route	Onset	Peak	Duration
P.O.	Unknown	3-6 hr	Unknown

ADVERSE REACTIONS
CNS: headache, dizziness, insomnia, asthenia, somnolence, *seizures.*
CV: prolonged QT interval, vasodilatation.
GI: dry mouth, taste perversion, nausea, diarrhea, vomiting, abdominal pain, dyspepsia, flatulence, pseudomembranous colitis.
GU: vaginal candidiasis.
Musculoskeletal: tendon rupture.
Skin: rash, photosensitivity, pruritus.
Other: hypersensitivity reactions, *anaphylaxis.*

INTERACTIONS
Drug-drug. *Antacids containing aluminum or magnesium, iron salts, sucralfate, zinc:* May interfere with GI absorption of levofloxacin. Give sparfloxacin 2 hours before or 6 hours after antacid.
Drugs that prolong the QT interval or cause torsades de pointes (including amiodarone, bepridil, class IA antiarrhythmics [such as procainamide and quinidine], class III drugs [such as sotalol and dofetilide], disopyramide, erythromycin, pentamidine, phenothiazines, TCAs): May cause torsades de pointes. Sparfloxacin is contraindicated in patients taking these drugs.
Drug-herb. *Dong quai, St. John's wort:* May cause photosensitivity. Advise patient to avoid excessive sunlight exposure.

Drug-lifestyle. *Sun exposure:* May cause photosensitivity. Advise patient to avoid excessive sunlight exposure.

EFFECTS ON LAB TEST RESULTS
● May increase ALT and AST levels.
● May increase WBC count.

CONTRAINDICATIONS
Contraindicated in patients with a history of hypersensitivity or photosensitivity reactions to drug and in those who can't avoid the sun. Don't give with drugs known to prolong the QT interval or cause torsades de pointes. Drug isn't recommended for patients with heart conditions that predispose them to arrhythmias.

NURSING CONSIDERATIONS
● Safety and efficacy of levofloxacin in pregnant and breast-feeding women and in patients younger than age 18 haven't been established.
● Use cautiously in patients with history of seizure disorders or other CNS diseases such as cerebral arteriosclerosis. If patient experiences symptoms of excessive CNS stimulation (restlessness, tremor, confusion, hallucinations), stop drug and notify prescriber. Then institute seizure precautions.
● Use cautiously and with dosage adjustment in patients with renal impairment. Monitor renal function.
● Obtain specimen for culture and sensitivity tests before starting therapy to determine if bacterial resistance has occurred.
● Drug may produce false-negative culture results for *Mycobacterium tuberculosis.*

PATIENT TEACHING
● Tell patient that drug may be taken with food, milk, or products that contain caffeine.
● Tell patient to take drug as prescribed, even if signs and symptoms disappear.
● Advise patient to take drug with plenty of fluids and to avoid antacids, sucralfate, and products containing iron or zinc for at least 4 hours after each dose.
● Warn patient to avoid hazardous tasks until adverse CNS effects of drug are known.
● *Alert:* Advise patient to avoid direct, indirect, and artificial ultraviolet light, even

---

Reactions may be *common,* uncommon, *life-threatening,* or COMMON AND LIFE-THREATENING.

with sunscreen on, during treatment and for 5 days after treatment. Patient should stop taking drug and notify prescriber if signs or symptoms of phototoxicity (skin burning, redness, swelling, blisters, rash, itching) occur.
• Tell patient to stop drug and notify prescriber if rash or other signs of hypersensitivity develop.
• Direct patient to stop drug and notify prescriber of pain or inflammation; tendon rupture can occur with drug use. He should rest and refrain from exercise until diagnosis is made.
• Instruct patient to notify prescriber about loose stools or diarrhea.

trovafloxacin mesylate
Trovan Tablets

alatrofloxacin mesylate
Trovan I.V.

Pregnancy risk category C

AVAILABLE FORMS
Injection: 5 mg/ml in 40-ml (200 mg) and 60-ml (300 mg) vials
Tablets: 100 mg, 200 mg

INDICATIONS & DOSAGES
➤ **Nosocomial pneumonia caused by** *Escherichia coli, Pseudomonas aeruginosa, Haemophilus influenzae,* **or** *Staphylococcus aureus*; **gynecologic and pelvic infections caused by** *E. coli, Bacteroides fragilis,* **viridans group streptococci,** *Enterococcus faecalis, Streptococcus agalactiae, Peptostreptococcus* **species,** *Prevotella species,* **or** *Gardnerella vaginalis*; **complicated intra-abdominal infections including postsurgical infections caused by** *E. coli, B. fragilis,* **viridans group streptococci,** *P. aeruginosa, Klebsiella pneumoniae, Peptostreptococcus species,* **or** *Prevotella* **species**—
Adults: 300 mg I.V. daily; then 200 mg P.O. daily for 7 to 14 days (10 to 14 days for pneumonia).
➤ **Community-acquired pneumonia caused by** *S. pneumoniae, H. influenzae, K. pneumoniae, S. aureus, Mycoplasma pneumoniae, Moraxella catarrhalis,*

Legionella pneumophila, **or** *Chlamydia pneumoniae*; **complicated skin and skin-structure infections including diabetic foot infections caused by** *S. aureus, S. agalactiae, P. aeruginosa, E. faecalis, E. coli,* **or** *Proteus mirabilis* **(not for treatment of osteomyelitis)**—
Adults: 200 mg P.O. or I.V. daily; then 200 mg P.O. daily for 7 to 14 days (10 to 14 days for complicated skin and skin-structure infections).
Adjust-a-dose: For patients with mild to moderate cirrhosis (Child-Pugh Class A and B), reduce 300-mg I.V. dose to 200 mg I.V. and 200-mg I.V. or P.O. dose to 100 mg I.V. or P.O.; no reduction is needed for 100-mg P.O. dose.

I.V. ADMINISTRATION
• Alatrofloxacin mesylate is supplied in single-use vials that must be further diluted with an appropriate solution (D_5W, half-normal saline solution) before administration. Don't dilute drug with normal saline solution or lactated Ringer's solution. Follow package insert for specific instructions regarding preparation of desired dosage.
• After dilution, administer alatrofloxacin mesylate by I.V. infusion over 60 minutes. Avoid rapid bolus or infusion. Don't administer drug and solutions containing multivalent cations (such as magnesium) through same I.V. line.

ACTION
Trovafloxacin is related to the fluoroquinolones with in vitro activity against a wide range of gram-positive and gram-negative aerobic and anaerobic microorganisms. Bactericidal action results from inhibition of DNA gyrase and topoisomerase IV, two enzymes involved in bacterial replication.

Route	Onset	Peak	Duration
I.V., P.O.	Unknown	1 hr	Unknown

ADVERSE REACTIONS
CNS: *dizziness,* light-headedness, headache, *seizures,* psychosis.
GI: diarrhea, nausea, vomiting, abdominal pain, *pseudomembranous colitis.*
GU: vaginitis.
Hepatic: *liver failure.*

Musculoskeletal: arthralgia, arthropathy, myalgia.
Skin: pruritus, rash, injection-site reaction, photosensitivity.

INTERACTIONS

Drug-drug. *Antacids containing aluminum, magnesium, or citric acid buffered with sodium citrate (Bicitra), I.V. morphine, preparations containing iron, sucralfate:* Bioavailability of trovafloxacin is significantly reduced following use with these drugs. Give antibiotic 2 hours before or 6 hours after antacids; avoid morphine I.V. for 4 hours if trovafloxacin is taken with food.
Drug-herb. *Dong quai, St. John's wort:* May cause photosensitivity. Advise patient to avoid excessive sunlight exposure.
Drug-lifestyle. *Sun exposure:* May cause photosensitivity. Advise patient to avoid excessive sunlight exposure.

EFFECTS ON LAB TEST RESULTS

• May increase BUN, creatinine, ALT, AST, and alkaline phosphatase levels.
• May increase platelet count. May decrease hemoglobin and hematocrit.

CONTRAINDICATIONS

Contraindicated in patients hypersensitive to drug, alatrofloxacin, other fluoroquinolones, or other components of these products.

NURSING CONSIDERATIONS

• Use cautiously in patients with CNS disorders (such as cerebral atherosclerosis or seizure disorders) and in those at increased risk for seizures. As with other quinolones, drug may cause neurologic complications, such as seizures, psychosis, or increased intracranial pressure. Monitor these patients closely.
• Safety and efficacy of drug haven't been established in children younger than age 18 and in breast-feeding women.
• Perform periodic assessment of liver function because of potential for increases in ALT, AST, and alkaline phosphatase levels.
• *Alert:* Using drug for longer than 2 weeks greatly increases the risk of serious liver injury. Liver injury also has been reported after reexposure to drug. Therefore, drug should be given only to patients with life- or limb-threatening infections who received their initial treatment as an inpatient in a hospital or long-term care nursing facility. Drug shouldn't be used if effective and safer alternative drugs are available.
• Drug can be given as a single daily dose without regard to food.
• Moderate to severe phototoxicity has occurred in patients exposed to direct sunlight.
• No dosage adjustment is necessary when switching from I.V. to oral form.
• If *P. aeruginosa* is the known or presumed pathogen, treatment with an aminoglycoside or aztreonam may be indicated.

PATIENT TEACHING

• Inform patient that drug may be taken without regard to meals. However, tell him to take antibiotic at least 2 hours before or 6 hours after products containing iron, aluminum, magnesium (vitamins, minerals, antacids), or sucralfate.
• Advise patient to take drug with meals or at bedtime if light-headedness or dizziness occurs.
• Advise patient to avoid activities that require mental alertness until CNS effects of drug are known.
• Warn patient to avoid excessive sunlight or artificial ultraviolet light and to use an effective sunscreen to prevent sunburn.
• Instruct patient to stop drug, refrain from exercise, and seek medical advice if pain, inflammation, or rupture of a tendon occurs.
• Advise patient to stop drug at first sign of rash, hives, difficulty swallowing or breathing, or other symptoms suggesting an allergic reaction, and to seek medical help immediately.
• Instruct patient to notify prescriber if severe diarrhea occurs; this may indicate pseudomembranous colitis.

Reactions may be *common*, uncommon, **life-threatening**, or COMMON AND LIFE-THREATENING.

abacavir sulfate
acyclovir sodium
amantadine hydrochloride
amprenavir
cidofovir
delavirdine mesylate
didanosine
efavirenz
famciclovir
fomivirsen sodium
foscarnet sodium
ganciclovir
indinavir sulfate
lamivudine
lamivudine/zidovudine
lopinavir/ritonavir
nelfinavir mesylate
nevirapine
oseltamivir phosphate
ribavirin
rimantadine hydrochloride
ritonavir
saquinavir
saquinavir mesylate
stavudine
tenofovir disoproxil fumarate
valacyclovir hydrochloride
valganciclovir
zalcitabine
zanamivir
zidovudine

COMBINATION PRODUCTS
None.

---

abacavir sulfate
Ziagen

Pregnancy risk category C

AVAILABLE FORMS
Oral solution: 20 mg/ml
Tablets: 300 mg

INDICATIONS & DOSAGES
➤ **HIV-1 infection—**
Adults: 300 mg P.O. b.i.d. with other antiretrovirals.

Children ages 3 months to 16 years: 8 mg/kg P.O. b.i.d. up to maximum of 300 mg P.O. b.i.d. with other antiretrovirals.

ACTION
Converted intracellularly to the active metabolite carbovir triphosphate, which inhibits activity of HIV-1 reverse transcriptase, terminating viral DNA growth.

Route	Onset	Peak	Duration
P.O.	Unknown	Unknown	Unknown

ADVERSE REACTIONS
CNS: insomnia and sleep disorders, headache.
GI: *nausea, vomiting, diarrhea, anorexia.*
Skin: rash.
Other: *hypersensitivity reaction,* fever.

INTERACTIONS
Drug-lifestyle. *Alcohol:* Decreased elimination of abacavir, increasing overall exposure to drug. Monitor alcohol consumption. Warn against using together.

EFFECTS ON LAB TEST RESULTS
● May increase GGT and triglyceride levels.

CONTRAINDICATIONS
Contraindicated in patients hypersensitive to drug or its components.

NURSING CONSIDERATIONS
● Use cautiously when administering drug to patients at risk for liver disease. Lactic acidosis and severe hepatomegaly with steatosis, including fatal cases, have been reported with the use of nucleoside analogues alone or in combination, including abacavir and other antiretrovirals.
● Women are more likely than men to experience lactic acidosis and severe hepatomegaly with steatosis. Obesity and prolonged nucleoside exposure may be risk factors.
● Discontinue treatment in patients who develop signs or symptoms of lactic aci-

---

dosis or pronounced hepatotoxicity, which may include hepatomegaly and steatosis even in absence of elevated transaminase levels.
• Use cautiously in pregnant women because no adequate studies of the effects of abacavir on pregnancy exist. Use during pregnancy only if the potential benefits outweigh the risk. Register pregnant women taking abacavir with the Antiretroviral Pregnancy Registry at 1-800-258-4263.
• *Alert:* Don't restart drug after a hypersensitivity reaction because severe signs and symptoms will recur within hours and may include life-threatening hypotension and death. To facilitate reporting of hypersensitivity reactions, register patients with the Abacavir Hypersensitivity Reaction Registry at 1-800-270-0425.
• *Alert:* Abacavir can cause fatal hypersensitivity reactions; as soon as patient develops signs or symptoms of hypersensitivity (such as fever, rash, fatigue, nausea, vomiting, diarrhea, or abdominal pain), stop drug and seek medical attention immediately.
• Always give drug with other antiretrovirals and never alone.
• Drug may cause mildly elevated glucose levels.
• *Alert:* Don't confuse abacavir with amprenavir.

PATIENT TEACHING
• Inform patient that abacavir can cause a life-threatening hypersensitivity reaction. Warn patient who develops signs or symptoms of hypersensitivity (such as fever, rash, severe tiredness, achiness, a generally ill feeling, nausea, vomiting, diarrhea, or stomach pain) to stop taking drug and notify prescriber immediately.
• Include information leaflet about drug with each new prescription and refill. Patient also should receive, and be instructed to carry, a warning card summarizing signs and symptoms of abacavir hypersensitivity reaction.
• Inform patient that this drug doesn't cure HIV infection. Tell patient that drug hasn't been shown to reduce the risk of transmission of HIV to others through sexual contact or blood contamination and that its long-term effects are unknown.

• Tell patient to take drug exactly as prescribed.
• Inform patient that drug can be taken with or without food.

---

acyclovir sodium
Avirax†, Zovirax

Pregnancy risk category C

AVAILABLE FORMS
Capsules: 200 mg
Injection: 500 mg/vial, 1 g/vial
Suspension: 200 mg/5 ml
Tablets: 400 mg, 800 mg

INDICATIONS & DOSAGES
➤ **Initial and recurrent episodes of mucocutaneous herpes simplex virus (HSV-1 and HSV-2) infections in immunocompromised patients; severe initial episodes of genital herpes in patients who aren't immunocompromised**—
Adults and children age 12 and older: 5 mg/kg given I.V. at a constant rate over 1 hour q 8 hours for 7 days. Give for 5 to 7 days for severe initial episode of genital herpes.
Children younger than age 12: 20 mg/kg given I.V. at a constant rate over 1 hour q 8 hours for 10 days.
➤ **Initial genital herpes**—
Adults: 200 mg P.O. q 4 hours while awake five times daily; or 400 mg P.O. q 8 hours. Continue for 7 to 10 days for treatment of initial genital herpes episodes.
➤ **Intermittent therapy for recurrent genital herpes**—
Adults: 200 mg P.O. q 4 hours while awake for total of five capsules daily. Treatment should continue for 5 days. Initiate therapy at first sign of recurrence.
➤ **Long-term suppressive therapy for recurrent genital herpes**—
Adults: 400 mg P.O. b.i.d. for up to 12 months. Or, 200 mg P.O. three to five times daily for up to 12 months.
➤ *Varicella* **(chickenpox) infections in immunocompromised patients**—
Adults and children age 12 and older: 10 mg/kg I.V. infused at a constant rate over 1 hour q 8 hours for 7 days. Dosage for obese patients is 10 mg/kg based on

ideal body weight q 8 hours for 7 days. Don't exceed maximum dosage equivalent of 500 mg/m² q 8 hours.

Children younger than age 12: 500 mg/m² I.V. infused at a constant rate over 1 hour q 8 hours for 7 days.

➤ *Varicella* **infection in immunocompetent patients—**

Adults and children weighing more than 40 kg (88 lb): 800 mg P.O. q.i.d. for 5 days.

Children age 2 and older, weighing less than 40 kg: 20 mg/kg (maximum 800 mg/ dose) P.O. q.i.d. for 5 days. Start therapy as soon as symptoms appear.

➤ **Acute** *herpes zoster* **infection in immunocompetent patients—**

Adults and children age 12 and older: 800 mg P.O. q 4 hours five times daily for 7 to 10 days.

➤ **Herpes simplex encephalitis—**

Adults and children age 12 and older: 10 mg/kg I.V. infused at a constant rate over 1 hour q 8 hours for 10 days. Or, in children ages 6 months to 12 years, 500 mg/m² I.V. infused at a constant rate over 1 hour q 8 hours for 10 days.

Children ages 3 months to 12 years: 20 mg/kg I.V. infused at a constant rate over 1 hour q 8 hours for 10 days.

Adjust-a-dose: For patients with renal failure, if creatinine clearance is more than 50 ml/minute, I.V. dose is 100% of dose q 8 hours; if clearance is 25 to 50 ml/ minute, 100% of dose q 12 hours; if clearance is 10 to 24 ml/minute, 100% of dose q 24 hours; if clearance is less than 10 ml/ minute, 50% of dose q 24 hours.

*P.O. dosage—*If normal dose is 200 mg q 4 hours five times daily and creatinine clearance is less than 10 ml/minute, 200 mg P.O. q 12 hours. If normal dose is 400 mg q 12 hours and clearance is less than 10 ml/minute, 200 mg q 12 hours. If normal dose is 800 mg q 4 hours five times daily and clearance is less than 10 ml/minute, 800 mg q 12 hours; and if clearance is 10 to 25 ml/minute, 800 mg q 8 hours.

I.V. ADMINISTRATION

● Administer I.V. infusion over at least 1 hour to prevent renal tubular damage. Don't give by bolus injection. Bolus injection, dehydration (decreased urine output),

renal disease, and use together with other nephrotoxic drugs increase the risk of renal toxicity.

● Concentrated solutions (7 mg/ml or more) may cause a higher risk of phlebitis.

● Encourage fluid intake because patient must be adequately hydrated during acyclovir infusion. Monitor intake and output, especially within the first 2 hours after I.V. administration.

ACTION

Interferes with DNA synthesis and inhibits viral multiplication.

Route	Onset	Peak	Duration
I.V.	Immediate	Immediate	Unknown
P.O.	Unknown	2.5 hr	Unknown

ADVERSE REACTIONS

CNS: *malaise, headache,* encephalopathic changes, including lethargy, obtundation, tremor, confusion, hallucinations, agitation, *seizures, coma.*

GI: *nausea, vomiting,* diarrhea.

GU: hematuria, *acute renal failure.*

Hematologic: *thrombocytopenia, leukopenia,* thrombocytosis.

Skin: rash, itching, urticaria.

Other: *inflammation, phlebitis at injection site.*

INTERACTIONS

Drug-drug. *Interferon:* May have synergistic effect. Monitor patient closely.

Probenecid: Increased acyclovir blood levels. Monitor patient for possible toxicity.

Zidovudine: May cause drowsiness or lethargy. Use together cautiously.

EFFECTS ON LAB TEST RESULTS

● May increase BUN and creatinine levels.

● May decrease WBC count. May increase or decrease platelet count.

CONTRAINDICATIONS

Contraindicated in patients hypersensitive to drug.

NURSING CONSIDERATIONS

● Use cautiously in patients with neurologic problems, renal disease, or dehydration and in those receiving other nephrotoxic drugs. Monitor renal function.

• *Alert:* Don't administer I.M. or S.C.
• Encephalopathic changes are more likely to occur in patients with neurologic disorders or in those who have had neurologic reactions to cytotoxic drugs.
• Because there are no adequate studies in pregnant women, acyclovir should be used during pregnancy only if potential benefits outweigh risks to fetus.

PATIENT TEACHING
• Tell patient to take drug as prescribed, even after he feels better.
• Tell patient that drug is effective in managing herpes infection but doesn't eliminate or cure it. Warn patient that acyclovir won't prevent spread of infection to others.
• Tell patient to avoid sexual contact while visible lesions are present.
• Teach patient about early signs and symptoms of herpes infection (such as tingling, itching, or pain). Tell him to notify prescriber and get a prescription for acyclovir before the infection fully develops. Early treatment is most effective.

---

amantadine hydrochloride
Symmetrel

Pregnancy risk category C

AVAILABLE FORMS
Capsules: 100 mg
Syrup: 50 mg/5 ml

INDICATIONS & DOSAGES
➤ **Prophylaxis or symptomatic treatment of influenza type A virus, respiratory tract illnesses—**
Adults up to age 65 with normal renal function: 200 mg P.O. daily in a single dose or 100 mg P.O. b.i.d.
Children ages 9 to 12: 100 mg P.O. b.i.d.
Children ages 1 to 9 or weighing less than 45 kg (99 lb): 4.4 to 8.8 mg/kg P.O. as a total daily dose given once daily or divided equally b.i.d. Maximum daily dose is 150 mg.
Elderly patients: 100 mg P.O. once daily in patients older than age 65 with normal renal function.

Begin treatment within 24 to 48 hours after symptoms appear and continue for 24

to 48 hours after symptoms disappear (usually 2 to 7 days of therapy). Start prophylaxis as soon as possible after initial exposure and continue for at least 10 days after exposure. May continue prophylactic treatment up to 90 days for repeated or suspected exposures if influenza vaccine is unavailable. If used with influenza vaccine, continue dose for 2 to 3 weeks until antibody response to vaccine has developed.
Adjust-a-dose: For patients with renal failure, if creatinine clearance is 30 to 50 ml/minute, give 200 mg the first day and 100 mg thereafter; if clearance is 15 to 29 ml/minute, give 200 mg the first day, then 100 mg on alternate days; if clearance is below 15 ml/minute, give 200 mg q 7 days.

ACTION
Unknown. Possibly inhibits the uncoating of the influenza A virus, preventing release of infection's viral nucleic acid into the host cell.

Route	Onset	Peak	Duration
P.O.	Unknown	1-4 hr	Unknown

ADVERSE REACTIONS
CNS: depression, fatigue, confusion, *dizziness,* hallucinations, anxiety, *irritability,* ataxia, *insomnia,* headache, *light-headedness.*
CV: peripheral edema, orthostatic hypotension, **heart failure.**
EENT: blurred vision.
GI: anorexia, *nausea,* constipation, vomiting, dry mouth.
Skin: livedo reticularis.

INTERACTIONS
Drug-drug. *Anticholinergics:* Increased anticholinergic effects. Use together cautiously; reduce dosage of anticholinergic before starting amantadine.
CNS stimulants: Increased CNS stimulation. Use together cautiously.
Drug-herb. *Jimsonweed:* May adversely affect CV function. Discourage use together.
Drug-lifestyle. *Alcohol:* Increased CNS effects. Discourage use together.

EFFECTS ON LAB TEST RESULTS
None reported.

Reactions may be *common*, uncommon, *life-threatening*, or COMMON AND LIFE-THREATENING.

CONTRAINDICATIONS
Contraindicated in patients hypersensitive to drug.

NURSING CONSIDERATIONS
● Use cautiously in elderly patients and in patients with seizure disorders, heart failure, peripheral edema, hepatic disease, mental illness, eczematoid rash, renal impairment, orthostatic hypotension, and CV disease. Monitor renal and liver function tests.
● Begin treatment within 24 to 48 hours after symptoms appear and continue for 24 to 48 hours after symptoms disappear (usually 2 to 7 days of therapy).
● Start prophylaxis as soon as possible after initial exposure and continue for at least 10 days after exposure. May continue prophylactic treatment up to 90 days for repeated or suspected exposures if influenza vaccine is unavailable. If used with influenza vaccine, continue dose for 2 to 3 weeks until antibody response to vaccine has developed.
● *Alert:* Elderly patients are more susceptible to adverse neurologic effects. Monitor patient for mental status changes.
● Suicidal ideation and attempts have been reported in patients both with and without prior psychiatric problems.
● Drug can exacerbate mental problems in patients with a history of psychiatric disorders or substance abuse.
● *Alert:* Don't confuse amantadine with rimantadine.

PATIENT TEACHING
● Tell patient to take drug exactly as prescribed. Taking more than prescribed can result in serious adverse reactions or death.
● If insomnia occurs, tell patient to take drug several hours before bedtime.
● If orthostatic hypotension occurs, instruct patient not to stand or change positions too quickly.
● Instruct patient to notify prescriber of adverse reactions, especially dizziness, depression, anxiety, nausea, and urine retention.
● Caution patient to avoid activities that require mental alertness until CNS effects of drug are known.

● Advise patient to avoid alcohol while taking drug.

amprenavir
Agenerase

Pregnancy risk category C

AVAILABLE FORMS
Capsules: 50 mg, 150 mg
Oral solution: 15 mg/ml

INDICATIONS & DOSAGES
➤ **HIV-1 infection (with other antiretrovirals)—**
Adults and adolescents ages 13 to 16 weighing more than or equal to 50 kg (110 lb): 1,200 mg (eight 150-mg capsules) P.O. b.i.d. with other antiretrovirals.
Children ages 4 to 12 and adolescents ages 13 to 16 weighing less than 50 kg:
Capsule—20 mg/kg P.O. b.i.d. or 15 mg/kg P.O. t.i.d. to maximum daily dose of 2,400 mg with other antiretrovirals.
Oral solution—22.5 mg/kg (1.5 ml/kg) P.O. b.i.d. or 17 mg/kg (1.1 ml/kg) P.O. t.i.d. to maximum daily dose of 2,800 mg with other antiretrovirals.
Adjust-a-dose: For patients with liver impairment and a Child-Pugh score from 5 to 8, reduce dose for capsules to 450 mg P.O. b.i.d. In patients with a Child-Pugh score from 9 to 12, reduce dose for capsules to 300 mg P.O. b.i.d.

ACTION
Inhibits HIV-1 protease by binding to the active site of HIV-1 protease, which causes immature noninfectious viral particles to form.

Route	Onset	Peak	Duration
P.O.	Unknown	1-2 hr	Unknown

ADVERSE REACTIONS
CNS: *oral and perioral paresthesia,* depression or mood disorders.
GI: *nausea, vomiting, diarrhea or loose stools,* taste disorders.
Metabolic: *hyperglycemia, hypertriglyceridemia,* hypercholesterolemia.
Skin: *rash,* **Stevens-Johnson syndrome.**

INTERACTIONS
Drug-drug. *Amiodarone, lidocaine, quinidine, tricyclic antidepressants:* Inhibited metabolism of these drugs. Monitor drug levels closely.

Antacids, didanosine: Decreased drug absorption. Separate administration times by at least 1 hour.

Anticonvulsants, such as carbamazepine, phenobarbital, and phenytoin: May decrease amprenavir levels. Monitor patient closely and adjust dosage, as needed.

Atorvastatin: Increased risk of myopathy, including rhabdomyolysis. Use together cautiously.

Bepridil, dihydroergotamine, ergotamine, midazolam, triazolam: Inhibited metabolism of these drugs, which may cause serious or life-threatening adverse reactions. Avoid using together.

Erythromycin: May increase plasma levels of both drugs. Monitor patient closely.

Indinavir, ritonavir, nelfinavir: Increased levels of amprenavir. Monitor patient closely.

Lovastatin, simvastatin: Increased plasma levels of these drugs, and risk of toxicity. Avoid using together.

Oral contraceptives: May reduce efficacy of contraceptives. Advise patient to use an alternative method of contraception.

Rifabutin: Decreased amprenavir levels and increased rifabutin levels. Reduce rifabutin dosage to at least half the recommended dosage. Monitor CBC weekly for neutropenia.

Rifampin: 90% reduced plasma amprenavir levels. Avoid using together.

Saquinavir: Decreased bioavailability of amprenavir, decreasing concentrations. Monitor patient closely.

Sildenafil: Increased sildenafil levels, which may increase frequency of adverse reactions caused by this drug, such as hypotension, visual changes, and priapism. Warn patient not to exceed 25 mg of sildenafil in 48 hours.

Warfarin: Inhibited metabolism of warfarin, which may cause serious or life-threatening adverse reactions. Monitor INR closely.

Drug-herb. *St. John's wort:* Reduced blood levels of indinavir by more than 50%; similar effects can be expected in other protease inhibitors. Discourage use together.

Drug-food. *High-fat foods:* Decreased absorption of drug. Tell patient to avoid taking drug with high-fat foods.

EFFECTS ON LAB TEST RESULTS
• May increase glucose, triglyceride, and cholesterol levels.

CONTRAINDICATIONS
Contraindicated in patients hypersensitive to drug or its components. Contraindicated in infants, children younger than 4 years of age, pregnant women, patients with liver or kidney failure, and patients treated with disulfuram (Antabuse) or metronidazole (Flagyl).

NURSING CONSIDERATIONS
• Use cautiously in patients with moderate or severe hepatic impairment, diabetes mellitus, a known sulfonamide allergy, or hemophilia A or B.
• Use cautiously in pregnant women because no adequate studies exist regarding the effects of amprenavir when administered during pregnancy. Use during pregnancy only if the potential benefits outweigh the risks. Register pregnant woman taking amprenavir with the Antiretroviral Pregnancy Registry by calling 1-800-258-4263.
• *Alert:* Drug can cause severe or life-threatening rash, including Stevens-Johnson syndrome. Stop therapy if patient develops a severe or life-threatening rash or a moderate rash accompanied by systemic signs and symptoms.
• *Alert:* Because amprenavir may interact with many drugs, obtain patient's complete drug history. Ask patient to show you the drugs he's taking.
• Patient shouldn't eat high-fat foods because they may decrease absorption of amprenavir.
• Amprenavir oral solution should only be used when the capsules or other protease inhibitor formulations are not therapeutic options.
• Monitor patient for adverse reactions. A patient taking a protease inhibitor may experience a redistribution of body fat, including central obesity, dorsocervical fat enlargement (buffalo hump), peripheral

wasting, breast enlargement, and cushin-goid appearance. The mechanism and long-term consequences of these effects are unknown.
• Drug provides high daily doses of vitamin E. Advise patient taking drug not to take supplemental vitamin E because high vitamin levels may exacerbate the blood coagulation defect of vitamin K deficiency that anticoagulant therapy or malabsorption causes.
• Protease inhibitors have caused spontaneous bleeding in some patients with hemophilia A or B. In some patients, additional factor VIII was needed. In many of the reported cases, treatment with protease inhibitors was continued or restarted.
• Amprenavir capsules aren't interchangeable with amprenavir oral solution on a milligram-per-milligram basis.
• *Alert:* Don't confuse amprenavir with abacavir.

PATIENT TEACHING
• Advise patient that drug doesn't cure HIV infection; patient may continue to develop opportunistic infections and other complications from the disease. Also, tell patient that drug doesn't reduce risk of HIV transmission through sexual contact.
• Tell patient that, although drug can be taken without regard to food, he shouldn't take it with a high-fat meal because of decreased drug absorption.
• Tell patient to report adverse reactions, especially rash.
• Advise patient to take drug daily, as prescribed, with other antiretrovirals. Dosage must not be altered or stopped without prescriber's approval.
• Inform patient to take an antacid or didanosine 1 hour before or after amprenavir to prevent a decrease in amprenavir absorption.
• If a dose is missed by more than 4 hours, advise patient to wait and take the next dose at the regularly scheduled time. If a dose is missed by less than 4 hours, advise him to take the dose as soon as possible and then take the next dose at the regularly scheduled time. If a dose is skipped, patient shouldn't double the dose.
• Advise patient using hormonal contraception to use another contraceptive method during drug therapy.

• Advise patient to notify prescriber if pregnancy occurs during therapy.
• Advise patient not to take supplemental vitamin E because drug contains a significant amount of the vitamin.

---

cidofovir
Vistide

Pregnancy risk category C

AVAILABLE FORMS
Injection: 75 mg/ml in 5-ml vial

INDICATIONS & DOSAGES
➤ **CMV retinitis in patients with AIDS—**
Adults: Initially, 5 mg/kg I.V. infused over 1 hour once weekly for 2 consecutive weeks; then maintenance dose of 5 mg/kg I.V. infused over 1 hour once q 2 weeks. Administer probenecid and prehydration with normal saline solution I.V. concomitantly; may reduce potential for nephrotoxicity.
Adjust-a-dose: For patients with renal failure, if serum creatinine increases 0.3 to 0.4 mg/dl above baseline, dose is reduced to 3 mg/kg at same rate and frequency. If serum creatinine increases 0.5 mg/dl or more above baseline, drug is discontinued.

I.V. ADMINISTRATION
• Because of the potential for increased nephrotoxicity, don't exceed recommended dosages or frequency or rate of administration.
• To prepare cidofovir for infusion, extract the appropriate amount of cidofovir from the vial using a syringe and transfer the dose to an infusion bag containing 100 ml of normal saline solution. Infuse the entire volume I.V. at a constant rate over a 1-hour period. Use a standard infusion pump for administration.
• Because of the mutagenic properties of cidofovir, drug should be prepared in a class II laminar flow biological safety cabinet. Personnel preparing drug should wear surgical gloves and a closed front surgical gown with knit cuffs.
• If drug contacts the skin, wash membranes and flush thoroughly with water. Excess drug and all other materials used

---

in the admixture preparation and administration should be placed in a leakproof, puncture-proof container. Recommended method of disposal is high temperature incineration.

• Cidofovir infusion admixtures should be administered within 24 hours of preparation; refrigerator or freezer storage shouldn't be used to extend this 24-hour period. If admixtures aren't used immediately, they may be refrigerated at 36° to 46° F (2° to 8° C) for longer than 24 hours. Allow cidofovir to reach room temperature before use.

• Don't add other drugs or supplements to admixture for concurrent administration.

• Compatibility with Ringer's solution, lactated Ringer's solution, or bacteriostatic infusion fluids hasn't been evaluated.

ACTION

A nucleotide analogue that suppresses CMV replication by selective inhibition of viral DNA synthesis.

Route	Onset	Peak	Duration
I.V.	Unknown	Unknown	Unknown

ADVERSE REACTIONS

CNS: *asthenia, headache,* amnesia, anxiety, confusion, **seizures,** depression, dizziness, abnormal gait, hallucinations, insomnia, neuropathy, paresthesia, somnolence, malaise.

CV: hypotension, orthostatic hypotension, pallor, syncope, tachycardia, vasodilation.

EENT: amblyopia, conjunctivitis, pharyngitis, eye disorders, *ocular hypotony,* iritis, retinal detachment, uveitis, abnormal vision, rhinitis, sinusitis.

GI: *nausea, vomiting, diarrhea, anorexia, abdominal pain,* dry mouth, colitis, constipation, tongue discoloration, dyspepsia, dysphagia, flatulence, gastritis, melena, oral candidiasis, rectal disorders, stomatitis, aphthous stomatitis, mouth ulcerations, taste perversion.

GU: **nephrotoxicity,** proteinuria, glycosuria, hematuria, urinary incontinence, urinary tract infection.

Hematologic: NEUTROPENIA, *anemia,* **thrombocytopenia.**

Hepatic: hepatomegaly.

Metabolic: weight loss, fluid imbalance, hyperglycemia, hyperlipemia, hypocalcemia, hypokalemia, decreased serum bicarbonate level.

Musculoskeletal: arthralgia; myasthenia; myalgia; pain in back, chest, or neck.

Respiratory: asthma, bronchitis, coughing, *dyspnea,* hiccups, increased sputum, lung disorders, pneumonia.

Skin: *rash, alopecia,* acne, skin discoloration, dry skin, pruritus, sweating, urticaria.

Other: *fever, infections, chills,* allergic reactions, herpes simplex, facial edema, **sarcoma, sepsis.**

INTERACTIONS

Drug-drug. *Nephrotoxic drugs (such as aminoglycosides, amphotericin B, foscarnet, I.V. pentamidine):* May increase nephrotoxicity. Avoid using together.

EFFECTS ON LAB TEST RESULTS

• May increase BUN, creatinine, alkaline phosphatase, ALT, AST, and LDH levels. May decrease creatinine clearance levels.

• May decrease hemoglobin and neutrophil and platelet counts.

CONTRAINDICATIONS

Contraindicated in patients hypersensitive to drug or with history of clinically severe hypersensitivity to probenecid or other sulfur-containing drugs. Also contraindicated in patients receiving drugs with nephrotoxic potential and in those with serum creatinine exceeding 1.5 mg/dl, a calculated creatinine clearance of 55 ml/minute or less, or a urine protein of 100 mg/dl or more (equivalent to 2+ proteinuria or more). Don't administer as a direct intraocular injection because it may be associated with significant decreases in intraocular pressure and vision impairment.

NURSING CONSIDERATIONS

• Use cautiously in patients with impaired renal function. Monitor renal function tests and patient's fluid balance.

• Cidofovir is indicated only for the treatment of CMV retinitis in patients with AIDS. Safety and efficacy of drug haven't been established for treating other CMV infections, congenital or neonatal CMV disease, or CMV disease in patients not infected with HIV.

• Cidofovir has been known to be carcinogenic and teratogenic and has caused hypospermia.
• Administer 1 L normal saline solution, usually over 1- to 2-hour period immediately before cidofovir infusion.
• Administer probenecid with cidofovir.
• Monitor renal function (serum creatinine and urine protein levels) before each dose. Dosage may be modified by a prescriber if changes in renal function occur.
• Fanconi's syndrome and decreased serum bicarbonate levels with renal tubular damage have been reported in patients receiving cidofovir. Monitor patient closely.
• Monitor WBC counts with differential before each dose.
• Granulocytopenia has been observed with drug treatment. Monitor neutrophil counts during therapy.
• Intraocular pressure, visual acuity, and ocular symptoms should be monitored periodically.
• Stop zidovudine therapy or reduce dosage by 50%, on the days cidofovir is administered; probenecid reduces metabolic clearance of zidovudine.
• Dosage adjustment may be necessary in elderly patients with renal impairment.
• Safety and effectiveness in children haven't been established.
• It's unknown if cidofovir appears in breast milk. Don't administer drug to breast-feeding women.

PATIENT TEACHING
• Inform patient that drug doesn't cure CMV retinitis and that regular ophthalmologic follow-up examinations are needed.
• Alert patient taking zidovudine that he'll need to obtain dosage guidelines on days cidofovir is administered.
• Tell patient that close monitoring of renal function will be needed and that abnormalities may require a change in cidofovir therapy.
• Stress importance of completing a full course of probenecid with each cidofovir dose. Tell patient to take probenecid after a meal to decrease nausea.
• Advise woman of childbearing age to use effective contraception during and for 1 month after treatment with cidofovir.

• Advise man to practice barrier contraception during and for 3 months after treatment with drug.
• Advise breast-feeding woman that it's unknown if cidofovir appears in breast milk.

delavirdine mesylate
Rescriptor

Pregnancy risk category C

AVAILABLE FORMS
Tablets: 100 mg

INDICATIONS & DOSAGES
➤ **HIV-1 infection when therapy is warranted—**
Adults: 400 mg P.O. t.i.d. with other appropriate antiretrovirals.

ACTION
A nonnucleoside reverse-transcriptase inhibitor of HIV-1. Drug binds directly to reverse transcriptase and blocks RNA- and DNA-dependent DNA polymerase activities.

Route	Onset	Peak	Duration
P.O.	Unknown	1 hr	Unknown

ADVERSE REACTIONS
CNS: abnormal coordination, agitation, amnesia, anxiety, change in dreams, cognitive impairment, confusion, depression, disorientation, dizziness, emotional lability, fatigue, hallucinations, headache, hyperesthesia, hyperreflexia, hypoesthesia, impaired concentration, lethargy, malaise, insomnia, manic symptoms, migraine, nervousness, neuropathy, nightmares, paralysis, paranoid symptoms, paresthesia, restlessness, somnolence, tetany, tingling, tremor, vertigo, weakness, asthenia.
CV: bradycardia, chest pain, edema, orthostatic hypotension, palpitations, syncope, tachycardia, vasodilation.
EENT: blepharitis, conjunctivitis, diplopia, dry eyes, ear pain, epistaxis, nystagmus, pharyngitis, photophobia, rhinitis, sinusitis, tinnitus.
GI: anorexia, aphthous stomatitis, bloody stools, colitis, constipation, decreased appetite, diarrhea, diverticulitis, duodenitis,

dry mouth, dyspepsia, dysphagia, enteritis, esophagitis, fecal incontinence, flatulence, gagging, gastritis, gastroesophageal reflux, GI bleeding, gingivitis, gum hemorrhage, increased thirst and appetite, increased saliva, mouth ulcer, *nausea,* nonspecific ***hepatitis, pancreatitis,*** rectal disorder, sialadenitis, stomatitis, tongue edema or ulceration, vomiting, abdominal cramps, distention, or pain, taste perversion.

GU: epididymitis, hematuria, hemospermia, impotence, renal calculi, renal pain, metrorrhagia, nocturia, polyuria, proteinuria, vaginal candidiasis.

Hematologic: eosinophilia, granulocytosis, anemia, ecchymosis, ***neutropenia, pancytopenia,*** petechiae, purpura, spleen disorder, ***thrombocytopenia.***

Hepatic: bilirubinemia.

Metabolic: weight gain or loss, alcohol intolerance, hyperkalemia, hyperuricemia, hypocalcemia, hyponatremia, hypophosphatemia, increased gamma glutamyl transpeptidase, lipase, serum alkaline phosphatase, serum amylase, serum CK, and serum creatinine levels.

Musculoskeletal: bone disorder, arthralgia or arthritis of single and multiple joints, bone pain, back pain, flank pain, leg cramps, muscle cramps, muscular weakness, myalgia, neck rigidity, tendon disorder, tenosynovitis.

Respiratory: chest congestion, bronchitis, dyspnea, laryngismus, cough, upper respiratory tract infection.

Skin: alopecia, dermal leukocytoblastic vasculitis, dermatitis, desquamation, diaphoresis, dry skin, epidermal cyst, erythema, ***erythema multiforme,*** folliculitis, fungal dermatitis, maculopapular rash, nail disorder, pallor, petechial rash, pruritus, *rash,* sebaceous cyst, seborrhea, skin nodule, ***Stevens-Johnson syndrome,*** urticaria, vesiculobullous rash.

Other: allergic reaction, breast enlargement, chills, decreased libido, fever, flu syndrome, lip edema, pain, trauma, peripheral edema, ***angioedema.***

INTERACTIONS
Drug-drug. *Amphetamines, benzodiazepines, calcium channel blockers, ergot alkaloid preparations, quinidine:* May cause serious or life-threatening adverse effects. Avoid using together.

Antacids: Reduced absorption of delavirdine. Separate doses by at least 1 hour.
Carbamazepine, phenobarbital, phenytoin, rifampin: Substantially decreased plasma delavirdine levels. Avoid using together.
Clarithromycin: Increased levels of both drugs. Adjust dosage, as needed.
Dapsone, warfarin: Delavirdine increases plasma levels of these drugs. Adjust dosage, as needed.
Didanosine: 20% decrease in absorption of both drugs. Separate administration times by at least 1 hour.
Fluoxetine, ketoconazole: Increased delavirdine trough levels. Monitor patient.
H₂-receptor antagonists: May reduce absorption of delavirdine. Avoid long-term use together.
Indinavir: Increased plasma levels of indinavir. May need to lower dosage of indinavir.
Rifabutin: Decreased delavirdine levels and increased rifabutin levels. Use together cautiously.
Saquinavir: Fivefold increase in systemic levels of saquinavir. Monitor AST and ALT levels frequently when used together.
Drug-herb. *St. John's wort:* May decrease serum levels of drug weakening its therapeutic effect. Discourage use together.

EFFECTS ON LAB TEST RESULTS
● May increase ALT and AST levels.
● May increase PTT and eosinophil count. May decrease hemoglobin and granulocyte, neutrophil, WBC, RBC, and platelet counts.

CONTRAINDICATIONS
Contraindicated in patients hypersensitive to drug or its components.

NURSING CONSIDERATIONS
● Use cautiously in patients with impaired hepatic function.
● Drug-induced rash is more common in patients with lower CD4⁺ cell counts and usually occurs within first 3 weeks of treatment. It's typically diffuse, maculopapular, erythematous, and often pruritic. It occurs commonly and its occurrence doesn't appear to be significantly reduced by adjusted drug doses.

• Rash occurs mainly on the upper body and proximal arms. Using diphenhydramine, hydroxyzine, or topical corticosteroids may relieve symptoms.

• Because drug's effects in patients with hepatic or renal impairment haven't been studied, monitor renal and liver function test results carefully.

• Drug hasn't been shown to reduce risk of transmission of HIV-1.

• Because resistance develops rapidly when used as monotherapy, always use drug with appropriate antiretroviral therapy.

• Monitor patient's fluid balance and weight.

PATIENT TEACHING

• Tell patient to stop drug and call prescriber if severe rash or such symptoms as fever, blistering, oral lesions, conjunctivitis, swelling, or muscle or joint aches occur.

• Inform patient that drug doesn't cure HIV-1 infection and that he may continue to acquire illnesses related to HIV-1 infection, including opportunistic infections. Therapy hasn't been shown to reduce the risk or frequency of such illnesses. Drug hasn't been shown to reduce transmission of HIV.

• Advise patient to remain under medical supervision when taking drug because the long-term effects aren't known.

• Tell patient to take drug as prescribed and not to alter doses without prescriber's approval. If a dose is missed, tell patient to take the next dose as soon as possible; he shouldn't double the next dose.

• Inform patient that drug may be dispersed in water before ingestion. Add tablets to at least 5 ounces (148 ml) of water, allow to stand for a few minutes, and stir until a uniform dispersion occurs. Tell patient to drink dispersion promptly, rinse glass, and swallow the rinse to ensure that entire dose is consumed.

• Tell patient that drug may be taken without regard to food.

• Instruct patient with achlorhydria to take drug with an acidic beverage, such as orange or cranberry juice.

• Instruct patient to take drug and antacids at least 1 hour apart.

• Advise patient to report use of other prescription or OTC drugs, including herbal remedies.

---

didanosine (ddI)
Videx, Videx EC

Pregnancy risk category B

AVAILABLE FORMS
Delayed-release capsules: 125 mg, 200 mg, 250 mg, 400 mg
Powder for oral solution (buffered): 100 mg/packet, 167 mg/packet, 250 mg/packet
Powder for oral solution (pediatric): 4-ounce, 8-ounce glass bottles containing 2 g and 4 g of Videx, respectively
Tablets (buffered, chewable): 25 mg, 50 mg, 100 mg, 150 mg, 200 mg

INDICATIONS & DOSAGES
➤ **HIV infection when antiretroviral therapy is warranted—**
Adults weighing 60 kg (132 lb) or more: 200 mg tablets P.O. q 12 hours or 400 mg P.O. once daily; or 250 mg buffered powder P.O. q 12 hours.
Adults weighing less than 60 kg: 125 mg tablets P.O. q 12 hours or 250 mg P.O. once daily; or 167 mg buffered powder P.O. q 12 hours.
Children: 120 mg/m² P.O. q 12 hours; Videx EC has not been studied in children.
Adjust-a-dose: Dialysis patients should receive 25% of usual dose. In adults who weigh 60 kg or more with creatinine clearance of 30 to 59 ml/minute, give 100-mg tablet b.i.d. or 200-mg tablet once daily or 200-mg capsule once daily or 100-mg oral solution b.i.d.; for clearance of 10 to 29 ml/minute, give 150-mg tablet once daily or 125-mg capsule once daily or 167-mg oral solution once daily; for clearance less than 10 ml/minute, give 100-mg tablet or 125-mg capsule once daily or 100-mg oral solution once daily.

In adults who weigh less than 60 kg with clearance of 30 to 59 ml/minute, give 75-mg tablet b.i.d. or 150-mg tablet once daily or 125-mg capsule once daily, or 100-mg oral solution b.i.d.; for clearance of 10 to 29 ml/minute, give 100-mg tablet

---

or 125-mg capsule once daily or 100-mg oral solution once daily. For clearance less than 10 ml/minute, give 75-mg tablet once daily or 100-mg oral solution once daily; capsule not indicated for these patients.

ACTION
Inhibits the enzyme HIV-RNA–dependent DNA polymerase (reverse transcriptase) and terminates DNA chain growth.

Route	Onset	Peak	Duration
P.O.	Unknown	0.5-1 hr	Unknown

ADVERSE REACTIONS
CNS: *headache, seizures,* confusion, anxiety, nervousness, abnormal thinking, twitching, depression, *peripheral neuropathy, dizziness,* asthenia, insomnia.
CV: hypertension, edema, ***heart failure.***
EENT: retinal changes, optic neuritis.
GI: *diarrhea, nausea, vomiting, abdominal pain, pancreatitis,* dry mouth, anorexia.
Hematologic: *leukopenia,* granulocytosis, ***thrombocytopenia,*** anemia.
Hepatic: *hepatic failure.*
Metabolic: hyperuricemia.
Musculoskeletal: myopathy.
Respiratory: dyspnea, pneumonia.
Skin: rash, pruritus, alopecia.
Other: pain, infection, *sarcoma,* allergic reactions, *chills, fever.*

INTERACTIONS
Drug-drug. *Amprenavir, delavirdine, indinavir, nelfinavir, ritonavir, saquinavir:* Altered pharmacokinetics of didanosine or these drugs. Separate administration times.
Antacids containing magnesium or aluminum hydroxides: Enhanced adverse effects of the antacid component (including diarrhea or constipation) when administered with didanosine tablets or pediatric suspension. Avoid using together.
Co-trimoxazole, pentamidine, other drugs linked to pancreatitis: Increased risk of pancreatic toxicity. Use together cautiously; consider temporarily stopping didanosine during administration of these drugs.
Dapsone, drugs that require gastric acid for adequate absorption, ketoconazole: Decreased absorption from buffering action. Administer these drugs 2 hours before didanosine.

Fluoroquinolones, tetracyclines: Decreased absorption from buffering products in didanosine tablets or antacids in pediatric suspension. Separate administration times by at least 2 hours.
Itraconazole: Decreased serum levels of itraconazole. Avoid using together.
Drug-herb. *St. John's wort:* Decreased drug serum levels decreasing the therapeutic effects. Warn patient about using together.
Drug-food. *Any food:* Decreased rate of absorption. Give drug on an empty stomach at least 30 minutes before a meal.

EFFECTS ON LAB TEST RESULTS
• May increase uric acid, AST, ALT, alkaline phosphatase, and bilirubin levels.
• May decrease hemoglobin and WBC, granulocyte, and platelet counts.

CONTRAINDICATIONS
Contraindicated in patients hypersensitive to drug or its components.

NURSING CONSIDERATIONS
• Use cautiously in patients with history of pancreatitis; fatalities have occurred. Also use cautiously in patients with peripheral neuropathy, renal or hepatic impairment, or hyperuricemia. Monitor liver and renal function tests.
• Administer didanosine on an empty stomach, regardless of dosage form used; giving drug with meals can decrease absorption by 50%.
• To administer single-dose packets containing buffered powder for oral solution, pour contents into 4 ounces (120 ml) of water. Don't use fruit juice or other beverages that may be acidic. Stir for 2 or 3 minutes until the powder dissolves completely. Give immediately.
• The powder for oral solution may cause diarrhea. The manufacturer suggests switching to the tablet formulation if diarrhea is a problem.
• *Alert:* The pediatric powder for oral solution must be prepared by a pharmacist before dispensing. It must be constituted with purified USP water and then diluted with an antacid (either Mylanta Double Strength Liquid or Maalox TC Suspension) to a final concentration of 10 mg/ml. The admixture is stable for 30 days if re-

frigerated (at 36° to 46° F [2° to 8° C]).
Shake the solution well before measuring
dose.
• **Alert:** Don't confuse drug with other antivirals that use abbreviations for identification.

PATIENT TEACHING
• Instruct patient to take drug on an empty
stomach.
• Because the tablets contain buffers that
raise stomach pH to levels that prevent
degradation of the active drug, instruct
patient to chew tablets thoroughly before
swallowing and drink at least 1 ounce
(30 ml) of water with each dose. Teach
patient how to prepare crushed tablets or
buffered powder form for ingestion, if appropriate.
• Inform patient on a sodium-restricted
diet that each two-tablet dose of didanosine contains 529 mg of sodium; each single packet of buffered powder for oral solution contains 1.38 g of sodium.
• Tell patient to report symptoms of pancreatitis, such as abdominal pain, nausea,
vomiting, diarrhea, or symptoms of
peripheral neuropathy.

---

efavirenz
Sustiva

Pregnancy risk category C

AVAILABLE FORMS
Capsules: 50 mg, 100 mg, 200 mg

INDICATIONS & DOSAGES
➤ **HIV-1 infection, with a protease
inhibitor or nucleoside analogue reverse
transcriptase inhibitors—**
*Adults and children age 3 and older
weighing 40 kg (88 lb) or more:* 600 mg
P.O. once daily.
*Children age 3 and older weighing 10 to
less than 15 kg (22 to under 33 lb):*
200 mg P.O. once daily.
*Children age 3 and older weighing 15 to
less than 20 kg (33 to under 44 lb):*
250 mg P.O. once daily.
*Children age 3 and older weighing 20 to
less than 25 kg (44 to under 55 lb):*
300 mg P.O. once daily.

*Children age 3 and older weighing 25 to
less than 33 kg (55 to under 72 lb):*
350 mg P.O. once daily.
*Children age 3 and older weighing 33 to
less than 40 kg (72 to under 88 lb):*
400 mg P.O. once daily.

ACTION
A nonnucleoside, reverse transcriptase inhibitor that inhibits the transcription of
HIV-1 RNA to DNA, a critical step in the
viral replication process.

Route	Onset	Peak	Duration
P.O.	Unknown	3-5 hr	Unknown

ADVERSE REACTIONS
CNS: abnormal dreams or thinking, agitation, amnesia, confusion, depersonalization, depression, *dizziness,* euphoria,
fatigue, hallucinations, headache, hypoesthesia, impaired concentration, insomnia,
somnolence, nervousness.
GI: abdominal pain, anorexia, *diarrhea,*
dyspepsia, flatulence, *nausea,* vomiting.
GU: hematuria, kidney stones.
Skin: increased sweating, *erythema multiforme, Stevens-Johnson syndrome, toxic epidermal necrolysis, rash,* pruritus.
Other: fever.

INTERACTIONS
Drug-drug. *Clarithromycin, indinavir:*
Decreased plasma levels. Consider alternative therapy; increase indinavir dosage
if used together.
*Drugs that induce the cytochrome P-450
enzyme system (phenobarbital, rifabutin,
rifampin):* Increased efavirenz clearance
resulting in lowered plasma levels. Clinical significance not known.
Ergot derivatives, midazolam, triazolam:
Competition for cytochrome P-450 enzyme system may result in inhibition of
the metabolism of these drugs and cause
serious or life-threatening adverse effects
such as arrhythmias, prolonged sedation,
or respiratory depression. Avoid using together.
Estrogens, ritonavir: Increased plasma
levels. Monitor patient.
Oral contraceptives: May interact with
oral contraceptives. Advise patient to use a
reliable method of barrier contraception in
addition to oral contraceptives.

Psychoactive drugs: Increased CNS effects. Avoid using together.

Saquinavir: Decreased plasma levels of saquinavir. Don't use with saquinavir as sole protease inhibitor.

Warfarin: May increase or decrease plasma levels and effects. Monitor INR.

Drug-food. *High-fat meals:* Increased absorption of drug. Instruct patient to maintain a proper low-fat diet.

Drug-lifestyle. *Alcohol:* Enhanced CNS effects. Discourage use together.

EFFECTS ON LAB TEST RESULTS
● May increase ALT, AST, and cholesterol levels.

CONTRAINDICATIONS
Contraindicated in patients hypersensitive to drug or its components.

NURSING CONSIDERATIONS
● Use cautiously in patients with hepatic impairment and in those receiving hepatotoxic drugs. Monitor liver function test results in patients with history of hepatitis B or C and in those taking ritonavir.
● Monitor cholesterol levels.
● Drug should be used with other antiretrovirals because resistant viruses emerge rapidly when used alone.
● *Alert:* Drug shouldn't be used as monotherapy or added on as a single drug to a failing regimen.
● Using drug with ritonavir may increase adverse effects (such as dizziness, nausea, paresthesia) and laboratory abnormalities (elevated liver enzyme levels).
● Give drug at bedtime to decrease CNS adverse effects.
● Drug therapy may cause false-positive urine cannabinoid test results.
● Pregnancy must be ruled out before starting therapy in women of childbearing age.
● Children may be more prone to adverse reactions, especially diarrhea, nausea, vomiting, and rash.

PATIENT TEACHING
● Instruct patient to take drug with water, juice, milk, or soda. It may be taken without regard to meals.

● Inform patient about need for scheduled blood tests to monitor liver function and cholesterol levels.
● Tell patient to use a reliable method of barrier contraception in addition to oral contraceptives and to notify prescriber immediately if pregnancy is suspected.
● Inform patient that drug doesn't cure HIV infection, that opportunistic infections and other complications of HIV infection may continue to occur, and that transmission of HIV to others through sexual contact or blood contamination is still possible.
● Instruct patient to take drug at the same time daily and always with other antiretrovirals.
● Tell patient to take drug exactly as prescribed and not to stop it without medical approval. Also instruct patient to report adverse reactions.
● Inform patient that rash is the most common adverse effect. Tell patient to report rash immediately because it may be serious (in rare cases).
● Advise patient to report use of other drugs.
● Advise patient that dizziness, difficulty sleeping or concentrating, drowsiness, or unusual dreams may occur during the first few days of therapy. Reassure him that these symptoms typically resolve after 2 to 4 weeks and may be less problematic if drug is taken at bedtime.
● Tell patient to avoid alcohol, driving, or operating machinery until the drug's CNS effects are known.

famciclovir
Famvir

Pregnancy risk category B

AVAILABLE FORMS
Tablets: 125 mg, 250 mg, 500 mg

INDICATIONS & DOSAGES
➤ **Acute herpes zoster infection (shingles)**—
Adults: 500 mg P.O. q 8 hours for 7 days.
Adjust-a-dose: For patients with reduced renal function, if creatinine clearance is 60 ml/minute or more, 500 mg P.O. q 8 hours; if clearance is 40 to 59 ml/minute,

500 mg P.O. q 12 hours; if 20 to 39 ml/minute, 500 mg P.O. q 24 hours; and if below 20 ml/minute, 250 mg P.O. q 24 hours. For hemodialysis patients, 250 mg P.O. after each hemodialysis session.

➤ **Recurrent episodes of genital herpes—**
Adults: 125 mg P.O. b.i.d. for 5 days. Begin therapy as soon as symptoms occur.
Adjust-a-dose: For patients with reduced renal function, if creatinine clearance is 40 ml/minute or more, 125 mg P.O. q 12 hours; if 20 to 39 ml/minute, 125 mg P.O. q 24 hours; if below 20 ml/minute, 125 mg P.O. q 48 hours. For hemodialysis patients, 125 mg P.O. after each hemodialysis session.

➤ **Recurrent mucocutaneous herpes simplex infections in HIV-infected patients—**
Adults: 500 mg P.O. b.i.d. for 7 days.
Adjust-a-dose: For patients with reduced renal function, if creatinine clearance is 40 ml/minute or more, 500 mg P.O. q 12 hours; if 20 to 39 ml/minute, 500 mg P.O. q 24 hours; and if below 20 ml/minute, 250 mg P.O. q 24 hours. For hemodialysis patients, 250 mg P.O. after each hemodialysis session.

ACTION
A guanosine nucleoside that's converted to penciclovir, which enters viral cells and inhibits DNA polymerase and viral DNA synthesis.

Route	Onset	Peak	Duration
P.O.	Unknown	1 hr	Unknown

ADVERSE REACTIONS
CNS: *headache,* fatigue, dizziness, paresthesia, somnolence.
EENT: pharyngitis, sinusitis.
GI: diarrhea, *nausea,* vomiting, constipation, anorexia, abdominal pain.
Musculoskeletal: back pain, arthralgia.
Skin: pruritus.
Other: fever, zoster-related signs, symptoms, and complications.

INTERACTIONS
Drug-drug. *Probenecid:* May increase plasma levels of penciclovir, the active metabolite of famciclovir. Monitor patient for increased adverse effects.

EFFECTS ON LAB TEST RESULTS
None reported.

CONTRAINDICATIONS
Contraindicated in patients hypersensitive to drug.

NURSING CONSIDERATIONS
● Use cautiously in patients with renal or hepatic impairment. Dosage adjustment may be needed. Monitor renal and liver function tests.
● Drug may be taken without regard to meals.

PATIENT TEACHING
● Inform patient that drug doesn't cure genital herpes but can decrease the length and severity of symptoms.
● Teach patient how to prevent spread of infection to others.
● Urge patient to recognize the early signs and symptoms of herpes infection, such as tingling, itching, and pain, and to report them. Treatment is more effective if therapy is started within 48 hours of rash onset.

---

fomivirsen sodium
Vitravene

Pregnancy risk category C

AVAILABLE FORMS
Intravitreal injection: Preservative-free, 0.25-ml, single-use vials containing 6.6 mg/ml

INDICATIONS & DOSAGES
➤ **Local treatment of CMV retinitis in patients with AIDS who are intolerant of or have a contraindication to other treatments or who were insufficiently responsive to previous treatment—**
Adults: Induction dose is 330 mcg (0.05 ml) by intravitreal injection every other week for two doses. Subsequent maintenance dose is 330 mcg (0.05 ml) by intravitreal injection once q 4 weeks after induction.

ACTION
A phosphorothioate oligonucleotide that inhibits human CMV replication by bind-

ing to the target mRNA and subsequently inhibiting virus replication.

Route	Onset	Peak	Duration
Intravitreal	Unknown	Unknown	Unknown

ADVERSE REACTIONS
CNS: asthenia, headache, abnormal thinking, depression, dizziness, neuropathy, pain.
CV: chest pain.
EENT: abnormal or blurred vision, anterior chamber inflammation, cataract, conjunctival hemorrhage, decreased visual acuity, desaturation of color vision, eye pain, floaters, increased intraocular pressure, photophobia, retinal detachment, retinal edema, retinal hemorrhage, retinal pigment changes, *uveitis, vitreitis,* application site reaction, conjunctival hyperemia, conjunctivitis, corneal edema, decreased peripheral vision, eye irritation, hypotony, keratic precipitates, optic neuritis, photopsia, retinal vascular disease, visual field defect, vitreous hemorrhage, vitreous opacity, sinusitis.
GI: abdominal pain, anorexia, diarrhea, nausea, vomiting, oral candidiasis, *pancreatitis.*
GU: catheter infection, *renal failure.*
Hematologic: anemia, lymphoma-like reaction, *neutropenia, thrombocytopenia.*
Metabolic: dehydration, weight loss.
Musculoskeletal: back pain.
Respiratory: bronchitis, dyspnea, increased cough, pneumonia.
Skin: rash, sweating.
Other: allergic reactions, cachexia, fever, flu syndrome, infection, *sepsis,* systemic CMV.

INTERACTIONS
None significant.

EFFECTS ON LAB TEST RESULTS
• May increase ALT, AST, GGT, and alkaline phosphatase levels.
• May decrease hemoglobin and neutrophil and platelet counts.

CONTRAINDICATIONS
Contraindicated in patients hypersensitive to drug or its components and in those who have recently (within 2 to 4 weeks) been treated with either I.V. or intravitreal cidofovir because of an increased risk of exaggerated ocular inflammation.

NURSING CONSIDERATIONS
• *Alert:* Drug is for ophthalmic use by intravitreal injection only.
• Drug provides localized therapy limited to the treated eye and doesn't provide treatment for systemic CMV disease. Monitor patient for extraocular CMV disease or disease in the other eye.
• Ocular inflammation (uveitis) is more common during induction dosing.
• Monitor light perception and optic nerve head perfusion postinjection.
• Watch for intraocular pressure. This is usually transient and returns to normal without treatment or with temporary use of topical drugs.

PATIENT TEACHING
• Inform patient that drug doesn't cure CMV retinitis, and that some patients continue to experience progression of retinitis during and after treatment.
• Tell patient that drug treats only the eye in which it has been injected, and that CMV may also exist in the body. Stress importance of follow-up visits to monitor progress and to check for additional infections.
• Instruct patient to also have regular ophthalmologic follow-up examinations.
• Advise HIV-infected patient to continue taking antiretroviral therapy, as indicated.

---

foscarnet sodium (phosphonoformic acid)
Foscavir

Pregnancy risk category C

AVAILABLE FORMS
Injection: 24 mg/ml in 250- and 500-ml bottles

INDICATIONS & DOSAGES
➤ **CMV retinitis in patients with AIDS—**
Adults: Initially, 60 mg/kg I.V. as an induction treatment in patients with normal renal function. Administer q 8 hours for 2 to 3 weeks, depending on clinical response. Follow with a maintenance infu-

Reactions may be *common*, uncommon, *life-threatening*, or COMMON AND LIFE-THREATENING.

sion of 90 to 120 mg/kg daily. Or, 90 mg/kg I.V. q 12 hours is used for induction.

➤ **Acyclovir-resistant herpes simplex virus infections—**
Adults: 40 mg/kg I.V. over 1 hour q 8 to 12 hours for 2 to 3 weeks or until healed.
Adjust-a-dose: Refer to package insert for specific dosage adjustments. Dosage must be adjusted when creatinine clearance is less than 1.5 ml/kg/minute. If clearance falls below 0.4 ml/kg/minute, stop drug.

I.V. ADMINISTRATION
• Drug may be infused via a central or peripheral vein that has adequate blood flow for rapid distribution and dilution into circulation.
• It isn't necessary to dilute the commercially available form (24 mg/ml) when infusing in a central vein; however, if giving drug by peripheral vein, the drug must be further diluted to a final concentration of 12 mg/ml with D_5W or normal saline solution before giving, to decrease risk of local irritation.
• Use an infusion pump to give foscarnet. To minimize renal toxicity, make sure patient is adequately hydrated before and during the infusion.
• Give induction treatment over 1 hour; maintenance infusions over 2 hours.
• *Alert:* Don't exceed the recommended dosage, infusion rate, or frequency of administration. All doses must be individualized according to patient's renal function.

ACTION
Inhibits all known herpes viruses in vitro by blocking the pyrophosphate binding site on DNA polymerases and reverse transcriptases.

Route	Onset	Peak	Duration
I.V.	Unknown	Immediate	Unknown

ADVERSE REACTIONS
CNS: cerebrovascular disorder, *headache, seizures, fatigue, malaise, asthenia, paresthesia, dizziness, hypoesthesia, neuropathy,* tremor, ataxia, generalized spasms, dementia, stupor, sensory disturbances, meningitis, aphasia, abnormal coordination, EEG abnormalities, depression, confusion, aggression, anxiety, insomnia,

somnolence, nervousness, amnesia, agitation, hallucinations.
CV: *hypertension, palpitations, ECG abnormalities, sinus tachycardia, first-degree AV block, hypotension, flushing,* edema, chest pain.
EENT: visual disturbances, eye pain, conjunctivitis, sinusitis, pharyngitis, rhinitis.
GI: taste perversion, *nausea, diarrhea, vomiting, abdominal pain, anorexia,* constipation, dysphagia, rectal hemorrhage, dry mouth, dyspepsia, melena, flatulence, ulcerative stomatitis, *pancreatitis.*
GU: *abnormal renal function,* albuminuria, dysuria, polyuria, urethral disorder, urine retention, urinary tract infections, *acute renal failure,* candidiasis.
Hematologic: *anemia, granulocytopenia, leukopenia, bone marrow suppression, thrombocytopenia,* platelet abnormalities, thrombocytosis, lymphadenopathy.
Hepatic: abnormal hepatic function.
Metabolic: *hypokalemia, hypomagnesemia, hypophosphatemia, hyperphosphatemia, hypocalcemia, hyponatremia.*
Musculoskeletal: leg cramps, arthralgia, myalgia, back pain.
Respiratory: *cough, dyspnea,* pneumonitis, respiratory insufficiency, pulmonary infiltration, stridor, pneumothorax, *bronchospasm,* hemoptysis.
Skin: *rash, diaphoresis,* pruritus, skin ulceration, erythematous rash, seborrhea, skin discoloration, facial edema.
Other: *fever,* pain, *sepsis,* rigors, inflammation and pain at infusion site, lymphoma-like disorder, *sarcoma,* bacterial or fungal infections, abscess, flulike symptoms.

INTERACTIONS
Drug-drug. *Nephrotoxic drugs (such as aminoglycosides, amphotericin B):* Increased risk of nephrotoxicity. Avoid using together.
Pentamidine: Increased risk of nephrotoxicity; severe hypocalcemia also has been reported. Monitor patient closely.
Zidovudine: Possible increased risk or severity of anemia. Monitor blood counts.

EFFECTS ON LAB TEST RESULTS
• May increase creatinine, phosphate, calcium, ALT, AST alkaline phosphatase, and bilirubin levels. May decrease calcium,

---

magnesium, phosphate, potassium, and sodium levels.
• May increase platelet count. May decrease hemoglobin and granulocyte, WBC, and platelet counts.

CONTRAINDICATIONS
Contraindicated in patients hypersensitive to drug.

NURSING CONSIDERATIONS
• Use cautiously and with reduced dosage in patients with abnormal renal function. Because drug is nephrotoxic, it can worsen renal impairment. Some degree of nephrotoxicity occurs in most patients treated with drug.
• Because drug is highly toxic and toxicity is probably dose-related, always use the lowest effective maintenance dose during therapy.
• Monitor patient's hemoglobin and hematocrit. Anemia occurs in up to 33% of patients treated with drug. It may be severe enough to require transfusions.
• Monitor creatinine clearance frequently during therapy because of drug's adverse effects on renal function. A baseline 24-hour creatinine clearance is recommended, then regular determinations two to three times weekly during induction and at least once every 1 to 2 weeks during maintenance.
• Because drug can alter serum electrolytes, monitor levels using a schedule similar to that established for creatinine clearance. Assess patient for tetany and seizures caused by abnormal electrolyte levels.
• Monitor patient's hemoglobin level and hematocrit. Anemia occurs in up to 33% of patients treated with drug. It may be severe enough to require transfusions.
• Drug administration may cause a dose-related transient decrease in ionized serum calcium, which may not always be reflected in patient's laboratory values.

PATIENT TEACHING
• Explain the importance of adequate hydration throughout therapy.
• Advise patient to report perioral tingling, numbness in the arms and legs, and paresthesia.

• Tell patient to alert nurse if discomfort occurs at I.V. insertion site.

---

ganciclovir
Cymevene§, Cytovene

Pregnancy risk category C

AVAILABLE FORMS
Capsules: 250 mg, 500 mg
Injection: 500 mg/vial

INDICATIONS & DOSAGES
➤ **CMV retinitis in immunocompromised individuals, including patients with AIDS and normal renal function—**
Adults and children older than age 3 months: Induction treatment is 5 mg/kg I.V. q 12 hours for 14 to 21 days. Maintenance treatment is 5 mg/kg daily or 6 mg/kg daily 5 times weekly. Or, for maintenance therapy, give 1,000 mg P.O. t.i.d. with food or 500 mg P.O. q 3 hours while awake (six times daily).
Adjust-a-dose: Refer to package insert for specific dosage adjustments. Adjust dosage for patients with impaired renal function based on creatinine clearance levels. Dosage adjustment is needed for patients with creatinine clearance less than 70 ml/minute.
➤ **Prevention of CMV disease in patients with advanced HIV infection and normal renal function—**
Adults: 1,000 mg P.O. t.i.d. with food.
➤ **Prevention of CMV disease in transplant recipients with normal renal function—**
Adults: 5 mg/kg I.V. (given at a constant rate over 1 hour) q 12 hours for 7 to 14 days; then 5 mg/kg daily or 6 mg/kg daily 5 times weekly. Duration of therapy depends on degree of immunosuppression.

I.V. ADMINISTRATION
• Reconstitute by adding 10 ml of sterile water for injection to vial containing 500 mg ganciclovir. Shake vial well to dissolve drug. Further dilute in 50 to 250 ml of compatible I.V. solution. If fluids are being restricted, dilute to a concentration not exceeding 10 mg/ml.

● Give infusion over at least 1 hour. Too-rapid infusions will result in toxicity. Use an infusion pump. Don't give as I.V. bolus.

ACTION
Inhibits binding of deoxyguanosine triphosphate to DNA polymerase, resulting in inhibition of DNA synthesis.

Route	Onset	Peak	Duration
I.V.	Unknown	Immediate	Unknown
P.O.	Unknown	1.8-3 hr	Unknown

ADVERSE REACTIONS
CNS: altered dreams, confusion, ataxia, headache, *seizures, coma,* dizziness, somnolence, tremor, abnormal thinking, agitation, amnesia, anxiety, neuropathy, paresthesia, asthenia.
EENT: retinal detachment in CMV retinitis patients.
GI: *nausea, vomiting, diarrhea, anorexia, abdominal pain,* flatulence, dyspepsia, dry mouth.
Hematologic: *agranulocytosis, thrombocytopenia, leukopenia,* anemia.
Respiratory: pneumonia.
Skin: *rash, sweating,* pruritus.
Other: *fever;* infection; chills; *sepsis;* inflammation, pain, and phlebitis at injection site.

INTERACTIONS
Drug-drug. *Amphotericin B, cyclosporine, other nephrotoxic drugs:* Increased risk of nephrotoxicity. Monitor renal function.
Cytotoxic drugs: Increased toxic effects, especially hematologic effects and stomatitis. Monitor patient closely.
Imipenem, cilastatin: Heightened seizure activity. Use together only if potential benefits outweigh risks.
Immunosuppressants (such as azathioprine, corticosteroids, cyclosporine): Enhanced immune and bone marrow suppression. Use together cautiously.
Probenecid: Increased ganciclovir blood levels. Monitor patient closely.
Zidovudine: Increased incidence of agranulocytosis with concurrent use. Use together cautiously; monitor hematologic function closely.

EFFECTS ON LAB TEST RESULTS
● May increase creatinine, ALT, AST, GGT, and alkaline phosphatase levels.
● May decrease hemoglobin and granulocyte, platelet, neutrophil, and WBC counts.

CONTRAINDICATIONS
Contraindicated in patients hypersensitive to drug or acyclovir and in those with an absolute neutrophil count below 500/mm^3 or a platelet count below 25,000/mm^3.

NURSING CONSIDERATIONS
● Use cautiously and reduce dosage in patients with renal dysfunction. Monitor renal function tests.
● Use caution when preparing ganciclovir solution, which is alkaline.
● *Alert:* Don't administer S.C. or I.M.
● Because of the frequency of agranulocytosis and thrombocytopenia, obtain neutrophil and platelet counts every 2 days during twice-daily ganciclovir dosing and at least weekly thereafter.

PATIENT TEACHING
● Explain importance of adequate hydration during therapy.
● Instruct patient to report adverse reactions promptly.
● Tell patient to report discomfort at I.V. insertion site.
● Advise patient that drug causes birth defects. Instruct women to use effective birth control methods during treatment; men should use barrier contraception during and for at least 90 days after treatment with ganciclovir.

---

indinavir sulfate
Crixivan

Pregnancy risk category C

AVAILABLE FORMS
Capsules: 100 mg, 200 mg, 333 mg, 400 mg

INDICATIONS & DOSAGES
➤ **HIV infection, with other antiretrovirals when antiretroviral therapy is warranted—**
Adults: 800 mg P.O. q 8 hours.

Adjust-a-dose: For patients with mild to moderate hepatic insufficiency from cirrhosis, reduce dosage to 600 mg P.O. q 8 hours.

ACTION

Inhibits HIV protease, enzyme required for the proteolytic cleavage of viral polyprotein precursors into individual functional proteins found in infectious HIV. Indinavir binds to the protease active site and inhibits activity of the enzyme, preventing cleavage of the viral polyproteins and resulting in formation of immature noninfectious viral particles.

Route	Onset	Peak	Duration
P.O.	Unknown	< 1 hr	Unknown

ADVERSE REACTIONS

CNS: headache, insomnia, dizziness, somnolence, asthenia, malaise, fatigue.
CV: chest pain, palpitations.
EENT: blurred vision, eye pain or swelling.
GI: abdominal pain, *nausea,* diarrhea, vomiting, acid regurgitation, anorexia, dry mouth, taste perversion.
GU: nephrolithiasis, hematuria.
Hematologic: *neutropenia, thrombocytopenia,* anemia.
Metabolic: *hyperbilirubinemia,* hyperglycemia.
Musculoskeletal: back pain.
Other: flank pain.

INTERACTIONS

Drug-drug. *Clarithromycin:* Increased serum levels of both drugs. Monitor patient closely.
Didanosine: May degrade didanosine, formulated with buffering products to increase pH. If used together, give at least 1 hour apart on an empty stomach; normal gastric pH (acidic) needed for optimum absorption of indinavir, but rapidly degrades didanosine.
Ketoconazole: Increased plasma level of indinavir. Consider dosage reduction of indinavir to 600 mg P.O. q 8 hours when used together.
Midazolam, triazolam: May inhibit the metabolism of these drugs because of competition for CYP3A4 by indinavir, creating potential for serious or life-

threatening events, such as arrhythmias or prolonged sedation. Avoid using together.
Rifabutin: Increased plasma levels. Reduce dosage of rifabutin by 50% if used together.
Rifampin: Markedly diminished plasma levels of indinavir. Avoid using together.
Ritonavir: Increased indinavir levels. Monitor patient closely.
Sildenafil: Increased sildenafil plasma concentrations; may increase sildenafil-associated adverse events, including hypotension, visual changes, and priapism. Patient shouldn't exceed 25 mg in 48 hours.
Drug-herb. *St. John's wort:* Reduced indinavir levels by more than 50%. Discourage use together.
Drug-food. *Any food:* Substantially decreased absorption of oral indinavir. Advise patient to take without food.

EFFECTS ON LAB TEST RESULTS

● May increase ALT, AST, bilirubin, amylase, and glucose levels.
● May decrease hemoglobin and neutrophil and platelet counts.

CONTRAINDICATIONS

Contraindicated in patients hypersensitive to drug or its components.

NURSING CONSIDERATIONS

● Use cautiously in patients with hepatic insufficiency from cirrhosis.
● Drug must be taken at 8-hour intervals.
● Drug may cause nephrolithiasis. If signs and symptoms of nephrolithiasis occur, prescriber may stop drug for 1 to 3 days during acute phases.
● To prevent nephrolithiasis, patient should maintain adequate hydration (at least 48 ounces or 1.5 L of fluids q 24 hours while on indinavir).
● Safety and effectiveness in children haven't been established.

PATIENT TEACHING

● Tell patient that drug doesn't cure HIV infection and that he may continue to develop opportunistic infections and other complications of HIV infection. Drug hasn't been shown to reduce the risk of HIV transmission.
● Advise patient to use barrier protection during sexual intercourse.

Reactions may be *common,* uncommon, *life-threatening*, or COMMON AND LIFE-THREATENING.

• Caution patient not to adjust dosage or stop indinavir therapy without first consulting prescriber.

• Advise patient that if a dose of indinavir is missed, he should take the next dose at the regularly scheduled time and shouldn't double the dose.

• Instruct patient to take drug on an empty stomach with water 1 hour before or 2 hours after a meal. Or, he may take it with other liquids (such as skim milk, juice, coffee, or tea) or a light meal. Inform patient that a meal high in fat, calories, and protein reduces absorption of drug.

• Instruct patient to store and use capsules in the original container and to keep desiccant in the bottle; capsules are sensitive to moisture.

• Tell patient to drink at least 48 ounces (1.5 L) of fluid daily.

• Advise woman to avoid breast-feeding because indinavir may appear in breast milk. Also, to prevent transmitting virus to infant, advise an HIV-positive woman not to breast-feed.

• Patients receiving sildenafil should be advised that they may be at an increased risk of sildenafil-associated adverse events including hypotension, visual changes, and priapism, and should promptly report any symptoms to their prescriber.

---

lamivudine
Epivir, Epivir-HBV

Pregnancy risk category C

AVAILABLE FORMS
Oral solution: 5 mg/ml, 10 mg/ml
Tablets: 100 mg, 150 mg

INDICATIONS & DOSAGES
➤ **HIV infection, with zidovudine—**
Adults weighing 50 kg (110 lb) or more and children age 12 and older: 150 mg P.O. b.i.d.
Adults weighing less than 50 kg: 2 mg/kg P.O. b.i.d.
Children ages 3 months to 12 years: 4 mg/kg P.O. b.i.d. Maximum dose is 150 mg b.i.d.
Adjust-a-dose: For patients with renal impairment, if creatinine clearance is 30 to 49 ml/minute, 150 mg P.O. daily. If

clearance is 15 to 29 ml/minute, 150 mg P.O. on day 1, then 100 mg daily; if 5 to 14 ml/minute, 150 mg on day 1, then 50 mg daily; if less than 5 ml/minute, 50 mg on day 1, then 25 mg daily.
➤ **Chronic hepatitis B with evidence of hepatitis B viral replication and active liver inflammation—**
Adults: 100 mg P.O. once daily (Epivir-HBV).
Children ages 2 to 17 years: 3 mg/kg P.O. once daily, up to a maximum dose of 100 mg daily. Optimum duration of treatment isn't known and safety and efficacy of treatment beyond 1 year haven't been established.
Adjust-a-dose: For adult patients with renal impairment, if creatinine clearance is 30 to 49 ml/minute, 100 mg first dose; then 50 mg P.O. once daily. If clearance is 15 to 29 ml/minute, 100 mg first dose; then 25 mg P.O. once daily. If clearance is 5 to 14 ml/minute, 35 mg first dose; then 15 mg P.O. once daily. If clearance is less than 5 ml/minute, 35 mg first dose; then 10 mg P.O. once daily.

ACTION
A synthetic nucleoside analogue that inhibits HIV and HBV reverse transcription via viral DNA chain termination. RNA- and DNA-dependent DNA polymerase activities also are inhibited.

Route	Onset	Peak	Duration
P.O.	Unknown	1-3 hr	Unknown

ADVERSE REACTIONS
Adverse reactions pertain to the combination therapy of lamivudine and zidovudine.
CNS: *headache, fatigue, neuropathy, malaise, dizziness, insomnia and other sleep disorders,* depressive disorders.
EENT: *nasal symptoms.*
GI: *nausea, diarrhea, vomiting, anorexia,* abdominal pain, abdominal cramps, dyspepsia, *pancreatitis.*
Hematologic: *neutropenia,* anemia, *thrombocytopenia.*
Musculoskeletal: *musculoskeletal pain,* myalgia, arthralgia.
Respiratory: *cough.*
Skin: rash.
Other: *fever, chills.*

INTERACTIONS
Drug-drug. *Trimethoprim/sulfamethoxazole:* May increase blood level of lamivudine because of decreased clearance of lamivudine. Monitor patient closely.
Zidovudine: Increased serum zidovudine level. Monitor patient closely.

EFFECTS ON LAB TEST RESULTS
● May increase ALT and bilirubin levels.
● May decrease hemoglobin and neutrophil and platelet counts.

CONTRAINDICATIONS
Contraindicated in patients hypersensitive to drug.

NURSING CONSIDERATIONS
● *Alert:* Drug should be used with extreme caution, if at all, in children with history of pancreatitis or other significant risk factors for development of pancreatitis. Stop lamivudine treatment immediately and notify prescriber if clinical signs, symptoms, or laboratory abnormalities suggest pancreatitis. Monitor serum amylase level.
● *Alert:* Lactic acidosis and hepatotoxicity have been reported. Notify prescriber if signs of lactic acidosis or hepatotoxicity occurs.
● Use cautiously in patients with renal impairment.
● Patient should discontinue breast-feeding if lamivudine is prescribed.
● Administer drug with zidovudine. It's not currently indicated for use alone unless for chronic hepatitis B virus infection.
● Safety and effectiveness of treatment with Epivir-HBV beyond 1 year haven't been established; optimum duration of treatment isn't known. Patients should be tested for HIV before starting treatment and during therapy because formulation and dosage of lamivudine in Epivir-HBV aren't appropriate for those infected with both hepatitis B virus and HIV. If lamivudine is administered to patients with hepatitis B virus and HIV, the higher dosage indicated for HIV therapy should be used as part of an appropriate combination regimen.
● Monitor patient's CBC, platelet count, renal and liver function studies. Report abnormalities.

● An Antiretroviral Pregnancy Registry has been established to monitor maternal-fetal outcomes of pregnant women exposed to lamivudine. To register a pregnant patient, the prescriber can call 1-800-258-4263.

PATIENT TEACHING
● Inform patient that long-term effects of lamivudine are unknown.
● Stress importance of taking lamivudine exactly as prescribed.
● Teach parents the signs and symptoms of pancreatitis. Advise them to report signs and symptoms immediately.

lamivudine/zidovudine
Combivir

Pregnancy risk category C

AVAILABLE FORMS
Tablets: 150 mg lamivudine and 300 mg zidovudine

INDICATIONS & DOSAGES
➤ **HIV infection—**
Adults and children age 12 and older, weighing more than 50 kg (110 lb): 1 tablet P.O. b.i.d.

ACTION
Inhibit reverse transcriptase via DNA chain termination. Both drugs are also weak inhibitors of DNA polymerase. Together, they have synergistic antiretroviral activity. Combination therapy with lamivudine and zidovudine is targeted at suppressing or delaying the emergence of resistant strains that can occur with retroviral monotherapy because dual resistance requires multiple mutations.

Route	Onset	Peak	Duration
P.O.	Unknown	Unknown	Unknown

ADVERSE REACTIONS
CNS: *headache, malaise, fatigue, insomnia, dizziness, neuropathy,* depression.
EENT: *nasal signs and symptoms.*
GI: *nausea, diarrhea, vomiting, anorexia,* abdominal pain, abdominal cramps, dyspepsia.
Hematologic: *neutropenia,* anemia.

Musculoskeletal: *musculoskeletal pain, myalgia, arthralgia.*
Respiratory: *cough.*
Skin: *rash.*
Other: *fever, chills.*

INTERACTIONS
Drug-drug. *Ganciclovir, interferon-alpha, other bone marrow suppressive or cytotoxic drugs:* May increase zidovudine's hematologic toxicity. Monitor patient.

EFFECTS ON LAB TEST RESULTS
● May increase ALT, AST, and amylase levels.
● May decrease hemoglobin and hematocrit and neutrophil count.

CONTRAINDICATIONS
Contraindicated in patients hypersensitive to drug or its components and in those younger than age 12, less than 50 kg, or with creatinine clearance below 50 ml/minute. Also contraindicated in patients experiencing dose-limiting adverse effects.

NURSING CONSIDERATIONS
● Use combination cautiously in patients with bone marrow suppression as evidenced by granulocyte count below 1,000 cells/mm³ or hemoglobin level below 9.5 g/dl.
● Lactic acidosis and severe hepatomegaly with steatosis have been reported in patients receiving lamivudine and zidovudine alone and in combination. Notify prescriber if signs of lactic acidosis or hepatotoxicity develop (abdominal pain, jaundice).
● Monitor patient for bone marrow toxicity with frequent blood counts, particularly in patients with advanced HIV infection. Monitor patients for signs and symptoms of lactic acidosis and hepatotoxicity.
● Assess patient's fine motor skills and peripheral sensation for evidence of peripheral neuropathies.
● An Antiretroviral Pregnancy Registry has been established to monitor maternal-fetal outcomes of pregnant women exposed to Combivir. To register a pregnant patient, prescriber can call 1-800-258-4263.

PATIENT TEACHING
● Advise patient that the lamivudine/zidovudine combination drug therapy doesn't cure HIV infection, and that he may continue to experience illness, including opportunistic infections.
● Warn patient that HIV transmission can still occur with drug therapy.
● Educate patient about using condoms when engaging in sexual activities to prevent disease transmission.
● Teach patient signs and symptoms of neutropenia and anemia (fever, chills, infection, fatigue) and instruct him to report such occurrences.
● Tell patient to have blood counts followed closely while on drug, especially if he has advanced disease.
● Advise patient to consult prescriber before taking other drugs.
● Warn patient to report abdominal pain immediately.
● Instruct patient to report signs and symptoms of myopathy or myositis (muscle inflammation, pain, weakness, decrease in muscle size).
● Stress importance of taking combination drug therapy exactly as prescribed, to reduce the development of resistance.
● Tell patient he may take drug combination with or without food.
● Inform woman that breast-feeding is contraindicated in HIV infection and during drug therapy.

✳ *NEW DRUG*

lopinavir/ritonavir
Kaletra

Pregnancy risk category C

AVAILABLE FORMS
Capsules: lopinavir 133.3 mg and ritonavir 33.3 mg
Solution: lopinavir 400 mg and ritonavir 100 mg per 5 ml (80 mg and 20 mg per ml)

INDICATIONS & DOSAGES
➤ **Treatment of HIV infection in combination with other antiretroviral agents—**
Adults and children older than age 12: 400 mg lopinavir and 100 mg ritonavir (3 capsules or 5 ml) P.O. b.i.d. with food.

Adjust-a-dose: In treatment-experienced patient also taking efavirenz or nevirapine, when reduced susceptibility to lopinavir is suspected, consider dosage of 533 mg lopinavir and 133 mg ritonavir (4 capsules or 6.5 ml) P.O. b.i.d. with food.
Children ages 6 months to 12 years weighing 15 to 40 kg (33 to 88 lb): 10 mg/kg (lopinavir content) P.O. b.i.d. with food up to a maximum of 400 mg lopinavir/100 mg ritonavir in children weighing more than 40 kg.
Adjust-a-dose: In treatment-experienced patient also taking efavirenz or nevirapine who weighs 15 to 50 kg (33 to 100 lb), when reduced susceptibility to lopinavir is suspected, consider dosage of 11 mg/kg (lopinavir content) P.O. b.i.d. Treatment-experienced children weighing more than 50 kg can receive adult dosage.
Children ages 6 months to 12 years, weighing 7 to 15 kg (15 to 33 lb): 12 mg/kg (lopinavir content) P.O. b.i.d. with food.
Adjust-a-dose: In treatment-experienced patients also taking efavirenz or nevirapine, when reduced susceptibility to lopinavir is suspected, consider dosage of 13 mg/kg (lopinavir content) P.O. b.i.d. with food.

ACTION

Lopinavir is an HIV protease inhibitor. Inhibition of HIV protease results in the production of immature, noninfectious viral particles. Ritonavir, also an HIV protease inhibitor, inhibits the metabolism of lopinavir, thereby increasing plasma levels of lopinavir.

Route	Onset	Peak	Duration
P.O.	Unknown	4 hr	5-6 hr

ADVERSE REACTIONS

CNS: asthenia, headache, insomnia, malaise, abnormal dreams, agitation, amnesia, anxiety, ataxia, confusion, depression, dizziness, dyskinesia, emotional lability, encephalopathy, hypertonia, nervousness, neuropathy, paresthesia, peripheral neuritis, somnolence, abnormal thinking, tremors.
CV: chest pain, *deep vein thrombosis,* hypertension, palpitations, thrombophlebitis, vasculitis, edema.

EENT: sinusitis, abnormal vision, eye disorder, otitis media, tinnitus.
GI: abdominal pain, abnormal stools, *diarrhea, nausea,* vomiting, anorexia, cholecystitis, constipation, dry mouth, dyspepsia, dysphagia, enterocolitis, eructation, esophagitis, fecal incontinence, flatulence, gastritis, gastroenteritis, GI disorder, hemorrhagic colitis, increased appetite, *pancreatitis,* sialadenitis, stomatitis, ulcerative stomatitis, taste perversion.
GU: abnormal ejaculation, hypogonadism, renal calculus, urine abnormality.
Hematologic: anemia, *leukopenia, neutropenia; thrombocytopenia* in children.
Hepatic: hyperbilirubinemia in children.
Metabolic: Cushing's syndrome, hypothyroidism, dehydration, decreased glucose tolerance, lactic acidosis, weight loss, hyperglycemia, hyperuricemia, hyponatremia in children.
Musculoskeletal: back pain, arthralgia, arthrosis, myalgia.
Respiratory: bronchitis, dyspnea, lung edema.
Skin: rash, acne, alopecia, dry skin, exfoliative dermatitis, furunculosis, nail disorder, pruritus, benign skin neoplasm, skin discoloration, sweating.
Other: gynecomastia, pain, chills, facial edema, fever, flu syndrome, viral infection, lymphadenopathy, peripheral edema, decreased libido.

INTERACTIONS

Drug-drug. *Amiodarone, bepridil, lidocaine, quinidine:* Increased levels of antiarrhythmics. Use together cautiously. Monitor blood levels of these drugs, if possible.
Amprenavir, indinavir, saquinavir: Increased levels of these drugs. Avoid using together.
Antiarrhythmics (flecainide, propafenone), pimozide: Increased risk of cardiac arrhythmias. Avoid using together.
Atorvastatin: Increased level of this drug. Use lowest possible dose and monitor patient carefully.
Atovaquone, methadone: Decreased levels of these drugs. Consider increased doses of these drugs.
Carbamazepine, dexamethasone, phenobarbital, phenytoin: Decreased lopinavir levels. Use together cautiously.

Reactions may be *common*, uncommon, *life-threatening*, or COMMON AND LIFE-THREATENING.

Clarithromycin: Increased clarithromycin levels in patients with renal impairment. Adjust clarithromycin dose.

Cyclosporine, rapamycin, tacrolimus: Increased levels of these drugs. Monitor therapeutic levels.

Delavirdine, ritonavir: Increased levels of lopinavir. Avoid using together.

Didanosine: Decreased absorption of didanosine because Kaletra is taken with food. Give didanosine 1 hour before or 2 hours after Kaletra.

Dihydroergotamine, ergonovine, ergotamine, methylergonovine: Increased risk of ergot toxicity characterized by peripheral vasospasm and ischemia. Avoid using together.

Disulfiram, metronidazole: Risk of disulfiram-like reaction. Avoid using together.

Efavirenz, nevirapine: Decreased lopinavir concentrations. Consider increased Kaletra dose.

Felodipine, nicardipine, nifedipine: Increased levels of these drugs. Use together cautiously. Monitor patient.

Itraconazole, ketoconazole: Increased levels of these drugs. Don't give more than 200 mg/day of these drugs.

Lovastatin, simvastatin: Increased risk of adverse reactions, such as myopathy, rhabdomyolysis. Avoid using together.

Midazolam, triazolam: Increased risk of prolonged or increased sedation or respiratory depression. Avoid using together.

Oral contraceptives (ethinyl estradiol): Decreased effectiveness of contraceptives. Recommend alternative contraception measures.

Rifabutin: Increased rifabutin levels. Decrease rifabutin dose by 75%. Monitor patient for adverse effects.

Rifampin: Decreased effectiveness of Kaletra. Avoid using together.

Sildenafil: Increased sildenafil levels and adverse effects of sildenafil, such as hypotension and priapism. Warn patient not to exceed 25 mg of sildenafil in 48 hours.

Warfarin: May affect warfarin concentration. Monitor PT and INR.

Drug-herb. *St. John's wort:* Loss of virologic response and possible resistance to Kaletra. Discourage use together.

Drug-food. *Any food:* Increased absorption of drug. Tell patient to take with food.

EFFECTS ON LAB TEST RESULTS
● May increase amylase, cholesterol, and triglyceride levels.
● May decrease hemoglobin and hematocrit and RBC, WBC, neutrophil, and platelet counts.

CONTRAINDICATIONS
Contraindicated in patients hypersensitive to drug or any of its components.

NURSING CONSIDERATIONS
● Use cautiously in patients with a history of pancreatitis or with hepatic impairment, hepatitis B or C, marked elevations in liver enzyme levels, or hemophilia.
● Use cautiously in elderly patients.
● To monitor maternal-fetal outcomes of pregnant women exposed to Kaletra, an Antiretroviral Pregnancy Registry has been established. Health care providers are encouraged to enroll patients by calling 1-800-258-4263.
● *Alert:* Be aware that many drug interactions are possible. Review current medications that patient is taking.
● Give drug with food.
● Refrigerated drug remains stable until expiration date on package. If stored at room temperature, drug should be used within 2 months.
● Monitor patient for signs of fat redistribution, including central obesity, buffalo hump, peripheral wasting, breast enlargement, and cushingoid appearance.
● Monitor total cholesterol and triglycerides before starting therapy and periodically thereafter.
● Monitor patient for signs of pancreatitis: nausea, vomiting, abdominal pain, increased lipase and amylase values.
● Monitor patient for signs of bleeding.

PATIENT TEACHING
● Tell patient to take drug with food.
● Tell patient also taking didanosine to take it 1 hour before or 2 hours after Kaletra.
● Advise patient to report side effects to prescriber.
● Tell patient to immediately report severe nausea, vomiting, or abdominal pain.
● Warn patient to tell prescriber about any other prescription or nonprescription med-

---

icine that he is taking, including herbal supplements.
• Tell patient that drug isn't a cure for HIV.

---

nelfinavir mesylate
Viracept

Pregnancy risk category B

AVAILABLE FORMS
Powder: 50 mg/g powder in 144-g bottle
Tablets: 250 mg

INDICATIONS & DOSAGES
➤ **HIV infection when antiretroviral therapy is warranted**—
Adults: 1,250 mg b.i.d. or 750 mg P.O. t.i.d. with meals or light snack.
Children ages 2 to 13: 20 to 30 mg/kg/ dose P.O. t.i.d. with meals or light snack; don't exceed 750 mg t.i.d. Recommended children's dose given t.i.d. is shown below.

Body weight (kg)	Level 1-g scoops	Level teaspoons	Tablets
7 to < 8.5	4	1	-
8.5 to < 10.5	5	1.25	-
10.5 to < 12	6	1.5	-
12 to < 14	7	1.75	-
14 to < 16	8	2	-
16 to < 18	9	2.25	-
18 to < 23	10	2.5	2
≥ 23	15	3.75	3

ACTION
An HIV-1 protease inhibitor, thereby preventing cleavage of the viral polyprotein, resulting in the production of immature, noninfectious virus.

Route	Onset	Peak	Duration
P.O.	Unknown	2-4 hr	Unknown

ADVERSE REACTIONS
CNS: anxiety, depression, dizziness, emotional lability, hyperkinesia, insomnia, migraine, headache, paresthesia, *seizures,* sleep disorders, malaise, somnolence, *suicidal ideation.*
CV: edema.
EENT: iritis, eye disorder, pharyngitis, rhinitis, sinusitis.

GI: nausea, *diarrhea,* flatulence, anorexia, dyspepsia, epigastric pain, GI bleeding, *pancreatitis,* mouth ulceration, vomiting.
GU: sexual dysfunction, renal calculus, urine abnormality.
Hematologic: anemia, *leukopenia, thrombocytopenia.*
Hepatic: *hepatitis,* jaundice, bilirubinemia.
Metabolic: dehydration, hyperglycemia, hyperlipidemia, hyperuricemia, hypoglycemia, metabolic acidosis.
Musculoskeletal: back pain, arthralgia, arthritis, cramps, myalgia, myasthenia, myopathy.
Respiratory: dyspnea, *bronchospasm.*
Skin: rash, dermatitis, folliculitis, fungal dermatitis, pruritus, sweating, urticaria.
Other: allergic reactions, fever, hypersensitivity reactions.

INTERACTIONS
Drug-drug. *Amiodarone, ergot derivatives, midazolam, quinidine, triazolam:* May increase plasma levels of these drugs, which may cause serious or life-threatening adverse effects. Avoid using together.
Carbamazepine, phenobarbital, phenytoin: May decrease nelfinavir plasma levels, which reduces the effectiveness. Monitor patient closely.
HIV protease inhibitors (indinavir, ritonavir): May increase nelfinavir plasma levels. Use together cautiously.
Oral contraceptives (ethinyl estradiol, norethindrone): Decreased plasma levels of these drugs. Advise patient to use alternative or additional contraceptive measures during nelfinavir therapy.
Rifabutin: Dramatically increased rifabutin plasma levels. Reduce dose of rifabutin to one-half the usual amount.
Rifampin: Decreased nelfinavir plasma levels. Avoid using together.
Sildenafil: May increase adverse effects of sildenafil. Warn patient not to exceed 25 mg of sildenafil in 48 hours.
Drug-herb. *St. John's wort:* Reduced blood levels of indinavir by more than 50%; similar effects can be expected in other protease inhibitors. Discourage use together.

Reactions may be *common*, uncommon, *life-threatening*, or COMMON AND LIFE-THREATENING.

EFFECTS ON LAB TEST RESULTS
● May increase ALT, AST, alkaline phosphatase, bilirubin, GGT, amylase, CPK, and lipid levels. May increase or decrease glucose levels.
● Decreased hemoglobin and WBC and platelet counts.

CONTRAINDICATIONS
Contraindicated in patients hypersensitive to drug or its components.

NURSING CONSIDERATIONS
● Use cautiously in patients with hepatic dysfunction or hemophilia types A and B. Monitor liver function test results.
● Drug dosage is the same whether used alone or with other antiretrovirals.
● Administer oral powder in children unable to take tablets. May mix oral powder with small amount of water, milk, formula, soy formula, soy milk, or dietary supplements. Patient should consume entire contents.
● Don't reconstitute with water in its original container.
● Use reconstituted powder within 6 hours.
● Mixing with acidic foods or juice isn't recommended because of bitter taste.
● It's not known if drug appears in breast milk. Because safety hasn't been established, HIV-infected women should be advised not to breast-feed, to avoid transmitting virus to the infant.
● *Alert:* Don't confuse nelfinavir with nevirapine.

PATIENT TEACHING
● Advise patient to take drug with food.
● Inform patient that drug doesn't cure HIV infection.
● Tell patient that long-term effects of drug are unknown and that there are no data stating that nelfinavir reduces risk of HIV transmission.
● Advise patient to take drug daily as prescribed and not to alter dose or stop drug without medical approval.
● If patient misses a dose, tell him to take it as soon as possible and then return to his normal schedule. Advise patient not to double the dose.

● Tell patient that diarrhea is the most common adverse effect and that it can be controlled with loperamide, if necessary.
● Instruct patient taking oral contraceptives to use alternative or additional contraceptive measures while taking nelfinavir.
● Warn patient with phenylketonuria that powder contains 11.2 mg phenylalanine per gram.
● Advise patient to report use of other prescribed or OTC drugs because of possible drug interactions.

nevirapine
Viramune

Pregnancy risk category C

AVAILABLE FORMS
Oral suspension: 50 mg/5 ml
Tablets: 200 mg

INDICATIONS & DOSAGES
➤ **Adjunct treatment in patients with HIV-1 infection who have experienced clinical or immunologic deterioration—**
Adults: 200 mg P.O. daily for the first 14 days, then 200 mg P.O. b.i.d. Used with nucleoside analogue antiretrovirals.
➤ **Adjunct treatment in children infected with HIV-1—**
Children ages 2 months to 8 years:
4 mg/kg P.O. once daily for first 14 days, then 7 mg/kg P.O. b.i.d. thereafter. Maximum daily dose is 400 mg.
Children age 8 and older: 4 mg/kg P.O. once daily for first 14 days; then 4 mg/kg P.O. b.i.d. thereafter. Maximum daily dose is 400 mg.

ACTION
A nonnucleoside reverse transcriptase inhibitor that binds directly to reverse transcriptase and blocks RNA-dependent and DNA-dependent DNA polymerase activities by causing a disruption of the enzyme's catalytic site.

Route	Onset	Peak	Duration
P.O.	Unknown	4 hr	Unknown

ADVERSE REACTIONS

CNS: headache, paresthesia.
GI: *nausea,* diarrhea, abdominal pain, ulcerative stomatitis.
Hematologic: *neutropenia.*
Hepatic: *hepatitis.*
Musculoskeletal: myalgia.
Skin: *rash, blistering,* **Stevens-Johnson syndrome.**
Other: *fever.*

INTERACTIONS

Drug-drug. *Drugs extensively metabolized by P-450 CYP3A:* May lower plasma levels of these drugs, requiring dosage adjustment. Monitor patient closely.
Protease inhibitors, oral contraceptives, other hormonal contraceptives: May decrease plasma levels of these drugs. Avoid using together.
Rifabutin, rifampin: More data needed to assess whether dosage adjustments are necessary. Monitor patient closely.
Drug-herb. *St. John's wort:* Decreased blood levels of drug. Discourage use together.

EFFECTS ON LAB TEST RESULTS

• May increase ALT, AST, GGT, and bilirubin levels.
• May decrease hemoglobin and neutrophil count.

CONTRAINDICATIONS

Contraindicated in patients hypersensitive to drug.

NURSING CONSIDERATIONS

• Use cautiously in patients with impaired renal and hepatic function; pharmacokinetics haven't been evaluated in those patients.
• Clinical chemistry tests, including renal and liver function tests, should be performed before starting drug therapy and regularly throughout therapy.
• Drug should be used with at least one other antiretroviral.
• **Alert:** Monitor patient for blistering, oral lesions, conjunctivitis, muscle or joint aches, or general malaise. Be especially alert for a severe rash or rash accompanied by fever. Report such signs and symptoms to prescriber. Patients who experience a rash during the initial 14 days

of therapy shouldn't have the dosage increased until the rash has resolved. Most rashes occur within the first 6 weeks of therapy.
• **Alert:** Moderate and severe liver function test abnormalities and hepatotoxicity may warrant temporarily stopping therapy; drug may be restarted at half the previous dose level.
• Patients who have nevirapine therapy interrupted for longer than 7 days should restart therapy as if receiving drug for the first time.
• Antiretroviral therapy may be changed if disease progresses while patient is receiving nevirapine.
• Safety and effectiveness in children haven't been established.
• Nevirapine appears in breast milk.
• **Alert:** Don't confuse nevirapine with nelfinavir.

PATIENT TEACHING

• Inform patient that nevirapine doesn't cure HIV and that illnesses associated with advanced HIV-1 infection still may occur. Explain that drug doesn't reduce risk of HIV-1 transmission.
• Instruct patient to report rash immediately and to stop drug until told to resume.
• Stress importance of taking drug exactly as prescribed. If a dose is missed, tell patient to take the next dose as soon as possible. Patient shouldn't double next dose.
• Tell patient not to use other drugs unless approved by prescriber.
• Advise woman of childbearing age that oral contraceptives and other hormonal methods of birth control shouldn't be used with nevirapine.
• Advise woman to avoid breast-feeding during drug therapy to reduce risk of postnatal HIV transmission.

oseltamivir phosphate
Tamiflu

Pregnancy risk category C

AVAILABLE FORMS

Capsules: 75 mg
Oral suspension: 12 mg/ml after reconstitution

Reactions may be *common,* uncommon, *life-threatening*, or COMMON AND LIFE-THREATENING.

INDICATIONS & DOSAGES
➤ **Uncomplicated, acute illness caused by influenza infection in patients who have had symptoms for 2 days or less—**
Adults: 75 mg P.O. b.i.d. for 5 days.
Adjust-a-dose: For patients with creatinine clearance less than 30 ml/minute, reduce dose to 75 mg P.O. once daily for 5 days.
✳ *NEW INDICATION:* **Prevention of influenza following close contact with infected person—**
Adults and adolescents age 13 and older: 75 mg P.O. once daily beginning within 2 days of exposure and lasting at least 7 days.
➤ **Prevention of influenza during a community outbreak—**
Adults and adolescents age 13 and older: 75 mg P.O. once daily for up to 6 weeks.
➤ **Treatment of influenza in children age 1 and older—**
Children who weigh more than 40 kg: 75 mg oral suspension P.O. b.i.d.
Children who weigh 23 to 40 kg (51 to 88 lb): 60 mg oral suspension P.O. b.i.d.
Children who weigh 15 to 23 kg (33 to 51 lb): 45 mg oral suspension P.O. b.i.d.
Children who weigh 15 kg (33 lb) or less: 30 mg oral suspension P.O. b.i.d.

ACTION
Inhibits influenza A and B virus enzyme neuraminidase, which is thought to play a role in viral particle aggregation and release from the host cell. Neuraminidase inhibition, therefore, appears to interfere with viral replication.

Route	Onset	Peak	Duration
P.O.	Unknown	Unknown	Unknown

ADVERSE REACTIONS
CNS: dizziness, insomnia, headache, vertigo, fatigue.
GI: abdominal pain, diarrhea, nausea, vomiting.
Respiratory: bronchitis, cough.

INTERACTIONS
None significant.

EFFECTS ON LAB TEST RESULTS
None reported.

CONTRAINDICATIONS
Contraindicated in patients hypersensitive to drug or its components.

NURSING CONSIDERATIONS
● Use cautiously in patients with chronic cardiac or respiratory diseases, or any medical condition that may require imminent hospitalization. Also use cautiously in patients with renal failure, especially those with creatinine clearance less than 10 ml/minute.
● No evidence supports drug use to treat viral infections other than influenza virus types A and B.
● Drug must be given within 2 days of onset of symptoms.
● Drug isn't a replacement for the annual influenza vaccination. Patients for whom vaccine is indicated should continue to receive the vaccine each fall.
● Safety and efficacy of repeated treatment courses haven't been established.
● Drug may be given with meals to decrease GI adverse effects.
● It's unknown if drug or its active metabolite appear in breast milk. Use only if potential benefits outweigh potential risks to infant.
● Store at controlled room temperature (59° to 86° F [15° to 30° C]).

PATIENT TEACHING
● Instruct patient to begin treatment as soon as possible after appearance of flu symptoms.
● Inform patient that drug may be taken with or without meals. If nausea or vomiting occurs, he can take drug with food or milk.
● Tell patient that, if a dose is missed, it should be taken as soon as possible. He should skip missed dose, however, if next dose is due within 2 hours, and take the next dose on schedule.
● Advise patient to complete the full 5 days of treatment, even if symptoms are resolved.
● Alert patient that drug isn't a replacement for the annual influenza vaccination.

Patients for whom vaccine is indicated should continue to receive the vaccine each fall.

---

ribavirin
Virazole

Pregnancy risk category X

AVAILABLE FORMS
Powder to be reconstituted for inhalation: 6 g in 100-ml glass vial

INDICATIONS & DOSAGES
➤ **Hospitalized infants and young children infected by respiratory syncytial virus (RSV)—**
Infants and young children: Solution in concentration of 20 mg/ml delivered via the Viratek Small Particle Aerosol Generator (SPAG-2) and mechanical ventilator or oxygen hood, face mask, or oxygen tent at a rate of about 12.5 L of mist/minute. Treatment is given for 12 to 18 hours/day for at least 3 days, and no longer than 7 days.

ACTION
Inhibits viral activity by an unknown mechanism, possibly by inhibiting RNA and DNA synthesis by depleting intracellular nucleotide pools.

Route	Onset	Peak	Duration
Inhalation	Unknown	Unknown	Unknown

ADVERSE REACTIONS
CV: *cardiac arrest,* hypotension, *bradycardia.*
EENT: conjunctivitis, rash or erythema of eyelids.
Hematologic: anemia, reticulocytosis.
Respiratory: *bronchospasm, pulmonary edema,* worsening respiratory state, *apnea,* bacterial pneumonia, pneumothorax.

INTERACTIONS
None significant.

EFFECTS ON LAB TEST RESULTS
• May increase ALT, AST, and bilirubin levels.
• May increase reticulocyte count. May decrease hemoglobin.

CONTRAINDICATIONS
Contraindicated in patients hypersensitive to drug. Although drug is used in children, manufacturer states that it's contraindicated in women who are or may become pregnant during treatment.

NURSING CONSIDERATIONS
• Administer ribavirin aerosol by the Viratek SPAG-2 only. Don't use any other aerosol-generating device.
• Use sterile USP water for injection, not bacteriostatic water. Water used to reconstitute this drug mustn't contain any antimicrobial product.
• Discard solutions placed in the SPAG-2 unit at least every 24 hours before adding newly reconstituted solution.
• *Alert:* The most frequent adverse effects reported in health care personnel exposed to aerosolized ribavirin include eye irritation and headache. Pregnant personnel should be advised of these effects.
• *Alert:* Monitor ventilator function frequently. Ribavirin may precipitate in ventilator apparatus, causing equipment malfunction with serious consequences.
• Store reconstituted solutions at room temperature for 24 hours.
• Ribavirin aerosol is indicated only for severe lower respiratory tract infection caused by RSV. Although treatment may begin while awaiting diagnostic test results, existence of RSV infection must be documented eventually.
• Most infants and children with RSV infection don't require treatment with antivirals because the disease is commonly mild and self-limiting. Premature infants or those with cardiopulmonary disease experience RSV in its severest form and benefit most from treatment with ribavirin aerosol.

PATIENT TEACHING
• Inform parents of need for drug, and answer any questions.
• Encourage parents to immediately report any subtle change in child.

Reactions may be *common*, uncommon, *life-threatening*, or COMMON AND LIFE-THREATENING.

rimantadine hydrochloride
Flumadine

Pregnancy risk category C

AVAILABLE FORMS
Syrup: 50 mg/5 ml
Tablets (film-coated): 100 mg

INDICATIONS & DOSAGES
➤ **Prevention of influenza A—**
Adults and adolescents: 100 mg P.O. b.i.d. beginning as soon as possible after initial exposure and continued through course of influenza A outbreak.
Children younger than age 10: 5 mg/kg P.O. in 1 or 2 divided doses. Maximum daily dose 150 mg.
Elderly patients: 100 mg P.O. daily beginning as soon as possible after initial exposure and continued through course of influenza A outbreak.
Adjust-a-dose: For patients with severe hepatic or renal dysfunction or those experiencing adverse effects with normal dosage, 100 mg P.O. daily.
➤ **Treatment of influenza A—**
Adults: 100 mg P.O. b.i.d. initiated within 24 to 48 hours after onset of symptoms and continued for 48 hours after symptoms disappear (usually 7-day total course).

ACTION
Unknown. Appears to prevent viral uncoating, an early step in virus reproductive cycle.

Route	Onset	Peak	Duration
P.O.	Unknown	6 hr	Unknown

ADVERSE REACTIONS
CNS: insomnia, headache, dizziness, nervousness, fatigue, asthenia.
GI: nausea, vomiting, anorexia, dry mouth, abdominal pain.

INTERACTIONS
Drug-drug. *Acetaminophen, aspirin:* Reduced level of rimantadine. Monitor patient for decreased effectiveness of rimantadine.
Cimetidine: May decrease clearance of rimantadine. Monitor patient for adverse reactions.

EFFECTS ON LAB TEST RESULTS
None reported.

CONTRAINDICATIONS
Contraindicated in patients hypersensitive to drug or amantadine.

NURSING CONSIDERATIONS
● Use cautiously in patients with renal or hepatic impairment and in patients with a history of seizures. Pregnant patients should consider the risks versus benefits before taking drug.
● Safety of therapy lasting longer than 6 weeks hasn't been established.
● Can be used for prophylaxis in children up to 6 weeks after first dose of influenza vaccine or until 2 weeks after second dose of vaccine.
● Consider the risk to contacts of treated patients who may be subject to morbidity from influenza A. Influenza A-resistant strains can emerge during therapy. Patients taking drug may still be able to spread the disease.
● *Alert:* Don't confuse rimantadine with amantadine.

PATIENT TEACHING
● Instruct patient to take drug several hours before bedtime to prevent insomnia.
● Inform patient that he may still be able to infect others with influenza A and to take infection-control precautions.

ritonavir
Norvir

Pregnancy risk category B

AVAILABLE FORMS
Capsules: 100 mg
Oral solution: 80 mg/ml

INDICATIONS & DOSAGES
➤ **HIV infection, with nucleoside analogues when antiretroviral therapy is warranted—**
Adults: 600 mg P.O. b.i.d with meals. If nausea occurs, gradually increasing dose may provide some relief: 300 mg b.i.d. for 1 day, 400 mg b.i.d. for 2 days, 500 mg

b.i.d. for 1 day, and then 600 mg b.i.d. thereafter.

ACTION
An HIV protease inhibitor with activity against HIV-1 and HIV-2 proteases. HIV protease is an enzyme required for the proteolytic cleavage of viral polyprotein precursors into the individual functional proteins in infectious HIV. Ritonavir binds to the protease active site and inhibits activity of the enzyme, preventing cleavage of the viral polyproteins and resulting in the formation of immature, noninfectious viral particles.

Route	Onset	Peak	Duration
P.O.	Unknown	2-4 hr	Unknown

ADVERSE REACTIONS
CNS: *asthenia,* headache, malaise, circumoral paresthesia, dizziness, insomnia, paresthesia, peripheral paresthesia, somnolence, thinking abnormality, migraine headache.
CV: vasodilation.
EENT: local throat irritation, blepharitis, diplopia, pharyngitis, photophobia.
GI: abdominal pain, anorexia, constipation, *diarrhea, nausea, vomiting,* dyspepsia, flatulence, cramping, *taste perversion.*
GU: dysuria, hematuria, nocturia, polyuria, pyelonephritis, urethritis.
Hematologic: *leukopenia, thrombocytopenia.*
Hepatic: jaundice.
Metabolic: hyperlipidemia, hyperglycemia, hyperkalemia, hyperuricemia.
Musculoskeletal: myalgia.
Skin: rash, sweating, urticaria.
Other: fever.

INTERACTIONS
Drug-drug. *Alprazolam, clorazepate, diazepam, dihydroergotamine, ergotamine, estazolam, flurazepam, midazolam, triazolam, zolpidem:* Significantly increased levels of these drugs. Because of risk of extreme sedation and respiratory depression, avoid using together.
Amiodarone, bepridil, bupropion, clozapine, flecainide, meperidine, piroxicam, propafenone, propoxyphene, quinidine, rifabutin: Significantly increased plasma levels of these drugs, which increases pa-

tient's risk of arrhythmias, hematologic abnormalities, seizures, or other potentially serious adverse effects. Avoid using together.
Clarithromycin: Reduced creatinine clearance. Patients with impaired renal function receiving drug with ritonavir require a 50% reduction in clarithromycin dose if creatinine clearance is 30 to 60 ml/minute and a 75% reduction if it's below 30 ml/minute. Monitor renal function closely.
Desipramine: Increased overall serum levels of desipramine. Adjust dosage when used together; monitor patient.
Directly glucuronidated drugs: May reduce therapeutic effects of these drugs; may need to adjust dosage of these drugs. Monitor therapeutic drug level and adverse effects, especially for drugs with narrow therapeutic margins, such as oral anticoagulants and immunosuppressants. May need to reduce dosage greater than 50% for drugs extensively metabolized by CYP3A.
Disulfiram or other drugs that produce disulfiram-like reactions such as metronidazole: Increased risk of disulfiram-like reactions. Ritonavir formulations contain alcohol that can produce reactions when used together. Monitor patient.
Drugs that increase CYP3A activity (such as carbamazepine, dexamethasone, phenobarbital, phenytoin, rifabutin, rifampin): May increase clearance of ritonavir, resulting in decreased ritonavir plasma levels. Monitor patient closely.
Oral contraceptives containing ethinyl estradiol: Decreased overall serum levels of the contraceptive. Advise patient that using together may require a dosage increase in the oral contraceptive or use of other contraceptive measures.
Saquinavir: Inhibited metabolism of saquinavir, resulting in greatly increased plasma levels. Safety of this combination hasn't been established. Monitor patient.
Theophylline: Decreased overall serum levels of theophylline. Increased theophylline dosage may be needed when administered with ritonavir. Monitor theophylline level.
Drug-herb. *St. John's wort:* Reduced blood levels of indinavir by more than 50%; similar effects can be expected in

---

other protease inhibitors. Discourage use together.
Drug-food. *Any food:* Increased absorption. Give drug with food.
Drug-lifestyle. *Smoking:* Decreased overall serum levels of ritonavir. Urge patients to avoid smoking.

EFFECTS ON LAB TEST RESULTS
• May increase ALT, AST, alkaline phosphatase, GGT, bilirubin, glucose, triglycerides, serum lipids, potassium, CK, and uric acid levels.
• May increase PT and INR. May decrease hemoglobin and hematocrit and WBC, platelet, neutrophil, and eosinophil counts.

CONTRAINDICATIONS
Contraindicated in patients hypersensitive to drug or its components.

NURSING CONSIDERATIONS
• Use cautiously in patients with hepatic insufficiency.
• Patients beginning combination regimens with ritonavir and nucleosides may improve GI tolerance by starting ritonavir alone and subsequently adding nucleosides before completing 2 weeks of ritonavir.
• Safety and effectiveness in children younger than age 12 haven't been established.
• It's unknown if ritonavir appears in breast milk.
• *Alert:* Do not confuse Norvir with Norvasc.

PATIENT TEACHING
• Inform patient that drug doesn't cure HIV infection. He may continue to develop opportunistic infections and other complications of HIV infection. Drug hasn't been shown to reduce the risk of transmitting HIV to others through sexual contact or blood contamination.
• Caution patient to take drug as prescribed and not to adjust dosage or stop therapy without first consulting prescriber.
• Tell patient that taste of ritonavir oral solution may be improved by mixing it with chocolate milk, Ensure, or Advera within 1 hour of the scheduled dose.

• Instruct patient to take drug with a meal to improve absorption.
• Tell patient that if a dose is missed, he should take the next dose as soon as possible. If a dose is skipped, he shouldn't double the next dose.
• Advise patient to report use of other drugs, including OTC drugs; ritonavir interacts with many drugs.
• Advise woman not to breast-feed to prevent transmission of infection.

---

saquinavir
Fortovase

saquinavir mesylate
Invirase

Pregnancy risk category B

AVAILABLE FORMS
saquinavir
Capsules (soft gelatin): 200 mg
saquinavir mesylate
Capsules (hard gelatin): 200 mg

INDICATIONS & DOSAGES
➤ **Adjunct treatment of advanced HIV infection in selected patients—**
Adults: 600 mg (Invirase) or 1,200 mg (Fortovase) P.O. t.i.d. taken within 2 hours after a full meal and with a nucleoside analogue such as zalcitabine at a dose of 0.75 mg P.O. t.i.d. or zidovudine at a dose of 200 mg P.O. t.i.d.

ACTION
Inhibits the activity of HIV protease and prevents the cleavage of HIV polyproteins, which are essential for HIV maturation.

Route	Onset	Peak	Duration
P.O.	Unknown	Unknown	Unknown

ADVERSE REACTIONS
CNS: paresthesia, headache, dizziness, asthenia, numbness, depression, insomnia, anxiety.
CV: chest pain.
GI: *diarrhea,* ulcerated buccal mucosa, abdominal pain, *nausea,* dyspepsia, *pancreatitis,* flatulence, vomiting, altered taste, constipation.

Hematologic: *pancytopenia, thrombo-cytopenia.*
Musculoskeletal: musculoskeletal pain.
Respiratory: bronchitis, cough.
Skin: rash.

INTERACTIONS

Drug-drug. *Ergot alkaloids, midazolam, triazolam and other drugs metabolized by the P-450 isoenzyme CYP3A4:* Decreased metabolism and increased plasma levels of these drugs, resulting in serious adverse effects. Avoid using together.
Ketoconazole, ritonavir: Increased serum saquinavir levels. Monitor patient closely.
Phenobarbital, phenytoin, rifabutin, rifampin: Reduced steady-state level of saquinavir. Use together cautiously.
Drug-herb. *St. John's wort:* Reduced blood levels of saquinavir by more than 50%; similar effects can be expected in other protease inhibitors. Discourage use together.
Drug-food. *Any food:* Increased absorption. Advise patient to take drug with food or within 2 hours of a full meal.
Grapefruit juice: Elevated levels of drug increasing the pharmacologic and adverse effects. Advise patient to take with liquid other than grapefruit juice.

EFFECTS ON LAB TEST RESULTS
● May decrease WBC, RBC, and platelet counts.

CONTRAINDICATIONS
Contraindicated in patients hypersensitive to drug or its components.

NURSING CONSIDERATIONS
● Safety of drug hasn't been established in pregnant or breast-feeding women or in children younger than age 16.
● *Alert:* Don't confuse the two forms of this drug because dosages are different.
● Invirase will be phased out over time and completely replaced by Fortovase.
● Evaluate CBC, platelets, electrolytes, uric acid, liver enzymes, and bilirubin before therapy begins and at appropriate intervals throughout therapy.
● If serious toxicity occurs during treatment, drug should be stopped until cause is identified or toxicity resolves. Drug

may be resumed with no dosage modifications.
● Monitor patient's hydration if adverse GI reactions occur.
● Monitor patient for adverse reactions to adjunct therapy (zidovudine or zalcitabine).

PATIENT TEACHING
● Advise patient to take drug with food or within 2 hours of a full meal to increase drug absorption.
● Inform patient that drug is usually given with other AIDS-related antivirals.
● Instruct patient to take drug around the clock, not missing any doses, to decrease the risk of developing HIV resistance.
● Inform patient that change from Invirase to Fortovase capsules should be made only under prescriber's supervision.
● Tell patient to store Fortovase capsules in the refrigerator; Invirase capsules can be kept at room temperature.

---

stavudine (2,3 didehydro-3-deoxythymidine, d4T)
Zerit

Pregnancy risk category C

AVAILABLE FORMS
Capsules: 15 mg, 20 mg, 30 mg, 40 mg
Oral solution: 1 mg/ml

INDICATIONS & DOSAGES
➤ **HIV-infected patients who have received prolonged prior zidovudine therapy—**
Adults and children weighing 60 kg (132 lb) or more: 40 mg P.O. q 12 hours.
Adults and children weighing 30 kg (66 lb) to 60 kg: 30 mg P.O. q 12 hours.
Children weighing less than 30 kg: 1 mg/kg P.O. q 12 hours.
Adjust-a-dose: For patients with renal impairment, if creatinine clearance is 26 to 50 ml/minute, adjust dosage to 20 mg (if weight exceeds 60 kg) or 15 mg (if weight is less than 60 kg) P.O. q 12 hours; if clearance is 10 to 25 ml/minute, 20 mg (if weight exceeds 60 kg) or 15 mg (if weight is less than 60 kg) P.O. q 24 hours.

ACTION
A thymidine nucleoside analogue that prevents replication of retroviruses, including HIV, by inhibiting the enzyme reverse transcriptase and causing termination of DNA chain growth.

Route	Onset	Peak	Duration
P.O.	Unknown	1 hr	Unknown

ADVERSE REACTIONS
CNS: peripheral neuropathy, headache, malaise, insomnia, anxiety, *asthenia,* depression, nervousness, dizziness.
CV: chest pain.
EENT: conjunctivitis.
GI: *abdominal pain, diarrhea, nausea, vomiting, anorexia,* dyspepsia, constipation, *pancreatitis.*
Hematologic: *neutropenia, thrombocytopenia,* anemia.
Hepatic: *hepatotoxicity.*
Metabolic: weight loss.
Musculoskeletal: *arthralgia, myalgia, back pain.*
Respiratory: *dyspnea.*
Skin: *rash, diaphoresis, pruritus,* maculopapular rash.
Other: *chills, fever.*

INTERACTIONS
None significant.

EFFECTS ON LAB TEST RESULTS
● May increase ALT and AST levels.
● May decrease hemoglobin and neutrophil and platelet counts.

CONTRAINDICATIONS
Contraindicated in patients hypersensitive to drug.

NURSING CONSIDERATIONS
● Use cautiously in patients with renal impairment or history of peripheral neuropathy. Adjust dosage as directed for creatinine clearance below 50 ml/minute; dosage adjustment or discontinuation is necessary in onset of peripheral neuropathy. Also use cautiously in pregnant women.
● *Alert:* Peripheral neuropathy appears to be the major dose-limiting adverse effect of stavudine. It may or may not resolve after drug is stopped.

● Monitor CBC results and creatinine, and AST, ALT, and alkaline phosphatase levels.

PATIENT TEACHING
● Tell patient that drug may be taken without regard to meals.
● Warn patient not to take other drugs for HIV or AIDS unless prescriber has approved them.
● Teach patient signs and symptoms of peripheral neuropathy (pain, burning, aching, weakness, or pins and needles in the limbs) and tell him to report these immediately.
● Tell patient to monitor weight patterns and report weight loss or gain.

✳ *NEW DRUG*

tenofovir disoproxil fumarate
Viread

Pregnancy risk category B

AVAILABLE FORMS
Tablets: 300 mg as the fumarate salt (equivalent to 245 mg of tenofovir disoproxil).

INDICATIONS & DOSAGES
➤ **HIV-1 infection, with other antiretroviral drugs—**
Adults: 300 mg P.O. once daily with a meal. When given with didanosine, give 2 hours before or 1 hour after didanosine.

ACTION
A prodrug that is hydrolyzed to produce tenofovir. Tenofovir, a nucleoside analog of adenosine monophosphate, undergoes sequential phosphorylations to yield tenofovir diphosphate. Tenofovir diphosphate is a competitive antagonist of HIV reverse transcriptase, via competition with the natural substrate and through DNA chain termination. These effects result in inhibition of HIV replication.

Route	Onset	Peak	Duration
P.O.	Unknown	1-2 hr	Unknown

ADVERSE REACTIONS
CNS: asthenia, headache.

GI: abdominal pain, anorexia, diarrhea, flatulence, *nausea,* vomiting.
GU: glycosuria.
Hematologic: *neutropenia.*
Metabolic: hyperglycemia.

INTERACTIONS
Drug-drug. *Didanosine (buffered formulation):* Increased didanosine bioavailability. Monitor patient for didanosine-related adverse effects, such as bone marrow suppression, GI distress, and peripheral neuropathy. Give tenofovir 2 hours before or 1 hour after didanosine.
Drugs that reduce renal function or compete for renal tubular secretion (acyclovir, cidofovir, ganciclovir, valacyclovir, valganciclovir): Increased levels of tenofovir or other renally eliminated drugs. Monitor patient for adverse effects.

EFFECTS ON LAB TEST RESULTS
• Increased amylase, AST, ALT, creatinine kinase, serum and urine glucose, and triglyceride levels.
• Decreased neutrophil count.

CONTRAINDICATIONS
Contraindicated in patients hypersensitive to any component of the drug. Don't use in patients with creatinine clearance less than 60 ml/minute.

NURSING CONSIDERATIONS
• Use very cautiously in patients with risk factors for liver disease or with hepatic impairment.
• Antiretrovirals, alone or combined, have been linked to lactic acidosis and severe (including fatal) hepatomegaly with steatosis. These effects may occur without elevated transaminase levels. Risk factors may include prolonged exposure to antiretrovirals, obesity, and being female. Monitor all patients for hepatotoxicity, including lactic acidosis and hepatomegaly with steatosis.
• Antiretrovirals have been linked to the accumulation and redistribution of body fat, resulting in central obesity, peripheral wasting, and development of a buffalo hump. The long-term effects of these changes are unknown. Monitor patients for changes in body fat.

• Tenofovir may be linked to bone abnormalities (osteomalacia and decreased bone mineral density) and renal toxicity (increased creatinine and phosphaturia levels). Monitor patient carefully during long-term treatment.
• Drug may lead to decreased HIV-1 RNA levels and CD4+ cell counts.
• The effects of tenofovir on the progression of HIV infection are unknown.
• Because the effects of tenofovir on pregnant women aren't known, give this drug to pregnant women only if its benefits clearly outweigh the risks.
• It isn't known whether tenofovir appears in breast milk, but mothers receiving tenofovir for HIV infection shouldn't breastfeed.
• Safety and efficacy haven't been studied in children.
• Use tenofovir cautiously in geriatric patients because these patients are more likely to have renal impairment and concurrent drug therapy.

PATIENT TEACHING
• Instruct patient to take tenofovir with a meal to enhance bioavailability.
• If patient takes tenofovir and didanosine (buffered form), instruct him to take tenofovir 2 hours before or 1 hour after didanosine.
• Tell patient to report adverse effects, including nausea, vomiting, diarrhea, flatulence, and headache.

---

valacyclovir hydrochloride
Valtrex

Pregnancy risk category B

AVAILABLE FORMS
Tablets: 500 mg, 1 g

INDICATIONS & DOSAGES
➤ **Herpes zoster infection (shingles)—**
Adults: 1 g P.O. t.i.d. for 7 days.
Adjust-a-dose: For renally impaired patients with creatinine clearance of 50 ml/minute or more, use regular dose; if 30 to 49 ml/minute, 1 g P.O. q 12 hours; if 10 to 29 ml/minute, 1 g P.O. q 24 hours; if below 10 ml/minute, 500 mg P.O. q 24

hours. For hemodialysis patients, 1 g P.O. after hemodialysis.

➤ **Initial episode of genital herpes—**
Adults: 1 g P.O. b.i.d. for 10 days.
Adjust-a-dose: For renally impaired patients with creatinine clearance of 30 ml/minute or more, dosage is 1 g P.O. q 12 hours; if 10 to 29 ml/minute, 1 g P.O. q 24 hours; if below 10 ml/minute, 500 mg P.O. q 24 hours. For hemodialysis patients, 1 g P.O. after hemodialysis.

➤ **Recurrent genital herpes in immunocompetent patients—**
Adults: 500 mg P.O. b.i.d. for 3 days, given at the first sign or symptom of an episode.

➤ **Chronic suppressive therapy in recurrent genital herpes—**
Adults: 1 g P.O. once daily. In patients with a history of nine or fewer recurrences per year, use alternative dose of 500 mg once daily.
Adjust-a-dose: For renally impaired patients with creatinine clearance of 30 ml/minute or more, dosage is 500 mg P.O. q 12 hours; if 29 ml/minute or less, 500 mg P.O. q 24 hours. For hemodialysis patients, 500 mg P.O. after hemodialysis.

ACTION

Rapidly converts to acyclovir, which in turn becomes incorporated into viral DNA, thereby terminating growth of the DNA chain; inhibits viral DNA polymerase, causing inhibition of viral replication.

Route	Onset	Peak	Duration
P.O.	30 min	Unknown	Unknown

ADVERSE REACTIONS

CNS: *headache,* asthenia, dizziness, depression.
GI: *nausea,* vomiting, diarrhea, constipation, abdominal pain, anorexia.
Musculoskeletal: arthralgia.

INTERACTIONS

Drug-drug. *Cimetidine, probenecid:* Reduced rate but not extent of conversion of valacyclovir to acyclovir and reduced renal clearance of acyclovir, thus increasing acyclovir blood levels. Monitor patient for acyclovir toxicity.

EFFECTS ON LAB TEST RESULTS

None reported.

CONTRAINDICATIONS

Contraindicated in patients hypersensitive to or intolerant of valacyclovir, acyclovir, or components of the formulation.

NURSING CONSIDERATIONS

● ***Alert:*** Valacyclovir isn't recommended for use in patients with HIV infection or in bone marrow or renal transplant recipients because of the occurrence of thrombotic thrombocytopenic purpura and hemolytic uremic syndrome in these patients at doses of 8 g/day.
● Use cautiously in elderly patients, those with renal impairment, and those receiving other nephrotoxic drugs. Monitor renal function test results.
● ***Alert:*** Don't confuse valacyclovir with valganciclovir.
● Safety and efficacy in children haven't been established.
● Use of drug during pregnancy should be considered only if the benefits outweigh the risks.
● If patient is breast-feeding, drug may need to be discontinued.
● Although there have been no reports of overdose, precipitation of acyclovir in renal tubules may occur when solubility (2.5 mg/ml) is exceeded in the intratubular fluid. With acute renal failure and anuria, the patient may benefit from hemodialysis until renal function is restored.

PATIENT TEACHING

● Inform patient that valacyclovir may be taken without regard to meals.
● Teach patient the signs and symptoms of herpes infection (rash, tingling, itching, and pain), and advise him to notify prescriber immediately if they occur. Treatment should begin as soon as possible after symptoms appear, preferably within 48 hours of the onset of zoster rash.
● Tell patient that valacyclovir isn't a cure for herpes but may decrease the length and severity of symptoms.

✳ *NEW DRUG*

valganciclovir
Valcyte

Pregnancy risk category C

AVAILABLE FORMS
Tablets: 450 mg

INDICATIONS & DOSAGES
➤ **Active cytomegalovirus (CMV) retinitis in patients with AIDS—**
Adults: 900 mg (two 450-mg tablets) P.O. b.i.d. with food for 21 days; maintenance dose is 900 mg (two 450-mg tablet) P.O. daily with food.
➤ **Inactive CMV retinitis—**
Adults: 900 mg (two 450-mg tablet) P.O. daily with food.
Adjust-a-dose: For patients with impaired renal function, if creatinine clearance is 40 to 59 ml/minute, induction dose is 450 mg b.i.d.; maintenance dose is 450 mg daily. If clearance is 25 to 39 ml/minute, induction dose is 450 mg daily; maintenance dose is 450 mg every 2 days. If clearance is 10 to 24 ml/minute, induction dose is 450 mg every 2 days; maintenance dose is 450 mg twice weekly.

ACTION
Drug is converted to the active drug ganciclovir, which inhibits replication of cytomegalovirus.

Route	Onset	Peak	Duration
P.O.	Unknown	1-3 hr	Unknown

ADVERSE REACTIONS
CNS: *headache, insomnia,* peripheral neuropathy, paresthesia, **seizures,** psychosis, hallucinations, confusion, agitation.
EENT: *retinal detachment.*
GI: *diarrhea, nausea, vomiting, abdominal pain.*
Hematologic: NEUTROPENIA, *anemia,* **thrombocytopenia, pancytopenia, bone marrow depression, aplastic anemia.**
Other: catheter-related infection, **sepsis,** local or systemic infections, *pyrexia,* hypersensitivity reactions.

INTERACTIONS
Drug-drug. *Didanosine:* May increase absorption of didanosine. Monitor patient closely for didanosine toxicity.
Immunosuppressants, zidovudine: May enhance neutropenia, anemia, thrombocytopenia, and bone marrow depression. Monitor CBC results.
Mycophenolate mofetil: May increase levels of both drugs in renally impaired patients. Use together carefully.
Probenecid: Decreased renal clearance of ganciclovir. Monitor patient for ganciclovir toxicity.
Drug-food. *Any food:* Increased absorption of drug. Give drug with food.

EFFECTS ON LAB TEST RESULTS
● May decrease hemoglobin and hematocrit and RBC, WBC, neutrophil, and platelet counts.

CONTRAINDICATIONS
Contraindicated in patients with hypersensitivity to valganciclovir or ganciclovir. Don't use in patients receiving hemodialysis.

NURSING CONSIDERATIONS
● Use cautiously in patients with preexisting cytopenias and in those who have received immunosuppressants or radiation.
● Be sure to adhere to dosing guidelines for valganciclovir because ganciclovir and valganciclovir aren't interchangeable and overdose may occur.
● Clinical toxicities include severe leukopenia, neutropenia, anemia, pancytopenia, bone marrow depression, aplastic anemia, and thrombocytopenia. Don't use if patient's absolute neutrophil count is less than 500 cells/mm³, platelets are less than 25,000/mm³, or hemoglobin is less than 8 g/dl.
● Monitor CBC, platelet counts, and creatinine levels or creatinine clearance values frequently during treatment.
● Cytopenia may occur at any time during treatment and increase with continued dosing. Cell counts usually recover 3 to 7 days after stopping drug.
● No drug interaction studies have been conducted with valganciclovir; however, because drug is converted to ganciclovir, it

---

Reactions may be *common,* uncommon, *life-threatening,* or COMMON AND LIFE-THREATENING.

can be assumed that drug interactions would be similar.
• Drug may cause temporary or permanent inhibition of spermatogenesis.

PATIENT TEACHING
• Tell patient to take drug with food.
• Tell patient to follow dosing instructions precisely. Ganciclovir capsules and valganciclovir tablets are not interchangeable on a one-to-one basis.
• Advise patient that blood tests are needed during treatment. Doses may need to be adjusted based on blood counts.
• Tell women of childbearing age to use contraception during treatment. Inform men that they should use barrier contraception during and for 90 days after treatment.
• Advise patient that ganciclovir is considered a potential carcinogen.
• Tell patient that CNS effects (seizures, ataxia, dizziness) can occur and to use care in driving or operating machinery.
• Advise patient that this drug isn't a cure for CMV retinitis and that the condition may recur. Tell patient to have ophthalmologic examinations at least every 4 to 6 weeks during treatment.

zalcitabine (ddC, dideoxycytidine)
Hivid

Pregnancy risk category C

AVAILABLE FORMS
Tablets: 0.375 mg, 0.75 mg

INDICATIONS & DOSAGES
➤ **Advanced HIV disease in patients who either can't tolerate zidovudine or who have disease progression while receiving zidovudine—**
Adults and children age 13 and older: 0.75 mg P.O. q 8 hours.
➤ **Therapy with zidovudine for treatment of advanced HIV disease (CD4+ cell count 300/mm³ or less)—**
Adults and children age 13 and older: 0.75 mg P.O. q 8 hours given with zidovudine 200 mg P.O. q 8 hours.
Adjust-a-dose: For renally impaired patients with creatinine clearance of 10 to

40 ml/minute, dosage is 0.75 mg P.O. q 12 hours; if clearance is below 10 ml/minute, 0.75 mg P.O. q 24 hours. If patient experiences moderate discomfort with signs and symptoms of peripheral neuropathy, stop drug temporarily. If symptoms improve after discontinuation, drug may be reintroduced at 0.375 mg P.O. q 8 hours.

ACTION
Nucleoside reverse transcriptase inhibitor that inhibits replication of HIV by blocking viral DNA synthesis.

Route	Onset	Peak	Duration
P.O.	Unknown	1-2 hr	Unknown

ADVERSE REACTIONS
CNS: *peripheral neuropathy, headache, fatigue,* dizziness, confusion, ***seizures,*** impaired concentration, amnesia, insomnia, mental depression, tremor, hypertonia, anxiety.
CV: cardiomyopathy, ***heart failure,*** chest pain.
EENT: pharyngitis, ocular pain, abnormal vision, ototoxicity, nasal discharge.
GI: nausea, vomiting, diarrhea, abdominal pain, anorexia, constipation, stomatitis, esophageal ulcer, glossitis, ***pancreatitis.***
Hematologic: anemia, ***neutropenia, leukopenia, thrombocytopenia.***
Metabolic: hypoglycemia.
Musculoskeletal: myalgia, arthralgia.
Respiratory: cough.
Skin: pruritus; night sweats; *erythematous, maculopapular, or follicular rash;* urticaria.
Other: *fever.*

INTERACTIONS
Drug-drug. *Aminoglycosides, amphotericin B, foscarnet, other drugs that may impair renal function:* Increased risk of nephrotoxicity. Monitor renal function.
Antacids containing aluminum or magnesium: Decreased bioavailability of zalcitabine. Separate administration times.
Chloramphenicol, cisplatin, dapsone, didanosine, disulfiram, ethionamide, glutethimide, gold salts, hydralazine, iodoquinol, isoniazid, metronidazole, nitrofurantoin, other drugs that can cause peripheral neuropathy, phenytoin, ribavirin, stavudine, vincristine: Increased

risk of peripheral neuropathy. Avoid using together.
Cimetidine, probenecid: Increased serum zalcitabine levels. Monitor patient closely.
Pentamidine: Increased risk of pancreatitis. Avoid using together.
Drug-food. *Any food:* Decreased rate of absorption. Give drug on an empty stomach.

EFFECTS ON LAB TEST RESULTS
• May increase glucose, alkaline phosphatase, ALT, and AST levels.
• May decrease hemoglobin and neutrophil, WBC, and platelet counts.

CONTRAINDICATIONS
Contraindicated in patients hypersensitive to drug or its components.

NURSING CONSIDERATIONS
• Use with extreme caution in patients with peripheral neuropathy.
• Use cautiously in patients with hepatic failure, history of pancreatitis or heart failure, or baseline cardiomyopathy. Monitor liver function test results and pancreatic enzymes.
• Toxic effects of drug may cause abnormalities in several laboratory tests, including CBC, hemoglobin, leukocyte, reticulocyte, granulocyte, and platelet counts; and AST, ALT, and alkaline phosphatase levels.
• Don't administer drug with food because it decreases the rate and extent of absorption.
• Assess patients for signs and symptoms of peripheral neuropathy, characterized by numbness and burning in the limbs, the drug's major toxic effects. If drug isn't withdrawn, peripheral neuropathy can progress to sharp shooting pain or severe continuous burning pain requiring opioid analgesics. The pain may or may not be reversible.
• *Alert:* Don't confuse drug with other antivirals identified by initials.

PATIENT TEACHING
• Instruct patient to take drug on an empty stomach.
• Make sure patient understands that the drug doesn't cure HIV infection and that opportunistic infections may occur despite continued use. Review safe sex practices with patient.
• Inform patient that peripheral neuropathy is the major toxic condition associated with drug and that pancreatitis is the major life-threatening toxic reaction. Review the signs and symptoms of these adverse reactions, and tell patient to call prescriber promptly if any appear.
• Advise patient of childbearing age to use an effective contraceptive while taking drug.

zanamivir
Relenza

Pregnancy risk category B

AVAILABLE FORMS
Powder for inhalation: 5 mg/blister

INDICATIONS & DOSAGES
➤ **Uncomplicated acute illness caused by influenza virus A and B in patients who have had symptoms for no longer than 2 days—**
Adults and children age 12 and older: 2 oral inhalations (one 5-mg blister per inhalation for total dose of 10 mg) b.i.d. using the Diskhaler inhalation device for 5 days. Two doses should be taken on first day of treatment, allowing at least 2 hours to elapse between doses. Subsequent doses should be about 12 hours apart (in the morning and evening) at about the same time each day.

ACTION
Likely exerts its antiviral action by inhibiting neuraminidase on the surface of the influenza virus, potentially altering virus particle aggregation and release.

Route	Onset	Peak	Duration
Inhalation	Unknown	1-2 hr	Unknown

ADVERSE REACTIONS
CNS: headache, dizziness.
EENT: nasal signs and symptoms; sinusitis; ear, nose, and throat infections.
GI: diarrhea, nausea, vomiting.
Respiratory: bronchitis, cough.

INTERACTIONS
None significant.

EFFECTS ON LAB TEST RESULTS
None reported.

CONTRAINDICATIONS
Contraindicated in patients hypersensitive to drug or its components.

NURSING CONSIDERATIONS
• Use cautiously in patients with severe or decompensated COPD, asthma, or other underlying respiratory disease.
• Patients with underlying respiratory disease should have a fast-acting bronchodilator available in case of wheezing while taking zanamivir. Patients scheduled to use an inhaled bronchodilator for asthma should use their bronchodilator before taking zanamivir.
• Safety and efficacy of drug haven't been established in patients who begin treatment after 48 hours of symptoms.
• Safety and efficacy of drug haven't been established for influenza prophylaxis. Use of drug shouldn't affect evaluation of patient for annual influenza vaccination.
• Lymphopenia, neutropenia, and a rise in liver enzyme and CK levels have been reported during zanamivir treatment.
• Monitor patient for bronchospasm and decline in lung function. Stop drug in such situations.

PATIENT TEACHING
• Tell patient to carefully read the instructions for the Diskhaler inhalation device to properly administer drug.
• Advise patient to keep the Diskhaler level when loading and inhaling zanamivir. Tell him to always check inside the mouthpiece of the Diskhaler before each use to make sure it's free of foreign objects.
• Tell patient to exhale fully before putting the mouthpiece in his mouth; then, keeping the Diskhaler level, to close his lips around the mouthpiece and breathe in steadily and deeply. Advise patient to hold his breath for a few seconds after inhaling to help drug stay in the lungs.
• Advise patient with respiratory disease who is scheduled to use an inhaled bronchodilator to do so before taking zana-

mivir. Tell patient to have a fast-acting bronchodilator available in case of wheezing while taking zanamivir.
• Advise patient that it's important to finish the entire 5-day course of treatment even if he starts to feel better and symptoms improve before the fifth day.
• Advise patient that the use of zanamivir hasn't been shown to reduce the risk of transmission of influenza virus to others.

---

zidovudine (azidothymidine, AZT)
Apo-Zidovudine†, Novo-AZT†, Retrovir

Pregnancy risk category C

AVAILABLE FORMS
Capsules: 100 mg
Injection: 10 mg/ml
Syrup: 50 mg/5 ml
Tablets: 300 mg

INDICATIONS & DOSAGES
➤ **Treatment of HIV infection—**
Adults and children age 12 and older:
300 mg P.O. q 12 hours, 200 mg P.O. q 8 hours, or 1 mg/kg I.V. five to six times daily.
Children ages 3 months to 12 years:
180 mg/m^2 P.O. q 6 hours (720 mg/m^2/ day), not to exceed 200 mg q 6 hours. Some prescribers recommend 160 mg/m^2 P.O. q 8 hours, 20 mg/m^2 I.V. q 6 hours, or 20 mg/m^2/hour continuous I.V. infusion.
➤ **Prevention of maternal-fetal transmission of HIV—**
Adults: 100 mg P.O. five times daily, given initially between 14 and 34 weeks' gestation and continued until onset of labor. During labor, give loading dose of 2 mg/ kg I.V. over 1 hour, then continuous I.V. infusion of 1 mg/kg/hour until umbilical cord is clamped.
Neonates: 2 mg/kg P.O. (syrup) q 6 hours for 6 weeks, beginning within 8 to 24 hours after birth. Or, 1.5 mg/kg I.V. infusion over 30 minutes q 6 hours.
➤ **Adjunctive therapy with zalcitabine or other antiretrovirals to treat advanced HIV disease—**
Adults and children age 13 and older:
200 mg P.O. q 8 hours or 300 mg (1 tablet)

P.O. q 12 hours given with zalcitabine 0.75 mg P.O. q 8 hours or other antiretrovirals.
Adjust-a-dose: For patient with end-stage renal disease or patient receiving hemodialysis or peritoneal dialysis, 100 mg P.O. or 1 mg/kg I.V. q 6 to 8 hours.

I.V. ADMINISTRATION
● Remove the calculated dose from the vial; add to D_5W to achieve a concentration that doesn't exceed 4 mg/ml.
● Infuse drug over 1 hour at a constant rate. Avoid rapid infusion or bolus injection. Don't add mixture to biological or colloidal fluids (for example, blood products, protein solutions).
● Protect undiluted vials from light.

ACTION
Nucleoside reverse transcriptase inhibitor that inhibits replication of HIV by blocking DNA synthesis.

Route	Onset	Peak	Duration
I.V., P.O.	Unknown	0.5-1.5 hr	Unknown

ADVERSE REACTIONS
CNS: headache, *seizures,* paresthesia, *malaise,* insomnia, *asthenia, dizziness,* somnolence.
GI: nausea, anorexia, abdominal pain, vomiting, constipation, diarrhea, taste perversion, dyspepsia, *pancreatitis.*
Hematologic: *severe bone marrow suppression, anemia, agranulocytosis, thrombocytopenia.*
Metabolic: lactic acidosis.
Musculoskeletal: myalgia.
Skin: *rash,* diaphoresis.
Other: *fever.*

INTERACTIONS
Drug-drug. *Acetaminophen, aspirin, indomethacin:* May impair hepatic metabolism of zidovudine, increasing drug's toxicity. Monitor patient closely.
Acyclovir: May cause seizures, lethargy, and fatigue. Use together cautiously.
Amphotericin B, dapsone, flucytosine, pentamidine: Increased risk of nephrotoxicity and bone marrow suppression. Monitor patient closely.

Fluconazole, methadone, valproic acid: Increased zidovudine level. Monitor patient for toxicity.
Ganciclovir, interferon alpha: Increased risk of hematologic toxicity. Monitor patient closely.
Other cytotoxic drugs: Additive adverse effects on bone marrow. Avoid using together.
Probenecid: May decrease the renal clearance of zidovudine. Avoid using together.
Ribavirin: Antagonized antiviral activity of zidovudine against HIV. Avoid using together.

EFFECTS ON LAB TEST RESULTS
● May increase ALT, AST, alkaline phosphatase, and LDH levels.
● May decrease hemoglobin and granulocyte and platelet counts.

CONTRAINDICATIONS
Contraindicated in patients hypersensitive to drug.

NURSING CONSIDERATIONS
● Use cautiously and with close monitoring in patients with advanced symptomatic HIV infection and in patients with severe bone marrow depression.
● Use with caution in patients with hepatomegaly, hepatitis, or other risk factors for liver disease and in those with renal insufficiency. Monitor renal and liver function tests.
● Monitor blood studies every 2 weeks to detect anemia or agranulocytosis. Patients may need dosage reduction or temporary discontinuation of drug.
● Drug may temporarily decrease morbidity and mortality in certain patients with AIDS.

PATIENT TEACHING
● Tell patient to take drug exactly as directed and not to share it with others.
● Instruct patient to take drug on an empty stomach. To avoid esophageal irritation, tell patient to take drug while sitting upright and with adequate fluids.
● Remind patient to comply with the dosage schedule. Suggest ways to avoid missing doses, perhaps by using an alarm clock.

Reactions may be *common,* uncommon, *life-threatening,* or COMMON AND LIFE-THREATENING.

- Advise patient that blood transfusions may be needed during treatment. Zidovudine frequently causes a low RBC count.
- Tell patient that gums may bleed. Recommend good mouth care with a soft toothbrush.
- Warn patient not to take other drugs for AIDS unless prescriber has approved them.
- Advise pregnant, HIV-infected patient that drug therapy only reduces the risk of HIV transmission to her newborn. Long-term risks to infants are unknown.
- Advise patient that monotherapy isn't recommended and to discuss any questions with prescriber.
- Advise health care worker considering zidovudine prophylaxis after occupational exposure (after needle-stick injury, for example) that drug's safety or efficacy hasn't yet been established.

azithromycin
clarithromycin
dirithromycin
erythromycin base
erythromycin estolate
erythromycin ethylsuccinate
erythromycin lactobionate
erythromycin stearate

COMBINATION PRODUCTS
ERYZOLE, PEDIAZOLE: erythromycin (200 mg) and sulfisoxazole (600 mg)/5 ml

---

azithromycin
Zithromax

Pregnancy risk category B

AVAILABLE FORMS
Oral suspension: 100 mg/5 ml, 200 mg/ 5 ml
Powder for injection: 500 mg
Single-dose powder for oral suspension: 1-g packet
Tablets: 250 mg, 600 mg

INDICATIONS & DOSAGES
➤ **Acute bacterial exacerbations of COPD caused by** *Haemophilus influenzae,* *Moraxella catarrhalis,* **or** *Streptococcus pneumoniae;* **uncomplicated skin and skin-structure infections caused by** *Staphylococcus aureus,* *Streptococcus pyogenes,* **or** *S. agalactiae;* **second-line therapy of pharyngitis or tonsillitis caused by** *S. pyogenes*—
Adults and adolescents age 16 and older: 500 mg P.O. as a single dose on day 1; then 250 mg daily on days 2 through 5. Total dose is 1.5 g.
➤ **Community-acquired pneumonia caused by** *Chlamydia pneumoniae,* *H. influenzae,* *Mycoplasma pneumoniae,* **or** *S. pneumoniae;* **or caused by** *Legionella pneumophila,* *M. catarrhalis,* **or** *S. aureus* **(I.V. form)**—
Adults and adolescents age 16 and older: 500 mg P.O. as a single dose on day 1; then 250 mg P.O. daily on days 2 through 5. Total dose is 1.5 g. For patients requiring initial I.V. therapy, 500 mg I.V. as a single daily dose for 2 days; then 500 mg P.O. as a single daily dose to complete a 7- to 10-day course of therapy. Switch from I.V. to P.O. therapy should be done at the prescriber's discretion and based on patient's clinical response.
➤ **Nongonococcal urethritis or cervicitis caused by** *C. trachomatis*—
Adults and adolescents age 16 and older: 1 g P.O. as a single dose.
➤ **Prevention of disseminated** *Mycobacterium avium* **complex disease in patients with advanced HIV infection**—
Adults: 1,200 mg P.O. once weekly, as indicated.
➤ **Urethritis and cervicitis caused by** *Neisseria gonorrhoeae*—
Adults: 2 g P.O. as a single dose.
➤ **Pelvic inflammatory disease caused by** *C. trachomatis, N. gonorrhoeae,* **or** *Mycoplasma hominis* **in patients who need initial I.V. therapy**—
Adults: 500 mg I.V. as a single daily dose for 1 to 2 days; then 250 mg P.O. daily to complete a 7-day course of therapy. Switch from I.V. to P.O. therapy should be at prescriber's discretion and based on patient's clinical response.
➤ **Genital ulcer disease in men caused by** *H. ducreyi* **(chancroid)**—
Adults: 1 g P.O. as a single dose.
➤ **Otitis media**—
Children older than age 6 months: 10 mg/kg (maximum 500 mg) P.O. on day 1; then 5 mg/kg (maximum 250 mg) on days 2 to 5.
➤ **Pharyngitis, tonsillitis**—
Children older than age 2: 12 mg/kg (maximum 500 mg) P.O. daily for 5 days.
➤ **Dental prophylaxis in patients allergic to penicillin**—
Adults: 500 mg P.O. 1 hour before procedure.
Children: 15 mg/kg P.O. 1 hour before procedure.

Reactions may be *common*, uncommon, *life-threatening*, or COMMON AND LIFE-THREATENING.

I.V. ADMINISTRATION
● Reconstitute drug in 500-mg vial with 4.8 ml of sterile water for injection and shake well until all the drug is dissolved (yields a concentration of 100 mg/ml).
● Dilute solution further in at least 250 ml of normal saline solution, half-normal saline solution, D_5W, or lactated Ringer's solution to yield a concentration range of 1 to 2 mg/ml.
● *Alert:* Infuse a 500-mg dose of azithromycin I.V. over 1 hour or more. Never give it as a bolus or an I.M. injection.

ACTION
Binds to the 50S subunit of bacterial ribosomes, blocking protein synthesis; bacteriostatic or bactericidal, depending on concentration.

Route	Onset	Peak	Duration
I.V.	Unknown	Unknown	Unknown
P.O.	Unknown	2.5-4.4 hr	Unknown

ADVERSE REACTIONS
CNS: dizziness, vertigo, headache, fatigue, somnolence.
CV: palpitations, chest pain.
GI: *nausea, vomiting, diarrhea, abdominal pain,* dyspepsia, flatulence, melena, cholestatic jaundice, pseudomembranous colitis.
GU: candidiasis, vaginitis, nephritis.
Skin: rash, photosensitivity.
Other: *angioedema.*

INTERACTIONS
Drug-drug. *Antacids containing aluminum and magnesium:* Lowered peak plasma levels of azithromycin. Separate administration times by at least 2 hours.
Carbamazepine, cyclosporine, phenytoin: May increase levels of these drugs. Monitor patient closely.
Digoxin: May cause elevated digoxin levels. Monitor patient closely.
Ergotamine: May cause acute ergotamine toxicity. Monitor patient closely.
Pimozide: May prolong QT interval and cause ventricular tachycardia. Monitor patient closely.
Theophylline: May increase plasma theophylline levels. Monitor theophylline levels carefully.

Triazolam: May decrease clearance of triazolam. Monitor patient closely.
Warfarin: May increase INR. Monitor INR carefully.
Drug-food. *Any food:* Decreased absorption of multidose oral suspension formulation. Give preparation on empty stomach.
Drug-lifestyle. *Sun exposure:* May cause photosensitivity. Tell patient to take precautions against sun exposure.

EFFECTS ON LAB TEST RESULTS
None reported.

CONTRAINDICATIONS
Contraindicated in patients hypersensitive to erythromycin or other macrolides.

NURSING CONSIDERATIONS
● Use cautiously in patients with impaired hepatic function.
● Obtain specimen for culture and sensitivity tests before giving first dose. Therapy may begin pending results.
● Give multidose oral suspension 1 hour before or 2 hours after meals; don't give with antacids. Tablets and single-dose packets for oral suspension can be taken with or without food.
● Monitor patient for superinfection. Drug may cause overgrowth of nonsusceptible bacteria or fungi.
● Single-dose, 1-g packets for suspension should be reconstituted with 2 ounces (60 ml) of water, mixed, and administered to patient. Patient should rinse glass with additional 2 ounces of water and drink to ensure he has consumed entire dose. Packets aren't for pediatric use.

PATIENT TEACHING
● Tell patient to take drug as prescribed, even after he feels better.

---

clarithromycin
Biaxin, Biaxin XL, Klaricid§

Pregnancy risk category C

AVAILABLE FORMS
Suspension: 125 mg/5 ml, 187.5 mg/5 ml
Tablets (extended-release): 500 mg
Tablets (film-coated): 250 mg, 500 mg

INDICATIONS & DOSAGES

➤ **Pharyngitis or tonsillitis caused by** *Streptococcus pyogenes*—
Adults: 250 mg P.O. q 12 hours for 10 days.
Children: 15 mg/kg/day P.O. in divided doses q 12 hours for 10 days.

➤ **Acute maxillary sinusitis caused by** *S. pneumoniae, Haemophilus influenzae,* **or** *Moraxella catarrhalis*—
Adults: 500 mg P.O. q 12 hours for 14 days. Or 1,000 mg P.O. extended-release tablets q 24 hours for 14 days.
Children: 15 mg/kg/day P.O. in divided doses q 12 hours for 10 days.

➤ **Acute exacerbations of chronic bronchitis caused by** *M. catarrhalis* **or** *S. pneumoniae;* **pneumonia caused by** *S. pneumoniae, Chlamydia pneumoniae,* **or** *Mycoplasma pneumoniae*—
Adults: 250 mg P.O. q 12 hours for 7 to 14 days. Or (for chronic bronchitis) 1,000 mg P.O. extended-release tablets q 24 hours for 7 days.

➤ **Acute exacerbations of chronic bronchitis caused by** *H. influenzae*—
Adults: 500 mg P.O. q 12 hours for 7 to 14 days. Or, 1,000 mg P.O. extended-release tablets q 24 hours for 7 days.

➤ **Uncomplicated skin and skin-structure infections caused by** *Staphylococcus aureus* **or** *S. pyogenes*—
Adults: 250 mg P.O. q 12 hours for 7 to 14 days.
Children: 15 mg/kg/day P.O. in divided doses q 12 hours for 10 days.

➤ **Acute otitis media caused by** *H. influenzae, M. catarrhalis,* **or** *S. pneumoniae*—
Children: 7.5 mg/kg P.O. q 12 hours for 10 days.

➤ ***Mycobacterium avium* complex (MAC) disease in patients with HIV infection**—
Adults: 500 mg P.O. q 12 hours, with other antimycobacterial drugs, for life.
Children: 7.5 mg/kg P.O. (maximum of 500 mg) q 12 hours, with other antimycobacterial drugs, for life.

➤ **Prophylaxis against MAC disease in patients with advanced HIV infection**—
Adults: 500 mg P.O. q 12 hours.
Children: 7.5 mg/kg P.O. (maximum of 500 mg) q 12 hours.

➤ **Active duodenal ulcer with** *Helicobacter pylori* **infection**—
Adults: 500 mg P.O. t.i.d. for 14 days with omeprazole 40 mg P.O. each morning. Omeprazole therapy should continue at a dose of 20 mg P.O. each morning for days 15 to 28. Or, 500 mg P.O. t.i.d. for 14 days with ranitidine bismuth citrate 400 mg P.O. b.i.d. Ranitidine bismuth citrate therapy continues for days 15 to 28. Or, 500 mg P.O. b.i.d. plus lansoprazole 30 mg P.O. b.i.d. and amoxicillin 1 g P.O. b.i.d. for 14 days.

➤ **Dental prophylaxis in patients allergic to penicillin**—
Adults: 500 mg P.O. 1 hour before procedure.
Children: 15 mg/kg P.O. 1 hour before procedure.

✹ *NEW INDICATION:* **Community-acquired pneumonia caused by** *Chlamydia pneumoniae, Mycoplasma pneumoniae, Streptococcus pneumoniae,* **or** *Haemophilus influenzae*—
Adults: 250 mg P.O. q 12 hours for 7 to 14 days or 1,000 mg P.O. extended-release tablets q 24 hours for 7 days.

ACTION

Binds to the 50S subunit of bacterial ribosomes, blocking protein synthesis; bacteriostatic or bactericidal, depending on concentration.

Route	Onset	Peak	Duration
P.O.	Unknown	2-4 hr	Unknown
P.O. (extended)	Unknown	5-6 hr	Unknown

ADVERSE REACTIONS

CNS: headache.
CV: *ventricular arrhythmias.*
GI: *diarrhea, nausea, abnormal taste,* dyspepsia, abdominal pain or discomfort, *pseudomembranous colitis.*
Hematologic: *leukopenia, thrombocytopenia.*
Skin: rash, *Stevens-Johnson syndrome,* urticaria.

INTERACTIONS

Drug-drug. *Carbamazepine:* May increase carbamazepine levels. Monitor blood levels.

Digoxin: May increase digoxin levels. Monitor patient for digitalis toxicity.
Fluconazole: Increased clarithromycin levels. Monitor patient closely.
Pimozide: Altered pimozide metabolism with prolongation of QT interval and ventricular tachycardia. Avoid using together.
Theophylline: Increased plasma theophylline levels. Monitor theophylline levels carefully.
Warfarin: Increased PT and INR possible with other macrolides; effect of clarithromycin is unknown. Monitor PT and INR carefully.
Zidovudine: Decreased zidovudine levels. Monitor effectiveness of zidovudine closely.

EFFECTS ON LAB TEST RESULTS
• May increase BUN, ALT, AST, alkaline phosphatase, bilirubin, GGT, and LDH levels.
• May increase PT and INR. May decrease WBC and platelet counts.

CONTRAINDICATIONS
Contraindicated in patients hypersensitive to erythromycin or other macrolides and in those receiving pimozide.

NURSING CONSIDERATIONS
• Use cautiously in patients with hepatic or renal impairment.
• *Alert:* The safety and efficacy of the extended-release formulation have not been established for treating other infections for which the original formulation has been approved.
• Obtain specimen for culture and sensitivity tests before giving first dose. Therapy may begin pending results.
• Monitor patient for superinfection. Drug may cause overgrowth of nonsusceptible bacteria or fungi.

PATIENT TEACHING
• Tell patient to take drug as prescribed, even after he feels better.
• Advise patient to report persistent adverse reactions.
• Inform patient that drug may be taken with or without food. He shouldn't refrigerate the suspension form. Discard unused portion after 10 days.

dirithromycin
Dynabac

Pregnancy risk category C

AVAILABLE FORMS
Tablets (enteric-coated): 250 mg

INDICATIONS & DOSAGES
➤ **Acute bacterial exacerbations of chronic bronchitis caused by *Moraxella catarrhalis*, *Streptococcus pneumoniae*, or *Haemophilus influenzae*; secondary bacterial infection of acute bronchitis caused by *M. catarrhalis* or *S. pneumoniae*; uncomplicated skin and skin-structure infections caused by *Staphylococcus aureus* (methicillin-susceptible strains) or *S. pyogenes*—**
Adults and children age 12 and older: 500 mg P.O. daily with food (or within 1 hour after eating) for 5 to 7 days.
➤ **Community-acquired pneumonia caused by *Legionella pneumophila*, *Mycoplasma pneumoniae*, or *S. pneumoniae*—**
Adults and children age 12 and older: 500 mg P.O. daily with food (or within 1 hour after eating) for 14 days.
➤ **Pharyngitis or tonsillitis caused by *S. pyogenes*—**
Adults and children age 12 and older: 500 mg P.O. daily with food (or within 1 hour after eating) for 10 days.

ACTION
Inhibits bacterial RNA-dependent protein synthesis by binding to the 50S subunit of the ribosome.

Route	Onset	Peak	Duration
P.O.	Unknown	4 hr	Unknown

ADVERSE REACTIONS
CNS: headache, dizziness, vertigo, asthenia, insomnia.
GI: abdominal pain, nausea, diarrhea, vomiting, dyspepsia, flatulence.
Metabolic: hyperkalemia.
Respiratory: increased cough, dyspnea.
Skin: rash, pruritus, urticaria.
Other: pain.

INTERACTIONS

Drug-drug. *Alfentanil, bromocriptine, carbamazepine, cyclosporine, digoxin, disopyramide, ergotamine, hexobarbital, lovastatin, oral anticoagulants, phenytoin, pimozide, triazolam, valproate:* Reported to interact with erythromycin products; it's unknown whether these drugs interact with dirithromycin. Use together cautiously.

Antacids, H₂-receptor antagonists: May slightly increase absorption of dirithromycin when it's administered immediately after these drugs. Avoid using together.

Theophylline: May alter steady-state plasma levels of theophylline. Monitor theophylline plasma levels. Dosage adjustments may be needed.

Drug-food. *Any food:* Increased absorption. Give drug with food.

EFFECTS ON LAB TEST RESULTS

● May increase potassium, CK, ALT, AST, alkaline phosphatase, bilirubin, GGT, and LDH levels.
● May increase platelet, eosinophil, and neutrophil counts.

CONTRAINDICATIONS

Contraindicated in patients hypersensitive to drug, erythromycin, or other macrolide antibiotics.

NURSING CONSIDERATIONS

● Use cautiously in patients with hepatic insufficiency and in breast-feeding women. Monitor liver function test results.
● Safety of drug in children younger than age 12 hasn't been established.
● Obtain results of culture and sensitivity tests to make sure organism is sensitive to dirithromycin. Drug isn't recommended for empiric use.
● Drug shouldn't be used in patients with known, suspected, or potential bacteremias because serum levels are inadequate to provide antibacterial coverage of organisms within the bloodstream.
● Give drug with food or within 1 hour of food intake.
● Monitor patient for superinfection. Drug may cause overgrowth of nonsusceptible bacteria or fungi.

PATIENT TEACHING

● Tell patient to take drug as prescribed, even after he feels better.
● Instruct patient to take drug with food or within 1 hour after eating and not to cut, chew, or crush tablet.

---

erythromycin base

Apo-Erythro Base†, E-Base, EMU-V Tablets‡, E-Mycin, Erybid†, Eryc, Ery-Tab, Erythromid†, Erythromycin Filmtab, Novo-Rythro Encap†, PCE Dispertab

erythromycin estolate

Ilosone, Novo-Rythro†

erythromycin ethylsuccinate

Apo-Erythro-ES†, E.E.S., EES-400‡, EES Granules‡, Erymin§, EryPed, EryPed 200, EryPed 400, Erythroped§, Erythroped A§, Novo-Rythro†

erythromycin lactobionate

Erythrocin, Erythromycin Lactobionate

erythromycin stearate

Apo-Erythro-S†, Erythrocin Stearate, Novo-Rythro†

Pregnancy risk category B

AVAILABLE FORMS

erythromycin base
Capsules (delayed-release): 250 mg
Tablets (enteric-coated): 250 mg, 333 mg, 500 mg
Tablets (filmtabs): 250 mg, 500 mg
erythromycin estolate
Capsules: 250 mg
Oral suspension: 125 mg/5 ml, 250 mg/5 ml
Tablets: 500 mg
erythromycin ethylsuccinate
Oral suspension: 200 mg/5 ml, 400 mg/5 ml, 100 mg/2.5 ml
Tablets (chewable): 200 mg
Tablets (film-coated): 400 mg
erythromycin lactobionate
Injection: 500-mg, 1-g vials

---

erythromycin stearate
Tablets (film-coated): 250 mg, 500 mg

INDICATIONS & DOSAGES
➤ **Acute pelvic inflammatory disease caused by *Neisseria gonorrhoeae*—**
Adults: 500 mg I.V. (lactobionate) q 6 hours for 3 days; then 250 mg (base, stearate) or 400 mg (ethylsuccinate) P.O. q 6 hours for 7 days.
➤ **Intestinal amebiasis caused by *Entamoeba histolytica*—**
Adults: 250 mg P.O. q.i.d. or 333 mg P.O. every 8 hours, or 500 mg delayed-release tablets P.O. every 12 hours for 10 to 14 days.
Children: 30 to 50 mg/kg P.O. daily, in divided doses, for 10 to 14 days.
➤ **Erythrasma—**
Adults: 250 mg P.O. t.i.d. for 21 days.
➤ **Rheumatic fever prophylaxis—**
Adults: 250 mg P.O. q 12 hours.
➤ **Mild to moderately severe respiratory tract, skin, and soft-tissue infections caused by sensitive group A beta-hemolytic streptococci, *Streptococcus pneumoniae*, *Mycoplasma pneumoniae*, *Corynebacterium diphtheriae*, or *Bordetella pertussis*—**
Adults: 250 to 500 mg (base, estolate, stearate) P.O. q 6 hours; or 400 to 800 mg (ethylsuccinate) P.O. q 6 hours; or 15 to 20 mg/kg I.V. daily, as continuous infusion or in divided doses q 6 hours for 10 days (3 weeks for *Mycoplasma* species infection).
Children: 30 to 50 mg/kg (oral erythromycin salts) P.O. daily, in divided doses q 6 hours; or 15 to 20 mg/kg I.V. daily, in divided doses q 4 to 6 hours for 10 days (3 weeks for *Mycoplasma* species infection).
➤ ***Listeria monocytogenes* infection—**
Adults: 250 mg P.O. q 6 hours or 500 mg P.O. q 12 hours.
➤ **Nongonococcal urethritis caused by *Ureaplasma urealyticum*—**
Adults: 500 mg P.O. q 6 hours for at least 7 days.
➤ **Syphilis in patients allergic to penicillin—**
Adults: 500 mg P.O. q.i.d. for 2 weeks.
➤ **Legionnaires' disease—**
Adults: 1 to 4 g P.O. daily in divided doses for 10 to 14 days alone or with rifampin.

I.V. route may be used initially in severe cases.
➤ **Uncomplicated urethral, endocervical, or rectal infections caused by *Chlamydia trachomatis* when tetracyclines are contraindicated—**
Adults: 500 mg (base) P.O. q.i.d. for at least 7 days or 666 mg P.O. q 8 hours for at least 7 days.
➤ **Urogenital *C. trachomatis* infections during pregnancy—**
Adults: 500 mg (base, estolate, stearate) P.O. q.i.d. for at least 7 days or 250 mg (base, estolate, stearate) or 400 mg (ethylsuccinate) P.O. q.i.d. for at least 14 days.
➤ **Conjunctivitis caused by *C. trachomatis* in neonates—**
Neonates: 50 mg/kg (base, estolate, stearate) P.O. daily in four divided doses for 14 days.
➤ **Pneumonia in infants caused by *C. trachomatis*—**
Infants: 50 mg/kg/day (base, estolate, stearate) P.O. in four divided doses for 21 days or 15 to 20 mg/kg/day (lactobionate) I.V. as a continuous infusion or in four divided doses.

I.V. ADMINISTRATION
● Reconstitute drug according to manufacturer's directions and dilute each 250 mg in at least 100 ml of normal saline solution. Infuse over 1 hour.
● *Alert:* Don't administer erythromycin lactobionate with other drugs.

ACTION
Inhibits bacterial protein synthesis by binding to the 50S subunit of the ribosome. Bacteriostatic or bactericidal, depending on concentration.

Route	Onset	Peak	Duration
I.V.	Unknown	Immediate	Unknown
P.O.	Unknown	1-4 hr	Unknown

ADVERSE REACTIONS
CV: *ventricular arrhythmias.*
EENT: hearing loss with high I.V. doses.
GI: *abdominal pain and cramping, nausea, vomiting, diarrhea.*
Hepatic: cholestatic jaundice with erythromycin estolate.
Skin: urticaria, rash, eczema.

Other: overgrowth of nonsusceptible bacteria or fungi, *anaphylaxis,* fever; *vein irritation, thrombophlebitis after I.V. injection.*

INTERACTIONS
Drug-drug. *Carbamazepine:* Increased carbamazepine blood levels and increased risk of toxicity. Monitor patient closely.
Clindamycin, lincomycin: May be antagonistic. Avoid using together.
Cyclosporine: Increased levels of cyclosporine. Monitor patient closely.
Digoxin: Increased serum digoxin levels. Monitor patient for digoxin toxicity.
Disopyramide: Increased disopyramide plasma levels, sometimes resulting in arrhythmias and prolonged QT intervals. Monitor ECG.
Midazolam, triazolam: Increased effects of these drugs. Monitor patient closely.
Oral anticoagulants: Increased anticoagulant effect. Monitor PT and INR closely.
Theophylline: Decreased erythromycin blood level and increased theophylline toxicity. Use together cautiously.
Drug-herb. *Pill-bearing spurge:* May inhibit CYP3A enzymes, affecting drug metabolism. Urge caution.

EFFECTS ON LAB TEST RESULTS
None reported.

CONTRAINDICATIONS
Contraindicated in patients hypersensitive to drug or other macrolides. Erythromycin estolate is contraindicated in patients with hepatic disease.

NURSING CONSIDERATIONS
● Use erythromycin salts cautiously in patients with impaired hepatic function. Monitor liver function test results.
● Erythromycin estolate isn't recommended during pregnancy because of the potential adverse effects on the mother and fetus.
● Drug appears in breast milk. Use cautiously in breast-feeding women.
● Drug isn't indicated for the treatment of neurosyphilis.
● Obtain urine specimen for culture and sensitivity tests before giving first dose. Therapy may begin pending results.

● Erythromycin may interfere with fluorometric determination of urine catecholamines. May interfere with colorimetric assays, resulting in falsely elevated AST and ALT levels.
● When administering suspension, note the concentration.
● Monitor patient for superinfection. Drug may cause overgrowth of nonsusceptible bacteria or fungi.
● Monitor hepatic function (increased serum levels of alkaline phosphatase, ALT, AST, and bilirubin may occur). Erythromycin estolate may cause serious hepatotoxicity in adults (reversible cholestatic jaundice). Other erythromycin salts cause hepatotoxicity to a lesser degree.
● Ototoxicity may occur, especially in patients with renal or hepatic insufficiency and in patients receiving high doses of drug.
● Coated tablets or encapsulated pellets cause less GI upset; they may be better tolerated by patients who can't tolerate erythromycin.

PATIENT TEACHING
● Tell patient to take drug as prescribed, even after he feels better.
● Instruct patient to take oral form of drug with full glass of water 1 hour before or 2 hours after meals for best absorption.
● Drug may be taken with food if GI upset occurs. Tell patient not to drink fruit juice with drug. Chewable erythromycin tablets shouldn't be swallowed whole.
● Instruct patient to report adverse reactions, especially nausea, abdominal pain, vomiting, and fever.

---

aztreonam
bacitracin
chloramphenicol sodium
   succinate
clindamycin hydrochloride
clindamycin palmitate
   hydrochloride
clindamycin phosphate
imipenem and cilastatin sodium
linezolid
meropenem
nitrofurantoin macrocrystals
nitrofurantoin microcrystals
quinupristin/dalfopristin
trimethoprim
vancomycin hydrochloride

COMBINATION PRODUCTS
MACROBID: nitrofurantoin macrocrystals
25 mg and nitrofurantoin monohydrate
75 mg

---

aztreonam
Azactam

Pregnancy risk category B

AVAILABLE FORMS
Injection: 500-mg vials, 1-g vials, 2-g
vials

INDICATIONS & DOSAGES
➤ **Urinary tract infections, lower respiratory tract infections, septicemia, skin
and skin-structure infections, intra-abdominal infections, surgical infections, and gynecologic infections caused
by susceptible strains of the following
gram-negative aerobic organisms:** *Escherichia coli, Klebsiella pneumoniae, Proteus mirabilis, Pseudomonas aeruginosa,
Enterobacter cloacae, K. oxytoca, Citrobacter* species, *Serratia marcescens;* **respiratory infections caused by** *Haemophilus influenzae—*
Adults: 500 mg to 2 g I.V. or I.M. q 8 to
12 hours. For severe systemic or life-threatening infections, 2 g q 6 to 8 hours
may be given. Maximum dose is 8 g daily.

Children ages 9 months to 15 years:
30 mg/kg q 6 to 8 hours I.V. Maximum
dose is 120 mg/kg/day.
Adjust-a-dose: For adults with renal impairment, if creatinine clearance is 10 to
30 ml/minute, dose is 1 to 2 g; then 50%
usual dose at usual interval. If clearance is
less than 10 ml/minute, dose is 500 mg to
2 g; then 25% usual dose at usual interval.
For adults with alcoholic cirrhosis, decrease dose by 20% to 25%.

ADVERSE REACTIONS
CNS: *seizures,* headache, insomnia, confusion.
CV: hypotension.
GI: diarrhea, nausea, vomiting,
pseudomembranous colitis.
Hematologic: *neutropenia,* anemia, *pancytopenia, thrombocytopenia,* leukocytosis, thrombocytosis.
Other: hypersensitivity reactions, thrombophlebitis, discomfort and swelling at
I.M. injection site.

I.V. ADMINISTRATION
● For direct injection, reconstitute with 6
to 10 ml of sterile water for injection and
immediately shake vial vigorously.
● To give a bolus, inject drug over 3 to 5
minutes, directly into a vein or I.V. tubing.
● For infusion, reconstitute with a compatible I.V. solution to yield a final concentration of 20 mg/ml or less.
● Thawed solutions should be given only
by I.V. infusion.
● Give infusions over 20 minutes to 1
hour.

ACTION
Inhibits bacterial cell-wall synthesis, ultimately causing cell-wall destruction; bactericidal.

Route	Onset	Peak	Duration
I.M.	Unknown	< 1 hr	Unknown
I.V.	Unknown	Immediate	Unknown

INTERACTIONS

Drug-drug. *Cefoxitin, imipenem:* May have antagonistic effect. Avoid using together.
Probenecid: Increased serum aztreonam levels. Avoid using together.

EFFECTS ON LAB TEST RESULTS

- May increase BUN, creatinine, ALT, AST, and LDH levels.
- May increase PT, PTT, and INR. May decrease neutrophil and RBC counts and hemoglobin. May increase or decrease WBC and platelet counts.

CONTRAINDICATIONS

Contraindicated in patients hypersensitive to drug or to ceftazidime.

NURSING CONSIDERATIONS

- Use cautiously in elderly patients and in those with impaired renal or hepatic function. Dosage adjustment may be needed. Monitor renal function tests.
- Obtain specimen for culture and sensitivity tests before giving first dose. Therapy may begin pending results.
- To prepare I.M. injection, add at least 3 ml of one of the following solutions per gram of aztreonam: sterile water for injection, bacteriostatic water for injection, normal saline solution, or bacteriostatic normal saline solution.
- Administer I.M. injections deep into a large muscle, such as the upper outer quadrant of the gluteus maximus or the lateral aspect of the thigh. Doses exceeding 1 g should be given I.V.
- *Alert:* Don't give I.M. injection to children.
- Drug therapy alters urine glucose determinations using cupric sulfate (Clinitest or Benedict's reagent). Coombs' test results may become positive during therapy.
- Observe patient for signs and symptoms of superinfection.
- Aztreonam is a narrow-spectrum antibiotic effective only against gram-negative organisms. Because drug is ineffective against gram-positive and anaerobic organisms, anticipate using it with other antibiotics for immediate treatment of life-threatening illnesses.

- Patients who are allergic to penicillins or cephalosporins may not be allergic to aztreonam. However, those who have had an immediate hypersensitivity reaction to these antibiotics, in particular to ceftazidime, should be monitored closely.

PATIENT TEACHING

- Warn patient receiving I.M. drug that pain and swelling may occur at injection site.
- Tell patient to report discomfort at I.V. insertion site.
- Instruct patient to report adverse reactions and signs and symptoms of superinfection promptly.

bacitracin
Baci-IM

Pregnancy risk category C

AVAILABLE FORMS

Injection: 50,000-unit vials

INDICATIONS & DOSAGES

➤ **Pneumonia or empyema caused by susceptible staphylococci—**
Infants weighing more than 2.5 kg (5.5 lb): 1,000 units/kg I.M. daily, divided q 8 to 12 hours for up to 12 days.
Infants weighing less than 2.5 kg: 900 units/kg I.M. daily, divided q 8 to 12 hours for up to 12 days.

ACTION

Hinders bacterial cell-wall synthesis, damaging the bacterial plasma membrane and making the cell more vulnerable to osmotic pressure.

Route	Onset	Peak	Duration
I.M.	Unknown	1-2 hr	Unknown

ADVERSE REACTIONS

EENT: ototoxicity.
GI: nausea, vomiting.
GU: *nephrotoxicity.*
Skin: urticaria, rash.
Other: injection site pain.

INTERACTIONS

Drug-drug. *Inhalation anesthetics, neuromuscular blockers:* Prolonged muscle

weakness. Monitor patient for excessive muscle weakness or respiratory distress.
Nephrotoxic drugs (such as aminoglycosides): Increased nephrotoxicity. Use together cautiously.

EFFECTS ON LAB TEST RESULTS
• May increase BUN and creatinine levels.

CONTRAINDICATIONS
Contraindicated in patients hypersensitive to drug and in those with impaired renal function. Because of significant risk of neurotoxicity, limit I.M. use to infants with staphylococcal pneumonia.

NURSING CONSIDERATIONS
• Use cautiously in patients with myasthenia gravis and neuromuscular disease.
• Obtain specimen for culture and sensitivity tests before giving first dose.
• Assess baseline renal function studies before and during therapy. Signs and symptoms of nephrotoxicity may include albuminuria, cylindruria, oliguria, anuria, and tubular and glomerular necrosis.
• Concentration of bacitracin should be between 5,000 and 10,000 units/ml. Reconstitute 50,000-unit vial with 9.8 ml of diluent. Store in refrigerator. Drug is inactivated if stored at room temperature.
• Administer by deep I.M. injection only.
• Urinary sediment tests may show increased protein and cast excretion.
• Maintain adequate fluid intake, and monitor urine output closely.
• Provide measures to keep urine pH above 6 to reduce risk of nephrotoxicity.
• Prolonged therapy may result in overgrowth of nonsusceptible organisms, especially *Candida albicans.*

PATIENT TEACHING
• Warn patient that injection may be painful.
• Instruct patient to report adverse reactions promptly.

chloramphenicol sodium succinate
Chloromycetin Sodium Succinate, Kemicetine§, Pentamycetin†

Pregnancy risk category C

AVAILABLE FORMS
Injection: 1-g vial; 1 g, 2 g premixed (frozen)

INDICATIONS & DOSAGES
➤ *Haemophilus influenzae* **meningitis, acute** *Salmonella typhi* **infection, and meningitis, bacteremia, or other severe infections caused by sensitive** *Salmonella* **species, Rickettsia, lymphogranuloma, psittacosis, or various sensitive gram-negative organisms—**
Adults: 50 to 100 mg/kg I.V. daily, divided q 6 hours. Maximum dose is 100 mg/kg daily.
Full-term infants older than age 2 weeks with normal metabolic processes: Up to 50 mg/kg I.V. daily, divided q 6 hours.
Premature infants, neonates age 2 weeks and younger, and children and infants with immature metabolic processes: 25 mg/kg I.V. once daily.

I.V. ADMINISTRATION
• Reconstitute 1-g vial of powder for injection with 10 ml of sterile water for injection. Concentration will be 100 mg/ml.
• Give I.V. slowly over at least 1 minute. Check injection site daily for phlebitis and irritation.
• Stable for 30 days at room temperature, but refrigeration recommended. Don't use cloudy solutions.

ACTION
Inhibits bacterial protein synthesis by binding to the 50S subunit of the ribosome; bacteriostatic.

Route	Onset	Peak	Duration
I.V.	Unknown	1-3 hr	Unknown

ADVERSE REACTIONS
CNS: headache, mild depression, confusion, delirium, peripheral neuropathy with prolonged therapy.

EENT: optic neuritis in patients with cystic fibrosis, decreased visual acuity.
GI: nausea, vomiting, stomatitis, diarrhea, enterocolitis, glossitis.
Hematologic: *aplastic anemia, hypoplastic anemia, granulocytopenia, thrombocytopenia.*
Hepatic: jaundice.
Other: hypersensitivity reactions, *anaphylaxis, gray syndrome in neonates.*

INTERACTIONS
Drug-drug. *Anticoagulants, barbiturates, hydantoins, iron salts, sulfonylureas:* Increased blood levels of these drugs. Monitor patient for toxicity.
Penicillins: May have synergistic effects in the treatment of certain microorganisms, but antagonism may also occur. Monitor patient for changes in effectiveness.
Rifampin: May reduce chloramphenicol levels. Monitor patient for changes in effectiveness.
Vitamin B₁₂: May decrease response of vitamin B in patients with pernicious anemia. Monitor patient closely.

EFFECTS ON LAB TEST RESULTS
• May decrease hemoglobin and granulocyte and platelet counts.

CONTRAINDICATIONS
Contraindicated in patients hypersensitive to drug.

NURSING CONSIDERATIONS
• Use cautiously in patients with impaired hepatic or renal function, acute intermittent porphyria, and G6PD deficiency; also use cautiously with other drugs that cause bone marrow suppression or blood disorders.
• *Alert:* Use cautiously in premature infants and newborns because potentially fatal gray syndrome may occur. Symptoms include abdominal distention, gray cyanosis, vasomotor collapse, respiratory distress, and death within a few hours of symptom onset.
• Obtain specimen for culture and sensitivity tests before giving first dose. Therapy may begin pending results.
• Obtain plasma levels. Maintain levels at 5 to 20 mcg/ml.

• Monitor CBC, platelets, iron, and reticulocytes before and every 2 days during therapy. Stop drug immediately if anemia, reticulocytopenia, leukopenia, or thrombocytopenia develops, and notify prescriber.
• Monitor patient for signs and symptoms of superinfection.
• False elevation of urine PABA levels result if chloramphenicol is given during a bentiromide test for pancreatic function. Treatment with chloramphenicol causes false-positive results on tests for urine glucose using cupric sulfate (Clinitest).

PATIENT TEACHING
• Instruct patient to notify prescriber if adverse reactions occur, especially nausea, vomiting, diarrhea, fever, confusion, sore throat, or mouth sores.
• Tell patient receiving drug I.V. to report discomfort at I.V. insertion site.
• Instruct patient to report signs and symptoms of superinfection.

---

clindamycin hydrochloride
Cleocin HCl, Dalacin C†‡

clindamycin palmitate hydrochloride
Cleocin Pediatric, Dalacin C Flavored Granules†

clindamycin phosphate
Cleocin Phosphate, Dalacin C†‡, Dalacin C Phosphate†‡

Pregnancy risk category B

AVAILABLE FORMS
clindamycin hydrochloride
Capsules: 75 mg, 150 mg, 300 mg
clindamycin palmitate hydrochloride
Granules for oral solution: 75 mg/5 ml
clindamycin phosphate
Injectable infusion (in D₅W): 300 mg (50 ml), 600 mg (50 ml), 900 mg (50 ml)
Injection: 150-mg base/ml, 300-mg base/ 2 ml, 600-mg base/4 ml, 900-mg base/ 6 ml, 9,000-mg base/60 ml

INDICATIONS & DOSAGES
➤ **Infections caused by sensitive staphylococci, streptococci, pneumococci, Bac-**

---

teroides, *Fusobacterium*, and *Clostridium perfringens*, and other sensitive aerobic and anaerobic organisms—
Adults: 150 to 450 mg P.O. q 6 hours; or 300 to 600 mg I.M. or I.V. q 6, 8, or 12 hours.
Children older than age 1 month: 8 to 20 mg/kg P.O. daily, in divided doses q 6 to 8 hours; or 15 to 40 mg/kg I.M. or I.V. daily, in divided doses q 6 or 8 hours.
➤ **Pelvic inflammatory disease—**
Adults: 900 mg I.V. q 8 hours with gentamicin. Continue at least 48 hours after improvement in symptoms; then switch to oral clindamycin 450 mg q.i.d. for total of 10 to 14 days or doxycycline 100 mg P.O. q 12 hours for total of 10 to 14 days.

I.V. ADMINISTRATION
● For I.V. infusion, dilute each 300 mg in 50-ml solution, and give no faster than 30 mg/minute (over 10 to 60 minutes). Never give undiluted as a bolus.
● When giving I.V., check site daily for phlebitis and irritation.

ACTION
Inhibits bacterial protein synthesis by binding to the 50S subunit of the ribosome.

Route	Onset	Peak	Duration
I.M.	Unknown	3 hr	Unknown
I.V.	Immediate	Immediate	Unknown
P.O.	Unknown	45-60 min	Unknown

ADVERSE REACTIONS
CV: thrombophlebitis.
GI: *nausea,* vomiting, abdominal pain, *diarrhea, pseudomembranous colitis.*
Hematologic: *transient leukopenia,* eosinophilia, *thrombocytopenia.*
Hepatic: jaundice.
Skin: maculopapular rash, urticaria.
Other: *anaphylaxis.*

INTERACTIONS
Drug-drug. *Erythromycin:* May block access of clindamycin to its site of action. Avoid using together.
Kaolin: Decreased absorption of oral clindamycin. Separate administration times.
Neuromuscular blockers: Increased neuromuscular blockade possible. Monitor patient closely.

Drug-food. *Diet foods with sodium cyclamate:* Decreased serum level of drug. Discourage use together.

EFFECTS ON LAB TEST RESULTS
● May increase bilirubin, AST, and alkaline phosphatase levels.
● May increase eosinophil count. May decrease WBC and platelet counts.

CONTRAINDICATIONS
Contraindicated in patients hypersensitive to drug or lincomycin.

NURSING CONSIDERATIONS
● Use cautiously in neonates and patients with renal or hepatic disease, asthma, history of GI disease, or significant allergies.
● Drug doesn't penetrate blood-brain barrier.
● Obtain specimen for culture and sensitivity tests before giving first dose. Therapy may begin pending results.
● For I.M. administration, inject deeply. Rotate sites. Don't exceed 600 mg per injection.
● I.M. injection may raise CK level in response to muscle irritation.
● Don't refrigerate reconstituted oral solution because it will thicken. Drug is stable for 2 weeks at room temperature.
● Monitor renal, hepatic, and hematopoietic functions during prolonged therapy.
● Observe patient for signs and symptoms of superinfection.
● *Alert:* Don't give opioid antidiarrheals to treat drug-induced diarrhea; they may prolong and worsen diarrhea.

PATIENT TEACHING
● Advise patient to take capsule form with a full glass of water to prevent esophageal irritation.
● Warn patient that I.M. injection may be painful.
● Tell patient to report discomfort at I.V. insertion site.
● Instruct patient to notify prescriber if adverse reactions, especially diarrhea, occur. Warn him not to treat such diarrhea himself because clindamycin therapy may cause severe, even life-threatening, colitis.

imipenem and cilastatin sodium
Primaxin I.M., Primaxin I.V.

Pregnancy risk category C

AVAILABLE FORMS
Powder for injection: 250 mg, 500 mg, 750 mg

INDICATIONS & DOSAGES
➤ **Serious lower respiratory, urinary tract, intra-abdominal, gynecologic, bone, joint, skin, and soft-tissue infections; endocarditis; bacterial septicemia. Most known microorganisms are susceptible:** *Acinetobacter, Enterococcus, Staphylococcus, Streptococcus, Escherichia coli, Haemophilus, Klebsiella, Morganella, Proteus, Enterobacter, Pseudomonas aeruginosa,* **and** *Bacteroides,* **including** *B. fragilis*—
Adults weighing more than 70 kg (154 lb): 250 mg to 1 g by I.V. infusion q 6 to 8 hours. Maximum daily dose is 50 mg/kg/day or 4 g/day, whichever is less. Or, 500 to 750 mg I.M. q 12 hours. Maximum daily dose is 1,500 mg.
Children age 3 months and older (except for CNS infections): 15 to 25 mg/kg I.V. q 6 hours. Maximum daily dose is 2 to 4 g.
Infants ages 4 weeks to 3 months, weighing 1.5 kg (3.3 lb) or more (except for CNS infections): 25 mg/kg I.V. q 6 hours.
Neonates ages 1 to 4 weeks, weighing 1.5 kg or more (except for CNS infections): 25 mg/kg I.V. q 8 hours.
Neonates younger than age 1 week, weighing 1.5 kg or more (except for CNS infections): 25 mg/kg I.V. q 12 hours.
Adjust-a-dose: For children older than age 12, patients weighing less than 70 kg, and those who are renally impaired, refer to package insert for dosage adjustments based on weight, creatinine clearance, and severity of infection.

I.V. ADMINISTRATION
● Reconstitute piggyback units with 100 ml of compatible I.V. solution to provide solution containing 2.5 to 5 mg/ml.
● When reconstituting powder, shake until the solution is clear. Solutions may range from colorless to yellow; variations of color within this range don't affect drug's potency.
● After reconstitution, solution is stable for 10 hours at room temperature and for 48 hours when refrigerated.
● Don't give by direct I.V. bolus injection.
● For adults, each 250- or 500-mg dose should be given by I.V. infusion over 20 to 30 minutes. Each 1-g dose should be infused over 40 to 60 minutes.
● For children, doses of 500 mg or less should be infused over 15 to 30 minutes. Doses greater than 500 mg should be infused over 40 to 60 minutes. If nausea occurs, the infusion may be slowed.

ACTION
Imipenem is bactericidal and inhibits bacterial cell-wall synthesis. Cilastatin inhibits the enzymatic breakdown of imipenem in the kidneys, thereby achieving adequate antibacterial levels of imipenem in the urine.

Route	Onset	Peak	Duration
I.M.	Unknown	1-2 hr	Unknown
I.V.	Immediate	Immediate	Unknown

ADVERSE REACTIONS
CNS: *seizures,* dizziness, somnolence.
CV: hypotension.
GI: nausea, vomiting, diarrhea, pseudomembranous colitis.
Hematologic: eosinophilia, *thrombocytopenia, leukopenia.*
Skin: rash, urticaria, pruritus.
Other: hypersensitivity reactions, *anaphylaxis,* fever; thrombophlebitis; injection site pain.

INTERACTIONS
Drug-drug. *Beta-lactam antibiotics:* May have antagonistic effect. Avoid using together.
Ganciclovir: May cause seizures. Avoid using together.
Probenecid: Increased cilastatin levels. May be used together for this effect.

EFFECTS ON LAB TEST RESULTS
● May increase BUN, creatinine, ALT, AST, alkaline phosphatase, bilirubin, and LDH.

Reactions may be *common,* uncommon, *life-threatening,* or COMMON AND LIFE-THREATENING.

• May increase eosinophil count. May decrease WBC and platelet counts.

CONTRAINDICATIONS

Contraindicated in patients hypersensitive to drug, in those with a history of hypersensitivity to local anesthetics of the amide type, and in those with severe shock or heart block.

NURSING CONSIDERATIONS

• Use cautiously in patients allergic to penicillins or cephalosporins because drug has similar properties.

• Use cautiously in patients with history of seizure disorders, especially if they also have compromised renal function.

• Use cautiously in children younger than age 3 months.

• **Alert:** Don't use for CNS infections in children because it increases the risk of seizures.

• Obtain specimen culture and sensitivity tests before giving first dose. Therapy may begin pending results.

• **Alert:** Don't give I.M. solution by I.V. route.

• Adjust dosage for patients with a creatinine clearance below 70 ml/minute. Monitor renal function tests.

• **Alert:** If seizures develop and persist despite anticonvulsant therapy, notify prescriber; then drug should be discontinued.

• Monitor patient for bacterial or fungal superinfections and resistant infections during and after therapy.

• Drug may interfere with glucose determination by Benedict's solution or Clinitest.

PATIENT TEACHING

• Instruct patient to report adverse reactions promptly.

• Tell patient to report discomfort at I.V. insertion site.

• Urge patient to notify prescriber about loose stools or diarrhea.

linezolid
Zyvox

Pregnancy risk category C

AVAILABLE FORMS

Injection: 2 mg/ml
Powder for oral suspension: 100 mg/5 ml when reconstituted
Tablets: 400 mg, 600 mg

INDICATIONS & DOSAGES

➤ **Vancomycin-resistant** *Enterococcus faecium* **infections, including those with concurrent bacteremia—**
Adults: 600 mg I.V. or P.O. q 12 hours for 14 to 28 days.

➤ **Nosocomial pneumonia caused by** *Staphylococcus aureus* **(methicillin-susceptible [MSSA] and methicillin-resistant [MRSA] strains) or** *Streptococcus pneumoniae* **(penicillin-susceptible strains only); complicated skin and skin-structure infections caused by** *Staphylococcus aureus* **(MSSA and MSRA),** *Streptococcus pyogenes,* **or** *S. agalactiae;* **community-acquired pneumonia caused by** *S. pneumoniae* **(penicillin-susceptible strains only), including those with concurrent bacteremia, or** *Staphylococcus aureus* **(MSSA only)—**
Adults: 600 mg I.V. or P.O. q 12 hours for 10 to 14 days.

➤ **Uncomplicated skin and skin-structure infections caused by** *S. aureus* **(MSSA only) or** *S. pyogenes—*
Adults: 400 mg P.O. q 12 hours for 10 to 14 days.

I.V. ADMINISTRATION

• Inspect for particulate matter and leaks.

• Linezolid is compatible with D_5W injection, normal saline solution for injection, and lactated Ringer's injection.

• Infuse over a period of 30 minutes to 2 hours. Don't infuse linezolid in a series connection.

• **Alert:** Don't inject additives into infusion bag. Administer other I.V. drugs separately or via a separate I.V. line to avoid incompatibilities. If single I.V. line is used, flush line before and after linezolid infusion with a compatible solution.

• Amphotericin B, chlorpromazine hydrochloride, diazepam, pentamidine isethionate, erythromycin lactobionate, phenytoin sodium, trimethoprim-sulfamethoxazole, and ceftriaxone sodium are incompatible with linezolid.
• Store drug at room temperature in its protective overwrap. Solution may turn yellow over time but this doesn't affect drug's potency.

ACTION
Prevents bacterial protein synthesis by interfering with DNA translation in the ribosomes. Also prevents formation of a functional 70S ribosomal subunit by binding to a site on the bacterial 50S ribosomal subunit.

Route	Onset	Peak	Duration
I.V.	Unknown	0.5 hr	Unknown
P.O.	Unknown	1 hr	Unknown

ADVERSE REACTIONS
CNS: headache, insomnia, dizziness.
GI: diarrhea, nausea, vomiting, constipation, elevated amylase and lipase, altered taste, tongue discoloration, oral candidiasis.
GU: vaginal candidiasis.
Hematologic: anemia, *leukopenia, neutropenia, mylosuppression, thrombocytopenia.*
Skin: rash.
Other: fever, fungal infection.

INTERACTIONS
Drug-drug. *Adrenergic drugs (such as dopamine, epinephrine, pseudoephedrine):* May cause hypertension. Monitor blood pressure and heart rate; start continuous infusions of dopamine and epinephrine at lower doses and titrate to response.
Serotoninergic drugs: May cause serotonin syndrome, including confusion, delirium, restlessness, tremors, blushing, diaphoresis, and hyperpyrexia. If signs and symptoms of serotonin syndrome are present, consider stopping serotoninergic drug.
Drug-food. *Foods and beverages high in tyramine (such as aged cheeses, air-dried meats, red wines, sauerkraut, soy sauce, tap beers):* May increase blood pressure when linezolid is used with diet high in

tyramine. Advise patient that tyramine content of meals shouldn't exceed 100 mg.

EFFECTS ON LAB TEST RESULTS
• May increase ALT, AST, bilirubin, alkaline phosphatase, and BUN levels.
• May decrease hemoglobin and WBC, neutrophil, and platelet counts.

CONTRAINDICATIONS
Contraindicated in patients hypersensitive to drug or its components.

NURSING CONSIDERATIONS
• Obtain specimen for culture and sensitivity tests before linezolid therapy. Sensitivity results should be used to guide subsequent therapy.
• No dosage adjustment is needed when switching from I.V. to P.O. forms.
• Reconstitute oral suspension according to manufacturer's instructions. Store reconstituted suspension at room temperature and use within 21 days.
• *Alert:* Safety and efficacy of drug for longer than 28 days haven't been studied.
• Drug may cause thrombocytopenia. Monitor platelet count in patients at increased risk for bleeding, in those with existing thrombocytopenia, in patients receiving drugs that may cause thrombocytopenia, and in patients receiving drug for longer than 14 days.
• Myelosuppression has been reported. Monitor CBC weekly in patients receiving linezolid.
• Pseudomembranous colitis or superinfection may occur. Consider these diagnoses and take appropriate measures in patients with persistent diarrhea or secondary infections.
• Inappropriate use of antibiotics may lead to development of resistant organisms; carefully consider alternative drugs before instituting linezolid therapy, especially in outpatient setting.

PATIENT TEACHING
• Tell patient that tablets and oral suspension may be taken with or without meals.
• Stress importance of completing entire course of therapy, even if patient feels better.

Reactions may be *common*, uncommon, *life-threatening*, or COMMON AND LIFE-THREATENING.

• Tell patient to alert prescriber if he has hypertension, is taking cough or cold preparations, or is being treated with selective serotonin reuptake inhibitors or other antidepressants.

• Inform patient with phenylketonuria that each 5 ml of linezolid oral suspension contains 20 mg of phenylalanine. Linezolid tablets and injection don't contain phenylalanine.

---

meropenem
Meronem§, Merrem IV

Pregnancy risk category B

AVAILABLE FORMS
Powder for injection: 500 mg, 1 g

INDICATIONS & DOSAGES
➤ **Complicated appendicitis and peritonitis caused by viridans group streptococci, *Escherichia coli*, *Klebsiella pneumoniae*, *Pseudomonas aeruginosa*, *B. fragilis*, *B. thetaiotaomicron*, and *Peptostreptococcus* species; bacterial meningitis (children only) caused by *Streptococcus pneumoniae*, *Haemophilus influenzae*, and *Neisseria meningitidis*—**
Adults: 1 g I.V. q 8 hours over 15 to 30 minutes as I.V. infusion or over 3 to 5 minutes as I.V. bolus injection (5 to 20 ml).
Children age 3 months and older, weighing less than 50 kg (110 lb): 20 mg/kg (intra-abdominal infection) or 40 mg/kg (bacterial meningitis) q 8 hours over 15 to 30 minutes as I.V. infusion or over 3 to 5 minutes as I.V. bolus injection (5 to 20 ml). Maximum dosage is 2 g I.V. q 8 hours.
Children weighing 50 kg or more: 1 g I.V. q 8 hours for intra-abdominal infections and 2 g I.V. q 8 hours for meningitis.
Adjust-a-dose: For patients with renal insufficiency or renal failure and creatinine clearance of 26 to 50 ml/minute, give usual dose q 12 hours; if clearance is 10 to 25 ml/minute, half the usual dose q 12 hours; and if below 10 ml/minute, half the usual dose q 24 hours.

I.V. ADMINISTRATION
• For I.V. bolus administration, add 10 ml of sterile water for injection to 500 mg/20-ml vial or 20 ml to 1 g/30-ml vial. Shake to dissolve, and let stand until clear.

• For I.V. infusion, infusion vials (500 mg/100 ml and 1 g/100 ml) may be directly reconstituted with a compatible infusion fluid. Or, an injection vial may be reconstituted, then the resulting solution added to an I.V. container and further diluted with an appropriate infusion fluid. Don't use ADD-Vantage vials for this purpose.

• For ADD-Vantage vials, constitute only with half-normal saline solution for injection, normal saline solution for injection, or 5% dextrose injection in 50-, 100-, or 250-ml Abbott ADD-Vantage flexible diluent containers. Follow manufacturer's guidelines closely when using ADD-Vantage vials.

• Don't mix meropenem with solutions containing other drugs.

• Use freshly prepared solutions of drug immediately whenever possible. Stability of drug varies with form of drug used (injection vial, infusion vial, or ADD-Vantage container). Consult manufacturer's literature for details.

ACTION
Inhibits cell-wall synthesis in bacteria. It readily penetrates cell wall of most gram-positive and -negative bacteria to reach penicillin–binding-protein targets.

Route	Onset	Peak	Duration
I.V.	Unknown	1 hr	Unknown

ADVERSE REACTIONS
CNS: *seizures,* headache.
GI: diarrhea, nausea, vomiting, constipation, pseudomembranous colitis, oral candidiasis, glossitis.
GU: presence of RBCs in urine.
Respiratory: *apnea,* dyspnea.
Skin: rash, pruritus.
Other: hypersensitivity reactions, *anaphylaxis,* inflammation, phlebitis, thrombophlebitis at injection site.

INTERACTIONS
Drug-drug. *Probenecid:* Decreased renal excretion of meropenem; probenecid com-

---

petes with meropenem for active tubular secretion, which significantly increases elimination half-life of meropenem and extent of systemic exposure. Avoid using together.

EFFECTS ON LAB TEST RESULTS
• May increase ALT, AST, bilirubin, alkaline phosphatase, LDH, creatinine, and BUN levels.
• May increase eosinophil count. May decrease hemoglobin and hematocrit and WBC count. May increase or decrease PT, PTT, and INR, and platelet count.

CONTRAINDICATIONS
Contraindicated in patients hypersensitive to components of drug or other drugs in same class and in patients who have had anaphylactic reactions to beta-lactams.

NURSING CONSIDERATIONS
• Use cautiously in elderly patients and in those with a history of seizure disorders or impaired renal function.
• Safety and effectiveness of drug haven't been established for patients younger than age 3 months.
• It's unknown whether meropenem appears in breast milk. Use drug cautiously in breast-feeding women.
• Drug isn't used to treat methicillin-resistant staphylococci.
• Obtain specimen for culture and sensitivity tests before giving first dose. Therapy may begin pending test results.
• **Alert:** Serious and occasionally fatal hypersensitivity reactions have been reported in patients receiving therapy with beta-lactams. Before therapy begins, determine whether previous hypersensitivity reactions to penicillins, cephalosporins, other beta-lactams, or other allergens have occurred.
• Stop drug and notify prescriber if an allergic reaction occurs. Serious anaphylactic reactions require immediate emergency treatment.
• Seizures and other CNS adverse reactions associated with meropenem therapy can occur in patients with CNS disorders, bacterial meningitis, and compromised renal function.

• If seizures occur during drug therapy, stop infusion and notify prescriber. Dosage adjustment may be needed.
• Monitor patient for signs and symptoms of superinfection. Drug may cause overgrowth of nonsusceptible bacteria or fungi.
• Periodic assessment of organ system functions, including renal, hepatic, and hematopoietic function, is recommended during prolonged therapy.
• Monitor patient's fluid balance and weight carefully.

PATIENT TEACHING
• Advise breast-feeding woman about risk of transmitting drug to infant through breast milk.
• Instruct patient to report adverse reactions or signs and symptoms of superinfection.

nitrofurantoin macrocrystals
Macrobid, Macrodantin

nitrofurantoin microcrystals
Apo-Nitrofurantoin†, Furadantin, Novo-Furantoin†

Pregnancy risk category B

AVAILABLE FORMS
nitrofurantoin macrocrystals
Capsules: 25 mg, 50 mg, 100 mg
nitrofurantoin microcrystals
Oral suspension: 25 mg/5 ml

INDICATIONS & DOSAGES
➤ **Urinary tract infections caused by susceptible *Escherichia coli*, *Staphylococcus aureus*, enterococci; or certain strains of *Klebsiella* and *Enterobacter* species**—
Adults and children older than age 12: 50 to 100 mg P.O. q.i.d. with meals and h.s.
Children ages 1 month to 12 years: 5 to 7 mg/kg P.O. daily, divided q.i.d.
➤ **Long-term suppression therapy**—
Adults: 50 to 100 mg P.O. daily h.s.
Children: 1 mg/kg P.O. daily in a single dose h.s. or divided into two doses given q 12 hours.

ACTION

Unknown. Appears to interfere with bacterial enzyme systems and possibly with bacterial cell-wall formation.

Route	Onset	Peak	Duration
P.O.	Unknown	Unknown	Unknown

ADVERSE REACTIONS

CNS: peripheral neuropathy, headache, dizziness, drowsiness, *ascending polyneuropathy with high doses or renal impairment.*
GI: *anorexia, nausea, vomiting,* abdominal pain, *diarrhea.*
GU: overgrowth of nonsusceptible organisms in urinary tract.
Hematologic: *hemolysis in patients with G6PD deficiency, agranulocytosis, thrombocytopenia.*
Hepatic: *hepatitis, hepatic necrosis.*
Metabolic: hypoglycemia.
Respiratory: *pulmonary sensitivity reactions, asthmatic attacks.*
Skin: maculopapular, erythematous, or eczematous eruption; transient alopecia; pruritus; urticaria; exfoliative dermatitis; *Stevens-Johnson syndrome.*
Other: hypersensitivity reactions, *anaphylaxis,* drug fever.

INTERACTIONS

Drug-drug. *Antacids containing magnesium:* Decreased nitrofurantoin absorption. Separate administration times by 1 hour.
Probenecid, sulfinpyrazone: Increased blood levels and decreased urine levels; possible increased toxicity and lack of therapeutic effect. Don't use together.
Drug-food. *Any food:* Increased absorption. Advise patient to take drug with food.

EFFECTS ON LAB TEST RESULTS

• May increase bilirubin and alkaline phosphatase levels. May decrease glucose level.
• May decrease granulocyte and platelet counts.

CONTRAINDICATIONS

Contraindicated in infants age 1 month and younger and in patients with moderate to severe renal impairment, anuria, oliguria, or creatinine clearance under 60 ml/minute. Also contraindicated in pregnant patients at term (38 to 42 weeks) and during labor and delivery.

NURSING CONSIDERATIONS

• Use cautiously in patients with renal impairment, anemia, diabetes mellitus, electrolyte abnormalities, vitamin B deficiency, debilitating disease, and G6PD deficiency. Drug may precipitate an asthma attack in patients with a history of asthma.
• Obtain urine specimen for culture and sensitivity tests before giving first dose. Repeat as needed. Therapy may begin pending results.
• Give drug with food or milk to minimize GI distress and improve absorption.
• Monitor fluid intake and output carefully. May turn urine brown or dark yellow.
• Monitor CBC and pulmonary status regularly.
• Monitor patient for signs and symptoms of superinfection. Use of nitrofurantoin may result in growth of nonsusceptible organisms, especially *Pseudomonas* species.
• Monitor patient for pulmonary sensitivity reactions, including cough, chest pain, fever, chills, dyspnea, and pulmonary infiltration with consolidation or effusions.
• *Alert:* Hypersensitivity may develop when drug is used for long-term therapy.
• Some patients may experience fewer adverse GI effects with nitrofurantoin macrocrystals.
• Dual-release capsules (25 mg nitrofurantoin macrocrystals combined with 75 mg nitrofurantoin monohydrate) enable patients to take drug only twice daily.
• Continue treatment for 3 days after sterile urine specimens have been obtained.
• Store drug in amber container. Keep away from metals other than stainless steel or aluminum to avoid precipitate formation.
• Nitrofurantoin may cause false-positive results in urine glucose tests using cupric sulfate (such as Benedict's reagent, Fehling's solution, or Chemstrip Ug).

PATIENT TEACHING

• Instruct patient to take drug for as long as prescribed, exactly as directed, even after he feels better.
• Tell patient to take drug with food or milk to minimize stomach upset.

• Instruct patient to report adverse reactions, especially peripheral neuropathy, which can become severe or irreversible.
• Alert patient that drug may turn urine dark yellow or brown color.
• Warn patient not to store drug in container made of metal other than stainless steel or aluminum.

---

quinupristin/dalfopristin
Synercid

Pregnancy risk category B

AVAILABLE FORMS
Injection: 500 mg/10 ml (150 mg quinupristin and 350 mg dalfopristin)

INDICATIONS & DOSAGES
➤ **Serious or life-threatening infections with vancomycin-resistant *Enterococcus faecium* (VREF) bacteremia—**
Adults and adolescents age 16 and older: 7.5 mg/kg I.V. infusion over 1 hour every 8 hours. Treatment duration should be determined by site and severity of infection.
➤ **Complicated skin and skin-structure infections caused by *Staphylococcus aureus* (methicillin susceptible) or *Streptococcus pyogenes*—**
Adults and adolescents age 16 and older: 7.5 mg/kg by I.V. infusion over 1 hour every 12 hours for at least 7 days.

I.V. ADMINISTRATION
• Reconstitute powder for injection by adding 5 ml of either sterile water for injection or D₅W and gently swirling vial by manual rotation to ensure dissolution; avoid shaking to limit foaming. Reconstituted solutions must be further diluted within 30 minutes.
• The appropriate dose, according to patient's weight, of reconstituted solution should be added to 250 ml of D₅W to make a final concentration of no more than 2 mg/ml. This diluted solution is stable for 5 hours at room temperature or 54 hours if refrigerated.
• Fluid-restricted patients with a central venous catheter may receive dose in 100 ml of D₅W. This concentration isn't recommended for peripheral venous administration.
• If moderate to severe peripheral venous irritation occurs, consider increasing infusion volume to 500 or 750 ml, changing injection site, or infusing by a central venous catheter.
• Administer all doses by I.V. infusion over 1 hour. An infusion pump or device may be used to control infusion rate.
• *Alert:* Quinupristin/dalfopristin is incompatible with saline and heparin solutions. Don't dilute drug with solutions containing saline or infuse into lines that contain saline or heparin. Flush line with D₅W before and after each dose.

ACTION
The two antibiotics work synergistically to inhibit or destroy susceptible bacteria through combined inhibition on protein synthesis in bacterial cells. Without the ability to manufacture new proteins, the bacterial cells are inactivated or die.

Route	Onset	Peak	Duration
I.V.	Unknown	Unknown	Unknown

ADVERSE REACTIONS
CNS: headache.
CV: thrombophlebitis.
GI: nausea, diarrhea, vomiting.
Musculoskeletal: arthralgia, myalgia.
Skin: rash, pruritus.
Other: *inflammation, pain, edema at infusion site; infusion site reaction.*

INTERACTIONS
Drug-drug. *Cyclosporine:* Reduced metabolism; may increase drug levels. Monitor cyclosporine levels.
Drugs metabolized by cytochrome P-450 3A4 (carbamazepine, delavirdine, diazepam, diltiazem, disopyramide, docetaxel, indinavir, lidocaine, lovastatin, methylprednisolone, midazolam, nevirapine, nifedipine, paclitaxel, ritonavir, tacrolimus, verapamil, vinblastine, and others): Increased plasma levels of these drugs that could increase both their therapeutic effects and adverse reactions. Use together cautiously.
Drugs metabolized by cytochrome P-450 3A4 that may prolong the QTc interval (such as quinidine): Decreased metabo-

lism of these drugs, resulting in prolongation of QTc interval. Avoid using together.

EFFECTS ON LAB TEST RESULTS
• Increased AST, ALT, and bilirubin levels.

CONTRAINDICATIONS
Contraindicated in patients hypersensitive to drug or other streptogramin antibiotics.

NURSING CONSIDERATIONS
• Drug isn't active against *Enterococcus faecalis*. Appropriate blood cultures are needed to avoid misidentifying *E. faecalis* as *E. faecium*.
• Because mild to life-threatening pseudomembranous colitis may occur with use of this drug, consider this diagnosis in patients who develop diarrhea during or after therapy.
• Adverse reactions, such as arthralgia and myalgia, may be reduced by decreasing dosage interval to every 12 hours.
• Because overgrowth of nonsusceptible organisms may occur, monitor patient closely for signs and symptoms of superinfection.
• Monitor liver function tests during therapy.

PATIENT TEACHING
• Advise patient to immediately report irritation at I.V. site, pain in joints or muscles, and diarrhea.
• Tell patient about importance of reporting persistent or worsening signs and symptoms of infection, such as pain or erythema.

---

trimethoprim
Ipral§, Monotrim§, Primsol, Proloprim, Trimopan§, Trimpex, Triprim‡

Pregnancy risk category C

AVAILABLE FORMS
Oral solution: 50 mg/5 ml
Tablets: 100 mg, 200 mg

INDICATIONS & DOSAGES
➤ **Uncomplicated urinary tract infections caused by susceptible strains of**
Escherichia coli, Proteus mirabilis, Klebsiella pneumoniae, Enterobacter **species, and coagulase-negative** *Staphylococcus,* **including** *S. saprophyticus—*
Adults: 200 mg P.O. daily as a single dose (as tablet or solution) or in divided doses q 12 hours for 10 days.
Adjust-a-dose: For patients with creatinine clearance of 15 to 30 ml/minute, give 50 mg P.O. q 12 hours; if clearance is below 15 ml/minute, don't use drug.
➤ **Acute otitis media caused by susceptible strains of** *S. pneumoniae* **and** *H. influenzae—*
Children 6 months of age and older:
10 mg/kg/day of Primsol, given in divided doses q 12 hours for 10 days.

ACTION
Interferes with the action of dihydrofolate reductase, inhibiting bacterial synthesis of folic acid.

Route	Onset	Peak	Duration
P.O.	Unknown	1-4 hr	Unknown

ADVERSE REACTIONS
GI: *epigastric distress, nausea, vomiting,* glossitis.
Hematologic: *thrombocytopenia, leukopenia,* megaloblastic anemia, methemoglobinemia.
Skin: *rash, pruritus.*
Other: fever.

INTERACTIONS
Drug-drug. *Phenytoin:* May decrease phenytoin metabolism and increase its serum levels. Monitor patient for toxicity.

EFFECTS ON LAB TEST RESULTS
• May increase BUN, creatinine, bilirubin, and aminotransferase levels.
• May decrease hemoglobin and platelet and WBC counts.

CONTRAINDICATIONS
Contraindicated in patients hypersensitive to drug and in those with documented megaloblastic anemia from folate deficiency.

NURSING CONSIDERATIONS
• Use cautiously in patients with impaired hepatic or renal function. Decrease dosage

in patients with severely impaired renal function. Also use cautiously in patients with possible folate deficiency. Monitor renal and liver function test results.
• Drug isn't recommended for children younger than age 12.
• Obtain urine specimen for culture and sensitivity tests before giving first dose. Therapy may begin pending results.
• Monitor CBC routinely. Sore throat, fever, pallor, or purpura may be early indications of serious blood disorders.
• Monitor patient's fluid balance.
• *Alert:* Prolonged use of trimethoprim at high doses may cause bone marrow suppression.
• Because resistance to trimethoprim develops rapidly when the drug is given alone, it's usually given with other drugs.
• *Alert:* Trimethoprim also is used with sulfamethoxazole; don't confuse the two products.

PATIENT TEACHING
• Instruct patient to take entire amount of drug, as prescribed, even after he feels better.
• Tell patient to report adverse reactions promptly, especially signs of infection or unusual bruising.
• Inform patient of the need for adequate hydration during therapy (2 to 3 L/day).

---

vancomycin hydrochloride
Vancocin, Vancoled

Pregnancy risk category C

AVAILABLE FORMS
Capsules: 125 mg, 250 mg
Powder for injection: 500-mg vials, 1-g vials, 5 g, 10 g
Powder for oral solution: 1-g bottles, 10-g bottles

INDICATIONS & DOSAGES
➤ **Serious or severe infections when other antibiotics are ineffective or contraindicated, including those caused by methicillin-resistant *Staphylococcus aureus*, *Staphylococcus epidermidis*, or diphtheroid organisms—**
Adults: 1 to 1.5 g I.V. q 12 hours.
Children: 10 mg/kg I.V. q 6 hours.

Neonates and young infants: 15 mg/kg I.V. loading dose, then 10 mg/kg I.V. q 12 hours if child is younger than age 1 week or 10 mg/kg I.V. q 8 hours if age is older than 1 week but younger than 1 month.
Elderly patients: 15 mg/kg I.V. loading dose. Subsequent doses are based on renal function and serum drug levels.
➤ **Antibiotic-related pseudomembranous (*Clostridium difficile*) and *S. enterocolitis*—**
Adults: 125 to 500 mg P.O. q 6 hours for 7 to 10 days.
Children: 40 mg/kg P.O. daily, in divided doses q 6 hours for 7 to 10 days. Maximum daily dose is 2 g.
➤ **Endocarditis prophylaxis for dental procedures—**
Adults: 1 g I.V. slowly over 1 to 2 hours, completing infusion 30 minutes before procedure.
Children: 20 mg/kg I.V. over 1 to 2 hours, completing infusion 30 minutes before procedure.
Adjust-a-dose: In patients with impaired renal function, give loading dose of 15 mg/kg I.V. Subsequent doses are based on renal function and serum drug levels. Daily dosage in mg can be calculated by multiplying the creatinine clearance in ml/minute by 15.

I.V. ADMINISTRATION
• For I.V. infusion, dilute in 200 ml normal saline solution for injection or D_5W, and infuse over 60 minutes; if dose is greater than 1 g, infuse over 90 minutes.
• Check site daily for phlebitis and irritation. Severe irritation and necrosis can result from extravasation.
• Refrigerate I.V. solution after reconstitution and use within 14 days.

ACTION
Hinders bacterial cell-wall synthesis, damaging the bacterial plasma membrane and making the cell more vulnerable to osmotic pressure. Also interferes with RNA synthesis.

Route	Onset	Peak	Duration
I.V.	Immediate	Immediate	Unknown
P.O.	Unknown	Unknown	Unknown

Reactions may be *common*, uncommon, *life-threatening*, or COMMON AND LIFE-THREATENING.

ADVERSE REACTIONS
CV: hypotension.
EENT: tinnitus, ototoxicity.
GI: nausea, pseudomembranous colitis.
GU: *nephrotoxicity.*
Hematologic: *neutropenia, leukopenia,* eosinophilia.
Respiratory: wheezing, dyspnea.
Skin: red-man syndrome (with rapid I.V. infusion).
Other: chills, fever, *anaphylaxis,* superinfection, pain, thrombophlebitis at injection site.

INTERACTIONS
Drug-drug. *Aminoglycosides, amphotericin B, cisplatin, pentamidine:* Increased risk of nephrotoxicity and ototoxicity. Monitor patient closely.

EFFECTS ON LAB TEST RESULTS
• May increase BUN and creatinine levels.
• May increase eosinophil counts. May decrease neutrophil and WBC counts.

CONTRAINDICATIONS
Contraindicated in patients hypersensitive to drug.

NURSING CONSIDERATIONS
• Use cautiously in patients receiving other neurotoxic, nephrotoxic, or ototoxic drugs; in patients older than age 60; and in those with impaired hepatic or renal function, preexisting hearing loss, or allergies to other antibiotics. Patients with renal dysfunction need dosage adjustment. Serum levels should be monitored to adjust I.V. dosage. Normal therapeutic levels of vancomycin are as follows: peak, 30 to 40 mg/L (drawn 1 hour after infusion ends); trough, 5 to 10 mg/L (drawn just before next dose is given).
• Obtain specimen for culture and sensitivity tests before giving first dose. Therapy may begin pending results.
• Obtain hearing evaluation and renal function studies before therapy.
• Monitor patient's fluid balance and watch for oliguria and cloudy urine.
• Monitor patient carefully for red-man syndrome, which can occur if drug is infused too rapidly. Signs and symptoms include maculopapular rash on face, neck, trunk, and limbs and pruritus and hypo-

tension caused by histamine release. If wheezing, urticaria, or pain and muscle spasm of the chest and back occur, stop infusion and notify prescriber.
• Don't give drug I.M.
• *Alert:* Oral administration is ineffective for systemic infections, and I.V. administration is ineffective for pseudomembranous (*C. difficile*) diarrhea.
• Oral preparation is stable for 2 weeks if refrigerated.
• Monitor renal function (BUN, creatinine, and creatinine clearance levels; urinalysis; and urine output) during therapy. Also monitor patient for signs and symptoms of superinfection.
• Have patient's hearing evaluated during prolonged therapy.
• When using drug to treat staphylococcal endocarditis, give for at least 4 weeks.

PATIENT TEACHING
• Tell patient to take entire amount of drug exactly as directed, even after he feels better.
• Instruct patient receiving drug I.V. to report discomfort at I.V. insertion site.
• Tell patient to report ringing in ears.

digoxin
inamrinone lactate
milrinone lactate

COMBINATION PRODUCTS
None.

---

digoxin
Digitek, Digoxin, Lanoxicaps, Lanoxin*

Pregnancy risk category C

AVAILABLE FORMS
Capsules: 0.05 mg, 0.1 mg, 0.2 mg
Elixir: 0.05 mg/ml
Injection: 0.05 mg/ml†, 0.1 mg/ml (pediatric), 0.25 mg/ml
Tablets: 0.125 mg, 0.25 mg

INDICATIONS & DOSAGES
➤ **Heart failure, paroxysmal supraventricular tachycardia, atrial fibrillation and flutter—**
Elderly patients: For patients older than age 65, 0.125 mg P.O. daily as maintenance dose. Frail or underweight elderly patients may need only 0.0625 mg daily or 0.125 mg every other day.
Adults: Loading dose is 0.5 to 1 mg I.V. or P.O. in divided doses over 24 hours; maintenance dose is 0.125 to 0.5 mg I.V. or P.O. daily (average is 0.25 mg). Depending on response, larger doses may be needed for arrhythmias.
Children older than age 2: Loading dose is 0.02 to 0.04 mg/kg P.O. daily, divided q 8 hours over 24 hours; I.V. loading dose is 0.025 to 0.035 mg/kg; maintenance dose is 0.012 mg/kg P.O. daily, divided q 12 hours.
Children ages 1 month to 2 years: Loading dose is 0.035 to 0.06 mg/kg P.O. in three divided doses over 24 hours; I.V. loading dose is 0.03 to 0.05 mg/kg; maintenance dose is 0.01 to 0.02 mg/kg P.O. daily, divided q 12 hours.
Neonates: Loading dose is 0.025 to 0.035 mg/kg P.O., divided q 8 hours over 24 hours; I.V. loading dose is 0.02 to 0.03 mg/kg; maintenance dose is 0.01 mg/kg P.O. daily, divided q 12 hours.
Premature neonates: Loading dose is 0.015 to 0.025 mg/kg I.V. in three divided doses over 24 hours; maintenance dose is 0.01 mg/kg daily, divided q 12 hours.
Adjust-a-dose: Give smaller loading and maintenance doses to patients with impaired renal function.

I.V. ADMINISTRATION
● Infuse drug slowly over at least 5 minutes.

ACTION
Inhibits sodium potassium-activated adenosine triphosphatase, thereby promoting movement of calcium from extracellular to intracellular cytoplasm and strengthening myocardial contraction. Also acts on CNS to enhance vagal tone, slowing conduction through the SA and AV nodes and providing an antiarrhythmic effect.

Route	Onset	Peak	Duration
I.V.	5-30 min	1-4 hr	3-4 days
P.O.	1.5-2 hr	2-6 hr	3-4 days

ADVERSE REACTIONS
CNS: *fatigue, generalized muscle weakness, agitation, hallucinations,* headache, malaise, dizziness, vertigo, stupor, paresthesia.
CV: *arrhythmias.*
EENT: yellow-green halos around visual images, blurred vision, light flashes, photophobia, diplopia.
GI: *anorexia, nausea,* vomiting, diarrhea.

INTERACTIONS
Drug-drug. *Amiloride:* Decreased digoxin effect and increased digoxin excretion. Monitor patient for altered digoxin effect. *Amiodarone, diltiazem, nifedipine, quinidine, verapamil:* Increased digoxin blood levels. Monitor patient for toxicity. *Amphotericin B, carbenicillin, corticosteroids, diuretics (such as chlorthalidone, loop diuretics, metolazone, thiazides),*

Reactions may be *common*, uncommon, *life-threatening*, or COMMON AND LIFE-THREATENING.

ticarcillin: Hypokalemia predisposing patient to digitalis toxicity. Monitor potassium levels.

Antacids, kaolin-pectin: Decreased absorption of oral digoxin. Separate doses as much as possible.

Antibiotics: Increased risk of toxicity because of altered intestinal flora. Monitor patient for toxicity.

Anticholinergics: May increase digoxin absorption of oral digoxin tablets. Monitor blood levels and observe for toxicity.

Cholestyramine, colestipol, metoclopramide: Decreased absorption of oral digoxin. Monitor patient for decreased digoxin effect and low blood levels. Give digoxin 1½ hours before or 2 hours after other drugs.

Parenteral calcium, thiazides: Hypercalcemia and hypomagnesemia predisposing patient to digitalis toxicity. Monitor calcium and magnesium levels.

Drug-herb. *Betel palm, fumitory, goldenseal, hawthorn, lily of the valley, motherwort, rue, shepherd's purse:* May increase cardiac effects. Discourage use together.

Gossypol, horsetail, licorice, oleander, Siberian ginseng, squill: May increase toxicity. Monitor patient closely.

Plantain, St. John's wort: May decrease effectiveness of digoxin. Dosage adjustment may be needed. Monitor patient for effect.

EFFECTS ON LAB TEST RESULTS
None reported.

CONTRAINDICATIONS
Contraindicated in patients hypersensitive to drug and in those with digitalis-induced toxicity, ventricular fibrillation, or ventricular tachycardia unless caused by heart failure.

NURSING CONSIDERATIONS
• Use with extreme caution in elderly patients and in those with acute MI, incomplete AV block, sinus bradycardia, PVCs, chronic constrictive pericarditis, hypertrophic cardiomyopathy, renal insufficiency, severe pulmonary disease, or hypothyroidism.

• Drug-induced arrhythmias may increase the severity of heart failure and hypotension.

• In children, cardiac arrythmias, including sinus bradycardia, are usually signs of early toxicity.

• Patients with hypothyroidism are extremely sensitive to cardiac glycosides and may need lower doses.

• Before administering loading dose, obtain baseline data (heart rate and rhythm, blood pressure, and electrolytes) and ask patient about use of cardiac glycosides within the previous 2 to 3 weeks.

• Loading dose is usually divided over the first 24 hours.

• Before giving drug, take apical-radial pulse for 1 minute. Record and notify prescriber of significant changes (sudden increase or decrease in pulse rate, pulse deficit, irregular beats and, particularly, regularization of a previously irregular rhythm). If these occur, check blood pressure and obtain a 12-lead ECG.

• Toxic effects on the heart may be life-threatening and require immediate attention.

• Absorption of digoxin from liquid-filled capsules is superior to absorption from tablets or elixir. Expect dosage reduction of 20% to 25% when changing from tablets or elixir to liquid-filled capsules or parenteral therapy.

• Monitor digoxin levels. Therapeutic levels range from 0.5 to 2 ng/ml. Obtain blood for digoxin levels at least 6 to 8 hours after last oral dose, preferably just before next scheduled dose.

• *Alert:* Excessive slowing of the pulse rate (60 beats per minute or less) may be a sign of digitalis toxicity. Withhold drug and notify prescriber.

• Monitor potassium levels carefully. Take corrective action before hypokalemia occurs.

• Withhold drug for 1 to 2 days before elective cardioversion. Adjust dosage after cardioversion.

• *Alert:* Don't confuse digoxin with doxepin.

PATIENT TEACHING
• Teach patient and a responsible family member about drug action, dosage regi-

men, how to take pulse, reportable signs, and follow-up care.

- Tell patient to report pulse below 60 beats/minute or above 110 beats/minute, or skipped beats or other rhythm changes.
- Instruct patient to report adverse reactions promptly. Nausea, vomiting, diarrhea, anorexia, and visual disturbances may be early indicators of toxicity.
- Encourage patient to eat potassium-rich foods.
- Tell patient not to substitute one brand of digoxin for another.

inamrinone lactate
Inocor

Pregnancy risk category C

AVAILABLE FORMS
Injection: 5 mg/ml in 20-ml ampules

INDICATIONS & DOSAGES
➤ **Short-term management of heart failure—**
Adults: Initially, 0.75 mg/kg I.V. bolus over 2 to 3 minutes. Then begin maintenance infusion of 5 to 10 mcg/kg/minute. May give additional bolus of 0.75 mg/kg 30 minutes after starting therapy. Don't exceed total daily dose of 10 mg/kg.

I.V. ADMINISTRATION
- Administer drug with an infusion pump and use as supplied, or dilute in half-normal saline solution or normal saline solution to a concentration of 1 to 3 mg/ml. Use diluted solution within 24 hours.
- Don't dilute with solutions containing dextrose because a slow chemical reaction occurs over 24 hours. Inamrinone can be injected into free-flowing dextrose infusions through a Y-connector or directly into tubing.
- *Alert:* Don't give furosemide or torsemide and inamrinone through the same I.V. line because precipitation occurs.
- Monitor blood pressure and heart rate throughout the infusion. If patient's blood pressure falls, slow or stop infusion and notify prescriber.

ACTION
Produces inotropic action by increasing cellular levels of cAMP. Produces vasodilation through a direct relaxant effect on vascular smooth muscle.

Route	Onset	Peak	Duration
I.V.	2-5 min	10 min	0.5-2 hr

ADVERSE REACTIONS
CV: *arrhythmias,* hypotension, chest pain.
GI: nausea, vomiting, anorexia, abdominal pain.
Hematologic: *thrombocytopenia.*
Metabolic: hypokalemia.
Other: burning at injection site, hypersensitivity reactions, fever.

INTERACTIONS
Drug-drug. *Cardiac glycosides:* Increased inotropic effect, which is a beneficial drug interaction. Monitor patient.
Disopyramide: Excessive hypotension. Monitor patient.

EFFECTS ON LAB TEST RESULTS
- May increase liver enzyme levels. May decrease potassium levels.
- May decrease platelet count.

CONTRAINDICATIONS
Contraindicated in patients hypersensitive to inamrinone or bisulfites. Drug shouldn't be used in patients with severe aortic or pulmonic valvular disease in place of surgical correction of the obstruction or during acute phase of MI.

NURSING CONSIDERATIONS
- Use cautiously in patients with hypertrophic cardiomyopathy.
- Inamrinone is prescribed primarily for patients who haven't responded to cardiac glycosides, diuretics, and vasodilators.
- Dosage depends on clinical response, including assessment of pulmonary wedge pressure and cardiac output.
- Anticipate that drug may be added to cardiac glycoside therapy in patients with atrial fibrillation and flutter because it slightly enhances AV conduction and increases ventricular response rate.
- Correct hypokalemia before or during therapy.

Reactions may be *common*, uncommon, *life-threatening*, or COMMON AND LIFE-THREATENING.

• Monitor platelet count. If it falls below 150,000/mm³, decrease dosage.
• Monitor patient for hypersensitivity reactions, such as pericarditis, ascites, myositis vasculitis, and pleuritis.
• Monitor intake and output and daily weight.
• Patients with end-stage cardiac disease may receive home treatment with an inamrinone drip while awaiting heart transplantation.
• **Alert:** Because of confusion with amiodarone, the generic name amrinone was changed to inamrinone.

PATIENT TEACHING
• Warn patient that burning may occur at injection site.
• Instruct home care patient and family on drug administration; tell them to report adverse reactions promptly.

---

milrinone lactate
Primacor

Pregnancy risk category C

AVAILABLE FORMS
Injection: 1 mg/ml
Injection (premixed): 200 mcg/ml in D₅W

INDICATIONS & DOSAGES
➤ **Short-term treatment of heart failure—**
Adults: Initial loading dose is 50 mcg/kg I.V., given slowly over 10 minutes; then continuous I.V. infusion of 0.375 to 0.75 mcg/kg/minute. Titrate infusion dose based on clinical and hemodynamic responses.

I.V. ADMINISTRATION
• Prepare I.V. infusion solution using half-normal saline solution, normal saline solution, or D₅W. Prepare the 100-mcg/ml solution by adding 180 ml of diluent per 20-mg (20-ml) vial, the 150-mcg/ml solution by adding 113 ml of diluent per 20-mg (20-ml) vial, and the 200-mcg/ml solution by adding 80 ml of diluent per 20-mg (20-ml) vial.

• **Alert:** If furosemide or torsemide is administered into an I.V. line that contains milrinone, a precipitate will form.

ACTION
Produces inotropic action by increasing cellular levels of cAMP. Produces vasodilation by directly relaxing vascular smooth muscle.

Route	Onset	Peak	Duration
I.V.	5-15 min	1-2 hr	3-6 hr

Adjust-a-dose: For patients with renal failure, if creatinine clearance is 50 ml/minute or less, titrate dosage to maximum clinical effect; don't exceed 1.13 mg/kg/day.

ADVERSE REACTIONS
CNS: headache.
CV: VENTRICULAR ARRHYTHMIAS, *ventricular ectopic activity,* nonsustained ventricular tachycardia, *sustained ventricular tachycardia, ventricular fibrillation.*

INTERACTIONS
None significant.

EFFECTS ON LAB TEST RESULTS
None reported.

CONTRAINDICATIONS
Contraindicated in patients hypersensitive to drug. Drug shouldn't be used in patients with severe aortic or pulmonic valvular disease in place of surgical correction of the obstruction or during acute phase of MI.

NURSING CONSIDERATIONS
• Use cautiously in patients with atrial flutter or fibrillation because drug slightly shortens AV node conduction time and may increase ventricular response rate. Give a cardiac glycoside, if ordered, before beginning milrinone therapy.
• Drug is typically given with digoxin and diuretics.
• Improved cardiac output may increase urine output. Expect dosage reduction in patient's diuretic therapy as heart failure improves. Potassium loss may predispose patient to digitalis toxicity.

• Monitor fluid and electrolyte status, blood pressure, heart rate, and renal function during therapy. Excessive decrease in blood pressure requires discontinuing or slowing rate of infusion. Correct hypokemia if it occurs during treatment.

PATIENT TEACHING
• Instruct patient to report adverse reactions promptly, especially angina.
• Tell patient that drug may cause headache, which can be treated with analgesics.
• Tell patient to report discomfort at I.V. insertion site.

19
Antiarrhythmics

adenosine
amiodarone hydrochloride
atropine sulfate
bretylium tosylate
diltiazem hydrochloride
   (See Chapter 20, ANTIANGINALS.)
disopyramide
disopyramide phosphate
dofetilide
esmolol hydrochloride
flecainide acetate
ibutilide fumarate
lidocaine hydrochloride
mexiletine hydrochloride
moricizine hydrochloride
phenytoin
   (See Chapter 28, ANTICONVULSANTS.)
phenytoin sodium
   (See Chapter 28, ANTICONVULSANTS.)
procainamide hydrochloride
propranolol hydrochloride
   (See Chapter 20, ANTIANGINALS.)
quinidine bisulfate
quinidine gluconate
quinidine polygalacturonate
quinidine sulfate
sotalol hydrochloride
tocainide hydrochloride
verapamil hydrochloride
   (See Chapter 20, ANTIANGINALS.)

COMBINATION PRODUCTS
None.

---

adenosine
Adenocard, Adenocor§

Pregnancy risk category C

AVAILABLE FORMS
Injection: 3 mg/ml in 2-ml and 5-ml vials

INDICATIONS & DOSAGES
➤ **Conversion of premature supraventricular tachycardia (PSVT) to sinus rhythm—**
Adults and children weighing 50 kg (110 lb) or more: 6 mg I.V. by rapid bolus injection over 1 to 2 seconds. If PSVT isn't eliminated in 1 to 2 minutes, 12 mg by rapid I.V. push may be given and repeated, if needed.
Children weighing less than 50 kg: Initially, 0.05 to 0.1 mg/kg I.V. by rapid bolus injection followed by a saline flush. If PSVT isn't eliminated in 1 to 2 minutes, additional bolus injections may be given in incrementally higher doses, increasing the amount given by 0.05 to 0.1 mg/kg followed by a saline flush. Continue, as needed, until conversion or a maximum single dose of 0.3 mg/kg is given.

I.V. ADMINISTRATION
● Give by rapid I.V. injection to ensure drug action.
● Give directly into a vein, if possible; when giving through an I.V. line, use the port closest to the patient.
● Flush immediately and rapidly with normal saline solution to ensure that drug quickly reaches the systemic circulation.
● Don't give single doses exceeding 12 mg.
● In adult patients, avoid giving the drug through a central line because more prolonged asystole may occur.

ACTION
A naturally occurring nucleoside that acts on the AV node to slow conduction and inhibit reentry pathways. Adenosine is also useful in treating PSVT, including those with accessory bypass tracts (Wolff-Parkinson-White syndrome).

Route	Onset	Peak	Duration
I.V.	Immediate	Immediate	Unknown

ADVERSE REACTIONS
CNS: dizziness, light-headedness, numbness, tingling in arms, headache.
CV: *facial flushing.*
GI: nausea.
Respiratory: chest pressure, *dyspnea, shortness of breath.*

INTERACTIONS
Drug-drug. *Carbamazepine:* May result in higher degrees of heart block. Use together cautiously.

Digoxin, verapamil: May cause ventricular fibrillation. Monitor patient closely.

Dipyridamole: May increase adenosine's effects. Smaller doses may be needed. Use with caution.

Methylxanthines: Antagonism of adenosine's effects. Patients receiving theophylline may require higher doses or may not respond to adenosine therapy. Monitor patient closely.

Drug-herb. *Guarana:* May decrease response. Monitor patient.

EFFECTS ON LAB TEST RESULTS
None reported.

CONTRAINDICATIONS
Contraindicated in patients hypersensitive to drug and in those with second- or third-degree heart block or sinus node disease (such as sick sinus syndrome or symptomatic bradycardia) unless an artificial pacemaker is present; adenosine decreases conduction through the AV node and may produce first-, second-, or third-degree heart block. Patients who develop high level heart block after a single dose of adenosine shouldn't receive additional doses.

NURSING CONSIDERATIONS
● *Alert:* Because new arrhythmias, including heart block or transient asystole, may develop, monitor cardiac rhythm and be prepared to give appropriate therapy.
● Use cautiously in patients with asthma, emphysema, or bronchitis because bronchoconstriction may occur.
● Crystals may form if solution is cold. If crystals are visible, gently warm solution to room temperature. Don't use solutions that aren't clear.
● Discard unused drug; adenosine lacks preservatives.

PATIENT TEACHING
● Instruct patient to report adverse reactions promptly.
● Tell patient to report discomfort at I.V. site.

● Inform patient that he may experience flushing or chest pain lasting 1 to 2 minutes.

---

amiodarone hydrochloride
Aratac‡, Cordarone, Cordarone X‡, Pacerone

Pregnancy risk category D

AVAILABLE FORMS
Injection: 50 mg/ml in 3-ml ampules
Tablets: 100 mg‡, 200 mg

INDICATIONS & DOSAGES
➤ **Recurrent ventricular fibrillation or recurrent hemodynamically unstable ventricular tachycardia unresponsive to adequate doses of other antiarrhythmics or when alternative drugs can't be tolerated—**
Adults: Loading dose is 800 to 1,600 mg P.O. daily divided b.i.d. for 1 to 3 weeks until initial therapeutic response occurs; then 600 to 800 mg P.O. daily for 1 month, followed by 200 to 600 mg P.O. daily for maintenance.

Or, give loading dose of 150 mg I.V. over 10 minutes (15 mg/minute); then 360 mg I.V. over next 6 hours (1 mg/minute), followed by 540 mg I.V. over next 18 hours (0.5 mg/minute). After first 24 hours, continue with maintenance I.V. infusion of 720 mg/24 hours (0.5 mg/minute).

➤ **Cardiac arrest, pulseless ventricular tachycardia, or ventricular fibrillation—**
Adults: 300 mg diluted in 20 to 30 mg of a compatible solution I.V. push.

I.V. ADMINISTRATION
● Drug may be given I.V. only in facilities where continuous ECG monitoring and electrophysiologic techniques are available. Mix initial dose of 150 mg in 100 ml of D₅W solution. Drug is incompatible with normal saline solution. Mix infusions planned for administration over 2 hours or longer in glass or polyolefin bottles. Give repeat doses through a central venous catheter.
● Give I.V. amiodarone whenever possible via a central line dedicated to that purpose.

Reactions may be *common*, uncommon, *life-threatening*, or COMMON AND LIFE-THREATENING.

• Use an in-line filter with I.V. administration.

• Continuously monitor cardiac status of patient receiving drug I.V. If hypotension occurs, reduce infusion rate.

• *Alert:* I.V. Cordarone can leech out plasticizers that can adversely affect male reproductive tract development in fetuses, infants, and toddlers.

ACTION

Effects result from blockade of potassium chloride leading to a prolongation of action potential duration.

Route	Onset	Peak	Duration
I.V.	Unknown	Unknown	Variable
P.O.	Variable	3-7 hr	Variable

ADVERSE REACTIONS

CNS: peripheral neuropathy, ataxia, paresthesia, *tremor,* insomnia, sleep disturbances, headache, *malaise, fatigue.*
CV: *bradycardia,* hypotension, ***arrhythmias, heart failure, heart block, sinus arrest,*** edema.
EENT: *asymptomatic corneal microdeposits,* optic neuropathy or neuritis resulting in visual impairment, abnormal smell, *visual disturbances.*
GI: abnormal taste, anorexia, *nausea, vomiting,* constipation, abdominal pain.
Hematologic: *coagulation abnormalities.*
Hepatic: hepatic dysfunction, ***hepatic failure.***
Metabolic: *hypothyroidism,* hyperthyroidism.
Respiratory: *adult respiratory distress syndrome,* SEVERE PULMONARY TOXICITY.
Skin: *photosensitivity,* solar dermatitis.

INTERACTIONS

Drug-drug. *Antiarrhythmics:* May reduce hepatic or renal clearance of certain antiarrhythmics, especially flecainide, procainamide, and quinidine. Use of amiodarone with other antiarrhythmics, especially mexiletine, propafenone, quinidine, disopyramide, and procainamide, may induce torsades de pointes. Avoid using together.
Antihypertensives: Increased hypotensive effect. Use together cautiously.

Beta blockers, calcium channel blockers: Increased cardiac depressant effects; may increase slowing of SA node and AV conduction. Use together cautiously.
Cyclosporine: Increased creatinine levels. Creatinine level can remain elevated even after cyclosporine dose is reduced. Monitor patient closely.
Digoxin: Increased digoxin levels (average of 70% to 100%). Monitor digoxin levels closely and adjust dosage. Digoxin dosage should be reduced by half or stopped upon initiation of amiodarone therapy.
Phenytoin: May decrease phenytoin metabolism. Monitor phenytoin levels and adjust dosage.
Theophylline: May increase theophylline levels and cause toxicity. Monitor theophylline levels.
Warfarin: Increased anticoagulant response with the potential for serious or fatal bleeding. Decrease warfarin dosage 33% to 50% when amiodarone is initiated. Monitor patient closely.
Drug-herb. *Pennyroyal:* May change the rate of formation of toxic metabolites of pennyroyal. Discourage use together.
Drug-lifestyle. *Sun exposure:* May cause photosensitivity reaction. Advise patient to take precautions to avoid excessive sunlight exposure.

EFFECTS ON LAB TEST RESULTS

• May increase ALT, AST, alkaline phosphatase, and GGT levels.
• May increase PT and INR.

CONTRAINDICATIONS

Contraindicated in patients hypersensitive to drug. Also contraindicated in those with cardiogenic shock, second- or third-degree AV block, severe SA node disease resulting in bradycardia unless an artificial pacemaker is present, and in those for whom bradycardia has caused syncope.

NURSING CONSIDERATIONS

• Use with extreme caution in patients receiving other antiarrhythmics.
• Use cautiously in patients with pulmonary, hepatic, or thyroid disease.
• Be aware of the high risk of adverse reactions.
• Obtain baseline pulmonary, liver, and thyroid function tests.

• Give loading doses in a hospital setting and with continuous ECG monitoring because of the slow onset of antiarrhythmic effect and the risk of life-threatening arrhythmias.

• Divide oral loading dose into two equal doses and give with meals to decrease GI intolerance. Maintenance dose may be given once daily, but may be divided into two doses taken with meals if GI intolerance occurs.

• **Alert:** Drug poses major and potentially life-threatening management problems in patients at risk for sudden death and should be used only in patients with documented, life-threatening, recurrent ventricular arrhythmias unresponsive to documented adequate doses of other antiarrhythmics or when alternative drugs can't be tolerated. Amiodarone can cause fatal toxicities, including hepatic and pulmonary toxicity.

• Watch carefully for pulmonary toxicity. Risk increases in patients receiving doses over 400 mg/day.

• Watch for evidence of pneumonitis—exertional dyspnea, nonproductive cough, and pleuritic chest pain. Monitor pulmonary function tests and chest X-ray.

• Monitor liver and thyroid function tests and electrolytes, particularly potassium and magnesium levels.

• Monitor PT and INR if patient takes warfarin and digoxin levels if patient takes digoxin.

• Instillation of methylcellulose ophthalmic solution is recommended during amiodarone therapy to minimize corneal microdeposits. About 1 to 4 months after beginning amiodarone therapy, most patients show corneal microdeposits on slit-lamp ophthalmic examination. However, 10% or less have actual vision disturbances.

• Monitor blood pressure and heart rate and rhythm frequently. Perform continuous ECG monitoring during initiation and alteration of dosage. Notify prescriber of significant change.

• A potentially fatal "gasping syndrome" may occur in neonates following administration of I.V. solutions containing benzyl alcohol.

• **Alert:** Don't confuse amiodarone with amiloride.

PATIENT TEACHING

• Advise patient to wear sunscreen or protective clothing to prevent photosensitivity reaction. Monitor patient for burning or tingling skin followed by erythema and possible skin blistering. A blue-gray discoloration of the exposed skin may occur.

• Tell patient to take oral drug with food if GI reactions occur.

• Inform patient that adverse effects of drug are more prevalent at high doses and become more frequent with treatment lasting over 6 months but are generally reversible when drug is stopped. Resolution of adverse reactions may take up to 4 months.

---

atropine sulfate

Pregnancy risk category C

AVAILABLE FORMS
Injection: 0.05 mg/ml, 0.1 mg/ml, 0.3 mg/ml, 0.4 mg/ml, 0.5 mg/ml, 0.8 mg/ml, 1 mg/ml
Tablets: 0.4 mg

INDICATIONS & DOSAGES
➤ **Symptomatic bradycardia, bradyarrhythmia (junctional or escape rhythm)—**
Adults: Usually 0.5 to 1 mg I.V. push, repeated q 3 to 5 minutes to maximum of 2 mg p.r.n.
Children: 0.01 mg/kg I.V.; may repeat q 4 to 6 hours; maximum dose is 0.4 mg or 0.3 mg/m².
➤ **Antidote for anticholinesterase insecticide poisoning—**
Adults: 2 to 3 mg I.V. repeated q 5 to 10 minutes until muscarinic signs and symptoms disappear or signs of atropine toxicity appear. Severe poisoning may require up to 6 mg hourly.
Children: 0.05 mg/kg I.M. or I.V. repeated q 10 to 30 minutes until muscarinic signs and symptoms disappear (may be repeated if they reappear) or until atropine toxicity occurs.
➤ **Preoperatively to diminish secretions and block cardiac vagal reflexes—**
Adults and children weighing 20 kg (44 lb) or more: 0.4 to 0.6 mg I.M. or S.C. 30 to 60 minutes before anesthesia.

Reactions may be *common*, uncommon, *life-threatening*, or COMMON AND LIFE-THREATENING.

Children weighing less than 20 kg:
0.01 mg/kg I.M. or S.C. up to maximum dose of 0.4 mg 30 to 60 minutes before anesthesia.
➤ **Adjunct treatment of peptic ulcer disease, treatment of functional GI disorders such as irritable bowel syndrome—**
Adults: 0.4 to 0.6 mg P.O. q 4 to 6 hours.
Children: 0.01 mg/kg or 0.3 mg/m² P.O. (not to exceed 0.4 mg) q 4 to 6 hours.

I.V. ADMINISTRATION

● Give I.V. into a large vein or into I.V. tubing over at least 1 minute.
● Slow I.V. administration may cause paradoxical slowing of the heart rate.

ACTION

An anticholinergic that inhibits acetylcholine at the parasympathetic neuroeffector junction, blocking vagal effects on the SA and AV nodes, thereby enhancing conduction through the AV node and increasing the heart rate.

Route	Onset	Peak	Duration
I.M.	5-40 min	20-60 min	4 hr
I.V.	Immediate	2-4 min	4 hr
P.O.	0.5-2 hr	1-2 hr	4 hr
S.C.	Unknown	Unknown	Unknown

ADVERSE REACTIONS

CNS: *headache, restlessness,* ataxia, disorientation, hallucinations, delirium, *insomnia, dizziness,* excitement, agitation, confusion.
CV: palpitations, **bradycardia,** tachycardia.
EENT: photophobia, *blurred vision, mydriasis,* cycloplegia, increased intraocular pressure.
GI: *dry mouth,* thirst, *constipation,* nausea, vomiting.
GU: urine retention, impotence.
Other: *anaphylaxis.*

INTERACTIONS

Drug-drug. *Antacids:* Decreased absorption of anticholinergics. Separate administration times by at least 1 hour.
Anticholinergics, drugs with anticholinergic effects (amantadine, antiarrhythmics, antiparkinsonians, glutethimide, meperidine, phenothiazines, TCAs): Increased

anticholinergic effects. Use together cautiously.
Ketoconazole, levodopa: Decreased absorption. Avoid using together.
Potassium chloride wax-matrix tablets: Increased risk of mucosal lesions. Use together cautiously.
Drug-herb. *Jaborandi tree, pill-bearing spurge:* Decreased effectiveness of drug. Discourage use together.
Jimsonweed: May adversely affect CV function. Discourage use together.
Squaw vine: Tannic acid may decrease metabolic breakdown. Monitor patient.

EFFECTS ON LAB TEST RESULTS

None reported.

CONTRAINDICATIONS

Contraindicated in patients hypersensitive to drug and in those with acute angle-closure glaucoma, obstructive uropathy, obstructive disease of GI tract, paralytic ileus, toxic megacolon, intestinal atony, unstable CV status in acute hemorrhage, tachycardia, myocardial ischemia, asthma, or myasthenia gravis.

NURSING CONSIDERATIONS

● Use cautiously in patients with Down syndrome because they may be more sensitive to drug.
● Many adverse reactions (such as dry mouth and constipation) vary with the dose.
● Monitor patients for paradoxical initial bradycardia, especially those receiving small doses (0.4 to 0.6 mg). This usually disappears within 2 minutes.
● *Alert:* Watch for tachycardia in cardiac patients because it may lead to ventricular fibrillation.
● Monitor fluid intake and urine output. Drug causes urine retention and urinary hesitancy.

PATIENT TEACHING

● Teach patient receiving oral form of drug how to handle distressing anticholinergic effects.
● Instruct patient to report serious or persistent adverse reactions promptly.
● Tell patient about potential for photophobia and suggest use of sunglasses.

---

*Liquid contains alcohol.   **May contain tartrazine.   †Canada   ‡Australia   §U.K.   ◇OTC

bretylium tosylate
Bretylate†

Pregnancy risk category C

AVAILABLE FORMS
Injection: 50 mg/ml in 10-ml ampules, vials, and syringes and in 20-ml vials

INDICATIONS & DOSAGES
➤ **Ventricular fibrillation (VF) or hemodynamically unstable ventricular tachycardia (VT) unresponsive to other antiarrhythmics—**
Adults: 5 mg/kg by I.V. push over 1 minute. If needed, dose may be increased to 10 mg/kg and repeated q 15 to 30 minutes until 30 to 35 mg/kg has been given. For continuous suppression, diluted solution given at 1 to 2 mg/minute continuously or 5 to 10 mg/kg diluted over more than 8 minutes q 6 hours.

I.V. ADMINISTRATION
• For maintenance therapy, dilute using dextrose or normal saline solution for injection before administration. Commercially prepared drug in solution of D_5W may be contraindicated in patients allergic to corn. Follow manufacturer's guidelines for specific dilution method (varies according to dosage).
• When giving as direct I.V. injection, use a 20G to 22G needle and inject over 1 minute into a vein or I.V. line containing a free-flowing, compatible solution.
• For intermittent I.V. administration, dilute and give over a period of 8 minutes or longer to minimize nausea and vomiting.

ACTION
Unknown. Considered a class III antiarrhythmic that initially exerts transient adrenergic stimulation through release of norepinephrine. Subsequent depletion of norepinephrine causes adrenergic blocking actions to predominate, prolonging repolarization and increasing duration of action potential and an effective refractory period.

Route	Onset	Peak	Duration
I.M.	5-40 min	1 hr	6-24 hr
I.V.	Immediate	Immediate	6-24 hr

ADVERSE REACTIONS
CNS: *vertigo, dizziness, light-headedness, syncope.*
CV: SEVERE HYPOTENSION, *bradycardia,* anginal pain, *transient arrhythmias,* transient hypertension, increased PVCs.
GI: severe nausea, vomiting.

INTERACTIONS
Drug-drug. *All antihypertensives:* May increase hypotension. Monitor blood pressure.
Digoxin: May aggravate digitalis toxicity. Make sure that arrhythmia doesn't stem from digitalis toxicity before giving bretylium.
Other antiarrhythmics: Increased or decreased antiarrhythmic effects. Monitor patient for additive toxicity.
Sympathomimetics: May increase effects of drugs given to correct hypotension. Monitor patient for effects.

EFFECTS ON LAB TEST RESULTS
None reported.

CONTRAINDICATIONS
Contraindicated in digitalized patients, unless arrhythmia is life-threatening and not caused by cardiac glycosides, and in those unresponsive to other antiarrhythmics.

NURSING CONSIDERATIONS
• Dosage adjustments may be necessary in patients with renal insufficiency.
• Drug isn't considered a first-line choice in the treatment of VT or VF.
• Use with extreme caution in patients with fixed cardiac output (aortic stenosis and pulmonary hypertension) to avoid severe and sudden drop in blood pressure.
• Keep patient supine until tolerance to hypotension develops.
• Monitor patient closely. The initial release of norepinephrine caused by bretylium may induce transient hypertension and arrhythmias.
• Monitor blood pressure, heart rate, and rhythm continuously. Immediately report significant change. If supine systolic blood pressure falls below 75 mm Hg, the prescriber may order norepinephrine, dopamine, or volume expanders.
• Observe for increased anginal pain in susceptible patients.

Reactions may be *common,* uncommon, *life-threatening,* or COMMON AND LIFE-THREATENING.

PATIENT TEACHING
• Instruct patient to report adverse reactions immediately.
• Tell patient to report discomfort at I.V. insertion site.
• Tell patient to avoid sudden postural changes.

---

disopyramide
Dirythmin SA§, Rythmodan†‡

disopyramide phosphate
Norpace, Norpace CR, Rythmodan Injection‡, Rythmodan-LA†

Pregnancy risk category C

AVAILABLE FORMS
disopyramide
Capsules: 100 mg†, 150 mg†
disopyramide phosphate
Capsules: 100 mg, 150 mg
Capsules (controlled-release): 100 mg, 150 mg
Injection: 10 mg/ml†‡§
Tablets (sustained-release): 250 mg†

INDICATIONS & DOSAGES
➤ **Ventricular tachycardia and ventricular arrhythmias believed to be life-threatening—**
P.O.
Adults weighing more than 50 kg (110 lb):
150 mg q 6 hours with conventional capsules or 300 mg q 12 hours with extended-release preparations.
Adults weighing 50 kg or less: Highly individualized.
Children ages 12 to 18: 6 to 15 mg/kg P.O. daily, divided into four doses (q 6 hours).
Children ages 4 to 12: 10 to 15 mg/kg P.O. daily, divided into four doses (q 6 hours).
Children ages 1 to 4: 10 to 20 mg/kg P.O. daily, divided into four doses (q 6 hours).
Children younger than age 1: 10 to 30 mg/kg P.O. daily, divided into four doses (q 6 hours).
Adjust-a-dose: For patients with advanced renal insufficiency, if creatinine clearance is 30 to 40 ml/minute, 100 mg q 8 hours; between 15 and 30 ml/minute, 100 mg q 12 hours; below 15 ml/minute, 100 mg q 24 hours.

I.V.
Adults: For parenteral use, initially give 2 mg/kg I.V. slowly (over not less than 15 minutes). Give until arrhythmias are eliminated or patient has received 150 mg. Repeat dosage if conversion is successful but arrhythmias return. Total I.V. dosage shouldn't exceed 300 mg in first hour. Follow with I.V. infusion of 0.4 mg/kg/hour (usually 20 to 30 mg/hour) to maximum of 800 mg/day.

I.V. ADMINISTRATION
• Add 200 mg to 200 to 500 ml of a compatible solution, such as normal saline solution or D₅W. Don't mix with other drugs.
• Give slowly, over at least 15 minutes.
• Switch to oral therapy as soon as possible.

ACTION
A class IA antiarrhythmic that depresses phase O and prolongs the action potential. All class I drugs have membrane-stabilizing effects.

Route	Onset	Peak	Duration
I.V.	Unknown	Unknown	Unknown
P.O.	0.5-3.5 hr	2-2.5 hr	1.5-8.5 hr

ADVERSE REACTIONS
CNS: dizziness, agitation, depression, fatigue, headache, nervousness, acute psychosis, syncope.
CV: *hypotension, heart failure, heart block,* edema, *arrhythmias,* shortness of breath, chest pain.
EENT: blurred vision, dry eyes or nose.
GI: *dry mouth,* nausea, vomiting, anorexia, bloating, gas, weight gain, abdominal pain, *constipation, diarrhea.*
GU: *urinary hesitancy.*
Hepatic: cholestatic jaundice.
Musculoskeletal: muscle weakness, aches, pain.
Skin: rash, pruritus, dermatosis.

INTERACTIONS
Drug-drug. *Antiarrhythmics:* Increased QRS complex or QT interval, which may predispose patient to other arrhythmias. Monitor patient closely.
Erythromycin: Increased disopyramide levels, resulting in arrhythmias. Monitor patient closely.

Phenytoin: Increased metabolism of disopyramide. Watch for decreased anti-arrhythmic effect.

Rifampin: May decrease disopyramide levels. Monitor patient closely.

Drug-herb. *Jimsonweed:* May adversely affect CV function. Discourage use together.

EFFECTS ON LAB TEST RESULTS
None reported.

CONTRAINDICATIONS
Contraindicated in patients hypersensitive to drug and in those with sick sinus syndrome, cardiogenic shock, congenital QT interval prolongation, or second- or third-degree heart block in the absence of an artificial pacemaker.

NURSING CONSIDERATIONS
● Use with extreme caution and avoid, if possible, in patients with heart failure. Use cautiously in patients with underlying conduction abnormalities, urinary tract diseases (especially prostatic hyperplasia), hepatic or renal impairment, myasthenia gravis, or acute angle-closure glaucoma.
● Correct electrolyte abnormalities before therapy begins.
● Patients with atrial fibrillation or flutter should be digitalized before starting disopyramide because of the risk of enhancing AV conduction.
● Check apical pulse before giving drug. Notify prescriber if pulse rate is slower than 60 beats/minute or faster than 120 beats/minute.
● Don't use sustained- or controlled-release preparations to control ventricular arrhythmias when therapeutic blood levels must be rapidly attained, in patients with cardiomyopathy or possible cardiac decompensation, or in those with severe renal impairment.
● For use in young children, pharmacist may prepare disopyramide suspension using 100-mg capsules and cherry syrup. Suspension should be dispensed in amber glass bottles and protected from light.
● Watch for recurrence of arrhythmias and check for adverse reactions; notify prescriber if any occur.
● Stop drug if heart block develops, if QRS complex widens by more than 25%,

or if QT interval lengthens by more than 25% above baseline.
● **Alert:** Don't confuse disopyramide with desipramine or dipyridamole.

PATIENT TEACHING
● Teach patient importance of taking drug on time and exactly as prescribed. This may require use of an alarm clock for nighttime doses.
● When transferring patient from immediate-release to sustained-release capsules, advise him to take the first sustained-release capsule 6 hours after taking the last immediate-release capsule.
● Tell patient not to crush or chew sustained-release capsules or tablets.
● If not contraindicated, advise patient to chew gum or hard candy to relieve dry mouth and to increase fiber and fluid intake to relieve constipation.

---

dofetilide
Tikosyn

Pregnancy risk category C

AVAILABLE FORMS
Distributed only to hospitals and other facilities that have received applicable dosing and treatment initiation programs. Inpatient and subsequent outpatient discharge and refill prescriptions are filled only after confirmation that prescriber has completed applicable dosing and treatment initiation programs.
Capsules: 125 mcg (0.125 mg), 250 mcg (0.25 mg), 500 mcg (0.5 mg)

INDICATIONS & DOSAGES
➤ **Maintenance of normal sinus rhythm in patients with symptomatic atrial fibrillation or atrial flutter of greater than 1 week's duration who have been converted to normal sinus rhythm; conversion of atrial fibrillation and atrial flutter to normal sinus rhythm—**
Adults: Dosage is individualized and is based on creatinine clearance and QTc interval, which must be determined before first dose (QT interval should be used if heart rate is less than 60 beats/minute). Usual recommended dosage is 500 mcg

P.O. b.i.d. for patients with creatinine clearance greater than 60 ml/minute.

Adjust-a-dose: If creatinine clearance is between 40 and 60 ml/minute, starting dose is 250 mcg P.O. b.i.d.; if between 20 and 39 ml/minute, starting dose is 125 mcg P.O. b.i.d. If clearance is less than 20 ml/minute, drug is contraindicated.

Determine QTc interval 2 to 3 hours after giving first dose. If QTc interval has increased by more than 15% compared with baseline or if it's more than 500 msec (550 msec in patients with ventricular conduction abnormalities), adjust dosage as follows: If starting dose based on creatinine clearance was 500 mcg P.O. b.i.d., give 250 mcg P.O. b.i.d. If starting dose based on clearance was 250 mcg P.O. b.i.d., give 125 mcg P.O. b.i.d. If starting dose based on clearance was 125 mcg P.O. b.i.d., give 125 mcg once a day.

Determine QTc interval 2 to 3 hours after each subsequent dose while patient is in hospital. If at any time after second dose the QTc interval is more than 500 msec (550 msec in patients with ventricular conduction abnormalities), stop drug.

ACTION

As a class III antiarrhythmic, dofetilide prolongs repolarization without affecting conduction velocity by blocking the cardiac ion channel carrying potassium current. It doesn't affect sodium channels, alpha-adrenergic receptors, or beta-adrenergic receptors.

Route	Onset	Peak	Duration
P.O.	Unknown	2-3 hr	Unknown

ADVERSE REACTIONS

CNS: *headache,* dizziness, insomnia, anxiety, migraine, cerebral ischemia, CVA, asthenia, paresthesia, syncope.
CV: *ventricular fibrillation, ventricular tachycardia, torsades de pointes, AV block,* bundle-branch block, *heart block, chest pain,* angina, atrial fibrillation, hypertension, palpitations, *bradycardia,* edema, *cardiac arrest, MI.*
GI: nausea, diarrhea, abdominal pain.
GU: urinary tract infection.
Hepatic: liver damage.

Musculoskeletal: back pain, arthralgia, facial paralysis.
Respiratory: respiratory tract infection, dyspnea, increased cough.
Skin: rash, sweating.
Other: flu syndrome, *angioedema,* peripheral edema.

INTERACTIONS

Drug-drug. *Amiloride, metformin, triamterene:* May increase dofetilide levels. Use together cautiously.
Amiodarone, diltiazem, macrolide antibiotics, nefazodone, norfloxacin, protease inhibitors, quinine, selected serotonin reuptake inhibitors, zafirlukast: May cause increased dofetilide plasma levels. Use together cautiously.
Cimetidine, ketoconazole, sulfamethoxazole, trimethoprim, verapamil: Increased plasma levels of dofetilide. Concomitant use is contraindicated.
Inhibitors of CYP3A4 (amiodarone, azole antifungals, cannabinoids, diltiazem, macrolide antibiotics, nefazodone, norfloxacin, protease inhibitors, quinine, selected serotonin reuptake inhibitors, zafirlukast): May decrease metabolism and increase dofetilide levels. Concomitant use is contraindicated.
Inhibitors of renal cationic secretion (megestrol, prochlorperazine): May increase dofetilide levels. Avoid using together.
Drug-food. *Grapefruit juice:* May decrease hepatic metabolism and increase plasma levels. Discourage use together.

EFFECTS ON LAB TEST RESULTS

None reported.

CONTRAINDICATIONS

Contraindicated in patients hypersensitive to drug and in those with congenital or acquired long QT interval syndromes. Don't use in patients with baseline QT or QTc interval greater than 440 msec (500 msec in patients with ventricular conduction abnormalities). Also contraindicated in patients with severe renal impairment (creatinine clearance less than 20 ml/minute).

NURSING CONSIDERATIONS

• Use cautiously in patient with severe hepatic impairment.

• Continuous ECG monitoring is needed for at least 3 days.
• Patient shouldn't be discharged within 12 hours of conversion to normal sinus rhythm.
• Monitor patient for prolonged diarrhea, sweating, and vomiting. Report these signs to prescriber because electrolyte imbalance may increase potential for arrhythmia development.
• Monitor renal function and QTc interval every 3 months.
• Hypokalemia and hypomagnesemia may occur with the administration of potassium-depleting diuretics, increasing the risk of torsades de pointes. Potassium levels should be within normal range before giving dofetilide and maintained in normal range.
• If patient doesn't convert to normal sinus rhythm within 24 hours of starting dofetilide, consider electrical conversion.
• Before starting dofetilide, previous antiarrhythmic therapy should be stopped under careful monitoring for a minimum of three plasma half-lives. Drug shouldn't be given after amiodarone therapy until amiodarone levels are below 0.3 mcg/ml or until amiodarone has been stopped for at least 3 months.
• If dofetilide must be stopped to allow dosing with interacting drugs, a washout period of at least 2 days is needed before starting other drug therapy.

PATIENT TEACHING
• Tell patient to report any change in OTC or prescription drug use or supplement or herb use.
• Inform patient that drug can be taken without regard to meals or antacid administration.
• Tell patient to immediately report excessive or prolonged diarrhea, sweating, vomiting, or loss of appetite or thirst.
• Inform patient not to take drug with grapefruit juice.
• Advise patient not to use OTC Tagamet-HB for ulcers or heartburn but instead to use antacids such as Zantac 75 mg, Pepcid, Prilosec, Axid, or Prevacid if needed.
• Instruct patient to tell prescriber if she becomes pregnant.
• Advise patient not to breast-feed while taking dofetilide.

• If a dose is missed, tell patient not to double a dose but to skip the dose and wait until the next dosing time for the regularly scheduled dose.

esmolol hydrochloride
Brevibloc

Pregnancy risk category C

AVAILABLE FORMS
Injection: 10 mg/ml in 10-ml vials, 250 mg/ml in 10-ml ampules
Premixed bags: 2,500 mg/250 ml normal saline solution

INDICATIONS & DOSAGES
➤ **Supraventricular tachycardia; to control ventricular rate in patients with atrial fibrillation or flutter in perioperative, postoperative, or other emergent circumstances; noncompensatory sinus tachycardia when heart rate requires specific interventions—**
Adults: 500 mcg/kg/minute as loading dose by I.V. infusion over 1 minute; then 4-minute maintenance infusion of 50 mcg/kg/minute. If adequate response doesn't occur within 5 minutes, repeat loading dose and follow with maintenance infusion of 100 mcg/kg/minute for 4 minutes. Repeat loading dose and increase maintenance infusion by increments of 50 mcg/kg/minute. Maximum maintenance infusion for tachycardia is 200 mcg/kg/minute.
➤ **Perioperative and postoperative tachycardia or hypertension—**
Adults: For perioperative treatment of tachycardia or hypertension, 80 mg (about 1 mg/kg) I.V. bolus over 30 seconds; then 150 mcg/kg/minute I.V. infusion, if needed. Titrate infusion rate, as needed, to maximum of 300 mcg/kg/minute.

I.V. ADMINISTRATION
• Don't give esmolol by I.V. push; use an infusion control device. The 10-mg/ml single-dose vials may be used without diluting, but the injection concentrate (250 mg/ml) must be diluted to maximum of 10 mg/ml before infusion. Remove 20 ml from 500 ml of D₅W, lactated Ringer's solution, half-normal or normal

saline solution and add two ampules of esmolol (final level 10 mg/ml). Don't mix in
sodium bicarbonate.
• Concentrations greater than 10 mg/ml
must be administered via a central line.

ACTION

A class II antiarrhythmic and ultrashort-
acting selective beta blocker that decreases heart rate, contractility, and blood pressure.

Route	Onset	Peak	Duration
I.V.	Immediate	30 min	30 min after infusion

ADVERSE REACTIONS

CNS: anxiety, depression, dizziness, somnolence, headache, agitation, fatigue, confusion.
CV: HYPOTENSION, peripheral ischemia.
GI: *nausea,* vomiting.
Skin: inflammation or induration at infusion site.

INTERACTIONS

Drug-drug. *Digoxin:* May increase digoxin levels by 10% to 20%. Monitor digoxin
levels.
Morphine: May increase esmolol blood
levels. Titrate esmolol carefully.
*Reserpine, other catecholamine-depleting
drugs:* May increase bradycardia and
hypotension. Titrate esmolol carefully.
Succinylcholine: Esmolol may prolong
neuromuscular blockade. Monitor patient
closely.

EFFECTS ON LAB TEST RESULTS

None reported.

CONTRAINDICATIONS

Contraindicated in patients with sinus
bradycardia, heart block greater than first-
degree, cardiogenic shock, or overt heart
failure.

NURSING CONSIDERATIONS

• Use cautiously if patient has renal impairment, diabetes, or bronchospasm.
• Esmolol solutions are incompatible with
diazepam, furosemide, sodium bicarbonate, and thiopental sodium.

• Dosage for postoperative treatment of
tachycardia and hypertension is same as
for supraventricular tachycardia.
• *Alert:* Monitor ECG and blood pressure
continuously during infusion. Up to 50%
of all patients treated with esmolol develop hypotension. Diaphoresis and dizziness
may accompany hypotension. Monitor patient closely, especially if pretreatment
blood pressure was low.
• Hypotension can usually be reversed
within 30 minutes by decreasing the dose
or, if needed, by stopping the infusion. Notify prescriber if this becomes necessary.
• If a local reaction develops at the infusion site, change to another site. Avoid using butterfly needles.
• Esmolol is recommended only for short-
term use, no longer than 48 hours. Avoid
extravasation.
• When patient's heart rate becomes stable, esmolol will be replaced by alternative (longer-acting) antiarrhythmics, such
as propranolol, digoxin, or verapamil. A
half-hour after the first dose of the alternative drug is given, reduce infusion rate by
50%. Monitor patient response and, if
heart rate is controlled for 1 hour after administration of the second dose of the alternative drug, stop esmolol infusion.

PATIENT TEACHING

• Instruct patient to report adverse reactions promptly.
• Tell patient to report discomfort at I.V.
site.

flecainide acetate
Tambocor

Pregnancy risk category C

AVAILABLE FORMS

Injection: 10 mg/ml‡
Tablets: 50 mg, 100 mg, 150 mg

INDICATIONS & DOSAGES

➤ **For the paroxysmal supraventricular
tachycardia, including AV nodal re-
entrant tachycardia and AV re-entrant
tachycardia, paroxysmal atrial fibrillation or flutter in patients without structural heart disease; life-threatening**

ventricular arrhythmias such as sustained ventricular tachycardia—
Adults: For paroxysmal supraventricular tachycardia, 50 mg P.O. q 12 hours. Increased in increments of 50 mg b.i.d. q 4 days. Maximum dose is 300 mg/day.

For life-threatening ventricular arrhythmias, 100 mg P.O. q 12 hours. Increase in increments of 50 mg b.i.d. q 4 days until efficacy occurs. Maximum dose is 400 mg daily for most patients.

Initial dosage for patients with heart failure is 50 mg P.O. q 12 hours.

Adjust-a-dose: For patients with renal impairment, if creatinine clearance is 35 ml/minute or less, initial dose is 100 mg once daily or 50 mg b.i.d.
Adults: 2 mg/kg I.V. push over not less than 10 minutes to maximum dose of 150 mg; or dilute dose and give as an infusion.

I.V. ADMINISTRATION
● When giving by I.V. push, give over at least 10 minutes. For I.V. infusion, mix only with D_5W.
● Because of drug's long half-life, full therapeutic effect may take 3 to 5 days. Give together with I.V. lidocaine for first several days.

ACTION
A class IC antiarrhythmic that decreases excitability, conduction velocity, and automaticity as a result of slowed atrial, AV node, His-Purkinje system, and intraventricular conduction; causes a slight but significant prolongation of refractory periods in these tissues.

Route	Onset	Peak	Duration
I.V.	Immediate	Immediate	Unknown
P.O.	Unknown	2-3 hr	Unknown

ADVERSE REACTIONS
CNS: *dizziness, headache,* fatigue, tremor, anxiety, insomnia, depression, malaise, paresthesia, ataxia, vertigo, *lightheadedness, syncope,* asthenia.
CV: **new or worsened arrhythmias,** chest pain, **heart failure, cardiac arrest,** palpitations, edema, flushing.
EENT: eye pain, eye irritation, *blurred vision and other visual disturbances.*
GI: nausea, constipation, abdominal pain, dyspepsia, vomiting, diarrhea, anorexia.

Respiratory: *dyspnea.*
Skin: rash.
Other: fever.

INTERACTIONS
Drug-drug. *Amiodarone, cimetidine:* Increased levels of flecainide. Watch for toxicity.
Digoxin: May increase digoxin levels by 15% to 25%. Monitor digoxin levels.
Disopyramide, verapamil: Increased negative inotropic properties. Avoid using together.
Propranolol, other beta blockers: Increased flecainide and propranolol levels by 20% to 30%. Watch for propranolol and flecainide toxicity.
Urine acidifying and alkalinizing drugs: Causes extremes of urine pH, which may alter flecainide excretion. Monitor patient for flecainide toxicity or decreased effectiveness.
Drug-lifestyle. *Smoking:* Decreased flecainide levels. Monitor patient closely.

EFFECTS ON LAB TEST RESULTS
None reported.

CONTRAINDICATIONS
Contraindicated in patients hypersensitive to drug and in those with second- or third-degree AV block or right bundle-branch block with a left hemiblock (in the absence of an artificial pacemaker), recent MI, or cardiogenic shock.

NURSING CONSIDERATIONS
● Use cautiously in patients with heart failure, cardiomyopathy, severe renal or hepatic disease, prolonged QT interval, sick sinus syndrome, or blood dyscrasia.
● When used to prevent ventricular arrhythmias, drug should be reserved for patients with documented life-threatening arrhythmias.
● Check that pacing threshold was determined 1 week before and after starting therapy in a patient with a pacemaker; flecainide can alter endocardial pacing thresholds.
● Correct hypokalemia or hyperkalemia before giving flecainide because these electrolyte disturbances may alter drug's effect.

Reactions may be *common*, uncommon, **life-threatening**, or COMMON AND LIFE-THREATENING.

• Monitor ECG rhythm for proarrhythmic effects.

• Most patients can be adequately maintained on an every-12-hour dosing schedule, but some need to receive flecainide every 8 hours.

• Make dosage adjustments only once every 3 to 4 days.

• Monitor flecainide levels, especially if patient has renal or heart failure. Therapeutic flecainide levels range from 0.2 to 1 mcg/ml. Risk of adverse effects increases when trough blood levels exceed 1 mcg/ml.

PATIENT TEACHING

• Stress importance of taking drug exactly as prescribed.

• Instruct patient to report adverse reactions promptly and to limit fluid and sodium intake to minimize fluid retention.

• Tell patient receiving drug I.V. to report discomfort at insertion site.

---

ibutilide fumarate
Corvert

Pregnancy risk category C

AVAILABLE FORMS
Injection: 0.1 mg/ml in 10-ml vials

INDICATIONS & DOSAGES
➤ **Rapid conversion of atrial fibrillation or atrial flutter of recent onset to sinus rhythm—**
Adults weighing 60 kg (132 lb) or more: 1 mg I.V. over 10 minutes.
Adults weighing less than 60 kg: 0.01 mg/ kg I.V. over 10 minutes.

I.V. ADMINISTRATION
• Drug may be given undiluted or diluted in 50 ml of diluent, and may be added to normal saline solution for injection or D_5W before infusion. Contents of 10-ml vial (0.1 mg/ml) may be added to 50-ml infusion bag to form admixture of about 0.017 mg/ml ibutilide. Use aseptic technique. Drug can be used with polyvinyl chloride plastic bags or polyolefin bags.
• Give drug over 10 minutes.

• *Alert:* Stop infusion if arrhythmia is terminated or patient develops ventricular tachycardia or marked prolongation of QT or QTc interval. If arrhythmia isn't terminated 10 minutes after infusion ends, may give a second 10-minute infusion of equal strength.

• Admixtures with approved diluents are stable for 24 hours at room temperature; 48 hours if refrigerated.

• Don't infuse parenteral products that contain particulate matter or are discolored.

ACTION
Prolongs action potential in isolated cardiac myocyte and increases atrial and ventricular refractoriness, namely class III electrophysiologic effects.

Route	Onset	Peak	Duration
I.V.	Unknown	Unknown	Unknown

ADVERSE REACTIONS
CNS: headache.
CV: ventricular extrasystoles, nonsustained ventricular tachycardia, hypotension, bundle-branch block, ***sustained polymorphic ventricular tachycardia, AV block, heart failure,*** hypertension, prolonged QT interval, ***bradycardia,*** palpitations, tachycardia.
GI: nausea.

INTERACTIONS
Drug-drug. *Class IA antiarrhythmics (disopyramide, procainamide, quinidine), other class III drugs (amiodarone, sotalol):* Increased potential for prolonged refractoriness. Don't give these drugs for at least 5 half-lives before and 4 hours after ibutilide dose.
Digoxin: Supraventricular arrhythmias may mask cardiotoxicity from excessive digoxin levels. Use cautiously.
H_1-receptor antagonist antihistamines, phenothiazines, tetracyclic antidepressants, TCAs, other drugs that prolong QT interval: Increased risk for proarrhythmia. Monitor patient closely.

EFFECTS ON LAB TEST RESULTS
None reported.

CONTRAINDICATIONS

Contraindicated in patients hypersensitive to drug or its components.

NURSING CONSIDERATIONS

• Drug isn't recommended in patients with history of polymorphic ventricular tachycardia and in breast-feeding women.
• Use cautiously in patients with hepatic or renal dysfunction.
• Safety of drug hasn't been established in children.
• Drug should be given only by skilled personnel. Cardiac monitor, intracardiac pacing, cardioverter or defibrillator, and medication for sustained ventricular tachycardia must be available.
• Before therapy, correct hypokalemia and hypomagnesemia to reduce proarrhythmia potential. Patients with atrial fibrillation of longer than 2 to 3 days' duration must be adequately anticoagulated, generally over at least 2 weeks.
• Monitor ECG continuously during administration and for at least 4 hours afterward or until QTc interval returns to baseline; drug can induce or worsen ventricular arrhythmias. Longer monitoring is required if ECG shows arrhythmia or in patients with hepatic insufficiency.
• Don't give class IA or other class III antiarrhythmics with ibutilide infusion or for 4 hours afterward.

PATIENT TEACHING

• Tell patient to report adverse reactions promptly.
• Instruct patient to alert nurse of discomfort at injection site.

---

lidocaine hydrochloride (lignocaine hydrochloride)
LidoPen Auto-Injector, Xylocaine, Xylocard†‡

Pregnancy risk category B

AVAILABLE FORMS

Infusion (premixed): 0.2% (2 mg/ml), 0.4% (4 mg/ml), 0.8% (8 mg/ml)
Injection (for direct I.V. use): 1% (10 mg/ml), 2% (20 mg/ml)
Injection (for I.M. use): 300 mg/3 ml automatic injection device

Injection (for I.V. admixtures): 4% (40 mg/ml), 10% (100 mg/ml), 20% (200 mg/ml)

INDICATIONS & DOSAGES

➤ **Ventricular arrhythmias caused by MI, cardiac manipulation, or cardiac glycosides—**
Adults: 50 to 100 mg (1 to 1.5 mg/kg) by I.V. bolus at 25 to 50 mg/minute. Bolus dose is repeated q 3 to 5 minutes until arrhythmias subside or adverse reactions develop. Don't exceed 300-mg total bolus during a 1-hour period. Simultaneously, constant infusion of 20 to 50 mcg/kg/minute (1 to 4 mg/minute) is begun. If single bolus has been given, smaller bolus dose may be repeated 15 to 20 minutes after start of infusion to maintain therapeutic level. Or, 200 to 300 mg I.M.; then second I.M. dose 60 to 90 minutes later, if needed.
Children: 0.5 to 1 mg/kg by I.V. bolus; then infusion of 10 to 50 mcg/kg/minute.
Elderly patients: Reduce dosage and rate of infusion by 50%.
Adjust-a-dose: For patients with heart failure, renal or liver disease, or who weigh less than 50 kg (110 lb), use reduced dosage.

I.V. ADMINISTRATION

• Lidocaine injections (additive syringes and single-use vials) containing 40, 100, or 200 mg/ml are for the preparation of I.V. infusion solutions only and must be diluted before use.
• Prepare I.V. infusion by adding 1 g of lidocaine hydrochloride (using 25 ml of 4% or 5 ml of 20% injection) to 1 L of D_5W injection to provide a solution containing 1 mg/ml.
• A more concentrated solution of up to 8 mg/ml may be used if patient is fluid restricted.
• Patients receiving infusions must be on a cardiac monitor and must be attended at all times. Use an infusion control device for giving infusion precisely. Don't exceed 4 mg/minute; faster rate greatly increases risk of toxicity.
• Injections containing preservatives shouldn't be given I.V.

ACTION
A class IB antiarrhythmic that decreases the depolarization, automaticity, and excitability in the ventricles during the diastolic phase by direct action on the tissues, especially the Purkinje network.

Route	Onset	Peak	Duration
I.M.	5-15 min	10 min	2 hr
I.V.	Immediate	Immediate	10-20 min

ADVERSE REACTIONS
CNS: *confusion, tremor,* lethargy, somnolence, *stupor, restlessness,* anxiety, hallucinations, nervousness, *light-headedness,* paresthesia, muscle twitching, *seizures.*
CV: *hypotension, bradycardia, new or worsened arrhythmias, cardiac arrest.*
EENT: *tinnitus, blurred or double vision.*
GI: vomiting.
Respiratory: *respiratory depression and arrest.*
Other: *anaphylaxis,* soreness at injection site, sensation of cold.

INTERACTIONS
Drug-drug. *Beta blockers, cimetidine:* Decreased metabolism of lidocaine. Monitor patient for toxicity.
Mexiletine, tocainide: Increased pharmacologic effects. Avoid using together.
Phenytoin, procainamide, propranolol, quinidine: Increased cardiac depressant effects. Monitor patient closely.
Succinylcholine: Prolonged neuromuscular blockade may occur. Monitor patient closely.
Drug-herb. *Pareira:* May increase the effects of neuromuscular blockade. Discourage use together.
Drug-lifestyle. *Smoking:* May increase metabolism of lidocaine. Monitor patient closely.

EFFECTS ON LAB TEST RESULTS
None reported.

CONTRAINDICATIONS
Contraindicated in patients hypersensitive to the amide-type local anesthetics and in those with Adams-Stokes syndrome, Wolff-Parkinson-White syndrome, and severe degrees of SA, AV, or intraventricular block in the absence of an artificial pacemaker.

NURSING CONSIDERATIONS
• Use cautiously and in reduced dosages in patients with complete or second-degree heart block or sinus bradycardia, in elderly patients, in those with heart failure or renal or hepatic disease, and in those weighing less than 110 lb (50 kg).
• Give I.M. injections in the deltoid muscle only.
• Monitor isoenzymes when using I.M. drug for suspected MI. A patient who has received I.M. lidocaine will show a seven-fold increase in CK level. Such an increase originates in the skeletal muscle, not the heart.
• Monitor levels. Therapeutic levels are 2 to 5 mcg/ml.
• **Alert:** Monitor patient for toxicity. In many severely ill patients, seizures may be the first sign of toxicity. However, severe reactions are usually preceded by somnolence, confusion, tremors, and paresthesia.
• If signs of toxicity such as dizziness occur, stop drug at once and notify prescriber. Continuing could lead to seizures and coma. Give oxygen via nasal cannula if not contraindicated. Keep oxygen and cardiopulmonary resuscitation equipment available.
• Monitor patient's response, especially blood pressure and electrolytes, BUN, and creatinine levels. Notify prescriber promptly if abnormalities develop.
• Stop infusion and notify prescriber if arrhythmias worsen or ECG changes, such as widening QRS complex or substantially prolonged PR interval, are evident.

PATIENT TEACHING
• Tell patient receiving lidocaine I.M. that drug may cause soreness at injection site. Tell him to report discomfort at the site.
• Tell patient to report adverse reactions promptly because toxicity can occur.

---

mexiletine hydrochloride
Mexitil

Pregnancy risk category C

AVAILABLE FORMS
Capsules: 50 mg‡, 100 mg†, 150 mg, 200 mg, 250 mg
Injection: 250 mg/10 ml‡

INDICATIONS & DOSAGES
➤ **Refractory life-threatening ventricular arrhythmias, including ventricular tachycardia and PVCs—**
Adults: 200 to 400 mg P.O.; then 200 mg q 8 hours. Dosage may be increased q 2 to 3 days to 400 mg q 8 hours if satisfactory control isn't obtained. Patients who respond well to a q-12-hour schedule may be given up to 450 mg q 12 hours.

Note: Where available, mexiletine may be given I.V.
Adults: Loading dose is 100 to 250 mg I.V. at 25 mg/minute. Then prepare an infusion solution of 250 mg mexiletine in 500 ml of D_5W, and give the first 120 ml (60 mg) over 1 hour. If clinical response is inadequate, give another bolus of 200 mg over 10 to 20 minutes. Maintenance dose is 0.5 mg/minute (1 ml/minute of prepared solution).

I.V. ADMINISTRATION
• Mexiletine injection is compatible with normal saline, D_5W, 5% sodium bicarbonate, 1/6 M sodium lactate, and 10% fructose (levulose) solutions.
• Give I.V. dose during continuous ECG monitoring.

ACTION
A class IB antiarrhythmic that blocks the fast sodium channel in cardiac tissues, especially the Purkinje network, without involving the autonomic nervous system. Drug reduces the rate of rise and amplitude of the action potential and decreases automaticity in the Purkinje fibers. It also shortens the duration of the action potential and, to a lesser extent, decreases the effective refractory period in the Purkinje fibers.

Route	Onset	Peak	Duration
I.V.	Immediate	Immediate	Unknown
P.O.	0.5-2 hr	2-3 hr	Unknown

ADVERSE REACTIONS
CNS: *tremor, dizziness,* confusion, *lightheadedness, incoordination,* changes in sleep habits, paresthesia, weakness, fatigue, speech difficulties, depression, *nervousness,* headache.

CV: NEW OR WORSENED ARRHYTHMIAS, palpitations, chest pain, nonspecific edema, angina.
EENT: blurred vision, diplopia, tinnitus.
GI: *nausea, vomiting, upper GI distress, heartburn,* diarrhea, constipation, dry mouth, changes in appetite, abdominal pain.
Skin: rash.

INTERACTIONS
Drug-drug. *Antacids, atropine, narcotics:* Slowed mexiletine absorption. Monitor patient.
Cimetidine: Increased or decreased mexiletine blood levels. Monitor patient.
Methylxanthines (such as caffeine, theophylline): Reduced clearance of methylxanthines, possibly resulting in toxicity. Monitor patient carefully.
Metoclopramide: Accelerated mexiletine absorption. Monitor patient for toxicity.
Phenobarbital, phenytoin, rifampin, urine acidifiers: Decreased mexiletine blood levels. Monitor patient carefully.
Urine alkalinizers: Increased mexiletine blood levels. Monitor patient carefully.

EFFECTS ON LAB TEST RESULTS
• May increase AST level.

CONTRAINDICATIONS
Contraindicated in patients with cardiogenic shock or second- or third-degree AV block in the absence of an artificial pacemaker.

NURSING CONSIDERATIONS
• Use cautiously in patients with first-degree heart block, a ventricular pacemaker, sinus node dysfunction, intraventricular conduction disturbances, hypotension, severe heart failure, or seizure disorder.
• *Alert:* When rapid control of ventricular arrhythmias is essential, use 400 mg P.O. initial loading dose.
• When changing from lidocaine to mexiletine, stop the lidocaine infusion when the first mexiletine dose is given. Keep the infusion line open, however, until the arrhythmia is satisfactorily controlled.
• Give oral dose with meals or antacids to lessen GI distress.

• If patient may be a good candidate for every-12-hour therapy, notify prescriber. Twice-daily dosage enhances compliance.
• Monitor therapeutic levels. Levels range from 0.5 to 2 mcg/ml.
• An early sign of mexiletine toxicity is tremor, usually a fine tremor of the hands, progressing to dizziness and then to ataxia and nystagmus as drug level in the blood increases. Watch for and ask patients about these symptoms.
• Monitor blood pressure and heart rate and rhythm frequently. Notify prescriber of significant change.

PATIENT TEACHING
• Tell patient to take drug exactly as prescribed and to take with food or antacids if GI reactions occur.
• Instruct patient to report adverse reactions promptly.
• Advise patient to notify prescriber if he develops jaundice, fever, or general tiredness; these symptoms may indicate liver damage.
• Tell patient receiving drug I.V. to report discomfort at insertion site.

moricizine hydrochloride
Ethmozine

Pregnancy risk category B

AVAILABLE FORMS
Tablets: 200 mg, 250 mg, 300 mg

INDICATIONS & DOSAGES
➤ **Life-threatening ventricular arrhythmias—**
Adults: Individualized dosage is based on clinical response and patient tolerance. Therapy should begin in the hospital. Most patients respond to 600 to 900 mg P.O. daily in divided doses q 8 hours. Daily dose may be increased q 3 days by 150 mg until desired effect is seen.
Adjust-a-dose: For patients with hepatic or renal impairment, 600 mg or less P.O. daily.

ACTION
A class I antiarrhythmic that reduces the fast inward current carried by sodium ions across myocardial cell membranes. Drug has potent local anesthetic activity and membrane-stabilizing effect.

Route	Onset	Peak	Duration
P.O.	Unknown	0.5-2 hr	10-24 hr

ADVERSE REACTIONS
CNS: *dizziness,* headache, fatigue, hyperesthesia, anxiety, asthenia, depression, nervousness, paresthesia, sleep disorders.
CV: *ventricular tachycardia, PVCs, supraventricular arrhythmias,* ECG abnormalities including conduction defects, sinus pause, junctional rhythm, and AV block, **heart failure,** palpitations, thrombophlebitis, chest pain, *cardiac death,* hypotension, hypertension, vasodilation, cerebrovascular events.
EENT: blurred vision.
GI: nausea, vomiting, abdominal pain, dyspepsia, diarrhea, dry mouth.
GU: urine retention, urinary frequency, dysuria.
Musculoskeletal: musculoskeletal pain.
Respiratory: dyspnea.
Skin: rash, diaphoresis.
Other: drug-induced fever.

INTERACTIONS
Drug-drug. *Cimetidine:* Increased plasma levels and decreased clearance of moricizine. Begin moricizine therapy at low dosage (not more than 600 mg daily), and monitor plasma levels and therapeutic effect closely.
Digoxin, propranolol: Additive prolongation of PR interval. Watch patient closely.
Theophylline: Increased clearance and reduced plasma levels of theophylline. Monitor plasma levels and therapeutic response; adjust theophylline dosage, as needed.

EFFECTS ON LAB TEST RESULTS
• May increase liver function test result values.

CONTRAINDICATIONS
Contraindicated in patients hypersensitive to drug, cardiogenic shock, or second- or third-degree AV block or right bundle-branch block with left hemiblock (bifascicular block) unless an artificial pacemaker is present.

NURSING CONSIDERATIONS
• Because drug appears in breast milk, the decision to stop breast-feeding or stop taking the drug depends on potential benefit of therapy to mother.
• Use with extreme caution in patients with sick sinus syndrome because drug may cause sinus bradycardia or sinus arrest. Also use with extreme caution in patients with coronary artery disease and left ventricular dysfunction because these patients may be at risk for sudden death when treated with the drug.
• Monitor patients with heart failure carefully for worsening of heart failure.
• Patients with hepatic or renal dysfunction will have decreased moricizine clearance. Give drug cautiously and monitor effects closely.
• When substituting moricizine for another antiarrhythmic, previous drug should be withdrawn for one to two of the drug's half-lives before moricizine is started. Patients who have shown a tendency to develop life-threatening arrhythmias after withdrawal of previous antiarrhythmic should be hospitalized during withdrawal and adjustment to moricizine. Guidelines for when to start moricizine therapy are as follows: disopyramide, 6 to 12 hours after last dose; flecainide, 12 to 24 hours after last dose; mexiletine, 8 to 12 hours after last dose; procainamide, 3 to 6 hours after last dose; propafenone, 8 to 12 hours after last dose; quinidine, 6 to 12 hours after last dose; and tocainide, 8 to 12 hours after last dose.
• Determine electrolyte status and correct imbalances before therapy, as prescribed. Hypokalemia, hyperkalemia, and hypomagnesemia may alter drug's effects.
• *Alert:* Don't confuse Ethmozine with Erythrocin.

PATIENT TEACHING
• Inform patient that he'll need to be hospitalized for start of therapy.
• Instruct patient to take drug exactly as prescribed and not to abruptly stop use.
• Tell patient to avoid hazardous activities if adverse CNS reactions or blurred vision occurs.
• Instruct patient to report persistent or serious adverse reactions promptly.

procainamide hydrochloride
Procanbid, Pronestyl**, Pronestyl-SR

Pregnancy risk category C

AVAILABLE FORMS
Capsules: 250 mg, 375 mg, 500 mg
Injection: 100 mg/ml, 500 mg/ml
Tablets: 250 mg, 375 mg, 500 mg
Tablets (extended-release): 250 mg, 500 mg, 750 mg, 1,000 mg

INDICATIONS & DOSAGES
➤ **Life-threatening ventricular arrhythmias—**
Adults: 50 to 100 mg by slow I.V. push q 5 minutes, no faster than 25 to 50 mg/ minute until arrhythmias disappear, adverse reactions develop, or 500 mg has been given. Or, give a loading dose I.V. infusion of 500 to 600 mg over 25 to 30 minutes. Usual effective dose is 500 to 600 mg. When arrhythmias disappear, give continuous infusion of 1 to 6 mg/ minute. If arrhythmias recur, repeat bolus as above and increase infusion rate. Or, give 50 mg/kg I.M. in divided doses q 3 to 6 hours until oral therapy begins.
For P.O. administration, give 50 mg/kg daily in divided doses q 3 hours (average is 250 to 500 mg q 3 hours); for extended-release tablets, give 50 mg/kg daily in divided doses q 6 hours. For Procanbid extended-release tablets, give 50 mg/kg daily in equally divided doses q 12 hours.
Adjust-a-dose: For patients with renal or hepatic dysfunction, decreased dosages or longer dosing intervals may be needed.

I.V. ADMINISTRATION
• Dilute with compatible I.V. solution such as D_5W injection and give with the patient in supine position at a rate not exceeding 25 to 50 mg/minute.
• Note that vials for I.V. injection contain 1 g of drug: 100 mg/ml (10 ml) or 500 mg/ml (2 ml).
• Attend patient receiving infusions at all times. Use an infusion control device to give infusion precisely.
• *Alert:* Monitor blood pressure and ECG continuously during I.V. administration. Watch for prolonged QT intervals and

---

Reactions may be *common,* uncommon, *life-threatening,* or COMMON AND LIFE-THREATENING.

QRS complexes, heart block, or increased arrhythmias. If they occur, withhold drug, obtain rhythm strip, and notify prescriber immediately.

• Keep patient in supine position during I.V. administration. If drug is given too rapidly, hypotension can occur. Watch closely for adverse reactions during infusion, and notify prescriber if they occur.

• Drug will invalidate bentiromide test results; discontinue at least 3 days before bentiromide test. Procainamide may alter edrophonium test results, and may cause positive antinuclear antibody (ANA) titers, positive direct antiglobulin (Coombs') tests, and ECG changes.

ACTION

A class IA antiarrhythmic that decreases excitability, conduction velocity, automaticity, and membrane responsiveness with prolonged refractory period. Larger than usual doses may induce AV block.

Route	Onset	Peak	Duration
I.M.	10-30 min	15-60 min	Unknown
I.V.	Immediate	Immediate	Unknown
P.O.	Unknown	90-120 min	Unknown

ADVERSE REACTIONS

CNS: hallucinations, psychosis, giddiness, confusion, *seizures,* depression, dizziness.
CV: hypotension, *bradycardia, AV block, ventricular fibrillation, ventricular asystole.*
GI: abdominal pain, nausea, vomiting, anorexia, diarrhea, bitter taste.
Skin: *maculopapular rash, urticaria, pruritus, flushing, angioneurotic edema.*
Other: *fever, lupuslike syndrome.*

INTERACTIONS

Drug-drug. *Amiodarone:* Increased procainamide levels and toxicity; additive effects on QT interval and QRS complex. Avoid using together.
Anticholinergics: Increased antivagal effects. Monitor patient closely.
Anticholinesterases: May decrease effect of anticholinesterases. Anticholinesterase dosage may need to be increased.

Beta blockers, cimetidine, ranitidine, trimethoprim: May increase procainamide blood levels. Watch for toxicity.
Neuromuscular blockers: Increased skeletal muscle relaxant effects. Monitor patient closely.
Drug-herb. *Jimsonweed:* May adversely affect CV function. Discourage use together.
Licorice: May prolong QT interval and be additive. Urge caution.
Drug-lifestyle. *Alcohol use:* Reduced drug levels. Discourage use together.

EFFECTS ON LAB TEST RESULTS

• May increase ALT, AST, alkaline phosphatase, LDH, and bilirubin levels.

CONTRAINDICATIONS

Contraindicated in patients hypersensitive to procaine and related drugs and in those with complete, second-, or third-degree heart block in the absence of an artificial pacemaker. Also contraindicated in those with myasthenia gravis, systemic lupus erythematosus, or atypical ventricular tachycardia (torsades de pointes).

NURSING CONSIDERATIONS

• Use with extreme caution when treating patients with ventricular tachycardia during coronary occlusion.

• Use cautiously in patients with heart failure or other conduction disturbances, such as bundle-branch heart block, sinus bradycardia, or digitalis intoxication, and in those with hepatic or renal insufficiency. Also use cautiously in patients with blood dyscrasias or bone marrow suppression.

• Monitor plasma levels of procainamide and its active metabolite NAPA. To suppress ventricular arrhythmias, therapeutic levels of procainamide are 4 to 8 mcg/ml; therapeutic levels of NAPA are 10 to 30 mcg/ml.

• Monitor QT interval closely in patients with renal failure.

• Hypokalemia predisposes patient to arrhythmias. Monitor electrolytes, especially potassium level.

• Elderly patients may be more likely to develop hypotension. Monitor blood pressure carefully.

● Monitor CBC frequently during first 3 months of therapy.
● Positive ANA titer is common in about 60% of patients who don't have symptoms of lupuslike syndrome. This response seems to be related to prolonged use, not dosage. May progress to systemic lupus erythematosus if drug isn't stopped.
● *Alert:* Don't confuse procainamide with probenecid.

PATIENT TEACHING
● Stress importance of taking drug exactly as prescribed. This may require use of an alarm clock for nighttime doses.
● Instruct patient to report fever, rash, muscle pain, diarrhea, bleeding, bruises, or pleuritic chest pain.
● Tell patient not to crush or break extended-release tablets.
● Reassure patient who is taking extended-release form that a wax-matrix "ghost" from the tablet may be passed in stools. Drug is completely absorbed before this occurs.

---

quinidine bisulfate
(66.4% quinidine base), Kinidin Durules‡

quinidine gluconate
(62% quinidine base) Quinaglute Dura-Tabs, Quinate†

quinidine polygalacturonate
(60.5% quinidine base) Cardioquin

quinidine sulfate
(83% quinidine base) Apo-Quinidine†, Cin-Quin, Novoquinidin†, Quinidex Extentabs, Quinora

Pregnancy risk category C

AVAILABLE FORMS
quinidine bisulfate
Tablets (extended-release): 250 mg†‡
quinidine gluconate
Injection: 80 mg/ml
Tablets (extended-release): 324 mg, 325 mg†

quinidine polygalacturonate
Tablets: 275 mg
quinidine sulfate
Injection: 200 mg/ml†
Tablets: 200 mg, 300 mg
Tablets (extended-release): 300 mg

INDICATIONS & DOSAGES
➤ **Atrial flutter or fibrillation—**
Adults: 300 to 400 mg quinidine sulfate or equivalent base P.O. q 6 hours. Or, 200 mg P.O. q 2 to 3 hours for 5 to 8 doses, increased daily until sinus rhythm is restored or toxic effects develop. Maximum, 3 to 4 g daily.
➤ **Paroxysmal supraventricular tachycardia—**
Adults: 400 to 600 mg P.O. gluconate q 2 to 3 hours until toxic adverse reactions develop or arrhythmia subsides.
➤ **Premature atrial and ventricular contractions, paroxysmal AV junctional rhythm, paroxysmal atrial tachycardia, paroxysmal ventricular tachycardia, maintenance after cardioversion of atrial fibrillation or flutter—**
Adults: Test dose is 200 mg P.O. or I.M. Quinidine sulfate or equivalent base 200 to 400 mg P.O. q 4 to 6 hours or 600 mg quinidine sulfate extended-release every 8 to 12 hours; or quinidine gluconate 800 mg (10 ml of commercially available solution) added to 40 ml of D_5W, infused I.V. at 2.5 mg/kg/minute.
➤ **Severe *Plasmodium falciparum* malaria—**
Adults: 10 mg/kg gluconate I.V. diluted in 250 ml normal saline solution and infused over 1 to 2 hours; then continuous infusion of 0.02 mg/kg/minute for 72 hours or until parasitemia is reduced to less than 1%.
Adjust-a-dose: Use reduced dosage for patients with impaired hepatic function or heart failure.

I.V. ADMINISTRATION
● For quinidine gluconate infusion to treat atrial fibrillation or flutter in adults, dilute 800 mg (10 ml of injection) with 40 ml D_5W and infuse at up to 0.25 mg/kg/minute.
● During infusion, continuously monitor patient's blood pressure and ECG.

Reactions may be *common*, uncommon, *life-threatening*, or COMMON AND LIFE-THREATENING.

• Titrate rate so that the arrhythmia is corrected without disturbing the normal mechanism of the heart beat.
• For quinidine gluconate infusion to treat malaria, dilute in 5 ml/kg (usually 250 ml) normal saline solution and infuse over 1 to 2 hours, followed by a continuous maintenance infusion.

ACTION
A class IA antiarrhythmic that has both direct and indirect (anticholinergic) effects on cardiac tissue. Drug decreases automaticity, conduction velocity, and membrane responsiveness. The effective refractory period is prolonged, and the anticholinergic action reduces vagal tone.

Route	Onset	Peak	Duration
I.M.	0.5-1.5 min	Unknown	Unknown
I.V.	Immediate	Immediate	Unknown
P.O.	1-3 hr	1-6 hr	6-8 hr

ADVERSE REACTIONS
CNS: *vertigo, headache,* ataxia, *lightheadedness,* confusion, depression, dementia.
CV: *PVCs, ventricular tachycardia, atypical ventricular tachycardia, hypotension, complete AV block,* tachycardia, *aggravated heart failure, ECG changes.*
EENT: *tinnitus,* blurred vision, diplopia, photophobia.
GI: *diarrhea, nausea, vomiting,* anorexia, excessive salivation, abdominal pain.
Hematologic: *hemolytic anemia, thrombocytopenia, agranulocytosis.*
Hepatic: *hepatotoxicity.*
Respiratory: acute asthmatic attack, *respiratory arrest.*
Skin: rash, petechial hemorrhage of buccal mucosa, pruritus, urticaria, lupus erythematosus, photosensitivity.
Other: *angioedema, fever, cinchonism.*

INTERACTIONS
Drug-drug. *Acetazolamide, antacids, sodium bicarbonate, thiazide diuretics:* May increase quinidine blood levels because of alkaline urine. Monitor patient for increased effect.
Amiodarone, cimetidine: Increased quinidine levels. Monitor patient for increased arrhythmias.

Barbiturates, phenytoin, rifampin: May lower blood levels of quinidine. Monitor patient for decreased effect.
Digoxin: Increased digoxin levels after initiating quinidine therapy. Monitor digoxin levels.
Fluvoxamine, nefazodone, TCAs: Increased blood levels of antidepressants with increased effect. Monitor patient closely.
Nifedipine: May decrease quinidine blood levels. Dosage adjustment may be needed.
Other antiarrhythmics (such as lidocaine, procainamide, propranolol): Increased risk of toxicity. Use together cautiously.
Verapamil: Decreased quinidine clearance. May cause hypotension, bradycardia, AV block, or pulmonary edema. Monitor blood pressure and heart rate.
Warfarin: Increased anticoagulant effect. Monitor patient closely.
Drug-herb. *Jimsonweed:* May adversely affect CV function. Discourage use together.
Licorice: May prolong QT interval and be additive. Advise caution.
Drug-food. *Grapefruit juice:* Inhibits metabolism. Tell patient not to take drug with grapefruit juice.

EFFECTS ON LAB TEST RESULTS
• May decrease hemoglobin and platelet and granulocyte counts.

CONTRAINDICATIONS
Contraindicated in patients with idiosyncrasy or hypersensitivity to quinidine or related cinchona derivatives and in those with myasthenia gravis, intraventricular conduction defects, digitalis toxicity when AV conduction is grossly impaired, abnormal rhythms caused by escape mechanisms, and history of prolonged QT interval syndrome. Also contraindicated in patients who developed thrombocytopenia after exposure to quinidine or quinine.

NURSING CONSIDERATIONS
• Use cautiously in patients with asthma, muscle weakness, or infection accompanied by fever because hypersensitivity reactions to drug may be masked.
• Also use cautiously in patients with hepatic or renal impairment because systemic accumulation may occur.

● Check apical pulse rate and blood pressure before therapy. If extremes in pulse rate are detected, withhold drug and notify prescriber at once.

● *Alert:* For atrial fibrillation or flutter, give quinidine only after AV node has been blocked with a beta blocker, digoxin, or a calcium channel blocker to avoid increasing AV conduction.

● Anticoagulant therapy is commonly advised before quinidine therapy in long-standing atrial fibrillation because restoration of normal sinus rhythm may result in thromboembolism caused by dislodgment of thrombi from atrial wall.

● Monitor patient for atypical ventricular tachycardia such as torsades de pointes and ECG changes, particularly widening of QRS complex, widened QT and PR intervals.

● *Alert:* When changing route of administration or oral salt form, prescriber should alter dosage to compensate for variations in quinidine base content.

● Never use discolored (brownish) quinidine solution.

● Quinidine gluconate I.M. is no longer recommended for treatment of arrhythmias because of erratic absorption.

● *Alert:* Patients with severe malaria should be hospitalized in an intensive-care setting. Continuous monitoring is needed. Decrease infusion rate if plasma quinidine level exceeds 6 mcg/ml, uncorrected QT interval exceeds 0.6 second, or QRS complex widening exceeds 25% of baseline.

● Monitor liver function test results during first 4 to 8 weeks of therapy.

● Monitor quinidine levels. Therapeutic plasma levels for antiarrhythmic effects are 2 to 5 mcg/ml.

● Monitor patient response carefully. If adverse GI reactions occur, especially diarrhea, notify prescriber. Check quinidine blood levels, which are toxic when greater than 8 mcg/ml. GI symptoms may be decreased by giving drug with meals or aluminum hydroxide antacids.

● Store drug away from heat and direct light.

● *Alert:* Don't confuse quinidine with quinine or clonidine.

PATIENT TEACHING

● Stress importance of taking drug exactly as prescribed and taking it with food if adverse GI reactions occur.

● Instruct patient not to crush or chew extended-release tablets.

● Tell patient to avoid grapefruit juice (inhibits metabolism) and significant changes in dietary salt intake (may affect quinidine absorption).

● Advise patient to report persistent or serious adverse reactions promptly, especially signs and symptoms of quinidine toxicity.

---

sotalol hydrochloride
Beta-Cardone§, Betapace, Betapace AF, Sotacort†‡

Pregnancy risk category B

AVAILABLE FORMS
Tablets: 80 mg, 120 mg, 160 mg, 240 mg (Betapace AF only)

INDICATIONS & DOSAGES
Betapace
➤ **Documented, life-threatening ventricular arrhythmias—**
Adults: Initially, 80 mg P.O. b.i.d. Dosage is increased q 2 to 3 days as needed and tolerated; most patients respond to daily dose of 160 to 320 mg. A few patients with refractory arrhythmias have received as much as 640 mg daily.
Adjust-a-dose: For patients with renal impairment, if creatinine clearance is more than 60 ml/minute, no adjustment in dosage interval is needed. If clearance is 30 to 60 ml/minute, dosage interval is increased to q 24 hours; if clearance is between 10 and 30 ml/minute, q 36 to 48 hours; and if clearance is less than 10 ml/minute, dosage must be individualized.
Betapace AF
➤ **Maintenance of normal sinus rhythm or delay in time to recurrence of atrial fibrillation or atrial flutter in patients with symptomatic atrial fibrillation or atrial flutter who are currently in sinus rhythm—**
Adults: 80 mg P.O. b.i.d. Dosage may be increased as needed to 120 mg P.O. b.i.d.

Reactions may be *common,* uncommon, *life-threatening,* or COMMON AND LIFE-THREATENING.

after 3 days if the QT interval is less than 500 msec. Maximum dose is 160 mg P.O. b.i.d.

Adjust-a-dose: In patients with creatinine clearance of 40 to 60 ml/minute, increase dosage interval to q 24 hours.

ACTION

A nonselective beta blocker that depresses sinus heart rate, slows AV conduction, decreases cardiac output, and lowers systolic and diastolic blood pressure.

Route	Onset	Peak	Duration
P.O.	Unknown	2.5-4 hr	Unknown

ADVERSE REACTIONS

CNS: *asthenia, headache, dizziness, weakness, fatigue,* sleep problems, *lightheadedness.*

CV: *bradycardia, arrhythmias, heart failure, AV block, proarrhythmic events (including polymorphic ventricular tachycardia, PVCs, ventricular fibrillation),* edema, *palpitations, chest pain,* ECG abnormalities, hypotension.

GI: *nausea, vomiting,* diarrhea, dyspepsia.

Metabolic: hyperglycemia.

Respiratory: *dyspnea, bronchospasm.*

INTERACTIONS

Drug-drug. *Antiarrhythmics:* Increased drug effects. Avoid using together.

Antihypertensives, catecholamine-depleting drugs (such as guanethidine, reserpine): Increased hypotensive effects. Monitor patient closely.

Calcium channel blockers: Increased myocardial depression. Avoid using together.

Clonidine: Beta blockers may enhance rebound effect after withdrawal of clonidine. Stop sotalol several days before withdrawing clonidine.

General anesthetics: May increase myocardial depression. Monitor patient closely.

Insulin, oral antidiabetics: May cause hyperglycemia. May mask signs and symptoms of hypoglycemia. Adjust dosage accordingly.

Drug-food. *Any food:* Decreased absorption by 20%. Give drug on empty stomach.

EFFECTS ON LAB TEST RESULTS

● May increase glucose level.

CONTRAINDICATIONS

Contraindicated in patients hypersensitive to drug and in those with severe sinus node dysfunction, sinus bradycardia, second- and third-degree AV block in the absence of an artificial pacemaker, congenital or acquired long QT interval syndrome, cardiogenic shock, uncontrolled heart failure, and bronchial asthma.

NURSING CONSIDERATIONS

● Use cautiously in patients with renal impairment or diabetes mellitus. Beta blockers may mask signs and symptoms of hypoglycemia.

● Because proarrhythmic events may occur at start of therapy and during dosage adjustments, patient should be hospitalized for a minimum of 3 days. Facilities and personnel should be available for cardiac rhythm monitoring and interpretation of ECG.

● Assess patient for new or worsened symptoms of heart failure.

● Although patients receiving I.V. lidocaine have started sotalol therapy without ill effect, other antiarrhythmics should be withdrawn before therapy with sotalol. Sotalol therapy typically is delayed until two or three half-lives of the withdrawn drug have elapsed. After withdrawal of amiodarone, sotalol shouldn't be given until the QT interval normalizes.

● Dosage should be adjusted slowly, allowing 2 to 3 days between dosage increments for adequate monitoring of QT intervals and for plasma levels of drug to reach a steady-state level.

● Drug may cause a false-positive catecholamine level.

● **Alert:** Don't substitute Betapace for Betapace AF.

● Monitor electrolytes regularly, especially if patient is receiving diuretics. Electrolyte imbalances, such as hypokalemia or hypomagnesemia, may enhance QT-interval prolongation and increase the risk of serious arrhythmias such as torsades de pointes.

● **Alert:** Don't confuse sotalol with Statrol or Stadol.

---

*Liquid contains alcohol. **May contain tartrazine. †Canada ‡Australia §U.K. ◊OTC

PATIENT TEACHING
• Explain to patient that he will need to be hospitalized for initiation of drug therapy.
• Stress need to take drug as prescribed, even when the patient is feeling well. Caution patient against stopping drug suddenly.
• Caution patient against using OTC drugs and decongestants while taking drug.
• Because food and antacids can interfere with absorption, tell patient to take drug on an empty stomach, 1 hour before or 2 hours after meals or antacids.

---

tocainide hydrochloride
Tonocard

Pregnancy risk category C

AVAILABLE FORMS
Tablets: 400 mg, 600 mg

INDICATIONS & DOSAGES
➤ **Suppression of symptomatic life-threatening ventricular arrhythmias—**
Adults: Initially, 400 mg P.O. q 8 hours. Usual dose is between 1,200 and 1,800 mg daily in three divided doses.
Adjust-a-dose: For patients with renal or hepatic impairment, a dose less than 1,200 mg daily may be adequate.

ACTION
A class IB antiarrhythmic that blocks the fast sodium channel in cardiac tissues, especially the Purkinje network, without involvement of the autonomic nervous system. It reduces the rate of rise and amplitude of the action potential and decreases automaticity in the Purkinje fibers. It shortens the duration of action potential and, to a lesser extent, decreases the effective refractory period in the Purkinje fibers.

Route	Onset	Peak	Duration
P.O.	Unknown	0.5-2 hr	8 hr

ADVERSE REACTIONS
CNS: ataxia, *light-headedness, tremor,* paresthesia, *dizziness, vertigo,* drowsiness, fatigue, confusion, headache.

CV: hypotension, *new or worsened arrhythmias, heart failure, bradycardia,* palpitations.
EENT: blurred vision, tinnitus.
GI: *nausea, vomiting,* diarrhea, anorexia.
Hematologic: *agranulocytosis, bone marrow depression, thrombocytopenia, aplastic anemia, neutropenia.*
Hepatic: *hepatitis.*
Respiratory: *pulmonary fibrosis,* pulmonary edema, interstitial pneumonitis, fibrosing alveolitis
Skin: rash, diaphoresis.

INTERACTIONS
Drug-drug. *Beta blockers:* Decreased myocardial contractility; increased CNS toxicity. Monitor patient closely.
Cimetidine: Reduced peak concentrations of tocainide. Monitor efficacy of tocainide.
Disopyramide, lidocaine, mexiletine, phenytoin, procainamide, quinidine: Increased pharmacologic effect and CV and CNS toxicity. Monitor patient.
Rifampin: Increased clearance of tocainide. Monitor efficacy of tocainide.

EFFECTS ON LAB TEST RESULTS
• May cause abnormal liver function test values. May decrease hemoglobin, hematocrit, and platelet and granulocyte counts.

CONTRAINDICATIONS
Contraindicated in patients hypersensitive to lidocaine or other amide-type local anesthetics and in those with second- or third-degree AV block in the absence of an artificial pacemaker.

NURSING CONSIDERATIONS
• Use cautiously in patients with heart failure or diminished cardiac reserve and in those with hepatic or renal impairment. These patients often may be treated effectively with a lower dose.
• Drug may ease transition from I.V. lidocaine to oral antiarrhythmic. Monitor patient carefully.
• Correct potassium deficits. Drug may be ineffective in hypokalemia.
• Monitor patient for tremor, which may indicate that maximum dosage has been reached.

Reactions may be *common,* uncommon, *life-threatening,* or COMMON AND LIFE-THREATENING.

• Notify prescriber if patient develops signs and symptoms of infection; a CBC should be performed immediately to rule out agranulocytosis.

PATIENT TEACHING
• Instruct patient to report immediately unusual bruising or bleeding or signs or symptoms of infection. Agranulocytosis and bone marrow suppression have been reported in patients taking usual doses of drug, typically within first 12 weeks of therapy.
• Advise patient to immediately report sudden onset of pulmonary symptoms, such as coughing, wheezing, or exertional dyspnea. Drug may cause serious pulmonary toxicity.
• Tell elderly patient to take safety precautions to reduce the risk of dizziness and falling.

amlodipine besylate
amyl nitrite
bepridil hydrochloride
diltiazem hydrochloride
isosorbide dinitrate
isosorbide mononitrate
nadolol
nicardipine hydrochloride
nifedipine
nitroglycerin
propranolol hydrochloride
verapamil
verapamil hydrochloride

COMBINATION PRODUCTS
LOTREL: amlodipine 2.5 mg and benazepril hydrochloride 10 mg, amlodipine 5 mg and benazepril hydrochloride 10 mg, amlodipine 5 mg and benazepril hydrochloride 20 mg

---

amlodipine besylate
Istin§, Norvasc

Pregnancy risk category C

AVAILABLE FORMS
Tablets: 2.5 mg, 5 mg, 10 mg

INDICATIONS & DOSAGES
➤ **Chronic stable angina, vasospastic angina (Prinzmetal's or variant angina)—**
Adults: Initially, 5 to 10 mg P.O. daily. Most patients need 10 mg daily.
Elderly patients: Initially, 5 mg P.O. daily.
Adjust-a-dose: For small, frail patients or those with hepatic insufficiency, initially 5 mg P.O. daily.
➤ **Hypertension—**
Adults: Initially, 2.5 to 5 mg P.O. daily. Dosage adjusted according to patient response and tolerance. Maximum daily dose is 10 mg.
Elderly patients: Initially, 2.5 mg P.O. daily.
Adjust-a-dose: For small, frail, patients, those currently receiving other antihypertensives, or those with hepatic insufficiency, initially 2.5 mg P.O. daily.

ACTION
Inhibits calcium ion influx across cardiac and smooth-muscle cells, thus decreasing myocardial contractility and oxygen demand; also dilates coronary arteries and arterioles.

Route	Onset	Peak	Duration
P.O.	Unknown	6-12 hr	24 hr

ADVERSE REACTIONS
CNS: *headache,* somnolence, fatigue, dizziness, light-headedness, paresthesia.
CV: *edema,* flushing, palpitations.
GI: nausea, abdominal pain.
GU: sexual difficulties.
Musculoskeletal: muscle pain.
Respiratory: dyspnea.
Skin: rash, pruritus.

INTERACTIONS
Drug-food. *Grapefruit juice:* Increased amlodipine levels, with increased effects. Avoid using together.

EFFECTS ON LAB TEST RESULTS
None reported.

CONTRAINDICATIONS
Contraindicated in patients hypersensitive to drug.

NURSING CONSIDERATIONS
• Use cautiously in patients receiving other peripheral vasodilators, especially those with severe aortic stenosis, and in those with heart failure. Because drug is metabolized by the liver, use cautiously and in reduced dosage in patients with severe hepatic disease.
• *Alert:* Monitor patient carefully. Some patients, especially those with severe obstructive coronary artery disease, have developed increased frequency, duration, or severity of angina or acute MI after initiation of calcium channel blocker therapy or at time of dosage increase.

Reactions may be *common,* uncommon, **life-threatening,** or COMMON AND LIFE-THREATENING.

• Monitor blood pressure frequently during initiation of therapy. Because drug-induced vasodilation has a gradual onset, acute hypotension is rare.

• Notify prescriber if signs of heart failure occur, such as swelling of hands and feet or shortness of breath.

• *Alert:* Don't confuse amlodipine with amiloride.

PATIENT TEACHING

• Caution patient to continue taking drug, even when feeling better.

• Tell patient S.L. nitroglycerin may be taken as needed when angina symptoms are acute. If patient continues nitrate therapy during adjustment of amlodipine dosage, urge continued compliance.

---

amyl nitrite

Pregnancy risk category X

AVAILABLE FORMS
Ampules (crushable): 0.3 ml

INDICATIONS & DOSAGES
➤ **Relief from angina pectoris—**
Adults and children: 0.3 ml by inhalation (one glass ampule), p.r.n.
➤ **Antidote for cyanide poisoning—**
Adults and children: 0.3 ml by inhalation for 15 to 60 seconds q 5 minutes until sodium nitrite infusion is available.

ACTION
Unknown. Effect probably results from dilation of arterial and venous beds. The net effect is a reduction in myocardial oxygen demand, improving perfusion to the ischemic myocardium. Drug converts hemoglobin to methemoglobin (which binds cyanide) to treat cyanide poisoning.

Route	Onset	Peak	Duration
Inhalation	30 sec	Unknown	3-5 min

ADVERSE REACTIONS
CNS: *headache, sometimes with throbbing;* dizziness; weakness; syncope.
CV: *orthostatic hypotension, tachycardia,* flushing, palpitations.
GI: nausea, vomiting.
Hematologic: methemoglobinemia.

Skin: cutaneous vasodilation, rash.
Other: hypersensitivity reactions.

INTERACTIONS
Drug-drug. *Calcium channel blockers:* Increased risk of symptomatic orthostatic hypotension. Monitor patient closely.
Sildenafil: Enhanced hypotensive effects of nitrates. Discourage use together.
Drug-lifestyle. *Alcohol use:* May cause severe hypotension and CV collapse. Warn against alcohol use.

EFFECTS ON LAB TEST RESULTS
None reported.

CONTRAINDICATIONS
Contraindicated in patients hypersensitive to nitrates; also contraindicated in those with severe anemia, angle-closure glaucoma, orthostatic hypotension, early MI, and increased intracranial pressure, and during pregnancy.

NURSING CONSIDERATIONS
• Use cautiously in patients with glaucoma (except angle-closure type, which is a contraindication), volume depletion, or hypotension.

• Extinguish all cigarettes before giving; ampule may ignite.

• Wrap ampule in cloth and crush. Hold near patient's nose and mouth so vapor is inhaled.

• Monitor patient for orthostatic hypotension.

• Store away from light.

• Drug alters the Zlatkis-Zak color reaction, causing a false decrease in cholesterol levels.

• Drug is claimed to have aphrodisiac benefits and is commonly abused. Street name is "Amy."

PATIENT TEACHING
• Show patient how to give drug. Stress importance of extinguishing all cigarettes before use.

• Tell patient to sit and avoid position changes while inhaling drug to prevent orthostatic hypotension.

• Advise patient to take a mild analgesic for drug-induced headache.

• Instruct patient that use of sildenafil with any nitrate may cause severe hypotension.

Patient should talk to prescriber before using these drugs together.

---

bepridil hydrochloride
Vascor

Pregnancy risk category C

AVAILABLE FORMS
Tablets: 200 mg, 300 mg, 400 mg

INDICATIONS & DOSAGES
➤ **Chronic stable angina in patients who can't tolerate or don't respond to other drugs—**
Adults: Initially, 200 mg P.O. daily. After 10 days, increase dosage based on response. Maintenance daily dose in most patients is 300 mg; maximum, 400 mg daily.

ACTION
A calcium channel blocker that inhibits calcium ion influx across cardiac and smooth-muscle cells, thereby dilating coronary arteries and peripheral arteries and arterioles. Drug may reduce heart rate, decrease myocardial contractility, and slow AV node conduction.

Route	Onset	Peak	Duration
P.O.	1 hr	2-3 hr	24 hr

ADVERSE REACTIONS
CNS: *dizziness,* drowsiness, *nervousness, headache,* insomnia, paresthesia, *asthenia,* tremor.
CV: edema, flushing, palpitations, **brady-cardia,** tachycardia, **ventricular arrhyth-mias (including torsades de pointes, ven-tricular tachycardia, ventricular fibrillation).**
EENT: tinnitus, sinusitis, rhinitis.
GI: anorexia, *nausea, diarrhea,* constipa-tion, abdominal discomfort, dry mouth.
Respiratory: dyspnea, shortness of breath.
Skin: rash, sweating.
Other: flu syndrome.

INTERACTIONS
Drug-drug. *Antiarrhythmics, cardiac gly-cosides, drugs that increase QT interval (TCAs):* May exaggerate prolongation of

the QT interval or depression of AV node with bepridil. Monitor patient closely.
Digoxin: May increase digoxin levels. Monitor patient.
Fentanyl: May cause severe hypotension. Monitor patient.

EFFECTS ON LAB TEST RESULTS
• May increase ALT levels.

CONTRAINDICATIONS
Contraindicated in patients hypersensitive to drug; also contraindicated in those with uncompensated cardiac insufficiency, sick sinus syndrome, second- or third-degree AV block unless pacemaker is present, hypotension (below 90 mm Hg systolic), congenital QT-interval prolongation, or history of serious ventricular arrhythmias. Don't use in patients receiving other drugs that prolong the QT interval.

NURSING CONSIDERATIONS
• Use cautiously if patient has left bundle-branch block, sinus bradycardia, impaired renal or hepatic function, or heart failure.
• Monitor patient for adverse reactions. Bepridil may cause severe ventricular ar-rhythmias, including torsades de pointes.
• Don't adjust dosage more frequently than every 10 to 14 days because of bepridil's long half-life and the time it takes to reach steady-state blood levels.
• *Alert:* Don't confuse bepridil with Pre-pidil.

PATIENT TEACHING
• Instruct patient to take drug exactly as directed.
• Tell patient that drug may be taken with food if GI upset occurs.
• Instruct patient to take potassium sup-plements or potassium-sparing diuretics as prescribed. Hypokalemia may increase the drug's tendency to promote arrhythmias.
• Advise patient to report adverse effects promptly.
• Tell patient to protect drug from light.

Reactions may be *common,* uncommon, *life-threatening,* or COMMON AND LIFE-THREATENING.

diltiazem hydrochloride
Adizem-SR§, Adizem-XL§, Angitil SR§, Apo-Diltiaz†, Calcicard CR§, Cardizem, Cardizem CD, Cardizem SR, CartiaXT, Diaclor XT, Dilacor XR, Diltia XT, Dilzem SR§, Dilzem XL§, Slozem§, Tiazac, Tildiem§, Tildiem LA§, Tildiem Retard§, Viazem XL§, Zemtard XL§

Pregnancy risk category C

AVAILABLE FORMS
Capsules (extended-release): 120 mg, 180 mg, 240 mg, 300 mg, 360 mg
Capsules (sustained-release): 60 mg, 90 mg, 120 mg, 180 mg, 240 mg, 300 mg, 360 mg, 420 mg
Injection: 5 mg/ml (25 mg and 50 mg)
Injection: 25 mg
Injection (for I.V. infusion only): 100 mg
Tablets: 30 mg, 60 mg, 90 mg, 120 mg

INDICATIONS & DOSAGES
➤ **Management of Prinzmetal's or variant angina or chronic stable angina pectoris—**
Adults: 30 mg P.O. q.i.d. before meals and h.s. Increase dose gradually to maximum of 360 mg/day divided into three to four doses, as indicated. Alternatively, give 120 or 180 mg (extended-release) P.O. once daily. Adjust over a 7- to 14-day period as needed and tolerated up to a maximum dose of 480 mg daily.
➤ **Hypertension—**
Adults: 60 to 120 mg P.O. b.i.d. (sustained-release). Adjust up to maximum recommended dose of 360 mg/day, p.r.n. Alternatively, give 180 to 240 mg (extended-release) P.O. once daily. Adjust dose based on patient response to a maximum dose of 480 mg/day.
➤ **Atrial fibrillation or flutter; paroxysmal supraventricular tachycardia—**
Adults: 0.25 mg/kg I.V. as a bolus injection over 2 minutes. Repeat after 15 minutes if response isn't adequate with a dose of 0.35 mg/kg I.V. over 2 minutes. Follow bolus with continuous I.V. infusion at 5 to 15 mg/hour (for up to 24 hours).

I.V. ADMINISTRATION
● For direct I.V. injection, no dilution of 5 mg/ml injection is needed.
● For continuous I.V. infusion, 5 mg/ml injection should be added to 100, 200, or 500 ml of normal saline solution, D₅W, or 5% dextrose and half-normal saline solution to produce a final concentration of 1, 0.83, or 0.45 mg/ml.
● Reconstitute drug in monovials labeled as containing 100 mg according to manufacturer's directions.
● For direct injection or continuous infusion, give slowly while continuously monitoring ECG and blood pressure.
● Don't give infusions lasting longer than 24 hours.

ACTION
A calcium channel blocker that inhibits calcium ion influx across cardiac and smooth-muscle cells, decreasing myocardial contractility and oxygen demand. Also dilates coronary arteries and arterioles.

Route	Onset	Peak	Duration
I.V.	Within 3 min	2-7 min	1-10 hr
P.O.	0.5-1 hr	2-3 hr	6-8 hr
P.O. (extended, sustained)	2-3 hr	10-14 hr	12-24 hr

ADVERSE REACTIONS
CNS: *headache,* dizziness, asthenia, somnolence.
CV: *edema,* **arrhythmias,** flushing, **bradycardia,** hypotension, conduction abnormalities, **heart failure, AV block,** abnormal ECG.
GI: *nausea, constipation,* abdominal discomfort.
Hepatic: *acute hepatic injury.*
Skin: *rash.*

INTERACTIONS
Drug-drug. *Anesthetics:* May increase effects of anesthetics. Monitor patient.
Carbamazepine: Increased levels of carbamazepine. Monitor carbamazepine levels, and watch for signs and symptoms of toxicity.
Cimetidine: May inhibit diltiazem metabolism, increasing additive AV node conduction slowing. Monitor patient for toxicity.

Cyclosporine: May increase cyclosporine levels, possibly by decreasing its metabolism, leading to increased risk of cyclosporine toxicity. Monitor cyclosporine levels with each dosage change.
Digoxin: May increase digoxin levels. Monitor patient for digoxin toxicity.
Furosemide: Forms a precipitate when mixed with diltiazem injection. Give through separate I.V. lines.
Propranolol, other beta blockers: May precipitate heart failure or prolong conduction time. Use together cautiously.

EFFECTS ON LAB TEST RESULTS
None reported.

CONTRAINDICATIONS
Contraindicated in patients hypersensitive to drug and in those with sick sinus syndrome or second- or third-degree AV block in the absence of an artificial pacemaker, ventricular tachycardia, systolic blood pressure below 90 mm Hg, acute MI, or pulmonary congestion (documented by X-ray). I.V. preparations are contraindicated in patients who have atrial fibrillation or flutter with an accessory bypass tract, as in Wolff-Parkinson-White syndrome or short PR interval syndrome.

NURSING CONSIDERATIONS
• Use cautiously in elderly patients and in those with heart failure or impaired hepatic or renal function.
• Monitor blood pressure and heart rate when starting therapy and during dosage adjustments.
• Maximum antihypertensive effect may not be seen for 14 days.
• If systolic blood pressure is below 90 mm Hg or heart rate is below 60 beats/minute, withhold dose and notify prescriber.
• *Alert:* Don't confuse Cardizem SR with Cardene SR.

PATIENT TEACHING
• Instruct patient to take medication as prescribed, even when feeling better.
• Advise patient to avoid hazardous activities during start of therapy.
• Stress patient compliance if nitrate therapy is prescribed during adjustment of diltiazem dosage. Tell patient that S.L. nitro-

glycerin may be taken with drug, as needed, when angina symptoms are acute.
• Tell patient to swallow extended-release capsules whole, and not to open, crush, or chew them.

---

isosorbide dinitrate
Apo-ISDN†, Cedocard Retard§, Cedocard SR†, Dilatrate-SR, Ismo Retard§, Isordil, Isordil Tembids, Isordil Titradose, Isotrate, Sorbid SA§, Sorbichew§, Sorbitrate

isosorbide mononitrate
Elantan§, Imdur, Isib 60XL§, ISMO, Isotrate§, Isotrate ER, Modisal XL§, Monit§, Mono-Cedocard§, Monoket, Monosorb XL 60§

Pregnancy risk category C

AVAILABLE FORMS
isosorbide dinitrate
Capsules (sustained-release): 40 mg
Tablets: 5 mg, 10 mg, 20 mg, 30 mg, 40 mg
Tablets (chewable): 5 mg, 10 mg
Tablets (S.L.): 2.5 mg, 5 mg, 10 mg
Tablets (sustained-release): 40 mg
isosorbide mononitrate
Tablets: 10 mg, 20 mg
Tablets (extended-release): 30 mg, 60 mg, 120 mg

INDICATIONS & DOSAGES
➤ **Acute anginal attacks (S.L. and chewable tablets of isosorbide dinitrate only), prophylaxis in situations likely to cause anginal attacks—**
S.L. form
Adults: 2.5 to 5 mg S.L. for prompt relief of angina, repeated q 5 to 10 minutes (maximum of three doses for each 30-minute period). For prophylaxis, 2.5 to 10 mg q 2 to 3 hours.
Chewable form
Adults: 5 to 10 mg, p.r.n., for acute attack or q 2 to 3 hours for prophylaxis, but only after initial test dose of 5 mg to determine risk of severe hypotension.

Reactions may be *common,* uncommon, **life-threatening**, or COMMON AND LIFE-THREATENING.

Oral form (isosorbide dinitrate)
Adults: 5 to 40 mg P.O. b.i.d. or t.i.d. for prophylaxis only (use smallest effective dose).

Oral form (isosorbide mononitrate using Imdur)
Adults: 30 to 60 mg P.O. once daily upon arising; increased to 120 mg once daily after several days, if needed.

Oral form (isosorbide mononitrate using ISMO or Monoket)
Adults: 20 mg b.i.d. with the two doses given 7 hours apart.

ACTION

Not completely known. Thought to reduce cardiac oxygen demand by decreasing preload and afterload. Drug also may increase blood flow through the collateral coronary vessels.

Route	Onset	Peak	Duration
P.O.	15-40 min	Unknown	4-6 hr
P.O. (chewable)	2-5 min	Unknown	2-2.5 hr
P.O. (extended)	0.5-4 hr	Unknown	12 hr
P.O. (S.L.)	2-5 min	Unknown	1.5 hr

ADVERSE REACTIONS

CNS: *headache,* dizziness, weakness.
CV: *orthostatic hypotension, tachycardia, palpitations, ankle edema,* fainting, *flushing.*
EENT: S.L. burning.
GI: nausea, vomiting.
Skin: cutaneous vasodilation, rash.

INTERACTIONS

Drug-drug. *Antihypertensives:* May increase hypotensive effects. Monitor patient closely during initial therapy.
Sildenafil: May increase hypotensive effects. Discourage use together.
Drug-lifestyle. *Alcohol use:* May increase hypotension. Discourage use together.

EFFECTS ON LAB TEST RESULTS

None reported.

CONTRAINDICATIONS

Contraindicated in patients with hypersensitivity or idiosyncrasy to nitrates and in those with severe hypotension, angle-closure glaucoma, increased intracranial

pressure, shock, or acute MI with low left ventricular filling pressure.

NURSING CONSIDERATIONS

● Use cautiously in patients with blood volume depletion (such as from diuretic therapy) or mild hypotension.
● To prevent development of tolerance, a nitrate-free interval of 8 to 12 hours per day is recommended. The regimen for isosorbide mononitrate (one tablet upon awakening with the second dose in 7 hours, or one extended-release tablet daily) is intended to minimize nitrate tolerance by providing a substantial nitrate-free interval.
● Monitor blood pressure and intensity and duration of drug response.
● Drug may cause headaches, especially at beginning of therapy. Dosage may be reduced temporarily, but tolerance usually develops. Treat headache with aspirin or acetaminophen.
● Methemoglobinemia has been seen with nitrates. Symptoms are those of impaired oxygen delivery despite adequate cardiac output and adequate arterial partial pressure of oxygen.
● May interfere with cholesterol determination tests using the Zlatkis-Zak color reaction, causing a falsely decreased value.
● *Alert:* Don't confuse Isordil with Isuprel or Inderal.

PATIENT TEACHING

● Caution patient to take drug regularly, as prescribed, and to keep it accessible at all times.
● *Alert:* Advise patient that stopping drug abruptly may cause coronary vasospasm with increased angina symptoms and potential risk of MI.
● Tell patient to take S.L. tablet at first sign of attack. The tablet should be wet with saliva and placed under the tongue until absorbed; the patient should sit down and rest. Dose may be repeated every 10 to 15 minutes for a maximum of three doses. If drug doesn't provide relief, tell patient to seek medical help promptly.
● Advise patient who complains of tingling sensation with S.L. drug to try holding tablet in buccal pouch.
● Warn patient not to confuse S.L. with P.O. form.

• Advise patient taking P.O. form of isosorbide dinitrate to take oral tablet on an empty stomach either 30 minutes before or 1 to 2 hours after meals, to swallow oral tablets whole, and to chew chewable tablets thoroughly before swallowing.

• Tell patient to minimize orthostatic hypotension by changing to upright position slowly. Advise him to go up and down stairs carefully and to lie down at first sign of dizziness.

• Caution patient to avoid alcohol because it may exacerbate hypotensive effects.

• Advise patient that use of sildenafil with any nitrate may cause severe hypotension. Patient should talk to his prescriber before using these drugs together.

• Instruct patient to store drug in a cool place, in a tightly closed container, and away from light.

---

nadolol
Corgard

Pregnancy risk category C

AVAILABLE FORMS
Tablets: 20 mg, 40 mg, 80 mg, 120 mg, 160 mg

INDICATIONS & DOSAGES
➤ **Angina pectoris—**
Adults: 40 mg P.O. once daily. Increased in 40- to 80-mg increments at 3- to 7-day intervals until optimum response occurs. Usual maintenance dose is 40 to 80 mg once daily; up to 240 mg once daily may be needed.
➤ **Hypertension—**
Adults: 40 mg P.O. once daily. Increased in 40- to 80-mg increments until optimum response occurs. Usual maintenance dose is 40 to 80 mg once daily. Doses of 320 mg may be needed.
Adjust-a-dose: For patients with renal impairment, dosage interval should be adjusted based on creatinine clearance. For creatinine clearance of over 50 ml/minute, give dose q 24 hours; for clearance of 31 to 50 ml/minute, q 24 to 36 hours; for clearance of 10 to 30 ml/minute, q 24 to 48 hours; and for clearance below 10 ml/minute, q 40 to 60 hours.

ACTION
A beta blocker that reduces cardiac oxygen demand by blocking catecholamine-induced increases in heart rate, blood pressure, and force of myocardial contraction. Depresses renin secretion.

Route	Onset	Peak	Duration
P.O.	Unknown	2-4 hr	Unknown

ADVERSE REACTIONS
CNS: fatigue, dizziness.
CV: *bradycardia,* hypotension, *heart failure,* peripheral vascular disease, rhythm and conduction disturbances.
GI: nausea, vomiting, diarrhea, abdominal pain, constipation, anorexia.
Respiratory: *increased airway resistance.*
Skin: rash.
Other: fever.

INTERACTIONS
Drug-drug. *Antihypertensives:* Increased antihypertensive effect. Monitor patient closely.
Cardiac glycosides: Excessive bradycardia and additive effects on AV conduction. Use together cautiously.
Epinephrine: Severe vasoconstriction and reflex bradycardia. Monitor blood pressure carefully.
Insulin, oral antidiabetics: May alter dosage requirements in previously stabilized diabetic patients. Monitor patient closely.
NSAIDs: Decreased antihypertensive effect. Monitor blood pressure and adjust dosage.
Phenothiazines: May increase hypotensive effects. Monitor patient closely.

EFFECTS ON LAB TEST RESULTS
None reported.

CONTRAINDICATIONS
Contraindicated in patients with bronchial asthma, sinus bradycardia and greater than first-degree heart block, and cardiogenic shock.

NURSING CONSIDERATIONS
• Use cautiously in patients with heart failure, chronic bronchitis, emphysema, or renal or hepatic impairment and in patients undergoing major surgery involving

---

general anesthesia. Also use cautiously in diabetic patients because beta blockers may mask certain signs and symptoms of hypoglycemia.
• Check apical pulse before giving drug. If slower than 60 beats/minute, withhold drug and call prescriber.
• Monitor blood pressure frequently. If patient develops severe hypotension, give a vasopressor, as prescribed.
• *Alert:* Abrupt discontinuation can worsen angina and cause MI. Dosage should be reduced gradually over 1 to 2 weeks.
• Drug masks signs and symptoms of shock and hyperthyroidism.

PATIENT TEACHING
• Explain importance of taking drug as prescribed, even when patient is feeling well.
• Teach patient how to check pulse rate and tell him to check it before each dose. If pulse rate is below 60 beats/minute, tell patient to notify prescriber.
• Warn patient not to stop drug suddenly.

---

nicardipine hydrochloride
Cardene, Cardene I.V., Cardene SR

Pregnancy risk category C

AVAILABLE FORMS
Capsules (immediate-release): 20 mg, 30 mg
Capsules (sustained-release): 30 mg, 45 mg, 60 mg
Injection: 2.5 mg/ml

INDICATIONS & DOSAGES
➤ **Chronic stable angina (used alone or with other antianginals)—**
Adults: Initially, 20 mg P.O. t.i.d. (immediate-release). Dosage adjusted based on patient response q 3 days. Usual range is 20 to 40 mg t.i.d.
➤ **Hypertension—**
Adults: Initially, 20 mg P.O. t.i.d. (immediate-release); range, 20 to 40 mg t.i.d. Or, 30 mg b.i.d. (sustained-release); range, 30 to 60 mg b.i.d. Dosage increased based on patient response. Or, for patients unable to take oral nicardipine, 50 ml/hour (5 mg/hour) I.V. infusion initially; then in-

creased by 25 ml/hour (2.5 mg/hour) q 15 minutes to maximum of 150 ml/hour (15 mg/hour).

I.V. ADMINISTRATION
• Dilute with compatible I.V. solution before administration. The drug is compatible with D_5W, D_5W in normal saline solution or half-normal saline solution, and normal saline solution or half-normal saline solution for 24 hours at room temperature.
• The drug is incompatible with sodium bicarbonate and lactated Ringer's solution.
• Give by slow I.V. infusion in a concentration of 0.1 mg/ml.
• Closely monitor blood pressure during and after completion of infusion.
• Titrate infusion rate if hypotension or tachycardia occurs.
• Change peripheral infusion site every 12 hours to minimize risk of venous irritation.
• When switching to oral therapy other than nicardipine, initiate therapy upon ending of infusion. If oral nicardipine is to be used, give first dose of t.i.d. regimen 1 hour before stopping infusion.

ACTION
A calcium channel blocker that inhibits calcium ion influx across cardiac and smooth-muscle cells, decreasing myocardial contractility and oxygen demand. Also dilates coronary arteries and arterioles.

Route	Onset	Peak	Duration
I.V.	Immediate	Immediate	Unknown
P.O. (immediate)	0.5-1.5 min	1-2 hr	Unknown
P.O. (sustained)	20 min	1-4 hr	12 hr

ADVERSE REACTIONS
CNS: *dizziness, light-headedness, headache, asthenia.*
CV: *peripheral edema, palpitations,* angina, tachycardia, *flushing.*
GI: nausea, abdominal discomfort, dry mouth.
Skin: rash.

INTERACTIONS
Drug-drug. *Antihypertensives:* Increased antihypertensive effect. Monitor patient closely.
Beta blockers: May increase cardiac depressant effects. Monitor patient closely.
Cimetidine: May decrease metabolism of calcium channel blockers. Monitor patient for increased pharmacologic effect.
Cyclosporine: May increase plasma levels of cyclosporine. Monitor patient for toxicity.
Theophylline: May increase pharmacologic effects of theophylline. Monitor patient for toxicity.

EFFECTS ON LAB TEST RESULTS
None reported.

CONTRAINDICATIONS
Contraindicated in patients hypersensitive to drug and in those with advanced aortic stenosis.

NURSING CONSIDERATIONS
• Use cautiously in patients with hypotension, heart failure, or impaired hepatic and renal function.
• Measure blood pressure frequently during initial therapy. Maximum blood pressure response occurs about 1 hour after dosing with the immediate-release form and 2 to 4 hours afterward with the sustained-release form. Check for potential orthostatic hypotension. Because large swings in blood pressure may occur based on blood level of drug, assess adequacy of antihypertensive effect 8 hours after dosing.
• Extended-release form is preferred because of improved medication adherence, fewer fluctuations in blood pressure, and increased risk in mortality with short-acting drugs.
• *Alert:* Don't confuse Cardene with Cardura or codeine. Don't confuse Cardene SR with Cardizem SR.

PATIENT TEACHING
• Tell patient to take oral form of drug exactly as prescribed.
• Advise patient to report chest pain immediately. Some patients may experience increased frequency, severity, or duration of chest pain at beginning of therapy or during dosage adjustments.

• Inform patient to get up from a sitting or lying position slowly in order to avoid dizziness caused by a decrease in blood pressure.

---

nifedipine
Adalat, Adalat CC, Adalat PA†, Adalat XL†, Apo-Nifed†, Cardilate MR§, Coracten§, Hypolar Retard 20§, Nifedotard 20 MR§, Nifelease§, Nifensar XL§, Novo-Nifedin†, Nu-Nifed†, Procardia, Procardia XL, Tensipine MR§, Unipine XL§

Pregnancy risk category C

AVAILABLE FORMS
Capsules: 10 mg, 20 mg
Tablets (extended-release): 30 mg, 60 mg, 90 mg

INDICATIONS & DOSAGES
➤ **Vasospastic angina (Prinzmetal's or variant angina), classic chronic stable angina pectoris—**
Adults: Initially, 10 mg P.O. t.i.d. Usual effective dosage range is 10 to 20 mg t.i.d. Some patients may require up to 30 mg q.i.d. Maximum daily dose is 180 mg. Adjust dose over 7 to 14 days to evaluate response.
➤ **Hypertension—**
Adults: 30 or 60 mg P.O. (extended-release form) once daily. Adjusted over 7 to 14 days. Doses larger than 90 mg (for Adalat CC) and 120 mg (for Procardia XL) aren't recommended.

ACTION
Unknown. Thought to inhibit calcium ion influx across cardiac and smooth-muscle cells, decreasing contractility and oxygen demand. Also may dilate coronary arteries and arterioles.

Route	Onset	Peak	Duration
P.O.	20 min	0.5-1 hr	4-8 hr
P.O. (extended)	20 min	6 hr	24 hr

ADVERSE REACTIONS
CNS: *dizziness, light-headedness, headache, weakness,* syncope, nervousness.

CV: *peripheral edema,* hypotension, palpitations, ***heart failure, MI,*** pulmonary edema, *flushing.*
EENT: nasal congestion.
GI: *nausea,* diarrhea, constipation, abdominal discomfort.
Metabolic: hypokalemia.
Musculoskeletal: muscle cramps.
Respiratory: dyspnea, cough.
Skin: rash, pruritus.

INTERACTIONS
Drug-drug. *Cimetidine, ranitidine:* Decreased nifedipine metabolism. Dosage may be adjusted.
Digoxin: May cause elevated digoxin levels. Monitor patient closely.
Fentanyl: May cause severe hypotension. Monitor patient closely.
Phenytoin: May reduce phenytoin metabolism. Monitor patient closely.
Propranolol, other beta blockers: May cause hypotension and heart failure. Use together cautiously.
Drug-herb. *Melatonin:* Interferes with antihypertensive effect. Discourage use together.
Drug-food. *Grapefruit juice:* Increased bioavailability of nifedipine. Discourage use together; monitor patient closely if used together.

EFFECTS ON LAB TEST RESULTS
● May increase ALT, AST, alkaline phosphatase, and LDH levels. May decrease potassium level.

CONTRAINDICATIONS
Contraindicated in patients hypersensitive to drug.

NURSING CONSIDERATIONS
● Use cautiously in patients with heart failure or hypotension and in elderly patients. Use extended-release tablets cautiously in patients with severe GI narrowing.
● Don't give immediate-release form within 1 week of acute MI or in acute coronary syndrome.
● *Alert:* Despite the previously widespread S.L. use of nifedipine capsules (or the "bite and swallow" method), avoid this route of administration. Excessive hypotension, MI, and death may result.

● Monitor blood pressure regularly, especially in patients who take beta blockers or antihypertensives.
● Watch for symptoms of heart failure.
● Although rebound effect hasn't been observed when drug is stopped, dosage should be reduced slowly under prescriber's supervision.
● *Alert:* Don't confuse nifedipine with nimodipine or nicardipine.

PATIENT TEACHING
● If patient is kept on nitrate therapy while nifedipine dosage is being adjusted, urge continued compliance. Patient may take S.L. nitroglycerin, as needed, for acute angina.
● Tell patient that angina may worsen briefly when beginning drug or when dosage is increased.
● Instruct patient to swallow extended-release tablets without breaking, crushing, or chewing them.
● Advise patient to avoid taking drug with grapefruit juice.
● Reassure patient who is taking the extended-release form that a wax-matrix "ghost" from the tablet may be passed in the stools. Drug is completely absorbed before this occurs.
● Warn patient not to switch brands. Procardia XL and Adalat CC aren't therapeutically equivalent because of major differences in their pharmacokinetics.
● Tell patient to protect capsules from direct light and moisture and to store at room temperature.

---

nitroglycerin (glyceryl trinitrate)
Anginine‡, Deponit, Minitran, Nitradisc‡, Nitro-Bid, Nitro-Bid IV, Nitrodisc, Nitro-Dur, Nitrogard, Nitrogard SR†, Nitroglyn, Nitrol, Nitrolingual, Nitrong, Nitrostat, Nitro-Time, NTS, Transderm-Nitro, Transiderm-Nitro‡, Tridil

Pregnancy risk category C

AVAILABLE FORMS
Aerosol (translingual): 0.4-mg metered spray

Capsules (sustained-release): 2.5 mg,
6.5 mg, 9 mg, 13 mg
Injection: 0.5 mg/ml, 5 mg/ml
Tablets (buccal): 1 mg, 2 mg, 3 mg
Tablets (S.L.): 0.15 mg (1/400 grain),
0.3 mg (1/200 grain), 0.4 mg (1/150 grain),
0.6 mg (1/100 grain)
Tablets (sustained-release): 2.6 mg,
6.5 mg, 9 mg, 13 mg
Topical: 2% ointment
Transdermal: 0.1 mg/hour, 0.2 mg/hour,
0.3 mg/hour, 0.4 mg/hour, 0.6 mg/hour,
0.8 mg/hour release rate

INDICATIONS & DOSAGES
➤ **Prophylaxis against chronic anginal attacks—**
Adults: 2.5 or 2.6 mg sustained-release
capsule or tablet q 8 to 12 hours, adjusted
upward to an effective dose in 2.5- or
2.6-mg increments b.i.d. to q.i.d. Or, use
2% ointment: Start dosage with ½-inch
ointment, increasing by ½-inch increments until desired results are achieved.
Range of dosage with ointment is ½ to 5
inches. Usual dose is 1 to 2 inches. Or,
transdermal disc or pad (Nitrodisc, Nitro-
Dur, or Transderm-Nitro) 0.2 to 0.4 mg/
hour once daily.
➤ **Acute angina pectoris, prophylaxis to
prevent or minimize anginal attacks
before stressful events—**
Adults: 1 S.L. tablet (1/400 grain, 1/200
grain, 1/150 grain, 1/100 grain) dissolved
under the tongue or in the buccal pouch
as soon as angina begins. Repeat q 5 minutes, if needed, for 15 minutes. Or, using
Nitrolingual spray, one or two sprays into
mouth, preferably onto or under the
tongue. Repeat q 3 to 5 minutes, if needed, to a maximum of three doses within a
15-minute period. Or, 1 to 3 mg transmu-
cosally q 3 to 5 hours during waking
hours.
➤ **Hypertension from surgery, heart
failure after MI, angina pectoris in
acute situations, to produce controlled
hypotension during surgery (by I.V. infusion)—**
Adults: Initial infusion rate is 5 mcg/
minute, increased p.r.n. by 5 mcg/minute q
3 to 5 minutes until response occurs. If a
20-mcg/minute rate doesn't produce a response, may increase dosage by as much

as 20 mcg/minute q 3 to 5 minutes. Up to
100 mcg/minute may be needed.

I.V. ADMINISTRATION
● Dilute with D₅W or normal saline solution for injection. Concentration shouldn't
exceed 400 mcg/ml.
● Always give with an infusion control device and titrate to desired response.
● Always mix in glass bottles, and avoid
use of I.V. filters because drug binds to
plastic. Regular polyvinyl chloride tubing
can bind up to 80% of drug, making it
necessary to infuse higher dosages.
● A special nonabsorbent polyvinyl chloride tubing is available from the manufacturer; patients receive more drug when
these infusion sets are used.
● Use the same type of infusion set when
changing I.V. lines.
● When changing the concentration of infusion, flush the I.V. administration set
with 15 to 20 ml of the new concentration
before use. This will clear the line of the
old drug solution.

ACTION
A nitrate that reduces cardiac oxygen demand by decreasing left ventricular end-
diastolic pressure (preload) and, to a lesser
extent, systemic vascular resistance (afterload). Also increases blood flow through
the collateral coronary vessels.

Route	Onset	Peak	Duration
Buccal	3 min	Unknown	3-5 hr
I.V.	Immediate	Immediate	3-5 min
P.O.	20-45 min	Unknown	3-8 hr
S.L.	1-3 min	Unknown	0.5-1 hr
Topical	30 min	Unknown	2-12 hr
Trans-dermal	30 min	Unknown	24 hr
Trans-lingual	2-4 min	Unknown	0.5-1 hr

ADVERSE REACTIONS
CNS: *headache, dizziness,* weakness.
CV: *orthostatic hypotension, tachycardia,
flushing, palpitations,* fainting.
EENT: S.L. burning.
GI: nausea, vomiting.
Skin: cutaneous vasodilation, contact der-
matitis, rash.
Other: hypersensitivity reactions.

Reactions may be *common,* uncommon, **_life-threatening_**, or **COMMON AND LIFE-THREATENING.**

INTERACTIONS
Drug-drug. *Antihypertensives:* May increase hypotensive effect. Monitor patient closely.
Heparin: I.V. nitroglycerin may interfere with anticoagulant effect of heparin. Monitor PTT.
Sildenafil: May increase risk of hypotension. Discourage use together.
Drug-lifestyle. *Alcohol use:* May increase hypotension. Discourage alcohol intake.

EFFECTS ON LAB TEST RESULTS
None reported.

CONTRAINDICATIONS
Contraindicated in patients with early MI, severe anemia, increased intracranial pressure, angle-closure glaucoma, orthostatic hypotension, allergy to adhesives (transdermal), or hypersensitivity to nitrates.
I.V. nitroglycerin is contraindicated in patients hypersensitive to I.V. form, cardiac tamponade, restrictive cardiomyopathy, or constrictive pericarditis.

NURSING CONSIDERATIONS
● Use cautiously in patients with hypotension or volume depletion.
● Closely monitor vital signs during infusion, particularly blood pressure, especially in a patient with an MI. Excessive hypotension may worsen the MI.
● To apply ointment, measure the prescribed amount on the application paper; then place the paper on any nonhairy area. Don't rub in. Cover with plastic film to aid absorption and to protect clothing. Remove all excess ointment from previous site before applying the next dose. Avoid getting ointment on fingers.
● Transdermal dosage forms can be applied to any nonhairy part of the skin except distal parts of the arms or legs (absorption won't be maximal at distal sites). Patch may cause contact dermatitis.
● Remove transdermal patch before defibrillation. Because of the aluminum backing on the patch, the electric current may cause arcing that can damage the paddles and burn the patient.
● When stopping transdermal treatment of angina, gradually reduce the dose and frequency of application over 4 to 6 weeks.

● Monitor blood pressure and intensity and duration of drug response.
● Drug may cause headaches, especially at beginning of therapy. Dosage may be reduced temporarily, but tolerance usually develops. Treat headache with aspirin or acetaminophen.
● Tolerance to drug can be minimized with a 10- to 12-hour nitrate-free interval. To achieve this, remove the transdermal system in the early evening and apply a new system the next morning or omit the last daily dose of a buccal, sustained-release, or ointment form. Check with the prescriber for alterations in dosage regimen if tolerance is suspected.
● Nitroglycerin may interfere with cholesterol determination tests using the Zlatkis-Zak color reaction, resulting in falsely decreased values.
● *Alert:* Don't confuse Nitro-Bid with Nicobid or nitroglycerin with nitroprusside.

PATIENT TEACHING
● Caution patient to take nitroglycerin regularly, as prescribed, and to have it accessible at all times.
● *Alert:* Advise patient that stopping drug abruptly causes coronary vasospasm.
● Teach patient how to give the prescribed form of nitroglycerin.
● Tell patient to take S.L. tablet at first sign of attack. The tablet should be wet with saliva and placed under the tongue until absorbed, and the patient should sit down and rest. Dose may be repeated every 5 minutes for a maximum of three doses. If drug doesn't provide relief, medical help should be obtained promptly.
● Advise patient who complains of a tingling sensation with S.L. drug to try holding tablet in buccal pouch.
● Tell patient to take oral tablets on an empty stomach either 30 minutes before or 1 to 2 hours after meals, to swallow oral tablets whole, and not to chew tablets.
● Remind patient using translingual aerosol form that he shouldn't inhale the spray, but should release it onto or under the tongue. Tell him to wait about 10 seconds or so before swallowing.
● Tell patient to place the buccal tablet between the lip and gum above the incisors

---

or between the cheek and gum. Tablets shouldn't be swallowed or chewed.
• Tell patient to take an additional dose before anticipated stress or at bedtime if angina is nocturnal.
• Instruct patient wearing transdermal patch to use caution when near a microwave oven. Leaking radiation may heat patch's metallic backing and cause burns.
• Urge patient using transdermal patches to dispose of them carefully because enough medication remains after normal use to be hazardous to children and pets.
• Advise patient to avoid alcohol.
• To minimize orthostatic hypotension, tell patient to change to upright position slowly. Advise him to go up and down stairs carefully and to lie down at the first sign of dizziness.
• Advise patient that use of sildenafil with any nitrate may cause severe hypotension. The patient should talk to his prescriber before considering use of these drugs together.
• Tell patient to store drug in cool, dark place in a tightly closed container. Tell him to remove cotton from container because it absorbs drug.
• Tell patient to store S.L. tablets in original container or other container specifically approved for this use and to carry the container in a jacket pocket or purse, not in a pocket close to the body.

---

propranolol hydrochloride
Apo-Propranolol†, Deralin‡, Inderal, Inderal LA, Novopranol†, PMS Propranolol†

Pregnancy risk category C

AVAILABLE FORMS
Capsules (extended-release): 60 mg, 80 mg, 120 mg, 160 mg
Injection: 1 mg/ml
Oral solution: 4 mg/ml, 8 mg/ml, 80 mg/ml (concentrate)
Tablets: 10 mg, 20 mg, 40 mg, 60 mg, 80 mg, 90 mg

INDICATIONS & DOSAGES
➤ **Angina pectoris—**
Adults: Total daily doses of 80 to 320 mg P.O. when given b.i.d., t.i.d., or q.i.d. Or,

one 80-mg extended-release capsule daily. Dosage increased at 3- to 7-day intervals.
➤ **Mortality reduction after MI—**
Adults: 180 to 240 mg P.O. daily in divided doses beginning 5 to 21 days after MI has occurred. Usually given t.i.d. or q.i.d.
➤ **Supraventricular, ventricular, and atrial arrhythmias; tachyarrhythmias caused by excessive catecholamine action during anesthesia, hyperthyroidism, or pheochromocytoma—**
Adults: 0.5 to 3 mg by slow I.V. push, not to exceed 1 mg/minute. After 3 mg have been given, another dose may be given in 2 minutes; subsequent doses, no sooner than q 4 hours. May be diluted and infused slowly. Usual maintenance dose is 10 to 30 mg P.O. t.i.d. or q.i.d.
➤ **Hypertension—**
Adults: Initially, 80 mg P.O. daily in two to four divided doses or extended-release form once daily. Increased at 3- to 7-day intervals to maximum daily dose of 640 mg. Usual maintenance dose is 160 to 480 mg daily.
➤ **Prevention of frequent, severe, uncontrollable, or disabling migraine or vascular headache—**
Adults: Initially, 80 mg P.O. daily in divided doses or one extended-release capsule daily. Usual maintenance dose is 160 to 240 mg daily, t.i.d. or q.i.d.
➤ **Essential tremor—**
Adults: 40 mg (tablets, oral solution) P.O. b.i.d. Usual maintenance dose is 120 to 320 mg daily in three divided doses.
➤ **Hypertrophic subaortic stenosis—**
Adults: 20 to 40 mg P.O. t.i.d. or q.i.d.; or 80 to 160 mg extended-release capsules once daily.
➤ **Adjunct therapy in pheochromocytoma—**
Adults: 60 mg P.O. daily in divided doses with an alpha blocker 3 days before surgery.

I.V. ADMINISTRATION
• For direct injection, give into a large vessel or into the tubing of a free-flowing, compatible I.V. solution; don't give by continuous I.V. infusion.
• For intermittent infusion, dilute drug with normal saline solution and give over

---

10 to 15 minutes in 0.1- to 0.2-mg increments.
• Drug is compatible with D_5W, half-normal saline solution, normal saline solution, and lactated Ringer's solution.
• Infusion rate shouldn't exceed 1 mg/minute.
• Double-check dose and route. I.V. doses are much smaller than oral doses.
• Monitor blood pressure, ECG, central venous pressure, and heart rate and rhythm frequently, especially during I.V. administration. If patient develops severe hypotension, notify prescriber; a vasopressor may be prescribed.
• For overdose, give I.V. isoproterenol, I.V. atropine, or glucagon; refractory cases may require a pacemaker.

ACTION
A nonselective beta blocker that reduces cardiac oxygen demand by blocking catecholamine-induced increases in heart rate, blood pressure, and force of myocardial contraction. Depresses renin secretion and prevents vasodilation of cerebral arteries.

Route	Onset	Peak	Duration
I.V.	Immediate	1 min	5 min
P.O.	30 min	1-1.5 hr	12 hr

ADVERSE REACTIONS
CNS: *fatigue, lethargy,* vivid dreams, hallucinations, mental depression, lightheadedness, insomnia.
CV: *bradycardia,* hypotension, *heart failure,* intermittent claudication, *intensification of AV block.*
GI: abdominal cramping, constipation, diarrhea, nausea, vomiting.
Hematologic: *agranulocytosis.*
Respiratory: *bronchospasm.*
Skin: rash.
Other: fever.

INTERACTIONS
Drug-drug. *Aminophylline:* Antagonized beta-blocking effects of propranolol. Use together cautiously.
Cardiac glycosides, diltiazem, verapamil: Hypotension, bradycardia, and increased depressant effect on myocardium. Use together cautiously.

Cimetidine: Inhibited metabolism of propranolol. Watch for increased beta-blocking effect.
Epinephrine: Severe vasoconstriction. Monitor blood pressure and observe patient carefully.
Glucagon, isoproterenol: Antagonized propranolol effect. May be used therapeutically and in emergencies.
Haloperidol: Cardiac arrest possible with concomitant therapy. Avoid use together.
Insulin, oral antidiabetics: Can alter requirements for these drugs in previously stabilized diabetics. Monitor patient for hypoglycemia.
Phenothiazines, reserpine: Additive effect. Use cautiously.
Drug-herb. *Betel palm:* Decreased temperature-elevating effects and enhanced CNS effects. Discourage use together.
Drug-lifestyle. *Cocaine use:* Increased angina-inducing potential of cocaine. Monitor patient carefully.

EFFECTS ON LAB TEST RESULTS
• May increase BUN, transaminase, alkaline phosphatase, and LDH levels.
• May decrease granulocyte count.

CONTRAINDICATIONS
Contraindicated in patients with bronchial asthma, sinus bradycardia and heart block greater than first-degree, cardiogenic shock, and heart failure (unless failure is secondary to a tachyarrhythmia that can be treated with propranolol).

NURSING CONSIDERATIONS
• Use cautiously in patients with hepatic or renal impairment, nonallergic bronchospastic diseases, or hepatic disease and in those taking other antihypertensives. Because drug blocks some symptoms of hypoglycemia, use cautiously in patients who have diabetes mellitus. Also use cautiously in patients with thyrotoxicosis because drug may mask some signs and symptoms of that disorder. Elderly patients may experience enhanced adverse reactions and may need dosage adjustment.
• Always check patient's apical pulse before giving drug. If extremes in pulse rates occur, withhold drug and notify prescriber immediately.

• Give drug consistently with meals. Food may increase absorption of propranolol.
• Drug masks common signs and symptoms of shock and hypoglycemia.
• *Alert:* Don't discontinue drug before surgery for pheochromocytoma. Before any surgical procedure, tell anesthesiologist that patient is receiving propranolol.
• Compliance may be improved by giving drug twice daily or as extended-release capsules. Check with prescriber.
• *Alert:* Don't confuse propranolol with Pravachol. Don't confuse Inderal with Inderide, Isordil, Adderall, or Imuran.

PATIENT TEACHING
• Caution patient to continue taking this drug as prescribed, even when he's feeling well.
• Instruct patient to take drug with food.
• *Alert:* Tell patient not to stop drug suddenly because this can exacerbate angina and precipitate MI.

---

verapamil
Apo-Verap†, Calan, Novo-Veramil†, Nu-Verap†

verapamil hydrochloride
Anpec‡, Calan, Calan SR, Cordilox‡, Cordilox SR‡, Half-Securon SR§, Isoptin SR, Novo-Veramil†, Securon§, Securon SR§, Univer§, Veracaps SR‡, Verapress MR§, Verelan, Verelan PM

Pregnancy risk category C

AVAILABLE FORMS
verapamil
Tablets: 40 mg, 80 mg, 120 mg
verapamil hydrochloride
Capsules (controlled- and extended-release): 100 mg, 200 mg, 300 mg
Capsules (sustained-release): 120 mg, 160 mg‡, 180 mg, 240 mg
Injection: 2.5 mg/ml
Tablets: 40 mg, 80 mg, 120 mg, 160 mg‡
Tablets (sustained-release): 120 mg, 180 mg, 240 mg

INDICATIONS & DOSAGES
➤ **Vasospastic angina (Prinzmetal's or variant angina); classic chronic, stable angina pectoris; chronic atrial fibrillation—**
Adults: Starting dose is 80 to 120 mg P.O. t.i.d. Increase dosage at daily or weekly intervals, p.r.n. Some patients may require up to 480 mg daily.
➤ **Prophylaxis for paroxysmal supraventricular tachycardia—**
Adults: 80 to 120 mg P.O. t.i.d. or q.i.d.
➤ **Supraventricular arrhythmias—**
Adults: 0.075 to 0.15 mg/kg (5 to 10 mg) by I.V. push over 2 minutes with ECG and blood pressure monitoring. Repeat dose in 30 minutes if no response occurs.
Children ages 1 to 15: 0.1 to 0.3 mg/kg as I.V. bolus over 2 minutes; not to exceed 5 mg.
Children younger than age 1: 0.1 to 0.2 mg/kg as I.V. bolus over 2 minutes with continuous ECG monitoring. Repeat dose in 30 minutes if no response occurs.
➤ **Digitalized patients with chronic atrial fibrillation or flutter—**
Adults: 240 to 320 mg P.O. daily divided t.i.d. or q.i.d.
➤ **Hypertension—**
Adults: 240 mg extended-release tablet P.O. once daily in the morning. If response isn't adequate, give an additional 120 mg in the evening or 240 mg q 12 hours or an 80-mg immediate-release tablet t.i.d.

I.V. ADMINISTRATION
• Give drug by direct injection into a vein or into the tubing of a free-flowing, compatible I.V. solution.
• Compatible solutions include D_5W, half-normal saline solution, normal saline solution, Ringer's solution, and lactated Ringer's solution.
• Give I.V. doses over at least 2 minutes (3 minutes in elderly patients) to minimize the risk of adverse reactions.
• Monitor ECG and blood pressure continuously in patient receiving I.V. verapamil.

ACTION
Not clearly defined. A calcium channel blocker that inhibits calcium ion influx across cardiac and smooth-muscle cells, thus decreasing myocardial contractility

---

and oxygen demand; it also dilates coronary arteries and arterioles.

Route	Onset	Peak	Duration
I.V.	Immediate	1-5 min	1-6 hr
P.O.	0.5 hr	1-2 hr	8-10 hr
P.O. (extended)	0.5 hr	5-9 hr	24 hr

ADVERSE REACTIONS
CNS: dizziness, headache, asthenia.
CV: *transient hypotension,* **heart failure,** pulmonary edema, **bradycardia, AV block, ventricular asystole, ventricular fibrillation,** peripheral edema.
GI: *constipation,* nausea.
Skin: rash.

INTERACTIONS
Drug-drug. *Antihypertensives, quinidine:* May cause hypotension. Monitor blood pressure.
Carbamazepine, cardiac glycosides: May increase levels of these drugs. Monitor patient for toxicity.
Cyclosporine: May increase cyclosporine levels. Monitor cyclosporine levels.
Disopyramide, flecainide, propranolol, other beta blockers (including ophthalmic timolol): May cause heart failure. Use together cautiously.
Lithium: May decrease or increase lithium levels. Monitor patient closely.
Rifampin: May decrease oral bioavailability of verapamil. Monitor patient for lack of effect.
Drug-herb. *Black catechu:* Causes additive effects. Discourage use together.
Yerba maté: May decrease clearance of yerba maté methylxanthines and cause toxicity. Urge caution.
Drug-food. *Any food:* Increased absorption. Advise patient to take drug with food.
Drug-lifestyle. *Alcohol use:* May enhance the effects of alcohol. Discourage use together.

EFFECTS ON LAB TEST RESULTS
● May increase ALT, AST, alkaline phosphatase, and bilirubin levels.

CONTRAINDICATIONS
Contraindicated in patients hypersensitive to drug and in those with severe left ventricular dysfunction, cardiogenic shock, second- or third-degree AV block or sick sinus syndrome except in presence of functioning pacemaker, atrial flutter or fibrillation and accessory bypass tract syndrome, severe heart failure (unless secondary to verapamil therapy), and severe hypotension. I.V. verapamil is contraindicated in patients receiving I.V. beta blockers and in those with ventricular tachycardia.

NURSING CONSIDERATIONS
● Use cautiously in elderly patients and in patients with increased intracranial pressure or hepatic or renal disease.
● Although drug should be taken with food, taking extended-release tablets with food may decrease rate and extent of absorption but allows smaller fluctuations of peak and trough blood levels.
● Pellet-filled capsules may be administered by carefully opening the capsule and sprinkling the pellets on a spoonful of applesauce. This should be swallowed immediately without chewing, followed by a glass of cool water to ensure all pellets are swallowed.
● Patients with severely compromised cardiac function or those receiving beta blockers should receive lower doses of verapamil. Monitor these patients closely.
● If verapamil is being used to terminate supraventricular tachycardia, prescriber may have the patient perform vagal maneuvers after receiving drug.
● Monitor blood pressure at the start of therapy and during dosage adjustments. Assist patient with walking because dizziness may occur.
● Notify prescriber if signs and symptoms of heart failure occur, such as swelling of hands and feet and shortness of breath.
● Monitor liver function during prolonged treatment.
● *Alert:* Don't confuse Verelan with Vivarin, Voltaren, or Virilon.

PATIENT TEACHING
● Instruct patient to take oral form of drug exactly as prescribed.
● Tell patient that long-acting forms shouldn't be crushed or chewed.
● Advise patient to take drug with food.

- Caution patient against abruptly stopping drug.
- If patient is kept on nitrate therapy during adjustment of oral verapamil dosage, urge continued compliance. S.L. nitroglycerin may be taken, as needed, when angina symptoms are acute.
- Encourage patient to increase fluid and fiber intake to combat constipation. Give a stool softener.
- Advise patient to avoid or severely limit alcohol consumption. Verapamil significantly inhibits alcohol elimination.

21

Antihypertensives

acebutolol hydrochloride
amlodipine besylate
(See Chapter 20, ANTIANGINALS.)
atenolol
benazepril hydrochloride
betaxolol hydrochloride
candesartan cilexetil
captopril
carteolol hydrochloride
carvedilol
clonidine
clonidine hydrochloride
diazoxide
diltiazem hydrochloride
(See Chapter 20, ANTIANGINALS.)
doxazosin mesylate
enalaprilat
enalapril maleate
eprosartan mesylate
felodipine
fenoldopam mesylate
fosinopril sodium
guanfacine hydrochloride
hydralazine hydrochloride
irbesartan
labetalol hydrochloride
lisinopril
losartan potassium
methyldopa
methyldopate hydrochloride
metoprolol succinate
metoprolol tartrate
minoxidil
nadolol
(See Chapter 20, ANTIANGINALS.)
nicardipine hydrochloride
(See Chapter 20, ANTIANGINALS.)
nifedipine
(See Chapter 20, ANTIANGINALS.)
nisoldipine
nitroprusside sodium
perindopril erbumine
pindolol
prazosin hydrochloride
propranolol hydrochloride
(See Chapter 20, ANTIANGINALS.)
quinapril hydrochloride
ramipril
telmisartan
terazosin hydrochloride

timolol maleate
trandolapril
valsartan
verapamil hydrochloride
(See Chapter 20, ANTIANGINALS.)

COMBINATION PRODUCTS

ALDOCLOR-150: chlorothiazide 150 mg and methyldopa 250 mg.
ALDOCLOR-250: chlorothiazide 250 mg and methyldopa 250 mg.
ALDORIL 15: hydrochlorothiazide 15 mg and methyldopa 250 mg.
ALDORIL 25: hydrochlorothiazide 25 mg and methyldopa 250 mg.
ALDORIL D30: hydrochlorothiazide 30 mg and methyldopa 500 mg.
ALDORIL D50: hydrochlorothiazide 50 mg and methyldopa 500 mg.
APRESAZIDE 25/25: hydrochlorothiazide 25 mg and hydralazine hydrochloride 25 mg.
APRESAZIDE 50/50: hydrochlorothiazide 50 mg and hydralazine hydrochloride 50 mg.
CAPOZIDE 25/15: hydrochlorothiazide 15 mg and captopril 25 mg.
CAPOZIDE 25/25: hydrochlorothiazide 25 mg and captopril 25 mg.
CAPOZIDE 50/15: hydrochlorothiazide 15 mg and captopril 50 mg.
CAPOZIDE 50/25: hydrochlorothiazide 25 mg and captopril 50 mg.
COMBIPRES 0.1: chlorthalidone 15 mg and clonidine hydrochloride 0.1 mg.
COMBIPRES 0.2: chlorthalidone 15 mg and clonidine hydrochloride 0.2 mg.
COMBIPRES 0.3: chlorthalidone 15 mg and clonidine hydrochloride 0.3 mg.
CORZIDE: nadolol 40 mg or 80 mg and bendroflumethiazide 5 mg.
DIURIGEN WITH RESERPINE: chlorothiazide 250 mg and reserpine 0.125 mg.
DIUTENSEN-R: methylclothiazide 2.5 mg and reserpine 0.1 mg.
ENDURONYL: methylclothiazide 5 mg and deserpidine 0.25 mg.
ENDURONYL FORTE: methylclothiazide 5 mg and deserpidine 0.5 mg.

---

*Liquid contains alcohol.   **May contain tartrazine.   †Canada   ‡Australia   §U.K.   ◇OTC

HYDROSERPINE: hydrochlorothiazide 25 or 50 mg and reserpine 0.125 mg.

HYZAAR: losartan 50 mg and hydrochlorothiazide 12.5 mg.

INDERIDE 40/25: propranolol hydrochloride 40 mg and hydrochlorothiazide 25 mg.

INDERIDE 80/25: propranolol hydrochloride 80 mg and hydrochlorothiazide 25 mg.

INDERIDE LA 80/50: propranolol hydrochloride 80 mg and hydrochlorothiazide 50 mg.

INDERIDE LA 120/50: propranolol hydrochloride 120 mg and hydrochlorothiazide 50 mg.

INDERIDE LA 160/50: propranolol hydrochloride 160 mg and hydrochlorothiazide 50 mg.

LEXXEL: enalapril maleate 5 mg and felodipine 5 mg.

LOPRESSOR HCT 50/25: metoprolol tartrate 50 mg and hydrochlorothiazide 25 mg.

LOPRESSOR HCT 100/25: metoprolol tartrate 100 mg and hydrochlorothiazide 25 mg.

LOPRESSOR HCT 100/50: metoprolol tartrate 100 mg and hydrochlorothiazide 50 mg.

MAXZIDE: triamterene 75 mg and hydrochlorothiazide 50 mg.

MINIZIDE 1: polythiazide 0.5 mg and prazosin hydrochloride 1 mg.

MINIZIDE 2: polythiazide 0.5 mg and prazosin hydrochloride 2 mg.

MINIZIDE 5: polythiazide 0.5 mg and prazosin hydrochloride 5 mg.

PRINZIDE 12.5: lisinopril 20 mg and hydrochlorothiazide 12.5 mg.

PRINZIDE 25: lisinopril 20 mg and hydrochlorothiazide 25 mg.

RAUZIDE**: bendroflumethiazide 4 mg and powdered rauwolfia serpentina 50 mg.

REGROTON: chlorthalidone 50 mg and reserpine 0.25 mg.

RENESE-R: polythiazide 2 mg and reserpine 0.25 mg.

SALUTENSIN-DEMI: hydroflumethiazide 25 mg and reserpine 0.125 mg.

SALUTENSIN TABLETS: hydroflumethiazide 50 mg and reserpine 0.125 mg.

SER-AP-ES: hydrochlorothiazide 15 mg, reserpine 0.1 mg, and hydralazine hydrochloride 25 mg.

TENORETIC 50: atenolol 50 mg and chlorthalidone 25 mg.

TENORETIC 100: atenolol 100 mg and chlorthalidone 25 mg.

TIMOLIDE 10-25: timolol maleate 10 mg and hydrochlorothiazide 25 mg.

TRI-HYDROSERPINE: hydrochlorothiazide 15 mg, hydralazine hydrochloride 25 mg, and reserpine 0.1 mg.

VASERETIC 10-25: enalapril maleate 10 mg and hydrochlorothiazide 25 mg.

ZESTORETIC: lisinopril 20 mg and hydrochlorothiazide 12.5 mg.

ZESTORETIC: lisinopril 20 mg and hydrochlorothiazide 25 mg.

ZIAC TABLETS: bisoprolol fumarate 2.5 mg, 5 mg, or 10 mg and hydrochlorothiazide 6.5 mg.

acebutolol hydrochloride
Monitan†, Sectral

Pregnancy risk category B

AVAILABLE FORMS
Capsules: 200 mg, 400 mg
Tablets: 100 mg†, 200 mg, 400 mg

INDICATIONS & DOSAGES
➤ **Hypertension**—
Adults: 400 mg P.O. either as a single daily dose or in divided doses b.i.d. Maximum daily dose is 1,200 mg.
➤ **Ventricular arrhythmias**—
Adults: 400 mg P.O. daily divided b.i.d. Dosage increased to provide an adequate clinical response. Usual dose is 600 to 1,200 mg daily.
Elderly patients: May need lower dosage; dose shouldn't exceed 800 mg daily.
Adjust-a-dose: For renally impaired patients with creatinine clearance of 25 to 50 ml/minute, reduce dosage by 50%; if clearance is below 25 ml/minute, reduce dosage by 75%.

ACTION
Unknown. Possible mechanisms include reduced cardiac output, decreased sympathetic outflow to peripheral vasculature, and inhibition of renin release. Drug de-

creases myocardial contractility and heart rate and has mild intrinsic sympathomimetic activity.

Route	Onset	Peak	Duration
P.O.	1-1.5 hr	2.5 hr	24 hr

ADVERSE REACTIONS
CNS: *fatigue,* headache, dizziness, insomnia, depression.
CV: chest pain, edema, ***bradycardia, heart failure,*** hypotension.
GI: nausea, constipation, diarrhea, dyspepsia, flatulence, vomiting.
GU: dysuria, impotence, nocturia, urinary frequency.
Musculoskeletal: arthralgia, myalgia.
Respiratory: dyspnea, ***bronchospasm,*** cough.
Skin: rash.

INTERACTIONS
Drug-drug. *Cardiac glycosides, diltiazem, verapamil:* Excessive bradycardia and increased depressant effect on myocardium. Use together cautiously.
Catecholamine-depleting drugs such as reserpine: Effects may be additive. Monitor patient closely.
Diuretics, other antihypertensives: Increased hypotensive effect. Use together cautiously.
Insulin, oral antidiabetics: Can alter dosage requirements in previously stabilized diabetic patients. Observe patient carefully.
NSAIDs: Decreased antihypertensive effect. Monitor blood pressure and adjust dosage.
Sympathomimetics: May antagonize effects. Expect to give greater-than-usual dosages of beta-adrenergic agonist bronchodilators.
Drug-food. *Grapefruit juice:* Increased levels of drug and risk of adverse effects. Advise patient to take with liquid other than grapefruit juice.

EFFECTS ON LAB TEST RESULTS
None reported.

CONTRAINDICATIONS
Contraindicated in patients with persistent severe bradycardia, second- and third-degree heart block, overt cardiac failure, and cardiogenic shock.

NURSING CONSIDERATIONS
• Use cautiously in patients with cardiac failure, peripheral vascular disease, bronchospastic disease, and diabetes.
• Check apical pulse before giving drug; if slower than 60 beats/minute, withhold drug and call prescriber. Also monitor blood pressure.
• Before surgery, tell anesthesiologist that patient is taking drug.
• Acebutolol may mask signs and symptoms of hyperthyroidism.
• Drug loses its selectivity for the beta₁ receptor at higher doses. Watch for peripheral effects.
• Drug may cause positive antinuclear antibody titers.
• *Alert:* Discontinue drug gradually over 2 weeks.
• Drug can mask signs and symptoms of hypoglycemia in diabetic patients.
• *Alert:* Don't confuse Sectral with Factrel or Septra.

PATIENT TEACHING
• Instruct patient to take drug exactly as prescribed.
• Tell patient to avoid taking OTC oral cold preparations or topical nasal decongestants because of risk of severe hypertensive reaction.
• Warn patient not to stop drug suddenly and to notify prescriber promptly of unpleasant adverse reactions.
• Teach patient how to take his pulse, and instruct him to withhold the dose and notify prescriber if pulse rate is below 60 beats/minute.
• Tell patient that drug may deplete body's stores of coenzyme Q10 and that he should discuss the need for supplements with prescriber.

---

atenolol
Anselol‡, Apo-Atenolol†, Noten‡, Tenormin, Tensig‡

Pregnancy risk category D

AVAILABLE FORMS
Injection: 5 mg/10 ml
Tablets: 25 mg, 50 mg, 100 mg

INDICATIONS & DOSAGES

➤ **Hypertension—**

Adults: Initially, 50 mg P.O. daily alone or in combination with a diuretic as a single dose, increased to 100 mg once daily after 7 to 14 days. Dosages of more than 100 mg are unlikely to produce further benefit.

➤ **Angina pectoris—**

Adults: 50 mg P.O. once daily, increased, p.r.n., to 100 mg daily after 7 days for optimal effect. Maximum dose is 200 mg daily.

➤ **To reduce CV mortality and risk of reinfarction in patients with acute MI—**

Adults: 5 mg I.V. over 5 minutes; then another 5 mg after 10 minutes. After an additional 10 minutes, 50 mg P.O.; then 50 mg P.O. in 12 hours. Thereafter, 100 mg P.O. daily (as a single dose or 50 mg b.i.d.) for at least 7 days.

Adjust-a-dose: For renally impaired patients with creatinine clearance of 15 to 35 ml/minute, maximum dose is 50 mg/day; if clearance is below 15 ml/minute, maximum dose is 25 mg/day.

Hemodialysis patients need 25 to 50 mg after each dialysis session.

I.V. ADMINISTRATION

• I.V. doses may be mixed with D_5W, normal saline, or dextrose and saline solutions. Solution is stable for 48 hours after mixing.

• Give by slow I.V. injection, not exceeding 1 mg/minute.

ACTION

A beta blocker that selectively blocks beta$_1$-adrenergic receptors; decreases cardiac output, peripheral resistance, and cardiac oxygen consumption; and depresses renin secretion.

Route	Onset	Peak	Duration
I.V.	5 min	5 min	12 hr
P.O.	1 hr	2-4 hr	24 hr

ADVERSE REACTIONS

CNS: *fatigue,* lethargy, vertigo, drowsiness, *dizziness.*

CV: **bradycardia,** *hypotension,* **heart failure,** intermittent claudication.

GI: nausea, diarrhea.

Musculoskeletal: leg pain.

Respiratory: dyspnea, **bronchospasm.**

Skin: rash.

Other: fever.

INTERACTIONS

Drug-drug. *Antihypertensives:* Increased hypotensive effect. Use together cautiously.

Cardiac glycosides, diltiazem, verapamil: Excessive bradycardia and increased depressant effect on myocardium. Use together cautiously.

Insulin, oral antidiabetics: Can alter dosage requirements in previously stabilized diabetic patient. Observe patient carefully.

Reserpine: May cause hypotension. Use together cautiously.

EFFECTS ON LAB TEST RESULTS

• May increase BUN, creatinine, potassium, uric acid, glucose, transaminase, alkaline phosphatase, and LDH levels. May decrease glucose level.

• May increase platelet count.

CONTRAINDICATIONS

Contraindicated in patients with sinus bradycardia, greater than first-degree heart block, overt cardiac failure, or cardiogenic shock.

NURSING CONSIDERATIONS

• Use cautiously in patients at risk for heart failure and in those with bronchospastic disease, diabetes, hyperthyroidism, and impaired renal or hepatic function.

• Check apical pulse before giving drug; if slower than 60 beats/minute, withhold drug and call prescriber.

• Monitor patient's blood pressure.

• Monitor hemodialysis patients closely because of risk of hypotension.

• Beta blockers may mask tachycardia caused by hyperthyroidism. In patients with suspected thyrotoxicosis, withdraw beta blocker gradually to avoid thyroid storm.

• Drug may mask signs and symptoms of hypoglycemia in diabetic patients.

• Calcium channel blockers may have additive effects.

• Drug may cause changes in exercise tolerance and ECG.

• **Alert:** Withdraw drug gradually over 2 weeks to avoid serious adverse reactions.

Reactions may be *common,* uncommon, **life-threatening,** or **COMMON AND LIFE-THREATENING.**

● *Alert:* Don't confuse atenolol with timolol or albuterol.

PATIENT TEACHING
● Instruct patient to take drug exactly as prescribed, at the same time every day.
● Caution patient not to stop drug suddenly, but to notify prescriber if unpleasant adverse reactions occur.
● Teach patient how to take his pulse. Tell him to withhold drug and call prescriber if pulse rate is below 60 beats/minute.
● Tell woman to notify prescriber about planned, suspected, or known pregnancy. Drug will need to be discontinued.
● Advise breast-feeding mother to contact prescriber; drug isn't recommended for breast-feeding women.
● Tell patient that drug may deplete body's stores of coenzyme Q10 and that he should discuss need for supplements with prescriber.

---

benazepril hydrochloride
Lotensin

Pregnancy risk category C (D in second and third trimesters)

AVAILABLE FORMS
Tablets: 5 mg, 10 mg, 20 mg, 40 mg

INDICATIONS & DOSAGES
➤ **Hypertension—**
Adults: For patients not receiving a diuretic, 10 mg P.O. daily initially. Dosage adjusted p.r.n. and as tolerated; most patients take 20 to 40 mg daily in one or two divided doses. For patients receiving a diuretic, initially, 5 mg P.O. daily.
Adjust-a-dose: For renally impaired patients with creatinine clearance below 30 ml/minute, 5 mg P.O. daily. Dose may be adjusted up to 40 mg/day.

ACTION
Drug and its active metabolite, benazeprilat, inhibit ACE, preventing conversion of angiotensin I to angiotensin II, a potent vasoconstrictor. Reduced formation of angiotensin II decreases peripheral arterial resistance, thus decreasing aldosterone secretion, which in turn reduces sodium and water retention and lowers blood pressure. Drug also exhibits antihypertensive activity in patients with low-renin hypertension.

Route	Onset	Peak	Duration
P.O.	1 hr	2-4 hr	24 hr

ADVERSE REACTIONS
CNS: headache, dizziness, drowsiness, fatigue, somnolence.
CV: symptomatic hypotension.
GI: nausea.
GU: impotence.
Metabolic: hyperkalemia.
Musculoskeletal: arthralgia, arthritis, myalgia.
Respiratory: dry, persistent, nonproductive cough.
Skin: increased diaphoresis.
Other: hypersensitivity reactions.

INTERACTIONS
Drug-drug. *Diuretics, other antihypertensives:* May cause excessive hypotension. Discontinue diuretic or lower dose of benazepril, as needed.
Lithium: Increased lithium levels and lithium toxicity. Use together cautiously; monitor lithium levels.
Potassium-sparing diuretics, potassium supplements: Risk of hyperkalemia. Monitor patient closely.
Drug-herb. *Capsaicin:* May cause cough. Discourage use together.
Drug-food. *Salt substitutes containing potassium:* May cause hyperkalemia. Monitor patient closely.

EFFECTS ON LAB TEST RESULTS
● May increase BUN, creatinine, and potassium levels.

CONTRAINDICATIONS
Contraindicated in patients hypersensitive to ACE inhibitors.

NURSING CONSIDERATIONS
● Use cautiously in patients with impaired hepatic or renal function.
● Safety and efficacy of dosages of more than 80 mg/day haven't been established.
● Monitor patient for hypotension. Excessive hypotension can occur when drug is given with diuretics. If possible, diuretic therapy should be stopped 2 to 3 days be-

---

fore starting benazepril to decrease potential for excessive hypotensive response. If drug doesn't adequately control blood pressure, diuretic may be reinstituted with care.

• Although ACE inhibitors reduce blood pressure in all races studied, this response is less in blacks who receive the drug as monotherapy. Therapy with a thiazide diuretic produces a more favorable response.

• ACE inhibitors appear to increase risk of angioedema in black patients.

• Measure blood pressure when drug levels are at peak (2 to 6 hours after administration) and at trough (just before a dose) to verify adequate blood pressure control.

• Assess renal and hepatic function before and periodically throughout therapy. Monitor potassium levels.

• *Alert:* Don't confuse benazepril with Benadryl or Lotensin with Loniten or lovastatin.

PATIENT TEACHING
• Instruct patient to avoid salt substitutes; these products may contain potassium, which can cause hyperkalemia in patients taking drug.

• Inform patient that light-headedness can occur, especially during first few days of therapy. Tell him to rise slowly to minimize this effect and to report dizziness to prescriber. If syncope occurs, he should stop drug and call prescriber immediately.

• Warn patient to use caution in hot weather and during exercise. Inadequate fluid intake, vomiting, diarrhea, and excessive perspiration can lead to light-headedness and syncope.

• Advise patient to report signs of infection, such as fever and sore throat. Tell him to call prescriber if the following signs or symptoms occur: easy bruising or bleeding; swelling of tongue, lips, face, eyes, mucous membranes, or extremities; difficulty swallowing or breathing; or hoarseness.

• Tell woman to notify prescriber if pregnancy occurs. Drug will need to be discontinued.

betaxolol hydrochloride
Kerlone

Pregnancy risk category C

AVAILABLE FORMS
Tablets: 10 mg, 20 mg

INDICATIONS & DOSAGES
➤ **Hypertension (used alone or with other antihypertensives)—**
Adults: Initially, 10 mg P.O. once daily; if desired response doesn't occur in 7 to 14 days, 20 mg P.O. once daily. Maximum, 40 mg daily.

ACTION
Unknown. A selective beta blocker that decreases blood pressure, possibly by slowing heart rate and decreasing cardiac output and peripheral resistance.

Route	Onset	Peak	Duration
P.O.	3 hr	2-4 hr	24-48 hr

ADVERSE REACTIONS
CNS: dizziness, fatigue, headache, insomnia, lethargy, anxiety.
CV: *bradycardia,* chest pain, *heart failure,* edema.
EENT: pharyngitis.
GI: nausea, diarrhea, dyspepsia.
GU: impotence.
Musculoskeletal: arthralgia.
Respiratory: dyspnea, *bronchospasm.*
Skin: rash.

INTERACTIONS
Drug-drug. *Calcium channel blockers:* May cause hypotension, left-sided heart failure, and AV conduction disturbances. Use I.V. calcium channel blockers with caution.
Catecholamine-depleting drugs, reserpine: May have an additive effect. Monitor patient closely.
General anesthetics: May cause hypotensive effects. Monitor patient carefully for excessive hypotension or bradycardia or orthostatic hypotension.
Lidocaine: May increase lidocaine's effects. Monitor patient.

EFFECTS ON LAB TEST RESULTS
None reported.

CONTRAINDICATIONS
Contraindicated in patients hypersensitive to drug; also contraindicated in those with severe bradycardia, greater than first-degree heart block, cardiogenic shock, or uncontrolled heart failure.

NURSING CONSIDERATIONS
• Use cautiously in patients with heart failure controlled by cardiac glycosides and diuretics because these patients may exhibit signs of cardiac decompensation with beta-blocker therapy.
• When discontinuing drug, withdraw gradually over 2 weeks.
• Monitor blood pressure closely.
• Monitor glucose levels regularly in patients with diabetes. Beta blockade may inhibit glycogenolysis as well as the signs and symptoms of hypoglycemia (such as tachycardia and blood pressure changes). Oral beta blockers may alter the results of glucose tolerance tests.
• Withdrawal of beta-blocker therapy before surgery is controversial. Withdrawal is sometimes advocated to prevent impairment of cardiac responsiveness to reflex stimuli and decreased responsiveness to administration of catecholamines. Advise anesthesiologist that patient is receiving a beta blocker so that isoproterenol or dobutamine can be readily available for reversal of drug's cardiac effects.
• Beta blockers may mask tachycardia caused by hyperthyroidism. In patients with suspected thyrotoxicosis, withdraw beta blocker gradually to avoid thyroid storm.

PATIENT TEACHING
• Instruct patient to take drug exactly as prescribed.
• *Alert:* Advise patient that abrupt discontinuation may precipitate angina pectoris in patients with unrecognized coronary artery disease.
• Emphasize importance of promptly reporting signs and symptoms of heart failure, including shortness of breath or difficulty breathing, unusually fast heartbeat, cough, and fatigue with exertion.

• Advise patient not to drive or do other tasks that require mental alertness until effects of drug are known.
• Tell patient that drug may deplete body's stores of coenzyme Q10 and that he should discuss need for supplements with prescriber.

---

candesartan cilexetil
Atacand

Pregnancy risk category C (D in second and third trimesters)

AVAILABLE FORMS
Tablets: 4 mg, 8 mg, 16 mg, 32 mg

INDICATIONS & DOSAGES
➤ **Hypertension (used alone or with other antihypertensives)—**
Adults: Initially, 16 mg P.O. once daily when used as monotherapy; usual range is 8 to 32 mg P.O. daily as a single dose or divided b.i.d.

ACTION
Inhibits vasoconstrictive action of angiotensin II by blocking angiotensin II receptor on the surface of vascular smooth muscle and other tissue cells.

Route	Onset	Peak	Duration
P.O.	Unknown	3-4 hr	24 hr

ADVERSE REACTIONS
CNS: dizziness, fatigue, headache.
CV: chest pain, peripheral edema.
EENT: pharyngitis, rhinitis, sinusitis.
GI: abdominal pain, diarrhea, nausea, vomiting.
GU: albuminuria.
Musculoskeletal: arthralgia, back pain.
Respiratory: coughing, bronchitis, upper respiratory tract infection.

INTERACTIONS
Drug-drug. *Potassium-sparing diuretics, potassium supplements:* May cause hyperkalemia. Monitor patient closely.
Drug-food. *Salt substitutes containing potassium:* May cause hyperkalemia. Monitor patient closely.

EFFECTS ON LAB TEST RESULTS
None reported.

CONTRAINDICATIONS
Contraindicated in patients hypersensitive to drug or its components.

NURSING CONSIDERATIONS
• Use cautiously in patients whose renal function depends on the renin-angiotensin-aldosterone system (such as patients with heart failure) because of risk of oliguria and progressive azotemia with acute renal failure or death.
• Use cautiously in patients who are volume- or salt-depleted because of potential for symptomatic hypotension. Start therapy with a lower dosage range and monitor blood pressure carefully.
• Drugs such as candesartan that act directly on the renin-angiotensin system can cause fetal and neonatal morbidity and death when given to pregnant women. These problems haven't been detected when exposure has been limited to first trimester. If pregnancy is suspected, notify prescriber because drug should be discontinued.
• If hypotension occurs after a dose of candesartan, place patient in the supine position and, if needed, give an I.V. infusion of normal saline.
• Most of drug's antihypertensive effect is present within 2 weeks. Maximal antihypertensive effect is obtained within 4 to 6 weeks. Diuretic may be added if blood pressure isn't controlled by drug alone.
• Carefully monitor therapeutic response and the occurrence of adverse reactions in elderly patients and in those with renal disease.

PATIENT TEACHING
• Inform woman of childbearing age of the consequences of second and third trimester exposure to drug. Advise her to notify prescriber immediately if pregnancy is suspected.
• Advise breast-feeding woman of the risk of adverse effects on the infant and the need to either stop breast-feeding or discontinue drug.
• Instruct patient to store drug at room temperature and to keep container tightly sealed.

• Inform patient to report adverse reactions without delay.
• Tell patient that drug may be taken without regard to meals.

captopril
Acenorm‡, Capoten, Enzace‡, Novo-Captoril†

Pregnancy risk category C (D in second and third trimesters)

AVAILABLE FORMS
Tablets: 12.5 mg, 25 mg, 50 mg, 100 mg

INDICATIONS & DOSAGES
➤ **Hypertension—**
Adults: Initially, 25 mg P.O. b.i.d. or t.i.d. If blood pressure isn't satisfactorily controlled in 1 to 2 weeks, increase dosage to 50 mg b.i.d. or t.i.d. If not satisfactorily controlled after another 1 to 2 weeks, expect a diuretic to be added. If further blood pressure reduction is needed, dosage may be raised to 150 mg t.i.d. while continuing diuretic. Maximum daily dose is 450 mg.
➤ **Heart failure, to reduce risk of death and to slow development of heart failure after MI—**
Adults: Initially, 6.25 to 12.5 mg P.O. t.i.d. Gradually increased to 50 mg t.i.d., p.r.n. Maximum daily dose is 450 mg.
➤ **Diabetic nephropathy—**
Adults: 25 mg P.O. t.i.d.

ACTION
Not clearly defined. Thought to inhibit ACE, preventing conversion of angiotensin I to angiotensin II, a potent vasoconstrictor. Reduced formation of angiotensin II decreases peripheral arterial resistance, decreasing aldosterone secretion, which reduces sodium and water retention and lowers blood pressure.

Route	Onset	Peak	Duration
P.O.	0.25-1 hr	1-1.5 hr	6-12 hr

ADVERSE REACTIONS
CNS: dizziness, fainting, headache, malaise, fatigue.
CV: *tachycardia, hypotension,* angina pectoris.

Reactions may be *common*, uncommon, **life-threatening**, or COMMON AND LIFE-THREATENING.

GI: abdominal pain, anorexia, constipation, diarrhea, dry mouth, dysgeusia, nausea, vomiting.

Hematologic: *leukopenia, agranulocytosis, pancytopenia,* anemia, *thrombocytopenia.*

Metabolic: hyperkalemia.

Respiratory: dyspnea; *dry, persistent, nonproductive cough.*

Skin: *urticarial rash, maculopapular rash,* pruritus, alopecia.

Other: fever, *angioedema of face and limbs.*

INTERACTIONS

Drug-drug. *Antacids:* Decreased captopril effect. Separate administration times.

Digoxin: May increase digoxin level by 15% to 30%. Monitor patient.

Diuretics, other antihypertensives: May cause excessive hypotension. Diuretic may need to be discontinued or captopril dosage lowered.

Insulin, oral antidiabetics: May cause hypoglycemia when captopril therapy is initiated. Monitor patient closely.

Lithium: Increased lithium levels and symptoms of toxicity possible. Monitor patient closely.

NSAIDs: May reduce antihypertensive effect. Monitor blood pressure.

Potassium-sparing diuretics, potassium supplements: May cause hyperkalemia. Avoid using together unless hypokalemic blood levels are confirmed.

Drug-herb. *Black catechu:* Additional hypotensive effect. Discourage use together.

Capsaicin: May cause cough. Discourage use together.

Drug-food. *Salt substitutes containing potassium:* May cause hyperkalemia. Monitor patient closely.

EFFECTS ON LAB TEST RESULTS

• May increase alkaline phosphatase, bilirubin, and potassium levels.

• May decrease hemoglobin and WBC, granulocyte, RBC, and platelet counts.

CONTRAINDICATIONS

Contraindicated in patients hypersensitive to drug or other ACE inhibitors.

NURSING CONSIDERATIONS

• Use cautiously in patients with impaired renal function or serious autoimmune disease, especially systemic lupus erythematosus, and in those who have been exposed to other drugs known to affect WBC counts or immune response.

• Monitor patient's blood pressure and pulse rate frequently.

• *Alert:* Elderly patients may be more sensitive to drug's hypotensive effects.

• Assess patient for signs of angioedema.

• Drug causes the most frequent occurrence of cough, compared with other ACE inhibitors.

• In patients with impaired renal function or collagen vascular disease, monitor WBC and differential counts before starting treatment, every 2 weeks for the first 3 months of therapy, and periodically thereafter.

• Drug may cause false-positive results for urinary acetone.

• *Alert:* Don't confuse captopril with Capitrol.

PATIENT TEACHING

• Instruct patient to take drug 1 hour before meals; food in the GI tract may reduce absorption.

• Inform patient that light-headedness is possible, especially during first few days of therapy. Tell him to rise slowly to minimize this effect and to report occurrence to prescriber. If syncope occurs, he should stop drug and call prescriber immediately.

• Tell patient to use caution in hot weather and during exercise. Inadequate fluid intake, vomiting, diarrhea, and excessive perspiration can lead to light-headedness and syncope.

• Advise patient to report signs and symptoms of infection, such as fever and sore throat.

• Tell woman to notify prescriber if pregnancy occurs. Drug will need to be discontinued.

• Urge patient to promptly report swelling of the face, lips, or mouth or difficulty breathing.

---

carteolol hydrochloride
Cartrol

Pregnancy risk category C

AVAILABLE FORMS
Tablets: 2.5 mg, 5 mg

INDICATIONS & DOSAGES
➤ **Hypertension—**
Adults: Initially, 2.5 mg P.O. as a single daily dose; gradually increased to 5 or 10 mg as a single daily dose, p.r.n. Doses that exceed 10 mg daily don't produce a greater response and may actually decrease it.
Adjust-a-dose: For patients with renal insufficiency, if creatinine clearance is between 20 and 60 ml/minute, dosage interval is 48 hours; if below 20 ml/minute, dosage interval is 72 hours.

ACTION
Unknown. A nonselective beta blocker with intrinsic sympathomimetic activity. Its antihypertensive effects are probably caused by decreased sympathetic outflow from the brain and decreased cardiac output. Drug doesn't have a consistent effect on renin output.

Route	Onset	Peak	Duration
P.O.	Unknown	1-3 hr	24 hr

ADVERSE REACTIONS
CNS: lassitude, fatigue, somnolence, *asthenia,* paresthesia.
CV: conduction disturbances, ***bradycardia.***
EENT: nasal congestion.
GI: diarrhea, nausea, abdominal pain.
Musculoskeletal: *muscle cramps,* arthralgia.
Skin: sweating, rash.

INTERACTIONS
Drug-drug. *Calcium channel blockers:* May cause hypotension, left-sided heart failure, and AV conduction disturbances. Use I.V. calcium channel blockers with caution.
Cardiac glycosides: May produce additive effects on slowing AV node conduction. Avoid using together.

Catecholamine-depleting drugs, reserpine: May have an additive effect. Monitor patient closely.
General anesthetics: May cause hypotensive effects. Observe carefully for excessive hypotension, bradycardia, or orthostatic hypotension.
Insulin, oral antidiabetics: May alter hypoglycemic response. Adjust dosage, as needed.

EFFECTS ON LAB TEST RESULTS
None reported.

CONTRAINDICATIONS
Contraindicated in patients with bronchial asthma, severe bradycardia, greater than first-degree heart block, cardiogenic shock, or uncontrolled heart failure.

NURSING CONSIDERATIONS
● Use cautiously in patients with heart failure controlled by cardiac glycosides and diuretics because these patients may exhibit signs of cardiac decompensation with beta-blocker therapy.
● Monitor blood pressure frequently.
● Beta blockade may inhibit glycogenolysis and the signs and symptoms of hypoglycemia (such as tachycardia and blood pressure changes). It may also attenuate insulin release. Monitor glucose levels frequently.
● *Alert:* Withdrawal of beta-blocker therapy before surgery is controversial. Withdrawal may be advocated to prevent impairment of cardiac responsiveness to reflex stimuli and decreased responsiveness to administration of catecholamines. However, the beta-blocking effects of carteolol may persist for weeks, and discontinuing drug before surgery may be impractical. Advise anesthesiologist that patient is receiving a beta blocker so that isoproterenol or dobutamine can be readily available for reversal of drug's cardiac effects.
● Beta blockers may mask tachycardia caused by hyperthyroidism. In patients with suspected thyrotoxicosis, gradually withdraw beta-blocker therapy to avoid thyroid storm.
● *Alert:* Patients with unrecognized coronary artery disease may exhibit signs of

---

Reactions may be *common,* uncommon, *life-threatening,* or COMMON AND LIFE-THREATENING.

angina pectoris on withdrawal of drug. Monitor patient closely.

PATIENT TEACHING
• Instruct patient to take drug exactly as prescribed.
• Tell patient not to stop drug suddenly but to notify prescriber and discuss unpleasant adverse reactions.
• Emphasize importance of reporting signs and symptoms of heart failure, including shortness of breath or difficulty breathing, unusually fast heartbeat, cough, or fatigue with exertion.

---

carvedilol
Coreg, Eucardic§

Pregnancy risk category C

AVAILABLE FORMS
Tablets: 3.125 mg, 6.25 mg, 12.5 mg, 25 mg

INDICATIONS & DOSAGES
➤ **Hypertension—**
Adults: Dosage highly individualized. Initially, 6.25 mg P.O. b.i.d. Measure standing blood pressure 1 hour after initial dose. If tolerated, continue dosage for 7 to 14 days. May increase to 12.5 mg P.O. b.i.d. for 7 to 14 days, following blood pressure monitoring protocol noted above. Maximum dose is 25 mg P.O. b.i.d. as tolerated.
➤ **Heart failure—**
Adults: Dosage highly individualized. Initially, 3.125 mg P.O. b.i.d. for 2 weeks; if tolerated, can increase to 6.25 mg P.O. b.i.d. Dosage may be doubled q 2 weeks as tolerated. Maximum dose for patients weighing less than 85 kg (187 lb) is 25 mg P.O. b.i.d.; for those weighing more than 85 kg, dose is 50 mg P.O. b.i.d.
Adjust-a-dose: In patient with pulse rate below 55 beats/minute, use reduced dosage.

ACTION
Nonselective beta blocker with alpha$_1$-blocking activity.

Route	Onset	Peak	Duration
P.O.	Unknown	1-2 hr	7-10 hr

ADVERSE REACTIONS
CNS: *dizziness, fatigue,* headache, hypoesthesia, insomnia, pain, paresthesia, somnolence, vertigo, syncope, malaise.
CV: aggravated angina pectoris, *AV block, bradycardia,* chest pain, fluid overload, hypertension, hypotension, orthostatic hypotension, peripheral edema, edema.
EENT: abnormal vision, pharyngitis, rhinitis, sinusitis.
GI: abdominal pain, *diarrhea,* melena, nausea, periodontitis, vomiting.
GU: abnormal renal function, albuminuria, hematuria, impotence, urinary tract infection.
Hematologic: purpura, *thrombocytopenia.*
Metabolic: dehydration, glycosuria, gout, hypercholesterolemia, *hyperglycemia,* hypertriglyceridemia, hypervolemia, hypovolemia, hyperuricemia, hypoglycemia, hyponatremia, weight gain.
Musculoskeletal: arthralgia, back pain, myalgia.
Respiratory: bronchitis, dyspnea, *upper respiratory tract infection.*
Other: allergic reaction, fever, viral infection.

INTERACTIONS
Drug-drug. *Calcium channel blockers:* Can cause isolated conduction disturbances. Monitor patient's heart rhythm and blood pressure.
Catecholamine-depleting drugs, such as MAO inhibitors, reserpine: May cause bradycardia or severe hypotension. Monitor patient closely.
Cimetidine: Increased bioavailability of carvedilol. Monitor vital signs closely.
Clonidine: May increase blood pressure and heart rate lowering effects. Monitor vital signs closely.
Digoxin: Increased levels of digoxin by about 15% when given together. Monitor digoxin levels.
Fluoxetine, paroxetine, propafenone, quinidine: Increased glucose levels of carvedilol by inhibiting metabolism. Monitor vital signs closely.
Insulin, oral antidiabetics: May enhance hypoglycemic properties. Monitor glucose levels.
Rifampin: Reduced plasma levels of carvedilol by 70%. Monitor vital signs closely.

Drug-food. *Any food:* Delayed rate of absorption of carvedilol with no change in bioavailability. Advise patient to take drug with food to minimize orthostatic effects.

EFFECTS ON LAB TEST RESULTS
• May increase BUN, ALT, AST, and alkaline phosphatase levels.
• May decrease platelet count, PT, and INR.

CONTRAINDICATIONS
Contraindicated in patients hypersensitive to drug and in those with New York Heart Association class IV decompensated cardiac failure requiring I.V. inotropic therapy. Also contraindicated in those with bronchial asthma or related bronchospastic conditions, second- or third-degree AV block, sick sinus syndrome (unless a permanent pacemaker is in place), cardiogenic shock, severe bradycardia, or symptomatic hepatic impairment.

NURSING CONSIDERATIONS
• Use cautiously in hypertensive patients with left-sided heart failure, perioperative patients who receive anesthetics that depress myocardial function (such as cyclopropane and trichloroethylene), diabetic patients receiving insulin or oral antidiabetics, and in those subject to spontaneous hypoglycemia. Also use with caution in patients with thyroid disease (may mask hyperthyroidism; withdrawal may precipitate thyroid storm or exacerbation of hyperthyroidism), pheochromocytoma, Prinzmetal's or variant angina, bronchospastic disease, or peripheral vascular disease (may precipitate or aggravate symptoms of arterial insufficiency). Also use cautiously in breast-feeding women.
• *Alert:* Patients receiving beta-blocker therapy who have a history of severe anaphylactic reaction to several allergens may be more reactive to repeated challenge (accidental, diagnostic, or therapeutic). They may be unresponsive to dosages of epinephrine typically used to treat allergic reactions.
• Mild hepatocellular injury may occur during therapy. At first sign of hepatic dysfunction, perform tests for hepatic injury or jaundice; if present, stop drug.

• If drug must be stopped, do so gradually over 1 to 2 weeks.
• Monitor patient with heart failure for worsened condition, renal dysfunction, or fluid retention; diuretics may need to be increased.
• Monitor diabetic patient closely; drug may mask signs of hypoglycemia, or hyperglycemia may be worsened.
• Observe patient for dizziness or lightheadedness for 1 hour after administration of each new dosage.
• Before initiation of carvedilol, dosages of digoxin, diuretics, and ACE inhibitors should be stabilized.
• Safety and efficacy in patients younger than age 18 haven't been established.
• Monitor elderly patients carefully; plasma levels are about 50% higher in elderly patients than in younger patients.

PATIENT TEACHING
• Tell patient not to interrupt or stop drug without medical approval.
• Inform patient that improvement of heart failure symptoms might take several weeks of drug therapy.
• Advise patient with heart failure to call prescriber if weight gain or shortness of breath occurs.
• Inform patient that he may experience low blood pressure when standing. If dizziness or fainting (rare) occurs, advise him to sit or lie down and to notify prescriber if symptoms persist.
• Caution patient against performing hazardous tasks during start of therapy.
• Advise diabetic patient to promptly report changes in glucose level.
• Inform patient who wears contact lenses that eyes may feel dry.

---

clonidine
Catapres-TTS

clonidine hydrochloride
Catapres, Dixarit†‡

Pregnancy risk category C

AVAILABLE FORMS
clonidine
Transdermal: TTS-1 (releases 0.1 mg/ 24 hours), TTS-2 (releases 0.2 mg/

24 hours), TTS-3 (releases 0.3 mg/
24 hours)
clonidine hydrochloride
Tablets: 0.025 mg†‡, 0.1 mg, 0.2 mg,
0.3 mg

INDICATIONS & DOSAGES
➤ **Essential and renal hypertension—**
Adults: Initially, 0.1 mg P.O. b.i.d.; then
increased by 0.1 to 0.2 mg daily on a
weekly basis. Usual range is 0.2 to 0.6 mg
daily in divided doses; infrequently,
dosages as high as 2.4 mg daily are used.

Or, a transdermal patch is applied to
a nonhairy area of intact skin on upper
arm or torso once q 7 days, starting with
0.1-mg system and adjusted with another
0.1-mg system or larger system.
Children: 50 to 400 mcg P.O. b.i.d.

ACTION
Unknown. Thought to stimulate alpha$_2$-
adrenergic receptors centrally and inhibit
the central vasomotor centers, thereby decreasing sympathetic outflow to the heart,
kidneys, and peripheral vasculature, resulting in decreased peripheral vascular
resistance, systolic and diastolic blood
pressure, and heart rate.

Route	Onset	Peak	Duration
P.O.	0.5-1 hr	2-4 hr	12-24 hr
Trans-dermal	2-3 days	2-3 days	7-8 days

ADVERSE REACTIONS
CNS: *drowsiness, dizziness,* fatigue, *seda-
tion, weakness,* malaise, agitation, depres-
sion.
CV: orthostatic hypotension, *bradycardia,
severe rebound hypertension.*
GI: *constipation, dry mouth,* nausea, vom-
iting, anorexia.
GU: urine retention, impotence.
Metabolic: weight gain.
Skin: *pruritus, dermatitis with transder-
mal patch,* rash.
Other: loss of libido.

INTERACTIONS
Drug-drug. *CNS depressants:* Increased
CNS depression. Use together cautiously.
Diuretics, other antihypertensives: In-
creased hypotensive effect. Monitor pa-
tient closely.

Levodopa: May reduce effectiveness of
levodopa. Monitor patient.
MAO inhibitors, prazosin, TCAs: May decrease antihypertensive effect. Use together cautiously.
Propranolol, other beta blockers: Paradoxical hypertensive response. Monitor
patient carefully.
Verapamil: May cause AV block and
severe hypotension. Monitor patient.
Drug-herb. *Capsicum:* May reduce antihypertensive effectiveness. Discourage
use together.

EFFECTS ON LAB TEST RESULTS
None reported.

CONTRAINDICATIONS
Contraindicated in patients hypersensitive
to drug. Transdermal form is contraindicated in patients hypersensitive to any
component of the adhesive layer of transdermal system.

NURSING CONSIDERATIONS
● Use cautiously in patients with severe
coronary insufficiency, recent MI, cerebrovascular disease, chronic renal failure,
or impaired liver function.
● Drug may be given to lower blood pressure rapidly in some hypertensive emergencies.
● Monitor blood pressure and pulse rate
frequently. Dosage is usually adjusted to
patient's blood pressure and tolerance.
● Elderly patients may be more sensitive
than younger ones to drug's hypotensive
effects.
● Observe patient for tolerance to drug's
therapeutic effects, which may require increased dosage.
● Noticeable antihypertensive effects of
transdermal clonidine may take 2 to 3
days. Oral antihypertensive therapy may
have to be continued in the interim.
● Clonidine may decrease urinary excretion of vanillylmandelic acid and catecholamines, and may cause a weakly positive Coombs' test.
● **Alert:** Remove transdermal patch before
defibrillation to prevent arcing.
● When stopping therapy in patients receiving both clonidine and a beta blocker,
gradually withdraw the beta blocker first
to minimize adverse reactions.

• Don't discontinue drug before surgery.
• *Alert:* Don't confuse clonidine with quinidine or clomiphene; or Catapres with Cetapred or Combipres.

PATIENT TEACHING
• Instruct patient to take drug exactly as prescribed.
• Advise patient that stopping drug abruptly may cause severe rebound hypertension. Tell him dosage must be reduced gradually over 2 to 4 days as instructed by prescriber.
• Tell patient to take the last dose immediately before bedtime.
• Reassure patient that the transdermal patch usually adheres despite showering and other routine daily activities. Instruct him on the use of the adhesive overlay to provide additional skin adherence, if needed. Also tell him to place patch at a different site each week.
• Caution patient that drug may cause drowsiness but that this adverse effect will usually diminish over 4 to 6 weeks.
• Inform patient that orthostatic hypotension can be minimized by rising slowly from a sitting or lying position and avoiding sudden position changes.

---

diazoxide
Eudemine§, Hyperstat IV

Pregnancy risk category C

AVAILABLE FORMS
Injection: 15 mg/ml in 20-ml ampules

INDICATIONS & DOSAGES
➤ **Hypertensive crisis—**
Adults and children: 1 to 3 mg/kg by I.V. bolus (to maximum of 150 mg) q 5 to 15 minutes until adequate response is seen (diastolic blood pressure less than 100 mm Hg). Repeat at 4- to 24-hour intervals, p.r.n.

I.V. ADMINISTRATION
• Protect I.V. solutions from light. Darkened I.V. solutions of diazoxide are subpotent and shouldn't be used.
• Give drug through peripheral vein only. Don't give I.M., S.C., or into body cavities.

• Monitor blood pressure and ECG continuously. Place patient supine or in Trendelenburg's position during infusion and for 1 hour afterward.
• Notify prescriber immediately if severe hypotension develops. Keep norepinephrine available.

ACTION
Unknown. Directly relaxes arteriolar smooth muscle and decreases peripheral vascular resistance.

Route	Onset	Peak	Duration
I.V.	1 min	2-5 min	2-12 hr

ADVERSE REACTIONS
CNS: *headache,* dizziness, lightheadedness, weakness, *seizures, paralysis,* euphoria, *cerebral ischemia.*
CV: *sodium and water retention,* orthostatic hypotension, flushing, warmth, angina pectoris, myocardial ischemia, *arrhythmias,* ECG changes, *shock, MI.*
EENT: optic nerve damage.
GI: *nausea, vomiting,* abdominal discomfort, dry mouth, constipation, diarrhea.
Metabolic: *hyperglycemia,* hyperuricemia.
Skin: inflammation and pain resulting from extravasation, diaphoresis.

INTERACTIONS
Drug-drug. *Antihypertensives such as beta blockers, hydralazine, methyldopa, minoxidil, nitrates, prazosin, reserpine:* May cause severe hypotension. Don't give within 6 hours of each other.
Hydantoins: May decrease levels of hydantoins, resulting in decreased anticonvulsant action. Monitor patient.
Sulfonylureas: May cause hyperglycemia. Monitor glucose levels.
Thiazide diuretics: May increase diazoxide's effects. Use together cautiously.

EFFECTS ON LAB TEST RESULTS
• May increase glucose and uric acid levels.

CONTRAINDICATIONS
Contraindicated in patients hypersensitive to drug, other thiazides, or other sulfonamide-derived drugs. Also contraindicated in those with compensatory hypertension (such as that from coarctation of the aorta or arteriovenous shunt).

Reactions may be *common,* uncommon, *life-threatening,* or COMMON AND LIFE-THREATENING.

NURSING CONSIDERATIONS

- Use cautiously in patients with impaired cerebral or cardiac function or uremia.
- Monitor patient's blood pressure frequently during bolus.
- Check patient's standing blood pressure before discontinuing close monitoring for hypotension.
- Monitor patient's fluid intake and output carefully. If fluid or sodium retention develops, prescriber may order diuretics.
- Weigh patient daily and notify prescriber of weight increase.
- Diazoxide may alter requirements for insulin, diet, or oral antidiabetics in patients with previously controlled diabetes. Monitor glucose level daily; watch for signs and symptoms of severe hyperglycemia or hyperosmolar hyperosmotic nonketotic syndrome. Insulin may be needed.
- Check uric acid levels frequently and report abnormalities to prescriber.
- Drug inhibits glucose-stimulated insulin release and may cause false-negative insulin response to glucagon. Drug may increase renin secretion and IgG, and decrease cortisol levels.
- *Alert:* Don't confuse diazoxide with Dyazide or diazepam, or Hyperstat with Nitrostat, Hyper-Tet, or HyperHep.

PATIENT TEACHING

- Inform patient that orthostatic hypotension can be minimized by rising slowly and avoiding sudden position changes. Tell patient to remain lying down for 60 minutes after injection.
- Tell patient to alert nurse if discomfort occurs at I.V. insertion site.

---

doxazosin mesylate
Cardura, Carduran‡

Pregnancy risk category C

AVAILABLE FORMS
Tablets: 1 mg, 2 mg, 4 mg, 8 mg

INDICATIONS & DOSAGES
➤ **Essential hypertension—**
Adults: Initially, 1 mg P.O. daily; determine effect on standing and supine blood pressure at 2 to 6 hours and 24 hours after dosing. If needed, dosage is increased to

2 mg daily. To minimize adverse reactions, dosage is adjusted slowly (dosage typically increased only q 2 weeks). If needed, dosage increased to 4 mg daily; then 8 mg. Maximum daily dose is 16 mg; however, doses over 4 mg daily raise the risk of adverse reactions.
➤ **BPH—**
Adults: Initially, 1 mg P.O. once daily in the morning or evening; may be increased to 2 mg and, thereafter, 4 mg and 8 mg once daily, p.r.n. Recommended adjustment interval is 1 to 2 weeks.

ACTION
An alpha$_1$-adrenergic blocker that acts on the peripheral vasculature to reduce peripheral vascular resistance and produce vasodilation.

Route	Onset	Peak	Duration
P.O.	1-2 hr	2-3 hr	24 hr

ADVERSE REACTIONS
CNS: *dizziness,* vertigo, somnolence, drowsiness, *asthenia, headache.*
CV: *orthostatic hypotension,* hypotension, edema, palpitations, **arrhythmias,** tachycardia.
EENT: rhinitis, pharyngitis, abnormal vision.
GI: nausea, vomiting, diarrhea, constipation.
Hematologic: *leukopenia, neutropenia.*
Musculoskeletal: arthralgia, myalgia.
Respiratory: dyspnea.
Skin: rash, pruritus.
Other: pain.

INTERACTIONS
Drug-herb. *Butcher's broom:* May decrease effect of doxazosin. Discourage use together.

EFFECTS ON LAB TEST RESULTS
- May decrease WBC and neutrophil counts.

CONTRAINDICATIONS
Contraindicated in patients hypersensitive to drug and quinazoline derivatives (including prazosin and terazosin).

NURSING CONSIDERATIONS
• Use cautiously in patients with impaired hepatic function.
• Monitor blood pressure closely.
• If syncope occurs, place patient in a recumbent position and treat supportively. A transient hypotensive response isn't considered a contraindication to continued therapy.
• **Alert:** Don't confuse doxazosin with doxapram, doxorubicin, or doxepin; or Cardura with Coumadin, K-Dur, Cardene, or Cordarone.

PATIENT TEACHING
• Instruct patient to take drug exactly as prescribed.
• **Alert:** Advise patient that he is susceptible to a first-dose effect (marked orthostatic hypotension with dizziness or syncope) similar to that produced by other alpha blockers. Orthostatic hypotension is most common after first dose but also can occur during dosage adjustment or interruption of therapy. Warn patient that dizziness or fainting may occur. Advise him to avoid driving and other hazardous activities until drug's CNS effects are known.

---

enalaprilat
Innovace§, Vasotec I.V.

enalapril maleate
Amprace‡, Renitec‡, Vasotec

Pregnancy risk category C (D in second and third trimesters)

AVAILABLE FORMS
enalaprilat
Injection: 1.25 mg/ml
enalapril maleate
Tablets: 2.5 mg, 5 mg, 10 mg, 20 mg

INDICATIONS & DOSAGES
➤ **Hypertension—**
Adults: In patients not taking diuretics, initially, 5 mg P.O. once daily; then adjusted based on response. Usual dosage range is 10 to 40 mg daily as a single dose or two divided doses. Or, 1.25 mg I.V. infusion over 5 minutes q 6 hours.
Adjust-a-dose: For patients taking diuretics, initially, 2.5 mg P.O. once daily. Or,

0.625 mg I.V. over 5 minutes, repeated in 1 hour, if needed; then 1.25 mg I.V. q 6 hours.
➤ **To convert from I.V. therapy to oral therapy—**
Adults: Initially, 2.5 mg P.O. once daily; if patient was receiving 0.625 mg I.V. q 6 hours, then 2.5 mg P.O once daily. Dosage is adjusted based on response.
➤ **To convert from oral therapy to I.V. therapy—**
Adults: 1.25 mg I.V. over 5 minutes q 6 hours. Higher dosages haven't shown greater efficacy.
Adjust-a-dose: For patients with renal impairment or hyponatremia, if creatinine level is more than 1.6 mg/dl or sodium level is below 130 mEq/L, start dosage at 2.5 mg P.O. daily and adjust slowly.
➤ **Management of symptomatic heart failure—**
Adults: Initially, 2.5 mg P.O. daily or b.i.d. increased gradually over several weeks. Maintenance is 5 to 20 mg daily, given in two divided doses. Maximum daily dose is 40 mg given in two divided doses.

I.V. ADMINISTRATION
• Compatible solutions include D₅W, normal saline solution for injection, dextrose 5% in lactated Ringer's injection, dextrose 5% in normal saline solution for injection, and Isolyte E.
• Inject drug slowly over at least 5 minutes, or dilute in 50 ml of a compatible solution and infuse over 15 minutes.

ACTION
Unknown. Thought to inhibit ACE, preventing conversion of angiotensin I to angiotensin II, a potent vasoconstrictor. Reduced formation of angiotensin II decreases peripheral arterial resistance, thus decreasing aldosterone secretion, thereby reducing sodium and water retention and lowering blood pressure.

Route	Onset	Peak	Duration
I.V.	15 min	1-4 hr	6 hr
P.O.	1 hr	4-6 hr	24 hr

ADVERSE REACTIONS
CNS: *headache, dizziness,* fatigue, vertigo, *asthenia,* syncope.

Reactions may be *common,* uncommon, **life-threatening,** or COMMON AND LIFE-THREATENING.

CV: *hypotension,* chest pain, angina pectoris.
GI: diarrhea, nausea, abdominal pain, vomiting.
GU: decreased renal function (in patients with bilateral renal artery stenosis or heart failure).
Hematologic: bone marrow depression.
Respiratory: dyspnea; *dry, persistent, tickling, nonproductive cough.*
Skin: rash.
Other: *angioedema.*

INTERACTIONS
Drug-drug. *Diuretics:* Excessive reduction of blood pressure. Use together cautiously.
Insulin, oral antidiabetics: May cause hypoglycemia, especially at start of enalapril therapy. Monitor patient closely.
Lithium: May cause lithium toxicity. Monitor lithium levels.
NSAIDs: May reduce antihypertensive effect. Monitor blood pressure.
Potassium-sparing diuretics, potassium supplements: May cause hyperkalemia. Avoid using together unless hypokalemic blood levels are confirmed.
Drug-herb. *Capsaicin:* May cause cough. Discourage use together.
Drug-food. *Salt substitutes containing potassium:* May cause hyperkalemia. Monitor patient closely.

EFFECTS ON LAB TEST RESULTS
● May increase BUN, creatinine, and potassium levels. May decrease sodium and bilirubin levels.
● May decrease liver function test values, hemoglobin, and hematocrit.

CONTRAINDICATIONS
Contraindicated in patients hypersensitive to drug and in those with a history of angioedema related to previous treatment with an ACE inhibitor.

NURSING CONSIDERATIONS
● Use cautiously in renally impaired patients or those with aortic stenosis or hypertrophic cardiomyopathy.
● Closely monitor blood pressure response to drug.
● *Alert:* Similar packaging and labeling of enalaprilat injection and pancuronium, a paralyzing drug, could result in a fatal

medication error. Check all labeling carefully.
● Monitor CBC with differential counts before and during therapy.
● Diabetic patients, those with impaired renal function or heart failure, and those receiving drugs that can increase potassium level may develop hyperkalemia. Monitor potassium intake and potassium level.
● *Alert:* Don't confuse enalapril with Anafranil or Eldepryl.

PATIENT TEACHING
● Instruct patient to report breathing difficulty or swelling of face, eyes, lips, or tongue. Angioedema (including laryngeal edema) may occur, especially after first dose.
● Advise patient to report signs of infection, such as fever and sore throat.
● Inform patient that light-headedness can occur, especially during first few days of therapy. Tell him to rise slowly to minimize this effect and to notify prescriber if symptoms develop. If syncope occurs, he should stop taking drug and call prescriber immediately.
● Tell patient to use caution in hot weather and during exercise. Inadequate fluid intake, vomiting, diarrhea, and excessive perspiration can lead to light-headedness and syncope.
● Advise patient to avoid salt substitutes; these products may contain potassium, which can cause hyperkalemia in patients taking this drug.
● Tell woman to notify prescriber if pregnancy occurs. Drug will need to be discontinued.

eprosartan mesylate
Teveten

Pregnancy risk category C (D in second and third trimesters)

AVAILABLE FORMS
Tablets: 400 mg, 600 mg

INDICATIONS & DOSAGES
➤ **Hypertension (alone or with other antihypertensives)—**
Adults: Initially, 600 mg P.O. daily. Dosage ranges from 400 to 800 mg daily,

given as single daily dose or two divided doses.

ACTION
An angiotensin II receptor antagonist that reduces blood pressure by blocking the vasoconstrictor and aldosterone-secreting effects of angiotensin II. Eprosartan selectively blocks the binding of angiotensin II to its receptor sites found in many tissues, such as vascular smooth muscle and the adrenal gland.

Route	Onset	Peak	Duration
P.O.	1-2 hr	1-3 hr	24 hr

ADVERSE REACTIONS
CNS: depression, fatigue, headache, dizziness.
CV: chest pain, dependent edema.
EENT: pharyngitis, rhinitis, sinusitis.
GI: abdominal pain, dyspepsia, diarrhea.
GU: urinary tract infection.
Hematologic: *neutropenia.*
Musculoskeletal: arthralgia, myalgia.
Respiratory: cough, upper respiratory tract infection, bronchitis.
Other: injury, viral infection.

INTERACTIONS
None significant.

EFFECTS ON LAB TEST RESULTS
• May increase BUN and triglyceride levels.
• May decrease neutrophil counts.

CONTRAINDICATIONS
Contraindicated in patients hypersensitive to eprosartan or its components.

NURSING CONSIDERATIONS
• Use cautiously in patients with an activated renin-angiotensin system, such as volume- or salt-depleted patients, and in patients whose renal function may depend on the activity of the renin-angiotensin-aldosterone system, such as patients with severe heart failure. Also use cautiously in patients with renal artery stenosis.
• Correct hypovolemia and hyponatremia before starting therapy, to reduce the risk of symptomatic hypotension.
• Monitor blood pressure closely for 2 hours during start of treatment. If hypo-

tension occurs, place patient in a supine position and, if needed, give an I.V. infusion of normal saline solution.
• A transient episode of hypotension isn't a contraindication to continued treatment. Drug may be restarted once patient's blood pressure has stabilized.
• Drug may be used alone or with other antihypertensives, such as diuretics and calcium channel blockers. Maximal blood pressure response may take 2 to 3 weeks.
• Monitor patient for facial or lip swelling because angioedema has occurred with other angiotensin II antagonists.
• Closely observe infants exposed to eprosartan in utero for hypotension, oliguria, and hyperkalemia.
• Safety and effectiveness in children haven't been established.

PATIENT TEACHING
• Advise woman of childbearing age to use a reliable form of contraception and to notify her prescriber immediately if pregnancy is suspected. Treatment may need to be discontinued under medical supervision.
• Advise patient to report facial or lip swelling and signs and symptoms of infection, such as fever and sore throat.
• Tell patient to notify prescriber before taking OTC medication to treat a dry cough.
• Inform patient that drug may be taken without regard to meals.
• Advise breast-feeding woman of potential for serious adverse reactions in breast-fed infants. A decision should be made to either discontinue drug or stop breast-feeding.
• Tell patient to store drug at 68° to 77° F (20° to 25° C).

---

felodipine
Agon SR‡, Plendil, Plendil ER‡, Renedil†

Pregnancy risk category C

AVAILABLE FORMS
Tablets (extended-release): 2.5 mg, 5 mg, 10 mg

INDICATIONS & DOSAGES
➤ **Hypertension—**
Adults: Initially, 5 mg P.O. daily. Adjust dosage based on patient response, usually at intervals not less than 2 weeks. Usual dose is 2.5 to 10 mg daily; maximum recommended dosage is 10 mg daily.
Elderly patients: 2.5 mg P.O. daily; adjust dosage as for adults. Maximum recommended dosage is 10 mg daily.
Adjust-a-dose: For patients with impaired hepatic function, 2.5 mg P.O. daily, adjusted as for adults. Maximum recommended dosage is 10 mg daily.

ACTION
Unknown. A dihydropyridine-derivative calcium channel blocker that prevents entry of calcium ions into vascular smooth-muscle and cardiac cells; shows some selectivity for smooth muscle compared with cardiac muscle.

Route	Onset	Peak	Duration
P.O.	2-5 hr	2.5-5 hr	24 hr

ADVERSE REACTIONS
CNS: *headache,* dizziness, paresthesia, asthenia.
CV: *peripheral edema,* chest pain, palpitations, flushing.
EENT: rhinorrhea, pharyngitis.
GI: abdominal pain, nausea, constipation, diarrhea.
Musculoskeletal: muscle cramps, back pain.
Respiratory: upper respiratory tract infection, cough.
Skin: rash.

INTERACTIONS
Drug-drug. *Anticonvulsants:* Decreased plasma level of felodipine. Avoid using together, if possible.
Cimetidine: Decreased clearance of felodipine. Reduce doses of felodipine.
Metoprolol: May alter pharmacokinetics of metoprolol. Monitor patient for adverse effects.
Theophylline: May slightly decrease theophylline levels. Monitor patient response closely.
Drug-food. *Grapefruit juice:* Increased drug bioavailability and effect. Discourage use together.

EFFECTS ON LAB TEST RESULTS
None reported.

CONTRAINDICATIONS
Contraindicated in patients hypersensitive to drug.

NURSING CONSIDERATIONS
● Use cautiously in patients with heart failure, particularly those receiving beta blockers, and in patients with impaired hepatic function.
● Monitor blood pressure for response.
● Monitor patient for peripheral edema, which appears to be both dose- and age-related. It's more common in patients taking higher doses, especially those older than age 60.
● *Alert:* Don't confuse Plendil with pindolol.

PATIENT TEACHING
● Tell patient to swallow tablets whole and not to crush or chew them.
● Tell patient drug may be taken without regard to meals.
● Advise patient not to take drug with grapefruit juice.
● Advise patient to continue taking drug even when he feels better, to watch his diet, and to check with prescriber or pharmacist before taking other drugs, including OTC drugs, nutritional supplements, or herbal remedies.
● Advise patient to observe good oral hygiene and to see a dentist regularly; use of drug may cause mild gingival hyperplasia.

fenoldopam mesylate
Corlopam

Pregnancy risk category B

AVAILABLE FORMS
Ampules: 10 mg/ml in single-dose ampules of 5 ml

INDICATIONS & DOSAGES
➤ **Short-term (up to 48 hours) hospital management of severe hypertension when rapid but quickly reversible reduction of blood pressure is indicated,**

---

including malignant hypertension with deteriorating end-organ function—
Adults: Give by continuous I.V. infusion. Start infusion rates at 0.025 to 0.3 mcg/kg/minute and titrate upward or downward no more frequently than q 15 minutes to achieve desired blood pressure. Recommended increments for titration are 0.05 to 0.1 mcg/kg/minute.

I.V. ADMINISTRATION
• Follow manufacturer's instructions for diluting drug. Diluted solution is stable at room temperature for at least 24 hours.
• Infuse drug with a calibrated mechanical infusion pump. Don't use a bolus dose.
• Infusion may be abruptly discontinued or gradually tapered.
• Oral antihypertensives can be added once blood pressure is stable during infusion or after infusion discontinuation.
• Monitor blood pressure frequently during infusions. Check blood pressure and heart rate every 15 minutes until patient is stable.

ACTION
Rapid-acting vasodilator. Drug is an agonist for D_1-like dopamine receptors and binds with moderate affinity to alpha$_2$ adrenoceptors.

Route	Onset	Peak	Duration
I.V.	15 min	20 min	Unknown

ADVERSE REACTIONS
CNS: dizziness, headache, insomnia.
CV: hypotension, palpitations, ***bradycardia,*** tachycardia, angina pectoris, *MI,* T-wave inversion, flushing, nonspecific chest pain.
EENT: nasal congestion.
GI: nausea, vomiting, abdominal pain, constipation, diarrhea.
GU: oliguria.
Hematologic: leukocytosis, bleeding.
Metabolic: hypokalemia.
Musculoskeletal: leg cramps, back pain.
Respiratory: dyspnea.
Other: pyrexia.

INTERACTIONS
Drug-drug. *Beta blockers:* May cause hypotension. Avoid using together.

EFFECTS ON LAB TEST RESULTS
• May increase BUN, glucose, LDH, and transaminase levels. May decrease potassium levels.

CONTRAINDICATIONS
No known contraindications.

NURSING CONSIDERATIONS
• Use with caution in patients with glaucoma or ocular hypertension because drug can cause dose-dependent increases in intraocular pressure. Drug may cause symptomatic hypotension; use particular caution when giving to patients who have sustained an acute cerebral infarction or hemorrhage. Use during pregnancy only if clearly needed. Drug may appear in breast milk; use cautiously in breast-feeding women.
• Safety and effectiveness in children haven't been established.
• Drug causes a dose-related tachycardia that diminishes over time but remains substantial at higher doses.
• *Alert:* Drug contains sodium metabisulfite, which may cause allergic-type reactions (including anaphylactic symptoms and severe asthmatic episodes in susceptible individuals). Sulfite sensitivity is more frequent in asthmatics than in nonasthmatics.
• Monitor electrolyte levels and watch for hypokalemia.

PATIENT TEACHING
• Tell patient that drug causes dose-related decreases in blood pressure and increases in heart rate. Advise patient to change positions slowly to avoid orthostatic symptoms.
• Encourage patient to report adverse reactions promptly.

---

fosinopril sodium
Monopril, Staril§

Pregnancy risk category C (D in second and third trimesters)

AVAILABLE FORMS
Tablets: 10 mg, 20 mg, 40 mg

Reactions may be *common,* uncommon, ***life-threatening**,* or COMMON AND LIFE-THREATENING.

INDICATIONS & DOSAGES
➤ **Hypertension—**
Adults: Initially, 10 mg P.O. daily; adjust dosage based on blood pressure response at peak and trough levels. Usual dosage is 20 to 40 mg daily; maximum is 80 mg daily. Dosage may be divided.
➤ **Heart failure—**
Adults: Initially, 10 mg P.O. once daily. Increase dosage over several weeks to a maximum of 40 mg P.O. daily, if needed.
Adjust-a-dose: For patients with moderate to severe renal failure or vigorous diuresis, start with 5 mg P.O. once daily.

ACTION
Antihypertensive action not clearly defined. Thought to inhibit ACE, preventing conversion of angiotensin I to angiotensin II, a potent vasoconstrictor. Reduced formation of angiotensin II decreases peripheral arterial resistance, thus decreasing aldosterone secretion, which reduces sodium and water retention and lowers blood pressure.

Route	Onset	Peak	Duration
P.O.	1 hr	3 hr	24 hr

ADVERSE REACTIONS
CNS: *CVA,* headache, dizziness, fatigue, syncope, paresthesia, sleep disturbance.
CV: chest pain, angina pectoris, *MI,* rhythm disturbances, palpitations, hypotension, orthostatic hypotension.
EENT: tinnitus, sinusitis.
GI: nausea, vomiting, diarrhea, *pancreatitis,* dry mouth, abdominal distention, abdominal pain, constipation.
GU: sexual dysfunction, renal insufficiency.
Hepatic: *hepatitis.*
Metabolic: hyperkalemia.
Musculoskeletal: arthralgia, musculoskeletal pain, myalgia.
Respiratory: *bronchospasm; dry, persistent, tickling, nonproductive cough.*
Skin: urticaria, rash, photosensitivity reactions, pruritus.
Other: *angioedema,* decreased libido, gout.

INTERACTIONS
Drug-drug. *Antacids:* May impair absorption. Separate administration times by at least 2 hours.

Diuretics, other antihypertensives: Excessive hypotension. Diuretic may need to be discontinued or fosinopril dosage lowered.
Lithium: Increased lithium levels and lithium toxicity. Monitor lithium levels.
Potassium-sparing diuretics, potassium supplements: Risk of hyperkalemia. Monitor patient closely.
Drug-herb. *Capsaicin:* May cause cough. Discourage use together.
Drug-food. *Salt substitutes containing potassium:* May cause hyperkalemia. Urge patient to avoid using together.

EFFECTS ON LAB TEST RESULTS
● May increase liver function test values and BUN, creatinine, and potassium levels.
● May decrease hemoglobin and hematocrit.

CONTRAINDICATIONS
Contraindicated in patients hypersensitive to drug or other ACE inhibitors and in breast-feeding women.

NURSING CONSIDERATIONS
● Use cautiously in patients with impaired renal or hepatic function.
● Monitor blood pressure for effect.
● Although ACE inhibitors reduce blood pressure in all races studied, this response is less in blacks who receive the drug as monotherapy. Therapy with a thiazide diuretic produces a more favorable response.
● ACE inhibitors appear to cause a higher risk of angioedema in black patients.
● Monitor potassium intake and potassium level. Diabetic patients, those with impaired renal function, and those receiving drugs that can increase potassium level may develop hyperkalemia.
● Other ACE inhibitors may cause agranulocytosis and neutropenia. Monitor CBC with differential counts before therapy and periodically thereafter.
● Assess renal and hepatic function before and periodically throughout therapy.
● Falsely low measurements of digoxin levels may result with the Digi-Tab radioimmunoassay kit for digoxin; other kits may be used.
● *Alert:* Don't confuse fosinopril with lisinopril or Monopril with Monurol.

PATIENT TEACHING
• Tell patient to avoid salt substitutes; these products may contain potassium that can cause hyperkalemia in patients taking drug.
• Instruct patient to contact prescriber if light-headedness or syncope occurs.
• Advise patient to report evidence of infection, such as fever and sore throat.
• Instruct patient to call prescriber if the following signs or symptoms occur: easy bruising or bleeding; swelling of tongue, lips, face, eyes, mucous membranes, or limbs; difficulty swallowing or breathing; and hoarseness.
• Urge patient to use caution in hot weather and during exercise. Inadequate fluid intake, vomiting, diarrhea, and excessive perspiration can lead to light-headedness and syncope.
• Tell woman to notify prescriber if pregnancy occurs. Drug will need to be discontinued.

---

guanfacine hydrochloride
Tenex

Pregnancy risk category B

AVAILABLE FORMS
Tablets: 1 mg, 2 mg

INDICATIONS & DOSAGES
➤ Hypertension—
Adults: Initially, 1 mg P.O. daily h.s. Dosage may be increased to 2 mg P.O. h.s. after 3 to 4 weeks, p.r.n. Dosage may be further increased to 3 mg P.O. h.s. after an additional 3 to 4 weeks, p.r.n. Average dose is 1 to 3 mg daily.

ACTION
Unknown. May inhibit the central vasomotor center, thereby decreasing sympathetic outflow to the heart, kidneys, and peripheral vasculature, and decreasing blood pressure.

Route	Onset	Peak	Duration
P.O.	Unknown	1-4 hr	24 hr

ADVERSE REACTIONS
CNS: *dizziness,* fatigue, headache, insomnia, *somnolence,* asthenia.
CV: *bradycardia.*

GI: *constipation,* diarrhea, nausea, *dry mouth.*
Skin: dermatitis, pruritus.

INTERACTIONS
Drug-drug. *CNS depressants:* May increase sedation. Use together cautiously.
TCAs: May inhibit antihypertensive effects. Monitor blood pressure.

EFFECTS ON LAB TEST RESULTS
None reported.

CONTRAINDICATIONS
Contraindicated in patients hypersensitive to drug.

NURSING CONSIDERATIONS
• Use cautiously in patients with severe coronary insufficiency, recent MI, cerebrovascular disease, or chronic renal or hepatic insufficiency.
• Monitor blood pressure frequently.
• Risk and severity of adverse reactions increase with higher dosages.
• Drug may be used alone or with a diuretic.
• Rebound hypertension may occur and will be noticeable within 2 to 4 days after therapy ends.
• *Alert:* Don't confuse guanfacine with guanidine, guaifenesin, or guanabenz or Tenex with Xanax, Entex, or Ten-K.

PATIENT TEACHING
• Tell patient not to stop therapy abruptly. Rebound hypertension may occur but is less common than that which occurs with similar drugs.
• Advise patient to avoid activities that require alertness until response to drug is established; drowsiness may occur.
• Warn patient that he may have less tolerance to alcohol and other CNS depressants.

---

hydralazine hydrochloride
Alphapress‡, Apresoline**, Novo-Hylazin†, Suprest†

Pregnancy risk category C

AVAILABLE FORMS
Injection: 20 mg/ml
Tablets: 10 mg, 25 mg, 50 mg, 100 mg

Reactions may be *common,* uncommon, *life-threatening,* or COMMON AND LIFE-THREATENING.

INDICATIONS & DOSAGES

➤ **Essential hypertension (orally, alone, or with other antihypertensives), severe essential hypertension (parenterally, to lower blood pressure quickly)—**

Adults: P.O.—Initially, 10 mg P.O. q.i.d.; gradually increased to 50 mg q.i.d., p.r.n. Maximum recommended dose is 200 mg daily, but some patients may need 300 to 400 mg daily.

I.V.—10 to 20 mg given slowly and repeated p.r.n., switching to oral antihypertensives as soon as possible.

I.M.—10 to 50 mg, repeated p.r.n., switching to oral form as soon as possible.

Children: P.O.—Initially, 0.75 mg/kg/day P.O. divided into four doses; gradually increased over 3 to 4 weeks to maximum of 7.5 mg/kg or 200 mg daily. Maximum initial P.O. dose is 25 mg.

I.V.—0.1 to 0.2 mg/kg I.V. q 4 to 6 hours, p.r.n. Maximum initial parenteral dose is 20 mg.

I.V. ADMINISTRATION

● Give drug slowly and repeat as needed, generally q 4 to 6 hours. Hydralazine will undergo color changes in most infusion solutions; these color changes don't indicate loss of potency.

● Drug is compatible with normal saline, Ringer's and lactated Ringer's solutions, and several other common I.V. solutions. Drug may undergo a reaction with dextrose. The manufacturer doesn't recommend mixing drug in infusion solutions. Check with pharmacist for additional compatibility information.

● Oral therapy should replace parenteral therapy as soon as possible.

ACTION

Unknown. A direct-acting vasodilator that mainly relaxes arteriolar smooth muscle.

Route	Onset	Peak	Duration
I.M.	10-30 min	1 hr	2-6 hr
I.V.	5-20 min	10-80 min	2-6 hr
P.O.	20-30 min	1-2 hr	2-4 hr

ADVERSE REACTIONS

CNS: peripheral neuritis, *headache,* dizziness.

CV: orthostatic hypotension, *tachycardia,* edema, *angina pectoris, palpitations.*

EENT: nasal congestion.

GI: *nausea, vomiting, diarrhea, anorexia,* constipation.

Hematologic: *neutropenia, leukopenia, agranulocytopenia, agranulocytosis, thrombocytopenia with or without purpura.*

Skin: rash.

Other: *lupus-like syndrome.*

INTERACTIONS

Drug-drug. *Diazoxide, MAO inhibitors:* May cause severe hypotension. Use together cautiously.

Diuretics, other hypotensive drugs: Excessive hypotension. Dosage adjustment may be needed.

Indomethacin: May decrease effects of hydralazine. Monitor blood pressure.

EFFECTS ON LAB TEST RESULTS

● May decrease hemoglobin and neutrophil, WBC, granulocyte, platelet, and RBC counts.

CONTRAINDICATIONS

Contraindicated in patients hypersensitive to drug and in those with coronary artery disease or mitral valvular rheumatic heart disease.

NURSING CONSIDERATIONS

● Use cautiously in patients with suspected cardiac disease, CVA, or severe renal impairment and in those taking other antihypertensives.

● Monitor patient's blood pressure, pulse rate, and body weight frequently. Hydralazine may be given with diuretics and beta blockers to decrease sodium retention and tachycardia and to prevent angina attacks.

● Elderly patients may be more sensitive than younger ones to drug's hypotensive effects.

● Monitor CBC, lupus erythematosus cell preparation, and antinuclear antibody titer determination before therapy and periodically during long-term therapy.

● *Alert:* Monitor patient closely for signs and symptoms of lupus-like syndrome (sore throat, fever, muscle and joint aches, rash). Notify prescriber immediately if these develop.

● Compliance may be improved by administering drug b.i.d. Check with prescriber.

• **Alert:** Don't confuse hydralazine with hydroxyzine or Apresoline with Apresazide.

PATIENT TEACHING
• Instruct patient to take oral form with meals to increase absorption.
• Inform patient that orthostatic hypotension can be minimized by rising slowly and avoiding sudden position changes.
• Tell woman to notify prescriber if she suspects pregnancy; drug should be stopped.
• Advise patient that the body's stores of vitamin B_6 (pyridoxine) and coenzyme Q10 may be depleted and that he should discuss supplements with prescriber.

---

irbesartan
Aprovel§, Avapro

Pregnancy risk category C (D in second and third trimesters)

AVAILABLE FORMS
Tablets: 75 mg, 150 mg, 300 mg

INDICATIONS & DOSAGES
➤ **Hypertension—**
Adults: Initially, 150 mg P.O. daily, increased to maximum of 300 mg daily if needed.
Adjust-a-dose: For volume- and salt-depleted patients, initially 75 mg P.O. daily.

ACTION
Produces antihypertensive effect by competitive antagonist activity at the angiotensin II receptor.

Route	Onset	Peak	Duration
P.O.	Unknown	1.5-2 hr	24 hr

ADVERSE REACTIONS
CNS: fatigue, anxiety, *dizziness, headache.*
CV: chest pain, edema, tachycardia.
EENT: pharyngitis, rhinitis, sinus abnormality.
GI: diarrhea, dyspepsia, abdominal pain, nausea, vomiting.
GU: urinary tract infection.
Musculoskeletal: musculoskeletal trauma or pain.

Respiratory: upper respiratory tract infection.
Skin: rash.

INTERACTIONS
None significant.

EFFECTS ON LAB TEST RESULTS
None reported.

CONTRAINDICATIONS
Contraindicated in patients hypersensitive to drug or its components.

NURSING CONSIDERATIONS
• Use cautiously in patients with impaired renal function, heart failure, and renal artery stenosis and in breast-feeding women.
• Use during pregnancy can cause injury and death to the developing fetus. When pregnancy is detected, stop drug as soon as possible.
• Drug may be administered with a diuretic or other antihypertensive, if needed, for control of hypertension.
• Symptomatic hypotension may occur in volume- or salt-depleted patients (vigorous diuretic use or dialysis). The cause of volume depletion should be corrected before administration or before a lower dose is used.
• If hypotension occurs, place patient in a supine position and give an I.V. infusion of normal saline solution, if needed. Once blood pressure has stabilized after a transient hypotensive episode, drug may be continued.

PATIENT TEACHING
• Warn woman of childbearing age of consequences of drug exposure to fetus. Tell her to call prescriber immediately if pregnancy is suspected.
• Tell patient that drug may be taken once daily without regard to food.

---

labetalol hydrochloride
Normodyne, Presolol‡, Trandate

Pregnancy risk category C

AVAILABLE FORMS
Injection: 5 mg/ml
Tablets: 100 mg, 200 mg, 300 mg

Reactions may be *common*, uncommon, ***life-threatening***, or COMMON AND LIFE-THREATENING.

INDICATIONS & DOSAGES

➤ **Hypertension—**
Adults: 100 mg P.O. b.i.d. with or without a diuretic. If needed, dosage is increased to 200 mg b.i.d. after 2 days. Further increases may be made q 2 to 3 days until optimum response is reached. Usual maintenance dose is 200 to 400 mg b.i.d.

➤ **Severe hypertension, hypertensive emergencies—**
Adults: 200 mg diluted in 160 ml of D_5W, infused at 2 mg/minute until satisfactory response is obtained; then infusion is stopped. May be repeated q 6 to 12 hours.

Or, administered by repeated I.V. injection: initially, 20 mg I.V. slowly over 2 minutes. Repeat injections of 40 to 80 mg q 10 minutes until maximum dose of 300 mg is reached, p.r.n.

I.V. ADMINISTRATION

● Drug may be given by slow, direct I.V. injection over 2 minutes at 10-minute intervals.

● For I.V. infusion, prepare by diluting with D_5W or normal saline solutions; for example, 200 mg of drug to 160 ml D_5W to yield 1 mg/ml.

● Administer labetalol infusion with an infusion control device.

● Monitor blood pressure closely every 5 minutes for 30 minutes, then every 30 minutes for 2 hours, then hourly for 6 hours.

● Patient should remain in a supine position for 3 hours after infusion. When administered I.V. for hypertensive emergencies, drug produces a rapid, predictable fall in blood pressure within 5 to 10 minutes.

ACTION

Unknown. May be related to reduced peripheral vascular resistance, as a result of alpha and beta blockade.

Route	Onset	Peak	Duration
I.V.	2-5 min	5 min	2-4 hr
P.O.	20 min	2-4 hr	8-12 hr

ADVERSE REACTIONS

CNS: vivid dreams, fatigue, headache, paresthesia, transient scalp tingling, *dizziness.*

CV: *orthostatic hypotension,* **ventricular arrhythmias,** syncope.
EENT: nasal congestion.
GI: nausea, vomiting.
GU: sexual dysfunction, urine retention.
Respiratory: dyspnea, **bronchospasm.**
Skin: rash.

INTERACTIONS

Drug-drug. *Beta-adrenergic agonists:* May blunt bronchodilator effect of these drugs in patients with bronchospasm. Increased dosages of these drugs may be needed.
Cimetidine: May enhance labetalol's effect. Use together cautiously.
Halothane: Increased hypotensive effect. Monitor blood pressure closely.
Insulin, oral antidiabetics: May alter dosage requirements in previously stabilized diabetic patient. Monitor patient closely.

EFFECTS ON LAB TEST RESULTS

● May increase transaminase and blood urea levels.

CONTRAINDICATIONS

Contraindicated in patients hypersensitive to drug and in those with bronchial asthma, overt cardiac failure, greater than first-degree heart block, cardiogenic shock, severe bradycardia, and other conditions that may cause severe and prolonged hypotension.

NURSING CONSIDERATIONS

● Use cautiously in patients with heart failure, hepatic failure, chronic bronchitis, emphysema, peripheral vascular disease, and pheochromocytoma.

● Monitor blood pressure frequently. Drug masks common signs and symptoms of shock.

● If dizziness occurs, ask prescriber if patient may take a dose at bedtime or take smaller doses t.i.d. to help minimize this adverse reaction.

● When switching from I.V. to P.O. form, begin P.O. regimen at 200 mg after blood pressure begins to rise; repeat dose with 200 to 400 mg in 6 to 12 hours. Adjust dosage according to blood pressure response.

• Monitor glucose levels in diabetic patients closely because beta blockers may mask certain signs and symptoms of hypoglycemia.
• Drug may cause a false-positive increase of urine free and total catecholamine levels when measured by a nonspecific trihydroxindole fluorometric method.
• *Alert:* Don't confuse Trandate with Trental or Tridrate.
• *Alert:* Sodium bicarbonate injection is incompatible with I.V. labetalol.

PATIENT TEACHING
• Tell patient that stopping drug abruptly can worsen angina and precipitate MI.
• Advise patient that dizziness is the most troublesome adverse reaction and tends to occur in the early stages of treatment, in patients also receiving diuretics, and in those receiving higher dosages. Inform patient that dizziness can be minimized by rising slowly and avoiding sudden position changes.
• Warn patient that transient scalp tingling may occur, especially at start of therapy, but is harmless.
• Tell patient that drug may deplete body's stores of coenzyme Q10 and that he should discuss the need for supplements with prescriber.

lisinopril
Carace§, Prinivil, Zestril

Pregnancy risk category C (D in second and third trimesters)

AVAILABLE FORMS
Tablets: 2.5 mg, 5 mg, 10 mg, 20 mg, 40 mg

INDICATIONS & DOSAGES
➤ **Hypertension—**
Adults: Initially, 10 mg P.O. daily for patients not taking a diuretic. Most patients are well controlled on 20 to 40 mg daily as a single dose. For patients taking a diuretic, initially, 5 mg P.O. daily.
Adjust-a-dose: For patients with renal impairment, dosage is based on creatinine clearance: if clearance is 10 to 30 ml/minute, give 5 mg P.O. daily; if clearance

is less than 10 ml/minute, give 2.5 mg P.O. daily.
➤ **Treatment adjunct in heart failure (with diuretics and cardiac glycosides)—**
Adults: Initially, 5 mg P.O. daily; increased p.r.n. to maximum of 20 mg P.O. daily.
Adjust-a-dose: For patients with sodium level less than 130 mEq/L or creatinine clearance less than 30 ml/minute, start treatment at 2.5 mg daily.
➤ **Hemodynamically stable patients within 24 hours of acute MI to improve survival—**
Adults: Initially, 5 mg P.O.; then 5 mg after 24 hours, 10 mg after 48 hours, followed by 10 mg once daily for 6 weeks.
Adjust-a-dose: For patients with low systolic blood pressure (120 mm Hg or less) when treatment is started or during first 3 days after an infarct, decrease dosage to 2.5 mg P.O. If hypotension occurs (systolic blood pressure 100 mm Hg or less), reduce daily maintenance dose of 5 mg to 2.5 mg if needed. If prolonged hypotension occurs (systolic blood pressure less than 90 mm Hg for longer than 1 hour), withdraw drug.

ACTION
Unknown. Thought to result primarily from suppression of the renin-angiotensin-aldosterone system.

Route	Onset	Peak	Duration
P.O.	1 hr	7 hr	24 hr

ADVERSE REACTIONS
CNS: *dizziness, headache,* fatigue, paresthesia.
CV: hypotension, *orthostatic hypotension,* chest pain.
EENT: *nasal congestion.*
GI: *diarrhea,* nausea, dyspepsia.
GU: impaired renal function, impotence.
Metabolic: hyperkalemia.
Respiratory: dyspnea; dry, persistent, tickling, nonproductive cough.
Skin: rash.

INTERACTIONS
Drug-drug. *Allopurinol:* May cause hypersensitivity reaction. Use together cautiously.

Diuretics, thiazide diuretics: Excessive hypotension with diuretics. Monitor blood pressure closely.

Indomethacin, phenothiazines: Attenuated hypotensive effect. Monitor blood pressure closely.

Insulin, oral antidiabetics: May cause hypoglycemia, especially at start of lisinopril therapy. Monitor glucose levels.

Potassium-sparing diuretics, potassium supplements: May cause hyperkalemia. Monitor laboratory values.

Drug-herb. *Capsaicin:* May cause ACE inhibitor–induced cough. Discourage use together.

Drug-food. *Potassium-containing salt substitutes:* May cause hyperkalemia. Monitor laboratory values.

EFFECTS ON LAB TEST RESULTS
● May increase BUN, creatinine, potassium, and bilirubin levels.
● May increase liver function test values.

CONTRAINDICATIONS
Contraindicated in patients hypersensitive to ACE inhibitors and in those with a history of angioedema related to previous treatment with ACE inhibitor.

NURSING CONSIDERATIONS
● Use cautiously in patients with impaired renal function; dosage adjustment is needed. Also use cautiously in patients at risk for hyperkalemia and in those with aortic stenosis or hypertrophic cardiomyopathy.
● When used in acute MI, patient should receive, as appropriate, the standard recommended treatment, such as thrombolytics, aspirin, and beta blockers.
● Although ACE inhibitors reduce blood pressure in all races studied, this response is less in blacks who receive the drug as monotherapy. Therapy with a thiazide diuretic produces a more favorable response.
● ACE inhibitors appear to increase risk of angioedema in black patients.
● Monitor blood pressure frequently. If drug doesn't adequately control blood pressure, diuretics may be added.
● Monitor WBC with differential counts before therapy, every 2 weeks for first 3 months of therapy, and periodically thereafter.

● **Alert:** Don't confuse lisinopril with fosinopril or Lioresal; Zestril with Zostrix; or Prinivil with Proventil or Prilosec.

PATIENT TEACHING
● **Alert:** Rarely, angioedema (including laryngeal edema) may occur, especially after first dose. Advise patient to report signs or symptoms, such as swelling of face, eyes, lips, or tongue; or breathing difficulty.
● Inform patient that light-headedness can occur, especially during first few days of therapy. Tell him to rise slowly to minimize this effect and to report symptoms to prescriber. If syncope occurs, advise patient to stop taking drug and call prescriber immediately.
● Tell patient not to stop drug suddenly but to notify prescriber if unpleasant adverse reactions occur.
● Advise patient to report signs and symptoms of infection, such as fever and sore throat.
● Tell woman to notify prescriber if pregnancy occurs. Drug will need to be discontinued.
● Instruct patient not to use salt substitutes that contain potassium without first consulting prescriber.

---

losartan potassium
Cozaar

Pregnancy risk category C (D in second and third trimesters)

AVAILABLE FORMS
Tablets: 25 mg, 50 mg, 100 mg

INDICATIONS & DOSAGES
➤ **Hypertension—**
Adults: Initially, 25 to 50 mg P.O. daily. Maximum daily dose is 100 mg in one or two divided doses.
Adjust-a-dose: For patients with impaired hepatic function and in those who are intravascularly volume-depleted (such as those taking diuretics), use lowest dosage (25 mg) initially.

ACTION
Inhibits vasoconstrictive and aldosterone-secreting action of angiotensin II by

blocking angiotensin II receptor on the surface of vascular smooth muscle and other tissue cells.

Route	Onset	Peak	Duration
P.O.	Unknown	1 hr	Unknown

ADVERSE REACTIONS
CNS: dizziness, insomnia.
EENT: nasal congestion, sinusitis.
GI: diarrhea, dyspepsia.
Musculoskeletal: muscle cramps, myalgia, back or leg pain.
Respiratory: cough, upper respiratory tract infection.

INTERACTIONS
Drug-drug. *Potassium-sparing diuretics, potassium supplements:* May cause hyperkalemia. Monitor patient closely.
Drug-food. *Salt substitutes containing potassium:* May cause hyperkalemia. Monitor patient closely.

EFFECTS ON LAB TEST RESULTS
None reported.

CONTRAINDICATIONS
Contraindicated in patients hypersensitive to drug.

NURSING CONSIDERATIONS
• Breast-feeding isn't recommended during losartan therapy.
• Use cautiously in patients with impaired renal or hepatic function.
• Drugs that act directly on the renin-angiotensin system (such as losartan) can cause fetal and neonatal morbidity and death when given to women in the second or third trimester of pregnancy. These problems haven't been detected when exposure was limited to the first trimester. If pregnancy is suspected, notify prescriber because drug should be discontinued.
• Drug can be used alone or with other antihypertensives.
• If antihypertensive effect measured by the trough level of drug, using once-daily dosing, is inadequate, a b.i.d. regimen using the same total daily dose or an increase in dose may give a more satisfactory response.

• Monitor patient's blood pressure closely to evaluate effectiveness of therapy. When losartan is used alone, the effect on blood pressure is notably less in black patients than in patients of other races.
• Monitor patients who are also taking diuretics for symptomatic hypotension.
• Regularly assess the patient's renal function (via creatinine and BUN levels).
• Patients with severe heart failure whose renal function depends on the angiotensin-aldosterone system have experienced acute renal failure during ACE inhibitor therapy. Manufacturer of losartan states that drug would be expected to have the same effect. Closely monitor patient, especially during first few weeks of therapy.
• *Alert:* Don't confuse Cozaar with Zocor.

PATIENT TEACHING
• Tell patient to avoid salt substitutes; these products may contain potassium, which can cause hyperkalemia in patients taking losartan.
• Inform woman of childbearing age about consequences of second- and third-trimester exposure to drug; instruct her to notify prescriber immediately if pregnancy is suspected.
• Advise patient to report swelling of face, eyes, lips, or tongue or any breathing difficulty immediately.

---

methyldopa
Aldomet, Aldopren‡, Apo-Methyldopa†, Dopamet†, Hydopa‡, Novo-Medopa†, Nu-Medopa†

methyldopate hydrochloride
Aldomet

Pregnancy risk category B (P.O.) or C (I.V.)

AVAILABLE FORMS
methyldopa
Oral suspension: 250 mg/5 ml
Tablets: 125 mg, 250 mg, 500 mg
methyldopate hydrochloride
Injection: 250 mg/5 ml (50 mg/ml in 5-ml and 10-ml vials)

INDICATIONS & DOSAGES

➤ **Hypertension, hypertensive crisis—**
Adults: Initially, 250 mg P.O. b.i.d. to t.i.d. in first 48 hours. Increase, p.r.n., q 2 days. May give entire daily dose in evening or h.s. Adjust dosages if other antihypertensives are added to or deleted from therapy. Maintenance dosage is 500 mg to 2 g daily in two to four divided doses. Maximum recommended dose is 3 g daily. Or, 250 to 500 mg I.V. q 6 hours. Maximum dosage is 1 g q 6 hours. Switch to oral antihypertensives as soon as possible.
Children: Initially, 10 mg/kg P.O. daily in two to four divided doses; or, 20 to 40 mg/kg I.V. daily in four divided doses. Increase dose daily until desired response occurs. Maximum daily dose is 65 mg/kg or 3 g, whichever is less.

I.V. ADMINISTRATION

● Dilute appropriate dose in 100 ml D_5W. Infuse slowly over 30 to 60 minutes.

ACTION

Unknown. Thought to inhibit the central vasomotor centers, thereby decreasing sympathetic outflow to the heart, kidneys, and peripheral vasculature.

Route	Onset	Peak	Duration
I.V.	Unknown	4-6 hr	10-16 hr
P.O.	Unknown	4-6 hr	12-48 hr

ADVERSE REACTIONS

CNS: *sedation, headache,* weakness, dizziness, *decreased mental acuity,* paresthesia, parkinsonism, involuntary choreoathetoid movements, psychic disturbances, depression, nightmares.
CV: *bradycardia, orthostatic hypotension,* aggravated angina, *myocarditis,* edema.
EENT: *nasal congestion.*
GI: nausea, vomiting, diarrhea, *pancreatitis, dry mouth,* constipation.
GU: galactorrhea.
Hematologic: hemolytic anemia, *thrombocytopenia, leukopenia, bone marrow depression.*
Hepatic: *hepatic necrosis, hepatitis.*
Musculoskeletal: arthralgia.
Skin: rash.
Other: drug-induced fever, gynecomastia.

INTERACTIONS

Drug-drug. *Amphetamines, nonselective beta blockers, norepinephrine, phenothiazines, TCAs:* May cause hypertensive effects. Monitor patient closely.
Anesthetics: May need lower doses of anesthetics. Use together cautiously.
Barbiturates: May decrease actions of methyldopa. Monitor patient closely.
Haloperidol: Psychomotor retardation, impaired memory, and difficulty concentrating in nonschizophrenic patients; increased sedation. Use together cautiously.
Levodopa: Increased hypotensive effects, which may increase adverse CNS reactions. Monitor patient closely.
Lithium: May increase lithium levels. Watch for increased lithium levels and signs and symptoms of toxicity.
Tolbutamide: May impair metabolism of tolbutamide. Monitor patient for hypoglycemic effect.
Drug-herb. *Capsicum:* May reduce antihypertensive effectiveness. Discourage use together.

EFFECTS ON LAB TEST RESULTS

● May increase creatinine level.
● May increase liver function test value. May decrease hemoglobin and platelet and WBC counts.

CONTRAINDICATIONS

Contraindicated in patients hypersensitive to drug and in those with active hepatic disease (such as acute hepatitis) or active cirrhosis. Also contraindicated if previous methyldopa therapy has caused liver problems.

NURSING CONSIDERATIONS

● Use cautiously in patients with history of impaired hepatic function or sulfite sensitivity and in breast-feeding women.
● Monitor patient's blood pressure regularly. Elderly patients are more likely than younger ones to experience hypotension and sedation.
● Occasionally tolerance may occur, usually between the second and third months of therapy. A diuretic may need to be added or a dosage adjustment may be necessary.

Notify prescriber of any significant changes in patient response.
● After dialysis, monitor patient for hypertension and notify prescriber, if needed. Patient may need an extra dose of methyldopa.
● Monitor CBC with differential counts before therapy and periodically thereafter.
● Patients who need blood transfusions should have direct and indirect Coombs' tests to prevent crossmatching problems.
● Monitor patient's Coombs' test results. In patients who have received drug for several months, positive reaction to direct Coombs' test indicates hemolytic anemia.
● Drug may cause falsely high levels of urine catecholamines, interfering with the diagnosis of pheochromocytoma.
● Observe for and report involuntary choreoathetoid movements. Drug may have to be discontinued.
● *Alert:* Don't confuse Aldomet with Aldoril or Anzemet.

PATIENT TEACHING
● Tell patient not to suddenly stop taking drug, but to notify prescriber if unpleasant adverse reactions occur.
● Instruct patient to report signs and symptoms of infection.
● Tell patient to check his weight daily and to notify prescriber of weight gain of more than 5 pounds. Sodium and water retention may occur but can be relieved with diuretics.
● Warn patient that drug may impair ability to perform tasks that require mental alertness, particularly at start of therapy. A once-daily dose at bedtime will minimize daytime drowsiness.
● Inform patient that orthostatic hypotension can be minimized by rising slowly and avoiding sudden position changes. Dry mouth can be relieved by chewing gum or sucking on hard candy or ice chips.
● Tell patient that urine may turn dark if left standing in toilet bowl or if toilet bowl has been treated with bleach.

metoprolol succinate
Toprol XL

metoprolol tartrate
Apo-Metoprolol†, Apo-Metoprolol (Type L)†, Betaloc††, Betaloc Durules†, Lopresor†, Lopresor SR†, Lopressor, Minax‡, Novo-Metoprol†, Nu-Metop†

Pregnancy risk category C

AVAILABLE FORMS
metoprolol succinate
Tablets (extended-release): 25 mg, 50 mg, 100 mg, 200 mg
metoprolol tartrate
Injection: 1 mg/ml in 5-ml ampules
Tablets: 50 mg, 100 mg
Tablets (extended-release): 100 mg†, 200 mg†

INDICATIONS & DOSAGES
➤ **Hypertension—**
Adults: Initially, 50 mg P.O. b.i.d. or 100 mg P.O. once daily; then up to 100 to 450 mg daily in two or three divided doses. Or, 50 to 100 mg of extended-release tablets (tartrate equivalent) once daily. Adjust dosage as needed and tolerated at intervals of not less than 1 week to maximum of 400 mg daily.
➤ **Early intervention in acute MI (metoprolol tartrate)—**
Adults: Three 5-mg I.V. boluses q 2 minutes. Then, beginning 15 minutes after last dose, 25 to 50 mg P.O. q 6 hours for 48 hours. Maintenance dose is 100 mg P.O. b.i.d. for 3 months to 3 years.
➤ **Angina pectoris—**
Adults: Initially, 100 mg P.O. daily as a single dose or in two equally divided doses; increased at weekly intervals until an adequate response or a pronounced decrease in heart rate is seen. Effects of daily dose beyond 400 mg aren't known. Or, give 100 mg of extended-release tablets (tartrate equivalent) once daily. Adjust dosage as needed and tolerated at intervals of not less than 1 week to maximum of 400 mg daily.
✷ **NEW INDICATION: Stable symptomatic heart failure (New York Heart Associa-**

tion class II) resulting from ischemia, hypertension, or cardiomyopathy—
Adults: 25 mg (Toprol XL) P.O. once daily for 2 weeks. Double the dose every 2 weeks, as tolerated, to a maximum of 200 mg daily.
Adjust-a-dose: In patients with more severe heart failure, start with 12.5 mg (Toprol XL) P.O. once daily for 2 weeks.

I.V. ADMINISTRATION
• Give drug undiluted by direct injection.
• Although mixing with other drugs should be avoided, metoprolol is compatible when mixed with meperidine hydrochloride or morphine sulfate or when administered with alteplase infusion at a Y-site connection.

ACTION
Unknown. A selective beta blocker that selectively blocks beta$_1$-adrenergic receptors; decreases cardiac output, peripheral resistance, and cardiac oxygen consumption; and depresses renin secretion.

Route	Onset	Peak	Duration
I.V.	5 min	20 min	5-8 hr
P.O.	15 min	1 hr	6-12 hr
P.O. (extended)	15 min	6-12 hr	24 hr

ADVERSE REACTIONS
CNS: *fatigue, dizziness,* depression.
CV: **bradycardia,** *hypotension,* **heart failure, AV block.**
GI: nausea, diarrhea.
Respiratory: dyspnea.
Skin: rash.

INTERACTIONS
Drug-drug. *Barbiturates, rifampin:* Increased metabolism of metoprolol. Watch for decreased effect.
Cardiac glycosides, diltiazem, verapamil: Excessive bradycardia and increased depressant effect on myocardium. Use together cautiously.
Catecholamine-depleting drugs such as H$_2$ antagonists, MAO inhibitors, reserpine: May have additive effect. Monitor patient for hypotension and bradycardia.
Chlorpromazine, cimetidine, verapamil: Decreased hepatic clearance. Watch for greater beta-blocking effect.

Indomethacin: Decreased antihypertensive effect. Monitor blood pressure and adjust dosage.
Insulin, oral antidiabetics: May alter dosage requirements in previously stabilized diabetic patients. Monitor patient closely.
Propafenone: May increase metoprolol levels. Monitor vital signs.
Terbutaline: May antagonize bronchodilatory effects of terbutaline. Monitor patient.
Drug-food. *Any food:* May increase absorption. Encourage patient to take drug with food.

EFFECTS ON LAB TEST RESULTS
• May increase transaminase, alkaline phosphatase, LDH, and uric acid levels.

CONTRAINDICATIONS
Contraindicated in patients hypersensitive to drug or other beta blockers. Also contraindicated in patients with sinus bradycardia, greater than first-degree heart block, cardiogenic shock, or overt cardiac failure when used to treat hypertension or angina. When used to treat MI, drug is contraindicated in patients with heart rate less than 45 beats/minute, greater than first-degree heart block, PR interval of 0.24 seconds or longer with first-degree heart block, systolic blood pressure less than 100 mm Hg, or moderate to severe cardiac failure.

NURSING CONSIDERATIONS
• Use cautiously in patients with heart failure, diabetes, or respiratory or hepatic disease.
• Always check patient's apical pulse rate before giving drug. If it's slower than 60 beats/minute, withhold drug and call prescriber immediately.
• Monitor glucose levels closely in diabetic patients because drug masks common signs and symptoms of hypoglycemia.
• Monitor blood pressure frequently; metoprolol masks common signs and symptoms of shock.
• Beta blockers may mask tachycardia caused by hyperthyroidism. In patients with suspected thyrotoxicosis, withdraw beta blocker gradually to avoid thyroid storm.

• When therapy is discontinued, reduce dose gradually over 1 to 2 weeks.
• Store drug at room temperature and protect from light. Discard solution if it's discolored or contains particles.
• Beta$_1$ selectivity is lost at higher doses. Watch for peripheral side effects.
• *Alert:* Don't confuse metoprolol with metaproterenol or metolazone.

PATIENT TEACHING
• Instruct patient to take drug exactly as prescribed and to take it with meals.
• Caution patient to avoid driving and other tasks requiring mental alertness until response to therapy has been established.
• Advise patient to inform dentist or prescriber about use of this drug before procedures or surgery.
• Tell patient to alert prescriber if shortness of breath occurs.
• Instruct patient not to stop drug suddenly but to notify prescriber about unpleasant adverse reactions. Inform him that drug must be withdrawn gradually over 1 to 2 weeks.
• Inform patient that use of metoprolol isn't advised in breast-feeding women.
• Tell patient that drug may deplete body's stores of coenzyme Q10 and that he should discuss the need for supplements with prescriber.

---

minoxidil
Loniten

Pregnancy risk category C

AVAILABLE FORMS
Tablets: 2.5 mg, 10 mg

INDICATIONS & DOSAGES
➤ **Severe hypertension—**
Adults: Initially, 2.5 to 5 mg P.O. as a single dose. Effective dosage range is usually 10 to 40 mg daily. Maximum dose is 100 mg daily.
Children younger than age 12: 0.2 mg/kg P.O. (maximum 5 mg) as a single daily dose. Effective dosage range is usually 0.25 to 1 mg/kg daily. Maximum dose is 50 mg daily.

ACTION
Unknown. Drug's predominant effect produces direct arteriolar vasodilation.

Route	Onset	Peak	Duration
P.O.	0.5 hr	2-3 hr	2-5 days

ADVERSE REACTIONS
CV: *edema, tachycardia, pericardial effusion and tamponade,* **heart failure,** ECG changes, rebound hypertension.
GI: nausea, vomiting.
Metabolic: weight gain.
Skin: rash, ***Stevens-Johnson syndrome.***
Other: *hypertrichosis,* breast tenderness.

INTERACTIONS
Drug-drug. *Antihypertensives:* Severe orthostatic hypotension. Advise patient to stand up slowly.

EFFECTS ON LAB TEST RESULTS
• May increase BUN, creatinine, and alkaline phosphatase levels.
• May decrease hemoglobin and hematocrit.

CONTRAINDICATIONS
Contraindicated in patients hypersensitive to drug and in those with pheochromocytoma.

NURSING CONSIDERATIONS
• Use cautiously in patients with impaired renal function and after acute MI.
• Closely monitor blood pressure and pulse rate at beginning of therapy.
• Elderly patients may be more sensitive than younger ones to drug's hypotensive effects.
• Drug is removed by hemodialysis. Be sure to administer dose after dialysis.
• Monitor fluid intake and urine output. Check for weight gain and edema.
• Monitor patient for hypertrichosis (elongation, thickening, and enhanced pigmentation of fine body hair).
• Minoxidil may elevate antinuclear antibody titers.
• *Alert:* Don't confuse Loniten with Lotensin.

PATIENT TEACHING
• Make sure patient receives and reads manufacturer's package insert that de-

---

Reactions may be *common*, uncommon, *life-threatening*, or COMMON AND LIFE-THREATENING.

scribes the drug and its adverse reactions. Also provide an oral explanation.

• Tell patient not to suddenly stop taking drug but to notify prescriber if unpleasant adverse effects occur.

• Make sure patient understands importance of compliance with total treatment regimen. Drug is usually prescribed with a beta blocker to control tachycardia and a diuretic to counteract fluid retention.

• Teach patient how to take his own pulse and to notify prescriber of increases of more than 20 beats/minute.

• Tell patient to weigh himself at least weekly and to report weight gain of more than 5 lb (2.3 kg).

• About 8 of 10 patients will experience hypertrichosis within 3 to 6 weeks of beginning treatment. Unwanted hair can be controlled with a depilatory or shaving. Assure patient that extra hair will disappear within 1 to 6 months of stopping minoxidil. Advise patient, however, not to stop drug without prescriber's approval.

• Advise woman to discuss drug therapy with prescriber if considering pregnancy or currently breast-feeding.

nisoldipine
Sular, Syscor MR§

Pregnancy risk category C

AVAILABLE FORMS
Tablets (extended-release): 10 mg, 20 mg, 30 mg, 40 mg

INDICATIONS & DOSAGES
➤ **Hypertension—**
Adults: Initially, 20 mg P.O. once daily; increased by 10 mg/week or at longer intervals, p.r.n. Usual maintenance dose is 20 to 40 mg/day. Doses of more than 60 mg/day aren't recommended.
Elderly patients: Initially, 10 mg P.O. once daily; dosage is adjusted as for adults.
Adjust-a-dose: For patients with impaired liver function, initially, 10 mg P.O. once daily; dosage is adjusted as for adults.

ACTION
Prevents calcium ions from entering vascular smooth-muscle cells, causing dilation of arterioles, which decreases peripheral vascular resistance.

Route	Onset	Peak	Duration
P.O.	Unknown	6-12 hr	24 hr

ADVERSE REACTIONS
CNS: *headache,* dizziness.
CV: vasodilation, palpitations, chest pain, *peripheral edema.*
EENT: sinusitis, pharyngitis.
GI: nausea.
Skin: rash.

INTERACTIONS
Drug-drug. *Cimetidine:* Increased bioavailability and peak levels of nisoldipine. Monitor blood pressure closely.
Quinidine: Decreased bioavailability of nisoldipine. Adjust dosage accordingly.
Drug-food. *Grapefruit juice:* Increased bioavailability and blood level of drug. Don't give together.
High-fat meal: Increased peak drug level. Monitor blood pressure closely.

EFFECTS ON LAB TEST RESULTS
None reported.

CONTRAINDICATIONS
Contraindicated in patients hypersensitive to dihydropyridine calcium channel blockers. Drug shouldn't be used in breast-feeding women.

NURSING CONSIDERATIONS
• Use cautiously in patients with heart failure or compromised ventricular function, particularly those receiving beta blockers and those with severe hepatic dysfunction.

• Monitor patient carefully. Some patients, especially those with severe obstructive coronary artery disease, have developed increased frequency, duration, or severity of angina or even acute MI after starting calcium channel blocker therapy or at time of dosage increase.

• Monitor blood pressure regularly, especially when starting therapy and during dosage adjustment.

PATIENT TEACHING
• Tell patient to take drug as prescribed, even if he feels better.

• Advise patient to swallow tablet whole and not to chew, divide, or crush it.
• Remind patient not to take drug with a high-fat meal or with grapefruit juice. Both may increase drug level in the body beyond intended amount.

---

nitroprusside sodium
Nipride†, Nitropress

Pregnancy risk category C

AVAILABLE FORMS
Injection: 50 mg/vial in 2-ml and 5-ml vials

INDICATIONS & DOSAGES
➤ **To lower blood pressure quickly in hypertensive emergencies, to produce controlled hypotension during anesthesia, to reduce preload and afterload in cardiac pump failure or cardiogenic shock (may be used with or without dopamine)—**
Adults and children: Begin infusion at 0.25 to 0.3 mcg/kg/minute I.V. and gradually titrate q few minutes to a maximum infusion rate of 10 mcg/kg/minute.
Adjust-a-dose: Patients taking other antihypertensives with nitroprusside are extremely sensitive to nitroprusside. Titrate dosage accordingly. Use with caution in patients with renal failure; reduce dosage as much as possible.

I.V. ADMINISTRATION
• Don't use bacteriostatic water for injection or sterile saline solution for reconstitution.
• Prepare solution by dissolving 50 mg in 2 to 3 ml of D_5W injection or according to manufacturer's instructions. Further dilute concentration in 250, 500, or 1,000 ml of D_5W to provide solutions with 200, 100, or 50 mcg/ml, respectively. Reconstitute ADD-Vantage vials labeled as containing 50 mg of drug according to manufacturer's directions.
• Because drug is sensitive to light, wrap I.V. solution in foil or other opaque material; it's not necessary to wrap the tubing. Fresh solution should have faint brownish tint. Discard if highly discolored after 24 hours.
• Infuse with an infusion pump. Drug is best given via piggyback through a peripheral line with no other drug. Don't titrate rate of main I.V. line while drug is being infused. Even a small bolus of nitroprusside can cause severe hypotension.
• Check blood pressure every 5 minutes at start of infusion and every 15 minutes thereafter.
• If severe hypotension occurs, discontinue nitroprusside infusion—effects of drug quickly reverse. Notify prescriber.
• If possible, start an arterial pressure line. Regulate drug flow to desired blood pressure response.
• ◆ *Alert:* Excessive doses or infusion at a rate greater than 10 mcg/kg/minute can cause cyanide toxicity. If these factors are present, check thiocyanate levels every 72 hours. Levels higher than 100 mcg/ml may be toxic. If profound hypotension, metabolic acidosis, dyspnea, headache, loss of consciousness, ataxia, or vomiting occurs, stop drug immediately and notify prescriber.

ACTION
Relaxes both arteriolar and venous smooth muscle.

Route	Onset	Peak	Duration
I.V.	Immediate	1-2 min	10 min

ADVERSE REACTIONS
CNS: *headache, dizziness,* loss of consciousness, apprehension, ***increased ICP,*** restlessness.
CV: ***bradycardia,*** hypotension, tachycardia, palpitations, ECG changes, flushing.
GI: *nausea, abdominal pain,* ileus.
Hematologic: ***methemoglobinemia.***
Metabolic: acidosis, hypothyroidism.
Musculoskeletal: *muscle twitching.*
Skin: pink color, rash, *diaphoresis.*
Other: ***thiocyanate toxicity, cyanide toxicity,*** venous streaking, irritation at infusion site.

INTERACTIONS
Drug-drug. *Antihypertensives:* May cause sensitivity to nitroprusside. Adjust dosage. *Ganglionic blocking drugs, general anesthetics, negative inotropic drugs, other antihypertensives:* Additive effects. Monitor blood pressure closely.

Reactions may be *common,* uncommon, *life-threatening,* or COMMON AND LIFE-THREATENING.

EFFECTS ON LAB TEST RESULTS
• May increase creatinine level.

CONTRAINDICATIONS
Contraindicated in patients hypersensitive to drug; also contraindicated in those with compensatory hypertension (such as in arteriovenous shunt or coarctation of the aorta), inadequate cerebral circulation, acute heart failure with reduced peripheral vascular resistance, congenital optic atrophy, or tobacco-induced amblyopia.

NURSING CONSIDERATIONS
• Use with extreme caution in patients with increased intracranial pressure. Use cautiously in patients with hypothyroidism, hepatic or renal disease, hyponatremia, or low vitamin B_{12} level.
• Obtain baseline vital signs before giving drug; find out parameters prescriber wants to achieve.
• Keep patient in the supine position when initiating or titrating drug.
• *Alert:* Don't confuse nitroprusside with nitroglycerin.

PATIENT TEACHING
• Instruct patient to report adverse reactions promptly.
• Tell patient to alert nurse if discomfort occurs at I.V. insertion site.

---

perindopril erbumine
Aceon

Pregnancy risk category C (D in second and third trimesters)

AVAILABLE FORMS
Tablets: 2 mg, 4 mg, 8 mg

INDICATIONS & DOSAGES
➤ **Essential hypertension—**
Adults: Initially, 4 mg P.O. once daily. Increase dosage until blood pressure is controlled or to maximum of 16 mg/day; usual maintenance dose is 4 to 8 mg once daily; may be given in two divided doses.
Elderly patients: Initially, 4 mg P.O. daily as one dose or in two divided doses. Dosage may be increased by more than 8 mg/day only under close medical supervision.

Adjust-a-dose: For patients with renal insufficiency, initially, 2 mg P.O. daily. Maximum maintenance dose is 8 mg/day. In patients taking diuretics, initially, 2 to 4 mg P.O. daily as single dose or in two divided doses, with close medical supervision for several hours and until blood pressure has stabilized. Adjust dosage based on patient's blood pressure response.

ACTION
A prodrug that's converted by the liver to the active metabolite perindoprilat, which inhibits ACE activity, thereby preventing conversion of angiotensin I to angiotensin II, a potent vasoconstrictor. Inhibition of ACE results in decreased vasoconstriction and decreased aldosterone activity, thus reducing sodium and water retention and lowering blood pressure.

Route	Onset	Peak	Duration
P.O.	Unknown	1 hr	Unknown

ADVERSE REACTIONS
CNS: dizziness, asthenia, sleep disorder, paresthesia, depression, somnolence, nervousness, *headache.*
CV: palpitations, edema, chest pain, abnormal ECG.
EENT: rhinitis, sinusitis, ear infection, pharyngitis, tinnitus.
GI: dyspepsia, diarrhea, abdominal pain, nausea, vomiting, flatulence.
GU: proteinuria, urinary tract infection, male sexual dysfunction, menstrual disorder.
Musculoskeletal: back pain, hypertonia, neck pain, joint pain, myalgia, arthritis, arm or leg pain.
Respiratory: *cough,* upper respiratory tract infection.
Skin: rash.
Other: viral infection, fever, injury, seasonal allergy.

INTERACTIONS
Drug-drug. *Diuretics:* Increased hypotensive effect. Monitor patient closely.
Lithium: Increased lithium level and risk of lithium toxicity. Use together cautiously; monitor lithium level.
Potassium-sparing diuretics (amiloride, spironolactone, triamterene), potassium supplements, other drugs capable of in-

---

creasing potassium level (cyclosporine, heparin, indomethacin): Increased hyperkalemic effect. Use together cautiously; monitor potassium level frequently.
Drug-herb. *Capsaicin:* May cause cough. Discourage use together.
Drug-food. *Salt substitutes containing potassium:* May cause hyperkalemia. Discourage use together.

EFFECTS ON LAB TEST RESULTS
• May increase ALT and triglyceride levels.

CONTRAINDICATIONS
Contraindicated in patients hypersensitive to drug or other ACE inhibitors and in those with a history of angioedema secondary to ACE inhibitors. Also contraindicated in pregnant women.

NURSING CONSIDERATIONS
• Use cautiously in patients with a history of angioedema unrelated to ACE inhibitor therapy. Also use cautiously in patients with impaired renal function, heart failure, ischemic heart disease, cerebrovascular disease or renal artery stenosis, and in patients with collagen vascular disease, such as systemic lupus erythematosus or scleroderma.
• Although ACE inhibitors reduce blood pressure in all races studied, this response is less in blacks who receive the drug as monotherapy. Therapy with a thiazide diuretic produces a more favorable response.
• ACE inhibitors appear to increase risk of angioedema in black patients.
• *Alert:* Angioedema involving the face, extremities, lips, tongue, glottis, and larynx may occur. Stop drug and observe patient until swelling disappears. If swelling is confined to face and lips, it will probably resolve without treatment, but antihistamines may be useful in relieving symptoms. Angioedema of the tongue, glottis, or larynx may be fatal because of airway obstruction. Appropriate therapy, such as S.C. epinephrine solution, should be promptly administered.
• Patients with a history of angioedema unrelated to ACE inhibitor therapy may be at increased risk for angioedema while receiving an ACE inhibitor.

• Other ACE inhibitors have caused agranulocytosis and neutropenia. Monitor CBC with differential before therapy, especially in renally impaired patients with systemic lupus erythematosus or scleroderma.
• Excessive hypotension can occur when drug is given with diuretics. If possible, discontinue diuretic 2 to 3 days before starting perindopril, to reduce the potential for excessive hypotensive response. If it isn't possible to discontinue the diuretic, consider starting perindopril with a lower dosage or decreasing dosage of diuretic.
• Monitor patient at risk for hypotension closely during initiation of therapy, for first 2 weeks of treatment, and whenever dosage of perindopril or concomitant diuretic is increased. If severe hypotension occurs, place patient in supine position and treat symptomatically.
• Hypotension can occur when starting therapy or adjusting dosage in patient who is volume- or salt-depleted from prolonged diuretic therapy, dietary salt restriction, dialysis, diarrhea, or vomiting. Volume and salt depletion should be corrected before starting drug.
• ACE inhibitors have rarely been linked to a syndrome of cholestatic jaundice, fulminant hepatic necrosis, and death. Discontinue drug in patient who develops jaundice or marked elevations of hepatic enzyme levels during therapy.
• Monitor renal function before and periodically throughout therapy. Don't use drug in patient with a creatinine clearance less than 30 ml/minute.
• Monitor potassium levels closely.

PATIENT TEACHING
• Inform patient that angioedema, including laryngeal edema, can occur during therapy, especially with the first dose. Advise patient to stop taking drug and immediately report any signs or symptoms of angioedema (swelling of face, extremities, eyes, lips, tongue, hoarseness or difficulty in swallowing or breathing).
• Advise patient to report promptly any sign or symptom of infection (sore throat, fever) or jaundice (yellowing of eyes or skin).
• Advise patient to avoid salt substitutes containing potassium unless instructed otherwise by prescriber.

Reactions may be *common*, uncommon, **life-threatening**, or COMMON AND LIFE-THREATENING.

• Caution patient that light-headedness may occur, especially during first few days of therapy. Advise patient to report light-headedness and, if fainting occurs, to discontinue drug and consult prescriber promptly.

• Caution patient that inadequate fluid intake or excessive perspiration, diarrhea, or vomiting can lead to an excessive drop in blood pressure.

• Advise woman of childbearing age of the consequences of second- and third-trimester exposure to drug. Advise her to notify prescriber immediately if she suspects pregnancy.

---

pindolol
Barbloc‡, Novo-Pindol†, Syn-Pindolol†, Visken

Pregnancy risk category B

AVAILABLE FORMS
Tablets: 5 mg, 10 mg, 15 mg‡

INDICATIONS & DOSAGES
➤ **Hypertension—**
Adults: Initially, 5 mg P.O. b.i.d. Dosage may be increased as needed and tolerated, to maximum of 60 mg daily.

ACTION
Unknown. A nonselective beta blocker that has intrinsic sympathomimetic activity. Possible mechanisms include reduced cardiac output, decreased sympathetic outflow to peripheral vasculature, and inhibition of renin release by the kidneys.

Route	Onset	Peak	Duration
P.O.	Unknown	1-2 hr	24 hr

ADVERSE REACTIONS
CNS: *insomnia, fatigue, dizziness, nervousness,* vivid dreams, weakness, paresthesia.
CV: *edema, **bradycardia, heart failure,*** chest pain.
GI: *nausea,* abdominal discomfort.
Musculoskeletal: *muscle pain, joint pain.*
Respiratory: *increased airway resistance,* dyspnea.
Skin: rash, pruritus.

INTERACTIONS
Drug-drug. *Cardiac glycosides, diltiazem, verapamil:* Excessive bradycardia and increased depression of AV node. Use together cautiously.
Catecholamine-depleting drugs such as reserpine: May have additive effects. Monitor patient for hypotension and bradycardia.
Epinephrine: Severe vasoconstriction. Monitor blood pressure and observe patient carefully.
Indomethacin: Decreased antihypertensive effect. Monitor blood pressure and adjust dosage.
Insulin, oral antidiabetics: May alter requirements for these drugs in previously stabilized diabetic patients. Monitor patient for hypoglycemia.

EFFECTS ON LAB TEST RESULTS
• May increase transaminase, alkaline phosphatase, LDH, and uric acid levels.

CONTRAINDICATIONS
Contraindicated in patients hypersensitive to drug and in those with bronchial asthma, severe bradycardia, greater than first-degree heart block, cardiogenic shock, or overt cardiac failure.

NURSING CONSIDERATIONS
• Use cautiously in patients with heart failure, nonallergic bronchospastic disease, diabetes, hyperthyroidism, and impaired renal or hepatic function.
• Always check patient's apical pulse rate before giving drug. If extremes in pulse rate are detected, withhold drug and call prescriber immediately.
• Monitor blood pressure frequently and notify prescriber if severe hypotension occurs. A vasopressor may be needed.
• Withdraw drug over 1 to 2 weeks after long-term therapy.
• Monitor glucose levels in diabetic patients closely because drug masks certain signs and symptoms of hypoglycemia.
• Beta blockers may mask tachycardia caused by hyperthyroidism. In patients with suspected thyrotoxicosis, withdraw beta blocker gradually to avoid thyroid storm.
• *Alert:* Don't confuse pindolol with Parlodel, Panadol, or Plendil; or Visken with Visine.

PATIENT TEACHING
● Advise patient to take drug exactly as prescribed.
● Tell patient not to stop drug suddenly but to notify prescriber to discuss unpleasant adverse drug reactions.
● Inform patient that drug may deplete body's stores of coenzyme Q10 and that he should discuss need for supplements with prescriber.

---

prazosin hydrochloride
Hypovase§, Minipress

Pregnancy risk category C

AVAILABLE FORMS
Capsules: 1 mg, 2 mg, 5 mg

INDICATIONS & DOSAGES
➤ **Mild to moderate hypertension, alone or with a diuretic or other antihypertensive—**
Adults: Test dose is 1 mg P.O. h.s. to prevent first-dose syncope (severe syncope with loss of consciousness). Initial dose is 1 mg P.O. b.i.d. or t.i.d. Dosage may be increased slowly. Maximum daily dose is 20 mg. Maintenance dose is 6 to 15 mg daily in three divided doses. Some patients need larger dosages (up to 40 mg daily). If other antihypertensives or diuretics are added to drug, prazosin is decreased to 1 to 2 mg t.i.d. and readjusted.

ACTION
Unknown. Drug's alpha$_1$-blocking activity is thought to account primarily for its effects.

Route	Onset	Peak	Duration
P.O.	0.5-1.5 hr	2-4 hr	7-10 hr

ADVERSE REACTIONS
CNS: *dizziness, headache,* drowsiness, nervousness, paresthesia, weakness, *first-dose syncope,* depression.
CV: orthostatic hypotension, *palpitations,* edema.
EENT: blurred vision, tinnitus, conjunctivitis, epistaxis, nasal congestion.
GI: vomiting, diarrhea, abdominal cramps, *nausea.*

GU: priapism, impotence, urinary frequency, incontinence.
Musculoskeletal: arthralgia, myalgia.
Respiratory: dyspnea.
Skin: pruritus.
Other: fever.

INTERACTIONS
Drug-drug. *Propranolol, other beta blockers:* Increased frequency of syncope with loss of consciousness. Advise patient to sit or lie down if dizziness occurs.
Verapamil: Increased prazosin levels. Monitor patient closely.
Drug-herb. *Butcher's broom:* May reduce effect. Discourage use together.

EFFECTS ON LAB TEST RESULTS
● May increase BUN and uric acid levels.
● May increase liver function test values.

CONTRAINDICATIONS
Contraindicated in patients hypersensitive to drug or other alpha$_1$ blockers.

NURSING CONSIDERATIONS
● Use cautiously in patients receiving other antihypertensives.
● Monitor patient's blood pressure and pulse rate frequently.
● Elderly patients may be more sensitive to drug's hypotensive effects.
● Compliance might be improved with twice-daily dosing. Discuss this dosing change with prescriber if compliance problems are suspected.
● Drug alters results of screening tests for pheochromocytoma and causes increases in levels of the urinary metabolite of norepinephrine and vanillylmandelic acid; it may cause positive antinuclear antibody titer.
● *Alert:* If initial dose is more than 1 mg, first-dose syncope may occur.

PATIENT TEACHING
● Warn patient that dizziness may occur with first dose. If he experiences dizziness, tell him to sit or lie down. Reassure him that this effect disappears with continued dosing.
● Caution patient to avoid driving or performing hazardous tasks for the first 24 hours after starting this drug or increasing the dose.

Reactions may be *common,* uncommon, **life-threatening,** or COMMON AND LIFE-THREATENING.

• Tell patient not to suddenly stop taking drug, but to notify prescriber if unpleasant adverse reactions occur.

• Advise patient to minimize orthostatic hypotension by rising slowly and avoiding sudden position changes. Dry mouth can be relieved by chewing gum or sucking on hard candy or ice chips.

---

quinapril hydrochloride
Accupril, Accupro§, Asig‡

Pregnancy risk category C (D in second and third trimesters)

AVAILABLE FORMS
Tablets: 5 mg, 10 mg, 20 mg, 40 mg

INDICATIONS & DOSAGES
➤ **Hypertension—**
Adults: Initially, 10 to 20 mg P.O. daily. Dosage may be adjusted based on patient response at intervals of about 2 weeks. Most patients are controlled at 20, 40, or 80 mg daily as a single dose or in two divided doses. If patient is taking a diuretic, initiate therapy with 5 mg daily.
Elderly patients: For patients older than age 65, initiate therapy at 10 mg P.O. daily.
➤ **Heart failure—**
Adults: Initially, 5 mg P.O. b.i.d. if patient is taking a diuretic and 10 to 20 mg P.O. b.i.d. if patient isn't taking a diuretic. Dosage may be increased at weekly intervals. Usual effective dose is 20 to 40 mg b.i.d. in equally divided doses.
Adjust-a-dose: For renally impaired patients with creatinine clearance of more than 60 ml/minute, give 10 mg daily; if clearance is 30 to 60 ml/minute, give 5 mg daily; and if clearance is 10 to 30 ml/minute, give 2.5 mg daily.

ACTION
Unknown. Thought to be involved with inhibiting conversion of angiotensin I to angiotensin II, a potent vasoconstrictor. Reduced formation of angiotensin II decreases peripheral arterial resistance, thus decreasing aldosterone secretion.

Route	Onset	Peak	Duration
P.O.	1 hr	2-6 hr	24 hr

ADVERSE REACTIONS
CNS: somnolence, vertigo, nervousness, *headache, dizziness, fatigue,* depression.
CV: palpitations, tachycardia, angina pectoris, hypertensive crisis, orthostatic hypotension, rhythm disturbances.
GI: dry mouth, abdominal pain, constipation, vomiting, nausea, ***hemorrhage.***
Metabolic: hyperkalemia.
Respiratory: dry, persistent, tickling, nonproductive cough.
Skin: pruritus, photosensitivity reactions, diaphoresis.

INTERACTIONS
Drug-drug. *Diuretics, other antihypertensives:* Excessive hypotension. Discontinue diuretic or lower dose of quinapril, as needed.
Lithium: Increased lithium levels and lithium toxicity. Monitor lithium levels.
Potassium-sparing diuretics, potassium supplements: May cause hyperkalemia. Monitor patient closely.
Tetracycline: Decreased absorption if taken with quinapril. Avoid using together.
Drug-herb. *Capsaicin:* May cause cough. Discourage use together.
Drug-food. *Salt substitutes containing potassium:* May cause hyperkalemia. Discourage use together.

EFFECTS ON LAB TEST RESULTS
• May increase potassium level.
• May increase liver function test values.

CONTRAINDICATIONS
Contraindicated in patients hypersensitive to ACE inhibitors and in those with a history of angioedema related to treatment with an ACE inhibitor.

NURSING CONSIDERATIONS
• Use cautiously in patients with impaired renal function.
• Assess renal and hepatic function before and periodically throughout therapy.
• Monitor blood pressure for effectiveness of therapy.
• Monitor potassium levels. Risk factors for the development of hyperkalemia include renal insufficiency, diabetes, and concomitant use of drugs that raise potassium level.

• Although ACE inhibitors reduce blood pressure in all races studied, this response is less in blacks who receive the drug as monotherapy. Therapy with a thiazide diuretic produces a more favorable response.

• ACE inhibitors appear to increase risk of angioedema in black patients.

• Other ACE inhibitors have caused agranulocytosis and neutropenia. Monitor CBC with differential counts before therapy and periodically thereafter.

PATIENT TEACHING

• Advise patient to report signs of infection, such as fever and sore throat.

• *Alert:* Angioedema (including laryngeal edema) may occur, especially after first dose. Advise patient to report signs or symptoms of angioedema, such as breathing difficulty or swelling of face, eyes, lips, or tongue.

• Light-headedness can occur, especially during first few days of therapy. Tell patient to rise slowly to minimize effect and to report signs and symptoms to prescriber. If syncope occurs, he should stop taking drug and call prescriber immediately.

• Inform patient that inadequate fluid intake, vomiting, diarrhea, and excessive perspiration can lead to light-headedness and syncope. Tell him to use caution in hot weather and during exercise.

• Tell patient to avoid salt substitutes. These products may contain potassium, which can cause hyperkalemia in patients taking quinapril.

• Advise woman to notify prescriber if pregnancy occurs. Drug will need to be discontinued.

---

ramipril
Altace, Ramace‡, Tritace‡

Pregnancy risk category C (D in second and third trimesters)

AVAILABLE FORMS
Capsules: 1.25 mg, 2.5 mg, 5 mg, 10 mg

INDICATIONS & DOSAGES
➤ **Hypertension—**
Adults: Initially, 2.5 mg P.O. once daily for patients not taking a diuretic, and 1.25 mg

P.O. once daily for patients taking a diuretic. Increase dosage p.r.n., based on patient response. Maintenance dose is 2.5 to 20 mg daily as a single dose or in divided doses.

Adjust-a-dose: For renally impaired patients with creatinine clearance less than 40 ml/minute, give 1.25 mg P.O. daily. Adjust dosage gradually based on response. Maximum daily dose is 5 mg.

➤ **Heart failure—**
Adults: Initially, 2.5 mg P.O. b.i.d. If hypotension occurs, decrease dosage to 1.25 mg P.O. b.i.d. Gradually increase dosage to maximum of 5 mg P.O. b.i.d., p.r.n.

Adjust-a-dose: For renally impaired patients with creatinine clearance less than 40 ml/minute, give 1.25 mg P.O. daily. Adjust dosage gradually based on response. Maximum daily dose is 2.5 mg b.i.d.

✱ **NEW INDICATION: Reduction in risk of MI, stroke, and death from CV causes—**
Adults age 55 and older: 2.5 mg P.O. once daily for 1 week, then 5 mg P.O. once daily for 3 weeks. Increase as tolerated to a maintenance dose of 10 mg P.O. once daily.

Adjust-a-dose: In patients who are hypertensive or who have recently had an MI, daily dose may be divided.

ACTION
Unknown. Thought to be involved with inhibiting conversion of angiotensin I to angiotensin II, a potent vasoconstrictor. Reduced formation of angiotensin II decreases peripheral arterial resistance, thus decreasing aldosterone secretion.

Route	Onset	Peak	Duration
P.O.	1-2 hr	1-3 hr	24 hr

ADVERSE REACTIONS
CNS: *headache, dizziness,* fatigue, asthenia, malaise, light-headedness, anxiety, amnesia, depression, insomnia, nervousness, neuralgia, neuropathy, paresthesia, somnolence, tremor, vertigo, syncope.
CV: *heart failure,* orthostatic hypotension, angina pectoris, chest pain, palpitations, *MI,* edema.
EENT: epistaxis, tinnitus.

Reactions may be *common,* uncommon, *life-threatening,* or COMMON AND LIFE-THREATENING.

GI: nausea, vomiting, abdominal pain, anorexia, constipation, diarrhea, dyspepsia, dry mouth, gastroenteritis.
GU: impotence.
Metabolic: hyperglycemia, hyperkalemia, weight gain.
Musculoskeletal: arthralgia, arthritis, myalgia.
Respiratory: dyspnea; dry, persistent, tickling, nonproductive cough.
Skin: rash, dermatitis, pruritus, photosensitivity reactions, increased diaphoresis.
Other: hypersensitivity reactions.

INTERACTIONS
Drug-drug. *Diuretics:* Excessive hypotension, especially at start of therapy. Discontinue diuretic at least 3 days before therapy begins, increase sodium intake, or reduce starting dose of ramipril.
Insulin, oral antidiabetics: May cause hypoglycemia, especially at start of ramipril therapy. Monitor patient closely.
Lithium: Increased lithium levels. Use together cautiously and monitor lithium levels.
Potassium-sparing diuretics, potassium supplements: May cause hyperkalemia; ramipril attenuates potassium loss. Monitor plasma potassium levels closely.
Drug-herb. *Capsaicin:* May cause cough. Discourage use together.
Drug-food. *Salt substitutes containing potassium:* May cause hyperkalemia; ramipril attenuates potassium loss. Discourage use of salt substitutes.

EFFECTS ON LAB TEST RESULTS
● May increase BUN, creatinine, bilirubin, liver enzymes, glucose, and potassium levels.
● May decrease hemoglobin and hematocrit.

CONTRAINDICATIONS
Contraindicated in patients hypersensitive to ACE inhibitors and in those with a history of angioedema related to treatment with an ACE inhibitor.

NURSING CONSIDERATIONS
● Use cautiously in patients with renal impairment.
● Monitor blood pressure regularly for drug effectiveness.

● Closely assess renal function in patients during first few weeks of therapy. Regular assessment of renal function is advisable. Patients with severe heart failure whose renal function depends on the renin-angiotensin-aldosterone system have experienced acute renal failure during ACE inhibitor therapy. Hypertensive patients with renal artery stenosis also may show signs of worsening renal function during first few days of therapy.
● Although ACE inhibitors reduce blood pressure in all races studied, this response is less in blacks who receive the drug as monotherapy. Therapy with a thiazide diuretic produces a more favorable response.
● ACE inhibitors appear to increase risk of angioedema in black patients.
● Monitor CBC with differential counts before therapy and periodically thereafter. Decreased WBC, RBC, platelet and hemoglobin counts may occur, especially in patients with impaired renal function or collagen vascular diseases (systemic lupus erythematosus or scleroderma).
● Monitor potassium levels. Risk factors for the development of hyperkalemia include renal insufficiency, diabetes, and concomitant use of drugs that raise potassium levels.

PATIENT TEACHING
● Tell patient to notify prescriber if any adverse reactions occur. Dosage adjustment or discontinuation of drug may be needed.
● *Alert:* Rarely, angioedema (including laryngeal edema) may occur, especially after first dose. Advise patient to report signs or symptoms of angioedema, such as breathing difficulty or swelling of face, eyes, lips, or tongue.
● Inform patient that light-headedness can occur, especially during the first few days of therapy. Tell him to rise slowly to minimize this effect and to report signs and symptoms to prescriber. If syncope occurs, patient should stop taking drug and call prescriber immediately.
● Tell patient that if he has difficulty swallowing capsules, he can open drug and sprinkle contents on a small amount of applesauce.

• Advise patient to report signs and symptoms of infection, such as fever and sore throat.

• Tell patient to avoid salt substitutes. These products may contain potassium, which can cause hyperkalemia in patients taking ramipril.

• Tell woman to notify prescriber if pregnancy occurs. Drug will need to be discontinued.

---

telmisartan
Micardis

Pregnancy risk category C (D in second and third trimesters)

AVAILABLE FORMS
Tablets: 40 mg, 80 mg

INDICATIONS & DOSAGES
➤ **Hypertension (used alone or with other antihypertensives)—**
Adults: 40 mg P.O. daily. Blood pressure response is dose-related over a range of 20 to 80 mg daily.

ACTION
Blocks the vasoconstricting and aldosterone-secreting effects of angiotensin II by selectively blocking the binding of angiotensin II to the angiotensin I receptor in many tissues, such as vascular smooth muscle and the adrenal gland.

Route	Onset	Peak	Duration
P.O.	Unknown	0.5-1 hr	24 hr

ADVERSE REACTIONS
CNS: *dizziness,* pain, fatigue, *headache.*
CV: chest pain, hypertension, peripheral edema.
EENT: pharyngitis, sinusitis.
GI: abdominal pain, diarrhea, dyspepsia, *nausea.*
GU: urinary tract infection.
Musculoskeletal: back pain, myalgia.
Respiratory: cough, upper respiratory tract infection.
Other: flulike symptoms.

INTERACTIONS
Drug-drug. *Digoxin:* Increased digoxin levels. Monitor digoxin levels closely.

Warfarin: Slightly decreased warfarin levels. Monitor INR.
Drug-food. *Salt substitutes containing potassium:* May cause hyperkalemia. Discourage use of salt substitutes.

EFFECTS ON LAB TEST RESULTS
• May increase liver enzyme levels.

CONTRAINDICATIONS
Contraindicated in patients hypersensitive to drug or its components.

NURSING CONSIDERATIONS
• Use cautiously in patients with biliary obstruction disorders or renal and hepatic insufficiency and in those with an activated renin-angiotensin system, such as volume- or salt-depleted patients (for example, those being treated with high doses of diuretics).

• Drugs such as telmisartan that act on the renin-angiotensin system can cause fetal and neonatal morbidity and death when given to pregnant women. These problems haven't been detected when exposure has been limited to the first trimester. If pregnancy is suspected, notify prescriber because drug should be discontinued.

• Monitor patient for hypotension after starting drug. Place patient in supine position if hypotension occurs and administer I.V. normal saline, if needed.

• Most of the antihypertensive effect occurs within 2 weeks. Maximal blood pressure reduction is usually reached after 4 weeks. Diuretic may be added if blood pressure isn't controlled by drug alone.

• For patients whose renal function may depend on the activity of the renin-angiotensin-aldosterone system (such as those with severe heart failure), treatment with ACE inhibitors and angiotensin receptor antagonists has caused oliguria or progressive azotemia and (rarely) acute renal failure or death.

• Drug isn't removed by hemodialysis. Patients undergoing dialysis may develop orthostatic hypotension. Closely monitor blood pressure.

PATIENT TEACHING
• Instruct patient to report suspected pregnancy to prescriber immediately.

Reactions may be *common,* uncommon, ***life-threatening***, or COMMON AND LIFE-THREATENING.

• Inform woman of childbearing age of the consequences of second- and third-trimester exposure to drug.

• Advise breast-feeding woman about risk of adverse drug effects in infant and the need to either discontinue drug or stop breast-feeding.

• Tell patient that, if transient hypotension occurs, he should lie down if feeling dizzy, rise slowly from a lying to standing position, and climb stairs slowly.

• Tell patient that drug may be taken without regard to meals.

• Tell patient that drug shouldn't be removed from blister-sealed packet until immediately before use.

---

terazosin hydrochloride
Hytrin

Pregnancy risk category C

AVAILABLE FORMS
Capsules: 1 mg, 2 mg, 5 mg, 10 mg
Tablets: 1 mg, 2 mg, 5 mg, 10 mg

INDICATIONS & DOSAGES
➤ **Hypertension**—
Adults: Initially, 1 mg P.O. h.s. Dosage may be increased gradually based on response. Usual dosage range is 1 to 5 mg daily. Maximum recommended dose is 20 mg daily.
➤ **Symptomatic BPH**—
Adults: Initially, 1 mg P.O. h.s. Dosage may be increased in a stepwise fashion to 2, 5, or 10 mg once daily to achieve optimal response. Most patients need 10 mg daily for optimal response.

ACTION
Decreases blood pressure by vasodilation produced in response to blockade of alpha$_1$-adrenergic receptors. It improves urine flow in patients with BPH by blocking alpha$_1$-adrenergic receptors in the smooth muscle of the bladder neck and prostate, thus relieving urethral pressure and reestablishing urine flow.

Route	Onset	Peak	Duration
P.O.	15 min	2-3 hr	24 hr

ADVERSE REACTIONS
CNS: asthenia, *dizziness, headache,* nervousness, paresthesia, somnolence.
CV: palpitations, orthostatic hypotension, tachycardia, *peripheral edema.*
EENT: *nasal congestion,* sinusitis, blurred vision.
GI: nausea.
GU: impotence.
Musculoskeletal: back pain, muscle pain.
Respiratory: dyspnea.

INTERACTIONS
Drug-drug. *Antihypertensives:* Excessive hypotension. Use together cautiously.
Clonidine: May decrease clonidine's antihypertensive effect. Monitor patient.
Drug-herb. *Butcher's broom:* May cause diminished effect of drug. Discourage use together.

EFFECTS ON LAB TEST RESULTS
• May decrease total protein and albumin levels.
• May decrease hematocrit, hemoglobin, and WBC count.

CONTRAINDICATIONS
Contraindicated in patients hypersensitive to drug.

NURSING CONSIDERATIONS
• Monitor blood pressure frequently.
• *Alert:* If terazosin is discontinued for several days, readjust dosage using initial dosing regimen (1 mg P.O. h.s.).

PATIENT TEACHING
• Tell patient not to stop drug suddenly, but to notify prescriber if adverse reactions occur.
• Warn patient to avoid hazardous activities that require mental alertness, such as driving or operating heavy machinery, for 12 hours after first dose.
• Tell patient that light-headedness can occur, especially during the first few days of therapy. Advise him to rise slowly to minimize this effect and to report signs and symptoms to prescriber.

---

*Liquid contains alcohol.   **May contain tartrazine.   †Canada   ‡Australia   §U.K.   ◊OTC

timolol maleate
Apo-Timol†, Betim§, Blocadren

Pregnancy risk category C

AVAILABLE FORMS
Tablets: 5 mg, 10 mg, 20 mg

INDICATIONS & DOSAGES
➤ **Hypertension—**
Adults: Initially, 10 mg P.O. b.i.d. Usual daily maintenance dose is 20 to 40 mg. Maximum daily dose is 60 mg. Allow at least 7 days between increases in dosage.
➤ **MI (long-term prophylaxis in patients who have survived acute phase)—**
Adults: 10 mg P.O. b.i.d.
➤ **Migraine headache prophylaxis—**
Adults: Initially, 10 mg P.O. b.i.d. Increase dosage as needed and tolerated to maximum of 30 mg daily as a divided dose. Discontinue treatment if no response occurs after 6 to 8 weeks at maximum dose.

ACTION
Unknown. In MI, drug may decrease myocardial oxygen requirements. For migraine headache prophylaxis, drug prevents arterial dilation through beta blockade.

Route	Onset	Peak	Duration
P.O.	15-30 min	1-2 hr	6-12 hr

ADVERSE REACTIONS
CNS: fatigue, lethargy, dizziness.
CV: *bradycardia,* hypotension, *heart failure,* peripheral vascular disease, *arrhythmias.*
GI: nausea, vomiting, diarrhea.
Metabolic: hyperkalemia, hyperglycemia.
Respiratory: dyspnea, *bronchospasm, increased airway resistance,* pulmonary edema.
Skin: pruritus.

INTERACTIONS
Drug-drug. *Cardiac glycosides, diltiazem, verapamil:* Excessive bradycardia and increased depressant effect on myocardium. Use together cautiously.
Catecholamine-depleting drugs such as reserpine: May have additive effect when given with beta blockers. Watch for hypotension and bradycardia.
Indomethacin: Decreased antihypertensive effect. Monitor blood pressure and adjust dosage.
Insulin, oral antidiabetics: May alter requirements for these drugs in previously stabilized diabetic patients. Monitor patient for hypoglycemia.

EFFECTS ON LAB TEST RESULTS
● May increase BUN, potassium, uric acid, and glucose levels.

CONTRAINDICATIONS
Contraindicated in patients hypersensitive to drug and in those with bronchial asthma, severe COPD, sinus bradycardia, and heart block greater than first-degree or cardiogenic shock.

NURSING CONSIDERATIONS
● Use cautiously in patients with hepatic, renal, or respiratory disease, diabetes, and hyperthyroidism.
● Although drug should be avoided in patient with overt heart failure, it may be used cautiously in patients with well-compensated heart failure.
● Check patient's apical pulse rate before giving drug. If extremes in pulse rates are detected, withhold drug and notify prescriber immediately.
● Monitor blood pressure frequently.
● Monitor glucose levels in diabetic patients; drug can mask signs and symptoms of hypoglycemia.
● Beta blockers may mask tachycardia caused by hyperthyroidism. In patients with suspected thyrotoxicosis, withdraw beta blocker gradually to avoid thyroid storm.
● *Alert:* Don't confuse timolol with atenolol.

PATIENT TEACHING
● Tell patient to take drug exactly as prescribed.
● Instruct patient not to stop drug suddenly, but to notify prescriber if adverse reactions occur. Tell patient that dosage should be reduced gradually over 1 to 2 weeks.
● Advise patient that drug may deplete body's stores of coenzyme Q10 and that

---

Reactions may be *common*, uncommon, ***life-threatening***, or COMMON AND LIFE-THREATENING.

he should discuss need for supplements with prescriber.

---

trandolapril
Gopten§, Mavik, Odrik§

Pregnancy risk category C (D in second and third trimesters)

AVAILABLE FORMS
Tablets: 1 mg, 2 mg, 4 mg

INDICATIONS & DOSAGES
➤ **Hypertension—**
Adults: For patients not taking a diuretic, initially, 1 mg P.O. for a nonblack patient and 2 mg P.O. for a black patient, once daily. If control isn't adequate, increase dosage at intervals of at least 1 week. Maintenance doses for most patients range from 2 to 4 mg daily. Some patients taking once-daily doses of 4 mg may need b.i.d. doses. For patients also taking a diuretic, initially, 0.5 mg P.O. once daily. Subsequent dosage adjustment is based on blood pressure response.
➤ **Heart failure or ventricular dysfunction after MI—**
Adults: Initially, 1 mg P.O. daily, adjusted to 4 mg P.O. daily. If patient can't tolerate 4 mg, continue at highest tolerated dose.
Adjust-a-dose: For patients with hepatic disease or renal impairment, if creatinine clearance is below 30 ml/minute, initial dose is 0.5 mg daily.

ACTION
Unknown. Thought to result primarily from inhibition of circulating and tissue ACE activity, thereby reducing angiotensin II formation, decreasing vasoconstriction and aldosterone secretion, and increasing plasma renin. Decreased aldosterone secretion leads to diuresis, natriuresis, and a small increase in potassium. Drug is converted in the liver to the prodrug, trandolaprilat.

Route	Onset	Peak	Duration
P.O.	Unknown	1-10 hr	24 hr

ADVERSE REACTIONS
CNS: *dizziness, headache,* fatigue, drowsiness, insomnia, paresthesia, vertigo, anxiety.
CV: chest pain, first-degree AV block, ***bradycardia,*** edema, flushing, hypotension, palpitations.
EENT: epistaxis, throat irritation.
GI: diarrhea, dyspepsia, abdominal distention, abdominal pain or cramps, constipation, vomiting, ***pancreatitis.***
GU: urinary frequency, impotence.
Hematologic: ***neutropenia, leukopenia.***
Metabolic: hyperkalemia, hyponatremia.
Respiratory: dyspnea; persistent, nonproductive cough; upper respiratory tract infection.
Skin: rash, pruritus, pemphigus.
Other: decreased libido.

INTERACTIONS
Drug-drug. *Diuretics:* Excessive hypotension. Discontinue diuretic or reduce initial dosage of trandolapril.
Lithium: Increased lithium levels and lithium toxicity. Avoid using together; monitor lithium levels.
Potassium-sparing diuretics, potassium supplements: May cause hyperkalemia. Monitor potassium level closely.
Drug-herb. *Capsaicin:* May cause cough. Discourage use together.
Drug-food. *Salt substitutes containing potassium:* May cause hyperkalemia. Discourage use of salt substitutes.

EFFECTS ON LAB TEST RESULTS
● May increase BUN, creatinine, potassium, and liver enzyme levels. May decrease sodium level.
● May decrease neutrophil and WBC counts.

CONTRAINDICATIONS
Contraindicated in patients hypersensitive to drug and in those with a history of angioedema related to previous treatment with an ACE inhibitor. Also contraindicated in pregnant patients.

NURSING CONSIDERATIONS
● Use cautiously in patients with impaired renal function, heart failure, or renal artery stenosis.
● Monitor potassium levels closely.

• Watch for hypotension. Excessive hypotension can occur when drug is given with diuretics. If possible, diuretic therapy should be discontinued 2 to 3 days before starting trandolapril to decrease potential for excessive hypotension response. If drug doesn't adequately control blood pressure, diuretic therapy may be started again cautiously.

• Assess patient's renal function before and periodically throughout therapy.

• Other ACE inhibitors have caused agranulocytosis and neutropenia. Monitor CBC with differential before therapy, especially in patients with collagen vascular disease and impaired renal function.

• Although ACE inhibitors reduce blood pressure in all races studied, this response is less in blacks who receive the drug as monotherapy. Therapy with a thiazide diuretic produces a more favorable response.

• *Alert:* Angioedema involving the tongue, glottis, or larynx may be fatal because of airway obstruction. Appropriate therapy should be ordered, including epinephrine 1:1,000 (0.3 to 0.5 ml) S.C.; have resuscitation equipment for maintaining a patent airway readily available. The risk of angioedema is higher in black patients than in nonblack patients.

• If patient develops jaundice, discontinue drug under prescriber's advice because, although rare, ACE inhibitors have been linked to a syndrome of cholestatic jaundice, fulminant hepatic necrosis, and death.

• Safety and effectiveness of drug in children haven't been established.

• It's unknown if drug appears in breast milk. Don't use drug in breast-feeding women.

PATIENT TEACHING

• Instruct patient to report jaundice.

• Advise patient to report fever and sore throat (signs of infection), easy bruising or bleeding; swelling of the tongue, lips, face, eyes, mucous membranes, or extremities; difficulty swallowing or breathing; hoarseness; and nonproductive, persistent cough.

• Tell patient to avoid salt substitutes during drug therapy. These products may contain potassium, which can cause hyperkalemia.

• Tell patient that light-headedness can occur, especially during first few days of therapy. Advise him to rise slowly to minimize this effect and to report it immediately.

• Advise patient to use caution in hot weather and during exercise. Inadequate fluid intake, vomiting, diarrhea, and excessive perspiration can lead to light-headedness and syncope.

• Tell woman to report suspected pregnancy immediately. Drug will need to be discontinued.

• Advise patient planning to undergo surgery or receive anesthesia to inform prescriber that he is taking this drug.

---

valsartan
Diovan

Pregnancy risk category C (D in second and third trimesters)

AVAILABLE FORMS
Capsules: 80 mg, 160 mg

INDICATIONS & DOSAGES
➤ **Hypertension (used alone or with other antihypertensives)—**
Adults: Initially, 80 mg P.O. once daily. Expect to see a reduction in blood pressure in 2 to 4 weeks. If additional antihypertensive effect is needed, dose may be increased to 160 or 320 mg daily, or a diuretic may be added. (Addition of a diuretic has a greater effect than dosage increases beyond 80 mg.) Usual dosage range is 80 to 320 mg daily.

ACTION
Blocks the binding of angiotensin II to receptor sites in vascular smooth muscle and the adrenal gland, which inhibits the pressor effects of the renin-angiotensin-aldosterone system.

Route	Onset	Peak	Duration
P.O.	2 hr	2-4 hr	24 hr

ADVERSE REACTIONS
CNS: *dizziness, headache,* insomnia, fatigue.
CV: edema.
EENT: rhinitis, sinusitis, pharyngitis.

Reactions may be *common,* uncommon, **life-threatening,** or COMMON AND LIFE-THREATENING.

GI: abdominal pain, diarrhea, nausea.
Hematologic: *neutropenia.*
Metabolic: hyperkalemia.
Musculoskeletal: arthralgia.
Respiratory: upper respiratory tract infection, cough.
Other: viral infection.

INTERACTIONS
Drug-drug. *Diuretics:* Excessive hypotension. Assess fluid status before starting concomitant therapy. Monitor patient closely.
Potassium-sparing diuretics, potassium: May cause hyperkalemia. Monitor potassium level closely.
Drug-food. *Any food:* Decreased peak levels. Give drug on an empty stomach.

EFFECTS ON LAB TEST RESULTS
● May increase potassium level.
● May decrease neutrophil count.

CONTRAINDICATIONS
Contraindicated in patients hypersensitive to drug. Use in pregnant and breastfeeding patients isn't recommended.

NURSING CONSIDERATIONS
● Use cautiously in patients with renal or hepatic disease.
● Watch for hypotension. Excessive hypotension can occur when drug is given with high doses of diuretics. Correct volume and salt depletions before starting drug.
● Drug can cause fetal or neonatal morbidity and death if given to a pregnant woman in the second or third trimester. Breastfeeding women shouldn't take drug.
● Safety and effectiveness of drug in children haven't been established.

PATIENT TEACHING
● Tell woman to notify prescriber if she becomes pregnant. Drug will need to be discontinued.
● Advise patient that drug may be taken without regard to food.

22

Antilipemics

atorvastatin calcium
cholestyramine
colesevelam hydrochloride
colestipol hydrochloride
fenofibrate (micronized)
fluvastatin sodium
gemfibrozil
lovastatin
niacin
   (See Chapter 88, VITAMINS AND
   MINERALS.)
pravastatin sodium
simvastatin

COMBINATION PRODUCTS
None.

---

atorvastatin calcium
Lipitor

Pregnancy risk category X

AVAILABLE FORMS
Tablets: 10 mg, 20 mg, 40 mg

INDICATIONS & DOSAGES
➤ **Adjunct to diet to reduce LDL and total cholesterol, apolipoprotein B (apo B), and triglyceride levels in patients with primary hypercholesterolemia and mixed dyslipidemia (Fredrickson types IIa and IIb); primary dysbetalipoproteinemia (Fredrickson type III) that doesn't respond adequately to diet; adjunct to diet for elevated triglyceride levels (Fredrickson type IV)—**
Adults: Initially, 10 mg P.O. once daily. Increase dosage, p.r.n., to maximum single dose of 80 mg daily. Dosage based on lipid levels drawn within 2 to 4 weeks after starting therapy.
➤ **Alone or as adjunct to lipid-lowering treatments such as LDL apheresis in patients with homozygous familial hypercholesterolemia—**
Adults: 10 to 80 mg P.O. once daily.
➤ **Adjunct to diet to increase HDL cholesterol levels in patients with primary hypercholesterolemia (heterozygous familial and nonfamilial) and mixed dyslipidemia (Fredrickson types IIa and IIb)—**
Adults: Initially, 10 mg P.O. daily. Adjust dosage based on lipid levels drawn within 2 to 4 weeks after starting therapy. Dosage range is 10 to 80 mg daily as single dose.

ACTION
Inhibits 3-hydroxy-3-methylglutaryl-coenzyme A (HMG-CoA) reductase, which is an early (and rate-limiting) step in cholesterol biosynthesis.

Route	Onset	Peak	Duration
P.O.	Unknown	1-2 hr	Unknown

ADVERSE REACTIONS
CNS: *headache,* asthenia, insomnia.
EENT: rhinitis, pharyngitis, sinusitis.
GI: abdominal pain, dyspepsia, flatulence, nausea, constipation, diarrhea.
GU: urinary tract infection.
Musculoskeletal: arthritis, arthralgia, myalgia.
Respiratory: bronchitis.
Skin: rash.
Other: infection, flu syndrome, allergic reactions, peripheral edema.

INTERACTIONS
Drug-drug. *Antacids:* May decrease plasma levels of drug. Monitor patient.
Azole antifungals, cyclosporine, erythromycin, fibric acid derivatives, niacin: May cause rhabdomyolysis. Avoid using together.
Colestipol: May decrease plasma levels of drug. Monitor patient.
Digoxin: May increase digoxin levels. Monitor digoxin levels and patient for evidence of toxicity.
Erythromycin: Increased plasma level of drug. Monitor patient.
Oral contraceptives: Increased levels of hormones. Consider when selecting an oral contraceptive.
Drug-herb. *Red yeast rice:* Theoretical increased risk of adverse reactions be-

cause herb contains compounds similar to those of statin drugs. Discourage use together.
Drug-food. *Grapefruit juice:* Elevated levels of drug, increasing the risk of side effects. Give with liquid other than grapefruit juice.

EFFECTS ON LAB TEST RESULTS
● May increase ALT and AST levels.

CONTRAINDICATIONS
Contraindicated in patients hypersensitive to drug and in those with active liver disease or unexplained persistent elevations of transaminase levels. Also contraindicated in pregnant and breast-feeding women and in women of childbearing potential.

NURSING CONSIDERATIONS
● Use cautiously in patients with history of liver disease or heavy alcohol use.
● Drug should be withheld or discontinued in patients at risk for renal failure caused by rhabdomyolysis resulting from trauma; in serious, acute conditions that suggest myopathy; and in major surgery, severe acute infection, hypotension, uncontrolled seizures, or severe metabolic, endocrine, or electrolyte disorders.
● Use of atorvastatin in children has been limited to those older than age 9 with homozygous familial hypercholesterolemia.
● Start drug therapy only after diet and other nonpharmacologic treatments prove ineffective. Patient should follow a standard low-cholesterol diet before and during therapy.
● Before starting treatment, secondary causes for hypercholesterolemia should be excluded and a baseline lipid profile done. Obtain periodic liver function test results and lipid levels before starting treatment and at 6 and 12 weeks after initiation, or after an increase in dosage and periodically thereafter.
● Drug may be given as a single dose at any time of day, with or without food.
● Watch for signs of myositis.
● *Alert:* Don't confuse Lipitor with Levatol.

PATIENT TEACHING
● Teach patient about proper dietary management, weight control, and exercise. Explain their importance in controlling elevated lipid levels.
● Warn patient to avoid alcohol.
● Tell patient to inform prescriber of adverse reactions, such as muscle pain, malaise, and fever.
● Advise patient that drug can be taken at any time of day, without regard to meals.
● Tell patient that the drug may deplete the body's stores of coenzyme Q10; he should discuss the need for supplements with prescriber.
● *Alert:* Inform woman that drug is contraindicated during pregnancy because of potential danger to the fetus. Advise her to notify prescriber immediately if pregnancy occurs or is suspected.

---

cholestyramine
LoCholest, LoCHOLEST Light, Prevalite, Questran**, Questran Light, Questran Lite‡

Pregnancy risk category C

AVAILABLE FORMS
Powder: 378-g cans, 9-g single-dose packets. Each scoop of powder or single-dose packet contains 4 g of cholestyramine resin.

INDICATIONS & DOSAGES
➤ **Primary hyperlipidemia or pruritus caused by partial bile obstruction, adjunct for reduction of elevated cholesterol levels in patients with primary hypercholesterolemia—**
Adults: 4 g once or twice daily. Maintenance dose is 8 to 16 g daily divided into two doses. Maximum daily dose is 24 g.

ACTION
A bile-acid sequestrant that combines with bile acid to form an insoluble compound that is excreted. The liver must synthesize new bile acid from cholesterol, which reduces LDL cholesterol levels.

Route	Onset	Peak	Duration
P.O.	Unknown	Unknown	2-4 wk

ADVERSE REACTIONS
CNS: *headache,* anxiety, *vertigo, dizziness,* insomnia, fatigue, syncope, tinnitus.
GI: *constipation, fecal impaction,* hemorrhoids, *abdominal discomfort,* flatulence, *nausea,* vomiting, steatorrhea, GI bleeding, diarrhea, anorexia.
GU: hematuria, dysuria.
Hematologic: anemia, bleeding tendencies, ecchymoses.
Metabolic: hyperchloremic acidosis.
Musculoskeletal: backache, muscle and joint pains, osteoporosis.
Skin: *rash;* irritation of skin, tongue, and perianal area.
Other: *vitamin A, D, E, and K deficiencies from decreased absorption.*

INTERACTIONS
Drug-drug. *Acetaminophen, beta blockers, cardiac glycosides, corticosteroids, estrogens, fat-soluble vitamins (A, D, E, and K), iron preparations, niacin, penicillin G, phenobarbital, progestins, tetracycline, thiazide diuretics, thyroid hormones, warfarin and other coumarin derivatives:* Absorption may be substantially decreased by cholestyramine. Give other drugs 1 hour before or 4 to 6 hours after cholestyramine.

EFFECTS ON LAB TEST RESULTS
● May increase alkaline phosphatase level.
● May decrease hemoglobin.

CONTRAINDICATIONS
Contraindicated in patients hypersensitive to bile-acid sequestering resins and in those with complete biliary obstruction.

NURSING CONSIDERATIONS
● Use cautiously in patients predisposed to constipation and in those with conditions aggravated by constipation, such as severe, symptomatic coronary artery disease.
● Monitor cholesterol and triglyceride levels regularly during therapy.
● Monitor levels of cardiac glycosides in patients receiving cardiac glycosides and cholestyramine together. If cholestyramine therapy is discontinued, adjust dosage of cardiac glycosides to avoid toxicity.

● Monitor bowel habits. Encourage a diet high in fiber and fluids. If severe constipation develops, decrease dosage, add a stool softener, or discontinue drug.
● Watch for hyperchloremic acidosis with long-term use or very high doses.
● Long-term use may lead to deficiencies of vitamins A, D, E, and K, and folic acid.
● Cholecystography using iopanoic acid will yield abnormal results because iopanoic acid is also bound by cholestyramine.
● *Alert:* Don't confuse Questran with Quarzan.

PATIENT TEACHING
● *Alert:* Tell patient never to take drug in its dry form; esophageal irritation or severe constipation may result.
● Tell patient to prepare drug in a large glass containing water, milk, or juice (especially pulpy fruit juice). Powder can be sprinkled on the surface of the preferred beverage; let the mixture stand for a few minutes, and then stir thoroughly. Avoid mixing with carbonated beverages because of excessive foaming. After drinking preparation, patient should swirl a small additional amount of liquid in the same glass and then drink again to ensure ingestion of the entire dose.
● Advise patient to take at mealtime, if possible.
● Advise patient to take all other drugs at least 1 hour before or 4 to 6 hours after cholestyramine to avoid blocking their absorption.
● Teach patient about proper dietary management of lipids. When appropriate, recommend weight-control, exercise, and smoking cessation programs.
● Tell patient that drug may deplete body stores of vitamins A, D, E, and K and folic acid. Patient should discuss need for supplements with prescriber.

✳ *NEW DRUG*

colesevelam hydrochloride
Welchol

Pregnancy risk category B

AVAILABLE FORMS
Tablets: 625 mg

INDICATIONS & DOSAGES
➤ **Adjunct to diet and exercise, either alone or with an HMG-CoA reductase inhibitor, to reduce elevated LDL cholesterol in patients with primary hypercholesterolemia (Fredrickson type IIa)—**
Adults: 3 tablets (1,875 mg) P.O. b.i.d. with meals and liquid or 6 tablets (3,750 mg) once daily with a meal and liquid. Maximum dosage is 7 tablets (4,375 mg) daily.

ACTION
Binds bile acids in the intestinal tract, impeding their absorption and causing their elimination in feces. In response to this bile acid depletion, LDL cholesterol levels decrease as the liver uses LDL cholesterol to replenish reduced bile acid stores.

Route	Onset	Peak	Duration
P.O.	Unknown	2 wk	Unknown

ADVERSE REACTIONS
CNS: *headache,* pain, asthenia.
EENT: pharyngitis, rhinitis, sinusitis.
GI: abdominal pain, *constipation,* diarrhea, dyspepsia, *flatulence,* nausea.
Musculoskeletal: myalgia, back pain.
Respiratory: increased cough.
Other: accidental injury, *infection,* flu syndrome.

INTERACTIONS
None reported.

EFFECTS ON LAB TEST RESULTS
None reported.

CONTRAINDICATIONS
Contraindicated in patients hypersensitive to drug or any of its components and in patients with bowel obstruction.

NURSING CONSIDERATIONS
• Use cautiously in patients susceptible to vitamin K or fat-soluble vitamin deficiencies and in patients with dysphagia, swallowing disorders, severe GI motility disorders, or major GI tract surgery.
• Use cautiously in patients with triglyceride levels greater than 300 mg/dl.

• Rule out secondary causes of hypercholesterolemia before starting drug, such as poorly controlled diabetes, hypothyroidism, nephrotic syndrome, dysproteinemias, obstructive liver disease, other drug therapy, and alcoholism.
• Give drug with a meal and a liquid.
• Store tablets at room temperature and protect them from moisture.
• Monitor patient's bowel habits. If severe constipation develops, decrease dosage, add a stool softener, or discontinue drug.
• Monitor the effects of concurrent drug therapy to identify possible drug interactions.
• Monitor total and LDL cholesterol and triglyceride levels periodically during therapy.
• Use only when clearly needed in breast-feeding patients because it's not known if drug appears in breast milk.

PATIENT TEACHING
• Instruct patient to take drug with a meal and a liquid.
• Teach patient to monitor bowel habits. Encourage a diet high in fiber and fluids. Instruct patient to notify prescriber promptly if severe constipation develops.
• Encourage patient to follow prescribed diet, exercise, and monitoring of lipid levels.
• Tell patient to notify prescriber if she is pregnant or breast-feeding.

colestipol hydrochloride
Colestid

Pregnancy risk category NR

AVAILABLE FORMS
Granules: 300-g and 500-g bottles; 5-g packets
Tablets: 1 g

INDICATIONS & DOSAGES
➤ **Primary hypercholesterolemia—**
Adults: Initially, 5 g P.O. daily or b.i.d., increased in 5-mg increments q 1 to 2 months, p.r.n. Usual dose is 5 to 30 g (granules) P.O. once daily or in divided doses. Or, 2 to 16 g (tablets) P.O. once daily or in divided doses.

ACTION

Combines with bile acid to form an insoluble compound that is excreted in feces. The liver must synthesize new bile acid from cholesterol; this leads to reduced LDL cholesterol levels.

Route	Onset	Peak	Duration
P.O.	1 mo	Unknown	1 mo

ADVERSE REACTIONS

CNS: *headache, dizziness,* anxiety, *vertigo,* insomnia, fatigue, syncope.
CV: angina pectoris, chest pain.
EENT: tinnitus.
GI: *constipation, fecal impaction,* hemorrhoids, abdominal discomfort, flatulence, nausea, vomiting, steatorrhea, GI bleeding, diarrhea, anorexia.
GU: dysuria, hematuria.
Hematologic: anemia, ecchymoses, bleeding tendencies.
Metabolic: hyperchloremic acidosis.
Musculoskeletal: backache, muscle and joint pain, osteoporosis.
Skin: rash, irritation of tongue and perianal area.
Other: vitamin A, D, E, and K deficiencies from decreased absorption.

INTERACTIONS

Drug-drug. *Chlorothiazide, furosemide, penicillin G, tetracycline:* Colestipol may decrease absorption. Separate administration times; give other drugs at least 1 hour before or 4 hours after colestipol.
Oral antidiabetics: May antagonize response to colestipol. Monitor lipids.

EFFECTS ON LAB TEST RESULTS

• May increase alkaline phosphatase, ALT, and AST levels.
• May decrease hemoglobin.

CONTRAINDICATIONS

Contraindicated in patients with hypersensitivity reactions to bile-acid sequestering resins.

NURSING CONSIDERATIONS

• Use cautiously in patients predisposed to constipation and in those with conditions aggravated by constipation, such as severe, symptomatic coronary artery disease.
• Monitor cholesterol and triglyceride levels regularly during therapy.
• Monitor bowel habits; if severe constipation develops, decrease dosage or add stool softener. Encourage a diet high in fiber and fluids.
• Monitor levels of cardiac glycosides in patients receiving cardiac glycosides and colestipol together. If colestipol therapy is discontinued, adjust dosage of cardiac glycosides to avoid toxicity.
• Long-term use may lead to deficiencies of vitamins A, D, E, and K, and folic acid.

PATIENT TEACHING

• *Alert:* Tell patient never to take drug in its dry form; esophageal irritation or severe constipation may result.
• Tell patient that the powder may be taken mixed with milk in hot or regular breakfast cereals, or even mixed in soups that have a high fluid content. It may also be added to pulpy fruits, such as crushed pineapple, pears, peaches, or fruit cocktail.
• Suggest that patient prepare drug in a large glass containing water, milk, or juice (especially pulpy fruit juice). The patient should sprinkle the powder on the surface of the preferred beverage, let the mixture stand a few minutes, and then stir thoroughly to obtain a uniform suspension. After drinking this preparation, patient should swirl a small additional amount of liquid in the same glass and then drink it to ensure ingestion of the entire dose.
• To enhance palatability, suggest that patient mix and refrigerate the next daily dose the previous evening.
• Instruct patient taking tablet form to swallow tablets whole and not to crush, cut, or chew them.
• Advise patient to take all other drugs at least 1 hour before or 4 to 6 hours after colestipol to avoid blocking their absorption.
• Teach patient about proper dietary management of lipids. When appropriate, recommend weight-control, exercise, and smoking cessation programs.
• Inform patient that long-term use may lead to deficiencies of vitamins A, D, E, and K, and folic acid. Instruct patient to

report any unusual signs or symptoms. Patient should discuss need for supplements with prescriber.

• Tell patient that vitamin K deficiency may increase bleeding tendencies. Patient should report abnormal bleeding or bruising.

---

fenofibrate (micronized)
Tricor

Pregnancy risk category C

AVAILABLE FORMS
Capsules: 67 mg, 134 mg, 200 mg

INDICATIONS & DOSAGES
➤ **Adjunct to diet for treatment of patients with very high triglyceride levels (types IV and V hyperlipidemia) who are at risk for pancreatitis and who don't respond adequately to a determined dietary effort—**
Adults: Initially, 67 mg P.O. daily. Dosage may be increased after repeat triglyceride estimations at 4- to 8-week intervals to maximum dose of 3 capsules daily (201 mg).
Adjust-a-dose: For patients with severe renal impairment, initially, 67 mg daily. Increase dosage only after effects on renal function and triglyceride levels have been evaluated at initial dose. No modification is needed for patients with moderate renal impairment.
➤ **Adjunct to diet for the reduction of LDL cholesterol, total cholesterol, triglycerides, and apolipoprotein B levels in patients with primary hypercholesterolemia or mixed dyslipidemia (Fredrickson types IIa and IIb)—**
Adults: 200 mg P.O. daily.
Adjust-a-dose: For elderly patients and those with renal impairment, initially, 67 mg daily. Increase dosage only after effects on renal function and lipid levels have been evaluated at initial dose.

ACTION
Unknown. Thought to lower triglyceride levels by inhibiting triglyceride synthesis, resulting in a decrease in the amount of very-LDLs released into the circulation.

Drug may stimulate breakdown of triglyceride-rich protein.

Route	Onset	Peak	Duration
P.O.	Unknown	6-8 hr	Unknown

ADVERSE REACTIONS
CNS: *dizziness,* localized pain, asthenia, fatigue, paresthesia, insomnia, increased appetite, *headache.*
CV: *arrhythmias.*
EENT: eye discomfort, eye floaters, earache, conjunctivitis, blurred vision, rhinitis, sinusitis.
GI: dyspepsia, eructation, flatulence, nausea, vomiting, abdominal pain, constipation, diarrhea.
GU: polyuria, vaginitis.
Musculoskeletal: arthralgia.
Respiratory: cough.
Skin: pruritus, rash.
Other: decreased libido, hypersensitivity reactions, *infection,* flu syndrome.

INTERACTIONS
Drug-drug. *Bile-acid sequestrants:* May bind and inhibit absorption of fenofibrate. Give drug 1 hour before or 4 to 6 hours after bile-acid sequestrants.
Coumarin-type anticoagulants: Potentiation of anticoagulant effect, prolonged PT and INR. Monitor PT and INR closely. Dosage of anticoagulant may need to be reduced.
Cyclosporine, immunosuppressants, nephrotoxic drugs: Induced renal dysfunction may compromise the elimination of fenofibrate. Use together cautiously.
3-Hydroxy-3-methylglutaryl coenzyme A (HMG-CoA) reductase inhibitors: No data available on use with fenofibrate. Because of risk of myopathy, rhabdomyolysis, and acute renal failure reported with concomitant use of HMG-CoA reductase inhibitors and gemfibrozil (another fibrate derivative), don't give these drugs together unless the benefit to the patient outweighs the risk.
Drug-food. *Any food:* Increased absorption of fenofibrate. Give drug with meals.
Drug-lifestyle. *Alcohol use:* May elevate triglyceride levels. Discourage use together.

EFFECTS ON LAB TEST RESULTS
• May increase BUN, creatinine, ALT, and AST levels. May decrease uric acid levels.
• May decrease hemoglobin, hematocrit, and WBC count.

CONTRAINDICATIONS
Contraindicated in patients hypersensitive to drug and in those with gallbladder disease, hepatic dysfunction, primary biliary cirrhosis, severe renal dysfunction, or unexplained persistent liver function abnormalities.

NURSING CONSIDERATIONS
• Use cautiously in patients with a history of pancreatitis.
• Obtain baseline lipid levels and liver function test results before starting therapy. Monitor liver function periodically for duration of drug therapy. Discontinue drug if enzyme levels persist above three times normal limit.
• Watch for signs and symptoms of pancreatitis, myositis, rhabdomyolysis, cholelithiasis, and renal failure. Monitor patient for muscle pain, tenderness, or weakness, especially with malaise or fever.
• If an adequate response hasn't been obtained after 2 months of treatment with maximum daily dose, therapy must be stopped.
• Drug lowers uric acid levels in patients with or without hyperuricemia by increasing uric acid excretion.
• Beta blockers, estrogens, and thiazide diuretics may increase plasma triglyceride levels; continued use of these drugs should be evaluated.
• Mild to moderate decreases in hemoglobin, hematocrit, and WBC count may occur when therapy starts, but they stabilize with long-term administration.

PATIENT TEACHING
• Inform patient that drug therapy doesn't reduce need for adhering to triglyceride-lowering diet.
• Advise patient to report promptly unexplained muscle weakness, pain, or tenderness, especially if accompanied by malaise or fever.
• Inform patient to take drug with meals to optimize drug absorption.
• Advise patient to continue weight-control measures, including diet and exercise, and to reduce alcohol intake before starting drug therapy.
• Instruct patient who is also taking a bile-acid resin to take fenofibrate 1 hour before or 4 to 6 hours after taking resin.
• Advise patient about potential for tumor growth.
• Tell women that a decision must be made to discontinue either breast-feeding or drug.

---

fluvastatin sodium
Lescol, Lescol XL

Pregnancy risk category X

AVAILABLE FORMS
Capsules: 20 mg, 40 mg
Tablets (extended-release): 80 mg

INDICATIONS & DOSAGES
➤ **Reduction of LDL and total cholesterol levels in patients with primary hypercholesterolemia (types IIa and IIb)—**
To slow progression of coronary atherosclerosis in patients with coronary artery disease—
Elevated triglyceride and apolipoprotein B levels in patients with primary hypercholesterolemia and mixed dyslipidemia whose response to dietary restriction and other nonpharmacologic measures has been inadequate—
Adults: Initially, 20 to 40 mg P.O. h.s., increased, p.r.n., to maximum of 80 mg daily (in divided doses) or 80 mg (Lescol XL) P.O. h.s.

ACTION
Inhibits 3-hydroxy-3-methylglutaryl coenzyme A reductase, which is an early (and rate-limiting) step in the synthetic pathway of cholesterol.

Route	Onset	Peak	Duration
P.O.	Unknown	1 hr	Unknown

ADVERSE REACTIONS
CNS: *headache,* fatigue, *dizziness,* insomnia.
EENT: sinusitis, rhinitis, pharyngitis.

Reactions may be *common*, uncommon, ***life-threatening***, or COMMON AND LIFE-THREATENING.

GI: dyspepsia, diarrhea, nausea, vomiting, abdominal pain, constipation, flatulence.
Hematologic: *thrombocytopenia,* hemolytic anemia, *leukopenia.*
Musculoskeletal: arthralgia, back pain, myalgia.
Respiratory: *upper respiratory tract infection,* cough, bronchitis.
Other: hypersensitivity reactions.

INTERACTIONS
Drug-drug. *Cholestyramine, colestipol:* May bind with fluvastatin in the GI tract and decrease absorption. Separate administration times by at least 4 hours.
Cimetidine, omeprazole, ranitidine: Decreased fluvastatin metabolism. Monitor patient for enhanced effects.
Cyclosporine and other immunosuppressants, erythromycin, gemfibrozil, niacin: May increase risk of polymyositis and rhabdomyolysis. Avoid using together.
Digoxin: May alter digoxin pharmacokinetics. Monitor digoxin levels carefully.
Rifampin: Enhanced fluvastatin metabolism and decreased plasma levels. Monitor patient for lack of effect.
Warfarin: Increased anticoagulant effect with bleeding. Monitor patient.
Drug-herb. *Red yeast rice:* Theoretical increased risk of adverse reactions because herb contains compounds similar to those of statin drugs. Discourage use together.
Drug-lifestyle. *Alcohol use:* Increased risk of hepatotoxicity. Discourage use together.

EFFECTS ON LAB TEST RESULTS
● May increase ALT, AST, and CK levels.
● May decrease hemoglobin and platelet and WBC counts.

CONTRAINDICATIONS
Contraindicated in patients hypersensitive to drug and in those with active liver disease or unexplained persistent elevations of transaminase levels; also contraindicated in pregnant and breast-feeding women and in women of childbearing potential.

NURSING CONSIDERATIONS
● Use cautiously in patients with severe renal impairment and history of liver disease or heavy alcohol use.
● Drug should be started only after diet and other nonpharmacologic therapies have proven ineffective. Patient should follow a standard low-cholesterol diet during therapy.
● Liver function tests should be performed at the start of therapy, at 12 weeks after the start of therapy, or an increase in dose, and then periodically.
● Watch for signs of myositis.
● *Alert:* Don't confuse fluvastatin with fluoxetine.

PATIENT TEACHING
● Tell patient that drug may be taken without regard to meals; however, efficacy is enhanced if drug is taken in the evening.
● Advise the patient who is also taking a bile-acid resin such as cholestyramine to take fluvastatin at bedtime, at least 4 hours after taking the resin.
● Teach patient about proper dietary management, weight control, and exercise. Explain their importance in controlling elevated lipid levels.
● Warn patient to avoid alcohol.
● Tell patient to notify prescriber of adverse reactions, particularly muscle aches and pains.
● Advise patient that it may take up to 4 weeks for full therapeutic effect to occur.
● Tell patient that drug may deplete body's stores of coenzyme Q10 and that he should discuss need for supplements with prescriber.
● *Alert:* Inform woman that drug is contraindicated during pregnancy. Advise her to stop drug and notify prescriber immediately if pregnancy occurs or is suspected. Inform patient that breast-feeding women shouldn't use this drug.

---

gemfibrozil
Apo-Gemfibrozil†, Lopid

Pregnancy risk category C

AVAILABLE FORMS
Tablets: 600 mg

INDICATIONS & DOSAGES
➤ **Types IV and V hyperlipidemia unresponsive to diet and other drugs, reduction of risk of coronary heart disease in patients with type IIb hyperlipidemia who can't tolerate or who are refractory to treatment with bile-acid sequestrants or niacin—**
Adults: 1,200 mg P.O. daily in two divided doses, 30 minutes before morning and evening meals.

ACTION
Inhibits peripheral lipolysis and reduces triglyceride synthesis in the liver. Lowers triglyceride levels and increases high-density-lipoprotein cholesterol levels.

Route	Onset	Peak	Duration
P.O.	2-5 days	4 wk	Unknown

ADVERSE REACTIONS
CNS: *headache,* fatigue, vertigo.
CV: atrial fibrillation.
GI: *abdominal and epigastric pain,* diarrhea, *nausea, vomiting, dyspepsia,* constipation, acute appendicitis.
Hematologic: anemia, *leukopenia,* eosinophilia, ***thrombocytopenia.***
Hepatic: bile duct obstruction.
Metabolic: hypokalemia.
Skin: rash, dermatitis, pruritus, eczema.

INTERACTIONS
Drug-drug. *Lovastatin:* May cause myopathy with rhabdomyolysis. Avoid using together.
Oral anticoagulants: May enhance effects of oral anticoagulants. Monitor patient closely.

EFFECTS ON LAB TEST RESULTS
• May increase ALT, AST, CK levels. May decrease potassium level.
• May decrease hemoglobin and eosinophil, WBC, and platelet counts.

CONTRAINDICATIONS
Contraindicated in patients hypersensitive to drug and in those with hepatic or severe renal dysfunction (including primary biliary cirrhosis) or gallbladder disease.

NURSING CONSIDERATIONS
• Periodic CBCs and liver function tests should be performed during the first 12 months of therapy.
• If drug has no beneficial effects after 3 months of therapy, expect prescriber to discontinue it.

PATIENT TEACHING
• Instruct patient to take drug 30 minutes before breakfast and dinner.
• Teach patient about proper dietary management of lipids. When appropriate, recommend weight-control, exercise, and smoking cessation programs.
• Because of possible dizziness and blurred vision, advise patient to avoid driving or other potentially hazardous activities until CNS effects of drug are known.
• Tell patient to observe bowel movements and to report evidence of steatorrhea or other signs of bile duct obstruction.

lovastatin (mevinolin)
Mevacor

Pregnancy risk category X

AVAILABLE FORMS
Tablets: 10 mg, 20 mg, 40 mg

INDICATIONS & DOSAGES
➤ **Reduction of LDL and total cholesterol levels in patients with primary hypercholesterolemia (types IIa and IIb), to slow the progression of coronary atherosclerosis with coronary artery disease—**
Adults: Initially, 20 mg P.O. once daily with evening meal. Recommended dosage range is 10 to 80 mg daily in one or two divided doses.
Adjust-a-dose: For patients receiving immunosuppressants, initially, 10 mg P.O. daily. Maximum, 20 mg daily. For patients receiving fibrates or niacin and in those with severe renal insufficiency (creatinine clearance < 30 ml/min), don't exceed 20 mg daily.
➤ **Primary prevention of coronary heart disease in patients without symptomatic CV disease, average to moderately elevated total cholesterol and LDL**

cholesterol, and below average HDL cholesterol—

Adults: Initially, 20 mg P.O. once daily with evening meal. Recommended range is 10 to 80 mg daily in one or two divided doses.

ACTION

Inhibits 3-hydroxy-3-methylglutaryl-coenzyme A reductase, which is an early (and rate-limiting) step in cholesterol biosynthesis.

Route	Onset	Peak	Duration
P.O.	Unknown	2 hr	Unknown

ADVERSE REACTIONS

CNS: *headache, dizziness,* peripheral neuropathy, insomnia.
CV: chest pain.
EENT: blurred vision.
GI: constipation, diarrhea, dyspepsia, flatulence, abdominal pain or cramps, heartburn, nausea, vomiting.
Musculoskeletal: muscle cramps, myalgia, myositis, ***rhabdomyolysis.***
Skin: rash, pruritus, alopecia.

INTERACTIONS

Drug-drug. *Azole antifungals, clarithromycin, cyclosporine or other immunosuppressants, erythromycin, gemfibrozil, nefazodone, niacin:* May cause polymyositis and rhabdomyolysis (maximum lovastatin dosage is 20 mg daily). Monitor patient closely.
Oral anticoagulants: Enhanced clinical effects of oral anticoagulants. Monitor patient closely.
Drug-herb. *Pectin:* Decreased effect of lovastatin. Discourage use together.
Red yeast rice: Theoretical increased risk of adverse reactions because herb contains compounds similar to those of statin drugs. Discourage use together.
Drug-food. *Grapefruit juice:* Elevated levels of drug, increasing the risk of side effects. Give with liquid other than grapefruit juice.
Drug-lifestyle. *Alcohol use:* Increased risk of hepatotoxicity. Discourage use together.

EFFECTS ON LAB TEST RESULTS
• May increase ALT, AST, and CK levels.

CONTRAINDICATIONS

Contraindicated in patients hypersensitive to drug and in those with active liver disease or unexplained persistent elevations of transaminase levels; also contraindicated in pregnant and breast-feeding women, in women of childbearing potential, and in patients taking mibefradil.

NURSING CONSIDERATIONS

• Use cautiously in patients who consume substantial quantities of alcohol or have a history of liver disease.
• In patients with severe renal insufficiency, the dosage shouldn't exceed 20 mg/day.
• Drug should be started only after diet and other nonpharmacologic therapies have proven ineffective. Patient should follow a standard low-cholesterol diet during therapy.
• Obtain liver function test results at the start of therapy, at 6 and 12 weeks after the start of therapy, and when increasing dose; then monitor results periodically.
• *Alert:* Don't confuse lovastatin with Lotensin, Leustatin, or Livostin; or Mevacor with Mivacron.

PATIENT TEACHING

• Instruct patient to take drug with the evening meal, when absorption is enhanced and cholesterol biosynthesis is greater.
• Teach patient about proper dietary management of lipids. When appropriate, recommend weight-control, exercise, and smoking cessation programs.
• Advise patient to have periodic eye examinations; related compounds cause cataracts.
• Instruct patient to store tablets at room temperature in a light-resistant container.
• Advise patient to promptly report unexplained muscle pain, tenderness, or weakness, particularly when accompanied by malaise or fever.
• Tell patient that drug may deplete body's stores of coenzyme Q10 and that he should discuss need for supplements with prescriber.
• *Alert:* Inform woman that drug is contraindicated during pregnancy. Advise her to immediately notify prescriber

---

about planned, suspected, or known pregnancy.

---

pravastatin sodium (eptastatin)
Lipostat§, Pravachol

Pregnancy risk category X

AVAILABLE FORMS
Tablets: 10 mg, 20 mg, 40 mg

INDICATIONS & DOSAGES
➤ **Adjunct to diet to reduce LDL, total cholesterol, and triglyceride levels in patients with primary hypercholesterolemia and mixed dyslipidemia (Fredrickson types IIa and IIb); primary prevention of coronary events in hypercholesterolemic patients without clinical evidence of heart disease—**
Adults: Initially, 10 or 20 mg P.O. h.s. Dosage adjusted q 4 weeks based on patient tolerance and response. Maximum, 40 mg daily.
Elderly patients: Initially, 10 mg P.O. h.s. Most patients respond to 20 mg daily or less.
➤ **Reduction of risk of acute coronary events or slowing progression of coronary atherosclerosis in hypercholesterolemic patients with clinical evidence of coronary artery disease, including prior MI; reduction of risk of undergoing myocardial revascularization procedure; reduction of risk of recurrent MI, CVA, or transient ischemic attacks in post-MI patients with normal cholesterol levels—**
Adults: Initially, 10 or 20 mg P.O. h.s. Dosage adjusted q 4 weeks based on patient tolerance and response. Maximum, 40 mg daily.
Elderly patients: Initially, 10 mg P.O. h.s. Most patients respond to 20 mg daily or less.
Adjust-a-dose: For patients taking immunosuppressants, initially, 10 mg P.O. daily. Maximum, 20 mg P.O. daily.
✷ **NEW INDICATION: To increase HDL cholesterol in patients with primary hypercholesterolemia and mixed dyslipidemia (Fredrickson types IIa and IIb)—**
Adults: 10 mg, 20 mg, or 40 mg P.O. once daily.
Adjust-a-dose: In patients with renal or hepatic dysfunction, start with 10 mg P.O. daily.

ACTION
Inhibits 3-hydroxy-3-methylglutaryl-coenzyme A (HMG-CoA) reductase, which is an early (and rate-limiting) step in cholesterol biosynthesis.

Route	Onset	Peak	Duration
P.O.	Unknown	1-1.5 hr	Unknown

ADVERSE REACTIONS
CNS: *headache, dizziness,* fatigue.
CV: chest pain.
EENT: rhinitis.
GI: *vomiting, diarrhea,* heartburn, abdominal pain, constipation, flatulence, *nausea.*
GU: *renal failure caused by myoglobinuria,* urinary abnormality.
Musculoskeletal: myositis, myopathy, *localized muscle pain,* myalgia, ***rhabdomyolysis.***
Respiratory: cough, influenza, common cold.
Skin: rash.
Other: flulike symptoms.

INTERACTIONS
Drug-drug. *Cholestyramine, colestipol:* Decreased plasma levels of pravastatin. Give pravastatin 1 hour before or 4 hours after these drugs.
Drugs that decrease levels or activity of endogenous steroids (such as cimetidine, ketoconazole, spironolactone): May cause endocrine dysfunction. No intervention is needed; obtain complete drug history in patients who develop endocrine dysfunction.
Erythromycin, fibric acid derivatives (such as clofibrate, gemfibrozil), immunosuppressants (such as cyclosporine), high doses (1 g or more daily) of niacin (nicotinic acid): May cause rhabdomyolysis. Monitor patient closely if use together can't be avoided.

Reactions may be *common,* uncommon, *life-threatening,* or COMMON AND LIFE-THREATENING.

Gemfibrozil: Decreased protein-binding and urinary clearance of pravastatin. Avoid using together.

Hepatotoxic drugs: Increased risk of hepatotoxicity. Avoid using together.

Drug-herb. *Red yeast rice:* Theoretical increased risk of adverse reactions because herb contains compounds similar to those of statin drugs. Discourage use together.

Drug-lifestyle. *Alcohol use:* Increased risk of hepatotoxicity. Discourage use together.

EFFECTS ON LAB TEST RESULTS
• May increase ALT, AST, CK, alkaline phosphatase, and bilirubin levels.
• May alter thyroid function test values.

CONTRAINDICATIONS
Contraindicated in patients hypersensitive to drug and in those with active liver disease or conditions that cause unexplained, persistent elevations of transaminase levels; also contraindicated in pregnant and breast-feeding women and in women of childbearing potential.

NURSING CONSIDERATIONS
• Use cautiously in patients who consume large quantities of alcohol or have history of liver disease.
• Drug should be started only after diet and other nonpharmacologic therapies prove ineffective. Patients should follow a standard low-cholesterol diet during therapy.
• Liver function tests should be performed at start of therapy and then periodically. A liver biopsy may be performed if elevated liver enzyme levels persist.
• *Alert:* Don't confuse Pravachol with Prevacid or propranolol.

PATIENT TEACHING
• Tell patient to take the prescribed dose in the evening, preferably at bedtime.
• Advise patient who is also taking a bile-acid resin such as cholestyramine to take provastatin at least 1 hour before or 4 hours after taking resin.
• Tell patient to notify prescriber of adverse reactions, particularly muscle aches and pains.

• Teach patient about proper dietary management of lipids. When appropriate, recommend weight-control, exercise, and smoking cessation programs.
• Inform patient that it will take up to 4 weeks for full therapeutic effect.
• *Alert:* Inform woman that drug is contraindicated during pregnancy. Advise her to immediately notify prescriber about planned, suspected, or known pregnancy.

---

simvastatin (synvinolin)
Lipex‡, Zocor

Pregnancy risk category X

AVAILABLE FORMS
Tablets: 5 mg, 10 mg, 20 mg, 40 mg, 80 mg

INDICATIONS & DOSAGES
➤ **Adjunct to diet for reduction of LDL and total cholesterol levels in patients with primary hypercholesterolemia (types IIa and IIb) and mixed dyslipidemia and in patients with coronary heart disease and hypercholesterolemia to reduce the risk of coronary death, nonfatal MI, CVA, transient ischemic attack, and undergoing myocardial revascularization procedures—**
Adults: Initially, 20 mg P.O. daily in the evening. Dosage adjusted q 4 weeks based on patient tolerance and response. Maximum, 80 mg daily.
Elderly patients: Initially, 5 mg P.O. daily in the evening. Maximum, 20 mg daily.
➤ **Reduction of total and LDL cholesterol in patients with homozygous familial hypercholesterolemia—**
Adults: 40 mg daily in the evening; or 80 mg daily given in three divided doses of 20 mg in morning, 20 mg in afternoon, and 40 mg in the evening.
➤ **To increase HDL cholesterol levels in patients with primary hypercholesterolemia and mixed dyslipidemia (Fredrickson types IIa and IIb); as an adjunct to diet to reduce elevated total and LDL cholesterol, apolipoprotein B, and triglyceride levels in patients with**

---

primary hypercholesterolemia and mixed dyslipidemia—
Adults: Initially, 20 mg P.O. daily in the evening. Adjust dosage at intervals of 4 weeks or more according to baseline LDL cholesterol levels, recommended goal of therapy, and patient response. Range is 5 to 80 mg daily.
➤ **Hypertriglyceridemia (Fredrickson type IV hyperlipidemia), primary dysbetalipoproteinemia (Fredrickson type III hyperlipidemia)—**
Adults: Initially, 20 mg P.O. daily in the evening. Adjust dosage every 4 weeks based on patient response and tolerance. Range is 5 to 80 mg daily as single dose in the evening.
Elderly patients: May be adequately treated with 20 mg daily or less.
Adjust-a-dose: For patients taking cyclosporine, initially, 5 mg P.O. daily; don't exceed 10 mg P.O. daily. In patients taking fibrates or niacin, maximum is 10 mg P.O. daily. In patients with severe renal insufficiency, initially, 5 mg P.O. daily.

ACTION
Inhibits 3-hydroxy-3-methylglutaryl-coenzyme A (HMG-CoA) reductase, which is an early (and rate-limiting) step in cholesterol biosynthesis.

Route	Onset	Peak	Duration
P.O.	Unknown	1.3-2.4 hr	Unknown

ADVERSE REACTIONS
CNS: *headache,* asthenia.
GI: abdominal pain, constipation, diarrhea, dyspepsia, flatulence, *nausea, vomiting.*
Respiratory: upper respiratory tract infection.

INTERACTIONS
Drug-drug. *Antifungals, clarithromycin, erythromycin, fibric acid derivatives (such as clofibrate, gemfibrozil), immunosuppressants (such as cyclosporine), nefazodone, high doses (1 g or more daily) of niacin (nicotinic acid):* May cause rhabdomyolysis. Monitor patient closely if use together can't be avoided. Limit daily dose of simvastatin to 10 mg if patient must take cyclosporine.

Digoxin: May slightly elevate digoxin levels. Closely monitor plasma digoxin levels at start of simvastatin therapy.
Drugs that decrease levels or activity of endogenous steroids (such as cimetidine, ketoconazole, spironolactone): May increase risk of endocrine dysfunction. No intervention is needed; obtain complete drug history in patients who develop endocrine dysfunction.
Hepatotoxic drugs: Increased risk of hepatotoxicity. Avoid using together.
Warfarin: Anticoagulant effect may be slightly enhanced. Monitor INR at start of therapy and during dosage adjustments.
Drug-herb. *Red yeast rice:* Theoretical increased risk of adverse reactions because herb contains compounds similar to those of statin drugs. Discourage use together.
Drug-food. *Grapefruit juice:* Elevated levels of drug, increasing the risk of side effects. Tell patient to take with liquid other than grapefruit juice.
Drug-lifestyle. *Alcohol use:* Increased risk of hepatotoxicity. Discourage use together.

EFFECTS ON LAB TEST RESULTS
• May increase ALT, AST, and CK levels.

CONTRAINDICATIONS
Contraindicated in patients hypersensitive to drug and in those with active liver disease or conditions that cause unexplained persistent elevations of transaminase levels. Also contraindicated in pregnant and breast-feeding women and in women of childbearing potential.

NURSING CONSIDERATIONS
• Use cautiously in patients who consume substantial quantities of alcohol or have a history of liver disease.
• Drug is started only after diet and other nonpharmacologic therapies prove ineffective. Patient should follow a standard low-cholesterol diet during therapy.
• Obtain liver function test results at start of therapy and then periodically. A liver biopsy may be performed if enzyme elevations persist.
• *Alert:* Don't confuse Zocor with Cozaar.

PATIENT TEACHING

• Instruct patient to take drug with the evening meal; absorption is enhanced and cholesterol biosynthesis is greater.

• Teach patient about proper dietary management of lipids. When appropriate, recommend weight-control, exercise, and smoking cessation programs.

• Tell patient to inform prescriber if adverse reactions occur, particularly muscle aches and pains.

• Tell patient that drug may deplete body's stores of coenzyme Q10 and that he should discuss need for supplements with prescriber.

• *Alert:* Inform woman that drug is contraindicated during pregnancy. Advise her to immediately notify prescriber about planned, suspected, or known pregnancy.

abciximab
alprostadil
arbutamine hydrochloride
cilostazol
clopidogrel bisulfate
dipyridamole
eptifibatide
midodrine hydrochloride
nesiritide
pentoxifylline
ticlopidine hydrochloride
tirofiban hydrochloride

COMBINATION PRODUCTS
None.

abciximab
ReoPro

Pregnancy risk category C

AVAILABLE FORMS
Injection: 2 mg/ml

INDICATIONS & DOSAGES
➤ **Adjunct to percutaneous transluminal coronary angioplasty (PTCA) or atherectomy for the prevention of acute cardiac ischemic complications in patients at high risk for abrupt closure of treated coronary vessel—**
Adults: 0.25 mg/kg as an I.V. bolus administered 10 to 60 minutes before start of PTCA or atherectomy; then a continuous I.V. infusion of 0.125 mcg/kg/minute to a maximum of 10 mcg/minute for 12 hours.
➤ **Patients with unstable angina not responding to conventional medical therapy who are to undergo percutaneous coronary intervention within 24 hours—**
Adults: 0.25 mg/kg as an I.V. bolus; then an 18- to 24-hour infusion of 10 mcg/minute, concluding 1 hour after percutaneous coronary intervention.

I.V. ADMINISTRATION
● Inspect solution for particulate matter before administration. If opaque particles are visible, discard solution and obtain new vial. Withdraw needed amount of drug for I.V. bolus through a sterile, nonpyrogenic, low-protein-binding, 0.2- or 0.22-micron filter into a syringe. Give I.V. bolus 10 to 60 minutes before procedure.
● Withdraw needed amount of drug for continuous I.V. infusion through a sterile, nonpyrogenic, low-protein-binding, 0.2- or 0.22-micron filter into a syringe. Inject into 250 ml of sterile normal saline solution or D_5W, and infuse at 0.125 mcg/kg/minute to a maximum of 10 mcg/minute for 12 hours via a continuous infusion pump equipped with an in-line filter. Discard unused portion at end of 12-hour infusion.
● Give drug in a separate I.V. line whenever possible; no other drug should be added to the infusion solution.

ACTION
Binds to the glycoprotein IIb/IIIa (GPIIb/IIIa) receptor of human platelets and inhibits platelet aggregation.

Route	Onset	Peak	Duration
I.V.	Immediate	Immediate	48 hr

ADVERSE REACTIONS
CNS: hyperesthesia, hypoesthesia, confusion, headache.
CV: *hypotension, bradycardia,* peripheral edema.
EENT: abnormal vision.
GI: *nausea,* vomiting, abdominal pain.
Hematologic: *bleeding, thrombocytopenia,* anemia, leukocytosis.
Respiratory: pleural effusion, pleurisy, pneumonia.
Other: pain.

INTERACTIONS
Drug-drug. *Antiplatelet drugs, dipyridamole, heparin, NSAIDs, other anticoagulants, thrombolytics, ticlopidine:* Increased risk of bleeding. Monitor patient closely.

Reactions may be *common,* uncommon, *life-threatening*, or COMMON AND LIFE-THREATENING.

EFFECTS ON LAB TEST RESULTS
• May decrease hemoglobin and platelet and WBC counts.

CONTRAINDICATIONS
Contraindicated in patients hypersensitive to drug, its ingredients, or murine proteins.

Also contraindicated in those with active internal bleeding, recent (within 6 weeks) GI or GU bleeding of clinical significance, CVA within past 2 years or with significant residual neurologic deficit, bleeding diathesis, thrombocytopenia (platelet count under 100,000/mm³), recent (within 6 weeks) major surgery or trauma, intracranial neoplasm, intracranial arteriovenous malformation, intracranial aneurysm, severe uncontrolled hypertension, or history of vasculitis.

Drug is contraindicated when oral anticoagulants have been administered within past 7 days unless PT is 1.2 times control or less, or when I.V. dextran is used before PTCA or is intended to be used during PTCA.

NURSING CONSIDERATIONS
• Use with caution in patients at increased risk for bleeding, including those weighing less than 165 lb (75 kg) or older than age 65, those who have a history of GI disease, and those who are receiving thrombolytics. Conditions that increase patient's risk of bleeding include PTCA within 12 hours of onset of symptoms for acute MI, prolonged PTCA (lasting longer than 70 minutes), or failed PTCA. Heparin used with drug also may contribute to the risk of bleeding.
• The risk of bleeding is reduced by using low-dose, weight-adjusted heparin, early sheath removal, and careful maintenance of access site immobility.
• Patients undergoing PTCA who have one or more of the following conditions should be considered candidates for drug therapy: unstable angina or a non–Q-wave MI, acute Q-wave MI within 12 hours of onset of symptoms, presence of two type B lesions in the artery to be dilated, presence of one type B lesion in the artery to be dilated in women older than age 65 or in diabetic patients, presence of one type C lesion in the artery to be dilated, or angioplasty of an infarct-related lesion within 7 days of MI.
• Review and monitor concomitant drugs; drug is intended for use with aspirin and heparin.
• *Alert:* Keep epinephrine, dopamine, theophylline, antihistamines, and corticosteroids readily available in case of anaphylaxis.
• Monitor patient closely for bleeding at the arterial access site used for cardiac catheterization and internal bleeding involving the GI or GU tract or retroperitoneal sites.
• Institute bleeding precautions. Maintain patient on bed rest for 6 to 8 hours after sheath removal or end of drug infusion, whichever is later. Minimize or avoid, if possible, arterial and venous punctures; I.M. injections; use of urinary catheters, nasogastric tubes, or automatic blood pressure cuffs; and nasotracheal intubation.
• Sheath may be removed during abciximab infusion, but only after heparin has been stopped and its effects largely reversed.
• Obtain platelet counts before treatment, 2 to 4 hours after the bolus dose, and at 24 hours or before discharge, whichever is first.
• Anticipate stopping abciximab and administering platelets for severe bleeding or thrombocytopenia.
• *Alert:* Don't confuse abciximab with arcitumomab.

PATIENT TEACHING
• Explain use and administration of drug to patient and family.
• Instruct patient to report adverse reactions immediately.

---

alprostadil
Prostin VR Pediatric

Pregnancy risk category NR

AVAILABLE FORMS
Injection: 500 mcg/ml

INDICATIONS & DOSAGES
➤ **Palliative therapy for temporary maintenance of patency of ductus**

arteriosus until surgery can be performed—

Infants: 0.05 to 0.1 mcg/kg/minute by I.V. infusion. When therapeutic response is achieved, reduce infusion rate to lowest dose that will maintain response. Maximum dose is 0.4 mcg/kg/minute. Or, drug can be given through umbilical artery catheter placed at ductal opening.

I.V. ADMINISTRATION

• Dilute drug before giving. Prepare fresh solution daily; discard solution after 24 hours.

• For infusion, 1 ml of concentrate labeled as containing 500 mcg is diluted in normal saline solution or D_5W injection to provide a solution containing 2 to 20 mcg/ml.

• When using a device with a volumetric infusion chamber, add appropriate volume of diluent to the chamber; then add 1 ml of alprostadil concentrate.

• During dilution, avoid direct contact between concentrate and wall of plastic volumetric infusion chamber because solution may become hazy. If this occurs, discard solution.

• Don't use diluents that contain benzyl alcohol. Fatal toxic syndrome may occur.

• Reduce infusion rate if fever or significant hypotension occurs.

• Drug isn't recommended for direct injection or intermittent infusion. Give by continuous infusion using an infusion pump. Infuse through a large peripheral or central vein or through an umbilical artery catheter placed at the level of the ductus arteriosus. If flushing from peripheral vasodilation occurs, reposition catheter.

ACTION

A prostaglandin derivative that relaxes the smooth muscle of the ductus arteriosus.

Route	Onset	Peak	Duration
I.V.	20 min	1-2 hr	Length of infusion

ADVERSE REACTIONS

CNS: *seizures.*
CV: *bradycardia,* hypotension, tachycardia, *cardiac arrest,* edema, flushing.
GI: diarrhea.

Hematologic: *disseminated intravascular coagulation.*
Metabolic: hypokalemia.
Respiratory: APNEA.
Other: fever, *sepsis.*

INTERACTIONS

None significant.

EFFECTS ON LAB TEST RESULTS

• May decrease potassium level.

CONTRAINDICATIONS

No known contraindications.

NURSING CONSIDERATIONS

• A differential diagnosis should be made between respiratory distress syndrome and cyanotic heart disease before drug is administered. Drug shouldn't be used in neonates who have respiratory distress syndrome.

• Use cautiously in neonates with bleeding tendencies because drug inhibits platelet aggregation.

• Keep respiratory support available.

• In infants with restricted pulmonary blood flow, measure drug's effectiveness by monitoring blood oxygenation. In infants with restricted systemic blood flow, measure drug's effectiveness by monitoring systemic blood pressure and blood pH.

• Monitor arterial pressure by umbilical artery catheter, auscultation, or Doppler transducer. Slow rate of infusion if arterial pressure falls significantly.

• Neonates receiving drug at recommended doses for longer than 120 hours should be carefully monitored for gastric outlet obstruction and antral hyperplasia.

• *Alert:* Apnea is most often seen in neonates weighing less than 4.5 lb (2 kg) at birth and usually appears during the first hour of drug infusion. CV and CNS adverse reactions occur more often in infants weighing less than 4.5 lb (2 kg) and in those receiving infusions for longer than 48 hours.

• *Alert:* Apnea and bradycardia may reflect drug overdose; if either occurs, stop infusion immediately.

• *Alert:* Don't confuse alprostadil with alprazolam.

PATIENT TEACHING
• Inform parents of the need for drug, and explain its use.
• Encourage parents to ask questions and express concerns.

arbutamine hydrochloride
GenESA

Pregnancy risk category B

AVAILABLE FORMS
Injection: 20-ml prefilled syringe containing 1 mg (0.05 mg/ml)

INDICATIONS & DOSAGES
➤ **Single-dose diagnostic aid in patients with suspected coronary artery disease who can't exercise adequately—**
Adults: 0.1 mcg/kg/minute for 1 minute via GenESA I.V. infusion system. The device adjusts dose until maximal heart rate limit (set by user) or maximal infusion rate of 0.8 mcg/kg/minute (maximum total dose, 10 mcg/kg) is achieved.

I.V. ADMINISTRATION
• Drug is manufactured with a prefilled glass syringe and plunger rod.
• *Alert:* Don't dilute drug before use. Drug should be administered only via the prefilled syringe using the GenESA system (a closed-loop, computer-controlled, I.V. infusion device).
• Before administration, inspect syringe for evidence of particulate matter or discoloration.

ACTION
A sympathomimetic that increases cardiac workload through both positive inotropic and chronotropic actions.

Route	Onset	Peak	Duration
I.V.	1 min	Unknown	Variable

ADVERSE REACTIONS
CNS: anxiety, *dizziness,* fatigue, *headache,* hypoesthesia, paresthesia, *tremor.*
CV: *angina pectoris,* **ARRHYTHMIAS,** chest pain, flushing, hot flashes, hypotension, palpitations, vasodilation.
GI: dry mouth, taste perversion, nausea.
Respiratory: dyspnea.

Skin: increased sweating.
Other: pain.

INTERACTIONS
Drug-drug. *Beta blockers:* May attenuate arbutamine's effects. Discontinue drug at least 48 hours before giving arbutamine.

EFFECTS ON LAB TEST RESULTS
None reported.

CONTRAINDICATIONS
Contraindicated in patients hypersensitive to drug and in those with idiopathic hypertrophic subaortic stenosis, a history of recurrent sustained ventricular tachycardia, or heart failure (New York Heart Association class III or IV). Also contraindicated in patients who have an implanted cardiac pacemaker or automated cardioverter or defibrillator and in those receiving digoxin, atropine, other anticholinergic drugs, or TCAs.

NURSING CONSIDERATIONS
• Use cautiously in patients with a known sulfite allergy. Arbutamine contains sodium metabisulfite, which may produce an allergic response in susceptible patients.
• Avoid use in patients with unstable angina, mechanical left ventricular outflow obstruction (such as severe valvular aortic stenosis), uncontrolled systemic hypertension, cardiac transplantation, history of cerebrovascular disease, peripheral vascular disorder resulting in cerebral or aortic aneurysm, narrow-angle glaucoma, supraventricular tachyarrhythmias or ventricular arrhythmias, or uncontrolled hyperthyroidism. Don't use in patients receiving class I antiarrhythmics, such as quinidine, lidocaine, or flecainide.
• Safety and efficacy of drug in patients with recent history (within 30 days) of MI haven't been evaluated; don't use in these patients.
• Don't give atropine to enhance drug-induced chronotropic response; taking these drugs together may lead to tachyarrhythmia.
• *Alert:* Before using the GenESA system, read and understand the manufacturer's directions.
• Monitor blood pressure, heart rate, and continuous ECG throughout drug infusion.

• Resuscitation equipment should be available by the bedside during drug administration.
• Transient prolongation of the corrected QT interval, as measured from a surface ECG, occurs with administration.
• Transient reductions in potassium levels may occur but rarely to hypokalemic levels.

PATIENT TEACHING
• Instruct patient to discontinue beta blockers at least 48 hours before undergoing cardiac stress testing with arbutamine.
• Inform patient that drug will temporarily increase heart rate, but that he will be closely monitored.
• Inform patient of potential adverse effects.

---

cilostazol
Pletal

Pregnancy risk category C

AVAILABLE FORMS
Tablets: 50 mg, 100 mg

INDICATIONS & DOSAGES
➤ **Reduction of symptoms of intermittent claudication—**
Adults: 100 mg P.O. b.i.d., at least 30 minutes before or 2 hours after breakfast and dinner.
Adjust-a-dose: Decrease dose to 50 mg P.O. b.i.d. when giving with drugs that may interact to cause an increase in cilostazol levels.

ACTION
A quinolinone derivative thought to inhibit the enzyme phosphodiesterase III, thus inhibiting platelet aggregation and causing vasodilation.

Route	Onset	Peak	Duration
P.O.	Unknown	2-4 hr	Unknown

ADVERSE REACTIONS
CNS: *headache, dizziness,* vertigo.
CV: *palpitations,* tachycardia, peripheral edema.
EENT: *pharyngitis, rhinitis.*

GI: *abnormal stools, diarrhea,* dyspepsia, abdominal pain, flatulence, nausea.
Musculoskeletal: back pain, myalgia.
Respiratory: increased cough.
Other: *infection.*

INTERACTIONS
Drug-drug. *Diltiazem:* Increased plasma cilostazol levels. Reduce cilostazol dosage to 50 mg b.i.d. when giving together.
Erythromycin, other macrolides: Increased cilostazol levels and levels of one of the metabolites. Reduce cilostazol dosage to 50 mg b.i.d. when giving together.
Omeprazole: Increased levels of active cilostazol metabolite. Reduce cilostazol dosage to 50 mg b.i.d. when giving together.
Strong inhibitors of CYP3A4 (such as fluconazole, fluoxetine, fluvoxamine, itraconazole, ketoconazole, miconazole, nefazodone, sertraline): May increase levels of cilostazol and its metabolites. Reduce cilostazol dosage to 50 mg b.i.d. when giving together.
Drug-food. *Grapefruit juice:* Increased drug levels. Discourage patient from drinking grapefruit juice during therapy.
Drug-lifestyle. *Smoking:* May decrease drug exposure. Discourage smoking.

EFFECTS ON LAB TEST RESULTS
None reported.

CONTRAINDICATIONS
Contraindicated in patients hypersensitive to drug or its components and in those with heart failure of any severity.

NURSING CONSIDERATIONS
• Use cautiously in patients with severe underlying heart disease; also use cautiously with other drugs having antiplatelet activity.
• *Alert:* Cilostazol, and similar drugs that inhibit the enzyme phosphodiesterase, decrease the likelihood of survival in patients with class III and IV heart failure.
• *Alert:* CV risk is unknown in patients who use drug on long-term basis and in those with severe underlying heart disease.

Reactions may be *common,* uncommon, *life-threatening,* or **COMMON AND LIFE-THREATENING.**

• Drug should be given at least 30 minutes before or 2 hours after breakfast and dinner.
• Beneficial effects of drug may not be seen for up to 12 weeks after start of therapy.
• Dosage can be reduced or discontinued without such rebound effects as platelet hyperaggregation.
• Drug may cause reduced triglyceride levels and increased HDL cholesterol level.

PATIENT TEACHING

• Instruct patient that drug should be taken on an empty stomach, at least 30 minutes before or 2 hours after breakfast and dinner.
• Tell patient that beneficial effect of drug on intermittent claudication isn't likely to be noticed for 2 to 4 weeks and that it may take as long as 12 weeks.
• Advise patient to avoid drinking grapefruit juice during drug therapy.
• Inform patient that CV risk is unknown in patients who use drug on a long-term basis and in those with severe underlying heart disease.
• Tell patient that drug may cause dizziness. Caution patient not to drive or perform other activities that require alertness until response to drug is known.

---

clopidogrel bisulfate
Plavix

Pregnancy risk category B

AVAILABLE FORMS
Tablets: 75 mg

INDICATIONS & DOSAGES
➤ **To reduce atherosclerotic events in patients with atherosclerosis documented by recent CVA, MI, or peripheral arterial disease—**
Adults: 75 mg P.O. daily.

ACTION
Inhibits platelet aggregation by inhibiting the binding of adenosine diphosphate (ADP) to its platelet receptor, inhibiting ADP-mediated activation and subsequent platelet aggregation. Because clopidogrel acts by irreversibly modifying the platelet

ADP receptor, platelets exposed to the drug are affected for their life span.

Route	Onset	Peak	Duration
P.O.	2 hr	Unknown	5 days

ADVERSE REACTIONS
CNS: *headache, dizziness,* fatigue, depression.
CV: edema, hypertension.
EENT: rhinitis, epistaxis.
GI: *hemorrhage,* abdominal pain, dyspepsia, gastritis, constipation, diarrhea, ulcers.
GU: urinary tract infection.
Hematologic: purpura.
Musculoskeletal: arthralgia.
Respiratory: bronchitis, coughing, dyspnea, upper respiratory tract infection.
Skin: *rash,* pruritus.
Other: flu syndrome, pain.

INTERACTIONS
Drug-drug. *Aspirin, NSAIDs:* May increase risk of GI bleeding. Use together cautiously.
Heparin, warfarin: Safety hasn't been established. Use together cautiously.
Drug-herb. *Red clover:* May increase risk of bleeding. Discourage use together.

EFFECTS ON LAB TEST RESULTS
• May decrease platelet count.

CONTRAINDICATIONS
Contraindicated in patients hypersensitive to drug or its components and in those with pathologic bleeding (such as peptic ulcer or intracranial hemorrhage).

NURSING CONSIDERATIONS
• Use cautiously in patients at risk for increased bleeding from trauma, surgery, or other pathologic conditions and in those with hepatic impairment.
• Platelet aggregation won't return to normal for at least 5 days after drug has been discontinued.
• Drug is usually used in patients hypersensitive or intolerant to aspirin or after stent placement.

PATIENT TEACHING
• Advise patient it may take longer than usual to stop bleeding. Tell him to refrain

---

from activities in which trauma and bleeding may occur, and encourage him to wear a seat belt when in a car.
• Instruct patient to notify prescriber if unusual bleeding or bruising occurs.
• Tell patient to inform all health care providers, including dentists, that he is taking drug before undergoing procedures or starting new drug therapy.
• Inform patient that drug may be taken without regard to meals.

---

dipyridamole
Apo-Dipyridamole FC†,
Novo-Dipiradol†, Persantin‡,
Persantine**

Pregnancy risk category B

AVAILABLE FORMS
Injection: 5 mg/ml in 2- and 10-ml vials
Tablets: 25 mg, 50 mg, 75 mg

INDICATIONS & DOSAGES
➤ **Inhibition of platelet adhesion in prosthetic heart valves (given together with warfarin or aspirin)—**
Adults: 75 to 100 mg P.O. q.i.d.
➤ **Alternative to exercise in evaluation of coronary artery disease during thallium myocardial perfusion scintigraphy—**
Adults: 0.57 mg/kg as an I.V. infusion at a constant rate over 4 minutes (0.142 mg/kg/minute).

I.V. ADMINISTRATION
• If giving as a diagnostic drug, dilute in half-normal or normal saline solution or D_5W in at least a 1:2 ratio for a total volume of 20 to 50 ml. Inject ^{201}Tl within 5 minutes after completing the 4-minute dipyridamole infusion.

ACTION
Unknown. Possibly involves drug's ability to increase adenosine, which is a coronary vasodilator and platelet aggregation inhibitor.

Route	Onset	Peak	Duration
I.V.	Unknown	2 min	Unknown
P.O.	Unknown	75 min	Unknown

ADVERSE REACTIONS
CNS: *headache, dizziness,* syncope.
CV: flushing, hypotension, angina pectoris, chest pain, ***ECG abnormalities,*** blood pressure lability, hypertension.
GI: *nausea,* vomiting, diarrhea, abdominal distress.
Skin: rash, irritation, pruritus.

INTERACTIONS
Drug-drug. *Heparin:* May increase risk of bleeding. Monitor patient closely.
Theophylline: May prevent the coronary vasodilation by I.V. dipyridamole; could lead to a false-negative thallium-imaging result. Avoid using together.

EFFECTS ON LAB TEST RESULTS
None reported.

CONTRAINDICATIONS
Contraindicated in patients hypersensitive to drug.

NURSING CONSIDERATIONS
• Use cautiously in patients with hypotension.
• If patient develops GI distress, administer drug 1 hour before meals or with meals.
• Observe for adverse reactions, especially with large doses. Monitor blood pressure.
• Observe for signs and symptoms of bleeding; note prolonged bleeding time (especially with large doses or long-term therapy).
• Dipyridamole's value as part of an antithrombotic regimen is controversial; its use may not provide significantly better results than aspirin alone.
• *Alert:* Don't confuse dipyridamole with disopyramide or Persantine with Periactin.

PATIENT TEACHING
• Instruct patient to take drug exactly as prescribed.
• Tell patient to report adverse reactions promptly.
• Tell patient receiving drug I.V. to report discomfort at insertion site.

---

eptifibatide
Integrilin

Pregnancy risk category B

AVAILABLE FORMS
Injection: 10-ml (2 mg/ml), 100-ml (0.75 mg/ml) vials

INDICATIONS & DOSAGES
➤ **Patients with acute coronary syndrome (unstable angina or non–Q-wave MI), including those who are to be managed medically and those undergoing percutaneous coronary intervention (PCI)—**
Adults: For patients with creatinine less than 2 mg/dl, I.V. bolus of 180 mcg/kg (maximum dose of 22.6 mg) as soon as possible after diagnosis; then a continuous I.V. infusion of 2 mcg/kg/minute (maximum infusion rate of 15 mg/hour) until hospital discharge or initiation of coronary artery bypass graft (CABG) surgery for up to 72 hours. If patient undergoes PCI, infusion should then be continued until hospital discharge or for an additional 18 to 24 hours after procedure for up to 96 hours.
Adjust-a-dose: For patients with a creatinine between 2 and 4 mg/dl, 180 mcg/kg I.V. bolus (maximum dose of 22.6 mg) as soon as possible after diagnosis; then a continuous I.V. infusion of 1 mcg/kg/minute (maximum infusion rate of 7.5 mg/hour).
➤ **PCI including intracoronary stenting—**
Adults: For patients with creatinine less than 2 mg/dl, I.V. bolus of 180 mcg/kg (maximum dose of 22.6 mg) immediately before PCI; then a continuous I.V. infusion of 2 mcg/kg/minute (maximum infusion rate of 15 mg/hour) and a second 180 mcg/kg I.V. bolus (maximum dose of 22.6 mg) 10 minutes after the first bolus. Infusion should then be continued until hospital discharge or for up to 18 to 24 hours. A minimum of 12 hours of infusion is recommended.
Adjust-a-dose: For patients with creatinine between 2 and 4 mg/dl, 180 mcg/kg I.V. bolus (maximum dose of 22.6 mg) immediately before PCI; then a continuous I.V. infusion of 1 mcg/kg/minute (maximum infusion rate of 7.5 mg/hour) and a second 180 mcg/kg I.V. bolus (maximum dose of 22.6 mg) 10 minutes after the first bolus.

I.V. ADMINISTRATION
● Withdraw bolus dose from 10-ml vial into a syringe and administer by I.V. push over 1 to 2 minutes. Give I.V. infusion undiluted directly from 100-ml vial using an infusion pump.
● Inspect solution for particulate matter before use. If particles are visible, the sterility is suspect; discard solution.
● Drug may be administered in same I.V. line as alteplase, atropine, dobutamine, heparin, lidocaine, meperidine, metoprolol, midazolam, morphine, nitroglycerin, or verapamil; and in the same I.V. line with normal saline or normal saline and D₅W. Main infusion may also contain up to 60 mEq/L of potassium chloride.
● Don't administer drug in same I.V. line as furosemide.

ACTION
Reversibly binds to the glycoprotein IIb/IIIa (GP IIb/IIIa) receptor on human platelets and inhibits platelet aggregation.

Route	Onset	Peak	Duration
I.V.	Immediate	Immediate	4-6 hr

ADVERSE REACTIONS
CV: hypotension.
GU: hematuria.
Hematologic: *bleeding, thrombocytopenia.*
Other: bleeding at femoral artery access site.

INTERACTIONS
Drug-drug. *Clopidogrel, dipyridamole, NSAIDs, oral anticoagulants (warfarin), thrombolytics, ticlopidine:* Increased risk of bleeding. Monitor patient closely.
Other inhibitors of platelet receptor IIb/IIIa: May cause serious bleeding. Avoid using together.

EFFECTS ON LAB TEST RESULTS
● May decrease platelet count.

CONTRAINDICATIONS

Contraindicated in patients hypersensitive to drug or its ingredients and in those with history of bleeding diathesis or evidence of active abnormal bleeding within previous 30 days; severe hypertension (systolic blood pressure higher than 200 mm Hg or diastolic blood pressure higher than 110 mm Hg) not adequately controlled with antihypertensives; major surgery within previous 6 weeks; history of CVA within 30 days or history of hemorrhagic CVA; current or planned use of another parenteral GP IIb/IIIa inhibitor; or platelet count less than 100,000/mm³; also contraindicated in patients whose creatinine is 4 mg/dl or higher and in patients who are dependent on renal dialysis.

NURSING CONSIDERATIONS

• Use cautiously in patients at increased risk for bleeding and in patients weighing more than 315 lb (143 kg).
• Drug is intended for use with heparin and aspirin.
• Discontinue eptifibatide and heparin and achieve sheath hemostasis by standard compressive techniques at least 4 hours before hospital discharge.
• The sheath may be removed during eptifibatide infusion, but only after heparin has been discontinued and its effects largely reversed.
• If patient is to undergo coronary artery bypass graft surgery, infusion should be stopped before surgery.
• Minimize use of arterial and venous punctures, I.M. injections, urinary catheters, and nasotracheal and nasogastric tubes.
• When obtaining I.V. access, avoid use of noncompressible sites (such as subclavian or jugular veins).
• Monitor patient for bleeding.
• If patient's platelet count is less than 100,000/mm³, discontinue eptifibatide and heparin.
• Perform baseline laboratory tests before start of drug therapy; also determine hemoglobin, hematocrit, PT, INR, APTT, platelet count, and creatinine level.
• Store vials in refrigerator at 36° to 46° F (2° to 8° C). The drug may be stored at room temperature for no longer than 2 months before use. Vials must be discarded if unused after 2 months of room temperature storage. Protect from light until administration.

PATIENT TEACHING

• Explain that drug is a blood thinner used to prevent chest pain and heart attack.
• Explain that benefits of drug far outweigh risk of serious bleeding.
• Tell patient to report chest discomfort or other adverse effects immediately.

---

midodrine hydrochloride
ProAmatine

Pregnancy risk category C

AVAILABLE FORMS
Tablets: 2.5 mg, 5 mg

INDICATIONS & DOSAGES
➤ **Symptomatic orthostatic hypotension unresponsive to standard clinical care—**
Adults: 10 mg P.O. t.i.d. Suggested dosing schedule: Dose 1 upon arising in the morning, dose 2 at midday, and dose 3 in late afternoon but no later than 6 p.m.
Adjust-a-dose: For patients with abnormal renal function, initial dose of 2.5 mg is recommended.

ACTION
Forms an active metabolite, desglymidodrine, which is an alpha$_1$-agonist. It increases blood pressure by activating alpha-adrenergic receptors in arteriolar and venous vasculature.

Route	Onset	Peak	Duration
P.O.	Unknown	1-2 hr	Unknown

ADVERSE REACTIONS
CNS: *paresthesia,* headache, confusion, anxiety.
CV: *supine hypertension, vasodilation.*
GI: dry mouth.
GU: urine retention, frequency and urgency; *dysuria.*
Skin: *piloerection, pruritus,* rash.
Other: pain, chills.

Reactions may be *common*, uncommon, **life-threatening**, or COMMON AND LIFE-THREATENING.

INTERACTIONS
Drug-drug. *Alpha-adrenergic agonists:*
Enhanced vasopressor effects. Monitor
blood pressure closely.
Alpha-adrenergic blockers: May antagonize drug effects. Avoid using together.
Beta blockers or cardiac glycosides: May
enhance or cause bradycardia, AV block,
or arrhythmias. Avoid using together.
Fludrocortisone: May increase risk of
supine hypertension. May also lead to increased intraocular pressure and worsened
glaucoma. Monitor patient closely.

EFFECTS ON LAB TEST RESULTS
None reported.

CONTRAINDICATIONS
Contraindicated in patients with severe
organic heart disease, persistent and excessive supine hypertension, acute renal
disease, urine retention, pheochromocytoma, or thyrotoxicosis.

NURSING CONSIDERATIONS
• Use cautiously in patients with history
of urine retention, visual problems, diabetes, or renal or hepatic impairment, and
in breast-feeding women.
• Drug should be used in pregnancy only
if benefit justifies potential risk to fetus.
• Safety and effectiveness of drug in children haven't been established.
• Monitor supine and sitting blood pressures closely, and notify prescriber if
supine blood pressure increases excessively.
• Drug should be taken during the day
when patient can be upright and performing activities of daily living. Space doses
at least 3 hours apart. Midodrine shouldn't
be given after the evening meal or within
4 hours of bedtime, to reduce risk of
supine hypertension during sleep.
• Drug should be continued only if symptoms improve during initial therapy.
• Perform renal and hepatic tests before
and during drug therapy.
• *Alert:* Don't confuse ProAmatine with
protamine.

PATIENT TEACHING
• Instruct patient about proper dosing intervals; tell him to take last dose of the
day 4 hours before bedtime.

• Instruct patient to stop drug and immediately notify prescriber about signs and
symptoms of supine hypertension (cardiac
awareness, pounding in ears, headache,
blurred vision).
• Tell patient to consult prescriber before
taking OTC drugs.

✳ **NEW DRUG**

nesiritide
Natrecor

Pregnancy risk category C

AVAILABLE FORMS
Injection: Single-dose vials of 1.5 mg
sterile, lyophilized powder

INDICATIONS & DOSAGES
➤ **Acutely decompensated heart failure
in patients with dyspnea at rest or with
minimal activity—**
Adults: 2 mcg/kg by I.V. bolus over 60
seconds followed by continuous infusion
of 0.01 mcg/kg/minute.
Adjust-a-dose: If hypotension develops
during administration, reduce dosage or
discontinue drug. Drug may be restarted
at a dosage reduced by 30% with no bolus
doses.

I.V. ADMINISTRATION
• Reconstitute one 1.5-mg vial with 5 ml
of diluent (such as D_5W, normal saline solution, 5% dextrose and 0.2% saline solution injection, or 5% dextrose and half-
normal saline solution) from a prefilled
250-ml I.V. bag.
• Gently rock (don't shake) vial until a
clear, colorless solution results.
• Withdraw contents of vial and add back
to the 250-ml I.V. bag to yield 6 mcg/ml.
Invert the bag several times to ensure
complete mixing, and use the solution
within 24 hours.
• Use the formulas below to calculate bolus volume (2 mcg/kg) and infusion flow
rate (0.01 mcg/kg/min):

$$\text{Bolus volume} = 0.33 \times \text{patient weight}$$
$$\text{(ml)} \qquad\qquad \text{(kg)}$$

$$\text{Infusion flow rate} = 0.1 \times \text{patient weight}$$
$$\text{(ml/hr)} \qquad\qquad \text{(kg)}$$

---

*Liquid contains alcohol.   **May contain tartrazine.   †Canada   ‡Australia   §U.K.   ◊OTC

- Before giving bolus dose, prime the I.V. tubing. Withdraw the bolus and administer over 60 seconds through an I.V. port in the tubing.
- Immediately after giving bolus, infuse drug at 0.1 m[g/h] to deliver 0.01 mcg/kg/minute.

ACTION

A human type natriuretic peptide, [bi]nds to receptors on vascular [mus]cle and endothelial cells, s[ignal]s to an increase in cGMP level, [relaxation o]f smooth muscles, and dilation [veins an]d arteries. Thus, the drug pro[duces do]se-dependent reduction in pul[monary cap]illary wedge pressure and sys[temic arteri]al pressure in patients with [heart failu]re.

Onset	Peak	Duration
15 min	1 hr	3 hr

ADVERSE REACTIONS

CNS: headache, confusion, somnolence, insomnia, dizziness, anxiety, paresthesia, tremor.
CV: *hypotension, ventricular tachycardia,* ventricular extrasystoles, angina, *bradycardia,* atrial fibrillation, AV node conduction abnormalities.
GI: nausea, vomiting, abdominal pain.
Hematologic: anemia, increased creatinine level.
Musculoskeletal: back pain, leg cramps.
Respiratory: *apnea,* cough.
Skin: injection site reactions, pain at the site, rash, sweating, pruritus.
Other: fever.

INTERACTIONS

Drug-drug. *ACE inhibitors:* Increased hypotension symptoms. Monitor blood pressure closely.

EFFECTS ON LAB TEST RESULTS

- May increase creatinine level more than 0.5 mg/dl above baseline.
- May decrease hemoglobin and hematocrit.

CONTRAINDICATIONS

Contraindicated in patients hypersensitive to drug or its components. Avoid using drug as primary therapy in patients with cardiogenic shock or patients with systolic blood pressure below 90 mm Hg; low cardiac filling pressures; conditions in which cardiac output is dependent on venous return; or conditions that make vasodilators inappropriate, such as valvular stenosis, restrictive or obstructive cardiomyopathy, constrictive pericarditis, or pericardial tamponade.

NURSING CONSIDERATIONS

- Because of possible hypotension, don't start drug at higher-than-recommended dosage. Dosage above the recommended range has been observed in few patients; infusion rate was increased by 0.005 mcg/kg/minute (preceded by a bolus of 1 mcg/kg), no more than every 3 hours, to a maximum of 0.03 mcg/kg/minute. Creatinine levels were elevated more often in these patients.
- *Alert:* May cause hypotension. Monitor patient's blood pressure closely, particularly if patient also takes an ACE inhibitor.
- *Alert:* Natrecor binds heparin and could bind the heparin lining of a heparin-coated catheter, decreasing the amount of nesiritide delivered. Don't give nesiritide through a central heparin-coated catheter.
- *Alert:* Drug is incompatible with injectable forms of bumetamide, enalaprilat, ethacrynate sodium, furosemide, heparin, hydralazine, and insulin. These drugs shouldn't be given through the same line with nesiritide.
- *Alert:* The preservative sodium metabisulfite is incompatible with nesiritide. Don't give injectable drugs with this preservative in the same line as nesiritide.
- Nesiritide may affect renal function in some people. In patients with severe heart failure whose renal function depends on the renin-angiotensin-aldosterone system, treatment may lead to azotemia.
- Experience in giving this drug for longer than 48 hours is limited.
- Store drug at a controlled room temperature.

PATIENT TEACHING

- Tell patient to report discomfort at I.V. site.
- Urge patient to report symptoms of hypotension, such as dizziness, lightheadedness, blurred vision, or sweating.

• Tell patient to report other adverse effects promptly.

pentoxifylline
Trental

Pregnancy risk category C

AVAILABLE FORMS
Tablets (extended-release): 400 mg

INDICATIONS & DOSAGES
➤ **Intermittent claudication from chronic occlusive vascular disease—**
Adults: 400 mg P.O. t.i.d. with meals. May decrease to 400 mg b.i.d. if GI and CNS adverse effects occur.

ACTION
Unknown. Improves capillary blood flow, probably by increasing RBC flexibility and lowering blood viscosity.

Route	Onset	Peak	Duration
P.O.	Unknown	1 hr	Unknown

ADVERSE REACTIONS
CNS: headache, dizziness.
GI: dyspepsia, nausea, vomiting.

INTERACTIONS
Drug-drug. *Anticoagulants:* Increased anticoagulant effect. Adjust anticoagulant dosage.
Antihypertensives: Increased hypotensive effect. May need to adjust dosage.
Theophylline: May increase theophylline level. Monitor patient closely.
Drug-lifestyle. *Smoking:* May cause vasoconstriction. Advise patient to avoid smoking because it may worsen his condition.

EFFECTS ON LAB TEST RESULTS
None reported.

CONTRAINDICATIONS
Contraindicated in patients intolerant to methylxanthines, such as caffeine, theophylline, and theobromine, and in those with recent cerebral or retinal hemorrhage.

NURSING CONSIDERATIONS
• Drug is useful in patients who aren't good surgical candidates.

• Elderly patients may be more sensitive to drug's effects.
• *Alert:* Don't confuse Trental with Trandate.

PATIENT TEACHING
• Advise patient to take drug with meals to minimize GI upset.
• Instruct patient to swallow tablet whole, without breaking, crushing, or chewing.
• Tell patient to report GI or CNS adverse reactions; prescriber may reduce dosage.
• Urge patient not to stop drug during the first 8 weeks of therapy unless directed by prescriber.

ticlopidine hydrochloride
Ticlid

Pregnancy risk category B

AVAILABLE FORMS
Tablets: 250 mg

INDICATIONS & DOSAGES
➤ **To reduce risk of thrombotic CVA in patients with history of CVA or who have experienced CVA precursors—**
Adults: 250 mg P.O. b.i.d. with meals.

ACTION
Unknown. An antiplatelet that probably blocks adenosine diphosphate-induced platelet-to-fibrinogen and platelet-to-platelet binding.

Route	Onset	Peak	Duration
P.O.	Unknown	2 hr	Unknown

ADVERSE REACTIONS
CNS: dizziness, peripheral neuropathy.
CV: vasculitis.
EENT: conjunctival hemorrhage.
GI: *diarrhea,* nausea, dyspepsia, abdominal pain, anorexia, vomiting, flatulence, bleeding.
GU: hematuria, dark-colored urine.
Hematologic: *neutropenia, pancytopenia, agranulocytosis, immune thrombocytopenia,* ecchymoses.
Musculoskeletal: arthropathy, myositis.
Respiratory: *allergic pneumonitis.*
Skin: rash, pruritus, *maculopapular rash,* urticaria, *thrombocytopenic purpura.*

Other: hypersensitivity reactions, postoperative bleeding.

INTERACTIONS

Drug-drug. *Antacids:* Decreased plasma ticlopidine levels. Separate administration times by at least 2 hours.
Aspirin: Increased effect of aspirin on platelets. Avoid using together.
Cimetidine: Decreased clearance of ticlopidine and increased risk of toxicity. Avoid using together.
Digoxin: Slight decrease in digoxin levels. Monitor digoxin levels.
Phenytoin: May cause elevation in phenytoin level. Monitor patient closely.
Theophylline: Decreased theophylline clearance and risk of toxicity. Monitor patient closely and adjust theophylline dosage.
Drug-herb. *Red clover:* May cause bleeding. Discourage use together.

EFFECTS ON LAB TEST RESULTS
● May increase ALT, AST, and alkaline phosphatase levels.
● May decrease neutrophil, WBC, RBC, platelet, and granulocyte counts.

CONTRAINDICATIONS
Contraindicated in patients hypersensitive to drug and in those with severe hepatic impairment, hematopoietic disorders, active pathologic bleeding from peptic ulceration, or active intracranial bleeding.

NURSING CONSIDERATIONS
● Use cautiously and with close monitoring of CBC and WBC differentials. Moderate to severe neutropenia and agranulocytosis have occurred in patients taking ticlopidine.
● Because of life-threatening adverse reactions, drug should be used only in patients who are allergic to, can't tolerate, or have failed aspirin therapy.
● Obtain baseline liver function test results before therapy.
● Determine CBC and WBC differentials at second week of therapy and repeat every 2 weeks until end of third month.
● Monitor liver function tests and repeat if dysfunction is suspected.
● Thrombocytopenia has occurred rarely. Discontinue drug in patients with platelet

count of 80,000/mm^3 or less. If needed, give methylprednisolone 20 mg I.V. to normalize bleeding time within 2 hours.
● When used preoperatively, drug may decrease risk of graft occlusion in patients receiving coronary artery bypass grafts and reduce severity of drop in platelet count in patients receiving extracorporeal hemoperfusion during open heart surgery.

PATIENT TEACHING
● Tell patient to take drug with meals.
● Warn patient to avoid aspirin and aspirin-containing products and to check with prescriber or pharmacist before taking OTC drugs.
● Explain that drug will prolong bleeding time and that unusual or prolonged bleeding should be reported. Advise patient to tell dentists and other health care providers that he takes ticlopidine.
● Stress importance of regular blood tests. Because neutropenia can result with increased risk of infection, tell patient to immediately report signs and symptoms of infection, such as fever, chills, or sore throat.
● If drug is being substituted for a fibrinolytic or anticoagulant, tell patient to discontinue those drugs before starting ticlopidine therapy.
● Advise patient to discontinue drug 10 to 14 days before undergoing elective surgery. Also tell patient to immediately report yellow skin or sclera, severe or persistent diarrhea, rashes, bleeding under the skin, light-colored stools, or dark urine.

---

tirofiban hydrochloride
Aggrastat

Pregnancy risk category B

AVAILABLE FORMS
Injection: 50-ml vials (250 mcg/ml), 250-ml and 500-ml premixed vials (50 mcg/ml)

INDICATIONS & DOSAGES
➤ Patients with acute coronary syndrome, with heparin or aspirin, including those who are to be managed medically and those undergoing percu-

taneous transluminal coronary angioplasty (PTCA) or atherectomy—
Adults: I.V. loading dose of 0.4 mcg/kg/minute for 30 minutes; then continuous I.V. infusion of 0.1 mcg/kg/minute. Continue infusion through angiography and for 12 to 24 hours after angioplasty or atherectomy.
Adjust-a-dose: For patients with renal insufficiency (creatinine clearance less than 30 ml/minute), use a loading dose of 0.2 mcg/kg/minute for 30 minutes; then continuous infusion of 0.05 mcg/kg/minute. Continue infusion through angiography and for 12 to 24 hours after angioplasty or atherectomy.

I.V. ADMINISTRATION
● Dilute 50-ml injection vials (250 mcg/ml) to same strength as 500-ml premixed vials (50 mcg/ml) as follows: Withdraw and discard 100 ml from a 500-ml bag of sterile normal saline solution or D_5W and replace this volume with 100 ml of tirofiban injection (from two 50-ml vials); or withdraw 50 ml from a 250-ml bag of sterile normal saline solution or D_5W and replace this volume with 50 ml of tirofiban injection, to yield 50 mcg/ml.
● Inspect solution for particulate matter before administration, and check for leaks by squeezing the inner bag firmly. If particles are visible or leaks occur, discard solution.
● Discard unused solution 24 hours after the start of infusion.
● Heparin and tirofiban can be administered through same I.V. catheter.

ACTION
Reversibly binds to the glycoprotein IIb/IIIa (GP IIb/IIIa) receptor on human platelets and inhibits platelet aggregation.

Route	Onset	Peak	Duration
I.V.	Immediate	Immediate	4-6 hr

ADVERSE REACTIONS
CNS: dizziness, headache.
CV: *bradycardia, coronary artery dissection,* edema, vasovagal reaction.
GI: nausea, *occult bleeding.*
Hematologic: *bleeding, thrombocytopenia.*
Musculoskeletal: leg pain.

Skin: sweating.
Other: fever, bleeding at arterial access site, pelvic pain.

INTERACTIONS
Drug-drug. *Clopidogrel, dipyridamole, NSAIDs, oral anticoagulants such as thrombolytics, ticlopidine, warfarin:* May cause bleeding. Monitor patient closely.
Levothyroxine, omeprazole: Increased tirofiban renal clearance. Monitor patient.

EFFECTS ON LAB TEST RESULTS
● May decrease hemoglobin and hematocrit, and platelet count.

CONTRAINDICATIONS
Contraindicated in patients hypersensitive to drug or its components. Also contraindicated in those with active internal bleeding or history of bleeding diathesis within the previous 30 days and in those with history of intracranial hemorrhage, intracranial neoplasm, arteriovenous malformation, aneurysm, thrombocytopenia after previous exposure to tirofiban, CVA within 30 days, or hemorrhagic CVA.

Drug is also contraindicated in those with history, symptoms, or findings suggestive of aortic dissection; severe hypertension (systolic blood pressure higher than 180 mm Hg or diastolic blood pressure higher than 110 mm Hg); acute pericarditis; major surgical procedure or severe physical trauma within previous month; or concomitant use of another parenteral GP IIb/IIIa inhibitor.

NURSING CONSIDERATIONS
● Use cautiously in patients with increased risk of bleeding, including those with hemorrhagic retinopathy or platelet count less than 150,000/mm^3.
● Monitor hemoglobin level, hematocrit, and platelet counts before starting therapy, 6 hours after loading dose, and at least daily during therapy.
● Monitor patient for bleeding.
● Minimize injection and avoid noncompatible I.V. sites.
● Give drug with aspirin and heparin.
● Safety and effectiveness of drug haven't been studied in patients younger than age 18.

• Notify prescriber if thrombocytopenia occurs.

• The most common adverse effect is bleeding at the arterial access site for cardiac catheterization.

• The risk of bleeding may be decreased by early sheath removal and by keeping the access site immobile. The sheath may be removed during tirofiban infusion, but only after heparin has been discontinued and its effects largely reversed.

• Minimize use of arterial and venous punctures, I.M. injections, urinary catheters, and nasotracheal and nasogastric tubes.

• When obtaining I.V. access, avoid use of noncompressible sites (such as subclavian or jugular veins).

• Store drug at room temperature. Protect from light.

PATIENT TEACHING

• Explain that drug is a blood thinner used to prevent chest pain and heart attack.

• Explain that risk of serious bleeding is far outweighed by the benefits of drug.

• Instruct patient to report chest discomfort or other adverse effects immediately.

• Tell patient that frequent blood sampling may be needed to evaluate therapy.

acetaminophen
aspirin
diflunisal

COMBINATION PRODUCTS

ALLEREST NO DROWSINESS ◇,
COLDRINE ◇, ORNEX CAPLETS ◇, SINUS-
RELIEF, SINUTAB MAXIMUM STRENGTH
WITHOUT DROWSINESS ◇: acetaminophen
325 mg and pseudoephedrine hydrochlo-
ride 30 mg.

FIORICET WITH CODEINE, ISOPAP, MEDI-
GESIC, REPAN, TRIAD: acetaminophen
325 mg, caffeine 40 mg, and butalbital
50 mg.

ASCRIPTIN, MAGNAPRIN: aspirin 325 mg,
magnesium hydroxide 50 mg, aluminum
hydroxide 50 mg, and calcium carbonate
50 mg ◇.

ASCRIPTIN A/D, MAGNAPRIN ARTHRITIS
STRENGTH: aspirin 325 mg, magnesium
hydroxide 75 mg, aluminum hydroxide
75 mg, and calcium carbonate 75 mg ◇.

BUFFERIN AF NITE TIME ◇, EXCEDRIN
P.M. ◇: acetaminophen 500 mg and
diphenhydramine citrate 38 mg.

CAMA ARTHRITIS PAIN RELIEVER: aspirin
500 mg, magnesium oxide 150 mg, and
aluminum hydroxide 150 mg.

EXCEDRIN EXTRA STRENGTH ◇: aspirin
250 mg, acetaminophen 250 mg, and caffeine 65 mg.

EXCEDRIN MIGRAINE: acetaminophen
250 mg, aspirin 250 mg, and caffeine
65 mg.

FIORINAL WITH CODEINE: aspirin
325 mg, caffeine 40 mg, and butalbital
50 mg.

MIDRIN: isometheptene mucate 65 mg,
dichloralphenazone 100 mg, and acetaminophen 325 mg.

P-A-C ANALGESIC ◇: aspirin 400 mg and
caffeine 32 mg.

SINUS EXCEDRIN EXTRA STRENGTH ◇:
acetaminophen 500 mg and pseudoephedrine hydrochloride 30 mg.

SINUTAB ◇: acetaminophen 325 mg,
chlorpheniramine maleate 2 mg, and pseudoephedrine hydrochloride 30 mg.

SINUTAB MAXIMUM STRENGTH
WITHOUT DROWSINESS ◇: acetaminophen
500 mg, pseudoephedrine hydrochloride
30 mg.

TECNAL†: aspirin 330 mg, caffeine 40 mg,
and butalbital 50 mg.

VANQUISH ◇: aspirin 227 mg, acetaminophen 194 mg, caffeine 33 mg, aluminum
hydroxide 25 mg, and magnesium hydroxide 50 mg.

acetaminophen (APAP, paracetamol)

Abenol† ◇; Acephen; Aceta ◇;
Acetaminophen ◇; Aceta ◇;
Actamin ◇; Aminofen ◇; Apacet ◇;
Apo-Acetaminophen† ◇;
Atasol† ◇; Banesin ◇; Dapa ◇;
Dymadon‡ ◇; Dymadon P‡ ◇;
Exdol† ◇; Feverall ◇; Genapap ◇;
Genebs ◇; Liquiprin ◇; Neopap ◇;
Oraphen-PD ◇; Panadol ◇;
Panamax‡ ◇; Paralgin‡ ◇;
Redutemp ◇; Robigesic† ◇;
Rounox† ◇; Snaplets-FR ◇;
St. Joseph Aspirin-Free Fever
Reducer for Children ◇;
Suppap ◇; Tapanol ◇; Tempra ◇;
Tylenol ◇; Valorin ◇

Pregnancy risk category B

AVAILABLE FORMS

Caplets: 160 mg, 500 mg ◇
Caplets (extended-release): 650 mg ◇
Capsules: 325 mg ◇, 500 mg ◇
Elixir: 80 mg/5 ml, 120 mg/5 ml, 160 mg/
5 ml* ◇, 325 mg/5 ml* ◇
Gelcaps: 500 mg ◇
Oral liquid: 160 mg/5 ml ◇, 500 mg/
15 ml ◇
Oral solution: 48 mg/ml ◇, 100 mg/ml ◇
Oral suspension: 80 mg/ml ◇, 120 mg/
5 ml‡, 160 mg/5 ml ◇
Oral syrup: 16 mg/ml ◇
Sprinkles: 80 mg/capsule, 160 mg/cap-
sule

---

*Liquid contains alcohol.   **May contain tartrazine.   †Canada   ‡Australia   §U.K.   ◇OTC

Suppositories: 80 mg ◇, 120 mg ◇,
125 mg ◇, 300 mg ◇, 325 mg ◇,
650 mg ◇
Tablets: 160 mg ◇, 325 mg ◇, 500 mg ◇,
650 mg ◇
Tablets (chewable): 80 mg ◇

INDICATIONS & DOSAGES
➤**Mild pain or fever—**
Adults: 325 to 650 mg P.O. q 4 to 6 hours;
or 1 g P.O. t.i.d. or q.i.d., p.r.n. Or, two
extended-release caplets P.O. q 8 hours.
Or, 650 mg P.R. q 4 to 6 hours, p.r.n. Max-
imum, 4 g daily (2.6 g daily for long-term
therapy).
P.O.
Children older than age 14: 650 mg P.O. q
4 to 6 hours, p.r.n.
Children ages 12 to 14: 640 mg P.O. q 4 to
6 hours, p.r.n.
Children age 11: 480 mg P.O. q 4 to 6
hours, p.r.n.
Children ages 9 to 10: 400 mg P.O. q 4 to
6 hours, p.r.n.
Children ages 6 to 8: 320 mg P.O. q 4 to 6
hours, p.r.n.
Children ages 4 to 5: 240 mg P.O. q 4 to 6
hours, p.r.n.
Children ages 2 to 3: 160 mg P.O. q 4 to 6
hours, p.r.n.
Children ages 12 to 23 months: 120 mg
P.O. q 4 to 6 hours, p.r.n.
Children ages 4 to 11 months: 80 mg P.O.
q 4 to 6 hours, p.r.n.
Children up to age 3 months: 40 mg P.O. q
4 to 6 hours, p.r.n.
P.R.
Children ages 6 to 12: 325 mg P.R. q 4 to
6 hours, p.r.n.
Children ages 3 to 6: 120 to 125 mg P.R. q
4 to 6 hours, p.r.n.
Children ages 1 to 3: 80 mg P.R. q 4 to 6
hours, p.r.n.
Children ages 3 to 11 months: 80 mg P.R.
q 6 hours, p.r.n.

ACTION
Unknown. Thought to produce analgesia
by blocking generation of pain impulses,
probably by inhibiting prostaglandin synthesis in the CNS or the synthesis or action of other substances that sensitize pain
receptors to mechanical or chemical stimulation. It's thought to relieve fever by

central action in the hypothalamic heat-
regulating center.

Route	Onset	Peak	Duration
P.O., P.R.	Unknown	1-3 hr	3-4 hr

ADVERSE REACTIONS
Hematologic: hemolytic anemia, *neu-
tropenia, leukopenia, pancytopenia.*
Hepatic: *liver damage,* jaundice.
Metabolic: hypoglycemia.
Skin: rash, urticaria.

INTERACTIONS
Drug-drug. *Barbiturates, carbamazepine,
hydantoins, rifampin, sulfinpyrazone:*
High doses or long-term use of these
drugs may reduce therapeutic effects and
enhance hepatotoxic effects of acetaminophen. Avoid using together.
Warfarin: May increase hypoprothrombinemic effects with long-term use with
high doses of acetaminophen. Monitor
INR closely.
Zidovudine: May increase risk of bone
marrow suppression because of impaired
zidovudine metabolism. Monitor patient
closely.
Drug-herb. *Watercress:* May inhibit
oxidative metabolism of acetaminophen.
Discourage use together.
Drug-food. *Caffeine:* May enhance analgesic effects of acetaminophen. This may
be a therapeutic advantage in combination
products.
Drug-lifestyle. *Alcohol use:* Increased
risk of hepatic damage. Discourage use
together.

EFFECTS ON LAB TEST RESULTS
● May decrease glucose level.
● May decrease hemoglobin and neu-
trophil, WBC, RBC, and platelet counts.

CONTRAINDICATIONS
Contraindicated in patients hypersensitive
to drug.

NURSING CONSIDERATIONS
● Use cautiously in patients with history
of chronic alcohol use because hepatotoxicity has occurred after therapeutic
doses.

Reactions may be *common*, uncommon, *life-threatening*, or COMMON AND LIFE-THREATENING.

• *Alert:* Many OTC products contain acetaminophen; be aware of this when calculating total daily dose.
• Use liquid form for children and patients who have difficulty swallowing.
• Acetaminophen may produce false-positive decreases in glucose levels in home monitoring systems; drug may cause a false-positive test result for urinary 5-hydroxyindoleacetic acid.

PATIENT TEACHING
• Tell parents to consult prescriber before giving drug to children younger than age 2.
• Advise patient that drug is only for short-term use and to consult prescriber if giving to children for longer than 5 days or adults for longer than 10 days.
• Tell patient not to use for marked fever (higher than 103.1° F [39.5° C]), fever persisting longer than 3 days, or recurrent fever unless directed by prescriber.
• *Alert:* Warn patient that high doses or unsupervised long-term use can cause hepatic damage. Excessive ingestion of alcohol may increase the risk of hepatotoxicity.
• Tell breast-feeding woman that acetaminophen appears in breast milk in low levels (less than 1% of dose). Drug may be used safely if therapy is short-term and doesn't exceed recommended doses.

---

aspirin (acetylsalicylic acid)
Artria S.R. ◇, ASA ◇,
Aspergum ◇, Aspro‡, Bayer
Aspirin ◇, Bex‡, Coryphen† ◇,
Easprin ◇, Ecotrin ◇, Empirin ◇,
Entrophen† ◇, Halfprin, Norwich
Extra-Strength ◇, Novasen† ◇,
Solprin‡, Vincent's Powders‡,
ZORprin ◇

Pregnancy risk category C (D in third trimester)

AVAILABLE FORMS
Chewing gum: 227.5 mg ◇
Suppositories: 120 mg ◇, 200 mg ◇, 300 mg ◇, 600 mg ◇
Tablets: 325 mg ◇, 500 mg ◇
Tablets (chewable): 81 mg ◇
Tablets (controlled-release): 800 mg

Tablets (enteric-coated): 165 mg, 325 mg ◇, 500 mg ◇, 650 mg ◇, 975 mg
Tablets (timed-release): 650 mg ◇

INDICATIONS & DOSAGES
➤ **Rheumatoid arthritis, osteoarthritis, or other polyarthritic or inflammatory conditions—**
Adults: Initially, 2.4 to 3.6 g P.O. daily in divided doses. Maintenance dosage is 3.2 to 6 g P.O. daily in divided doses.
➤ **Juvenile rheumatoid arthritis—**
Children: 60 to 110 mg/kg/day P.O. divided q 6 to 8 hours.
➤ **Mild pain or fever—**
Adults and children older than age 11: 325 to 650 mg P.O. or P.R. q 4 hours, p.r.n.
Children ages 2 to 11: 10 to 15 mg/kg/dose P.O. or P.R. q 4 hours up to 80 mg/kg/day.
➤ **Prevention of thrombosis—**
Adults: 1.3 g P.O. daily in two to four divided doses.
➤ **Reduction of risk of MI in patients with previous MI or unstable angina—**
Adults: 75 to 325 mg P.O. daily.
➤ **Kawasaki syndrome (mucocutaneous lymph node syndrome)—**
Adults: 80 to 180 mg/kg P.O. daily in four divided doses during febrile phase. When fever subsides, decreased to 10 mg/kg once daily and adjusted according to salicylate level.
➤ **Acute rheumatic fever—**
Adults: 5 to 8 g P.O. daily.
Children: 100 mg/kg/day P.O. for 2 weeks; then 75 mg/kg/day P.O. for 4 to 6 weeks.

ACTION
Aspirin and other salicylates are thought to produce analgesia by blocking generation of pain impulses, probably by inhibiting prostaglandin synthesis in the CNS or the synthesis or action of other substances that sensitize pain receptors to mechanical or chemical stimulation. It's thought to relieve fever by central action in the hypothalamic heat-regulating center. Exerts its anti-inflammatory effect by inhibiting prostaglandin synthesis; also may inhibit the synthesis or action of other mediators of the inflammatory response. In low doses, aspirin also appears to impede

---

clotting by blocking prostaglandin synthesis, which prevents formation of the platelet-aggregating substance, thromboxane A_2.

Route	Onset	Peak	Duration
P.O. (buffered)	5-30 min	1-2 hr	1-4 hr
P.O. (enteric-coated)	5-30 min	Variable	1-4 hr
P.O. (extended)	5-30 min	1-4 hr	1-4 hr
P.O. (solution)	5-30 min	15-40 min	1-4 hr
P.O. (tablet)	5-30 min	25-40 min	1-4 hr
P.R.	Unknown	3-4 hr	Unknown

ADVERSE REACTIONS
EENT: *tinnitus, hearing loss.*
GI: *nausea*, GI distress, occult bleeding, dyspepsia, **GI bleeding.**
Hematologic: *leukopenia, thrombocytopenia, prolonged bleeding time.*
Hepatic: *hepatitis.*
Skin: *rash*, bruising, urticaria.
Other: *angioedema,* hypersensitivity reactions, *Reye's syndrome.*

INTERACTIONS
Drug-drug. *ACE inhibitors:* May decrease antihypertensive effects. Monitor blood pressure closely.
Ammonium chloride, other urine acidifiers: Increased levels of aspirin products. Watch for aspirin toxicity.
Antacids in high doses, other urine alkalinizers: Decreased levels of aspirin products. Watch for decreased aspirin effect.
Anticoagulants: Increased risk of bleeding. Avoid using together.
Beta blockers: Decreased antihypertensive effect. Avoid long-term aspirin use if patient is taking antihypertensives.
Corticosteroids: Enhanced salicylate elimination. Watch for decreased salicylate effect.
Methotrexate: Increased risk of methotrexate toxicity. Avoid using together.
Nizatidine: May increase risk of salicylate toxicity in patients receiving high doses of aspirin. Monitor patient closely.
NSAIDs: Altered pharmacokinetics of these drugs, leading to lowered levels and decreased effectiveness. Avoid using together.
NSAIDs, corticosteroids: Increased risk of GI bleeding. Avoid using together.
Oral antidiabetics: Increased hypoglycemic effect. Monitor patient closely.
Probenecid, sulfinpyrazone: Decreased uricosuric effect. Avoid aspirin during therapy with these drugs.
Valproic acid: May increase valproic acid levels. Avoid using together.
Drug-herb. *Dong quai, feverfew, ginkgo, horse chestnut, kelpware, red clover:* May increase risk of bleeding. Monitor patient closely for increased effects. Discourage use together.
White willow: Herb contains compounds similar to aspirin, theoretically increasing risk of adverse effects. Discourage use together.
Drug-food. *Caffeine:* May increase the absorption of aspirin. Watch for increased effects.
Drug-lifestyle. *Alcohol use:* Increased risk of GI bleeding. Discourage use together.

EFFECTS ON LAB TEST RESULTS
• May increase liver function test values. May decrease WBC and platelet counts.

CONTRAINDICATIONS
Contraindicated in patients hypersensitive to drug and in those with NSAID-induced sensitivity reactions, G6PD deficiency, or bleeding disorders, such as hemophilia, von Willebrand's disease, or telangiectasia.

NURSING CONSIDERATIONS
• Use cautiously in patients with GI lesions, impaired renal function, hypoprothrombinemia, vitamin K deficiency, thrombocytopenia, thrombotic thrombocytopenic purpura, or severe hepatic impairment.
• *Alert:* Because of epidemiologic link to Reye's syndrome, the Centers for Disease Control and Prevention recommend not giving salicylates to children or teenagers with chickenpox or flulike illness.
• For inflammatory conditions, rheumatic fever, and thrombosis, aspirin is administered on a schedule rather than p.r.n.

Reactions may be *common*, uncommon, *life-threatening*, or COMMON AND LIFE-THREATENING.

• Because enteric-coated and sustained-release tablets are slowly absorbed, they aren't suitable for rapid relief of acute pain, fever, or inflammation. They cause less GI bleeding and may be better suited for long-term therapy, such as treatment of arthritis.

• For patient with swallowing difficulties, crush nonenteric-coated aspirin and dissolve in soft food or liquid. Administer liquid immediately after mixing because drug will break down rapidly.

• For patients who can't tolerate oral drugs, ask prescriber about using aspirin rectal suppositories. Watch for rectal mucosal irritation or bleeding.

• Febrile, dehydrated children can develop toxicity rapidly.

• Monitor elderly patients closely because they may be more susceptible to aspirin's toxic effects.

• Monitor salicylate levels, as indicated. Therapeutic salicylate level in arthritis is 10 to 30 mg/100 ml. Tinnitus may occur at plasma levels of 30 mg/100 ml and above, but this isn't a reliable indicator of toxicity, especially in very young patients and those older than age 60. With long-term therapy, mild toxicity may occur at plasma levels of 20 mg/100 ml.

• During prolonged therapy, hematocrit, hemoglobin, PT, INR, and renal function should be assessed periodically.

• Aspirin interferes with urinary glucose analysis performed with Diastix, Chemstrip uG, Clinitest, and Benedict's solution, and with urinary 5-hydroxyindoleacetic acid and vanillylmandelic acid tests. Aspirin may also interfere with the Gerhardt's test for urine acetoacetic acid.

• Aspirin irreversibly inhibits platelet aggregation. It should be discontinued 5 to 7 days before elective surgery to allow time for production and release of new platelets.

• Monitor patient for hypersensitivity reactions such as anaphylaxis or asthma.

• *Alert:* Don't confuse aspirin with Asendin or Afrin.

PATIENT TEACHING
• Tell patient who is allergic to tartrazine dye to avoid aspirin.

• Advise patient on a sodium-restricted diet that 1 tablet of buffered aspirin contains 553 mg of sodium.

• Advise patient to take drug with food, milk, antacid, or large glass of water to reduce adverse GI reactions.

• Tell patient that sustained-release or enteric-coated forms shouldn't be crushed or chewed but should be swallowed whole.

• Instruct patient to discard aspirin tablets that have a strong vinegar-like odor.

• Tell patient to consult prescriber if giving drug to children for longer than 5 days or adults for longer than 10 days.

• Advise patient receiving prolonged treatment with large doses of aspirin to watch for petechiae, bleeding gums, and signs of GI bleeding, and to maintain adequate fluid intake. Encourage use of a soft-bristled toothbrush.

• Because of many possible drug interactions involving aspirin, warn patient taking prescription drugs to check with prescriber or pharmacist before taking aspirin or OTC products containing aspirin.

• Urge pregnant woman to avoid aspirin during last trimester of pregnancy unless specifically directed by prescriber.

• Aspirin is a leading cause of poisoning in children. Caution parents to keep drug out of reach of children. Encourage use of child-resistant containers.

---

diflunisal
Dolobid

Pregnancy risk category C

AVAILABLE FORMS
Tablets: 250 mg, 500 mg

INDICATIONS & DOSAGES
➤ **Osteoarthritis, rheumatoid arthritis—**
Adults: 500 to 1,000 mg P.O. daily in two divided doses, usually q 12 hours. Maximum, 1,500 mg daily.
Elderly patients: In patients older than age 65, one-half usual adult dosage.
➤ **Mild to moderate pain—**
Adults: 1 g P.O., then 500 mg q 8 to 12 hours. A lower dosage of 500 mg P.O., then 250 mg q 8 to 12 hours may be appropriate.

ACTION
Unknown. Probably related to inhibition of prostaglandin synthesis.

Route	Onset	Peak	Duration
P.O.	1 hr	2-3 hr	8-12 hr

ADVERSE REACTIONS
CNS: dizziness, somnolence, insomnia, headache, fatigue.
EENT: tinnitus.
GI: nausea, dyspepsia, GI pain, diarrhea, vomiting, constipation, flatulence, stomatitis.
GU: renal impairment, hematuria, *interstitial nephritis.*
Skin: rash, pruritus, sweating, *erythema multiforme, Stevens-Johnson syndrome.*

INTERACTIONS
Drug-drug. *Acetaminophen, hydrochlorothiazide, indomethacin:* May substantially increase levels of these drugs, increasing risk of toxicity. Avoid using together.
Antacids, aspirin: Decreased diflunisal levels. Monitor patient for reduced therapeutic effect.
Anticoagulants, thrombolytics: May enhance pharmacologic effects of these drugs. Use together cautiously.
Cyclosporine: May enhance the nephrotoxicity of cyclosporine. Avoid using together.
Methotrexate: May enhance the toxicity of methotrexate. Avoid using together.
Sulindac: Decreased levels of sulindac's active metabolite. Monitor patient for reduced effect.

EFFECTS ON LAB TEST RESULTS
None reported.

CONTRAINDICATIONS
Contraindicated in patients hypersensitive to drug and in those for whom acute asthmatic attacks, urticaria, or rhinitis are precipitated by aspirin or other NSAIDs.

NURSING CONSIDERATIONS
• Use cautiously in patients with GI bleeding, history of peptic ulcer disease, renal impairment, compromised cardiac function, hypertension, or other conditions predisposing patient to fluid retention.

• **Alert:** Because of the epidemiologic link to Reye's syndrome, the Centers for Disease Control and Prevention recommend not giving salicylates to children and teenagers with chickenpox or flulike illness.

PATIENT TEACHING
• Advise patient to take with water, milk, or meals.
• Tell patient that tablets must be swallowed whole.
• Instruct patient to avoid aspirin or acetaminophen while using diflunisal, unless ordered.
• Inform breast-feeding woman that drug appears in breast milk and that a decision should be made to stop breast-feeding or discontinue drug.

Reactions may be *common*, uncommon, *life-threatening*, or COMMON AND LIFE-THREATENING.

celecoxib
diclofenac potassium
diclofenac sodium
etodolac
fenoprofen calcium
flurbiprofen
ibuprofen
indomethacin
indomethacin sodium
  trihydrate
ketoprofen
ketorolac tromethamine
meloxicam
nabumetone
naproxen
naproxen sodium
oxaprozin
piroxicam
rofecoxib
sulindac

COMBINATION PRODUCTS
ADVIL COLD AND SINUS CAPLETS ◊,
DIMETAPP SINUS CAPLETS, DRISTAN
SINUS CAPLETS ◊, SINE-AID IB CAPLETS:
pseudoephedrine hydrochloride 30 mg and
ibuprofen 200 mg.
ARTHROTEC: diclofenac 50 mg and miso-
prostol 200 mcg.
ARTHROTEC: diclofenac 75 mg and miso-
prostol 200 mcg.

---

celecoxib
Celebrex

Pregnancy risk category C

AVAILABLE FORMS
Capsules: 100 mg, 200 mg

INDICATIONS & DOSAGES
➤ **Relief from signs and symptoms of
osteoarthritis—**
Adults: 200 mg P.O. daily as a single dose
or divided equally b.i.d.
➤ **Relief from signs and symptoms of
rheumatoid arthritis—**
Adults: 100 to 200 mg P.O. b.i.d.

Adjust-a-dose: For patients weighing less
than 50 kg (110 lb), start at lowest recommended dosage. For patients with moderate hepatic impairment (Child-Pugh Class
II), start therapy with reduced dosage.
➤ **Adjunct to treatment for familial
adenomatous polyposis to reduce the
number of adenomatous colorectal
polyps—**
Adults: 400 mg P.O. b.i.d. with food for up
to 6 months.

ACTION
Thought to inhibit prostaglandin synthesis, primarily via inhibition of cyclooxyge-
nase-2 (COX-2), thereby producing anti-
inflammatory, analgesic, and antipyretic
effects.

Route	Onset	Peak	Duration
P.O.	Unknown	3 hr	Unknown

ADVERSE REACTIONS
CNS: dizziness, *headache,* insomnia.
CV: peripheral edema.
EENT: pharyngitis, rhinitis, sinusitis.
GI: abdominal pain, diarrhea, dyspepsia,
flatulence, nausea.
Metabolic: hyperchloremia.
Musculoskeletal: back pain.
Respiratory: upper respiratory tract in-
fection.
Skin: rash.
Other: accidental injury.

INTERACTIONS
Drug-drug. *ACE inhibitors:* Diminished
antihypertensive effects. Monitor patient's
blood pressure.
*Aluminum- and magnesium-containing
antacids:* Reduced celecoxib levels. Separate administration times.
Aspirin: Increased risk of ulcers; low aspirin dosages can be used safely to prevent
CV events. Monitor patient for signs and
symptoms of GI bleeding.
Fluconazole: Increased celecoxib levels.
Reduce dosage of celecoxib to minimal
effective dose.

---

*Liquid contains alcohol.   **May contain tartrazine.   †Canada   ‡Australia   §U.K.   ◊OTC

Furosemide: NSAIDs can reduce sodium excretion caused by diuretics, leading to sodium retention. Monitor patient for swelling and increased blood pressure.

Lithium: Increased lithium level. Monitor plasma lithium levels closely during treatment.

Warfarin: Increased PT and bleeding complications. Monitor PT and INR, and check for signs and symptoms of bleeding.

Drug-herb. *Dong quai, feverfew, garlic, ginger, horse chestnut, red clover:* Based on the known effects or components, possible increased risk of bleeding. Discourage use together.

White willow: Herb contains components similar to those of aspirin. Discourage use with NSAIDs.

Drug-lifestyle. *Long-term alcohol use, smoking:* May cause GI irritation or bleeding. Check for signs and symptoms of bleeding.

EFFECTS ON LAB TEST RESULTS
• May increase BUN, ALT, AST, and chloride levels. May decrease phosphate levels.

CONTRAINDICATIONS
Contraindicated in patients hypersensitive to drug, sulfonamides, aspirin, or other NSAIDs and in those with severe hepatic impairment; also contraindicated in pregnant women in the third trimester.

NURSING CONSIDERATIONS
• Use cautiously in patients with history of ulcers or GI bleeding, advanced renal disease, dehydration, anemia, symptomatic liver disease, hypertension, edema, heart failure, or asthma and in those with known or suspected history as poor P-450 2C9 metabolizers. Also use cautiously in elderly or debilitated patients.

• *Alert:* Patients may be allergic to drug if they are allergic and have had anaphylactic reactions to sulfonamides, aspirin, or other NSAIDs.

• Patient with history of ulcers or GI bleeding is at higher risk for GI bleeding while taking NSAIDs such as celecoxib. Other risk factors for GI bleeding include treatment with corticosteroids or anticoag-

ulants, longer duration of NSAID treatment, smoking, alcoholism, older age, and poor overall health.

• Although drug may be used with low aspirin dosages, the combination may increase risk of GI bleeding.

• Watch for signs and symptoms of overt and occult bleeding.

• NSAIDs such as celecoxib can cause fluid retention; monitor patient with hypertension, edema, or heart failure.

• Drug may be hepatotoxic; watch for signs and symptoms of liver toxicity.

• Before starting drug therapy, rehydrate patient who is dehydrated.

• Drug can be given without regard to meals, but food may decrease GI upset.

• *Alert:* Don't confuse Celebrex with Cerebyx or Celexa.

PATIENT TEACHING
• Tell patient to report history of allergic reactions to sulfonamides, aspirin, or other NSAIDs before starting therapy.

• Instruct patient to promptly report signs of GI bleeding, such as bloody vomitus, blood in urine or stool, and black, tarry stools.

• Advise patient to immediately report rash, unexplained weight gain, or edema.

• Tell woman to notify prescriber if she becomes pregnant or is planning to become pregnant during drug therapy.

• Instruct patient to take drug with food if stomach upset occurs.

• Teach patient that all NSAIDs, including celecoxib, may adversely affect the liver. Signs and symptoms of liver toxicity include nausea, fatigue, lethargy, itching, jaundice, right upper quadrant tenderness, and flu syndrome. Advise patient to stop therapy and seek immediate medical advice if he experiences these signs or symptoms.

• Inform patient that it may take several days before he feels consistent pain relief.

diclofenac potassium
Cataflam

diclofenac sodium
Diclomax Retard§, Fenac‡,
Voltaren, Voltaren-XR, Voltaren
Rapide†, Voltaren SR†, Voltarol§

Pregnancy risk category B

AVAILABLE FORMS
Suppositories: 50 mg†, 100 mg†
Tablets: 50 mg
Tablets (enteric-coated): 25 mg, 50 mg,
75 mg
Tablets (extended-release): 100 mg

INDICATIONS & DOSAGES
➤ **Ankylosing spondylitis—**
Adults: 25 mg P.O. q.i.d. (and h.s., p.r.n.)
➤ **Osteoarthritis—**
Adults: 50 mg P.O. b.i.d. or t.i.d. Or,
75 mg P.O. b.i.d. Maintenance dose is
100 mg P.O. daily (extended-release diclofenac sodium only).
➤ **Rheumatoid arthritis—**
Adults: 50 mg P.O. t.i.d. or q.i.d. Or,
75 mg P.O. b.i.d. (diclofenac sodium
only), 100 mg P.O. daily (extended-release
form), or 50 to 100 mg P.R. (where available) h.s. as substitute for last oral dose of
the day. Not to exceed 225 mg daily.
➤ **Analgesia, primary dysmenorrhea—**
Adults: 50 mg P.O. t.i.d. (diclofenac potassium only).

ACTION
Unknown. Produces anti-inflammatory,
analgesic, and antipyretic effects, possibly
by inhibiting prostaglandin synthesis.

Route	Onset	Peak	Duration
P.O. (enteric)	30 min	2-3 hr	8 hr
P.O., P.R.	10 min	1 hr	8 hr

ADVERSE REACTIONS
CNS: anxiety, depression, dizziness,
drowsiness, insomnia, irritability, headache, *aseptic meningitis.*
CV: *heart failure,* hypertension, edema,
fluid retention.
EENT: tinnitus, *laryngeal edema,*
swelling of the lips and tongue, blurred
vision, eye pain, night blindness, epistaxis,
reversible hearing loss.
GI: abdominal pain or cramps, constipation, diarrhea, indigestion, nausea, abdominal distention, flatulence, taste disorder,
peptic ulceration, *bleeding,* melena,
bloody diarrhea, appetite change, colitis.
GU: proteinuria, *acute renal failure,* oliguria, interstitial nephritis, papillary necrosis, *nephrotic syndrome,* fluid retention.
Hepatic: jaundice, *hepatitis, hepatotoxicity.*
Metabolic: hypoglycemia, hyperglycemia.
Musculoskeletal: back, leg, or joint pain.
Respiratory: asthma.
Skin: rash, pruritus, urticaria, eczema,
dermatitis, alopecia, photosensitivity reactions, bullous eruption, *Stevens-Johnson
syndrome,* allergic purpura.
Other: *anaphylaxis, anaphylactoid reactions, angioedema.*

INTERACTIONS
Drug-drug. *Anticoagulants, including
warfarin:* May cause bleeding. Monitor
patient closely.
Aspirin: May decrease effectiveness of
diclofenac and increase GI toxicity. Avoid
using together.
Beta blockers: May blunt antihypertensive
effects. Monitor patient closely.
*Cyclosporine, digoxin, lithium, methotrex-
ate:* May reduce renal clearance of these
drugs and increase risk of toxicity. Monitor patient closely.
Diuretics: Decreased effectiveness of
diuretics. Avoid using together.
Insulin, oral antidiabetics: May alter
requirements for antidiabetics. Monitor
patient closely.
Potassium-sparing diuretics: Enhanced
potassium retention and increased potassium levels. Monitor potassium level.
Drug-herb. *Dong quai, feverfew, garlic,
ginger, horse chestnut, red clover:* Based
on the known effects or components, may
cause bleeding. Discourage use together.
White willow: Herb contains components
similar to those of aspirin. Advise patients
to avoid use with NSAIDs.
Drug-lifestyle. *Sun exposure:* May cause
photosensitivity reactions. Tell patient to
take precautions.

---

*Liquid contains alcohol.   **May contain tartrazine.   †Canada   ‡Australia   §U.K.   ◊OTC

EFFECTS ON LAB TEST RESULTS
• May increase ALT, AST, and bilirubin levels. May increase or decrease glucose level.

CONTRAINDICATIONS
Contraindicated in patients hypersensitive to drug and in those with hepatic porphyria or history of asthma, urticaria, or other allergic reactions after taking aspirin or other NSAIDs. Drug isn't recommended for use during late pregnancy or breast-feeding.

NURSING CONSIDERATIONS
• Use cautiously in patients with history of peptic ulcer disease, hepatic dysfunction, cardiac disease, hypertension, fluid retention, or impaired renal function.
• Because NSAIDs impair the synthesis of renal prostaglandins, they can decrease renal blood flow and lead to reversible renal impairment, especially in patients with renal or heart failure or liver dysfunction, in elderly patients, and in those taking diuretics. Monitor these patients closely.
• Liver function test values may become elevated during therapy. Monitor transaminase, especially ALT levels, periodically in patients undergoing long-term therapy. The first transaminase measurement should be no later than 8 weeks after therapy begins.
• Because of their antipyretic and anti-inflammatory actions, NSAIDs may mask the signs and symptoms of infection.
• *Alert:* Don't confuse diclofenac with Diflucan or Duphalac.

PATIENT TEACHING
• Tell patient to take drug with milk or meals to minimize GI distress.
• Instruct patient not to crush, break, or chew enteric-coated tablets.
• Serious GI toxicity, including peptic ulceration and bleeding, can occur in patients taking NSAIDs despite absence of GI symptoms. Teach patient signs and symptoms of GI bleeding, and tell the patient to contact prescriber immediately if these occur.
• Teach patient the signs and symptoms of hepatotoxicity, including nausea, fatigue, lethargy, pruritus, jaundice, right upper quadrant tenderness, and flulike symp-

toms. Tell the patient to contact prescriber immediately if these symptoms occur.
• Advise patient to avoid consumption of alcohol or aspirin during drug therapy.
• Tell patient to wear sunscreen or protective clothing because drug may cause photosensitivity reactions.
• Warn patient to avoid hazardous activities that require alertness until adverse CNS effects of drug are known.
• Tell pregnant woman to avoid use of drug during last trimester.

---

etodolac
Lodine, Lodine XL

Pregnancy risk category C

AVAILABLE FORMS
Capsules: 200 mg, 300 mg
Tablets: 400 mg, 500 mg
Tablets (extended-release): 400 mg, 500 mg, 600 mg

INDICATIONS & DOSAGES
➤ **Acute pain—**
Adults: 200 to 400 mg P.O. q 6 to 8 hours, p.r.n., not to exceed 1,200 mg daily. In patients weighing 60 kg (132 lb) or less, don't exceed total daily dose of 20 mg/kg.
➤ **Acute and long-term management of osteoarthritis and rheumatoid arthritis—**
Adults: 600 to 1,000 mg P.O. daily, divided into two or three doses. Maximum dose is 1,200 mg/day. For extended-release product, 400 to 1,000 mg P.O. daily. Maximum dose is 1,200 mg/day.

ACTION
Unknown. Produces anti-inflammatory, analgesic, and antipyretic effects, possibly by inhibiting prostaglandin synthesis.

Route	Onset	Peak	Duration
P.O.	30 min	1-2 hr	4-12 hr
P.O. (extended)	Unknown	3-12 hr	6-12 hr

ADVERSE REACTIONS
CNS: asthenia, malaise, dizziness, depression, drowsiness, nervousness, insomnia, syncope.

Reactions may be *common,* uncommon, *life-threatening,* or COMMON AND LIFE-THREATENING.

CV: hypertension, *heart failure,* flushing, palpitations, edema, fluid retention.
EENT: blurred vision, tinnitus, photophobia.
GI: *dyspepsia,* flatulence, abdominal pain, diarrhea, nausea, constipation, gastritis, melena, vomiting, anorexia, *peptic ulceration with or without GI bleeding or perforation,* ulcerative stomatitis, thirst, dry mouth.
GU: dysuria, urinary frequency, *renal failure.*
Hematologic: anemia, *leukopenia,* hemolytic anemia.
Hepatic: *hepatitis.*
Metabolic: weight gain.
Respiratory: asthma.
Skin: pruritus, rash, *Stevens-Johnson syndrome.*
Other: chills, fever.

INTERACTIONS
Drug-drug. *Antacids:* May decrease peak levels of drug. Watch for decreased effect of etodolac.
Aspirin: Reduced protein-binding of etodolac without altering its clearance. Clinical significance unknown. May increase GI toxicity. Avoid using together.
Beta blockers, diuretics: Effects may be blunted. Monitor patient closely.
Cyclosporine: Impaired elimination and increased risk of nephrotoxicity. Avoid using together.
Digoxin, lithium, methotrexate: Etodolac may impair elimination of these drugs, resulting in increased levels and risk of toxicity. Monitor levels.
Phenytoin: Increased levels of phenytoin. Monitor patient for toxicity.
Warfarin: Etodolac decreases the protein-binding of warfarin but doesn't change its clearance. Although no dosage adjustment is needed, monitor INR closely and watch for bleeding.
Drug-herb. *Dong quai, feverfew, garlic, ginger, horse chestnut, red clover:* Based on the known effects or components, possible increased risk of bleeding. Discourage use together.
White willow: Herb contains components similar to those of aspirin. Advise patients to avoid use with NSAIDs.

Drug-lifestyle. *Alcohol use:* Increased chance of adverse effects. Discourage use together.
Sun exposure: May cause photosensitivity reactions. Tell patient to take precautions.

EFFECTS ON LAB TEST RESULTS
• May decrease hemoglobin and WBC count.

CONTRAINDICATIONS
Contraindicated in patients hypersensitive to drug and in those with history of aspirin- or NSAID-induced asthma, rhinitis, urticaria, or other allergic reactions.

NURSING CONSIDERATIONS
• Use cautiously in patients with history of renal or hepatic impairment or GI bleeding, ulceration, and perforation.
• Because NSAIDs impair the synthesis of renal prostaglandins, they can decrease renal blood flow and lead to reversible renal impairment, especially in patients with renal or heart failure or liver dysfunction, in elderly patients, and in those taking diuretics. Monitor these patients closely.
• A false-positive test for urinary bilirubin may be caused by phenolic metabolites.
• *Alert:* Drug appears to cause fewer GI problems than most NSAIDs. Minimal GI blood loss has been reported at doses up to 1,200 mg daily.
• *Alert:* Don't confuse Lodine with codeine, iodine, or Iopidine.

PATIENT TEACHING
• Tell patient to take drug with milk or meals to minimize GI discomfort.
• Serious GI toxicity, including peptic ulceration and bleeding, can occur in patients taking NSAIDs despite absence of GI symptoms. Teach patient signs and symptoms of GI bleeding, and tell him to contact prescriber immediately if they occur.
• Advise patient to avoid consumption of alcohol or aspirin while taking drug.
• Warn patient to avoid hazardous activities that require alertness until adverse CNS effects of drug are known.
• Teach patient signs and symptoms of hepatotoxicity, including nausea, fatigue, lethargy, pruritus, jaundice, right upper quadrant tenderness, and flulike symp-

toms. Tell him to contact prescriber immediately if any of these symptoms occur.
● Because of possibility of photosensitivity reactions, advise patient to use a sunblock, wear protective clothing, and avoid prolonged exposure to sunlight.
● Tell pregnant woman to avoid use of drug during last trimester.

fenoprofen calcium
Fenopron§, Nalfon

Pregnancy risk category NR

AVAILABLE FORMS
Capsules: 200 mg, 300 mg
Tablets: 600 mg

INDICATIONS & DOSAGES
➤ **Rheumatoid arthritis, osteoarthritis—**
Adults: 300 to 600 mg P.O. t.i.d. or q.i.d.
Maximum dose is 3.2 g daily.
➤ **Mild to moderate pain—**
Adults: 200 mg P.O. q 4 to 6 hours, p.r.n.

ACTION
Unknown. Produces anti-inflammatory, analgesic, and antipyretic effects, possibly by inhibiting prostaglandin synthesis.

Route	Onset	Peak	Duration
P.O.	15-30 min	2 hr	4-6 hr

ADVERSE REACTIONS
CNS: *headache,* dizziness, *somnolence,* fatigue, nervousness, asthenia, tremor, confusion.
CV: peripheral edema, palpitations.
EENT: tinnitus, blurred vision, decreased hearing, nasopharyngitis.
GI: epigastric distress, nausea, GI bleeding, vomiting, occult blood loss, peptic ulceration, constipation, anorexia, dyspepsia, flatulence.
GU: oliguria, interstitial nephritis, proteinuria, cystitis, hematuria.
Hematologic: prolonged bleeding time, anemia, bruising, hemolytic anemia.
Hepatic: *hepatitis.*
Metabolic: hyperkalemia.
Respiratory: dyspnea, upper respiratory tract infection.

Skin: pruritus, rash, urticaria, increased diaphoresis.
Other: *angioedema.*

INTERACTIONS
Drug-drug. *Aspirin:* Decreased fenoprofen half-life; may increase GI toxicity. Avoid using together.
Corticosteroids: Increased risk of adverse GI reactions. Avoid using together.
Diuretics: Decreased diuretic effectiveness. Monitor patient closely.
Oral anticoagulants, sulfonylureas: Fenoprofen enhances pharmacologic effects of these drugs. Use together cautiously.
Phenobarbital: Enhanced metabolism of fenoprofen. Watch for lack of fenoprofen effectiveness.
Drug-herb. *Dong quai, feverfew, garlic, ginger, horse chestnut, red clover:* Based on the known effects or components, possible increased risk of bleeding. Discourage use together.
White willow: Herb contains components similar to those of aspirin. Advise patients to avoid use with NSAIDs.
Drug-lifestyle. *Alcohol use:* Increased risk of adverse GI reactions. Discourage use together.

EFFECTS ON LAB TEST RESULTS
● May increase BUN, creatinine, ALT, AST, LDH, alkaline phosphatase, and potassium levels.
● May increase bleeding time. May decrease hemoglobin.

CONTRAINDICATIONS
Contraindicated in patients hypersensitive to drug and in those with history of aspirin- or NSAID-induced asthma, urticaria or rhinitis, or significantly impaired renal function; also contraindicated during pregnancy.

NURSING CONSIDERATIONS
● Use cautiously in elderly patients and in those with history of serious GI events or peptic ulcer disease, compromised cardiac function, or hypertension.
● Safety of drug hasn't been established in pregnant women. Use during pregnancy isn't recommended.
● Because NSAIDs impair the synthesis of renal prostaglandins, they can decrease re-

---

Reactions may be *common*, uncommon, *life-threatening*, or COMMON AND LIFE-THREATENING.

nal blood flow and lead to reversible renal impairment, especially in patients with renal or heart failure or liver dysfunction, in elderly patients, and in those taking diuretics. Monitor these patients closely during therapy.

• Because of their antipyretic and anti-inflammatory actions, NSAIDs may mask the signs and symptoms of infection.

• Renal, hepatic, ocular, and auditory function should be checked periodically in long-term therapy. Drug should be stopped if abnormalities occur.

• Drug or its metabolite may cross-react with the antibody used in the Amerlex-M assay. Limited data suggest that drug may alter free and total T_3 levels determined by the Corning method.

• Drug isn't recommended for use in children.

• *Alert:* Don't confuse Nalfon with Naldecon.

PATIENT TEACHING
• Tell patient that full therapeutic effect for arthritis may be delayed for 2 to 3 weeks.

• Urge patient to take drug 30 minutes before or 2 hours after meals. If adverse GI reactions occur, tell him that drug may be taken with milk or meals.

• Serious GI toxicity, including peptic ulceration and bleeding, can occur in patients taking NSAIDs despite the absence of GI symptoms. Teach patient the signs and symptoms of GI bleeding, and tell him to contact prescriber immediately if they occur.

• Advise patient to avoid consumption of alcohol or aspirin while taking drug.

• Warn patient to avoid hazardous activities that require alertness until adverse CNS effects of drug are known.

• Teach patient signs and symptoms of hepatotoxicity, including nausea, fatigue, lethargy, pruritus, jaundice, right upper quadrant tenderness, and flulike symptoms. Tell him to contact prescriber immediately if any of these symptoms occur.

• Advise patient with impaired hearing to have periodic tests of auditory function during prolonged therapy.

flurbiprofen
Ansaid, Apo-Flurbiprofen†, Froben†, Froben SR†, Ocufen Ophthalmic

Pregnancy risk category C

AVAILABLE FORMS
Capsules (extended-release): 200 mg†
Ophthalmic solution: 0.03%
Tablets: 50 mg, 100 mg

INDICATIONS & DOSAGES
➤ **Rheumatoid arthritis, osteo-arthritis—**
Adults: 200 to 300 mg P.O. daily, divided b.i.d. to q.i.d. Patients maintained on 200 mg daily may switch to one 200-mg extended-release capsule (where available) P.O. daily taken in the evening after food. Doses over 300 mg/day aren't recommended.
Elderly patients: May need lower dosage. Monitor patient closely.
Adjust-a-dose: For debilitated patients and those with hepatic or renal dysfunction, reduced dosage may be needed. Monitor patient closely.
➤ **Inhibition of intraoperative miosis—**
Adults: 1 drop in eye undergoing surgery beginning 2 hours before surgery and repeated at 30-minute intervals for total of 4 drops per affected eye.

ACTION
Unknown. Produces anti-inflammatory, analgesic, and antipyretic effects, possibly by inhibiting prostaglandin synthesis.

Route	Onset	Peak	Duration
Ophthalmic	Unknown	Unknown	Unknown
P.O.	Unknown	1.5 hr	Unknown

ADVERSE REACTIONS
CNS: headache, anxiety, insomnia, dizziness, increased reflexes, tremors, amnesia, asthenia, drowsiness, malaise, depression.
CV: edema, *heart failure,* hypertension, vasodilation.
EENT: rhinitis, tinnitus, visual changes, epistaxis (oral form); ocular stinging or burning, ocular discomfort, itching, foreign body sensation, tearing, dry eyes,

---

dull eye pain, photophobia (ophthalmic form).
GI: dyspepsia, diarrhea, abdominal pain, nausea, constipation, *bleeding,* flatulence, vomiting.
GU: urinary tract infection, hematuria, interstitial nephritis, *renal failure.*
Hematologic: *thrombocytopenia, neutropenia,* anemia, *aplastic anemia.*
Hepatic: jaundice.
Metabolic: weight changes.
Respiratory: asthma.
Skin: rash, photosensitivity reactions, urticaria.
Other: *angioedema.*

INTERACTIONS
Drug-drug. *Anticoagulants:* May cause bleeding. Monitor patient closely.
Aspirin: Decreased flurbiprofen levels. May increase GI toxicity. Avoid using together.
Beta blockers: May impair antihypertensive effect of beta blockers. Monitor blood pressure.
Cyclosporine: May cause nephrotoxicity. Avoid using together.
Diuretics: May reduce diuretic effect. Monitor patient closely.
Lithium: May increase lithium levels. Avoid using together.
Methotrexate: May cause methotrexate toxicity. Monitor patient closely.
Drug-herb. *Dong quai, feverfew, garlic, ginger, horse chestnut, red clover:* Based on the known effects or components, may increase risk of bleeding. Discourage use together.
White willow: Herb contains components similar to those of aspirin. Advise patients to avoid use with NSAIDs.
Drug-lifestyle. *Alcohol use:* May cause adverse GI reactions. Discourage use together.
Sun exposure: May cause photosensitivity reactions. Tell patient to take precautions.

EFFECTS ON LAB TEST RESULTS
• May increase ALT and AST levels.
• May decrease hemoglobin and neutrophil and platelet counts.

CONTRAINDICATIONS
Contraindicated in patients hypersensitive to drug and in those with a history of aspirin- or NSAID-induced asthma, urticaria, or other allergic-type reactions. Ophthalmic form should be used cautiously in patients with history of herpes simplex keratitis.

NURSING CONSIDERATIONS
• Use cautiously in patients with history of peptic ulcer disease, hepatic dysfunction, cardiac disease, or other conditions that cause fluid retention or impaired renal function.
• Safety and effectiveness of drug use in children haven't been established.
• Drug isn't recommended during last trimester of pregnancy.
• Elderly or debilitated patients and patients with hepatic or renal dysfunction may be at risk for renal toxicity, jaundice, or toxic hepatitis. Periodically monitor renal and hepatic function.
• Because NSAIDs impair synthesis of renal prostaglandins, they can decrease renal blood flow and lead to reversible renal impairment, especially in patients with renal or heart failure or liver dysfunction, in elderly patients, and in those taking diuretics. Monitor these patients closely during therapy.
• Patients receiving long-term therapy should have periodic liver function studies, eye examinations, and hematocrit determinations.
• Ophthalmic solution may be absorbed systemically, causing systemic adverse reactions. Monitor patient closely.

PATIENT TEACHING
• Instruct patient to take drug with food, milk, or antacid if GI upset occurs.
• Tell patient taking extended-release capsules to swallow them whole and not to crush, chew, or break open capsules.
• Serious GI toxicity, including peptic ulceration and bleeding, can occur in patients taking NSAIDs despite absence of GI symptoms. Teach patient signs and symptoms of GI bleeding, and tell him to notify prescriber immediately if they occur.
• Advise patient to avoid consumption of alcohol or aspirin while taking drug.
• Warn patient to avoid hazardous activities that require mental alertness until CNS effects are known.

Reactions may be *common,* uncommon, *life-threatening,* or **COMMON AND LIFE-THREATENING.**

ibuprofen
ACT-3‡, Actiprofen‡, Advil◇,
Apo-Ibuprofen†, Bayer Select
Ibuprofen Pain Relief Formula,
Brufen‡, Children's Advil,
Children's Motrin◇, Excedrin IB◇,
Genpril◇, Haltran◇, Ibu-Tab◇,
Junifen Sugar Free§, Medipren◇,
Menadol, Midol IB, Motrin,
Motrin-IB◇, Novo-Profen†,
Nuprin◇, Nurofen‡, Nurofen
Junior‡, Pamprin-IB, Rafen‡,
Rufen, Saleto-200, Trendar◇

Pregnancy risk category NR

AVAILABLE FORMS
Oral drops: 40 mg/ml
Oral suspension: 100 mg/5 ml
Tablets: 100 mg, 200 mg◇, 300 mg,
400 mg, 600 mg, 800 mg
Tablets (chewable): 50 mg, 100 mg

INDICATIONS & DOSAGES
➤ **Rheumatoid arthritis, osteoarthritis,
arthritis—**
Adults: 300 to 800 mg P.O. t.i.d. or q.i.d.,
not to exceed 3.2 g daily.
➤ **Mild to moderate pain, dysmenorrhea—**
Adults: 400 mg P.O. q 4 to 6 hours, p.r.n.
➤ **Fever—**
Adults: 200 to 400 mg P.O. q 4 to 6 hours.
Don't exceed 1.2 g daily or give longer
than 3 days.
Children ages 6 months to 12 years: If
fever is below 102.5° F (39.2° C), the recommended dose is 5 mg/kg P.O. q 6 to 8
hours. Treat higher fevers with 10 mg/kg q
6 to 8 hours. Don't exceed 40 mg/kg daily.
➤ **Juvenile arthritis—**
Children: 30 to 40 mg/kg/day P.O. in three
or four divided doses. Maximum dose is
50 mg/kg/day.

ACTION
Unknown. Produces anti-inflammatory,
analgesic, and antipyretic effects, possibly
by inhibiting prostaglandin synthesis.

Route	Onset	Peak	Duration
P.O.	Variable	1-2 hr	4-6 hr

ADVERSE REACTIONS
CNS: headache, dizziness, nervousness,
aseptic meningitis.
CV: peripheral edema, fluid retention,
edema.
EENT: tinnitus.
GI: epigastric distress, nausea, occult
blood loss, peptic ulceration, diarrhea,
constipation, dyspepsia, flatulence, heart-
burn, decreased appetite.
GU: *acute renal failure,* azotemia, cysti-
tis, hematuria.
Hematologic: prolonged bleeding time,
anemia, *neutropenia, pancytopenia,
thrombocytopenia, aplastic anemia,
leukopenia, agranulocytosis.*
Metabolic: hypoglycemia, hyperkalemia.
Respiratory: *bronchospasm.*
Skin: pruritus, rash, urticaria, *Stevens-
Johnson syndrome.*

INTERACTIONS
Drug-drug. *Antihypertensives, furose-
mide, thiazide diuretics:* May decrease the
effectiveness of diuretics or antihyperten-
sives. Monitor patient closely.
Aspirin: May decrease levels of ibuprofen.
Avoid using together.
Aspirin, corticosteroids: May cause adverse GI reactions. Avoid using together.
Cyclosporine: May increase nephrotoxicity of both drugs. Avoid using together.
Digoxin, lithium, oral anticoagulants:
May increase plasma levels or effects of
these drugs. Monitor patient toxicity.
Methotrexate: Decreased methotrexate
clearance and increased toxicity. Use together cautiously.
Drug-herb. *Dong quai, feverfew, garlic,
ginger, ginkgo biloba, horse chestnut, red
clover:* Based on the known effects or
components, possible increased risk of
bleeding. Discourage use together.
White willow: Herb contains components
similar to those of aspirin. Advise patients
to avoid use with NSAIDs.
Drug-lifestyle. *Alcohol use:* Adverse GI
reactions may occur. Discourage use together.
Sun exposure: May cause photosensitivity
reactions. Tell patient to take precautions.

---

*Liquid contains alcohol.   **May contain tartrazine.   †Canada   ‡Australia   §U.K.   ◇OTC

EFFECTS ON LAB TEST RESULTS
• May increase BUN, creatinine, ALT, AST, and potassium levels. May decrease glucose level.
• May decrease hemoglobin and neutrophil, WBC, RBC, platelet, and granulocyte counts.

CONTRAINDICATIONS
Contraindicated in patients hypersensitive to drug and in those with angioedema, syndrome of nasal polyps, or bronchospastic reaction to aspirin or other NSAIDs.

NURSING CONSIDERATIONS
• Use cautiously in patients with GI disorders, history of peptic ulcer disease, hepatic or renal disease, cardiac decompensation, hypertension, or known intrinsic coagulation defects.
• Don't use drug in pregnant women.
• Check renal and hepatic function periodically in patients on long-term therapy. Stop drug if abnormalities occur and notify prescriber.
• Because of their antipyretic and antiinflammatory actions, NSAIDs may mask signs and symptoms of infection.
• Blurred or diminished vision and changes in color vision have occurred.
• It may take 1 to 2 weeks before full antiinflammatory effects occur.
• *Alert:* Don't confuse Trendar with Trandate.

PATIENT TEACHING
• Tell patient to take with meals or milk to reduce adverse GI reactions.
• *Alert:* Drug is available OTC in several brands. Instruct patient not to exceed 1.2 g daily, give to children younger than age 12, or take for extended periods without consulting prescriber.
• Tell patient that full therapeutic effect for arthritis may be delayed for 2 to 4 weeks. Although analgesic effect occurs at low dosage levels, anti-inflammatory effect doesn't occur at dosages less than 400 mg q.i.d.
• Caution patient that use with aspirin, alcohol, or corticosteroids may increase risk of GI adverse reactions.
• Serious GI toxicity, including peptic ulceration and bleeding, can occur in patients taking NSAIDs despite absence of GI symptoms. Teach patient signs and symptoms of GI bleeding, and tell him to notify prescriber immediately if they occur.
• Tell patient to contact prescriber before using this drug if fluid intake hasn't been adequate or if fluids have been lost as a result of vomiting or diarrhea.
• Warn patient to avoid hazardous activities that require mental alertness until CNS effects are known.
• Advise patient to wear sunscreen to avoid photosensitivity reactions.

---

indomethacin
Apo-Indomethacin†, Arthrexin‡, Indocid†‡, Indocid SR†, Indocin, Indocin SR, Novo-Methacin†

indomethacin sodium trihydrate
Apo-Indomethacin†, Indocin I.V., Novo-Methacin†

Pregnancy risk category NR

AVAILABLE FORMS
indomethacin
Capsules: 25 mg, 50 mg
Capsules (sustained-release): 75 mg
Oral suspension: 25 mg/5 ml
Suppositories: 50 mg
indomethacin sodium trihydrate
Injection: 1-mg vials

INDICATIONS & DOSAGES
➤ **Moderate to severe rheumatoid arthritis or osteoarthritis, ankylosing spondylitis—**
Adults: 25 mg P.O. or P.R. b.i.d. or t.i.d. with food or antacids; increase daily dose by 25 or 50 mg q 7 days, up to 200 mg daily. Or, sustained-release capsules (75 mg): 75 mg P.O. to start, in morning or h.s. followed, if needed, by 75 mg b.i.d.
➤ **Acute gouty arthritis—**
Adults: 50 mg P.O. t.i.d. Dose reduced as soon as possible; then discontinued.
➤ **Acute painful shoulders (bursitis or tendinitis)—**
Adults: 75 to 150 mg P.O. daily in divided doses t.i.d. or q.i.d. for 7 to 14 days.

Reactions may be *common*, uncommon, *life-threatening*, or COMMON AND LIFE-THREATENING.

➤ **To close a hemodynamically signifi-cant patent ductus arteriosus in prema-ture neonates (I.V. form only)—**
Neonates younger than age 48 hours:
0.2 mg/kg I.V.; then two doses of 0.1 mg/kg at 12- to 24-hour intervals.
Neonates ages 2 to 7 days: 0.2 mg/kg I.V.; then two doses of 0.2 mg/kg at 12- to 24-hour intervals.
Neonates older than age 7 days: 0.2 mg/kg I.V.; then two doses of 0.25 mg/kg at 12- to 24-hour intervals.

I.V. ADMINISTRATION
• Reconstitute powder for injection with sterile water or normal saline solution. For each 1-mg vial, add 1 ml of diluent for a solution containing 1 mg/ml. Administer over 20 to 30 minutes.
• *Alert:* Use only preservative-free sterile saline solution or sterile water to prepare I.V. injection. Never use diluents contain-ing benzyl alcohol because it has been linked to toxicity in newborns. Because injection contains no preservatives, recon-stitute drug immediately before use, and discard unused solution.
• Withhold administration of second or third scheduled I.V. dose if anuria or marked oliguria is evident; notify pre-scriber.
• Watch carefully for bleeding and for re-duced urine output with I.V. administra-tion.

ACTION
Unknown. Produces anti-inflammatory, analgesic, and antipyretic effects, possibly by inhibiting prostaglandin synthesis.

Route	Onset	Peak	Duration
I.V.	Immediate	Immediate	4-6 hr
P.O.	0.5 hr	1-4 hr	4-6 hr
P.R.	Unknown	Unknown	4-6 hr

ADVERSE REACTIONS
P.O. and P.R.
CNS: *headache,* dizziness, depression, drowsiness, confusion, somnolence, fa-tigue, peripheral neuropathy, psychic dis-turbances, syncope, *vertigo.*
CV: hypertension, edema.
EENT: blurred vision, corneal and retinal damage, hearing loss, tinnitus.

GI: nausea, anorexia, diarrhea, peptic ulceration, GI bleeding, constipation, dys-pepsia, *pancreatitis.*
GU: hematuria.
Hematologic: iron deficiency anemia.
Metabolic: hyperkalemia.
Skin: pruritus, urticaria, *Stevens-Johnson syndrome.*
Other: hypersensitivity reactions.
I.V.
GU: hematuria, proteinuria, interstitial nephritis.

INTERACTIONS
Drug-drug. *Aminoglycosides, cyclospor-ine, methotrexate:* May enhance toxicity of these drugs. Avoid using together.
Anticoagulants: May cause bleeding. Monitor patient closely.
Antihypertensives: Reduced antihyperten-sive effect. Monitor patient closely.
Antihypertensives, furosemide, thiazide diuretics: Impaired response to both drugs. Avoid using together, if possible.
Aspirin: Decreased levels of in-domethacin. Avoid using together.
Aspirin, corticosteroids: Increased risk of GI toxicity. Avoid using together.
Diflunisal, probenecid: Decreased in-domethacin excretion. Watch for increased indomethacin adverse reactions.
Digoxin: May prolong half-life of digoxin. Use together cautiously.
Dipyridamole: Enhanced fluid retention. Avoid using together.
Lithium: Increased plasma lithium levels. Monitor patient for toxicity.
Penicillamine: May increase bioavail-ability of penicillamine. Monitor patient closely.
Phenytoin: May increase phenytoin levels. Monitor patient closely.
Triamterene: May cause nephrotoxicity. Monitor patient closely.
Drug-herb. *Dong quai, feverfew, garlic, ginger, horse chestnut, red clover:* Based on the known effects or components, may cause bleeding. Discourage use together.
Senna: Blocked diarrheal effects. Discour-age use together.
White willow: Herb contains components similar to those of aspirin. Advise patients to avoid use with NSAIDs.
Drug-lifestyle. *Alcohol use:* GI toxicity may occur. Discourage use together.

---

*Liquid contains alcohol. **May contain tartrazine. †Canada ‡Australia §U.K. ◇OTC

EFFECTS ON LAB TEST RESULTS
• May increase potassium level.
• May decrease hemoglobin.

CONTRAINDICATIONS
Contraindicated in patients hypersensitive to drug and in those with a history of aspirin- or NSAID-induced asthma, rhinitis, or urticaria. Also contraindicated in pregnant or breast-feeding women and in neonates with untreated infection, active bleeding, coagulation defects or thrombocytopenia, congenital heart disease for whom patency of the ductus arteriosus is needed, necrotizing enterocolitis, or significant renal impairment. Suppositories are contraindicated in patients with history of proctitis or recent rectal bleeding.

NURSING CONSIDERATIONS
• Use cautiously in patients with epilepsy, parkinsonism, hepatic or renal disease, CV disease, infection, and mental illness or depression. Also use cautiously in elderly patients and patients with history of GI disease.
• Because of its high risk of adverse effects during long-term use, indomethacin shouldn't be used routinely as an analgesic or antipyretic.
• Sustained-release capsules shouldn't be used for treatment of acute gouty arthritis.
• Don't use drug in pregnant women.
• Give oral dose with food, milk, or antacid to prevent GI upset.
• If ductus arteriosus reopens, a second course of one to three doses may be given. If ineffective, surgery may be needed.
• Watch for bleeding in patients receiving anticoagulants, patients with coagulation defects, and neonates.
• Because NSAIDs impair synthesis of renal prostaglandins, they can decrease renal blood flow and lead to reversible renal impairment, especially in patients with renal failure, heart failure, or liver dysfunction; in elderly patients; and in those taking diuretics. Monitor these patients closely.
• Drug causes sodium retention; watch for weight gain (especially in elderly patients) and increased blood pressure in patients with hypertension.
• Monitor patient for rash and respiratory distress, which may indicate a hypersensitivity reaction.

• Because of their antipyretic and anti-inflammatory actions, NSAIDs may mask signs and symptoms of infection.

PATIENT TEACHING
• Tell patient to take oral drug with food, milk, or antacid to prevent GI upset.
• Alert patient that use of oral form with aspirin, alcohol, or corticosteroids may increase risk of adverse GI reactions.
• Serious GI toxicity, including peptic ulceration and bleeding, can occur in patients taking oral NSAIDs despite absence of GI symptoms. Teach patient signs and symptoms of GI bleeding, and tell him to notify prescriber immediately if they occur.
• Warn patient to avoid hazardous activities that require mental alertness until CNS effects are known.
• Tell patient to notify prescriber immediately if visual or hearing changes occur. Monitor patient on long-term oral therapy for toxicity by conducting regular eye examinations, hearing tests, CBC, and renal function tests.

---

ketoprofen
Actron, Apo-Keto†, Apo-Keto-E†, Novo-Keto-EC†, Orudis, Orudis E†, Orudis KT, Orudis SR‡, Oruvail, Rhodis†, Rhodis-EC†

Pregnancy risk category B

AVAILABLE FORMS
Capsules: 25 mg, 50 mg, 75 mg
Capsules (extended-release): 100 mg, 150 mg, 200 mg
Suppositories: 100 mg†
Tablets: 12.5 mg ◊
Tablets (enteric-coated): 50 mg†, 100 mg†
Tablets (extended-release): 200 mg†

INDICATIONS & DOSAGES
➤**Rheumatoid arthritis, osteoarthritis—**
Adults: 75 mg t.i.d. or 50 mg q.i.d. or 200 mg as an extended-release tablet once daily. Maximum dose is 300 mg daily or 200 mg daily for extended-release capsules. Or, where suppository is available,

---

100 mg P.R. b.i.d.; or one suppository h.s. (with oral ketoprofen during the day).
Elderly patients: Reduce initial dose to between one-third and one-half of normal initial dose.
➤ **Mild to moderate pain, dysmenorrhea—**
Adults: 25 to 50 mg P.O. q 6 to 8 hours, p.r.n.
Elderly patients: Reduce initial dose to between one-third and one-half of normal initial dose.
➤ **Minor aches and pain or fever—**
Adults: 12.5 mg q 4 to 6 hours. Don't exceed 25 mg in a 4- to 6-hour period or 75 mg in 24 hours.
Elderly patients: Reduce initial dose to between one-third and one-half of normal initial dose.
Adjust-a-dose: For patients with impaired renal function, reduce initial dose to between one-third and one-half of normal initial dose.

ACTION
Unknown. Produces anti-inflammatory, analgesic, and antipyretic effects, possibly by inhibiting prostaglandin synthesis.

Route	Onset	Peak	Duration
P.O., P.R.	1-2 hr	0.5-2 hr	3-4 hr

ADVERSE REACTIONS
CNS: headache, dizziness, CNS excitation or depression.
EENT: tinnitus, visual disturbances.
GI: nausea, abdominal pain, diarrhea, constipation, flatulence, peptic ulceration, *dyspepsia,* anorexia, vomiting, stomatitis.
GU: *nephrotoxicity.*
Hematologic: prolonged bleeding time.
Respiratory: dyspnea.
Skin: rash, photosensitivity reactions.
Other: peripheral edema.

INTERACTIONS
Drug-drug. *Aspirin, corticosteroids:* Increased risk of adverse GI reactions. Avoid using together.
Aspirin, probenecid: Increased plasma levels of ketoprofen. Avoid using together.
Cyclosporine: Increased nephrotoxicity. Avoid using together.

Hydrochlorothiazide, other diuretics: Decreased diuretic effectiveness. Monitor patient for lack of effect.
Lithium, methotrexate, phenytoin: Increased levels of these drugs, leading to toxicity. Monitor patient closely.
Warfarin: Increased risk of bleeding. Monitor patient closely.
Drug-herb. *Dong quai, feverfew, garlic, ginger, horse chestnut, red clover:* Based on the known effects or components, may cause bleeding. Discourage use together.
White willow: Herb contains components similar to those of aspirin. Advise patients to avoid use with NSAIDs.
Drug-lifestyle. *Alcohol use:* May cause GI toxicity. Discourage use together.
Sun exposure: May cause photosensitivity reactions. Tell patient to take precautions.

EFFECTS ON LAB TEST RESULTS
● May increase BUN, ALT, and AST levels.
● May increase bleeding time.

CONTRAINDICATIONS
Contraindicated in patients hypersensitive to drug and in those with history of aspirin- or NSAID-induced asthma, urticaria, or other allergic reactions.

NURSING CONSIDERATIONS
● Use cautiously in patients with history of peptic ulcer disease, renal dysfunction, hypertension, heart failure, or fluid retention.
● Avoid use during last trimester of pregnancy.
● Sustained-release form isn't recommended for patients in acute pain.
● Because NSAIDs impair synthesis of renal prostaglandins, they can decrease renal blood flow and lead to reversible renal impairment, especially in patients with renal or heart failure or liver dysfunction, in elderly patients, and in those taking diuretics. Monitor these patients closely.
● Check renal and hepatic function every 6 months or as indicated.
● Drug decreases platelet adhesion and aggregation, and can prolong bleeding time about 3 to 4 minutes from baseline.

• In vitro interactions with glucose determinations have been reported with glucose oxidase and peroxidase methods. Drug may interfere with iron determinations (false increases or decreases depending on method used) and produce false increases in bilirubin levels. These interactions were reported with drug levels above 60 mg/ml.

• NSAIDs may mask signs and symptoms of infection because of their antipyretic and anti-inflammatory actions.

• Drug isn't recommended for children or breast-feeding women.

PATIENT TEACHING

• **Alert:** Drug is available OTC. Instruct patient not to exceed 75 mg/day.

• Tell patient to take drug 30 minutes before or 2 hours after meals. If adverse GI reactions occur, patient may take drug with milk or meals.

• Tell patient that full therapeutic effect may be delayed for 2 to 4 weeks.

• Serious GI toxicity, including peptic ulceration and bleeding, can occur in patient taking NSAIDs despite absence of GI symptoms. Teach patient evidence of GI bleeding, and tell him to notify prescriber immediately if it occurs.

• Alert patient that use with aspirin, alcohol, or corticosteroids may increase risk of adverse GI reactions.

• Warn patient to avoid hazardous activities that require mental alertness until CNS effects are known.

• Because of possibility of photosensitivity reactions, advise patient to use a sunblock, wear protective clothing, and avoid prolonged exposure to sunlight.

• Instruct patient to report visual or auditory adverse reactions immediately.

• Tell patient to protect drug from direct light and excessive heat and humidity.

---

ketorolac tromethamine
Toradol

Pregnancy risk category C

AVAILABLE FORMS
Injection: 15 mg/ml, 30 mg/ml
Tablets: 10 mg

INDICATIONS & DOSAGES
➤ **Short-term management of moderately severe, acute pain for single-dose treatment—**
Adults: For patients younger than age 65, 60 mg I.M. or 30 mg I.V.
Elderly patients: In patients age 65 and older, 30 mg I.M. or 15 mg I.V.
Adjust-a-dose: For renally impaired patients or those weighing less than 50 kg (110 lb), 30 mg I.M. or 15 mg I.V.
➤ **Short-term management of moderately severe, acute pain for multiple-dose treatment—**
Adults: In patients younger than age 65, 30 mg I.M. or I.V. q 6 hours. Maximum daily dose is 120 mg.
Elderly patients: In patients age 65 and older, 15 mg I.M. or I.V. q 6 hours. Maximum daily dose is 60 mg.
Adjust-a-dose: For renally impaired patients or those weighing less than 50 kg (110 lb), 15 mg I.M. or I.V. q 6 hours. Maximum daily dose is 60 mg.
➤ **Short-term management of moderately severe, acute pain when switching from parenteral to oral administration (oral therapy is indicated only as continuation of parenterally administered drug and should never be given without patient first having received parenteral therapy)—**
Adults: For patients younger than age 65, 20 mg P.O. as single dose; then 10 mg P.O. q 4 to 6 hours. Maximum daily dose is 40 mg.
Elderly patients: For patients age 65 and older, 10 mg P.O. as single dose; then 10 mg P.O. q 4 to 6 hours. Maximum daily dose is 40 mg.
Adjust-a-dose: For renally impaired patients or those weighing less than 50 kg (110 lb), 10 mg P.O. as single dose; then 10 mg P.O. q 4 to 6 hours. Maximum daily dose is 40 mg.

I.V. ADMINISTRATION
• Don't mix with morphine sulfate, meperidine hydrochloride, promethazine hydrochloride, or hydroxyzine hydrochloride. Ketorolac will precipitate out in solution.
• Dilute with normal saline solution, D_5W, 5% dextrose and normal saline solution,

---

Reactions may be *common*, uncommon, *life-threatening*, or COMMON AND LIFE-THREATENING.

Ringer's solution, lactated Ringer's solution, or Plasma-Lyte A.
● Give I.V. injection in no fewer than 15 seconds.

ACTION
Unknown. Produces anti-inflammatory, analgesic, and antipyretic effects, possibly by inhibiting prostaglandin synthesis.

Route	Onset	Peak	Duration
I.M.	10 min	0.5-1 hr	6-8 hr
I.V.	Immediate	Immediate	6-8 hr
P.O.	0.5-1 hr	0.5-1 hr	6-8 hr

ADVERSE REACTIONS
CNS: drowsiness, sedation, dizziness, headache.
CV: edema, hypertension, palpitations, *arrhythmias.*
GI: *nausea, dyspepsia, GI pain,* diarrhea, peptic ulceration, vomiting, constipation, flatulence, stomatitis.
Hematologic: decreased platelet adhesion, purpura, prolonged bleeding time.
Skin: pruritus, rash, diaphoresis.
Other: pain at injection site.

INTERACTIONS
Drug-drug. *ACE inhibitors:* May cause renal impairment, particularly in volume-depleted patients. Avoid using together in volume-depleted patients.
Anticoagulants, salicylates: May increase levels of free (unbound) salicylates or anticoagulants in the blood. Use together with extreme caution and monitor patient closely.
Antihypertensives, diuretics: Decreased effectiveness. Monitor patient closely.
Lithium: Increased lithium levels. Monitor patient closely.
Methotrexate: Decreased methotrexate clearance and increased toxicity. Avoid using together.
Drug-herb. *Dong quai, feverfew, garlic, ginger, horse chestnut, red clover:* Based on the known effects or components, may cause bleeding. Discourage use together.
White willow: Herb contains components similar to those of aspirin. Advise patients to avoid use with NSAIDs.

EFFECTS ON LAB TEST RESULTS
● May increase ALT and AST levels.
● May increase bleeding time.

CONTRAINDICATIONS
Contraindicated in patients hypersensitive to drug and in those with active peptic ulcer disease, recent GI bleeding or perforation, advanced renal impairment, risk for renal impairment from volume depletion, suspected or confirmed cerebrovascular bleeding, hemorrhagic diathesis, incomplete hemostasis, or high risk of bleeding. Also contraindicated in patients with history of peptic ulcer disease or GI bleeding, past allergic reactions to aspirin or other NSAIDs, and during labor and delivery or breast-feeding. Also contraindicated as prophylactic analgesic before major surgery or intraoperatively when hemostasis is critical; and in patients currently receiving aspirin, an NSAID, or probenecid. Don't administer drug epidurally or intrathecally because of alcohol content.

NURSING CONSIDERATIONS
● Ketorolac isn't recommended for children.
● Use cautiously in patients with hepatic or renal impairment or cardiac decompensation.
● Correct hypovolemia before treatment with ketorolac.
● **Alert:** The maximum combined duration of therapy (parenteral and oral) is 5 days.
● I.M. administration may cause pain at injection site. Holding pressure over site for 15 to 30 seconds after injection may minimize local effects. Give deep I.M.
● Carefully observe patients with coagulopathies and those taking anticoagulants. Ketorolac inhibits platelet aggregation and can prolong bleeding time. This effect will disappear within 48 hours of discontinuing drug. It won't alter platelet count, INR, PTT, or PT.
● NSAIDs may mask signs and symptoms of infection because of their antipyretic and anti-inflammatory actions.
● **Alert:** Don't confuse Toradol with Tegretol.

PATIENT TEACHING
● Warn patient receiving drug I.M. that pain may occur at injection site.

• Serious GI toxicity, including peptic ulceration and bleeding, can occur in patient taking NSAIDs despite absence of GI symptoms. Teach patient signs and symptoms of GI bleeding, and tell him to notify prescriber immediately if they occur.

---

meloxicam
Mobic

Pregnancy risk category C

AVAILABLE FORMS
Tablets: 7.5 mg

INDICATIONS & DOSAGES
➤ **Relief from signs and symptoms of osteoarthritis—**
Adults: 7.5 mg P.O. once daily. May increase p.r.n. to maximum dose of 15 mg daily.

ACTION
Unknown. Produces anti-inflammatory, analgesic, and antipyretic effects, possibly by inhibiting prostaglandin synthesis.

Route	Onset	Peak	Duration
P.O.	Unknown	Unknown	Unknown

ADVERSE REACTIONS
CNS: dizziness, headache, insomnia, fatigue, *seizures,* paresthesia, tremor, vertigo, anxiety, confusion, depression, nervousness, somnolence, malaise, syncope.
CV: *arrhythmias,* palpitations, tachycardia, angina pectoris, *heart failure,* hypertension, hypotension, *MI,* edema.
EENT: pharyngitis, abnormal vision, conjunctivitis, tinnitus, taste perversion.
GI: abdominal pain, diarrhea, dyspepsia, flatulence, nausea, constipation, colitis, dry mouth, duodenal ulcer, esophagitis, gastric ulcer, gastritis, gastroesophageal reflux, *hemorrhage, pancreatitis,* vomiting, increased appetite.
GU: albuminuria, hematuria, urinary frequency, *renal failure,* urinary tract infection.
Hematologic: anemia, *leukopenia,* purpura, *thrombocytopenia.*
Hepatic: *hepatitis.*
Metabolic: dehydration, weight increase or decrease.

Musculoskeletal: arthralgia, back pain.
Respiratory: upper respiratory tract infection, asthma, *bronchospasm,* dyspnea, coughing.
Skin: rash, pruritus, alopecia, bullous eruption, photosensitivity reactions, sweating, urticaria.
Other: accidental injury, allergic reaction, fever, *angioedema,* flulike symptoms.

INTERACTIONS
Drug-drug. *ACE inhibitors:* Decreased antihypertensive effects. Monitor blood pressure.
Aspirin: May cause adverse effects. Avoid using together.
Furosemide, thiazide diuretics: NSAIDs can reduce sodium excretion caused by diuretics, leading to sodium retention. Monitor patient for edema and increased blood pressure.
Lithium: Increased lithium levels. Monitor lithium levels closely.
Warfarin: Increased PT and INR and increased risk of bleeding complications. Monitor PT and INR, and check for signs and symptoms of bleeding.
Drug-lifestyle. *Alcohol use:* May cause GI irritation and bleeding. Discourage use together.
Smoking: May cause GI irritation and bleeding. Discourage use together.

EFFECTS ON LAB TEST RESULTS
• May increase BUN, creatinine, ALT, AST, and bilirubin levels.
• May decrease hemoglobin and WBC and platelet counts.

CONTRAINDICATIONS
Contraindicated in patients hypersensitive to drug and in those who have experienced asthma, urticaria, or allergic-type reactions after taking aspirin or other NSAIDs. Also contraindicated in patients late in pregnancy.

NURSING CONSIDERATIONS
• Use with extreme caution in patients with history of ulcers or GI bleeding. Use cautiously in patients with dehydration, anemia, hepatic disease, renal disease, hypertension, fluid retention, heart failure, or asthma. Also use cautiously in elderly and

---

debilitated patients because of increased risk of fatal GI bleeding.
- **Alert:** Patients may be allergic to meloxicam, and the drug can produce allergic-like reactions in patients hypersensitive to aspirin and other NSAIDs.
- Patients with a history of ulcers or GI bleeding are at higher risk for GI bleeding while taking NSAIDs. Other risk factors for GI bleeding include treatment with corticosteroids or anticoagulants, longer duration of NSAID treatment, smoking, alcoholism, older age, and poor overall health.
- Watch for signs and symptoms of overt and occult bleeding.
- NSAIDs can cause fluid retention; closely monitor patients who have hypertension, edema, or heart failure.
- Drug may be hepatotoxic. Watch for elevated ALT and AST levels. If signs and symptoms consistent with liver disease develop, or if systemic signs and symptoms such as eosinophilia rash occur, stop drug and call prescriber.
- Rehydrate patients who are dehydrated before starting drug.

PATIENT TEACHING
- Tell patient to report history of allergic reactions to aspirin or other NSAIDs before starting therapy.
- Advise patient to report signs and symptoms of GI ulcerations and bleeding (vomiting blood, blood in stool, and black, tarry stools) and to contact prescriber if they occur.
- Instruct patient to report any skin rash, weight gain, or edema.
- Advise patient to report warning signs of hepatotoxicity (nausea, fatigue, lethargy, pruritus, jaundice, right upper quadrant tenderness, and flulike symptoms).
- Warn patient with history of asthma that asthma may recur while taking drug. Tell him to stop drug and contact prescriber if it does.
- Tell woman to notify prescriber if she becomes pregnant or is planning to become pregnant while taking drug.
- Inform patient that it may take several days to achieve consistent pain relief.

nabumetone
Relafen, Relifex§

Pregnancy risk category C

AVAILABLE FORMS
Tablets: 500 mg, 750 mg

INDICATIONS & DOSAGES
➤ **Rheumatoid arthritis, osteoarthritis—**
Adults: Initially, 1,000 mg P.O. daily as a single dose or in divided doses b.i.d. Maximum, 2,000 mg daily.

ACTION
Unknown. Produces anti-inflammatory, analgesic, and antipyretic effects, possibly by inhibiting prostaglandin synthesis.

Route	Onset	Peak	Duration
P.O.	Unknown	2-4 hr	Unknown

ADVERSE REACTIONS
CNS: dizziness, headache, fatigue, insomnia, nervousness, somnolence.
CV: vasculitis, edema.
EENT: tinnitus.
GI: *diarrhea, dyspepsia, abdominal pain,* constipation, flatulence, nausea, dry mouth, gastritis, stomatitis, anorexia, vomiting, ***bleeding,*** ulceration.
Respiratory: dyspnea, pneumonitis.
Skin: pruritus, rash, increased diaphoresis.

INTERACTIONS
Drug-drug. *Diuretics:* NSAIDs may decrease diuretic effectiveness. Monitor patient closely.
Warfarin, other highly protein-bound drugs: May cause adverse effects from displacement of drugs by nabumetone. Use together cautiously.
Drug-herb. *Dong quai, feverfew, garlic, ginger, horse chestnut, red clover:* Based on the known effects or components, may cause bleeding. Discourage use together.
White willow: Herb contains components similar to those of aspirin. Advise patient to avoid use with NSAIDs.
Drug-food. *Any food:* Increased absorption. Give drug with food.

Drug-lifestyle. *Alcohol use:* Increased risk of additive GI toxicity. Discourage use together.

EFFECTS ON LAB TEST RESULTS
None reported.

CONTRAINDICATIONS
Contraindicated in patients with hypersensitivity reactions and history of aspirin- or NSAID-induced asthma, urticaria, or other allergic-type reactions.

NURSING CONSIDERATIONS
• Use cautiously in patients with renal or hepatic impairment; heart failure, hypertension, or other conditions that may predispose patient to fluid retention; or a history of peptic ulcer disease.
• Use of drug isn't recommended during third trimester of pregnancy.
• Because NSAIDs impair synthesis of renal prostaglandins, they can decrease renal blood flow and lead to reversible renal impairment, especially in patients with renal or heart failure or liver dysfunction, in elderly patients, and in those taking diuretics. Monitor these patients closely.
• During long-term therapy, periodically monitor renal and liver function, CBC, and hematocrit; assess patients for signs and symptoms of GI bleeding.
• Serious GI toxicity, including peptic ulceration and bleeding, can occur in patient taking NSAIDs despite absence of GI symptoms.
• Drug isn't recommended for use in children.

PATIENT TEACHING
• Instruct patient to take drug with food, milk, or antacids. Drug is absorbed more rapidly when taken with food or milk.
• Advise patient to limit alcohol intake because of additive GI toxicity risk.
• Teach patient signs and symptoms of GI bleeding, and tell him to notify prescriber immediately if they occur.
• Warn patient against hazardous activities that require mental alertness until CNS effects are known.

naproxen
Apo-Naproxen†, EC-Naprosyn, Naprosyn, Naprosyn-E†, Naprosyn-SR, Naxent†, Novo-Naprox†, Nu-Naprox†, Nycopren§

naproxen sodium
Aleve◇, Anaprox, Anaprox DS, Apo-Napro-Na†, Naprelan, Naprogesic‡, Novo-Naprox Sodium†, Synflex†

Pregnancy risk category B

AVAILABLE FORMS
naproxen
Oral suspension: 125 mg/5 ml
Suppositories: 500 mg‡
Tablets: 250 mg, 375 mg, 500 mg
Tablets (delayed-release): 375 mg, 500 mg
Tablets (extended-release): 750 mg, 1,000 mg
naproxen sodium
Tablets (controlled-release): 421.5 mg, 550 mg
Tablets (film-coated): 220 mg◇, 275 mg, 550 mg
  Note: 275 mg of naproxen sodium contains 250 mg of naproxen.

INDICATIONS & DOSAGES
➤ **Rheumatoid arthritis, osteoarthritis, ankylosing spondylitis, pain, dysmenorrhea, tendinitis, bursitis—**
Adults: 250 to 500 mg (naproxen) b.i.d.; maximum, 1.5 g daily for a limited time. Or, 375 to 500 mg delayed-release (EC-Naprosyn) b.i.d. Or, 750 to 1,000 mg controlled-release (Naprelan) daily. Or, 275 to 550 mg naproxen sodium b.i.d.
➤ **Juvenile arthritis—**
Children: 10 mg/kg P.O. in two divided doses.
➤ **Acute gout—**
Adults: 750 mg (naproxen) P.O.; then 250 mg q 8 hours until attack subsides. Or, 825 mg naproxen sodium; then 275 mg q 8 hours until attack subsides. Or, 1,000 to 1,500 mg/day controlled-release (Naprelan) on first day; then 1,000 mg daily until attack subsides.

➤ **Mild to moderate pain, primary dysmenorrhea—**
Adults: 500 mg (naproxen) P.O.; then 250 mg q 6 to 8 hours up to 1.25 g/day. Or, 550 mg naproxen sodium; then 275 mg q 6 to 8 hours up to 1,375 mg/day. Or, 1,000 mg controlled-release (Naprelan) once daily.
Elderly patients: In patients older than age 65, don't exceed 400 mg/day.

ACTION

Unknown. Produces anti-inflammatory, analgesic, and antipyretic effects, possibly by inhibiting prostaglandin synthesis.

Route	Onset	Peak	Duration
P.O.	1 hr	2-4 hr	7 hr
P.R.	Unknown	Unknown	Unknown

ADVERSE REACTIONS

CNS: headache, drowsiness, dizziness, vertigo.
CV: edema, palpitations.
EENT: visual disturbances, *tinnitus,* auditory disturbances.
GI: epigastric pain, occult blood loss, nausea, peptic ulceration, constipation, dyspepsia, heartburn, diarrhea, stomatitis, thirst.
Hematologic: increased bleeding time, ecchymoses.
Metabolic: hyperkalemia.
Respiratory: dyspnea.
Skin: pruritus, rash, urticaria, diaphoresis, purpura.

INTERACTIONS

Drug-drug. *ACE inhibitors:* May cause renal impairment. Use together cautiously.
Antihypertensives, diuretics: Decreased effect of these drugs. Monitor patient closely.
Aspirin, corticosteroids: May cause adverse GI reactions. Avoid using together.
Methotrexate: May cause toxicity. Monitor patient closely.
Oral anticoagulants, other sulfonylureas, highly protein-bound drugs: May cause toxicity. Monitor patient closely.
Probenecid: Decreased elimination of naproxen. Monitor patient for toxicity.
Drug-herb. *Dong quai, feverfew, garlic, ginger, horse chestnut, red clover:* Based

on the known effects or components, may cause bleeding. Discourage use together.
White willow: Herb contains components similar to those of aspirin. Advise patient to avoid use with NSAIDs.
Drug-lifestyle. *Alcohol use:* May cause adverse GI reactions. Discourage use together.

EFFECTS ON LAB TEST RESULTS

● May increase BUN, creatinine, ALT, AST, and potassium levels.
● May increase bleeding time.

CONTRAINDICATIONS

Contraindicated in patients hypersensitive to drug and in those with the syndrome of asthma, rhinitis, and nasal polyps.

NURSING CONSIDERATIONS

● Use cautiously in elderly patients and in patients with renal disease, CV disease, GI disorders, hepatic disease, or history of peptic ulcer disease.
● Drug should be avoided during last trimester of pregnancy.
● Because NSAIDs impair synthesis of renal prostaglandins, they can decrease renal blood flow and lead to reversible renal impairment, especially in patients with renal failure, heart failure, or liver dysfunction; in elderly patients; and in those taking diuretics. Monitor these patients closely.
● Monitor CBC and renal and hepatic function every 4 to 6 months during long-term therapy.
● Drug and its metabolite may interfere with urinary 5-hydroxyindoleacetic acid and 17-hydroxycorticosteroid determinations.
● Serious GI toxicity, including peptic ulceration and bleeding, can occur in patient taking NSAIDs despite absence of GI symptoms.
● Because of their antipyretic and anti-inflammatory actions, NSAIDs may mask signs and symptoms of infection.

PATIENT TEACHING

● *Alert:* Drug is available OTC (naproxen sodium, 200 mg). Instruct patient not to exceed 600 mg in 24 hours. Dosage in patient older than age 65 shouldn't exceed 400 mg/day.

• Advise patient to take drug with food or milk to minimize GI upset. A full glass of water or other liquid should be taken with each dose.
• Tell patient taking prescription doses of naproxen for arthritis that full therapeutic effect may be delayed 2 to 4 weeks.
• Warn patient against taking naproxen and naproxen sodium at the same time; both circulate in the blood as the naproxen anion.
• Teach patient signs and symptoms of GI bleeding, and tell him to notify prescriber immediately if they occur.
• Caution patient that use with aspirin, alcohol, or corticosteroids may increase risk of adverse GI reactions.
• Warn patient against hazardous activities that require mental alertness until CNS effects are known.

---

oxaprozin
Daypro

Pregnancy risk category C

AVAILABLE FORMS
Caplets: 600 mg

INDICATIONS & DOSAGES
➤ **Osteoarthritis, rheumatoid arthritis—**
Adults: Initially, 1,200 mg P.O. daily. Then, individualized to smallest effective dose to minimize adverse reactions. Smaller patients and those with mild symptoms may need only 600 mg daily. Maximum, 1,800 mg or 26 mg/kg daily, whichever is lower, in divided doses.

ACTION
Unknown. Produces anti-inflammatory, analgesic, and antipyretic effects, possibly by inhibiting prostaglandin synthesis.

Route	Onset	Peak	Duration
P.O.	Unknown	3-5 hr	Unknown

ADVERSE REACTIONS
CNS: depression, sedation, somnolence, confusion, sleep disturbances.
EENT: tinnitus, blurred vision.
GI: nausea, dyspepsia, diarrhea, constipation, abdominal pain or distress, anorexia,
flatulence, vomiting, *hemorrhage,* stomatitis.
GU: dysuria, urinary frequency.
Hematologic: prolonged bleeding time, anemia.
Hepatic: severe hepatic dysfunction.
Skin: *rash,* photosensitivity reactions.

INTERACTIONS
Drug-drug. *Antihypertensives, diuretics:* Decreased effect. Monitor patient closely and adjust dosage.
Aspirin: Oxaprozin displaces salicylates from plasma protein-binding sites, increasing risk of salicylate toxicity. Avoid using together.
Aspirin, corticosteroids: May cause adverse GI reactions. Avoid using together.
Cyclosporine: Nephrotoxicity may be increased. Avoid using together.
Lithium, phenytoin: Levels of these drugs may be increased. Avoid using together.
Methotrexate: Methotrexate toxicity. Avoid using together.
Oral anticoagulants: Although problems haven't been reported, may cause bleeding. Use together cautiously.
Drug-herb. *Dong quai, feverfew, garlic, ginger, horse chestnut, red clover:* Based on the known effects or components, may cause bleeding. Discourage use together.
White willow: Herb contains components similar to those of aspirin. Advise patient to avoid use with NSAIDs.
Drug-lifestyle. *Alcohol use:* Adverse GI reactions may result. Discourage use together.
Sun exposure: May cause photosensitivity reactions. Tell patient to take precautions.

EFFECTS ON LAB TEST RESULTS
• May increase ALT and AST levels.
• May increase bleeding time. May decrease hemoglobin.

CONTRAINDICATIONS
Contraindicated in patients hypersensitive to drug and in those with the syndrome of nasal polyps, angioedema, and bronchospastic reaction to aspirin or other NSAIDs.

NURSING CONSIDERATIONS
• Use cautiously in patients with history of peptic ulcer disease, hepatic or renal

dysfunction, hypertension, CV disease, or conditions predisposing patient to fluid retention.
• Because renal prostaglandins play a role in the maintenance of renal perfusion, patients with conditions that reduce renal blood flow may experience renal toxicity with NSAID therapy. Patients at greatest risk are the elderly, those taking diuretics, and those with impaired renal, hepatic, or cardiac function. Closely monitor renal function in these patients, and discontinue NSAID therapy if problems develop.
• Elevations of liver function test values can occur after long-term use. These abnormal findings may persist, worsen, or resolve with continued therapy. Rarely, patients may progress to severe hepatic dysfunction. Periodically obtain liver function test results in patients receiving long-term therapy, and closely monitor patients whose test results are abnormal.
• Serious GI toxicity, including peptic ulceration and bleeding, can occur in patient taking NSAIDs despite absence of GI symptoms.
• Because of their antipyretic and anti-inflammatory actions, NSAIDs may mask signs and symptoms of infection.
• *Alert:* Don't confuse oxaprozin with oxazepam.

PATIENT TEACHING
• Tell patient to take drug 30 minutes before or 2 hours after meals. If adverse GI reactions occur, drug may be taken with milk or meals.
• Inform patient that full therapeutic effects may be delayed for 2 to 4 weeks.
• Teach patient signs and symptoms of GI bleeding, and tell him to notify prescriber immediately if they occur.
• Tell patient to report adverse visual or auditory reactions immediately.
• Warn patient against hazardous activities that require mental alertness until CNS effects are known.
• Because of possibility of photosensitivity reactions, advise patient to use a sunblock, wear protective clothing, and avoid prolonged exposure to sunlight.

piroxicam
Apo-Piroxicam†, Feldene,
Novo-Pirocam†, Pirox‡

Pregnancy risk category B (D in third trimester or near delivery)

AVAILABLE FORMS
Capsules: 10 mg, 20 mg

INDICATIONS & DOSAGES
➤ **Osteoarthritis, rheumatoid arthritis—**
Adults: 20 mg P.O. daily. If desired, dose may be divided b.i.d.

ACTION
Unknown. Produces anti-inflammatory, analgesic, and antipyretic effects, possibly by inhibiting prostaglandin synthesis.

Route	Onset	Peak	Duration
P.O.	1 hr	3-5 hr	48-72 hr

ADVERSE REACTIONS
CNS: headache, drowsiness, dizziness, somnolence, vertigo.
CV: peripheral edema.
EENT: auditory disturbances.
GI: epigastric distress, nausea, occult blood loss, peptic ulceration, *severe GI bleeding,* diarrhea, constipation, abdominal pain, dyspepsia, flatulence, anorexia, stomatitis.
GU: *nephrotoxicity.*
Hematologic: prolonged bleeding time, anemia, *leukopenia, agranulocytosis,* eosinophilia.
Metabolic: hyperkalemia, hypoglycemia in diabetic patients.
Respiratory: *bronchospasm.*
Skin: pruritus, rash, urticaria, *photosensitivity reactions.*

INTERACTIONS
Drug-drug. *Antihypertensives, diuretics:* Decreased effects. Avoid using together.
Aspirin, corticosteroids: May cause GI toxicity. Decreased plasma levels of piroxicam. Avoid using together.
Cyclosporine, methotrexate: Increased toxicity. Monitor patient closely.
Lithium: Increased plasma lithium levels. Monitor patient for toxicity.

Oral anticoagulants, other highly protein-bound drugs: Toxicity may result. Monitor patient closely.
Oral antidiabetics: Enhanced antidiabetic effects. Monitor patient closely.
Drug-herb. *Dong quai, feverfew, garlic, ginger, horse chestnut, red clover:* Based on the known effects or components, may cause bleeding. Discourage use together.
St. John's wort: Photosensitivity reaction may occur. Advise patient to take precautions.
White willow: Herb contains components similar to those of aspirin. Advise patient to avoid use with NSAIDs.
Drug-lifestyle. *Alcohol use:* May cause GI toxicity. Decreased plasma levels of piroxicam. Discourage use together.
Sun exposure: May cause photosensitivity reactions. Tell patient to take precautions.

EFFECTS ON LAB TEST RESULTS
● May increase BUN, creatinine, liver enzyme, and potassium levels. May decrease glucose levels.
● May decrease hemoglobin and WBC, granulocyte, and eosinophil counts.

CONTRAINDICATIONS
Contraindicated in patients hypersensitive to drug and in those with bronchospasm or angioedema precipitated by aspirin or NSAIDs. Also contraindicated in pregnant or breast-feeding patients.

NURSING CONSIDERATIONS
● Use cautiously in elderly patients and in patients with GI disorders, history of renal or peptic ulcer disease, cardiac disease, hypertension, or conditions predisposing to fluid retention.
● Because NSAIDs impair the synthesis of renal prostaglandins, they can decrease renal blood flow and lead to reversible renal impairment, especially in elderly patients, in patients taking diuretics, and in patients with renal failure, heart failure, or liver dysfunction. Monitor these patients closely.
● Check renal, hepatic, and auditory function and CBC periodically during prolonged therapy. Discontinue drug and notify prescriber if abnormalities occur.
● Serious GI toxicity, including peptic ulceration and bleeding, can occur in patient

taking NSAIDs despite absence of GI symptoms.
● NSAIDs may mask signs and symptoms of infection because of their antipyretic and anti-inflammatory actions.

PATIENT TEACHING
● Tell patient to take drug with milk, antacids, or meals if adverse GI reactions occur.
● Inform patient that full therapeutic effects may be delayed for 2 to 4 weeks.
● Teach patient signs and symptoms of GI bleeding and tell him when to report them to prescriber.
● Warn patient against hazardous activities that require mental alertness until CNS effects are known.
● Because drug causes adverse skin reactions more often than other drugs in its class, advise patient to use a sunblock, wear protective clothing, and avoid prolonged exposure to sunlight. Photosensitivity reactions are the most common.

rofecoxib
Vioxx

Pregnancy risk category C

AVAILABLE FORMS
Oral suspension: 12.5 mg/5 ml, 25 mg/5 ml
Tablets: 12.5 mg, 25 mg, 50 mg

INDICATIONS & DOSAGES
➤ **Relief from signs and symptoms of osteoarthritis—**
Adults: Initially, 12.5 mg P.O. once daily, increased, p.r.n., to maximum of 25 mg P.O. once daily.
➤ **Management of acute pain, treatment of primary dysmenorrhea—**
Adults: 50 mg P.O. once daily, p.r.n., for up to 5 days.

ACTION
Unknown. Produces anti-inflammatory, analgesic, and antipyretic effects, possibly by inhibiting prostaglandin synthesis.

Route	Onset	Peak	Duration
P.O.	Unknown	2-3 hr	Unknown

ADVERSE REACTIONS

CNS: headache, asthenia, fatigue, dizziness.
CV: hypertension, leg edema.
EENT: sinusitis.
GI: diarrhea, dyspepsia, epigastric discomfort, heartburn, nausea, abdominal pain.
GU: urinary tract infection.
Musculoskeletal: back pain.
Respiratory: bronchitis, upper respiratory tract infection.
Other: flu syndrome.

INTERACTIONS

Drug-drug. *ACE inhibitors:* Decreased antihypertensive effects of ACE inhibitors. Monitor blood pressure closely.
Aspirin: Increased rate of GI ulceration and other complications. Avoid using together, if possible. If used together, monitor patient closely for GI bleeding.
Furosemide, thiazide diuretics: Reduced efficacy of these drugs. Monitor patient closely.
Lithium: Increased lithium levels and decreased lithium clearance. Monitor patient for toxic reaction to lithium.
Methotrexate: Increased methotrexate levels. Monitor patient closely for toxic reaction to methotrexate.
Rifampin: Decreased rofecoxib levels by about 50%. Initiate therapy with a higher dosage of rofecoxib.
Warfarin: Increased effects of warfarin. Monitor INR more frequently in first few days after therapy is initiated or dosage is changed.
Drug-herb. *Dong quai, feverfew, garlic, ginger, horse chestnut, red clover:* Based on the known effects or components, may cause bleeding. Discourage use together.
White willow: Herb contains components similar to those of aspirin. Advise patients to avoid use with NSAIDs.
Drug-lifestyle. *Long-term alcohol use, smoking:* May cause GI bleeding. Monitor patient closely.

EFFECTS ON LAB TEST RESULTS

None reported.

CONTRAINDICATIONS

Contraindicated in patients hypersensitive to drug or its components and in those who have experienced asthma, urticaria, or allergic reactions after taking aspirin or other NSAIDs. Also contraindicated in patients with advanced kidney disease or moderate or severe hepatic insufficiency and in pregnant women because drug may cause ductus arteriosus to close prematurely.

NURSING CONSIDERATIONS

● *Alert:* NSAIDs may cause serious GI toxicity. Signs and symptoms include bleeding, ulceration, and perforation of the stomach, small intestine, and large intestine. Such toxicity can occur any time, with or without warning. To minimize risk of an adverse GI event, use lowest effective dose for the shortest possible duration. Monitor patient for GI bleeding.
● Use cautiously in patients with history of ulcer disease or GI bleeding and in those taking such drugs as oral corticosteroids and anticoagulants. Also use cautiously in patients with conditions such as older age, alcoholism, poor general health, and addiction to smoking that may increase risk of GI bleeding.
● Use cautiously in patient who is considerably dehydrated. Rehydration is recommended before therapy begins.
● In patient with fluid retention, hypertension, or heart failure, use cautiously and start therapy at the lowest recommended dosage. Monitor blood pressure and check patient for fluid retention or worsening heart failure.
● In patient older than age 65, start therapy at the lowest recommended dosage.
● Patient may be allergic to drug if he has an allergy to aspirin or other NSAIDs.
● Drug may be hepatotoxic. Monitor patient for signs and symptoms of liver toxicity. Drug should be discontinued if signs and symptoms consistent with liver disease develop.
● Oral suspension should be shaken well before it's administered.
● Patient undergoing long-term treatment should have his hemoglobin level and hematocrit checked if he experiences signs or symptoms of anemia or blood loss.
● Drug isn't recommended for use in breast-feeding women.

PATIENT TEACHING

● Warn patient that he may experience signs and symptoms of GI bleeding, in-

cluding bloody vomitus, blood in urine and stool, and black, tarry stools. Advise patient to call prescriber if they occur.
• Advise patient to report rash, unexplained weight gain, or edema.
• Tell patient to avoid aspirin and aspirin-containing products unless prescriber has instructed him otherwise.
• Urge patient to avoid OTC anti-inflammatories such as ibuprofen (Advil) unless prescriber has instructed him otherwise.
• Tell patient that all NSAIDs, including rofecoxib, may adversely affect the liver. Signs and symptoms of liver toxicity include nausea, fatigue, lethargy, itching, jaundice, right upper quadrant tenderness, and flu syndrome. Advise him to stop therapy and call prescriber immediately if he experiences these signs or symptoms.
• Instruct woman to inform prescriber if she becomes pregnant or is planning to become pregnant while taking drug.
• Tell patient that drug may be taken without regard to food, although taking it with food may decrease GI upset.
• Tell patient that the most common adverse effects of drug are dyspepsia, epigastric discomfort, heartburn, and nausea. Advise him that taking drug with food may help minimize these effects.

sulindac
Aclin‡, Apo-Sulin†, Clinoril, Novo-Sundac†, Saldac‡

Pregnancy risk category NR

AVAILABLE FORMS
Tablets: 100 mg‡, 150 mg, 200 mg

INDICATIONS & DOSAGES
➤ **Osteoarthritis, rheumatoid arthritis, ankylosing spondylitis—**
Adults: Initially, 150 mg P.O. b.i.d.; increased to 200 mg b.i.d., p.r.n. Maximum dose is 400 mg daily.
➤ **Acute subacromial bursitis or supraspinatus tendinitis, acute gouty arthritis—**
Adults: 200 mg P.O. b.i.d. for 7 to 14 days. Dosage reduced as symptoms subside. Maximum dose is 400 mg daily.

ACTION
Unknown. Produces anti-inflammatory, analgesic, and antipyretic effects, possibly by inhibiting prostaglandin synthesis.

Route	Onset	Peak	Duration
P.O.	Unknown	2-4 hr	Unknown

ADVERSE REACTIONS
CNS: dizziness, headache, nervousness, psychosis.
CV: hypertension, *heart failure,* palpitations, edema.
EENT: tinnitus, transient visual disturbances.
GI: *epigastric distress,* peptic ulceration, occult blood loss, nausea, constipation, dyspepsia, flatulence, anorexia, GI bleeding.
GU: interstitial nephritis.
Hematologic: prolonged bleeding time.
Metabolic: hyperkalemia.
Skin: rash, pruritus.
Other: drug fever, *anaphylaxis, angioedema,* hypersensitivity reactions.

INTERACTIONS
Drug-drug. *Anticoagulants:* May cause bleeding. Monitor PT and INR closely.
Aspirin: Decreased sulindac level and increased risk of GI adverse reactions. Avoid using together.
Cyclosporine: Increased nephrotoxicity of cyclosporine. Avoid using together.
Diflunisal, dimethyl sulfoxide: Decreased metabolism of sulindac to its active metabolite, reducing its effectiveness. Avoid using together.
Methotrexate: Increased methotrexate toxicity. Avoid using together.
Probenecid: Increased levels of sulindac and its active metabolite. Monitor patient for toxicity.
Sulfonamides, sulfonylureas, other highly protein-bound drugs: May cause displacement of these drugs from plasma protein-binding sites, leading to increased toxicity. Monitor patient closely.
Drug-herb. *Dong quai, feverfew, garlic, ginger, horse chestnut, red clover:* Based on the known effects or components, may cause bleeding. Discourage use together.
White willow: Herb contains components similar to those of aspirin. Advise patients to avoid use with NSAIDs.

Reactions may be *common,* uncommon, *life-threatening,* or COMMON AND LIFE-THREATENING.

EFFECTS ON LAB TEST RESULTS
• May increase BUN, creatinine, ALT, AST, and potassium levels.

CONTRAINDICATIONS
Contraindicated in patients hypersensitive to drug and in those for whom aspirin or NSAIDs precipitate acute asthmatic attacks, urticaria, or rhinitis.

NURSING CONSIDERATIONS
• Use cautiously in patients with a history of ulcers and GI bleeding, renal dysfunction, compromised cardiac function, hypertension, or conditions predisposing to fluid retention.
• Don't use drug in pregnant women.
• Periodically monitor hepatic and renal function and CBC in patient receiving long-term therapy.
• Serious GI toxicity, including peptic ulceration and bleeding, can occur in patient taking NSAIDs despite absence of GI symptoms.
• NSAIDs may mask signs and symptoms of infection.

PATIENT TEACHING
• Tell patient to take drug with food, milk, or antacids.
• Teach patient signs and symptoms of GI bleeding, including fatigue, weakness, coffee ground emesis, and black, tarry stool, and tell him to contact prescriber immediately if they occur.
• *Alert:* Tell patient to notify prescriber immediately if easy bruising or prolonged bleeding occurs.
• Advise patient to avoid hazardous activities that require mental alertness until CNS effects are known.
• Instruct patient to report edema and have blood pressure checked monthly. Drug causes sodium retention but is thought to have less effect on the kidneys than other NSAIDs.
• Advise patient to notify prescriber and have complete eye examination if visual disturbances occur.

anil hydrochloride
norphine hydrochloride
hanol tartrate
e phosphate
e sulfate
citrate
transdermal system
transmucosal
morphine hydrochloride
dine hydrochloride
done hydrochloride
ine hydrochloride
hine sulfate
phine tartrate
uphine hydrochloride
codone hydrochloride
xycodone pectinate
xymorphone hydrochloride
xymorcine hydrochloride
pentazocine hydrochloride
pentazocine hydrochloride and
naloxone hydrochloride
pentazocine lactate
propoxyphene hydrochloride
propoxyphene napsylate
remifentanil hydrochloride
tramadol hydrochloride

COMBINATION PRODUCTS

222†: aspirin 375 mg, codeine phosphate 8 mg, and caffeine citrate 30 mg.
282 MEP†: aspirin 375 mg, codeine phosphate 15 mg, and caffeine citrate 30 mg.
292†: aspirin 375 mg, codeine phosphate 30 mg, and caffeine citrate 30 mg.
692†: aspirin 375 mg, propoxyphene hydrochloride 65 mg, and caffeine 30 mg.
ACETA WITH CODEINE, EMPRACET-30†, EMTEC-30†: acetaminophen 300 mg and codeine phosphate 30 mg.
ANACIN WITH CODEINE†: aspirin 325 mg, codeine phosphate 8 mg, and caffeine 32 mg.
ANEXSIA 5/500: hydrocodone bitartrate 5 mg and acetaminophen 500 mg.
CAPITAL WITH CODEINE, TYLENOL WITH CODEINE ELIXIR*: acetaminophen 120 and codeine phosphate 12 mg/5 ml.
COCET-N 50: acetaminophen 325 mg and propoxyphene napsylate 50 mg.

DARVOCET-N 100, PROPACET 100: acetaminophen 650 mg and propoxyphene napsylate 100 mg.
DARVON COMPOUND-65†: aspirin 389 mg, propoxyphene hydrochloride 65 mg, and caffeine 32.4 mg.
DARVON-N COMPOUND†: aspirin 375 mg, propoxyphene napsylate 100 mg, and caffeine 30 mg.
DARVON-N WITH A.S.A.†: aspirin 325 mg and propoxyphene napsylate 100 mg.
E-LOR, WYGESIC: acetaminophen 650 mg and propoxyphene hydrochloride 65 mg.
EMPIRIN WITH CODEINE NO. 3, PHENAPHEN WITH CODEINE NO. 3: aspirin 325 mg and codeine phosphate 30 mg.
EMPIRIN WITH CODEINE NO. 4, PHENAPHEN WITH CODEINE NO. 4: aspirin 325 mg and codeine phosphate 60 mg.
EMPRACET-60†: acetaminophen 300 mg and codeine phosphate 60 mg.
ENDOCET, OXYCOCET†, PERCOCET, ROXICET: acetaminophen 325 mg and oxycodone hydrochloride 5 mg.
ENDODAN†, OXYCODAN†, PERCODAN†: aspirin 325 mg and oxycodone hydrochloride 5 mg.
FIORICET WITH CODEINE CAPSULES: acetaminophen 325 mg, butalbital 50 mg, caffeine 40 mg, and codeine phosphate 30 mg.
FIORINAL WITH CODEINE CAPSULES: aspirin 325 mg, butalbital 50 mg, caffeine 40 mg, and codeine 30 mg.
INNOVAR: droperidol 2.5 mg and fentanyl citrate 0.05 mg/ml.
LENOLTEC WITH CODEINE NO. 1†,
LORCET 10/650 tablets: acetaminophen 650 mg and hydrocodone bitartrate 10 mg.
LORCET PLUS TABLETS: acetaminophen 650 mg and hydrocodone bitartrate 7.5 mg.
LORTAB 2.5/500 TABLETS: acetaminophen 500 mg and hydrocodone bitartrate 2.5 mg.
LORTAB 5/500 TABLETS: acetaminophen 500 mg and hydrocodone bitartrate 5 mg.

be common, uncommon, *life-threatening*, or **COMMON AND LIFE-THREATENING.**

LORTAB 7.5/500 TABLETS: acetaminophen 500 mg and hydrocodone bitartrate 7.5 mg.

NOVO-GESIC C8†: acetaminophen 300 mg, codeine phosphate 8 mg, and caffeine 15 mg.

PERCODAN-DEMI TABLETS: aspirin 325 mg, oxycodone hydrochloride 2.25 mg, and oxycodone terephthalate 0.19 mg.

PERCODAN-DEMI†: aspirin 325 mg and oxycodone hydrochloride 2.5 mg.

PERCODAN, ROXIPRIN TABLETS: aspirin 325 mg, oxycodone hydrochloride 4.5 mg, and oxycodone terephthalate 0.38 mg.

ROXICET 5/500 CAPLETS, TYLOX CAPSULES: acetaminophen 500 mg and oxycodone hydrochloride 5 mg.

ROXICET ORAL SOLUTION*: acetaminophen 325 mg and oxycodone hydrochloride 5 mg/5 ml.

TALACEN: acetaminophen 650 mg and pentazocine hydrochloride 25 mg.

TALWIN COMPOUND: aspirin 325 mg and pentazocine hydrochloride 12.5 mg.

TYLENOL WITH CODEINE NO. 1: acetaminophen 300 mg and codeine phosphate 7.5 mg.

TYLENOL WITH CODEINE NO. 2: acetaminophen 300 mg and codeine phosphate 15 mg.

TYLENOL WITH CODEINE NO. 3: acetaminophen 300 mg and codeine phosphate 30 mg.

TYLENOL WITH CODEINE NO. 4: acetaminophen 300 mg and codeine phosphate 60 mg.

ULTRACET: acetaminophen 325 mg and tramadol hydrochloride 37.5 mg.

VICODIN: acetaminophen 500 mg and hydrocodone bitartrate 5 mg.

VICODIN ES: acetaminophen 750 mg and hydrocodone bitartrate 7.5 mg.

alfentanil hydrochloride
Alfenta, CD Rapifen§

Pregnancy risk category C
Controlled substance schedule II

AVAILABLE FORMS
Injection: 500 mcg/ml

INDICATIONS & DOSAGES
➤ **Adjunct to general anesthetic—**
Adults: Initially, 8 to 50 mcg/kg I.V.; then increments of 3 to 15 mcg/kg I.V. q 5 to 20 minutes.
➤ **As a primary anesthetic—**
Adults: Initially, 130 to 245 mcg/kg I.V.; then 0.5 to 1.5 mcg/kg/minute I.V.
➤ **Monitored anesthesia care—**
Adults: Initially, 3 to 8 mcg/kg I.V.; then 3 to 5 mcg/kg I.V. q 5 to 20 minutes or 0.25 to 1 mcg/kg/minute I.V. Total dose is 3 to 40 mcg/kg I.V.
Adjust-a-dose: For debilitated patients, dosage should be reduced. In obese patients, dosage is based on lean body weight.

I.V. ADMINISTRATION
● Drug is compatible with D_5W, D_5W in lactated Ringer's solution, and normal saline solution. Infusions containing 25 to 80 mcg/ml are used most frequently.
● Discontinue infusion at least 10 to 15 minutes before end of surgery.
● Drug should be administered only by persons specifically trained in use of I.V. anesthetics.
● Keep narcotic antagonist (naloxone) and resuscitation equipment available when giving drug I.V.

ACTION
Unknown. Binds with opiate receptors in the CNS, altering both perception of and emotional response to pain.

Route	Onset	Peak	Duration
I.V.	1 min	1.5-2 min	5-10 min

ADVERSE REACTIONS
CNS: anxiety, headache, confusion, dizziness, sleepiness, sedation.
CV: *hypotension, hypertension,* BRADYCARDIA, *tachycardia,* ARRHYTHMIAS.
EENT: blurred vision.
GI: *nausea, vomiting.*
Musculoskeletal: skeletal muscle movements.
Respiratory: *chest wall rigidity, bronchospasm, respiratory depression,* hypercapnia, *respiratory arrest, laryngospasm.*
Skin: pruritus, urticaria.

INTERACTIONS
Drug-drug. *Cimetidine:* CNS toxicity. Monitor patient closely.
CNS depressants: Additive effects. Use together cautiously.
Diazepam: CV depression and decreased blood pressure with high doses of alfentanil. Monitor patient closely.
Drug-lifestyle. *Alcohol use:* Additive effects. Discourage use together.

EFFECTS ON LAB TEST RESULTS
● May increase amylase and lipase levels.

CONTRAINDICATIONS
Contraindicated in patients hypersensitive to drug.

NURSING CONSIDERATIONS
● Use cautiously in patients with head injury, pulmonary disease, decreased respiratory reserve, or hepatic or renal impairment.
● Clearance is reduced by about 30% in patients age 65 and older, leading to a prolonged half-life. Dosage should be reduced in these patients.
● *Alert:* To administer small volumes of alfentanil accurately, use a tuberculin syringe.
● Accidental skin contact should be treated by rinsing the area with water.
● Periodically monitor postoperative vital signs and bladder function. Because drug decreases both rate and depth of respirations, monitoring arterial oxygen saturation may aid in assessing respiratory depression.
● *Alert:* Don't confuse alfentanil with Anafranil, fentanyl, or sufentanil; or Alfenta with Sufenta.

PATIENT TEACHING
● Explain anesthetic effect of drug and preoperative and postoperative care measures.
● Inform patient that another analgesic will be available to relieve pain after effects of drug have worn off.

---

buprenorphine hydrochloride
Buprenex, Temgesic‡

Pregnancy risk category C
Controlled substance schedule V

AVAILABLE FORMS
Injection: 0.324 mg (equivalent to 0.3 mg base/ml)

INDICATIONS & DOSAGES
➤ **Moderate to severe pain—**
Adults and children age 13 and older:
0.3 mg I.M. or slow I.V. q 6 hours, p.r.n., or around the clock; dose repeated (up to 0.3 mg), p.r.n., 30 to 60 minutes after initial dose.
Children ages 2 to 12: 2 to 6 mcg/kg I.M. or I.V. q 4 to 6 hours.
Elderly patients: Reduce dose by one-half.
Adjust-a-dose: Reduce dose by one-half in high-risk patients, such as debilitated patients.

I.V. ADMINISTRATION
● Give drug by direct I.V. injection, slowly into a vein or through tubing of a free-flowing, compatible I.V. solution over not less than 2 minutes.
● When mixed in a 1:1 volume ratio, drug is compatible with atropine sulfate, diphenhydramine hydrochloride, droperidol, glycopyrrolate, haloperidol lactate, hydroxyzine hydrochloride, promethazine hydrochloride, scopolamine hydrochloride, D_5W, 5% dextrose and normal saline solution, sodium chloride, lactated Ringer's solution, and normal saline solution injections.

ACTION
Unknown. Binds with opiate receptors in the CNS, altering both perception of and emotional response to pain.

Route	Onset	Peak	Duration
I.M.	15 min	1 hr	6 hr
I.V.	Immediate	2 min	6 hr

ADVERSE REACTIONS
CNS: *dizziness, sedation,* headache, confusion, nervousness, euphoria, *vertigo,* **increased intracranial pressure.**

CV: hypotension, ***bradycardia,*** tachycardia, hypertension.
EENT: *miosis,* blurred vision.
GI: *nausea,* vomiting, constipation, dry mouth.
GU: urine retention.
Respiratory: *respiratory depression,* hypoventilation, dyspnea.
Skin: pruritus, diaphoresis.

INTERACTIONS
Drug-drug. *CNS depressants, MAO inhibitors:* Additive effects. Use together cautiously.
Drug-lifestyle. *Alcohol use:* Additive effects. Discourage use together.

EFFECTS ON LAB TEST RESULTS
None reported.

CONTRAINDICATIONS
Contraindicated in patients hypersensitive to drug.

NURSING CONSIDERATIONS
• Use cautiously in elderly or debilitated patients and in those with head injury, intracranial lesions, and increased intracranial pressure; severe respiratory, liver, or kidney impairment; CNS depression or coma; thyroid irregularities; adrenal insufficiency; and prostatic hyperplasia, urethral stricture, acute alcoholism, delirium tremens, or kyphoscoliosis.
• S.C. administration isn't recommended.
• Buprenorphine 0.3 mg is equal to 10 mg of morphine and 75 mg of meperidine in analgesic potency. It has longer duration of action than morphine or meperidine.
• *Alert:* Naloxone won't completely reverse the respiratory depression caused by buprenorphine overdose; an overdose may necessitate mechanical ventilation. Larger than customary doses of naloxone (more than 0.4 mg) and doxapram also may be ordered.
• Accidental skin exposure should be treated by removing exposed clothing and rinsing skin with water.
• *Alert:* Drug's narcotic antagonist properties may precipitate withdrawal syndrome in narcotic-dependent patients.
• If dependence occurs, withdrawal symptoms may appear up to 14 days after drug is stopped.

• *Alert:* Don't confuse Buprenex with Bumex.

PATIENT TEACHING
• Caution ambulatory patient about getting out of bed or walking.
• When drug is used postoperatively, encourage patient to turn, cough, and breathe deeply to prevent atelectasis.

---

butorphanol tartrate
Stadol, Stadol NS

Pregnancy risk category C
Controlled substance schedule IV

AVAILABLE FORMS
Injection: 1 mg/ml, 2 mg/ml
Nasal spray: 10 mg/ml

INDICATIONS & DOSAGES
➤ **Moderate to severe pain—**
Adults: 1 to 4 mg I.M. q 3 to 4 hours, p.r.n., or around the clock. Not to exceed 4 mg per dose. Or, 0.5 to 2 mg I.V. q 3 to 4 hours, p.r.n. or around the clock. Or, 1 mg by nasal spray q 3 to 4 hours (1 spray in one nostril); repeated in 60 to 90 minutes if pain relief is inadequate. For severe pain, 2 mg (1 spray in each nostril) q 3 to 4 hours.
Elderly patients: One-half usual dose at twice the interval for I.V. use; for nasal use, allow 1 to 2 hours to elapse before repeating dose.
Adjust-a-dose: For patients with renal or hepatic impairment, increase dosage interval to 6 to 8 hours.
➤ **Labor for patients at full term and in early labor—**
Adults: 1 to 2 mg I.V. or I.M.; repeat after 4 hours, p.r.n.
➤ **Preoperative anesthesia or preanesthesia—**
Adults: 2 mg I.M. 60 to 90 minutes before surgery.
➤ **Adjunct to balanced anesthesia—**
Adults: 2 mg I.V. shortly before induction, or 0.5 to 1 mg I.V. in increments during anesthesia.
Elderly patients: One-half usual dose at twice the interval for I.V. use.

---

*Liquid contains alcohol. **May contain tartrazine. †Canada ‡Australia §U.K. ◊OTC

I.V. ADMINISTRATION
• Give by direct injection into a vein or into the tubing of a free-flowing I.V. solution.
• Compatible solutions include D₅W and normal saline solutions.

ACTION
Unknown. Binds with opiate receptors in the CNS, altering both perception of and emotional response to pain.

Route	Onset	Peak	Duration
I.M.	10-15 min	30-60 min	3-4 hr
I.V.	2-3 min	30-60 min	3-4 hr
Nasal	15 min	1-2 hr	4-5 hr

ADVERSE REACTIONS
CNS: confusion, nervousness, lethargy, headache, *somnolence, dizziness, insomnia,* anxiety, paresthesia, euphoria, hallucinations, flushing, ***increased intracranial pressure.***
CV: palpitations, vasodilation, hypotension.
EENT: blurred vision, *nasal congestion,* tinnitus.
GI: *nausea, vomiting,* constipation, anorexia, *unpleasant taste.*
Respiratory: *respiratory depression.*
Skin: rash, hives, clamminess, excessive diaphoresis.
Other: sensation of heat.

INTERACTIONS
Drug-drug. *CNS depressants:* Additive effects. Use together cautiously.
Drug-lifestyle. *Alcohol use:* Additive effects. Discourage use together.

EFFECTS ON LAB TEST RESULTS
None reported.

CONTRAINDICATIONS
Contraindicated in patients hypersensitive to drug or to preservative, benzethonium chloride, and in those with narcotic addiction; may precipitate withdrawal syndrome.

NURSING CONSIDERATIONS
• Use cautiously in patients with head injury, increased intracranial pressure, acute MI, ventricular dysfunction, coronary insufficiency, respiratory disease or depression, and renal or hepatic dysfunction. Also administer cautiously to patients who have recently received repeated doses of narcotic analgesic.
• Don't give by S.C. route.
• Respiratory depression apparently doesn't increase with larger dosage.
• Psychological and physical addiction may occur.
• Periodically monitor postoperative vital signs and bladder function. Because drug decreases both rate and depth of respirations, monitoring of arterial oxygen saturation may aid in assessing respiratory depression.
• Watch for nasal congestion with nasal spray use.
• ***Alert:*** Don't confuse Stadol with sotalol.

PATIENT TEACHING
• Caution ambulatory patient about getting out of bed or walking. Warn outpatient to avoid driving and other hazardous activities that require mental alertness until drug's CNS effects are known.
• Teach patient how to administer and store nasal spray, if applicable.
• Instruct patient to avoid alcohol during therapy.

---

codeine phosphate
Paveral†

codeine sulfate

Pregnancy risk category C
Controlled substance schedule II

AVAILABLE FORMS
codeine phosphate
Injection: 30 mg/ml, 60 mg/ml
Oral solution: 15 mg/5 ml, 10 mg/ml†
Tablets (soluble): 30 mg, 60 mg
codeine sulfate
Tablets: 15 mg, 30 mg, 60 mg
Tablets (soluble): 15 mg, 30 mg, 60 mg

INDICATIONS & DOSAGES
➤ **Mild to moderate pain—**
Adults: 15 to 60 mg P.O. or 15 to 60 mg (phosphate) S.C., I.M., or I.V. q 4 to 6 hours, p.r.n. Maximum dose is 360 mg/day.

Reactions may be *common,* uncommon, ***life-threatening,*** or COMMON AND LIFE-THREATENING.

Children older than age 1: 0.5 mg/kg P.O., S.C., or I.M. q 4 hours, p.r.n. *Don't use I.V. in children.*

➤ **Nonproductive cough—**
Adults: 10 to 20 mg P.O. q 4 to 6 hours. Maximum dose is 120 mg/day.
Children ages 6 to 12: 5 to 10 mg P.O. q 4 to 6 hours. Maximum dose is 60 mg/day.
Children ages 2 to 6: 2.5 to 5 mg P.O. q 4 to 6 hours. Don't exceed 30 mg/day.

I.V. ADMINISTRATION
● Give drug by direct injection into a large vein. Administer very slowly.

ACTION
Unknown. Binds with opiate receptors in the CNS, altering both perception of and emotional response to pain. Drug also suppresses the cough reflex by direct action on the cough center in the medulla.

Route	Onset	Peak	Duration
I.M.	10-30 min	0.5-1 hr	4-6 hr
I.V.	Immediate	Immediate	4-6 hr
P.O.	30-45 min	1-2 hr	4-6 hr
S.C.	10-30 min	Unknown	4-6 hr

ADVERSE REACTIONS
CNS: *sedation, clouded sensorium,* euphoria, dizziness, light-headedness, physical dependence.
CV: hypotension, **bradycardia,** flushing.
GI: nausea, vomiting, *constipation,* dry mouth, ileus.
GU: urine retention.
Respiratory: *respiratory depression.*
Skin: pruritus, *diaphoresis.*

INTERACTIONS
Drug-drug. *CNS depressants, general anesthetics, hypnotics, MAO inhibitors, other narcotic analgesics, sedatives, tranquilizers, TCAs:* Additive effects. Use together with extreme caution. Monitor patient response.
Drug-lifestyle. Alcohol use: Additive effects. Discourage use together.

EFFECTS ON LAB TEST RESULTS
● May increase amylase and lipase levels.

CONTRAINDICATIONS
Contraindicated in patients hypersensitive to drug.

NURSING CONSIDERATIONS
● Use with extreme caution in elderly or debilitated patients and in those with head injury, increased intracranial pressure, increased CSF pressure, hepatic or renal disease, hypothyroidism, Addison's disease, acute alcoholism, seizures, severe CNS depression, bronchial asthma, COPD, respiratory depression, and shock.
● *Alert:* Don't mix with other solutions because codeine phosphate is incompatible with many drugs.
● Don't administer discolored solution.
● Codeine and aspirin or acetaminophen are commonly prescribed together to provide enhanced pain relief.
● For full analgesic effect, administer drug before patient has intense pain.
● Drug is an antitussive and shouldn't be used when cough is a valuable diagnostic sign or is beneficial (as after thoracic surgery).
● Monitor cough type and frequency.
● Monitor respiratory and circulatory status.
● Opiates may cause constipation. Assess bowel function and need for stool softeners or laxatives.
● Codeine may delay gastric emptying, increase biliary tract pressure from contraction of the sphincter of Oddi, and interfere with hepatobiliary imaging studies.
● *Alert:* Don't confuse codeine with Cardene, Lodine, or Cordran.

PATIENT TEACHING
● Advise patient that GI distress caused by oral administration can be minimized by taking with milk or meals.
● Instruct patient to ask for or to take drug before pain is intense.
● Caution ambulatory patient about getting out of bed or walking. Warn outpatient to avoid driving and other hazardous activities that require mental alertness until drug's CNS effects are known.
● Advise patient to avoid alcohol during therapy.

fentanyl citrate
Sublimaze

fentanyl transdermal system
Duragesic-25, Duragesic-50,
Duragesic-75, Duragesic-100

fentanyl transmucosal
Actiq, Fentanyl Oralet

Pregnancy risk category C
Controlled substance schedule II

AVAILABLE FORMS
Injection: 50 mcg/ml
Transdermal system: Patches designed to release 25 mcg, 50 mcg, 75 mcg, or 100 mcg of fentanyl per hour
Transmucosal: (Oralets) 100 mcg, 200 mcg, 300 mcg, 400 mcg; (Actiq) 200 mcg, 400 mcg, 600 mcg, 800 mcg, 1,200 mcg, 1,600 mcg

INDICATIONS & DOSAGES
➤ **Adjunct to general anesthetic—**
Adults: For low-dose therapy, 2 mcg/kg I.V. For moderate-dose therapy, 2 to 20 mcg/kg I.V.; then 25 to 100 mcg I.V., p.r.n. For high-dose therapy, 20 to 50 mcg/kg I.V.; then 25 mcg to one-half initial loading dose I.V., p.r.n.
➤ **Adjunct to regional anesthesia—**
Adults: 50 to 100 mcg I.M. or slowly I.V. over 1 to 2 minutes, p.r.n.
➤ **Induction and maintenance of anesthesia—**
Children ages 2 to 12: 2 to 3 mcg/kg I.V.
➤ **Postoperatively—**
Adults: 50 to 100 mcg I.M. q 1 to 2 hours, p.r.n.
➤ **Preoperatively—**
Adults: 50 to 100 mcg I.M. 30 to 60 minutes before surgery. Or, 5 mcg/kg dispensed as Oralet unit, 20 to 40 minutes before need of desired effects.
➤ **Management of chronic pain—**
Adults: One transdermal system applied to a portion of the upper torso on an area of skin that isn't irritated and hasn't been irradiated. Therapy initiated with the 25-mcg/hour system; dosage adjusted as needed and tolerated. Each system may be worn for 72 hours, although some patients may need systems to be applied q 48

hours. Upward adjustment may be done q 3 days after initial dose; then 6 days thereafter.
➤ **Management of breakthrough cancer pain in patients who are already receiving and are tolerant to opioid therapy for their underlying persistent cancer pain (Actiq ONLY)—**
Adults: 200 mcg initially; may give second Actiq dose 15 minutes after completion of the first (30 minutes after first lozenge placed in mouth). Maximum dose is 2 lozenges per breakthrough episode. If several episodes of breakthrough pain occur requiring 2 lozenges, dose may be increased to the next available strength. Once a successful dosage has been reached, patient should limit use of lozenges to no more than 4 daily.

I.V. ADMINISTRATION
● Only staff trained in administration of I.V. anesthetics and management of their potential adverse effects should administer I.V. fentanyl. Inject slowly over 1 to 2 minutes.
● Drug is often used I.V. with droperidol to produce neuroleptanalgesia.
● Keep narcotic antagonist (naloxone) and resuscitation equipment available when giving drug I.V.

ACTION
Unknown. Binds with opiate receptors in the CNS, altering both perception of and emotional response to pain.

Route	Onset	Peak	Duration
I.M.	7-15 min	20-30 min	1-2 hr
I.V.	1-2 min	3-5 min	0.5-1 hr
Transdermal	12-24 hr	1-3 days	Variable
Transmucosal	5-15 min	20-30 min	Unknown

ADVERSE REACTIONS
CNS: *sedation, somnolence, clouded sensorium, euphoria,* dizziness, headache, *confusion, asthenia,* nervousness, hallucinations, anxiety, depression, *seizures.*
CV: hypotension, hypertension, *arrhythmias,* chest pain.
GI: nausea, vomiting, constipation, ileus, abdominal pain, dry mouth, anorexia, diarrhea, dyspepsia.

Reactions may be *common,* uncommon, *life-threatening,* or COMMON AND LIFE-THREATENING.

GU: urine retention.
Respiratory: *respiratory depression,* hypoventilation, dyspnea, *apnea.*
Skin: reaction at application site, *pruritus, diaphoresis.*
Other: physical dependence.

INTERACTIONS
Drug-drug. *CNS depressants, general anesthetics, hypnotics, MAO inhibitors, other narcotic analgesics, sedatives, TCAs:* Additive effects. Use together with extreme caution. Reduce fentanyl dose by one-quarter to one-third; also give above drugs in reduced dosages.
Diazepam: CV depression when given with high doses of fentanyl. Monitor patient closely.
Droperidol: Hypotension and decreased pulmonary arterial pressure. Use together cautiously.
Drug-lifestyle. *Alcohol use:* Additive effects. Discourage use together.

EFFECTS ON LAB TEST RESULTS
None reported.

CONTRAINDICATIONS
Contraindicated in patients with known intolerance to drug. Fentanyl patch is contraindicated for pain management after surgery, mild or intermittent pain that can be managed with nonnarcotic drugs, or in doses exceeding 25 mcg/hour initially. Actiq is contraindicated in management of acute or postoperative pain.

NURSING CONSIDERATIONS
• Use with caution in patients with head injury, increased CSF pressure, COPD, decreased respiratory reserve, potentially compromised respirations, hepatic or renal disease, and cardiac bradyarrhythmias. Also use with caution in elderly or debilitated patients.
• For better analgesic effect, give drug before patient has intense pain.
• *Alert:* High doses can produce muscle rigidity, which can be reversed with neuromuscular blockers; however, patient must be artificially ventilated.
• Monitor circulatory and respiratory status and urinary function carefully. Drug may cause respiratory depression, hypotension, urine retention, nausea, vomiting,

ileus, or altered level of consciousness without regard to route of administration.
• Periodically monitor postoperative vital signs and bladder function. Because drug decreases both rate and depth of respirations, monitoring of arterial oxygen saturation (SaO_2) may help assess respiratory depression. Immediately report respiratory rate below 12 breaths/minute, decreased respiratory volume, or decreased SaO_2.
Transdermal form
• Transdermal fentanyl isn't recommended for postoperative pain.
• Don't give transdermal fentanyl to patients younger than age 12 or those younger than age 18 who weigh less than 110 lb (50 kg).
• Dosage equivalent charts are available to calculate the fentanyl transdermal dose based on the daily morphine intake; for example, for every 90 mg of oral morphine or 15 mg of I.M. morphine per 24 hours, 25 mcg/hour of transdermal fentanyl is needed.
• Dosage adjustments in patient using the transdermal system should be made gradually. Reaching steady-state levels of a new dosage may take up to 6 days; delay dosage adjustment until after at least two applications.
• Monitor patient who develops adverse reactions to the transdermal system for at least 12 hours after removal. Fentanyl levels drop gradually and may take as long as 17 hours to decline by 50%.
• Most patients experience good control of pain for 3 days while wearing the transdermal system, but a few may need a new application after 48 hours.
• Because serum fentanyl level rises for the first 24 hours after application, analgesic effect can't be evaluated on the first day. Be sure patient has adequate supplemental analgesic to prevent breakthrough pain.
• When reducing opiate therapy or switching to a different analgesic, the transdermal system should be withdrawn gradually. Because fentanyl's serum level drops gradually after removal, give half of the equianalgesic dose of the new analgesic 12 to 18 hours after removal.
Transmucosal form
• *Alert:* Actiq is only indicated for management of breakthrough cancer pain in

patients who are already receiving and are tolerant to opioid therapy for their underlying persistent cancer pain.
● Remove foil overwrap of Fentanyl Oralet just before administration.
● Have patient place the Fentanyl Oralet in mouth and suck (not chew or swallow) it.
● Remove Fentanyl Oralet unit (using the handle) after it has been consumed, when patient shows adequate effect, or if patient shows signs of respiratory depression. Place any remaining portion in the plastic overwrap provided, and dispose accordingly for Schedule II drugs.
● Use of Actiq is similar; lozenge is placed between the cheek and gum and may occasionally be moved from side to side using the stick. The Actiq lozenge should be consumed over about 15 minutes.
● *Alert:* Don't confuse fentanyl with alfentanil.

PATIENT TEACHING
● When using drug for pain control, instruct patient to ask for drug before pain becomes intense.
● When drug is used postoperatively, encourage patient to turn, cough, and breathe deeply to prevent atelectasis.
● Instruct patient to avoid hazardous activities until CNS effects subside.
● Tell home care patient to avoid drinking alcohol or taking other CNS-type drugs while receiving fentanyl because additive effects can occur.
● Teach patient about proper application of prescribed transdermal patch. Tell patient to clip hair at application site, but not to use a razor, which may irritate skin. Wash area with clear water, if needed, but not with soaps, oils, lotions, alcohol, or other substances that may irritate skin or prevent adhesion. Dry area completely before application.
● Tell patient to remove transdermal system from package just before applying, hold in place for 30 seconds, and be sure the edges of patch adhere to skin.
● Teach patient to dispose of the transdermal patch by folding so the adhesive side adheres to itself and then flushing it down the toilet.
● Tell patient that, if another patch is needed after 48 to 72 hours, he should apply it to a new site.

● Inform patient that heat from fever or environment, such as from heating pads, electric blankets, heat lamps, hot tubs, or water beds, may increase transdermal delivery and cause toxicity requiring dosage adjustment. Instruct patient to notify prescriber if fever occurs or if he'll be spending time in a hot climate.
● *Alert:* Warn patient and patient's family that the amount of fentanyl in one Actiq lozenge can be fatal to a child.
● Keep well secured and out of children's reach.

---

hydromorphone hydrochloride (dihydromorphinone hydrochloride)
CD Palladone§, CD Palladone SR§, Dilaudid, Dilaudid-5, Dilaudid-HP

Pregnancy risk category C
Controlled substance schedule II

AVAILABLE FORMS
Injection: 1 mg/ml, 2 mg/ml, 3 mg/ml, 4 mg/ml, 10 mg/ml
Liquid: 5 mg/5 ml
Suppositories: 3 mg
Syrup: 1 mg/5 ml**
Tablets: 1 mg, 2 mg, 3 mg, 4 mg, 8 mg

INDICATIONS & DOSAGES
➤ **Moderate to severe pain—**
Adults: 2 to 4 mg P.O. q 4 to 6 hours, p.r.n. Or, 1 to 4 mg I.M., S.C., or I.V. (slowly over at least 2 to 5 minutes) q 4 to 6 hours, p.r.n. Or, 3 mg P.R. suppository q 6 to 8 hours, p.r.n.
➤ **Cough—**
Adults and children older than age 12: 1 tsp (5 ml) P.O. q 3 to 4 hours, p.r.n.

I.V. ADMINISTRATION
● Give by direct injection over no less than 2 minutes.
● For infusion, drug may be mixed in D_5W, normal saline solution, dextrose 5% in normal saline solution, dextrose 5% in half-normal saline solution, or Ringer's or lactated Ringer's solutions.

Reactions may be *common*, uncommon, *life-threatening*, or COMMON AND LIFE-THREATENING.

• Respiratory depression and hypotension can occur with I.V. administration. Give very slowly, and monitor patient constantly. Keep resuscitation equipment available.

ACTION
Unknown. Binds with opiate receptors in the CNS, altering both perception of and emotional response to pain. Also suppresses the cough reflex by direct action on the cough center in the medulla.

Route	Onset	Peak	Duration
I.M.	15 min	0.5-1 hr	4-5 hr
I.V.	10-15 min	15-30 min	2-3 hr
P.O.	30 min	1.5-2 hr	4 hr
P.R.	Unknown	Unknown	4 hr
S.C.	15 min	0.5-1.5 hr	4 hr

ADVERSE REACTIONS
CNS: sedation, somnolence, clouded sensorium, dizziness, euphoria.
CV: hypotension, *bradycardia.*
EENT: blurred vision, diplopia, nystagmus.
GI: nausea, vomiting, constipation, ileus.
GU: urine retention.
Respiratory: *respiratory depression, bronchospasm.*
Other: induration with repeated S.C. injections, physical dependence.

INTERACTIONS
Drug-drug. *CNS depressants, general anesthetics, hypnotics, MAO inhibitors, other narcotic analgesics, sedatives, tranquilizers, TCAs:* Additive effects. Use together with extreme caution. Reduce hydromorphone dose and monitor patient response.
Drug-lifestyle. *Alcohol use:* Additive effects. Advise patient to use together cautiously.

EFFECTS ON LAB TEST RESULTS
• May increase amylase and lipase levels.

CONTRAINDICATIONS
Contraindicated in patients hypersensitive to drug and in those with intracranial lesions that cause increased intracranial pressure; also contraindicated whenever ventilator function is depressed, such as in

status asthmaticus, COPD, cor pulmonale, emphysema, and kyphoscoliosis.

NURSING CONSIDERATIONS
• Use with extreme caution in elderly or debilitated patients and in those with hepatic or renal disease, hypothyroidism, Addison's disease, prostatic hyperplasia, or urethral stricture.
• For better analgesic effect, give drug before patient has intense pain.
• Dilaudid-HP, a highly concentrated form (10 mg/ml), may be administered in smaller volumes to prevent the discomfort of large-volume I.M. or S.C. injections. Check dosage carefully.
• Rotate injection sites to avoid induration with S.C. injection.
• Monitor respiratory and circulatory status and bowel function.
• Keep narcotic antagonist (naloxone) available.
• Drug may delay gastric emptying; increased biliary tract pressure resulting from contraction of the sphincter of Oddi may interfere with hepatobiliary imaging studies.
• Drug may worsen or mask gallbladder pain.
• Drug is a commonly abused narcotic.
• *Alert:* Don't confuse hydromorphone with morphine or Dilaudid with Dilantin.

PATIENT TEACHING
• Instruct patient to ask for or take drug before pain becomes intense.
• Tell patient to store suppositories in refrigerator.
• Advise patient to take drug with food if GI upset occurs.
• When drug is used postoperatively, encourage patient to turn, cough, and deep-breathe to avoid atelectasis.
• Caution ambulatory patient about getting out of bed or walking. Warn outpatient to avoid hazardous activities that require mental alertness until drug's CNS effects are known.
• Advise patient to avoid alcohol during therapy.

meperidine hydrochloride (pethidine hydrochloride)
CD Pamergan-P 100§, CD Pathidine§, Demerol

Pregnancy risk category B (D if used for prolonged periods or in high doses at term)
Controlled substance schedule II

Route	Onset	Peak	Duration
I.M.	10-15 min	30-50 min	2-4 hr
I.V.	1 min	5-7 min	2-4 hr
P.O.	15 min	1-1.5 hr	2-4 hr
S.C.	10-15 min	40-60 min	2-4 hr

AVAILABLE FORMS
Injection: 10 mg/ml, 25 mg/ml, 50 mg/ml, 75 mg/ml, 100 mg/ml
Syrup: 50 mg/5 ml
Tablets: 50 mg, 100 mg

INDICATIONS & DOSAGES
➤ **Moderate to severe pain—**
Adults: 50 to 150 mg P.O., I.M., or S.C. q 3 to 4 hours, p.r.n.
Children: 1.1 to 1.8 mg/kg P.O., I.M., or S.C. q 3 to 4 hours. Maximum, 100 mg q 4 hours, p.r.n.
➤ **Preoperatively—**
Adults: 50 to 100 mg I.M. or S.C. 30 to 90 minutes before surgery.
Children: 1 to 2 mg/kg I.M. or S.C. up to the adult dose 30 to 90 minutes before surgery.
➤ **Adjunct to anesthesia—**
Adults: Repeated slow I.V. injections of fractional doses (10 mg/ml). Or, continuous I.V. infusion of a more dilute solution (1 mg/ml) titrated to patient's needs.
➤ **Obstetric analgesia—**
Adults: 50 to 100 mg I.M. or S.C. when pain becomes regular; repeated at 1- to 3-hour intervals.

I.V. ADMINISTRATION
● Keep narcotic antagonist (naloxone) available when giving this drug I.V.
● Give drug slowly by direct I.V. injection.
● Meperidine also may be given by slow continuous I.V. infusion. Drug is compatible with most I.V. solutions, including D_5W, normal saline solution, and Ringer's or lactated Ringer's solutions.

ACTION
Unknown. Binds with opiate receptors in the CNS, altering both perception of and emotional response to pain.

ADVERSE REACTIONS
CNS: physical dependence, *sedation, somnolence, clouded sensorium, euphoria,* paradoxical anxiety, tremor, *dizziness, seizures,* headache, hallucinations, syncope, *light-headedness.*
CV: hypotension, **bradycardia,** tachycardia, **cardiac arrest, shock.**
GI: constipation, ileus, dry mouth, *nausea, vomiting,* biliary tract spasms.
GU: urine retention.
Musculoskeletal: muscle twitching.
Respiratory: *respiratory depression,* respiratory arrest.
Skin: pruritus, urticaria, *diaphoresis.*
Other: phlebitis after I.V. delivery, pain at injection site, local tissue irritation, induration.

INTERACTIONS
Drug-drug. *Aminophylline, barbiturates, heparin, methicillin, morphine sulfate, phenytoin, sodium bicarbonate, sulfonamides:* Incompatible when mixed in same I.V. container. Avoid using together. *CNS depressants, general anesthetics, hypnotics, other narcotic analgesics, phenothiazines, sedatives, TCAs:* May cause respiratory depression, hypotension, profound sedation, or coma. Use together with extreme caution. Reduce meperidine dosage.
MAO inhibitors: Increased CNS excitation or depression that can be severe or fatal. Avoid using together.
Phenytoin: Decreased blood meperidine levels. Watch for decreased analgesia.
Drug-lifestyle. *Alcohol use:* Additive effects. Discourage use together.

EFFECTS ON LAB TEST RESULTS
● May increase amylase and lipase levels.

CONTRAINDICATIONS
Contraindicated in patients hypersensitive to drug and in those who have received MAO inhibitors within past 14 days.

Reactions may be *common*, uncommon, **life-threatening**, or COMMON AND LIFE-THREATENING.

NURSING CONSIDERATIONS

• Use with extreme caution in elderly or debilitated patients and in those with increased intracranial pressure, head injury, asthma and other respiratory conditions, supraventricular tachycardias, seizures, acute abdominal conditions, hepatic or renal disease, hypothyroidism, Addison's disease, urethral stricture, and prostatic hyperplasia.

• Drug may be used in some patients who are allergic to morphine.

• S.C. injection isn't recommended because it's very painful. However, it may be suitable for occasional use.

• *Alert:* Oral dose is less than half as effective as parenteral dose. Give I.M., if possible. When changing from parenteral to oral route, dosage should be increased.

• Monitor patient for pain at injection site, local tissue irritation, and induration after S.C. injection.

• Syrup has local anesthetic effect. Give with full glass of water.

• Drug and its active metabolite, normeperidine, accumulate in the body. Watch for increased toxic effect, especially in patients with impaired renal function.

• Because drug toxicity frequently appears after several days of treatment, drug isn't recommended for treatment of chronic pain.

• Monitor respirations of neonates exposed to drug during labor. Have resuscitation equipment and naloxone available.

• Monitor respiratory and CV status carefully. Don't give if respirations are below 12 breaths/minute, if respiratory rate or depth is decreased, or if change in pupils is noted.

• Watch for withdrawal symptoms if drug is stopped abruptly after long-term use.

• Monitor bladder function in postoperative patients.

• Monitor bowel function. Patient may need a laxative or stool softener.

• *Alert:* Don't confuse Demerol with Demulen.

PATIENT TEACHING

• When drug is used postoperatively, encourage patient to turn, cough, and deep-breathe and to use an incentive spirometer to prevent atelectasis.

• Caution ambulatory patient about getting out of bed or walking. Warn outpatient to avoid driving and other potentially hazardous activities that require mental alertness until drug's CNS effects are known.

• Advise patient to avoid alcohol during therapy.

methadone hydrochloride
Dolophine, Methadose, Physeptone‡

Pregnancy risk category C
Controlled substance schedule II

AVAILABLE FORMS
Dispersible tablets (for methadone maintenance therapy): 40 mg
Injection: 10 mg/ml
Oral solution: 5 mg/5 ml, 10 mg/5 ml, 10 mg/10 ml, 10 mg/ml (concentrate)
Tablets: 5 mg, 10 mg

INDICATIONS & DOSAGES
➤ **Severe pain—**
Adults: 2.5 to 10 mg P.O., I.M., or S.C. q 3 to 4 hours, p.r.n.
➤ **Narcotic withdrawal syndrome—**
Adults: 15 to 20 mg P.O. daily (highly individualized—some patients may require up to 40 mg). Maintenance dose is 20 to 120 mg P.O. daily. Dosage adjusted, p.r.n.

ACTION
Unknown. Binds with opiate receptors in the CNS, altering both perception of and emotional response to pain.

Route	Onset	Peak	Duration
I.M., S.C.	10-20 min	1-2 hr	4-5 hr
P.O.	0.5-1 hr	1.5-2 hr	4-6 hr

ADVERSE REACTIONS
CNS: *sedation, somnolence, clouded sensorium,* euphoria, *dizziness,* choreic movements, **seizures,** headache, insomnia, agitation, *light-headedness,* syncope.
CV: hypotension, **bradycardia, shock, cardiac arrest,** palpitations, edema.
EENT: visual disturbances.
GI: *nausea, vomiting,* constipation, ileus, dry mouth, anorexia, biliary tract spasm.
GU: urine retention.

Respiratory: *respiratory depression, respiratory arrest.*
Skin: diaphoresis, pruritus, urticaria.
Other: physical dependence, pain at injection site, tissue irritation, induration, decreased libido.

INTERACTIONS
Drug-drug. *Ammonium chloride, other urine acidifiers, phenytoin:* May reduce methadone effect. Watch for decreased pain control.
CNS depressants, general anesthetics, hypnotics, MAO inhibitors, sedatives, tranquilizers, TCAs: May cause respiratory depression, hypotension, profound sedation, or coma. Use together with extreme caution. Monitor patient response.
Rifampin: Withdrawal symptoms; reduced blood levels of methadone. Use together cautiously.
Drug-lifestyle. *Alcohol use:* Additive effects. Discourage use together.

EFFECTS ON LAB TEST RESULTS
● May increase amylase levels.

CONTRAINDICATIONS
Contraindicated in patients hypersensitive to drug.

NURSING CONSIDERATIONS
● Use with extreme caution in elderly or debilitated patients and in those with acute abdominal conditions, severe hepatic or renal impairment, hypothyroidism, Addison's disease, prostatic hyperplasia, urethral stricture, head injury, increased intracranial pressure, asthma, and other respiratory conditions.
● When used in narcotic withdrawal syndrome, daily doses of more than 120 mg require special state and federal approval.
● Oral liquid form legally required in maintenance programs. Completely dissolve tablets in one-half cup of orange juice or powdered citrus drink.
● For parenteral use, I.M. injection is preferred. Rotate injection sites.
● Monitor patient for pain at injection site, tissue irritation, and induration after S.C. injection.
● Oral dose is half as potent as injected dose.

● An around-the-clock regimen is needed to manage severe, chronic pain.
● Patient treated for narcotic withdrawal syndrome usually will need an additional analgesic if pain control is needed.
● Monitor patient closely because drug has cumulative effect; marked sedation can occur after repeated doses.
● Monitor circulatory and respiratory status and bladder and bowel function. Patient may need a laxative.
● When used as an adjunct in the treatment of narcotic addiction (maintenance), withdrawal usually will be delayed and mild.

PATIENT TEACHING
● Caution ambulatory patient about getting out of bed or walking. Warn outpatient to avoid hazardous activities that require mental alertness until drug's CNS effects are known.
● Instruct patient to increase fluid and fiber in diet, if not contraindicated, to combat constipation.
● Advise patient to avoid alcohol during therapy.

---

morphine hydrochloride
Morphitec†, M.O.S.†, M.O.S.-S.R.†

morphine sulfate
Anamorph‡, Astramorph PF, CD Morcap SR§, CD MST Continus§, CD Sevredol§, CD Zomorph§, Duramorph, Epimorph†, Infumorph, Infumorph 500, Morphine H.P.†, MS Contin, MSIR, MS/L, OMS Concentrate, Oramorph SR, RMS Uniserts, Roxanol, Roxanol 100, Roxanol Rescudose, Roxanol UD, Statex

morphine tartrate‡

Pregnancy risk category C
Controlled substance schedule II

AVAILABLE FORMS
morphine hydrochloride
Oral solution: 1 mg/ml†, 5 mg/ml†, 10 mg/ml†, 20 mg/ml†, 50 mg/ml†
Suppositories: 10 mg†, 20 mg†, 30 mg†

Syrup: 1 mg/ml†, 5 mg/ml†, 10 mg/ml†, 20 mg/ml†, 50 mg/ml†
Tablets: 10 mg†, 20 mg†, 40 mg†, 60 mg†
Tablets (extended-release): 30 mg†, 60 mg†
morphine sulfate
Injection (with preservative): 0.5 mg/ml, 1 mg/ml, 2 mg/ml, 3 mg/ml, 4 mg/ml, 5 mg/ml, 8 mg/ml, 10 mg/ml, 15 mg/ml, 25 mg/ml, 50 mg/ml
Injection (without preservative): 0.5 mg/ml, 1 mg/ml, 10 mg/ml, 25 mg/ml
Oral solution: 10 mg/5 ml, 20 mg/5 ml, 20 mg/ml (concentrate), 100 mg/5 ml
Soluble tablets: 10 mg, 15 mg, 30 mg
Suppositories: 5 mg, 10 mg, 20 mg, 30 mg
Syrup: 1 mg/ml, 5 mg/ml
Tablets: 15 mg, 30 mg
Tablets (extended-release): 15 mg, 30 mg, 60 mg, 100 mg, 200 mg
morphine tartrate
Injection: 80 mg/ml‡

INDICATIONS & DOSAGES
➤ **Severe pain—**
Adults: 5 to 20 mg S.C. or I.M. or 2.5 to 15 mg I.V. q 4 hours, p.r.n. Or, 10 to 30 mg P.O. or 10 to 20 mg P.R. q 4 hours, p.r.n. When given by continuous I.V. infusion, a loading dose of 15 mg I.V. may be followed by a continuous infusion of 0.8 to 10 mg/hour. Fifteen- to 30-mg extended-release tablets P.O. q 8 to 12 hours may also be given. As an epidural injection, 5 mg by epidural catheter; then, if adequate pain relief not obtained within 1 hour, additional doses of 1 to 2 mg given at intervals sufficient to assess efficacy. Maximum total epidural dose shouldn't exceed 10 mg/24 hours. As an intrathecal injection, a single dose of 0.2 to 1 mg may provide pain relief for 24 hours (only in the lumbar area). Repeat injections not recommended.
Children: 0.1 to 0.2 mg/kg S.C. or I.M. q 4 hours. Maximum single dose is 15 mg.

I.V. ADMINISTRATION
● When given by direct injection, 2.5 to 15 mg may be diluted in 4 or 5 ml of sterile water for injection and given over 4 to 5 minutes.

● For continuous infusion, drug may be mixed with D_5W to a concentration of 0.1 to 1 mg/ml and administered by a continuous infusion device.
● Morphine sulfate is compatible with most common I.V. solutions.

ACTION
Unknown. Binds with opiate receptors in the CNS, altering both perception of and emotional response to pain.

Route	Onset	Peak	Duration
Epidural	15-60 min	15-60 min	24 hr
I.M.	10-30 min	30-60 min	4-5 hr
Intrathecal	15-60 min	30-60 min	24 hr
I.V.	5 min	20 min	4-5 hr
P.O.	1 hr	1-2 hr	4-12 hr
P.R.	20-30 min	20-60 min	4-5 hr
S.C.	10-30 min	50-90 min	4-5 hr

ADVERSE REACTIONS
CNS: *sedation, somnolence, clouded sensorium, euphoria, **seizures,** dizziness, nightmares,* physical dependence, *lightheadedness,* hallucinations, nervousness, depression, syncope.
CV: hypotension, ***bradycardia, shock, cardiac arrest,*** tachycardia, hypertension.
GI: *nausea, vomiting, constipation,* ileus, dry mouth, biliary tract spasms, anorexia.
GU: urine retention.
Hematologic: ***thrombocytopenia.***
Respiratory: ***respiratory depression, apnea, respiratory arrest.***
Skin: pruritus and skin flushing, diaphoresis, edema.
Other: decreased libido.

INTERACTIONS
Drug-drug. *CNS depressants, general anesthetics, hypnotics, MAO inhibitors, other narcotic analgesics, sedatives, tranquilizers, TCAs:* May cause respiratory depression, hypotension, profound sedation, or coma. Use together with extreme caution. Reduce morphine dose and monitor patient response.
Drug-lifestyle. *Alcohol use:* Additive effects. Advise patient to use together cautiously.

EFFECTS ON LAB TEST RESULTS
● May increase amylase levels.
● May decrease platelet count.

CONTRAINDICATIONS
Contraindicated in patients hypersensitive to drug and in those with conditions that would preclude administration of opioids by I.V. route (acute bronchial asthma or upper airway obstruction).

NURSING CONSIDERATIONS
• Use with extreme caution in elderly or debilitated patients and in those with head injury, increased intracranial pressure, seizures, chronic pulmonary disease, prostatic hyperplasia, severe hepatic or renal disease, acute abdominal conditions, hypothyroidism, Addison's disease, and urethral stricture.
• Keep narcotic antagonist (naloxone) and resuscitation equipment available.
• Oral solutions of various concentrations and an intensified oral solution (20 mg/ml) are available. Carefully note the strength administered.
• Don't crush, break, or chew extended-release tablets.
• Oral capsules may be carefully opened and the entire bead contents poured into cool, soft foods, such as water, orange juice, applesauce, or pudding; mixture should be consumed immediately.
• S.L. administration may be ordered. Measure oral solution with tuberculin syringe. Administer dose a few drops at a time to allow maximal S.L. absorption and minimize swallowing.
• Refrigeration of rectal suppository isn't needed. In some patients, rectal and oral absorption may not be equivalent.
• Preservative-free preparations are available for epidural and intrathecal administration.
• When given epidurally, monitor patient closely for respiratory depression up to 24 hours after the injection. Check respiratory rate and depth every 30 to 60 minutes for 24 hours.
• Watch for pruritus and skin flushing with epidural administration.
• Morphine is drug of choice in relieving MI pain; may cause transient decrease in blood pressure.
• An around-the-clock regimen best manages severe, chronic pain.
• Morphine may worsen or mask gallbladder pain.

• Monitor circulatory, respiratory, bladder, and bowel functions carefully. Drug may cause respiratory depression, hypotension, urine retention, nausea, vomiting, ileus, or altered level of consciousness regardless of the route used. Withhold dose and notify prescriber if respirations are below 12 breaths/minute.
• Constipation is commonly severe with maintenance dose. Ensure that stool softener or other laxative is ordered.
• *Alert:* Don't confuse morphine with hydromorphone.

PATIENT TEACHING
• When drug is used postoperatively, encourage patient to turn, cough, and deep-breathe and to use incentive spirometer to prevent atelectasis.
• Caution ambulatory patient about getting out of bed or walking. Warn outpatient to avoid driving and other potentially hazardous activities that require mental alertness until drug's adverse CNS effects are known.
• Advise patient to avoid alcohol during therapy.

---

nalbuphine hydrochloride
Nubain

Pregnancy risk category B

AVAILABLE FORMS
Injection: 10 mg/ml, 20 mg/ml

INDICATIONS & DOSAGES
➤ **Moderate to severe pain—**
Adults: For an average-weight (70-kg [154 lb]) person, 10 to 20 mg S.C., I.M., or I.V. q 3 to 6 hours, p.r.n. Maximum, 160 mg daily.
➤ **Adjunct to balanced anesthesia—**
Adults: 0.3 mg/kg to 3.0 mg/kg I.V. over 10 to 15 minutes; then maintenance doses of 0.25 to 0.50 mg/kg in single I.V. dose, p.r.n.

I.V. ADMINISTRATION
• Inject slowly over at least 2 to 3 minutes into a vein or into an I.V. line containing a compatible, free-flowing I.V. solution, such as D_5W, normal saline solution, or lactated Ringer's solution.

Reactions may be *common*, uncommon, *life-threatening*, or COMMON AND LIFE-THREATENING.

• Respiratory depression can be reversed with naloxone. Keep resuscitation equipment available, particularly when administering I.V.

ACTION

Unknown. Binds with opiate receptors in the CNS, altering both perception of and emotional response to pain.

Route	Onset	Peak	Duration
I.M.	15 min	1 hr	3-6 hr
I.V.	2-3 min	30 min	3-6 hr
S.C.	15 min	Unknown	3-6 hr

ADVERSE REACTIONS

CNS: *headache, sedation, dizziness, vertigo,* nervousness, depression, restlessness, crying, euphoria, hostility, unusual dreams, confusion, hallucinations, speech disorders, delusions.
CV: hypertension, hypotension, tachycardia, *bradycardia.*
EENT: blurred vision, dry mouth.
GI: cramps, dyspepsia, bitter taste, nausea, vomiting, constipation, biliary tract spasms.
GU: urinary urgency.
Respiratory: *respiratory depression,* dyspnea, asthma, *pulmonary edema.*
Skin: pruritus, burning, urticaria, clamminess.

INTERACTIONS

Drug-drug. *CNS depressants, general anesthetics, hypnotics, MAO inhibitors, sedatives, tranquilizers, TCAs:* May cause respiratory depression, hypertension, profound sedation, or coma. Use together with extreme caution. Monitor patient response.
Narcotic analgesics: May decrease analgesic effect. Avoid using together.
Drug-lifestyle. *Alcohol use:* Additive effects. Discourage use together.

EFFECTS ON LAB TEST RESULTS

None reported.

CONTRAINDICATIONS

Contraindicated in patients hypersensitive to drug.

NURSING CONSIDERATIONS

• Use cautiously in patients with history of drug abuse and in those with emotional instability, head injury, increased intracranial pressure, impaired ventilation, MI accompanied by nausea and vomiting, upcoming biliary surgery, and hepatic or renal disease.
• Drug acts as a narcotic antagonist; may precipitate withdrawal syndrome. For patients who have received opiates longterm, administer 25% of the usual dose initially. Watch for signs of withdrawal.
• *Alert:* Drug causes respiratory depression, which at 10 mg is equal to respiratory depression produced by 10 mg of morphine.
• Monitor circulatory and respiratory status and bladder and bowel function. Withhold dose and notify prescriber if respirations are shallow or rate is below 12 breaths/minute.
• Constipation is often severe with maintenance therapy. Make sure stool softener or other laxative is ordered.
• Psychological and physical dependence may occur with prolonged use.
• *Alert:* Don't confuse Nubain with Navane.

PATIENT TEACHING

• Caution ambulatory patient about getting out of bed or walking. Warn outpatient to avoid driving and other hazardous activities that require mental alertness until drug's CNS effects are known.
• Teach patient how to manage troublesome adverse effects such as constipation.

---

oxycodone hydrochloride
Endocodone, Endone‡, OxyContin, OxyIR, Roxicodone, Roxicodone Intensol, Supeudol†

oxycodone pectinate
Proladone‡

Pregnancy risk category C
Controlled substance schedule II

AVAILABLE FORMS
oxycodone hydrochloride
Capsules: 5 mg

Oral solution: 5 mg/5 ml, 20 mg/ml (concentrate)
Suppositories: 10 mg†, 20 mg†
Tablets: 5 mg
Tablets (controlled-release): 10 mg, 20 mg, 40 mg, 80 mg, 160 mg
oxycodone pectinate
Suppositories: 30 mg‡

INDICATIONS & DOSAGES
➤ **Moderate to severe pain—**
Adults: 5 mg P.O. q 6 hours, p.r.n. Or, 1 to 3 suppositories P.R. daily, p.r.n. Or, 10 mg (controlled-release tablets) P.O. q 12 hours, p.r.n., for patients not currently receiving opiates.

ACTION
Unknown. Binds with opiate receptors in the CNS, altering both perception of and emotional response to pain.

Route	Onset	Peak	Duration
P.O.	10-15 min	1 hr	3-6 hr
P.R.	Unknown	Unknown	Unknown

ADVERSE REACTIONS
CNS: sedation, somnolence, clouded sensorium, euphoria, dizziness, lightheadedness, physical dependence.
CV: hypotension, ***bradycardia.***
GI: *nausea, vomiting,* constipation, ileus.
GU: urine retention.
Respiratory: *respiratory depression.*
Skin: diaphoresis, pruritus.

INTERACTIONS
Drug-drug. *Anticoagulants:* Oxycodone hydrochloride products containing aspirin may increase anticoagulant effect. Monitor clotting times. Use together cautiously.
CNS depressants, general anesthetics, hypnotics, MAO inhibitors, other narcotic analgesics, sedatives, tranquilizers, TCAs: Additive effects. Use together with extreme caution. Reduce oxycodone dose and monitor patient response.
Drug-lifestyle. *Alcohol use:* Additive effects. Advise patient to use together cautiously.

EFFECTS ON LAB TEST RESULTS
• May increase amylase and lipase levels.

CONTRAINDICATIONS
Contraindicated in patients hypersensitive to drug and in those suspected of having paralytic ileus.

NURSING CONSIDERATIONS
• Use with extreme caution in elderly and debilitated patients and in those with head injury, increased intracranial pressure, seizures, asthma, COPD, prostatic hyperplasia, severe hepatic or renal disease, acute abdominal conditions, urethral stricture, hypothyroidism, Addison's disease, and arrhythmias.
• For full analgesic effect, administer drug before patient has intense pain.
• To minimize GI upset, administer drug after meals or with milk.
• Single-drug oxycodone solution or tablets are especially useful for patients who shouldn't take aspirin or acetaminophen.
• Monitor circulatory and respiratory status. Withhold dose and notify prescriber if respirations are shallow or if respiratory rate falls below 12 breaths/minute.
• Monitor patient's bladder and bowel patterns. Patient may need a laxative because drug has a constipating effect.
• The 80-mg controlled-release tablet should be reserved for opioid-dependent patients who are taking daily doses of 160 mg or more.
• For patients who are taking more than 60 mg daily, dosing should be tapered when discontinued to prevent withdrawal.

PATIENT TEACHING
• Instruct patient to ask for drug before pain is intense.
• Tell patient to take drug with milk or after eating.
• Advise patient to swallow extended-release tablets whole.
• Caution ambulatory patient about getting out of bed or walking. Warn outpatient to avoid driving and other hazardous activities that require mental alertness until drug's CNS effects are known.
• Advise patient to avoid alcohol during therapy.
• Tell patient not to stop drug abruptly.

---

oxymorphone hydrochloride
Numorphan

Pregnancy risk category C (D if used for prolonged periods or high doses at term)
Controlled substance schedule II

AVAILABLE FORMS
Injection: 1 mg/ml, 1.5 mg/ml
Suppositories: 5 mg

INDICATIONS & DOSAGES
➤ **Moderate to severe pain—**
Adults: 1 to 1.5 mg I.M. or S.C. q 4 to 6 hours, p.r.n. Or, 0.5 mg I.V. q 4 to 6 hours, p.r.n. Or, 5 mg P.R. q 4 to 6 hours, p.r.n.
➤ **Analgesia during labor—**
Adults: 0.5 to 1 mg I.M.

I.V. ADMINISTRATION
• Give drug by direct I.V. injection. If necessary, drug may be diluted in normal saline solution.

ACTION
Unknown. Binds with opiate receptors in the CNS, altering both perception of and emotional response to pain.

Route	Onset	Peak	Duration
I.M.	10-15 min	0.5-1.5 hr	3-6 hr
I.V.	5-10 min	15-30 min	3-4 hr
P.R.	15-30 min	2 hr	3-6 hr
S.C.	10-20 min	1-1.5 hr	3-6 hr

ADVERSE REACTIONS
CNS: *sedation, somnolence, clouded sensorium, euphoria,* dizziness, **seizures,** physical dependence, light-headedness, headache.
CV: *hypotension,* **bradycardia.**
GI: *nausea, vomiting, constipation,* ileus.
GU: *urine retention.*
Respiratory: *respiratory depression.*
Skin: pruritus.

INTERACTIONS
Drug-drug. *CNS depressants, general anesthetics, MAO inhibitors, phenothiazines, sedative hypnotics, TCAs:* Additive effects. Use together with extreme caution.

Drug-lifestyle. *Alcohol use:* Additive effects. Discourage use together.

EFFECTS ON LAB TEST RESULTS
• May increase amylase levels.

CONTRAINDICATIONS
Contraindicated in patients hypersensitive to drug and in those with acute asthma attacks, severe respiratory depression, upper airway obstruction, or paralytic ileus. Don't use to treat pulmonary edema caused by a respiratory irritant.

NURSING CONSIDERATIONS
• Use with extreme caution in elderly or debilitated patients and in those with head injury, increased intracranial pressure, seizures, asthma, COPD, acute abdominal conditions, prostatic hyperplasia, severe hepatic or renal disease, urethral stricture, respiratory depression, hypothyroidism, Addison's disease, and arrhythmias.
• Keep narcotic antagonist (naloxone) and resuscitation equipment available.
• Drug isn't for mild pain. May worsen gallbladder pain.
• For better effect, administer drug before patient has intense pain.
• Monitor CV and respiratory status. Withhold dose and notify prescriber if respirations decrease or rate is below 12 breaths/minute.
• Monitor patient's bladder and bowel function. Patient may need laxative.
• *Alert:* Don't confuse oxymorphone with oxymetholone.

PATIENT TEACHING
• Instruct patient to ask for drug before pain is intense.
• When drug is used postoperatively, encourage patient to turn, cough, and deep-breathe and to use incentive spirometer to avoid atelectasis.
• Caution ambulatory patient about getting out of bed or walking. Warn outpatient to avoid driving and other hazardous activities that require mental alertness until drug's CNS effects are known.
• Instruct patient to store suppositories in refrigerator.
• Advise patient to avoid alcohol during therapy.

---

*Liquid contains alcohol.   **May contain tartrazine.   †Canada   ‡Australia   §U.K.   ◊OTC

pentazocine hydrochloride
Fortral†‡, Talwin†

**pentazocine hydrochloride
and naloxone hydrochloride**
Talwin NX

pentazocine lactate
Fortral‡, Talwin

Pregnancy risk category C
Controlled substance schedule IV

AVAILABLE FORMS
pentazocine hydrochloride
Tablets: 25 mg‡, 50 mg†‡
**pentazocine hydrochloride and nalox-
one hydrochloride**
Tablets: 50 mg pentazocine hydrochloride
and 500 mcg naloxone hydrochloride
pentazocine lactate
Injection: 30 mg/ml

INDICATIONS & DOSAGES
➤ **Moderate to severe pain—**
Adults: 50 to 100 mg P.O. q 3 to 4 hours,
p.r.n. Maximum oral dose is 600 mg/day.
Or, 30 mg I.M., I.V., or S.C. q 3 to 4 hours,
p.r.n. Maximum parenteral dose is 360
mg/day. Single doses above 30 mg I.V. or
60 mg I.M. or S.C. aren't recommended.
➤ **Labor—**
Adults: 30 mg I.M. or 20 mg I.V. q 2 to 3
hours when contractions become regular.

I.V. ADMINISTRATION
• Give drug by direct I.V. injection slowly.
Don't mix in syringe with aminophylline,
barbiturates, or other alkaline substances.
• Talwin NX, the oral pentazocine available in the United States, contains the narcotic antagonist naloxone. This discour-
ages illicit I.V. use.

ACTION
Unknown. Binds with opiate receptors in
the CNS, altering both perception of and
emotional response to pain.

Route	Onset	Peak	Duration
I.M., S.C.	10-20 min	30-60 min	2-3 hr
I.V.	2-3 min	15-30 min	2-3 hr
P.O.	15-30 min	1-3 hr	2-3 hr

ADVERSE REACTIONS
CNS: *sedation,* visual disturbances, hallucinations, drowsiness, *dizziness, light-
headedness,* confusion, *euphoria,* headache, psychotomimetic effects.
CV: circulatory depression, **shock,** hypertension.
EENT: dry mouth.
GI: *nausea, vomiting,* constipation.
GU: urine retention.
Respiratory: *respiratory depression,* dyspnea, **apnea.**
Skin: induration, nodules, sloughing,
sclerosis at injection site; diaphoresis;
pruritus.
Other: hypersensitivity reactions, **anaphylaxis,** physical and psychological dependence.

INTERACTIONS
Drug-drug. *CNS depressants:* Additive
effects. Use together cautiously.
Fluoxetine: Additive effects resulting in
serotonin syndrome. Use together cautiously.
Narcotic analgesics: May decrease analgesic effect. Avoid using together.
Drug-lifestyle. *Alcohol use:* Additive
effects. Discourage use together.
Smoking: May increase requirements for
pentazocine. Monitor drug's effectiveness.

EFFECTS ON LAB TEST RESULTS
None reported.

CONTRAINDICATIONS
Contraindicated in patients hypersensitive to drug or its components. It isn't
recommended for children younger than
age 12.

NURSING CONSIDERATIONS
• Use cautiously in patients with hepatic
or renal disease, acute MI, head injury, increased intracranial pressure, and respiratory depression.
• Have naloxone readily available. Respiratory depression can be reversed with
naloxone.
• **Alert:** When giving by S.C. or I.M. injection, rotate injection sites to minimize tissue irritation. If possible, avoid giving by
S.C. route.

Reactions may be *common,* uncommon, *life-threatening,* or COMMON AND LIFE-THREATENING.

• Drug has narcotic antagonist properties. May precipitate withdrawal syndrome in narcotic-dependent patients.
• Psychological and physical dependence may occur with prolonged use.
• Drug may interfere with certain laboratory tests for urinary 17-hydroxycorticosteroids.

PATIENT TEACHING
• Instruct patient to ask for drug before pain is intense.
• Caution ambulatory patient about getting out of bed or walking. Warn outpatient to avoid driving and other hazardous activities that require mental alertness until drug's CNS effects are known.
• Advise patient to avoid alcohol during therapy.
• Instruct patient or family to report skin rash, disorientation, or confusion to prescriber.

---

propoxyphene hydrochloride (dextropropoxyphene hydrochloride)
Darvon, 642†

propoxyphene napsylate (dextropropoxyphene napsylate)
Darvon N, Doloxene‡

Pregnancy risk category C
Controlled substance schedule IV

AVAILABLE FORMS
propoxyphene hydrochloride
Capsules: 32 mg, 65 mg
propoxyphene napsylate
Oral suspension: 10 mg/ml
Tablets: 100 mg

INDICATIONS & DOSAGES
➤ **Mild to moderate pain—**
Adults: 65 mg (hydrochloride) P.O. q 4 hours, p.r.n. Maximum dose is 390 mg/day. Or, 100 mg (napsylate) P.O. q 4 hours, p.r.n. Maximum dose is 600 mg/day.
Adjust-a-dose: For patients with hepatic or renal dysfunction, reduce dosage.

ACTION
Unknown. Binds with opiate receptors in the CNS, altering both perception of and emotional response to pain.

Route	Onset	Peak	Duration
P.O.	15-60 min	2-2.5 hr	4-6 hr

ADVERSE REACTIONS
CNS: *dizziness,* headache, *sedation,* euphoria, light-headedness, weakness, hallucinations, psychological and physical dependence.
GI: *nausea, vomiting,* constipation, abdominal pain.
Respiratory: *respiratory depression.*

INTERACTIONS
Drug-drug. *Carbamazepine:* May increase carbamazepine levels. Monitor patient closely.
CNS depressants: Additive effects. Use together cautiously.
TCAs (such as doxepin): Inhibited antidepressant metabolism. Monitor patient for toxicity.
Warfarin: May increase anticoagulant effect. Monitor PT and INR.
Drug-lifestyle. *Alcohol use:* Additive effects. Discourage use together.
Smoking: Increased metabolism of propoxyphene. Monitor patient closely.

EFFECTS ON LAB TEST RESULTS
• Altered liver function test values.

CONTRAINDICATIONS
Contraindicated in patients hypersensitive to drug.

NURSING CONSIDERATIONS
• Use cautiously in hepatic or renal disease, emotional instability, or history of drug or alcohol abuse.
• Sixty-five milligrams of propoxyphene hydrochloride equals 100 mg of propoxyphene napsylate.
• Drug is considered a mild narcotic analgesic, but pain relief is equivalent to that provided by aspirin. Tolerance and physical dependence may occur. Drug is used with aspirin or acetaminophen to maximize analgesia.
• Smokers may need increased dosage because smoking may induce liver enzymes

---

responsible for the metabolism of the drug, thereby decreasing its efficacy.

PATIENT TEACHING
• Advise patient to take drug with food or milk to minimize GI upset.
• Warn patient not to exceed recommended dosage. Respiratory depression, hypotension, profound sedation, and coma may result if used in excessive doses or with other CNS depressants. Advise patient to avoid alcohol or other CNS-type drugs when taking propoxyphene.
• Caution ambulatory patient about getting out of bed or walking. Warn outpatient to avoid driving and other hazardous activities that require mental alertness until drug's CNS effects are known.

---

remifentanil hydrochloride
Ultiva

Pregnancy risk category C
Controlled substance schedule II

AVAILABLE FORMS
Injection (vials): 1 mg/3 ml, 2 mg/5 ml, 5 mg/10 ml

INDICATIONS & DOSAGES
➤ **Induction of anesthesia through intubation—**
Adults: 0.5 to 1 mcg/kg/minute with hypnotic or volatile drug; may load with 1 mcg/kg over 30 to 60 seconds if endotracheal intubation is to occur less than 8 minutes after start of drug infusion.
➤ **Maintenance of anesthesia—**
Adults: 0.25 to 0.4 mcg/kg/minute, dependent on concomitant anesthetics (nitrous oxide, isoflurane, propofol). Increase doses by 25% to 100% and decrease by 25% to 50% q 2 to 5 minutes, p.r.n. If rate exceeds 1 mcg/kg/minute, concomitant anesthetics may be increased. May supplement with 1 mcg/kg boluses over 30 to 60 seconds q 2 to 5 minutes, p.r.n.
➤ **Continuation as analgesic immediately postoperatively—**
Adults: Initially, 0.1 mcg/kg/minute. Adjust rate by 0.025-mcg/kg/minute increments q 5 minutes, p.r.n. Rates over 0.2 mcg/kg/minute may cause respiratory depression (less than 8 breaths/minute).

➤ **Monitored anesthesia care—**
Adults: As single I.V. dose, 0.5 to 1 mcg/kg over 30 to 60 seconds starting 90 seconds before placement of local or regional anesthetic. As continuous I.V. infusion, 0.1 mcg/kg/minute beginning 5 minutes before giving local anesthetic; after placement of local anesthetic, titrate rate to 0.05 mcg/kg/minute. Titrate rate by 0.025 mcg/kg/minute q 5 minutes, p.r.n. Rates over 0.2 mcg/kg/minute may cause respiratory depression (less than 8 breaths/minute).
Elderly patients: Decrease initial dose by 50%.
Adjust-a-dose: For obese patients (more than 30% over ideal body weight), base starting dose on ideal body weight.

I.V. ADMINISTRATION
• To reconstitute solution, add 1 ml of diluent per mg of drug. Shake well to dissolve. Reconstituted solution contains 1 mg/ml and should be clear and colorless.
• Further dilute to 25, 50, or 250 mcg/ml before administration. Drug is stable at room temperature for 24 hours when in final concentration in D_5W, D_5W in normal saline solution, normal saline solution, half-normal saline solution, or D_5W in lactated Ringer's solution. Drug is stable for 4 hours when mixed in lactated Ringer's solution.
• Continuous infusion of drug must be administered by infusion device. When the drug is stopped, clear I.V. tubing to avoid inadvertently giving drug later.
• Hypotension may occur and can be treated by decreasing rate of infusion or administering I.V. fluids or catecholamine.
• I.V. bolus administration should be used only during maintenance of general anesthesia. In nonintubated patients, single doses should be administered over 30 to 60 seconds.

ACTION
Unknown. Binds with μ-opiate receptors in the CNS, altering both perception of and emotional response to pain.

Route	Onset	Peak	Duration
I.V.	Immediate	Unknown	5-10 min

Reactions may be *common*, uncommon, *life-threatening*, or COMMON AND LIFE-THREATENING.

ADVERSE REACTIONS
CNS: agitation, dizziness, headache.
CV: *bradycardia,* hypertension, *hypotension,* tachycardia.
EENT: visual disturbances.
GI: *nausea, vomiting.*
Musculoskeletal: *muscle rigidity.*
Respiratory: *apnea, hypoxia, respiratory depression.*
Skin: flushing, pain at injection site, pruritus, sweating.
Other: chills, fever, postoperative pain, shivering, warm sensation.

INTERACTIONS
Drug-drug. *Benzodiazepine, hypnotics, inhaled anesthetics:* Synergistic effect. Monitor patient closely.

EFFECTS ON LAB TEST RESULTS
None reported.

CONTRAINDICATIONS
Contraindicated in patients hypersensitive to fentanyl analogues. Don't use via epidural or intrathecal routes because of presence of glycine in preparation.

NURSING CONSIDERATIONS
● Use cautiously in breast-feeding women because fentanyl analogues appear in breast milk.
● Monitor vital signs and oxygenation continually during drug administration.
● Don't use as a single drug in general anesthesia.
● When giving drug during monitored anesthesia care, decrease dose by 50% if given with 2 mg midazolam. Bolus doses administered simultaneously with continuously infusing remifentanil to spontaneously breathing patients aren't recommended.
● Manage respiratory depression in spontaneously breathing patients by decreasing infusion rate by 50% or by temporarily discontinuing infusion.
● Skeletal muscle rigidity may occur. To treat, either stop or decrease the rate of infusion in spontaneously breathing patients.
● Effects of long-term (longer than 16 hours) use in intensive care settings aren't known.

● Bradycardia has been reported and responds to ephedrine, atropine, and glycopyrrolate.
● Interruption of drug infusion results in rapid reversal (no residual opioid effects within 5 to 10 minutes of infusion discontinuation) of effects; adequate postoperative anesthesia should first be established.
● Drug shouldn't be used outside the monitored anesthesia care setting. Keep narcotic antagonist (naloxone) and resuscitation equipment available. Naloxone may be used to manage severe respiratory depression.
● Drug is incompatible with blood products.
● Obtain history from patient regarding previous adverse anesthesia reactions in patient or patient's family.

PATIENT TEACHING
● Reassure patient that appropriate monitoring will occur during anesthesia administration.

---

tramadol hydrochloride
Ultram, Zamadol§, Zydol§

Pregnancy risk category C

AVAILABLE FORMS
Tablets: 50 mg

INDICATIONS & DOSAGES
➤ **Moderate to moderately severe pain**—
Adults: 50 to 100 mg P.O. q 4 to 6 hours, p.r.n. Maximum, 400 mg daily.
Elderly patients: For patients older than age 75, maximum is 300 mg daily in divided doses.
Adjust-a-dose: For renally impaired patients with creatinine clearance below 30 ml/minute, increase dose interval to q 12 hours; maximum is 200 mg daily. For patients with cirrhosis, give 50 mg q 12 hours.

ACTION
Unknown. A centrally acting synthetic analgesic compound not chemically related to opiates. Drug is thought to bind to

---

opioid receptors and inhibit reuptake of norepinephrine and serotonin.

Route	Onset	Peak	Duration
P.O.	Unknown	2 hr	Unknown

ADVERSE REACTIONS
CNS: *dizziness, vertigo, headache, somnolence,* CNS stimulation, asthenia, anxiety, confusion, coordination disturbance, euphoria, nervousness, sleep disorder, *seizures,* malaise.
CV: vasodilation.
EENT: visual disturbances.
GI: *nausea, constipation, vomiting,* dyspepsia, dry mouth, diarrhea, abdominal pain, anorexia, flatulence.
GU: urine retention, urinary frequency, menopausal symptoms, proteinuria.
Musculoskeletal: hypertonia.
Respiratory: *respiratory depression.*
Skin: pruritus, diaphoresis, rash.

INTERACTIONS
Drug-drug. *Carbamazepine:* Increased tramadol metabolism. Patients receiving long-term carbamazepine therapy at up to 800 mg daily may need up to twice the recommended dose of tramadol.
CNS depressants: Additive effects. Use together with caution. Dosage of tramadol may need to be reduced.
Cyclobenzaprine, MAO inhibitors, neuroleptics, selective serotonin reuptake inhibitors, TCAs: Increased risk of seizures. Monitor patient closely.
Quinidine: Increased levels of tramadol. Monitor patient closely.
Selective serotonin reuptake inhibitors (sertraline, paroxetine): Increased risk of serotonin syndrome. Monitor patient for adverse effects.

EFFECTS ON LAB TEST RESULTS
• May increase liver enzyme levels.
• May decrease hemoglobin.

CONTRAINDICATIONS
Contraindicated in patients hypersensitive to drug and in those with acute intoxication from alcohol, hypnotics, centrally acting analgesics, opioids, or psychotropic drugs.

NURSING CONSIDERATIONS
• Use cautiously in patients at risk for seizures or respiratory depression; in increased intracranial pressure or head injury, acute abdominal conditions, or renal or hepatic impairment; and in physical dependence on opioids.
• Monitor CV and respiratory status. Withhold dose and notify prescriber if respirations decrease or rate is below 12 breaths/minute.
• Monitor bowel and bladder function. Anticipate need for laxative.
• For better analgesic effect, give drug before onset of intense pain.
• Monitor patients at risk for seizures. Drug may reduce seizure threshold.
• Monitor patient for drug dependence. Drug can produce dependence similar to that of codeine or dextropropoxyphene and thus has potential for abuse.

PATIENT TEACHING
• Tell patient to take drug as prescribed and not to increase dose or dosage interval unless ordered by prescriber.
• Caution ambulatory patient to be careful when rising and walking. Warn outpatient to avoid driving and other potentially hazardous activities that require mental alertness until drug's CNS effects are known.
• Advise patient to check with prescriber before taking OTC drugs; drug interactions can occur.

27

Sedative-hypnotics

chloral hydrate
dexmedetomidine hydrochloride
estazolam
flurazepam hydrochloride
pentobarbital
pentobarbital sodium
phenobarbital sodium
(See Chapter 28, ANTICONVULSANTS.)
secobarbital sodium
temazepam
triazolam
zaleplon
zolpidem tartrate

COMBINATION PRODUCTS

TUINAL 100 mg PULVULES: amobarbital sodium 50 mg and secobarbital sodium 50 mg.
TUINAL 200 mg PULVULES: amobarbital sodium 100 mg and secobarbital sodium 100 mg.

---

chloral hydrate
Aquachloral Supprettes,
Novo-Chlorhydrate†

Pregnancy risk category C
Controlled substance schedule IV

AVAILABLE FORMS
Capsules: 250 mg, 500 mg
Suppositories: 324 mg, 500 mg, 648 mg
Syrup: 250 mg/5 ml, 500 mg/5 ml

INDICATIONS & DOSAGES
➤ Sedation—
Adults: 250 mg P.O. or P.R. t.i.d. after meals.
Children: 25 mg/kg/day P.O. or P.R. Maximum daily dose is 500 mg per single dose; doses may be divided.
➤ Insomnia—
Adults: 500 mg to 1 g P.O. or P.R. 15 to 30 minutes before bedtime.
Children: 50 mg/kg P.O. or P.R. 15 to 30 minutes before bedtime. Maximum single dose is 1 g.

➤ Preoperatively to produce sedation and relieve anxiety—
Adults: 500 mg to 1 g P.O. or P.R. 30 minutes before surgery.
➤ Premedication for EEG—
Children: 20 to 25 mg/kg P.O. or P.R.

ACTION
Unknown. Sedative effects may be caused by drug's main metabolite, trichloroethanol.

Route	Onset	Peak	Duration
P.O.	0.5 hr	Unknown	4-8 hr
P.R.	Unknown	Unknown	4-8 hr

ADVERSE REACTIONS
CNS: drowsiness, nightmares, dizziness, ataxia, paradoxical excitement, hangover, somnolence, disorientation, delirium, light-headedness, hallucinations, confusion, vertigo, malaise, physical and psychological dependence.
GI: *nausea, vomiting, diarrhea,* flatulence.
Hematologic: eosinophilia, *leukopenia.*
Skin: hypersensitivity reactions.

INTERACTIONS
Drug-drug. *CNS depressants, including narcotic analgesics:* Excessive CNS depression or vasodilation reaction. Use together cautiously.
Furosemide I.V.: Sweating, flushes, variable blood pressure, nausea, and uneasiness. Use together cautiously or use a different hypnotic drug.
Oral anticoagulants: Increased risk of bleeding. Monitor patient closely.
Phenytoin: Decreased phenytoin levels. Monitor patient closely.
Drug-lifestyle. *Alcohol use:* Excessive CNS and respiratory depression. Advise patient to avoid use together.

EFFECTS ON LAB TEST RESULTS
• May increase eosinophil count. May decrease WBC count.

---

*Liquid contains alcohol. **May contain tartrazine. †Canada ‡Australia §U.K. ◊OTC

CONTRAINDICATIONS

Contraindicated in patients hypersensitive to drug and in those with hepatic or renal impairment or severe cardiac disease. Oral administration contraindicated in patients with gastric disorders.

NURSING CONSIDERATIONS

• Use with extreme caution in patients with severe cardiac disease. Use cautiously in patients with mental depression, suicidal tendencies, or history of drug abuse.
• *Alert:* Note two strengths of oral liquid form. Double-check dose, especially when giving to children. Fatal overdoses have occurred.
• To minimize unpleasant taste and stomach irritation, dilute or give with liquid. Drug should be taken after meals.
• Take precautions to prevent hoarding or self-overdosing by patients who are depressed, suicidal, or drug-dependent or who have history of drug abuse.
• Long-term use isn't recommended; drug loses its effectiveness in promoting sleep after 14 days of continued use. Long-term use may cause drug dependence, and patient may experience withdrawal symptoms if drug is suddenly stopped.
• Monitor BUN levels; large doses may raise BUN levels.
• Drug therapy may produce false-positive results for urine glucose with tests using cupric sulfate, such as Benedict's reagent. It doesn't interfere with Diastix or Chemstrip uG results. Drug may interfere with Reddy-Jenkins-Thorn test for urinary 17-hydroxycorticosteroids. It may also cause a false-positive phentolamine test result.
• Don't give drug for 48 hours before fluorometric test.

PATIENT TEACHING

• Instruct patient to take capsule with a full glass of water or juice and to swallow capsule whole.
• Tell patient to avoid alcohol during drug therapy.
• Caution patient to avoid performing activities that require mental alertness or physical coordination.
• Advise patient to store drug in dark container; store suppositories in refrigerator.

dexmedetomidine hydrochloride
Precedex

Pregnancy risk category C

AVAILABLE FORMS
Injection: 100 mcg/ml in 2-ml vials and 2-ml ampules

INDICATIONS & DOSAGES
➤ **Sedation of initially intubated and mechanically ventilated patients in intensive care unit (ICU) setting—**
Adults: Loading infusion of 1 mcg/kg I.V. over 10 minutes; then maintenance infusion of 0.2 to 0.7 mcg/kg/hr for up to 24 hours, titrated to achieve desired level of sedation.

I.V. ADMINISTRATION
• Dexmedetomidine must be diluted in normal saline solution before administration. To prepare infusion, withdraw 2 ml of drug and add to 48 ml of normal saline injection to total of 50 ml. Shake gently to mix well.
• Don't administer through same I.V. catheter with blood or plasma; physical compatibility hasn't been established.
• Infusion is compatible with lactated Ringer's solution, D_5W, normal saline solution in water, and 20% mannitol. It's also compatible with thiopental sodium, etomidate, vecuronium bromide, pancuronium bromide, succinylcholine, atracurium besylate, mivacurium chloride, glycopyrrolate bromide, phenylephrine hydrochloride, atropine sulfate, midazolam, morphine sulfate, fentanyl citrate, and plasma substitute.
Alert: Don't administer infusion for longer than 24 hours.

ACTION
Sedation produced by selective stimulation of alpha$_2$-adrenergic receptors in CNS.

Route	Onset	Peak	Duration
I.V.	Unknown	Unknown	Unknown

ADVERSE REACTIONS
CV: *hypotension, **bradycardia, arrhythmias.***
GI: *nausea,* thirst.
GU: oliguria.
Hematologic: anemia, leukocytosis.
Respiratory: *hypoxia,* pleural effusion, pulmonary edema.
Other: pain, infection.

INTERACTIONS
Drug-drug. *Anesthetics, hypnotics, opioids, sedatives:* May enhance effects of dexmedetomidine. May need to reduce dexmedetomidine dose.

EFFECTS ON LAB TEST RESULTS
• May decrease hemoglobin and WBC count.

CONTRAINDICATIONS
No known contraindications.

NURSING CONSIDERATIONS
• Use cautiously in patients with advanced heart block or renal or hepatic impairment and in elderly patients.
• Drug should be administered only by health care professionals skilled in management of patients in the ICU setting where cardiac status can be continuously monitored.
• *Alert:* Administer using controlled infusion device at rate calculated for body weight.
• Determine renal and hepatic function before administration, and consider dosage adjustments in patients with renal or hepatic impairment and in elderly patients.
• Some patients receiving drug are able to awaken when stimulated. This alone shouldn't be considered evidence of lack of efficacy in absence of other signs and symptoms.
• Drug has been continuously infused in mechanically ventilated patients before, during, and after extubation. It isn't necessary to stop drug before extubation.

PATIENT TEACHING
• Tell patient he will be sedated while drug is being given but that he may awaken when stimulated.

• Reassure patient that he will be closely monitored and attended while sedated.

---

estazolam
ProSom

Pregnancy risk category X
Controlled substance schedule IV

AVAILABLE FORMS
Tablets: 1 mg, 2 mg

INDICATIONS & DOSAGES
➤ **Insomnia—**
Adults: 1 mg P.O. h.s. Some patients may need 2 mg.
Elderly patients: 1 mg P.O. h.s. Use higher doses with extreme care. Frail, elderly, or debilitated patients may take 0.5 mg, but this low dose may be only marginally effective.

ACTION
Unknown. Thought to act on the limbic system and thalamus of CNS by binding to specific benzodiazepine receptors.

Route	Onset	Peak	Duration
P.O.	Unknown	1-3 hr	Unknown

ADVERSE REACTIONS
CNS: fatigue, dizziness, daytime drowsiness, *somnolence, asthenia,* hypokinesia, abnormal thinking.
GI: dyspepsia, abdominal pain.
Musculoskeletal: back pain, stiffness.

INTERACTIONS
Drug-drug. *Cimetidine, disulfiram, isoniazid, oral contraceptives:* May impair metabolism and clearance of benzodiazepines and prolong their plasma half-life. Watch for increased CNS depression.
CNS depressants, including antihistamines, opiate analgesics, other benzodiazepines: Increased CNS depression. Avoid using together.
Digoxin: May cause increased digoxin levels, resulting in toxicity. Monitor patient closely.
Phenytoin: May cause increased phenytoin levels, resulting in toxicity. Monitor patient closely.

---

*Liquid contains alcohol.   **May contain tartrazine.   †Canada   ‡Australia   §U.K.   ◇OTC

Rifampin: May increase metabolism and clearance and decrease plasma half-life. Watch for decreased effectiveness.
Theophylline: Pharmacologic antagonism. Watch for decreased effectiveness of estazolam.
Drug-herb. *Calendula, hops, kava, lemon balm, passion flower, skullcap, valerian:* May enhance sedative effect of drug. Advise patient to avoid using together.
Drug-lifestyle. *Alcohol use:* Excessive CNS and respiratory depression. Advise patient to use cautiously.
Smoking: May increase metabolism and clearance. Advise patient to watch for signs of decreased effectiveness.

EFFECTS ON LAB TEST RESULTS
● May increase AST levels.

CONTRAINDICATIONS
Contraindicated in pregnant patients and in those hypersensitive to drug.

NURSING CONSIDERATIONS
● Use cautiously in patients with depression, suicidal tendencies, or hepatic, renal, or pulmonary disease.
● Check liver and renal function and CBC before and periodically during long-term therapy.
● Take precautions to prevent hoarding by depressed, suicidal, or drug-dependent patients or those with history of drug abuse.
● Patients who receive prolonged treatment with benzodiazepines may experience withdrawal symptoms if drug is suddenly stopped (possibly after 6 weeks of continuous therapy).
● *Alert:* Don't confuse ProSom with Proscar, Prozac, or Psorcon E.

PATIENT TEACHING
● Advise patient to notify prescriber about planned, suspected, or known pregnancy during therapy.
● Tell patient not to increase dosage but to inform prescriber if he thinks that drug is no longer effective.
● Caution patient to avoid performing activities that require mental alertness or physical coordination.

● Warn patient that additive depressant effects can occur if alcohol is consumed while taking drug or within 24 hours after taking drug.
● Warn patient not to abruptly stop use after taking drug for 1 month or longer.
● Tell breast-feeding patient to avoid using drug.

---

flurazepam hydrochloride
Apo-Flurazepam†, Dalmane, Novo-Flupam†

Pregnancy risk category X
Controlled substance schedule IV

AVAILABLE FORMS
Capsules: 15 mg, 30 mg

INDICATIONS & DOSAGES
➤ **Insomnia—**
Adults: 15 to 30 mg P.O. h.s. Dose repeated once, p.r.n.
Elderly patients: Initiate with 15-mg dose until response determined.

ACTION
Unknown. A benzodiazepine that is thought to act on the limbic system, thalamus, and hypothalamus of CNS to produce hypnotic effects.

Route	Onset	Peak	Duration
P.O.	Unknown	0.5-1 hr	Unknown

ADVERSE REACTIONS
CNS: *daytime sedation, dizziness, drowsiness, disturbed coordination,* lethargy, confusion, physical or psychological dependence, *headache,* light-headedness, nervousness, hallucinations, staggering, ataxia, disorientation, *coma.*
GI: nausea, vomiting, heartburn, diarrhea, abdominal pain.

INTERACTIONS
Drug-drug. *Cimetidine:* Increased sedation. Monitor patient carefully.
CNS depressants, including narcotic analgesics: Excessive CNS depression. Use together cautiously.
Digoxin: May increase digoxin levels, resulting in toxicity. Monitor patient closely.

Disulfiram, isoniazid, oral contraceptives:
Decreased metabolism of benzodiazepines, leading to toxicity. Monitor patient
closely.
Phenytoin: Increased phenytoin levels.
Watch for toxicity.
Rifampin: Enhanced metabolism of benzodiazepines. Watch for decreased effectiveness of benzodiazepine.
Theophylline: Antagonist with flurazepam. Watch for decreased effectiveness of
flurazepam.
Drug-herb. *Calendula, hops, kava,
lemon balm, passion flower, skullcap,
valerian:* May enhance sedative effect of
drug. Advise patient to avoid using together.
Drug-lifestyle. *Alcohol use:* Excessive
CNS and respiratory depression. Advise
patient to avoid use together.
Smoking: May increase metabolism and
clearance and decrease plasma half-life.
Advise patient to watch for signs of decreased effectiveness.

EFFECTS ON LAB TEST RESULTS
● May increase AST, ALT, total and direct
bilirubin, and alkaline phosphatase levels.

CONTRAINDICATIONS
Contraindicated in patients hypersensitive
to drug and during pregnancy.

NURSING CONSIDERATIONS
● Use cautiously in patients with impaired
hepatic or renal function, chronic pulmonary insufficiency, mental depression,
suicidal tendencies, or history of drug
abuse.
● Check hepatic and renal function and
CBC before and periodically during long-
term therapy.
● Minor changes in EEG patterns (usually
low-voltage, fast activity) may occur during and after flurazepam therapy.
● Assess mental status before starting therapy. Elderly patients are more sensitive to
drug's adverse CNS reactions.
● Take precautions to prevent hoarding or
self-overdosing by patients who are depressed, suicidal, or drug-dependent or
who have history of drug abuse.
● Physical and psychological dependence
is possible with long-term use.

● *Alert:* Don't confuse Dalmane with
Dialume or Demulen.

PATIENT TEACHING
● Inform patient that drug is more effective on second, third, and fourth nights of
treatment because active metabolite accumulates.
● Warn patient not to abruptly stop after
taking drug for 1 month or longer.
● Tell patient to avoid alcohol while taking
drug.
● Caution patient to avoid performing activities that require mental alertness or
physical coordination.

---

pentobarbital
Nembutal*†**

pentobarbital sodium
Nembutal Sodium*, Nova Rectal†,
NovoPentobarb†

*Pregnancy risk category D
Controlled substance schedule II (III
for suppositories)*

AVAILABLE FORMS
pentobarbital
Elixir: 18.2 mg/5 ml
pentobarbital sodium
Capsules: 50 mg, 100 mg
Injection: 50 mg/ml
Suppositories: 30 mg, 60 mg, 120 mg,
200 mg

INDICATIONS & DOSAGES
➤ **Sedation—**
Adults: 20 mg P.O. t.i.d. or q.i.d.
Children: 2 to 6 mg/kg P.O. daily in three
divided doses. Maximum daily dose is
100 mg.
➤ **Insomnia—**
Adults: 100 to 200 mg P.O. h.s. Or, 150 to
200 mg deep I.M. Or, 100 mg initially
I.V., with additional small doses up to total
of 500 mg. Or, 120 or 200 mg P.R.
Children: 2 to 6 mg/kg or 125 mg/m² I.M.
Maximum dose is 100 mg.
Children ages 12 to 14: 60 or 120 mg P.R.
Children ages 5 to 11: 60 mg P.R.
Children ages 1 to 4: 30 or 60 mg P.R.

Children ages 2 months to 1 year: 30 mg
P.R.
➤ **Preoperative sedation—**
Adults: 150 to 200 mg I.M.
Children age 10 and older: 5 mg/kg P.O.
or I.M.
Children younger than age 10: 5 mg/kg
I.M. or P.R.

I.V. ADMINISTRATION
● I.V. administration of barbiturates may
cause severe respiratory depression,
laryngospasm, or hypotension. Have
emergency resuscitation equipment available.
● To minimize deterioration, use I.V. injection solution within 30 minutes after
opening container. Don't use cloudy solution.
● Reserve I.V. injection for emergency
treatment, which should be given under
close supervision. Administer slowly at no
more than 50 mg/minute.
● Parenteral solution is alkaline. Local tissue reactions and injection site pain may
follow I.V. use. Avoid extravasation. Assess patency of I.V. site before and during
administration.
● Don't mix in syringe or in I.V. solutions
or lines with other drugs.

ACTION
Unknown. Probably interferes with transmission of impulses from the thalamus to
the cortex of the brain.

Route	Onset	Peak	Duration
I.M.	10-25 min	Unknown	Unknown
I.V.	Immediate	Immediate	15 min
P.O.	20 min	0.5-1 hr	1-4 hr
P.R.	20 min	Unknown	1-4 hr

ADVERSE REACTIONS
CNS: *drowsiness, lethargy, hangover,*
paradoxical excitement in elderly patients,
somnolence, physical and psychological
dependence.
GI: nausea, vomiting.
Hematologic: exacerbation of porphyria.
Respiratory: *respiratory depression.*
Skin: rash, urticaria, ***Stevens-Johnson
syndrome.***
Other: *angioedema.*

INTERACTIONS
Drug-drug. *CNS depressants, including
narcotic analgesics:* Excessive CNS and
respiratory depression. Use together cautiously.
*Corticosteroids, digitoxin, doxycycline, es-
trogens and oral contraceptives, oral anticoagulants, theophylline, verapamil:* May
enhance metabolism of these drugs. Watch
for decreased effect of pentobarbital.
Griseofulvin: Decreased absorption of
griseofulvin. Monitor effectiveness of
griseofulvin.
MAO inhibitors: Inhibited metabolism of
barbiturates; may cause prolonged CNS
depression. Reduce barbiturate dosage.
Rifampin: May decrease barbiturate levels. Watch for decreased effect of pentobarbital.
Drug-herb. *Kava:* May cause additive
effects. Advise patient to avoid using together.
Drug-lifestyle. *Alcohol use:* Excessive
CNS and respiratory depression. Advise
patient to avoid using together.

EFFECTS ON LAB TEST RESULTS
None reported.

CONTRAINDICATIONS
Contraindicated in patients hypersensitive
to barbiturates and in those with porphyria.

NURSING CONSIDERATIONS
● Use cautiously in elderly or debilitated
patients and in patients with acute or
chronic pain, mental depression, suicidal
tendencies, history of drug abuse, or
hepatic impairment.
● Assess mental status before starting therapy, and use reduced doses. Elderly patients are more sensitive to drug's adverse
CNS effects.
● *Alert:* Administer I.M. injection deeply
with no more than 5 ml of drug at any one
site. Superficial injection may cause pain,
sterile abscess, and sloughing.
● To ensure accurate dosage, don't divide
suppositories.
● Take precautions to prevent hoarding or
overdosing by patients who are depressed,
suicidal, or drug-dependent or who have a
history of drug abuse.

Reactions may be *common*, uncommon, *life-threatening*, or COMMON AND LIFE-THREATENING.

• Watch for signs of barbiturate toxicity: coma, pupillary constriction, cyanosis, clammy skin, and hypotension. Overdose can be fatal.

• Inspect patient's skin. Skin eruptions may precede potentially fatal reactions to barbiturate therapy. Stop drug when skin reactions occur and call prescriber. In some patients, high fever, stomatitis, headache, or rhinitis may precede skin reactions.

• Drug has no analgesic effect and may cause restlessness or delirium in patients with pain.

• Long-term use isn't recommended; drug loses its effectiveness in promoting sleep after 14 days of continuous use. Long-term high dosage may cause drug dependence, and patient may experience withdrawal symptoms if drug is suddenly discontinued. Withdraw barbiturates gradually.

• Drug may cause a false-positive phentolamine test result. Physiologic effects of the drug may impair absorption of cyanocobalamin Co 57.

• Drug may decrease bilirubin levels in neonates, epileptic patients, and patients with congenital, nonhemolytic, unconjugated hyperbilirubinemia.

• EEG patterns show a change in low-voltage fast activity; changes persist after discontinuation of therapy.

• **Alert:** Don't confuse pentobarbital with phenobarbital.

PATIENT TEACHING
• Inform patient that morning hangover is common after hypnotic dose, which suppresses REM sleep. Patient may experience increased dreaming after drug is discontinued.

• Caution patient to avoid performing activities that require mental alertness or physical coordination.

• Tell patient to avoid alcohol while taking drug.

• Instruct patient using oral contraceptives to consider alternative birth control methods because drug may decrease oral contraceptive's effect.

secobarbital sodium
Novosecobarb†, Seconal Sodium

Pregnancy risk category D
Controlled substance schedule II

AVAILABLE FORMS
Capsules: 100 mg
Injection: 50 mg/ml

INDICATIONS & DOSAGES
➤ **Preoperative sedation—**
Adults: 200 to 300 mg P.O. 1 to 2 hours before surgery. Or, 1 mg/kg I.M. 10 to 15 minutes before surgery.
Children: 2 to 6 mg/kg P.O. 1 to 2 hours before surgery. Maximum single dose is 100 mg P.O. or 4 to 5 mg/kg I.M.
➤ **Insomnia—**
Adults: 100 to 200 mg P.O. or I.M. or 50 to 250 mg I.V.
Children: 3 to 5 mg/kg I.M. or 125 mg/m². Maximum, 100 mg, with no more than 5 ml injected in any one site.
➤ **Acute tetanus seizure—**
Adults and children: 5.5 mg/kg I.M. or slow I.V., repeated q 3 to 4 hours, if needed. Maximum I.V. injection rate, 50 mg/ 15 seconds.
➤ **Status epilepticus—**
Children: 15 to 20 mg/kg I.V. over 15 minutes.

I.V. ADMINISTRATION
• I.V. injection is reserved for emergency treatment; it should be given under close supervision by direct injection and administered slowly at a rate not exceeding 50 mg/15 seconds. May be administered as supplied or diluted with sterile water for injection, normal saline solution, or Ringer's injection solution. Don't use lactated Ringer's injection solution.

• I.V. administration of barbiturates may cause severe respiratory depression, laryngospasm, or hypotension. Have emergency resuscitation equipment readily available.

• Continue close observation for at least 30 minutes after administration.

• Don't add to acidic solutions because precipitate will form.

• Local tissue reactions and injection-site pain have been noted with I.V. use. Assess

---

patency of I.V. site before and during administration.

ACTION
Unknown. Probably interferes with transmission of impulses from the thalamus to the cortex of the brain.

Route	Onset	Peak	Duration
I.M.	Unknown	7-10 min	Unknown
I.V.	Immediate	1-3 min	15 min
P.O.	15 min	15-30 min	1-4 hr

ADVERSE REACTIONS
CNS: *drowsiness, lethargy, hangover,* paradoxical anxiety, somnolence.
CV: hypotension with I.V. use.
GI: nausea, vomiting.
Hematologic: exacerbation of porphyria.
Respiratory: *respiratory depression.*
Skin: rash, urticaria, ***Stevens-Johnson syndrome,*** tissue reactions, injection-site pain.
Other: *angioedema,* physical and psychological dependence.

INTERACTIONS
Drug-drug. *Chloramphenicol, MAO inhibitors, valproic acid:* Inhibited metabolism of barbiturates; may cause prolonged CNS depression. Reduce barbiturate dosage.
CNS depressants, including narcotic analgesics: Excessive CNS and respiratory depression. Use together cautiously.
Corticosteroids, digitoxin, doxycycline, estrogens and oral contraceptives, oral anticoagulants, theophylline, TCAs, verapamil: May enhance metabolism of these drugs. Watch for decreased effect.
Griseofulvin: Decreased absorption of griseofulvin. Monitor effectiveness of griseofulvin.
Rifampin: May decrease barbiturate levels. Watch for decreased effect.
Drug-lifestyle. *Alcohol use:* Excessive CNS and respiratory depression. Advise patient to avoid use together.

EFFECTS ON LAB TEST RESULTS
None reported.

CONTRAINDICATIONS
Contraindicated in patients hypersensitive to barbiturates and in those with marked liver impairment, respiratory disease in which dyspnea or obstruction is evident, or porphyria.

NURSING CONSIDERATIONS
• Use cautiously in elderly or debilitated patients and in patients with acute or chronic pain, depression, suicidal tendencies, history of drug abuse, or hepatic or renal impairment.
• Assess mental status before starting therapy. Elderly patients are more sensitive to drug's adverse CNS effects. Watch for paradoxical excitement in this population.
• Use injection solution within 30 minutes after opening container to minimize deterioration. Don't use cloudy solution.
• **Alert:** Give I.M. injection deeply, and inject no more than 5 ml of drug at any one site. Superficial injection may cause pain, sterile abscess, and sloughing. Don't give drug S.C.
• Take precautions to prevent hoarding or overdosing by patients who are depressed, suicidal, or drug-dependent or who have history of drug abuse.
• Watch for signs of barbiturate toxicity: coma, pupillary constriction, cyanosis, clammy skin, and hypotension. Overdose can be fatal.
• Inspect patient's skin. Skin eruptions may precede potentially fatal reactions to barbiturate therapy. Discontinue drug when skin reactions occur and notify prescriber. In some patients, high fever, stomatitis, headache, or rhinitis may precede skin reactions.
• Long-term use isn't recommended; drug loses its effectiveness in promoting sleep after 14 days of continued use.
• Drug may cause a false-positive phentolamine test result. The physiologic effects of drug may impair the absorption of cyanocobalamin Co 57.
• Drug may decrease bilirubin levels in neonates, epileptic patients, and patients with congenital, nonhemolytic, unconjugated hyperbilirubinemia.
• EEG patterns are altered, with a change in low-voltage fast activity; changes persist for a time after discontinuation of therapy.

PATIENT TEACHING
• Tell patient that morning hangover is common after hypnotic dose, which sup-

presses REM sleep. Patient may experience increased dreaming after drug is discontinued.
• Advise patient to avoid alcohol while taking drug.
• Caution patient to avoid performing activities that require mental alertness or physical coordination.
• Tell patient using oral contraceptives to consider a different birth control method.

---

temazepam
Euhypnos 10‡, Euhypnos 20‡, Nomapam‡, Normison‡, Restoril, Temaze‡, Temtabs‡

Pregnancy risk category X
Controlled substance schedule IV

AVAILABLE FORMS
Capsules: 7.5 mg, 10 mg‡, 15 mg, 20 mg‡, 30 mg

INDICATIONS & DOSAGES
➤ **Insomnia—**
Adults: 15 to 30 mg P.O. h.s.
Patients older than age 65: 15 mg P.O. h.s.

ACTION
Unknown. A benzodiazepine that probably acts on the limbic system, thalamus, and hypothalamus of the CNS to produce hypnotic effects.

Route	Onset	Peak	Duration
P.O.	Unknown	1-2 hr	Unknown

ADVERSE REACTIONS
CNS: drowsiness, dizziness, lethargy, disturbed coordination, daytime sedation, confusion, nightmares, vertigo, euphoria, weakness, headache, fatigue, nervousness, anxiety, depression, minor changes in EEG patterns (usually low-voltage fast activity).
EENT: blurred vision.
GI: diarrhea, nausea, dry mouth.
Other: physical and psychological dependence.

INTERACTIONS
Drug-drug. *CNS depressants:* Increased CNS depression. Use together cautiously.

Drug-herb. *Calendula, hops, kava, lemon balm, passion flower, skullcap, valerian:* May enhance sedative effect of drug. Advise patient to avoid using together.
Drug-lifestyle. *Alcohol use:* Increased CNS depression. Advise patient to avoid using together.

EFFECTS ON LAB TEST RESULTS
• May increase liver function test values.

CONTRAINDICATIONS
Contraindicated in pregnant patients and those hypersensitive to drug or other benzodiazepines.

NURSING CONSIDERATIONS
• Use cautiously in patients with chronic pulmonary insufficiency, impaired hepatic or renal function, severe or latent mental depression, suicidal tendencies, and history of drug abuse.
• Assess mental status before starting therapy. Elderly patients are more sensitive to drug's adverse CNS effects.
• Take precautions to prevent hoarding or overdosing by patients who are depressed, suicidal, or drug-dependent or who have history of drug abuse.
• **Alert:** Don't confuse Restoril with Vistaril.

PATIENT TEACHING
• Tell patient to avoid alcohol during therapy.
• Caution patient to avoid performing activities that require mental alertness or physical coordination.
• Warn patient not to stop drug abruptly if taken for 1 month or longer.
• Tell patient that onset of drug's effects may take as long as 2 to 2½ hours.

---

triazolam
Apo-Triazo†, Halcion, Novo-Triolam†

Pregnancy risk category X
Controlled substance schedule IV

AVAILABLE FORMS
Tablets: 0.125 mg, 0.25 mg

INDICATIONS & DOSAGES
➤ Insomnia—
Adults: 0.125 to 0.5 mg P.O. h.s.
Elderly patients: 0.125 mg P.O. h.s.; increased, p.r.n., to 0.25 mg P.O. h.s.

ACTION
Unknown. A benzodiazepine that probably acts on the limbic system, thalamus, and hypothalamus of the CNS to produce hypnotic effects.

Route	Onset	Peak	Duration
P.O.	Unknown	1-2 hr	Unknown

ADVERSE REACTIONS
CNS: *drowsiness,* dizziness, headache, rebound insomnia, amnesia, lack of coordination, mental confusion, depression, nervousness, ataxia, physical or psychological dependence.
GI: nausea, vomiting.

INTERACTIONS
Drug-drug. *Azole antifungal agents, cimetidine, erythromycin, fluoxetine, fluvoxamine, isoniazid, nefazodone, ranitidine:* May cause prolonged triazolam blood levels. Don't give drug with azole antifungal agents or nefazodone. Watch for increased sedation if used together.
CNS depressants: Excessive CNS depression. Use together cautiously.
Drug-herb. *Calendula, hops, kava, lemon balm, passion flower, skullcap, valerian:* May enhance sedative effect of drug. Advise patient to avoid using together.
Drug-food. *Grapefruit juice:* Increased triazolam blood levels. Tell patient not to take drug with grapefruit juice.
Drug-lifestyle. *Alcohol use:* Excessive CNS depression. Advise patient to avoid use together.

EFFECTS ON LAB TEST RESULTS
● May increase liver function test values.

CONTRAINDICATIONS
Contraindicated in pregnant patients and those hypersensitive to benzodiazepines.

NURSING CONSIDERATIONS
● Use cautiously in patients with impaired hepatic or renal function, chronic pulmonary insufficiency, sleep apnea, mental depression, suicidal tendencies, or history of drug abuse. Also use cautiously in breast-feeding women.
● Assess mental status before starting therapy. Elderly patients are more sensitive to drug's CNS effects.
● Take precautions to prevent hoarding or overdosing by patients who are depressed, suicidal, or drug-dependent or who have history of drug abuse.
● Minor changes in EEG patterns (usually low-voltage fast activity) may occur during and after therapy.
● *Alert:* Don't confuse Halcion with Haldol or halcinonide.

PATIENT TEACHING
● Warn patient not to take more than prescribed amount; overdose can occur at total daily dose of 2 mg (or four times highest recommended amount).
● Tell patient to avoid alcohol while taking drug.
● Warn patient not to stop drug abruptly after taking for 2 weeks or longer.
● Caution patient to avoid performing activities that require mental alertness or physical coordination.
● Inform patient that drug doesn't tend to cause morning drowsiness.
● Tell patient that rebound insomnia may occur for 1 or 2 nights after stopping therapy.

zaleplon
Sonata

Pregnancy risk category C
Controlled substance schedule IV

AVAILABLE FORMS
Capsules: 5 mg, 10 mg

INDICATIONS & DOSAGES
➤ Insomnia—
Adults: 10 mg P.O. daily h.s.; may increase to 20 mg, if needed. Low-weight adults may respond to 5-mg dose.
Elderly patients: Initially, 5 mg P.O. daily h.s.; doses of more than 10 mg aren't recommended.
Adjust-a-dose: For debilitated patients, initially, 5 mg P.O. daily h.s.; doses of more than 10 mg aren't recommended.

Reactions may be *common,* uncommon, *life-threatening,* or COMMON AND LIFE-THREATENING.

For patients with mild to moderate hepatic impairment or those also taking cimetidine, 5 mg P.O. daily h.s.

ACTION

A hypnotic with chemical structure unrelated to benzodiazepines that interacts with the gamma-aminobutyric acid BZ receptor complex in the CNS. Modulation of this complex is thought to be responsible for sedative, anxiolytic, muscle relaxant, and anticonvulsant effects of benzodiazepines.

Route	Onset	Peak	Duration
P.O.	1 hr	1 hr	3-4 hr

ADVERSE REACTIONS

CNS: *headache,* amnesia, dizziness, somnolence, depression, hypertonia, nervousness, depersonalization, hallucinations, vertigo, difficulty concentrating, anxiety, paresthesia, hypesthesia, tremor, asthenia, migraine, malaise.
CV: chest pain, peripheral edema.
EENT: abnormal vision, conjunctivitis, eye discomfort, ear discomfort, hyperacusis, epistaxis, smell alteration.
GI: constipation, dry mouth, anorexia, dyspepsia, nausea, abdominal pain, colitis.
GU: dysmenorrhea.
Musculoskeletal: arthritis, myalgia, back pain.
Respiratory: bronchitis.
Skin: pruritus, rash, photosensitivity reactions.
Other: fever.

INTERACTIONS

Drug-drug. *Carbamazepine, phenobarbital, phenytoin, rifampin, other CYP3A4:* May reduce bioavailability and peak levels of zaleplon by about 80%. Consider an alternative hypnotic.
Cimetidine: Increased zaleplon bioavailability and peak levels by 85%. For patient taking cimetidine, use an initial zaleplon dose of 5 mg.
CNS depressants (imipramine, thioridazine): May cause additive CNS effects. Use together cautiously.
Drug-food. *High-fat foods, heavy meals:* Prolonged absorption, delaying peak zaleplon levels by about 2 hours; may delay

sleep onset. Advise patient to avoid taking with meals.
Drug-lifestyle. *Alcohol use:* Concurrent use may increase CNS effects. Advise patient to avoid using together.

EFFECTS ON LAB TEST RESULTS

None reported.

CONTRAINDICATIONS

Contraindicated in patients with severe hepatic impairment.

NURSING CONSIDERATIONS

● Use cautiously in elderly and debilitated patients, in those with compromised respiratory function, and in those with evidence of depression.
● Drug isn't recommended in breast-feeding women.
● Because drug works rapidly, it should only be given immediately before bedtime or after patient has gone to bed and has experienced difficulty falling asleep.
● Don't give drug with or after a high-fat or heavy meal.
● Closely monitor patients who have compromised respiratory function caused by illness or who are elderly or debilitated because they are more sensitive to respiration depression.
● Zaleplon may be used up to 5 weeks. Reevaluate patient if hypnotics are to be taken for longer than 2 to 3 weeks.
● Initiate treatment only after careful evaluation of patient because sleep disturbances may be a symptom of an underlying physical or psychiatric disorder.
● Adverse reactions are usually dose-related. Notify prescriber about a dose reduction if adverse reactions are bothersome to patient.

PATIENT TEACHING

● Advise patient that drug works rapidly and should only be taken immediately before bedtime or after he has gone to bed and has experienced difficulty falling asleep.
● Advise patient to take drug only if he will be able to sleep for at least 4 undisturbed hours.
● Caution patient that drowsiness, dizziness, light-headedness, and difficulty with

---

*Liquid contains alcohol.   **May contain tartrazine.   †Canada   ‡Australia   §U.K.   ◊OTC

coordination most frequently occur within 1 hour after taking drug.

• Advise patient to avoid performing activities that require mental alertness until CNS effects of drug are known.

• Advise patient to avoid alcohol while taking drug and to notify prescriber before taking other prescription or OTC drugs.

• Tell patient not to take drug after a high-fat or heavy meal.

• Advise patient to report sleep problems that continue despite use of drug.

• Notify patient that dependence can occur and that drug is recommended for short-term use only.

• Warn patient not to abruptly stop drug because withdrawal symptoms, including unpleasant feelings, stomach and muscle cramps, vomiting, sweating, shakiness, and seizures, may occur.

• Notify patient that insomnia may recur for a few nights after stopping drug, but should resolve on its own.

• Warn patient that drug may cause changes in behavior and thinking, including outgoing or aggressive behavior, loss of personal identity, confusion, strange behavior, agitation, hallucinations, worsening of depression, or suicidal thoughts. Tell patient to notify prescriber immediately if these symptoms occur.

---

zolpidem tartrate
Ambien, Stilnoct§

Pregnancy risk category B
Controlled substance schedule IV

AVAILABLE FORMS
Tablets: 5 mg, 10 mg

INDICATIONS & DOSAGES
➤ **Short-term management of insomnia—**
Adults: 10 mg P.O. immediately before bedtime.
Elderly patients: 5 mg P.O. immediately before bedtime. Maximum daily dose is 10 mg.
Adjust-a-dose: For debilitated patients and those with hepatic insufficiency, 5 mg P.O. immediately before bedtime. Maximum daily dose is 10 mg.

ACTION
Although drug interacts with one of three identified gamma-aminobutyric acid-benzodiazepine receptor complexes, it isn't a benzodiazepine. It exhibits hypnotic activity and minimal muscle relaxant and anticonvulsant properties.

Route	Onset	Peak	Duration
P.O.	Rapid	0.5-2 hr	Unknown

ADVERSE REACTIONS
CNS: daytime drowsiness, light-headedness, change in dreams, amnesia, dizziness, *headache,* hangover, sleep disorder, lethargy, depression.
CV: palpitations.
EENT: sinusitis, pharyngitis.
GI: nausea, vomiting, dry mouth, diarrhea, dyspepsia, constipation, abdominal pain.
Musculoskeletal: myalgia, arthralgia.
Skin: rash.
Other: back or chest pain, flu syndrome, hypersensitivity reactions.

INTERACTIONS
Drug-drug. *CNS depressants:* Excessive CNS depression. Use together cautiously.
Rifampin: Decreased effects of zolpidem. Avoid using together, if possible. Consider alternative hypnotic.
Drug-lifestyle. *Alcohol use:* Excessive CNS depression. Advise patient to avoid use together.

EFFECTS ON LAB TEST RESULTS
None reported.

CONTRAINDICATIONS
No known contraindications.

NURSING CONSIDERATIONS
• Use cautiously in patients with compromised respiratory status.

• Hypnotics should be used only for short-term management of insomnia, usually 7 to 10 days.

• The smallest effective dose should be used in all patients.

• Take precautions to prevent hoarding or overdosing by patients who are depressed, suicidal, or drug-dependent or who have history of drug abuse.

Reactions may be *common,* uncommon, *life-threatening,* or COMMON AND LIFE-THREATENING.

● **Alert:** Don't confuse Ambien with
Amen.

PATIENT TEACHING
● For rapid sleep onset, instruct patient not
to take drug with or immediately after
meals.
● Instruct patient to take drug immediately
before going to bed; onset of action is
rapid.
● Tell patient to avoid alcohol during drug
therapy.
● Caution patient to avoid performing activities that require mental alertness or
physical coordination during therapy.

28

Anticonvulsants

acetazolamide sodium
(See Chapter 60, DIURETICS.)
carbamazepine
clonazepam
clorazepate dipotassium
(See Chapter 30, ANXIOLYTICS.)
diazepam
(See Chapter 30, ANXIOLYTICS.)
divalproex sodium
fosphenytoin sodium
gabapentin
lamotrigine
levetiracetam
magnesium sulfate
oxcarbazepine
phenobarbital
phenobarbital sodium
phenytoin
phenytoin sodium
phenytoin sodium (extended)
primidone
tiagabine hydrochloride
topiramate
valproate sodium
valproic acid
zonisamide

COMBINATION PRODUCTS
None.

---

carbamazepine
Apo-Carbamazepine†, Atretol,
Carbatrol, Epitol, Novo-
Carbamaz†, Tegretol, Tegretol
CR†, Tegretol-XR, Teril‡

Pregnancy risk category D

AVAILABLE FORMS
Capsules (extended-release): 200 mg,
300 mg
Oral suspension: 100 mg/5 ml
Tablets: 200 mg
Tablets (chewable): 100 mg
Tablets (extended-release)†: 100 mg,
200 mg, 400 mg

INDICATIONS & DOSAGES
➤ **Generalized tonic-clonic and
complex partial seizures, mixed seizure
patterns—**
Adults and children older than age 12:
Initially, 200 mg P.O. b.i.d. (tablets), or
100 mg P.O. q.i.d. of suspension with
meals. May be increased weekly by
200 mg P.O. daily in divided doses at 6-
to 8-hour intervals, adjusted to minimum
effective level. Maximum, 1 g daily in
children ages 12 to 15, and 1.2 g daily in
patients older than age 15. Usual maintenance dosage is 800 to 1,200 mg/day.
Children ages 6 to 12: Initially, 100 mg
P.O. b.i.d. or 50 mg of suspension P.O.
q.i.d. with meals, increased at weekly intervals by 100 mg P.O. daily. Maximum,
1 g daily. Usual maintenance dosage is
400 to 800 mg/day.
➤ **Trigeminal neuralgia—**
Adults: Initially, 100 mg P.O. b.i.d. or ½
teaspoon of suspension q.i.d. with meals,
increased by 100 mg q 12 hours for tablets
or ½ teaspoon of suspension q.i.d. until
pain is relieved. Maximum, 1.2 g daily.
Maintenance dosage is 200 to 400 mg P.O.
b.i.d.

ACTION
Unknown. Thought to stabilize neuronal
membranes and limit seizure activity by
either increasing efflux or decreasing influx of sodium ions across cell membranes
in the motor cortex during generation of
nerve impulses.

Route	Onset	Peak	Duration
P.O.	Unknown	1.5-12 hr	Unknown

ADVERSE REACTIONS
CNS: *dizziness, vertigo, drowsiness,*
fatigue, *ataxia,* **worsening of seizures,**
confusion, headache, syncope.
CV: *heart failure,* hypertension, hypotension, aggravation of coronary artery disease, *arrhythmias, AV block.*
EENT: conjunctivitis, dry pharynx,
blurred vision, diplopia, nystagmus.

Reactions may be *common,* uncommon, *life-threatening,* or COMMON AND LIFE-THREATENING.

GI: dry mouth, *nausea, vomiting,* abdominal pain, diarrhea, anorexia, stomatitis, glossitis.

GU: urinary frequency, urine retention, impotence, albuminuria, glycosuria.

Hematologic: *aplastic anemia, agranulocytosis,* eosinophilia, leukocytosis, *thrombocytopenia.*

Hepatic: *hepatitis.*

Metabolic: SIADH.

Respiratory: pulmonary hypersensitivity.

Skin: rash, urticaria, *erythema multiforme, Stevens-Johnson syndrome,* excessive diaphoresis.

Other: fever, chills.

INTERACTIONS

Drug-drug. *Cimetidine, danazol, diltiazem, fluoxetine, fluvoxamine, isoniazid, macrolides such as erythromycin, propoxyphene, valproic acid, verapamil:* May increase carbamazepine blood levels. Use together cautiously.

Doxycycline, felbamate, haloperidol, oral contraceptives, phenytoin, theophylline, tiagabine, topiramate, valproate, warfarin: May decrease blood levels of these drugs. Watch for decreased effect.

Lithium: Increased CNS toxicity of lithium. Avoid using together.

MAO inhibitors: Increased depressant and anticholinergic effects. Avoid using together.

Phenobarbital, phenytoin, primidone: May decrease carbamazepine levels. Watch for decreased effect.

Drug-herb. *Plantains (psyllium seed):* May inhibit GI absorption of drug. Discourage use together.

EFFECTS ON LAB TEST RESULTS

• May increase BUN levels.

• May increase liver function test values and eosinophil count. May decrease thyroid function test values, hemoglobin, and granulocyte, WBC, and platelet counts.

CONTRAINDICATIONS

Contraindicated in patients hypersensitive to carbamazepine or TCAs and in those with a history of previous bone marrow suppression; also contraindicated in those who have taken an MAO inhibitor within 14 days of therapy.

NURSING CONSIDERATIONS

• Use cautiously in patients with mixed seizure disorders because they may experience an increased risk of seizures.

• Use with caution in patients with hepatic dysfunction.

• Watch for worsening of seizures, especially in patients with mixed seizure disorders, including atypical absence seizures.

• Obtain baseline determinations of urinalysis, BUN level, liver function, CBC, platelet and reticulocyte counts, and iron level. Monitor periodically thereafter.

• Shake oral suspension well before measuring dose.

• Contents of extended-release capsules may be sprinkled over applesauce if patient has difficulty swallowing capsules. Capsules and tablets shouldn't be crushed or chewed, unless labeled as chewable form.

• When administering by nasogastric tube, mix dose with an equal volume of water, normal saline solution, or D_5W. Flush tube with 100 ml of diluent after administering dose.

• Never stop drug suddenly when treating seizures. Notify prescriber immediately if adverse reactions occur.

• Drug may interfere with some pregnancy tests.

• Adverse reactions may be minimized by gradually increasing dosage.

• Therapeutic carbamazepine blood level is 4 to 12 mcg/ml. Monitor blood levels and effects closely. Ask patient when last dose was taken to better evaluate blood levels.

• When managing seizures, take appropriate precautions.

• *Alert:* Watch for signs of anorexia or subtle appetite changes, which may indicate excessive blood levels.

• *Alert:* Don't confuse Tegretol with Toradol or Tegopen; or Carbatrol with carvedilol.

PATIENT TEACHING

• Instruct patient to take drug with food to minimize GI distress. Tell patient taking suspension form to shake container well before measuring dose.

• Tell patient not to crush or chew extended-release form and not to take broken or chipped tablets.

• Tegretol-XR tablet coating may appear in stool because it isn't absorbed.

• Advise patient to keep tablets in the original container and to keep the container tightly closed and away from moisture. Some formulations may harden when exposed to excessive moisture, resulting in decreased bioavailability and loss of seizure control.

• Inform patient that, when drug is used for trigeminal neuralgia, an attempt to decrease dosage or withdraw drug is usually done every 3 months.

• Advise patient to notify prescriber immediately if fever, sore throat, mouth ulcers, or easy bruising or bleeding occurs.

• Tell patient that drug may cause mild to moderate dizziness and drowsiness when first taken. Advise him to avoid hazardous activities until effects disappear, usually within 3 to 4 days.

• Advise patient that periodic eye examinations are recommended.

• Advise woman of risks to fetus should pregnancy occur while taking carbamazepine.

• Advise woman that breast-feeding isn't recommended during therapy.

---

clonazepam
Klonopin, Paxam‡, Rivotril†

Pregnancy risk category D
Controlled substance schedule IV

AVAILABLE FORMS
Drops: 2.5 mg/ml‡
Injection: 1 mg/ml‡
Tablets: 0.5 mg, 1 mg, 2 mg

INDICATIONS & DOSAGES
➤ **Lennox-Gastaut syndrome, atypical absence seizures, akinetic and myoclonic seizures—**
Adults: Initially, not to exceed 1.5 mg P.O. daily in three divided doses. May be increased by 0.5 to 1 mg q 3 days until seizures are controlled. If given in unequal doses, largest dose given h.s. Maximum recommended daily dose is 20 mg.
Children up to age 10 or 30 kg (66 lb): Initially, 0.01 to 0.03 mg/kg P.O. daily (not to exceed 0.05 mg/kg daily) in two or three divided doses. Increased by 0.25 to 0.5 mg q third day to maximum maintenance dose of 0.1 to 0.2 mg/kg daily, p.r.n.

➤ **Status epilepticus (where parenteral form is available)—**
Adults: 1 mg by slow I.V. infusion.
Children: 0.5 mg by slow I.V. infusion.
➤ **Panic disorder—**
Adults: Initially, 0.25 mg P.O. b.i.d.; increase to target dose of 1 mg/day after 3 days. Some patients may benefit from doses up to maximum of 4 mg/day. To achieve 4 mg/day, dosage increased in increments of 0.125 to 0.25 mg b.i.d. q 3 days, as tolerated, until panic disorder is controlled. Discontinue drug gradually with decrease of 0.125 mg b.i.d. q 3 days until drug is stopped.

I.V. ADMINISTRATION
• Mix solutions in glass bottles because drug binds to polyvinyl chloride plastic. If polyvinyl chloride infusion bags are used, administer immediately and infuse at 60 ml/hour or faster.
• Give slowly by direct injection or by slow I.V. infusion. Drug may be diluted with D₅W, dextrose 2.5% in water, or normal or half-normal saline solution.

ACTION
Unknown. A benzodiazepine that probably acts by facilitating the effects of the inhibitory neurotransmitter gamma-aminobutyric acid.

Route	Onset	Peak	Duration
I.V.	Unknown	Unknown	Unknown
P.O.	Unknown	1-2 hr	Unknown

ADVERSE REACTIONS
CNS: *drowsiness,* ataxia, behavioral disturbances, slurred speech, tremor, confusion, agitation, depression.
CV: palpitations.
EENT: nystagmus, abnormal eye movements.
GI: sore gums, constipation, gastritis, change in appetite, nausea, anorexia, diarrhea.
GU: dysuria, enuresis, nocturia, urine retention.
Hematologic: *leukopenia, thrombocytopenia,* eosinophilia.
Respiratory: *respiratory depression,* chest congestion, shortness of breath.
Skin: rash.

Reactions may be *common,* uncommon, *life-threatening,* or COMMON AND LIFE-THREATENING.

INTERACTIONS
Drug-drug. *Carbamazepine, phenobarbital, phenytoin:* Lowered plasma clonazepam levels. Monitor patient closely.
CNS depressants: Increased CNS depression. Avoid using together.
Drug-lifestyle. *Alcohol use:* Increased CNS depression. Discourage use together.

EFFECTS ON LAB TEST RESULTS
• May increase liver function test values and eosinophil counts. May decrease WBCs and platelet counts.

CONTRAINDICATIONS
Contraindicated in patients hypersensitive to benzodiazepines and in those with significant hepatic disease or acute angle-closure glaucoma.

NURSING CONSIDERATIONS
• Use cautiously in patients with mixed-type seizures because drug may cause generalized tonic-clonic seizures. Also use cautiously in children and in patients with chronic respiratory disease or open-angle glaucoma.
• Watch for behavioral disturbances, especially in children.
• Never withdraw drug suddenly because seizures may worsen. Call prescriber at once if adverse reactions develop.
• Assess elderly patient's response closely. Elderly patients are more sensitive to drug's CNS effects.
• Monitor patient for oversedation.
• Monitor CBCs and liver function tests.
• Withdrawal symptoms are similar to those of barbiturates.
• To reduce inconvenience of somnolence when drug is used for panic disorder, administration of one dose at bedtime may be desirable.

PATIENT TEACHING
• Advise patient to avoid driving and other hazardous activities that require mental alertness until drug's CNS effects are known.
• Instruct parent to monitor child's school performance because drug may interfere with attentiveness in school.
• Tell patient and parents not to stop drug abruptly because seizures may occur.

• Advise patient that drug isn't for use during pregnancy or breast-feeding.

fosphenytoin sodium
Cerebyx

Pregnancy risk category D

AVAILABLE FORMS
Injection: 2 ml (150 mg fosphenytoin sodium equivalent to 100 mg phenytoin sodium), 10 ml (750 mg fosphenytoin sodium equivalent to 500 mg phenytoin sodium)

INDICATIONS & DOSAGES
➤ **Status epilepticus—**
Adults: 15 to 20 mg phenytoin sodium equivalent (PE)/kg I.V. at 100 to 150 mg PE/minute as loading dose; then 4 to 6 mg PE/kg/day I.V. as maintenance dose.
➤ **Prevention and treatment of seizures during neurosurgery (nonemergent loading or maintenance dosing)—**
Adults: Loading dose of 10 to 20 mg PE/kg I.M. or I.V. at infusion rate not exceeding 150 mg PE/minute. Maintenance dose is 4 to 6 mg PE/kg/day I.V. or I.M.
➤ **Short-term substitution for oral phenytoin therapy—**
Adults: Same total daily dose equivalent as oral phenytoin sodium therapy given as a single daily dose I.M. or I.V. at infusion rate not exceeding 150 mg PE/minute. Some patients may need more frequent dosing.
Elderly patients: Phenytoin clearance is decreased slightly in elderly patients; lower or less frequent dosing may be required.

I.V. ADMINISTRATION
• Before I.V. infusion, dilute fosphenytoin in D_5W or normal saline solution for injection to a level ranging from 1.5 to 25 mg PE/ml. Don't administer at a rate exceeding 150 mg PE/minute.
• For status epilepticus, administer dose of I.V. fosphenytoin at a maximum rate of 150 mg PE/minute. Typical infusion to a 50-kg patient takes 5 to 7 minutes. (An infusion of an identical molar dose of phenytoin can't be accomplished in less than 15 to 20 minutes because of adverse CV effects that accompany direct I.V. ad-

ministration of phenytoin at rates above 50 mg/minute.) Don't use fosphenytoin I.M. for status epilepticus because therapeutic phenytoin levels may not be reached as rapidly as with I.V. administration.

• Patients receiving 20 mg PE/kg of drug at 150 mg PE/minute typically experience discomfort, most often in the groin. Occurrence and intensity of discomfort can be lessened by slowing or temporarily stopping infusion.

• If rapid phenytoin loading is a primary goal, I.V. administration of drug is preferred because it takes longer to achieve therapeutic plasma phenytoin levels after I.M. injection than after I.V. infusion.

• Monitor patient's ECG, blood pressure, and respirations continuously during maximal phenytoin levels—about 10 to 20 minutes after end of fosphenytoin infusions. Severe CV complications are most commonly encountered in elderly or gravely ill patients. Reducing the rate of administration or discontinuing drug may be necessary.

ACTION

Drug is a prodrug of phenytoin, so its anticonvulsant action is that of phenytoin. Phenytoin is thought to stabilize neuronal membranes and limit seizure activity by modulation of voltage-dependent sodium channels of neurons, inhibition of calcium flux across neuronal membranes, modulation of voltage-dependent calcium channels of neurons, and enhancement of sodium-potassium ATPase activity of neurons and glial cells.

Route	Onset	Peak	Duration
I.M.	Unknown	30 min	Unknown
I.V.	Unknown	End of infusion	Unknown

ADVERSE REACTIONS

CNS: increased or decreased reflexes, speech disorders, asthenia, ***intracranial hypertension,*** thinking abnormalities, nervousness, hypesthesia, dysarthria, extrapyramidal syndrome, ***brain edema,*** headache, *nystagmus, dizziness, somnolence, ataxia,* stupor, incoordination, paresthesia, tremor, agitation, vertigo.
CV: hypertension, vasodilation, tachycardia, hypotension.

GI: constipation, taste perversion.
Metabolic: hypokalemia, hyperglycemia.
Musculoskeletal: pelvic pain, back pain, myasthenia.
Respiratory: pneumonia.
Skin: rash, ecchymoses, *pruritus.*
Other: lymphadenopathy, accidental injury, injection site reaction and pain, infection, chills, decreased folate levels.

INTERACTIONS

Drug-drug. *Amiodarone, chloramphenicol, chlordiazepoxide, cimetidine, diazepam, dicumarol, disulfiram, estrogens, ethosuximide, fluoxetine, H_2 antagonists, halothane, isoniazid, methylphenidate, phenothiazines, phenylbutazone, salicylates, succinimides, sulfonamides, tolbutamide, trazodone:* May increase plasma phenytoin levels and its therapeutic effects. Use together cautiously.
Carbamazepine, reserpine: May decrease plasma phenytoin levels. Monitor patient.
Corticosteroids, coumarin, digitoxin, doxycycline, estrogens, furosemide, oral contraceptives, quinidine, rifampin, theophylline, vitamin D: Efficacy may be decreased by phenytoin as a result of increased hepatic metabolism. Monitor patient closely.
Phenobarbital, valproate sodium, valproic acid: May increase or decrease plasma phenytoin levels. Similarly, the effects of phenytoin on levels of these drugs are unpredictable. Monitor patient.
TCAs: May lower seizure threshold and require adjustments in phenytoin dosage. Use cautiously.
Drug-lifestyle. *Alcohol use:* May increase plasma phenytoin level and its therapeutic effects. Advise caution.
Long-term alcohol use: May decrease plasma phenytoin levels. Monitor patient.

EFFECTS ON LAB TEST RESULTS

• May increase alkaline phosphatase, GGT, and glucose levels. May decrease potassium and T_4 levels.

CONTRAINDICATIONS

Contraindicated in patients hypersensitive to drug or its components, phenytoin, or other hydantoins; also contraindicated in those with sinus bradycardia, SA block,

---

Reactions may be *common,* uncommon, ***life-threatening***, or COMMON AND LIFE-THREATENING.

second- or third-degree AV block, or Adams-Stokes syndrome.

NURSING CONSIDERATIONS
• Use cautiously in patients with porphyria and in those with history of hypersensitivity to similarly structured drugs, such as barbiturates, oxazolidinediones, and succinimides.
• Most significant drug interactions are those commonly seen with phenytoin.
• *Alert:* Fosphenytoin should always be prescribed and dispensed in phenytoin sodium equivalent units (PE). Don't make adjustments in the recommended doses when substituting fosphenytoin for phenytoin, and vice versa.
• In status epilepticus, phenytoin may be used instead of fosphenytoin as maintenance, using the appropriate dose.
• Phosphate load provided by fosphenytoin (0.0037 mmol phosphate/mg PE fosphenytoin) must be taken into consideration when treating patients who need phosphate restriction, such as those with severe renal impairment. Monitor laboratory values.
• Discontinue drug and notify prescriber if rash appears. If rash is exfoliative, purpuric, or bullous, or if lupus erythematosus, Stevens-Johnson syndrome, or toxic epidermal necrolysis is suspected, drug should be discontinued and alternative therapy considered. If rash is mild (measleslike or scarlatiniform), therapy may be resumed after rash disappears. If rash recurs when therapy is resumed, further fosphenytoin or phenytoin administration is contraindicated. Document that patient is allergic to drug.
• Drug should be stopped in patients with acute hepatotoxicity.
• I.M. administration generates systemic phenytoin levels similar enough to oral phenytoin sodium to allow essentially interchangeable use.
• After fosphenytoin administration, phenytoin levels shouldn't be monitored until conversion to phenytoin is essentially complete—about 2 hours after the end of an I.V. infusion or 4 hours after I.M. administration.
• Interpret total phenytoin plasma levels cautiously in patients with renal or hepatic disease or hypoalbuminemia caused by an increased fraction in unbound phenytoin.

It may be more useful to monitor unbound phenytoin levels in these patients. When giving drug I.V., monitor patients with renal and hepatic disease because they are at increased risk for more frequent and severe adverse reactions.
• Drug may produce artificially low results in dexamethasone or metyrapone tests.
• Monitor glucose closely in diabetic patients; drug may cause hyperglycemia.
• Abrupt withdrawal of drug may precipitate status epilepticus.
• Store drug under refrigeration. Don't store at room temperature longer than 48 hours. Discard vials that develop particulate matter.
• *Alert:* Don't confuse Cerebyx with Cerezyme, Celexa, or Celebrex.

PATIENT TEACHING
• Warn patient that sensory disturbances may occur with I.V. administration.
• Instruct patient to immediately report adverse reactions, especially rash.
• Warn patient never to stop drug abruptly or adjust dosage without discussing with prescriber.
• Advise woman to discuss drug therapy with prescriber if she's considering pregnancy.
• Advise woman that breast-feeding isn't recommended during therapy.

---

gabapentin
Neurontin

Pregnancy risk category C

AVAILABLE FORMS
Capsules: 100 mg, 300 mg, 400 mg

INDICATIONS & DOSAGES
➤ **Adjunctive treatment of partial seizures with and without secondary generalization in adults with epilepsy—**
Adults: Initially, 300 mg P.O. h.s. on day 1; 300 mg P.O. b.i.d. on day 2; then 300 mg P.O. t.i.d. on day 3. Dosage increased as needed and tolerated to 1,800 mg daily in divided doses. Doses up to 3,600 mg daily have been well tolerated.
Adjust-a-dose: For patients with renal impairment with creatinine clearance higher than 60 ml/minute, give 400 mg P.O. t.i.d.;

if clearance is between 30 and 60 ml/minute, 300 mg P.O. b.i.d.; between 15 and 30 ml/minute, 300 mg P.O. daily; and if clearance is less than 15 ml/minute, 300 mg P.O. every other day. Patients on dialysis should receive a loading dose of 300 to 400 mg P.O.; then 200 to 300 mg P.O. q 4 hours during hemodialysis.

✴ **NEW INDICATION: Adjunctive therapy for the control of partial seizures in children—**
Starting dosage, children ages 3 to 12: 10 to 15 mg/kg/day P.O. in three divided doses, adjusting over 3 days to reach effective dosage.
Effective dosage, children ages 5 to 12: 25 to 35 mg/kg/day P.O. in three divided doses.
Effective dosage, children ages 3 to 4: 40 mg/kg/day P.O. in three divided doses.

ACTION

Unknown. Although structurally related to gamma-aminobutyric acid (GABA), drug doesn't interact with GABA receptors and isn't converted metabolically into GABA or a GABA agonist. It doesn't inhibit GABA reuptake and doesn't prevent degradation.

Route	Onset	Peak	Duration
P.O.	Unknown	Unknown	Unknown

ADVERSE REACTIONS

CNS: *fatigue, somnolence, dizziness, ataxia,* nystagmus, tremor, nervousness, dysarthria, amnesia, depression, abnormal thinking, twitching, incoordination.
CV: peripheral edema, vasodilation.
EENT: diplopia, rhinitis, pharyngitis, dry throat, amblyopia.
GI: nausea, vomiting, dyspepsia, dry mouth, constipation, increased appetite, dental abnormalities.
GU: impotence.
Hematologic: *leukopenia.*
Metabolic: weight gain.
Musculoskeletal: back pain, myalgia, fractures.
Respiratory: coughing.
Skin: pruritus, abrasion.

INTERACTIONS

Drug-drug. *Antacids:* Decreased absorption of gabapentin. Separate administration times by at least 2 hours.

EFFECTS ON LAB TEST RESULTS
● May decrease WBC count.

CONTRAINDICATIONS
Contraindicated in patients hypersensitive to drug.

NURSING CONSIDERATIONS
● First dose should be given at bedtime to minimize drowsiness, dizziness, fatigue, and ataxia.
● If drug therapy is discontinued or alternative drug is substituted, do so gradually over at least 1 week, to minimize risk of precipitating seizures.
● *Alert:* Don't suddenly withdraw other anticonvulsants in patients starting gabapentin therapy.
● Routine monitoring of plasma drug levels isn't necessary. Drug doesn't appear to alter plasma levels of other anticonvulsants.
● Drug causes false-positive results with the Ames-N-Multistix SG dipstick test for urinary protein when added to other antiepileptic drugs. The more specific sulfosalicylic acid precipitation procedure is recommended to determine the presence of urine protein.

PATIENT TEACHING
● Advise patient that drug may be taken without regard to meals.
● Instruct patient to take first dose at bedtime to minimize adverse reactions.
● Warn patient to avoid driving and operating heavy machinery until drug's CNS effects are known.
● Advise patient not to stop drug abruptly.
● Advise woman to discuss drug therapy with prescriber if she's considering pregnancy.

lamotrigine
Lamictal

Pregnancy risk category C

AVAILABLE FORMS
Tablets: 25 mg, 100 mg, 150 mg, 200 mg
Tablets (chewable dispersible): 5 mg, 25 mg

INDICATIONS & DOSAGES
➤ **Adjunct therapy in treatment of partial seizures caused by epilepsy—**
Adults and children older than age 16: For patients taking valproic acid with other enzyme-inducing antiepileptics, 25 mg P.O. every other day for 2 weeks; then 25 mg P.O. daily for 2 weeks. Continue to increase, p.r.n., by 25 to 50 mg/day q 1 to 2 weeks. Maximum, 150 mg P.O. daily in two divided doses.

For patients receiving enzyme-inducing antiepileptics but not valproic acid, 50 mg P.O. daily for 2 weeks; then 100 mg P.O. daily in two divided doses for 2 weeks. Increase, p.r.n., by 100 mg daily q 1 to 2 weeks. Usual maintenance dosage is 300 to 500 mg P.O. daily in two divided doses.
Adjust-a-dose: Use lower maintenance dosage for patients with severe renal impairment.
➤ **Adjunctive treatment of generalized seizures of Lennox-Gastaut syndrome—**
Adults and children older than age 12: For patients on an antiepileptic drug regimen with valproic acid, 25 mg P.O. every other day for 2 weeks; then 25 mg P.O. daily for 2 weeks. Thereafter, usual maintenance dosage is 100 to 400 mg P.O. daily in one or two divided doses.

For patients taking enzyme-inducing antiepileptics but not valproic acid, 50 mg P.O. daily for 2 weeks; then 100 mg P.O. daily in two divided doses for 2 weeks. Thereafter, usual maintenance dosage is 300 to 500 mg P.O. daily in two divided doses.
Children ages 2 to 12, weighing more than 17 kg (37 lb): For patients on antiepileptic drug regimen with valproic acid, 0.15 mg/kg/day P.O. in one or two divided doses (rounded down to nearest 5 mg) for 2 weeks. If calculated daily dose of lamotrigine is 2.5 to 5 mg, then 5 mg of lamotrigine should be taken on alternate days; then 0.3 mg/kg/day P.O. in one or two doses rounded down to nearest 5 mg for 2 weeks. Thereafter, usual maintenance dosage is 1 to 5 mg/kg/day (maximum, 200 mg daily in one to two divided doses).

For patients on an antiepileptic drug regimen without valproic acid, 0.6 mg/kg/day P.O. in two divided doses rounded down to nearest 5 mg for 2 weeks; then 1.2 mg/kg/day P.O. in two divided doses

rounded down to nearest 5 mg for 2 weeks. Thereafter, usual maintenance dosage is 5 to 15 mg/kg/day (maximum, 400 mg daily in two divided doses).

ACTION
Unknown. May inhibit release of glutamate and aspartate (excitatory neurotransmitters) in the brain via an action at voltage-sensitive sodium channels.

Route	Onset	Peak	Duration
P.O.	Unknown	1.4-4.8 hr	Unknown

ADVERSE REACTIONS
CNS: *dizziness, headache, ataxia, somnolence,* incoordination, insomnia, tremor, depression, anxiety, *seizures,* irritability, speech disorder, decreased memory, aggravated reaction, concentration disturbance, sleep disorder, emotional lability, vertigo, mind racing, dysarthria, malaise.
CV: palpitations.
EENT: *diplopia, blurred vision,* vision abnormality, nystagmus, *rhinitis,* pharyngitis.
GI: *nausea, vomiting,* diarrhea, dyspepsia, abdominal pain, constipation, anorexia, dry mouth.
GU: dysmenorrhea, vaginitis, amenorrhea.
Musculoskeletal: muscle spasm, neck pain.
Respiratory: cough, dyspnea.
Skin: *rash, Stevens-Johnson syndrome, toxic epidermal necrolysis,* pruritus, hot flashes, alopecia, acne.
Other: flu syndrome, fever, infection, chills, tooth disorder.

INTERACTIONS
Drug-drug. *Acetaminophen:* May decrease therapeutic effects. Monitor patient.
Carbamazepine, phenobarbital, phenytoin, primidone: Decrease in lamotrigine's steady-state levels. Monitor patient closely.
Folate inhibitors, such as co-trimoxazole and methotrexate: Lamotrigine inhibits dihydrofolate reductase, an enzyme involved in folic acid synthesis. May have an additive effect. Monitor patient.
Valproic acid: Decreased clearance of lamotrigine, which increases the drug's steady-state levels. Also decreases val-

proic acid levels. Monitor patient for toxicity.

Drug-lifestyle. *Sun exposure.* Photosensitivity reactions may occur. Urge patient to take precautions against sun exposure.

EFFECTS ON LAB TEST RESULTS
None reported.

CONTRAINDICATIONS
Contraindicated in patients hypersensitive to drug or its components.

NURSING CONSIDERATIONS
• Use cautiously in patients with renal, hepatic, or cardiac impairment.
• Drug shouldn't be discontinued abruptly because of possibility of increased seizure frequency. Instead, drug should be tapered over at least 2 weeks.
• *Alert:* Drug should be stopped at first sign of rash unless rash isn't drug-related.
• Lamotrigine dose should be lowered if drug is added to a multidrug regimen that includes valproic acid.
• Chewable dispersible tablets may be swallowed whole, chewed, or dispersed in water or diluted fruit juice. If tablets are chewed, a small amount of water or diluted fruit juice should be given to aid in swallowing.
• Safety and efficacy of drug in children younger than age 16 (other than those with Lennox-Gastaut syndrome) haven't been established. Children weighing less than 37 lb (17 kg) shouldn't receive drug because therapy can't be initiated using dosing guidelines and currently available tablet strength.
• Patients should be evaluated for changes in seizure activity. Adjunct anticonvulsant's serum levels should be checked.
• *Alert:* Don't confuse lamotrigine with lamivudine or Lamictal with Lamisil.

PATIENT TEACHING
• Inform patient that drug may cause rash. Combination therapy of valproic acid and lamotrigine may cause a serious rash. Tell patient to report rash or signs or symptoms of hypersensitivity promptly to prescriber because they may warrant drug discontinuation.

• Warn patient not to engage in hazardous activity until drug's CNS effects are known.
• Warn patient that photosensitivity reactions may occur and to take precautions until tolerance is determined.
• Warn patient not to stop drug abruptly.
• Advise woman to discuss drug therapy with prescriber if she's considering pregnancy.
• Advise woman that breast-feeding isn't recommended during therapy.

levetiracetam
Keppra

Pregnancy risk category C

AVAILABLE FORMS
Tablets: 250 mg, 500 mg, 750 mg

INDICATIONS & DOSAGES
➤ **Adjunctive therapy for partial seizures—**
Adults: Initially, 500 mg b.i.d. Dosage can be increased by 500 mg b.i.d., p.r.n., for seizure control at 2-week intervals to maximum of 1,500 mg b.i.d.
Adjust-a-dose: For patients with renal impairment, if creatinine clearance is more than 80 ml/minute, give 500 to 1,500 mg q 12 hours; if clearance is 50 to 80 ml/minute, give 500 to 1,000 mg q 12 hours; if clearance is 30 to 50 ml/minute, give 250 to 750 mg q 12 hours; if clearance is less than 30 ml/minute, give 250 to 500 mg q 12 hours. For dialysis patients, give 500 to 1,000 mg q 24 hours. A 250- to 500-mg dose should be given after dialysis.

ACTION
May act by inhibiting simultaneous neuronal firing that leads to seizure activity.

Route	Onset	Peak	Duration
P.O.	1 hr	1 hr	12 hr

ADVERSE REACTIONS
CNS: *asthenia, headache, somnolence,* dizziness, depression, vertigo, paresthesia, nervousness, hostility, emotional lability, ataxia, amnesia, anxiety.

Reactions may be *common*, uncommon, **life-threatening**, or COMMON AND LIFE-THREATENING.

EENT: diplopia, pharyngitis, rhinitis, sinusitis.
GI: anorexia.
Hematologic: *leukopenia, neutropenia.*
Musculoskeletal: pain.
Respiratory: cough, infection.

INTERACTIONS
Drug-drug. *Antihistamines, benzodiazepines, narcotics, other drugs that cause drowsiness, TCAs:* May lead to severe sedation. Avoid using together.
Drug-lifestyle. *Alcohol:* May lead to severe sedation. Discourage use together.

EFFECTS ON LAB TEST RESULTS
• May decrease WBC and neutrophil counts.

CONTRAINDICATIONS
Contraindicated in patients hypersensitive to drug.

NURSING CONSIDERATIONS
• Patients with poor renal function need dosage adjustment.
• Leukopenia and neutropenia have been reported with drug use. Use cautiously in immunocompromised patients, such as those with cancer or HIV infection.
• Drug can be taken with or without food.
• Use drug only with other anticonvulsants; it's not recommended for monotherapy.
• Seizures can occur if drug is stopped abruptly. Tapering is recommended.
• Monitor patients closely for such adverse reactions as dizziness, which may lead to falls.

PATIENT TEACHING
• Warn patient to use extra care when sitting or standing to avoid falling.
• Advise patient to call prescriber and not to stop drug suddenly if adverse reactions occur.
• Tell patient to take with other prescribed seizure drugs.
• Inform patient that drug can be taken with or without food.

magnesium sulfate

Pregnancy risk category A

AVAILABLE FORMS
Injection: 4%, 8%, 10%, 12.5%, 25%, 50%
Injection solution: 1% in D_5W, 2% in D_5W

INDICATIONS & DOSAGES
➤ **Prevention or control of seizures in preeclampsia or eclampsia—**
Women: Initially, 4 g I.V. in 250 ml D_5W and 4 to 5 g deep I.M. into each buttock; then 4 to 5 g deep I.M. into alternate buttock q 4 hours, p.r.n. Or, 4 g I.V. loading dose; then 1 to 2 g hourly as I.V. infusion. Total dose shouldn't exceed 30 or 40 g daily.
➤ **Hypomagnesemia—**
Adults: For mild deficiency, 1 g I.M. q 6 hours for four doses; for severe deficiency, 5 g in 1,000 ml D_5W or normal saline solution infused over 3 hours.
➤ **Seizures, hypertension, and encephalopathy with acute nephritis in children—**
Children: 0.2 ml/kg of 50% solution I.M. q 4 to 6 hours, p.r.n. For severe symptoms, 100 to 200 mg/kg I.V. slowly over 1 hour with 50% of dose administered in first 15 to 20 minutes. Dosage titrated according to blood magnesium levels and seizure response.
➤ **Management of paroxysmal atrial tachycardia—**
Adults: 3 to 4 g I.V. over 30 seconds.
➤ **Management of life-threatening ventricular arrhythmias, such as sustained ventricular tachycardia or torsades de pointes—**
Adults: 2 to 6 g I.V. over several minutes; then continuous I.V. infusion of 3 to 20 mg/ minute for 5 to 48 hours. Dosage and duration of therapy are based on patient response and magnesium levels.

I.V. ADMINISTRATION
• If necessary, dilute to maximum level of 20%. Infuse no faster than 150 mg/minute (1.5 ml/minute of a 10% solution or

0.75 ml/minute of a 20% solution). Drug is compatible with D_5W.
• Maximum infusion rate is 150 mg/minute. Too-rapid infusion will induce uncomfortable feeling of heat.
• Monitor vital signs every 15 minutes when giving drug I.V.

ACTION

May decrease acetylcholine released by nerve impulses, but its anticonvulsant mechanism is unknown.

Route	Onset	Peak	Duration
I.M.	1 hr	Unknown	3-4 hr
I.V.	1-2 min	Rapid	30 min

ADVERSE REACTIONS

CNS: drowsiness, *depressed reflexes,* flaccid paralysis, hypothermia.
CV: *hypotension, flushing,* **circulatory collapse,** depressed cardiac function.
Metabolic: hypocalcemia.
Respiratory: *respiratory paralysis.*
Skin: diaphoresis.

INTERACTIONS

Drug-drug. *Anesthetics, CNS depressants:* May cause additive CNS depression. Use cautiously.
Cardiac glycosides: Concomitant use may exacerbate arrhythmias. Use together cautiously.
Neuromuscular blockers: May cause increased neuromuscular blockade. Use cautiously.

EFFECTS ON LAB TEST RESULTS

• May increase magnesium levels. May decrease calcium levels.

CONTRAINDICATIONS

Parenteral administration of drug contraindicated in patients with heart block or myocardial damage. Don't give in toxemia of pregnancy during 2 hours preceding delivery.

NURSING CONSIDERATIONS

• Use cautiously in patients with impaired renal function. Also use cautiously in women who are in labor.
• If used to treat seizures, take appropriate seizure precautions.

• **Alert:** Watch for respiratory depression and signs and symptoms of heart block.
• Keep I.V. calcium gluconate available to reverse magnesium intoxication; however, use cautiously in patients undergoing digitalization because of danger of arrhythmias.
• Check blood magnesium levels after repeated doses. Disappearance of knee-jerk and patellar reflexes is sign of impending magnesium toxicity.
• Signs of hypermagnesemia begin to appear at blood levels of 4 mEq/L.
• Monitor fluid intake and output. Urine output should be 100 ml or more in 4-hour period before each dose.
• Observe neonates for signs of magnesium toxicity, including neuromuscular or respiratory depression, when giving I.V. form of drug to toxemic mothers within 24 hours before delivery.
• **Alert:** Don't confuse magnesium sulfate with manganese sulfate.

PATIENT TEACHING

• Inform patient of short-term need for drug and answer any questions and address concerns.
• Review potential adverse reactions and instruct patient to promptly report any occurrences. Reassure patient that, although adverse reactions can occur, frequent monitoring of vital signs, reflexes, and blood levels will be done to ensure safety.

oxcarbazepine
Trileptal

Pregnancy risk category C

AVAILABLE FORMS

Oral suspension: 300 mg/5 ml (60 mg/ml)
Tablets (film-coated): 150 mg, 300 mg, 600 mg

INDICATIONS & DOSAGES

➤ **Adjunctive therapy for treatment of partial seizures in patients with epilepsy—**
Adults: Initially, 300 mg P.O. b.i.d. Increase by a maximum of 600 mg/day (300 mg P.O. b.i.d.) at weekly intervals. Recommended daily dose is 1,200 mg P.O. divided b.i.d.

Children ages 4 to 16: Initially, 8 to 10 mg/kg/day P.O. divided b.i.d., not to exceed 600 mg/day. The target maintenance dose depends on patient's weight and should be divided b.i.d. If patient weighs between 20 and 29 kg (44 and 64 lb), then target maintenance dose is 900 mg/day. If between 29 and 39 kg (64 and 86 lb), target maintenance dose is 1,200 mg/day. If more than 39 kg, target maintenance dose is 1,800 mg/day. Target doses should be achieved over 2 weeks.

➤ **Conversion to monotherapy for treatment of partial seizures in patients with epilepsy—**
Adults: Initially, 300 mg P.O. b.i.d., with simultaneous reduction in dose of concomitant antiepileptics. Increase oxcarbazepine by a maximum of 600 mg/day at weekly intervals over 2 to 4 weeks. Recommended daily dose is 2,400 mg P.O. divided b.i.d. Concomitant antiepileptics should be completely withdrawn over 3 to 6 weeks.

➤ **Initiation of monotherapy for treatment of partial seizures in patients with epilepsy—**
Adults: Initially, 300 mg P.O. b.i.d. Increase dosage by 300 mg/day every third day to a daily dose of 1,200 mg divided b.i.d.
Adjust-a-dose: For adults with creatinine clearance less than 30 ml/minute, initiate therapy at 150 mg P.O. b.i.d. (one-half usual starting dose), and increase slowly to achieve desired response.

ACTION
Unknown. Antiseizure activity is thought to occur through blockade of voltage-sensitive sodium channels, which ultimately may prevent seizure spread in the brain. Increased potassium conductance and modulation of high-voltage activated calcium channels may also contribute to anticonvulsant effects.

Route	Onset	Peak	Duration
P.O.	Unknown	Variable	Unknown

ADVERSE REACTIONS
CNS: *fatigue,* asthenia, feeling abnormal, *headache, dizziness, somnolence, ataxia, abnormal gait,* insomnia, *tremor,* nervousness, agitation, abnormal coordination, speech disorder, confusion, anxiety, amnesia, *aggravated seizures,* hypesthesia, emotional lability, impaired concentration, *vertigo.*
CV: hypotension, edema, chest pain.
EENT: *nystagmus, diplopia, abnormal vision,* abnormal accommodation, rhinitis, sinusitis, pharyngitis, epistaxis, ear pain.
GI: *nausea, vomiting, abdominal pain,* diarrhea, dyspepsia, constipation, gastritis, anorexia, dry mouth, *rectal hemorrhage,* taste perversion, thirst.
GU: urinary tract infection, urinary frequency, vaginitis.
Metabolic: hyponatremia, weight increase.
Musculoskeletal: muscular weakness, back pain.
Respiratory: *upper respiratory tract infection,* coughing, bronchitis, chest infection.
Skin: acne, hot flushes, purpura, rash, bruising, increased sweating.
Other: toothache, fever, allergic reaction, lymphadenopathy, infection.

INTERACTIONS
Drug-drug. *Carbamazepine, valproic acid, verapamil:* Decreased levels of active metabolite of oxcarbazepine. Monitor patient and serum levels closely.
Felodipine: Decreased felodipine level. Monitor patient closely.
Hormonal contraceptives: Decreased plasma levels of ethynylestradiol and levonorgestrel, rendering oral contraceptives less effective. Women of childbearing age should use alternative forms of contraception.
Phenobarbital: Decreased levels of active metabolite of oxcarbazepine; increased phenobarbital level. Monitor patient closely.
Phenytoin: Decreased levels of active metabolite of oxcarbazepine; may increase phenytoin level in adults receiving high doses of oxcarbazepine. Monitor phenytoin levels closely when initiating therapy in these patients.
Drug-lifestyle. *Alcohol:* Increased CNS depression. Discourage use together.

EFFECTS ON LAB TEST RESULTS
● May decrease sodium and thyroxine levels.

CONTRAINDICATIONS
Contraindicated in patients hypersensitive to drug or its components.

NURSING CONSIDERATIONS
• *Alert:* Between 25% and 30% of patients with history of hypersensitivity reaction to carbamazepine may develop hypersensitivities to oxcarbazepine. Question patient about carbamazepine hypersensitivity and stop drug immediately if signs or symptoms of hypersensitivity occur.
• Shake oral suspension well. Suspension can be mixed with water or swallowed directly from syringe.
• Oral suspension and tablets may be interchanged at equal doses.
• *Alert:* Withdraw drug gradually to minimize potential for increased seizure frequency.
• Watch for signs and symptoms of hyponatremia, including nausea, malaise, headache, lethargy, confusion, and decreased sensation.
• Monitor sodium levels in patients receiving oxcarbazepine for maintenance treatment, especially patients receiving other therapies that may decrease sodium levels.
• Oxcarbazepine use has been linked to several nervous system-related adverse reactions, including psychomotor slowing, difficulty with concentration, speech or language problems, somnolence, fatigue, and coordination abnormalities, such as ataxia and gait disturbances.

PATIENT TEACHING
• Drug may be taken with or without food.
• Tell patient to contact prescriber before interrupting or stopping drug.
• Advise patient to report signs and symptoms of hyponatremia, such as nausea, malaise, headache, lethargy, and confusion.
• Caution patient to avoid driving and other potentially hazardous activities that require mental alertness until effects of drug are known.
• Instruct woman using oral contraceptives to use alternative form of contraception while taking drug.
• Tell patient to avoid alcohol while taking drug.

• Advise patient to inform prescriber if he has ever experienced hypersensitivity reaction to carbamazepine.

---

phenobarbital (phenobarbitone)
Barbita, Solfoton

phenobarbital sodium
Luminal Sodium

Controlled substance schedule IV
Pregnancy risk category D

AVAILABLE FORMS
Capsules: 16 mg
Elixir*: 15 mg/5 ml, 20 mg/5 ml
Injection: 30 mg/ml, 60 mg/ml, 65 mg/ml, 130 mg/ml
Tablets: 15 mg, 16 mg, 30 mg, 60 mg, 100 mg

INDICATIONS & DOSAGES
➤ **All forms of epilepsy, febrile seizures—**
Adults: 60 to 200 mg P.O. daily in divided doses t.i.d. or as single dose h.s.
Children: 3 to 6 mg/kg P.O. daily, usually divided q 12 hours. Drug can be administered once daily, usually h.s.
➤ **Status epilepticus—**
Adults: 200 to 600 mg I.V.
Children: 100 to 400 mg I.V. Don't exceed 50 mg/minute.
➤ **Sedation—**
Adults: 30 to 120 mg P.O. daily in two or three divided doses.
Children: 3 to 5 mg/kg P.O. daily in divided doses t.i.d.
➤ **Insomnia—**
Adults: 100 to 200 mg P.O. or I.M. h.s.
➤ **Preoperative sedation—**
Adults: 100 to 200 mg I.M. 60 to 90 minutes before surgery.
Children: 16 to 100 mg I.M. or 1 to 3 mg/kg I.V., I.M., or P.O. 60 to 90 minutes before surgery.

I.V. ADMINISTRATION
• I.V. injection is reserved for emergency treatment. Give slowly under close supervision. Monitor respirations closely. When administering, don't give more than

---

60 mg/minute. Have resuscitation equipment available.
- **Alert:** Inadvertent intra-arterial injection can cause spasm of the artery and severe pain, and may even lead to gangrene.
- Don't mix parenteral form with acidic solutions; precipitation may result.
- Dilute drug in half-normal or normal saline, D₅W, lactated Ringer's, or Ringer's solution.

ACTION
Unknown. A barbiturate that probably depresses monosynaptic and polysynaptic transmission in CNS and increases threshold for seizure activity in motor cortex. As a sedative, drug probably interferes with transmission of impulses from thalamus to cortex of brain.

Route	Onset	Peak	Duration
I.M.	> 5 min	> 30 min	4-10 hr
I.V.	5 min	30 min	4-10 hr
P.O.	1 hr	8-12 hr	10-12 hr

ADVERSE REACTIONS
CNS: *drowsiness, lethargy, hangover,* paradoxical excitement in elderly patients, somnolence, changes in EEG patterns, physical and psychological dependence.
CV: *bradycardia,* hypotension.
GI: nausea, vomiting.
Hematologic: exacerbation of porphyria.
Respiratory: *respiratory depression, apnea.*
Skin: rash, *erythema multiforme, Stevens-Johnson syndrome,* urticaria, pain, swelling, thrombophlebitis, necrosis, nerve injury at injection site.
Other: *angioedema.*

INTERACTIONS
Drug-drug. *Chloramphenicol, MAO inhibitors, valproic acid:* Potentiated barbiturate effect. Monitor patient for increased CNS and respiratory depression.
CNS depressants, including narcotic analgesics: Excessive CNS depression. Monitor patient closely.
Corticosteroids, digitoxin, doxycycline, estrogens and oral contraceptives, oral anticoagulants, TCAs: May enhance metabolism of these drugs. Watch for decreased effect.

Diazepam: Increased effects of both drugs. Use together cautiously.
Griseofulvin: Decreased absorption of griseofulvin. Monitor effectiveness of griseofulvin.
Mephobarbital, primidone: Excessive phenobarbital blood levels. Monitor patient closely.
Rifampin: May decrease barbiturate levels. Watch for decreased effect.
Valproic acid: Increased phenobarbital levels. Watch for toxicity.
Drug-herb. *Evening primrose oil:* May increase anticonvulsant dosage requirement. Discourage use together.
Drug-lifestyle. *Alcohol use:* Excessive CNS depression. Discourage use together.

EFFECTS ON LAB TEST RESULTS
- May decrease bilirubin level.

CONTRAINDICATIONS
Contraindicated in patients hypersensitive to barbiturates and in those with history of manifest or latent porphyria; also contraindicated in patients with hepatic dysfunction, respiratory disease with dyspnea or obstruction, or nephritis.

NURSING CONSIDERATIONS
- Use cautiously in patients with acute or chronic pain, depression, suicidal tendencies, history of drug abuse, blood pressure alterations, CV disease, shock, or uremia, and in elderly or debilitated patients.
- Don't use injectable solution if it contains a precipitate.
- Give I.M. injection deeply. Superficial injection may cause pain, sterile abscess, and tissue sloughing.
- Elderly patients are more sensitive to drug's effects.
- **Alert:** Watch for signs of barbiturate toxicity: coma, cyanosis, asthmatic breathing, clammy skin, and hypotension. Overdose can be fatal.
- Therapeutic blood levels are 15 to 40 mcg/ml.
- Don't stop drug abruptly because seizures may worsen. Call prescriber immediately if adverse reactions develop.
- EEG patterns show a change in low-voltage fast activity. Changes persist for a time after therapy ends.

- Drug may decrease bilirubin levels in neonates, epileptics, and in patients with congenital nonhemolytic, unconjugated hyperbilirubinemia.
- Drug may cause a false-positive phentolamine test.
- The physiologic effects of drug may impair the absorption of cyanocobalamin Co 57.
- *Alert:* Don't confuse phenobarbital with pentobarbital.

PATIENT TEACHING

- Ensure that patient is aware that phenobarbital is available in different milligram strengths and sizes. Advise him to check prescription and refills closely.
- Inform patient that full therapeutic effects aren't seen for 2 to 3 weeks, except when loading dose is used.
- Advise patient to avoid driving and other potentially hazardous activities that require mental alertness until drug's CNS effects are known.
- Warn patient and parents not to stop drug abruptly.
- Tell patient using oral contraceptives to consider alternative method because drug may decrease effect of contraceptive.

phenytoin
(diphenylhydantoin)
Dilantin 125, Dilantin Infatabs, Epanutin§

phenytoin sodium
Dilantin, Phenytex

phenytoin sodium (extended)
Dilantin Kapseals

Pregnancy risk category D

AVAILABLE FORMS
phenytoin
Oral suspension: 125 mg/5 ml
Tablets (chewable): 50 mg
phenytoin sodium
Capsules: 100 mg (92-mg base)
Injection: 50 mg/ml (46-mg base)
phenytoin sodium (extended)
Capsules: 30 mg (27.6-mg base), 100 mg (92-mg base)

INDICATIONS & DOSAGES
➤ **Control of tonic-clonic (grand mal) and complex partial (temporal lobe) seizures—**
Adults: Highly individualized. Initially, 100 mg P.O. t.i.d., increased in increments of 100 mg P.O. q 2 to 4 weeks until desired response is obtained. Usual range is 300 to 600 mg daily. If patient is stabilized with extended-release capsules, once-daily dosing with 300-mg extended-release capsules is possible as an alternative.
Children: 5 mg/kg or 250 mg/m^2 P.O. divided b.i.d. or t.i.d. Maximum daily dose is 300 mg.
➤ **For patient requiring a loading dose—**
Adults: Initially, 1 g P.O. daily divided into three doses and administered at 2-hour intervals. Or, 10 to 15 mg/kg I.V. at a rate not exceeding 50 mg/minute. Normal maintenance dose is started 24 hours later.
Children: 5 mg/kg/day P.O. in two or three equally divided doses with subsequent dose individualized to maximum of 300 mg daily.
➤ **Prevention and treatment of seizures occurring during neurosurgery—**
Adults: 100 to 200 mg I.M. q 4 hours during surgery and continued during postoperative period.
➤ **Status epilepticus—**
Adults: Loading dose of 10 to 15 mg/kg I.V. (1 to 1.5 g may be needed) at a rate not exceeding 50 mg/minute; then maintenance doses of 100 mg P.O. or I.V. q 6 to 8 hours.
Children: Loading dose of 15 to 20 mg/kg I.V., at a rate not exceeding 1 to 3 mg/kg/minute; then highly individualized maintenance doses.
Elderly patients: May need lower dosages.

I.V. ADMINISTRATION
- Administer slowly (50 mg/minute) as I.V. bolus. If giving as an infusion, don't mix drug with D$_5$W because it will precipitate. Clear I.V. tubing first with normal saline solution. Never use cloudy solution. May mix with normal saline solution, if needed, and give as an infusion over 30 minutes to 1 hour, when possible. Infusion must begin within 1 hour after preparation

and should run through an in-line filter. Discard 4 hours after preparation.
• *Alert:* Check patency of I.V. catheter before administering. Extravasation has caused severe local tissue damage.
• If possible, don't administer phenytoin by I.V. push into veins on back of hand, to avoid discoloration (purple-glove syndrome). Inject into larger veins or central venous catheter, if available.
• Check vital signs, blood pressure, and ECG during I.V. administration.

ACTION
Unknown. A hydantoin derivative that probably stabilizes neuronal membranes and limits seizure activity by either increasing efflux or decreasing influx of sodium ions across cell membranes in the motor cortex during generation of nerve impulses.

Route	Onset	Peak	Duration
I.M.	Unknown	Unknown	Unknown
I.V.	Immediate	1-2 hr	Unknown
P.O.	Unknown	1.5-12 hr	Unknown

ADVERSE REACTIONS
CNS: *ataxia, slurred speech,* dizziness, insomnia, nervousness, twitching, headache, *mental confusion, decreased coordination.*
CV: periarteritis nodosa.
EENT: *nystagmus, diplopia,* blurred vision.
GI: *gingival hyperplasia, nausea, vomiting,* constipation.
Hematologic: *thrombocytopenia, leukopenia, agranulocytosis, pancytopenia,* macrocythemia, megaloblastic anemia.
Hepatic: *toxic hepatitis.*
Metabolic: hyperglycemia.
Musculoskeletal: osteomalacia.
Skin: scarlatiniform or morbilliform rash; bullous or purpuric dermatitis; exfoliative dermatitis; *Stevens-Johnson syndrome;* lupus erythematosus; *toxic epidermal necrolysis;* photosensitivity reactions; pain, necrosis, inflammation at injection site; discoloration of skin if given by I.V. push in back of hand; hypertrichosis.
Other: *hirsutism,* lymphadenopathy.

INTERACTIONS
Drug-drug. *Amiodarone, antihistamines, chloramphenicol, cimetidine, cycloserine, diazepam, disulfiram, isoniazid, phenylbutazone, salicylates, sulfamethizole, valproate:* May increase phenytoin activity and toxicity. Monitor patient.
Barbiturates, carbamazepine, dexamethasone, diazoxide, folic acid, rifampin: Decreased phenytoin activity. Monitor levels.
Carbamazepine, cardiac glycosides, oral contraceptives, quinidine, theophylline, valproic acid: Effects may be decreased by phenytoin. Monitor patient.
Drug-food. *Enteral tube feedings:* May interfere with absorption of oral phenytoin. Stop enteral feedings for 2 hours before and 2 hours after phenytoin administration.
Drug-lifestyle. *Long-term alcohol use:* Decreased phenytoin activity. Inform patient that heavy alcohol use may diminish drug's benefits.

EFFECTS ON LAB TEST RESULTS
• May increase alkaline phosphatase, GGT, and glucose levels.
• May decrease hemoglobin and platelet, WBC, RBC, and granulocyte counts.

CONTRAINDICATIONS
Contraindicated in patients hypersensitive to hydantoin and in those with sinus bradycardia, SA block, second- or third-degree AV block, or Adams-Stokes syndrome.

NURSING CONSIDERATIONS
• Use cautiously in patients with hepatic dysfunction, hypotension, myocardial insufficiency, diabetes, or respiratory depression; in elderly or debilitated patients; and in those receiving other hydantoin derivatives.
• Elderly patients tend to metabolize phenytoin slowly and may need reduced dosages.
• Phenytoin requirements usually increase during pregnancy.
• Use only clear solution for injection. A slight yellow color is acceptable. Don't refrigerate.
• Don't give I.M. unless dosage adjustments are made; drug may precipitate at

injection site, cause pain, and be absorbed erratically.

• Divided doses given with or after meals may decrease adverse GI reactions.

• Stop drug if rash appears. If rash is scarlatiniform or morbilliform, drug may be resumed after rash clears. If rash reappears, therapy should be discontinued. If rash is exfoliative, purpuric, or bullous, drug won't be resumed.

• Don't withdraw drug suddenly because seizures may worsen. Call prescriber at once if adverse reactions develop.

• Monitor blood levels of drug. Therapeutic phenytoin blood level is 10 to 20 mcg/ml.

• Allow at least 7 to 10 days to elapse between dosage changes.

• Monitor CBC and calcium level every 6 months, and periodically monitor hepatic function. If megaloblastic anemia is evident, prescriber may order folic acid and vitamin B_{12}.

• If using to treat seizures, take appropriate safety precautions.

• Mononucleosis may decrease phenytoin levels. Watch for increased seizures.

• Watch for gingival hyperplasia, especially in children.

• Drug may cause reduced protein-bound iodine and free thyroxine levels without evidence of hypothyroidism; a slight decrease in urinary 17-hydroxysteroid and 17-ketosteroid levels; increased urine 6-hydroxycortisol excretion; and decreased values for dexamethasone suppression or metyrapone tests.

• *Alert:* Doubling the dose doesn't result in twice initial serum levels but may result in toxic serum levels. Consult pharmacist for specific dosing recommendations.

• *Alert:* Don't confuse phenytoin with mephenytoin or fosphenytoin or Dilantin with Dilaudid.

PATIENT TEACHING
• Tell patient to notify prescriber if skin rash develops.

• Advise patient to avoid driving and other potentially hazardous activities that require mental alertness until drug's CNS effects are known.

• Advise patient not to change brands or dosage forms once he's stabilized on therapy.

• Dilantin capsules are the only oral form that can be given once daily. Toxic levels may result if any other brand or form is given once daily. Dilantin tablets and oral suspension should never be taken once daily.

• Advise patient to avoid alcohol.

• Warn patient and parents not to stop drug abruptly.

• Stress importance of good oral hygiene and regular dental examinations. Gingivectomy may be needed periodically if dental hygiene is poor.

• Caution patient that drug may color urine pink, red, or reddish brown.

primidone
Apo-Primidone†, Mysoline, PMS Primidone†, Sertan†

Pregnancy risk category NR

AVAILABLE FORMS
Oral suspension: 250 mg/5 ml
Tablets: 50 mg, 250 mg

INDICATIONS & DOSAGES
➤ **Tonic-clonic, complex partial, and simple partial seizures—**
Adults and children age 8 and older: Initially, 100 to 125 mg P.O. h.s. on days 1 to 3; then 100 to 125 mg P.O. b.i.d. on days 4 to 6; then 100 to 125 mg P.O. t.i.d. on days 7 to 9, followed by maintenance dose of 250 mg P.O. t.i.d. Maintenance dose may be increased to 250 mg q.i.d., if needed. Dosage may be increased to maximum of 2 g daily in divided doses.
Children younger than age 8: Initially, 50 mg P.O. h.s. for 3 days; then 50 mg P.O. b.i.d. for days 4 to 6; then 100 mg P.O. b.i.d. for days 7 to 9, followed by maintenance dose of 125 to 250 mg P.O. t.i.d. or 10 to 25 mg/kg/day in divided doses.

ACTION
Unknown. Some activity may be caused by phenylethylmalonamide and phenobarbital, which are active metabolites.

Route	Onset	Peak	Duration
P.O.	Unknown	3-4 hr	Unknown

ADVERSE REACTIONS
CNS: *drowsiness, ataxia,* emotional disturbances, vertigo, hyperirritability, fatigue, paranoid symptoms.
EENT: *diplopia,* nystagmus.
GI: anorexia, *nausea, vomiting.*
GU: impotence, polyuria.
Hematologic: megaloblastic anemia, *thrombocytopenia.*
Skin: morbilliform rash.

INTERACTIONS
Drug-drug. *Acetazolamide, succinimide:* May decrease primidone levels. Monitor levels.
Carbamazepine: Increased carbamazepine levels and decreased primidone and phenobarbital levels. Watch for toxicity.
Isoniazid: Increased primidone level. Monitor levels.
Phenytoin: Stimulated conversion of primidone to phenobarbital. Watch for increased phenobarbital effect.

EFFECTS ON LAB TEST RESULTS
• May decrease hemoglobin and platelet count. May alter liver function test values.

CONTRAINDICATIONS
Contraindicated in patients hypersensitive to phenobarbital and in those with porphyria.

NURSING CONSIDERATIONS
• Shake liquid suspension well.
• Don't withdraw drug suddenly because seizures may worsen. Notify prescriber immediately if adverse reactions develop.
• Therapeutic blood level of primidone is 5 to 12 mcg/ml. Therapeutic blood level of phenobarbital is 15 to 40 mcg/ml.
• Monitor CBC and routine blood chemistry every 6 months.
• Brand interchange isn't recommended because of documented bioequivalence problems for primidone products marketed by different manufacturers.
• *Alert:* Don't confuse primidone with prednisone or prinivil.

PATIENT TEACHING
• Advise patient to avoid driving and other potentially hazardous activities that require mental alertness until drug's CNS effects are known.

• Warn patient and parents not to stop drug therapy suddenly.
• Tell patient that full therapeutic response may take 2 weeks or longer.
• Advise woman to discuss drug therapy with prescriber if she's considering pregnancy.
• Caution woman that breast-feeding is contraindicated while taking this drug.

---

tiagabine hydrochloride
Gabitril

Pregnancy risk category C

AVAILABLE FORMS
Tablets: 4 mg, 12 mg, 16 mg, 20 mg

INDICATIONS & DOSAGES
➤ **Adjunctive therapy in treatment of partial seizures—**
Adults: Initially, 4 mg P.O. once daily. Total daily dose may be increased by 4 to 8 mg at weekly intervals until clinical response or up to 56 mg/day. Total daily dose should be given in divided doses b.i.d. to q.i.d.
Children ages 12 to 18: Initially, 4 mg P.O. once daily. Total daily dose may be increased by 4 mg at beginning of week 2 and thereafter by 4 to 8 mg/week until clinical response or up to 32 mg/day. Total daily dose should be given in divided doses b.i.d. to q.i.d.
Adjust-a-dose: For patients with hepatic impairment, reduced initial and maintenance doses or longer dosing intervals may be required.

ACTION
Unknown. May act by facilitating the effects of the inhibitory neurotransmitter gamma aminobutyric acid (GABA).
Drug binds to recognition sites associated with the GABA uptake carrier and may thus permit more GABA to be available for binding to receptors on postsynaptic cells.

Route	Onset	Peak	Duration
P.O.	Rapid	45 min	7-9 hr

ADVERSE REACTIONS
CNS: *dizziness, asthenia, somnolence, nervousness,* tremor, difficulty with concentration and attention, insomnia, ataxia, confusion, speech disorder, difficulty with memory, paresthesia, depression, emotional lability, abnormal gait, hostility, language problems, agitation.
CV: vasodilation.
EENT: nystagmus, pharyngitis.
GI: abdominal pain, *nausea,* diarrhea, vomiting, increased appetite, mouth ulceration.
Musculoskeletal: generalized weakness, pain, myasthenia.
Respiratory: increased cough.
Skin: rash, pruritus.

INTERACTIONS
Drug-drug. *Carbamazepine, phenobarbital, phenytoin:* Increased tiagabine clearance. Monitor patient closely.
CNS depressants: Enhanced CNS effects. Use together cautiously.
Drug-lifestyle. *Alcohol use:* Enhanced CNS effects. Advise patient to use together cautiously.

EFFECTS ON LAB TEST RESULTS
None reported.

CONTRAINDICATIONS
Contraindicated in patients hypersensitive to drug or its components.

NURSING CONSIDERATIONS
• Use cautiously in breast-feeding women.
• Never withdraw drug suddenly because seizures may occur more frequently. Withdraw drug gradually unless safety concerns require a more rapid withdrawal.
• *Alert:* Status epilepticus and sudden unexpected death in epilepsy have occurred in patients receiving antiepileptics, including tiagabine.
• Patients who aren't receiving at least one enzyme-inducing antiepileptic when starting tiagabine may need lower doses or a slower dosage adjustment.
• Moderately severe to incapacitating generalized weakness has occurred in patients receiving tiagabine. Weakness resolves after dosage reduction or discontinuation of drug.

PATIENT TEACHING
• Advise patient to take drug only as prescribed.
• Tell patient to take drug with food.
• Warn patient that drug may cause dizziness, somnolence, and other signs and symptoms of CNS depression. Advise patient to avoid driving and other potentially hazardous activities that require mental alertness until drug's CNS effects are known.
• Tell woman to call prescriber if she becomes pregnant or plans to become pregnant during therapy.
• Instruct woman to notify prescriber if planning to breast-feed because drug may appear in breast milk.

---

topiramate
Topamax

Pregnancy risk category C

AVAILABLE FORMS
Capsules, sprinkles: 15 mg, 25 mg, 50 mg
Tablets: 25 mg, 100 mg, 200 mg

INDICATIONS & DOSAGES
➤ **Adjunctive therapy for adults with partial onset seizures—**
Adults: Initially, 25 to 50 mg P.O. daily, increased gradually in increments of 25 to 50 mg/week until an effective daily dose is reached. Adjust up to maximum daily dose of 400 mg P.O. in divided doses b.i.d.
➤ **Adjunctive therapy for partial onset seizures in children—**
Children ages 2 to 16: Initially, 25 mg (or less based on range of 1 to 3 mg/kg/day) P.O. nightly for first week. Increase dosage based on response at 1- to 2-week intervals by increments of 1 to 3 mg/kg/day given in two divided doses. Recommended total daily dose is 5 to 9 mg/kg/day P.O. in two divided doses.
➤ **Adjunctive therapy for primary generalized tonic-clonic seizures—**
Adults: 50 mg P.O. daily in evening for first week; then adjust to maximum daily dose of 400 mg given in two divided doses. Adjustment schedule is as follows: Week 1, 50 mg P.O. in evening; week 2, 50 mg P.O. b.i.d. (in morning and even-

ing); week 3, 50 mg P.O. in morning and 100 mg P.O. in evening; week 4, 100 mg P.O. b.i.d. (in morning and evening); week 5, 100 mg P.O. in morning and 150 mg P.O. in evening; week 6, 150 mg P.O. b.i.d. (in morning and evening); week 7, 150 mg P.O. in morning and 200 mg P.O. in evening; week 8, 200 mg P.O. b.i.d. (in morning and evening).

Children ages 2 to 16: 1 to 3 mg/kg P.O. daily in evening for first week; then increase dose at 1- or 2-week intervals by increments of 1 to 3 mg/kg/day. Dosage range is 5 to 9 mg/kg/day given in two divided doses. Adjust dosage based on response.

➤ **Lennox-Gastaut syndrome—**
Children ages 2 to 16: Initially, 25 mg (or less based on range of 1 to 3 mg/kg/day) P.O. nightly for first week. Increase dosage based on response at 1- to 2-week intervals by increments of 1 to 3 mg/kg/day given in two divided doses. Recommended total daily dose is 5 to 9 mg/kg/day P.O. in two divided doses. Adjust up to maximum daily dose of 400 mg P.O. in divided doses b.i.d.

Adjust-a-dose: For renally impaired patients with creatinine clearance less than 70 ml/minute, reduce dosage by 50%. For patients on hemodialysis, supplemental doses may be needed to avoid rapid drops in drug levels during prolonged dialysis treatment.

ACTION

Unknown. Suggestive of a sodium channel blocking action. May also potentiate the activity of gamma-aminobutyrate (GABA) and antagonize the ability of kainate to activate the kainate/alpha-amino-3-hydroxy-5-methylisoxazole-4-propionic acid subtype of excitatory amino acid (glutamate) receptor.

Route	Onset	Peak	Duration
P.O.	Unknown	2 hr	Unknown

ADVERSE REACTIONS

CNS: abnormal coordination, aggressive reaction, agitation, apathy, asthenia, *ataxia, confusion,* depression, depersonalization, *difficulty with memory, dizziness,* emotional lability, euphoria, *generalized tonic-clonic seizures,* hallucination, hyperkinesia, hypertonia, hypoesthesia, hypokinesia, insomnia, mood problems, *nervousness, paresthesia,* personality disorder, *psychomotor slowing,* psychosis, *somnolence, speech disorders,* stupor, *suicide attempts, tremor,* vertigo, malaise, *fatigue,* difficulty with concentration, attention, or language.

CV: chest pain, palpitations, vasodilation, edema.

EENT: *abnormal vision,* conjunctivitis, *diplopia,* eye pain, epistaxis, hearing problems, tinnitus, pharyngitis, sinusitis, *nystagmus.*

GI: abdominal pain, anorexia, constipation, diarrhea, dry mouth, dyspepsia, flatulence, gastroenteritis, gingivitis, *nausea,* vomiting, taste perversion.

GU: amenorrhea, dysuria, dysmenorrhea, hematuria, impotence, intermenstrual bleeding, menstrual disorder, menorrhagia, micturition frequency, renal calculi, urinary incontinence, urinary tract infection, vaginitis, leukorrhea.

Hematologic: anemia, *leukopenia.*

Metabolic: increased or decreased weight.

Musculoskeletal: arthralgia, back or leg pain, muscle weakness, myalgia, rigors.

Respiratory: bronchitis, coughing, dyspnea, *upper respiratory tract infection.*

Skin: acne, alopecia, increased sweating, pruritus, rash.

Other: decreased libido, breast pain, body odor, fever, flu syndrome, hot flashes, lymphadenopathy.

INTERACTIONS

Drug-drug. *Carbamazepine:* Decreased topiramate levels. Monitor patient.

Carbonic anhydrase inhibitors (acetazolamide, dichlorphenamide): May cause renal calculus formation. Avoid using together.

CNS depressants: Possible topiramate-induced CNS depression as well as other adverse cognitive and neuropsychiatric events. Use with caution.

Oral contraceptives: Decreased efficacy. Report changes in bleeding patterns.

Phenytoin: Decreased topiramate levels and increased phenytoin levels. Monitor levels.

Valproic acid: Decrease in valproic acid and topiramate levels. Monitor patient.

Drug-lifestyle. *Alcohol use:* Possible topiramate-induced CNS depression as well as other adverse cognitive and neuropsychiatric events. Advise caution.

EFFECTS ON LAB TEST RESULTS
● May increase liver enzyme levels.
● May decrease hemoglobin and WBC count.

CONTRAINDICATIONS
Contraindicated in patients hypersensitive to drug or its components.

NURSING CONSIDERATIONS
● Use with caution in breast-feeding or pregnant women and in those with hepatic impairment.
● If necessary, withdraw antiepileptics (including topiramate) gradually to minimize risk of increased seizure activity.
● Monitoring plasma levels of topiramate isn't necessary.
● Drug is rapidly cleared by dialysis. A prolonged period of dialysis may result in low drug levels and seizures. A supplemental dose may be required.

PATIENT TEACHING
● Tell patient to maintain adequate fluid intake during therapy to minimize risk of forming renal calculi.
● Advise patient not to drive or operate hazardous machinery until CNS effects of drug are known. Drug can cause somnolence, dizziness, confusion, and difficulty concentrating.
● Tell woman that drug may decrease effectiveness of oral contraceptives. Advise woman taking oral contraceptives to report change in her bleeding patterns.
● Tell patient to avoid crushing or breaking tablets because of bitter taste.
● Inform patient that drug can be taken without regard to food.
● Tell patient that sprinkle capsules may either be swallowed whole or carefully opened and contents sprinkled on a teaspoonful of soft food. This should be swallowed immediately without chewing.

valproate sodium
Depacon, Depakene, Epilim‡, Valpro‡

valproic acid
Convulex§, Depakene

divalproex sodium
Depakote, Depakote ER, Depakote Sprinkle, Epival†

Pregnancy risk category D

AVAILABLE FORMS
valproate sodium
Syrup: 250 mg/5 ml
valproic acid
Capsules: 250 mg
Syrup: 200 mg/5 ml‡
Tablets (crushable): 100 mg‡
Tablets (enteric-coated): 200 mg‡, 500 mg‡
divalproex sodium
Capsules (containing coated particles): 125 mg
Injection: 500-mg vial
Tablets (delayed-release): 125 mg, 250 mg, 500 mg

INDICATIONS & DOSAGES
➤ **Simple and complex absence seizures, mixed seizure types (including absence seizures)—**
Adults and children: Initially, 15 mg/kg P.O. or I.V. daily; then increase by 5 to 10 mg/kg daily at weekly intervals up to maximum of 60 mg/kg daily.
➤ **Mania (divalproex sodium only)—**
Adults and children: Initially, 750 mg daily in divided doses. Adjust dosage based on patient's response; maximum dose is 60 mg/kg/day.
➤ **Prophylaxis for migraine headache (divalproex sodium only)—**
Adults: Initially, 250 mg P.O. b.i.d. Some patients may need up to 1,000 mg/day. Or, 500 mg (Depakote ER) P.O. daily for 1 week; then 1,000 mg P.O. daily.
Elderly patients: Start at lower dosage, using Depakote delayed-release tablets. Increase dosage more slowly and with regular monitoring for fluid and nutritional intake, dehydration, somnolence, and other adverse events.

➤ **Complex partial seizures—**
Adults and children age 10 and older: 10 to 15 mg/kg P.O. or I.V. daily; then increase by 5 to 10 mg/kg daily at weekly intervals, up to 60 mg/kg/day.
Elderly patients: Reduce initial dose.

I.V. ADMINISTRATION
● I.V. use is indicated only in patients who can't take drug orally. Switch patient to oral form as soon as clinically feasible; effects of using I.V. dosage for longer than 14 days are unknown.
● Dilute valproate sodium injection with at least 50 ml of a compatible diluent. It's physically compatible and chemically stable in D_5W, normal saline, and lactated Ringer's solution for 24 hours.
● Administer drug as a 60-minute I.V. infusion (but not more than 20 mg/minute) with the same frequency as oral dosage.
● Monitoring of plasma levels and dosage adjustment may be needed.

ACTION
Unknown. Probably facilitates the effects of the inhibitory neurotransmitter gamma-aminobutyric acid.

Route	Onset	Peak	Duration
I.V.	Unknown	1 hr	Unknown
P.O.	Unknown	15 min-4 hr	Unknown

ADVERSE REACTIONS
CNS: asthenia, *sedation,* emotional upset, depression, psychosis, aggressiveness, hyperactivity, behavioral deterioration, muscle weakness, tremor, ataxia, *headache, dizziness,* incoordination.
EENT: nystagmus, *diplopia.*
GI: nausea, vomiting, indigestion, *diarrhea,* abdominal cramps, constipation, increased appetite, anorexia, *pancreatitis.*
Hematologic: *thrombocytopenia,* increased bleeding time, petechiae, bruising, eosinophilia, *hemorrhage, leukopenia, bone marrow suppression.*
Hepatic: *toxic hepatitis.*
Metabolic: weight gain.
Skin: rash, alopecia, pruritus, photosensitivity reactions, *erythema multiforme.*

INTERACTIONS
Drug-drug. *Aspirin, chlorpromazine, cimetidine, erythromycin, felbamate:* May

cause valproic acid toxicity. Use together cautiously and monitor blood levels of drug.
Benzodiazepines, other CNS depressants: Excessive CNS depression. Avoid using together.
Lamotrigine: Increased lamotrigine levels, decreased valproate levels. Monitor levels closely.
Phenobarbital: Increased phenobarbital levels. Monitor patient closely.
Phenytoin: Increased or decreased phenytoin levels, decreased valproate levels. Monitor patient closely.
Rifampin: May decrease valproate levels. Monitor levels.
Warfarin: Valproic acid may displace warfarin from binding sites. Monitor PT and INR.
Drug-lifestyle. *Alcohol use:* Excessive CNS depression. Discourage use together.

EFFECTS ON LAB TEST RESULTS
● May increase ALT, AST, and bilirubin levels.
● May increase eosinophil count and bleeding time. May decrease platelet and WBC counts.

CONTRAINDICATIONS
Contraindicated in patients hypersensitive to drug and in those with hepatic disease or significant hepatic dysfunction.

NURSING CONSIDERATIONS
● Obtain liver function test results, platelet count, and PT and INR before starting drug and monitor periodically.
● Don't administer syrup to patients who need sodium restriction. Check with prescriber.
● Adverse reactions may not be caused by valproic acid alone because it's usually used with other anticonvulsants.
● Divalproex sodium has a lower risk of adverse GI reactions.
● Never withdraw drug suddenly because sudden withdrawal may worsen seizures. Call prescriber at once if adverse reactions develop.
● *Alert:* Serious or fatal hepatotoxicity may follow nonspecific symptoms, such as malaise, fever, and lethargy. If these symptoms occur, notify prescriber at once because drug will need to be discontinued

in the presence of suspected or apparent substantial hepatic dysfunction.

• Patients at high risk for hepatotoxicity include those with congenital metabolic disorders, mental retardation, or organic brain disease; those taking multiple anticonvulsants; and children younger than age 2.

• Notify prescriber if tremors occur; a dosage reduction may be needed.

• Monitor blood levels of drug. Therapeutic blood level is 50 to 100 mcg/ml.

• Use caution when converting patients from a brand to a generic product because breakthrough seizures are possible.

• Drug may cause false-positive results for urine ketones.

PATIENT TEACHING

• Tell patient to take drug with food or milk to reduce adverse GI effects.

• Advise patient not to chew capsules; irritation of mouth and throat may result.

• Tell patient that sprinkle capsules may be either swallowed whole or carefully opened and contents sprinkled on a teaspoonful of soft food. This should be swallowed immediately without chewing.

• Tell patient and parents that syrup shouldn't be mixed with carbonated beverages; mixture may be irritating to mouth and throat.

• Tell patient and parents to keep drug out of children's reach.

• Warn patient and parents not to stop drug therapy abruptly.

• Advise patient to avoid driving and other potentially hazardous activities that require mental alertness until drug's CNS effects are known.

• Instruct patient or parents to call prescriber if malaise, weakness, lethargy, facial edema, anorexia, or vomiting occurs.

• Tell woman to call prescriber if she becomes pregnant or plans to become pregnant during therapy.

---

zonisamide
Zonegran

Pregnancy risk category C

AVAILABLE FORMS
Capsules: 100 mg

INDICATIONS & DOSAGES
➤ **Adjunct therapy for treatment of partial seizures in adults with epilepsy—**
Adults and children older than age 16:
Initially, 100 mg P.O. as a single daily dose for 2 weeks. Then, dose may be increased to 200 mg/day for at least 2 weeks. Dose can be increased to 300 mg and 400 mg P.O. daily, with the dose stable for at least 2 weeks to achieve steady state at each level. Doses can be given once or twice daily except for the daily dose of 100 mg at start of therapy. Maximum dose is 600 mg/day.
Adjust-a-dose: Use cautiously in patients with hepatic and renal disease; these patients may need slower adjustment and more frequent monitoring. Don't use if glomerular filtration rate is less than 50 ml/minute.

ACTION
Unknown. May stabilize neuronal membranes and suppress neuronal hypersynchronization, which prevents seizures.

Route	Onset	Peak	Duration
P.O.	Unknown	2-6 hr	Unknown

ADVERSE REACTIONS
CNS: *headache, dizziness,* ataxia, nystagmus, paresthesia, confusion, difficulties in concentration or memory, mental slowing, agitation or irritability, depression, insomnia, anxiety, nervousness, schizophrenic or schizophreniform behavior, *somnolence,* fatigue, asthenia, speech disorders, difficulties in verbal expression, hyperesthesia, incoordination, tremor, *seizures, status epilepticus.*
EENT: taste perversion, diplopia, amblyopia, tinnitus, rhinitis, pharyngitis.
GI: *anorexia,* nausea, vomiting, diarrhea, dyspepsia, constipation, dry mouth, abdominal pain.
GU: kidney stones.
Hematologic: ecchymoses.
Metabolic: weight loss.
Respiratory: cough.
Skin: rash, pruritus.
Other: flu syndrome, accidental injury.

Reactions may be *common*, uncommon, *life-threatening*, or COMMON AND LIFE-THREATENING.

INTERACTIONS

Drug-drug. *Drugs that induce or inhibit CYP3A4:* Altered levels of zonisamide. Clearance of zonisamide is increased by phenytoin, carbamazepine, phenobarbital, and valproate. Monitor patient closely.

EFFECTS ON LAB TEST RESULTS

• May increase BUN and creatinine levels.

CONTRAINDICATIONS

Contraindicated in patients hypersensitive to drug or to sulfonamides.

NURSING CONSIDERATIONS

• Use cautiously in patients with renal and hepatic dysfunction. If glomerular filtration rate is less than 50 ml/minute, don't use. If patient develops acute renal failure or a significant sustained increase in creatinine or BUN level, discontinue drug and notify prescriber.

• *Alert:* Rarely, fatalities have occurred in patients receiving sulfonamides because of severe reactions such as Stevens-Johnson syndrome, fulminant hepatic necrosis, aplastic anemia, otherwise unexplained rashes, and agranulocytosis. If signs and symptoms of hypersensitivity or other serious reactions occur, discontinue drug immediately and notify prescriber.

• It may take 2 weeks to achieve steady-state levels.

• Monitor patient for signs and symptoms of hypersensitivity.

• Monitor body temperature, especially in summer, because decreased sweating has occurred (especially in patients ages 17 and younger), resulting in heatstroke and dehydration.

• Abrupt withdrawal of zonisamide may precipitate increased frequency of seizures or status epilepticus; reduce dosage or discontinue drug gradually.

• Increase fluid intake and urine output to help prevent kidney stones, especially in patients with predisposing factors.

• Monitor renal function periodically.

PATIENT TEACHING

• Tell patient to take drug with or without food and not to bite or break capsule.

• Advise patient to call prescriber immediately if rash develops or seizures worsen.

• Tell patient to contact prescriber immediately if he develops sudden back pain, abdominal pain, pain when urinating, bloody or dark urine, fever, sore throat, mouth sores or easy bruising, decreased sweating, rise in body temperature, depression, or speech or language problems.

• Tell patient to drink 6 to 8 glasses of water a day.

• Caution patient that this drug can cause drowsiness and not to drive or operate dangerous machinery until drug's effects are known.

• Advise patient not to stop taking drug without prescriber's approval.

• Instruct woman to call prescriber if she is pregnant or breast-feeding or plans to become pregnant or breast-feed.

• Advise woman of childbearing potential to use contraceptives while taking drug.

29

Antidepressants

amitriptyline hydrochloride
amitriptyline pamoate
amoxapine
bupropion hydrochloride
citalopram hydrobromide
clomipramine hydrochloride
desipramine hydrochloride
doxepin hydrochloride
fluoxetine hydrochloride
imipramine hydrochloride
imipramine pamoate
mirtazapine
nefazodone hydrochloride
nortriptyline hydrochloride
paroxetine hydrochloride
phenelzine sulfate
sertraline hydrochloride
tranylcypromine sulfate
trazodone hydrochloride
trimipramine maleate
venlafaxine hydrochloride

COMBINATION PRODUCTS
ETRAFON: perphenazine 2 mg and
amitriptyline hydrochloride 25 mg.
ETRAFON 2-10: perphenazine 2 mg and
amitriptyline hydrochloride 10 mg.
ETRAFON-A: perphenazine 4 mg and
amitriptyline hydrochloride 10 mg.
ETRAFON-FORTE: perphenazine 4 mg and
amitriptyline hydrochloride 25 mg.
LIMBITROL DS: chlordiazepoxide 10 mg
and amitriptyline hydrochloride 25 mg.
TRIAVIL 2-10, TRIAVIL 4-10, TRIAVIL 2-25,
TRIAVIL 4-25 are products identical to the
Etrafon products listed above. Triavil is
also available as TRIAVIL 4-50 (perphenazine 4 mg and amitriptyline hydrochloride
50 mg).

amitriptyline hydrochloride
Apo-Amitriptyline†, Elavil, Endep,
Levate†, Novotriptyn†, Tryptanol‡,
Tryptine‡

amitriptyline pamoate
Elavil Plus†

Pregnancy risk category C

AVAILABLE FORMS
amitriptyline hydrochloride
Injection: 10 mg/ml
Tablets: 10 mg, 25 mg, 50 mg, 75 mg,
100 mg, 150 mg
amitriptyline pamoate†
Syrup: 10 mg/5 ml*†

INDICATIONS & DOSAGES
➤ **Depression—**
Adults: Initially, 50 to 100 mg P.O. h.s.,
increasing to 150 mg daily. Maximum,
300 mg daily, if needed. Maintenance, 50
to 100 mg daily. Or, 20 to 30 mg I.M.
q.i.d.
Elderly patients and adolescents: 10 mg
P.O. t.i.d. and 20 mg h.s. daily.

ACTION
Unknown. A TCA that increases the
amount of norepinephrine, serotonin, or
both in the CNS by blocking their reuptake by the presynaptic neurons.

Route	Onset	Peak	Duration
I.M., P.O.	Unknown	2-12 hr	Unknown

ADVERSE REACTIONS
CNS: *coma, seizures, CVA,* hallucinations, delusions, disorientation, ataxia,
tremor, peripheral neuropathy, anxiety, insomnia, restlessness, drowsiness, dizziness, weakness, fatigue, headache, extrapyramidal reactions.
CV: *MI, arrhythmias, heart block, orthostatic hypotension, tachycardia,* ECG
changes, hypertension, edema.
EENT: blurred vision, tinnitus, mydriasis,
increased intraocular pressure.

Reactions may be *common,* uncommon, *life-threatening,* or **COMMON AND LIFE-THREATENING.**

GI: *dry mouth,* nausea, vomiting, anorexia, epigastric pain, diarrhea, constipation, paralytic ileus.

GU: urine retention.

Hematologic: *agranulocytosis, thrombocytopenia, leukopenia,* eosinophilia.

Metabolic: hypoglycemia, hyperglycemia.

Skin: rash, urticaria, photosensitivity reactions, diaphoresis.

Other: hypersensitivity reactions.

INTERACTIONS

Drug-drug. *Barbiturates, CNS depressants:* Enhanced CNS depression. Avoid using together.

Cimetidine, fluoxetine, fluvoxamine, oral contraceptives, paroxetine, sertraline: Increased TCA blood levels. Watch for increased antidepressant adverse effects.

Clonidine: May reduce effectiveness of clonidine. Avoid using together, if possible. Monitor blood pressure.

Epinephrine, norepinephrine: Increased hypertensive effect. Use together cautiously.

MAO inhibitors: May cause severe excitation, hyperpyrexia, or seizures, usually with high doses. Avoid using together.

Drug-herb. *Evening primrose:* May cause additive or synergistic effect, resulting in lower seizure threshold and increasing the risk of seizure. Discourage use together.

St. John's wort, SAM-e, yohimbe: May cause serotonin syndrome, which is a toxic hyperserotonergic state, characterized by euphoria, drowsiness, overreactive reflexes, jaw clenching, sweating, high body temperature, unconsciousness, and even death. Discourage use together.

Drug-lifestyle. *Alcohol use:* Enhanced CNS depression. Discourage use together.

Smoking: May lower drug levels. Watch for lack of effect.

Sun exposure: Increased risk of photosensitivity reactions. Advise patient to avoid excessive sunlight exposure.

EFFECTS ON LAB TEST RESULTS

● May increase or decrease glucose levels.

● May increase eosinophil count and liver function test values. May decrease granulocyte, platelet, and WBC counts.

CONTRAINDICATIONS

Contraindicated in patients hypersensitive to drug and in those who have received an MAO inhibitor within the past 14 days; also contraindicated during acute recovery phase of MI.

NURSING CONSIDERATIONS

● Use cautiously in patients with history of seizures, urine retention, angle-closure glaucoma, or increased intraocular pressure; in those with hyperthyroidism, CV disease, diabetes, or impaired liver function; and in those receiving thyroid drugs.

● Use with caution if patient is receiving electroshock therapy.

● *Alert:* Parenteral form of drug is for I.M. administration only. Drug shouldn't be given I.V.

● Amitriptyline has strong anticholinergic effects and is one of the most sedating TCAs. Anticholinergic effects have rapid onset even though therapeutic effect is delayed for weeks.

● If signs or symptoms of psychosis occur or increase, expect prescriber to reduce dosage. Record mood changes. Monitor patient for suicidal tendencies and allow only minimum supply of drug.

● Because hypertensive episodes have occurred during surgery in patients receiving TCAs, drug should be discontinued gradually several days before surgery.

● Monitor glucose levels.

● Watch for nausea, headache, and malaise after abrupt withdrawal of long-term therapy; however, these symptoms don't indicate addiction.

● Don't withdraw drug abruptly.

● *Alert:* Don't confuse amitriptyline with nortriptyline or aminophylline, Elavil with Equanil or Mellaril, or Endep with Depen.

PATIENT TEACHING

● Whenever possible, advise patient to take full dose at bedtime, but warn him of possible morning orthostatic hypotension.

● Tell patient to avoid alcohol during drug therapy.

● Advise patient to consult prescriber before taking other drugs.

● Warn patient to avoid activities that require alertness and good psychomotor coordination until CNS effects of drug are

known. Drowsiness and dizziness usually subside after a few weeks.
• Inform patient that dry mouth may be relieved with sugarless hard candy or gum. Saliva substitutes may be useful.
• To prevent photosensitivity reactions, advise patient to use a sunblock, wear protective clothing, and avoid prolonged exposure to strong sunlight.
• Warn patient not to stop drug therapy abruptly.
• Advise patient that it may take as long as 30 days to achieve full therapeutic effect.

amoxapine
Asendin

Pregnancy risk category C

AVAILABLE FORMS
Tablets: 25 mg, 50 mg, 100 mg, 150 mg

INDICATIONS & DOSAGES
➤ Depression—
Adults: Initially, 50 mg P.O. b.i.d. or t.i.d. Increased to 100 mg b.i.d. or t.i.d. by end of week 1 of therapy, if tolerated. Increases above 300 mg daily are made only if 300 mg daily has been ineffective during trial period of at least 2 weeks. Maximum recommended dose is 400 mg daily for outpatients and 600 mg daily for hospitalized patients without a seizure history. When effective dose is established, entire dose (not to exceed 300 mg) may be given h.s.
Elderly patients: Initially, 25 mg P.O. b.i.d. or t.i.d. If tolerated by end of week 1, increase to 50 mg b.i.d. or t.i.d. Carefully increase up to 300 mg daily.

ACTION
Unknown. A TCA that increases the amount of norepinephrine, serotonin, or both in the CNS by blocking their reuptake by the presynaptic neurons.

Route	Onset	Peak	Duration
P.O.	Unknown	1.5 hr	Unknown

ADVERSE REACTIONS
CNS: *drowsiness, dizziness,* excitation, tremor, weakness, confusion, anxiety, insomnia, restlessness, nightmares, ataxia, fatigue, headache, nervousness, tardive dyskinesia, EEG changes, *seizures,* extrapyramidal reactions, *neuroleptic malignant syndrome.*
CV: *orthostatic hypotension, tachycardia,* hypertension, palpitations, edema, ECG changes.
EENT: blurred vision.
GI: *dry mouth,* constipation, nausea, excessive appetite.
GU: urine retention, *acute renal failure.*
Metabolic: hypoglycemia, hyperglycemia.
Skin: rash, diaphoresis.

INTERACTIONS
Drug-drug. *Barbiturates:* Decreased TCA blood levels. Watch for decreased antidepressant effect.
Cimetidine, fluoxetine, fluvoxamine, paroxetine, sertraline: May increase amoxapine levels. Watch for increased adverse effects.
Clonidine: May reduce the effectiveness of clonidine. Avoid using together, if possible. Monitor blood pressure.
CNS depressants: Enhanced CNS depression. Avoid using together.
Epinephrine, norepinephrine: Increased hypertensive effect. Use together cautiously.
MAO inhibitors: May cause severe excitation, hyperpyrexia, or seizures, usually with high doses. Avoid using together.
Drug-herb. *Evening primrose:* Additive or synergistic effects resulting in lower seizure threshold and increasing the risk of seizure. Discourage use together.
St. John's wort, SAM-e, yohimbe: May cause serotonin syndrome. Discourage use together.
Drug-lifestyle. *Alcohol use:* Enhanced CNS depression. Discourage use together.
Sun exposure: Increased risk of photosensitivity reactions. Advise patient to avoid excessive sunlight exposure.

EFFECTS ON LAB TEST RESULTS
• May increase or decrease glucose levels.
• May increase liver function test values.

CONTRAINDICATIONS
Contraindicated in patients hypersensitive to drug and in those who have received an MAO inhibitor within the past 14 days; also contraindicated during acute recovery phase of MI.

Reactions may be *common,* uncommon, *life-threatening,* or COMMON AND LIFE-THREATENING.

NURSING CONSIDERATIONS

• Use cautiously in patients with history of urine retention, angle-closure glaucoma, or increased intraocular pressure and in patients with CV disease. Use with extreme caution in patients with history of seizure disorders.
• Safe use of drug in children younger than age 16 hasn't been determined.
• Monitor patient for nausea, headache, and malaise after abrupt withdrawal of long-term therapy; these symptoms don't indicate addiction.
• Don't withdraw drug abruptly.
• Because hypertensive episodes have occurred during surgery in patients receiving TCAs, drug should be gradually discontinued several days before surgery.
• Expect delay of 2 weeks or longer before noticeable effect. Full effect may take 4 weeks or longer. However, adverse anticholinergic effects can occur rapidly.
• If signs or symptoms of psychosis occur or increase, expect prescriber to reduce dosage. Record mood changes. Monitor patient for suicidal tendencies and allow only a minimum supply of drug.
• Watch for signs and symptoms of tardive dyskinesia, especially in elderly women.
• Watch for acute renal failure in case of overdose.
• Drug therapy has been linked to neuroleptic malignant syndrome (high fever, tachycardia, tachypnea, profuse diaphoresis), a rare but life-threatening syndrome usually seen with use of phenothiazines. Stop drug immediately and institute appropriate therapy if symptoms occur.
• Relieve dry mouth with sugarless hard candy or gum. Saliva substitutes may be needed.
• *Alert:* Don't confuse amoxapine with amoxicillin, or Asendin with aspirin.

PATIENT TEACHING

• Whenever possible, tell patient to take full dose at bedtime.
• Caution patient not to stop drug therapy abruptly.
• Warn patient to avoid activities that require alertness and good psychomotor coordination until CNS effects of drug are known. Drowsiness and dizziness usually subside after a few weeks.

• To prevent photosensitivity reactions, advise patient to use sunblock, wear protective clothing, and avoid prolonged exposure to strong sunlight.
• Instruct patient to report presence of any involuntary movements to prescriber.

---

bupropion hydrochloride
Wellbutrin, Wellbutrin SR

Pregnancy risk category B

AVAILABLE FORMS
Tablets: 75 mg, 100 mg
Tablets (sustained-release): 100 mg, 150 mg

INDICATIONS & DOSAGES
➤ **Depression—**
Adults: For conventional tablets, 100 mg P.O. b.i.d. initially, increased after 3 days to 100 mg P.O. t.i.d., if needed. If no response occurs after several weeks of therapy, dosage increased to 150 mg t.i.d. No single dose should exceed 150 mg. For sustained-release tablets, initially, 150 mg P.O. q morning; increased to target dose of 150 mg P.O. b.i.d. as tolerated as early as day 4 of dosing. Maximum, 450 mg daily.

ACTION
Unknown. Drug is neither a TCA nor an MAO inhibitor, but is a weak inhibitor of norepinephrine, dopamine, and serotonin reuptake.

Route	Onset	Peak	Duration
P.O.	Unknown	2 hr	Unknown
P.O. (sustained)	Unknown	3 hr	Unknown

ADVERSE REACTIONS
CNS: *headache, seizures,* anxiety, confusion, delusions, euphoria, hostility, impaired sleep quality, *insomnia, sedation, tremor,* akinesia, akathisia, *agitation, dizziness,* fatigue, syncope.
CV: *arrhythmias,* hypertension, hypotension, palpitations, *tachycardia.*
EENT: *auditory disturbances,* blurred vision.
GI: *dry mouth,* taste disturbance, increased appetite, *constipation,* dyspepsia, *nausea, vomiting, anorexia,* diarrhea.

GU: impotence, menstrual complaints, urinary frequency, urine retention.
Metabolic: *weight loss, weight gain.*
Musculoskeletal: arthritis.
Skin: pruritus, rash, cutaneous temperature disturbance, *excessive diaphoresis.*
Other: fever and chills, decreased libido.

INTERACTIONS
Drug-drug. *Levodopa, phenothiazines, TCAs; recent and rapid withdrawal of benzodiazepines:* May cause adverse reactions, including seizures. Monitor patient closely.
MAO inhibitors: Altered seizure threshold. Avoid using together.
Drug-lifestyle. *Alcohol use:* Altered seizure threshold. Discourage use together.
Sun exposure: Increased risk of photosensitivity reactions. Advise patient to avoid excessive sunlight exposure.

EFFECTS ON LAB TEST RESULTS
None reported.

CONTRAINDICATIONS
Contraindicated in patients hypersensitive to drug, in those who have taken MAO inhibitors within previous 14 days, and in those with seizure disorders or history of bulimia or anorexia nervosa because of a higher risk of seizures. Don't use with Zyban or other drugs containing bupropion and used for smoking cessation.

NURSING CONSIDERATIONS
• Use cautiously in patients with recent history of MI, unstable heart disease, or renal or hepatic impairment.
• Many patients experience a period of increased restlessness, especially at start of therapy. This may include agitation, insomnia, and anxiety.
• **Alert:** Risk of seizure may be minimized by not exceeding 450 mg/day and by administering daily dose in three to four equally divided doses. Increases in doses shouldn't exceed 100 mg/day in a 3-day period. Patients who experience seizures often have predisposing factors, including history of head trauma, prior seizures, or CNS tumors, or they may be taking a drug that lowers seizure threshold.

• Closely monitor patient with history of bipolar disorder. Antidepressants can cause manic episodes during the depressed phase of bipolar disorder. However, this may be less likely to occur with bupropion than with other antidepressants.
• **Alert:** Don't confuse bupropion with buspirone or Wellbutrin with Wellcovorin or Wellferon.

PATIENT TEACHING
• Advise patient to take drug as scheduled and to take each day's dose in three divided doses (conventional tablets) to minimize risk of seizures.
• Advise patient to consult prescriber before taking other prescription or OTC drugs.
• Tell patient to avoid alcohol while taking drug because it may contribute to development of seizures.
• Advise patient to avoid hazardous activities that require alertness and good psychomotor coordination until CNS effects of drug are known.
• Advise patient that this drug has the same ingredients as Zyban, used to aid smoking cessation, and that the two shouldn't be used together.
• Tell patient that it may take 4 weeks to reach full therapeutic effect of drug.
• Tell patient to protect drug from light and moisture.

---

citalopram hydrobromide
Celexa

Pregnancy risk category C

AVAILABLE FORMS
Tablets: 20 mg, 40 mg

INDICATIONS & DOSAGES
➤ **Depression**—
Adults: Initially, 20 mg P.O. once daily, increasing to 40 mg daily after no less than 1 week. Maximum recommended dose is 40 mg daily.
Elderly patients: 20 mg/day P.O. with adjustment to 40 mg/day only for nonresponding patients.
Adjust-a-dose: For patients with hepatic impairment, use 20 mg/day P.O. with ad-

---

Reactions may be *common*, uncommon, *life-threatening*, or COMMON AND LIFE-THREATENING.

justment to 40 mg/day only for nonresponding patients.

ACTION
A selective serotonin reuptake inhibitor whose action is presumed to be linked to potentiation of serotonergic activity in the CNS resulting from inhibition of neuronal reuptake of serotonin.

Route	Onset	Peak	Duration
P.O.	Unknown	4 hr	Unknown

ADVERSE REACTIONS
CNS: tremor, *somnolence, insomnia,* anxiety, agitation, dizziness, paresthesia, migraine, impaired concentration, amnesia, depression, apathy, **suicide attempt,** confusion, fatigue.
CV: tachycardia, orthostatic hypotension, hypotension.
EENT: rhinitis, sinusitis, abnormal accommodation.
GI: *dry mouth, nausea,* diarrhea, anorexia, dyspepsia, vomiting, abdominal pain, taste perversion, increased saliva, flatulence, increased appetite.
GU: dysmenorrhea, amenorrhea, ejaculation disorder, impotence, polyuria.
Metabolic: decreased and increased weight.
Musculoskeletal: arthralgia, myalgia.
Respiratory: upper respiratory tract infection, coughing.
Skin: rash, pruritus, *increased sweating.*
Other: fever, yawning, decreased libido.

INTERACTIONS
Drug-drug. *Carbamazepine:* May increase citalopram clearance. Monitor patient for effects.
CNS drugs: Additive effects. Use together cautiously.
Drugs that inhibit cytochrome P-450 isoenzymes 3A4 and 2C19: May cause decreased clearance of citalopram. Monitor patient for increased adverse effects.
Imipramine, other TCAs: Level of imipramine metabolite desipramine increased by about 50%. Use together cautiously.
Lithium: May enhance serotonergic effect of citalopram. Use with caution, and monitor lithium levels.

MAO inhibitors: Serious, sometimes fatal, reactions may occur. Don't use drug within 14 days of MAO inhibitor use.
Drug-lifestyle. *Alcohol use:* May increase CNS effects. Discourage use together.

EFFECTS ON LAB TEST RESULTS
None reported.

CONTRAINDICATIONS
Contraindicated in patients hypersensitive to drug or its inactive components and in those taking MAO inhibitors; also contraindicated within 14 days of stopping MAO inhibitor therapy.

NURSING CONSIDERATIONS
• Use cautiously in patients with history of mania, seizures, suicidal ideation, or hepatic or renal impairment.
• Safety and effectiveness of drug haven't been established in children.
• Although drug hasn't been shown to impair psychomotor performance, any psychoactive drug has the potential to impair judgment, thinking, or motor skills.
• The possibility of a suicide attempt is inherent in depression and may persist until significant remission occurs. Closely supervise high-risk patients at start of drug therapy. Reduce risk of overdose by limiting amount of drug available per refill.
• At least 14 days should elapse between MAO inhibitor therapy and citalopram therapy.
• **Alert:** Don't confuse Celexa with Celebrex or Cerebyx.

PATIENT TEACHING
• Tell patient that drug may be taken in the morning or evening without regard to meals. If drowsiness occurs, he should take drug in evening.
• Caution patient against use of MAO inhibitors while taking citalopram.
• Inform patient that, although improvement may take 1 to 4 weeks, he should continue therapy as prescribed.
• Instruct patient to exercise caution when driving or operating hazardous machinery; drug may impair judgment, thinking, and motor skills.
• Advise patient to consult prescriber before taking other prescription or OTC drugs.

• Advise woman to consult prescriber before breast-feeding.
• Warn patient to avoid alcohol during drug therapy.
• Instruct woman of childbearing potential to use contraceptives during drug therapy and to notify prescriber immediately if pregnancy is suspected.

clomipramine hydrochloride
Anafranil, Placil‡

Pregnancy risk category C

AVAILABLE FORMS
Capsules: 25 mg, 50 mg, 75 mg

INDICATIONS & DOSAGES
➤ **Obsessive-compulsive disorder—**
Adults: Initially, 25 mg P.O. daily with meals, gradually increased to 100 mg daily in divided doses during first 2 weeks. Thereafter, increased to maximum dose of 250 mg daily in divided doses with meals, p.r.n. After adjustment, give total daily dose h.s.
Children and adolescents: Initially, 25 mg P.O. daily with meals, gradually increased over first 2 weeks to daily maximum of 3 mg/kg or 100 mg P.O. in divided doses, whichever is smaller. Maximum daily dose is 3 mg/kg or 200 mg, whichever is smaller; give h.s. after adjustment. Reassess and adjust dosage periodically.

ACTION
Unknown. A TCA that selectively inhibits reuptake of norepinephrine at the presynaptic neuron.

Route	Onset	Peak	Duration
P.O.	≥ 2 wk	2-6 hr	Unknown

ADVERSE REACTIONS
CNS: *somnolence, tremor, dizziness, headache, insomnia, nervousness, myoclonus, fatigue,* EEG changes, **seizures.**
CV: orthostatic hypotension, palpitations, tachycardia.
EENT: *pharyngitis, rhinitis, visual changes.*
GI: *dry mouth, constipation, nausea, dyspepsia, increased appetite,* diarrhea, *anorexia, abdominal pain.*

GU: *urinary hesitancy,* urinary tract infection, *dysmenorrhea, ejaculation failure, impotence.*
Hematologic: purpura.
Metabolic: *weight gain.*
Musculoskeletal: *myalgia.*
Skin: *diaphoresis,* rash, pruritus, dry skin.
Other: *altered libido.*

INTERACTIONS
Drug-drug. *Barbiturates:* Decreased TCA blood levels. Watch for decreased antidepressant effect.
Cimetidine, fluoxetine, fluvoxamine, paroxetine, sertraline: Increased TCA blood levels. Watch for enhanced antidepressant effect.
Clonidine: May reduce the effectiveness of clonidine. Avoid using together, if possible. Monitor blood pressure.
CNS depressants: Enhanced CNS depression. Avoid using together.
Epinephrine, norepinephrine: Increased hypertensive effect. Use together cautiously.
MAO inhibitors: May cause hyperpyretic crisis, seizures, coma, or death. Avoid using together.
Drug-herb. *Evening primrose oil:* May cause additive or synergistic effect, resulting in lower seizure threshold and increasing the risk of seizure. Discourage use together.
St. John's wort, SAM-e, yohimbe: May cause serotonin syndrome. Discourage use together.
Drug-food. *Grapefruit juice:* Elevated levels of clomipramine and reduced levels of the metabolite, desmethylclomipramine. Advise patient to avoid fluctuations in ingestion of grapefruit juice while taking the drug unless instructed by a prescriber to take clomipramine with grapefruit juice.
Drug-lifestyle. *Alcohol use:* Enhanced CNS depression. Discourage use together.
Sun exposure: Increased risk of photosensitivity reactions. Advise patient to avoid excessive sunlight exposure.

EFFECTS ON LAB TEST RESULTS
None reported.

Reactions may be *common,* uncommon, **life-threatening,** or COMMON AND LIFE-THREATENING.

CONTRAINDICATIONS

Contraindicated in patients hypersensitive to drug or other TCAs, in those who have taken MAO inhibitors within previous 14 days, and in patients in acute recovery period after MI.

NURSING CONSIDERATIONS

• Use cautiously in patients with history of seizure disorders or with brain damage of varying cause; in patients receiving other seizure threshold-lowering drugs; in patients at risk for suicide; in patients with history of urine retention or angle-closure glaucoma, increased intraocular pressure, CV disease, impaired hepatic or renal function, or hyperthyroidism; in patients with tumors of the adrenal medulla; in patients receiving thyroid drug or electroconvulsive therapy; and in those undergoing elective surgery.

• Monitor mood and watch for suicidal tendencies. Allow patient to have only minimal amount of drug.

• Don't withdraw drug abruptly.

• Because hypertensive episodes have occurred during surgery in patients receiving TCAs, drug should be gradually discontinued several days before surgery.

• Relieve dry mouth with sugarless candy or gum. Saliva substitutes may be needed.

• *Alert:* Don't confuse clomipramine with chlorpromazine or clomiphene, or Anafranil with enalapril, nafarelin, or alfentanil.

PATIENT TEACHING

• Warn patient to avoid hazardous activities requiring alertness and good psychomotor coordination, especially during adjustment. Daytime sedation and dizziness may occur.

• Tell patient to avoid alcohol during drug therapy.

• Warn patient not to stop drug suddenly.

• Advise patient to use sunblock, wear protective clothing, and avoid prolonged exposure to strong sunlight to prevent photosensitivity reactions.

desipramine hydrochloride
Norpramin**, Pertofran‡, Pertofrane†

Pregnancy risk category NR

AVAILABLE FORMS
Capsules: 25 mg, 50 mg
Tablets: 10 mg, 25 mg, 50 mg, 75 mg, 100 mg, 150 mg

INDICATIONS & DOSAGES
➤ **Depression—**
Adults: 100 to 200 mg P.O. daily in divided doses, increased to maximum of 300 mg daily. Or, entire dose can be given h.s.
Adolescents and elderly patients: 25 to 100 mg P.O. daily in divided doses, increased gradually to maximum of 150 mg daily, if needed.

ACTION
Unknown. A TCA that increases amount of norepinephrine, serotonin, or both in the CNS by blocking their reuptake by the presynaptic neurons.

Route	Onset	Peak	Duration
P.O.	Unknown	4-6 hr	Unknown

ADVERSE REACTIONS
CNS: *drowsiness, dizziness,* excitation, tremor, weakness, confusion, anxiety, restlessness, agitation, headache, nervousness, EEG changes, *seizures,* extrapyramidal reactions.
CV: orthostatic hypotension, *tachycardia,* ECG changes, hypertension.
EENT: *blurred vision,* tinnitus, mydriasis.
GI: *dry mouth,* constipation, nausea, vomiting, anorexia, paralytic ileus.
GU: urine retention.
Metabolic: hypoglycemia, hyperglycemia.
Skin: rash, urticaria, photosensitivity reactions, diaphoresis.
Other: hypersensitivity reactions, *sudden death in children.*

INTERACTIONS
Drug-drug. *Barbiturates, CNS depressants:* Enhanced CNS depression. Avoid using together.
Cimetidine, fluvoxamine, fluoxetine, paroxetine, sertraline: May increase de-

sipramine levels. Monitor patient for adverse reactions.

Clonidine: Decreased effects of clonidine. Avoid using together, if possible. Monitor blood pressure.

Epinephrine, norepinephrine: Increased hypertensive effect. Use together cautiously.

MAO inhibitors: May cause severe excitation, hyperpyrexia, or seizures, usually with high doses. Avoid using together.

Drug-herb. *Evening primrose oil:* May cause additive or synergistic effect, resulting in lower seizure threshold and increasing the risk of seizure. Discourage use together.

St. John's wort, SAM-e, yohimbe: May cause serotonin syndrome. Discourage use together.

Drug-lifestyle. *Alcohol use:* Enhanced CNS depression. Discourage use together.

Smoking: May lower plasma desipramine levels. Monitor patient for lack of effect.

Sun exposure: Increased risk of photosensitivity reactions. Advise patient to avoid excessive sunlight exposure.

EFFECTS ON LAB TEST RESULTS
• May increase or decrease glucose levels.
• May increase liver function test values.

CONTRAINDICATIONS
Contraindicated in patients hypersensitive to drug, in those who have taken MAO inhibitors within previous 14 days, and in patients in acute recovery phase after MI.

NURSING CONSIDERATIONS
• Use with extreme caution in patients with CV disease; in those with history of urine retention, glaucoma, seizure disorders, or thyroid disease; and in those taking thyroid drug.
• Monitor patient for nausea, headache, and malaise after abrupt withdrawal of long-term therapy; these symptoms don't indicate addiction.
• Don't withdraw drug abruptly.
• Because hypertensive episodes have occurred during surgery in patients receiving TCAs, drug should be gradually discontinued several days before surgery.
• If signs or symptoms of psychosis occur or increase, expect prescriber to reduce dosage. Record mood changes. Monitor

patient for suicidal tendencies, and allow only a minimum supply of drug.
• Because desipramine produces fewer anticholinergic effects than other TCAs, it's often prescribed for cardiac patients.
• Recommend sugarless hard candy or gum to relieve dry mouth. Saliva substitutes may be needed.
• **Alert:** Don't confuse desipramine with disopyramide or imipramine.

PATIENT TEACHING
• Advise patient to take full dose at bedtime, whenever possible.
• Warn patient to avoid hazardous activities that require alertness and good psychomotor coordination until CNS effects of drug are known. Drowsiness and dizziness usually subside after a few weeks.
• Advise patient to call prescriber if fever and sore throat occur. Leukocyte and differential counts may need to be obtained.
• Tell patient to avoid alcohol during drug therapy because it may antagonize effects of desipramine.
• Tell patient to consult prescriber before taking other prescription or OTC drugs.
• Warn patient not to stop drug suddenly.
• To prevent photosensitivity reactions, advise patient to use sunblock, wear protective clothing, and avoid prolonged exposure to strong sunlight.

---

doxepin hydrochloride
Deptran‡, Novo-Doxepin†, Sinequan, Triadapin†

Pregnancy risk category NR

AVAILABLE FORMS
Capsules: 10 mg, 25 mg, 50 mg, 75 mg, 100 mg, 150 mg
Oral concentrate: 10 mg/ml

INDICATIONS & DOSAGES
➤ **Depression—**
Adults: Initially, 25 to 75 mg P.O. daily in divided doses to maximum of 300 mg daily. Or, entire maintenance dose may be given once daily with maximum dose of 150 mg.

ACTION

Unknown. A TCA that increases amount of norepinephrine, serotonin, or both in the CNS by blocking their reuptake by the presynaptic neurons.

Route	Onset	Peak	Duration
P.O.	Unknown	2 hr	Unknown

ADVERSE REACTIONS

CNS: *drowsiness, dizziness,* confusion, numbness, hallucinations, paresthesia, ataxia, weakness, headache, *seizures,* extrapyramidal reactions.
CV: *orthostatic hypotension, tachycardia,* ECG changes.
EENT: *blurred vision,* tinnitus.
GI: *dry mouth, constipation,* nausea, vomiting, anorexia.
GU: urine retention.
Metabolic: hypoglycemia, hyperglycemia.
Skin: rash, urticaria, photosensitivity reactions, *diaphoresis.*
Other: hypersensitivity reactions.

INTERACTIONS

Drug-drug. *Barbiturates, CNS depressants:* Enhanced CNS depression. Avoid using together.
Cimetidine, fluoxetine, fluvoxamine, paroxetine, sertraline: May increase doxepin levels. Watch for increased adverse reactions.
Clonidine: Decreased effects of clonidine. Avoid using together, if possible. Monitor blood pressure.
Epinephrine, norepinephrine: Increased hypertensive effect. Use together cautiously.
MAO inhibitors: May cause severe excitation, hyperpyrexia, or seizures, usually with high dosage. Avoid using together.
Drug-herb. *Evening primrose oil:* May cause additive or synergistic effect, resulting in lower seizure threshold and increasing the risk of seizure. Discourage use together.
St. John's wort, SAM-e, yohimbe: May cause serotonin syndrome. Discourage use together.
Drug-lifestyle. *Alcohol use:* Enhanced CNS depression. Discourage use together.
Sun exposure: Increased risk of photosensitivity reactions. Advise patient to avoid excessive sunlight exposure.

EFFECTS ON LAB TEST RESULTS

- May increase or decrease glucose levels.
- May increase liver function test values.

CONTRAINDICATIONS

Contraindicated in patients hypersensitive to drug and in those with glaucoma or tendency toward urine retention; also contraindicated in those who have received an MAO inhibitor within past 14 days and during acute recovery phase of an MI.

NURSING CONSIDERATIONS

- Don't withdraw drug abruptly.
- Monitor patient for nausea, headache, and malaise after abrupt withdrawal of long-term therapy; these symptoms don't indicate addiction.
- *Alert:* Because hypertensive episodes may occur during surgery in patients receiving TCAs, drug should be gradually discontinued several days before surgery.
- If signs or symptoms of psychosis occur or increase, expect prescriber to reduce dosage. Record mood changes. Monitor patient for suicidal tendencies and allow only a minimum supply of drug.
- Doxepin has strong anticholinergic effects and is one of the most sedating TCAs. Adverse anticholinergic effects can occur rapidly.
- Recommend use of sugarless hard candy or gum to relieve dry mouth.
- *Alert:* Don't confuse doxepin with doxazosin, digoxin, doxapram, or Doxidan; don't confuse Sinequan with saquinavir.

PATIENT TEACHING

- Tell patient to dilute oral concentrate with 4 ounces (120 ml) of water, milk, or juice (orange, grapefruit, tomato, prune, or pineapple, but not grape); preparation is incompatible with carbonated beverages.
- Tell patient to take full dose at bedtime whenever he can, but warn him of possible morning orthostatic hypotension.
- Advise patient to consult prescriber before taking other prescription or OTC drugs.
- Warn patient to avoid hazardous activities that require alertness and good psychomotor coordination until CNS effects of drug are known. Drowsiness and dizziness usually subside after a few weeks.

• Tell patient to avoid alcohol during drug therapy.
• Tell patient that maximum antidepressant effect may not be evident for 2 to 3 weeks.
• Warn patient not to stop drug suddenly.
• To prevent photosensitivity reactions, advise patient to use sunblock, wear protective clothing, and avoid prolonged exposure to strong sunlight.

---

fluoxetine hydrochloride
Erocap‡, Lovan‡, Prozac,
Prozac-20‡, Prozac Weekly,
Sarafem, Zactin‡

Pregnancy risk category C

AVAILABLE FORMS
Capsules: 90 mg
Oral solution: 20 mg/5 ml
Pulvules: 10 mg, 20 mg
Tablets: 10 mg

INDICATIONS & DOSAGES
➤ **Prozac: Depression, obsessive-compulsive disorder—**
Adults: Initially, 20 mg P.O. in the morning; dosage increased based on patient response. Maximum dose is 80 mg/day.
➤ **Depression in elderly patients—**
Adults age 65 and older: Initially, 20 mg P.O. daily in the morning. Increase dose based on response. Doses may be given b.i.d., morning and noon. Maximum dose is 80 mg/day. A lower dosage or less frequent dosing should be considered in these patients, especially those with systemic illness and those who are receiving drugs for other illnesses.
✱ *NEW INDICATION:* **Prozac Weekly Maintenance therapy for depression in stabilized patients (not for newly diagnosed depression)—**
Adults: 90 mg P.O. once weekly. Initiate once weekly dosing 7 days after the last daily dose of Prozac 20 mg.
➤ **Binge-eating and vomiting behavior in patients with moderate to severe bulimia nervosa—**
Adults: 60 mg P.O. in the morning.
Adjust-a-dose: For patients with renal or hepatic impairment, a lower dosage or less frequent dosing is recommended.

✱ *NEW INDICATION:* **Sarafem Premenstrual dysphoric disorder—**
Adults: 20 mg P.O. daily. Maximum dose, 80 mg daily.
Adjust-a-dose: For patients with hepatic impairment or concurrent disease and in those taking multiple drugs at the same time, use reduced or less frequent dose.

ACTION
Unknown. Thought to be linked to drug's inhibition of CNS neuronal uptake of serotonin.

Route	Onset	Peak	Duration
P.O.	Unknown	6-8 hr	Unknown

ADVERSE REACTIONS
CNS: *nervousness, anxiety, insomnia, headache, drowsiness,* fatigue, *tremor, dizziness, asthenia.*
CV: palpitations, hot flashes.
EENT: nasal congestion, pharyngitis, sinusitis.
GI: *nausea, diarrhea, dry mouth, anorexia,* dyspepsia, constipation, abdominal pain, vomiting, flatulence, increased appetite.
GU: sexual dysfunction.
Metabolic: weight loss.
Musculoskeletal: muscle pain.
Respiratory: upper respiratory tract infection, cough, respiratory distress.
Skin: rash, pruritus, diaphoresis.
Other: flu syndrome, fever.

INTERACTIONS
Drug-drug. *Carbamazepine, flecainide, vinblastine:* Increased serum levels of these drugs. Monitor serum levels and monitor patient for adverse effects.
Cyproheptadine: May reverse or decrease pharmacologic effect. Monitor patient closely.
Insulin, oral antidiabetics: Altered glucose levels; may also alter antidiabetic requirements. Adjust dosage.
Lithium, TCAs: Risk of increased adverse CNS effects. Monitor patient closely.
Phenytoin: Increased plasma phenytoin levels and risk of toxicity. Monitor phenytoin levels and adjust dosage.
Tryptophan: Increased agitation, restlessness, and GI adverse effects. Use together cautiously.

Reactions may be *common,* uncommon, **life-threatening,** or COMMON AND LIFE-THREATENING.

Warfarin, other highly protein-bound drugs: May increase plasma levels of fluoxetine or other highly protein-bound drugs. Monitor patient closely.

Drug-herb. *St. John's wort:* May increase serotonin reuptake inhibition. Discourage use together.

Drug-lifestyle. *Alcohol use:* Increased CNS depression. Discourage use together.

EFFECTS ON LAB TEST RESULTS
None reported.

CONTRAINDICATIONS
Contraindicated in patients hypersensitive to drug and in those taking MAO inhibitors within 14 days of starting therapy. MAO inhibitors shouldn't be started within 5 weeks of stopping fluoxetine therapy. Thioridazine shouldn't be administered with Sarafem or within a minimum of 5 weeks after Sarafem has been discontinued.

NURSING CONSIDERATIONS
• Use cautiously in patients at high risk for suicide and in those with history of hepatic, renal, or CV disease; diabetes mellitus; or seizures.
• Use antihistamines or topical corticosteroids to treat rashes or pruritus.
• Watch for weight change during therapy, particularly in underweight or bulimic patients.
• Record mood changes. Watch for suicidal tendencies.
• **Alert:** Don't confuse fluoxetine with fluvoxamine or fluvastatin, or Prozac with Proscar, Prilosec, or ProSom.

PATIENT TEACHING
• Tell patient to avoid taking drug in the afternoon whenever possible, because fluoxetine commonly causes nervousness and insomnia.
• Drug may cause dizziness or drowsiness. Warn patient to avoid driving and other hazardous activities that require alertness and good psychomotor coordination until CNS effects of drug are known.
• Tell patient to consult prescriber before taking other prescription or OTC drugs.
• Advise patient that full therapeutic effect may not be seen for 4 weeks or longer.

imipramine hydrochloride
Apo-Imipramine†, Impril†, Melipramine‡, Norfranil, Novopramine†, Tipramine, Tofranil**

imipramine pamoate
Tofranil-PM**

Pregnancy risk category D

AVAILABLE FORMS
imipramine hydrochloride
Injection: 12.5 mg/ml
Tablets: 10 mg, 25 mg, 50 mg
imipramine pamoate
Capsules: 75 mg, 100 mg, 125 mg, 150 mg

INDICATIONS & DOSAGES
➤ **Depression**—
Adults: 75 to 100 mg P.O. or I.M. daily in divided doses, increased in 25- to 50-mg increments. Maximum dose for outpatients is 200 mg daily; 300 mg daily may be used for hospitalized patients. Entire dose may be given h.s.
Adolescents and elderly patients: Initially, 30 to 40 mg daily; it usually isn't necessary to exceed 100 mg daily.
➤ **Childhood enuresis**—
Children age 5 and older: 25 mg P.O. 1 hour before bedtime. If no response within 1 week, increase dose to 50 mg if child is younger than age 12; increase dose to 75 mg for children age 12 and older. In either case, maximum dose is 2.5 mg/kg/day.

ACTION
Unknown. A TCA that increases norepinephrine, serotonin, or both in the CNS by blocking their reuptake by the presynaptic neurons.

Route	Onset	Peak	Duration
I.M.	Unknown	30 min	Unknown
P.O.	Unknown	1-2 hr	Unknown

ADVERSE REACTIONS
CNS: *CVA, drowsiness, dizziness,* excitation, tremor, confusion, hallucinations, anxiety, ataxia, paresthesia, nervousness,

EEG changes, *seizures,* extrapyramidal reactions.
CV: *orthostatic hypotension, tachycardia, ECG changes,* hypertension, *MI, arrhythmias, heart block,* precipitation of heart failure.
EENT: *blurred vision,* tinnitus, mydriasis.
GI: *dry mouth, constipation,* nausea, vomiting, anorexia, paralytic ileus, abdominal cramps.
GU: *urine retention.*
Metabolic: hypoglycemia, hyperglycemia.
Skin: rash, urticaria, photosensitivity reactions, pruritus, diaphoresis.
Other: hypersensitivity reactions.

INTERACTIONS
Drug-drug. *Barbiturates, CNS depressants:* Enhanced CNS depression. Avoid using together.
Cimetidine, fluoxetine, sertraline: May increase imipramine levels. Monitor patient for adverse reactions.
Clonidine: Decreased effects of clonidine. Avoid using together, if possible. Monitor blood pressure.
Epinephrine, norepinephrine: Increased hypertensive effect. Use together cautiously.
MAO inhibitors: May cause hyperpyretic crisis, severe seizures, and death. Avoid using together.
Drug-herb. *Evening primrose oil:* May cause additive or synergistic effect, resulting in lower seizure threshold and increasing the risk of seizure. Discourage use together.
St. John's wort, SAM-e, yohimbe: May cause serotonin syndrome. Discourage use together.
Drug-lifestyle. *Alcohol use:* Enhanced CNS depression. Discourage use together.
Smoking: May lower plasma levels of imipramine. Monitor patient for lack of effect.
Sun exposure: Increased risk of photosensitivity reactions. Advise patient to avoid excessive sunlight exposure.

EFFECTS ON LAB TEST RESULTS
● May increase or decrease glucose levels.
● May increase liver function test values.

CONTRAINDICATIONS
Contraindicated in patients hypersensitive to drug and in those receiving MAO inhibitors; also contraindicated during acute recovery phase of MI.

NURSING CONSIDERATIONS
● Use with extreme caution in patients at risk for suicide; in patients with history of urine retention, angle-closure glaucoma, or seizure disorders; in patients with increased intraocular pressure, CV disease, impaired hepatic function, hyperthyroidism, or impaired renal function; and in patients receiving thyroid drugs. Injectable form contains sulfites, which may cause allergic reactions in hypersensitive patients.
● Monitor patient for nausea, headache, and malaise after abrupt withdrawal of long-term therapy; these symptoms don't indicate addiction.
● Don't withdraw drug abruptly.
● Because of hypertensive episodes during surgery in patients receiving TCAs, drug should be gradually discontinued several days before surgery.
● If signs or symptoms of psychosis occur or increase, expect prescriber to reduce dosage. Record mood changes. Monitor patient for suicidal tendencies, and allow only a minimum supply of drug.
● To prevent relapse in children receiving drug for enuresis, drug should be withdrawn gradually.
● Recommend sugarless hard candy or gum to relieve dry mouth. Saliva substitutes may be useful.
● *Alert:* Don't confuse imipramine with desipramine.

PATIENT TEACHING
● Tell patient to take full dose at bedtime whenever possible, but warn him of possible morning orthostatic hypotension.
● If child is an early night bedwetter, tell parents it may be more effective to divide dose and give the first dose earlier in day.
● Tell patient to avoid alcohol while taking this drug.
● Advise patient to consult prescriber before taking other prescription or OTC drugs.
● Warn patient to avoid hazardous activities that require alertness and good psy-

---

Reactions may be *common,* uncommon, *life-threatening,* or COMMON AND LIFE-THREATENING.

chomotor coordination until CNS effects of the drug are known. Drowsiness and dizziness usually subside after a few weeks.

• Warn patient not to stop drug suddenly.
• To prevent photosensitivity reactions, advise patient to use sunblock, wear protective clothing, and avoid prolonged exposure to strong sunlight.

---

mirtazapine
Remeron, Remeron Soltab, Zispin§

Pregnancy risk category C

AVAILABLE FORMS
Tablets: 15 mg, 30 mg, 45 mg
Tablets (orally disintegrating): 15 mg, 30 mg, 45 mg

INDICATIONS & DOSAGES
➤ Depression—
Adults: Initially, 15 mg P.O. h.s. Maintenance dose ranges from 15 to 45 mg daily. Dosage adjustments should be made at intervals of no less than 1 to 2 weeks.

ACTION
Thought to be caused by enhancement of central noradrenergic and serotonergic activity.

Route	Onset	Peak	Duration
P.O.	Unknown	2 hr	Unknown

ADVERSE REACTIONS
CNS: *somnolence,* dizziness, asthenia, abnormal dreams, abnormal thinking, tremors, confusion.
CV: edema.
GI: nausea, *increased appetite, dry mouth, constipation.*
GU: urinary frequency.
Metabolic: *weight gain.*
Musculoskeletal: back pain, myalgia.
Respiratory: dyspnea.
Other: flu syndrome, peripheral edema.

INTERACTIONS
Drug-drug. *Diazepam, other CNS depressants:* May cause additive CNS effects. Avoid using together.

MAO inhibitors: Sometimes fatal reactions. Avoid using together.
Drug-lifestyle. *Alcohol use:* May cause additive CNS effects. Discourage use together.

EFFECTS ON LAB TEST RESULTS
• May increase ALT levels.

CONTRAINDICATIONS
Contraindicated in patients hypersensitive to drug. Drug shouldn't be used with MAO inhibitor or within 14 days of initiating or discontinuing therapy with MAO inhibitor.

NURSING CONSIDERATIONS
• Use cautiously in patients with CV or cerebrovascular disease, seizure disorders, suicidal ideations, hepatic or renal impairment, or history of mania or hypomania.
• At least 14 days should elapse after stopping mirtazapine and before starting an MAO inhibitor.
• Record mood changes. Watch for suicidal tendencies.
• Use cautiously in patients with conditions that predispose them to hypotension, such as dehydration, hypovolemia, or treatment with antihypertensives.
• Although agranulocytosis occurs rarely, discontinue drug and monitor patient closely if he develops a sore throat, fever, stomatitis, or other signs and symptoms of infection with a low WBC count.
• Monitor patient closely for signs and symptoms of dependence.
• Give drug cautiously to elderly patients; decreased clearance has occurred in this age group.
• Lower dosages tend to be more sedating than higher dosages.

PATIENT TEACHING
• Caution patient not to perform hazardous activities if somnolence occurs.
• Tell patient to report signs and symptoms of infection, such as fever, chills, sore throat, mucous membrane ulceration, or flu syndrome.
• Instruct patient not to use alcohol or other CNS depressants while taking drug.
• Stress importance of compliance with therapy.

---

*Liquid contains alcohol.   **May contain tartrazine.   †Canada   ‡Australia   §U.K.   ◇OTC

• Instruct patient not to take other drugs without prescriber's approval.
• Tell woman of childbearing potential to report suspected pregnancy immediately and to notify prescriber if she is breast-feeding.
• Instruct patient to remove orally disintegrating tablets from blister pack and place immediately on tongue.
• Advise patient not to break or split tablet.

---

nefazodone hydrochloride
Dutonin§, Serzone

Pregnancy risk category C

AVAILABLE FORMS
Tablets: 50 mg, 100 mg, 150 mg, 300 mg

INDICATIONS & DOSAGES
➤ **Depression—**
Adults: Initially, 200 mg/day P.O. in two divided doses. Dosage may be increased in increments of 100 to 200 mg/day at intervals of no less than 1 week, p.r.n. Usual dosage range is 300 to 600 mg/day.
Elderly patients: Initially, 100 mg/day P.O. in two divided doses.
Adjust-a-dose: For debilitated patients, initially 100 mg/day P.O. in two divided doses.

ACTION
Unknown. Thought to be linked to drug's inhibition of CNS neuronal uptake of serotonin (5-HT$_2$) and norepinephrine; it also occupies serotonin and alpha$_1$-adrenergic receptors in the CNS.

Route	Onset	Peak	Duration
P.O.	Unknown	1 hr	Unknown

ADVERSE REACTIONS
CNS: *headache, somnolence, dizziness, asthenia, insomnia, light-headedness, confusion,* memory impairment, paresthesia, vasodilation, abnormal dreams, decreased concentration, ataxia, incoordination, psychomotor retardation, tremor, hypertonia.
CV: orthostatic hypotension, hypotension, peripheral edema.

EENT: blurred vision, abnormal vision, tinnitus, visual field defect, pharyngitis.
GI: *dry mouth, nausea, constipation,* taste perversion, dyspepsia, diarrhea, increased appetite, vomiting.
GU: urinary frequency, urinary tract infection, urine retention, vaginitis.
Metabolic: hypernatremia.
Musculoskeletal: neck rigidity, arthralgia.
Respiratory: cough.
Skin: pruritus, rash.
Other: infection, flu syndrome, chills, fever, breast tenderness, thirst.

INTERACTIONS
Drug-drug. *Alprazolam, triazolam:* Potentiated effects of these drugs. Avoid using together; however, if necessary, dosage of alprazolam and triazolam can be greatly reduced.
CNS drugs: May alter CNS activity. Use together cautiously.
Cyclosporine: May cause cyclosporine toxicity. Monitor cyclosporine level.
Digoxin: May increase digoxin level. Use together cautiously and monitor digoxin level.
MAO inhibitors: May cause severe excitation, hyperpyrexia, seizures, delirium, or coma. Avoid using together.
Other highly protein-bound drugs: May increase risk and severity of adverse reactions. Monitor patient closely.
Drug-lifestyle. *Alcohol use:* Enhanced CNS depression. Discourage use together.

EFFECTS ON LAB TEST RESULTS
• May decrease sodium levels.

CONTRAINDICATIONS
Contraindicated in patients hypersensitive to drug or other phenylpiperazine antidepressants; also contraindicated within 14 days of MAO inhibitor therapy.

NURSING CONSIDERATIONS
• Use cautiously in patients with CV or cerebrovascular disease that could be exacerbated by hypotension (such as history of MI, angina, or CVA) and conditions that would predispose patients to hypotension (such as dehydration, hypovolemia, and treatment with antihypertensives). Also use cautiously in patients with a history of mania.

Reactions may be *common,* uncommon, *life-threatening,* or COMMON AND LIFE-THREATENING.

• At least 1 week should elapse between stopping nefazodone and starting MAO inhibitor therapy, and at least 14 days should elapse before patient begins taking nefazodone after MAO inhibitor therapy has been discontinued.

• *Alert:* Drug may cause severe liver failure. Watch closely for signs and symptoms of liver failure.

• Record mood changes. Monitor patient for suicidal tendencies, and allow only minimum supply of drug.

• *Alert:* Don't confuse Serzone with Seroquel.

PATIENT TEACHING
• Warn patient not to engage in hazardous activity until CNS effects of drug are known.

• *Alert:* Instruct men who experience prolonged or inappropriate erections to stop drug immediately and notify prescriber.

• Instruct woman to notify prescriber if she becomes pregnant or is planning pregnancy during therapy or if she's breastfeeding.

• *Alert:* Warn patient to immediately report jaundice, anorexia, GI complaints, and malaise to prescriber.

• Tell patient to notify prescriber if rash, hives, or related allergic reactions occur.

• Instruct patient to avoid alcohol during therapy.

• Tell patient to notify prescriber before taking OTC drugs.

• Inform patient that several weeks of therapy may be needed to obtain full antidepressant effect. Once improvement occurs, advise him not to stop drug until directed by prescriber.

---

nortriptyline hydrochloride
Allegron‡, Pamelor*

Pregnancy risk category NR

AVAILABLE FORMS
Capsules: 10 mg, 25 mg, 50 mg, 75 mg
Oral solution: 10 mg/5 ml*
Tablets: 10 mg‡, 25 mg‡

INDICATIONS & DOSAGES
➤ **Depression—**
Adults: 25 mg P.O. t.i.d. or q.i.d., gradually increased to maximum of 150 mg daily. Entire dose may be given h.s. Monitor plasma levels when doses above 100 mg/day are given.
Adolescents and elderly patients: 30 to 50 mg daily given once or in divided doses.

ACTION
Unknown. A TCA that increases the amount of norepinephrine, serotonin, or both in the CNS by blocking their reuptake by the presynaptic neurons.

Route	Onset	Peak	Duration
P.O.	Unknown	7-8.5 hr	Unknown

ADVERSE REACTIONS
CNS: *drowsiness, dizziness, seizures,* tremor, weakness, confusion, headache, nervousness, EEG changes, *CVA,* extrapyramidal syndrome, insomnia, nightmares, hallucinations, paresthesia, ataxia, agitation.
CV: ECG changes, *tachycardia,* hypertension, hypotension, *MI, heart block.*
EENT: *blurred vision,* tinnitus, mydriasis.
GI: dry mouth, *constipation,* nausea, vomiting, anorexia, paralytic ileus.
GU: *urine retention.*
Hematologic: bone marrow depression, *agranulocytosis,* eosinophilia, *thrombocytopenia.*
Metabolic: hypoglycemia, hyperglycemia.
Skin: rash, urticaria, photosensitivity reactions, diaphoresis.
Other: hypersensitivity reactions.

INTERACTIONS
Drug-drug. *Barbiturates, CNS depressants:* Enhanced CNS depression. Avoid using together.
Cimetidine, fluoxetine, sertraline: May increase nortriptyline levels. Watch for adverse reactions.
Clonidine: Decreased effects of clonidine. Avoid using together, if possible. Monitor blood pressure.
Epinephrine, norepinephrine: Increased hypertensive effect. Use together cautiously.

MAO inhibitors: May cause severe excitation, hyperpyrexia, or seizures, usually with high doses. Avoid using together.

Drug-herb. *Evening primrose oil:* May cause additive or synergistic effect, resulting in lower seizure threshold and increasing the risk of seizure. Discourage use together.

St. John's wort, SAM-e, yohimbe: May cause serotonin syndrome. Discourage use together.

Drug-lifestyle. *Alcohol use:* Enhanced CNS depression. Discourage use together.

Smoking: May lower plasma levels of nortriptyline. Monitor patient for lack of effect.

Sun exposure: Increased risk of photosensitivity reactions. Advise patient to avoid excessive sunlight exposure.

EFFECTS ON LAB TEST RESULTS
● May increase or decrease glucose levels.
● May increase liver function test values and eosinophil count. May decrease granulocyte and platelet counts.

CONTRAINDICATIONS
Contraindicated in patients hypersensitive to drug and during acute recovery phase of MI; also contraindicated within 14 days of MAO therapy.

NURSING CONSIDERATIONS
● Use with extreme caution in patients with glaucoma, suicidal tendency, history of urine retention or seizures, CV disease, or hyperthyroidism and in those receiving thyroid drugs.
● Monitor patient for nausea, headache, and malaise after abrupt withdrawal of long-term therapy; however, these symptoms don't indicate addiction.
● Because hypertensive episodes have occurred during surgery in patients receiving TCAs, dosage should be gradually discontinued several days before surgery.
● If signs or symptoms of psychosis occur or increase, expect prescriber to reduce dosage. Record mood changes. Monitor patient for suicidal tendencies and allow him only a minimum supply of drug.
● Recommend use of sugarless hard candy or gum to relieve dry mouth. Saliva substitutes may be needed.

● **Alert:** Don't confuse nortriptyline with amitriptyline.

PATIENT TEACHING
● Advise patient to take full dose at bedtime whenever possible, to reduce risk of orthostatic hypotension.
● Warn patient to avoid activities that require alertness and good psychomotor coordination until CNS effects of drug are known. Drowsiness and dizziness usually subside after a few weeks.
● Tell patient to consult prescriber before taking other prescription or OTC drugs.
● Warn patient not to stop drug suddenly.
● To prevent photosensitivity reactions, advise patient to use sunblock, wear protective clothing, and avoid prolonged exposure to strong sunlight.

---

paroxetine hydrochloride
Aropax‡, Paxil, Paxil CR, Seroxat§

Pregnancy risk category C

AVAILABLE FORMS
Suspension: 10 mg/5 ml
Tablets: 10 mg, 20 mg, 30 mg, 40 mg
Tablets (controlled-release): 12.5 mg, 25 mg

INDICATIONS & DOSAGES
➤ **Depression**—
Adults: Initially, 20 mg P.O. daily, preferably in morning, as indicated. If patient doesn't respond after full antidepressant effect has occurred (usually 1 to 4 weeks), dosage may be increased in 10-mg/day increments at weekly intervals, to maximum of 50 mg daily. If using controlled-release formulation, initially 25 mg P.O. daily. Dose may be increased in 12.5-mg/day increments at weekly intervals, to maximum of 62.5 mg/day.
Elderly patients: Initially, 10 mg P.O. daily, preferably in morning, as indicated. If patient doesn't respond after full antidepressant effect has occurred (usually 1 to 4 weeks), dose may be increased in 10-mg/day increments at weekly intervals, to maximum of 40 mg daily. If using controlled-release formulation, start ther-

---

apy at 12.5 mg P.O. daily. Don't exceed 50 mg/day.

➤ **Obsessive-compulsive disorder**—
Adults: Initially, 20 mg P.O. daily, preferably in morning. Dose may be increased in 10-mg/day increments at weekly intervals. Recommended daily dose is 40 mg. Maximum dose is 60 mg/day.

➤ **Panic disorder**—
Adults: Initially, 10 mg P.O. daily. Dose may be increased in 10-mg increments at no less than weekly intervals, to maximum of 60 mg/day.

➤ **Social anxiety disorder**—
Adults: Initially, 20 mg P.O. daily, preferably in morning. Dosage range is 20 to 60 mg/day. Adjust dosage to maintain patient on lowest effective dose.

✸ *NEW INDICATION:* **Generalized anxiety disorder**—
Adults: 20 mg P.O. daily initially, increasing by 10 mg/day weekly up to 50 mg daily.

Adjust-a-dose: For debilitated patients or those with renal or hepatic failure taking immediate-release formulation, initially, 10 mg P.O. daily, preferably in morning. If patient doesn't respond after full antidepressant effect has occurred, dosage may be increased in 10-mg/day increments at weekly intervals, to maximum of 40 mg daily. If using controlled-release formulation, start therapy at 12.5 mg/day. Don't exceed 50 mg daily.

ACTION
Unknown. Thought to be linked to drug's inhibition of CNS neuronal uptake of serotonin.

Route	Onset	Peak	Duration
P.O.	Unknown	2-8 hr	Unknown

ADVERSE REACTIONS
CNS: *somnolence, dizziness, insomnia, tremor, nervousness,* anxiety, paresthesia, confusion, *headache,* agitation, *asthenia.*
CV: palpitations, vasodilation, orthostatic hypotension.
EENT: lump or tightness in throat.
GI: *dry mouth, nausea, constipation, diarrhea,* flatulence, vomiting, dyspepsia, dysgeusia, increased appetite, abdominal pain.

GU: ejaculatory disturbances, sexual dysfunction, urinary frequency, other urinary disorders.
Musculoskeletal: myopathy, myalgia, myasthenia.
Skin: rash, pruritus, *diaphoresis.*
Other: yawning, decreased libido.

INTERACTIONS
Drug-drug. *Cimetidine:* Decreased hepatic metabolism of paroxetine, leading to risk of toxicity. Dosage adjustments may be needed.
Digoxin: May decrease digoxin levels. Monitor patient closely.
MAO inhibitors: May increase risk of serious, sometimes fatal, adverse reactions. Avoid using together.
Phenobarbital, phenytoin: May alter pharmacokinetics of both drugs. Dosage adjustments may be needed.
Procyclidine: May increase procyclidine levels. Watch for excessive anticholinergic effects.
Theophylline: Decreased clearance. Dosage reductions are needed.
Tryptophan: May cause adverse reactions, such as diaphoresis, headache, nausea, and dizziness. Avoid using together.
Warfarin: May cause bleeding. Use together cautiously.
Drug-herb. *St. John's wort:* May cause sedative-hypnotic intoxication. Discourage use together.
Drug-lifestyle. *Alcohol use:* May alter psychomotor function. Tell patient to avoid use together.

EFFECTS ON LAB TEST RESULTS
None reported.

CONTRAINDICATIONS
Contraindicated in patients hypersensitive to drug and in those taking MAO inhibitors; also contraindicated within 14 days of discontinuing MAO inhibitor therapy.

NURSING CONSIDERATIONS
● Use cautiously in patients with history of seizure disorders or mania and in those with other severe, systemic illness.
● Controlled-release formulation indicated for depression only.

• Use cautiously in patients at risk for volume depletion and monitor them appropriately.
• If signs or symptoms of psychosis occur or increase, expect prescriber to reduce dosage. Record mood changes. Monitor patient for suicidal tendencies, and allow only a minimum supply of drug.
• Monitor patient for complaints of sexual dysfunction. In men, they include anorgasmy, erectile difficulties, delayed ejaculation or orgasm, or impotence; in women, they include anorgasmy or difficulty with orgasm.
• *Alert:* Don't confuse paroxetine with paclitaxel, or Paxil with Doxil, paclitaxel, or Taxol.

PATIENT TEACHING
• Tell patient that drug may be taken with or without food, usually in morning.
• Tell patient not to break, crush, or chew controlled-release tablets.
• Warn patient to avoid activities that require alertness and good psychomotor coordination until CNS effects of drug are known.
• Advise woman to contact prescriber if she becomes pregnant or plans to become pregnant during therapy, or if she's currently breast-feeding.
• Tell patient to avoid alcohol and to consult prescriber before taking other prescription or OTC drugs or herbal medicines.
• Advise patient to continue therapy.
• Instruct patient not to stop taking medication abruptly.

---

phenelzine sulfate
Nardil

Pregnancy risk category C

AVAILABLE FORMS
Tablets: 15 mg

INDICATIONS & DOSAGES
➤ Depression—
Adults: 15 mg P.O. t.i.d., increased rapidly to 60 mg daily. Maximum dose is 90 mg daily; dose can usually be reduced to 15 mg daily.

ACTION
Unknown. An MAO inhibitor that probably promotes accumulation of neurotransmitters by inhibiting their metabolism.

Route	Onset	Peak	Duration
P.O.	Unknown	2-4 hr	≤ 10 days

ADVERSE REACTIONS
CNS: *dizziness, vertigo, headache,* hyperreflexia, tremor, muscle twitching, *insomnia,* drowsiness, weakness, fatigue.
CV: *orthostatic hypotension,* edema.
GI: dry mouth, *anorexia,* nausea, *constipation.*
Metabolic: weight gain.
Skin: diaphoresis.

INTERACTIONS
Drug-drug. *Amphetamines, antihistamines, buspirone, ephedrine, levodopa, meperidine, metaraminol, methylphenidate, phenylephrine, sympathomimetics:* Enhanced pressor effects. Avoid using together.
Antihypertensives containing thiazide diuretics, barbiturates, dextromethorphan, methotrimeprazine, narcotics, other sedatives, serotonin reuptake inhibitors, spinal anesthetics, TCAs: Unpredictable interaction. Use these drugs with caution and in reduced dosages.
Insulin, oral antidiabetics: May cause hypoglycemia. Use with caution and in reduced dosages.
Drug-herb. *Cacao:* Potential vasopressor effects. Discourage use together.
Ephedra: May cause severe reactions including hypertensive crisis. Discourage use together.
Ginseng: May cause headache, tremors, or mania. Discourage use together.
Drug-food. *Foods high in caffeine, tryptophan, tyramine:* May precipitate hypertensive crisis. Discourage use together; watch for adverse effects.
Drug-lifestyle. *Alcohol use:* May precipitate hypertensive crisis. Discourage use together.

EFFECTS ON LAB TEST RESULTS
• May increase ALT and AST levels.

Reactions may be *common*, uncommon, *life-threatening*, or COMMON AND LIFE-THREATENING.

CONTRAINDICATIONS

Contraindicated in patients hypersensitive to drug and in those with heart failure, pheochromocytoma, hypertension, significant renal impairment, cerebrovascular defect, liver disease, and CV disease. Also contraindicated during therapy with other MAO inhibitors (isocarboxazid, tranylcypromine) or within 10 days of such therapy or within 10 days of elective surgery requiring general anesthesia, cocaine use, or local anesthesia containing sympathomimetic vasoconstrictors.

NURSING CONSIDERATIONS

• Use cautiously with antihypertensives containing thiazide diuretics, with spinal anesthetics, and in patients at risk for suicide, diabetes, or seizure disorders.
• Obtain baseline blood pressure, heart rate, CBC, and liver function test results before therapy, and continue to monitor them throughout treatment.
• Drug therapy elevates urinary catecholamine levels.
• Discontinue MAO inhibitors 14 days before elective surgery to avoid drug interactions that may occur during anesthesia.
• Monitor patient closely for suicidal tendencies and allow only a minimum supply of drug.
• If patient develops symptoms of overdose (severe hypotension, palpitations, or frequent headaches), withhold dose and notify prescriber.
• **Alert:** Have phentolamine available to combat severe hypertension.
• Continue precautions 14 days after stopping phenelzine because drug has long-lasting effects.

PATIENT TEACHING

• Advise patient to consult prescriber before taking other prescription or OTC drugs. Severe adverse effects can occur if MAO inhibitors are taken with OTC cold, hay fever, or diet preparations.
• Warn patient about probability of orthostatic hypotension. Supervise walking. Tell patient to get out of bed slowly, sitting up first for 1 minute.
• Because MAO inhibitors may suppress chest pain in patients with angina, warn such patients to engage only in moderate activities and to avoid overexertion.
• Advise patient to avoid anchovies, avocados, bananas, broad beans, canned figs, caviar, cheese, chocolate, dry sausage, liver, meat extract, meat prepared with tenderizers, pickled herring, raisins, sauerkraut, sour cream, soy sauce, yeast extract, yogurt, and any pickled, fermented, or smoked foods. These foods have a high tyramine content, which may interact with the drug and cause a hypertensive crisis.
• Tell patient to avoid alcohol.

---

sertraline hydrochloride
Lustral§, Zoloft

Pregnancy risk category C

AVAILABLE FORMS

Capsules†: 25 mg, 50 mg, 100 mg
Oral concentrate: 20 mg/ml
Tablets: 50 mg, 100 mg

INDICATIONS & DOSAGES

➤ **Depression**—
Adults: 50 mg P.O. daily. Dosage adjusted as needed and tolerated; doses of 50 to 200 mg daily have been given.
➤ **Obsessive-compulsive disorder**—
Adults: 50 mg P.O. once daily. If no response, dose may be increased to maximum of 200 mg/day.
Children ages 6 to 17: Initially, 25 mg P.O. daily in children ages 6 to 12, or 50 mg P.O. daily in children ages 13 to 17. May increase dosage, p.r.n., up to 200 mg/day at intervals of no less than 1 week.
➤ **Panic disorder**—
Adults: Initially, 25 mg P.O. daily. After 1 week, increase dose to 50 mg P.O. daily. If no response, dose may be increased to maximum of 200 mg/day.
Adjust-a-dose: For patients with hepatic disease, lower or less frequent doses should be used.
➤ **Posttraumatic stress disorder**—
Adults: Initially, 25 mg P.O. once daily. Increase dosage to 50 mg P.O. once daily after 1 week. Dosage may be increased at weekly intervals to a maximum of 200 mg daily. Maintain patient on lowest effective dose.

ACTION
Unknown. Thought to be linked to drug's inhibition of CNS neuronal uptake of serotonin.

Route	Onset	Peak	Duration
P.O.	Unknown	4.5-8.5 hr	Unknown

ADVERSE REACTIONS
CNS: *headache, tremor, dizziness, insomnia, somnolence,* paresthesia, hypesthesia, *fatigue,* nervousness, anxiety, agitation, hypertonia, twitching, confusion.
CV: palpitations, chest pain, hot flashes.
GI: *dry mouth, nausea, diarrhea, loose stools, dyspepsia,* vomiting, constipation, thirst, flatulence, anorexia, abdominal pain, increased appetite.
GU: *male sexual dysfunction.*
Musculoskeletal: myalgia.
Skin: rash, pruritus, diaphoresis.

INTERACTIONS
Drug-drug. *Benzodiazepines, tolbutamide:* Decreased clearance of these drugs. Significance unknown; monitor patient for increased drug effects.
Cimetidine: Decreased clearance of sertraline. Monitor patient closely.
Disulfiram: Oral concentrate contains alcohol that could cause a reaction. Avoid use.
MAO inhibitors: May cause serotonin syndrome, a serious, sometimes fatal, reaction, including myoclonus rigidity, mental status changes, hyperthermia, autonomic nervous system instability, rapid fluctuations of vital signs, delirium, coma, and death. Avoid using together.
Warfarin, other highly protein-bound drugs: May increase plasma levels of sertraline or other highly protein-bound drug. PT or INR may increase by 8% with use of warfarin. Monitor patient closely.

EFFECTS ON LAB TEST RESULTS
• May increase ALT and AST levels.

CONTRAINDICATIONS
Contraindicated in patients taking MAO inhibitors or within 14 days of discontinuing MAO inhibitor therapy.

NURSING CONSIDERATIONS
• Use cautiously in patients at risk for suicide and in those with seizure disorders, major affective disorder, or diseases or conditions that affect metabolism or hemodynamic responses.
• Administer sertraline once daily, either in morning or evening. May be given with or without food.
• Dosage adjustments should be made at intervals of no less than 1 week.
• Record mood changes. Monitor patient for suicidal tendencies and allow only a minimum supply of drug.
• Avoid using the oral concentrate dropper, which is made of rubber, in a patient with a latex allergy.

PATIENT TEACHING
• Advise patient to use caution when performing hazardous tasks that require alertness.
• Tell patient to avoid alcohol and to consult prescriber before taking OTC drugs.
• Advise patient to mix the oral concentrate with 4 ounces (½ cup) of water, ginger ale, lemon or lime soda, lemonade, or orange juice only, and to take the dose right away.
• Instruct patient to avoid stopping the medication abruptly.

---

tranylcypromine sulfate
Parnate

Pregnancy risk category C

AVAILABLE FORMS
Tablets: 10 mg

INDICATIONS & DOSAGES
➤ **Depression**—
Adults: 10 mg P.O. t.i.d. Increase dose by 10 mg P.O. daily at 1- to 3-week intervals to maximum of 60 mg daily, if needed, after 2 weeks of therapy.

ACTION
Unknown. An MAO inhibitor that probably promotes accumulation of neurotransmitters by inhibiting their metabolism.

Route	Onset	Peak	Duration
P.O.	Unknown	1-3.5 hr	≤ 10 days

ADVERSE REACTIONS

CNS: *dizziness, headache,* anxiety, agitation, paresthesia, drowsiness, weakness, numbness, tremor, jitters, confusion, *vertigo.*

CV: *orthostatic hypotension, tachycardia,* paradoxical hypertension, palpitations, *edema.*

EENT: blurred vision, tinnitus.

GI: dry mouth, *anorexia,* nausea, diarrhea, constipation, abdominal pain.

GU: impotence, urine retention, impaired ejaculation.

Hematologic: anemia, *leukopenia, agranulocytosis, thrombocytopenia.*

Hepatic: *hepatitis.*

Metabolic: SIADH.

Musculoskeletal: muscle spasm, myoclonic jerks.

Skin: rash.

Other: chills.

INTERACTIONS

Drug-drug. *Amphetamines, antihistamines, antihypertensives, diuretics, ephedrine, levodopa, meperidine, metaraminol, methylphenidate, phenylephrine, sympathomimetics:* Enhanced pressor effects of these drugs. Avoid using together.

Antiparkinsonians, barbiturates, dextromethorphan, methotrimeprazine, narcotics, other sedatives, selective serotonin reuptake inhibitors, spinal anesthetics, TCAs: Enhanced adverse CNS effects. Avoid using together. If necessary, use with caution and in reduced dosage.

Buspirone: May elevate blood pressure. Monitor patient closely.

Insulin, oral antidiabetics: May cause hypoglycemia. Use with caution and in reduced dosages.

Drug-herb. *Cacao:* Potential vasopressor effects. Discourage use together.

Ephedra: May cause severe reactions including hypertensive crisis. Discourage use together.

Ginseng: May cause headache, tremors, or mania. Monitor patient for effects.

Licorice: May cause increase in tranylcypromine activity. Discourage use together.

Tryptophan: May cause additive effect leading to serotonin syndrome, which is a toxic hyperserotonergic state, characterized by euphoria, drowsiness, overreactive reflexes, jaw clenching, sweating, high body temperature, unconsciousness, and even death. Avoid using together.

Drug-food. *Foods high in caffeine, tryptophan, tyramine:* May cause hypertensive crisis. Discourage use together.

Drug-lifestyle. *Alcohol use:* Enhanced CNS effects. Discourage use together.

EFFECTS ON LAB TEST RESULTS
• May increase ALT and AST levels.
• May decrease hemoglobin and WBC, granulocyte, and platelet counts.

CONTRAINDICATIONS

Contraindicated in patients hypersensitive to drug and in those with pheochromocytoma, cerebrovascular or CV disease, confirmed or suspected cerebrovascular defect, hypertension, heart failure, hepatic disease, significant renal impairment, or history of headache.

Also contraindicated in patients receiving MAO inhibitors or dibenzazepine derivatives within 2 weeks, in those undergoing elective surgery, and debilitated patients.

NURSING CONSIDERATIONS
• Use cautiously in patients with renal disease, diabetes, seizure disorders, Parkinson's disease, or hyperthyroidism, and in those at risk for suicide.
• Obtain baseline blood pressure, heart rate, CBC, and liver function test results before therapy, and continue to monitor them throughout treatment.
• Drug therapy elevates urinary catecholamine levels.
• Dosage usually is reduced to maintenance level as soon as possible.
• Don't withdraw drug abruptly.
• Discontinue MAO inhibitors 14 days before elective surgery, to avoid drug interactions that may occur during anesthesia.
• Monitor patient for suicidal tendencies and allow only a minimum supply of drug.
• If patient develops signs or symptoms of overdose (palpitations, severe hypotension, or frequent headaches), withhold dose and notify prescriber.
• *Alert:* Have phentolamine available to combat severe hypertension.

---

*Liquid contains alcohol.   **May contain tartrazine.   †Canada   ‡Australia   §U.K.   ◊OTC

• Continue precautions for 10 days after stopping drug because it has long-lasting effects.

PATIENT TEACHING
• Warn patient to avoid foods high in tyramine, tryptophan, or caffeine. Tranylcypromine is the MAO inhibitor most frequently reported to cause hypertensive crisis with ingestion of tyramine-rich foods, including aged cheese, Chianti wine, beer, avocados, chicken livers, chocolate, bananas, soy sauce, meat tenderizers, salami, and bologna.
• Tell patient to avoid alcohol during therapy.
• Advise patient to consult prescriber before taking other prescription or OTC drugs.
• To prevent dizziness resulting from orthostatic hypotension, tell patient to get out of bed slowly, sitting up first for 1 minute.
• Because MAO inhibitors may suppress anginal pain, warn patient to perform only moderate activities and to avoid overexertion.
• Warn patient not to stop drug suddenly.
• Advise patient to avoid anchovies, avocados, bananas, broad beans, canned figs, caviar, cheese, chocolate, dry sausage, liver, meat extract, meat prepared with tenderizers, pickled herring, raisins, sauerkraut, sour cream, soy sauce, yeast extract, yogurt, and any pickled, fermented, or smoked foods. These foods have a high tyramine content, which may interact with the drug and cause a hypertensive crisis.

---

trazodone hydrochloride
Desyrel, Molipaxin§

Pregnancy risk category C

AVAILABLE FORMS
Tablets: 50 mg, 100 mg, 150 mg, 300 mg

INDICATIONS & DOSAGES
➤ **Depression—**
Adults: Initially, 150 mg P.O. daily in divided doses; then increased by 50 mg daily q 3 to 4 days, p.r.n. Dose ranges from 150 to 400 mg daily. Maximum,

600 mg daily for inpatients and 400 mg daily for outpatients.

ACTION
Unknown. Inhibits CNS neuronal uptake of serotonin; not a tricyclic derivative.

Route	Onset	Peak	Duration
P.O.	Unknown	1-2 hr	Unknown

ADVERSE REACTIONS
CNS: *drowsiness, dizziness,* nervousness, fatigue, confusion, tremor, weakness, hostility, anger, nightmares, vivid dreams, headache, insomnia, syncope.
CV: orthostatic hypotension, tachycardia, hypertension, shortness of breath, ECG changes.
EENT: blurred vision, tinnitus, nasal congestion.
GI: dry mouth, dysgeusia, constipation, nausea, vomiting, anorexia.
GU: urine retention; priapism possibly leading to impotence; hematuria.
Hematologic: anemia.
Skin: rash, urticaria, diaphoresis.
Other: decreased libido.

INTERACTIONS
Drug-drug. *Antihypertensives:* Increased hypotensive effect of trazodone. Antihypertensive dosage may need to be decreased.
Clonidine, CNS depressants: Enhanced CNS depression. Avoid using together.
Digoxin, phenytoin: May increase serum levels of these drugs. Watch for toxicity.
MAO inhibitors: Effects unknown. Use together with extreme caution.
Drug-herb. *Ginkgo biloba:* May cause sedation. Discourage use together.
St. John's wort: May cause serotonin syndrome, which is a toxic hyperserotonergic state, characterized by euphoria, drowsiness, overreactive reflexes, jaw clenching, sweating, high body temperature, unconsciousness, and even death. Discourage use together.
Drug-lifestyle. *Alcohol use:* Enhanced CNS depression. Discourage use together.

EFFECTS ON LAB TEST RESULTS
• May increase ALT and AST levels.
• May decrease hemoglobin.

Reactions may be *common,* uncommon, *life-threatening,* or COMMON AND LIFE-THREATENING.

CONTRAINDICATIONS
Contraindicated in patients hypersensitive to drug.

NURSING CONSIDERATIONS
• Use cautiously in patients with cardiac disease or in the initial recovery phase of MI and in patients at risk for suicide.
• Give drug after meals or a light snack for optimal absorption and to decrease risk of dizziness.
• Record mood changes. Monitor patient for suicidal tendencies and allow only minimum supply of drug.

PATIENT TEACHING
• *Alert:* Priapism, a persistent, painful erection, may occur in men taking trazodone. Tell patient to report it immediately because he may need surgery.
• Warn patient to avoid activities that require alertness and good psychomotor coordination until CNS effects of drug are known. Drowsiness and dizziness usually subside after few weeks.
• Teach caregivers how to recognize signs and symptoms of suicidal tendency or suicidal ideation.

---

trimipramine maleate
Apo-Trimip†, Novo-Tripramine†,
Rhotrimine†, Surmontil

Pregnancy risk category C

AVAILABLE FORMS
Capsules: 25 mg, 50 mg, 100 mg
Tablets: 25 mg‡

INDICATIONS & DOSAGES
➤ **Depression—**
Adults: 75 to 100 mg P.O. daily in divided doses, increased to 200 to 300 mg daily. Doses of more than 300 mg daily not recommended in hospitalized patients, or more than 200 mg in outpatients. Total dose requirement may be given h.s.
Adolescents and elderly patients: Initially, 50 mg/day, gradually increased to 100 mg/day.

ACTION
Unknown. A TCA that increases amount of norepinephrine, serotonin, or both in the CNS by blocking their reuptake by the presynaptic neurons.

Route	Onset	Peak	Duration
P.O.	Unknown	2 hr	Unknown

ADVERSE REACTIONS
CNS: *drowsiness, dizziness,* paresthesia, ataxia, hallucinations, delusions, anxiety, agitation, insomnia, tremor, weakness, confusion, headache, EEG changes, *seizures, CVA,* extrapyramidal syndrome.
CV: *orthostatic hypotension, tachycardia,* hypertension, *arrhythmias, heart block, MI,* ECG changes.
EENT: *blurred vision,* tinnitus, mydriasis.
GI: *dry mouth, constipation,* nausea, vomiting, anorexia, paralytic ileus.
GU: *urine retention.*
Metabolic: altered glucose levels.
Skin: rash, urticaria, photosensitivity reactions, *diaphoresis.*
Other: hypersensitivity reactions.

INTERACTIONS
Drug-drug. *Barbiturates:* Decreased TCA blood levels. Watch for decreased antidepressant effect.
Cimetidine, fluoxetine, fluvoxamine, paroxetine, sertraline: May increase trimipramine levels. Watch for increased adverse reactions.
Clonidine: Decreased effects of clonidine. Avoid using together, if possible. Monitor blood pressure.
CNS depressants: Enhanced CNS depression. Avoid using together.
Epinephrine, norepinephrine: Increased hypertensive effect. Use together cautiously.
MAO inhibitors: May cause severe excitation, hyperpyrexia, or seizures, usually with high doses. Avoid using together.
Drug-herb. *St. John's wort, SAM-e, yohimbe:* May cause serotonin syndrome, which is a toxic hyperserotonergic state, characterized by euphoria, drowsiness, overreactive reflexes, jaw clenching, sweating, high body temperature, unconsciousness, and even death. Discourage use together.
Drug-lifestyle. *Alcohol use:* Enhanced CNS depression. Discourage use together.

---

*Liquid contains alcohol. **May contain tartrazine. †Canada ‡Australia §U.K. ◇OTC

Sun exposure: Increased risk of photosensitivity reactions. Advise patient to avoid excessive sunlight exposure.

EFFECTS ON LAB TEST RESULTS
• May increase ALT and AST levels. May increase or decrease glucose levels.

CONTRAINDICATIONS
Contraindicated in patients hypersensitive to drug, in patients in acute recovery phase after MI, and in patients receiving MAO inhibitor therapy within 14 days.

NURSING CONSIDERATIONS
• Use with extreme caution in patients with CV disease, history of urine retention or angle-closure glaucoma, increased intraocular pressure, hyperthyroidism, impaired hepatic function, or history of seizures, and in those receiving thyroid medications, guanethidine, or similar drugs.
• Watch for nausea, headache, and malaise after abrupt withdrawal of long-term therapy; however, these symptoms don't indicate addiction.
• *Alert:* Because hypertensive episodes have occurred during surgery in patients receiving TCAs, dosage should be gradually discontinued several days before surgery.
• If signs or symptoms of psychosis occur or increase, expect prescriber to reduce dosage. Record mood changes. Monitor patient for suicidal tendencies and allow only a minimum supply of drug.
• Recommend use of sugarless hard candy or gum to relieve dry mouth. Saliva substitutes may be needed.
• *Alert:* Don't confuse trimipramine with triamterene.

PATIENT TEACHING
• Tell patient to take full dose at bedtime whenever possible, to avoid daytime sedation. Warn him about possible morning orthostatic hypotension.
• Tell patient to avoid alcohol and to consult prescriber before taking other prescription or OTC drugs.
• Warn patient to avoid hazardous activities that require alertness and good psychomotor coordination until CNS effects

of drug are known. Drowsiness and dizziness usually subside after a few weeks.
• Warn patient not to stop drug suddenly.
• To prevent photosensitivity reactions, advise patient to use sunblock, wear protective clothing, and avoid prolonged exposure to strong sunlight.

venlafaxine hydrochloride
Efexor‡, Effexor, Effexor XR

Pregnancy risk category C

AVAILABLE FORMS
Capsules (extended-release): 37.5 mg, 75 mg, 150 mg
Tablets: 25 mg, 37.5 mg, 50 mg, 75 mg, 100 mg

INDICATIONS & DOSAGES
➤ **Depression—**
Adults: Initially, 75 mg P.O. daily in two or three divided doses with food. Increase as tolerated and needed in increments of 75 mg/day at intervals of no less than 4 days. For moderately depressed outpatients, usual maximum is 225 mg daily; in certain severely depressed patients, dose may be as high as 375 mg daily. For extended-release capsules, 75 mg P.O. daily in a single dose. For some patients, it may be desirable to start at 37.5 mg P.O. daily for 4 to 7 days before increasing to 75 mg daily. Dosage may be increased at increments of 75 mg/day q 4 days to maximum of 225 mg/day.
➤ **Generalized anxiety disorder—**
Adults: Initially, 75 mg of Effexor XR P.O. daily in a single dose. For some patients, it may be desirable to start at 37.5 mg P.O. daily for 4 to 7 days before increasing to 75 mg daily. May be increased at increments of 75 mg/day q 4 days to maximum of 225 mg/day.
Adjust-a-dose: For renally impaired patients, reduce daily amount by 25%. For patients undergoing hemodialysis, reduce daily amount by 50% and withhold dose until dialysis is completed. For patients with hepatic impairment, reduce daily amount by 50%.

ACTION

Increases the amount of norepinephrine, serotonin, or both in the CNS by blocking their reuptake by the presynaptic neurons.

Route	Onset	Peak	Duration
P.O.	Unknown	Unknown	Unknown

ADVERSE REACTIONS

CNS: *headache, somnolence, dizziness, nervousness, insomnia,* anxiety, tremor, abnormal dreams, paresthesia, agitation, *asthenia.*
CV: hypertension, tachycardia, vasodilation.
EENT: blurred vision.
GI: *nausea, constipation,* vomiting, *dry mouth, anorexia,* diarrhea, dyspepsia, flatulence, vomiting.
GU: *abnormal ejaculation,* impotence, urinary frequency, impaired urination.
Metabolic: weight loss.
Skin: *diaphoresis,* rash.
Other: yawning, chills, infection.

INTERACTIONS

Drug-drug. *MAO inhibitors:* May cause a syndrome similar to neuroleptic malignant syndrome (high fever, tachycardia, tachypnea, and profuse diaphoresis). Avoid using together.
Drug-herb. *Yohimbe:* Additive stimulation. Advise patient to use cautiously.

EFFECTS ON LAB TEST RESULTS

None reported.

CONTRAINDICATIONS

Contraindicated in patients hypersensitive to drug or within 14 days of MAO inhibitor therapy.

NURSING CONSIDERATIONS

● Use cautiously in patients with renal impairment, diseases or conditions that could affect hemodynamic responses or metabolism, and in those with history of mania or seizures.
● Monitor patient for suicidal tendencies. Provide only a minimal supply of drug.
● Carefully monitor blood pressure. Drug therapy may cause sustained, dose-dependent increases in blood pressure. Greatest increases (averaging about 7 mm

Hg above baseline) occur in patients taking 375 mg daily.
● Monitor patient's weight, particularly underweight, depressed patients.

PATIENT TEACHING

● If medication is to be discontinued, inform patient who has received drug for 6 weeks or longer that drug should be gradually discontinued by tapering dosage over a 2-week period as instructed by prescriber.
● Warn patient to avoid hazardous activities that require alertness and good psychomotor coordination until CNS effects of drug are known.
● Tell patient to avoid alcohol and to consult prescriber before taking other prescription or OTC drugs.
● Advise woman to contact prescriber if she becomes pregnant or intends to become pregnant during therapy or if she's breast-feeding.

---

alprazolam
buspirone hydrochloride
chlordiazepoxide
chlordiazepoxide hydrochloride
clorazepate dipotassium
diazepam
doxepin hydrochloride
(See Chapter 29, ANTIDEPRESSANTS.)
hydroxyzine embonate
hydroxyzine hydrochloride
hydroxyzine pamoate
lorazepam
meprobamate
midazolam hydrochloride
oxazepam

COMBINATION PRODUCTS
EQUAGESIC: meprobamate 200 mg and aspirin 325 mg.
LIBRAX: chlordiazepoxide hydrochloride 5 mg and clidinium bromide 2.5 mg.
LIMBITROL DS: chlordiazepoxide 10 mg and amitriptyline hydrochloride 25 mg.

---

alprazolam
Apo-Alpraz†, Kalma‡, Novo-Alprazol†, Nu-Alpraz†, Ralozam‡, Xanax

Pregnancy risk category D
Controlled substance schedule IV

AVAILABLE FORMS
Oral solution: 0.5 mg/5 ml, 1 mg/ml (concentrate)
Tablets: 0.25 mg, 0.5 mg, 1 mg, 2 mg

INDICATIONS & DOSAGES
➤ **Anxiety—**
Adults: Usual initial dose, 0.25 to 0.5 mg P.O. t.i.d. Maximum, 4 mg daily in divided doses.
Elderly patients: Usual initial dose, 0.25 mg P.O. b.i.d. or t.i.d. Maximum, 4 mg daily in divided doses.
➤ **Panic disorders—**
Adults: 0.5 mg P.O. t.i.d., increased at intervals of 3 to 4 days in increments of no

more than 1 mg. Maximum, 10 mg daily in divided doses.
Adjust-a-dose: For debilitated patients or those with advanced hepatic disease, usual initial dose is 0.25 mg P.O. b.i.d. or t.i.d. Maximum, 4 mg daily in divided doses.

ACTION
Unknown. A benzodiazepine that probably potentiates the effects of gamma-aminobutyric acid, an inhibitory neurotransmitter, and depresses the CNS at the limbic and subcortical levels of the brain.

Route	Onset	Peak	Duration
P.O.	Unknown	1-2 hr	Unknown

ADVERSE REACTIONS
CNS: *drowsiness, light-headedness,* headache, confusion, tremor, dizziness, syncope, *depression,* insomnia, memory impairment, nervousness, minor changes in EEG patterns.
CV: hypotension, tachycardia.
EENT: blurred vision, nasal congestion.
GI: *dry mouth,* nausea, vomiting, *diarrhea, constipation,* increased salivation.
Metabolic: weight gain or loss.
Musculoskeletal: muscle rigidity.
Skin: dermatitis.

INTERACTIONS
Drug-drug. *Azole antifungal agents:* Decreased alprazolam clearance and increased risk of adverse reactions. Avoid using together.
Cimetidine, fluoxetine, fluvoxamine, paroxetine, sertraline: Decreased alprazolam clearance and increased risk of adverse reactions. Monitor patient carefully.
CNS depressants: Increased CNS depression. Use together cautiously.
Digoxin: May increase digoxin levels, increasing toxicity. Monitor patient closely.
TCAs: Increased plasma levels of TCAs. Monitor patient for toxicity.
Drug-herb. *Kava:* May increase sedation. Discourage use together.

Reactions may be *common,* uncommon, *life-threatening,* or COMMON AND LIFE-THREATENING.

Drug-food. *Grapefruit juice:* Increased alprazolam concentrations. Advise patient to take drug with liquid other than grapefruit juice.

Drug-lifestyle. *Alcohol use:* Increased CNS depression. Discourage use together. *Smoking:* Decreased effectiveness of benzodiazepines. Monitor patient closely.

EFFECTS ON LAB TEST RESULTS
• May increase ALT and AST levels.

CONTRAINDICATIONS
Contraindicated in patients hypersensitive to drug or other benzodiazepines and in those with acute angle-closure glaucoma.

NURSING CONSIDERATIONS
• Use cautiously in patients with hepatic, renal, or pulmonary disease.
• Drug isn't for daily stress or long-term use. Further study is needed to determine the optimum duration of therapy.
• *Alert:* Don't withdraw drug abruptly; withdrawal symptoms, including seizures, may occur. Abuse or addiction is possible.
• Monitor hepatic, renal, and hematopoietic function periodically in patients receiving repeated or prolonged therapy.
• *Alert:* Don't confuse alprazolam with alprostadil or Xanax with Zantac or Tenex.

PATIENT TEACHING
• Warn patient to avoid hazardous activities that require alertness and good psychomotor coordination until CNS effects of drug are known.
• Tell patient to avoid alcohol while taking drug.
• Advise patient that smoking may decrease drug's effectiveness.
• Warn patient not to stop drug abruptly because withdrawal symptoms or seizures may occur.

---

buspirone hydrochloride
BuSpar

Pregnancy risk category B

AVAILABLE FORMS
Tablets: 5 mg, 10 mg, 15 mg, 30 mg

INDICATIONS & DOSAGES
➤ **Anxiety disorders, short-term relief of anxiety—**
Adults: Initially, 10 to 15 mg daily in two or three divided doses. Increase dosage by 5-mg increments at 2- to 4-day intervals. Usual maintenance dosage is 15 to 30 mg daily in divided doses. Don't exceed 60 mg daily.

ACTION
Unknown. May inhibit neuronal firing and reduce serotonin turnover in cortical, amygdaloid, and septohippocampal tissue.

Route	Onset	Peak	Duration
P.O.	Unknown	40-90 min	Unknown

ADVERSE REACTIONS
CNS: *dizziness, drowsiness,* nervousness, insomnia, *headache,* light-headedness, fatigue, numbness.
CV: tachycardia, nonspecific chest pain.
EENT: blurred vision.
GI: dry mouth, nausea, diarrhea, abdominal distress.

INTERACTIONS
Drug-drug. *CNS depressants:* Increased CNS depression. Use together cautiously.
Drugs metabolized by CYP-450 3A4 (erythromycin, itraconazole, nefazodone): Increased buspirone concentrations. Monitor patient; a decrease in buspirone dosage may be needed.
MAO inhibitors: May elevate blood pressure. Avoid using together.
Drug-food. *Grapefruit juice:* Elevated levels of buspirone, increasing the pharmacologic and adverse effects. Give with liquid other than grapefruit juice.
Drug-lifestyle. *Alcohol use:* Increased CNS depression. Discourage use together.

EFFECTS ON LAB TEST RESULTS
None reported.

CONTRAINDICATIONS
Contraindicated in patients hypersensitive to drug; also contraindicated within 14 days of MAO inhibitor therapy.

NURSING CONSIDERATIONS
• Drug isn't recommended for patients with severe hepatic or renal impairment.

• Monitor patient closely for adverse CNS reactions. Buspirone is less sedating than other anxiolytics. However, CNS effects may be unpredictable.

• **Alert:** Before starting buspirone therapy in a patient already receiving a benzodiazepine, don't stop the benzodiazepine abruptly; a withdrawal reaction may occur.

• Drug has shown no potential for abuse and hasn't been classified as a controlled substance; however, it isn't recommended for relief of daily stress.

• **Alert:** Don't confuse buspirone with bupropion.

PATIENT TEACHING

• Warn patient to avoid hazardous activities that require alertness and good psychomotor coordination until CNS effects of drug are known.

• Remind patient that drug effects may not be noticeable for several weeks.

• Warn patient not to abruptly stop a benzodiazepine because of risk of withdrawal symptoms.

• Tell patient to avoid alcohol during drug therapy.

---

chlordiazepoxide
Libritabs

chlordiazepoxide hydrochloride
Apo-Chlordiazepoxide†, Librium, Novo-Poxide†

Pregnancy risk category NR
Controlled substance schedule IV

AVAILABLE FORMS
chlordiazepoxide
Tablets: 10 mg, 25 mg
chlordiazepoxide hydrochloride
Capsules: 5 mg, 10 mg, 25 mg
Powder for injection: 100-mg ampule

INDICATIONS & DOSAGES
➤ **Mild to moderate anxiety—**
Adults: 5 to 10 mg P.O. t.i.d. or q.i.d.
Children older than age 6: 5 mg P.O. b.i.d. to q.i.d. Maximum, 10 mg P.O. b.i.d. or t.i.d.
➤ **Severe anxiety—**
Adults: 20 to 25 mg P.O. t.i.d. or q.i.d.

Elderly patients: 5 mg P.O. b.i.d. to q.i.d.
Adjust-a-dose: For debilitated patients, 5 mg P.O. b.i.d. to q.i.d.
➤ **Withdrawal symptoms of acute alcoholism—**
Adults: 50 to 100 mg P.O., I.M., or I.V. Repeated in 2 to 4 hours, p.r.n. Maximum, 300 mg daily.
➤ **Preoperative apprehension and anxiety—**
Adults: 5 to 10 mg P.O. t.i.d. or q.i.d. on day before surgery; or 50 to 100 mg I.M. 1 hour before surgery.

I.V. ADMINISTRATION
• Parenteral form isn't recommended in children younger than age 12.

• Use 5 ml of normal saline solution or sterile water for injection as diluent for an ampule containing 100 mg of drug. Don't give prepackaged diluent I.V. because air bubbles may form. Administer over 1 minute.

• When giving drug I.V., make sure equipment and staff needed for emergency airway management are available. Monitor respirations every 5 to 15 minutes and before each I.V. dose.

ACTION
Unknown. A benzodiazepine that probably potentiates the effects of gamma-aminobutyric acid, an inhibitory neurotransmitter. Depresses the CNS at the limbic and subcortical levels of the brain and suppresses the spread of seizure activity produced by epileptogenic foci in the cortex, thalamus, and limbic structures.

Route	Onset	Peak	Duration
I.M.	Unknown	Unknown	Unknown
I.V.	1-5 min	Unknown	15-60 min
P.O.	Unknown	0.5-4 hr	Unknown

ADVERSE REACTIONS
CNS: *drowsiness, lethargy,* ataxia, confusion, extrapyramidal reactions, minor changes in EEG patterns.
CV: edema.
GI: nausea, constipation.
GU: menstrual irregularities.
Hematologic: *agranulocytosis.*
Hepatic: jaundice.

Reactions may be *common,* uncommon, *life-threatening,* or COMMON AND LIFE-THREATENING.

Skin: *swelling and pain at injection site,* skin eruptions.
Other: altered libido.

INTERACTIONS
Drug-drug. *Cimetidine:* Decreased chlordiazepoxide clearance and increased risk of adverse reactions. Monitor patient carefully.
CNS depressants: Increased CNS depression. Use together cautiously.
Digoxin: Increased digoxin levels and risk of toxicity. Monitor patient closely.
Disulfiram: Reduced plasma clearance and increased plasma half-life of chlordiazepoxide. Monitor patient for enhanced effects. Consider dosage adjustment.
Levodopa: Decreased control of parkinsonian symptoms in patients with Parkinson's disease. Use together cautiously.
Drug-herb. *Kava:* May increase sedation. Discourage use together.
Drug-lifestyle. *Alcohol use:* Increased CNS depression. Discourage use together.
Smoking: Decreased effectiveness of benzodiazepines. Monitor patient closely.

EFFECTS ON LAB TEST RESULTS
● May increase liver function test values. May decrease granulocyte count.

CONTRAINDICATIONS
Contraindicated in patients hypersensitive to drug.

NURSING CONSIDERATIONS
● Use cautiously in patients with mental depression, porphyria, or hepatic or renal disease.
● Drug should be avoided during pregnancy, especially during first trimester.
● Drug shouldn't be prescribed regularly for daily stress.
● **Alert:** Chlordiazepoxide 5-mg and 25-mg unit-dose capsules may look similar in color when viewed through the package. When using unit doses of this or any product, verify contents and read label carefully.
● Injectable form (as hydrochloride) comes in two types of ampules—as diluent and as powdered drug. Read directions carefully.
● Keep powder refrigerated and away from light; mix just before use and discard remainder.

● For I.M. use, add 2 ml of diluent to powder and agitate gently until clear. Use immediately. I.M. form may be absorbed erratically.
● Monitor hepatic, renal, and hematopoietic function periodically in patients receiving repeated or prolonged therapy.
● Possibility of abuse and addiction exists. Don't withdraw drug abruptly after long-term administration; withdrawal symptoms may occur.
● Drug may cause a false-positive pregnancy test, depending on method used. It also may alter urinary 17-ketosteroids (Zimmerman reaction), urine alkaloid determination (Frings thin-layer chromatography method), and urinary glucose determinations (with Chemstrip uG and Diastix).

PATIENT TEACHING
● Warn patient to avoid hazardous activities that require alertness and good psychomotor coordination until CNS effects of drug are known.
● Tell patient to avoid alcohol while taking drug.
● Notify patient that smoking may decrease drug's effectiveness.
● Warn patient not to abruptly stop the drug because withdrawal symptoms may occur.
● Caution woman to avoid use during pregnancy.

---

clorazepate dipotassium
Apo-Clorazepate†, Gen-Xene,
Novo-Clopate†, Tranxene,
Tranxene-SD

Pregnancy risk category D
Controlled substance schedule IV

AVAILABLE FORMS
Capsules: 3.75 mg, 7.5 mg, 15 mg
Tablets: 3.75 mg, 7.5 mg, 11.25 mg, 15 mg, 22.5 mg

INDICATIONS & DOSAGES
➤ **Acute alcohol withdrawal**—
Adults: Day 1, 30 mg P.O. initially; then 30 to 60 mg P.O. in divided doses. Day 2, 45 to 90 mg P.O. in divided doses. Day 3, 22.5 to 45 mg P.O. in divided doses. Day

4, 15 to 30 mg P.O. in divided doses. Then gradually reduce dosage to 7.5 to 15 mg daily. Maximum recommended dosage is 90 mg daily.
➤ **Anxiety—**
Adults: 15 to 60 mg P.O. daily.
Elderly patients: Initially, 7.5 to 15 mg daily in divided doses or a single dose h.s.
Adjust-a-dose: For debilitated patients, initially, 7.5 to 15 mg daily in divided doses or a single dose h.s.
➤ **Adjunct in partial seizure disorder—**
Adults and children older than age 12: Maximum recommended initial dose is 7.5 mg P.O. t.i.d. Dosage increases shouldn't exceed 7.5 mg weekly. Maximum, 90 mg daily.
Children ages 9 to 12: Maximum recommended initial dose is 7.5 mg P.O. b.i.d. Dosage increases shouldn't exceed 7.5 mg weekly. Maximum, 60 mg daily.

ACTION
Unknown. A benzodiazepine that probably potentiates the effects of gamma-aminobutyric acid, an inhibitory neurotransmitter. Depresses the CNS at the limbic and subcortical levels of the brain and suppresses the spread of seizure activity produced by epileptogenic foci in the cortex, thalamus, and limbic structures.

Route	Onset	Peak	Duration
P.O.	Unknown	0.5-2 hr	Unknown

ADVERSE REACTIONS
CNS: *drowsiness, dizziness,* nervousness, confusion, headache, insomnia, depression, irritability, tremor, minor changes in EEG patterns.
CV: hypotension.
EENT: blurred vision, diplopia.
GI: nausea, vomiting, abdominal discomfort, dry mouth.
GU: urine retention, incontinence.
Skin: rash.

INTERACTIONS
Drug-drug. *Cimetidine:* Decreased clorazepate clearance and increased risk of adverse reactions. Monitor patient carefully.
CNS depressants: Increased CNS depression. Use together cautiously.

Digoxin: May increase digoxin levels and risk of toxicity. Monitor patient closely.
Drug-herb. *Kava:* May cause increased sedation. Discourage use together.
Drug-lifestyle. *Alcohol use:* Increased CNS depression. Discourage use together.
Smoking: Decreased benzodiazepine effectiveness. Monitor patient closely.

EFFECTS ON LAB TEST RESULTS
● May increase liver function test values.

CONTRAINDICATIONS
Contraindicated in patients hypersensitive to drug and in those with acute angle-closure glaucoma.

NURSING CONSIDERATIONS
● Use cautiously in patients with suicidal tendencies, renal or hepatic impairment, pulmonary disease, or history of drug abuse.
● Drug should be avoided during pregnancy, especially during first trimester.
● *Alert:* Monitor hepatic, renal, and hematopoietic function periodically in patients receiving repeated or prolonged therapy.
● The possibility of abuse and addiction exists. Don't withdraw drug abruptly after prolonged use because withdrawal symptoms may occur.
● Drug isn't recommended for children younger than age 9.
● *Alert:* Don't confuse clorazepate with clofibrate.

PATIENT TEACHING
● Warn patient to avoid activities that require alertness and good psychomotor coordination until CNS effects of drug are known.
● Tell patient to avoid alcohol while taking drug.
● Advise patient that smoking may decrease drug's effectiveness.
● Warn patient not to stop drug abruptly because withdrawal symptoms may occur.
● Caution woman to avoid use during pregnancy.
● Inform patient that sugarless chewing gum or hard candy can relieve dry mouth.

Reactions may be *common*, uncommon, ***life-threatening***, or **COMMON AND LIFE-THREATENING**.

diazepam

Antenex‡, Apo-Diazepam†,
Diastat, Diazemuls†‡, Diazepam
Intensol, Ducene‡, Novo-Dipam†,
PMS-Diazepam†, Valium, Vivol†

Pregnancy risk category D
Controlled substance schedule IV

AVAILABLE FORMS

Capsules (extended-release): 15 mg
Injection: 5 mg/ml
Oral solution: 5 mg/5 ml, 5 mg/ml
Rectal gel twin packs: 2.5 mg, 5 mg,
10 mg, 15 mg, 20 mg
Sterile emulsion for injection: 5 mg/ml
Tablets: 2 mg, 5 mg, 10 mg

INDICATIONS & DOSAGES

➤ **Anxiety**—
Adults: Depending on severity, 2 to
10 mg P.O. b.i.d. to q.i.d. or 15 to 30 mg
extended-release capsules P.O. once daily.
Or, 2 to 10 mg I.M. or I.V. q 3 to 4 hours,
p.r.n.
Children age 6 months and older: 1 to
2.5 mg P.O. t.i.d. or q.i.d., increased gradually, as needed and tolerated.
Elderly patients: Initially, 2 to 2.5 mg
once daily or b.i.d.; increased gradually.
➤ **Acute alcohol withdrawal**—
Adults: 10 mg P.O. t.i.d. or q.i.d. first 24
hours; reduced to 5 mg P.O. t.i.d. or q.i.d.,
p.r.n. Or, initially, 10 mg I.M. or I.V. Then,
5 to 10 mg I.M. or I.V. q 3 to 4 hours,
p.r.n.
➤ **Before endoscopic procedures**—
Adults: I.V. dose titrated to desired sedative response (up to 20 mg). Or, 5 to
10 mg I.M. 30 minutes before procedure.
➤ **Muscle spasm**—
Adults: 2 to 10 mg P.O. b.i.d. to q.i.d. Or,
15 to 30 mg extended-release capsules
once daily. Or, 5 to 10 mg I.M. or I.V. initially; then 5 to 10 mg I.M. or I.V. q 3 to 4
hours, p.r.n. For tetanus, larger doses may
be needed.
Children ages 1 month to 5 years: 1 to
2 mg I.M. or I.V. slowly, repeated q 3 to 4
hours, p.r.n.
Children age 5 and older: 5 to 10 mg I.M.
or I.V. q 3 to 4 hours, p.r.n.

➤ **Preoperative sedation**—
Adults: 10 mg I.M. (preferred) or I.V. be-
fore surgery.
➤ **Cardioversion**—
Adults: 5 to 15 mg I.V. within 5 to 10 min-
utes before procedure.
➤ **Adjunct in seizure disorders**—
Adults: 2 to 10 mg P.O. b.i.d. to q.i.d.
Children age 6 months and older: 1 to
2.5 mg P.O. t.i.d. or q.i.d. initially; increased as needed and tolerated.
➤ **Status epilepticus, severe recurrent
seizures**—
Adults: 5 to 10 mg I.V. or I.M. initially.
Use I.M. route only if I.V. access is unavailable. Repeated q 10 to 15 minutes,
p.r.n., up to maximum dose of 30 mg. Repeated q 2 to 4 hours, if needed.
Children ages 1 month to 5 years: 0.2 to
0.5 mg I.V. slowly q 2 to 5 minutes up to
maximum of 5 mg. Repeated q 2 to 4
hours, if needed.
Children age 5 and older: 1 mg I.V. q 2 to
5 minutes up to maximum of 10 mg. Repeated q 2 to 4 hours, if needed.
➤ **Patients on stable regimens of
antiepileptic drugs who need intermittent use of diazepam to control bouts of
increased seizure activity**—
Adults and children age 12 and older:
0.2 mg/kg P.R. A second dose may be
given 4 to 12 hours after first.
Children ages 6 to 11: 0.3 mg/kg P.R. A
second dose may be given 4 to 12 hours
after first.
Children ages 2 to 5: 0.5 mg/kg P.R. A
second dose may be given 4 to 12 hours
after first.
Adjust-a-dose: For elderly and debilitated
patients, reduce dosage to decrease the
likelihood of ataxia and oversedation.

I.V. ADMINISTRATION

● Give I.V. at no more than 5 mg/minute.
When injecting, administer directly into a
large vein. If this is impossible, inject
slowly through infusion tubing as near to
the insertion site as possible. Watch closely for phlebitis at injection site.
● Don't inject into small veins.
● *Alert:* Monitor respirations every 5 to 15
minutes and before each I.V. dose. Keep
emergency resuscitation equipment and
oxygen at bedside.

---

*Liquid contains alcohol.   **May contain tartrazine.   †Canada   ‡Australia   §U.K.   ◇OTC

• I.V. route is the most reliable parenteral route; I.M. administration isn't recommended because absorption is variable and injection is painful.

ACTION

Unknown. A benzodiazepine that probably potentiates the effects of gamma-aminobutyric acid, an inhibitory neurotransmitter. Depresses the CNS at the limbic and subcortical levels of the brain and suppresses the spread of seizure activity produced by epileptogenic foci in the cortex, thalamus, and limbic structures.

Route	Onset	Peak	Duration
I.M.	Unknown	2 hr	Unknown
I.V.	1-5 min	1-5 min	15-60 min
P.O.	0.5 hr	2 hr	3-8 hr
P.R.	Unknown	1.5 hr	Unknown

ADVERSE REACTIONS

CNS: *drowsiness,* dysarthria, slurred speech, tremor, transient amnesia, fatigue, ataxia, headache, insomnia, paradoxical anxiety, hallucinations, minor changes in EEG patterns.
CV: hypotension, *CV collapse, bradycardia.*
EENT: diplopia, blurred vision, nystagmus.
GI: nausea, constipation, diarrhea with rectal form.
GU: incontinence, urine retention.
Hematologic: *neutropenia.*
Hepatic: jaundice.
Respiratory: *respiratory depression, apnea.*
Skin: rash.
Other: altered libido, physical or psychological dependence, *pain, phlebitis at injection site.*

INTERACTIONS

Drug-drug. *Cimetidine:* Decreased clearance of diazepam and increased risk of adverse effects. Monitor patient carefully.
CNS depressants: Increased CNS depression. Use together cautiously.
Digoxin: May increase digoxin levels and risk of toxicity. Monitor patient closely.
Phenobarbital: Increased effects of both drugs. Use together cautiously.
Drug-herb. *Kava:* May cause increased sedation. Discourage use together.

Drug-lifestyle. *Alcohol use:* Increased CNS depression. Discourage use together. *Smoking:* Decreased effectiveness of benzodiazepines. Monitor patient closely.

EFFECTS ON LAB TEST RESULTS

• May increase liver function test values. May decrease neutrophil count.

CONTRAINDICATIONS

Contraindicated in patients hypersensitive to drug or soy protein; in patients experiencing shock, coma, or acute alcohol intoxication (parenteral form); and in children younger than age 6 months (oral form). Diastat rectal gel is contraindicated in patients with acute angle-closure glaucoma.

NURSING CONSIDERATIONS

• Use cautiously in patients with liver or renal impairment, depression, or chronic open-angle glaucoma.
• Use cautiously in elderly and debilitated patients.
• Drug should be avoided during pregnancy, especially during first trimester.
• Use Diastat rectal gel to treat no more than five episodes per month and no more than one episode every 5 days because tolerance may develop.
• Don't mix injectable diazepam with other drugs, and don't store parenteral solution in plastic syringes.
• When using oral concentrate solution, dilute dose just before administering.
• Parenteral emulsion—a stabilized oil-in-water emulsion—should appear milky white and uniform. Avoid mixing with any other drugs or solutions, and avoid infusion sets or containers made from polyvinyl chloride. If dilution is needed, drug may be mixed with I.V. fat emulsion. Use admixture within 6 hours.
• *Alert:* Diastat rectal gel should be given only by caregivers who can distinguish the distinct cluster of seizures or events from the patient's ordinary seizure activity, who have been instructed and can give the treatment competently, who understand which seizures may or may not be treated with Diastat, and who can monitor the clinical response and recognize when immediate professional medical evaluation is needed.

Reactions may be *common,* uncommon, *life-threatening,* or COMMON AND LIFE-THREATENING.

• Monitor periodic hepatic, renal, and hematopoietic function studies in patients receiving repeated or prolonged therapy.
• Possibility of abuse and addiction exists. Don't withdraw drug abruptly after long-term use; withdrawal symptoms may occur.
• *Alert:* Don't confuse diazepam with diazoxide.

PATIENT TEACHING
• Warn patient to avoid activities that require alertness and good psychomotor coordination until CNS effects of drug are known.
• Tell patient to avoid alcohol while taking drug.
• Notify patient that smoking may decrease drug's effectiveness.
• Warn patient not to abruptly stop drug because withdrawal symptoms may occur.
• Caution woman to avoid use during pregnancy.
• Instruct patient's caregiver on the proper administration of Diastat rectal gel.

hydroxyzine embonate‡
Atarax

hydroxyzine hydrochloride
Anx, Apo-Hydroxyzine†, Atarax*, Hydroxacen, Hyzine-50, Multipax†, Novo-Hydroxyzin†, QYS, Ucerax§, Vistacon-50, Vistaject-50, Vistaril

hydroxyzine pamoate
Vistaril

Pregnancy risk category NR

AVAILABLE FORMS
hydroxyzine embonate‡
Capsules: 25 mg, 50 mg
hydroxyzine hydrochloride
Capsules: 10 mg†‡, 25 mg†‡, 50 mg†‡
Injection: 25 mg/ml, 50 mg/ml
Syrup: 10 mg/5 ml
Tablets: 10 mg, 25 mg, 50 mg, 100 mg
hydroxyzine pamoate
Capsules: 25 mg, 50 mg, 100 mg
Oral suspension: 25 mg/5 ml

INDICATIONS & DOSAGES
➤ **Anxiety—**
Adults: 50 to 100 mg P.O. q.i.d.
Children age 6 and older: 50 to 100 mg P.O. daily in divided doses.
Children younger than age 6: 50 mg P.O. daily in divided doses.
➤ **Preoperative and postoperative adjunctive therapy—**
Adults: 25 to 100 mg I.M. q 4 to 6 hours.
Children: 1.1 mg/kg I.M. q 4 to 6 hours.
➤ **Pruritus from allergies—**
Adults: 25 mg P.O. t.i.d. or q.i.d.
Children age 6 and older: 50 to 100 mg P.O. daily in divided doses.
Children younger than age 6: 50 mg P.O. daily in divided doses.
➤ **Psychiatric and emotional emergencies, including acute alcoholism—**
Adults: 50 to 100 mg I.M. q 4 to 6 hours, p.r.n.
➤ **Nausea and vomiting (excluding nausea and vomiting of pregnancy)—**
Adults: 25 to 100 mg I.M.
Children: 1.1 mg/kg I.M.
➤ **Antepartum and postpartum adjunctive therapy—**
Adults: 25 to 100 mg I.M.

ACTION
Unknown. A piperazine antihistamine whose action may result from suppression of activity in certain key regions of the subcortical area of the CNS.

Route	Onset	Peak	Duration
I.M.	Unknown	Unknown	4-6 hr
P.O.	15-30 min	2 hr	4-6 hr

ADVERSE REACTIONS
CNS: *drowsiness,* involuntary motor activity.
GI: *dry mouth.*
Other: pain at I.M. injection site, hypersensitivity reactions.

INTERACTIONS
Drug-drug. *Anticholinergics:* Additive anticholinergic effects. Use together cautiously.
CNS depressants: Increased CNS depression. Use together cautiously; dosage adjustments may be needed.

Epinephrine: Inhibited and reversed vasopressor effects of epinephrine. Avoid using together.
Drug-lifestyle. *Alcohol use:* Increased CNS depression. Discourage use together.

EFFECTS ON LAB TEST RESULTS
None reported.

CONTRAINDICATIONS
Contraindicated in patients hypersensitive to drug, patients in early pregnancy, and breast-feeding women.

NURSING CONSIDERATIONS
• Parenteral form (hydroxyzine hydrochloride) is for I.M. use only, preferably by Z-track injection. Never give drug I.V. or S.C.
• Aspirate I.M. injection carefully to prevent inadvertent intravascular injection. Inject deeply into a large muscle mass.
• If patient takes other CNS drugs, observe for oversedation.
• Drug falsely elevates urinary 17-hydroxycorticosteroid levels. It also may cause false-negative skin allergen tests by attenuating or inhibiting the cutaneous response to histamine.
• *Alert:* Don't confuse hydroxyzine with hydroxyurea or hydralazine.

PATIENT TEACHING
• Warn patient to avoid hazardous activities that require alertness and good psychomotor coordination until CNS effects of drug are known.
• Tell patient to avoid alcohol while taking drug.
• Advise patient to use sugarless hard candy or gum to relieve dry mouth.
• Warn woman to avoid use during pregnancy and breast-feeding.

---

lorazepam
Apo-Lorazepam†, Ativan, Lorazepam Intensol, Novo-Lorazem†, Nu-Loraz† ◊

Pregnancy risk category D
Controlled substance schedule IV

AVAILABLE FORMS
Injection: 2 mg/ml, 4 mg/ml
Oral solution (concentrated): 2 mg/ml
Tablets: 0.5 mg, 1 mg, 2 mg
Tablets (S.L.): 0.5 mg†, 1 mg†, 2 mg

INDICATIONS & DOSAGES
➤ **Anxiety—**
Adults: 2 to 6 mg P.O. daily in divided doses. Maximum, 10 mg daily.
Elderly patients: 1 to 2 mg P.O. daily in divided doses. Maximum, 10 mg daily.
➤ **Insomnia from anxiety—**
Adults: 2 to 4 mg P.O. h.s.
➤ **Preoperative sedation—**
Adults: 0.05 mg/kg I.M. 2 hours before procedure. Total dose shouldn't exceed 4 mg. Or, 2 mg I.V. total or 0.044 mg/kg I.V., whichever is smaller. Larger doses up to 0.05 mg/kg I.V., to total of 4 mg, may be needed.

I.V. ADMINISTRATION
• Dilute with an equal volume of sterile water for injection, normal saline solution for injection, or D_5W. Give slowly at no more than 2 mg/minute.
• *Alert:* Monitor respirations every 5 to 15 minutes and before each I.V. dose. Keep emergency resuscitation equipment and oxygen available.

ACTION
Unknown. A benzodiazepine that probably potentiates the effects of the inhibitory neurotransmitter gamma-aminobutyric acid and depresses the CNS at the limbic and subcortical levels of the brain.

Route	Onset	Peak	Duration
I.M.	15-30 min	1-1.5 hr	6-8 hr
I.V.	5 min	1-1.5 hr	6-8 hr
P.O.	1 hr	2 hr	12-24 hr

ADVERSE REACTIONS
CNS: *drowsiness,* amnesia, insomnia, agitation, *sedation,* dizziness, weakness, unsteadiness, disorientation, depression, headache.
CV: hypotension.
EENT: visual disturbances.
GI: abdominal discomfort, nausea, change in appetite.

INTERACTIONS
Drug-drug. *CNS depressants:* Increased CNS depression. Use together cautiously.

Reactions may be *common,* uncommon, *life-threatening*, or COMMON AND LIFE-THREATENING.

Digoxin: May increase digoxin levels and risk of toxicity. Monitor patient closely.
Drug-herb. *Kava:* May cause increased sedation. Discourage use together.
Drug-lifestyle. *Alcohol use:* Increased CNS depression. Discourage use together.
Smoking: Decreased benzodiazepine effectiveness. Monitor patient closely.

EFFECTS ON LAB TEST RESULTS
● May increase liver function test values.

CONTRAINDICATIONS
Contraindicated in patients hypersensitive to drug, other benzodiazepines, or the vehicle used in parenteral dosage form. Also contraindicated in those with acute angle-closure glaucoma.

NURSING CONSIDERATIONS
● Drug should be avoided during pregnancy, especially during first trimester.
● Use cautiously in patients with pulmonary, renal, or hepatic impairment. Also, use cautiously in elderly, acutely ill, or debilitated patients.
● For I.M. administration, inject deeply into a muscle mass. Don't dilute.
● Refrigerate parenteral form to prolong shelf life.
● Monitor hepatic, renal, and hematopoietic function periodically in patients receiving repeated or prolonged therapy.
● *Alert:* Possibility of abuse and addiction exists. Don't withdraw drug abruptly after long-term use because withdrawal symptoms may occur.
● *Alert:* Don't confuse lorazepam with alprazolam.

PATIENT TEACHING
● As a premedication for surgery, lorazepam provides substantial preoperative amnesia. Patient teaching requires extra care to ensure adequate recall. Provide written materials or inform a family member, if possible.
● Warn patient to avoid hazardous activities that require alertness or good psychomotor coordination until CNS effects of drug are known.
● Tell patient to avoid alcohol while taking drug.
● Notify patient that smoking may decrease drug's effectiveness.

● Warn patient not to abruptly stop drug because withdrawal symptoms may occur.
● Caution woman to avoid drug during pregnancy.

meprobamate
Apo-Meprobamate†, Equanil**, Miltown-200, Miltown-400, Miltown-600, Neuramate, Probate, Trancot

Pregnancy risk category D
Controlled substance schedule IV

AVAILABLE FORMS
Tablets: 200 mg, 400 mg, 600 mg

INDICATIONS & DOSAGES
➤ **Anxiety—**
Adults: 1.2 to 1.6 g P.O. daily in three or four equally divided doses. Maximum, 2.4 g daily.
Children ages 6 to 12: 200 to 600 mg P.O. in two or three divided doses.

ACTION
Unknown. Appears to act at multiple sites in the CNS.

Route	Onset	Peak	Duration
P.O.	Unknown	Unknown	Unknown

ADVERSE REACTIONS
CNS: *drowsiness, ataxia,* dizziness, slurred speech, headache, vertigo, *seizures,* syncope.
CV: palpitations, tachycardia, hypotension, *arrhythmias.*
GI: nausea, vomiting, diarrhea, anorexia.
Hematologic: *aplastic anemia, thrombocytopenia, agranulocytosis.*
Skin: pruritus, urticaria, erythematous maculopapular rash.
Other: hypersensitivity reactions.

INTERACTIONS
Drug-drug. *CNS depressants:* Increased CNS depression. Use together cautiously.
Drug-lifestyle. *Alcohol use:* Increased CNS depression. Discourage use together.

EFFECTS ON LAB TEST RESULTS
● May decrease hemoglobin and platelet and granulocyte counts.

CONTRAINDICATIONS
Contraindicated in patients hypersensitive to drug or related compounds (such as carisoprodol, mebutamate, tybamate, and carbromal); also contraindicated in those with porphyria.

NURSING CONSIDERATIONS
• Use cautiously in patients with hepatic or renal impairment, seizure disorders, or suicidal tendencies.
• Drug should be avoided during pregnancy, especially during first trimester.
• Miltown-600 isn't recommended for children.
• Give drug with meals to reduce GI distress.
• Possibility of abuse and addiction exists with long-term use. Withdraw drug gradually over 2 weeks to avoid withdrawal symptoms.
• *Alert:* After abrupt withdrawal of long-term therapy, severe generalized tonic-clonic seizures may occur.
• Periodically monitor CBC and renal and liver function tests in patients receiving high doses.
• Drug may falsely elevate urinary 17-ketosteroids, 17-ketogenic steroids (Zimmerman reaction), and 17-hydroxy-corticosteroid levels (Glenn-Nelson technique).
• *Alert:* Don't confuse Miltown with Milontin.

PATIENT TEACHING
• Advise patient to take drug with meals and not to crush or chew sustained-release capsules but to swallow them whole.
• Warn patient to avoid hazardous activities that require alertness and good psychomotor coordination until CNS effects of drug are known.
• Tell patient to avoid alcohol while taking drug.
• Advise patient to report unusual bruising, bleeding, fever, or sore throat, which may indicate serious hematologic toxicity.
• Warn patient not to abruptly stop drug because withdrawal symptoms may occur.
• Caution woman to avoid use during pregnancy.

midazolam hydrochloride
Hypnovel‡, Versed, Versed Syrup

Pregnancy risk category D
Controlled substance schedule IV

AVAILABLE FORMS
Injection: 1 mg/ml, 5 mg/ml
Syrup: 2 mg/ml

INDICATIONS & DOSAGES
➤ **Preoperative sedation (to induce sleepiness or drowsiness and relieve apprehension)—**
Adults: 0.07 to 0.08 mg/kg I.M. about 1 hour before surgery.
➤ **Conscious sedation before short diagnostic or endoscopic procedures—**
Adults younger than age 60: Initially, small dose not to exceed 2.5 mg I.V. administered slowly; repeated in 2 minutes, if needed, in small increments of initial dose over at least 2 minutes to achieve desired effect. Total dose of up to 5 mg may be used. Additional doses to maintain desired level of sedation may be given by slow titration in increments of 25% of dose used to first reach the sedative end point.
Elderly patients: 1.5 mg or less I.V. over at least 2 minutes. If additional titration is needed, give at rate not exceeding 1 mg over 2 minutes. Total doses exceeding 3.5 mg aren't usually needed.
➤ **To induce sleepiness and amnesia and to relieve apprehension before anesthesia or before or during procedures in pediatric patients—**
I.M.
Children: 0.1 to 0.15 mg/kg I.M. Doses up to 0.5 mg/kg can be used for more anxious patients.
I.V.
Children ages 12 to 16: Initially, small dose not to exceed 2.5 mg I.V. administered slowly; repeated in 2 minutes, if needed, in small increments of initial dose over at least 2 minutes to achieve desired effect. Total dose of up to 10 mg may be used. Additional doses to maintain desired level of sedation may be given by slow titration in increments of 25% of dose used to first reach the sedative end point.

Reactions may be *common*, uncommon, *life-threatening*, or COMMON AND LIFE-THREATENING.

Children ages 6 to 12: 0.025 to 0.05 mg/kg I.V. over 2 to 3 minutes. Additional doses may be given in small increments after 2 to 3 minutes. Total dose of up to 0.4 mg/kg, not to exceed 10 mg, may be used.

Children ages 6 months to 5 years: 0.05 to 0.1 mg/kg I.V. over 2 to 3 minutes. Additional doses may be given in small increments after 2 to 3 minutes. Total dose of up to 0.6 mg/kg, not to exceed 6 mg, may be used.

P.O.

Children ages 6 to 16 and cooperative patients: 0.25 to 0.5 mg/kg P.O. as a single dose, up to 20 mg.

Infants and children ages 6 months to 5 years and less cooperative patients: 0.25 to 1 mg/kg P.O. as a single dose, up to 20 mg.

Adjust-a-dose: For obese children, base dose on ideal body weight; high-risk or debilitated children and children receiving other sedatives need lower doses.

➤ **Induction of general anesthesia—**
Adults older than age 55: 0.3 mg/kg I.V. over 20 to 30 seconds if patient hasn't received premedication, or 0.2 mg/kg I.V. over 20 to 30 seconds if patient has received sedative or narcotic premedication. Additional increments of 25% of initial dose may be needed to complete induction.

Adults younger than age 55: 0.3 to 0.35 mg/kg I.V. over 20 to 30 seconds if patient hasn't received premedication, or 0.25 mg/kg I.V. over 20 to 30 seconds if patient has received sedative or narcotic premedication. Additional increments of 25% of initial dose may be needed to complete induction.

Adjust-a-dose: For debilitated patients, initially, 0.2 to 0.25 mg/kg. As little as 0.15 mg/kg may be needed.

➤ **Continuous infusion for sedation of intubated patients in the critical care setting—**
Adults: Initially, 0.01 to 0.05 mg/kg may be given I.V. over several minutes, repeated at 10- to 15-minute intervals until adequate sedation is achieved. For maintenance of sedation, usual initial infusion rate is 0.02 to 0.10 mg/kg/hour. Higher loading dose or infusion rates may be needed in some patients. Use the lowest effective rate.

Children: Initially, 0.05 to 0.2 mg/kg may be given I.V. over 2 to 3 minutes or longer; then continuous infusion at rate of 0.06 to 0.12 mg/kg/hour. Increase or decrease infusion to maintain desired effect.

Neonates more than 32 weeks' gestational age: Initially, 0.06 mg/kg/hour. Adjust rate, p.r.n., using lowest possible rate.

Neonates less than 32 weeks' gestational age: Initially, 0.03 mg/kg/hour. Adjust rate, p.r.n., using lowest possible rate.

I.V. ADMINISTRATION
● When mixing infusion, use 5-mg/ml vial, dilute to 0.5 mg/ml with D_5W or normal saline solution.
● Administer slowly over at least 2 minutes and wait at least 2 minutes when titrating doses to effect.

ACTION
Unknown. May depress CNS at the limbic and subcortical levels of the brain by potentiating the effects of gamma-aminobutyric acid.

Route	Onset	Peak	Duration
I.M.	15 min	15-60 min	2-6 hr
I.V.	1.5-5 min	Rapid	2-6 hr
P.O.	10-20 min	45-60 min	2-6 hr

ADVERSE REACTIONS
CNS: headache, *oversedation, drowsiness,* amnesia, involuntary movements, nystagmus, paradoxical behavior or excitement.
CV: variations in blood pressure and pulse rate.
GI: *nausea,* vomiting.
Respiratory: *decreased respiratory rate,* APNEA, *hiccups.*
Other: *pain at injection site.*

INTERACTIONS
Drug-drug. *CNS depressants:* May cause apnea. Use together cautiously. Prepare to adjust dosage of midazolam if used with opiates or other CNS depressants.
Diltiazem, verapamil: Increased midazolam levels. Monitor patient closely.
Erythromycin: May alter metabolism of midazolam. Use together cautiously.
Oral contraceptives: Prolonged half-life of midazolam. Use together cautiously.

---

*Liquid contains alcohol.   **May contain tartrazine.   †Canada   ‡Australia   §U.K.   ◇OTC

Rifampin: Decreased midazolam levels. Monitor for effectiveness of midazolam.
Theophylline: Sedative effects of midazolam may be antagonized by theophylline. Use together cautiously.
Drug-food. *Grapefruit juice:* Increased bioavailability of P.O. midazolam. Discourage use together.
Drug-lifestyle. *Alcohol use:* May increase risk of apnea. Discourage use together.

EFFECTS ON LAB TEST RESULTS
None reported.

CONTRAINDICATIONS
Contraindicated in patients hypersensitive to drug and in those with acute angle-closure glaucoma, shock, coma, or acute alcohol intoxication.

NURSING CONSIDERATIONS
• Use cautiously in patients with uncompensated acute illness and in elderly or debilitated patients.
• *Alert:* Before administering, have oxygen and resuscitation equipment available in case of severe respiratory depression. Excessive amounts and rapid infusion have been linked to respiratory arrest. Continuously monitor patients who have received midazolam, including children who have received midazolam syrup, to detect potentially life-threatening respiratory depression.
• May be mixed in the same syringe with morphine sulfate, meperidine, atropine, or scopolamine.
• When injecting I.M., give deeply into a large muscle mass.
• Monitor blood pressure, heart rate and rhythm, respirations, airway integrity, and arterial oxygen saturation during procedure.
• *Alert:* Don't confuse Versed with VePesid.

PATIENT TEACHING
• Because drug's beneficial amnesic effect diminishes patient's recall of perioperative events, provide written information, family member instruction, and follow-up contact to make sure patient has adequate information.
• Warn patient to avoid hazardous activities that require alertness or good psychomotor coordination until CNS effects of drug are known.
• Tell patient to avoid alcohol while taking drug.
• Tell patient not to take P.O. form with grapefruit juice.

---

oxazepam
Alepam‡, Apo-Oxazepam†, Murelax‡, Novoxapam†, Serax**, Serepax‡

Pregnancy risk category D
Controlled substance schedule IV

AVAILABLE FORMS
Capsules, tablets: 10 mg, 15 mg, 30 mg

INDICATIONS & DOSAGES
➤ **Alcohol withdrawal, severe anxiety—**
Adults: 15 to 30 mg P.O. t.i.d. or q.i.d.
➤ **Mild to moderate anxiety—**
Adults: 10 to 15 mg P.O. t.i.d. or q.i.d.
Elderly patients: Initially, 10 mg t.i.d.; increased to 15 mg t.i.d. to q.i.d.

ACTION
Unknown. May stimulate gamma-aminobutyric acid receptors in the ascending reticular activating system.

Route	Onset	Peak	Duration
P.O.	Unknown	3 hr	Unknown

ADVERSE REACTIONS
CNS: *drowsiness, lethargy,* dizziness, vertigo, headache, syncope, tremor, slurred speech, changes in EEG patterns.
CV: edema.
GI: nausea.
Hepatic: *hepatic dysfunction.*
Skin: rash.
Other: altered libido.

INTERACTIONS
Drug-drug. *CNS depressants:* Increased CNS depression. Use together cautiously.
Digoxin: May increase digoxin levels and risk of toxicity. Monitor patient closely.
Drug-herb. *Kava:* May increase sedation. Discourage use together.
Drug-lifestyle. *Alcohol use:* Increased CNS depression. Discourage use together.

Smoking: Decreased effectiveness of benzodiazepines. Monitor patient closely.

EFFECTS ON LAB TEST RESULTS
None reported.

CONTRAINDICATIONS
Contraindicated in patients hypersensitive to drug and in those with psychoses.

NURSING CONSIDERATIONS
• Use cautiously in elderly patients and in those with history of drug abuse or in whom a decrease in blood pressure might lead to cardiac problems.
• Drug should be avoided during pregnancy, especially during first trimester.
• Monitor hepatic, renal, and hematopoietic function periodically in patients receiving repeated or prolonged therapy.
• *Alert:* Possibility of abuse and addiction exists. Don't stop drug abruptly because withdrawal symptoms may occur.
• *Alert:* Don't confuse oxazepam with oxaprozin.

PATIENT TEACHING
• Warn patient to avoid hazardous activities that require alertness or good psychomotor coordination until CNS effects of drug are known.
• Tell patient to avoid alcohol while taking drug.
• Notify patient that smoking may decrease drug's effectiveness.
• Warn patient not to stop drug abruptly because withdrawal symptoms may occur.
• Caution woman to avoid use during pregnancy.

---

chlorpromazine hydrochloride
clozapine
fluphenazine decanoate
fluphenazine enanthate
fluphenazine hydrochloride
haloperidol
haloperidol decanoate
haloperidol lactate
loxapine hydrochloride
loxapine succinate
mesoridazine besylate
olanzapine
perphenazine
pimozide
prochlorperazine
   (See Chapter 49, ANTIEMETICS.)
quetiapine fumarate
risperidone
thioridazine hydrochloride
thiothixene
thiothixene hydrochloride
trifluoperazine hydrochloride
ziprasidone

COMBINATION PRODUCTS

ETRAFON: perphenazine 2 mg and amitriptyline hydrochloride 25 mg.
ETRAFON 2-10: perphenazine 2 mg and amitriptyline hydrochloride 10 mg.
ETRAFON-A: perphenazine 4 mg and amitriptyline hydrochloride 10 mg.
ETRAFON-FORTE: perphenazine 4 mg and amitriptyline hydrochloride 25 mg.
TRIAVIL 2-10, TRIAVIL 4-10, TRIAVIL 2-25, TRIAVIL 4-25 are identical to Etrafon products above. Triavil also is available as TRIAVIL 4-50 (perphenazine 4 mg and amitriptyline hydrochloride 50 mg).

---

chlorpromazine hydrochloride
Chlorpromanyl-20†,
Chlorpromanyl-40†, Largactil†‡,
Novo-Chlorpromazine†, Thorazine

Pregnancy risk category C

AVAILABLE FORMS

Capsules (extended-release): 30 mg, 75 mg, 150 mg
Injection: 25 mg/ml
Oral concentrate: 30 mg/ml, 100 mg/ml
Suppositories: 25 mg, 100 mg
Syrup: 10 mg/5 ml
Tablets: 10 mg, 25 mg, 50 mg, 100 mg, 200 mg

INDICATIONS & DOSAGES

➤ **Psychosis, mania—**
Adults: For hospitalized patients with acute disease, 25 mg I.M.; may give an additional 25 to 50 mg I.M. in 1 hour if needed. Increase over several days to 400 mg q 4 to 6 hours. Switch to oral therapy as soon as possible. Or, 25 mg P.O. t.i.d. initially; then gradually increase to 400 mg daily in divided doses. For outpatients, 30 to 75 mg daily in two to four divided doses. Increase dosage by 20 to 50 mg twice weekly until symptoms are controlled.
Children age 6 months and older: 0.55 mg/kg P.O. q 4 to 6 hours or I.M. q 6 to 8 hours. Or, 1.1 mg/kg P.R. q 6 to 8 hours. Maximum I.M. dose in children younger than age 5 or weighing less than 22.7 kg (50 lb) is 40 mg. Maximum I.M. dose in children ages 5 to 12 or weighing 22.7 to 45.4 kg (50 to 100 lb) is 75 mg.
➤ **Nausea and vomiting—**
Adults: 10 to 25 mg P.O. q 4 to 6 hours, p.r.n. Or, 50 to 100 mg P.R. q 6 to 8 hours, p.r.n. Or, 25 mg I.M. initially. If no hypotension occurs, 25 to 50 mg I.M. q 3 to 4 hours may be given, p.r.n., until vomiting stops.
Children age 6 months and older: 0.55 mg/kg P.O. q 4 to 6 hours or I.M. q 6 to 8 hours. Or, 1.1 mg/kg P.R. q 6 to 8 hours. Maximum I.M. dose in children younger than age 5 or weighing less than 22.7 kg (50 lb) is 40 mg. Maximum I.M. dose in children ages 5 to 12 or weighing 22.7 to 45.4 kg (50 to 100 lb) is 75 mg.
➤ **Acute intermittent porphyria, intractable hiccups—**
Adults: 25 to 50 mg P.O. t.i.d. or q.i.d. If symptoms persist for 2 to 3 days, 25 to 50 mg I.M. For hiccups, if symptoms still persist, 25 to 50 mg diluted in 500 to

---

Reactions may be *common*, uncommon, **life-threatening**, or COMMON AND LIFE-THREATENING.

1,000 ml of normal saline solution and infused slowly with patient in supine position.

➤ **Tetanus—**
Adults: 25 to 50 mg I.V. or I.M. t.i.d. or q.i.d.
Children age 6 months and older: 0.55 mg/kg I.M. or I.V. q 6 to 8 hours. Maximum parenteral dosage in children weighing less than 22.7 kg (50 lb) is 40 mg daily; for children weighing 22.7 to 45.4 kg (50 to 100 lb), 75 mg, except in severe cases.

➤ **Surgery—**
Adults: Preoperatively, 25 to 50 mg P.O. 2 to 3 hours before surgery or 12.5 to 25 mg I.M. 1 to 2 hours before surgery; during surgery, 12.5 mg I.M., repeated in 30 minutes, if needed, or fractional 2-mg doses I.V. at 2-minute intervals to maximum dose of 25 mg; postoperatively, 10 to 25 mg P.O. q 4 to 6 hours or 12.5 to 25 mg I.M., repeated in 1 hour, if needed.
Children age 6 months and older: Preoperatively, 0.55 mg/kg P.O. 2 to 3 hours before surgery or I.M. 1 to 2 hours before surgery. During surgery, 0.275 mg/kg I.M., repeated in 30 minutes if needed, or fractional doses I.V. at 2-minute intervals to maximum of 0.275 mg/kg. May repeat fractional I.V. regimen in 30 minutes if needed. Postoperatively, 0.55 mg/kg P.O. or I.M. q 4 to 6 hours (oral dose) or 1 hour (I.M. dose), if needed and if hypotension doesn't occur.
Elderly patients: Lower dosages are sufficient; dosage increments should be more gradual than in adults.

I.V. ADMINISTRATION
● Chlorpromazine is compatible with most common I.V. solutions, including D₅W, Ringer's injection, lactated Ringer's injection, and normal saline solution for injection.
● For direct injection, drug may be diluted with normal saline solution for injection and administered into a large vein or through the tubing of a free-flowing I.V. solution. Don't exceed 1 mg/minute for adults or 0.5 mg/minute for children.
● For intermittent I.V. infusion, dilute with 50 or 100 ml of a compatible solution and infuse over 30 minutes.

ACTION
Unknown. A piperidine phenothiazine that probably blocks postsynaptic dopamine receptors in the brain.

Route	Onset	Peak	Duration
I.M., I.V.	Unknown	Unknown	Unknown
P.O.	0.5-1 hr	Unknown	4-6 hr
P.O. (extended)	0.5-1 hr	Unknown	10-12 hr
P.R.	> 1 hr	Unknown	3-4 hr

ADVERSE REACTIONS
CNS: *extrapyramidal reactions,* drowsiness, *sedation,* **seizures,** *tardive dyskinesia, pseudoparkinsonism,* dizziness, **neuroleptic malignant syndrome.**
CV: *orthostatic hypotension,* tachycardia, quinidine-like ECG effects.
EENT: ocular changes, blurred vision, nasal congestion.
GI: *dry mouth, constipation,* nausea.
GU: *urine retention,* menstrual irregularities, inhibited ejaculation, priapism.
Hematologic: **leukopenia, agranulocytosis,** eosinophilia, hemolytic anemia, **aplastic anemia, thrombocytopenia.**
Hepatic: jaundice.
Skin: *mild photosensitivity reactions,* allergic reactions, *pain at I.M. injection site,* sterile abscess, skin pigmentation.
Other: gynecomastia, lactation.

INTERACTIONS
Drug-drug. *Antacids:* Inhibited absorption of oral phenothiazines. Separate antacid and phenothiazine doses by at least 2 hours.
Anticholinergics such as antidepressants, antiparkinsonians: Increased anticholinergic activity, aggravated parkinsonian symptoms. Use together cautiously.
Anticonvulsants: May lower seizure threshold. Monitor patient closely.
Barbiturates, lithium: May decrease phenothiazine effect. Monitor patient.
Centrally acting antihypertensives: Decreased antihypertensive effect. Monitor blood pressure.
CNS depressants: Increased CNS depression. Use together cautiously.
Electroconvulsive therapy, insulin: May precipitate severe reactions. Monitor patient closely.

Lithium: Possible increase in neurologic effects. Monitor patient closely.

Propranolol: Increased levels of both propranolol and chlorpromazine. Monitor patient closely.

Warfarin: Decreased effect of oral anticoagulants. Monitor PT and INR.

Drug-herb. *Kava:* May cause dystonic reactions. Discourage use together.

St. John's wort: May cause photosensitivity reactions. Advise patient to avoid excessive sunlight exposure.

Yohimbe: May cause yohimbe toxicity. Discourage use together.

Drug-lifestyle. *Alcohol use:* Increased CNS depression. Discourage use together.

Sun exposure: Increased risk of photosensitivity reactions. Advise patient to avoid excessive sunlight exposure.

EFFECTS ON LAB TEST RESULTS
• May increase liver function test values and eosinophil count. May decrease hemoglobin and WBC, granulocyte, and platelet counts.

CONTRAINDICATIONS
Contraindicated in patients hypersensitive to drug and in those with CNS depression, bone marrow suppression, subcortical damage, or coma.

NURSING CONSIDERATIONS
• Use cautiously in elderly or debilitated patients and in patients with hepatic or renal disease, severe CV disease (may cause sudden decrease in blood pressure), respiratory disorders, hypocalcemia, glaucoma, or prostatic hyperplasia. Also use cautiously in those exposed to extreme heat or cold (including antipyretic therapy) or organophosphate insecticides.

• Use cautiously in acutely ill or dehydrated children.

• Obtain baseline blood pressure measurements before starting therapy, and monitor them regularly. Watch for orthostatic hypotension, especially with parenteral administration. Monitor blood pressure before and after I.M. administration; keep patient supine for 1 hour afterward and have him get up slowly.

• Wear gloves when preparing solutions and avoid contact with skin and clothing.

Oral liquid and parenteral forms can cause contact dermatitis.

• Slight yellowing of injection or concentrate is common and doesn't affect potency. Discard markedly discolored solutions.

• Protect liquid concentrate from light. Dilute with fruit juice, milk, or semisolid food just before administration.

• Give deep I.M. only in upper outer quadrant of buttocks. Consider giving injection by Z-track method. Massage slowly afterward to prevent sterile abscess. Injection stings. Rotate injection sites.

• Monitor patient for tardive dyskinesia, which may occur after prolonged use. It may not appear until months or years later and may disappear spontaneously or persist for life, despite stopping drug.

• After abrupt withdrawal of long-term therapy, gastritis, nausea, vomiting, dizziness, or tremor may occur.

• *Alert:* Watch for evidence of neuroleptic malignant syndrome (extrapyramidal effects, hyperthermia, autonomic disturbance), which is rare but usually fatal. It may not be related to length of drug use or type of neuroleptic; however, more than 60% of affected patients are men.

• Monitor therapy with weekly bilirubin tests during first month, periodic blood tests (CBCs and liver function tests), and ophthalmic tests (long-term use).

• Drug causes false-positive test results for urinary porphyrins, urobilinogen, amylase, and 5-hydroxyindoleacetic acid because of darkening of urine by metabolites; it also causes false-positive results for urine pregnancy tests that use human chorionic gonadotropin.

• Withhold dose and notify prescriber if jaundice, symptoms of blood dyscrasia (fever, sore throat, infection, cellulitis, weakness), or persistent extrapyramidal reactions (longer than a few hours) develop, or if such reactions occur in children or pregnant women.

• Don't withdraw drug abruptly unless necessitated by severe adverse reactions.

• *Alert:* Don't confuse chlorpromazine with chlorpropamide, a hypoglycemic. Make sure that any drug administered is appropriate for patient's treatment.

• *Alert:* Don't confuse chlorpromazine with clomipramine.

PATIENT TEACHING
● Warn patient to avoid activities that require alertness or good psychomotor coordination until CNS effects of drug are known. Drowsiness and dizziness usually subside after first few weeks.
● Tell patient to avoid alcohol while taking drug.
● Have patient report signs of urine retention or constipation.
● Tell patient to use sunblock and to wear protective clothing to avoid photosensitivity reactions. Chlorpromazine is more likely to cause photosensitivity reactions than any other drug in its class.
● Tell patient to relieve dry mouth with sugarless gum or hard candy.
● Advise patient receiving drug parenterally to remain supine for 1 hour afterward and to rise slowly.

---

clozapine
Clozaril

Pregnancy risk category B

AVAILABLE FORMS
Tablets: 25 mg, 100 mg

INDICATIONS & DOSAGES
➤ **Schizophrenia in severely ill patients unresponsive to other therapies—**
Adults: Initially, 12.5 mg P.O. once daily or b.i.d., adjusted upward by 25 to 50 mg daily (if tolerated) to 300 to 450 mg daily by end of 2 weeks. Individual dosage is based on clinical response, patient tolerance, and adverse reactions. Subsequent dosage shouldn't be increased more than once or twice weekly, and shouldn't exceed 50- to 100-mg increments. Many patients respond to dosages of 200 to 600 mg daily, but some may need as much as 900 mg daily. Don't exceed 900 mg daily.

ACTION
Unknown. Binds selectively to dopaminergic receptors (D_1 and D_2) in the limbic system of the CNS and may interfere with adrenergic, cholinergic, histaminergic, and serotonergic receptors.

Route	Onset	Peak	Duration
P.O.	Unknown	2.5 hr	4-12 hr

ADVERSE REACTIONS
CNS: *drowsiness, sedation, **seizures**, dizziness,* syncope, *vertigo, headache,* tremor, disturbed sleep or nightmares, restlessness, hypokinesia or akinesia, agitation, rigidity, akathisia, confusion, fatigue, insomnia, hyperkinesia, weakness, lethargy, ataxia, slurred speech, depression, myoclonus, anxiety.
CV: *tachycardia,* hypotension, hypertension, chest pain, ECG changes, orthostatic hypotension.
EENT: visual disturbances.
GI: dry mouth, *constipation,* nausea, vomiting, *excessive salivation,* heartburn, diarrhea.
GU: urinary frequency or urgency, urine retention, incontinence, abnormal ejaculation.
Hematologic: *leukopenia, agranulocytosis, granulocytopenia.*
Metabolic: weight gain.
Musculoskeletal: muscle pain or spasm, muscle weakness.
Skin: rash, diaphoresis.
Other: fever.

INTERACTIONS
Drug-drug. *Anticholinergics:* May potentiate anticholinergic effects of clozapine. Use together cautiously.
Antihypertensives: May potentiate hypotensive effects. Monitor blood pressure.
Bone marrow suppressants: May increase bone marrow toxicity. Don't use together.
Digoxin, other highly protein-bound drugs, warfarin: May increase serum levels of these drugs. Monitor patient closely for adverse reactions.
Phenytoin: Decreased clozapine levels and breakthrough psychosis. Monitor patient for psychosis and adjust clozapine dosage as directed.
Psychoactive drugs: May produce additive effects. Use together cautiously.
Drug-herb. *Nutmeg:* May reduce effectiveness of drug therapy. Discourage use together.
St. John's wort: May decrease clozapine levels. Discourage use together.
Drug-food. *Caffeine-containing beverages:* May inhibit antipsychotic effects of clozapine. Monitor patient closely.
Drug-lifestyle. *Alcohol use:* Increased CNS depression. Discourage use together.

Smoking: May decrease clozapine levels. Monitor patient for effectiveness, and adjust dosage as directed.

EFFECTS ON LAB TEST RESULTS
● May decrease WBC and granulocyte counts.

CONTRAINDICATIONS
Contraindicated in patients with uncontrolled epilepsy, history of clozapine-induced agranulocytosis, WBC count below 3,500/mm³, severe CNS depression or coma, and myelosuppressive disorders. Also contraindicated in patients taking other drugs that suppress bone marrow function.

NURSING CONSIDERATIONS
● Use cautiously in patients with prostatic hyperplasia or angle-closure glaucoma because drug has potent anticholinergic effects.
● Use cautiously in patients with hepatic, renal, or cardiac disease and in those receiving general anesthesia.
● *Alert:* Clozapine carries significant risk of agranulocytosis. If possible, patient should receive at least two trials of drug therapy with a standard antipsychotic before clozapine therapy begins. Baseline WBC and differential counts are needed before therapy. Monitor WBC counts weekly for at least 4 weeks after clozapine therapy ends.
● When administering clozapine, ensure that WBC counts and blood tests are performed weekly and that no more than a 1-week supply of drug is dispensed at a time for first 6 months of therapy. If WBC count stays at 3,000/mm³ or more and absolute neutrophil count stays at 1,500/mm³ or more during first 6 months of continuous therapy, frequency of monitoring blood counts may be reduced to every other week.
● If WBC count drops below 3,500/mm³ after therapy begins or if it drops substantially from baseline, monitor patient closely for signs and symptoms of infection. If WBC count is 3,000 to 3,500/mm³ and granulocyte count is above 1,500/mm³, perform WBC and differential count twice weekly. If WBC count drops below 3,000/mm³ and granulocyte count drops

below 1,500/mm³, interrupt therapy, notify prescriber, and monitor patient for signs and symptoms of infection. Therapy may be restarted cautiously if WBC count returns to above 3,000/mm³ and granulocyte count returns to above 1,500/mm³. Continue monitoring WBC and differential counts twice weekly until WBC count exceeds 3,500/mm³.
● If WBC count drops below 2,000/mm³ and granulocyte count drops below 1,000/mm³, patient may need protective isolation. If infection develops, prepare cultures according to institutional policy and give antibiotics. Bone marrow aspiration may be needed to assess bone marrow function. Future clozapine therapy is contraindicated in such situations.
● Seizures may occur, especially in patients receiving high doses.
● Some patients experience transient fever with temperature above 100.4° F (38° C), especially in the first 3 weeks of therapy. Monitor these patients closely.
● After abrupt withdrawal of long-term therapy, abrupt recurrence of psychotic symptoms is possible.
● If clozapine therapy must be discontinued, withdraw drug gradually over 1 to 2 weeks. If changes in patient's medical condition (including development of leukopenia) necessitate abrupt discontinuation of drug, monitor patient closely for recurrence of psychotic symptoms.
● If therapy is reinstated in patient withdrawn from drug, follow usual guidelines for dosage increase. However, reexposure of patient to drug may increase severity and risk of adverse reactions. If therapy was terminated because WBC counts were below 2,000/mm³ or granulocyte counts were below 1,000/mm³, don't expect drug to be continued.
● *Alert:* Don't confuse clozapine with clonidine, clofazimine, or Klonopin.

PATIENT TEACHING
● Tell patient about need for weekly blood tests to check for agranulocytosis. Advise him to report flulike symptoms, fever, sore throat, lethargy, malaise, or other signs of infection.
● Warn patient to avoid hazardous activities that require alertness and good psychomotor coordination while taking drug.

Reactions may be *common*, uncommon, *life-threatening*, or COMMON AND LIFE-THREATENING.

• Tell patient to check with prescriber before taking alcohol or OTC drugs.
• Advise patient that smoking may decrease drug effectiveness.
• Tell patient to rise slowly to avoid orthostatic hypotension.
• Inform patient that ice chips or sugarless candy or gum may help relieve dry mouth.

---

fluphenazine decanoate
Modecate†‡, Modecate Concentrate†, Prolixin Decanoate

fluphenazine enanthate
Moditen Enanthate†, Prolixin Enanthate

fluphenazine hydrochloride
Anatensol‡*, Apo-Fluphenazine†, Moditen HCl†, Permitil*†**, Permitil Concentrate, Prolixin*†**, Prolixin Concentrate

Pregnancy risk category C

AVAILABLE FORMS
fluphenazine decanoate
Depot injection: 25 mg/ml
fluphenazine enanthate
Depot injection: 25 mg/ml
fluphenazine hydrochloride
Elixir: 2.5 mg/5 ml*
I.M. injection: 2.5 mg/ml
Oral concentrate: 5 mg/ml*
Tablets: 1 mg, 2.5 mg, 5 mg, 10 mg

INDICATIONS & DOSAGES
➤ **Psychotic disorders—**
Adults: Initially, 0.5 to 10 mg fluphenazine hydrochloride P.O. daily in divided doses q 6 to 8 hours; may increase cautiously to 20 mg. Higher doses (50 to 100 mg) have been given. Maintenance dose is 1 to 5 mg P.O. daily. I.M. doses are one-third to one-half of oral doses. Usual I.M. dose is 1.25 mg. Give more than 10 mg/day with caution.
Or, 12.5 to 25 mg of long-acting esters (decanoate or enanthate) I.M. or S.C. q 1 to 6 weeks; maintenance dose is 25 to 100 mg, p.r.n.
Elderly patients: Use lower dosages, 1 to 2.5 mg daily.

ACTION
Unknown. A piperazine phenothiazine that probably blocks postsynaptic dopamine in the brain.

Route	Onset	Peak	Duration
I.M.	24-72 hr	Unknown	1-6 wk
I.M. (HCl)	< 1 hr	1.5-2 hr	6-8 hr
P.O.	< 1 hr	0.5 hr	6-8 hr
S.C.	Unknown	Unknown	Unknown

ADVERSE REACTIONS
CNS: *extrapyramidal reactions, tardive dyskinesia,* sedation, *pseudoparkinsonism,* EEG changes, drowsiness, *seizures,* dizziness, *neuroleptic malignant syndrome.*
CV: orthostatic hypotension, tachycardia, ECG changes.
EENT: ocular changes, *blurred vision,* nasal congestion.
GI: *dry mouth, constipation,* increased appetite.
GU: *urine retention,* dark urine, menstrual irregularities, inhibited ejaculation.
Hematologic: *leukopenia, agranulocytosis,* eosinophilia, hemolytic anemia, *aplastic anemia, thrombocytopenia.*
Hepatic: cholestatic jaundice.
Metabolic: weight gain.
Skin: *mild photosensitivity reactions,* allergic reactions.
Other: gynecomastia.

INTERACTIONS
Drug-drug. *Antacids:* Inhibited absorption of oral phenothiazines. Separate antacid and phenothiazine doses by at least 2 hours.
Anticholinergics: Increased anticholinergic effects. Use together cautiously.
Barbiturates, lithium: May decrease phenothiazine effect and increase neurologic adverse effects. Observe patient.
Centrally acting antihypertensives: Decreased antihypertensive effect. Monitor blood pressure.
CNS depressants: Increased CNS depression. Use together cautiously.
Drug-herb. *Kava:* Increased risk of dystonic reactions. Discourage use together.
St. John's wort: Increased risk of photosensitivity reactions. Advise patient to avoid excessive sunlight exposure.
Yohimbe: Increased risk of yohimbe toxicity. Discourage use together.

---

*Liquid contains alcohol.   **May contain tartrazine.   †Canada   ‡Australia   §U.K.   ◇OTC

Drug-lifestyle. *Alcohol use:* Increased CNS depression. Discourage use together. *Sun exposure:* Increased risk of photosensitivity reactions. Advise patient to avoid excessive sunlight exposure.

EFFECTS ON LAB TEST RESULTS
• May increase liver function test values and eosinophil count. May decrease hemoglobin and WBC, granulocyte, and platelet counts.

CONTRAINDICATIONS
Contraindicated in patients hypersensitive to drug and in those with coma, CNS depression, bone marrow suppression or other blood dyscrasia, subcortical damage, or liver damage.

NURSING CONSIDERATIONS
• Use cautiously in elderly or debilitated patients and in those with pheochromocytoma, severe CV disease (may cause sudden drop in blood pressure), peptic ulcer, respiratory disorder, hypocalcemia, seizure disorder (may lower seizure threshold), severe reactions to insulin or electroconvulsive therapy, mitral insufficiency, glaucoma, or prostatic hyperplasia. Also use cautiously in those exposed to extreme heat or cold (including antipyretic therapy) or phosphorus insecticides. Use parenteral form cautiously in asthmatic patients and in those allergic to sulfites.
• Prolixin Concentrate and Permitil Concentrate are 10 times more concentrated than Prolixin elixir (5 mg/ml versus 0.5 mg/ml). Check dosage order carefully.
• Oral liquid and parenteral forms can cause contact dermatitis. Wear gloves when preparing solutions, and avoid contact with skin and clothing.
• Protect drug from light. Slight yellowing of injection or concentrate is common and doesn't affect potency. Discard markedly discolored solutions.
• Dilute liquid concentrate with water, fruit juice, milk, or semisolid food just before administration.
• For long-acting forms (decanoate and enanthate), which are oil preparations, use a dry needle of at least 21G. Allow 24 to 96 hours for onset of action. Note and report adverse reactions in patients taking these drug forms.

• Monitor patient for tardive dyskinesia, which may occur after prolonged use. It may not appear until months or years later and may disappear spontaneously or persist for life, despite ending drug.
• *Alert:* Watch for evidence of neuroleptic malignant syndrome (extrapyramidal effects, hyperthermia, autonomic disturbance), which is rare but commonly fatal. It may not be related to length of drug use or type of neuroleptic; however, more than 60% of affected patients are men.
• Monitor therapy with weekly bilirubin tests during first month, periodic blood tests (CBCs and liver function tests), and periodic renal function and ophthalmic tests (long-term use).
• Drug causes false-positive test results for urinary porphyrins, urobilinogen, amylase, and 5-hydroxyindoleacetic acid because of darkening of urine by metabolites; it also causes false-positive results for urine pregnancy tests that use human chorionic gonadotropin.
• Withhold dose and notify prescriber if symptoms of blood dyscrasia (fever, sore throat, infection, cellulitis, weakness) or persistent extrapyramidal reactions (longer than a few hours) develop, especially in children and pregnant women.
• Don't withdraw drug abruptly unless serious adverse reactions occur.
• After abrupt withdrawal of long-term therapy, gastritis, nausea, vomiting, dizziness, tremor, feeling of warmth or cold, diaphoresis, tachycardia, headache, or insomnia may occur.

PATIENT TEACHING
• Warn patient to avoid activities that require alertness and good psychomotor coordination until CNS effects of drug are known. Drowsiness and dizziness usually subside after first few weeks.
• Warn patient to avoid alcohol while taking drug.
• Tell patient to relieve dry mouth with sugarless gum or hard candy.
• Have patient report signs of urine retention or constipation.
• Advise patient to use sunblock and wear protective clothing to avoid photosensitivity reactions.
• Tell patient that drug may discolor urine.

Reactions may be *common,* uncommon, *life-threatening*, or COMMON AND LIFE-THREATENING.

haloperidol
Apo-Haloperidol†, Dozic§,
Haldol**, Novo-Peridol†, Peridol†,
Serenace§‡

haloperidol decanoate
Haldol Decanoate, Haldol LA†

haloperidol lactate
Haldol, Haldol Concentrate,
Haloperidol Intensol

Pregnancy risk category C

AVAILABLE FORMS
haloperidol
Tablets: 0.5 mg, 1 mg, 2 mg, 5 mg, 10 mg,
20 mg
haloperidol decanoate
Injection: 50 mg/ml, 100 mg/ml
haloperidol lactate
Injection: 5 mg/ml
Oral concentrate: 2 mg/ml

INDICATIONS & DOSAGES
➤ **Psychotic disorders—**
Adults and children age 12 and older:
Dosage varies for each patient. Initial
range, 0.5 to 5 mg P.O. b.i.d. or t.i.d. Or,
2 to 5 mg I.M. q 4 to 8 hours, although
hourly administration may be needed until
control is obtained. Maximum, 100 mg
P.O. daily.
Children ages 3 to 12: 0.05 mg/kg to
0.15 mg/kg P.O. daily. Severely disturbed
children may need higher doses.
➤ **Chronic psychosis requiring
prolonged therapy—**
Adults: 50 to 100 mg I.M. decanoate q 4
weeks.
➤ **Nonpsychotic behavior disorders—**
Children ages 3 to 12: 0.05 mg/kg P.O.
daily. Maximum, 6 mg daily.
➤ **Tourette syndrome—**
Adults: 0.5 to 5 mg P.O. b.i.d., t.i.d., or
p.r.n.
Children ages 3 to 12: 0.05 to 0.075 mg/
kg P.O. daily in two or three divided doses.
Elderly patients: 0.5 to 2 mg P.O. b.i.d. or
t.i.d., increased gradually, p.r.n.
Adjust-a-dose: For debilitated patients,
give 0.5 to 2 mg P.O. b.i.d. or t.i.d., in-
creased gradually, p.r.n.

ACTION
Unknown. A butyrophenone that probably
exerts antipsychotic effects by blocking
postsynaptic dopamine receptors in the
brain.

Route	Onset	Peak	Duration
I.M. (decanoate)	Unknown	3-9 days	Unknown
I.M. (lactate)	Unknown	10-20 min	Unknown
I.V.	Unknown	Unknown	Unknown
P.O.	Unknown	3-6 hr	Unknown

ADVERSE REACTIONS
CNS: *severe extrapyramidal reactions,
tardive dyskinesia,* sedation, drowsiness,
lethargy, headache, insomnia, confusion,
vertigo, *seizures, neuroleptic malignant
syndrome.*
CV: tachycardia, hypotension, hypertension, ECG changes, *torsades de pointes*
with I.V. use.
EENT: blurred vision.
GI: dry mouth, anorexia, constipation, diarrhea, nausea, vomiting, dyspepsia.
GU: urine retention, menstrual irregularities, priapism.
Hematologic: *leukopenia,* leukocytosis.
Hepatic: jaundice.
Skin: rash, other skin reactions, diaphoresis.
Other: gynecomastia.

INTERACTIONS
Drug-drug. *Anticholinergics:* Increased
anticholinergic effects and glaucoma. Use
together cautiously.
CNS depressants: Increased CNS depres-
sion. Use together cautiously.
Lithium: Lethargy and confusion after
high doses. Monitor patient.
Drug-herb. *Nutmeg:* May reduce effec-
tiveness of or interfere with drug therapy.
Discourage use together.
Drug-lifestyle. *Alcohol use:* Increased
CNS depression. Discourage use together.

EFFECTS ON LAB TEST RESULTS
● May increase liver function test values.
May increase or decrease WBC count.

CONTRAINDICATIONS

Contraindicated in patients hypersensitive to drug and in those with parkinsonism, coma, or CNS depression.

NURSING CONSIDERATIONS

• Use cautiously in elderly and debilitated patients; in patients with history of seizures or EEG abnormalities, severe CV disorders, allergies, glaucoma, or urine retention; and in those taking anticonvulsants, anticoagulants, antiparkinsonians, or lithium.

• Protect drug from light. Slight yellowing of injection or concentrate is common and doesn't affect potency. Discard markedly discolored solutions.

• When changing from tablets to decanoate injection, patient should be given 10 to 15 times the oral dose once a month (maximum 100 mg).

• Dilute oral dose with water or a beverage, such as orange juice, apple juice, tomato juice, or cola, immediately before administration.

• *Alert:* Don't administer decanoate form I.V.

• Monitor patient for tardive dyskinesia, which may occur after prolonged use. It may not appear until months or years later and may disappear spontaneously or persist for life, despite ending drug.

• *Alert:* Watch for evidence of neuroleptic malignant syndrome (extrapyramidal effects, hyperthermia, autonomic disturbance), which is rare but commonly fatal. It may not be related to length of drug use or type of neuroleptic; however, more than 60% of affected patients are men.

• Don't withdraw drug abruptly unless required by severe adverse reactions.

• *Alert:* Don't confuse Haldol with Halcion or Halog.

PATIENT TEACHING

• Although drug is the least sedating of the antipsychotics, warn patient to avoid activities that require alertness and good psychomotor coordination until CNS effects of drug are known. Drowsiness and dizziness usually subside after a few weeks.

• Warn patient to avoid alcohol while taking drug.

• Tell patient to relieve dry mouth with sugarless gum or hard candy.

loxapine hydrochloride
Loxapac†, Loxitane C, Loxitane IM

loxapine succinate
Loxapac†, Loxitane

Pregnancy risk category NR

AVAILABLE FORMS
loxapine hydrochloride
Injection: 50 mg/ml
Oral concentrate: 25 mg/ml
loxapine succinate
Capsules: 5 mg, 10 mg, 25 mg, 50 mg
Tablets: 5 mg†, 10 mg†, 25 mg†, 50 mg†

INDICATIONS & DOSAGES
➤ Psychotic disorders—
Adults: 10 mg P.O. b.i.d. to q.i.d., rapidly increasing to 60 to 100 mg P.O. daily for most patients; dosage varies. If patient can't take oral dose, give 12.5 to 50 mg I.M. q 4 to 6 hours or longer; dosage and interval depend on patient response. Dosages exceeding 250 mg/day aren't recommended.
Elderly patients: Initially, 3 to 5 mg P.O. b.i.d. Adjust dosage as needed and tolerated.

ACTION
Unknown. A dibenzoxazepine that probably exerts antipsychotic effects by blocking postsynaptic dopamine receptors in the brain.

Route	Onset	Peak	Duration
I.M., P.O.	30 min	1.5-3 hr	12 hr

ADVERSE REACTIONS
CNS: *extrapyramidal reactions, sedation,* drowsiness, **seizures,** numbness, confusion, syncope, *tardive dyskinesia,* pseudoparkinsonism, EEG changes, dizziness, **neuroleptic malignant syndrome.**
CV: orthostatic hypotension, tachycardia, ECG changes, hypertension.
EENT: *blurred vision,* nasal congestion.
GI: *dry mouth, constipation,* nausea, vomiting, paralytic ileus.

Reactions may be *common,* uncommon, *life-threatening,* or COMMON AND LIFE-THREATENING.

GU: *urine retention,* menstrual irregularities.
Hematologic: *leukopenia, agranulocytosis, thrombocytopenia.*
Hepatic: jaundice.
Metabolic: weight gain.
Skin: allergic reactions, rash, pruritus.
Other: gynecomastia.

INTERACTIONS
Drug-drug. *Anticholinergics:* Increased anticholinergic effects. Use together cautiously.
CNS depressants: Increased CNS depression. Use together cautiously.
Epinephrine: Inhibited vasopressor effects of epinephrine. Avoid using together.
Drug-lifestyle. *Alcohol use:* Increased CNS depression. Discourage use together.

EFFECTS ON LAB TEST RESULTS
• May increase liver function test values. May decrease WBC, granulocyte, and platelet counts.

CONTRAINDICATIONS
Contraindicated in patients hypersensitive to dibenzoxazepines and in those with coma, severe CNS depression, or drug-induced depressed states.

NURSING CONSIDERATIONS
• Use with extreme caution in patients with seizure disorder, CV disorder, glaucoma, or history of urine retention.
• Obtain baseline blood pressure measurements before starting therapy and monitor pressure regularly.
• Dilute liquid concentrate with orange or grapefruit juice just before giving it.
• Monitor patient for tardive dyskinesia, which may occur after prolonged use. It may not appear until months or years later and may disappear spontaneously or persist for life, despite ending drug.
• Loxapine causes false-positive test results for urinary porphyrins, urobilinogen, amylase, and 5-hydroxyindoleacetic acid because of darkening of urine by metabolites; it also causes false-positive results for urine pregnancy tests that use human chorionic gonadotropin.
• *Alert:* Watch for evidence of neuroleptic malignant syndrome (extrapyramidal effects, hyperthermia, autonomic distur-

bance), which is rare but commonly fatal. It may not be related to length of drug use or type of neuroleptic; however, more than 60% of affected patients are men.

PATIENT TEACHING
• Warn patient to avoid activities that require alertness and good psychomotor coordination until CNS effects of drug are known. Drowsiness and dizziness usually subside after first few weeks.
• Advise patient to report bruising, fever, or sore throat immediately.
• Tell patient to avoid alcohol while taking drug.
• Advise patient to get up slowly to avoid orthostatic hypotension.
• Tell patient to relieve dry mouth with sugarless gum or hard candy.
• Recommend periodic eye examinations.

---

mesoridazine besylate
Serentil*, Serentil Concentrate

Pregnancy risk category NR

AVAILABLE FORMS
Injection: 25 mg/ml
Oral concentrate: 25 mg/ml (0.6% alcohol)*
Tablets: 10 mg, 25 mg, 50 mg, 100 mg

INDICATIONS & DOSAGES
➤ **Schizophrenic patients who don't show an acceptable response to adequate treatment with other antipsychotic drugs—**
Adults: Initially, 50 mg P.O. t.i.d. or 25 mg I.M. repeated in 30 to 60 minutes, p.r.n. Maximum, 400 mg P.O. daily or 200 mg I.M. daily.

ACTION
Unknown. A piperidine phenothiazine and the major sulfoxide metabolite of thioridazine that probably exerts antipsychotic effects by blocking postsynaptic dopamine receptors in the brain.

Route	Onset	Peak	Duration
I.M., P.O.	Unknown	Unknown	Unknown

ADVERSE REACTIONS
CNS: *extrapyramidal reactions, tardive dyskinesia, sedation,* drowsiness, tremor, rigidity, weakness, EEG changes, dizziness, **neuroleptic malignant syndrome.**
CV: *hypotension,* tachycardia, **prolonged QTc interval, torsades de pointes,** ECG changes.
EENT: *ocular changes, blurred vision,* retinitis pigmentosa, nasal congestion.
GI: *dry mouth, constipation,* nausea, vomiting.
GU: *urine retention,* menstrual irregularities, inhibited ejaculation.
Hematologic: *leukopenia, agranulocytosis, aplastic anemia,* eosinophilia, **thrombocytopenia.**
Hepatic: jaundice.
Metabolic: weight gain.
Skin: *mild photosensitivity reactions,* allergic reactions, pain at I.M. injection site, sterile abscess, rash.
Other: gynecomastia.

INTERACTIONS
Drug-drug. *Antacids:* Inhibited absorption of oral phenothiazines. Separate antacid and phenothiazine doses by at least 2 hours.
Anticholinergics: May increase anticholinergic effects. Use together cautiously.
Barbiturates: May decrease phenothiazine effect. Observe patient.
CNS depressants: Increased CNS depression. Use together cautiously.
Lithium: Increased neurologic adverse effects. Monitor patient closely.
Other drugs that prolong the QTc interval (disopyramide, procainamide, and quinidine): Increased risk of arrhythmias. Avoid using together.
Drug-herb. *Kava:* May cause dystonic reactions. Discourage use together.
St. John's wort: May cause photosensitivity reactions. Tell patient to take precautions to avoid excessive sunlight exposure.
Yohimbe: May cause yohimbe toxicity. Discourage use together.
Drug-lifestyle. *Alcohol use:* Increased CNS depression. Discourage use together.
Sun exposure: Increased risk of photosensitivity reactions. Advise patient to avoid excessive sunlight exposure.

EFFECTS ON LAB TEST RESULTS
• May increase liver function test values and eosinophil count. May decrease hemoglobin and WBC, granulocyte, and platelet counts.

CONTRAINDICATIONS
Contraindicated in patients hypersensitive to drug and in those with severe CNS depression or coma. Don't use this drug in combination with other drugs known to prolong the QTc interval and in patients with congenital long QT syndrome or a history of cardiac arrhythmias.

NURSING CONSIDERATIONS
• Protect drug from light. Slight yellowing of injection or concentrate is common and doesn't affect potency. Discard markedly discolored solutions.
• Oral liquid and parenteral forms may cause contact dermatitis. Wear gloves when preparing solutions and avoid contact with skin and clothing.
• *Alert:* Before treatment, obtain baseline ECG and measure serum potassium levels. Serum potassium should be normalized before starting treatment and patient with a QTc interval above 450 msec shouldn't receive Serentil. Patients with a QTc interval above 500 msec should discontinue use.
• Obtain baseline blood pressure measurements before starting therapy and monitor them regularly. Watch for orthostatic hypotension, especially with parenteral administration.
• Give deeply I.M. only in upper outer quadrant of buttocks. Massage slowly afterward to prevent sterile abscess. Injection may sting.
• Monitor patient for tardive dyskinesia, which may occur after prolonged use. It may not appear until months or years later and may disappear spontaneously or persist for life, despite ending drug.
• *Alert:* Watch for evidence of neuroleptic malignant syndrome (extrapyramidal effects, hyperthermia, autonomic disturbance), which is rare but commonly fatal. It may not be related to length of drug use or type of neuroleptic; however, more than 60% of affected patients are men.
• Monitor therapy with weekly bilirubin tests during first month, periodic blood

---

Reactions may be *common*, uncommon, *life-threatening*, or **COMMON AND LIFE-THREATENING**.

tests (CBCs and liver function tests), and ophthalmic tests (long-term use).

• Drug causes false-positive test results for urinary porphyrins, urobilinogen, amylase, and 5-hydroxyindoleacetic acid because of darkening of urine by metabolites. It also causes false-positive results for urine pregnancy tests that use human chorionic gonadotropin.

• Withhold dose and notify prescriber if jaundice, symptoms of blood dyscrasia (fever, sore throat, infection, cellulitis, weakness), or persistent extrapyramidal reactions (longer than a few hours) develop, especially in children or pregnant women.

• Don't withdraw drug abruptly unless severe adverse reactions make it necessary.

• After abrupt withdrawal of long-term therapy, gastritis, nausea, vomiting, dizziness, tremor, feeling of warmth or cold, diaphoresis, tachycardia, headache, or insomnia may occur.

• **Alert:** Don't confuse Serentil with Serevent or Aventyl.

PATIENT TEACHING

• Warn patient to avoid activities that require alertness and good psychomotor coordination until CNS effects of drug are known. Drowsiness and dizziness usually subside after a few weeks.

• Advise patient to report symptoms of dizziness, palpitations, or syncope.

• Tell patient to change positions slowly.

• Warn patient to avoid alcohol while taking drug.

• Have patient report signs of urine retention or constipation.

• Tell patient that drug may discolor urine.

• Instruct patient to relieve dry mouth with sugarless gum or hard candy.

• Advise patient to use sunblock and wear protective clothing to avoid photosensitivity reactions.

olanzapine
Zyprexa, Zyprexa Zydis

Pregnancy risk category C

AVAILABLE FORMS
Tablets: 2.5 mg, 5 mg, 7.5 mg, 10 mg, 15 mg, 20 mg

Tablets (orally disintegrating): 5 mg, 10 mg, 15 mg, 20 mg

INDICATIONS & DOSAGES
➤ **Schizophrenia—**
Adults: Initially, 5 to 10 mg P.O. once daily. Dosage adjustments in 5-mg daily increments should occur at intervals of not less than 1 week. Most patients respond to 10 mg/day. Don't exceed 20 mg/day.
➤ **Long-term treatment of schizophrenia—**
Adults: Initially, 5 to 10 mg P.O. daily. Goal is 10 mg P.O. daily within several days of starting therapy. Dosage may be increased weekly in increments of 5 mg daily to a maximum of 20 mg daily. However, clinical assessment is recommended for dosages that exceed 10 mg daily.
Elderly patients age 65 and older: Start therapy at low end of dosage range. Adjust carefully.
Adjust-a-dose: Initially, give 5 mg to patients who are debilitated, predisposed to hypotension, pharmacologically sensitive to drug, or those who may metabolize olanzapine slowly, such as nonsmoking women age 65 and older.
➤ **Short-term treatment of acute manic episodes from bipolar I disorder—**
Adults: Initially, 10 to 15 mg P.O. daily. Adjust dosage p.r.n. in increments of 5 mg daily at intervals of 24 hours or more. Maximum, 20 mg P.O. daily. Duration of treatment is 3 to 4 weeks.

ACTION
Unknown. May block dopamine and 5-HT$_2$ receptors.

Route	Onset	Peak	Duration
P.O.	Unknown	6 hr	Unknown

ADVERSE REACTIONS
CNS: *somnolence, agitation, insomnia, headache, nervousness, hostility,* parkinsonism, *dizziness,* anxiety, personality disorder, akathisia, hypertonia, tremor, amnesia, articulation impairment, euphoria, stuttering, tardive dyskinesia, ***neuroleptic malignant syndrome.***
CV: orthostatic hypotension, tachycardia, chest pain, hypotension, edema.
EENT: amblyopia, blepharitis, corneal lesion, *rhinitis,* pharyngitis.

GI: constipation, dry mouth, abdominal pain, increased appetite, increased salivation, nausea, vomiting, thirst.
GU: premenstrual syndrome, hematuria, metrorrhagia, urinary incontinence, urinary tract infection.
Hematologic: asymptomatic increases in eosinophil count, *leukopenia.*
Metabolic: weight gain or loss.
Musculoskeletal: joint pain, extremity pain, back pain, neck rigidity, twitching.
Respiratory: increased cough, dyspnea.
Skin: vesiculobullous rash.
Other: fever.

INTERACTIONS
Drug-drug. *Antihypertensives:* May potentiate hypotensive effects. Monitor blood pressure closely.
Carbamazepine, omeprazole, rifampin: Increased clearance of olanzapine. Monitor patient.
Diazepam: Increased CNS effects. Monitor patient.
Dopamine agonists, levodopa: Antagonized activity of these drugs. Monitor patient.
Drug-herb. *Nutmeg:* May reduce effectiveness or interfere with drug therapy. Discourage use together.
St. John's wort: May decrease blood levels of olanzapine. Discourage use together.
Drug-lifestyle. *Alcohol use:* Increased CNS effects. Discourage use together.

EFFECTS ON LAB TEST RESULTS
• May increase AST, ALT, GGT, CK, and serum prolactin levels.
• May increase eosinophil count.

CONTRAINDICATIONS
Contraindicated in patients hypersensitive to drug.

NURSING CONSIDERATIONS
• Use cautiously in patients with heart disease, cerebrovascular disease, conditions that predispose patient to hypotension, history of seizures or conditions that might lower the seizure threshold, and hepatic impairment. Also use cautiously in elderly patients, those with a history of paralytic ileus, and those at risk for aspiration pneumonia, prostatic hyperplasia, or angle-closure glaucoma.

• Drug should be used in pregnancy only if benefit justifies risk to the fetus. Women taking drug shouldn't breast-feed.
• Safety and effectiveness of drug in patients younger than age 18 haven't been established.
• Obtain baseline and periodic liver function tests; especially in patients with hepatic disorders.
• Monitor patient's weight gain.
• *Alert:* Watch for evidence of neuroleptic malignant syndrome (hyperpyrexia, muscle rigidity, altered mental status, autonomic instability), which is rare but commonly fatal. Drug should be stopped immediately and patient monitored and treated as needed.
• Monitor patient for tardive dyskinesia, which may occur after prolonged use. It may not appear until months or years later and may disappear spontaneously or persist for life, despite discontinuing drug.
• *Alert:* Don't confuse olanzapine with olsalazine, or Zyprexa with Zyrtec.

PATIENT TEACHING
• Warn patient to avoid hazardous tasks until full CNS effects of drug are known.
• Warn patient against exposure to extreme heat; drug may impair body's ability to reduce core temperature.
• Advise patient to avoid alcohol.
• Tell patient to rise slowly to avoid orthostatic hypotension.
• Instruct patient to relieve dry mouth with ice chips or sugarless candy or gum.
• Urge woman to notify prescriber if she becomes pregnant or if pregnancy is planned or suspected. Tell her not to breast-feed during therapy.

---

perphenazine
Apo-Perphenazine†, Fentazin§, PMS Perphenazine†, Trilafon, Trilafon Concentrate

Pregnancy risk category NR

AVAILABLE FORMS
Injection: 5 mg/ml
Oral concentrate: 16 mg/5 ml
Syrup: 2 mg/5 ml†
Tablets: 2 mg, 4 mg, 8 mg, 16 mg

Reactions may be *common*, uncommon, *life-threatening*, or COMMON AND LIFE-THREATENING.

INDICATIONS & DOSAGES

➤ **Psychosis in nonhospitalized patients—**
Adults and children older than age 12:
Initially, 4 to 8 mg P.O. t.i.d., reduced as soon as possible to minimum effective dose.

➤ **Psychosis in hospitalized patients—**
Adults and children older than age 12:
Initially, 8 to 16 mg P.O. b.i.d., t.i.d., or q.i.d., increased to 64 mg daily, p.r.n. Or, 5 to 10 mg I.M. q 6 hours, p.r.n. Maximum dose, 30 mg.

➤ **Severe nausea and vomiting—**
Adults: 8 to 16 mg P.O. daily in divided doses to maximum of 24 mg. Or, 5 to 10 mg I.M., p.r.n. May be given I.V., diluted to 0.5 mg/ml with saline solution. Dose given I.V. shouldn't exceed 5 mg.

ACTION

Unknown. Probably exerts antipsychotic effects by blocking postsynaptic dopamine receptors in the brain.

Route	Onset	Peak	Duration
I.M., I.V., P.O.	Unknown	Unknown	Unknown

ADVERSE REACTIONS

CNS: *extrapyramidal reactions, tardive dyskinesia,* sedation, pseudoparkinsonism, dizziness, *seizures,* drowsiness, *neuroleptic malignant syndrome.*
CV: *orthostatic hypotension,* tachycardia, ECG changes.
EENT: ocular changes, *blurred vision,* nasal congestion.
GI: *dry mouth, constipation,* nausea, vomiting, diarrhea.
GU: *urine retention,* dark urine, menstrual irregularities, inhibited ejaculation.
Hematologic: *leukopenia, agranulocytosis,* eosinophilia, hemolytic anemia, *thrombocytopenia.*
Hepatic: cholestatic jaundice.
Metabolic: weight gain.
Skin: *mild photosensitivity reactions,* allergic reactions, pain at I.M. injection site, sterile abscess.
Other: gynecomastia.

INTERACTIONS

Drug-drug. *Antacids:* Inhibited absorption of oral phenothiazines. Separate antacid and phenothiazine doses by at least 2 hours.
Barbiturates: May decrease phenothiazine effect. Monitor patient.
CNS depressants: Increased CNS depression. Use together cautiously.
Lithium: Increased neurologic adverse effects. Monitor patient closely.
Drug-herb. *Kava:* May cause dystonic reactions. Discourage use together.
St. John's wort: May cause photosensitivity reactions. Tell patient to take precautions to avoid excessive sunlight exposure.
Yohimbe: May cause yohimbe toxicity. Discourage use together.
Drug-lifestyle. *Alcohol use:* Increased CNS depression. Discourage use together.
Sun exposure: Increased risk of photosensitivity reactions. Advise patient to avoid excessive sunlight exposure.

EFFECTS ON LAB TEST RESULTS

• May increase liver function test values and eosinophil count. May decrease hemoglobin and WBC, granulocyte, and platelet counts.

CONTRAINDICATIONS

Contraindicated in patients hypersensitive to drug and in those with CNS depression, blood dyscrasia, bone marrow depression, liver damage, or subcortical damage; also contraindicated in those experiencing coma or receiving large doses of CNS depressants.

NURSING CONSIDERATIONS

• Use cautiously in elderly or debilitated patients and in those taking other CNS depressants or anticholinergics.
• Use cautiously in patients with alcohol withdrawal, psychotic depression, suicidal tendency, severe adverse reactions to other phenothiazines, renal impairment, CV disease, or respiratory disorders.
• Obtain baseline blood pressure measurements before starting therapy and monitor pressure regularly. Watch for orthostatic hypotension, especially with parenteral administration. Keep patient supine for 1 hour after giving drug; tell him to change positions slowly.
• Protect drug from light. Slight yellowing of injection or concentrate is common and

doesn't affect potency. Discard markedly discolored solutions.
● Prevent contact dermatitis by keeping drug away from skin and clothes. Wear gloves when preparing liquid forms.
● Dilute liquid concentrate with fruit juice, milk, carbonated beverage, or semisolid food just before giving. Don't use colas, black coffee, grape juice, apple juice, or tea because turbidity or precipitation may result.
● Give by deep I.M. injection only in upper outer quadrant of buttocks. Massage slowly afterward to prevent sterile abscess. Injection may sting.
● Monitor patient for tardive dyskinesia, which may occur after prolonged use. It may not appear until months or years later and may disappear spontaneously or persist for life, despite ending drug.
● *Alert:* Watch for evidence of neuroleptic malignant syndrome (extrapyramidal effects, hyperthermia, autonomic disturbance), which is rare but commonly fatal. It may not be related to length of drug use or type of neuroleptic; however, more than 60% of affected patients are men.
● Monitor therapy with weekly bilirubin tests during first month, periodic blood tests (CBCs and liver function tests), and ophthalmic tests (long-term use).
● Drug causes false-positive test results for urinary porphyrins, urobilinogen, amylase, and 5-hydroxyindoleacetic acid because of darkening of urine by metabolites. It also causes false-positive results for urine pregnancy tests that use human chorionic gonadotropin.
● Withhold dose and notify prescriber if jaundice, symptoms of blood dyscrasia (fever, sore throat, infection, cellulitis, weakness), or persistent extrapyramidal reactions (longer than a few hours) develop.
● Don't withdraw drug abruptly unless severe adverse reactions make it necessary.
● After abrupt withdrawal of long-term therapy, gastritis, nausea, vomiting, dizziness, tremor, feeling of warmth or cold, diaphoresis, tachycardia, headache, or insomnia may occur.

PATIENT TEACHING
● Tell patient which beverages to use to dilute oral concentrate.

● Warn patient to avoid activities that require alertness or good psychomotor coordination until CNS effects of drug are known. Drowsiness and dizziness usually subside after a few weeks.
● Tell patient to avoid alcohol while taking drug.
● Advise patient to report signs of urine retention or constipation.
● Tell patient to use sunblock and wear protective clothing to avoid photosensitivity reactions.
● Advise patient to relieve dry mouth with sugarless gum or hard candy.

pimozide
Orap

Pregnancy risk category C

AVAILABLE FORMS
Tablets: 2 mg, 4 mg†, 10 mg

INDICATIONS & DOSAGES
➤ **Suppression of motor and phonic tics in patients with Tourette syndrome refractory to first-line therapy—**
Adults and children older than age 12: Initially, 1 to 2 mg P.O. daily in divided doses; then increased every other day, p.r.n. Maintenance dose is less than 0.2 mg/kg/day or 10 mg/day, whichever is less. Maximum, 10 mg daily.

ACTION
Unknown. May block dopamine nonselectively at both presynaptic and postsynaptic receptors on neurons in the CNS.

Route	Onset	Peak	Duration
P.O.	Unknown	4-12 hr	Unknown

ADVERSE REACTIONS
CNS: *parkinsonian-like symptoms,* drowsiness, headache, insomnia, other extrapyramidal symptoms, *tardive dyskinesia, sedation,* **neuroleptic malignant syndrome.**
CV: *prolonged QT interval,* hypotension, hypertension, tachycardia.
EENT: visual disturbances.
GI: *dry mouth, constipation,* excessive salivation.
GU: impotence, urinary frequency.

Musculoskeletal: muscle rigidity.
Skin: rash, diaphoresis.

INTERACTIONS
Drug-drug. *Antiarrhythmics, azole antifungal agents, macrolide antibiotics, phenothiazines, protease inhibitors, TCAs:* May cause ECG abnormalities. Avoid using together.
CNS depressants: Increased CNS depression. Use together cautiously.
Drug-food. *Grapefruit juice:* Inhibited metabolism of pimozide. Advise patient to avoid taking drug with grapefruit juice.
Drug-lifestyle. *Alcohol use:* Increased CNS depression. Discourage use together.

EFFECTS ON LAB TEST RESULTS
None reported.

CONTRAINDICATIONS
Contraindicated in patients hypersensitive to drug and in those with severe toxic CNS depression, congenital long QT syndrome, coma, or a history of arrhythmias. Also contraindicated for use with other drugs known to cause motor and phonic tics and for treatment of simple tics or tics other than those related to Tourette syndrome.

NURSING CONSIDERATIONS
● Use cautiously in patients with hepatic or renal dysfunction, glaucoma, prostatic hyperplasia, seizure disorder, or EEG abnormalities.
● *Alert:* Obtain an ECG before treatment begins and periodically thereafter. Watch for prolonged QT interval.
● Monitor patient for extrapyramidal symptoms such as dystonia, akathisia, hyperreflexia, opisthotonos, and oculogyric crisis.
● Avoid administration together with other drugs that prolong the QT interval, such as antiarrhythmics.
● Monitor patient for tardive dyskinesia, which may occur after prolonged use. It may not appear until months or years later, and may disappear spontaneously or persist for life, despite discontinuing drug.
● *Alert:* Watch for evidence of neuroleptic malignant syndrome (extrapyramidal effects, hyperthermia, autonomic disturbance), which is rare but commonly fatal. It may not be related to length of drug use

or type of neuroleptic; however, more than 60% of affected patients are men.
● If patient also takes an anticonvulsant, watch for increased seizure activity. Pimozide may lower the seizure threshold.

PATIENT TEACHING
● Warn patient not to stop taking drug abruptly and not to exceed prescribed dosage.
● Tell patient to avoid alcohol and grapefruit juice while taking drug.
● Advise patient to use sugarless hard candy, gum, and liquids to relieve dry mouth.

---

quetiapine fumarate
Seroquel

Pregnancy risk category C

AVAILABLE FORMS
Tablets: 25 mg, 100 mg, 200 mg

INDICATIONS & DOSAGES
➤ **Management of signs and symptoms of psychotic disorders—**
Adults: Initially, 25 mg P.O. b.i.d., with increases in increments of 25 to 50 mg b.i.d. or t.i.d. on days 2 and 3, as tolerated. Target range is 300 to 400 mg daily divided into two or three doses by day 4. Further dosage adjustments, if indicated, should generally occur at intervals of not less than 2 days. Dosage can be increased or decreased by 25 to 50 mg b.i.d. Antipsychotic effect generally occurs at 150 to 750 mg/day. Safety of dosages of more than 800 mg/day hasn't been evaluated.
Elderly patients: Give lower dosages, adjust more slowly, and monitor patient carefully in initial dosing period.
Adjust-a-dose: For debilitated patients and those with hepatic impairment or hypotension, consider lower dosages and slower adjustment.

ACTION
Unknown. A dibenzoxazepine that may block dopamine D_2 receptors and serotonin 5-HT_2 receptors in the brain.

Route	Onset	Peak	Duration
P.O.	Unknown	1.5 hr	Unknown

ADVERSE REACTIONS

CNS: *dizziness, headache, somnolence,* hypertonia, dysarthria, asthenia, ***neuroleptic malignant syndrome.***
CV: orthostatic hypotension, tachycardia, palpitations, peripheral edema.
EENT: ear pain, pharyngitis, rhinitis.
GI: dry mouth, dyspepsia, abdominal pain, constipation, anorexia.
Hematologic: *leukopenia.*
Metabolic: *weight gain.*
Musculoskeletal: back pain.
Respiratory: increased cough, dyspnea.
Skin: rash, diaphoresis.
Other: flu syndrome.

INTERACTIONS

Drug-drug. *Antihypertensives:* Increased effects. Monitor blood pressure.
Carbamazepine, glucocorticoids, phenobarbital, phenytoin, rifampin: Increased quetiapine clearance. Adjust quetiapine dosage, as directed.
CNS depressants: Increased CNS effects. Use together cautiously.
Erythromycin, fluconazole, itraconazole, ketoconazole: Decreased quetiapine clearance. Use together cautiously.
Lorazepam: Decreased lorazepam clearance. Monitor patient for increased CNS effects.
Drug-lifestyle. *Alcohol use:* Increased CNS effects. Discourage use together.

EFFECTS ON LAB TEST RESULTS

● May increase liver enzyme, cholesterol, and triglyceride levels. May decrease T_4 and thyroid-stimulating hormone levels.
● May decrease WBC count.

CONTRAINDICATIONS

Contraindicated in patients hypersensitive to drug or its ingredients.

NURSING CONSIDERATIONS

● Use cautiously in patients with CV disease, cerebrovascular disease, conditions that predispose to hypotension, a history of seizures or conditions that lower the seizure threshold, and conditions in which core body temperature may be elevated.
● Dispense lowest appropriate quantity of drug to reduce risk of overdose.
● *Alert:* Watch for evidence of neuroleptic malignant syndrome (extrapyramidal ef-

fects, hyperthermia, autonomic disturbance), which is rare but commonly fatal. It may not be related to length of drug use or type of neuroleptic; however, more than 60% of affected patients are men.
● Monitor patient for tardive dyskinesia, which may occur after prolonged use. It may not appear until months or years later and may disappear spontaneously or persist for life, despite ending drug.
● Monitor patient for weight gain.
● Cataract formation is possible. Obtain ophthalmologic examinations every 6 months.
● *Alert:* Don't confuse Seroquel with Serzone.

PATIENT TEACHING

● Advise patient about risk of orthostatic hypotension. The risk is greatest during the 3- to 5-day period of initial dosage adjustment, when resuming treatment, and when increasing dosages.
● Tell patient to avoid becoming overheated or dehydrated.
● Warn patient to avoid activities that require mental alertness until CNS effects of drug are known, especially during initial dosage adjustment or dosage increases.
● Remind patient to have an eye examination at start of therapy and every 6 months during therapy to check for cataract formation.
● Tell patient to notify prescriber about other drugs (prescription or OTC) he is taking or plans to take.
● Tell woman to notify prescriber about planned, suspected, or known pregnancy. Advise her not to breast-feed during therapy.
● Advise patient to avoid alcohol while taking drug.

risperidone
Risperdal

Pregnancy risk category C

AVAILABLE FORMS

Solution: 1 mg/ml
Tablets: 0.25 mg, 0.5 mg, 1 mg, 2 mg, 3 mg, 4 mg

Reactions may be *common,* uncommon, *life-threatening,* or COMMON AND LIFE-THREATENING.

INDICATIONS & DOSAGES
➤ **Psychosis—**
Adults: Initially, 1 mg P.O. b.i.d. Increased in increments of 1 mg b.i.d. on days 2 and 3 of treatment to a target dose of 3 mg b.i.d. At least 1 week must pass before dosage is adjusted further. Maintenance doses are generally 4 to 8 mg/day and can be given once daily or as two divided doses. Safety of dosages exceeding 16 mg/day hasn't been evaluated.
Elderly patients: Initially, 0.5 mg P.O. b.i.d. Increased in increments of 0.5 mg b.i.d. on days 2 and 3 of treatment to a target dose of 1.5 mg P.O. b.i.d. At least 1 week must pass before dosage is increased further.
Adjust-a-dose: For debilitated patients or those with severe renal impairment, hepatic impairment, or hypotension, start with 0.5 mg P.O. b.i.d. Increase in increments of 0.5 mg b.i.d. on days 2 and 3 of treatment to a target dosage of 1.5 mg P.O. b.i.d. At least 1 week must pass before dosage is increased further.

ACTION
Blocks dopamine and 5-HT$_2$ receptors in the brain.

Route	Onset	Peak	Duration
P.O.	Unknown	1 hr	Unknown

ADVERSE REACTIONS
CNS: somnolence, *extrapyramidal reactions,* headache, *insomnia, agitation, anxiety,* tardive dyskinesia, aggressiveness, ***neuroleptic malignant syndrome.***
CV: tachycardia, chest pain, orthostatic hypotension, ***prolonged QT interval.***
EENT: *rhinitis,* sinusitis, pharyngitis, abnormal vision.
GI: *constipation, nausea, vomiting, dyspepsia.*
Musculoskeletal: arthralgia, back pain.
Respiratory: coughing, upper respiratory tract infection.
Skin: rash, dry skin, photosensitivity reactions.
Other: fever.

INTERACTIONS
Drug-drug. *Carbamazepine:* Increased risperidone clearance and decreased effectiveness. Monitor patient closely.

Clozapine: Decreased risperidone clearance, increasing toxicity. Monitor patient closely.
CNS depressants: Additive CNS depression. Use together cautiously.
Levodopa: Antagonized effects of levodopa. Use together cautiously.
Drug-lifestyle. *Alcohol use:* Additive CNS depression. Discourage use together.
Sun exposure: Increased risk of photosensitivity reactions. Advise patient to avoid excessive sunlight exposure.

EFFECTS ON LAB TEST RESULTS
• May increase serum prolactin levels.

CONTRAINDICATIONS
Contraindicated in patients hypersensitive to drug and in breast-feeding women.

NURSING CONSIDERATIONS
• Use cautiously in patients with prolonged QT interval, CV disease, cerebrovascular disease, dehydration, hypovolemia, history of seizures, or conditions that could affect metabolism or hemodynamic responses; also, use cautiously in those exposed to extreme heat.
• *Alert:* Obtain baseline blood pressure measurements before starting therapy, and monitor pressure regularly. Watch for orthostatic hypotension, especially during initial dosage adjustment.
• Monitor patient for tardive dyskinesia, which may occur after prolonged use. It may not appear until months or years later and may disappear spontaneously or persist for life, despite ending drug.
• Monitor patient for weight gain.
• *Alert:* Watch for evidence of neuroleptic malignant syndrome (extrapyramidal effects, hyperthermia, autonomic disturbance), which is rare but commonly fatal. It may not be related to length of drug use or type of neuroleptic; however, more than 60% of patients are men.
• *Alert:* Don't confuse risperidone with reserpine.

PATIENT TEACHING
• Warn patient to avoid activities that require alertness until CNS effects of drug are known.

• Warn patient to rise slowly, avoid hot showers, and use extra caution during first few days of therapy to avoid fainting.
• Advise patient to use caution in hot weather to prevent heatstroke.
• Tell patient to avoid alcohol.
• Tell patient to use sunblock and wear protective clothing outdoors.
• Advise woman to notify prescriber if she is or plans to become pregnant during therapy.

---

thioridazine hydrochloride
Aldazine‡, Apo-Thioridazine†, Mellaril*, Mellaril Concentrate, Novo-Ridazine†, PMS Thioridazine†

Pregnancy risk category C

AVAILABLE FORMS
Oral concentrate: 30 mg/ml, 100 mg/ml (3% to 4.2% alcohol)
Oral suspension: 25 mg/5 ml, 100 mg/5 ml
Tablets: 10 mg, 15 mg, 25 mg, 50 mg, 100 mg, 150 mg, 200 mg

INDICATIONS & DOSAGES
➤ **Schizophrenic patients who don't show an acceptable response to treatment with other antipsychotic drugs—**
Adults: Initially, 50 to 100 mg P.O. t.i.d., increased gradually to 800 mg daily in divided doses, if needed. Dosage varies.
Children: Initially, 0.5 mg/kg/day in divided doses. Increase gradually to optimum therapeutic effect; maximum dose is 3 mg/kg/day.

ACTION
Unknown. A piperidine phenothiazine that probably blocks postsynaptic dopamine receptors in the brain.

Route	Onset	Peak	Duration
P.O.	Unknown	Unknown	Unknown

ADVERSE REACTIONS
CNS: *tardive dyskinesia, sedation,* EEG changes, dizziness, *neuroleptic malignant syndrome.*

CV: *orthostatic hypotension,* tachycardia, *prolonged QTc interval, torsades de pointes,* ECG changes.
EENT: *ocular changes, blurred vision,* retinitis pigmentosa.
GI: *dry mouth, constipation,* increased appetite.
GU: *urine retention,* dark urine, menstrual irregularities, inhibited ejaculation.
Hematologic: *transient leukopenia, agranulocytosis,* hyperprolactinemia.
Hepatic: cholestatic jaundice.
Metabolic: weight gain.
Skin: *mild photosensitivity reactions,* allergic reactions.
Other: gynecomastia.

INTERACTIONS
Drug-drug. *Antacids:* Inhibited absorption of oral phenothiazines. Separate antacid and phenothiazine doses by at least 2 hours.
Barbiturates: May decrease phenothiazine effect. Monitor patient.
Centrally acting antihypertensives: Decreased antihypertensive effect. Monitor blood pressure.
Fluoxetine, fluvoxamine, pindolol, propranolol; other drugs that inhibit the cytochrome P450 2D6 enzyme; drugs known to prolong the QTc interval (disopyramide, procainamide, and quinidine): Inhibited metabolism of thioridazine; may cause arrhythmias resulting from QTc interval prolongation. Avoid using together.
Lithium: May decrease phenothiazine effect and increase neurologic adverse effects. Monitor patient closely.
Other CNS depressants: Increased CNS depression. Use together cautiously.
Drug-herb. *Kava:* May cause dystonic reactions. Discourage use together.
St. John's wort: May cause photosensitivity reactions. Tell patient to take precautions to avoid excessive sunlight exposure.
Yohimbe: May cause yohimbe toxicity. Discourage use together.
Drug-lifestyle. *Alcohol use:* Increased CNS depression. Discourage use together.
Sun exposure: Increased risk of photosensitivity reactions. Advise patient to avoid excessive sunlight exposure.

EFFECTS ON LAB TEST RESULTS
• May increase liver enzyme levels.

Reactions may be *common,* uncommon, *life-threatening,* or COMMON AND LIFE-THREATENING.

● May decrease granulocyte and WBC counts.

CONTRAINDICATIONS

Contraindicated in patients hypersensitive to drug and in those with CNS depression, coma, or severe hypertensive or hypotensive cardiac disease. Don't use thioridazine with fluvoxamine, propranolol, pindolol, fluoxetine, and any drug that inhibits the cytochrome P450 2D6 enzyme and agents known to prolong the QTc interval. Also contraindicated in patients with reduced levels of cytochrome P450 2D6 isoenzyme, patients with congenital long QT syndrome, or patients with a history of cardiac arrhythmias.

NURSING CONSIDERATIONS

● Use cautiously in elderly or debilitated patients and in patients with hepatic disease, CV disease, respiratory disorders, hypocalcemia, seizure disorders, or severe reactions to insulin or electroconvulsive therapy; also, use cautiously in those exposed to extreme heat or cold (including antipyretic therapy) or organophosphate insecticides.

● *Alert:* Before starting treatment, obtain baseline ECG and potassium level. Patients with a QTc interval greater than 450 msec shouldn't receive Mellaril. Patients with a QTc greater than 500 msec should discontinue use.

● *Alert:* Drug isn't used in initial treatment of schizophrenia.

● *Alert:* Different liquid formulations have different concentrations. Check dosage carefully.

● Prevent contact dermatitis by keeping drug away from skin and clothes. Wear gloves when preparing liquid forms.

● Dilute liquid concentrate with water or fruit juice just before giving.

● Shake suspension well before using.

● Monitor patient for tardive dyskinesia, which may occur after prolonged use. It may not appear until months or years later and may disappear spontaneously or persist for life, despite ending drug.

● *Alert:* Watch for evidence of neuroleptic malignant syndrome (extrapyramidal effects, hyperthermia, autonomic disturbance), which is rare but commonly fatal. It may not be related to length of drug use

or type of neuroleptic; however, more than 60% of patients are men.

● Monitor therapy with weekly bilirubin tests during first month, periodic blood tests (CBCs and liver function tests), and ophthalmic tests (long-term use).

● Drug causes false-positive test results for urinary porphyrins, urobilinogen, amylase, and 5-hydroxyindoleacetic acid because of darkening of urine by metabolites; it also causes false-positive results for urine pregnancy tests that use human chorionic gonadotropin.

● Withhold dose and notify prescriber if jaundice, blood dyscrasia (fever, sore throat, infection, cellulitis, weakness), or persistent extrapyramidal reactions develop, especially in children or pregnant women.

● Don't stop drug abruptly unless required by severe adverse reactions.

● After abrupt withdrawal of long-term therapy, gastritis, nausea, vomiting, dizziness, tremor, feeling of warmth or cold, diaphoresis, tachycardia, headache, or insomnia may occur.

● *Alert:* Don't confuse thioridazine with Thorazine or Mellaril with Elavil.

PATIENT TEACHING

● Tell patient to shake suspension before use.

● Warn patient to avoid activities that require alertness until CNS effects of drug are known.

● Tell patient to watch for orthostatic hypotension, especially with parenteral administration. Advise patient to change positions slowly.

● Instruct patient to report symptoms of dizziness, palpitations, or syncope to prescriber.

● Tell patient to avoid alcohol.

● Have patient report signs of urine retention, constipation, or blurred vision.

● Tell patient that drug may discolor the urine.

● Advise patient to relieve dry mouth with sugarless gum or hard candy.

● Instruct patient to use sunblock and to wear protective clothing outdoors.

---

thiothixene
Navane

thiothixene hydrochloride
Navane*

Pregnancy risk category C

AVAILABLE FORMS
thiothixene
Capsules: 1 mg, 2 mg, 5 mg, 10 mg, 20 mg
thiothixene hydrochloride
Injection: 2 mg/ml, 5 mg/ml
Oral concentrate: 5 mg/ml*

INDICATIONS & DOSAGES
➤ **Mild to moderate psychosis—**
Adults: Initially, 2 mg P.O. t.i.d. Increased gradually to 15 mg daily, p.r.n.
➤ **Severe psychosis—**
Adults: Initially, 5 mg P.O. b.i.d. Increased gradually to 20 to 30 mg daily, p.r.n. Maximum recommended dose is 60 mg daily. Or, 4 mg I.M. b.i.d. to q.i.d. Maximum, 30 mg I.M. daily. Switch to oral form as soon as possible.

ACTION
Unknown. A thioxanthene that probably blocks dopamine receptors in the brain.

Route	Onset	Peak	Duration
I.M., P.O.	Unknown	Unknown	Unknown

ADVERSE REACTIONS
CNS: *extrapyramidal reactions, drowsiness,* restlessness, agitation, insomnia, *tardive dyskinesia,* sedation, EEG changes, pseudoparkinsonism, dizziness, **neuroleptic malignant syndrome.**
CV: *hypotension,* tachycardia, ECG changes.
EENT: ocular changes, *blurred vision,* nasal congestion.
GI: *dry mouth, constipation.*
GU: *urine retention,* menstrual irregularities, inhibited ejaculation.
Hematologic: *transient leukopenia,* leukocytosis, **agranulocytosis.**
Hepatic: jaundice.
Metabolic: weight gain.

Skin: *mild photosensitivity reactions,* allergic reactions, pain at I.M. injection site, sterile abscess, exfoliative dermatitis.
Other: gynecomastia.

INTERACTIONS
Drug-drug. *CNS depressants:* Increased CNS depression. Use together cautiously.
Drug-herb. *Nutmeg:* May reduce effectiveness or interfere with drug therapy. Discourage use together.
Drug-lifestyle. *Alcohol use:* Increased CNS depression. Discourage use together. *Sun exposure:* Increased risk of photosensitivity reactions. Advise patient to avoid excessive sunlight exposure.

EFFECTS ON LAB TEST RESULTS
• May increase liver enzyme levels.
• May decrease WBC and granulocyte counts.

CONTRAINDICATIONS
Contraindicated in patients hypersensitive to drug and in those with CNS depression, circulatory collapse, coma, or blood dyscrasia.

NURSING CONSIDERATIONS
• Use with extreme caution in patients with history of seizure disorder and in those undergoing alcohol withdrawal.
• Use cautiously in elderly or debilitated patients and in those with CV disease (may cause sudden drop in blood pressure), hepatic disease, heat exposure, glaucoma, or prostatic hyperplasia.
• Prevent contact dermatitis by keeping drug off skin and clothes. Wear gloves when preparing liquid forms.
• Dilute liquid concentrate with fruit juice, milk, or semisolid food just before administering.
• Slight yellowing of injection or concentrate is common and doesn't affect potency. Discard markedly discolored solutions.
• Give I.M. only in upper outer quadrant of buttocks or midlateral thigh. Massage slowly afterward to prevent sterile abscess. Injection may sting.
• Monitor patient for tardive dyskinesia, which may occur after prolonged use; it may not appear until months or years later, and may disappear spontaneously or persist for life, despite ending drug.

Reactions may be *common,* uncommon, **life-threatening,** or **COMMON AND LIFE-THREATENING.**

• **Alert:** Watch for evidence of neuroleptic malignant syndrome (extrapyramidal effects, hyperthermia, autonomic disturbance), which is rare but commonly fatal. It may not be related to length of drug use or type of neuroleptic; however, more than 60% of patients are men.

• Monitor therapy with weekly bilirubin tests during first month, periodic blood tests (CBCs and liver function tests), and ophthalmic tests (long-term use).

• Drug causes false-positive test results for urinary porphyrins, urobilinogen, amylase, and 5-hydroxyindoleacetic acid because of darkening of urine by metabolites; it also causes false-positive results for urine pregnancy tests that use human chorionic gonadotropin.

• Watch for orthostatic hypotension, especially with parenteral administration. Keep patient supine for 1 hour after drug administration, and tell him to change positions slowly.

• Withhold dose and notify prescriber if jaundice, blood dyscrasia (fever, sore throat, infection, cellulitis, weakness), or persistent extrapyramidal reactions develop, especially in pregnant women.

• Don't withdraw drug abruptly unless severe adverse reactions make it necessary.

• After abrupt withdrawal of long-term therapy, gastritis, nausea, vomiting, dizziness, tremor, feeling of warmth or cold, diaphoresis, tachycardia, headache, or insomnia may occur.

• **Alert:** Don't confuse Navane with Nubain or Norvasc.

PATIENT TEACHING
• Warn patient to avoid activities that require alertness until CNS effects of drug are known.

• Tell patient to watch for orthostatic hypotension. Advise him to change positions slowly.

• Instruct patient to dilute liquid appropriately.

• Tell patient to avoid alcohol during therapy.

• Have patient report signs of urine retention, constipation, or blurred vision.

• Instruct patient to use sunblock and to wear protective clothing outdoors.

---

trifluoperazine hydrochloride
Apo-Trifluoperazine†, Novo-Trifluzine†, PMS Trifluoperazine†, Stelazine, Stelazine Concentrate

Pregnancy risk category NR

AVAILABLE FORMS
Injection: 2 mg/ml
Oral concentrate: 10 mg/ml
Tablets (regular and film-coated): 1 mg, 2 mg, 5 mg, 10 mg

INDICATIONS & DOSAGES
➤ **Anxiety states—**
Adults: 1 to 2 mg P.O. b.i.d. Maximum, 6 mg daily. Don't give drug for longer than 12 weeks for this indication.
➤ **Schizophrenia, other psychotic disorders—**
Adults: 2 to 5 mg P.O. b.i.d., gradually increased until therapeutic response occurs. Or, 1 to 2 mg deeply I.M. q 4 to 6 hours, p.r.n. Most patients respond to 15 to 20 mg P.O. daily, although some may need 40 mg/day or more. More than 6 mg I.M. in 24 hours is rarely needed.
Children ages 6 to 12: 1 mg P.O. daily or b.i.d.; may increase gradually to 15 mg daily, if needed.

ACTION
Unknown. A piperazine phenothiazine that probably blocks dopamine receptors in the brain.

Route	Onset	Peak	Duration
I.M., P.O.	Unknown	Unknown	Unknown

ADVERSE REACTIONS
CNS: *extrapyramidal reactions, tardive dyskinesia,* pseudoparkinsonism, dizziness, drowsiness, insomnia, fatigue, headache, *neuroleptic malignant syndrome.*
CV: *orthostatic hypotension,* tachycardia, ECG changes.
EENT: ocular changes, *blurred vision.*
GI: *dry mouth, constipation,* nausea.
GU: *urine retention,* menstrual irregularities, inhibited ejaculation.
Hematologic: *transient leukopenia, agranulocytosis.*
Hepatic: cholestatic jaundice.
Metabolic: weight gain.

Skin: *photosensitivity reactions,* allergic reactions, pain at I.M. injection site, sterile abscess, rash.
Other: gynecomastia.

INTERACTIONS
Drug-drug. *Antacids:* Inhibited absorption of oral phenothiazines. Separate antacid and phenothiazine doses by at least 2 hours.
Barbiturates, lithium: May decrease phenothiazine effect. Monitor patient.
Centrally acting antihypertensives: Decreased antihypertensive effect. Monitor blood pressure.
CNS depressants: Increased CNS depression. Use together cautiously.
Propranolol: Increased levels of both propranolol and trifluoperazine. Monitor patient.
Warfarin: Decreased effect of oral anticoagulants. Monitor PT and INR.
Drug-herb. *Kava:* Increased risk of dystonic reactions. Discourage use together.
St. John's wort: May cause photosensitivity reactions. Tell patient to take precautions to avoid excessive sunlight exposure.
Yohimbe: May cause yohimbe toxicity. Discourage use together.
Drug-lifestyle. *Alcohol use:* Increased CNS depression. Discourage use together.
Sun exposure: Increased risk of photosensitivity reactions. Advise patient to avoid excessive sunlight exposure.

EFFECTS ON LAB TEST RESULTS
• May increase liver enzyme levels.
• May decrease WBC and granulocyte counts.

CONTRAINDICATIONS
Contraindicated in patients hypersensitive to phenothiazines and in those with CNS depression, coma, bone marrow suppression, or liver damage.

NURSING CONSIDERATIONS
• Use cautiously in elderly or debilitated patients and in patients with CV disease (may decrease blood pressure), seizure disorder, glaucoma, or prostatic hyperplasia; also, use cautiously in those exposed to extreme heat.

• Use in children should be reserved for those who are hospitalized or under close supervision.
• Wear gloves when preparing liquid forms.
• Dilute liquid concentrate with 60 ml of tomato or fruit juice, carbonated beverage, coffee, tea, milk, water, or semisolid food just before giving.
• Protect drug from light. Slight yellowing of injection or concentrate is common and doesn't affect potency. Discard markedly discolored solutions.
• Give deeply I.M. only in upper outer quadrant of buttocks. Massage slowly afterward to prevent sterile abscess. Injection may sting.
• Watch for orthostatic hypotension, especially with parenteral administration. Keep patient supine for 1 hour after drug administration and tell him to change positions slowly.
• Monitor patient for tardive dyskinesia, which may occur after prolonged use. It may not appear until months or years later and may disappear spontaneously or persist for life, despite ending drug.
• *Alert:* Watch for evidence of neuroleptic malignant syndrome (extrapyramidal effects, hyperthermia, autonomic disturbance), which is rare but commonly fatal. It may not be related to length of drug use or type of neuroleptic; however, more than 60% of patients are men.
• Monitor therapy with weekly bilirubin tests during first month, periodic blood tests (CBCs and liver function tests), and ophthalmic tests (long-term use).
• Drug causes false-positive test results for urinary porphyrins, urobilinogen, amylase, and 5-hydroxyindoleacetic acid because of darkening of urine by metabolites; it also causes false-positive results for urine pregnancy tests that use human chorionic gonadotropin.
• Withhold dose and notify prescriber if jaundice, symptoms of blood dyscrasia (fever, sore throat, infection, cellulitis, weakness), or persistent extrapyramidal reactions (longer than a few hours) develop, especially in children or pregnant women.
• Don't withdraw drug abruptly unless severe adverse reactions occur.

Reactions may be *common,* uncommon, *life-threatening*, or COMMON AND LIFE-THREATENING.

• After abrupt withdrawal of long-term therapy, gastritis, nausea, vomiting, dizziness, tremor, feeling of warmth or cold, diaphoresis, tachycardia, headache, insomnia, anorexia, muscle rigidity, altered mental status, or evidence of autonomic instability may occur.
• **Alert:** Don't confuse trifluoperazine with triflupromazine.

PATIENT TEACHING
• Warn patient to avoid activities that require alertness until CNS effects of drug are known.
• Tell patient to avoid alcohol while taking drug.
• Instruct patient to properly dilute liquid.
• Tell patient to report signs of urine retention or constipation.
• Tell patient to use sunblock and to wear protective clothing outdoors.
• Advise patient to relieve dry mouth with sugarless gum or hard candy.

✳ NEW DRUG

ziprasidone
Geodon

Pregnancy risk category C

AVAILABLE FORMS
Capsules: 20 mg, 40 mg, 60 mg, 80 mg

INDICATIONS & DOSAGES
➤ **Symptomatic treatment of schizophrenia—**
Adults: Initially, 20 mg b.i.d. with food. Dosages are highly individualized. Dosage adjustments, if necessary, should occur no more frequently than q 2 days, but to allow for lowest possible doses, the interval should be several weeks to assess symptom response. Effective dosage range is usually 20 to 80 mg b.i.d. Maximum recommended dosage is 100 mg b.i.d.

ACTION
May inhibit dopamine and serotonin-2 receptors, leading to a decrease in symptoms associated with schizophrenia.

Route	Onset	Peak	Duration
P.O.	1-3 days	6-8 hr	12 hr

ADVERSE REACTIONS
CNS: *somnolence,* akathisia, dizziness, extrapyramidal reactions, dystonia, hypertonia, asthenia.
CV: tachycardia, orthostatic hypotension.
EENT: rhinitis, abnormal vision.
GI: *nausea,* constipation, dyspepsia, diarrhea, dry mouth, anorexia.
Musculoskeletal: myalgia.
Respiratory: cough.
Skin: rash.

INTERACTIONS
Drug-drug. *Carbamazepine:* May decrease levels of ziprasidone. May need to increase dose of ziprasidone to achieve desired effect.
Drugs that increase dopamine, such as levodopa and dopamine agonists: May have antagonistic effect on ziprasidone. Use cautiously together.
Drugs that lower serum potassium or magnesium, such as diuretics: May increase risk of arrhythmias. Monitor potassium and magnesium levels if using these drugs together.
Drugs that prolong QT interval, such as dofetilide, moxifloxacin, pimozide, quinidine, sotalol, sparfloxacin, thioridazine: May increase risk of arrhythmias when used together. Avoid using together.
Ketoconazole: May increase levels of ziprasidone. May need to reduce dose of ziprasidone to achieve desired effect.

EFFECTS ON LAB TEST RESULTS
None reported.

CONTRAINDICATIONS
Contraindicated in patients hypersensitive to drug and in those with history of prolonged QT interval, congenital long QT syndrome, recent MI, or uncompensated heart failure. Also contraindicated in those taking other drugs that prolong QT interval.

NURSING CONSIDERATIONS
• Use cautiously in patients with history of bradycardia, hypokalemia, or hypomagnesemia and in those with acute diarrhea.
• Don't give drug to patients with a history of QT prolongation or congenital QT syndrome. Drug can increase QT interval, particularly when given with other drugs that prolong QT interval. Stop drug in pa-

tients with a QT interval more than 500 msec.

• Dizziness, palpitations, or syncope may be symptoms of a life-threatening arrhythmia such as torsades de pointes. Further CV evaluation and monitoring are needed in patients who experience these symptoms.

• Electrolyte disturbances, such as hypokalemia or hypomagnesemia, increase the risk of developing an arrhythmia. Don't give drug under these circumstances.

• Patient taking antipsychotic drugs is at risk for developing neuroleptic malignant syndrome or tardive dyskinesia. Hyperpyrexia, muscle rigidity, altered mental status, and autonomic instability are signs of neuroleptic malignant syndrome, which can be fatal. Perform abnormal involuntary movement scale before initiating therapy, at dosage changes, and periodically thereafter to monitor patient for tardive dyskinesia.

• Symptoms may not improve for 4 to 6 weeks.

• Always give drug with food for optimal effect.

• Don't use drug in breast-feeding patients.

PATIENT TEACHING

• Tell patient to take drug with food.

• Tell patient to immediately report to prescriber signs or symptoms of dizziness, fainting, irregular heartbeat, or relevant cardiac problems.

• Advise patient to also report any recent episodes of diarrhea, abnormal movements, sudden fever, muscle rigidity, or change in mental status.

amphetamine sulfate
caffeine
dextroamphetamine sulfate
doxapram hydrochloride
methamphetamine hydrochloride
methylphenidate hydrochloride
modafinil
pemoline
phentermine hydrochloride

COMBINATION PRODUCTS

ADDERALL 5 MG: amphetamine aspartate 1.25 mg, amphetamine sulfate 1.25 mg, dextroamphetamine saccharate 1.25 mg, dextroamphetamine sulfate 1.25 mg, total amphetamine base equivalence 3.13 mg.

ADDERALL 10 MG: amphetamine aspartate 2.5 mg, amphetamine sulfate 2.5 mg, dextroamphetamine saccharate 2.5 mg, dextroamphetamine sulfate 2.5 mg, total amphetamine base equivalence 6.3 mg.

ADDERALL 20 MG: amphetamine aspartate 5 mg, amphetamine sulfate 5 mg, dextroamphetamine saccharate 5 mg, dextroamphetamine sulfate 5 mg, total amphetamine base equivalence 12.6 mg.

ADDERALL 30 MG: amphetamine aspartate 7.5 mg, amphetamine sulfate 7.5 mg, dextroamphetamine saccharate 7.5 mg, dextroamphetamine sulfate 7.5 mg, total amphetamine base equivalence 18.8 mg.

ADDERALL XR 10 mg: dextroamphetamine saccharate 2.5 mg, amphetamine aspartate monohydrate 2.5 mg, dextroamphetamine sulfate USP 2.5 mg, amphetamine sulfate USP 2.5 mg. Total amphetamine equivalence 6.3 mg.

ADDERALL XR 20 mg: dextroamphetamine saccharate 5 mg, amphetamine aspartate monohydrate 5 mg, dextroamphetamine sulfate USP 5 mg, amphetamine sulfate USP 5 mg. Total amphetamine equivalence 12.5 mg.

ADDERALL XR 30 mg: dextroamphetamine saccharate 7.5 mg, amphetamine aspartate monohydrate 7.5 mg, dextroamphetamine sulfate USP 7.5 mg, amphetamine sulfate USP 7.5 mg. Total amphetamine equivalence 18.8 mg.

amphetamine sulfate

Pregnancy risk category C
Controlled substance schedule II

AVAILABLE FORMS
Tablets: 5 mg, 10 mg

INDICATIONS & DOSAGES
➤ **Attention deficit hyperactivity disorder—**
Children ages 3 to 5: 2.5 mg P.O. daily, with dosage increases in 2.5-mg increments weekly, p.r.n.
Children age 6 and older: 5 mg P.O. daily to b.i.d., with dosage increases in 5-mg increments weekly, p.r.n. Give first dose on awakening; additional doses (one or two) given at intervals of 4 to 6 hours. Dosage rarely exceeds 40 mg/day.
➤ **Narcolepsy—**
Adults and children age 12 and older: 10 mg P.O. daily. Increase dosage in 10-mg increments weekly, p.r.n. Daily dosage may be divided, with first dose given on awakening; additional doses given at intervals of 4 to 6 hours.
Children ages 6 to 12: 5 mg P.O. daily. Increase dosage in 5-mg increments weekly, p.r.n. Daily dosage may be divided, with first dose given on awakening; additional doses given at intervals of 4 to 6 hours.
➤ **Short-term adjunct in exogenous obesity—**
Adults: 5 to 30 mg P.O. daily in divided doses 30 to 60 minutes before meals.

ACTION
Unknown. Probably promotes nerve impulse transmission by releasing stored norepinephrine from nerve terminals in the brain. Main sites of activity appear to be the cerebral cortex and the reticular activating system.

Route	Onset	Peak	Duration
P.O.	Unknown	Unknown	Unknown

---

*Liquid contains alcohol.   **May contain tartrazine.   †Canada   ‡Australia   §U.K.   ◇OTC

ADVERSE REACTIONS
CNS: *restlessness,* tremor, *hyperactivity, talkativeness, insomnia,* irritability, dizziness, headache, chills, dysphoria, euphoria, *nervousness.*
CV: *tachycardia, palpitations,* hypertension, **arrhythmias.**
GI: dry mouth, metallic taste, diarrhea, constipation, anorexia.
GU: impotence.
Metabolic: weight loss.
Skin: urticaria.
Other: increased libido.

INTERACTIONS
Drug-drug. *Acetazolamide, antacids, sodium bicarbonate:* Increased renal reabsorption. Watch for enhanced effect.
Ammonium chloride, ascorbic acid: Decreased levels and increased renal excretion of amphetamine. Monitor patient for decreased amphetamine effect.
Antihypertensives: Reversal of antihypertensive action. Monitor blood pressure.
Haloperidol, phenothiazines, TCAs: Altered CNS effect. Avoid using together.
Insulin, oral antidiabetics: May decrease antidiabetic requirements. Monitor glucose level.
MAO inhibitors: May cause severe hypertension or hypertensive crisis. Don't use together or within 14 days of MAO inhibitor therapy.
Drug-food. *Caffeine:* May increase amphetamine and related amine effects. Discourage use together.

EFFECTS ON LAB TEST RESULTS
• May increase plasma corticosteroid levels.

CONTRAINDICATIONS
Contraindicated in patients who are hypersensitive to sympathomimetic amines or have idiosyncratic reactions to them, in agitated patients, and in those with symptomatic CV disease, hyperthyroidism, moderate to severe hypertension, glaucoma, advanced arteriosclerosis, or history of drug abuse. Also contraindicated within 14 days of MAO inhibitor therapy.

NURSING CONSIDERATIONS
• Use cautiously in elderly, debilitated, or hyperexcitable patients and in those with psychopathic personalities or a history of suicidal or homicidal tendencies.
• Drug isn't recommended for first-line treatment of obesity or for treatment of obesity in children younger than age 12. Use as an anorexigenic is prohibited in some states.
• Drug shouldn't be used to combat fatigue.
• Obtain baseline ECG. Drug isn't recommended for patients with baseline arrhythmias.
• Obese patient should follow a weight-reduction program. Give drug 30 to 60 minutes before meals. Monitor dietary intake and count calories, if needed.
• If tolerance to anorexigenic effect develops, stop drug and notify prescriber.

PATIENT TEACHING
• To avoid sleep interference, tell patient to take drug at least 6 hours before bedtime.
• Warn patient to avoid activities that require alertness or good psychomotor coordination until CNS effects of drug are known.
• Tell patient to report signs and symptoms of excessive stimulation.
• Inform patient that fatigue may result as drug effects wear off.
• Advise patient to avoid caffeine while taking drug.
• Warn patient with seizure disorder that drug may decrease seizure threshold. Instruct him to notify prescriber if seizure occurs.

---

caffeine
Caffedrine Caplets ◇ , Dexitac ◇ ,
NoDoz ◇ , Quick Pep ◇ , Vivarin ◇

Pregnancy risk category C

AVAILABLE FORMS
Capsules (timed-release): 200 mg ◇
Injection: caffeine (250 mg/ml) with sodium benzoate (250 mg/ml)
Tablets: 100 mg ◇ , 150 mg ◇ , 200 mg ◇
Tablets (timed-release): 200 mg ◇

INDICATIONS & DOSAGES
➤ **CNS stimulant—**
Adults: 100 to 200 mg anhydrous caffeine P.O. q 3 to 4 hours, p.r.n. Or, 500 mg to

1 g I.M. or slow I.V. Total daily dose should seldom exceed 2.5 g.

I.V. ADMINISTRATION
• Caffeine may be given I.V. in emergencies.
• Caffeine citrate may be given by slow I.V. infusion using a syringe infusion pump.
• Caffeine and sodium benzoate may be given by slow I.V. injection.

ACTION
Inhibits phosphodiesterase, the enzyme that degrades cAMP.

Route	Onset	Peak	Duration
I.M., I.V.	Unknown	Unknown	Unknown
P.O.	Unknown	50-75 min	Unknown

ADVERSE REACTIONS
CNS: *insomnia,* restlessness, *nervousness,* headache, excitement, agitation, muscle tremor, twitching.
CV: *tachycardia, palpitations,* extrasystoles.
EENT: tinnitus.
GI: nausea, vomiting, diarrhea, stomach pain.
GU: *diuresis.*

INTERACTIONS
Drug-drug. *Beta-adrenergic agonists, cimetidine, fluoroquinolones, oral contraceptives, theophylline:* Excessive CNS stimulation. Avoid using together.
Drug-herb. *Ephedra:* Increased CNS effects. Discourage use together.
Drug-food. *Caffeine-containing beverages:* Excessive CNS stimulation. Advise patient to use cautiously.

EFFECTS ON LAB TEST RESULTS
• May increase glucose levels.

CONTRAINDICATIONS
Contraindicated in patients hypersensitive to drug.

NURSING CONSIDERATIONS
• Use cautiously in patients with history of peptic ulcer, symptomatic arrhythmias, or palpitations. Also use cautiously during the first several days to weeks after an acute MI.

• Caffeine doesn't reverse alcohol intoxication or CNS depressant effects of alcohol. Overly vigorous therapy with caffeine may aggravate depression in an already depressed patient.
• Caffeine may increase glucose levels and cause false-positive urate levels; it also may cause false-positive test results for pheochromocytoma or neuroblastoma by increasing urinary catecholamines.
• **Alert:** A single dose shouldn't exceed 1 g. High doses are related to decreased seizure threshold.
• Watch for signs and symptoms of overdose, such as GI pain, mild delirium, insomnia, diuresis, dehydration, and fever. Treat with short-acting barbiturates, gastric emesis, or lavage, as directed.
• Monitor patient for tolerance or psychological dependence.
• After abrupt withdrawal, sudden headache and irritability may occur.

PATIENT TEACHING
• Stress importance of not exceeding recommended dosage.
• Instruct patient to stop taking caffeine if increased or abnormal heart rate, dizziness, or palpitations occur.
• Inform patient that caffeine isn't a substitute for sleep.
• Advise patient to minimize use of caffeine-containing beverages while taking drug.
• Tell patient to take drug at least 6 hours before bedtime to avoid sleep interference.
• Warn patient with seizure disorder that drug may decrease seizure threshold. Urge him to notify prescriber if seizure occurs.

dextroamphetamine sulfate
Dexedrine* **, Dexedrine Spansule

Pregnancy risk category C
Controlled substance schedule II

AVAILABLE FORMS
Capsules (extended-release): 5 mg, 10 mg, 15 mg
Tablets: 5 mg, 10 mg

INDICATIONS & DOSAGES
➤ **Narcolepsy—**
Adults: 5 to 60 mg P.O. daily in divided doses.
Children ages 6 to 12: 5 mg P.O. daily. Increase dosage in 5-mg increments weekly, p.r.n.
Children age 12 and older: 10 mg P.O. daily. Increase dosage in 10-mg increments weekly, p.r.n. Give first dose on awakening; additional doses (one or two) given at intervals of 4 to 6 hours.
➤ **Short-term adjunct in exogenous obesity—**
Adults and children age 12 and older: 5 to 30 mg P.O. daily 30 to 60 minutes before meals in divided doses of 5 to 10 mg. Or, one 10- or 15-mg extended-release capsule daily as a single dose in the morning.
➤ **Attention deficit hyperactivity disorder—**
Children ages 3 to 5: 2.5 mg P.O. daily. Increase dosage in 2.5-mg increments weekly, p.r.n.
Children age 6 and older: 5 mg P.O. once daily or b.i.d. Increase dosage in 5-mg increments weekly, p.r.n. Only rarely is it necessary to exceed 40 mg/day.

ACTION
Unknown. Probably promotes nerve impulse transmission by releasing stored norepinephrine from nerve terminals in the brain. Main sites of activity appear to be the cerebral cortex and the reticular activating system. In children with hyperkinesis, dextroamphetamine has a paradoxical calming effect.

Route	Onset	Peak	Duration
P.O.	Unknown	2 hr	Unknown
P.O. (extended)	Unknown	8-10 hr	Unknown

ADVERSE REACTIONS
CNS: *restlessness,* tremor, *insomnia,* dizziness, headache, chills, overstimulation, dysphoria, euphoria, *nervousness.*
CV: *tachycardia, palpitations,* hypertension, ***arrhythmias.***
GI: dry mouth, unpleasant taste, diarrhea, constipation, anorexia, other GI disturbances.
GU: impotence.

Metabolic: weight loss.
Skin: urticaria.
Other: increased libido.

INTERACTIONS
Drug-drug. *Acetazolamide, alkalizing drugs, antacids, sodium bicarbonate:* Increased renal reabsorption. Monitor patient for enhanced amphetamine effects.
Acidifying drugs, ammonium chloride, ascorbic acid: Decreased blood levels and increased renal clearance of dextroamphetamine. Monitor patient for decreased amphetamine effects.
Adrenergic blockers: Inhibited by amphetamines. Avoid using together.
Chlorpromazine: Inhibits central stimulant effects of amphetamines. Can be used to treat amphetamine poisoning.
Haloperidol, phenothiazines, TCAs: Increased CNS effects. Avoid using together.
Insulin, oral antidiabetics: May decrease antidiabetic requirements. Monitor glucose levels.
Lithium carbonate: May inhibit antiobesity and stimulating effects of amphetamines. Monitor patient closely.
MAO inhibitors: May cause severe hypertension, possibly hypertensive crisis. Don't use together or within 14 days of MAO inhibitor therapy.
Meperidine: Amphetamines potentiate analgesic effect. Use together cautiously.
Methenamine: Increased urinary excretion of amphetamines and reduced efficacy. Monitor effects.
Norepinephrine: Enhanced adrenergic effect of norepinephrine. Monitor patient.
Phenobarbital, phenytoin: Amphetamines may delay absorption of these drugs. Monitor patient closely.
Drug-food. *Caffeine:* May increase amphetamine and related amine effects. Advise patient to use together cautiously.

EFFECTS ON LAB TEST RESULTS
● May increase plasma corticosteroid levels.

CONTRAINDICATIONS
Contraindicated in patients hypersensitive to sympathomimetic amines, in those with idiosyncratic reactions to them, and in those with hyperthyroidism, moderate to

---

severe hypertension, symptomatic CV disease, glaucoma, advanced arteriosclerosis, or history of drug abuse. Also contraindicated within 14 days of MAO inhibitor therapy.

NURSING CONSIDERATIONS
• Use cautiously in agitated patients and patients with motor tics, phonic tics, or Tourette syndrome.
• Drug isn't recommended for first-line treatment of obesity. Use as an anorexigenic is prohibited in some states.
• Drug shouldn't be used to prevent fatigue.
• Obese patient should follow a weight-reduction program.
• Drug may cause dependence.
• *Alert:* Overdose may cause seizures.
• If tolerance to anorexigenic effect develops, stop drug and notify prescriber.
• *Alert:* Don't confuse Dexedrine with dextran or Excedrin.

PATIENT TEACHING
• Tell patient to take drug 30 to 60 minutes before meals if used for weight reduction and at least 6 hours before bedtime to avoid sleep interference.
• Warn patient to avoid activities that require alertness or good psychomotor coordination until CNS effects of drug are known.
• Tell patient that fatigue may result as drug effects wear off.
• Ask patient to report signs and symptoms of excessive stimulation.
• Advise patient to consume caffeine-containing products cautiously.
• Warn patient with seizure disorder that drug may decrease seizure threshold. Instruct him to notify prescriber if seizure occurs.

---

doxapram hydrochloride
Dopram

Pregnancy risk category B

AVAILABLE FORMS
Injection: 20 mg/ml (benzyl alcohol 0.9%)

INDICATIONS & DOSAGES
➤ **Postanesthesia respiratory stimulation—**
Adults: 0.5 to 1 mg/kg as a single I.V. injection (not to exceed 1.5 mg/kg) or as multiple injections q 5 minutes, total not to exceed 2 mg/kg. Or, 250 mg in 250 ml of normal saline solution or D₅W infused at initial rate of 5 mg/minute I.V. until satisfactory response is achieved. Maintain at 1 to 3 mg/minute. Recommended total dose for infusion shouldn't exceed 4 mg/kg.
➤ **Drug-induced CNS depression—**
Adults: For injection, priming dose of 2 mg/kg I.V., repeated in 5 minutes and again q 1 to 2 hours until patient awakens (and if relapse occurs). Maximum daily dose is 3 g.

For infusion, priming dose of 2 mg/kg I.V., repeated in 5 minutes and again in 1 to 2 hours, if needed. If response occurs, give I.V. infusion (1 mg/ml) at 1 to 3 mg/minute until patient awakens. Don't infuse for longer than 2 hours or give more than 3 g/day. May resume I.V. infusion after rest period of 30 minutes to 2 hours, if needed.
➤ **Chronic pulmonary disease related to acute hypercapnia—**
Adults: 1 to 2 mg/minute by I.V. infusion using 2 mg/ml solution. Maximum, 3 mg/minute for a maximum duration of 2 hours.

I.V. ADMINISTRATION
• Give slowly; rapid infusion may cause hemolysis. Doxapram is physically incompatible with strongly alkaline drugs, such as thiopental sodium, aminophylline, and sodium bicarbonate. Drug is compatible with D₅W, dextrose 10% in water, and normal saline solution.
• Avoid extravasation, which may lead to thrombophlebitis and local skin irritation.

ACTION
Not clearly defined. Directly stimulates the central respiratory centers in the medulla and may indirectly act on carotid, aortic, or other peripheral chemoreceptors.

Route	Onset	Peak	Duration
I.V.	20-40 sec	1-2 min	5-12 min

ADVERSE REACTIONS
CNS: *seizures, headache, dizziness,* apprehension, disorientation, hyperactivity, bilateral Babinski's signs, paresthesia.
CV: *chest pain and tightness, variations in heart rate, hypertension, arrhythmias,* T-wave depression on ECG, flushing.
EENT: sneezing, *laryngospasm.*
GI: nausea, vomiting, diarrhea.
GU: urine retention, bladder stimulation with incontinence, albuminuria.
Musculoskeletal: muscle spasms.
Respiratory: cough, *bronchospasm,* dyspnea, rebound hypoventilation, hiccups.
Skin: pruritus, diaphoresis.

INTERACTIONS
Drug-drug. *General anesthetics:* Risk of self-limiting arrhythmias. Don't give doxapram within 10 minutes of an anesthetic known to sensitize the myocardium to catecholamines.
MAO inhibitors, sympathomimetics: Potentiated adverse CV effects. Use together cautiously.

EFFECTS ON LAB TEST RESULTS
● May increase BUN levels.
● May decrease hemoglobin, hematocrit, and erythrocyte, WBC, and RBC counts.

CONTRAINDICATIONS
Contraindicated in patients with seizure disorders; head injury; CV disorders; frank, uncompensated heart failure; severe hypertension; CVA; respiratory failure or incompetence secondary to neuromuscular disorders, muscle paresis, flail chest, obstructed airway, pulmonary embolism, pneumothorax, restrictive respiratory disease, acute bronchial asthma, or extreme dyspnea; or hypoxia not related to hypercapnia.

NURSING CONSIDERATIONS
● Use cautiously in patients with bronchial asthma, severe tachycardia or arrhythmias, cerebral edema, increased intracranial pressure, hyperthyroidism, pheochromocytoma, or metabolic disorders.
● Drug is used only in surgical or emergency department situations.
● Separate discontinuation of anesthetics and start of doxapram by at least 10 minutes.

● **Alert:** Establish an adequate airway before giving drug. Prevent patient from aspirating vomitus by placing him on his side.
● Monitor blood pressure, heart rate, deep tendon reflexes, and arterial blood gases before giving drug and every 30 minutes afterward.
● Monitor patient for evidence of overdose, such as hypertension, tachycardia, arrhythmias, skeletal muscle hyperactivity, and dyspnea. Hold drug and notify prescriber if patient needs mechanical ventilation or shows signs of increased arterial carbon dioxide or oxygen tension.
● **Alert:** Don't confuse doxapram with doxorubicin, doxepin, doxacurium, or doxazosin.

PATIENT TEACHING
● Inform family and patient, if alert, about patient's need for drug.
● Answer patient's questions and address his concerns.

---

methamphetamine hydrochloride
Desoxyn, Desoxyn Gradumet

Pregnancy risk category C
Controlled substance schedule II

AVAILABLE FORMS
Tablets: 5 mg
Tablets (extended-release): 5 mg, 10 mg, 15 mg**

INDICATIONS & DOSAGES
➤ **Attention deficit hyperactivity disorder—**
Children age 6 and older: 2.5 to 5 mg P.O. once daily or b.i.d. Increase dosage by 5-mg increments weekly, p.r.n. Usual effective dose is 20 to 25 mg daily.
➤ **Short-term adjunct in exogenous obesity—**
Adults: 2.5 to 5 mg P.O. b.i.d. or t.i.d. 30 minutes before meals. Or, 10- to 15-mg long-acting tablet daily before breakfast.

ACTION
Unknown. Probably promotes nerve impulse transmission by releasing stored norepinephrine from nerve terminals in

---

Reactions may be *common*, uncommon, *life-threatening*, or COMMON AND LIFE-THREATENING.

the brain. Main sites of activity appear to be the cerebral cortex and the reticular activating system. In children with hyperkinesis, methamphetamine has a paradoxical calming effect.

Route	Onset	Peak	Duration
P.O.	Unknown	Unknown	24 hr

ADVERSE REACTIONS
CNS: *nervousness, insomnia,* irritability, *talkativeness,* dizziness, headache, hyperexcitability, tremor, euphoria.
CV: hypertension, *tachycardia, palpitations,* **arrhythmias.**
EENT: blurred vision, mydriasis.
GI: dry mouth, metallic taste, diarrhea, constipation, anorexia.
GU: impotence.
Skin: urticaria.
Other: increased libido.

INTERACTIONS
Drug-drug. *Acetazolamide, antacids, sodium bicarbonate:* Increased renal reabsorption. Monitor patient for enhanced effects.
Ammonium chloride, ascorbic acid: Decreased levels and increased renal excretion of methamphetamine. Monitor patient for decreased methamphetamine effects.
Haloperidol, phenothiazines, TCAs: Altered CNS effects. Avoid using together.
Insulin, oral antidiabetics: May decrease antidiabetic requirements. Monitor glucose levels.
MAO inhibitors: May cause severe hypertension, possibly hypertensive crisis. Don't use together or within 14 days of MAO inhibitor therapy.
Drug-herb. *Melatonin:* Enhanced monoaminergic effects of methamphetamine; may worsen insomnia. Discourage use together.
Drug-food. *Caffeine-containing beverages:* May increase amphetamine and related amine effects. Discourage use together.

EFFECTS ON LAB TEST RESULTS
• May increase plasma corticosteroid levels.

CONTRAINDICATIONS
Contraindicated in patients hypersensitive to sympathomimetic amines, in those with idiosyncratic reactions to them, in agitated patients, and in those with moderate to severe hypertension, hyperthyroidism, symptomatic CV disease, advanced arteriosclerosis, glaucoma, or history of drug abuse. Also contraindicated within 14 days of MAO inhibitor therapy.

NURSING CONSIDERATIONS
• Use cautiously in patients with a history of suicidal or homicidal tendencies and in those who are elderly, debilitated, asthenic, or psychopathic.
• Drug isn't recommended for first-line treatment of obesity. Use as an anorexigenic is prohibited in some states.
• When used for obesity, make sure patient is on a weight-reduction program.
• Monitor patient for tolerance or dependence.
• *Alert:* Don't confuse Desoxyn with digitoxin or digoxin.

PATIENT TEACHING
• Tell patient to take drug at least 6 hours before bedtime to avoid sleep interference.
• Warn patient about high risk of abuse. Advise him that drug shouldn't be used to prevent fatigue.
• If tolerance to anorexigenic effect develops, notify prescriber because drug will need to be discontinued.
• Tell patient never to crush extended-release tablets.
• Warn patient to avoid activities that require alertness or good psychomotor coordination until CNS effects of drug are known.
• Tell patient to avoid caffeine-containing products, which increase the effects of amphetamines and related amines. Ask him to report evidence of excessive stimulation.
• Warn patient with seizure disorder that drug may decrease seizure threshold. Urge him to notify prescriber if seizure occurs.

methylphenidate hydrochloride
Concerta, Metadate CD,
Metadate ER, Methylin ER,
PMS Methylphenidate†, Ritalin,
Ritalin-SR

Pregnancy risk category NR (C for Concerta and Metadate CD)
Controlled substance schedule II

AVAILABLE FORMS
Capsules (extended-release): 20 mg
Tablets: 5 mg, 10 mg, 20 mg
Tablets (extended-release): 10 mg, 18 mg, 20 mg, 36 mg, 54 mg
Tablets (sustained-release): 20 mg

INDICATIONS AND DOSAGES
➤ **Attention deficit hyperactivity disorder (Metadate, Methylin, Ritalin)—**
Children age 6 and older: Initially, 5 mg P.O. daily before breakfast and lunch, increased in 5- to 10-mg increments weekly, p.r.n., until an optimum daily dose of 2 mg/kg is reached, not to exceed 60 mg daily.
➤ **Attention deficit hyperactivity disorder (Concerta)—**
Children age 6 and older who aren't taking methylphenidate or are taking stimulants other than methylphenidate: 18 mg P.O. (extended-release) once daily in the morning. Adjust dosage by 18 mg at weekly intervals to a maximum of 54 mg daily taken once daily in the morning.
Children age 6 and older who are taking methylphenidate: If the previous methylphenidate daily dose was 5 mg b.i.d. or t.i.d., or 20 mg sustained release, the recommended dose of Concerta is 18 mg P.O. q morning. If the previous methylphenidate daily dose was 10 mg b.i.d. or t.i.d., or 40 mg sustained release, the recommended dose of Concerta is 36 mg P.O. every morning. If the previous methylphenidate daily dose is 15 mg b.i.d. or t.i.d. or 60 mg sustained release, the recommended dose of Concerta is 54 mg P.O. every morning. Maximum daily dose is 54 mg.
➤ **Attention deficit hyperactivity disorder (Metadate CD)—**
Children age 6 and older: 20 mg P.O. once daily before breakfast, increased in

20-mg increments weekly to a maximum of 60 mg/day.
➤ **Narcolepsy (Methylin, Ritalin)—**
Adults: 10 mg P.O. b.i.d. or t.i.d. 30 to 45 minutes before meals. Dosage varies with patient needs; average dose is 40 to 60 mg daily.

When using sustained-release tablets, calculate regular dose in q 8-hour intervals and give as such.

ACTION
Unknown. Probably promotes nerve impulse transmission by releasing stored norepinephrine from nerve terminals in the brain. Main site of activity appears to be the cerebral cortex and the reticular activating system. In children with hyperkinesis, methylphenidate has a paradoxical calming effect.

Route	Onset	Peak	Duration
P.O.	Unknown	2-5 hr	Unknown

ADVERSE REACTIONS
CNS: *nervousness, insomnia,* Tourette syndrome, dizziness, *headache,* akathisia, dyskinesia, *seizures,* drowsiness.
CV: *palpitations,* angina, *tachycardia,* changes in blood pressure and heart rate, *arrhythmias.*
EENT: pharyngitis, sinusitis.
GI: nausea, abdominal pain, anorexia, vomiting.
Hematologic: *thrombocytopenia, thrombocytopenic purpura, leukopenia,* anemia.
Metabolic: weight loss.
Respiratory: cough, upper respiratory tract infection.
Skin: rash, urticaria, *exfoliative dermatitis, erythema multiforme.*

INTERACTIONS
Drug-drug. *Centrally acting antihypertensives:* Decreased antihypertensive effect. Monitor blood pressure.
Coumarin anticoagulants, anticonvulsants (such as phenobarbital, phenytoin, primidone), and some antidepressants (selective serotonin reuptake inhibitors and TCAs): May inhibit the metabolism of these drugs. May need to reduce dosage of these drugs when given together with methylphenidate.

MAO inhibitors: May cause severe hypertension, possibly hypertensive crisis. Don't use together or within 14 days of MAO inhibitor therapy.

TCAs: Increased levels of these drugs. Avoid using together.

Drug-food. *Beverages containing caffeine:* May increase amphetamine and related amine effects. Discourage use together.

EFFECTS ON LAB TEST RESULTS
• May decrease hemoglobin and platelet and WBC counts.

CONTRAINDICATIONS
Contraindicated in patients hypersensitive to drug and in those with glaucoma, motor tics, family history or diagnosis of Tourette syndrome, or history of marked anxiety, tension, or agitation. Also contraindicated in patients with severe GI narrowing (such as small bowel inflammatory disease, short-gut syndrome caused by adhesions or decreased transit time, history of peritonitis, cystic fibrosis, chronic intestinal pseudoobstruction, or Meckel's diverticulum) and during and for 2 weeks after treatment with an MAO inhibitor.

NURSING CONSIDERATIONS
• Use cautiously in patients with a history of seizures, EEG abnormalities, or hypertension, and in patients whose underlying medical conditions might be compromised by increases in blood pressure or heart rate, such as those with preexisting hypertension, heart failure, recent MI, or hyperthyroidism. Also use cautiously in patients who are emotionally unstable or have a history of drug dependence or alcoholism.
• Don't use drug to prevent fatigue or to treat severe depression.
• Drug may precipitate Tourette syndrome in children. Monitor patient, especially at start of therapy.
• Observe patient for signs of excessive stimulation. Monitor blood pressure.
• Monitor results of periodic CBC, differential, and platelet counts with long-term use.
• Monitor height and weight in children on long-term therapy. Drug may delay growth spurt, but children will attain normal height when drug is stopped.

• Monitor patient for tolerance or psychological dependence.
• *Alert:* Don't confuse Ritalin with Rifadin.

PATIENT TEACHING
• Tell patient to take drug at least 6 hours before bedtime to prevent insomnia and after meals to reduce appetite-suppressant effects.
• Warn patient against chewing sustained-release tablets.
• Caution patient to avoid activities that require alertness or good psychomotor coordination until CNS effects of drug are known.
• Warn patient with seizure disorder that drug may decrease seizure threshold. Urge him to notify prescriber if seizure occurs.
• Inform patient that he'll need more rest as drug effects wear off.
• Advise patient to avoid caffeine-containing beverages while taking drug.

---

modafinil
Provigil

Pregnancy risk category C
Controlled substance schedule IV

AVAILABLE FORMS
Tablets: 100 mg, 200 mg

INDICATIONS & DOSAGES
➤ **Improvement of wakefulness in patients with excessive daytime sleepiness and narcolepsy—**
Adults: 200 mg P.O. daily, given as a single dose in the morning.
Adjust-a-dose: In patients with severe hepatic impairment, 100 mg P.O. daily, given as a single dose in the morning.

ACTION
Unknown. Drug's wake-promoting actions are similar to those of sympathomimetics, including amphetamines, but drug is structurally distinct from amphetamines and doesn't appear to alter release of either dopamine or norepinephrine to produce CNS stimulation.

Route	Onset	Peak	Duration
P.O.	Unknown	2-4 hr	Unknown

ADVERSE REACTIONS
CNS: *headache, nervousness, dizziness,* depression, anxiety, cataplexy, *insomnia,* paresthesia, dyskinesia, hypertonia, confusion, syncope, amnesia, emotional lability, ataxia, tremor.
CV: hypotension, hypertension, vasodilation, *arrhythmias,* chest pain.
EENT: *rhinitis,* pharyngitis, epistaxis, amblyopia, abnormal vision.
GI: *nausea,* diarrhea, dry mouth, anorexia, vomiting, mouth ulcer, gingivitis, thirst.
GU: abnormal urine, urine retention, abnormal ejaculation, albuminuria.
Hematologic: eosinophilia.
Metabolic: hyperglycemia.
Musculoskeletal: joint disorder, neck pain, neck rigidity.
Respiratory: lung disorder, dyspnea, asthma.
Skin: dry skin.
Other: herpes simplex, chills, fever.

INTERACTIONS
Drug-drug. *Carbamazepine, phenobarbital, rifampin, and other inducers of CYP3A4:* Altered levels of modafinil. Monitor patient closely.
Cyclosporine, theophylline: Reduced levels of these drugs. Use together cautiously.
Diazepam, phenytoin, propranolol, and other drugs metabolized by CYP2C19: Modafinil is a reversible inhibitor of cytochrome P-450 isoenzyme CYP2C19 and thus may lead to increases in levels of drugs metabolized by this enzyme. Use together cautiously; adjust dosage, as needed.
Hormonal contraceptives: Reduced contraceptive effectiveness. Recommend alternative or additional method of contraception during modafinil therapy and for 1 month after drug is discontinued.
Itraconazole, ketoconazole, other inhibitors of CYP3A4: Altered levels of modafinil. Monitor patient closely.
Methylphenidate: One-hour delay in absorption of modafinil when given together. Separate administration times.
Phenytoin, warfarin: Level-dependent inhibition of CYP2C9 activity and increased levels of phenytoin and warfarin. Monitor patient closely for signs of toxicity.

TCAs (such as clomipramine, desipramine): Increased TCA levels. Reduce dosage of these drugs, as needed.

EFFECTS ON LAB TEST RESULTS
• May increase glucose, GGT, and AST levels.
• May increase eosinophil count.

CONTRAINDICATIONS
Contraindicated in patients hypersensitive to drug and in those with a history of left ventricular hypertrophy or ischemic ECG changes, chest pain, arrhythmias, or other evidence of mitral valve prolapse linked to CNS stimulant use.

NURSING CONSIDERATIONS
• Use cautiously in patients with recent MI or unstable angina and in those with history of psychosis. Use cautiously and give reduced dosage to patients with severe hepatic impairment, with or without cirrhosis. Also, use cautiously in patients taking MAO inhibitors.
• Safety and efficacy in patients with severe renal impairment haven't been determined.
• Monitor hypertensive patients closely.
• Although single, daily, 400-mg doses have been well tolerated, the larger dose offers no additional benefit beyond that of the 200-mg dose.
• Food has no effect on overall bioavailability, although it may delay absorption of drug by 1 hour.

PATIENT TEACHING
• Advise woman to notify prescriber about planned, suspected, or known pregnancy or if she's breast-feeding.
• Caution patient that use of hormonal contraceptives (including depot or implantable contraceptives) together with modafinil tablets may reduce contraceptive effectiveness. Recommend an alternative method of contraception during modafinil therapy and for 1 month after drug is discontinued.
• Instruct patient to confer with prescriber before taking prescription or OTC drugs to avoid drug interactions.
• Tell patient to avoid alcohol while taking drug.

Reactions may be *common,* uncommon, *life-threatening,* or COMMON AND LIFE-THREATENING.

• Tell patient to notify prescriber if rash, hives, or related allergic reaction develops.
• Warn patient to avoid activities that require alertness or good psychomotor coordination until CNS effects of drug are known.

pemoline
Cylert, Cylert Chewable

Pregnancy risk category B
Controlled substance schedule IV

AVAILABLE FORMS
Tablets: 18.75 mg, 37.5 mg, 75 mg
Tablets (chewable): 37.5 mg

INDICATIONS & DOSAGES
➤ **Attention deficit hyperactivity disorder—**
Children age 6 and older: Initially, 37.5 mg P.O. in the morning, with daily dose raised by 18.75 mg weekly, p.r.n. Usual effective dose is 56.25 to 75 mg daily; maximum is 112.5 mg daily.

ACTION
Unknown. Probably promotes nerve impulse transmission by releasing stored norepinephrine from nerve terminals in the brain. Main sites of activity appear to be the cerebral cortex and the reticular activating system.

Route	Onset	Peak	Duration
P.O.	Unknown	2-4 hr	Unknown

ADVERSE REACTIONS
CNS: *insomnia,* dyskinetic movements, irritability, fatigue, mild depression, dizziness, headache, drowsiness, hallucinations, **seizures,** *Tourette syndrome,* abnormal oculomotor function.
CV: tachycardia.
GI: anorexia, abdominal pain, nausea.
GU: prostatic enlargement.
Hematologic: *aplastic anemia.*
Hepatic: *acute hepatic failure, hepatitis,* jaundice.
Skin: rash.

INTERACTIONS
Drug-drug. *CNS stimulants:* Increased CNS effects. Monitor patient closely.

Insulin, oral antidiabetics: May decrease antidiabetic requirements. Monitor glucose levels.

EFFECTS ON LAB TEST RESULTS
• May increase liver enzyme and prostate-specific antigen levels.
• May decrease hemoglobin.

CONTRAINDICATIONS
Contraindicated in patients hypersensitive to drug, in those with idiosyncratic reactions to drug, and in those with hepatic dysfunction.

NURSING CONSIDERATIONS
• Use cautiously in patients with renal impairment.
• Obtain liver function tests before starting and periodically during therapy; however, they may not predict onset of acute hepatic failure. Treatment should be started only in patients without hepatic disease and with normal baseline liver function test results.
• Closely monitor patients on long-term therapy for possible blood or hepatic function abnormalities and for growth suppression.
• **Alert:** Discontinue drug if patient experiences significant hepatic dysfunction during therapy.
• Drug is structurally dissimilar to amphetamines or methylphenidate; however, it may produce similar adverse reactions. Drug has greater risk of abuse and dependence than previously thought.
• Drug may precipitate Tourette syndrome in children. Monitor patient, especially at start of therapy.
• **Alert:** Don't confuse pemoline with Pelamine.

PATIENT TEACHING
• Tell patient to take drug at least 6 hours before bedtime to avoid sleep interference.
• Tell patient to avoid activities that require alertness or good psychomotor coordination until CNS effects of drug are known.
• Warn patient with seizure disorder that drug may decrease seizure threshold. Urge him to notify prescriber if seizure occurs.

phentermine hydrochloride
Adipex-P, Duromine‡, Fastin,
Ionamin, Obe-Nix, Phentercot,
Phentride

Pregnancy risk category NR
Controlled substance schedule IV

AVAILABLE FORMS
Capsules: 15 mg, 18.75 mg, 30 mg,
37.5 mg
Capsules (resin complex, sustained-release): 15 mg, 30 mg
Tablets: 8 mg, 30 mg, 37.5 mg

INDICATIONS & DOSAGES
➤ **Short-term adjunct in exogenous obesity—**
Adults: 8 mg P.O. t.i.d. 30 minutes before meals. Or, 15 to 37.5 mg or 15 to 30 mg (as resin complex) P.O. daily as a single dose in the morning.

ACTION
Unknown. Drug probably promotes nerve impulse transmission by releasing stored norepinephrine from nerve terminals in the brain. Main sites of activity appear to be the cerebral cortex and the reticular activating system.

Route	Onset	Peak	Duration
P.O.	Unknown	Unknown	12-14 hr

ADVERSE REACTIONS
CNS: overstimulation, headache, euphoria, dysphoria, dizziness, *insomnia.*
CV: *palpitations, tachycardia,* increased blood pressure.
GI: dry mouth, dysgeusia, constipation, diarrhea, unpleasant taste, other GI disturbances.
GU: impotence.
Skin: urticaria.
Other: altered libido.

INTERACTIONS
Drug-drug. *Acetazolamide, antacids, sodium bicarbonate:* Increased renal reabsorption. Monitor patient for enhanced effects.
Ammonium chloride, ascorbic acid: Decreased levels and increased renal excre-

tion of phentermine. Monitor patient for decreased phentermine effects.
Haloperidol, phenothiazines, TCAs: Altered CNS effects. Avoid using together.
Insulin, oral antidiabetics: May alter antidiabetic requirements. Monitor glucose levels.
MAO inhibitors: May cause severe hypertension, possibly hypertensive crisis. Don't use together or within 14 days of MAO inhibitor therapy.
Drug-food. *Caffeine:* May increase CNS stimulation. Discourage use together.

EFFECTS ON LAB TEST RESULTS
None reported.

CONTRAINDICATIONS
Contraindicated in patients hypersensitive to sympathomimetic amines, in those with idiosyncratic reactions to them, in agitated patients, and in those with hyperthyroidism, moderate to severe hypertension, advanced arteriosclerosis, symptomatic CV disease, or glaucoma. Also contraindicated within 14 days of MAO inhibitor therapy.

NURSING CONSIDERATIONS
• Use cautiously in patients with mild hypertension.
• Use drug with a weight-reduction program.
• Monitor patient for tolerance or dependence.
• *Alert:* Don't confuse phentermine with phentolamine.

PATIENT TEACHING
• Tell patient to take drug at least 10 hours before bedtime to avoid sleep interference.
• Advise patient to avoid caffeine-containing products. Tell him to report evidence of excessive stimulation.
• Warn patient that fatigue may result as drug effects wear off and that he'll need more rest.
• Warn patient that drug may lose its effectiveness over time.

Reactions may be *common,* uncommon, *life-threatening,* or COMMON AND LIFE-THREATENING.

amantadine hydrochloride
(See Chapter 15, ANTIVIRALS.)
benztropine mesylate
bromocriptine mesylate
entacapone
levodopa
levodopa-carbidopa
pergolide mesylate
pramipexole dihydrochloride
ropinirole hydrochloride
selegiline hydrochloride
tolcapone
trihexyphenidyl hydrochloride

COMBINATION PRODUCTS
MADOPAR‡: levodopa 200 mg and benserazide 50 mg.
MADOPAR HBS‡: levodopa 100 mg and benserazide 25 mg.
MADOPAR Q‡: levodopa 50 mg and benserazide 12.5 mg.
SINEMET 10-100: carbidopa 10 mg and levodopa 100 mg.
SINEMET 25-100: carbidopa 25 mg and levodopa 100 mg.
SINEMET 25-250: carbidopa 25 mg and levodopa 250 mg.
SINEMET CR: carbidopa 50 mg and levodopa 200 mg, in extended-release tablets.

---

benztropine mesylate
Apo-Benztropine†, Cogentin, PMS Benztropine†

Pregnancy risk category NR

AVAILABLE FORMS
Injection: 1 mg/ml in 2-ml ampules
Tablets: 0.5 mg, 1 mg, 2 mg

INDICATIONS & DOSAGES
➤ **Drug-induced extrapyramidal disorders (except tardive dyskinesia)—**
Adults: 1 to 4 mg P.O. or I.M. once or twice daily.
➤ **Acute dystonic reaction—**
Adults: 1 to 2 mg I.V. or I.M.; then 1 to 2 mg P.O. b.i.d. to prevent recurrence.

➤ **Parkinsonism—**
Adults: 0.5 to 6 mg P.O. or I.M. daily. Initial dose is 0.5 mg to 1 mg, increased by 0.5 mg q 5 to 6 days. Adjust dosage to meet individual requirements. Maximum, 6 mg daily.

I.V. ADMINISTRATION
● The I.V. route is seldom used because no clinically significant difference exists between it and the I.M. route.

ACTION
Unknown. May block central cholinergic receptors, helping to balance cholinergic activity in the basal ganglia.

Route	Onset	Peak	Duration
I.M., I.V.	15 min	Unknown	24 hr
P.O.	1-2 hr	Unknown	24 hr

ADVERSE REACTIONS
CNS: disorientation, hallucinations, depression, toxic psychosis, confusion, memory impairment, nervousness, depression.
CV: tachycardia.
EENT: dilated pupils, blurred vision.
GI: *dry mouth, constipation,* nausea, vomiting, paralytic ileus.
GU: urine retention, dysuria.
Skin: decreased sweating.

INTERACTIONS
Drug-drug. *Phenothiazines, TCAs:* Additive anticholinergic adverse reactions, such as confusion and hallucinations. Reduce dosage before giving.
Drug-herb. *Jimsonweed:* May adversely affect CV function. Discourage use together.

EFFECTS ON LAB TEST RESULTS
None reported.

CONTRAINDICATIONS
Contraindicated in patients hypersensitive to drug or its components, in those with angle-closure glaucoma, and in children younger than age 3.

---

*Liquid contains alcohol.   **May contain tartrazine.   †Canada   ‡Australia   §U.K.   ◇OTC

NURSING CONSIDERATIONS

• Use cautiously in hot weather, in patients with mental disorders, and in children age 3 and older. Also, use cautiously in patients with prostatic hyperplasia, arrhythmias, and seizure disorders.
• Monitor vital signs carefully. Watch closely for adverse reactions, especially in elderly or debilitated patients. Call prescriber promptly if they occur.
• Some adverse reactions may result from atropine-like toxicity and are dose-related.
• Drug produces atropine-like adverse reactions and may aggravate tardive dyskinesia.
• Watch for intermittent constipation and abdominal distention and pain; these symptoms may indicate onset of paralytic ileus.
• *Alert:* Never stop drug abruptly. Reduce dosage gradually.
• *Alert:* Don't confuse benztropine with bromocriptine.

PATIENT TEACHING

• Warn patient to avoid activities that require alertness until CNS effects of drug are known.
• If patient takes a single daily dose, tell him to do so at bedtime.
• Advise patient to report signs and symptoms of urinary hesitancy or urine retention.
• Tell patient to relieve dry mouth with cool drinks, ice chips, sugarless gum, or hard candy.
• Advise patient to limit hot weather activities because drug-induced anhidrosis may cause hyperthermia.

---

bromocriptine mesylate
Parlodel

Pregnancy risk category B

AVAILABLE FORMS
Capsules: 5 mg
Tablets: 2.5 mg

INDICATIONS & DOSAGES
➤ **Parkinson's disease—**
Adults: 1.25 mg P.O. b.i.d. with meals. Dosage increased by 2.5 mg/day q 14 to 28 days, up to 100 mg daily.

➤ **Amenorrhea and galactorrhea from hyperprolactinemia; female infertility; macroprolactinoma—**
Adults: 1.25 to 2.5 mg P.O. daily, increased by 2.5 mg daily at 3- to 7-day intervals until desired effect occurs. Therapeutic daily dose is 2.5 to 15 mg. Safety and efficacy of doses exceeding 100 mg daily haven't been established.
➤ **Acromegaly—**
Adults: 1.25 to 2.5 mg P.O. with h.s. snack for 3 days. Another 1.25 to 2.5 mg may be added q 3 to 7 days until patient experiences therapeutic benefit. Maximum, 100 mg daily.

ACTION
Inhibits secretion of prolactin and acts as a dopamine-receptor agonist by activating postsynaptic dopamine receptors.

Route	Onset	Peak	Duration
P.O.	2 hr	8 hr	24 hr

ADVERSE REACTIONS
CNS: *CVA, dizziness, headache, fatigue,* mania, light-headedness, drowsiness, delusions, nervousness, insomnia, depression, *seizures.*
CV: *hypotension,* **acute MI.**
EENT: nasal congestion, blurred vision.
GI: *nausea,* vomiting, *abdominal cramps,* constipation, diarrhea, anorexia.
GU: urine retention, urinary frequency.
Skin: coolness and pallor of fingers and toes.

INTERACTIONS
Drug-drug. *Amitriptyline, haloperidol, imipramine, loxapine, MAO inhibitors, methyldopa, metoclopramide, phenothiazines, reserpine:* Interferes with bromocriptine's effects. Bromocriptine dosage may need to be increased.
Antihypertensives: Increased hypotensive effects. Adjust dosage of antihypertensive.
Erythromycin: Increased bromocriptine levels and risk of adverse reactions. Use together cautiously.
Estrogens, oral contraceptives, progestins: Interfere with effects of bromocriptine. Avoid using together.
Levodopa: May have additive effects. Adjust dosage of levodopa, if needed.

Reactions may be *common*, uncommon, *life-threatening*, or COMMON AND LIFE-THREATENING.

Drug-lifestyle. *Alcohol use:* Disulfiram-like reaction. Discourage use together.

EFFECTS ON LAB TEST RESULTS
• May increase BUN, alkaline phosphatase, uric acid, AST, ALT, and CK levels.

CONTRAINDICATIONS
Contraindicated in patients hypersensitive to ergot derivatives and in those with uncontrolled hypertension, toxemia of pregnancy, severe ischemic heart disease, or peripheral vascular disease.

NURSING CONSIDERATIONS
• Use cautiously in patients with impaired renal or hepatic function and in those with a history of MI with residual arrhythmias.
• For Parkinson's disease, bromocriptine usually is given with either levodopa or levodopa-carbidopa. The levodopa-carbidopa dose may need to be reduced.
• Adverse reactions may be minimized if drug is given in the evening with food.
• *Alert:* Monitor patient for adverse reactions. They occur in 68% of patients, particularly at start of therapy, but most are mild to moderate, with nausea the most common. Minimize adverse reactions by gradually adjusting dosages to effective levels. Adverse reactions are more common when drug is used for Parkinson's disease.
• Baseline and periodic evaluations of cardiac, hepatic, renal, and hematopoietic function are recommended during prolonged therapy.
• Drug may lead to early postpartum conception. Test for pregnancy every 4 weeks or whenever period is missed after menses resumes.
• *Alert:* Don't confuse bromocriptine with benztropine or brimonidine, or Parlodel with pindolol.

PATIENT TEACHING
• Instruct patient to take drug with meals.
• Advise patient to use contraceptive methods other than oral contraceptives or subdermal implants during treatment.
• Instruct patient to avoid dizziness and fainting by rising slowly to an upright position and avoiding sudden position changes.

• Inform patient that it may take 8 weeks or longer for menses to resume and galactorrhea to be suppressed.
• Advise patient to avoid alcohol while taking drug.

entacapone
Comtan

Pregnancy risk category C

AVAILABLE FORMS
Tablets: 200 mg

INDICATIONS & DOSAGES
➤ **Adjunct to levodopa-carbidopa for treatment of idiopathic Parkinson's disease in patients with signs and symptoms of end-of-dose wearing-off—**
Adults: 200 mg P.O. with each dose of levodopa-carbidopa to maximum of eight times daily. Maximum, 1,600 mg daily. May need to reduce daily levodopa dose or extend the interval between doses to optimize patient's response.

ACTION
A reversible catechol-O-methyltransferase (COMT) inhibitor that's given with levodopa-carbidopa. Giving together is thought to result in higher levels of levodopa and optimal control of parkinsonian symptoms.

Route	Onset	Peak	Duration
P.O.	1 hr	1 hr	6 hr

ADVERSE REACTIONS
CNS: *dyskinesia, hyperkinesia,* hypokinesia, dizziness, anxiety, somnolence, agitation, fatigue, asthenia, hallucinations.
GI: *nausea, diarrhea,* abdominal pain, constipation, vomiting, dry mouth, dyspepsia, flatulence, gastritis, taste perversion.
GU: *urine discoloration.*
Hematologic: purpura.
Musculoskeletal: back pain.
Respiratory: dyspnea.
Skin: sweating.
Other: bacterial infection.

INTERACTIONS
Drug-drug. *Ampicillin, chloramphenicol, cholestyramine, erythromycin, probene-*

cid: May block biliary excretion, resulting in higher levels of entacapone. Use together cautiously.

CNS depressants: Additive effect. Use together cautiously.

Drugs metabolized by COMT (bitolterol, dobutamine, dopamine, epinephrine, isoetharine, isoproterenol, norepinephrine): May cause higher levels of these drugs, resulting in increased heart rate, changes in blood pressure, or possibly arrhythmias. Use together cautiously.

Nonselective MAO inhibitors (such as phenelzine, tranylcypromine): May inhibit normal catecholamine metabolism. Avoid using together.

Drug-lifestyle. *Alcohol use:* May cause additive CNS effects. Discourage use together.

EFFECTS ON LAB TEST RESULTS
None reported.

CONTRAINDICATIONS
Contraindicated in patients hypersensitive to drug.

NURSING CONSIDERATIONS
● Use cautiously in patients with hepatic impairment, biliary obstruction, or orthostatic hypotension.
● Drug should be used only with levodopa-carbidopa; no antiparkinsonian effects occur when drug is given as monotherapy.
● Levodopa-carbidopa dosage requirements are usually lower when drug is given with entacapone; levodopa-carbidopa dose should be lowered or dosing interval increased to avoid adverse effects.
● Drug may cause or worsen dyskinesia, despite reduction of levodopa dose.
● Hallucinations may occur or worsen during therapy with this drug.
● Monitor blood pressure closely, and watch for orthostatic hypotension.
● Diarrhea most commonly begins within 4 to 12 weeks of starting therapy, but may begin as early as 1 week or as late as many months after starting treatment.
● Drug may discolor urine.
● Rarely, rhabdomyolysis has occurred with drug use.
● Rapid withdrawal or abrupt reduction in dose could lead to signs and symptoms of Parkinson's disease; it may also lead to

hyperpyrexia and confusion, a symptom complex resembling neuroleptic malignant syndrome. Discontinue drug slowly and monitor patient closely. Adjust other dopaminergic treatments, as needed.
● Drug can be given with immediate or sustained-release levodopa-carbidopa and can be taken with or without food.

PATIENT TEACHING
● Instruct patient not to crush or break tablet and to take it at same time as levodopa-carbidopa.
● Warn patient to avoid hazardous activities until CNS effects of drug are known.
● Advise patient to avoid alcohol during treatment.
● Instruct patient to use caution when standing after a prolonged period of sitting or lying down because dizziness may occur. This effect is more common during initial therapy.
● Warn patient that hallucinations, increased dyskinesia, nausea, and diarrhea could occur.
● Inform patient that drug may cause urine to turn brownish orange.
● Advise patient to notify prescriber about planned, suspected, or known pregnancy. Also, tell her to notify prescriber if she's breast-feeding.

---

levodopa
Larodopa

Pregnancy risk category NR

AVAILABLE FORMS
Capsules: 100 mg**, 250 mg**, 500 mg**
Tablets: 100 mg, 250 mg, 500 mg

INDICATIONS & DOSAGES
➤ **Idiopathic parkinsonism, postencephalitic parkinsonism, and symptomatic parkinsonism after carbon monoxide or manganese intoxication or with cerebral arteriosclerosis—**
Adults and children older than age 12:
Initially, 0.5 to 1 g P.O. daily, divided in two or more doses with food; increased by no more than 0.75 g daily q 3 to 7 days until maximum response is achieved. Don't exceed 8 g daily. Dosage adjusted to

patient requirements, tolerance, and response. Higher dosage needs close supervision.

ACTION

Unknown. May be decarboxylated to dopamine, countering the depletion of striatal dopamine in extrapyramidal centers; this depletion is thought to produce parkinsonism.

Route	Onset	Peak	Duration
P.O.	Unknown	1-3 hr	5 hr

ADVERSE REACTIONS

CNS: *aggressive behavior; choreiform, dystonic, and dyskinetic movements; involuntary grimacing, head movements, myoclonic body jerks,* **seizures,** *ataxia, tremor, muscle twitching; bradykinetic episodes; psychiatric disturbances; mood changes, nervousness, anxiety, disturbing dreams, euphoria, malaise, fatigue; severe depression,* **suicidal tendencies,** *dementia, delirium, hallucinations.*
CV: *orthostatic hypotension,* cardiac irregularities.
EENT: blepharospasm, blurred vision, diplopia, mydriasis or miosis, activation of latent Horner's syndrome, oculogyric crises.
GI: dry mouth, bitter taste, *nausea, vomiting, anorexia,* constipation, flatulence, diarrhea, abdominal pain, excessive salivation.
GU: urinary frequency, urine retention, incontinence, darkened urine, priapism.
Hematologic: *leukopenia,* hemolytic anemia, **agranulocytosis.**
Hepatic: *hepatotoxicity.*
Metabolic: transient elevations in protein-bound iodine levels, weight loss.
Respiratory: hiccups, hyperventilation.
Skin: dark perspiration.
Other: phlebitis.

INTERACTIONS

Drug-drug. *Antacids:* Increased absorption of levodopa. Give antacids 1 hour after levodopa.
Furazolidone, MAO inhibitors, procarbazine: Risk of severe hypertension. Avoid using together.

Inhaled anesthetics, sympathomimetics: Increased risk of arrhythmias. Monitor patient closely.
Metoclopramide: Accelerated gastric emptying of levodopa. Give metoclopramide 1 hour after levodopa.
Papaverine, phenothiazines, other antipsychotics, phenytoin, rauwolfia alkaloids: Decreased levodopa effect. Avoid using together.
Pyridoxine: Reversal of antiparkinsonian effects. Check vitamin preparations and nutritional supplements for pyridoxine (vitamin B_6) content. Avoid using together.
Drug-herb. *Jimsonweed:* May adversely affect CV function. Discourage use together.
Kava: Increased parkinsonian symptoms. Discourage use together.
Drug-food. *Foods high in protein:* Decreased levodopa absorption. Discourage use together.
Drug-lifestyle. *Cocaine use:* Increased risk of arrhythmias. Inform patient of this interaction.

EFFECTS ON LAB TEST RESULTS

● May increase BUN, ALT, AST, alkaline phosphatase, LDH, and bilirubin levels.
● May decrease hemoglobin and WBC and granulocyte counts.

CONTRAINDICATIONS

Contraindicated in patients hypersensitive to drug and in those with acute angle-closure glaucoma, melanoma, or undiagnosed skin lesions; also contraindicated within 14 days of MAO inhibitor therapy.

NURSING CONSIDERATIONS

● Use cautiously in patients with severe CV, renal, hepatic, and pulmonary disorders; peptic ulcer; psychiatric illness; MI with residual arrhythmias; bronchial asthma; emphysema; and endocrine disease.
● Patients who need surgery should continue levodopa therapy as long as oral intake is permitted, usually until 6 to 24 hours before surgery. Resume therapy as soon as patient can take drug orally.
● Levodopa-carbidopa typically decreases amount of levodopa needed by 75%, reducing risk of adverse reactions.
● Monitor vital signs, especially while adjusting dosage. Report changes.

• Coombs' test occasionally becomes positive during extended therapy. Drug may falsely elevate colorimetric test for uric acid. Copper-reduction method has shown false-positive results for urine glucose; glucose oxidase method has shown false-negative results. Levodopa also may interfere with tests for urine ketones. Levodopa interferes with urine screening tests for phenylketonuria, falsely elevates urinary catecholamine levels, and may falsely decrease urinary vanillylmandelic acid levels.

• **Alert:** Watch for muscle twitching and blepharospasm, which may be early signs of drug overdose; report immediately.

• **Alert:** Hallucinations may require reduction or withdrawal of drug.

• An accurate measure for urine glucose can be obtained if paper strip is partially immersed in the urine sample. Urine migrates up the strip, as with an ascending chromatographic system. Read only the top of the strip.

• Patients receiving long-term therapy should be tested regularly for diabetes and acromegaly; also, periodically monitor renal, hepatic, and hematopoietic function.

PATIENT TEACHING

• Tell patient to take drug with food to minimize GI upset. However, high-protein meals can impair absorption and reduce effectiveness.

• If patient has trouble swallowing pills, tell him or caregiver to crush tablets and mix with applesauce or pureed fruit.

• Warn patient or caregiver not to increase dosage unless ordered. Daily dosage shouldn't exceed 8 g.

• Tell patient to protect drug from heat, light, and moisture. If preparation darkens, it has lost potency and should be discarded.

• Warn patient about possible dizziness and orthostatic hypotension, especially at start of therapy. Tell him to change positions slowly and dangle legs before rising. Elastic stockings may control these adverse reactions.

• Advise patient and caregivers that multivitamin preparations, fortified cereals, and certain OTC drugs may contain pyridoxine (vitamin B_6), which can block the effects of levodopa by enhancing its peripheral metabolism.

levodopa-carbidopa
Sinemet, Sinemet CR

Pregnancy risk category C

AVAILABLE FORMS
Tablets: carbidopa 10 mg with levodopa 100 mg (Sinemet 10-100), carbidopa 25 mg with levodopa 100 mg (Sinemet 25-100), carbidopa 25 mg with levodopa 250 mg (Sinemet 25-250)
Tablets (extended-release): carbidopa 50 mg with levodopa 200 mg (Sinemet CR); carbidopa 25 mg with levodopa 100 mg

INDICATIONS & DOSAGES
➤ **Idiopathic Parkinson's disease, postencephalitic parkinsonism, and symptomatic parkinsonism resulting from carbon monoxide or manganese intoxication—**
Adults: 1 tablet of 25 mg carbidopa and 100 mg levodopa P.O. t.i.d.; then increased by 1 tablet daily or every other day, p.r.n., to maximum daily dose of 8 tablets. Substitute 25-mg carbidopa and 250-mg levodopa or 10-mg carbidopa and 100-mg levodopa tablets, as directed, to obtain maximum response. Optimum daily dose must be determined by careful adjustment for each patient.

Patients given conventional tablets may receive extended-release tablets; dosage is calculated on current levodopa intake. Initially, extended-release tablets should provide 10% more levodopa daily, increased p.r.n. and as tolerated to 30% more levodopa daily. Give in divided doses at intervals of 4 to 8 hours.

ACTION
Levodopa is converted to dopamine in the CNS, increasing dopamine levels in the brain. Carbidopa inhibits the peripheral decarboxylation of levodopa without affecting levodopa's metabolism in the CNS. Therefore, more levodopa is available to be decarboxylated to dopamine in the brain.

Route	Onset	Peak	Duration
P.O.	Unknown	40-150 min	Unknown

ADVERSE REACTIONS

CNS: *choreiform, dystonic, dyskinetic movements; involuntary grimacing, head movements, myoclonic body jerks, ataxia,* tremor, muscle twitching; bradykinetic episodes; psychiatric disturbances, anxiety, disturbing dreams, euphoria, malaise, fatigue; severe depression, *suicidal tendencies,* dementia, delirium, hallucinations, confusion, insomnia, agitation.
CV: *orthostatic hypotension, cardiac irregularities,* phlebitis.
EENT: blepharospasm, blurred vision, diplopia, mydriasis or miosis, oculogyric crises, excessive salivation.
GI: *dry mouth,* bitter taste, *nausea, vomiting, anorexia,* constipation, flatulence, diarrhea, abdominal pain.
GU: urinary frequency, urine retention, urinary incontinence, darkened urine, priapism.
Hematologic: hemolytic anemia, *thrombocytopenia, leukopenia, agranulocytosis.*
Hepatic: *hepatotoxicity.*
Metabolic: weight loss.
Respiratory: hiccups, hyperventilation.
Skin: dark perspiration.

INTERACTIONS

Drug-drug. *Antihypertensives:* Additive hypotensive effects. Use together cautiously.
Iron salts: May reduce bioavailability of levodopa and carbidopa. Give iron 1 hour before or 2 hours after Sinemet.
MAO inhibitors: Risk of severe hypertension. Avoid using together.
Papaverine, phenytoin: Antagonism of antiparkinsonian actions. Avoid using together.
Phenothiazines, other antipsychotics: May antagonize antiparkinsonian actions. Use together cautiously.
Drug-herb. *5-HTP:* May cause harmful skin changes. Discourage use together.
Kava: May cause decreased action of drug. Discourage use together.
Octacosanol: May worsen dyskinesias. Discourage use together.
Drug-food. *Foods high in protein:* Decreased levodopa absorption. Don't give levodopa with high-protein foods.

EFFECTS ON LAB TEST RESULTS

• May increase uric acid, ALT, AST, alkaline phosphatase, LDH, and bilirubin levels.
• May decrease hemoglobin and WBC, granulocyte, and platelet counts.

CONTRAINDICATIONS

Contraindicated in patients hypersensitive to drug and in those with angle-closure glaucoma, melanoma, or undiagnosed skin lesions; also contraindicated within 14 days of MAO inhibitor therapy.

NURSING CONSIDERATIONS

• Use cautiously in patients with severe CV, renal, hepatic, endocrine, or pulmonary disorders; history of peptic ulcer; psychiatric illness; MI with residual arrhythmias; bronchial asthma; emphysema; and well-controlled, chronic open-angle glaucoma.
• If patient takes levodopa, discontinue drug at least 8 hours before starting levodopa-carbidopa.
• Levodopa-carbidopa typically decreases amount of levodopa needed by 75%, reducing risk of adverse reactions.
• Therapeutic and adverse reactions occur more rapidly with levodopa-carbidopa than with levodopa alone. Observe patient and monitor vital signs, especially while adjusting dosage. Report significant changes.
• Hallucinations may require reduction or withdrawal of drug.
• Drug elevates serum and urinary uric acid levels in colorimetric tests; it may produce false-positive test results for urinary glucose when cupric sulfate reagent is used and false-negative results in tests using glucose oxidase. False-positive results may occur for urine ketone tests using sodium nitroprusside reagent. Levodopa interferes with urine screening tests for phenylketonuria, falsely elevates urinary catecholamine levels, and may falsely decrease urinary vanillylmandelic acid levels.
• An accurate measure for urine glucose can be obtained if the paper strip is only partially immersed in the urine sample. Urine migrates up the strip, as with an ascending chromatographic system. Read only the top of the strip.

• **Alert:** Muscle twitching and blepharospasm may be early signs of drug overdose; report immediately.

• Patients receiving long-term therapy should be tested regularly for diabetes and acromegaly and should have periodic tests of hepatic, renal, and hematopoietic function.

PATIENT TEACHING

• Tell patient to take drug with food to minimize GI upset. Inform patient that high-protein meals can impair absorption and reduce effectiveness.

• Tell patient not to chew or crush extended-release form.

• Warn patient and caregivers not to increase dosage without prescriber's orders.

• Caution patient about possible dizziness and orthostatic hypotension, especially at start of therapy. Tell him to change positions slowly and dangle his legs before getting out of bed. Elastic stockings may control these adverse reactions in some patients.

• Instruct patient to report adverse reactions and therapeutic effects.

• Inform patient that pyridoxine (vitamin B_6) doesn't reverse beneficial effects of levodopa-carbidopa. Multivitamins can be taken without reversal of levodopa's effects.

pergolide mesylate
Celance§, Permax

Pregnancy risk category B

AVAILABLE FORMS
Tablets: 0.05 mg, 0.25 mg, 1 mg

INDICATIONS & DOSAGES
➤ **Adjunctive treatment with levodopa-carbidopa in management of symptoms in Parkinson's disease—**
Adults: Initially, 0.05 mg P.O. daily for first 2 days; then increased by 0.1 to 0.15 mg q third day over 12 days. Subsequent dosage increased by 0.25 mg q third day, if needed, until optimum response occurs. Drug usually is given in divided doses t.i.d. Gradual reduction in levodopa-carbidopa dosage may be needed during dosage adjustment.

ACTION
Dopamine agonist that directly stimulates dopamine receptors in the nigrostriatal system.

Route	Onset	Peak	Duration
P.O.	Unknown	Unknown	Unknown

ADVERSE REACTIONS
CNS: headache, asthenia, *dyskinesia, dizziness, hallucinations, dystonia, confusion, somnolence,* insomnia, anxiety, depression, tremor, abnormal dreams, personality disorder, psychosis, abnormal gait, akathisia, extrapyramidal syndrome, incoordination, akinesia, hypertonia, neuralgia, speech disorder, syncope, twitching, paresthesia.
CV: *orthostatic hypotension,* vasodilation, palpitations, hypotension, hypertension, *arrhythmias, MI.*
EENT: *rhinitis,* epistaxis, abnormal vision, diplopia, eye disorder.
GI: dry mouth, taste perversion, abdominal pain, *nausea, constipation,* diarrhea, dyspepsia, anorexia, vomiting.
GU: urinary frequency, urinary tract infection, hematuria.
Metabolic: weight gain.
Musculoskeletal: chest, neck, and back pain; arthralgia; bursitis; myalgia.
Respiratory: dyspnea.
Skin: rash, diaphoresis.
Other: flu syndrome; chills; infection; facial, peripheral, or generalized edema.

INTERACTIONS
Drug-drug. *Butyrophenones, dopamine antagonists, metoclopramide, phenothiazines, thioxanthenes:* May antagonize effects of pergolide. Avoid using together.

EFFECTS ON LAB TEST RESULTS
None reported.

CONTRAINDICATIONS
Contraindicated in patients hypersensitive to drug or to ergot alkaloids.

NURSING CONSIDERATIONS
• Use cautiously in patients prone to arrhythmias.
• **Alert:** Monitor blood pressure. Symptomatic orthostatic or sustained hypotension may occur, especially at start of therapy.

PATIENT TEACHING

• Inform patient about possible adverse reactions, especially hallucinations and confusion.

• Warn patient to avoid activities that could result in injury from orthostatic hypotension and syncope.

• Advise patient to take drug with food.

---

pramipexole dihydrochloride
Mirapex

Pregnancy risk category C

AVAILABLE FORMS
Tablets: 0.125 mg, 0.25 mg, 0.5 mg, 1 mg, 1.5 mg

INDICATIONS & DOSAGES
➤ Signs and symptoms of idiopathic Parkinson's disease—

Adults: Initially, 0.375 mg P.O. daily in three divided doses; don't increase more often than q 5 to 7 days. Maintenance dosage is 1.5 to 4.5 mg daily in three divided doses.

Adjust-a-dose: For patients with creatinine clearance over 60 ml/minute, initial dosage is 0.125 mg P.O. t.i.d., up to 1.5 mg t.i.d. For those with creatinine clearance between 35 and 59 ml/minute, initial dosage is 1.25 mg P.O. b.i.d., up to 1.5 mg b.i.d. For those with creatinine clearance between 15 and 34 ml/minute, initial dosage is 0.125 mg P.O. daily, up to 1.5 mg daily.

ACTION
Unknown. Non–ergot-derivative dopamine receptor agonist that's thought to stimulate dopamine (D_2) receptors in striatum.

Route	Onset	Peak	Duration
P.O.	Rapid	2 hr	8-12 hr

ADVERSE REACTIONS
CNS: akathisia, amnesia, *asthenia, confusion,* delusions, *dizziness, dream abnormalities,* drowsiness, *dyskinesia,* dystonia, *extrapyramidal syndrome,* gait abnormalities, *hallucinations,* hypoesthesia, hypertonia, *insomnia,* myoclonus, paranoid re-

action, malaise, *somnolence,* sleep disorders, thought abnormalities.

CV: chest pain, peripheral edema, *orthostatic hypotension.*

EENT: accommodation abnormalities, diplopia, rhinitis, vision abnormalities.

GI: dry mouth, anorexia, *constipation,* dysphagia, *nausea.*

GU: impotence, urinary frequency, urinary tract infection, urinary incontinence.

Metabolic: weight loss.

Musculoskeletal: arthritis, bursitis, myasthenia, twitching.

Respiratory: dyspnea, pneumonia.

Skin: skin disorders.

Other: decreased libido, *accidental injury,* general edema, fever.

INTERACTIONS
Drug-drug. *Butyrophenones, metoclopramide, phenothiazines, thioxanthenes:* May diminish the effectiveness of pramipexole. Monitor patient closely. *Cimetidine, diltiazem, quinidine, quinine, ranitidine, triamterene, verapamil:* Decreased clearance of pramipexole. Adjust dosage, as needed.

EFFECTS ON LAB TEST RESULTS
None reported.

CONTRAINDICATIONS
Contraindicated in patients hypersensitive to drug or its components.

NURSING CONSIDERATIONS
• Dosage may need to be adjusted in patients with renal impairment.

• No data exist to demonstrate whether drug appears in breast milk. Use with caution.

• If drug must be discontinued, withdraw over 1 week.

• Drug may cause orthostatic hypotension, especially during dosage increases. Monitor patient carefully.

• Adjust dosage gradually. Increase to achieve maximum therapeutic effect, balanced against the main adverse effects of dyskinesia, hallucinations, somnolence, and dry mouth.

---

*Liquid contains alcohol.   **May contain tartrazine.   †Canada   ‡Australia   §U.K.   ◇OTC

PATIENT TEACHING
• Instruct patient not to rise rapidly after sitting or lying down because of risk of orthostatic hypotension.
• Caution patient to avoid hazardous activities until CNS response to drug is known.
• Tell patient to use caution before taking drug with other CNS depressants.
• Tell patient (especially elderly patient) that hallucinations may occur.
• Advise patient to take drug with food if nausea develops.
• Tell woman to notify prescriber if she is breast-feeding or intends to do so.
• Advise patient that it may take 4 weeks for effects of drug to be noticed because of slow adjustment schedule.

---

ropinirole hydrochloride
Requip

Pregnancy risk category C

AVAILABLE FORMS
Tablets: 0.25 mg, 0.5 mg, 1 mg, 2 mg, 3 mg, 4 mg, 5 mg

INDICATIONS & DOSAGES
➤ **Idiopathic Parkinson's disease—**
Adults: Initially, 0.25 mg P.O., t.i.d. After week 4, dosage may be increased by 1.5 mg daily, on a weekly basis, up to 9 mg daily; then dosage may be increased weekly by up to 3 mg daily, to maximum of 24 mg daily.
Elderly patients: Clearance is reduced in patients older than age 65; dosages are individually adjusted to clinical response.

ACTION
Unknown. Non–ergot-derivative dopamine receptor agonist that's thought to stimulate dopamine (D_2) receptors in striatum.

Route	Onset	Peak	Duration
P.O.	Unknown	1-2 hr	6 hr

ADVERSE REACTIONS
Early Parkinson's disease (without levodopa)
CNS: hallucinations, *dizziness,* aggravated Parkinson's disease, *somnolence,* head-ache, confusion, hyperkinesia, hypoesthesia, vertigo, amnesia, impaired concentration, *syncope, fatigue,* malaise, asthenia.
CV: orthostatic hypotension, orthostatic symptoms, hypertension, edema, chest pain, extrasystoles, atrial fibrillation, palpitations, tachycardia, flushing.
EENT: pharyngitis, abnormal vision, eye abnormality, xerophthalmia, rhinitis, sinusitis.
GI: dry mouth, *nausea, vomiting, dyspepsia,* flatulence, abdominal pain, anorexia, constipation.
GU: urinary tract infection, impotence.
Respiratory: bronchitis, dyspnea.
Other: *viral infection,* pain, increased sweating, yawning, peripheral ischemia.
Advanced Parkinson's disease (with levodopa)
CNS: *dizziness,* aggravated parkinsonism, *somnolence, headache,* insomnia, *hallucinations,* abnormal dreaming, confusion, tremor, anxiety, nervousness, amnesia, paresis, paresthesia, syncope.
CV: hypotension.
EENT: diplopia.
GI: *nausea,* abdominal pain, dry mouth, vomiting, constipation, diarrhea, dysphagia, flatulence, increased saliva.
GU: urinary tract infection, pyuria, urinary incontinence.
Hematologic: anemia.
Metabolic: weight decrease, suppressed prolactin.
Musculoskeletal: arthralgia, arthritis, *dyskinesia,* hypokinesia.
Respiratory: upper respiratory tract infection, dyspnea.
Skin: increased sweating.
Other: injury, *falls,* viral infection, pain.

INTERACTIONS
Drug-drug. *Ciprofloxacin, inhibitors or substrates of cytochrome P-450 1A2:* Altered clearance of ropinirole. Adjust ropinirole dose if other drugs are started or stopped during treatment.
CNS depressants: Increased CNS effects. Use together cautiously.
Dopamine agonists (neuroleptics) or metoclopramide: May diminish effects of ropinirole. Avoid using together.
Estrogens: Reduced ropinirole clearance. Adjust ropinirole dosage if estrogens are started or stopped during treatment.

Reactions may be *common,* uncommon, **life-threatening**, or **COMMON AND LIFE-THREATENING**.

Drug-lifestyle. *Alcohol use:* Increased sedative effects. Advise patient to use cautiously.
Smoking: May increase ropinirole clearance. Discourage use together.

EFFECTS ON LAB TEST RESULTS
• May increase BUN and alkaline phosphatase levels.
• May decrease hemoglobin.

CONTRAINDICATIONS
Contraindicated in patients hypersensitive to drug.

NURSING CONSIDERATIONS
• Use cautiously in patients with severe hepatic or renal impairment.
• *Alert:* Monitor patient carefully for orthostatic hypotension, especially during dosage increases.
• Drug may potentiate the dopaminergic adverse effects of levodopa and may cause or worsen dyskinesia. Dosage may be decreased.
• Other adverse reactions reported with dopaminergic therapy could occur with ropinirole (but haven't been reported): withdrawal-emergent hyperpyrexia and confusion (fever, muscle rigidity, altered consciousness, and autonomic instability), which may occur with rapid dosage reduction or withdrawal of medication; fibrotic complications.
• Patient may have syncope, with or without bradycardia. Monitor patient carefully, especially for 4 weeks after start of therapy and with dosage increases.
• Withdraw drug gradually over 7 days.

PATIENT TEACHING
• Advise patient to take drug with food if nausea occurs.
• Inform patient (especially elderly patient) that hallucinations can occur.
• Instruct patient not to rise rapidly after sitting or lying down because of risk of orthostatic hypotension, which may occur more frequently early in therapy or when dosage increases.
• Somnolence can occur early in therapy. Warn patient to minimize hazardous activities until CNS effects of drug are known.
• Advise patient to avoid alcohol.

• Tell woman to notify prescriber about planned, suspected, or known pregnancy; also tell her to inform prescriber if she's breast-feeding.

selegiline hydrochloride (L-deprenyl hydrochloride)
Eldepryl

Pregnancy risk category C

AVAILABLE FORMS
Capsules: 5 mg

INDICATIONS & DOSAGES
➤ **Adjunctive treatment with levodopa-carbidopa in managing symptoms of Parkinson's disease—**
Adults: 10 mg P.O. daily, 5 mg at breakfast and 5 mg at lunch. After 2 or 3 days, gradual decrease of levodopa-carbidopa dosage may be needed.

ACTION
Unknown. May selectively inhibit MAO type B (found mostly in the brain) and dopamine metabolism. At higher-than-recommended doses, it's a nonselective inhibitor of MAO, including MAO type A (found in the GI tract). May also directly increase dopaminergic activity by decreasing the reuptake of dopamine into nerve cells.

Route	Onset	Peak	Duration
P.O.	Unknown	0.5-2 hr	Unknown

ADVERSE REACTIONS
CNS: *dizziness,* increased tremor, chorea, loss of balance, restlessness, increased bradykinesia, facial grimacing, stiff neck, dyskinesia, involuntary movements, twitching, increased apraxia, behavioral changes, fatigue, headache, confusion, hallucinations, vivid dreams, anxiety, insomnia, lethargy, malaise, syncope.
CV: orthostatic hypotension, hypertension, hypotension, *arrhythmias,* palpitations, new or increased angina, tachycardia, peripheral edema.
EENT: blepharospasm.
GI: dry mouth, *nausea,* vomiting, constipation, abdominal pain, anorexia or poor appetite, dysphagia, diarrhea, heartburn.

GU: slow urination, transient nocturia, prostatic hyperplasia, urinary hesitancy, urinary frequency, urine retention, sexual dysfunction.
Metabolic: weight loss.
Skin: rash, hair loss, diaphoresis.

INTERACTIONS
Drug-drug. *Adrenergics:* May cause increased pressor response, particularly in patients who have taken an overdose of selegiline. Use together cautiously.
MAO inhibitors: May cause hypertensive crisis. Avoid using together.
Meperidine: May cause stupor, muscle rigidity, severe agitation, and fever. Avoid using together.
TCAs and selective serotonin reuptake inhibitors: May cause mental status change. Avoid using together.
Drug-herb. *Cacao:* May cause vasopressor effects. Discourage use together.
Ginseng: Adverse reactions including headache, tremors, mania. Discourage use together.
Drug-food. *Foods high in tyramine:* May cause hypertensive crisis. Monitor blood pressure.

EFFECTS ON LAB TEST RESULTS
None reported.

CONTRAINDICATIONS
Contraindicated in patients hypersensitive to drug and in those receiving meperidine.

NURSING CONSIDERATIONS
• *Alert:* Some patients experience increased adverse reactions to levodopa when it's used with selegiline and need a 10% to 30% reduction of carbidopa-levodopa dosage.
• *Alert:* Don't confuse selegiline with Stelazine or Eldepryl with enalapril.
• *Alert:* Severe adverse reactions may occur if used with antidepressants.

PATIENT TEACHING
• Warn patient to move cautiously at start of therapy because he may become dizzy.
• Advise patient not to take more than 10 mg daily. A larger amount may increase adverse reactions.

---

tolcapone
Tasmar

Pregnancy risk category C

AVAILABLE FORMS
Tablets: 100 mg, 200 mg

INDICATIONS & DOSAGES
➤ **Adjunct to levodopa and carbidopa for treating signs and symptoms of idiopathic Parkinson's disease in patients who have symptom fluctuation or haven't responded to other adjunctive treatment—**
Adults: Initially, 100 mg P.O. t.i.d. with levodopa-carbidopa. Recommended daily dose is 100 mg P.O. t.i.d. Reduction of levodopa dosage by 20% to 30% may be needed to minimize risk of dyskinesias. Maximum, 600 mg daily. Discontinue drug if patient shows no benefit within 3 weeks.

ACTION
Unknown. May reversibly inhibit catechol-O-methyltransferase when given with levodopa-carbidopa, resulting in increased levodopa bioavailability, which causes a more constant dopaminergic stimulation in the brain.

Route	Onset	Peak	Duration
P.O.	Unknown	2 hr	Unknown

ADVERSE REACTIONS
CNS: *dyskinesia, sleep disorder, dystonia, excessive dreaming, somnolence,* dizziness, *confusion, headache, hallucinations,* hyperkinesia, hypertonia, fatigue, falling, syncope, balance loss, depression, tremor, speech disorder, paresthesia, agitation, irritability, mental deficiency, hyperactivity, hypokinesia.
CV: *orthostatic complaints,* chest pain, chest discomfort, palpitations, hypotension.
EENT: pharyngitis, tinnitus, sinus congestion.
GI: *nausea, anorexia, diarrhea,* flatulence, *vomiting,* constipation, abdominal pain, dyspepsia, dry mouth.
GU: urinary tract infection, urine discoloration, hematuria, micturition disorder, urinary incontinence, impotence.

Reactions may be *common*, uncommon, **life-threatening**, or **COMMON AND LIFE-THREATENING**.

Hematologic: bleeding.
Hepatic: *hepatotoxicity.*
Musculoskeletal: *muscle cramps,* stiffness, arthritis, neck pain.
Respiratory: bronchitis, dyspnea, upper respiratory tract infection.
Skin: increased sweating, rash.
Other: fever, influenza.

INTERACTIONS
Drug-drug. *CNS depressants:* Additive effects. Monitor patient closely.
Desipramine, selective serotonin reuptake inhibitors, TCAs: Increased risk of adverse effects. Use together cautiously.
Nonselective MAO inhibitors (phenelzine, tranylcypromine): May cause hypertensive crisis. Avoid using together.
Warfarin: May cause increased warfarin levels. Monitor INR, and adjust warfarin dosage, as needed.

EFFECTS ON LAB TEST RESULTS
• May increase liver function test values.

CONTRAINDICATIONS
Contraindicated in patients hypersensitive to drug or its components and in those with hepatic disease, elevated ALT or AST levels, or history of drug-related confusion and nontraumatic rhabdomyolysis or hyperpyrexia. Also contraindicated in those who were withdrawn from tolcapone because of evidence of drug-induced hepatocellular injury.

NURSING CONSIDERATIONS
• Use cautiously in patients with severe renal impairment and in breast-feeding women.
• Because of risk of liver toxicity, stop treatment if patient shows no benefit within 3 weeks.
• Use drug only in patients taking levodopa-carbidopa who don't respond to or who aren't appropriate candidates for other adjunctive therapies because of risk of fatal hepatic failure.
• *Alert:* Make sure patient provides written informed consent before using drug.
• Monitor liver function test results before starting drug, every 2 weeks for first year of therapy, every 4 weeks for next 6 months, and every 8 weeks thereafter.

Stop drug if results are outside normal limits or if patient appears jaundiced.
• Because of highly protein-bound nature of tolcapone, drug isn't significantly removed during dialysis.
• Monitor patient for orthostatic hypotension and syncope.
• Give first dose of the day with first daily dose of levodopa-carbidopa.
• Diarrhea is common, sometimes occurring 2 to 12 weeks after therapy begins. Although it usually resolves when therapy stops, patient rarely may need hospitalization.

PATIENT TEACHING
• Advise patient to take drug exactly as prescribed.
• Teach patient the signs and symptoms of liver injury (jaundice, fatigue, loss of appetite, persistent nausea, pruritus, dark urine, or right upper quadrant tenderness), and instruct him to report them immediately.
• Warn patient about risk of orthostatic hypotension; tell him to use caution when rising from a seated or recumbent position.
• Advise patient to avoid hazardous activities until CNS effects of drug are known.
• Tell patient that nausea may occur early in therapy.
• Advise patient about risk of increased dyskinesia or dystonia.
• Inform patient that hallucinations may occur.
• Tell woman to notify prescriber about planned, suspected, or known pregnancy.
• Tell patient to report adverse effects, including diarrhea, to prescriber. Inform patient that diarrhea may occur from 2 to 12 weeks after therapy starts.
• Inform patient that drug may be taken without regard to meals.

---

trihexyphenidyl hydrochloride
Apo-Trihex†, Artane*, Artane
Sequels, Trihexane, Trihexy

Pregnancy risk category NR

AVAILABLE FORMS
Capsules (sustained-release): 5 mg
Elixir: 2 mg/5 ml
Tablets: 2 mg, 5 mg

INDICATIONS & DOSAGES
➤ **All forms of parkinsonism, including drug-induced parkinsonism; adjunctive treatment to levodopa in management of parkinsonism—**
Adults: 1 mg P.O. on day 1, 2 mg on day 2; then increased in 2-mg increments q 3 to 5 days up to total of 6 to 10 mg daily. Usually given t.i.d. with meals; sometimes given q.i.d. (last dose h.s.) or switched to extended-release form b.i.d.

Patients with postencephalitic parkinsonism may need total daily dose of 12 to 15 mg.

ACTION
Unknown. Drug blocks central cholinergic receptors, helping to balance cholinergic activity in the basal ganglia.

Route	Onset	Peak	Duration
P.O.	1 hr	Unknown	6-12 hr

ADVERSE REACTIONS
CNS: nervousness, dizziness, headache, hallucinations, drowsiness, weakness.
CV: tachycardia.
EENT: blurred vision, mydriasis, increased intraocular pressure.
GI: *dry mouth,* constipation, *nausea,* vomiting.
GU: urinary hesitancy, urine retention.

INTERACTIONS
Drug-drug. *Amantadine:* Additive anticholinergic adverse reactions, such as confusion and hallucinations. Reduce dose of trihexyphenidyl before giving.
Levodopa: Decreased total bioavailability of levodopa. May require lower doses of both drugs.
Drug-lifestyle. *Alcohol use:* Increased sedative effects. Discourage use together.

EFFECTS ON LAB TEST RESULTS
None reported.

CONTRAINDICATIONS
Contraindicated in patients hypersensitive to drug.

NURSING CONSIDERATIONS
• Use cautiously in patients with glaucoma, cardiac disorders, hepatic disorders,

renal disorders, obstructive GI or GU disorders, and prostatic hyperplasia.
• Dosage may need to be gradually increased in patients who develop tolerance to drug.
• Monitor patient. Adverse reactions are dose-related and transient.
• *Alert:* Make sure gonioscopic evaluation is performed and intraocular pressure is monitored, especially in patients older than age 40.
• *Alert:* Don't confuse Artane with Anturane or Altace.

PATIENT TEACHING
• Tell patient that drug may cause nausea if taken before meals.
• Tell patient to avoid activities that require alertness until CNS effects of drug are known.
• Advise patient to report signs and symptoms of urinary hesitancy or urine retention.
• Tell patient to relieve dry mouth with cool drinks, ice chips, or sugarless gum or hard candy.
• Advise patient to avoid alcohol while taking drug.
• Advise patient to avoid OTC sleep aids or cold medicines because of possibility of increased anticholinergic effects.

34

Miscellaneous central nervous system drugs

almotriptan
bupropion hydrochloride
donepezil hydrochloride
droperidol
fluvoxamine maleate
galantamine hydrobromide
lithium carbonate
lithium citrate
naratriptan hydrochloride
nicotine polacrilex
nicotine transdermal system
propofol
rivastigmine tartrate
rizatriptan benzoate
sibutramine hydrochloride
  monohydrate
sumatriptan succinate
tacrine hydrochloride
zolmitriptan

COMBINATION PRODUCTS
None.

❋ *NEW DRUG*

almotriptan
Axert

Pregnancy risk category C

AVAILABLE FORMS
Tablets: 6.25 mg, 12.5 mg

INDICATIONS & DOSAGES
➤ **Acute migraine with or without aura—**
Adults: 6.25-mg or 12.5-mg tablet P.O., with one additional dose after 2 hours if headache is unresolved or recurs. Maximum, two doses within 24 hours.
Adjust-a-dose: For patients with hepatic or renal impairment, initially 6.25 mg, with maximum daily dose of 12.5 mg.

ACTION
Drug inhibits cranial vasoconstriction through serotonin-1 agonist activity.

Route	Onset	Peak	Duration
P.O.	1-3 hr	1-3 hr	3-4 hr

ADVERSE REACTIONS
CNS: paresthesia, headache, dizziness, somnolence.
GI: nausea, dry mouth.

INTERACTIONS
Drug-drug. *CYP2D6 inhibitors, MAO inhibitors:* May increase levels of almotriptan. Although no adverse clinical effects have been reported, monitor patient for potential adverse reaction. May need to reduce dosage.
CYP3A4 inhibitors such as ketoconazole: May increase levels of almotriptan. Monitor patient for potential adverse reaction. May need to reduce dosage.
Ergot-containing drugs: May cause additive effects. Avoid using together.
Selective serotonin reuptake inhibitors: May cause additive serotonin effects, resulting in weakness, hyperreflexia, or incoordination. Monitor patient closely.
5-HT$_{1B/1D}$ agonists: May cause additive effects. Use together within 24 hours of each other is contraindicated.

EFFECTS ON LAB TEST RESULTS
None reported.

CONTRAINDICATIONS
Contraindicated in patients hypersensitive to drug. Also contraindicated in those with angina pectoris, history of MI, silent ischemia, coronary artery vasospasm, Prinzmetal's variant angina, or other CV disease; uncontrolled hypertension; and hemiplegic or basilar migraine. Don't give within 24 hours after treatment with other 5-HT$_{1B/1D}$ agonists or ergotamine drugs.

NURSING CONSIDERATIONS
● Use cautiously in patients with renal or hepatic impairment and in those with cataracts because of the potential for corneal opacities. Use cautiously also in patients with risk factors for coronary artery disease (CAD), such as obesity, diabetes, and family history of CAD.

• Reduce dosage in patients with poor renal or hepatic function.
• Repeat dose after 2 hours, if needed.
• Don't give more than 2 doses within 24 hours.

PATIENT TEACHING
• Tell patient that drug can be taken with or without food.
• Advise patient to take drug only when he's having a migraine and that drug isn't taken on a regular schedule.
• Advise patient to use only one repeat dose within 24 hours and that repeat dose should be taken no sooner than 2 hours after initial dose.
• Advise patient that other commonly prescribed migraine medications can interact with almotriptan.
• Tell patient with history of heart disease or uncontrolled high blood pressure not to take drug.
• Advise patient to report chest or throat tightness, pain, or heaviness.
• Teach patient to avoid possible migraine triggers such as cheese, chocolate, citrus fruits, caffeine, and alcohol.

---

bupropion hydrochloride
Zyban

Pregnancy risk category B

AVAILABLE FORMS
Tablets (sustained-release): 150 mg

INDICATIONS & DOSAGES
➤ **Aid to smoking cessation treatment—**
Adults: 150 mg P.O. daily for 3 days; increased to maximum of 300 mg P.O. daily in two divided doses at least 8 hours apart.

ACTION
Unknown. Relatively weak inhibitor of the neuronal uptake of norepinephrine, serotonin, and dopamine. Drug doesn't inhibit MAO.

Route	Onset	Peak	Duration
P.O.	Unknown	3 hr	Unknown

ADVERSE REACTIONS
CNS: agitation, asthenia, depression, *dizziness,* headache, *insomnia,* irritability, somnolence, tremor, thinking or dream abnormalities, disturbed concentration, anxiety, nervousness.
CV: *complete AV block,* hypertension, hypotension, *tachycardia,* palpitations, hot flashes.
EENT: amblyopia, epistaxis, *pharyngitis,* sinusitis, tinnitus, *rhinitis, blurred vision.*
GI: *anorexia,* dyspepsia, increased appetite, abdominal pain, *nausea, constipation,* diarrhea, flatulence, *vomiting, dry mouth,* taste perversion, mouth ulcer.
GU: urinary frequency.
Musculoskeletal: arthralgia, leg cramps and twitching, myalgia, neck pain.
Respiratory: bronchitis, increased cough, dyspnea.
Skin: dry skin, pruritus, rash, urticaria, *excessive sweating.*
Other: allergic reactions, injury, fever.

INTERACTIONS
Drug-drug. *Antidepressants, antipsychotics, systemic corticosteroids, theophylline:* May lower seizure threshold. Use cautiously.
Carbamazepine, phenobarbital, phenytoin: May induce metabolism of bupropion and decrease its effect. Monitor patient closely.
Cimetidine: May inhibit metabolism of bupropion and lead to increased levels. Monitor patient closely.
Levodopa: May increase risk of adverse reactions. If used together, give small initial doses of bupropion and increase dosage gradually.
MAO inhibitors (phenelzine): Increased toxicity. Separate administration by at least 2 weeks.
Other drugs containing bupropion (Wellbutrin, Wellbutrin SR): Contain same active ingredient as Zyban. Avoid using together.
Drug-lifestyle. *Alcohol:* May increase risk of seizures. Discourage use together.
Sun exposure: Photosensitivity reactions may occur. Urge patient to take precautions against sun exposure.

EFFECTS ON LAB TEST RESULTS
None reported.

CONTRAINDICATIONS
Contraindicated in patients allergic to drug or its components, in those with seizure disorders or a current or prior diagnosis of bulimia or anorexia nervosa, and in those being treated with other drugs containing bupropion (such as Wellbutrin and Wellbutrin SR). Also contraindicated within 14 days of MAO inhibitor therapy.

NURSING CONSIDERATIONS
• Use cautiously in patients with recent MI or unstable heart disease. Also, use cautiously in patients with history of seizures, head trauma, or other predisposition to seizures, and in those being treated with drugs that lower seizure threshold.

• *Alert:* Excessive use of alcohol, abrupt withdrawal from alcohol or other sedatives, and addiction to cocaine, opiates, or stimulants may increase risk of seizures. Seizure risk is also linked to OTC stimulants and anorectics. Diabetic patients being treated with oral antidiabetics or insulin are also at risk for seizures.

• To reduce seizure risk, don't exceed 300 mg daily. Divide dose (150 mg twice daily) so that no single dose exceeds 150 mg.

• Therapy should stop if patient hasn't made progress toward abstinence by week 7 of therapy.

• Dose doesn't need tapering before ending treatment.

• *Alert:* Therapy should begin while patient is still smoking; about 1 week is needed to achieve steady-state plasma drug levels.

• *Alert:* Don't confuse bupropion with buspirone.

PATIENT TEACHING
• Stress importance of combining behavioral interventions, counseling, and support services with drug therapy.

• Advise patient to take doses at least 8 hours apart. If insomnia occurs, tell him not to take dose at bedtime.

• Tell patient not to chew, divide, or crush tablets.

• Tell patient that it may take 1 week for effects of drug to appear. Also, tell him to set a target date for smoking cessation during the second week of therapy.

• Tell patient that treatment usually lasts 7 to 12 weeks.

• Inform patient that tablets may have a characteristic odor.

• Advise patient to avoid alcohol while taking drug.

• Tell patient to avoid hazardous activities that require mental alertness until drug's CNS effects are known.

• Warn patient not to use drug with nicotine patches unless directed by prescriber. Doing so may increase blood pressure.

• Inform patient that risk of seizures increases if he has a seizure or eating disorder, exceeds the recommended dosage, or takes other drugs that contain bupropion or that lower seizure threshold.

• Advise patient to read accompanying patient information before starting drug.

• Advise patient to notify prescriber about planned, suspected, or known pregnancy.

---

donepezil hydrochloride
Aricept

Pregnancy risk category C

AVAILABLE FORMS
Tablets: 5 mg, 10 mg

INDICATIONS & DOSAGES
➤ **Mild to moderate dementia of the Alzheimer's type—**
Adults: Initially, 5 mg P.O. daily h.s. After 4 to 6 weeks, dosage may be increased to 10 mg daily.

ACTION
Thought to increase acetylcholine concentration by inhibiting hydrolysis of cholinesterase enzyme. Drug may improve cognitive function in patients with Alzheimer's disease.

Route	Onset	Peak	Duration
P.O.	Unknown	3-4 hr	Unknown

ADVERSE REACTIONS
CNS: *headache, insomnia,* dizziness, fatigue, depression, abnormal dreams, somnolence, *seizures,* tremor, irritability,

paresthesia, aggression, vertigo, ataxia, restlessness, abnormal crying, nervousness, aphasia, syncope, pain.
CV: chest pain, hypertension, vasodilation, atrial fibrillation, hot flashes, hypotension.
EENT: cataract, blurred vision, eye irritation, sore throat.
GI: *nausea, diarrhea,* vomiting, anorexia, fecal incontinence, GI bleeding, bloating, epigastric pain.
GU: urinary frequency.
Hematologic: ecchymosis.
Metabolic: weight loss, dehydration.
Musculoskeletal: muscle cramps, arthritis, bone fracture.
Respiratory: dyspnea, bronchitis.
Skin: pruritus, urticaria, diaphoresis.
Other: toothache, influenza, increased libido.

INTERACTIONS
Drug-drug. *Anticholinergics:* May reduce the effects of donepezil. Avoid using together.
Anticholinesterases, cholinomimetics: Synergistic effect. Monitor patient closely.
Bethanechol, succinylcholine: Additive effects. Monitor patient closely.
Carbamazepine, dexamethasone, phenobarbital, phenytoin, rifampin: May increase rate of donepezil elimination. Monitor patient.
Drug-herb. *Jaborandi tree:* May cause additive effects. Discourage use together to avoid risk of toxicity.
Pill-bearing spurge: May cause additive effects and increased risk of toxicity. Discourage use together.

EFFECTS ON LAB TEST RESULTS
None reported.

CONTRAINDICATIONS
Contraindicated in patients hypersensitive to drug or piperidine derivatives.

NURSING CONSIDERATIONS
• Use cautiously in patients who take NSAIDs or have CV disease, asthma, obstructive pulmonary disease, urinary outflow impairment, or history of ulcer disease.

• Drug should be used during pregnancy only if benefit justifies risk to fetus. Breast-feeding should be avoided.
• Monitor patient for evidence of active or occult GI bleeding.
• *Alert:* Don't confuse Aricept with Ascriptin.

PATIENT TEACHING
• Stress that drug doesn't alter underlying degenerative disease but can temporarily stabilize or relieve symptoms. Effectiveness relies on taking drug at regular intervals.
• Tell caregiver to give drug just before patient's bedtime.
• Advise patient and caregiver to immediately report significant adverse effects or changes in overall health status and to inform health care team that patient is taking drug before he receives anesthesia.
• Tell patient to avoid OTC cold or sleep remedies because of risk of increased anticholinergic effects.

droperidol
Droleptan§, Inapsine

Pregnancy risk category C

AVAILABLE FORMS
Injection: 2.5 mg/ml in 1-, 2-, and 5-ml ampules, and 2-, 5-, and 10-ml vials

INDICATIONS & DOSAGES
➤ **Premedication—**
Adults and children older than age 12: 2.5 to 10 mg I.M. 30 to 60 minutes preoperatively.
Children ages 2 to 12: 0.088 to 0.165 mg/kg I.M. or I.V.
Elderly patients: Reduce dosage.
Adjust-a-dose: For debilitated patients and those who have received other depressant drugs, give reduced dosage.
➤ **For induction as an adjunct to general anesthesia—**
Adults and children older than age 12: 0.22 to 0.275 mg/kg I.M. or I.V. given with general anesthesia
Children ages 2 to 12: 0.088 to 0.165 mg/kg I.M. or I.V.

➤ **For use without a general anesthetic in diagnostic procedures—**
Adults and children older than age 12: 2.5 to 10 mg I.M. 30 to 60 minutes before procedure. Additional doses of 1.25 to 2.5 mg, usually I.V., may be given.
➤ **Adjunct to regional anesthesia when additional sedation is needed—**
Adults: 2.5 to 5 mg I.M. or slow I.V.

I.V. ADMINISTRATION
● Give I.V. doses slowly.
● For high-risk patients, dilute calculated dose in D$_5$W or lactated Ringer's injection and give as a slow I.V. infusion.

ACTION
Unknown. Produces marked tranquilization, sedation, and antiemetic effects while allowing for reflex alertness. It also causes mild alpha blockade.

Route	Onset	Peak	Duration
I.M., I.V.	3-10 min	30 min	2-4 hr

ADVERSE REACTIONS
CNS: *drowsiness,* restlessness, hyperactivity, anxiety, extrapyramidal symptoms, dizziness, hallucinations, dysphoria, *neuroleptic malignant syndrome.*
CV: hypotension, tachycardia.
Respiratory: *laryngospasm, bronchospasm.*
Other: chills, shivering.

INTERACTIONS
Drug-drug. *CNS depressants:* Additive CNS effects. Adjust dosage, p.r.n.
Fentanyl citrate: May cause hypertension and respiratory depression. Use together cautiously.

EFFECTS ON LAB TEST RESULTS
None reported.

CONTRAINDICATIONS
Contraindicated in patients hypersensitive to drug. Drug isn't recommended for patients at high risk for arrhythmias.

NURSING CONSIDERATIONS
● Use cautiously in patients with hepatic or renal dysfunction and in breast-feeding patients.

● Use with caution in patients with suspected or diagnosed pheochromocytoma because severe hypertension and tachycardia can occur.
● When used for induction of general anesthesia, give drug with an analgesic.
● If used in procedures such as bronchoscopy, appropriate topical anesthesia is still needed.
● *Alert:* Keep fluids and other measures to manage hypotension readily available.
● Monitor vital signs routinely.
● *Alert:* Monitor patient for signs and symptoms of neuroleptic malignant syndrome (fever, altered consciousness, extrapyramidal symptoms, tachycardia).
● *Alert:* Don't confuse droperidol with dronabinol.

PATIENT TEACHING
● Warn patient to rise slowly to minimize orthostatic hypotension.
● Advise patient to avoid alcohol for 24 hours after receiving droperidol.

---

fluvoxamine maleate
Faverin§, Luvox

Pregnancy risk category C

AVAILABLE FORMS
Tablets: 50 mg, 100 mg

INDICATIONS & DOSAGES
➤ **Obsessive-compulsive disorder (OCD)—**
Adults: Initially, 50 mg P.O. daily h.s., increased in 50-mg increments q 4 to 7 days until maximum benefit achieved. Maximum, 300 mg daily. Total daily amounts above 100 mg should be given in two divided doses.

ACTION
Unknown. Selectively inhibits the presynaptic neuronal uptake of serotonin, which is thought to improve OCDs.

Route	Onset	Peak	Duration
P.O.	Unknown	3-8 hr	Unknown

ADVERSE REACTIONS
CNS: *headache, asthenia, somnolence, insomnia, nervousness,* dizziness, tremor,

---

anxiety, hypertonia, *agitation,* depression, CNS stimulation.
CV: palpitations, vasodilation.
EENT: amblyopia.
GI: *nausea, diarrhea, constipation, dyspepsia,* anorexia, *vomiting,* flatulence, dysphagia, *dry mouth,* taste perversion.
GU: abnormal ejaculation, urinary frequency, impotence, anorgasmia, urine retention.
Respiratory: upper respiratory tract infection, dyspnea, yawning.
Skin: sweating.
Other: tooth disorder, flu syndrome, chills, decreased libido.

INTERACTIONS

Drug-drug. *Benzodiazepines, theophylline, warfarin:* Reduced clearance of these drugs. Use together cautiously (except for diazepam, which shouldn't be given with fluvoxamine). Adjust dosage, as needed.
Carbamazepine, clozapine, methadone, metiprolol, propranolol, TCAs: Elevated levels of these drugs. Use together cautiously, and monitor patient closely for adverse reactions. Dosage adjustments may be needed.
Diltiazem: Bradycardia may occur. Monitor heart rate.
Lithium, tryptophan: May enhance effects of fluvoxamine. Use together cautiously.
MAO inhibitors: May cause severe excitation, hyperpyrexia, myoclonus, delirium, and coma. Avoid using together.
Drug-lifestyle. *Smoking:* Decreased drug effectiveness. Urge patient to stop smoking.

EFFECTS ON LAB TEST RESULTS
None reported.

CONTRAINDICATIONS
Contraindicated in patients hypersensitive to drug or to other phenyl piperazine antidepressants and within 14 days of MAO inhibitor therapy.

NURSING CONSIDERATIONS
● Use cautiously in patients with hepatic dysfunction, other conditions that may affect hemodynamic responses or metabolism, or history of mania or seizures.

●*Alert:* Record mood changes. Monitor patient for suicidal tendencies, and provide only a minimum supply of drug.
●*Alert:* Don't confuse Luvox with Lasix or fluvoxamine with fluoxetine.

PATIENT TEACHING
● Warn patient to avoid hazardous activities until CNS effects of drug are known.
● Tell woman to notify prescriber about planned, suspected, or known pregnancy.
● Tell patient who develops a rash, hives, or a related allergic reaction to notify prescriber.
● Inform patient that several weeks of therapy may be needed to obtain full antidepressant effect. Once improvement occurs, advise patient not to stop drug until directed by prescriber.
● Advise patient to check with prescriber before taking OTC drugs; drug interactions can occur.

✳ *NEW DRUG*

galantamine hydrobromide
Reminyl

Pregnancy risk category B

AVAILABLE FORMS
Oral solution: 4 mg/ml
Tablets: 4 mg, 8 mg, 12 mg

INDICATIONS AND DOSAGES
➤ **Mild to moderate dementia of Alzheimer's type—**
Adults: Initially, 4 mg b.i.d., preferably with morning and evening meals. If dose is well tolerated after minimum of 4 weeks of therapy, increase dose to 8 mg b.i.d. A further increase to 12 mg b.i.d. may be attempted but only after at least 4 weeks of therapy at the previous dosage. Recommended dosage range is 16 to 24 mg daily in two divided doses.
Adjust-a-dose: For patients with moderate hepatic impairment (Child-Pugh score of 7 to 9), dosage usually shouldn't exceed 16 mg daily. For patients with severe hepatic impairment (Child-Pugh score of 10 to 15), drug isn't recommended. For patients with moderate renal impairment, dosage usually shouldn't exceed 16 mg daily. For patients with severe renal im-

pairment (creatinine clearance < 9 ml/min), drug isn't recommended.

ACTION
Exact mechanism of action is unknown. Drug is a competitive and reversible inhibitor of acetylcholinesterase, which is believed to enhance cholinergic function by increasing the level of acetylcholine in the brain.

Route	Onset	Peak	Duration
P.O.	Unknown	1 hr	Unknown

ADVERSE REACTIONS
CNS: depression, dizziness, headache, tremor, insomnia, somnolence, fatigue, syncope.
CV: *bradycardia.*
EENT: rhinitis.
GI: *nausea, vomiting,* anorexia, *diarrhea,* abdominal pain, dyspepsia, anorexia.
GU: urinary tract infection, hematuria.
Hematologic: anemia.
Metabolic: weight loss.

INTERACTIONS
Drug-drug. *Amitriptyline, fluoxetine, fluvoxamine, quinidine:* Decreased galantamine clearance. Monitor patient closely.
Anticholinergics: May antagonize anticholinergic activity. Monitor patient.
Cholinergics (such as bethanechol, succinylcholine): Synergistic effect. Monitor patient closely. May need to avoid use before procedures using general anesthesia with succinylcholine-type neuromuscular blockers.
Cimetidine, erythromycin, ketoconazole, paroxetine: Increased galantamine bioavailability. Monitor patient closely.

EFFECTS ON LAB TEST RESULTS
None reported.

CONTRAINDICATIONS
Contraindicated in patients hypersensitive to drug or its components.

NURSING CONSIDERATIONS
• Use cautiously in patients with supraventricular cardiac conduction disorders and in those taking other drugs that significantly slow heart rate. Use cautiously during or before procedures involving anesthesia using succinylcholine-type or similar neuromuscular blockers. Also use cautiously in patients with history of peptic ulcer disease and in those taking NSAIDs. Because of the potential for cholinomimetic effects, use cautiously in patients with bladder outflow obstruction, seizures, asthma, or COPD.
• Bradycardia and heart block may occur in patients with and without underlying cardiac conduction abnormalities. Consider all patients at risk for adverse effects on cardiac conduction.
• Give drug with food and antiemetics and ensure adequate fluid intake to decrease the risk of nausea and vomiting.
• Use proper technique when dispensing the oral solution with the pipette. Dispense measured amount in a nonalcoholic beverage and give right away.
• If drug is stopped for several days or longer, it should be restarted at the lowest dose and gradually increased, at 4-week or longer intervals, to the previous dosage level.
• Because of the risk of increased gastric acid secretion, monitor patients closely for symptoms of active or occult GI bleeding, especially those with an increased risk of developing ulcers.
• Safety and efficacy in children haven't been established.

PATIENT TEACHING
• Advise patient to take drug with morning and evening meals.
• Inform patient that nausea and vomiting are common adverse effects.
• Teach caregiver the proper technique when measuring the oral solution with the pipette. Place measured amount in a nonalcoholic beverage and have patient drink right away.
• Urge patient or caregiver to report slow heartbeat immediately.
• Advise patient that drug is believed to enhance cognitive function, but there's no evidence that it alters the underlying disease process.

---

lithium carbonate
Camcolit§, Carbolith†, Duralith†, Eskalith, Eskalith CR, Lithane**, Lithicarb‡, Lithizine†, Lithobid, Lithonate, Lithotabs, Priadel§

lithium citrate
Cibalith-S*

Pregnancy risk category D

AVAILABLE FORMS
lithium carbonate
Capsules: 150 mg, 300 mg, 600 mg
Tablets: 250 mg‡, 300 mg (300 mg equals 8.12 mEq lithium)
Tablets (controlled-release): 300 mg, 400 mg‡, 450 mg
lithium citrate
Syrup (sugarless): 8 mEq (lithium)/5 ml
  Note: 5 ml of lithium citrate (liquid) contains 8 mEq lithium, equal to 300 mg lithium carbonate.

INDICATIONS & DOSAGES
➤ **Prevention or control of mania—**
Adults: 300 to 600 mg P.O. up to q.i.d. Or, 900 mg controlled-release tablets P.O. q 12 hours. Increase dosage based on blood levels to achieve optimal dosage. Recommended therapeutic lithium levels are 1.5 mEq/L for acute mania, 0.6 to 1.2 mEq/L for maintenance therapy, and 2 mEq/L maximum.

ACTION
Unknown. Probably alters chemical transmitters in the CNS, possibly by interfering with ionic pump mechanisms in brain cells, and may compete with or replace sodium ions.

Route	Onset	Peak	Duration
P.O.	Unknown	0.5-3 hr	Unknown

ADVERSE REACTIONS
CNS: tremors, drowsiness, headache, confusion, restlessness, dizziness, psychomotor retardation, *lethargy,* **coma,** blackouts, **epileptiform seizures,** EEG changes, worsened organic mental syndrome, impaired speech, ataxia, incoordination, *fatigue.*
CV: reversible ECG changes, *arrhythmias,* hypotension, **bradycardia.**

EENT: tinnitus, blurred vision.
GI: dry mouth, metallic taste, nausea, *vomiting, anorexia, diarrhea, thirst,* abdominal pain, flatulence, indigestion.
GU: *polyuria,* glycosuria, decreased creatinine clearance, albuminuria, *renal toxicity* with long-term use.
Hematologic: *leukocytosis with leukocyte count of 14,000 to 18,000/mm³.*
Metabolic: transient hyperglycemia; goiter; hypothyroidism, hyponatremia.
Musculoskeletal: *muscle weakness.*
Skin: pruritus, rash, diminished or absent sensation, drying and thinning of hair, psoriasis, acne, alopecia.
Other: ankle and wrist edema.

INTERACTIONS
Drug-drug. *ACE inhibitors:* Increased plasma lithium levels. Monitor lithium levels; adjust lithium dosage, as needed.
Aminophylline, sodium bicarbonate, urine alkalinizers: Increased lithium excretion. Avoid excessive salt, and monitor lithium levels.
Calcium channel blockers (verapamil): May decrease lithium levels and increase risk of neurotoxicity. Use together cautiously.
Carbamazepine, fluoxetine, methyldopa, NSAIDs, probenecid: Increased effect of lithium. Monitor patient for lithium toxicity.
Diuretics: Increased reabsorption of lithium by kidneys, with possible toxic effect. Use with extreme caution, and monitor lithium and electrolyte levels (especially sodium).
Neuroleptics: May cause encephalopathy. Watch for signs and symptoms (lethargy, tremor, extrapyramidal symptoms), and stop drug if encephalopathy occurs.
Neuromuscular blockers: May cause prolonged paralysis or weakness. Monitor patient closely.
Thyroid hormones: May induce hypothyroidism. Monitor thyroid function.
Drug-herb. *Ispaghula, plantain, psyllium seed:* May decrease GI absorption of lithium, reducing the pharmacologic effect. Discourage use together.
Parsley: May promote or produce serotonin syndrome. Discourage use together.
Drug-food. *Caffeine:* Decreased lithium plasma levels; may reduce pharmacologic

---

effect. Tell patient who ingests large amounts of caffeine to tell prescriber before stopping caffeine. Adjust lithium dosage, as needed.

EFFECTS ON LAB TEST RESULTS
• May increase glucose level. May decrease sodium, T_3, T_4, and protein-bound iodine levels.
• May increase ^{131}I uptake and WBC and neutrophil counts.

CONTRAINDICATIONS
Contraindicated if therapy can't be closely monitored.

NURSING CONSIDERATIONS
• Don't give to pregnant patient unless benefits outweigh risks to fetus.
• Use with extreme caution in patients receiving neuroleptics, neuromuscular blockers, and diuretics; in elderly or debilitated patients; and in patients with thyroid disease, seizure disorder, infection, renal or CV disease, severe debilitation or dehydration, or sodium depletion.
• *Alert:* Determination of lithium level is crucial to safe use of drug. Don't use drug in patients who can't have regular tests. Monitor lithium level 8 to 12 hours after first dose, the morning before second dose is given, two or three times weekly for the first month, then weekly to monthly during maintenance therapy.
• When levels of lithium are below 1.5 mEq/L, adverse reactions are usually mild.
• Monitor baseline ECG, thyroid studies, renal studies, and electrolyte levels.
• Check fluid intake and output, especially when surgery is scheduled.
• Weigh patient daily; check for edema or sudden weight gain.
• Adjust fluid and salt ingestion to compensate if excessive loss occurs from protracted diaphoresis or diarrhea. Under normal conditions, patient should have fluid intake of 2½ to 3 L daily and a balanced diet with adequate salt intake.
• Check urine specific gravity and report level below 1.005, which may indicate diabetes insipidus.
• Drug alters glucose tolerance in diabetics. Monitor glucose level closely.

• Perform outpatient follow-up of thyroid and renal functions every 6 to 12 months. Palpate thyroid to check for enlargement.
• *Alert:* Don't confuse Lithobid with Levbid, Lithonate with Lithostat, or Lithotabs with Lithobid or Lithostat.

PATIENT TEACHING
• Tell patient to take drug with plenty of water and after meals to minimize GI upset.
• Explain that lithium has a narrow therapeutic margin of safety. A level that's even slightly high can be dangerous.
• Warn patient and caregivers to expect transient nausea, polyuria, thirst, and discomfort during first few days of therapy and to watch for evidence of toxicity (diarrhea, vomiting, tremor, drowsiness, muscle weakness, ataxia).
• Instruct patient to withhold one dose and call prescriber if signs and symptoms of toxicity appear, but not to stop drug abruptly.
• Warn patient to avoid hazardous activities that require alertness and good psychomotor coordination until CNS effects of drug are known.
• Tell patient not to switch brands of lithium or take other prescription or OTC drugs without prescriber's guidance.
• Tell patient to wear or carry medical identification at all times.

---

naratriptan hydrochloride
Amerge

Pregnancy risk category C

AVAILABLE FORMS
Tablets: 1 mg, 2.5 mg

INDICATIONS & DOSAGES
➤ **Acute migraine attacks with or without aura—**
Adults: 1 or 2.5 mg P.O. as a single dose. If headache returns or responds only partially, dose may be repeated after 4 hours. Maximum, 5 mg in 24 hours.
Adjust-a-dose: For patients with mild to moderate renal or hepatic impairment, a lower initial dose is recommended. Maximum, 2.5 mg in 24 hours.

ACTION

May selectively activate serotonin receptors in intracranial blood vessels, resulting in vasoconstriction and migraine headache relief. Or the inhibition of neuropeptide release may reduce pain transmission in the trigeminal pathways.

Route	Onset	Peak	Duration
P.O.	Unknown	2-3 hr	Unknown

ADVERSE REACTIONS

CNS: paresthesia, dizziness, drowsiness, malaise, fatigue, vertigo, syncope.
CV: palpitations, increased blood pressure, *tachyarrhythmias, abnormal ECG changes, coronary vasospasm.*
EENT: ear, nose, and throat infections; photophobia.
GI: nausea, hyposalivation, vomiting.
Other: sensations of warmth, cold, pressure, tightness, or heaviness.

INTERACTIONS

Drug-drug. *Ergot-containing or ergot-type drugs (dihydroergotamine, methysergide), other 5-HT₁ agonists:* Prolonged vasospastic reactions. Don't give within 24 hours of naratriptan.
Oral contraceptives: Slightly increased levels of naratriptan. Monitor patient.
Selective serotonin reuptake inhibitors (fluoxetine, fluvoxamine, paroxetine, sertraline): May cause weakness, hyperreflexia, and incoordination. Monitor patient.
Drug-herb. *St. John's wort:* Increased serotonergic effect. Discourage use together.
Drug-lifestyle. *Smoking:* Increased clearance of naratriptan. Discourage use together.

EFFECTS ON LAB TEST RESULTS

None reported.

CONTRAINDICATIONS

Contraindicated in patients hypersensitive to drug or its components and in those with a history or evidence of cardiac ischemia and cerebrovascular or peripheral vascular syndromes or a history of uncontrolled hypertension. Also, contraindicated in elderly patients, patients with severe renal impairment (creatinine clearance below 15 ml/minute), patients with severe hepatic impairment (Child-Pugh grade C), and patients who have received ergot-containing, ergot-type, or other 5-HT₁ agonists during the previous 24 hours.

NURSING CONSIDERATIONS

• Use cautiously in patients with risk factors for coronary artery disease, such as hypertension, hypercholesterolemia, obesity, diabetes, or strong family history of coronary artery disease. Also, use cautiously in women with surgical or physiologic menopause, in men older than age 40, and in patients who smoke unless a CV evaluation has shown patient to be free from cardiac disease. If patient has cardiac risk factors but a satisfactory CV evaluation, monitor him closely after first dose.
• Use cautiously in patients with renal or hepatic impairment.
• Assess cardiac status in patients who develop risk factors for coronary artery disease.
• *Alert:* Drug can cause coronary artery vasospasm and increased risk of cerebrovascular events.
• Drug isn't intended to prevent migraines or manage hemiplegic or basilar migraine.
• Safety and effectiveness of drug haven't been established for treating cluster headaches or more than four headaches in a 30-day period.
• Use drug after a definite diagnosis of migraine has been established.

PATIENT TEACHING

• Instruct patient to take drug only as prescribed and to read the accompanying patient instruction leaflet before using drug.
• Tell patient that drug is intended to relieve, not prevent, migraines.
• Instruct patient to take dose soon after headache starts. If no response occurs with first tablet, tell patient to seek medical approval before taking second tablet. Tell patient that if more relief is needed after first tablet (if a partial response occurs or headache returns), and prescriber has approved a second dose, patient may take a second tablet but not sooner than 4 hours after first tablet. Tell him not to exceed two tablets within 24 hours.

- Advise patient to increase fluid intake.
- Advise patient not to use drug if she suspects or knows that she's pregnant.
- Tell patient to alert prescriber about bothersome adverse effects.

---

nicotine polacrilex (nicotine-polacrilin resin complex)
Nicorette ◊ , Nicotinell§

Pregnancy risk category X

AVAILABLE FORMS
Chewing gum: 2 mg/square, 4 mg/square

INDICATIONS & DOSAGES
➤ **Relief from nicotine withdrawal symptoms in patients undergoing smoking cessation—**
Adults: Initially, one 2-mg square; highly dependent patients should start treatment with 4-mg squares. Patient should chew 1 piece of gum slowly and intermittently for 30 minutes whenever the urge to smoke occurs. Most patients need 9 to 12 pieces of gum daily during the first month. For patients using 4-mg squares, maximum dose is 20 pieces daily. For patients using 2-mg squares, maximum dose is 30 pieces daily.

ACTION
Provides nicotine, which stimulates nicotinic acetylcholine receptors in the CNS, neuromuscular junction, autonomic ganglia, and adrenal medulla.

Route	Onset	Peak	Duration
P.O.	Unknown	15-30 min	Unknown

ADVERSE REACTIONS
CNS: dizziness, light-headedness, irritability, insomnia, headache.
CV: atrial fibrillation.
EENT: *throat soreness.*
GI: nausea, vomiting, indigestion, eructation, anorexia, excessive salivation.
Musculoskeletal: *jaw muscle ache from chewing.*
Respiratory: *hiccups.*

INTERACTIONS
Drug-drug. *Beta blockers, methylxanthines, propoxyphene, propranolol:* De-

creased metabolism of these drugs, increasing therapeutic effects. Dosage adjustments of these drugs may be needed.
Drug-lifestyle. *Smoking:* Reduced effectiveness of drug. Warn patient to avoid smoking while taking drug.

EFFECTS ON LAB TEST RESULTS
None reported.

CONTRAINDICATIONS
Contraindicated in nonsmokers and in patients with recent MI, life-threatening arrhythmias, severe or worsening angina pectoris, or active temporomandibular joint disease; also contraindicated during pregnancy.

NURSING CONSIDERATIONS
- Use cautiously in patients with hyperthyroidism, pheochromocytoma, type 1 diabetes mellitus, peptic ulcer disease, history of esophagitis, oral or pharyngeal inflammation, or dental conditions that might be exacerbated by chewing gum.
- Smokers most likely to benefit from nicotine gum are those with high physical nicotine dependence—those who smoke more than 15 cigarettes daily, prefer brands of cigarettes with high nicotine levels, usually inhale the smoke, smoke the first cigarette within 30 minutes of rising, find the first morning cigarette the hardest to give up, smoke most frequently during the morning, find it difficult to refrain from smoking in places where it's forbidden, or smoke even when ill and confined to bed.
- *Alert:* Don't confuse Nicorette with Nordette.

PATIENT TEACHING
- Instruct patient to chew gum slowly and intermittently (chew several times; then place between cheek and gum) for about 30 minutes to promote slow and even buccal absorption of nicotine. Gum must be chewed to release nicotine. Swallowing gum is ineffective. Fast chewing tends to produce more adverse reactions.
- Make sure patient reads and understands instructions included in the package.
- Stress importance of withdrawing gum gradually.

• Tell patient to gradually withdraw gum usage after 3 months. Use of gum for longer than 6 months isn't recommended. For gradual withdrawal, tell patient to cut gum in halves or quarters and mix with other sugarless gum.

---

nicotine transdermal system
Habitrol ◇ , Nicoderm, Nicotrol ◇
ProStep

Pregnancy risk category D

AVAILABLE FORMS
Transdermal system: designed to release nicotine at a fixed rate
Habitrol ◇ —7 mg/day, 14 mg/day,
21 mg/day
Nicoderm—7 mg/day, 14 mg/day,
21 mg/day
Nicotrol ◇ —5 mg/16 hours, 10 mg/
16 hours, 15 mg/16 hours
ProStep—11 mg/day, 22 mg/day

INDICATIONS & DOSAGES
➤ **Relief from nicotine withdrawal symptoms in patients undergoing smoking cessation—**
Adults: Initially, one transdermal system, delivering the largest available dose of nicotine in its dosage series, applied once daily to nonhairy part of body. For Habitrol, Nicoderm, and ProStep, patch should be kept on for 24 hours, then removed and a new system applied to an alternate skin site. For Nicotrol, patch should be applied upon awakening and removed h.s. After 4 to 12 weeks, depending on brand used, dose is tapered to next lowest available level in its dosage series, followed in 2 to 4 weeks by lowest nicotine dosage system in series. Drug is then stopped in 2 to 4 weeks.

ACTION
Provides nicotine, which stimulates nicotinic acetylcholine receptors in the CNS, neuromuscular junction, autonomic ganglia, and adrenal medulla.

Route	Onset	Peak	Duration
Trans-dermal	Unknown	3-9 hr	Unknown

ADVERSE REACTIONS
CNS: somnolence, dizziness, *headache, insomnia,* paresthesia, abnormal dreams, nervousness.
CV: hypertension.
EENT: pharyngitis, sinusitis.
GI: abdominal pain, constipation, dyspepsia, nausea, diarrhea, vomiting, dry mouth.
GU: dysmenorrhea.
Musculoskeletal: back pain, myalgia.
Respiratory: increased cough.
Skin: *local or systemic erythema, pruritus, burning at application site,* cutaneous hypersensitivity, rash, diaphoresis.

INTERACTIONS
Drug-drug. *Acetaminophen, imipramine, oxazepam, pentazocine, propranolol, theophylline:* May decrease induction of hepatic enzymes that help metabolize certain drugs. Dosage reductions may be needed.
Adrenergic agonists such as isoproterenol and phenylephrine: May decrease circulating catecholamines. Dosage increases may be needed.
Adrenergic antagonists such as labetalol and prazosin: May decrease circulating catecholamines. Dosage reductions may be needed.
Insulin: May increase amount of S.C. insulin absorbed. Dosage reductions may be needed.
Drug-herb. *Blue cohash:* Increased effects of nicotine. Discourage use together.
Drug-food. *Caffeine:* May decrease induction of hepatic enzymes that help metabolize certain drugs. Dosage reductions may be needed.

EFFECTS ON LAB TEST RESULTS
None reported.

CONTRAINDICATIONS
Contraindicated in patients hypersensitive to nicotine or any component of transdermal system. Also, contraindicated in nonsmokers and in patients with recent MI, life-threatening arrhythmias, or severe or worsening angina pectoris.

NURSING CONSIDERATIONS
• Use cautiously in patients with hyperthyroidism, pheochromocytoma, hypertension, type 1 diabetes mellitus, or peptic ulcer disease.

Reactions may be *common*, uncommon, *life-threatening*, or COMMON AND LIFE-THREATENING.

• Health care workers' exposure to nicotine in transdermal systems is probably minimal; however, avoid unnecessary contact with system. Wash hands with water alone because soap may enhance absorption.

• *Alert:* Don't confuse Nicoderm with Nitro-Derm.

PATIENT TEACHING

• Inform patient that using transdermal system for longer than 3 months isn't recommended. Warn patient that long-term nicotine consumption by any route can be dangerous and habit forming.

• *Alert:* Warn patient not to smoke. If he continues to smoke while using system, he may experience serious adverse effects because peak nicotine levels will be substantially higher than those achieved by smoking alone.

• Make sure patient reads and understands information dispensed with drug.

• Advise patient to apply patch promptly because nicotine can evaporate from transdermal system once it's removed from its protective packaging. Patch shouldn't be folded or cut before application and shouldn't be stored at temperatures above 86° F (30° C).

• Teach patient proper disposal of transdermal system. After removal, fold patch in half, bringing adhesive sides together. If patch came in a protective pouch, place used patch in same pouch. Careful disposal is needed to prevent accidental poisoning of children or pets.

• Tell patient with persistent or severe local skin reactions or generalized rash to immediately stop using patch and notify prescriber.

• Inform patient that those who can't stop smoking during first 4 weeks of therapy probably won't benefit from continued use of drug. Such patients may benefit from counseling to identify factors that led to treatment failure. Encourage patient to minimize or eliminate factors contributing to treatment failure and to try again, possibly after some time has passed.

propofol
Diprivan

Pregnancy risk category B

AVAILABLE FORMS
Injection: 10 mg/ml in 20-ml ampules; 50-ml prefilled syringes; 50-ml and 100-ml infusion vials

INDICATIONS & DOSAGES
➤ **Induction of general anesthesia—**
Adults younger than age 55: 40 mg or 2 to 2.5 mg/kg I.V. q 10 seconds until induction onset. In patients receiving cardiac anesthesia, 20 mg or 0.5 to 1.5 mg/kg q 10 seconds until induction onset. In neurosurgical patients, 20 mg or 1 to 2 mg/kg q 10 seconds until induction onset.
Children age 3 and older: In healthy children, 2.5 to 3.5 mg/kg given over 20 to 30 seconds.
Elderly patients: 20 mg or 1 to 1.5 mg/kg q 10 seconds until induction onset.
Adjust-a-dose: For debilitated patients or patients considered class III or IV by the American Society of Anesthesiologists (ASA), 20 mg or 1 to 1.5 mg/kg q 10 seconds until induction onset.
➤ **Maintenance of general anesthesia: infusion—**
Adults younger than age 55: 100 to 200 mcg/kg/minute. In patients receiving cardiac anesthesia, 50 to 150 mcg/kg/minute. In neurosurgical patients, 100 to 200 mcg/kg/minute.
Children age 3 and older: In healthy children, 125 to 300 mcg/kg/minute.
Elderly patients: 50 to 100 mcg/kg/minute.
Adjust-a-dose: For debilitated or ASA class III or IV patients, 50 to 100 mcg/kg/minute.
➤ **Maintenance of general anesthesia: intermittent bolus—**
Adults younger than age 55: Increments of 20 to 50 mg I.V., p.r.n.
➤ **Initiation of monitored anesthesia care sedation—**
Adults younger than age 55: Dosage individualized; 100 to 150 mcg/kg/minute infusion for 3 to 5 minutes. Or, slow injection of 0.5 mg/kg over 3 to 5 minutes followed immediately by I.V. infusion.

➤ **Maintenance of monitored anesthesia care sedation—**

Adults younger than age 55: 25 to 75 mcg/kg/minute infusion or incremental bolus doses of 10 to 20 mg I.V.

Elderly patients: 80% of healthy adult dose.

Adjust-a-dose: For debilitated, neurosurgical, or ASA class III or IV patients, 80% of healthy adult dose.

➤ **Initiation and maintenance of sedation in intubated, mechanically ventilated patients in intensive care unit (ICU)—**

Adults: Dosage individualized; initial infusion usually 5 mcg/kg/minute for 5 minutes. May increase rate at 5- to 10-minute intervals in increments of 5 to 10 mcg/kg/minute until desired level of sedation occurs. Rates of 5 to 50 mcg/kg/minute or higher may be needed.

I.V. ADMINISTRATION
● Maintain strict aseptic technique when handling the solution.
● Allow an adequate time interval (3 to 5 minutes) between dosage adjustments to assess effects.
● Protect drug from light. Shake well. Dilute only with D_5W. Don't dilute to less than 2 g/ml. Don't infuse through a filter with a pore size smaller than 5 microns. Give via larger veins in arms to decrease injection site pain.
● Drug shouldn't be mixed with other therapeutic drugs before infusion.
● Don't give drug in same I.V. line with blood or plasma.

ACTION
Unknown. Rapidly acting I.V. sedative-hypnotic.

Route	Onset	Peak	Duration
I.V.	< 40 sec	Unknown	10-15 min

ADVERSE REACTIONS
CNS: movement.
CV: *bradycardia, hypotension,* hypertension, decreased cardiac output.
Metabolic: hyperlipemia.
Respiratory: APNEA, respiratory acidosis.
Skin: rash.
Other: *burning or stinging at injection site.*

INTERACTIONS
Drug-drug. *Inhaled anesthetics (such as enflurane, halothane, isoflurane), opioids (fentanyl, meperidine, morphine), sedatives (such as barbiturates, benzodiazepines, chloral hydrate, droperidol):* May increase anesthetic and sedative effects and may result in a more pronounced decrease in blood pressure and cardiac output. Monitor patient closely.

EFFECTS ON LAB TEST RESULTS
● May increase lipid levels.

CONTRAINDICATIONS
Contraindicated in patients hypersensitive to drug or its components (including egg lecithin, soybean oil, and glycerol) or when general anesthesia or sedation is contraindicated.

NURSING CONSIDERATIONS
● Use cautiously in patients who are hemodynamically unstable or who have seizures, disorders of lipid metabolism, or increased intracranial pressure.
● Drug isn't recommended for obstetric use because it crosses the placenta and may cause neonatal depression.
● Because drug appears in breast milk, it isn't recommended in breast-feeding patients.
● Urine may turn green if drug is used for prolonged sedation in ICU.
● Always use strict aseptic technique during handling. Drug can support the growth of microorganisms; don't use if contamination is suspected. Discard tubing and unused portions of drug after 12 hours.
● Don't use if phases of emulsion show evidence of separation.
● Titrate drug daily to maintain minimum effective level.
● For general anesthesia or monitored anesthesia care sedation, drug should be given by trained staff not involved in the surgical or diagnostic procedure. For ICU sedation, drug should be given by persons skilled in managing critically ill patients and trained in cardiopulmonary resuscitation and airway management.
● Continuously monitor vital signs.
● Monitor patient at risk of hyperlipidemia for increases in triglyceride levels.

Reactions may be *common*, uncommon, *life-threatening*, or COMMON AND LIFE-THREATENING.

• Drug contains 0.1 g of fat (1.1 kcal)/ml. A reduction in lipids given together is needed.

• Propofol contains ethylenediamine-tetraacetic acid, a strong metal chelator. Consider supplemental zinc during prolonged therapy.

• When drug is given in the ICU, assess patient's CNS function daily to determine minimum dose needed.

• Drug should be discontinued slowly to prevent abrupt awakening and increased agitation.

PATIENT TEACHING

• Advise patient that performance of activities requiring mental alertness may be impaired for some time after drug use.

---

rivastigmine tartrate
Exelon

Pregnancy risk category B

AVAILABLE FORMS
Capsules: 1.5 mg, 3 mg, 4.5 mg, 6 mg

INDICATIONS & DOSAGES
➤ **Symptomatic treatment of patients with mild to moderate Alzheimer's disease—**
Adults: Initially, 1.5 mg P.O. b.i.d. with food. If tolerated, may be increased to 3 mg b.i.d after 2 weeks. Further increases to 4.5 mg b.i.d. and 6 mg b.i.d may be implemented as tolerated after 2 weeks at the previous dose. Effective dosage range is 6 to 12 mg daily; maximum recommended amount, 12 mg daily.

ACTION
Thought to increase acetylcholine concentration by reversibly inhibiting hydrolysis of the cholinesterase enzyme. This may result in some memory improvement.

Route	Onset	Peak	Duration
P.O.	Unknown	1 hr	12 hr

ADVERSE REACTIONS
CNS: syncope, fatigue, asthenia, malaise, *dizziness, headache,* somnolence, tremor, insomnia, confusion, depression, anxiety, hallucinations, aggressive reaction, vertigo, agitation, nervousness, delusion, paranoid reaction.
CV: hypertension, chest pain, peripheral edema.
EENT: rhinitis, pharyngitis.
GI: *nausea, vomiting, diarrhea, anorexia, abdominal pain,* dyspepsia, constipation, flatulence, eructation.
GU: urinary tract infection, urinary incontinence.
Metabolic: weight loss.
Musculoskeletal: back pain, arthralgia, bone fracture.
Respiratory: upper respiratory tract infection, cough, bronchitis.
Skin: increased sweating, rash.
Other: *accidental trauma,* flulike symptoms, pain.

INTERACTIONS
Drug-drug. *Anticholinergics:* May decrease effectiveness. Avoid using together. *Bethanechol, succinylcholine, other neuromuscular blocking drugs or cholinergic antagonists:* May have a synergistic effect with rivastigmine. Monitor patient closely.
Drug-lifestyle. *Nicotine:* Increased rivastigmine clearance. Ask patient about nicotine use.

EFFECTS ON LAB TEST RESULTS
None reported.

CONTRAINDICATIONS
Contraindicated in patients hypersensitive to drug, other carbamate derivatives, or other components of the drug.

NURSING CONSIDERATIONS
• Expect significant GI adverse effects (such as nausea, vomiting, anorexia, and weight loss). These effects are less common during maintenance doses.
• Monitor patient for evidence of active or occult GI bleeding.
• Dramatic memory improvement is unlikely. As disease progresses, the benefits of rivastigmine may decline.
• Monitor patient for severe nausea, vomiting, and diarrhea, which may lead to dehydration and weight loss.
• Carefully monitor patient with a history of GI bleeding, NSAID use, arrhythmias, seizures, or pulmonary conditions for adverse effects.

• No data exist to demonstrate whether drug appears in breast milk, and there's no indication for use in breast-feeding women.

PATIENT TEACHING

• Tell patient to take rivastigmine with food in the morning and evening.
• Advise patient that memory improvement may be subtle and that a more likely result of taking rivastigmine will be a slower decline in memory loss.
• Tell patient to report nausea, vomiting, or diarrhea.
• Urge patient to consult prescriber before taking OTC medications.

---

rizatriptan benzoate
Maxalt, Maxalt-MLT

Pregnancy risk category C

AVAILABLE FORMS
Tablets: 5 mg, 10 mg
Tablets (orally disintegrating): 5 mg, 10 mg

INDICATIONS & DOSAGES
➤ **Acute migraine headaches with or without aura—**
Adults: Initially, 5 or 10 mg P.O. If first dose is ineffective, another dose can be given at least 2 hours after first. Maximum, 30 mg in a 24-hour period. For patients receiving propranolol, 5 mg P.O. up to maximum of 15 mg in 24 hours.

ACTION
May act as an agonist at serotonin receptors on extracerebral intracranial blood vessels, which results in vasoconstriction of the affected vessels, inhibition of neuropeptide release, and reduction of pain transmission in the trigeminal pathways.

Route	Onset	Peak	Duration
P.O.	Unknown	1-1.5 hr	Unknown

ADVERSE REACTIONS
CNS: dizziness, headache, somnolence, paresthesia, asthenia, fatigue, decreased mental acuity, euphoria, tremor, pain.
CV: chest pain, pressure, or heaviness; palpitations; flushing.
EENT: neck, throat, and jaw pain.
GI: dry mouth, nausea, diarrhea, vomiting.
Respiratory: dyspnea.
Other: hot flashes, warm or cold feelings.

INTERACTIONS
Drug-drug. *Ergot-containing or ergot-type drugs (dihydroergotamine, methysergide), other 5-HT$_1$ agonists:* Prolonged vasospastic reactions. Don't use within 24 hours of rizatriptan.
MAO inhibitors (moclobemide), nonselective MAO inhibitors (types A and B; isocarboxazid, phenelzine, tranylcypromine): Increased plasma rizatriptan levels. Avoid using together and allow at least 14 days between ending MAO inhibitor and beginning rizatriptan.
Propranolol: Increased rizatriptan levels. Reduce rizatriptan dose to 5 mg.
Selective serotonin reuptake inhibitors (fluoxetine, fluvoxamine, paroxetine, sertraline): Weakness, hyperreflexia, incoordination may occur. Monitor patient.

EFFECTS ON LAB TEST RESULTS
None reported.

CONTRAINDICATIONS
Contraindicated in patients hypersensitive to drug or its inactive ingredients and in those with ischemic heart disease (angina pectoris, history of MI, or documented silent ischemia) or symptoms or findings consistent with ischemic heart disease, coronary artery vasospasm (Prinzmetal's variant angina), or other significant underlying CV disease. Also, contraindicated in patients with uncontrolled hypertension or within 24 hours of treatment with another 5-HT$_1$ agonist or ergotamine-containing or ergot-type drug, such as dihydroergotamine or methysergide. Don't use within 2 weeks of stopping an MAO inhibitor.

NURSING CONSIDERATIONS
• Use cautiously in patients with hepatic or renal impairment.
• Use cautiously in patients with risk factors for coronary artery disease (hypertension, hypercholesterolemia, smoking, obesity, diabetes, strong family history of coronary artery disease, women with surgical or physiologic menopause, or men

---

Reactions may be *common*, uncommon, **life-threatening**, or COMMON AND LIFE-THREATENING.

older than age 40), unless a cardiac evaluation provides evidence that patient is free from cardiac disease. Monitor patient closely after first dose.

• Use cautiously in patients with hepatic or renal impairment.

• Assess CV status in patients who develop risk factors for coronary artery disease during treatment.

• Drug should be used only after a definite diagnosis of migraine is established.

• Don't use drug to prevent migraines or to treat hemiplegic or basilar migraine or cluster headaches.

• Safety of treating more than four headaches in a 30-day period hasn't been established.

• Safety and effectiveness of drug haven't been evaluated in children younger than age 18.

• The orally disintegrating tablets contain phenylalanine.

PATIENT TEACHING

• Inform patient that drug doesn't prevent migraine headache.

• For Maxalt-MLT, tell patient to remove blister pack from pouch and remove drug from blister pack immediately before use. Tablet shouldn't be popped out of blister pack; pack should be carefully peeled away with dry hands and tablet placed on tongue and allowed to dissolve. Tablet is then swallowed with saliva. No water is needed or recommended. Tell patient that orally dissolving tablet doesn't relieve headache more quickly.

• Advise patient that, if headache returns after initial dose, a second dose may be taken with medical approval at least 2 hours after the first dose. Warn against taking more than 30 mg in a 24-hour period.

• Inform patient that drug may cause somnolence and dizziness, and warn him to avoid hazardous activities until effects are known.

• Tell patient that food may delay onset of drug action.

• Advise patient to notify prescriber about suspected or known pregnancy.

• Instruct patient not to breast-feed during therapy because effects on the infant are unknown.

sibutramine hydrochloride monohydrate
Meridia

Pregnancy risk category C
Controlled substance schedule IV

AVAILABLE FORMS
Capsules: 5 mg, 10 mg, 15 mg

INDICATIONS & DOSAGES
➤ **Management of obesity—**
Adults: 10 mg P.O. given once daily with or without food. May increase to 15 mg P.O. daily after 4 weeks if weight loss is inadequate. Patients who don't tolerate 10 mg daily may receive 5 mg P.O. daily. Doses above 15 mg daily aren't recommended.

ACTION
Inhibits reuptake of norepinephrine, serotonin, and dopamine.

Route	Onset	Peak	Duration
P.O.	Unknown	3-4 hr	Unknown

ADVERSE REACTIONS
CNS: *headache, insomnia,* dizziness, nervousness, anxiety, depression, paresthesia, somnolence, CNS stimulation, emotional lability, asthenia, migraine.
CV: tachycardia, vasodilation, hypertension, palpitations, chest pain.
EENT: *rhinitis, pharyngitis,* sinusitis, ear disorder, ear pain.
GI: thirst, *anorexia, constipation,* increased appetite, nausea, dyspepsia, gastritis, vomiting, *dry mouth,* taste perversion, abdominal pain, rectal disorder.
GU: dysmenorrhea, urinary tract infection, vaginal candidiasis, metrorrhagia.
Musculoskeletal: arthralgia, myalgia, tenosynovitis, joint disorder, neck or back pain.
Respiratory: increased cough, laryngitis.
Skin: rash, sweating, acne.
Other: herpes simplex, flu syndrome, injury, accident, allergic reaction, generalized edema.

INTERACTIONS
Drug-drug. *CNS depressants:* May enhance CNS depression. Use together cautiously.

---

*Liquid contains alcohol.   **May contain tartrazine.   †Canada   ‡Australia   §U.K.   ◇OTC

Dextromethorphan, dihydroergotamine, fentanyl, fluoxetine, fluvoxamine, lithium, MAO inhibitors, meperidine, paroxetine, pentazocine, sertraline, sumatriptan, tryptophan, venlafaxine: May cause hyperthermia, tachycardia, and loss of consciousness. Avoid use together.
Ephedrine, pseudoephedrine: May increase blood pressure or heart rate. Use together cautiously.
Drug-lifestyle. *Alcohol use:* Enhanced CNS depression. Discourage use together.

EFFECTS ON LAB TEST RESULTS
● May increase ALT, AST, GGT, LDH, alkaline phosphatase, and bilirubin levels.

CONTRAINDICATIONS
Contraindicated in patients hypersensitive to drug or its active ingredients, in those taking MAO inhibitors or other centrally acting appetite suppressants, and in those with anorexia nervosa. Don't give to patients with severe renal or hepatic dysfunction, history of hypertension, coronary artery disease, heart failure, arrhythmias, or CVA.

NURSING CONSIDERATIONS
● Use cautiously in patients with history of seizures or angle-closure glaucoma.
● *Alert:* Sumatriptan is no longer recommended for use in elderly patients. Current precautions report that this population is more susceptible to decreased hepatic function, higher risk of coronary artery disease, and increased blood pressure when treated with the drug.
● Drug is recommended for obese patients with an initial body mass index of 30 kg/m^2 or more (27 kg/m^2 or more if patient has other risk factors, such as hypertension, diabetes, or dyslipidemia).
● Rule out organic causes of obesity before starting therapy.
● Measure blood pressure and pulse before starting therapy, with dosage changes, and at regular intervals during therapy.
● Separate drug therapy and MAO inhibitor therapy by at least 2 weeks.

PATIENT TEACHING
● Advise patient to report rash, hives, or other allergic reactions immediately.

● Instruct patient to notify prescriber before taking other prescription or OTC drugs.
● Advise patient to have blood pressure and pulse monitored at regular intervals. Stress importance of regular follow-up visits with health care provider.
● Advise patient to follow a reduced-calorie diet.
● Tell patient that weight loss can cause gallstone formation. Teach signs and symptoms, and tell patient to notify prescriber promptly if they occur.

---

sumatriptan succinate
Imigran§, Imitrex

Pregnancy risk category C

AVAILABLE FORMS
Injection: 6 mg/0.5 ml (12 mg/ml) in 0.5-ml prefilled syringes and vials
Nasal solution: 5 mg/0.1 ml, 20 mg/ 0.1 ml
Tablets: 25 mg, 50 mg, 100 mg (base)†

INDICATIONS & DOSAGES
➤ **Acute migraine attacks with or without aura—**
Adults: 6 mg S.C. Maximum recommended dose is two 6-mg injections daily with at least 1 hour between injections. Or, initially 25 to 100 mg P.O. and a second dose of up to 100 mg in 2 hours, if needed. Additional doses may be given q 2 hours, p.r.n., to maximum P.O. dosage of 300 mg daily. Intranasal dose is 5 to 20 mg sprayed into one nostril. If a 10-mg dose is needed, 5 mg is sprayed into each nostril. If needed, dosing may be repeated after 2 hours, to maximum of 40 mg daily.

ACTION
May act as an agonist at serotonin receptors on extracerebral intracranial blood vessels, which results in vasoconstriction of the affected vessels, inhibition of neuropeptide release, and reduction of pain transmission in the trigeminal pathways.

Route	Onset	Peak	Duration
Intranasal	Rapid	1-2 hr	Unknown
P.O.	0.5 hr	1.5 hr	Unknown
S.C.	10 min	12 min	Unknown

Reactions may be *common*, uncommon, *life-threatening*, or COMMON AND LIFE-THREATENING.

ADVERSE REACTIONS

CNS: *dizziness, vertigo,* drowsiness, headache, anxiety, malaise, fatigue, feeling of strangeness, tight feeling in head.
CV: pressure or tightness in chest, atrial fibrillation, *ventricular fibrillation, ventricular tachycardia, MI,* flushing.
EENT: discomfort of throat, nasal cavity, sinus, mouth, jaw, or tongue; altered vision.
GI: abdominal discomfort, dysphagia.
Musculoskeletal: myalgia, muscle cramps, neck pain.
Skin: diaphoresis.
Other: *injection site reaction; sensations of tingling, warmth, heat, burning, cold, or pressure; feelings of heaviness or tightness.*

INTERACTIONS

Drug-drug. *Ergot and ergot derivatives:* Prolonged vasospastic effects. Don't use these drugs and sumatriptan in the same 24-hour period.
MAO inhibitors: Increased sumatriptan effects. Avoid use within 2 weeks of MAO inhibitor therapy.
Selective serotonin reuptake inhibitors: May cause weakness, hyperreflexia, and incoordination. Monitor patient.
Drug-herb. *Horehound:* May enhance serotonergic effects. Discourage use together.

EFFECTS ON LAB TEST RESULTS
None reported.

CONTRAINDICATIONS
Contraindicated in patients hypersensitive to drug and in those with uncontrolled hypertension, ischemic heart disease (such as angina pectoris, Prinzmetal's angina, history of MI, or documented silent ischemia), or hemiplegic or basilar migraine. Also, contraindicated in those taking ergotamine or within 14 days of MAO inhibitor therapy.

NURSING CONSIDERATIONS
• Use cautiously in patient who is or intends to become pregnant.
• Also, use cautiously in patients who may have unrecognized coronary artery disease (such as postmenopausal women, men older than age 40, or patients with

such risk factors as hypertension, hypercholesterolemia, obesity, diabetes, smoking, or family history of coronary artery disease).
• *Alert:* When giving drug to patient at risk for unrecognized coronary artery disease, consider giving first dose in presence of other medical personnel. Serious adverse cardiac effects can follow S.C. administration of drug, but such events are rare.
• After S.C. injection, most patients experience relief in 1 to 2 hours.
• Redness or pain at injection site should subside within 1 hour after injection.
• *Alert:* Don't confuse sumatriptan with somatropin.

PATIENT TEACHING
• Inform patient that drug is intended only to treat migraine attacks, not to prevent them or reduce their occurrence.
• If patient is pregnant or intends to become pregnant, tell her not to use drug. Advise her to discuss with prescriber the risks and benefits of using drug during pregnancy.
• Tell patient that drug may be taken any time during a migraine attack, but should be taken as soon as signs or symptoms appear.
• Review information about drug's injectable form, which is available in a spring-loaded injector system that facilitates patient use. Make sure patient understands how to load the injector, give the injection, and dispose of used syringes.
• *Alert:* Tell patient to notify prescriber immediately about persistent or severe chest pain. Warn him to stop using drug and to call prescriber if he develops pain or tightness in the throat, wheezing, heart throbbing, rash, lumps, hives, or swollen eyelids, face, or lips.

---

tacrine hydrochloride
Cognex

Pregnancy risk category C

AVAILABLE FORMS
Capsules: 10 mg, 20 mg, 30 mg, 40 mg

INDICATIONS & DOSAGES
➤ **Mild to moderate dementia of the Alzheimer's type—**
Adults: Initially, 10 mg P.O. q.i.d. After 6 weeks, if patient tolerates treatment and has no elevations in transaminase levels, dosage increased to 20 mg q.i.d. After 6 weeks, dosage adjusted upward to 30 mg q.i.d. If still tolerated, dosage increased to 40 mg q.i.d. after another 6 weeks.

ACTION
Reversibly inhibits the enzyme cholinesterase in the CNS, preventing or blocking the breakdown of acetylcholine and thereby temporarily improving cognitive function in patients with Alzheimer's disease.

Route	Onset	Peak	Duration
P.O.	Unknown	0.5-3 hr	Unknown

ADVERSE REACTIONS
CNS: agitation, ataxia, insomnia, abnormal thinking, somnolence, depression, anxiety, *headache,* fatigue, *dizziness,* confusion.
CV: chest pain.
EENT: rhinitis.
GI: *nausea, vomiting, diarrhea,* dyspepsia, loose stools, changes in stool color, anorexia, abdominal pain, flatulence, constipation.
Metabolic: weight loss.
Musculoskeletal: myalgia.
Respiratory: upper respiratory tract infection, cough.
Skin: rash, jaundice, facial flushing.

INTERACTIONS
Drug-drug. *Anticholinergics:* May lessen the effects of tacrine. Avoid using together.
Cholinergics such as bethanechol, anticholinesterases: Additive effects. Monitor patient for toxicity.
Succinylcholine: Enhanced neuromuscular blockade and prolonged duration of action. Monitor patient closely.
Theophylline: Increased plasma theophylline levels and prolonged theophylline half-life. Carefully monitor plasma theophylline levels and adjust dosage.
Drug-food. *Any food:* Delayed drug absorption. Give drug 1 hour before meals.
Drug-lifestyle. *Smoking:* Decreased plasma drug levels. Ask patient about nicotine use, and monitor him closely.

EFFECTS ON LAB TEST RESULTS
● May increase ALT and AST levels.

CONTRAINDICATIONS
Contraindicated in patients hypersensitive to drug or to acridine derivatives. Also, contraindicated in patients for whom tacrine-related jaundice has previously developed and has been confirmed with a total bilirubin level of more than 3 mg/dl.

NURSING CONSIDERATIONS
● Use cautiously in patients with sick sinus syndrome or bradycardia, in patients at risk for peptic ulceration (including those taking NSAIDs or those with history of peptic ulcer), and in those with a history of hepatic disease. Also, use cautiously in patients with renal disease, asthma, prostatic hyperplasia, or other urine outflow impairment.
● Monitor ALT levels weekly during first 18 weeks of therapy. If ALT is modestly elevated (twice the upper limit of normal range) after first 18 weeks, continue weekly monitoring. If no problems are detected, frequency of serum level determinations is decreased to once every 3 months. On each occasion that dosage is increased, resume weekly monitoring for at least 6 weeks.
● If drug is discontinued for 4 weeks or longer, full dosage adjustment and monitoring schedule must be restarted.

PATIENT TEACHING
● Stress that drug doesn't alter the underlying degenerative disease but can stabilize or alleviate symptoms. Effect of therapy depends on drug administration at regular intervals.
● *Alert:* Remind caregiver that dosage adjustment is an integral part of the safe use of drug. Abrupt discontinuation or a large reduction in daily dosage (80 mg daily or more) may cause behavioral disturbances and a decline in cognitive function.
● Tell caregiver to give drug between meals whenever possible. If GI upset becomes a problem, drug may be taken with meals, although doing so may reduce plasma levels by 30% to 40%.
● Advise patient and caregiver to immediately report significant adverse reactions or changes in status.

Reactions may be *common,* uncommon, *life-threatening,* or COMMON AND LIFE-THREATENING.

zolmitriptan
Zomig, Zomig ZMT

Pregnancy risk category C

AVAILABLE FORMS
Tablets (immediate-release): 2.5 mg, 5 mg
Tablets (oral disintegrating): 2.5 mg, 5 mg

INDICATIONS & DOSAGES
➤ **Acute migraine headaches—**
Adults: Initially, 2.5 mg or less P.O., increased to 5 mg per dose, p.r.n. Or, disintegrating tablets: initially, 2.5 mg P.O. Don't break tablets in half. If headache returns after initial dose, a second dose may be given after 2 hours. Maximum dose is 10 mg in 24-hour period.
Adjust-a-dose: In patients with hepatic disease, use doses under 2.5 mg. Don't use orally disintegrating tablets because they shouldn't be broken in half.

ACTION
May act as an agonist at serotonin receptors on extracerebral intracranial blood vessels, which results in vasoconstriction of the affected vessels, inhibition of neuropeptide release, and reduction of pain transmission in the trigeminal pathways.

Route	Onset	Peak	Duration
P.O.	Unknown	2 hr	3 hr
S.L.	Unknown	2 hr	Unknown

ADVERSE REACTIONS
CNS: somnolence, vertigo, hyperesthesia, paresthesia, asthenia, *dizziness,* syncope.
CV: pain or heaviness in chest, ***arrhythmias,*** hypertension.
GI: dyspepsia, dysphagia, nausea.
Metabolic: hyperglycemia.
Musculoskeletal: myalgia.
Other: warm or cold sensations; *pain, tightness, or pressure in the neck, throat, or jaw.*

INTERACTIONS
Drug-drug. *Cimetidine:* Doubles half-life of zolmitriptan. Monitor patient.
Ergot-containing drugs: May cause additive vasospastic reactions. Avoid using together.

Fluoxetine, fluvoxamine, paroxetine, sertraline: May cause weakness, hyperreflexia, and incoordination. Use cautiously.
MAO inhibitors: Increased effects of zolmitriptan. Avoid using together.

EFFECTS ON LAB TEST RESULTS
● May increase glucose levels.

CONTRAINDICATIONS
Contraindicated in patients hypersensitive to drug and in those with ischemic heart disease, other significant heart disease (including Wolff-Parkinson-White syndrome), or uncontrolled hypertension. Don't give within 24 hours of ergot-containing drugs or within 2 weeks of discontinuing MAO inhibitor therapy.

NURSING CONSIDERATIONS
● Use cautiously in patients with liver disease.
● Drug isn't intended for preventing migraines or treating hemiplegic or basilar migraines.
● Safety of drug hasn't been established for cluster headaches.
● Don't give drug to patient who is or may be pregnant; also, don't give drug to breast-feeding patient.

PATIENT TEACHING
● Tell patient that drug is intended to relieve, not prevent, signs and symptoms of migraine.
● Advise patient to take drug as prescribed and not to take a second dose unless instructed by prescriber. Tell patient if a second dose is indicated and permitted, he should take it 2 hours after initial dose.
● Instruct patient not to release the orally disintegrating tablets from their blister pack until just before taking. Open the pack and dissolve on tongue.
● Advise patient not to break the orally disintegrating tablets in half.
● Advise patient to immediately report pain or tightness in the chest or throat, heart throbbing, rash, skin lumps, or swelling of the face, lips, or eyelids.
● Tell patient not to take drug if she plans to become or suspects or knows that she's pregnant.

35

Cholinergics (parasympathomimetics)

bethanechol chloride
cevimeline hydrochloride
edrophonium chloride
neostigmine bromide
neostigmine methylsulfate
physostigmine salicylate
pyridostigmine bromide

COMBINATION PRODUCTS
None.

---

bethanechol chloride
Duvoid, Myotonachol, Myotonine§,
Urabeth, Urecholine, Urocarb‡

Pregnancy risk category C

AVAILABLE FORMS
Injection: 5 mg/ml
Tablets: 5 mg, 10 mg, 25 mg, 50 mg

INDICATIONS & DOSAGES
➤**Acute postoperative and postpartum nonobstructive (functional) urine retention, neurogenic atony of urinary bladder with urine retention—**
Adults: 10 to 50 mg P.O. t.i.d. to q.i.d. Or, 2.5 to 5 mg S.C. Never give I.M. or I.V. When drug is used for urine retention, some patients may need 50 to 100 mg P.O. per dose. Use such doses with extreme caution.

Test dose is 2.5 mg S.C., repeated at 15- to 30-minute intervals to total of four doses to determine the minimal effective dose; then, minimal effective dose used q 6 to 8 hours. All doses must be adjusted individually.

ACTION
Directly stimulates primarily muscarinic cholinergic receptors, mimicking the action of acetylcholine, increasing tone and peristalsis in the GI tract, and increasing contraction of the detrusor muscle of the urinary bladder.

Route	Onset	Peak	Duration
P.O.	30-90 min	1 hr	6 hr
S.C.	5-15 min	15-30 min	2 hr

ADVERSE REACTIONS
CNS: headache, malaise.
CV: *bradycardia,* profound hypotension with reflexive tachycardia, flushing.
EENT: lacrimation, miosis.
GI: *abdominal cramps, diarrhea,* excessive salivation, nausea, belching, borborygmus.
GU: urinary urgency.
Respiratory: *bronchoconstriction,* increased bronchial secretions.
Skin: diaphoresis.

INTERACTIONS
Drug-drug. *Anticholinergics, atropine, procainamide, quinidine:* May reverse cholinergic effects. Observe patient for lack of drug effect.
Anticholinesterases, cholinergic agonists: May cause additive effects or increase toxicity. Avoid using together.
Ganglionic blockers: May cause critical decrease in blood pressure, usually preceded by severe abdominal pain. Avoid using together.

EFFECTS ON LAB TEST RESULTS
• May increase liver enzyme, amylase, and lipase levels.

CONTRAINDICATIONS
Contraindicated in patients hypersensitive to drug or its components and in those with uncertain strength or integrity of bladder wall, mechanical obstruction of GI or urinary tract, hyperthyroidism, peptic ulceration, latent or active bronchial asthma, obstructive pulmonary disease, pronounced bradycardia or hypotension, vasomotor instability, cardiac or coronary artery disease, hypertension, seizure disorder, Parkinson's disease, spastic GI disturbances, acute inflammatory lesions of the GI tract, peritonitis, or marked vago-

---

tonia. Also contraindicated for I.M. or I.V. use and when increased muscular activity of the GI or urinary tract is harmful.

NURSING CONSIDERATIONS
• Use cautiously in pregnant patient.
• Give drug on empty stomach; otherwise, it may cause nausea and vomiting.
• Adverse effects are rare with P.O. dosing.
• *Alert:* Never give I.M. or I.V. because of possible circulatory collapse, hypotension, severe abdominal cramping, bloody diarrhea, shock, or cardiac arrest.
• Monitor vital signs frequently, especially respirations. Always have atropine injection available, and be prepared to give 0.6 mg S.C. or by slow I.V. push. Provide respiratory support, if needed.
• Watch for toxicity, especially with S.C. administration. Edrophonium isn't effective against muscle relaxation caused by bethanechol.
• Watch closely for adverse reactions that may indicate drug toxicity.
• Oral drug absorption is poor and variable, requiring larger oral doses. Oral and S.C. doses aren't interchangeable.

PATIENT TEACHING
• Tell patient to take oral form on an empty stomach and at regular intervals.
• Inform patient that drug is usually effective 30 to 90 minutes after oral use and 5 to 15 minutes after S.C. administration.

---

cevimeline hydrochloride
Evoxac

Pregnancy risk category C

AVAILABLE FORMS
Tablets: 30 mg

INDICATIONS & DOSAGES
➤ **Treatment of dry mouth in patients with Sjögren's syndrome—**
Adults: 30 mg P.O. t.i.d.

ACTION
Helps counteract dry mouth caused by Sjögren's syndrome by stimulating the muscarinic receptors of the saliva-producing glands.

Route	Onset	Peak	Duration
P.O.	Unknown	1.5-2 hr	Unknown

ADVERSE REACTIONS
CNS: anxiety, depression, dizziness, fatigue, *headache,* hypoesthesia, insomnia, migraine, pain, tremor, vertigo.
CV: chest pain, palpitations, peripheral edema.
EENT: abnormal vision, conjunctivitis, earache, epistaxis, eye infection, eye pain, otitis media, pharyngitis, *rhinitis, sinusitis,* xeropthalmia, eye abnormality.
GI: abdominal pain, anorexia, constipation, *diarrhea,* dry mouth, eructation, excessive salivation, flatulence, gastroesophageal reflux, *nausea,* salivary gland enlargement and pain, sialoadenitis, ulcerative stomatitis, vomiting, dyspepsia, increased amylase.
GU: cystitis, candidiasis, urinary tract infection, vaginitis.
Hematologic: anemia.
Musculoskeletal: arthralgia, back pain, hypertonia, hyporeflexia, leg cramps, myalgia, rigors, skeletal pain, tooth disorder, toothache.
Respiratory: *upper respiratory tract infection,* bronchitis, pneumonia, coughing, hiccups.
Skin: rash, pruritus, skin disorder, erythematous rash, *excessive sweating.*
Other: fever, fungal infections, flulike symptoms, injury, hot flushes, postoperative pain, allergic reaction, infection, abscess.

INTERACTIONS
Drug-drug. *Beta blockers:* May cause conduction disturbances. Use together cautiously.
Drugs with parasympathomimetic effects: Additive effects. Use together cautiously.
Drugs that inhibit CYP2D6, CYP3A4, CYP3A3: Inhibited metabolism of cevimeline. Monitor patient closely.

EFFECTS ON LAB TEST RESULTS
• May increase amylase levels.
• May decrease hemoglobin.

CONTRAINDICATIONS

Contraindicated in patients hypersensitive to drug and in those for whom miosis is undesirable (as in those who have acute iritis or narrow-angle glaucoma). Also contraindicated in patients with uncontrolled asthma.

NURSING CONSIDERATIONS

● Use cautiously in patients with significant CV disease (such as angina pectoris or MI) because drug may alter cardiac conduction and heart rate.

● Because drug may cause bronchial constriction and increase bronchial secretions, it should be used cautiously in patients with controlled asthma, chronic bronchitis, or COPD.

● In patients with a history of nephrolithiasis, drug should be used with caution because an increase in ureteral smooth muscle tone could cause renal colic or ureteral reflux.

● Use cautiously in patients with cholelithiasis because contractions of the gallbladder or biliary smooth muscle could cause cholecystitis, cholangitis, and biliary obstruction.

● Monitor patients with a history of asthma, COPD, or chronic bronchitis for an increase in signs or symptoms, such as wheezing, increased sputum production, or cough.

● Monitor patients with a history of cardiac disease for changes in heart rate or increased frequency, severity, or duration of angina.

● Monitor elderly patients closely because they have an increased risk of decreased renal, hepatic, and cardiac function and a greater likelihood of contracting disease together with drug or therapy.

PATIENT TEACHING

● Tell patient not to interrupt or stop treatment without consulting prescriber.

● Tell patient that sweating is a common drug effect. Urge adequate fluid intake to prevent dehydration.

● Inform patient that drug may cause visual disturbances, especially at night, which can impair driving ability.

---

edrophonium chloride
Enlon, Reversol, Tensilon

Pregnancy risk category C

AVAILABLE FORMS
Injection: 10 mg/ml in 1-ml ampules or in 10-ml or 15-ml vials

INDICATIONS & DOSAGES
➤**As curare antagonist to reverse nondepolarizing neuromuscular blocking action—**
Adults: 10 mg I.V. given over 30 to 45 seconds. Dose may be repeated, p.r.n., to maximum of 40 mg. Larger amounts may potentiate curare effect.

➤**Diagnostic aid in myasthenia gravis (Tensilon test)—**
Adults: 1 to 2 mg I.V. over 15 to 30 seconds; then 8 mg if no response occurs. Or, 10 mg I.M. If cholinergic reaction occurs, 2 mg I.M. is given 30 minutes later to rule out false-negative response.
Children weighing more than 34 kg (75 lb): 2 mg I.V. If no response within 45 seconds, 1 mg q 45 seconds to maximum of 10 mg. Or, 5 mg I.M.
Children weighing 34 kg or less: 1 mg I.V. If no response within 45 seconds, 1 mg q 45 seconds to maximum of 5 mg. Or, 2 mg I.M.

➤**To differentiate myasthenic crisis from cholinergic crisis—**
Adults: 1 mg I.V. If no response in 1 minute, repeat dose once. Increased muscle strength confirms myasthenic crisis; no increase or exaggerated weakness confirms cholinergic crisis.

I.V. ADMINISTRATION
● For easier administration, use tuberculin syringe with an I.V. needle.

● *Alert:* Monitor vital signs frequently, especially respirations. Always have atropine injection available, and be prepared to give 0.5 to 1 mg by S.C. route or slow I.V. push. Provide respiratory support, as needed.

● If using drug to distinguish myasthenic crisis from cholinergic crisis and patient is apneic, secure controlled ventilation before giving drug.

ACTION
Rapidly, reversibly inhibits acetylcholinesterase, thus blocking destruction of acetylcholine released from the parasympathetic and somatic efferent nerves. Acetylcholine accumulates, promoting increased stimulation of the receptors.

Route	Onset	Peak	Duration
I.M.	2-10 min	Unknown	10-40 min
I.V.	< 1 min	Unknown	5-20 min

ADVERSE REACTIONS
CNS: *seizures,* weakness, dysarthria, dysphonia, dizziness, drowsiness, headache, syncope.
CV: hypotension, *bradycardia,* flushing, *AV block, cardiac arrest.*
EENT: excessive lacrimation, diplopia, miosis, conjunctival hyperemia.
GI: nausea, vomiting, *diarrhea, abdominal cramps,* excessive salivation, dysphagia.
GU: urinary frequency, incontinence.
Musculoskeletal: muscle cramps, muscle fasciculation.
Respiratory: *paralysis of respiratory muscles, central respiratory paralysis, bronchospasm, laryngospasm,* increased bronchial secretions, *respiratory depression, respiratory arrest,* dyspnea.
Skin: rash, diaphoresis.

INTERACTIONS
Drug-drug. *Aminoglycosides:* Prolonged or enhanced muscle weakness. Monitor patient closely.
Cardiac glycosides: May increase sensitivity of heart to edrophonium. Use together cautiously.
Cholinergics: Increased effects of cholinergics mimicking myasthenic weakness. Stop all other cholinergics before giving drug.
Corticosteroids, magnesium, procainamide, quinidine: May antagonize cholinergic effects. Watch for lack of drug effect.
Depolarizing muscle relaxants (succinylcholine): Increased neuromuscular blocking effects, prolonged respiratory depression. Monitor patient closely.
Local and general anesthetics: May antagonize cholinergic effects. Watch for lack of drug effect.

Drug-herb. *Jaborandi tree, pill-bearing spurge:* May have additive effect. Ask patient about alternative medicine remedies, and recommend caution.

EFFECTS ON LAB TEST RESULTS
None reported.

CONTRAINDICATIONS
Contraindicated in patients hypersensitive to anticholinesterases and in those with mechanical obstruction of the intestine or urinary tract.

NURSING CONSIDERATIONS
● Use cautiously in patients with bronchial asthma or cardiac arrhythmias.
● *Alert:* Watch closely for adverse reactions; they may indicate toxicity.
● Drug isn't effective against neuromuscular block induced by decamethonium bromide and succinylcholine chloride.
● Because this cholinergic has the most rapid onset but shortest duration, it isn't used to treat myasthenia gravis.
● When giving drug to differentiate myasthenic crisis from cholinergic crisis, observe patient's muscle strength closely.
● I.M. route may be used in children because of difficulty with I.V. route. Expect same reactions as with I.V. test, but these appear after 2- to 10-minute delay.

PATIENT TEACHING
● Urge patient to report adverse reactions promptly.
● Tell patient to report discomfort at I.V. site.

---

neostigmine bromide
Prostigmin

neostigmine methylsulfate
Prostigmin

Pregnancy risk category C

AVAILABLE FORMS
neostigmine bromide
Tablets: 15 mg
neostigmine methylsulfate
Injection: 0.25 mg/ml, 0.5 mg/ml, 1 mg/ml

INDICATIONS & DOSAGES
➤**Myasthenia gravis—**
Adults: Initially, 15 mg P.O. t.i.d.; increase gradually, p.r.n. Range is 15 to 375 mg/day. Average dosage is 150 mg/day with intervals individualized. Or, 0.5 to 2.5 mg S.C. or I.M.; subsequent parenteral doses should be based on patient's response.
Children: 7.5 to 15 mg P.O. t.i.d. or q.i.d. or 0.01 to 0.04 mg/kg/dose I.M. or S.C. q 2 to 3 hours, p.r.n.
➤**Diagnosis of myasthenia gravis—**
Adults: 0.022 mg/kg I.M. 30 minutes after 0.011 mg/kg of atropine sulfate I.M.
Children: 0.025 to 0.04 mg/kg I.M. after 0.011 mg/kg of atropine sulfate S.C.
➤**Postoperative abdominal distention and bladder atony—**
Adults: For treatment, 0.5 to 1 mg I.M. or S.C. q 3 hours for 5 doses after bladder has emptied. For prevention, 0.25 mg I.M. or S.C. q 4 to 6 hours for 2 to 3 days.
➤**Antidote for nondepolarizing neuromuscular blockers—**
Adults: 0.5 to 2.5 mg I.V. slowly. Repeat, p.r.n., to total of 5 mg. Before antidote dose, give 0.6 to 1.2 mg atropine sulfate I.V. if patient is bradycardic.

I.V. ADMINISTRATION
• Give at a slow, controlled rate, not exceeding 1 mg/minute in adults.
• If patient's muscle weakness is severe, prescriber will determine whether severity is caused by drug-induced toxicity or worsening of myasthenia gravis. Test dose of edrophonium I.V. will aggravate drug-induced weakness but will temporarily relieve disease-induced weakness.

ACTION
Competitively inhibits acetylcholinesterase, thus blocking the destruction of acetylcholine released from the parasympathetic and somatic efferent nerves. Acetylcholine accumulates, promoting increased stimulation of the receptors.

Route	Onset	Peak	Duration
I.M., S.C.	20-30 min	1-2 hr	2-4 hr
I.V.	4-8 min	1-2 hr	2-4 hr
P.O.	45-75 min	1-2 hr	2-4 hr

ADVERSE REACTIONS
CNS: dizziness, headache, muscle weakness, loss of consciousness, drowsiness, syncope, *seizures.*
CV: *bradycardia,* hypotension, tachycardia, *AV block,* flushing, *cardiac arrest.*
EENT: blurred vision, lacrimation, miosis.
GI: *nausea, vomiting, diarrhea, abdominal cramps,* excessive salivation, flatulence, increased peristalsis.
GU: urinary frequency.
Musculoskeletal: *muscle cramps,* muscle fasciculations, arthralgia.
Respiratory: *bronchospasm,* dyspnea, *respiratory depression, respiratory arrest,* increased secretions, *laryngospasm, paralysis of respiratory muscles, central respiratory paralysis.*
Skin: rash, urticaria, diaphoresis.
Other: hypersensitivity reactions, *anaphylaxis.*

INTERACTIONS
Drug-drug. *Aminoglycosides, anticholinergics, atropine, corticosteroids, local and general anesthetics, magnesium sulfate, procainamide, quinidine:* May reverse cholinergic effects; watch for lack of drug effect. Stop all other cholinergics before giving this drug.
Succinylcholine: May worsen blockade produced by succinylcholine when used to reverse the effects of nondepolarizing neuromuscular blockers in patients who have undergone surgery. Monitor patient.

EFFECTS ON LAB TEST RESULTS
None reported.

CONTRAINDICATIONS
Contraindicated in patients hypersensitive to cholinergics or bromides and in those with peritonitis or mechanical obstruction of the intestinal or urinary tract.

NURSING CONSIDERATIONS
• Use cautiously in patients with bronchial asthma, bradycardia, seizure disorders, recent coronary occlusion, vagotonia, hyperthyroidism, arrhythmias, and peptic ulcer.
• Dosage for the treatment of myasthenia gravis must be highly individualized, depending on response and tolerance of ad-

verse effects. Therapy may be needed day and night.
● In myasthenia gravis, schedule doses before periods of fatigue. For example, if patient has dysphagia, schedule dose 30 minutes before each meal.
● *Alert:* Monitor vital signs frequently, especially respirations. Keep atropine injection available, and be prepared to provide respiratory support, as needed.
● Monitor and document patient's response after each dose. Optimum dosage is difficult to judge. Watch closely for improvement in strength, vision, and ptosis 45 to 60 minutes after each dose.
● Neostigmine I.M. may be used instead of edrophonium to diagnose myasthenia gravis and may be preferable to edrophonium for lengthy procedures to test limb strength.
● When drug is used to prevent abdominal distention and GI distress, insertion of a rectal tube may help passage of gas.
● When drug is given for postoperative abdominal distention and bladder atony, mechanical obstruction should be ruled out before doses are given. If no response within 1 hour after first dose, patient should be catheterized.
● Patients sometimes develop resistance to neostigmine.
● If appropriate, obtain order for hospitalized patient to have bedside supply of tablets. Many patients with long-standing disease insist on self-administration.

PATIENT TEACHING
● Tell patient to take drug with food or milk to reduce adverse GI reactions.
● When giving drug for myasthenia gravis, explain that it will relieve ptosis, double vision, trouble chewing and swallowing, and trunk and limb weakness. Stress the importance of taking drug exactly as ordered, including nighttime doses. Explain that patient may need to take drug for life.
● Teach patient how to observe and record variations in muscle strength.
● Advise patient to wear or carry medical identification that identifies his myasthenia gravis.

physostigmine salicylate (eserine salicylate)
Antilirium

Pregnancy risk category C

AVAILABLE FORMS
Injection: 1 mg/ml

INDICATIONS & DOSAGES
➤ **To reverse CNS toxicity from clinical or toxic dosages of drugs capable of producing anticholinergic syndrome—**
Adults: 0.5 to 2 mg I.M. or I.V. or 1 mg/ minute I.V. repeated q 20 minutes p.r.n. until patient responds or adverse cholinergic effects occur. Additional doses of 1 to 4 mg I.M. or I.V. q 30 to 60 minutes may be given if life-threatening problems such as coma, seizures, and arrhythmias recur.
Children: Reserved for life-threatening situations. Give 0.02 mg/kg I.M. or slow I.V., repeated q 5 to 10 minutes until response occurs. Maximum dose is 2 mg.

I.V. ADMINISTRATION
● Give I.V. at controlled rate; use direct injection at no more than 1 mg/minute in adults or 0.5 mg/minute in children.
● Monitor vital signs frequently, especially respirations. Position patient to ease breathing. Keep atropine injection available, and be prepared to give 0.5 mg S.C. or by slow I.V. push. Provide respiratory support, as needed. Best given in presence of prescriber.

ACTION
Reversibly inhibits acetylcholinesterase, thus blocking the destruction of acetylcholine released from the parasympathetic and somatic efferent nerves. Acetylcholine accumulates, promoting increased stimulation of the receptor.

Route	Onset	Peak	Duration
I.M.	3-5 min	20-30 min	0.5-5 hr
I.V.	3-5 min	5 min	0.5-5 hr

ADVERSE REACTIONS
CNS: *seizures,* muscle weakness, *restlessness, excitability.*
CV: *bradycardia,* hypotension.
EENT: miosis.

GI: nausea, vomiting, epigastric pain, *diarrhea, excessive salivation.*
GU: urinary urgency.
Respiratory: *bronchospasm, bronchial constriction,* dyspnea, *respiratory paralysis.*
Skin: diaphoresis.

INTERACTIONS
Drug-drug. *Anticholinergics, atropine, local and general anesthetics, procainamide, quinidine:* May reverse cholinergic effects. Observe patient for lack of drug effect.
Ganglionic blockers: May decrease blood pressure. Avoid using together.
Neuromuscular blockers (succinylcholine): Increased neuromuscular blockade, respiratory depression. Use together cautiously.
Drug-herb. *Jaborandi tree, pill-bearing spurge:* May have additive effect. Ask patient about use of herbal remedies, and recommend caution.

EFFECTS ON LAB TEST RESULTS
None reported.

CONTRAINDICATIONS
Contraindicated in patients with mechanical obstruction of the intestine or urogenital tract; in patients with asthma, gangrene, diabetes, CV disease, or vagotonia; and in patients receiving choline esters or depolarizing neuromuscular blockers.

NURSING CONSIDERATIONS
● Use cautiously in pregnant patients and patients with epilepsy, parkinsonian syndrome, or bradycardia.
● Use only clear solution. Darkening may indicate loss of potency.
● *Alert:* Watch closely for adverse reactions, particularly CNS disturbances. Raise side rails of bed if patient becomes restless or hallucinates. Adverse reactions may indicate drug toxicity.
● Effectiveness is typically immediate and dramatic but it may be transient. Patient may need repeated doses.

PATIENT TEACHING
● Inform patient of need for drug, explain its use and adverse reactions, and answer any questions or concerns.

● Tell patient to report adverse reactions promptly.
● Instruct patient to report discomfort at I.V. site.

---

pyridostigmine bromide
Mestinon*, Mestinon-SR†, Mestinon Timespans, Regonol

Pregnancy risk category C

AVAILABLE FORMS
Injection: 5 mg/ml in 2-ml ampules or 5-ml vials
Syrup: 60 mg/5 ml
Tablets: 60 mg
Tablets (extended-release): 180 mg

INDICATIONS & DOSAGES
➤**Antidote for nondepolarizing neuromuscular blockers—**
Adults: 10 to 20 mg I.V., preceded by atropine sulfate 0.6 to 1.2 mg I.V.
➤**Myasthenia gravis—**
Adults: 60 to 120 mg P.O. q 3 or 4 hours. Usual dose is 600 mg daily but doses up to 1,500 mg daily may be needed. For I.M. or I.V. use, give ¹⁄₃₀ of oral dose. Dosage must be adjusted for each patient, based on response and tolerance. Or, 180 to 540 mg extended-release tablets P.O. b.i.d., with at least 6 hours between doses.
Children: 7 mg/kg or 200 mg/m² daily in five or six divided doses.
➤**Supportive treatment of neonates born to myasthenic mothers—**
Neonates: 0.05 to 0.15 mg/kg I.M. q 4 to 6 hours. Dosage decreased daily until drug can be withdrawn.

I.V. ADMINISTRATION
● *Alert:* Give I.V. injection no faster than 1 mg/minute. Rapid I.V. infusion may cause bradycardia and seizures. Monitor vital signs frequently, especially respirations. Position patient to ease breathing. Keep atropine injection available, and be prepared to give it; provide respiratory support, as needed.
● If patient's muscle weakness is severe, prescriber will determine whether severity is caused by drug-induced toxicity or worsening of myasthenia gravis. Test dose of edrophonium I.V. will aggravate drug-

---

induced weakness, but will temporarily relieve disease-induced weakness.

ACTION
Competitively inhibits acetylcholin-esterase, thus blocking the destruction of acetylcholine released from the parasym-pathetic and somatic efferent nerves. Acetylcholine accumulates, promoting in-creased stimulation of the receptors.

Route	Onset	Peak	Duration
I.M.	15 min	Unknown	2-4 hr
I.V.	2-5 min	Unknown	2-4 hr
P.O.	20-30 min	1-2 hr	3-6 hr
P.O. (extended)	30-60 min	1-2 hr	6-12 hr

ADVERSE REACTIONS
CNS: headache with high doses, weak-ness, syncope.
CV: *bradycardia,* hypotension, *cardiac arrest,* thrombophlebitis.
EENT: miosis.
GI: abdominal cramps, *nausea, vomiting,* diarrhea, excessive salivation, increased peristalsis.
Musculoskeletal: muscle cramps, muscle fasciculations.
Respiratory: *bronchospasm, broncho-constriction,* increased bronchial secre-tions.
Skin: rash, diaphoresis.

INTERACTIONS
Drug-drug. *Aminoglycosides:* Prolonged or enhanced muscle weakness. Use to-gether cautiously.
Anticholinergics, atropine, corticoste-roids, general or local anesthetics, magne-sium, procainamide, quinidine: May an-tagonize cholinergic effects. Observe patient for lack of drug effect.
Ganglionic blockers: Increased risk of hypotension. Monitor patient closely.

EFFECTS ON LAB TEST RESULTS
None reported.

CONTRAINDICATIONS
Contraindicated in patients hypersensitive to anticholinesterases or bromides and in those with mechanical obstruction of the intestinal or urinary tract.

NURSING CONSIDERATIONS
● Use cautiously in patients with bronchial asthma, bradycardia, arrhythmias, epilep-sy, recent coronary occlusion, vagotonia, hyperthyroidism, or peptic ulcer. Also use cautiously in pregnant women.
● Stop all other cholinergics before giving this drug.
● Don't crush extended-release tablets.
● When using sweet syrup for patients who have trouble swallowing, give over ice chips if patient can't tolerate flavor.
● Monitor and document patient's re-sponse after each dose. Optimum dosage is difficult to judge.
● *Alert:* In the United States, Regonol con-tains benzyl ethanol preservative, which may cause toxicity in neonates if given in high doses. The Canadian formulation of this drug doesn't contain benzyl ethanol.
● If appropriate, obtain order for hospital-ized patient to have bedside supply of tablets. Many patients with long-standing disease insist on self-administration.
● *Alert:* Don't confuse Mestinon with Mesantoin or Metatensin.

PATIENT TEACHING
● When giving drug for myasthenia gravis, stress importance of taking it exactly as ordered, on time, in evenly spaced doses. If using extended-release tablets, explain that patient must take tablets at same time each day, at least 6 hours apart.
● Advise patient not to crush or chew extended-release tablets.
● Explain that patient may have to take drug for life.
● Advise patient to wear or carry medical identification that identifies his myasthe-nia gravis.

36

Anticholinergics

atropine sulfate
(See Chapter 19, ANTIARRHYTHMICS.)
dicyclomine hydrochloride
glycopyrrolate
hyoscyamine
hyoscyamine sulfate
scopolamine
scopolamine butylbromide
scopolamine hydrobromide

COMBINATION PRODUCTS
BARBIDONNA No. 2 TABLETS: atropine sulfate 0.025 mg, scopolamine hydrobromide 0.0074 mg, hyoscyamine hydrobromide or sulfate 0.1286 mg, and phenobarbital 32 mg.
BARBIDONNA TABLETS: atropine sulfate 0.025 mg, scopolamine hydrobromide 0.0074 mg, hyoscyamine hydrobromide or sulfate 0.1286 mg, and phenobarbital 16 mg.
DONNATAL CAPSULES AND TABLETS: atropine sulfate 0.0194 mg, scopolamine hydrobromide 0.0065 mg, hyoscyamine hydrobromide or sulfate 0.1037 mg, and phenobarbital 16.2 mg.
DONNATAL ELIXIR*: atropine sulfate 0.0194 mg/5 ml, scopolamine hydrobromide 0.0065 mg/5 ml, ethanol 23%, hyoscyamine hydrobromide or sulfate 0.1037 mg/5 ml, and phenobarbital 16 mg/5 ml.
DONNATAL EXTENTABS: atropine sulfate 0.0582 mg, scopolamine hydrobromide 0.0195 mg, hyoscyamine sulfate 0.3111 mg, and phenobarbital 48.6 mg.

---

dicyclomine hydrochloride
Antispas, A-Spas, Bentyl, Bentylol†, Byclomine, Dibent, Di-Spaz, Formulex†, Lominet†, Merbentyl‡, Or-Tyl, Spasmoban†

Pregnancy risk category B

AVAILABLE FORMS
Capsules: 10 mg, 20 mg
Injection: 10 mg/ml

Syrup: 5 mg/5 ml‡, 10 mg/5 ml
Tablets: 10 mg‡, 20 mg

INDICATIONS & DOSAGES
➤ **Irritable bowel syndrome, other functional GI disorders—**
Adults: Initially, 20 mg P.O. q.i.d., increased to 40 mg q.i.d. Or, 20 mg I.M. q.i.d.

ACTION
Inhibits action of acetylcholine on postganglionic, parasympathetic muscarinic receptors, decreasing GI motility. Also, possesses local anesthetic properties that may be partly responsible for spasmolysis.

Route	Onset	Peak	Duration
I.M., P.O.	Unknown	1-1.5 hr	Unknown

ADVERSE REACTIONS
CNS: *headache; dizziness;* insomnia; light-headedness; drowsiness; nervousness, confusion, and excitement in elderly patients.
CV: *palpitations,* tachycardia.
EENT: blurred vision, increased intraocular pressure, mydriasis, photophobia.
GI: nausea, vomiting, *constipation, dry mouth, thirst,* abdominal distention, heartburn, paralytic ileus.
GU: *urinary hesitancy, urine retention,* impotence.
Skin: urticaria, decreased sweating or possible anhidrosis, local irritation.
Other: fever, allergic reactions.

INTERACTIONS
Drug-drug. *Amantadine, antihistamines, antiparkinsonians, disopyramide, glutethimide, meperidine, phenothiazines, procainamide, quinidine, TCAs:* Additive adverse effects. Avoid using together.
Antacids: Decreased absorption of oral anticholinergics. Separate administration times by 2 to 3 hours.
Ketoconazole: Anticholinergics may interfere with ketoconazole absorption.

Reactions may be *common*, uncommon, ***life-threatening***, or COMMON AND LIFE-THREATENING.

Separate administration times by 2 to 3 hours.

Methotrimeprazine: Anticholinergics may enhance risk of extrapyramidal reactions. Avoid using together.

EFFECTS ON LAB TEST RESULTS
None reported.

CONTRAINDICATIONS
Contraindicated in patients hypersensitive to anticholinergics and in those with obstructive uropathy, obstructive disease of the GI tract, reflux esophagitis, severe ulcerative colitis, toxic megacolon, myasthenia gravis, unstable CV status in acute hemorrhage, tachycardia secondary to cardiac insufficiency or thyrotoxicosis, or glaucoma; also contraindicated in breast-feeding patients and in children younger than age 6 months.

NURSING CONSIDERATIONS
• Use cautiously in patients with autonomic neuropathy, hyperthyroidism, coronary artery disease, arrhythmias, heart failure, hypertension, hiatal hernia, hepatic or renal disease, prostatic hyperplasia, known or suspected GI infection, and ulcerative colitis. Also, use cautiously in patients in hot or humid environments. Drug-induced heat stroke can develop.
• Give drug 30 to 60 minutes before meals and at bedtime. Bedtime dose can be larger; give at least 2 hours after last meal of day.
• *Alert:* Don't give S.C. or I.V.
• Adjust dosage based on patient's needs and response. Doses up to 40 mg P.O. q.i.d. have been used in adults, but safety and efficacy for longer than 2 weeks haven't been established.
• Dicyclomine is a synthetic tertiary derivative that may have atropine-like adverse reactions.
• *Alert:* Overdose may cause curarelike effects, such as respiratory paralysis. Keep emergency equipment available.
• Monitor patient's vital signs and urine output carefully.
• *Alert:* The dicyclomine labeling may be misleading. The ampule label reads 10 mg/ml but doesn't indicate that the ampule contains 2 ml of solution and, therefore, 20 mg of drug.

• *Alert:* Don't confuse dicyclomine with dyclonine or doxycycline; don't confuse Bentyl with Aventyl or Benadryl.

PATIENT TEACHING
• Tell patient when to take drug, and stress importance of doing so on time and at evenly spaced intervals.
• Advise patient to avoid driving and other hazardous activities if drowsiness, dizziness, or blurred vision occurs; to drink plenty of fluids to help prevent constipation; and to report rash or other skin eruption.

---

glycopyrrolate
Robinul, Robinul Forte

Pregnancy risk category B

AVAILABLE FORMS
Injection: 0.2 mg/ml
Tablets: 1 mg, 2 mg

INDICATIONS & DOSAGES
➤ **Blockade of adverse cholinergic effects caused by anticholinesterases used to reverse neuromuscular blockade—**
Adults and children: 0.2 mg I.V. for each 1 mg of neostigmine or 5 mg of pyridostigmine. May be given I.V. without dilution or may be added to dextrose injection and given by infusion.
➤ **Preoperatively to diminish secretions and block cardiac vagal reflexes—**
Adults and children 2 and older: 0.0044 mg/kg I.M. 30 to 60 minutes before anesthesia.
Children younger than age 2: 0.0088 mg/kg I.M. 30 to 60 minutes before anesthesia.
➤ **Adjunctive therapy in peptic ulcerations and other GI disorders—**
Adults: 1 to 2 mg P.O. t.i.d. or 0.1 to 0.2 mg I.M. or I.V. t.i.d. or q.i.d. Dosage must be individualized. Maximum oral dose, 8 mg daily.

I.V. ADMINISTRATION
• Give by direct injection without dilution. Or, inject into tubing of a free-flowing I.V. solution.

● Don't mix with I.V. solutions that contain sodium bicarbonate or alkaline solutions with a pH higher than 6. Alkaline drugs, such as barbiturates, chloramphenicol, dexamethasone, diazepam, dimenhydrinate, methylprednisolone, and pentazocine, are incompatible.

ACTION
Inhibits cholinergic (muscarinic) actions of acetylcholine on autonomic effectors innervated by postganglionic cholinergic nerves.

Route	Onset	Peak	Duration
I.M., S.C.	15-30 min	30-45 min	3-7 hr
I.V.	1 min	Unknown	3-7 hr
P.O.	Unknown	Unknown	8-12 hr

ADVERSE REACTIONS
CNS: weakness, nervousness, insomnia, drowsiness, dizziness, headache, confusion, excitement.
CV: palpitations, tachycardia.
EENT: *dilated pupils, blurred vision,* photophobia, increased intraocular pressure.
GI: *constipation, dry mouth,* nausea, loss of taste, abdominal distention, vomiting, epigastric distress.
GU: urinary hesitancy, urine retention, impotence.
Skin: urticaria, decreased sweating or anhidrosis.
Other: allergic reactions, *anaphylaxis,* fever.

INTERACTIONS
Drug-drug. *Amantadine, antihistamines, antiparkinsonians, disopyramide, glutethimide, meperidine, phenothiazines, procainamide, quinidine, TCAs:* Additive adverse effects. Avoid using together.
Antacids: Decreased absorption of oral anticholinergics. Separate administration times by 2 to 3 hours.
Ketoconazole: Anticholinergics may interfere with ketoconazole absorption. Separate administration times by 2 to 3 hours.
Methotrimeprazine: Anticholinergics may increase risk of extrapyramidal reactions. Avoid using together.

EFFECTS ON LAB TEST RESULTS
None reported.

CONTRAINDICATIONS
Contraindicated in patients hypersensitive to drug and in those with glaucoma, obstructive uropathy, obstructive disease of the GI tract, myasthenia gravis, paralytic ileus, intestinal atony, unstable CV status in acute hemorrhage, tachycardia secondary to cardiac insufficiency or thyrotoxicosis, severe ulcerative colitis, toxic megacolon, or known or suspected GI infection.

NURSING CONSIDERATIONS
● Use cautiously in patients with autonomic neuropathy, hyperthyroidism, coronary artery disease, arrhythmias, heart failure, hypertension, hiatal hernia, hepatic or renal disease, ulcerative colitis, and known or suspected GI infection. Also, use cautiously in patients in hot or humid environments. Drug-induced heat stroke is possible.
● Give oral form 30 to 60 minutes before meals.
● *Alert:* Check all dosages carefully; slight overdose can lead to toxicity.
● *Alert:* Overdose may cause curarelike effects, such as respiratory paralysis. Keep emergency equipment available.
● Monitor vital signs carefully. Watch closely for adverse reactions, especially in elderly or debilitated patients. Call prescriber promptly if they occur.
● Elderly patients may be more susceptible to adverse effects and typically receive smaller doses.

PATIENT TEACHING
● Tell patient to take oral drug 30 to 60 minutes before meals.
● Warn patient to avoid activities that require alertness until drug's CNS effects are known.
● Advise patient to report signs and symptoms of urinary hesitancy or urine retention.

---

hyoscyamine
Cystospaz

hyoscyamine sulfate
Anaspaz, Cystospaz,
Cystospaz-M, Gastrosed,
Levbid, Levsin*, Levsin Drops*,
Levsin SL, Levsinex Timecaps,
Neoquess

Pregnancy risk category C

AVAILABLE FORMS
hyoscyamine
Tablets: 0.15 mg
hyoscyamine sulfate
Capsules (extended-release): 0.375 mg
Elixir: 0.125 mg/5 ml
Injection: 0.5 mg/ml
Oral solution: 0.125 mg/ml
Tablets: 0.125 mg, 0.13 mg, 0.15 mg

INDICATIONS & DOSAGES
➤ **GI tract disorders caused by spasm;
to diminish secretions and block cardiac vagal reflexes preoperatively; as
adjunctive therapy for peptic ulcerations, cystitis, renal colic; as drying
agent to relieve symptoms of allergic
rhinitis—**
Adults and children age 12 and older:
0.125 to 0.25 mg P.O. or S.L. t.i.d. or
q.i.d. before meals and h.s. Or, 0.375 to
0.75 mg extended-release form P.O. q 8 to
12 hours. Or, 0.25 to 0.5 mg or 1 or 2 ml
I.M., I.V., or S.C. b.i.d. to q.i.d. Oral drug
is substituted when symptoms are controlled. Maximum, 1.5 mg daily.
Children younger than age 12: Dosage individualized according to weight.

I.V. ADMINISTRATION
• I.V. form used when oral or S.L. therapy
isn't feasible or when rapid effect is
needed.

ACTION
Competitively blocks the action of acetylcholine at muscarinic receptors, which decreases GI motility and inhibits gastric
acid secretion.

Route	Onset	Peak	Duration
I.M., S.C.	Unknown	15-30 min	4-12 hr
I.V.	2 min	15-30 min	4 hr
P.O.	20-30 min	0.5-1 hr	4-12 hr
P.O. (extended)	20-30 min	40-90 min	12 hr
S.L.	5-20 min	0.5-1 hr	4 hr

ADVERSE REACTIONS
CNS: headache, insomnia, drowsiness,
dizziness, *confusion or excitement in
elderly patients,* nervousness, weakness.
CV: *palpitations,* tachycardia.
EENT: *blurred vision,* mydriasis, increased intraocular pressure, cycloplegia,
photophobia.
GI: *dry mouth,* dysphagia, *constipation,*
heartburn, loss of taste, nausea, vomiting,
paralytic ileus.
GU: *urinary hesitancy, urine retention,*
impotence.
Skin: urticaria, decreased or lack of
sweating.
Other: fever, hypersensitivity reactions.

INTERACTIONS
Drug-drug. *Amantadine, antihistamines,
antiparkinsonians, disopyramide, glutethimide, meperidine, phenothiazines, procainamide, quinidine, TCAs:* Additive adverse effects. Avoid using together.
Antacids: Decreased absorption of oral
anticholinergics. Separate administration
times by 2 to 3 hours.
Ketoconazole: Anticholinergics may interfere with ketoconazole absorption.
Separate administration times by 2 to 3
hours.
Methotrimeprazine: Anticholinergics may
increase risk of extrapyramidal reactions.
Avoid using together.
Drug-herb. *Jimsonweed:* May adversely
affect CV function system. Discourage
use together.

EFFECTS ON LAB TEST RESULTS
None reported.

CONTRAINDICATIONS
Contraindicated in patients hypersensitive
to anticholinergics and in those with glaucoma, obstructive uropathy, obstructive
disease of the GI tract, severe ulcerative
colitis, myasthenia gravis, paralytic ileus,

intestinal atony, unstable CV status in acute hemorrhage, tachycardia secondary to cardiac insufficiency of thyrotoxicosis, or toxic megacolon.

NURSING CONSIDERATIONS
• Use cautiously in patients with autonomic neuropathy, hyperthyroidism, coronary artery disease, arrhythmias, heart failure, hypertension, hiatal hernia with reflux esophagitis, hepatic or renal disease, known or suspected GI infection, and ulcerative colitis. Also use cautiously in patients in hot or humid environments. Drug-induced heat stroke can develop.
• Give drug 30 minutes to 1 hour before meals and at bedtime. Bedtime dose can be larger; give at least 2 hours after last meal of day.
• *Alert:* Overdose may cause curarelike effects, such as respiratory paralysis. Keep emergency equipment available.
• Monitor patient's vital signs and urine output carefully.
• Injection contains sodium metabisulfite, which may cause allergic reaction in certain people.

PATIENT TEACHING
• Urge patient to take drug as prescribed.
• Caution patient not to crush or chew extended-release tablets.
• Advise patient to avoid driving and other hazardous activities if drowsiness, dizziness, or blurred vision occurs; to drink plenty of fluids to help prevent constipation; and to report rash or other skin eruption.

---

scopolamine (hyoscine)
Transderm-Scop, Transderm-V

scopolamine butylbromide (hyoscine butylbromide)
Buscopan†

scopolamine hydrobromide (hyoscine hydrobromide)
Scopolamine Hydrobromide Injection

Pregnancy risk category C

AVAILABLE FORMS
scopolamine
Transdermal patch: 1.5 mg/2.5 cm² (1 mg/ 72 hours)
scopolamine butylbromide
Capsules: 0.25 mg
Suppositories: 10 mg†
Tablets: 10 mg†
scopolamine hydrobromide
Injection: 0.3 mg, 0.4 mg, 0.5 mg, 0.6 mg, and 1 mg/ml in 1-ml vials and ampules; 0.86 mg/ml in 0.5-ml ampules

INDICATIONS & DOSAGES
➤ **Spastic states—**
Adults: 10 to 20 mg P.O. t.i.d. or q.i.d. or 10 mg P.R. t.i.d. or q.i.d. Adjust dosage, p.r.n. Or, 10 to 20 mg butylbromide S.C., I.M., or I.V., t.i.d. or q.i.d.
➤ **Delirium, preanesthetic sedation, and obstetric amnesia with analgesics—**
Adults: 0.3 to 0.65 mg I.M., S.C., or I.V. Dilute solution with sterile water for injection before giving I.V.
Children: 0.006 mg/kg I.M., S.C., or I.V. Maximum dose, 0.3 mg. Dilute solution with sterile water for injection before giving I.V.
➤ **Prevention of nausea and vomiting from motion sickness—**
Adults: One Transderm-Scop or one Transderm-V patch, a circular flat unit, programmed to deliver 0.5 mg scopolamine daily over 3 days, applied to the skin behind the ear at least 4 hours before antiemetic is needed. Or, 300 to 600 mcg hydrobromide S.C., I.M., or I.V.
Children: 6 mcg/kg or 200 mcg/m² hydrobromide S.C., I.M., or I.V.

I.V. ADMINISTRATION
• Intermittent and continuous infusions aren't recommended. For direct injection, dilute with sterile water and inject diluted drug at ordered rate through patent I.V. line.
• Protect I.V. solutions from freezing and light, and store at room temperature.

ACTION
Inhibits muscarinic actions of acetylcholine on autonomic effectors innervated by postganglionic cholinergic neurons. Also may affect neural pathways originat-

---

ing in the labyrinth (inner ear) to inhibit nausea and vomiting.

Route	Onset	Peak	Duration
I.M., P.O.	1 hr	1-2 hr	4-6 hr
I.V.	10 min	50-80 min	2 hr
P.R., S.C.	Unknown	Unknown	Unknown
Transdermal	4 hr	Unknown	72 hr

ADVERSE REACTIONS

CNS: disorientation, restlessness, irritability, dizziness, drowsiness, headache, confusion, hallucinations, delirium.
CV: palpitations, tachycardia, *paradoxical bradycardia,* flushing.
EENT: dilated pupils, blurred vision, photophobia, increased intraocular pressure, difficulty swallowing.
GI: *constipation, dry mouth, nausea, vomiting, epigastric distress.*
GU: urinary hesitancy, urine retention.
Respiratory: bronchial plugging, depressed respirations.
Skin: rash, dryness, contact dermatitis with transdermal patch.
Other: fever.

INTERACTIONS

Drug-drug. *Amantadine, antihistamines, antiparkinsonians, disopyramide, glutethimide, meperidine, phenothiazines, procainamide, quinidine, TCAs:* Increased risk of adverse CNS reactions. Avoid using together.
Antacids: Decreased oral absorption of anticholinergics. Separate administration times by 2 to 3 hours.
CNS depressants: Increased risk of CNS depression. Monitor patient closely.
Digoxin: Increased digoxin levels. Monitor patient for digoxin toxicity.
Ketoconazole: Anticholinergics may interfere with ketoconazole absorption. Separate administration times by 2 to 3 hours.
Methotrimeprazine: Increased risk of extrapyramidal reactions. Avoid using together.
Drug-herb. *Jaborandi tree:* May decrease drug effects. Discourage use together.
Pill-bearing spurge: Choline may decrease effect of scopolamine. Inform patient of this interaction.
Squaw vine: Tannic acid may decrease metabolic breakdown. Ask patient about

use of alternative remedies, and recommend caution.
Drug-lifestyle. *Alcohol use:* Increased risk of CNS depression. Discourage use together.

EFFECTS ON LAB TEST RESULTS
None reported.

CONTRAINDICATIONS
Contraindicated in patients with angle-closure glaucoma, obstructive uropathy, obstructive disease of the GI tract, asthma, chronic pulmonary disease, myasthenia gravis, paralytic ileus, intestinal atony, unstable CV status in acute hemorrhage, tachycardia secondary to cardiac insufficiency, or toxic megacolon.

NURSING CONSIDERATIONS
• Use cautiously in patients with autonomic neuropathy, hyperthyroidism, coronary artery disease, arrhythmias, heart failure, hypertension, hiatal hernia with reflux esophagitis, hepatic or renal disease, known or suspected GI infection, or ulcerative colitis. Also use cautiously in children younger than age 6. And use cautiously in patients in hot or humid environments. Drug-induced heat stroke is possible.
• Raise side rails as a precaution because some patients become temporarily excited or disoriented and some develop amnesia or become drowsy. Reorient patient, as needed.
• Tolerance may develop when therapy is prolonged.
• Adverse reactions may be caused by pending atropine-like toxicity and are dose-related. Individual tolerance varies greatly.
• *Alert:* Overdose may cause curarelike effects, such as respiratory paralysis. Keep emergency equipment available.

PATIENT TEACHING
• Advise patient to apply patch the night before a planned trip. Transdermal method releases a controlled therapeutic amount of scopolamine. Transderm-Scop is effective if applied 2 to 3 hours before experiencing motion but is more effective if applied 12 hours before.

• Instruct patient to wash and dry hands thoroughly before and after applying the transdermal patch (on dry skin behind the ear) and before touching the eye because pupil may dilate. Tell patient to discard patch after removing it and to wash hands and application site thoroughly.

• Tell patient that, if patch becomes displaced, he should remove it and apply another patch on a fresh skin site behind the ear.

• Alert patient to possible withdrawal signs or symptoms (nausea, vomiting, headache, dizziness) when transdermal system is used for longer than 72 hours.

• Advise patient that eyes may be more sensitive to light while wearing patch.

• Warn patient to avoid activities that require alertness until CNS effects of drug are known.

• Instruct patient to ask pharmacist for brochure that comes with the transdermal product.

• Urge patient to report urinary hesitancy or urine retention.

dobutamine hydrochloride
dopamine hydrochloride
metaraminol bitartrate
norepinephrine bitartrate
phenylephrine hydrochloride
pseudoephedrine hydrochloride
pseudoephedrine sulfate

COMBINATION PRODUCTS
ENTEX PSE: pseudoephedrine 120 mg and guaifenesin 600 mg.
SEMPREX-D: acrivastine 8 mg and pseudoephedrine hydrochloride 60 mg.

dobutamine hydrochloride
Dobutrex

Pregnancy risk category B

AVAILABLE FORMS
Injection: 12.5 mg/ml in 20-ml vials (parenteral)

INDICATIONS & DOSAGES
➤ **Increased cardiac output in short-term treatment of cardiac decompensation caused by depressed contractility, such as during refractory heart failure; adjunct in cardiac surgery—**
Adults: 2.5 to 15 mcg/kg/minute I.V. infusion. Rarely, rates up to 40 mcg/kg/minute may be needed.

I.V. ADMINISTRATION
● Dilute concentrate for injection before giving it. Compatible solutions include D_5W, half-normal or normal saline solution for injection, and lactated Ringer's injection. Contents of one vial (250 mg) diluted with 1,000 ml of solution yields 250 mcg/ml. Diluting with 500 ml yields 500 mcg/ml. Diluting with 250 ml yields 1,000 mcg/ml. Don't exceed maximum of 5 mg/ml.
● Oxidation of drug may slightly discolor admixtures containing dobutamine. This doesn't indicate a significant loss of potency provided drug is used within 24 hours of reconstitution.

● Give through a central venous catheter or large peripheral vein. Titrate infusion according to prescriber's orders and patient's condition. Use an infusion pump. Infusions for up to 72 hours produce no more adverse effects than shorter infusions.
● Avoid extravasation; it may cause an inflammatory response. Change I.V. sites regularly to avoid phlebitis.
● Don't give through same I.V. line with other drugs. Drug is incompatible with heparin, hydrocortisone sodium succinate, cefazolin, cefamandole, neutral cephalothin, penicillin, sodium bicarbonate, and ethacrynate sodium.
● I.V. solutions remain stable for 24 hours.

ACTION
Directly stimulates $beta_1$ receptors of heart to increase myocardial contractility and stroke volume. At therapeutic dosages, drug decreases peripheral vascular resistance (afterload), reduces ventricular filling pressure (preload), and may facilitate AV node conduction. Net result is increased cardiac output.

Route	Onset	Peak	Duration
I.V.	1-2 min	10 min	< 5 min after infusion ends

ADVERSE REACTIONS
CNS: headache.
CV: *increased heart rate, hypertension,* PVCs, angina, nonspecific chest pain, palpitations, hypotension.
GI: nausea, vomiting.
Respiratory: shortness of breath, *asthmatic episodes.*
Other: phlebitis, hypersensitivity reactions, *anaphylaxis.*

INTERACTIONS
Drug-drug. *Beta blockers:* May antagonize dobutamine effects. Avoid using together.

Bretylium: May potentiate action of vasopressors on adrenergic receptors. Monitor patient closely for arrhythmias.
General anesthetics: Greater risk of ventricular arrhythmias. Monitor ECG closely.
Guanethidine, oxytocic drugs: May increase pressor response, possibly resulting in severe hypertension. Monitor blood pressure closely.
TCAs: May increase pressor response. Use with caution.
Drug-herb. *Rue:* Increased inotropic potential. Discourage use together.

EFFECTS ON LAB TEST RESULTS
None reported.

CONTRAINDICATIONS
Contraindicated in patients hypersensitive to drug or its ingredients and in those with idiopathic hypertrophic subaortic stenosis.

NURSING CONSIDERATIONS
• Use cautiously in patients with history of hypertension. Drug may cause exaggerated pressor response. Also, use cautiously in patients with history of sulfite sensitivity.
• Before starting therapy with dobutamine, correct hypovolemia with plasma volume expanders.
• Give a cardiac glycoside before dobutamine. Because drug increases AV node conduction, patients with atrial fibrillation may develop a rapid ventricular rate.
• Continuously monitor ECG, blood pressure, pulmonary artery wedge pressure, cardiac output, and urine output.
• Monitor electrolytes. Drug may lower potassium levels.
• *Alert:* Don't confuse dobutamine with dopamine.

PATIENT TEACHING
• Tell patient to report adverse reactions promptly, especially dyspnea and drug-induced headache.
• Instruct patient to report discomfort at I.V. insertion site.

dopamine hydrochloride
Intropin, Revimine†

Pregnancy risk category C

AVAILABLE FORMS
Injection: 40 mg/ml, 80 mg/ml, 160 mg/ml parenteral concentrate for injection for I.V. infusion; 0.8 mg/ml (200 or 400 mg) in D_5W; 1.6 mg/ml (400 or 800 mg) in D_5W; 3.2 mg/ml (800 mg) in D_5W parenteral injection for I.V. infusion

INDICATIONS & DOSAGES
➤ **To treat shock and correct hemodynamic imbalances, to improve perfusion to vital organs, to increase cardiac output, to correct hypotension—**
Adults: Initially, 1 to 5 mcg/kg/minute by I.V. infusion. Titrate dosage to desired hemodynamic or renal response. Infusion may be increased by 1 to 4 mcg/kg/minute at 10- to 30-minute intervals.

I.V. ADMINISTRATION
• Dilute with D_5W, normal saline solution, or a combination of D_5W and normal saline solution. Mix just before use.
• Use a continuous infusion pump to regulate flow rate. Patient response depends on dosage and pharmacologic effects. Dosages of 0.5 to 2 mcg/kg/minute predominantly stimulate dopamine receptors and produce vasodilation of the renal vasculature. Dosages of 2 to 10 mcg/kg/minute stimulate beta receptors for a positive inotropic effect. Higher dosages also stimulate alpha receptors, causing vasoconstriction and increased blood pressure. Most patients are satisfactorily maintained on dosages of less than 20 mcg/kg/minute.
• Use a central line or large vein, as in the antecubital fossa, to minimize risk of extravasation. Watch infusion site carefully for signs of extravasation; if it occurs, stop infusion immediately and call prescriber. Extravasation may require treatment by infiltration of the area with 5 to 10 mg phentolamine in 10 to 15 ml normal saline solution.
• Don't mix other drugs in I.V. container with dopamine. Don't give alkaline drugs, oxidizing drugs, or iron salts through I.V. line containing dopamine.

Reactions may be *common*, uncommon, *life-threatening*, or COMMON AND LIFE-THREATENING.

• Discard after 24 hours (dopamine solutions deteriorate after 24 hours), or earlier if solution is discolored.

ACTION
Stimulates dopaminergic and alpha and beta receptors of the sympathetic nervous system. Action is dose-related; large doses cause mainly alpha stimulation.

Route	Onset	Peak	Duration
I.V.	5 min	Unknown	< 10 min after infusion ends

ADVERSE REACTIONS
CNS: headache.
CV: ectopic beats, tachycardia, angina, palpitations, *hypotension.*
GI: nausea, vomiting.
GU: elevated urinary catecholamine levels.
Metabolic: azotemia, hyperglycemia.
Respiratory: dyspnea, asthmatic episodes.
Skin: necrosis and tissue sloughing with extravasation, piloerection.
Other: *anaphylactic reactions.*

INTERACTIONS
Drug-drug. *Alpha-adrenergic blockers, beta blockers:* May antagonize dopamine effects. Monitor patient closely.
Ergot alkaloids: Extreme elevations in blood pressure. Avoid using together.
Inhaled anesthetics: Increased risk of arrhythmias or hypertension. Monitor patient closely.
MAO inhibitors: May cause hypertensive crisis. Avoid using together.
Oxytocics: May cause severe, persistent hypertension. Use together cautiously.
Phenytoin: May cause seizures, severe hypotension, and bradycardia. Monitor patient carefully.
TCAs: Decreased pressor response. Higher doses of dopamine may be needed.

EFFECTS ON LAB TEST RESULTS
• May increase glucose and nitrogenous compound (urea) levels.

CONTRAINDICATIONS
Contraindicated in patients with uncorrected tachyarrhythmias, pheochromocytoma, or ventricular fibrillation.

NURSING CONSIDERATIONS
• Use cautiously in patients with occlusive vascular disease, cold injuries, diabetic endarteritis, and arterial embolism; in pregnant patients; in those with a history of sulfite sensitivity; and in those taking MAO inhibitors.
• Drug isn't a substitute for blood or fluid volume deficit. If deficit exists, replace fluid before giving vasopressors.
• During infusion, frequently monitor ECG, blood pressure, cardiac output, central venous pressure, pulmonary artery wedge pressure, pulse rate, urine output, and color and temperature of limbs.
• If diastolic pressure rises disproportionately (a marked decrease in pulse pressure) in a patient receiving dopamine, decrease infusion rate, and watch carefully for further evidence of predominant vasoconstrictor activity, unless such an effect is desired.
• Observe patient closely for adverse reactions; prescriber may adjust dosage or discontinue drug.
• Check urine output often. If urine flow decreases without hypotension, notify prescriber because dosage may need to be reduced.
• **Alert:** After drug is stopped, watch closely for sudden decrease in blood pressure. Taper dosage slowly to evaluate stability of blood pressure.
• Acidosis decreases effectiveness of dopamine.
• **Alert:** Don't confuse dopamine with dobutamine.

PATIENT TEACHING
• Tell patient to report adverse reactions promptly.
• Instruct patient to report discomfort at I.V. insertion site.

---

metaraminol bitartrate
Aramine

Pregnancy risk category D

AVAILABLE FORMS
Injection: 10 mg/ml

INDICATIONS & DOSAGES
➤ **Prevention of hypotension from spinal anesthesia—**
Adults: 2 to 10 mg I.M. or S.C.
➤ **Hypotension from spinal anesthesia, hemorrhage, drug reaction, surgical complications, or shock from brain damage caused by trauma or tumor—**
Adults: 0.5 to 5 mg by direct I.V. injection; then I.V. infusion titrated to maintain blood pressure.
Children: 0.01 mg/kg as single I.V. injection; 1 mg/25 ml of D_5W as I.V. infusion. Rate titrated to maintain blood pressure within normal range. Or, 0.1 mg/kg I.M. as single dose, p.r.n. At least 10 minutes should elapse before dosage is increased because maximum effect isn't immediately apparent.

I.V. ADMINISTRATION
• To prepare an I.V. infusion, mix 15 to 100 mg in 500 ml of normal saline solution or D_5W. Aramine may be added to less than 500 ml of fluid if a smaller volume is desired. Titrate rate to maintain blood pressure.
• Use a central venous catheter or large vein, as in the antecubital fossa, to minimize risk of extravasation. Use a continuous infusion pump to regulate infusion flow rate and a piggyback setup so I.V. line remains open if drug is stopped. Watch infusion site carefully for signs of extravasation. If they appear, stop infusion immediately and notify prescriber.
• To treat extravasation, infiltrate site promptly with 10 to 15 ml of normal saline solution for injection containing 5 to 10 mg phentolamine. Use a fine needle.
• When stopping drug, gradually slow infusion rate. Continue monitoring vital signs, watching for possible severe drop in blood pressure. Keep equipment nearby to resume drug, if needed. Don't reinstate vasopressor therapy until systolic blood pressure falls below 70 to 80 mm Hg.

ACTION
Stimulates alpha and $beta_1$ receptors in the sympathetic nervous system, causing an increase in both systolic and diastolic blood pressure as a result of vasoconstriction.

Route	Onset	Peak	Duration
I.M.	10 min	Unknown	< 90 min
I.V.	1-2 min	Unknown	20 min
S.C.	5-20 min	Unknown	< 90 min

ADVERSE REACTIONS
CNS: apprehension, dizziness, headache, tremor.
CV: hypertension; hypotension; palpitations; flushing; ***arrhythmias,*** including sinus or ***ventricular tachycardia; cardiac arrest.***
GI: nausea.
Skin: diaphoresis; abscess, necrosis, and sloughing with extravasation.

INTERACTIONS
Drug-drug. *Beta blockers:* Mutual inhibition of drug effects with possible hypertension, bradycardia, and heart block. Avoid using together.
Cardiac glycosides, doxapram, ergot alkaloids, general anesthetics, levodopa, maprotiline, other sympathomimetics, thyroid hormones, TCAs: Increased risk of adverse cardiac effects. Monitor patient closely.
Furazolidone, MAO inhibitors, procarbazine: May cause severe hypertension (hypertensive crisis) and increase action of metaraminol. Avoid using together.
Guanadrel, guanethidine: Metaraminol may decrease hypotensive effect of these drugs; guanadrel and guanethidine may enhance pressor effect of metaraminol. Avoid using together.
Oxytocics: May cause severe, persistent hypertension. Use together cautiously.
Drug-lifestyle. *Cocaine use:* Increased risk of adverse cardiac effects. Inform patient of this interaction.

EFFECTS ON LAB TEST RESULTS
None reported.

CONTRAINDICATIONS
Contraindicated in patients hypersensitive to drug and in those receiving anesthesia with cyclopropane and halogenated hydrocarbon anesthetics.

Reactions may be *common,* uncommon, *life-threatening,* or COMMON AND LIFE-THREATENING.

NURSING CONSIDERATIONS
● Use cautiously in patients receiving cardiac glycosides and in patients with heart disease, hypertension, peripheral vascular disease, thyroid disease, diabetes, cirrhosis, history of malaria, or sulfite sensitivity.
● Drug isn't a substitute for blood or fluid volume deficit. If deficit exists, replace fluid before giving vasopressors.
● Don't mix metaraminol with other drugs.
● During infusion, check blood pressure every 5 minutes until stabilized; then check every 15 minutes. Frequently monitor ECG, blood pressure, cardiac output, central venous pressure, pulmonary artery wedge pressure, pulse rate, urine output, and color and temperature of limbs. Titrate infusion rate according to findings and prescriber's guidelines.
● *Alert:* Blood pressure should be raised to slightly less than the patient's normal level. Avoid excessive blood pressure response. Headache may be a symptom of hypertension. Rapidly induced hypertensive response can cause acute pulmonary edema, arrhythmias, and cardiac arrest.
● Allow at least 10 minutes between doses. Drug effects aren't always immediately apparent.
● Because of prolonged action, a cumulative effect is possible. With an excessive vasopressor response, elevated blood pressure may persist after drug is stopped.
● Observe patient closely for adverse effects; prescriber may adjust dosage or discontinue drug.
● Keep emergency drugs on hand to reverse effects of metaraminol: atropine for reflex bradycardia, phentolamine to decrease vasopressor effects, and propranolol for arrhythmias.
● Urine output may decrease initially and then increase as blood pressure returns to normal level. Report persistently decreased urine output.
● Closely monitor patient with diabetes; insulin dosage may need to be adjusted.
● Keep solution in light-resistant container, away from heat. Use within 24 hours.

PATIENT TEACHING
● Tell patient to report adverse reactions promptly.
● Instruct patient to report discomfort at I.V. site.

norepinephrine bitartrate (levarterenol bitartrate, noradrenaline acid tartrate)
Levophed

Pregnancy risk category C

AVAILABLE FORMS
Injection: 1 mg/ml

INDICATIONS & DOSAGES
➤ **To restore blood pressure in acute hypotensive states—**
Adults: Initially, 8 to 12 mcg/minute by I.V. infusion; then titrated to maintain normal blood pressure. Average maintenance dose is 2 to 4 mcg/minute.
Children: 2 mcg/m^2/minute by I.V. infusion; adjust dosage based on patient response.
➤ **Severe hypotension during cardiac arrest—**
Children: Initial I.V. infusion rate is 0.1 mcg/kg/minute. Titrate infusion rate based on patient response.

I.V. ADMINISTRATION
● Use a central venous catheter or large vein, as in the antecubital fossa, to minimize risk of extravasation. Give in D$_5$W in normal saline solution for injection; normal saline solution for injection alone isn't recommended. Use continuous infusion pump to regulate infusion flow rate and a piggyback setup so I.V. line stays open if norepinephrine is stopped.
● Check site frequently for signs of extravasation. If they appear, stop infusion immediately and call prescriber. As ordered, infiltrate area with 5 to 10 mg phentolamine in 10 to 15 ml of normal saline solution to counteract effect of extravasation. Also, check for blanching along course of infused vein, which may progress to superficial sloughing.
● Protect drug from light. Discard discolored solutions or solutions that contain a precipitate. Norepinephrine solutions deteriorate after 24 hours.
● Avoid mixing with alkaline solutions, oxidizing drugs, or iron salts.
● If prolonged I.V. therapy is needed, change injection site frequently.

ACTION
Stimulates alpha and beta$_1$ receptors in the sympathetic nervous system, causing vasoconstriction and cardiac stimulation.

Route	Onset	Peak	Duration
I.V.	Immediate	Immediate	1-2 min after infusion ends

ADVERSE REACTIONS
CNS: *headache,* anxiety, weakness, dizziness, tremor, restlessness, insomnia.
CV: *bradycardia, severe hypertension, arrhythmias.*
Respiratory: respiratory difficulties, *asthmatic episodes.*
Skin: irritation with extravasation, necrosis and gangrene secondary to extravasation.
Other: *anaphylaxis.*

INTERACTIONS
Drug-drug. *Alpha-adrenergic blockers:* May antagonize drug effects. Avoid using together.
Antihistamines, ergot alkaloids, guanethidine, MAO inhibitors, methyldopa, oxytocics, TCAs: When given with sympathomimetics, may cause severe hypertension (hypertensive crisis). Avoid using together.
Bretylium, inhaled anesthetics: Increased risk of arrhythmias. Watch patient closely.

EFFECTS ON LAB TEST RESULTS
None reported.

CONTRAINDICATIONS
Contraindicated in patients with mesenteric or peripheral vascular thrombosis, profound hypoxia, hypercarbia, or hypotension resulting from blood volume deficit. Also contraindicated during cyclopropane and halothane anesthesia.

NURSING CONSIDERATIONS
• Use with extreme caution in patients receiving MAO inhibitors or triptyline- or imipramine-type antidepressants. Use cautiously in patients with sulfite sensitivity.
• Drug isn't a substitute for blood or fluid replacement therapy. If patient has volume deficit, replace fluids before giving vasopressors.
• *Alert:* Never leave patient unattended during infusion. Check blood pressure

every 2 minutes until stabilized; then check every 5 minutes. In previously hypertensive patients, blood pressure should be raised no higher than 40 mm Hg below baseline systolic pressure.
• During infusion, frequently monitor ECG, cardiac output, central venous pressure, pulmonary artery wedge pressure, pulse rate, urine output, and color and temperature of limbs. Titrate infusion rate based on findings and prescriber guidelines.
• Keep emergency drugs on hand to reverse effects of norepinephrine: atropine for reflex bradycardia, phentolamine to decrease vasopressor effects, and propranolol for arrhythmias.
• Notify prescriber immediately of decreased urine output.
• When stopping drug, gradually slow infusion rate. Continue monitoring vital signs, watching for possible severe drop in blood pressure.
• *Alert:* Don't confuse norepinephrine with epinephrine.

PATIENT TEACHING
• Tell patient to report adverse reactions promptly.
• Advise patient to report discomfort at I.V. insertion site.

---

phenylephrine hydrochloride
Neo-Synephrine

Pregnancy risk category C

AVAILABLE FORMS
Injection: 10 mg/ml

INDICATIONS & DOSAGES
➤ **Hypotensive emergencies during spinal anesthesia—**
Adults: Initially, 0.2 mg I.V.; subsequent doses shouldn't exceed the preceding dose by more than 0.2 mg. Maximum single dose is 0.5 mg.
➤ **Maintenance of blood pressure during spinal or inhaled anesthesia—**
Adults: 2 to 3 mg S.C. or I.M. 3 to 4 minutes before anesthesia.
Children: 0.044 mg to 0.088 mg/kg S.C. or I.M.

Reactions may be *common,* uncommon, ***life-threatening,*** or **COMMON AND LIFE-THREATENING.**

➤ **Prolongation of spinal anesthesia—**
Adults: 2 to 5 mg added to anesthetic solution.
➤ **Vasoconstrictor for regional anesthesia—**
Adults: 1 mg phenylephrine added to 20 ml local anesthetic.
➤ **Mild to moderate hypotension—**
Adults: 2 to 5 mg S.C. or I.M.; repeated in 1 to 2 hours as needed and tolerated. Initial dose shouldn't exceed 5 mg. Or, 0.1 to 0.5 mg slow I.V., not to be repeated more often than 10 to 15 minutes.
Children: 0.1 mg/kg I.M. or S.C.; repeated in 1 to 2 hours as needed and tolerated.
➤ **Severe hypotension and shock (including drug-induced)—**
Adults: 10 mg in 250 to 500 ml of D₅W or normal saline solution for injection. I.V. infusion started at 100 to 180 mcg/minute; then decreased to maintenance infusion of 40 to 60 mcg/minute when blood pressure stabilizes.
➤ **Paroxysmal supraventricular tachycardia—**
Adults: Initially, 0.5 mg rapid I.V.; subsequent doses shouldn't exceed preceding dose by more than 0.1 to 0.2 mg and shouldn't exceed 1 mg.

I.V. ADMINISTRATION

• For direct injection, dilute 10 mg (1 ml) with 9 ml sterile water for injection to provide 1 mg/ml. Infusions are usually prepared by adding 10 mg of drug to 500 ml of D₅W or normal saline solution for injection. The initial I.V. infusion rate is usually 100 to 180 mcg/minute; maintenance rate is usually 40 to 60 mcg/minute.
• Use a central venous catheter or large vein, as in the antecubital fossa, to minimize risk of extravasation. Use a continuous infusion pump to regulate infusion flow rate.
• To treat extravasation, infiltrate site promptly with 10 to 15 ml of normal saline solution for injection containing 5 to 10 mg phentolamine. Use a fine needle.
• During infusion, frequently monitor ECG, blood pressure, cardiac output, central venous pressure, pulmonary artery wedge pressure, pulse rate, urine output, and color and temperature of limbs. Titrate infusion rate according to findings and prescriber guidelines. Maintain blood

pressure slightly below patient's normal level. In previously normotensive patients, maintain systolic blood pressure at 80 to 100 mm Hg; in previously hypertensive patients, maintain systolic blood pressure at 30 to 40 mm Hg below usual level. Avoid abrupt withdrawal after prolonged I.V. infusions.

ACTION
Stimulates alpha receptors in the sympathetic nervous system, causing vasoconstriction.

Route	Onset	Peak	Duration
I.M.	10-15 min	Unknown	0.5-2 hr
I.V.	Immediate	Unknown	15-20 min
S.C.	10-15 min	Unknown	50-60 min

ADVERSE REACTIONS
CNS: *headache,* excitability.
CV: *bradycardia, arrhythmias,* hypertension.
Respiratory: *asthmatic episodes.*
Skin: tissue sloughing with extravasation.
Other: tachyphylaxis and decreased organ perfusion with continued use, *anaphylaxis.*

INTERACTIONS
Drug-drug. *Alpha-adrenergic blockers, phenothiazines:* Decreased vasopressor response. Monitor patient closely.
Beta blockers: Blocked cardiostimulatory effects. Monitor patient closely.
Bretylium, halogenated hydrocarbon anesthetics, sympathomimetics: May cause serious arrhythmias. Use together with extreme caution.
Guanethidine, oxytocics, TCAs: Increased pressor response. Observe patient.
MAO inhibitors: May cause severe hypertension (hypertensive crisis). Avoid using together.

EFFECTS ON LAB TEST RESULTS
None reported.

CONTRAINDICATIONS
Contraindicated in patients hypersensitive to drug and in those with severe hypertension or ventricular tachycardia.

NURSING CONSIDERATIONS
• Use with extreme caution in elderly patients and in patients with heart disease,

hyperthyroidism, severe atherosclerosis, bradycardia, partial heart block, myocardial disease, or sulfite sensitivity.
● Drug causes little or no CNS stimulation.
● Drug may lower intraocular pressure in normal eyes or in open-angle glaucoma. It also may cause false-normal tonometry readings.
● Drug is incompatible with butacaine sulfate, alkalis, ferric salts, and oxidizing drugs.
● Also used in eyedrops and OTC cold preparations for decongestant effects.

PATIENT TEACHING
● Tell patient to report adverse reactions promptly.
● Instruct patient to report discomfort at I.V. insertion site.

---

pseudoephedrine
hydrochloride
Allermed ◇, Cenafed ◇,
Children's Congestion Relief ◇,
Congestion Relief ◇, Decofed ◇,
DeFed-60 ◇, Dorcol Children's
Decongestant Liquid ◇, Drixoral
Non-Drowsy Formula ◇,
Efidac/24 ◇, Eltor 120† ◇,
Galpseud§, Genaphed ◇,
Halofed ◇, Halofed Adult
Strength ◇, Maxenal† ◇,
Myfedrine ◇, Novafed ◇,
Ornex ◇, PediaCare Infants'
Decongestant ◇, PediaCare
Infants' Oral Decongestant
Drops ◇, Pseudo ◇,
Pseudogest ◇, Seudotabs ◇,
Sinufed Timecelles ◇, Sinustop
Pro ◇, Sudafed ◇, Sudafed 12
Hour ◇, Sufedrin ◇

pseudoephedrine sulfate
Afrin ◇, Drixoral†, Drixoral Non-
Drowsy Formula ◇

Pregnancy risk category C

AVAILABLE FORMS
pseudoephedrine hydrochloride
Capsules: 60 mg
Capsules (extended-release): 120 mg
Oral solution: 7.5 mg/0.8 ml ◇, 15 mg/
5 ml ◇, 30 mg/5 ml ◇

Syrup: 30 mg/5 ml
Tablets: 30 mg ◇, 60 mg ◇
Tablets (extended-release): 120 mg ◇,
240 mg ◇
pseudoephedrine sulfate
Tablets (extended-release): 120 mg
(60 mg immediate-release, 60 mg
delayed-release) ◇

INDICATIONS & DOSAGES
➤ **Nasal and eustachian tube
decongestion—**
Adults: 60 mg P.O. q 4 hours. Maximum, 240 mg daily. Or, 120 mg extended-release tablet P.O. q 12 hours. Or, 240 mg extended-release Efidac/24 once daily.
Children older than age 12: 60 mg P.O. q 4 to 6 hours. Maximum, 240 mg daily. Or, 120 mg extended-release tablet P.O. q 12 hours or 240 mg extended-release Efidac/24 once daily.
Children ages 6 to 12: 30 mg P.O. regular-release form q 4 to 6 hours. Maximum, 120 mg daily.
Children ages 2 to 6: 15 mg P.O. regular-release form q 4 to 6 hours. Maximum, 60 mg daily.
Children ages 1 to 2: 7 drops or 0.2 ml/kg P.O. q 4 to 6 hours, up to four doses daily.
Children ages 3 to 12 months: 3 drops/kg P.O. q 4 to 6 hours, up to four doses daily.

ACTION
Stimulates alpha receptors in the respiratory tract, producing vasoconstriction, shrinking swollen nasal mucous membranes, increasing airway patency, and reducing tissue hyperemia, edema, and nasal congestion.

Route	Onset	Peak	Duration
P.O.	0.5 hr	0.5-1 hr	4-12 hr

ADVERSE REACTIONS
CNS: *anxiety,* transient stimulation, tremor, dizziness, headache, insomnia, *nervousness.*
CV: *arrhythmias, palpitations,* tachycardia, *CV collapse.*
GI: anorexia, nausea, vomiting, dry mouth.
GU: difficulty urinating.
Respiratory: respiratory difficulties.
Skin: pallor.

Reactions may be *common,* uncommon, *life-threatening,* or COMMON AND LIFE-THREATENING.

INTERACTIONS

Drug-drug. *Antihypertensives:* May attenuate hypotensive effect. Monitor blood pressure closely.

MAO inhibitors: May cause severe hypertension (hypertensive crisis). Avoid using together.

Methyldopa: May increase pressor response. Monitor patient closely.

EFFECTS ON LAB TEST RESULTS

None reported.

CONTRAINDICATIONS

Contraindicated in patients with severe hypertension or severe coronary artery disease, in those receiving MAO inhibitors, and in breast-feeding women. Extended-release forms are contraindicated in children younger than age 12.

NURSING CONSIDERATIONS

● Use cautiously in patients with hypertension, cardiac disease, diabetes, glaucoma, hyperthyroidism, and prostatic hyperplasia.

● Elderly patients are more sensitive to drug's effects. Extended-release tablets shouldn't be given to elderly patients until safety with short-acting preparations has been established.

PATIENT TEACHING

● Tell patient not to crush or break extended-release forms.

● Warn against using OTC products containing other sympathomimetics.

● Instruct patient not to take drug within 2 hours of bedtime because it can cause insomnia.

● Tell patient to stop drug and notify prescriber if he becomes unusually restless.

38

Adrenergic blockers (sympatholytics)

dihydroergotamine mesylate
methysergide maleate
propranolol hydrochloride
(See Chapter 20, ANTIANGINALS.)

COMBINATION PRODUCTS
HYDERGINE: dihydroergocornine mesylate 0.167 mg, dihydroergocristine mesylate 0.167 mg, and dihydroergocryptine mesylate 0.167 mg.

---

dihydroergotamine mesylate
D.H.E. 45, Dihydergot‡, Dihydroergotamine-Sandoz†, Migranal

Pregnancy risk category X

AVAILABLE FORMS
Injection: 1 mg/ml
Intranasal solution: 0.5 mg/metered spray (4 mg/ml)

INDICATIONS & DOSAGES
➤ **To prevent or abort vascular or migraine headache—**
Adults: 1 mg I.M. or I.V. repeated q 1 to 2 hours, p.r.n., up to total of 2 mg I.V. or 3 mg I.M. per attack. Maximum, 6 mg weekly. For nasal spray, 1 spray into each nostril to total of 1 mg initially, repeated in 15 minutes for a total dose of 2 mg.

I.V. ADMINISTRATION
• Directly inject solution into the vein over 3 minutes. Continuous and intermittent infusions aren't recommended.
• Protect ampules from heat and light. Discard if solution is discolored.

ACTION
Causes peripheral vasoconstriction primarily by stimulating alpha receptors; may abort vascular headaches by direct vasoconstriction of dilated carotid artery bed with a decline in amplitude of pulsa-tions. Also, causes antagonistic effect of serotonin 5-HT_2 receptors.

Route	Onset	Peak	Duration
I.M.	15-30 min	30 min	3-4 hr
Intranasal	Rapid	0.5-1 hr	Unknown
I.V.	5 min	15 min	8 hr

ADVERSE REACTIONS
CV: transient tachycardia or ***bradycardia,*** precordial distress and pain, increased arterial pressure.
GI: *nausea, vomiting.*
GU: uterine contractions.
Musculoskeletal: weakness in legs, muscle pain in arms and legs, numbness and tingling in fingers and toes.
Skin: itching.
Other: localized edema, injection site irritation.

INTERACTIONS
Drug-drug. *Erythromycin, other macrolides:* May cause symptoms of ergot toxicity (severe peripheral vasospasm with possible ischemia, cyanosis, and numbness). Vasodilators (nifedipine, nitroprusside, or prazosin) may be ordered to treat such an attack. Monitor patient closely.
Propranolol, other beta blockers: Blocked natural pathway for vasodilation in patients receiving ergot alkaloids; may result in excessive vasoconstriction and cold arms and legs. Watch closely if drugs are used together.
Selective serotonin reuptake inhibitors: Increased risk of weakness, hyperflexion, and incoordination. Monitor patient closely.
Sumatriptan: Additive effect, causing an increased risk of coronary vasospasm. Don't give within 24 hours of each other.
Vasoconstrictors: Additive effect, causing an increased risk of high blood pressure. Monitor blood pressure.
Drug-lifestyle. *Nicotine:* Can have additive effect leading to vasoconstriction. Discourage use together.

Reactions may be *common,* uncommon, *life-threatening,* or COMMON AND LIFE-THREATENING.

EFFECTS ON LAB TEST RESULTS
None reported.

CONTRAINDICATIONS
Contraindicated in patients hypersensitive to drug and in those with ischemic heart disease, coronary artery spasm including Prinzmetal's angina, hemiplegic or basilar migraine, peripheral and occlusive vascular disease, coronary artery disease, uncontrolled hypertension, severe hepatic or renal dysfunction, malnutrition, severe pruritus, or sepsis; also, contraindicated in pregnant and breast-feeding patients.

NURSING CONSIDERATIONS
• Drug is most effective when used at first sign of migraine or soon after onset.
• Avoid prolonged use; don't exceed recommended dosage. Adjust to most effective minimal dosage, for best results.
• Intranasal solution isn't intended for prolonged daily use.
• *Alert:* Watch for ergotamine rebound, or an increase in frequency and duration of headache, which may occur when drug is stopped.

PATIENT TEACHING
• Instruct patient to lie down and relax in a quiet, low-light environment after taking drug.
• Tell patient to report feeling of coldness in arms and legs or of tingling in fingers and toes. Severe vasoconstriction may result in tissue damage. Keep arms and legs warm and give vasodilators.
• Help patient evaluate underlying causes of stress, which may precipitate attacks.
• Advise patient to notify prescriber if she's pregnant or plans to become pregnant.

---

methysergide maleate
Deseril‡, Sansert**

Pregnancy risk category X

AVAILABLE FORMS
Tablets: 1 mg‡, 2 mg

INDICATIONS & DOSAGES
➤ **Prevention of frequent, severe, uncontrollable, or disabling migraine or other vascular headaches—**
Adults: 4 to 8 mg P.O. daily with meals. Patient must have a drug-free interval of 3 to 4 weeks after each 6-month course of treatment.

ACTION
Unknown. Specifically blocks serotonin in the peripheral nervous system. In CNS, drug may act as a serotonin agonist.

Route	Onset	Peak	Duration
P.O.	1-2 days	Unknown	1-2 days after initiation

ADVERSE REACTIONS
CNS: insomnia, drowsiness, *euphoria, vertigo,* ataxia, *light-headedness,* hyperesthesia, weakness, hallucinations or feelings of dissociation, rapid speech, lethargy.
CV: *fibrotic thickening of cardiac valves, aorta, inferior vena cava, and common iliac branches;* vasoconstriction, causing chest pain, vascular insufficiency of legs; cold, numb, painful arms and legs with or without paresthesia and diminished or absent pulses; orthostatic hypotension; flushing; tachycardia; peripheral edema; murmurs; bruits.
GI: abdominal pain, nausea, vomiting, diarrhea, constipation, heartburn.
Hematologic: *neutropenia,* eosinophilia.
Metabolic: weight gain.
Musculoskeletal: arthralgia, myalgia.
Respiratory: *pulmonary fibrosis.*
Skin: hair loss, rash.

INTERACTIONS
Drug-drug. *Beta blockers:* May result in peripheral ischemia, cold arms and legs, and possible gangrene. Monitor patient closely.

EFFECTS ON LAB TEST RESULTS
• May increase eosinophil count. May decrease neutrophil count.

CONTRAINDICATIONS
Contraindicated in debilitated or pregnant patients and in patients with severe hyper-

tension or arteriosclerosis, peripheral vascular insufficiency, renal or hepatic disease, coronary artery disease, pulmonary disease, serious infection, phlebitis or cellulitis of the legs, collagen diseases, fibrotic processes, or valvular heart disease.

NURSING CONSIDERATIONS

• Use cautiously in patients with peptic ulcerations or suspected coronary artery disease. Ensure ECG and cardiac status evaluation before giving drug to patients older than age 40. Also, use cautiously in patients sensitive to aspirin or tartrazine.

• *Alert:* Drug is indicated only for patients unresponsive to other drugs and who can have close medical supervision.

• Gradually introduce drug, and give with meals to prevent adverse GI effects.

• Give drug for 3 weeks before evaluating effectiveness. If patient shows no response after 3 weeks, drug is unlikely to be beneficial.

• Pulmonary fibrosis may occur with drug use, causing dyspnea, tightness and pain in chest, pleural friction rubs, and effusion.

• Monitor laboratory studies of cardiac and renal function, CBC, and erythrocyte sedimentation rate before and during therapy.

• Drug shouldn't be used for migraine, vascular headache, or tension (muscle contraction) headache.

• Drug may be withdrawn gradually every 6 months and then restarted after at least 3 weeks.

PATIENT TEACHING

• Tell patient to take drug with meals.

• Instruct patient to keep daily weight record and to report unusually rapid weight gain. Teach patient to check for peripheral edema. Explain and suggest low-sodium diet, if needed.

• Stress importance of keeping regular medical appointments as scheduled.

• Tell patient not to stop drug abruptly but to do so gradually over 2 to 3 weeks; abrupt withdrawal may cause rebound headaches.

• Instruct patient to promptly notify prescriber if these symptoms occur: cold, numb, or painful hands and feet; leg cramps when walking; and pelvic, chest, or flank pain.

• Advise patient to notify prescriber if she becomes pregnant or plans to become pregnant.

39

Skeletal muscle relaxants

baclofen
carisoprodol
chlorzoxazone
cyclobenzaprine hydrochloride
dantrolene sodium
methocarbamol
tizanidine hydrochloride

COMBINATION PRODUCTS
NORGESIC: orphenadrine citrate 25 mg, aspirin 385 mg, and caffeine 30 mg.
NORGESIC FORTE: orphenadrine citrate 50 mg, aspirin 770 mg, and caffeine 60 mg.
ROBAXISAL: methocarbamol 400 mg and aspirin 325 mg.
SOMA COMPOUND: carisoprodol 200 mg and aspirin 325 mg.
SOMA COMPOUND WITH CODEINE: carisoprodol 200 mg, aspirin 325 mg, and codeine phosphate 16 mg.

---

baclofen
Clofen‡, Lioresal, Lioresal Intrathecal

Pregnancy risk category C

AVAILABLE FORMS
Intrathecal injection: 500 mcg/ml, 2,000 mcg/ml
Tablets: 10 mg, 20 mg, 25 mg‡

INDICATIONS & DOSAGES
➤ **Spasticity in multiple sclerosis; spinal cord injury—**
Adults: Initially, 5 mg P.O. t.i.d. for 3 days; then 10 mg t.i.d. for 3 days, 15 mg t.i.d. for 3 days, 20 mg t.i.d. for 3 days. Dosage increase based on response, up to maximum of 80 mg daily.
➤ **Management of severe spasticity in patients who don't respond to or can't tolerate oral baclofen therapy—**
*Adults: Screening phase—*After test dose to check responsiveness, give drug via implantable infusion pump. Give test dose of 1 ml of 50-mcg/ml dilution into intrathecal space by barbotage over 1 minute or longer. Significantly decreased severity or frequency of muscle spasm or reduced muscle tone should appear within 4 to 8 hours. If response is inadequate, give second test dose of 75 mcg/1.5 ml 24 hours after the first. If response is still inadequate, give final test dose of 100 mcg/2 ml after 24 hours. Patients unresponsive to the 100-mcg dose shouldn't be considered candidates for implantable pump.
*Maintenance therapy—*Adjust initial dose based on screening dose that elicited an adequate response. Double this effective dose and give over 24 hours. However, if screening dose efficacy was maintained for 12 hours or longer, don't double the dose. After the first 24 hours, increase dose slowly as needed and tolerated by 10% to 30% daily. During prolonged maintenance therapy, daily dose may be increased by 10% to 40% if needed; if patient experiences adverse effects, dosage may be decreased by 10% to 20%. Maintenance doses have ranged from 12 mcg to 2,000 mcg daily; however, experience with dosages over 1,000 mcg daily is limited. Most patients need 300 to 800 mcg daily.
Adjust-a-dose: For patients with impaired renal function, oral and intrathecal doses are decreased.

ACTION
Hyperpolarizes fibers to reduce impulse transmission. Appears to reduce transmission of impulses from the spinal cord to skeletal muscle, thus decreasing the frequency and amplitude of muscle spasms in patients with spinal cord lesions.

Route	Onset	Peak	Duration
Intrathecal	0.5-1 hr	4 hr	4-8 hr
P.O.	Unknown	2-3 hr	Unknown

ADVERSE REACTIONS
CNS: *drowsiness, dizziness,* headache, *weakness, fatigue,* hypotonia, *confusion,* insomnia, dysarthria, ***seizures with intrathecal use.***
CV: hypotension, hypertension.

---

*Liquid contains alcohol.   **May contain tartrazine.   †Canada   ‡Australia   §U.K.   ◇OTC

EENT: blurred vision, nasal congestion, slurred speech.
GI: *nausea,* constipation, *vomiting.*
GU: urinary frequency.
Metabolic: hyperglycemia, weight gain.
Respiratory: dyspnea.
Skin: rash, pruritus, excessive sweating.

INTERACTIONS
Drug-drug. *CNS depressants:* Increased CNS depression. Avoid using together.
Drug-lifestyle. *Alcohol use:* Increased CNS depression. Discourage use together.

EFFECTS ON LAB TEST RESULTS
● May increase AST, alkaline phosphatase, and glucose levels.

CONTRAINDICATIONS
Contraindicated in patients hypersensitive to drug.

NURSING CONSIDERATIONS
● Use cautiously in patients with impaired renal function or seizure disorder or when spasticity is used to maintain motor function.
● Give oral form with meals or with milk to prevent GI distress.
● *Alert:* Don't use oral drug to treat muscle spasm caused by rheumatic disorders, cerebral palsy, Parkinson's disease, or CVA because efficacy hasn't been established. Don't give intrathecal injection by I.V., I.M., S.C., or epidural route.
● Watch for sensitivity reactions, such as fever, skin eruptions, and respiratory distress.
● Expect an increased risk of seizures in patients with seizure disorder.
● The amount of relief determines whether dosage (and drowsiness) can be reduced.
● Don't withdraw drug abruptly after long-term use unless severe adverse reactions demand it; doing so may precipitate hallucinations or rebound spasticity.
● Experience with long-term intrathecal use suggests that about 5% of patients may develop tolerance to drug. In some cases, it may be treated by hospitalizing patient and slowly withdrawing drug over a 2-week period.
● *Alert:* Don't confuse baclofen with Bactroban.

PATIENT TEACHING
● Instruct patient to take oral form with meals or milk.
● Tell patient to avoid activities that require alertness until CNS effects of drug are known. Drowsiness usually is transient.
● Tell patient to avoid alcohol and OTC antihistamines while taking drug.
● Advise patient to follow prescriber's orders regarding rest and physical therapy.

---

carisoprodol
Carisoma§, Soma, Vanadom

Pregnancy risk category C

AVAILABLE FORMS
Tablets: 350 mg

INDICATIONS & DOSAGES
➤ **As an adjunct in acute, painful musculoskeletal conditions—**
Adults: 350 mg P.O. t.i.d. and h.s.

ACTION
Unknown. Appears to modify central perception of pain without modifying pain reflexes. Muscle relaxant effects may be related to sedative properties.

Route	Onset	Peak	Duration
P.O.	0.5 hr	4 hr	4-6 hr

ADVERSE REACTIONS
CNS: *drowsiness, dizziness,* vertigo, ataxia, tremor, agitation, irritability, headache, depressive reactions, insomnia.
CV: *orthostatic hypotension,* tachycardia, facial flushing.
GI: nausea, vomiting, epigastric distress.
Hematologic: eosinophilia.
Respiratory: *asthmatic episodes,* hiccups.
Skin: rash, *erythema multiforme,* pruritus.
Other: fever, *angioedema, anaphylaxis.*

INTERACTIONS
Drug-drug. *CNS depressants:* Increased CNS depression. Avoid using together.
Drug-lifestyle. *Alcohol use:* Increased CNS depression. Discourage use together.

EFFECTS ON LAB TEST RESULTS
● May increase eosinophil count.

Reactions may be *common*, uncommon, *life-threatening*, or COMMON AND LIFE-THREATENING.

CONTRAINDICATIONS

Contraindicated in patients hypersensitive to related compounds (such as meprobamate or tybamate) and in those with intermittent porphyria.

NURSING CONSIDERATIONS

• Use cautiously in patients with impaired hepatic or renal function.
• *Alert:* Watch for idiosyncratic reactions after first to fourth doses (weakness, ataxia, visual and speech difficulties, fever, skin eruptions, and mental changes) and for severe reactions, including bronchospasm, hypotension, and anaphylactic shock. Withhold dose and notify prescriber immediately about unusual reactions.
• Record amount of relief to help prescriber determine whether dosage can be reduced.
• Don't stop drug abruptly; mild withdrawal effects, such as insomnia, headache, nausea, and abdominal cramps, may result.
• Safety and efficacy in children younger than age 12 haven't been established.
• Drug may be habit forming.

PATIENT TEACHING

• Warn patient to avoid activities that require alertness until CNS effects of drug are known. Drowsiness is transient.
• Advise patient to avoid combining drug with alcohol or other CNS depressants.
• Tell patient to ask prescriber before using OTC cold or hay fever remedies.
• Instruct patient to follow prescriber's orders regarding rest and physical therapy.
• Advise patient to avoid sudden changes in posture if dizziness occurs.
• Tell patient to take drug with food or milk if GI upset occurs.

---

chlorzoxazone
Paraflex, Parafon Forte DSC, Remular-S

Pregnancy risk category C

AVAILABLE FORMS
Caplets: 250 mg, 500 mg
Tablets: 250 mg, 500 mg

INDICATIONS & DOSAGES
➤ **As an adjunct in acute, painful musculoskeletal conditions—**
Adults: 250 to 750 mg P.O. t.i.d. or q.i.d.

ACTION
Unknown. Appears to modify central perception of pain without modifying pain reflexes.

Route	Onset	Peak	Duration
P.O.	1 hr	1-2 hr	3-4 hr

ADVERSE REACTIONS
CNS: *drowsiness, dizziness, lightheadedness,* malaise, headache, overstimulation, tremor.
GI: anorexia, nausea, vomiting, heartburn, abdominal distress, constipation, diarrhea.
GU: orange or purple-red urine discoloration.
Hepatic: hepatic dysfunction.
Skin: urticaria, redness, pruritus, petechiae, bruising.

INTERACTIONS
Drug-drug. *CNS depressants:* Increased CNS depression. Avoid using together.
Drug-herb. *Watercress:* Elevated chlorzoxazone levels, increasing therapeutic and adverse effects. Discourage use together.
Drug-lifestyle. *Alcohol use:* Increased CNS depression. Discourage use together.

EFFECTS ON LAB TEST RESULTS
• May increase AST, ALT, alkaline phosphatase, and bilirubin levels.

CONTRAINDICATIONS
Contraindicated in patients hypersensitive to drug and in those with hepatic impairment.

NURSING CONSIDERATIONS
• Use cautiously in patients with history of drug allergies.
• The amount of relief determines whether dosage (and drowsiness) can be reduced.
• *Alert:* Monitor patient's liver enzyme levels. Watch for early signs of hepatic dysfunction or abnormal liver enzyme levels. If they occur, withhold dose and notify prescriber. Serious (including fatal)

---

hepatocellular toxicity has been reported in patients receiving drug.

PATIENT TEACHING
• Tell patient to take drug with meals or milk.
• Warn patient to avoid activities that require alertness until CNS effects of drug are known.
• Instruct patient to immediately notify prescriber about fever, rash, anorexia, nausea, vomiting, fatigue, right upper quadrant pain, dark urine, or jaundice because these may indicate hepatocellular toxicity, which warrants stopping drug immediately.
• Warn patient to avoid alcohol and other CNS depressants; using together with drug may increase risk of hepatocellular toxicity.
• Tell patient that drug may discolor urine orange or purple-red.
• Advise patient to follow prescriber's orders regarding physical activity.

---

cyclobenzaprine hydrochloride
Flexeril

Pregnancy risk category B

AVAILABLE FORMS
Tablets: 10 mg

INDICATIONS & DOSAGES
➤ **Short-term treatment of muscle spasm—**
Adults: 10 mg P.O. t.i.d. for 2 to 3 weeks.

ACTION
Unknown. Relieves skeletal muscle spasm of local origin without disrupting muscle function.

Route	Onset	Peak	Duration
P.O.	1 hr	3-8 hr	12-24 hr

ADVERSE REACTIONS
CNS: *drowsiness,* headache, insomnia, fatigue, asthenia, nervousness, confusion, paresthesia, *dizziness,* depression, *seizures,* dysarthria, ataxia, syncope.
CV: tachycardia, *arrhythmias,* palpitations, hypotension, vasodilation.

EENT: visual disturbances, blurred vision.
GI: dyspepsia, abnormal taste, constipation, *dry mouth,* nausea.
GU: urine retention, urinary frequency.
Skin: rash, urticaria, pruritus.

INTERACTIONS
Drug-drug. *Anticholinergics:* Additive anticholinergic effects. Avoid using together.
CNS depressants: Increased CNS depression. Avoid using together.
MAO inhibitors: Hyperpyretic crisis, seizures, and death have occurred when MAO inhibitors are combined with TCAs; may also occur with cyclobenzaprine. Don't give within 14 days after discontinuing MAO inhibitors.
Drug-lifestyle. *Alcohol use:* Increased CNS depression. Discourage use together.

EFFECTS ON LAB TEST RESULTS
None reported.

CONTRAINDICATIONS
Contraindicated in patients hypersensitive to drug and in those with hyperthyroidism, heart block, arrhythmias, conduction disturbances, or heart failure; also contraindicated in those who have received MAO inhibitors within 14 days and those who are in the acute recovery phase of an MI.

NURSING CONSIDERATIONS
• Use cautiously in elderly patients, debilitated patients, and patients with a history of urine retention, acute angle-closure glaucoma, or increased intraocular pressure.
• Cyclobenzaprine may cause toxic reactions similar to TCAs. Observe precautions as you would when giving TCAs.
• Monitor patient for nausea, headache, and malaise, which may occur if drug is stopped abruptly after long-term use.
• *Alert:* Watch for signs and symptoms of overdose, including cardiac toxicity. Notify prescriber immediately.
• Safety and efficacy in children younger than age 15 haven't been established.
• *Alert:* Don't confuse Flexeril with Floxin or Flaxedil.

PATIENT TEACHING
● Advise patient to report urinary hesitancy or urine retention. If constipation is a problem, suggest that he increase fluid intake and use a stool softener.
● Warn patient to avoid activities that require alertness until CNS effects of drug are known.
● Warn patient not to combine with alcohol or other CNS depressants, including OTC cold or allergy remedies.

---

dantrolene sodium
Dantrium, Dantrium Intravenous

Pregnancy risk category C

AVAILABLE FORMS
Capsules: 25 mg, 50 mg, 100 mg
Injection: 20 mg/vial

INDICATIONS & DOSAGES
➤ **Spasticity and sequelae from severe chronic disorders, such as multiple sclerosis, cerebral palsy, spinal cord injury, CVA—**
Adults: 25 mg P.O. daily. Increased gradually in 25-mg increments up to 100 mg b.i.d. to q.i.d. Maximum, 400 mg daily. Maintain each dosage level for 4 to 7 days to determine response.
Children: Initially, 0.5 mg/kg P.O. b.i.d.; increased to t.i.d. then q.i.d. Dosage increased, p.r.n., by 0.5 mg/kg daily up to 3 mg/kg b.i.d. to q.i.d. Maximum, 100 mg q.i.d.
➤ **Management of malignant hyperthermic crisis—**
Adults and children: 1 mg/kg I.V. push initially. Repeated, p.r.n., up to cumulative dose of 10 mg/kg.
➤ **Prevention or attenuation of malignant hyperthermic crisis in susceptible patients who need surgery—**
Adults: 4 to 8 mg/kg P.O. daily in three to four divided doses for 1 to 2 days before procedure. Final dose given 3 to 4 hours before procedure.
➤ **Prevention of recurrence of malignant hyperthermic crisis—**
Adults: 4 to 8 mg/kg/day P.O. in four divided doses for up to 3 days after hyperthermic crisis.

I.V. ADMINISTRATION
● Give as soon as malignant hyperthermia reaction is recognized.
● Reconstitute drug by adding 60 ml of sterile water for injection and shaking vial until clear. Don't use a diluent that contains a bacteriostatic drug.
● Protect contents from light, and use within 6 hours.

ACTION
Acts directly on skeletal muscle to decrease excitation and contraction coupling and reduce muscle strength by interfering with intracellular calcium movement.

Route	Onset	Peak	Duration
I.V.	Unknown	Unknown	3 hr after infusion ends
P.O.	Unknown	5 hr	Unknown

ADVERSE REACTIONS
CNS: *drowsiness, dizziness,* headache, light-headedness, *malaise, fatigue,* confusion, nervousness, insomnia, *seizures.*
CV: tachycardia, blood pressure changes, phlebitis, thrombophlebitis.
EENT: excessive lacrimation, speech disturbance, diplopia, visual disturbances.
GI: anorexia, constipation, cramping, dysphagia, metallic taste, severe diarrhea, GI bleeding.
GU: urinary frequency, hematuria, incontinence, nocturia, dysuria, crystalluria, difficult erection, urine retention.
Hepatic: *hepatitis.*
Musculoskeletal: myalgia, back pain, *muscle weakness.*
Respiratory: pleural effusion with pericarditis, pulmonary edema.
Skin: eczematous eruption, pruritus, urticaria, abnormal hair growth, diaphoresis.
Other: chills, fever.

INTERACTIONS
Drug-drug. *Clofibrate, warfarin:* May decrease plasma protein binding of dantrolene. Use together cautiously.
CNS depressants: Increased CNS depression. Avoid using together.
Estrogens: May increase risk of hepatotoxicity. Use together cautiously.
I.V. verapamil: May result in CV collapse. Stop verapamil before giving I.V. dantrolene.

Drug-lifestyle. *Alcohol use:* Increased CNS depression. Discourage use together. *Sun exposure:* May cause photosensitivity reactions. Advise patient to avoid excessive sunlight exposure.

EFFECTS ON LAB TEST RESULTS
• May increase BUN, ALT, AST, and bilirubin levels.

CONTRAINDICATIONS
Contraindicated for spasms in rheumatic disorders and when spasticity is used to maintain motor function. Also contraindicated in breast-feeding patients and patients with upper motor neuron disorders or active hepatic disease.

NURSING CONSIDERATIONS
• Use cautiously in women, patients older than age 35, and patients with hepatic disease or severely impaired cardiac or pulmonary function.
• Because of risk of liver damage with long-term use, therapy should be discontinued within 45 days if benefits aren't seen.
• Obtain liver function test results at start of therapy.
• Prepare oral suspension for single dose by dissolving capsule contents in juice or other liquid. For multiple doses, use acid vehicle, and refrigerate. Use within several days.
• *Alert:* Watch for hepatitis (fever and jaundice), severe diarrhea, severe weakness, and sensitivity reactions (fever and skin eruptions). Withhold dose and notify prescriber.
• The amount of relief obtained determines whether dosage (and drowsiness) can be reduced.
• *Alert:* Don't confuse Dantrium with Daraprim.

PATIENT TEACHING
• Instruct patient to take drug with meals or milk in four divided doses.
• Tell patient to use caution when eating to avoid choking. Some patients may have trouble swallowing during therapy.
• Warn patient to avoid driving and other hazardous activities until CNS effects of drug are known.

• Advise patient to avoid combining drug with alcohol and other CNS depressants.
• Advise patient to notify prescriber if skin or eyes turn yellow, skin is itchy, or fever develops.
• Tell patient to avoid photosensitivity reactions by using sunblock and wearing protective clothing, to report abdominal discomfort or GI problems immediately, and to follow prescriber's orders regarding rest and physical therapy.

---

methocarbamol
Carbacot, Robaxin, Robaxin-750, Skelex

Pregnancy risk category C

AVAILABLE FORMS
Injection: 100 mg/ml
Tablets: 500 mg, 750 mg

INDICATIONS & DOSAGES
➤ **As an adjunct in acute, painful musculoskeletal conditions—**
Adults: 1.5 g P.O. q.i.d. for 2 to 3 days, then 1 g P.O. q.i.d. Or, not more than 500 mg or 5 ml I.M. into each gluteal region, repeated q 8 hours, p.r.n. Or, 1 to 3 g or 10 to 30 ml daily I.V. directly into vein at 3 ml/minute. Or, 10 ml may be added to no more than 250 ml of D_5W or normal saline solution. Maximum I.V. or I.M. dose is 3 g daily for not longer than 3 days.
➤ **Supportive therapy in tetanus management—**
Adults: 1 to 2 g by direct I.V. or 1 to 3 g as infusion q 6 hours until nasogastric tube can be inserted; then give oral doses through nasogastric tube. Maximum, 24 g daily.
Children: 15 mg/kg I.V. q 6 hours.

I.V. ADMINISTRATION
• Dilute 10 ml of drug in no more than 250 ml of solution. Use D_5W or normal saline solution for injection. Infuse slowly; maximum rate is 300 mg (3 ml)/minute.
• Drug irritates veins and may cause phlebitis, aggravate seizures, and cause fainting if injected rapidly. Make sure patient stays supine during infusion. Drug is an irritant; avoid extravasation.

Reactions may be *common*, uncommon, **life-threatening**, or COMMON AND LIFE-THREATENING.

ACTION

Unknown. Probably modifies central perception of pain through sedative effects without modifying pain reflexes.

Route	Onset	Peak	Duration
I.M.	Unknown	Unknown	Unknown
I.V.	Immediate	Immediate	Unknown
P.O.	0.5 hr	2 hr	Unknown

ADVERSE REACTIONS

CNS: *drowsiness, dizziness,* headache, *light-headedness,* syncope, mild muscular incoordination with I.M. or I.V. use, *seizures* with I.V. use, vertigo.
CV: hypotension, *bradycardia* with I.M. or I.V. use, thrombophlebitis, flushing.
EENT: blurred vision, conjunctivitis, nystagmus, diplopia.
GI: nausea, GI upset, metallic taste.
GU: hematuria with I.V. use, discoloration of urine.
Skin: urticaria, pruritus, rash.
Other: extravasation with I.V. use, fever, *anaphylactic reactions* with I.M. or I.V. use.

INTERACTIONS

Drug-drug. *CNS depressants:* Increased CNS depression. Avoid using together.
Drug-lifestyle. *Alcohol use:* Increased CNS depression. Discourage use together.

EFFECTS ON LAB TEST RESULTS

None reported.

CONTRAINDICATIONS

Contraindicated in patients hypersensitive to drug and in those with impaired renal function (injectable form) or seizure disorder (injectable form).

NURSING CONSIDERATIONS

• For nasogastric tube administration, prepare liquid by crushing tablets into water or saline solution.
• In tetanus management, methocarbamol is used with tetanus antitoxin, penicillin, tracheotomy, and aggressive supportive care. Long course of I.V. methocarbamol therapy is needed.
• Give I.M. deeply, only into upper outer quadrant of buttocks, with maximum of 5 ml in each buttock.
• Don't give by S.C. route.

• Drug therapy causes false-positive laboratory test results for urine 5-hydroxyindoleacetic acid using quantitative method of Udenfriend. Also causes false-positive results in Gitlow screening test for urine vanillylmandelic acid (no false-positive in quantitative method of Sunderman).
• Watch for orthostatic hypotension, especially with parenteral use. Keep patient in a supine position for 15 minutes afterward, and supervise ambulation. Have patient rise slowly.
• Watch for sensitivity reactions, such as fever and skin eruptions.
• Keep epinephrine, antihistamines, and corticosteroids available.
• **Alert:** Don't confuse methocarbamol with mephobarbital.

PATIENT TEACHING

• Instruct patient to take drug with food or milk at evenly spaced intervals.
• Tell patient that a metallic taste may develop and that urine may turn green, black, or brown.
• Advise patient to follow prescriber's orders regarding physical activity.
• Warn patient to avoid activities that require alertness until CNS effects of drug are known.
• Advise patient not to combine drug with alcohol or other CNS depressants.

---

tizanidine hydrochloride
Zanaflex

Pregnancy risk category C

AVAILABLE FORMS

Tablets: 2 mg, 4 mg

INDICATIONS & DOSAGES

➤ **Acute and intermittent management of increased muscle tone with spasticity**—
Adults: Initially, 4 mg P.O. q 6 to 8 hours, p.r.n., to maximum of three doses in 24 hours. Dosage can be increased gradually in 2- to 4-mg increments. Maximum, 36 mg daily.
Adjust-a-dose: For patients with renal failure, reduce dosage. If higher dosages are needed, increase individual doses rather than frequency.

ACTION
Unknown. Acts as an alpha$_2$ agonist. May reduce spasticity by increasing presynaptic inhibition of motor neurons at the level of the spinal cord.

Route	Onset	Peak	Duration
P.O.	Unknown	1-2 hr	3-6 hr

ADVERSE REACTIONS
CNS: *somnolence, sedation, asthenia, dizziness,* speech disorder, dyskinesia, nervousness, hallucinations.
CV: *hypotension.*
EENT: amblyopia, pharyngitis, rhinitis.
GI: *dry mouth,* constipation, vomiting.
GU: *urinary tract infection,* urinary frequency.
Hepatic: hepatic injury.
Other: infection, flu syndrome.

INTERACTIONS
Drug-drug. *Antihypertensives, other alpha$_2$ agonists such as clonidine:* May cause hypotension; monitor patient closely. Don't use with other alpha$_2$ agonists.
Baclofen, benzodiazepines, other CNS depressants: Additive CNS depressant effects. Avoid using together.
Oral contraceptives: Decreased clearance of tizanidine. Dosage of tizanidine may be reduced.
Drug-lifestyle. *Alcohol use:* Increased CNS depression. Discourage use together.

EFFECTS ON LAB TEST RESULTS
• May increase AST and ALT levels.

CONTRAINDICATIONS
Contraindicated in patients hypersensitive to drug.

NURSING CONSIDERATIONS
• Use cautiously in patients who are taking antihypertensives, in those with renal and hepatic impairment, and in elderly patients.
• Drug should be used during pregnancy only if benefit justifies risk to fetus.
• Women taking drug shouldn't breastfeed.
• Safety and effectiveness in children haven't been established.

• Obtain liver function test results before treatment; during treatment at 1, 3, and 6 months; and then periodically thereafter.

PATIENT TEACHING
• Caution patient to avoid alcohol and activities that require alertness. Drug may cause drowsiness.
• Inform patient that orthostatic hypotension can be minimized by rising slowly and avoiding sudden position changes.

atracurium besylate
cisatracurium besylate
doxacurium chloride
mivacurium chloride
pancuronium bromide
rocuronium bromide
succinylcholine chloride
tubocurarine chloride
vecuronium bromide

COMBINATION PRODUCTS
None.

---

atracurium besylate
Tracrium

Pregnancy risk category C

AVAILABLE FORMS
Injection: 10 mg/ml

INDICATIONS & DOSAGES
➤ **Adjunct to general anesthesia to facilitate endotracheal intubation and relax skeletal muscles during surgery or mechanical ventilation—**
Adults and children older than age 2: 0.4 to 0.5 mg/kg by I.V. bolus. Maintenance dose of 0.08 to 0.1 mg/kg within 20 to 45 minutes should be given during prolonged surgery. Maintenance doses may be given q 12 to 25 minutes in patients receiving balanced anesthesia. For prolonged procedures, a constant infusion of 5 to 9 mcg/kg/minute may be used.
Children ages 1 month to 2 years: Initial dose, 0.3 to 0.4 mg/kg. Frequent maintenance doses may be needed.

I.V. ADMINISTRATION
• Use drug only under direct supervision by medical staff skilled in using neuromuscular blockers and maintaining patent airway. Keep emergency respiratory support (endotracheal equipment, ventilator, oxygen, atropine, edrophonium, neostigmine, and epinephrine) available.
• Give sedatives or general anesthetics before neuromuscular blockers, which don't

obtund consciousness or alter pain threshold.
• Drug usually is given by rapid I.V. bolus injection but may be given by intermittent infusion or continuous infusion. At concentrations of 0.2 mg/ml to 0.5 mg/ml, atracurium is compatible for 24 hours in D_5W, normal saline solution for injection, or dextrose 5% in normal saline solution for injection.
• Don't use lactated Ringer's solution. In lactated Ringer's injection, atracurium is stable for 8 hours at 0.5 mg/ml. However, because of increased degradation in this solution, it isn't recommended.
• Don't mix with alkaline solutions, such as barbiturates, because precipitates may form.
• Stable if undiluted for 6 weeks.
• Store in refrigerator. Don't freeze. Once removed, use within 14 days.

ACTION
A nondepolarizing drug that keeps acetylcholine from binding to receptors on motor end plate, thus blocking neuromuscular transmission.

Route	Onset	Peak	Duration
I.V.	2 min	3-5 min	35-70 min

ADVERSE REACTIONS
CV: *bradycardia,* hypotension, tachycardia.
Respiratory: *prolonged, dose-related apnea;* wheezing; increased bronchial secretions; dyspnea; *bronchospasm; laryngospasm.*
Skin: *skin flushing,* erythema, pruritus, urticaria, rash.
Other: *anaphylaxis.*

INTERACTIONS
Drug-drug. *Aminoglycoside antibiotics (amikacin, gentamicin, kanamycin, neomycin, streptomycin), clindamycin, general anesthetics (enflurane, halothane, isoflurane), polymyxin antibiotics (colistin, polymyxin B sulfate), procainamide, quinidine, quinine, thiazide and loop diuretics,*

---

*Liquid contains alcohol.   **May contain tartrazine.   †Canada   ‡Australia   §U.K.   ◇OTC

trimethaphan, verapamil: Enhanced neuromuscular blockade, leading to increased skeletal muscle relaxation and prolonged effect of atracurium. Use together cautiously during and after surgery.

Carbamazepine, phenytoin, theophylline: Resistance to or reversal of neuromuscular blockade. Monitor patient closely.

Corticosteroids: May cause prolonged weakness. Monitor patient closely.

Edrophonium, neostigmine, pyridostigmine: Inhibition of drug and reversed neuromuscular block. Monitor patient closely.

General anesthetics (cyclopropane, enflurane, halothane, methoxyflurane): Potentiated effects of atracurium. Consider reduced dosage of inhaled anesthetic.

Lithium, magnesium salts, opioid analgesics: Enhanced neuromuscular blockade, leading to increased skeletal muscle relaxation and possible respiratory paralysis. Reduce atracurium dosage.

Succinylcholine: Quicker onset of atracurium; may increase depth of neuromuscular blockade. Monitor patient.

EFFECTS ON LAB TEST RESULTS
None reported.

CONTRAINDICATIONS
Contraindicated in patients hypersensitive to drug.

NURSING CONSIDERATIONS
• Use cautiously in elderly or debilitated patients and in those with CV disease; severe electrolyte disorder; bronchogenic carcinoma; hepatic, renal, or pulmonary impairment; neuromuscular disease; or myasthenia gravis.
• Dosage depends on anesthetic used, individual needs, and response. Recommended dosages are only representative.
• Give analgesics for pain. Patient may have pain but not be able to express it.
• Don't give drug by I.M. injection.
• Once spontaneous recovery starts, be prepared to reverse atracurium-induced neuromuscular blockade with an anticholinesterase (such as neostigmine or edrophonium). Usually given together with an anticholinergic (such as atropine). Complete reversal of neuromuscular blockade is usually achieved within 8 to

10 minutes after use of an anticholinesterase.
• Monitor respirations and vital signs closely until patient has fully recovered from neuromuscular blockade, as evidenced by tests of muscle strength (hand grip, head lift, and ability to cough).
• A nerve stimulator and train-of-four monitoring are recommended to confirm antagonism of neuromuscular blockade and recovery of muscle strength. Evidence of spontaneous recovery should be seen before attempting reversal with neostigmine.
• Prior use of succinylcholine doesn't prolong duration of action but quickens onset and may deepen neuromuscular blockade.
• *Alert:* Careful dosage calculation is essential. Always verify dosage with another health care professional.

PATIENT TEACHING
• Explain all events and procedures to patient because he can still hear.

---

cisatracurium besylate
Nimbex

Pregnancy risk category B

AVAILABLE FORMS
Injection: 2 mg/ml, 10 mg/ml

INDICATIONS & DOSAGES
➤ **Adjunct to general anesthesia to facilitate endotracheal intubation and relax skeletal muscles during surgery—**
Adults: Initial dose of 0.15 mg/kg I.V., then maintenance doses of 0.03 mg/kg I.V. q 40 to 50 minutes, p.r.n. Or, initial dose of 0.2 mg/kg I.V., then maintenance doses of 0.03 mg/kg I.V. q 50 to 60 minutes, p.r.n. Or, after initial dose, a maintenance infusion may be given at 3 mcg/kg/minute, reduced to 1 to 2 mcg/kg/minute, p.r.n.
Children ages 2 to 12: 0.1 mg/kg I.V. over 5 to 10 seconds. After initial dose, a maintenance infusion may be given at 3 mcg/kg/minute, reduced to 1 to 2 mcg/kg/minute, p.r.n.

➤ **Maintenance of neuromuscular blockade during mechanical ventilation in intensive care unit (ICU)—**
Adults: Principles for infusion in operating room apply to use in ICU. After initial dose, give 3 mcg/kg/minute by I.V. infusion. Range, 0.5 to 10.2 mcg/kg/minute.
Adjust-a-dose: In patients with neuromuscular disease such as myasthenia gravis and Eaton-Lambert syndrome, a dose of no more than 0.02 mg/kg is recommended. Patients with burns may need increased amount.

I.V. ADMINISTRATION
● Use only under direct supervision by medical staff skilled in using neuromuscular blockers and maintaining airway patency. Don't use unless resources for intubation, mechanical ventilation, and oxygen therapy are within reach.
● Drug has no known effect on consciousness, pain threshold, or cerebration. To avoid patient distress, don't induce neuromuscular block before unconsciousness.
● The 20-ml vial is intended for use only in ICU. Drug isn't compatible with propofol injection or ketorolac injection for Y-site use. Drug is acidic and may not be compatible with an alkaline solution of more than 8.5 pH (such as barbiturate solutions for Y-site use). Drug shouldn't be diluted in lactated Ringer's injection because of chemical instability.
● Drug is colorless to slightly yellow to green-yellow. Inspect vials for particulates and discoloration before use. Unclear solutions or those with visible particulates shouldn't be used.

ACTION
Nondepolarizing drug that binds to cholinergic receptors on the motor end plate, antagonizing acetylcholine and blocking neuromuscular transmission.

Route	Onset	Peak	Duration
I.V.	1-2 min	2-5 min	25-44 min

ADVERSE REACTIONS
CV: *bradycardia,* hypotension, flushing.
Respiratory: *bronchospasm, prolonged apnea.*
Skin: rash.

INTERACTIONS
Drug-drug. *Aminoglycosides, bacitracin, clindamycin, colistimethate sodium, colistin, lincomycin, lithium, local anesthetics, magnesium salts, polymyxins, procainamide, quinidine, quinine, tetracyclines:* May enhance neuromuscular blocking action of cisatracurium. Use together cautiously.
Carbamazepine, phenytoin: May cause slightly shorter duration of neuromuscular block, requiring higher infusion rate. Monitor patient closely.
Enflurane or isoflurane given with nitrous oxide or oxygen: May prolong cisatracurium duration of action. Patient may need less frequent maintenance dosing, lower maintenance doses, or reduced infusion rate of cisatracurium.
Succinylcholine: Shorter time to onset of maximum neuromuscular block. Monitor patient.

EFFECTS ON LAB TEST RESULTS
None reported.

CONTRAINDICATIONS
Contraindicated in patients hypersensitive to drug, other bis-benzylisoquinolinium drugs, or benzyl alcohol (found in 10-ml vial).

NURSING CONSIDERATIONS
● Drug isn't recommended for rapid-sequence endotracheal intubation because of its intermediate onset.
● Use cautiously in pregnant or breast-feeding women.
● Dosage requirements vary widely among patients.
● Monitor neuromuscular function with nerve stimulator while giving. If stimulation doesn't elicit a response, stop infusion until response returns.
● To avoid inaccurate dosing, perform neuromuscular monitoring on a nonparetic limb in patients with hemiparesis or paraparesis.
● In patients with neuromuscular disease (myasthenia gravis and myasthenic syndrome [Eaton-Lambert syndrome]), prolonged neuromuscular block is possible. Use of a peripheral nerve stimulator and a dose of no more than 0.02 mg/kg is recommended to assess the level of neuro-

muscular block and to monitor dosage requirements.
• Monitor acid-base balance and electrolyte levels. Abnormalities may potentiate or antagonize the action of cisatracurium.
• Monitor patient for malignant hyperthermia.
• Give analgesics, if appropriate. Patient can feel pain but can't indicate its presence.
• *Alert:* Careful dosage calculation is essential. Always verify dosage with another health care professional.

PATIENT TEACHING
• Explain purpose of drug.
• Assure patient that monitoring will be continuous.
• Explain all procedures and events because patient can still hear.

---

doxacurium chloride
Neuromax

Pregnancy risk category C

AVAILABLE FORMS
Injection: 1 mg/ml

INDICATIONS & DOSAGES
➤ **Adjunct to general anesthesia to relax skeletal muscles during surgery—**
Adults: 0.05 mg/kg rapid I.V. produces adequate conditions for endotracheal intubation in 5 minutes in about 90% of patients when used as part of a thiopental-narcotic induction technique. Lower doses may need longer delay before intubation is possible. Neuromuscular blockade at this dose lasts for an average of 100 minutes.
Children older than age 2: An initial dose of 0.03 mg/kg I.V. given during halothane anesthesia produces effective blockade in 7 minutes with duration of 30 minutes. Under the same conditions, 0.05 mg/kg produces blockade in 4 minutes with duration of 45 minutes.
➤ **Maintenance of neuromuscular blockade during long procedures—**
Adults: After initial dose of 0.05 mg/kg I.V., maintenance doses of 0.005 to 0.01 mg/kg will prolong neuromuscular blockade for an average of 30 to 45 minutes.

Adjust-a-dose: Patients with renal or hepatic insufficiency may need dosage adjustment. In obese patients 30% or more above their ideal weight, dosage should be adjusted to ideal body weight to avoid prolonged neuromuscular blockade. In patients with severe burns and in some patients with severe liver disease, higher initial doses may be needed. Doses of 0.8 mg/kg will produce intubating conditions more rapidly, within 4 minutes, with neuromuscular blockade for 160 minutes or longer. Consequently, these higher doses should be reserved for long procedures. Administration during steady-state anesthesia with enflurane, halothane, or isoflurane may allow 33% reduction of dose.

I.V. ADMINISTRATION
• Use drug only under direct supervision by medical staff skilled in using neuromuscular blockers and maintaining patent airway. Don't use unless an antagonist and resources for mechanical ventilation, oxygen therapy, and intubation are within reach.
• To avoid patient distress, don't give drug until patient's consciousness is obtunded by general anesthetic. Drug has no effect on consciousness or pain threshold.
• Prepare drug for I.V. use with D_5W, normal saline solution for injection, dextrose 5% in normal saline solution for injection, lactated Ringer's injection, or dextrose 5% in lactated Ringer's injection.
• Give product immediately after reconstitution. Diluted solutions are stable for 24 hours at room temperature; however, because reconstitution dilutes the preservative, risk of contamination increases. Discard unused solutions after 8 hours.
• When diluted as directed, drug is compatible with alfentanil, fentanyl, and sufentanil.

ACTION
Nondepolarizing neuromuscular blocker that competes with acetylcholine for receptor sites at the motor end plate; because this action may be antagonized by anticholinesterases, doxacurium is considered a competitive antagonist.

Route	Onset	Peak	Duration
I.V.	Variable	Variable	Variable

Reactions may be *common*, uncommon, *life-threatening*, or COMMON AND LIFE-THREATENING.

ADVERSE REACTIONS
Musculoskeletal: prolonged muscle weakness.
Respiratory: dyspnea, *respiratory depression, respiratory insufficiency or apnea.*

INTERACTIONS
Drug-drug. *Alkaline solutions:* Physically incompatible; precipitate may form. Don't give through same I.V. line.
Aminoglycosides (gentamicin, kanamycin, neomycin, streptomycin), bacitracin, clindamycin, colistimethate sodium, colistin, lincomycin, polymyxin B sulfate, tetracyclines: Enhanced neuromuscular blockade, leading to increased skeletal muscle relaxation and prolonged effect of doxacurium. Use together cautiously.
Beta blockers, lithium, local anesthetics, magnesium salts, procainamide, quinidine, quinine: May enhance neuromuscular blockade. Monitor patient for excessive weakness.
Carbamazepine, phenytoin: May prolong the time to maximal block or shorten the duration of block with neuromuscular blockers. Monitor patient.
Inhalation anesthetics: May enhance or prolong action of nondepolarizing neuromuscular blockers. Monitor patient.

EFFECTS ON LAB TEST RESULTS
None reported.

CONTRAINDICATIONS
Contraindicated in patients hypersensitive to drug; also contraindicated in neonates because drug contains benzyl alcohol, which has been linked to neonatal deaths.

NURSING CONSIDERATIONS
● Use cautiously, possibly at reduced dosage, in elderly or debilitated patients; in patients with metastatic cancer, severe electrolyte disturbances, renal or hepatic impairment, or neuromuscular diseases; and in those for whom potentiation or difficulty in reversal of neuromuscular blockade is anticipated. Patients with myasthenia gravis or myasthenic syndrome (Eaton-Lambert syndrome) are particularly sensitive to the effects of nondepolarizing relaxants. Shorter-acting drugs are recommended for use in such patients.
● Because of lack of data supporting drug's safety, drug isn't recommended for patients who need prolonged mechanical ventilation in the intensive care unit. Also not recommended before or after use of nondepolarizing neuromuscular blockers or during cesarean section.
● Dosage is highly individualized. All times of onset and duration are averages; considerable individual variation is normal.
● Drug isn't metabolized; it's excreted in urine and bile. Patients with renal or hepatic insufficiency may need dosage adjustment.
● A nerve stimulator and train-of-four monitoring are recommended to document antagonism of neuromuscular blockade and recovery of muscle strength. Before attempting pharmacologic reversal with neostigmine, some evidence of spontaneous recovery should be present.
● Because drug has minimal vagolytic action, monitor patient for bradycardia, which may occur during anesthesia.
● Monitor respirations until patient recovers fully from neuromuscular blockade, as evidenced by tests of muscle strength (hand grip, head lift, and ability to cough).
● Acid-base and electrolyte balance may influence the actions of nondepolarizing neuromuscular blockers. Alkalosis may counteract paralysis; acidosis may enhance it.
● *Alert:* Careful dosage calculation is essential. Always verify dosage with another health care professional.
● *Alert:* Don't confuse doxacurium with doxapram or doxorubicin.

PATIENT TEACHING
● Explain drug's purpose.
● Assure patient that monitoring will be continuous.
● Explain all procedures and events because patient can still hear.

---

mivacurium chloride
Mivacron

Pregnancy risk category C

AVAILABLE FORMS
Infusion: 0.5 mg/ml in 50 ml of D_5W
Injection: 2 mg/ml in 5-ml and 10-ml vials

INDICATIONS & DOSAGES
➤ **Adjunct to general anesthesia to facilitate endotracheal intubation and relax skeletal muscles during surgery or mechanical ventilation—**
Adults: Dosage is highly individualized. Usually, 0.15 mg/kg by I.V. push over 5 to 15 seconds provides adequate muscle relaxation in 2½ to 3 minutes for endotracheal intubation. Supplemental doses of 0.1 mg/kg I.V. q 15 minutes are usually sufficient to maintain muscle relaxation. Or, maintain neuromuscular blockade with a continuous infusion of 4 mcg/kg/minute begun simultaneously with the initial dose. Or, 9 to 10 mcg/kg/minute started after evidence of spontaneous recovery caused by the initial dose. When used with isoflurane or enflurane anesthesia, dosage is usually reduced up to 40%.
Children ages 2 to 12: 0.2 mg/kg by I.V. push given over 5 to 15 seconds. Neuromuscular blockade is usually evident in less than 2 minutes. Maintenance doses are usually needed more frequently in children.
Or, neuromuscular blockade can be maintained with a continuous I.V. infusion titrated to effect. Most children respond to 5 to 31 mcg/kg/minute (average, 14 mcg/kg/minute).
Adjust-a-dose: In obese patients 30% or more above their ideal weight, dosage should be adjusted to ideal body weight to avoid prolonged neuromuscular blockade.

I.V. ADMINISTRATION
• Use only under direct supervision by medical staff skilled in using neuromuscular blockers and maintaining patent airway. Don't use unless an antagonist and resources for mechanical ventilation, oxygen therapy, and intubation are within reach.
• To avoid patient distress, don't give until patient's consciousness is obtunded by general anesthetic because drug has no effect on consciousness or pain threshold.
• Prepare drug for I.V. use with D_5W, normal saline solution for injection, dextrose 5% in normal saline solution for injection, lactated Ringer's injection, or dextrose 5% in lactated Ringer's injection. Diluted solutions are stable for 24 hours at room temperature.
• For drug available as premixed infusion in D_5W, remove the protective outer wrap, and then check container for minor leaks by squeezing the bag before giving. Don't add other drugs to the container, and don't use the container in series connections.
• When diluted as directed, mivacurium is compatible with alfentanil, fentanyl, sufentanil, droperidol, and midazolam.
• Alkaline solutions, such as barbiturate solutions, are physically incompatible; precipitate may form. Don't give through same I.V. line.

ACTION
Nondepolarizing drug that competes with acetylcholine for receptor sites at the motor end plate, blocking neuromuscular transmission. Because this action may be antagonized by anticholinesterases, mivacurium is considered a competitive antagonist. Drug is a mixture of three stereoisomers, each with neuromuscular blocking activity.

Route	Onset	Peak	Duration
I.V.	1-2 min	2-5 min	20-35 min

ADVERSE REACTIONS
CNS: dizziness.
CV: *flushing,* tachycardia, **bradycardia, arrhythmias,** hypotension, phlebitis.
Musculoskeletal: prolonged muscle weakness, muscle spasms.
Respiratory: *bronchospasm,* wheezing, *respiratory insufficiency or apnea.*
Skin: rash, urticaria, erythema.

INTERACTIONS
Drug-drug. *Aminoglycosides (gentamicin, kanamycin, neomycin, streptomycin), bacitracin, clindamycin, colistimethate sodium, colistin, lincomycin,*

polymyxin B sulfate, tetracyclines: Enhanced neuromuscular blockade, leading to increased skeletal muscle relaxation and prolonged effect of mivacurium. Use together cautiously.

Beta blockers, lithium, local anesthetics, magnesium salts, procainamide, quinidine, quinine: May enhance neuromuscular blockade. Monitor patient for excessive weakness.

Carbamazepine, phenytoin: May prolong time to maximal blockade or shorten duration of blockade with neuromuscular blockers. Monitor patient.

Inhaled anesthetics (enflurane, isoflurane): May enhance or prolong action of nondepolarizing neuromuscular blockers. Monitor patient for excessive weakness.

EFFECTS ON LAB TEST RESULTS
None reported.

CONTRAINDICATIONS
Contraindicated in patients hypersensitive to drug, other bis-benzylisoquinolinium drugs, or benzyl alcohol.

NURSING CONSIDERATIONS
● Use cautiously in patients with significant CV disease and in those who may be adversely affected by histamine release (such as asthmatic patients). To avoid hypotension, use lower initial dose or give drug over longer period (60 seconds).
● Use cautiously, possibly at reduced dosage, in debilitated patients; in those with metastatic cancer, severe electrolyte disturbances, or neuromuscular diseases; and in those for whom potentiation or difficulty in reversing neuromuscular blockade is anticipated. Patients with myasthenia gravis or myasthenic syndrome (Eaton-Lambert syndrome) are particularly sensitive to effects of nondepolarizing relaxants. Test dose of 0.015 to 0.02 mg/kg may be used to assess patient's sensitivity to drug.
● *Alert:* Use cautiously, if at all, in patients who are homozygous for the atypical plasma pseudocholinesterase gene. Drug is metabolized to inactive compound by plasma pseudocholinesterase.
● Give a test dose to assess patient's sensitivity to drug. Patients with severe burns can develop resistance to nondepolarizing

neuromuscular blockers; however, they also may have reduced plasma pseudocholinesterase activity.
● Like other neuromuscular blockers, dosage requirements for children are higher on a milligram per kilogram basis than those for adults. Onset and recovery of neuromuscular blockade occur more rapidly in children.
● A nerve stimulator and train-of-four monitoring are recommended to document antagonism of neuromuscular blockade and recovery of muscle strength. Before attempting pharmacologic reversal with neostigmine or edrophonium, some signs of spontaneous recovery should be evident.
● Monitor respirations closely until patient recovers fully from neuromuscular blockade, as evidenced by tests of muscle strength (hand grip, head lift, and ability to cough).
● Experimental evidence suggests that acid-base and electrolyte balances may influence the actions of nondepolarizing neuromuscular blockers. Alkalosis may counteract the paralysis; acidosis may enhance it.
● Duration of drug effect is increased about 150% in patients with end-stage renal disease and 300% in patients with hepatic dysfunction.
● *Alert:* Careful dosage calculation is essential. Always verify dosage with another health care professional.
● *Alert:* Don't confuse Mivacron with Mevacor.

PATIENT TEACHING
● Explain purpose of drug.
● Assure patient that monitoring will be continuous.
● Explain all procedures and events because patient can still hear.

pancuronium bromide

Pregnancy risk category C

AVAILABLE FORMS
Injection: 1 mg/ml, 2 mg/ml

INDICATIONS & DOSAGES
➤ **Adjunct to anesthesia to relax skeletal muscle, facilitate intubation, assist with mechanical ventilation—**
Adults and children age 1 month and older: Initially, 0.04 to 0.1 mg/kg I.V.; then 0.01 mg/kg q 30 to 60 minutes.
Neonates: Individualized.

I.V. ADMINISTRATION
• Give sedatives or general anesthetics before neuromuscular blockers. Neuromuscular blockers don't obtund consciousness or alter the pain threshold.
• Keep emergency respiratory support equipment (endotracheal equipment, ventilator, oxygen, atropine, edrophonium, epinephrine, and neostigmine) immediately available.
• Don't mix with alkaline solutions, such as barbiturate solutions, because precipitate will form; use only fresh solutions.
• Store in refrigerator. Don't store in plastic containers or syringes, although plastic syringes may be used for administration.

ACTION
Nondepolarizing drug that prevents acetylcholine from binding to receptors on the motor end plate, thus blocking neuromuscular transmission.

Route	Onset	Peak	Duration
I.V.	30-45 sec	3-4.5 min	35-65 min

ADVERSE REACTIONS
CV: tachycardia, increased blood pressure.
EENT: excessive salivation.
Musculoskeletal: residual muscle weakness.
Respiratory: *prolonged respiratory insufficiency or apnea.*
Skin: transient rashes.
Other: *allergic or idiosyncratic hypersensitivity reactions.*

INTERACTIONS
Drug-drug. *Aminoglycoside antibiotics (including amikacin, gentamicin, kanamycin, neomycin, streptomycin), beta blockers, clindamycin, general anesthetics (such as enflurane, halothane, isoflurane), lincomycin, magnesium sulfate, polymyxin antibiotics (colistin, polymyxin B sulfate),*
quinidine, quinine: Enhanced neuromuscular blockade, leading to increased skeletal muscle relaxation and prolonged effect of pancuronium. Use together cautiously during and after surgery.
Azathioprine: May reverse neuromuscular blockade induced by pancuronium. Monitor patient.
Lithium, opioid analgesics: Enhanced neuromuscular blockade, leading to increased skeletal muscle relaxation and possible respiratory paralysis. Use with extreme caution, and reduce dose of pancuronium.
Succinylcholine: Increased intensity and duration of neuromuscular blockade. Allow effects of succinylcholine to subside before giving pancuronium.

EFFECTS ON LAB TEST RESULTS
None reported.

CONTRAINDICATIONS
Contraindicated in patients hypersensitive to bromides, those with tachycardia, and those for whom even a minor increase in heart rate is undesirable.

NURSING CONSIDERATIONS
• Use cautiously in elderly or debilitated patients; in patients with renal, hepatic, or pulmonary impairment; and in those with respiratory depression, myasthenia gravis, myasthenic syndrome related to lung cancer, dehydration, thyroid disorders, CV disease, collagen diseases, porphyria, electrolyte disturbances, hyperthermia, and toxemic states. Also, use large doses cautiously in patients undergoing cesarean section.
• Dosage depends on anesthetic used, individual needs, and response. Dosages are representative.
• Drug should be used only by staff skilled in airway management.
• Allow succinylcholine effects to subside before giving pancuronium.
• Monitor baseline electrolyte determinations (electrolyte imbalance can potentiate neuromuscular effects) and vital signs, especially respirations and heart rate.
• Measure fluid intake and output; renal dysfunction may prolong duration of action because 25% of drug is excreted unchanged in the urine.

• A nerve stimulator and train-of-four monitoring are recommended to confirm antagonism of neuromuscular blockade and recovery of muscle strength. Before attempting pharmacologic reversal with neostigmine, some evidence of spontaneous recovery should be present.

• Monitor respirations closely until patient recovers fully from neuromuscular blockade, as evidenced by tests of muscle strength (hand grip, head lift, and ability to cough).

• Once spontaneous recovery starts, pancuronium-induced neuromuscular blockade may be reversed with an anticholinesterase (such as neostigmine or edrophonium), which is usually given with an anticholinergic (such as atropine).

• Drug doesn't cause histamine release or hypotension, but it may raise heart rate and blood pressure.

• Give analgesics for pain.

• *Alert:* Careful dosage calculation is essential. Always verify dosage with another health care professional.

• *Alert:* Don't confuse pancuronium with pipecuronium or Pavulon with Peptavlon.

PATIENT TEACHING
• Explain all events and procedures to patient because he can still hear.

---

rocuronium bromide
Zemuron

Pregnancy risk category C

AVAILABLE FORMS
Injection: 10 mg/ml

INDICATIONS & DOSAGES
➤ **Adjunct to general anesthesia to facilitate endotracheal intubation and relax skeletal muscles during surgery or mechanical ventilation—**
Adults: Initially, 0.6 mg/kg I.V. bolus. In most patients, tracheal intubation may be performed within 2 minutes; muscle paralysis should last about 31 minutes. A maintenance dose of 0.1 mg/kg should provide an additional 12 minutes of muscle relaxation; 0.15 mg/kg will add 17 minutes; or 0.2 mg/kg will add 24 minutes to the duration of effect.

I.V. ADMINISTRATION
• Give sedatives or general anesthetics before neuromuscular blockers. Neuromuscular blockers don't obtund consciousness or alter the pain threshold.

• Give by rapid I.V. injection. Or, give by continuous I.V. infusion. Infusion rates are highly individualized. Compatible solutions include D_5W, normal saline solution for injection, dextrose 5% in normal saline solution for injection, sterile water for injection, and lactated Ringer's injection.

• Keep airway clear. Keep emergency respiratory support (endotracheal equipment, ventilator, oxygen, atropine, edrophonium, epinephrine, and neostigmine) available.

• Store vials at room temperature for up to 30 days. Use diluted infusion solutions within 24 hours.

ACTION
Nondepolarizing drug that prevents acetylcholine from binding to receptors on the motor end plate, thus blocking neuromuscular transmission.

Route	Onset	Peak	Duration
I.V.	1 min	2 min	22-67 min

ADVERSE REACTIONS
CV: tachycardia, abnormal ECG, transient hypotension, hypertension, edema.
GI: nausea, vomiting.
Respiratory: asthma, hiccups, *respiratory insufficiency, apnea.*
Skin: rash, pruritus.

INTERACTIONS
Drug-drug. *Aminoglycoside antibiotics (amikacin, gentamicin, kanamycin, neomycin, streptomycin), anticonvulsants, beta blockers, clindamycin, general anesthetics (enflurane, halothane, isoflurane), magnesium salts, opiate analgesics, polymyxin antibiotics (colistin, polymyxin B sulfate), quinidine, quinine, succinylcholine, tetracyclines:* Enhanced neuromuscular blockade, leading to increased skeletal muscle relaxation and potentiated effect. Use together cautiously during and after surgery.

EFFECTS ON LAB TEST RESULTS
None reported.

CONTRAINDICATIONS
Contraindicated in patients hypersensitive to drug or to bromides.

NURSING CONSIDERATIONS
• Use cautiously in patients with hepatic disease, severe obesity, bronchogenic carcinoma, electrolyte disturbances, neuromuscular disease, and an altered circulation time caused by CV disease, old age, or edema.

• Drug isn't recommended for use during rapid sequence induction for cesarean section.

• Dosage depends on anesthetic used, individual needs, and response. Recommended dosages are representative and must be adjusted.

• Drug should be used only by staff skilled in airway management.

• Rocuronium provides conditions for intubation within 3 minutes.

• A nerve stimulator and train-of-four monitoring are recommended to confirm antagonism of neuromuscular blockade and recovery of muscle strength. Before attempting pharmacologic reversal with neostigmine, some evidence of spontaneous recovery should be present.

• Prior use of succinylcholine may enhance neuromuscular blocking effect and duration of action.

• Monitor patients with liver disease because they may need higher doses to achieve adequate muscle relaxation. However, such patients have prolonged drug effects.

• Monitor respirations closely until patient recovers fully from neuromuscular blockade, as evidenced by tests of muscle strength (hand grip, head lift, and ability to cough).

• Rocuronium is well tolerated in patients with renal failure.

• Give analgesics for pain.

• **Alert:** Careful drug calculation is essential. Always verify dosage with another health care professional.

PATIENT TEACHING
• Explain all events and procedures to patient because he can still hear.

succinylcholine chloride (suxamethonium chloride)
Anectine, Anectine Flo-Pack, Quelicin, Scoline‡, Sucostrin

Pregnancy risk category C

AVAILABLE FORMS
Injection: 20 mg/ml, 50 mg/ml, 100 mg/ml, 100-mg vial, 500-mg vial, 1-g vial

INDICATIONS & DOSAGES
➤ **Adjunct to anesthesia to relax skeletal muscles for surgery and orthopedic manipulations; to facilitate intubation and assist with mechanical ventilation; to lessen muscle contractions in pharmacologically or electrically induced seizures—**
Adults: 0.6 mg/kg I.V. given over 10 to 30 seconds. For longer response, give continuous infusion at 0.5 to 10 mg/minute, or give 0.04 to 0.07 mg/kg intermittently, p.r.n., to maintain relaxation.
Children: 1 to 2 mg/kg I.V. or 3 to 4 mg/kg I.M. Maximum I.M. dose is 150 mg.

I.V. ADMINISTRATION
• Give sedatives or general anesthetics before neuromuscular blockers, which don't obtund consciousness or alter the pain threshold.

• Give test dose (5 to 10 mg I.V.) after patient has been anesthetized. Normal response (no respiratory depression or transient depression for up to 5 minutes) indicates patient can metabolize drug and it may be given. Don't give if patient develops respiratory paralysis sufficient to permit endotracheal intubation. (Recovery should occur within 30 to 60 minutes.)

ACTION
Binds with a high affinity to cholinergic receptors, prolonging depolarization of the motor end plate and ultimately producing muscle paralysis.

Route	Onset	Peak	Duration
I.M.	2-3 min	Unknown	10-30 min
I.V.	0.5-1 min	1-2 min	4-10 min

ADVERSE REACTIONS
CV: *bradycardia,* tachycardia, hypertension, hypotension, *arrhythmias,* flushing, *cardiac arrest.*
EENT: increased intraocular pressure.
GI: excessive salivation.
Musculoskeletal: muscle fasciculation, *postoperative muscle pain.*
Respiratory: *prolonged respiratory depression, apnea, bronchoconstriction.*
Skin: rash.
Other: *malignant hyperthermia, allergic or idiosyncratic hypersensitivity reactions, anaphylaxis.*

INTERACTIONS
Drug-drug. *Aminoglycoside antibiotics (including amikacin, gentamicin, kanamycin, neomycin, streptomycin), anticholinesterases (such as echothiophate, edrophonium, neostigmine, physostigmine, pyridostigmine), general anesthetics (such as enflurane, halothane, isoflurane), polymyxin antibiotics (colistin, polymyxin B sulfate):* Enhanced neuromuscular blockade, leading to increased skeletal muscle relaxation and potentiated effect. Use together cautiously during and after surgery.
Cardiac glycosides: May cause arrhythmias. Use together cautiously.
Cyclophosphamide, lithium, MAO inhibitors: Prolonged apnea. Use together cautiously.
Methotrimeprazine, opioid analgesics: Enhanced neuromuscular blockade, leading to increased skeletal muscle relaxation and possible respiratory paralysis. Use together with extreme caution.
Parenteral magnesium sulfate: Enhanced neuromuscular blockade, increased skeletal muscle relaxation, and possible respiratory paralysis. Use together cautiously, preferably at reduced doses.
Drug-herb. *Melatonin:* Potentiated blocking properties of succinylcholine. Ask patient about use of herbal remedies, and recommend caution.

EFFECTS ON LAB TEST RESULTS
• May increase myoglobin and potassium levels.

CONTRAINDICATIONS
Contraindicated in patients hypersensitive to drug and in those with abnormally low plasma pseudocholinesterase, angle-closure glaucoma, personal or family history of malignant hyperthermia, myopathies with elevated CK, or penetrating eye injuries.

NURSING CONSIDERATIONS
• Use cautiously in elderly or debilitated patients; in patients receiving quinidine or cardiac glycoside therapy; in patients with hepatic, renal, or pulmonary impairment; in those with respiratory depression, severe burns or trauma, electrolyte imbalances, hyperkalemia, paraplegia, spinal CNS injury, CVA, degenerative or dystrophic neuromuscular disease, myasthenia gravis, myasthenic syndrome related to lung cancer, dehydration, thyroid disorders, collagen diseases, porphyria, fractures, muscle spasms, eye surgery, and pheochromocytoma. Also, use large doses cautiously in patients undergoing cesarean section.
• Dosage depends on anesthetic used, individual needs, and response. Recommended dosages are representative.
• Children may be less sensitive to succinylcholine than adults.
• Succinylcholine is the drug of choice for short procedures (less than 3 minutes) and for orthopedic manipulations; use cautiously with fractures or dislocations.
• Succinylcholine should be used only by staff skilled in airway management.
• When giving drug by I.M. route, inject deeply, preferably high into deltoid muscle.
• Store injectable form in refrigerator. Store powder form at room temperature in tightly closed container. Use immediately after reconstitution. Don't mix with alkaline solutions (thiopental sodium, sodium bicarbonate, or barbiturates).
• Monitor baseline electrolyte determinations and vital signs. Check respirations every 5 to 10 minutes during infusion.
• Monitor respirations closely until patient recovers fully from neuromuscular blockade, as evidenced by tests of muscle strength (hand grip, head lift, and ability to cough).
• *Alert:* Don't use reversing drugs. Unlike nondepolarizing drugs, neostigmine or edrophonium may worsen neuromuscular blockade.

● Repeated or continuous infusions of succinylcholine aren't advisable; they may cause reduced response or prolonged muscle relaxation and apnea.

● Give analgesics for pain.

● Keep airway clear. Have emergency respiratory support equipment (endotracheal equipment, ventilator, oxygen, atropine, and epinephrine) immediately available.

● *Alert:* Careful dosage calculation is essential. Always verify dosage with another health care professional.

PATIENT TEACHING

● Explain all events and procedures to patient because he can still hear.

● Reassure patient that postoperative stiffness is normal and will soon subside.

---

tubocurarine chloride

Pregnancy risk category C

AVAILABLE FORMS
Injection: 3 mg (20 units)/ml

INDICATIONS & DOSAGES

➤ **Adjunct to anesthesia to relax skeletal muscles; to facilitate intubation and orthopedic manipulations; adjunct during pharmacologically or electrically induced convulsive therapy—**
Adults: 1.1 units/kg or 0.165 mg/kg I.V. slowly over 60 to 90 seconds. Average dose is initially 40 to 60 units I.V. May give 20 to 30 units in 3 to 5 minutes. For longer procedures, give 20 units, p.r.n.

➤ **To assist with mechanical ventilation—**
Adults and children: Initially, 0.0165 mg/kg I.V. (average, 1 mg or 7 units); then adjust subsequent doses to patient response.

➤ **To lessen muscle contractions in pharmacologically or electrically induced seizures—**
Adults and children: 1.1 units/kg or 0.165 mg/kg over 60 to 90 seconds. As a precaution, initial dose should be 20 units (3 mg) less than calculated dose.

➤ **Diagnosis of myasthenia gravis—**
Adults: 4 to 33 mcg/kg as a single I.V. dose.

I.V. ADMINISTRATION

● Give sedatives or general anesthetics before neuromuscular blockers, which don't obtund consciousness or alter the pain threshold.

● Keep airway clear. Have emergency respiratory support (endotracheal equipment, ventilator, oxygen, atropine, edrophonium, epinephrine, and neostigmine) available.

● Allow succinylcholine effects to subside before giving tubocurarine.

● Give I.V. over 60 to 90 seconds.

● Don't mix with barbiturates or other alkaline solutions because a precipitate will form. Use only fresh solutions, and discard if discolored.

ACTION
Nondepolarizing neuromuscular blocker that prevents acetylcholine from binding to receptors on the motor end plate, thus blocking neuromuscular transmission.

Route	Onset	Peak	Duration
I.V.	1 min	2-5 min	25-90 min

ADVERSE REACTIONS
CV: hypotension, *arrhythmias, cardiac arrest, bradycardia.*
GI: increased salivation.
Musculoskeletal: profound and prolonged muscle relaxation, residual muscle weakness.
Respiratory: *respiratory depression or apnea, bronchospasm.*
Other: hypersensitivity reactions.

INTERACTIONS
Drug-drug. *Aminoglycoside antibiotics (amikacin, gentamicin, kanamycin, neomycin, streptomycin), clindamycin, general anesthetics (enflurane, halothane, isoflurane), lincomycin, magnesium salts, polymyxin antibiotics (colistin, polymyxin B sulfate):* Enhanced neuromuscular blockade, leading to increased skeletal muscle relaxation and potentiated effect. Use together cautiously during and after surgery.
Amphotericin B, ethacrynic acid, furosemide, methotrimeprazine, opioid analgesics, propranolol, thiazide diuretics, verapamil: Enhanced neuromuscular blockade, leading to increased skeletal muscle relaxation and possible respiratory

paralysis. Use together with extreme caution during and after surgery.

Quinidine, quinine: Prolonged neuromuscular blockade. Use together cautiously. Monitor patient closely.

EFFECTS ON LAB TEST RESULTS

None reported.

CONTRAINDICATIONS

Contraindicated in patients hypersensitive to drug and in those for whom histamine release is a hazard (such as patients with asthma).

NURSING CONSIDERATIONS

• Use cautiously in elderly or debilitated patients and in those with hepatic or pulmonary impairment, hypothermia, respiratory depression, myasthenia gravis, myasthenic syndrome related to lung cancer, sulfite sensitivity, dehydration, thyroid disorders, collagen diseases, porphyria, electrolyte disturbances, fractures, and muscle spasms. Also, use large doses cautiously in patients undergoing cesarean section.

• Dosage depends on anesthetic used, individual needs, and response. Recommended dosages are representative and must be adjusted.

• Only staff skilled in airway management should give tubocurarine.

• Assess baseline electrolyte determinations because electrolyte imbalance can potentiate neuromuscular blocking effects.

• Check vital signs every 15 minutes. Notify prescriber at once of changes.

• Measure fluid intake and output; renal dysfunction prolongs duration of action because much of drug is excreted unchanged in urine.

• A nerve stimulator and train-of-four monitoring are recommended to confirm antagonism of neuromuscular blockade and recovery of muscle strength. Before attempting pharmacologic reversal with neostigmine, some evidence of spontaneous recovery should be present.

• Large doses produce a factor that interferes with detection of urinary catecholamines by fluorometric measures in patients with tetanus.

• Monitor respirations closely until patient recovers fully from neuromuscular blockade, as evidenced by tests of muscle strength (hand grip, head lift, and ability to cough).

• Give analgesics for pain.

• Premedication with an antihistamine will reduce the risk of histamine-related hypotension.

• *Alert:* Careful dosage calculation is essential. Always verify dosage with another health care professional.

PATIENT TEACHING

• Explain all events and procedures to patient because he can still hear.

---

vecuronium bromide
Norcuron

Pregnancy risk category C

AVAILABLE FORMS

Injection: 10-mg, 20-mg vials

INDICATIONS & DOSAGES

➤ **Adjunct to general anesthesia to facilitate endotracheal intubation and relax skeletal muscles during surgery or mechanical ventilation—**

Adults and children older than age 9: Initially, 0.08 to 0.1 mg/kg I.V. bolus. Maintenance doses of 0.01 to 0.015 mg/kg within 25 to 40 minutes of initial dose should be given during prolonged surgical procedures. Maintenance doses may be given q 12 to 15 minutes in patients receiving balanced anesthesia.

Children ages 1 to 9: May need a slightly higher initial dose and may need supplementation slightly more often than adults. Or, drug may be given by continuous I.V. infusion of 1 mcg/kg/minute initially, then 0.8 to 1.2 mcg/kg/minute.

Children ages 7 weeks to 1 year: Doses comparable to those used in adults are appropriate, but less frequent use of maintenance doses may be needed.

I.V. ADMINISTRATION

• Give sedatives or general anesthetics before neuromuscular blockers, which don't obtund consciousness or alter the pain threshold.

• Keep airway clear. Have emergency respiratory support (endotracheal equipment,

---

ventilator, oxygen, atropine, edrophonium, epinephrine, and neostigmine) available.
• Allow succinylcholine effects to subside before giving tubocurarine.
• Give I.V. over 60 to 90 seconds.
• Don't mix with barbiturates or other alkaline solutions because a precipitate will form. Use only fresh solutions, and discard if discolored.

ACTION
Nondepolarizing drug that prevents acetylcholine from binding to receptors on the motor end plate, thus blocking neuromuscular transmission.

Route	Onset	Peak	Duration
I.V.	1 min	3-5 min	15-25 min

ADVERSE REACTIONS
Musculoskeletal: skeletal muscle weakness.
Respiratory: *prolonged respiratory insufficiency or apnea.*

INTERACTIONS
Drug-drug. *Aminoglycoside antibiotics (amikacin, gentamicin, kanamycin, neomycin, streptomycin), bacitracin, beta blocker, clindamycin, general anesthetics (enflurane, halothane, isoflurane), magnesium salts, other skeletal muscle relaxants, polymyxin antibiotics (colistin, polymyxin B sulfate), quinidine, quinine, succinylcholine, tetracyclines:* Enhanced neuromuscular blockade, leading to increased skeletal muscle relaxation and potentiated effect. Use together cautiously during and after surgery.
Opioid analgesics: Enhanced neuromuscular blockade, leading to increased skeletal muscle relaxation and possible respiratory paralysis. Use together with extreme caution, and reduce vecuronium dose.

EFFECTS ON LAB TEST RESULTS
None reported.

CONTRAINDICATIONS
Contraindicated in patients hypersensitive to drug or to bromides.

NURSING CONSIDERATIONS
• Use cautiously in elderly patients; in patients with altered circulation caused by CV disease or edema; and in those with hepatic disease, severe obesity, bronchogenic carcinoma, electrolyte disturbances, and neuromuscular disease.
• Dosage depends on anesthetic used, individual needs, and response. Recommended dosages are representative and must be adjusted.
• Drug should be used only by staff skilled in airway management.
• A nerve stimulator and train-of-four monitoring are recommended to confirm antagonism of neuromuscular blockade and recovery of muscle strength. Before attempting pharmacologic reversal with neostigmine, some evidence of spontaneous recovery should be present.
• Monitor respirations closely until patient recovers fully from neuromuscular blockade, as evidenced by tests of muscle strength (hand grip, head lift, and ability to cough).
• Prior use of succinylcholine may enhance the neuromuscular blocking effect and duration of action.
• Vecuronium is well tolerated in patients with renal failure.
• Give analgesics for pain.
• *Alert:* Careful dosage calculation is essential. Always verify dosage with another health care professional.

PATIENT TEACHING
• Explain all events and procedures to patient because he can still hear.

41

Antihistamines

brompheniramine maleate
cetirizine hydrochloride
chlorpheniramine maleate
clemastine fumarate
cyproheptadine hydrochloride
diphenhydramine hydrochloride
fexofenadine hydrochloride
loratadine
promethazine hydrochloride
promethazine theoclate

COMBINATION PRODUCTS

ALLEGRA-D: fexofenadine hydrochloride 60 mg and pseudoephedrine sulfate 120 mg.

ALLEREST MAXIMUM STRENGTH TABLETS ◊: pseudoephedrine hydrochloride 30 mg and chlorpheniramine maleate 2 mg.

BROMFED CAPSULES: brompheniramine maleate 12 mg and pseudoephedrine 120 mg.

BROMFED DM COUGH SYRUP: brompheniramine maleate 2 mg, pseudoephedrine 30 mg and dextromethorphan 10 mg per 5 ml.

BROMFED PD CAPSULES: brompheniramine maleate 6 mg and pseudoephedrine 60 mg.

CHLOR-TRIMETON ALLERGY 4-HOUR DECONGESTANT ◊: chlorpheniramine maleate 4 mg and pseudoephedrine sulfate 60 mg.

CHLOR-TRIMETON 12 HOUR RELIEF TABLETS ◊: chlorpheniramine maleate 8 mg and pseudoephedrine sulfate 120 mg.

CLARITIN-D: loratadine 5 mg and pseudoephedrine sulfate 120 mg.

CONTAC SEVERE COLD & FLU CAPLETS ◊: acetaminophen 500 mg, dextromethorphan hydrobromide 15 mg, pseudoephedrine hydrochloride 30 mg, and chlorpheniramine maleate 2 mg.

CORICIDIN D COLD, FLU, & SINUS ◊: chlorpheniramine maleate 2 mg, acetaminophen 325 mg, and pseudoephedrine sulfate 30 mg.

CORICIDIN D TABLETS ◊: chlorpheniramine maleate 2 mg and acetaminophen 325 mg.

DECONAMINE: pseudoephedrine hydrochloride 60 mg and chlorpheniramine maleate 4 mg.

DIMETAPP COLD & ALLERGY ELIXIR ◊: brompheniramine maleate 1 mg and pseudoephedrine 15 mg per 5 ml.

DIMETAPP DM ELIXIR ◊: brompheniramine maleate 1 mg, dextromethorphan 5 mg, and pseudoephedrine 15 mg per 5 ml.

FEDAHIST: pseudoephedrine hydrochloride 60 mg and chlorpheniramine maleate 4 mg.

NOVAFED A: pseudoephedrine hydrochloride 120 mg and chlorpheniramine maleate 8 mg.

NOVAHISTINE ELIXIR ◊*: phenylephrine 5 mg, chlorpheniramine maleate 2 mg, and alcohol 5% per 5 ml.

P-V-TUSSIN SYRUP*: chlorpheniramine maleate 2 mg/5 ml, phenindamine tartrate 5 mg/5 ml, phenylephrine hydrochloride 5 mg/5 ml, and pyrilamine maleate 6 mg/5 ml.

SUDAFED PLUS ◊: pseudoephedrine hydrochloride 60 mg and chlorpheniramine maleate 4 mg.

TRIAMINIC COLD & ALLERGY ◊: pseudoephedrine hydrochloride 15 mg and chlorpheniramine maleate 1 mg.

TRIAMINIC COLD & COUGH ◊: pseudoephedrine hydrochloride 15 mg, dextromethorphan hydrobromide 5 mg, and chlorpheniramine maleate 1 mg.

TRIAMINIC COLD & NIGHTTIME COUGH ◊: pseudoephedrine hydrochloride 15 mg, dextromethorphan hydrobromide 7.5 mg, and chlorpheniramine maleate 1 mg.

TRINALIN REPETABS: azatadine maleate 1 mg and pseudoephedrine sulfate 120 mg.

ZYRTEC-D 12 HOUR EXTENDED-RELEASE TABLETS: cetirizine 5 mg and pseudoephedrine 120 mg.

---

*Liquid contains alcohol.   **May contain tartrazine.   †Canada   ‡Australia   §U.K.   ◊OTC

brompheniramine maleate
Bromphen*◊, Chlorphed◊,
Codimal-L.A., Dimotane§,
Nasahist B, ND-Stat

Pregnancy risk category C

AVAILABLE FORMS
Elixir: 2 mg/5 ml*◊
Injection: 10 mg/ml
Tablets: 4 mg◊, 8 mg, 12 mg
Tablets (extended-release): 8 mg◊, 12 mg◊

INDICATIONS & DOSAGES
➤ Rhinitis, allergy symptoms—
Adults and children older than age 12: 4 to 8 mg P.O. t.i.d. or q.i.d. Or, 8 to 12 mg extended-release P.O. b.i.d. or t.i.d. Maximum oral dosage is 24 mg daily. Or, 5 to 20 mg q 6 to 12 hours I.M., I.V., or S.C. Maximum parenteral dosage is 40 mg daily.
Children ages 6 to 12: 2 to 4 mg P.O. t.i.d. or q.i.d. Or, 8 to 12 mg extended-release P.O. q 12 hours. Or, 0.5 mg/kg I.M., I.V., or S.C. daily in divided doses t.i.d. or q.i.d. Maximum oral dose is 12 mg daily.
Children younger than age 6: 0.5 mg/kg P.O., I.M., I.V., or S.C. daily in divided doses t.i.d. or q.i.d.

I.V. ADMINISTRATION
● Injectable form containing 10 mg/ml can be given undiluted or diluted with D_5W or normal saline solution very slowly I.V., preferably with the patient in supine position.

ACTION
Competes with histamine for H_1-receptor sites on effector cells. Prevents, but doesn't reverse, histamine-mediated responses.

Route	Onset	Peak	Duration
I.M., I.V., S.C.	Unknown	Unknown	Unknown
P.O.	15-60 min	2-5 hr	3-24 hr

ADVERSE REACTIONS
CNS: dizziness, tremors, irritability, insomnia, syncope, *drowsiness, stimulation.*
CV: hypotension, palpitations.
GI: anorexia, nausea, vomiting, *dry mouth and throat.*
GU: urine retention.
Hematologic: *thrombocytopenia, agranulocytosis.*
Skin: urticaria, rash, diaphoresis after parenteral use.
Other: local stinging.

INTERACTIONS
Drug-drug. *CNS depressants:* Increased sedation. Use together cautiously.
MAO inhibitors: Increased anticholinergic effects. Avoid using together.
Drug-lifestyle. *Alcohol use:* Increased CNS depression. Discourage use together.

EFFECTS ON LAB TEST RESULTS
● May decrease platelet and granulocyte counts.

CONTRAINDICATIONS
Contraindicated in patients hypersensitive to drug's ingredients and in those with acute asthma, severe hypertension, coronary artery disease, angle-closure glaucoma, urine retention, symptomatic prostatic hyperplasia, pyloroduodenal obstruction, or peptic ulcer; also contraindicated within 14 days of MAO inhibitor therapy.

NURSING CONSIDERATIONS
● Use cautiously in elderly patients and those with increased intraocular pressure, diabetes, ischemic heart disease, hyperthyroidism, hypertension, bronchial asthma, and prostatic hyperplasia.
● Children younger than age 12 should use drug only as directed by prescriber.
● Discontinue drug 4 days before performing diagnostic skin tests. May reduce or mask positive test response.
● Monitor blood count during long-term therapy; watch for signs of blood dyscrasias.

PATIENT TEACHING
● Instruct patient to reduce GI distress by taking drug with food or milk.
● Warn patient to avoid alcohol and activities that require alertness until CNS effects of drug are known.
● Advise patient to notify prescriber about unusual bleeding or bruising.

Reactions may be *common*, uncommon, *life-threatening*, or **COMMON AND LIFE-THREATENING.**

• Tell patient that coffee or tea may reduce drowsiness, although drug causes less drowsiness than some other antihistamines. Urge caution if palpitations develop.
• Inform patient that sugarless gum, hard candy, or ice chips may relieve dry mouth.
• Tell patient to notify prescriber if tolerance develops because a different antihistamine may need to be prescribed.

---

cetirizine hydrochloride
Zyrtec

Pregnancy risk category B

AVAILABLE FORMS
Oral solution: 5 mg/5 ml
Tablets: 5 mg, 10 mg

INDICATIONS & DOSAGES
➤ **Seasonal allergic rhinitis, perennial allergic rhinitis, chronic urticaria—**
Adults and children age 12 and older: 5 or 10 mg P.O. daily depending on symptom severity.
Children ages 6 to 11: 5 or 10 mg or 1 or 2 tsp P.O. once daily depending on symptom severity.
Children ages 2 to 5: 2.5 to 5 mg P.O. once daily depending on symptom severity.
Adjust-a-dose: Give 5 mg P.O. daily to renally impaired patients with creatinine clearance of 11 to 31 ml/minute, those on dialysis with creatinine clearance less than 7 ml/minute, and those with hepatic impairment.

ACTION
A long-acting nonsedating antihistamine that selectively inhibits peripheral H_1 receptors.

Route	Onset	Peak	Duration
P.O.	20-60 min	0.5-1.5 hr	24 hr

ADVERSE REACTIONS
CNS: *somnolence,* fatigue, dizziness, headache.
EENT: pharyngitis.
GI: dry mouth, nausea, vomiting, abdominal distress.

INTERACTIONS
Drug-drug. *CNS depressants:* Possible additive effect. Avoid using together.
Theophylline: May decrease cetirizine clearance. Monitor patient closely.
Drug-lifestyle. *Alcohol use:* Possible additive effect. Discourage using together.

EFFECTS ON LAB TEST RESULTS
None reported.

CONTRAINDICATIONS
Contraindicated in patients hypersensitive to drug or to hydroxyzine.

NURSING CONSIDERATIONS
• Use cautiously in patients with renal or liver impairment.
• Drug isn't recommended for breast-feeding women.
• Discontinue drug 4 days before patient undergoes diagnostic skin tests. Drug can prevent, reduce, or mask positive skin test response.
• *Alert:* Don't confuse Zyrtec with Zyprexa or Zantac.

PATIENT TEACHING
• Warn patient not to perform hazardous activities until CNS effects of drug are known. Somnolence is a common adverse reaction.
• Advise patient not to use alcohol or other CNS depressants while taking drug.
• Tell patient that coffee or tea may reduce drowsiness.
• Inform patient that sugarless gum, hard candy, or ice chips may relieve dry mouth.

---

chlorpheniramine maleate
Aller-Chlor* ◇, Chlo-Amine ◇, Chlorate ◇, Chlor-Trimeton* ◇, Chlor-Trimeton 12 Hour Relief ◇, Chlor-Tripolon† ◇, Gen-Allerate ◇, Novo-Pheniram† ◇, Phenetron*, Piriton§, Telachlor, Teldrin ◇

Pregnancy risk category B

AVAILABLE FORMS
Capsules (timed-release): 6 mg ◇, 8 mg ◇, 12 mg ◇
Injection: 10 mg/ml, 100 mg/ml

Syrup: 2 mg/5 ml* ◇
Tablets: 4 mg ◇, 8 mg ◇, 12 mg ◇
Tablets (chewable): 2 mg ◇
Tablets (timed-release): 8 mg ◇, 12 mg ◇

INDICATIONS & DOSAGES
➤ **Rhinitis, allergy symptoms—**
Adults and children older than age 12:
4 mg P.O. q 4 to 6 hours, not to exceed
24 mg daily. Or, 8 to 12 mg timed-release
P.O. q 8 to 12 hours, not to exceed 24 mg
daily. Or, 5 to 20 mg I.M., I.V., or S.C. as
a single dose. Maximum recommended
parenteral dosage is 40 mg per 24 hours.
Children ages 6 to 12: 2 mg P.O. q 4 to 6
hours, not to exceed 12 mg daily. Or, may
give 8 mg timed-release P.O. h.s.
Children ages 2 to 5: 1 mg P.O. q 4 to 6
hours, not to exceed 4 mg daily.
Children younger than age 2: 0.35 mg/kg
daily in divided doses q 4 to 6 hours.

I.V. ADMINISTRATION
• Drug is available in 10-mg/ml ampules
for I.V. use. It's compatible with most I.V.
solutions. Check with pharmacist before
mixing with I.V. solutions to verify specific compatibilities. Give injection over 1
minute.
• *Alert:* Don't give the 100 mg/ml strength
I.V.

ACTION
Competes with histamine for H_1-receptor
sites on effector cells. It prevents, but
doesn't reverse, histamine-mediated responses.

Route	Onset	Peak	Duration
I.M., S.C.	15-60 min	Unknown	24 hr
I.V.	Immediate	Immediate	24 hr
P.O.	15-60 min	2-6 hr	24 hr

ADVERSE REACTIONS
CNS: *stimulation,* sedation, *drowsiness,*
excitability in children.
CV: hypotension, palpitations, weak
pulse.
GI: epigastric distress, *dry mouth.*
GU: urine retention.
Respiratory: thick bronchial secretions.
Skin: rash, urticaria, pallor.
Other: local stinging, burning sensation
after parenteral use.

INTERACTIONS
Drug-drug. *CNS depressants:* Increased
sedation. Use together cautiously.
MAO inhibitors: Increased anticholinergic
effects. Avoid using together.
Drug-lifestyle. *Alcohol use:* Increased
CNS depression. Discourage use together.

EFFECTS ON LAB TEST RESULTS
None reported.

CONTRAINDICATIONS
Contraindicated in patients having acute
asthmatic attacks and in those with angle-
closure glaucoma, symptomatic prostatic
hyperplasia, pyloroduodenal obstruction,
or bladder neck obstruction; also contraindicated in those taking MAO inhibitors.
Antihistamines aren't recommended for
breast-feeding women because small
amounts of drug appear in breast milk.

NURSING CONSIDERATIONS
• Use cautiously in elderly patients and in
those with increased intraocular pressure,
hyperthyroidism, CV or renal disease, hypertension, bronchial asthma, urine retention, prostatic hyperplasia, and stenosing
peptic ulcerations.
• Injectable form contains benzyl alcohol.
Avoid use in infants.
• Discontinue drug 4 days before performing diagnostic skin tests. Antihistamines
can prevent, reduce, or mask positive skin
test response.
• If symptoms occur during or after parenteral dose, discontinue drug and notify
prescriber.

PATIENT TEACHING
• Warn patient to avoid alcohol and hazardous activities that require alertness until CNS effects of drug are known.
• Tell patient that coffee or tea may reduce
drowsiness.
• Inform patient that sugarless gum, hard
candy, or ice chips may relieve dry
mouth.
• Instruct patient to notify prescriber if
tolerance develops because a different
antihistamine may need to be prescribed.
• Tell parent that drug, including
extended-release products, shouldn't be

Reactions may be *common,* uncommon, *life-threatening,* or COMMON AND LIFE-THREATENING.

used in children younger than age 12 unless directed by prescriber.

---

clemastine fumarate
Antihist-1 ◇ , Tavist ◇ , Tavist-1 ◇

Pregnancy risk category B

AVAILABLE FORMS
Syrup: 0.67 mg/5 ml*
Tablets: 1.34 mg ◇ , 2.68 mg

INDICATIONS & DOSAGES
➤ **Rhinitis, allergy symptoms—**
Adults and children age 12 and older:
1.34 mg P.O. q 12 hours or 2.68 mg P.O. once daily to t.i.d., p.r.n. Don't exceed 8.04 mg daily.
Children ages 6 to 11: 0.67 to 1.34 mg P.O. b.i.d. Don't exceed 4.02 mg daily.

ACTION
Competes with histamine for H_1-receptor sites on effector cells. It prevents, but doesn't reverse, histamine-mediated responses.

Route	Onset	Peak	Duration
P.O.	15-60 min	5-7 hr	12 hr

ADVERSE REACTIONS
CNS: *sedation, drowsiness,* **seizures,** nervousness, tremor, confusion, restlessness, vertigo, headache, *sleepiness, dizziness, incoordination,* fatigue.
CV: hypotension, palpitations, tachycardia.
GI: *epigastric distress,* anorexia, diarrhea, nausea, vomiting, constipation, *dry mouth.*
GU: urine retention, urinary frequency.
Hematologic: hemolytic anemia, **thrombocytopenia, agranulocytosis.**
Respiratory: *thick bronchial secretions.*
Skin: rash, urticaria, photosensitivity, diaphoresis.
Other: *anaphylactic shock.*

INTERACTIONS
Drug-drug. *CNS depressants:* Increased sedation. Use together cautiously.
MAO inhibitors: Increased anticholinergic effects. Avoid using together.
Drug-lifestyle. *Alcohol use:* Increased CNS depression. Discourage use together.

Sun exposure: Photosensitivity reactions may occur. Advise patient to avoid prolonged or unprotected sun exposure.

EFFECTS ON LAB TEST RESULTS
● May decrease hemoglobin and platelet and granulocyte counts.

CONTRAINDICATIONS
Contraindicated in patients hypersensitive to drug or other antihistamines of similar chemical structure and in those with acute asthma, angle-closure glaucoma, stenosing peptic ulcer, symptomatic prostatic hyperplasia, bladder neck obstruction, or pyloroduodenal obstruction. Also contraindicated in neonates, premature infants, and breast-feeding women. Avoid use in those taking MAO inhibitors.

NURSING CONSIDERATIONS
● Use cautiously in elderly patients and in those with increased intraocular pressure, hyperthyroidism, CV disease, hypertension, bronchial asthma, and prostatic hyperplasia.
● Children younger than age 12 should use drug only as directed by prescriber.
● Discontinue drug 4 days before patient undergoes diagnostic skin tests. Antihistamines can prevent, reduce, or mask positive skin test response.
● Monitor blood counts during long-term therapy; observe for signs of blood dyscrasias.

PATIENT TEACHING
● Warn patient to avoid alcohol and hazardous activities that require alertness until CNS effects of drug are known.
● Tell patient that coffee or tea may reduce drowsiness. Urge caution if palpitations develop.
● Inform patient that sugarless gum, hard candy, or ice chips may relieve dry mouth.
● Warn patient of possible photosensitivity reactions. Advise use of a sunblock.
● Tell patient to notify prescriber if tolerance develops because a different antihistamine may need to be prescribed.

---

*Liquid contains alcohol.   **May contain tartrazine.   †Canada   ‡Australia   §U.K.   ◇OTC

cyproheptadine hydrochloride
Periactin

Pregnancy risk category B

AVAILABLE FORMS
Syrup: 2 mg/5 ml
Tablets: 4 mg

INDICATIONS & DOSAGES
➤ **Allergy symptoms, pruritus—**
Adults and children older than age 14: 4 to 20 mg P.O. daily in divided doses. Maximum, 0.5 mg/kg daily.
Children ages 7 to 14: 4 mg P.O. b.i.d. or t.i.d. Maximum, 16 mg daily.
Children ages 2 to 6: 2 mg P.O. b.i.d. or t.i.d. Maximum, 12 mg daily.
Children younger than age 2: 0.25 mg/kg/day in two or three divided doses.

ACTION
Competes with histamine for H_1-receptor sites on effector cells. It prevents, but doesn't reverse, histamine-mediated responses; also has antiserotonergic activity.

Route	Onset	Peak	Duration
P.O.	15-60 min	6-9 hr	Unknown

ADVERSE REACTIONS
CNS: *drowsiness,* dizziness, headache, fatigue, sedation, sleepiness, incoordination, confusion, restlessness, insomnia, nervousness, tremor, *seizures.*
CV: hypotension, palpitations, tachycardia.
GI: nausea, vomiting, epigastric distress, *dry mouth,* diarrhea, constipation.
GU: urine retention, urinary frequency.
Hematologic: hemolytic anemia, *leukopenia, agranulocytosis, thrombocytopenia.*
Metabolic: weight gain.
Skin: rash, urticaria, photosensitivity.
Other: *anaphylactic shock.*

INTERACTIONS
Drug-drug. *CNS depressants:* Increased sedation. Use together cautiously.
MAO inhibitors: Increased anticholinergic effects. Avoid using together.
Drug-lifestyle. *Alcohol use:* Increased CNS depression. Discourage use together.

Sun exposure: Photosensitivity reactions may occur. Advise patient to avoid prolonged or unprotected sun exposure.

EFFECTS ON LAB TEST RESULTS
● May decrease hemoglobin and WBC, platelet, and granulocyte counts.

CONTRAINDICATIONS
Contraindicated in patients hypersensitive to drug or other drugs of similar chemical structure and in those with acute asthma, angle-closure glaucoma, stenosing peptic ulcer, symptomatic prostatic hyperplasia, bladder-neck obstruction, or pyloroduodenal obstruction. Also contraindicated in those taking MAO inhibitors, in neonates or premature infants, in elderly or debilitated patients, and in breast-feeding women.

NURSING CONSIDERATIONS
● Use cautiously in patients with increased intraocular pressure, hyperthyroidism, CV disease, hypertension, or bronchial asthma.
● Children younger than age 14 should use drug only as directed by prescriber.
● Discontinue drug 4 days before patient undergoes diagnostic skin tests. Antihistamines can prevent, reduce, or mask positive skin test response.
● *Alert:* Don't confuse cyproheptadine with cyclobenzaprine.

PATIENT TEACHING
● Tell patient that GI distress can be reduced by taking drug with food or milk.
● Warn patient to avoid alcohol and hazardous activities that require alertness until CNS effects of drug are known.
● Tell patient that coffee or tea may reduce drowsiness. Urge caution if palpitations develop.
● Inform patient that sugarless gum, hard candy, or ice chips may relieve dry mouth.
● Warn patient of possible photosensitivity reactions. Advise use of a sunblock.
● Instruct patient to notify prescriber if tolerance develops because a different antihistamine may need to be prescribed.

diphenhydramine hydrochloride

Allerdryl† ◇, AllerMax Allergy and Cough Formula, AllerMax Caplets ◇, Allermed ◇, Banophen ◇, Banophen Caplets ◇, Benadryl ◇, Benadryl Allergy, Benylin Cough ◇, Bydramine Cough ◇, Compoz ◇, Diphen Cough ◇, Diphenadryl ◇, Diphenhist ◇, Diphenhist Captabs ◇, Dormarex 2 ◇, Genahist ◇, Hydramine ◇, Hydramine Cough ◇, Hyrexin-50, Nervine Nighttime Sleep-Aid ◇, Nordryl Cough ◇, Sleep-eze 3 ◇, Sominex ◇, Tusstat ◇, Twilite Caplets ◇, Uni-Bent Cough ◇

Pregnancy risk category B

AVAILABLE FORMS

Capsules: 25 mg ◇, 50 mg ◇
Elixir: 12.5 mg/5 ml * ◇
Injection: 10 mg/ml, 50 mg/ml
Liquid: 6.25 mg/5 ml
Syrup: 12.5 mg/5 ml* ◇
Tablets: 25 mg ◇, 50 mg ◇
Tablets (chewable): 12.5 mg ◇

INDICATIONS & DOSAGES

➤ **Rhinitis, allergy symptoms, motion sickness, Parkinson's disease—**
Adults and children age 12 and older: 25 to 50 mg P.O. t.i.d. or q.i.d. Maximum P.O. dose is 300 mg daily. Or, 10 to 50 mg deep I.M. or I.V. Maximum by I.M. or I.V. route, 400 mg daily.
Children younger than age 12: 5 mg/kg/ day P.O., deep I.M., or I.V. in divided doses q.i.d. Maximum, 300 mg daily.
➤ **Sedation—**
Adults: 25 to 50 mg P.O. or deep I.M., p.r.n.
➤ **Nighttime sleep aid—**
Adults: 25 to 50 mg P.O. h.s.
➤ **Nonproductive cough—**
Adults and children age 12 and older: 25 mg P.O. q 4 to 6 hours. Don't exceed 150 mg daily.
Children ages 6 to 11: 12.5 mg P.O. q 4 to 6 hours. Don't exceed 75 mg daily.
Children ages 2 to 5: 6.25 mg P.O. q 4 to 6 hours. Don't exceed 25 mg daily.

I.V. ADMINISTRATION

● I.V. use shouldn't exceed 25 mg/min.
● Make sure I.V. site is patent. Drug given perivascularly causes tissue irritation.

ACTION

Competes with histamine for H_1-receptor sites on effector cells. Prevents, but doesn't reverse, histamine-mediated responses, particularly the effects of histamine on the smooth muscle of the bronchial tubes, GI tract, uterus, and blood vessels. Structurally related to local anesthetics, diphenhydramine provides local anesthesia by preventing initiation and transmission of nerve impulses. Also suppresses cough reflex by a direct effect in the medulla.

Route	Onset	Peak	Duration
I.M.	Unknown	1-4 hr	6-8 hr
I.V.	Immediate	1-4 hr	6-8 hr
P.O.	15 min	1-4 hr	6-8 hr

ADVERSE REACTIONS

CNS: *drowsiness,* confusion, insomnia, headache, vertigo, *sedation, sleepiness, dizziness, incoordination,* fatigue, restlessness, tremor, nervousness, **seizures.**
CV: palpitations, hypotension, tachycardia.
EENT: diplopia, blurred vision, nasal congestion, tinnitus.
GI: *nausea,* vomiting, diarrhea, *dry mouth,* constipation, *epigastric distress,* anorexia.
GU: dysuria, urine retention, urinary frequency.
Hematologic: hemolytic anemia, **thrombocytopenia, agranulocytosis.**
Respiratory: *thickening of bronchial secretions.*
Skin: urticaria, photosensitivity, rash.
Other: *anaphylactic shock.*

INTERACTIONS

Drug-drug. *CNS depressants:* Increased sedation. Use together cautiously.
MAO inhibitors: Increased anticholinergic effects. Avoid using together.
Drug-lifestyle. *Alcohol use:* Increased CNS depression. Discourage use together.
Sun exposure: Photosensitivity reactions may occur. Advise patient to avoid prolonged or unprotected sun exposure.

EFFECTS ON LAB TEST RESULTS
• May decrease hemoglobin and platelet and granulocyte counts.

CONTRAINDICATIONS
Contraindicated in patients hypersensitive to drug, in newborns, in premature neonates, in breast-feeding women, and in patients with angle-closure glaucoma, stenosing peptic ulcer, symptomatic prostatic hyperplasia, bladder neck obstruction, or pyloroduodenal obstruction; also contraindicated during acute asthmatic attacks. Avoid use in patients taking MAO inhibitors.

NURSING CONSIDERATIONS
• Use with extreme caution in patients with prostatic hyperplasia, asthma, COPD, increased intraocular pressure, hyperthyroidism, CV disease, and hypertension.
• Children younger than age 12 should use drug only as directed by prescriber.
• Discontinue drug 4 days before patient undergoes diagnostic skin tests. Antihistamines can prevent, reduce, or mask positive skin test response.
• Alternate injection sites to prevent irritation. Give I.M. injection deeply into large muscle.
• *Alert:* Don't confuse diphenhydramine with dimenhydrinate; don't confuse Benadryl with Bentyl, Benylin, or benazepril.

PATIENT TEACHING
• Instruct patient to take drug 30 minutes before travel to prevent motion sickness.
• Tell patient to take diphenhydramine with food or milk to reduce GI distress.
• Warn patient to avoid alcohol and hazardous activities that require alertness until CNS effects of drug are known.
• Tell patient that coffee or tea may reduce drowsiness. Urge caution if palpitations develop.
• Inform patient that sugarless gum, hard candy, or ice chips may relieve dry mouth.
• Tell patient to notify prescriber if tolerance develops because a different antihistamine may need to be prescribed.
• Diphenhydramine is contained in many OTC sleep and cold products. Advise patient to consult prescriber before using these products.

• Warn patient of possible photosensitivity reactions. Advise use of a sunblock.

---

fexofenadine hydrochloride
Allegra, Telfast‡

Pregnancy risk category C

AVAILABLE FORMS
Tablets: 30 mg, 60 mg, 180 mg

INDICATIONS & DOSAGES
➤ **Seasonal allergic rhinitis—**
Adults and children age 12 and older:
60 mg P.O. b.i.d or 180 mg P.O. once daily.
Adjust-a-dose: For patients with impaired renal function or a need for dialysis, 60 mg daily.
Children ages 6 to 11: 30 mg P.O. b.i.d.
➤ **Chronic idiopathic urticaria—**
Children age 12 and older: 60 mg P.O. b.i.d.
Children ages 6 to 11: 30 mg P.O. b.i.d.
Adjust-a-dose: In patients with creatinine clearance less than 80 ml/minute, increase dosage interval to every 24 hours.

ACTION
A long-acting nonsedating antihistamine that selectively inhibits peripheral H_1 receptors.

Route	Onset	Peak	Duration
P.O.	Unknown	3 hr	14 hr

ADVERSE REACTIONS
CNS: fatigue, drowsiness.
GI: nausea, dyspepsia.
GU: dysmenorrhea.
Other: viral infection.

INTERACTIONS
Drug-lifestyle. *Alcohol use:* Increased CNS depression. Discourage use together.

EFFECTS ON LAB TEST RESULTS
None reported.

CONTRAINDICATIONS
Contraindicated in patients hypersensitive to drug or its components.

Reactions may be *common*, uncommon, *life-threatening*, or COMMON AND LIFE-THREATENING.

NURSING CONSIDERATIONS

• Use cautiously in patients with impaired renal function.

• Discontinue drug 4 days before patient undergoes diagnostic skin tests. Drug can prevent, reduce, or mask positive skin test response.

• Safety and effectiveness in children younger than age 12 haven't been established.

• No data exist to demonstrate whether drug appears in breast milk; use caution when giving drug to breast-feeding woman. Advise woman taking drug to avoid breast-feeding.

PATIENT TEACHING

• Instruct patient not to exceed prescribed dosage and to take drug only when needed.

• Warn patient to avoid alcohol and hazardous activities that require alertness until CNS effects of drug are known. Explain that drug may cause drowsiness.

• Inform patient that sugarless gum, hard candy, or ice chips may relieve dry mouth.

---

loratadine
Claratyne‡, Clarinase‡, Claritin, Claritin Reditabs

Pregnancy risk category B

AVAILABLE FORMS
Syrup: 1 mg/ml
Tablets: 10 mg
Tablets (rapidly disintegrating): 10 mg

INDICATIONS & DOSAGES
➤ **Symptomatic treatment of seasonal allergic rhinitis, chronic urticaria—**
Adults and children age 6 and older: 10 mg P.O. daily.
Children ages 2 to 5: 5 mg (1 tsp) of syrup P.O. once daily.
Adjust-a-dose: For adults and children age 6 and older who are renally impaired with glomerular filtration rate below 30 ml/minute and for those with hepatic failure, initial dose is 10 mg every other day.
➤ **Relief of nasal and other symptoms of seasonal allergic rhinitis and of**

chronic idiopathic urticaria in children ages 2 to 5 years—
Children ages 2 to 5: 5 mg P.O. daily.

ACTION
Blocks effects of histamine at H_1-receptor sites. Loratadine is a nonsedating antihistamine; its chemical structure prevents entry into the CNS.

Route	Onset	Peak	Duration
P.O.	1-3 hr	8-10 hr	24 hr

ADVERSE REACTIONS
CNS: headache, somnolence, fatigue.
GI: dry mouth.
Skin: photosensitivity reactions.

INTERACTIONS
Drug-drug. *Cimetidine, ketoconazole, macrolide antibiotics (clarithromycin, erythromycin, troleandomycin):* Increased plasma loratadine levels. Monitor patient closely.
Drug-herb. *Licorice:* May prolong the QT interval and may be additive. Discourage use together.
Drug-lifestyle. *Alcohol use:* Increased CNS depression. Discourage use together.
Sun exposure: Photosensitivity reactions may occur. Advise patient to avoid prolonged or unprotected sun exposure.

EFFECTS ON LAB TEST RESULTS
None reported.

CONTRAINDICATIONS
Contraindicated in patients hypersensitive to drug.

NURSING CONSIDERATIONS
• Use cautiously in patients with liver or renal impairment and in breast-feeding patients.

• Discontinue drug 4 days before patient undergoes diagnostic skin tests. Drug can prevent, reduce, or mask positive skin test response.

PATIENT TEACHING
• Make sure patient understands that drug should be taken once daily. If symptoms persist or worsen, tell him to contact prescriber.

• Advise patient taking Claritin Reditabs to place tablet on the tongue where it disintegrates within a few seconds. It can be swallowed with or without water.
• Warn patient to avoid alcohol and hazardous activities that require alertness until CNS effects of drug are known.
• Warn patient about possible photosensitivity reactions. Advise use of a sunblock.
• Tell patient that dry mouth can be relieved with sugarless gum, hard candy, or ice chips.

---

promethazine hydrochloride
Anergan 25, Anergan 50, Histantil†, Pentazine, Phencen-50, Phenergan*, Phenergan Fortis*, Phenergan Plain*, Phenoject-50, Pro-50, Promethegan, Prorex-25, Prorex-50, Prothazine*, Prothazine Plain, V-Gan-25, V-Gan-50

promethazine theoclate
Avomine‡

Pregnancy risk category C

AVAILABLE FORMS
promethazine hydrochloride
Injection: 25 mg/ml, 50 mg/ml
Suppositories: 12.5 mg, 25 mg, 50 mg
Syrup: 5 mg/5 ml‡*, 6.25 mg/5 ml*, 10 mg/5 ml†*, 25 mg/5 ml*
Tablets: 12.5 mg, 25 mg, 50 mg
promethazine theoclate
Tablets: 25 mg‡

INDICATIONS & DOSAGES
➤ **Motion sickness—**
Adults: 25 mg P.O. b.i.d.
Children: 12.5 to 25 mg P.O. or P.R. b.i.d. Or, 0.5 mg/kg 30 minutes to 1 hour before departure.
➤ **Nausea—**
Adults: 12.5 to 25 mg P.O., I.M., or P.R. q 4 to 6 hours, p.r.n.
Children: 12.5 to 25 mg P.O. or P.R. q 4 to 6 hours, p.r.n. Or, 0.25 to 1 mg/kg q 4 to 6 hours, p.r.n. Or, 6.25 to 12.5 mg I.M. q 4 to 6 hours, p.r.n.
➤ **Rhinitis, allergy symptoms—**
Adults: 12.5 mg P.O. q.i.d.; or 25 mg P.O. h.s.

Children: 6.25 to 12.5 mg P.O. t.i.d. Or, 25 mg P.O. or P.R. h.s. Or, 0.1 mg/kg q 6 hours during the day and 0.5 mg/kg h.s.
➤ **Sedation—**
Adults: 25 to 50 mg P.O. or I.M. h.s. or p.r.n.
Children: 12.5 to 25 mg P.O., I.M., or P.R. h.s. Or, 0.5 to 1 mg/kg q 6 hours, p.r.n.
➤ **Routine preoperative or postoperative sedation, adjunct to analgesics—**
Adults: 25 to 50 mg I.M., I.V., or P.O.
Children: 12.5 to 25 mg I.M., I.V., or P.O.

I.V. ADMINISTRATION
• Don't give at a concentration above 25 mg/ml or a rate above 25 mg/minute. Shield I.V. infusion from direct light.
• Discard injection if solution is discolored or contains a precipitate.

ACTION
Phenothiazine derivative that competes with histamine for H_1-receptor sites on effector cells. Prevents, but doesn't reverse, histamine-mediated responses. At high doses, it also has local anesthetic effects.

Route	Onset	Peak	Duration
I.M., P.R.	20 min	Unknown	< 12 hr
I.V.	3-5 min	Unknown	< 12 hr
P.O.	15-60 min	Unknown	< 12 hr

ADVERSE REACTIONS
CNS: *sedation,* confusion, sleepiness, dizziness, disorientation, extrapyramidal symptoms, *drowsiness.*
CV: hypotension, hypertension.
EENT: blurred vision.
GI: nausea, vomiting, *dry mouth.*
GU: urine retention.
Hematologic: *leukopenia, agranulocytosis, thrombocytopenia.*
Metabolic: hyperglycemia.
Skin: photosensitivity, rash.

INTERACTIONS
Drug-drug. *Anticholinergics, phenothiazines, TCAs:* Increased anticholinergic effects. Don't give together.
CNS depressants: Increased sedation. Use together cautiously.
Epinephrine: May block or reverse effects of epinephrine. Use other pressor drugs instead.

Reactions may be *common*, uncommon, *life-threatening*, or **COMMON AND LIFE-THREATENING**.

Levodopa: May decrease antiparkinsonian action of levodopa. Avoid using together.
Lithium: May reduce GI absorption or enhance renal elimination of lithium. Avoid using together.
MAO inhibitors: Increased extrapyramidal effects. Avoid using together.
Drug-herb. *Yohimbe:* Increased risk of yohimbe toxicity. Ask patient about use of herbal remedies, and recommend caution.
Drug-lifestyle. *Alcohol use:* Increased sedation. Discourage use together.
Sun exposure: Photosensitivity reactions may occur. Advise patient to avoid prolonged and unprotected sun exposure.

EFFECTS ON LAB TEST RESULTS
● May increase hemoglobin.
● May decrease WBC, platelet, and granulocyte counts.

CONTRAINDICATIONS
Contraindicated in patients hypersensitive to drug and in those with intestinal obstruction, prostatic hyperplasia, bladder-neck obstruction, angle-closure glaucoma, seizure disorders, coma, CNS depression, and stenosing or peptic ulcerations. Also contraindicated in newborns, premature neonates, breast-feeding women, and acutely ill or dehydrated children.

NURSING CONSIDERATIONS
● Use cautiously in patients with asthma or pulmonary, hepatic, or CV disease.
● Discontinue drug 4 days before patient undergoes diagnostic skin tests. Antihistamines can prevent, reduce, or mask positive skin test response.
● Pronounced sedative effect limits use in many ambulatory patients.
● Promethazine is used as an adjunct to analgesics (usually to increase sedation); it has no analgesic activity.
● Reduce GI distress by giving drug with food or milk.
● Drug may cause either false-positive or false-negative pregnancy test results. It may also interfere with blood grouping in the ABO system.
● Inject deep I.M. into large muscle mass. Rotate injection sites.
● *Alert:* Don't give by S.C. route.
● Drug may be mixed with meperidine in same syringe.

● In patients scheduled for a myelogram, discontinue drug 48 hours before procedure. Don't resume drug until 24 hours after procedure, because of the risk of seizures.
● *Alert:* Don't confuse promethazine with promazine.

PATIENT TEACHING
● Tell patient to take oral form with food or milk.
● When treating motion sickness, tell patient to take first dose 30 to 60 minutes before travel. On succeeding days of travel, patient should take dose upon rising and with evening meal.
● Warn patient to avoid alcohol and hazardous activities that require alertness until CNS effects of drug are known.
● Inform patient that sugarless gum, hard candy, or ice chips may relieve dry mouth.
● Warn patient about possible photosensitivity reactions. Advise use of a sunblock.

albuterol
albuterol sulfate
aminophylline
atropine sulfate
(See Chapter 19, ANTIARRHYTHMICS.)
ephedrine sulfate
epinephrine
epinephrine bitartrate
epinephrine hydrochloride
formoterol fumarate inhalation
powder
ipratropium bromide
isoproterenol
isoproterenol hydrochloride
isoproterenol sulfate
levalbuterol hydrochloride
metaproterenol sulfate
oxtriphylline
pirbuterol acetate
salmeterol xinafoate
terbutaline sulfate
theophylline

COMBINATION PRODUCTS
Inhalants
ADVAIR: salmeterol xinafoate 50 mcg and fluticasone propionate 100 mcg, salmeterol xinafoate 50 mcg and fluticasone propionate 250 mcg, salmeterol xinafoate 50 mcg and fluticasone propionate 500 mcg.
COMBIVENT: ipratropium bromide 18 mcg and albuterol sulfate 103 mcg.
Oral bronchodilators
BRONCHIAL CAPSULES: theophylline 150 mg and guaifenesin 90 mg.
DILOR-G TABLETS: dyphylline 200 mg and guaifenesin 200 mg.
DYFLEX-G TABLETS: dyphylline 200 mg and guaifenesin 200 mg.
DYLINE-GG TABLETS: dyphylline 200 mg and guaifenesin 200 mg.
GLYCERYL-T CAPSULES: theophylline 150 mg and guaifenesin 90 mg.
MARAX*: theophylline 130 mg, ephedrine sulfate 25 mg, and hydroxyzine hydrochloride 10 mg.
MUDRANE GG-2 TABLETS: theophylline 111 mg and guaifenesin 100 mg.

QUIBRON CAPSULES: theophylline 150 mg and guaifenesin 90 mg.
SLO-PHYLLIN GG SYRUP: theophylline 150 mg and guaifenesin 90 mg.
SYNOPHYLATE-GG SYRUP*: guaifenesin 33.3 mg/5 ml and theophylline sodium glycinate 100 mg/5 ml.
Decongestants
ELIXOPHYLLIN KI ELIXIR: theophylline 80 mg and potassium iodide 130 mg.
MARAX-DF SYRUP: theophylline 97.5 mg, ephedrine sulfate 18.75 mg, hydroxyzine hydrochloride 7.5 mg.

---

albuterol (salbutamol)
Asmol‡, Proventil, Ventolin

albuterol sulfate (salbutamol sulfate)
Aerolin Autoinhaler Airomir§, Proventil, Proventil Repetabs, Respolin Autohaler‡, Respolin Inhaler‡, Respolin Respirator Solution‡, Steri-Neb Salamol§, Ventolin, Ventolin HFA, Ventolin Obstetric Injection‡, Ventolin Rotacaps, Volmax

Pregnancy risk category C

AVAILABLE FORMS
albuterol
Aerosol inhaler: 90 mcg/metered spray, 100 mcg/metered spray‡
albuterol sulfate
Capsules for inhalation: 200 mcg
Injection: 1 mg/ml‡
Solution for inhalation: 0.083%, 0.5%, 0.63 mg/ml, 1.25 mg/3 ml
Syrup: 2 mg/5 ml
Tablets: 2 mg, 4 mg
Tablets (extended-release): 4 mg, 8 mg

INDICATIONS & DOSAGES
➤ **To prevent or treat bronchospasm in patients with reversible obstructive airway disease—**
Adults and children age 4 and older: Dosage and frequency vary with drug form.

Reactions may be *common*, uncommon, *life-threatening*, or COMMON AND LIFE-THREATENING.

Aerosol inhalation—1 or 2 inhalations q 4 to 6 hours. More frequent use and more inhalations aren't recommended.

Capsules for inhalation—200 mcg inhaled q 4 to 6 hours using a Rotahaler inhalation device. Some patients may need 400 mcg q 4 to 6 hours.

Adults and children age 12 and older: Solution for inhalation—2.5 mg t.i.d. or q.i.d. by nebulizer. To prepare solution, use 0.5 ml of 0.5% solution diluted with 2.5 ml of normal saline solution. Or, use 3 ml of 0.083% solution.

Children ages 2 to 12: Solution for inhalation—initially, 0.1 to 0.15 mg/kg by nebulizer, with subsequent dosing titrated to response. Don't exceed 2.5 mg t.i.d. or q.i.d. by nebulization.

Adults and children age 14 and older: Syrup—2 to 4 mg (1 to 2 tsp) P.O. t.i.d. or q.i.d. Maximum, 8 mg q.i.d.

Children ages 6 to 14: Syrup—2 mg (1 tsp) P.O. t.i.d. or q.i.d. Maximum, 24 mg daily in divided doses.

Children ages 2 to 6: Syrup—initially, 0.1 mg/kg P.O. t.i.d. Starting dose shouldn't exceed 2 mg (1 tsp) t.i.d. Maximum, 4 mg (2 tsp) t.i.d.

Adults and children age 12 and older: Oral tablets—2 to 4 mg P.O. t.i.d. or q.i.d. Maximum, 8 mg q.i.d.

Extended-release tablets—4 to 8 mg P.O. q 12 hours. Maximum, 16 mg b.i.d.

Children ages 6 to 12: Oral tablets—2 mg P.O. t.i.d. or q.i.d. Maximum, 6 mg q.i.d.

Extended-release tablets—4 mg P.O. q 12 hours. Maximum, 12 mg b.i.d.

Elderly patients: 2 mg P.O. t.i.d. or q.i.d. as oral tablets or syrup. Maximum, 8 mg t.i.d. or q.i.d.

Adjust-a-dose: For those sensitive to beta stimulators, 2 mg P.O. t.i.d. or q.i.d. as oral tablets or syrup. Maximum, 8 mg t.i.d. or q.i.d.

➤ **Prevention of exercise-induced bronchospasm—**

Adults and children age 4 and older: 2 aerosol inhalations 15 to 30 minutes before exercise. Or, 200 mcg (capsule for inhalation) inhaled using a Rotahaler inhalation device 15 minutes before exercise.

I.V. ADMINISTRATION

● Where available, I.V. form may be used to prevent premature labor. To prepare infusion, use saline solution, D_5W for injection, or saline solution and dextrose for injection. Don't give drug without dilution. Don't mix with other drugs. Discard unused diluted solution after 24 hours.

● After uterine contractions have stopped, maintain drip rate for 1 hour; then gradually taper at 50% increments in six hourly intervals. Don't continue infusions for longer than 48 hours. If therapy must continue for longer than 48 hours, prescriber may specify 4 to 8 mg P.O. q.i.d.

ACTION

Relaxes bronchial, uterine, and vascular smooth muscle by stimulating $beta_2$ receptors.

Route	Onset	Peak	Duration
Inhalation	5-15 min	0.5-2 hr	2-6 hr
I.V.	Variable	Unknown	4-6 hr
P.O.	15-30 min	2-3 hr	6-12 hr
P.O. (extended)	Unknown	Unknown	12 hr

ADVERSE REACTIONS

CNS: *tremor, nervousness,* dizziness, insomnia, *headache, hyperactivity,* weakness, CNS stimulation, malaise.

CV: *tachycardia, palpitations,* hypertension.

EENT: dry and irritated nose and throat with inhaled form, nasal congestion, epistaxis, hoarseness.

GI: heartburn, *nausea, vomiting,* anorexia, bad taste, increased appetite.

Metabolic: hypokalemia.

Musculoskeletal: muscle cramps.

Respiratory: *bronchospasm,* cough, wheezing, dyspnea, bronchitis, increased sputum.

Other: hypersensitivity reactions.

INTERACTIONS

Drug-drug. *CNS stimulants:* Increased CNS stimulation. Avoid using together.

Digoxin: Digoxin levels may be decreased. Monitor digoxin level closely.

MAO inhibitors, TCAs: Increased adverse CV effects. Monitor patient closely.

Propranolol, other beta blockers: Mutual antagonism. Monitor patient carefully.

EFFECTS ON LAB TEST RESULTS
• May decrease potassium level.

CONTRAINDICATIONS
Contraindicated in patients hypersensitive to drug or its ingredients.

NURSING CONSIDERATIONS
• Use cautiously in patients with CV disorders (including coronary insufficiency and hypertension), hyperthyroidism, or diabetes mellitus and in those who are unusually responsive to adrenergics.
• Give extended-release tablets cautiously to patients with GI narrowing.
• Albuterol may decrease sensitivity of spirometry used for diagnosis of asthma.
• When switching from regular-release to extended-release tablets, remember that a regular-release 2-mg tablet every 6 hours is equivalent to an extended-release 4-mg tablet every 12 hours.
• Syrup may be taken by children as young as age 2; it contains no alcohol or sugar.
• Rarely, erythema multiforme and Stevens-Johnson syndrome have been linked to use of syrup in children.
• Aerosol form may be used 15 minutes before exercise to prevent exercise-induced bronchospasm.
• Ventolin HFA is a new version of the Ventolin metered-dose inhaler (MDI) for asthma and other obstructive lung diseases. Ventolin HFA uses the propellant hydrofluoroalkane as an alternative to chlorofluorocarbons to propel the medication.
• *Alert:* Patient may use tablets and aerosol together. Monitor him closely for toxicity.
• If drug is used to prevent premature labor, monitor maternal heart rate closely. It shouldn't exceed 140 beats/minute.
• *Alert:* Don't confuse albuterol with atenolol or Albutein or Flomax with Volmax.

PATIENT TEACHING
• Warn patient about possibility of paradoxical bronchospasm. Tell him to stop drug immediately if it occurs.

• Teach patient to perform oral inhalation correctly. Give the following instructions for using metered-dose inhaler:
–Shake the inhaler.
–Clear nasal passages and throat.
–Breathe out, expelling as much air from lungs as possible.
–Place mouthpiece well into mouth, seal lips around mouthpiece, and inhale deeply as you release a dose from inhaler. Or, you may hold inhaler about 1 inch (two finger widths) from your open mouth; inhale while dose is released.
–Hold breath for several seconds, remove mouthpiece, and exhale slowly.
• If prescriber orders more than 1 inhalation, tell patient to wait at least 2 minutes before repeating procedure.
• Tell patient that use with an AeroChamber may improve drug delivery to the lungs.
• If patient is also using a corticosteroid inhaler, instruct him to use the bronchodilator first and then wait about 5 minutes before using the corticosteroid. This allows the bronchodilator to open the air passages for maximum effectiveness of the corticosteroid.
• Tell patient to remove canister and wash inhaler with warm, soapy water at least once a week.
• Advise patient not to chew or crush extended-release tablets and not to mix them with food.

---

aminophylline (theophylline ethylenediamine)
Aminophylline, Pecram§, Phyllocontin, Phyllocontin Continus§, Phyllocontin-350, Truphylline

Pregnancy risk category C

AVAILABLE FORMS
Injection: 250 mg/10 ml, 500 mg/20 ml, 100 mg/100 ml in half-normal saline solution, 200 mg/100 ml in half-normal saline solution
Oral liquid: 105 mg/5 ml
Rectal suppositories: 250 mg, 500 mg
Tablets: 100 mg, 200 mg
Tablets (extended-release): 225 mg, 350 mg†

INDICATIONS & DOSAGES
➤ **Symptomatic relief of bronchospasm (aminophylline doses)—**
Patients not currently receiving theophylline products who need rapid relief from symptoms: Loading dose is 6 mg/kg (equivalent to 4.7 mg/kg anhydrous theophylline) I.V. at 25 mg/minute or less; then maintenance infusion.
Nonsmoking adults and adolescents older than age 16: 0.7 mg/kg/hour I.V. for 12 hours; then 0.5 mg/kg/hour.
Children ages 9 to 16: 1 mg/kg/hour I.V. for 12 hours; then 0.8 mg/kg/hour.
Children ages 6 months to 9 years: 1.2 mg/kg/hour for 12 hours; then 1 mg/kg/hour.
Elderly patients: 0.6 mg/kg/hour I.V. for 12 hours; then 0.3 mg/kg/hour.
Adjust-a-dose: For otherwise healthy adult smokers, 1 mg/kg/hour I.V. for 12 hours; then 0.8 mg/kg/hour. For adults with cor pulmonale, 0.6 mg/kg/hour I.V. for 12 hours; then 0.3 mg/kg/hour. For adults with heart failure or liver disease, 0.5 mg/kg/hour I.V. for 12 hours; then 0.1 to 0.2 mg/kg/hour.
Patients currently receiving theophylline products: First determine time, amount, route of administration, and dosage form of patient's last theophylline dose. Aminophylline infusions of 0.63 mg/kg (0.5 mg/kg anhydrous theophylline) will increase plasma levels of theophylline by 1 mcg/ml. Some prescribers recommend a dose of 3.1 mg/kg (2.5 mg/kg anhydrous theophylline) if no obvious signs or symptoms of theophylline toxicity are present.
➤ **Chronic bronchial asthma—**
Adults and children: Dosage is highly individualized. Dosage by P.R. route is the same as that recommended for P.O. route. Doses reflect anhydrous theophylline equivalents: 100 mg aminophylline hydrous = 78.9 mg theophylline anhydrous (tablets, suppositories, and parental injection); 100 mg aminophylline hydrous = 85.7 mg theophylline anhydrous.
Usual initial P.O. dose is 16 mg/kg or 400 mg (whichever is less) daily in three or four divided doses q 6 to 8 hours if using rapidly absorbed dosage forms. Dosage may be increased, if tolerated, in increments of 25% q 2 to 3 days. Or, if using extended-release preparations, 12 mg/kg or 400 mg (whichever is less)

P.O. daily in two to three divided doses q 8 to 12 hours. Dosage may be increased, if tolerated, by 2 to 3 mg/kg daily q 3 days.
Regardless of dosage form, the following are recommended maximum doses. For adults and children age 16 and older, 13 mg/kg daily or 900 mg/day, whichever is less; children ages 12 to 16, 18 mg/kg daily; children ages 9 to 12, 20 mg/kg daily; and children ages 1 to 8, 24 mg/kg daily.
When recommended maximum dosage is reached, dosage adjustment is based on measurement of peak theophylline levels. Target theophylline levels are generally between 10 and 20 mcg/ml.

I.V. ADMINISTRATION
● I.V. drug use can cause burning; dilute with compatible I.V. solution, and inject at no more than 25 mg/minute. Drug is compatible with most I.V. solutions except invert sugar, fructose, and fat emulsions.

ACTION
Inhibits phosphodiesterase, the enzyme that degrades cAMP, resulting in relaxation of smooth muscle of the bronchial airways and pulmonary blood vessels.

Route	Onset	Peak	Duration
I.V.	15 min	Immediate	Variable
P.O. (extended)	Variable	Variable	Variable
P.O. (solution)	15-60 min	1-7 hr	Variable
P.R.	Unknown	Unknown	Unknown

ADVERSE REACTIONS
CNS: *nervousness, restlessness,* headache, *insomnia, seizures,* muscle twitching, irritability, *dizziness.*
CV: *palpitations, sinus tachycardia,* extrasystoles, flushing, marked hypotension, *arrhythmias.*
GI: *nausea, vomiting,* diarrhea, epigastric pain, hematemesis, irritation with rectal suppositories.
Metabolic: hyperglycemia.
Respiratory: tachypnea, *respiratory arrest.*
Skin: urticaria.
Other: fever, hypersensitivity reactions.

INTERACTIONS

Drug-drug. *Adenosine:* Decreased anti-arrhythmic effectiveness. Higher adenosine doses may be needed.

Alkali-sensitive drugs: Reduced activity. Don't add to I.V. fluids containing aminophylline.

Barbiturates, nicotine, phenytoin, rifampin: Enhanced metabolism and decreased theophylline levels. Monitor patient for decreased aminophylline effect.

Beta blockers: Antagonism; nadolol and propranolol, especially, may cause bronchospasm in sensitive patients. Use together cautiously.

Calcium channel blockers, cimetidine, disulfiram, influenza virus vaccine, interferon, macrolide antibiotics (such as erythromycin), methotrexate, oral contraceptives, quinolone antibiotics (ciprofloxacin): Decreased hepatic clearance of theophylline; elevated theophylline levels. Monitor patient for signs and symptoms of toxicity.

Carbamazepine, isoniazid, loop diuretics: May increase or decrease theophylline levels. Monitor theophylline levels closely.

Ephedrine, other sympathomimetics: Theophylline may exhibit synergistic toxicity with these drugs, predisposing patient to arrhythmias. Monitor patient closely.

Lithium: May increase lithium excretion. Monitor patient closely.

Drug-herb. *Cayenne:* Increased risk of theophylline toxicity. Ask patient about use of herbal remedies, and recommend caution.

Ipriflavone: May increase risk of theophylline toxicity. Urge caution.

St. John's wort: May lower levels of theophylline. Monitor theophylline levels and discourage use together.

Drug-lifestyle. *Smoking:* Increased elimination of theophylline, increasing dosing requirements. Monitor theophylline response and serum levels.

EFFECTS ON LAB TEST RESULTS

• May increase glucose and free fatty acid levels.

CONTRAINDICATIONS

Contraindicated in patients hypersensitive to xanthine compounds (caffeine, theobromine) and ethylenediamine and in those with active peptic ulcer disease and seizure disorders (unless they receive adequate anticonvulsant therapy). Rectal suppositories are contraindicated in patients who have an irritation or infection of the rectum or lower colon.

NURSING CONSIDERATIONS

• Use cautiously in neonates, infants, young children, and elderly patients; also, use cautiously in patients with heart failure, other cardiac or circulatory impairment, COPD, cor pulmonale, renal or hepatic disease, hyperthyroidism, diabetes mellitus, glaucoma, peptic ulcer, severe hypoxemia, or hypertension.

• Relieve GI symptoms by giving oral drug with full glass of water at meals, although food in stomach delays absorption. No evidence exists that antacids reduce adverse GI reactions. Enteric-coated tablets may delay and impair absorption.

• *Alert:* Before giving loading dose, make sure patient hasn't had recent theophylline therapy.

• Aminophylline may alter the assay for uric acid, depending on method used. Theophylline levels are falsely elevated in the presence of furosemide, phenylbutazone, probenecid, theobromine, caffeine, tea, chocolate, cola beverages, and acetaminophen, depending on type of assay used.

• Suppositories are slowly and erratically absorbed. Give rectal suppository if patient can't take drug orally. Schedule dose after bowel evacuation, if possible; may be retained better if given before a meal. Have patient remain recumbent 15 to 20 minutes after insertion.

• Monitor vital signs; measure and record fluid intake and output. Expect improved quality of pulse and respirations.

• Aminophylline is a soluble salt of theophylline. Dosage is adjusted by monitoring response, tolerance, pulmonary function, and theophylline levels. Drug levels should range from 10 to 20 mcg/ml; toxicity has been reported with levels above 20 mcg/ml.

• *Alert:* Evidence of toxicity includes tachycardia, anorexia, nausea, vomiting, diarrhea, restlessness, irritability, and headache. Check theophylline levels, and adjust dosage as directed.

Reactions may be *common*, uncommon, **life-threatening**, or COMMON AND LIFE-THREATENING.

● Patients who develop urticaria may tolerate other theophylline preparations. Urticaria may be caused by the ethylenediamine salt.

● *Alert:* Don't confuse aminophylline with amitriptyline or ampicillin.

PATIENT TEACHING

● Provide dosage schedule and instructions for home use of prescribed form. Some patients may need an around-the-clock dosage schedule.

● Warn elderly patient that dizziness is common at start of therapy.

● Warn patient to check with prescriber before combining aminophylline with other drugs. Prescription or OTC remedies may contain ephedrine and theophylline salts; excessive CNS stimulation may result.

● Caution patient not to switch brands without first checking with prescriber.

● If patient smokes, tell him to notify prescriber if he quits.

ephedrine sulfate
Pretz-D ◊

Pregnancy risk category C

AVAILABLE FORMS

Capsules: 25 mg, 50 mg
Injection: 25 mg/ml, 30 mg/ml‡, 50 mg/ml
Nasal spray: 0.25% ◊

INDICATIONS & DOSAGES

➤ **To correct hypotension—**
Adults: 25 mg one to four times daily P.O. Or, 25 to 50 mg I.M. or S.C. Or, 10 to 25 mg I.V., p.r.n., to maximum of 150 mg/ 24 hours.
Children: 3 mg/kg or 25 to 100 mg/m² S.C. or I.V. daily, in four to six divided doses.

➤ **Bronchodilation, nasal decongestion—**
Adults and children older than age 12: 12.5 to 50 mg P.O. q 3 to 4 hours, p.r.n., not to exceed 150 mg in 24 hours. As a nasal decongestant, 2 to 3 sprays in each nostril not more often than q 4 hours.
Children older than age 2: 2 to 3 mg/kg or 100 mg/m² P.O. daily in four to six divid-

ed doses. Or, for children ages 6 to 12, 6.25 to 12.5 mg P.O. q 4 hours, not to exceed 75 mg in 24 hours. As a nasal decongestant, 1 to 2 sprays in each nostril not more often than q 4 hours.

I.V. ADMINISTRATION

● Give 10 to 25 mg by I.V. injection slowly; repeat in 5 to 10 minutes, if needed. Compatible with most common I.V. solutions.

ACTION

Relaxes bronchial smooth muscle by stimulating beta₂ receptors; also, stimulates alpha and beta receptors and is a direct- and indirect-acting sympathomimetic.

Route	Onset	Peak	Duration
I.M., S.C.	10-20 min	Unknown	0.5-1 hr
I.V.	5 min	Unknown	1 hr
P.O.	15-60 min	Unknown	3-5 hr

ADVERSE REACTIONS

CNS: *insomnia, nervousness,* dizziness, headache, muscle weakness, euphoria, confusion, delirium, tremor, ***cerebral hemorrhage.***
CV: *palpitations,* tachycardia, hypertension, precordial pain, ***arrhythmias.***
EENT: dry nose and throat.
GI: nausea, vomiting, anorexia.
GU: urine retention, painful urination caused by visceral sphincter spasm.
Skin: diaphoresis.

INTERACTIONS

Drug-drug. *Acetazolamide:* Increased ephedrine levels. Monitor patient for toxicity.
Alpha-adrenergic blockers: Unopposed beta-adrenergic effects, resulting in hypotension. Avoid using together.
Antihypertensives: Decreased effects. Monitor blood pressure.
Beta blockers: Unopposed alpha-adrenergic effects, resulting in hypertension. Monitor blood pressure.
Cardiac glycosides, general anesthetics (halogenated hydrocarbons): Increased risk of ventricular arrhythmias. Monitor ECG closely.
Ergot alkaloids: Decreased vasoconstrictor activity. Monitor patient closely.

Guanadrel, guanethidine: Decreased pressor effects of ephedrine. Monitor patient closely.

Levodopa: Enhanced risk of ventricular arrhythmias. Monitor ECG closely.

MAO inhibitors, TCAs: When given with sympathomimetics, may cause severe hypertension (hypertensive crisis). Monitor patient and blood pressure closely.

Methyldopa, reserpine: May inhibit ephedrine effects. Use together cautiously.

EFFECTS ON LAB TEST RESULTS
None reported.

CONTRAINDICATIONS
Contraindicated in patients hypersensitive to ephedrine and other sympathomimetics and in those with porphyria, severe coronary artery disease, arrhythmias, angle-closure glaucoma, psychoneurosis, angina pectoris, substantial organic heart disease, or CV disease. Also, contraindicated in those receiving MAO inhibitors or general anesthesia with cyclopropane or halothane.

NURSING CONSIDERATIONS
● Use with extreme caution in elderly patients and in those with hypertension, hyperthyroidism, nervous or excitable states, diabetes, or prostatic hyperplasia.

● *Alert:* Hypoxia, hypercapnia, and acidosis must be identified and corrected before or during ephedrine therapy because they may reduce effectiveness or increase adverse reactions.

● Drug isn't a substitute for blood or fluid volume replenishment. Volume deficit must be corrected before giving vasopressors.

● To prevent insomnia, avoid giving drug within 2 hours of bedtime.

● Effectiveness decreases after 2 to 3 weeks as tolerance develops. Prescriber may increase dosage. Drug isn't addictive.

● Ephedrine should be used in children younger than age 12 only under direction of prescriber.

● Rebound congestion and tachyphylaxis may occur with topical decongestant formulations.

● *Alert:* Don't confuse ephedrine with epinephrine.

PATIENT TEACHING
● Tell patient taking oral form of drug at home to take last dose of day at least 2 hours before bedtime.

● Warn patient not to take OTC drugs or herbs that contain ephedrine without consulting prescriber.

epinephrine (adrenaline)
Bronkaid Mist◇, Bronkaid Mistometer†, Primatene Mist◇

epinephrine bitartrate
AsthmaHaler Mist◇, Bronkaid Mist◇, Primatene Mist*

epinephrine hydrochloride
Adrenalin Chloride, AsthmaNefrin◇, EpiPen, EpiPen Jr., MicroNefrin◇, Nephron◇, Sus-Phrine, Vaponefrin

Pregnancy risk category C

AVAILABLE FORMS
Aerosol inhaler: 160 mcg◇, 200 mcg◇, 220 mcg◇, 250 mcg/metered spray◇
Injection: 0.01 mg/ml (1:100,000), 0.1 mg/ml (1:10,000), 0.5 mg/ml (1:2,000), 1 mg/ml (1:1,000) parenteral; 5 mg/ml (1:200) parenteral suspension
Nebulizer inhaler: 1% (1:100)†◇, 1.25%†◇, 2.25%†◇

INDICATIONS & DOSAGES
➤ **Bronchospasm, hypersensitivity reactions, anaphylaxis—**
Adults: 0.1 to 0.5 ml of 1:1,000 solution S.C. or I.M. Repeated q 10 to 15 minutes, p.r.n. Or, 0.1 to 0.25 ml of 1:1,000 solution I.V. slowly over 5 to 10 minutes (1 to 2.5 ml of a commercially available 1:10,000 injection or of a 1:10,000 dilution prepared by diluting 1 ml of a commercially available 1:1,000 injection with 10 ml of water for injection or normal saline solution for injection). This may be repeated q 5 to 15 minutes, p.r.n., or followed by a continuous I.V. infusion, starting at 1 mcg/minute and increasing to 4 mcg/minute, p.r.n.
Children: 0.01 ml/kg (10 mcg) of 1:1,000 solution S.C.; repeated q 20 minutes to 4 hours, p.r.n. Maximum single dose

shouldn't exceed 0.5 mg. Or, 0.004 to 0.005 ml/kg of 1:200 Sus-Phrine S.C.; repeated q 8 to 12 hours, p.r.n. Maximum single dose shouldn't exceed 0.75 mg.

➤ **Hemostasis—**
Adults: 1:50,000 to 1:1,000, sprayed or applied topically.

➤ **Acute asthma attacks—**
Adults and children age 4 and older: 160 to 250 mcg metered aerosol, which is equivalent to 1 inhalation, repeated once if needed after at least 1 minute; subsequent doses shouldn't be used for at least 3 hours. Or, 1% (1:100) solution of epinephrine or 2.25% solution of racepinephrine used with a hand-bulb nebulizer as 1 to 3 deep inhalations, repeated q 3 hours, p.r.n.

➤ **To prolong local anesthetic effect—**
Adults and children: With local anesthetics, may be used in concentrations of 1:500,000 to 1:50,000. The most commonly used concentration is 1:200,000.

➤ **To restore cardiac rhythm in cardiac arrest—**
Adults: Usual adult dose is 0.5 to 1 mg I.V. Doses may be repeated q 3 to 5 minutes, if needed. Higher dose epinephrine may be used if 1-mg doses fail: 3 to 5 mg (about 0.1 mg/kg) of epinephrine repeated q 3 to 5 minutes.
Children: Usual dose is 0.01 mg/kg (0.1 ml/kg of 1:10,000 injection) I.V. Initial endotracheal dose is 0.1 mg/kg (0.1 ml/kg of a 1:1,000 injection) diluted in 1 to 2 ml of half-normal or normal saline solution. Subsequent I.V. or intratracheal doses range from 0.1 to 0.2 mg/kg (0.1 to 0.2 ml/kg of a 1:1,000 injection). I.V. or intratracheal doses may be repeated q 3 to 5 minutes, if needed.

I.V. ADMINISTRATION
● Don't mix with alkaline solutions. Use D_5W, normal saline solution for injection, lactated Ringer's injection, or combinations of dextrose in saline solution. Mix just before use.
● Monitor blood pressure, heart rate, and ECG when therapy starts and frequently thereafter.

ACTION
Relaxes bronchial smooth muscle by stimulating beta$_2$ receptors; also stimulates alpha and beta receptors in the sympathetic nervous system.

Route	Onset	Peak	Duration
I.M.	Variable	Unknown	1-4 hr
Inhalation	1-5 min	Unknown	1-3 hr
I.V.	Immediate	5 min	Short
S.C.	5-15 min	0.5 hr	1-4 hr

ADVERSE REACTIONS
CNS: *nervousness, tremor,* vertigo, pain, *headache,* disorientation, agitation, *drowsiness,* fear, dizziness, weakness, *cerebral hemorrhage.*
CV: *palpitations;* widened pulse pressure; hypertension; tachycardia; *ventricular fibrillation; shock;* anginal pain; altered ECG, including a decreased T-wave amplitude, *CVA.*
GI: *nausea, vomiting.*
Respiratory: dyspnea.
Skin: urticaria, hemorrhage at injection site, pallor.
Other: tissue necrosis.

INTERACTIONS
Drug-drug. *Alpha-adrenergic blockers:* Hypotension from unopposed beta-adrenergic effects. Avoid using together.
Antihistamines, thyroid hormones, TCAs: When given with sympathomimetics, may cause severe adverse cardiac effects. Avoid using together.
Beta blockers such as propranolol: May cause vasoconstriction and reflex bradycardia. Monitor patient carefully.
Cardiac glycosides, general anesthetics (halogenated hydrocarbons): Increased risk of ventricular arrhythmias. Monitor ECG closely.
Doxapram, mazindol, methylphenidate: Enhanced CNS stimulation or pressor effects. Monitor patient closely.
Ergot alkaloids: Decreased vasoconstrictor activity. Monitor patient closely.
Guanadrel, guanethidine: Enhanced pressor effects of epinephrine. Monitor patient closely.
Levodopa: Enhanced risk of arrhythmias. Monitor ECG closely.
MAO inhibitors: Increased risk of hypertensive crisis. Monitor blood pressure closely.

EFFECTS ON LAB TEST RESULTS
• May increase BUN, glucose, and lactic acid levels.

CONTRAINDICATIONS
Contraindicated in patients with angle-closure glaucoma, shock (other than anaphylactic shock), organic brain damage, cardiac dilation, arrhythmias, coronary insufficiency, or cerebral arteriosclerosis. Also, contraindicated in patients receiving general anesthesia with halogenated hydrocarbons or cyclopropane and in patients in labor (may delay second stage).

Some commercial products contain sulfites and are contraindicated in patients with sulfite allergies except when epinephrine is being used to treat serious allergic reactions or other emergency situations.

With local anesthetics, epinephrine is contraindicated for use in fingers, toes, ears, nose, or genitalia.

NURSING CONSIDERATIONS
• Use with extreme caution in patients with long-standing bronchial asthma or emphysema who have developed degenerative heart disease. Also use cautiously in elderly patients and in those with hyperthyroidism, CV disease, hypertension, psychoneurosis, and diabetes.
• In patients with Parkinson's disease, drug increases rigidity and tremor.
• Epinephrine therapy interferes with tests for urinary catecholamines.
• One mg equals 1 ml of 1:1,000 solution or 10 ml of 1:10,000 solution.
• Epinephrine is drug of choice in emergency treatment of acute anaphylactic reactions.
• Discard epinephrine solution after 24 hours or if it's discolored or contains precipitate. Keep solution in light-resistant container, and don't remove before use.
• *Alert:* Avoid I.M. use of parenteral suspension into buttocks. Gas gangrene may occur because epinephrine reduces oxygen tension of the tissues, encouraging the growth of contaminating organisms.
• Massage site after I.M. injection to counteract possible vasoconstriction. Repeated local injection can cause necrosis resulting from vasoconstriction at injection site.

• Observe patient closely for adverse reactions. Notify prescriber if adverse reactions develop; dosage adjustment or drug discontinuation may be warranted.
• If blood pressure increases sharply, rapid-acting vasodilators, such as nitrates or alpha-adrenergic blockers, can be given to counteract the marked pressor effect of large doses of epinephrine.
• Epinephrine is rapidly destroyed by oxidizing products, such as iodine, chromates, nitrites, oxygen, and salts of easily reducible metals (such as iron).
• *Alert:* Don't confuse epinephrine with ephedrine or norepinephrine.
• When treating reactions caused by other drugs which were given I.M. or S.C., epinephrine may be injected into the site where the other drug was given to minimize further absorption.

PATIENT TEACHING
• Teach patient to perform oral inhalation correctly. Give the following instructions for using a metered-dose inhaler:
–Shake canister.
–Clear nasal passages and throat.
–Breathe out, expelling as much air from lungs as possible.
–Place mouthpiece well into mouth, and inhale deeply as you release dose from inhaler. Or, hold inhaler about 1 inch (two finger widths) from open mouth, and inhale while releasing dose.
–Hold breath for several seconds, remove mouthpiece, and exhale slowly.
• If more than 1 inhalation is prescribed, advise patient to wait at least 2 minutes before repeating procedure.
• Tell patient that use with an AeroChamber may improve drug delivery to the lungs.
• If patient is also using a corticosteroid inhaler, instruct him to use the bronchodilator first and then to wait about 5 minutes before using the corticosteroid. This allows the bronchodilator to open the air passages for maximum effectiveness.
• Instruct patient to remove canister and wash inhaler with warm, soapy water at least once weekly.
• If patient has acute hypersensitivity reactions, such as to bee stings, you may need to teach him to self-inject epinephrine.

Reactions may be *common*, uncommon, *life-threatening*, or COMMON AND LIFE-THREATENING.

✳ NEW DRUG

formoterol fumarate inhalation powder
Foradil Aerolizer

Pregnancy risk category C

AVAILABLE FORMS
Available by prescription only.
Capsules for inhalation: 12 mcg

INDICATIONS & DOSAGES
➤ **Maintenance treatment and prevention of bronchospasm in patients with reversible obstructive airway disease or nocturnal asthma, who usually require treatment with short-acting inhaled beta$_2$-adrenergic agonists—**
Adults and children age 5 and older: One 12-mcg capsule by inhalation via Aerolizer inhaler q 12 hours. Total daily dose shouldn't exceed 1 capsule b.i.d. (24 mcg/day). If symptoms are present between doses, use a short-acting beta$_2$-adrenergic agonist for immediate relief.
➤ **Prevention of exercise-induced bronchospasm—**
Adults and children age 12 and older: One 12-mcg capsule by inhalation via Aerolizer inhaler at least 15 minutes before exercise given occasionally on a p.r.n. basis. Don't give additional doses within 12 hours of first dose.

ACTION
Long-acting selective beta$_2$-adrenergic agonist that causes bronchodilation. It ultimately increases cAMP, leading to relaxation of bronchial smooth muscle and inhibition of mediator release from mast cells.

Route	Onset	Peak	Duration
Inhalation	≤ 15 min	1-3 hr	12 hr

ADVERSE REACTIONS
CNS: tremor, dizziness, insomnia, nervousness, headache, fatigue, malaise.
CV: chest pain, angina, hypertension, hypotension, tachycardia, *arrhythmias*, palpitations.
EENT: dry mouth, tonsillitis, dysphonia.
GI: nausea.

Metabolic: hypokalemia, hyperglycemia, metabolic acidosis.
Musculoskeletal: muscle cramps.
Respiratory: bronchitis, chest infection, dyspnea.
Skin: rash.
Other: viral infection.

INTERACTIONS
Drug-drug. *Adrenergics:* May potentiate sympathetic effects of formoterol. Use together cautiously.
Beta blockers: May antagonize effects of beta-adrenergic agonists, causing bronchospasm in asthmatic patients. Avoid use except when benefit outweighs risks. Use cardioselective beta blockers with caution to minimize risk of bronchospasm.
Diuretics, steroids, xanthine derivatives: May potentiate hypokalemic effect of formoterol. Use together cautiously.
MAO inhibitors, TCAs, other drugs that prolong QT interval: May increase risk of ventricular arrhythmias. Use together cautiously.
Non–potassium-sparing diuretics (such as loop or thiazide diuretics): May worsen ECG changes or hypokalemia. Use together cautiously, and monitor for toxicity.

EFFECTS ON LAB TEST RESULTS
● May increase glucose level. May decrease potassium level.

CONTRAINDICATIONS
Contraindicated in patients hypersensitive to drug or its components.

NURSING CONSIDERATIONS
● Use cautiously in patients with CV disease, particularly coronary insufficiency, cardiac arrhythmias, and hypertension, and in those who are unusually responsive to sympathomimetic amines.
● Use cautiously in patients with preexisting diabetes mellitus because instances of hyperglycemia and ketoacidosis have occurred rarely with the use of beta-adrenergic agonists.
● Use cautiously in patients with seizure disorders or thyrotoxicosis.
● Drug isn't indicated for patients who can control asthma symptoms with just occasional use of inhaled, short-acting beta$_2$-adrenergic agonists or for treatment of

---

*Liquid contains alcohol. **May contain tartrazine. †Canada ‡Australia §U.K. ◇OTC

acute bronchospasm requiring immediate reversal with short-acting beta₂-adrenergic agonists.

• Drug may be used along with short-acting beta₂-adrenergic agonists, inhaled corticosteroids, and theophylline therapy for asthma management.

• Patients using drug twice daily shouldn't use additional doses for prevention of exercise-induced bronchospasm.

• Don't use as a substitute for short-acting beta₂-adrenergic agonists for immediate relief of bronchospasm, or as a substitute for inhaled or oral corticosteroids.

• Don't begin use in patients with rapidly deteriorating or significantly worsening asthma.

• If usual dose doesn't control symptoms of bronchoconstriction, and patient's short-acting beta₂-adrenergic agonist becomes less effective, reevaluate patient and treatment regimen.

• For patients formerly using regularly scheduled short-acting beta₂-adrenergic agonists, decrease use of the short-acting drug to an as-needed basis when starting long-acting formoterol.

• As with all beta-2 agonists, formoterol may produce life-threatening paradoxical bronchospasm. If bronchospasm occurs, discontinue formoterol immediately and use an alternative drug.

• Monitor patient for tachycardia, hypertension and other CV adverse effects. If these occur, drug may need to be discontinued.

• Watch for immediate hypersensitivity reactions, such as anaphylaxis, urticaria, angioedema, rash, and bronchospasm.

• Foradil capsules should only be given via oral inhalation and used only with the Aerolizer inhaler. They aren't for oral ingestion. Patient shouldn't exhale into the device. Capsules should remain in the unopened blister until administration time and only be removed immediately before use.

• Before dispensing, store drug in refrigerator. Once dispensed to patient, drug may be stored at room temperature.

• Don't use Foradil Aerolizer with a spacer device.

• Pierce capsules only once. In rare instances, the gelatin capsule may break into small pieces and get delivered to the mouth or throat upon inhalation. The Aerolizer contains a screen that should catch any broken pieces before they leave the device. To minimize the possibility of shattering the capsule, strictly follow storage and use instructions.

• No overall differences in safety or efficacy have been observed in elderly patients. However, increased sensitivity of some elderly patients is possible.

• It's unknown if drug appears in breast milk. Use cautiously in breast-feeding women.

PATIENT TEACHING

• Tell patient not to increase the dosage or frequency of use without medical advice.

• Warn patient not to stop or reduce other medication taken for asthma.

• Advise patient that drug isn't to be used for acute asthmatic episodes. A short-acting beta₂-adrenergic agonist should be prescribed for this use.

• Advise patient to report worsening symptoms or if treatment becomes less effective or use of short-acting beta₂-adrenergic agonists increases.

• Tell patient to report nausea, vomiting, shakiness, headache, fast or irregular heartbeat, or sleeplessness.

• Warn patient not to exceed the recommended daily dosage.

• Tell patient being treated for exercise-induced bronchospasm to take drug at least 15 minutes before exercise and that additional doses can't be taken for 12 hours.

• Tell patient that side effects, such as palpitations, chest pain, rapid heart rate, tremor, and nervousness, may occur.

• Tell patient not to use the Foradil Aerolizer with a spacer device or to exhale or blow into the Aerolizer inhaler.

• Advise patient to avoid washing the Aerolizer and to always keep it dry. A new device comes with each refill. The new device should replace the old one.

• Tell patient to avoid exposing capsules to moisture and to handle them only with dry hands.

• Advise woman to notify prescriber if she becomes pregnant or is breast-feeding.

---

ipratropium bromide
Atrovent

Pregnancy risk category B

AVAILABLE FORMS
Inhaler: each metered dose supplies 18 mcg
Nasal spray: 0.03% (each metered dose supplies 21 mcg), 0.06% (each metered dose supplies 42 mcg)
Solution (for inhalation): 0.02% (500 mcg/vial)
Solution (for nebulizer): 0.025% (250 mcg/ml)‡

INDICATIONS AND DOSAGES
➤ **Bronchospasm in chronic bronchitis and emphysema—**
Adults: Usually, 2 inhalations (36 mcg) q.i.d.; patient may take additional inhalations, p.r.n., but shouldn't exceed 12 inhalations in 24 hours or 500 mcg q 6 to 8 hours via oral nebulizer.
➤ **Rhinorrhea associated with allergic and nonallergic perennial rhinitis—**
0.03% nasal spray
Adults and children age 6 and older: 2 sprays (42 mcg) per nostril b.i.d. or t.i.d.
➤ **Rhinorrhea associated with the common cold—**
0.06% nasal spray
Adults and children age 12 and older: 2 sprays (84 mcg) per nostril t.i.d. or q.i.d.
Children ages 5 to 11: 2 sprays (84 mcg) per nostril t.i.d.

ACTION
Inhibits vagally mediated reflexes by antagonizing acetylcholine at muscarinic receptors on bronchial smooth muscle.

Route	Onset	Peak	Duration
Inhalation	5-15 min	1-2 hr	3-6 hr

ADVERSE REACTIONS
CNS: dizziness, pain, headache, nervousness.
CV: palpitations, hypertension, chest pain.
EENT: blurred vision, rhinitis, pharyngitis, sinusitis, epistaxis.
GI: nausea, GI distress, dry mouth.
Musculoskeletal: back pain.

Respiratory: *upper respiratory tract infection, bronchitis,* cough, dyspnea, ***bronchospasm,*** increased sputum.
Skin: rash.
Other: flu symptoms, hypersensitivity reactions.

INTERACTIONS
Drug-drug. *Anticholinergics:* Increased anticholinergic effects. Avoid using together.
Drug-herb. *Jaborandi tree:* May decrease effects of ipratropium when used together. Advise patient to use cautiously.
Pill-bearing spurge: Choline, a chemical component of the herb, may decrease effect of ipratropium. Ask patient about use of herbal remedies, and recommend caution.

EFFECTS ON LAB TEST RESULTS
None reported.

CONTRAINDICATIONS
Contraindicated in patients hypersensitive to drug, atropine, or its derivatives and in those hypersensitive to soy lecithin or related food products, such as soybeans and peanuts.

NURSING CONSIDERATIONS
● Use cautiously in patients with angle-closure glaucoma, prostatic hyperplasia, or bladder-neck obstruction.
● If using a face mask for a nebulizer, take care to avoid leakage around the mask; eye pain or temporary blurring of vision may occur.
● Safety and efficacy of use beyond 4 days in patients with the common cold haven't been established.
● *Alert:* A patient with a severe peanut allergy could have an anaphylactic reaction after using Atrovent inhalation aerosol (metered-dose inhaler). Take a thorough allergy history from patient before giving any drug.
● *Alert:* Don't confuse Atrovent with Alupent.

PATIENT TEACHING
● Warn patient that drug isn't effective for treating acute episodes of bronchospasm when rapid response is needed.

• Teach patient to perform oral inhalation correctly. Give the following instructions for using a metered-dose inhaler:
–Shake canister.
–Clear nasal passages and throat.
–Breathe out, expelling as much air from lungs as possible.
–Place mouthpiece well into mouth, and inhale deeply as you release dose from inhaler. (Patient may want to close eyes.)
–Hold breath for several seconds, remove mouthpiece, and exhale slowly.

• Inform patient that use of AeroChamber with metered-dose inhaler may improve drug delivery to lungs.

• Warn patient to avoid accidentally spraying drug into eyes. Temporary blurring of vision may result.

• If more than 1 inhalation is ordered, tell patient to wait at least 2 minutes before repeating procedure.

• Instruct patient to remove canister and wash inhaler in warm, soapy water at least once weekly.

• If patient also uses a corticosteroid inhaler, tell him to use ipratropium first, and then wait about 5 minutes before using the corticosteroid. This method allows the bronchodilator to open air passages for maximum effectiveness of the corticosteroid.

---

isoproterenol (isoprenaline)
Isuprel, Medihaler-Iso

isoproterenol hydrochloride
Isuprel, Isuprel Mistometer

isoproterenol sulfate
Medihaler-Iso

Pregnancy risk category C

AVAILABLE FORMS
isoproterenol
Nebulizer inhaler: 0.25%, 0.5%, 1%
isoproterenol hydrochloride
Aerosol inhaler: 131 mcg/metered spray
Injection: 20 mcg/ml, 200 mcg/ml
isoproterenol sulfate
Aerosol inhaler: 80 mcg/metered spray

INDICATIONS & DOSAGES
➤ **Bronchospasm—**
Adults and children: For acute dyspneic episodes, initially 1 inhalation of sulfate form. Repeat, if needed, after 2 to 5 minutes. Maintenance dosage is 1 to 2 inhalations four to six times daily. No more than 6 inhalations should be taken during any single hour in a 24-hour period.
➤ **Bronchospasm in COPD—**
Given via IPPB or nebulizer by compressed air or oxygen.
Adults: 2 ml of 0.125% or 2.5 ml of 0.1% solution up to five times daily. Prepared by diluting 0.5 ml of 0.5% solution to 2 or 2.5 ml, respectively, or by diluting 0.25 ml of 1% solution to 2 or 2.5 ml, respectively, with water or half-normal or normal saline solution.
Adults: 2 ml of a 0.0625% solution or 2.5 ml of 0.05% solution up to five times daily. Prepared by diluting 0.25 ml of 0.5% solution to 2 or 2.5 ml, respectively, with water or half-normal or normal saline solution.
➤ **Heart block, ventricular arrhythmias—**
Adults: Initially, 0.02 to 0.06 mg hydrochloride I.V. Subsequent doses 0.01 to 0.2 mg I.V. or 5 mcg/minute I.V. Or, 0.2 mg I.M. initially, then 0.02 to 1 mg, p.r.n.
Children: I.V. infusion of 2.5 mcg/minute or 0.1 mcg/kg/minute hydrochloride. Dosage is adjusted based on patient's response.
➤ **Shock—**
Adults and children: 0.5 to 5 mcg/minute hydrochloride by continuous I.V. infusion. Usual concentration is 1 mg or 5 ml in 500 ml D_5W. Titrate infusion rate according to heart rate, central venous pressure, blood pressure, and urine flow.

I.V. ADMINISTRATION
• Give by direct injection or I.V. infusion. For infusion, drug may be diluted with most common I.V. solutions. However, don't use with sodium bicarbonate injection; drug decomposes rapidly in alkaline solutions.

• When giving I.V. isoproterenol to treat shock, closely monitor blood pressure, central venous pressure, ECG, arterial blood gas measurements, and urine output. Carefully titrate infusion rate according to these measurements. Use a continuous infusion pump to regulate flow rate.

ACTION
Relaxes bronchial smooth muscle by stimulating beta₂ receptors. As a cardiac stimulant, acts on beta₁ receptors in the heart.

Route	Onset	Peak	Duration
Inhalation	2-5 min	Unknown	0.5-2 hr
I.V.	Immediate	Unknown	< 1 hr

ADVERSE REACTIONS
CNS: *headache, mild tremor,* weakness, dizziness, *nervousness,* insomnia, ***Stokes-Adams seizures.***
CV: *palpitations, tachycardia, angina,* ***arrhythmias, cardiac arrest,*** *rapid rise and fall in blood pressure.*
EENT: pharyngitis.
GI: *nausea, vomiting, heartburn.*
Metabolic: hyperglycemia.
Respiratory: ***bronchospasm,*** bronchitis, increased sputum, pulmonary edema.
Skin: diaphoresis.
Other: swelling of parotid glands with prolonged use.

INTERACTIONS
Drug-drug. *Epinephrine, other sympathomimetics:* Increased risk of arrhythmias. Use together cautiously.
Halogenated general anesthetics or cyclopropane: Increased risk of arrhythmias. Avoid using together.
Propranolol, other beta blockers: Blocked bronchodilating effect of isoproterenol. Monitor patient carefully.

EFFECTS ON LAB TEST RESULTS
• May increase glucose levels.

CONTRAINDICATIONS
Contraindicated in patients with tachycardia or AV block caused by digoxin intoxication, arrhythmias (other than those that may respond to treatment with isoproterenol), angina pectoris, or angle-closure glaucoma. Also, contraindicated when used with general anesthetics with halogenated drugs or cyclopropane.

NURSING CONSIDERATIONS
• Use cautiously in elderly patients and in those with renal or CV disease, coronary

insufficiency, diabetes, hyperthyroidism, or history of sensitivity to sympathomimetic amines.
• Drug isn't a substitute for blood or fluid volume deficit. Volume deficit should be corrected before giving vasopressors.
• Don't use injection or inhalation solution if it's discolored or contains precipitate. Drug may reduce sensitivity of spirometry in the diagnosis of asthma.
• *Alert:* If heart rate exceeds 110 beats/minute with I.V. infusion, notify prescriber. Doses sufficient to increase the heart rate to more than 130 beats/minute may induce ventricular arrhythmias.
• If drug is given via inhalation with oxygen, make sure oxygen level won't suppress respiratory drive.
• Follow same instructions for metered powder nebulizer, although deep inhalation isn't needed.
• Drug may aggravate ventilation-perfusion abnormalities; although ease of breathing is improved, arterial oxygen tension may fall paradoxically.
• Isoproterenol may cause a slight increase in systolic blood pressure and a slight to marked decrease in diastolic blood pressure.
• Monitor patient for adverse reactions.
• *Alert:* Don't confuse Isuprel with Ismelin or Isordil.

PATIENT TEACHING
• Teach patient to perform oral inhalation correctly. Give the following instructions for using a metered-dose inhaler:
–Shake canister.
–Clear nasal passages and throat.
–Breathe out, expelling as much air from lungs as possible.
–Place mouthpiece well into mouth, and inhale deeply as you release dose from inhaler. Or, hold inhaler about 1 inch (two finger widths) from open mouth, and inhale as dose is released.
–Hold breath for several seconds, remove mouthpiece, and exhale slowly.
• If more than 1 inhalation is ordered, tell patient to wait at least 2 minutes before repeating procedure.
• Tell patient that use of an AeroChamber may improve drug delivery to the lungs.
• If patient is also using a corticosteroid inhaler, instruct him to use the bron-

chodilator first and then wait about 5 minutes before using the corticosteroid. This method allows the bronchodilator to open the air passages for maximum effectiveness of the corticosteroid.

- Instruct patient to remove canister and wash inhaler with warm, soapy water at least once weekly.
- Warn patient that oral inhalant may turn sputum and saliva pink.
- Tell patient not to use drug at bedtime, if possible; it interrupts sleep patterns.
- Urge patient to stop drug immediately and notify prescriber if he develops precordial distress, angina, or increased chest tightness or dyspnea.
- Warn patient against overuse; tolerance may develop.

---

levalbuterol hydrochloride
Xopenex

Pregnancy risk category C

AVAILABLE FORMS
Solution for inhalation: 0.63 mg or 1.25 mg in 3-ml vials

INDICATIONS & DOSAGES
➤ **To prevent or treat bronchospasm in patients with reversible obstructive airway disease—**
Adults and adolescents age 12 and older: 0.63 mg given t.i.d. q 6 to 8 hours, by oral inhalation via a nebulizer. Patients with more severe asthma who don't respond adequately to 0.63 mg t.i.d. may benefit from 1.25 mg t.i.d.

ACTION
Relaxes bronchial smooth muscle by stimulating beta$_2$ receptors; also, inhibits release of mediators from mast cells in the airway.

Route	Onset	Peak	Duration
Inhalation	10-17 min	1.5 hr	5-8 hr

ADVERSE REACTIONS
CNS: dizziness, migraine, nervousness, pain, tremor, anxiety.
CV: tachycardia.
EENT: *rhinitis,* sinusitis, turbinate edema.
GI: dyspepsia.

Musculoskeletal: leg cramps.
Respiratory: increased cough.
Other: flu syndrome, accidental injury, *viral infection.*

INTERACTIONS
Drug-drug. *Beta blockers:* Blocked pulmonary effect of the drug and possibly severe bronchospasm. Don't use together, if possible. If use together is necessary, consider a cardioselective beta blocker but give with caution.
Digoxin: Decreased digoxin levels (up to 22%). Monitor digoxin levels.
Loop or thiazide diuretics: ECG changes and hypokalemia from administration together of these non–potassium-sparing diuretics. Use together cautiously.
MAO inhibitors, TCAs: Potentiated action of levalbuterol on the vascular system. Give with extreme caution to patients being treated with MAO inhibitors or TCAs, or within 2 weeks of stopping these drugs.
Other short-acting sympathomimetic aerosol bronchodilators, epinephrine: Increased adrenergic adverse effects. To avoid serious CV effects, additional adrenergics should be used with caution.

EFFECTS ON LAB TEST RESULTS
None reported.

CONTRAINDICATIONS
Contraindicated in patients hypersensitive to drug or to racemic albuterol.

NURSING CONSIDERATIONS
- Use cautiously in patients with CV disorders, especially coronary insufficiency, hypertension, and arrhythmias. Also, use cautiously in patients with seizure disorders, hyperthyroidism, or diabetes mellitus and in patients who are unusually responsive to sympathomimetic amines.
- *Alert:* Like other inhaled beta-adrenergic agonists, levalbuterol can produce paradoxical bronchospasm, which may be life-threatening. If this occurs, discontinue drug immediately and start alternative therapy.
- *Alert:* Like all other beta-adrenergic agonists, levalbuterol can produce significant CV effects in some patients. Although such effects are uncommon at recom-

---

Reactions may be *common,* uncommon, *life-threatening,* or COMMON AND LIFE-THREATENING.

mended doses, you should discontinue drug as directed if they occur.
● Drug may worsen diabetes mellitus and ketoacidosis.
● Potassium levels may be transiently decreased, but potassium supplementation is usually unnecessary.
● The compatibility, efficacy, and safety of levalbuterol mixed with other drugs in a nebulizer haven't been established.

PATIENT TEACHING
● Warn patient that he may experience paradoxical bronchospasm (worsened breathing). Tell him to stop drug and contact prescriber immediately if this occurs.
● Tell patient not to increase dosage without consulting prescriber.
● Urge patient to seek medical attention immediately if levalbuterol becomes less effective, if signs and symptoms become worse, or if he's using levalbuterol more frequently than usual.
● Tell patient that the effects of levalbuterol may last up to 8 hours.
● Tell patient not to double the next dose if he misses a dose. Doses should be at least 6 hours apart.
● Advise patient to use other inhalations and antiasthmatics only as directed while taking levalbuterol.
● Inform patient that common adverse reactions include palpitations, rapid heart rate, headache, dizziness, tremor, and nervousness.
● Encourage patient to contact prescriber if she becomes pregnant or is breast-feeding.
● Tell patient to keep unopened vials in foil pouch. Once the foil pouch is opened, vials should be used within 2 weeks. Inform patient that vials removed from the pouch, if not used immediately, should be protected from light and excessive heat and used within 1 week.
● Teach patient to correctly give drug by oral inhalation via a nebulizer.
● Instruct patient to breathe as calmly, deeply, and evenly as possible until no more mist is formed in the nebulizer reservoir (5 to 15 minutes).

metaproterenol sulfate
Alupent, Arm-a-Med
Metaproterenol, Dey-Lute
Metaproterenol

Pregnancy risk category C

AVAILABLE FORMS
Aerosol inhaler: 0.65 mg/metered spray
Nebulizer inhaler: 0.4%, 0.6%, 5% solution
Syrup: 10 mg/5 ml
Tablets: 10 mg, 20 mg

INDICATIONS & DOSAGES
➤ **Acute episodes of bronchial asthma—**
Adults and children age 12 and older: 2 to 3 inhalations q 3 to 4 hours. Don't exceed 12 inhalations daily.
➤ **Bronchial asthma and reversible bronchospasm—**
Adults: 20 mg P.O. q 6 to 8 hours.
Children older than age 9, or weighing more than 27 kg (60 lb): 20 mg P.O. q 6 to 8 hours.
Children ages 6 to 9, or weighing less than 27 kg: 10 mg P.O. q 6 to 8 hours.
Children younger than age 6: 1.3 to 2.6 mg/kg/day in divided doses of syrup.
For IPPB or nebulizer
Adults and children age 12 and older: 0.2 to 0.3 ml of 5% solution diluted in about 2.5 ml of half-normal or normal saline solution. Or, 2.5 ml of a commercially available 0.4% or 0.6% solution q 4 hours, p.r.n.
Children ages 6 to 12: 0.1 to 0.2 ml of a 5% solution diluted in normal saline solution to final volume of 3 ml q 4 hours, p.r.n.

ACTION
Relaxes bronchial smooth muscle by stimulating beta$_2$ receptors.

Route	Onset	Peak	Duration
Inhalation	1 min	1 hr	1-2.5 hr
Nebulizer	5-30 min	1 hr	1-2.5 hr
P.O.	15 min	1 hr	1-4 hr

ADVERSE REACTIONS
CNS: *nervousness,* weakness, drowsiness, *tremor,* vertigo, headache.

CV: *tachycardia,* hypertension, palpitations, *cardiac arrest with excessive use.*
EENT: dry and irritated throat.
GI: *vomiting, nausea,* heartburn, dry mouth.
Respiratory: *paradoxical bronchiolar constriction with excessive use,* cough.
Skin: rash, hypersensitivity reactions.

INTERACTIONS
Drug-drug. *Epinephrine, other sympathomimetics:* Increased risk of arrhythmias. Use together cautiously.
MAO inhibitors, TCAs: May potentiate the effect of metaproterenol on the vascular system. Use together cautiously.
Propranolol, other beta blockers: Blocked bronchodilating effect of metaproterenol. Monitor patient carefully.

EFFECTS ON LAB TEST RESULTS
None reported.

CONTRAINDICATIONS
Contraindicated in patients hypersensitive to its ingredients and in those with tachycardia, arrhythmias linked to tachycardia, peripheral or mesenteric vascular thrombosis, profound hypoxia or hypercapnia. Also, contraindicated in those receiving general anesthesia with cyclopropane or halogenated hydrocarbon anesthetics.

NURSING CONSIDERATIONS
● Use cautiously in patients receiving cardiac glycosides and in patients with hypertension, hyperthyroidism, heart disease, diabetes, or cirrhosis.
● Patients may use tablets and aerosol together. Watch closely for toxicity.
● Drug may reduce the sensitivity of spirometry in the diagnosis of asthma.
● Inhalant solution can be given by IPPB with drug diluted in normal saline solution or with a hand nebulizer at full strength.
● *Alert:* Don't confuse metaproterenol with metoprolol or metipranolol; don't confuse Alupent with Atrovent.

PATIENT TEACHING
● Teach patient to perform oral inhalation correctly. Give the following instructions for using a metered-dose inhaler:
–Shake canister.

–Clear nasal passages and throat.
–Breathe out, expelling as much air from lungs as possible.
–Place mouthpiece well into mouth, and inhale deeply as you release dose from inhaler. Or, hold inhaler about 1 inch (two finger widths) from open mouth; inhale while dose is released.
–Hold breath for several seconds, remove mouthpiece, and exhale slowly. Allow 2 minutes between inhalations.
● Inform patient that use of AeroChamber with metered-dose inhaler may improve drug delivery to lungs.
● Advise patient to store drug in light-resistant container.
● Tell patient who is also using a corticosteroid inhaler to use bronchodilator first, and then wait about 5 minutes before using the corticosteroid. This method allows bronchodilator to open air passages for maximum effectiveness of the corticosteroid.
● Tell patient to remove canister and wash inhaler in warm, soapy water at least once weekly.
● Warn patient to stop drug immediately and notify prescriber if paradoxical bronchospasm occurs.
● Warn patient to notify prescriber if he has no response to drug.

---

oxtriphylline (choline salt of theophyllinate)
Choledyl SA

Pregnancy risk category C

AVAILABLE FORMS
Elixir*: 100 mg/5 ml
Syrup: 50 mg/5 ml
Tablets: 100 mg, 200 mg
Tablets (extended-release): 400 mg, 600 mg

INDICATIONS & DOSAGES
➤ **Acute bronchial asthma and reversible bronchospasm from chronic bronchitis and emphysema—**
Adult nonsmokers: 4.7 mg/kg P.O. q 8 hours. If total daily maintenance dose is established at 800 to 1,200 mg, may substitute 1 sustained-action tablet q 12 hours.

Reactions may be *common,* uncommon, *life-threatening,* or **COMMON AND LIFE-THREATENING.**

Adult smokers and children ages 9 to 16: 4.7 mg/kg q 6 hours. If total daily maintenance dose is established at 800 to 1,200 mg, may substitute 1 sustained-action tablet q 12 hours.

Children ages 1 to 9: 6.2 mg/kg P.O. q 6 hours. If total daily maintenance dose is established at 800 to 1,200 mg, may substitute 1 sustained-action tablet q 12 hours.

Adjust-a-dose: Reduce dosage in elderly patients and those with heart failure, cor pulmonale, or hepatic disease.

ACTION

Inhibits phosphodiesterase, the enzyme that degrades cAMP, resulting in relaxation of smooth muscle of the bronchial airways and pulmonary blood vessels. Oxtriphylline is equivalent to 64% anhydrous theophylline.

Route	Onset	Peak	Duration
P.O.	Unknown	2 hr	Unknown
P.O. (extended)	Variable	Variable	Variable

ADVERSE REACTIONS

CNS: *restlessness, dizziness,* headache, *insomnia,* irritability, **seizures,** muscle twitching.

CV: *palpitations, sinus tachycardia,* extrasystoles, flushing, marked hypotension, **arrhythmias.**

GI: *nausea, vomiting,* epigastric pain, diarrhea.

Respiratory: tachypnea, **respiratory arrest.**

INTERACTIONS

Drug-drug. *Adenosine:* Decreased antiarrhythmic effectiveness. Higher adenosine doses may be needed.

Allopurinol (high-dose): Increased theophylline levels. Monitor patient for theophylline toxicity.

Barbiturates, nicotine, phenytoin, rifampin: Enhanced metabolism and decreased theophylline levels. Monitor patient for decreased effect.

Beta blockers (nadolol and propranolol): May cause bronchospasm in sensitive patients. Use together cautiously.

Calcium channel blockers, cimetidine, influenza virus vaccine, macrolide anti-

biotics (such as erythromycin), oral contraceptives, quinolone antibiotics (such as ciprofloxacin): Decreased hepatic clearance of theophylline; elevated theophylline levels. Monitor patient for signs and symptoms of toxicity.

Carbamazepine, isoniazid, loop diuretics: May increase or decrease theophylline levels. Monitor theophylline levels.

Lithium: Increased renal excretion of lithium. Monitor patient for decreased effect.

Drug-herb. *Cayenne:* Increased risk of theophylline toxicity. Ask patient about use of herbal remedies, and advise patient to use together cautiously.

Ipriflavone: May increase risk of theophylline toxicity. Advise patient to use together cautiously.

St. John's wort: May lower levels of theophylline. Monitor theophylline levels, and discourage use together.

Drug-lifestyle. *Smoking:* Increased elimination of oxtriphylline. Increase dose, as ordered; monitor response and serum levels.

EFFECTS ON LAB TEST RESULTS

None reported.

CONTRAINDICATIONS

Contraindicated in patients hypersensitive to xanthines (caffeine, theobromine) and in those with arrhythmias (especially tachyarrhythmias), active peptic ulcer disease, or poorly controlled seizure disorders.

NURSING CONSIDERATIONS

● Use cautiously in young children, elderly patients, and patients with peptic ulceration, COPD, heart failure, cor pulmonale, renal or hepatic impairment, glaucoma, severe hypoxemia, hypertension, compromised cardiac or circulatory function, angina, acute MI, sulfite sensitivity, hyperthyroidism, or diabetes.

● *Alert:* Don't combine with products containing ephedrine; excessive CNS stimulation (nervousness, tremor, akathisia) may result.

● Give drug after meals and at bedtime.

● Drug may falsely elevate uric acid levels measured by colorimetric methods. Theophylline levels may be falsely elevated in

INTERACTIONS
Drug-drug. *Beta-adrenergic agonists, other methylxanthines, theophylline:* May cause adverse cardiac effects with excessive use. Monitor patient.
MAO inhibitors: Risk of severe adverse CV effects. Avoid use within 14 days of MAO therapy.
TCAs: Risk of moderate to severe adverse CV effects. Use together with extreme caution.

EFFECTS ON LAB TEST RESULTS
None reported.

CONTRAINDICATIONS
Contraindicated in patients hypersensitive to drug or its ingredients.

NURSING CONSIDERATIONS
• Use cautiously in patients unusually responsive to sympathomimetics and those with coronary insufficiency, arrhythmias, hypertension, other CV disorders, thyrotoxicosis, or seizure disorders.
• Drug isn't indicated for acute bronchospasm.
• *Alert:* Monitor patient for rash and urticaria, which may signal a hypersensitivity reaction.
• *Alert:* Don't confuse Serevent with Serentil.

PATIENT TEACHING
• Remind patient to take drug at about 12-hour intervals for optimum effect and to take drug even when feeling better.
• If patient is taking drug to prevent exercise-induced bronchospasm, tell him to take it 30 to 60 minutes before exercise.
• *Alert:* Tell patient that, although drug is a beta-adrenergic agonist, it shouldn't be used to treat acute bronchospasm. He must be provided with a short-acting beta-adrenergic agonist such as albuterol to treat exacerbations.
• Tell patient to contact prescriber if the short-acting agonist no longer provides sufficient relief or if he needs more than 4 inhalations daily. This may be a sign that the asthma symptoms are worsening. Tell him not to increase the dosage of salmeterol.

• If patient takes an inhaled corticosteroid, he should continue to use it on a regular basis. Warn patient not to take other drugs without prescriber's consent.
• If patient takes the inhalation powder (Diskus device), instruct him not to exhale into the device. It should only be activated and used in a level, horizontal position.
• Tell patient not to use Diskus with a spacer.
• Instruct patient never to wash the mouthpiece or any part of the Diskus; it must be kept dry.

---

terbutaline sulfate
Brethine, Bricanyl

Pregnancy risk category B

AVAILABLE FORMS
Injection: 1 mg/ml
Tablets: 2.5 mg, 5 mg

INDICATIONS & DOSAGES
➤ **Bronchospasm in patients with reversible obstructive airway disease—**
Adults and children age 12 and older: Dosage varies with form.
*Injection—*0.25 mg S.C. May be repeated in 15 to 30 minutes, p.r.n. Maximum, 0.5 mg in 4 hours.
*Tablets in adults—*2.5 to 5 mg P.O. q 6 hours t.i.d. during waking hours. Maximum, 15 mg daily.
*Tablets in children ages 12 to 15—*2.5 mg P.O. q 6 hours t.i.d. during waking hours. Maximum, 7.5 mg daily.

ACTION
Relaxes bronchial smooth muscle by stimulating beta$_2$ receptors and relaxes uterine smooth muscle.

Route	Onset	Peak	Duration
P.O.	30 min	2-3 hr	4-8 hr
S.C.	15 min	30 min	1.5-4 hr

ADVERSE REACTIONS
CNS: *nervousness, tremor, drowsiness, dizziness, headache,* weakness.
CV: *palpitations,* tachycardia, ***arrhythmias,*** flushing.
GI: *vomiting, nausea,* heartburn.
Metabolic: hypokalemia.

Reactions may be *common,* uncommon, ***life-threatening,*** or COMMON AND LIFE-THREATENING.

Respiratory: *paradoxical bronchospasm with prolonged use,* dyspnea.
Skin: diaphoresis.

INTERACTIONS
Drug-drug. *Cardiac glycosides, cyclopropane, halogenated inhaled anesthetics, levodopa:* Increased risk of arrhythmias. Monitor patient closely, and avoid using together with levodopa.
CNS stimulants: Increased CNS stimulation. Avoid using together.
MAO inhibitors: When given with sympathomimetics, may cause severe hypertension (hypertensive crisis). Avoid using together.
Propranolol, other beta blockers: Blocked bronchodilating effects of terbutaline. Avoid using together.

EFFECTS ON LAB TEST RESULTS
• May decrease potassium levels.

CONTRAINDICATIONS
Contraindicated in patients hypersensitive to drug or sympathomimetic amines.

NURSING CONSIDERATIONS
• Use cautiously in patient with CV disorders, hyperthyroidism, diabetes, or seizure disorders.
• Give S.C. injections in lateral deltoid area.
• Protect injection from light. Don't use if discolored.
• Terbutaline may reduce the sensitivity of spirometry for the diagnosis of bronchospasm.
• *Alert:* Don't confuse terbutaline with tolbutamide or terbinafine.

PATIENT TEACHING
• Make sure patient and caregivers understand why patient needs drug.

theophylline
Immediate-release liquids:
Accurbron*, Aerolate, Aquaphyllin, Asmalix*, Bronkodyl*, Elixomin*, Elixophyllin*, Lanophyllin*, Slo-Phyllin, Theoclear-80, Theolair Liquid, Theostat 80*

Immediate-release tablets and capsules:
Bronkodyl, Elixophyllin, Nuelin‡, Quibron T Dividose, Slo-Phyllin

Timed-release tablets:
Lasma§, Quibron-T/SR, Respbid, Sustaire, Theochron, Theolair-SR, Theo-Sav, Theo-Time, T-Phyl, Uniphyl, Uniphyllin Continus§

Timed-release capsules:
Aerolate, Elixophyllin, Nuelin-SR‡, Slo-bid Gyrocaps, Slo-Phyllin, Theobid Duracaps, Theochron, Theoclear L.A., Theo-Dur Sprinkle, Theospan-SR, Theo-24, Theovent Long-Acting

Pregnancy risk category C

AVAILABLE FORMS
Capsules: 100 mg, 200 mg
Capsules (extended-release): 50 mg, 60 mg, 65 mg, 75 mg, 100 mg, 125 mg, 130 mg, 200 mg, 250 mg, 260 mg, 300 mg
D_5W injection: 200 mg in 50 ml or 100 ml; 400 mg in 100 ml, 250 ml, 500 ml, or 1,000 ml; 800 mg in 500 ml or 1,000 ml
Elixir: 27 mg/5 ml*, 50 mg/5 ml*
Oral solution: 27 mg/5 ml, 50 mg/5 ml
Syrup: 27 mg/5 ml, 50 mg/5 ml
Tablets: 100 mg, 125 mg, 200 mg, 250 mg, 300 mg
Tablets (chewable): 100 mg
Tablets (extended-release): 100 mg, 200 mg, 250 mg, 300 mg, 400 mg, 500 mg, 600 mg

INDICATIONS & DOSAGES
Extended-release preparations shouldn't be used to treat acute bronchospasm.
➤**Oral theophylline for acute bronchospasm in patients not currently receiving theophylline—**
Adult nonsmokers and children older than age 16: 5 mg/kg P.O., then 3 mg/kg q 6 hours for two doses. Maintenance dosage is 3 mg/kg q 8 hours.
Children ages 9 to 16: 5 mg/kg P.O.; then 3 mg/kg q 4 hours for three doses. Maintenance dosage is 3 mg/kg q 6 hours.

Children ages 6 months to 9 years: 5 mg/kg P.O.; then 4 mg/kg q 4 hours for three doses. Maintenance dosage is 4 mg/kg q 6 hours.

Adjust-a-dose: For otherwise healthy adult smokers, 5 mg/kg P.O.; then 3 mg/kg q 4 hours for three doses. Maintenance dosage is 3 mg/kg q 6 hours.

For older adults and patients with cor pulmonale, 5 mg/kg P.O.; then 2 mg/kg q 6 hours for two doses. Maintenance dosage is 2 mg/kg q 8 hours.

For adults with heart failure or liver disease, 5 mg/kg P.O.; then 2 mg/kg q 8 hours for two doses. Maintenance dosage is 1 to 2 mg/kg q 12 hours.

➤ **Parenteral theophylline for patients not currently receiving theophylline—**
Loading dose: 4.7 mg/kg I.V. slowly; then maintenance infusion.

Adult nonsmokers and children older than age 16: 0.55 mg/kg/hour I.V. for 12 hours; then 0.39 mg/kg/hour.

Children ages 9 to 16: 0.79 mg/kg/hour I.V. for 12 hours; then 0.63 mg/kg/hour.

Children ages 6 months to 9 years: 0.95 mg/kg/hour I.V. for 12 hours; then 0.79 mg/kg/hour.

Adjust-a-dose: For otherwise healthy adult smokers, 0.79 mg/kg/hour I.V. for 12 hours; then 0.63 mg/kg/hour.

For older adults and patients with cor pulmonale, 0.47 mg/kg/hour I.V. for 12 hours; then 0.24 mg/kg/hour.

For adults with heart failure or liver disease, 0.39 mg/kg/hour I.V. for 12 hours; then 0.08 to 0.16 mg/kg/hour.

➤ **Oral and parenteral theophylline for acute bronchospasm in patients currently receiving theophylline—**
Adults and children: Ideally, dose is based on current theophylline level. Each 0.5 mg/kg I.V. or P.O. loading dose will increase plasma levels by 1 mcg/ml. In emergency situations, some clinicians recommend a 2.5 mg/kg P.O. dose of rapidly absorbed form if patient has no obvious signs or symptoms of theophylline toxicity.

➤ **Chronic bronchospasm—**
Adults and children: Initially, 16 mg/kg or 400 mg P.O. daily, whichever is less, given in three or four divided doses at 6- to 8-hour intervals. Or, 12 mg/kg or 400 mg P.O. daily, whichever is less, in

an extended-release preparation given in two or three divided doses at 8- or 12-hour intervals. Dosage may be increased, as tolerated, at 2- to 3-day intervals to following maximums: adults and children ages 16 and older, 13 mg/kg or 900 mg P.O. daily, whichever is less; children ages 12 to 16, 18 mg/kg P.O. daily; children ages 9 to 12, 20 mg/kg P.O. daily; children younger than age 9, 24 mg/kg P.O. daily.

I.V. ADMINISTRATION
● Use commercially available infusion solution, or mix in D_5W solution.
● Use infusion pump for continuous infusion.

ACTION
Inhibits phosphodiesterase, the enzyme that degrades cAMP, resulting in relaxation of smooth muscle of the bronchial airways and pulmonary blood vessels.

Route	Onset	Peak	Duration
I.V.	15 min	15-30 min	Unknown
P.O.	15-60 min	1-2 hr	Unknown
P.O. (extended)	15-60 min	4-7 hr	Unknown

ADVERSE REACTIONS
CNS: *restlessness, dizziness,* headache, *insomnia,* irritability, **seizures,** muscle twitching.
CV: *palpitations, sinus tachycardia,* extrasystoles, flushing, marked hypotension, **arrhythmias.**
GI: *nausea, vomiting,* diarrhea, epigastric pain.
Metabolic: urinary catecholamines.
Respiratory: tachypnea, **respiratory arrest.**

INTERACTIONS
Drug-drug. *Adenosine:* Decreased antiarrhythmic effectiveness. Higher doses of adenosine may be needed.
Allopurinol, calcium channel blockers, cimetidine, disulfiram, influenza virus vaccine, interferon, macrolide antibiotics (such as erythromycin), methotrexate, oral contraceptives, quinolone antibiotics (such as ciprofloxacin): Decreased hepatic clearance of theophylline; elevated theophylline

levels. Monitor patient for evidence of toxicity.

Barbiturates, nicotine, phenytoin, rifampin: Enhanced metabolism and decreased theophylline levels. Monitor patient for decreased effect.

Beta blockers: Antagonism; nadolol and propranolol, especially, may cause bronchospasm in sensitive patients. Use together cautiously.

Carbamazepine, isoniazid, loop diuretics: May increase or decrease theophylline levels. Monitor theophylline levels.

Ephedrine, other sympathomimetics: May exhibit synergistic toxicity with these drugs, predisposing patient to arrhythmias. Monitor patient closely.

Lithium: May increase lithium excretion. Monitor patient closely.

Drug-herb. *Cacao tree:* Possible inhibition of theophylline metabolism. Advise patient to avoid using together.

Cayenne: Increased risk of theophylline toxicity. Ask patient about use of herbal remedies, and advise him to use together cautiously.

Ephedra: May increase risk of adverse reactions. Discourage use together.

Guarana: May cause additive CNS and CV effects. Discourage use together.

Ipriflavone: May increase risk of theophylline toxicity. Advise patient to use together cautiously.

St. John's wort: May lower levels of theophylline. Discourage use together.

Drug-food. *Any food:* Accelerated release of theophylline from extended-release products. Tell patient to take Theo-24 on an empty stomach.

Caffeine: Decreased hepatic clearance of theophylline; elevated theophylline levels. Monitor patient for evidence of toxicity.

Drug-lifestyle. *Smoking:* Increased elimination of theophylline, increasing dosage requirements. Monitor theophylline response and serum levels.

EFFECTS ON LAB TEST RESULTS

● May increase plasma free fatty acid levels.

CONTRAINDICATIONS

Contraindicated in patients hypersensitive to xanthine compounds (caffeine, theobromine) and in those with active peptic ulcer or poorly controlled seizure disorders.

NURSING CONSIDERATIONS

● Use cautiously in young children, infants, neonates, elderly patients, and those with COPD, cardiac failure, cor pulmonale, renal or hepatic disease, peptic ulceration, hyperthyroidism, diabetes mellitus, glaucoma, severe hypoxemia, hypertension, compromised cardiac or circulatory function, angina, acute MI, or sulfite sensitivity.

● *Alert:* Don't confuse extended-release forms with regular-release forms.

● Dosage may need to be increased in cigarette smokers and in habitual marijuana smokers because smoking causes drug to be metabolized faster.

● Give drug around-the-clock, using extended-release product at bedtime.

● Depending on assay used, theophylline levels may be falsely elevated in the presence of furosemide, phenylbutazone, probenecid, theobromine, caffeine, tea, chocolate, cola beverages, and acetaminophen.

● Monitor vital signs; measure and record fluid intake and output. Expect improved quality of pulse and respirations.

● People metabolize xanthines at different rates; dosage is determined by monitoring response, tolerance, pulmonary function, and theophylline levels. Theophylline levels should range from 10 to 20 mcg/ml; toxicity has been reported at levels above 20 mcg/ml.

● *Alert:* Evidence of toxicity includes tachycardia, anorexia, nausea, vomiting, diarrhea, restlessness, irritability, and headache. The presence of any of these signs in patients taking theophylline warrants checking theophylline levels and adjusting dosage, as indicated.

● *Alert:* Don't confuse Theolair with Thyrolar.

PATIENT TEACHING

● Supply instructions for home care and dosage schedule.

● Warn patient not to dissolve, crush, or chew extended-release products. Small children unable to swallow these can ingest (without chewing) the contents of capsules sprinkled over soft food.

• Tell patient to relieve GI symptoms by taking oral drug with full glass of water after meals, although food in stomach delays absorption.

• Warn patient to take drug regularly, only as directed. Patients tend to want to take extra "breathing pills."

• Inform elderly patient that dizziness is common at start of therapy.

• Urge patient to tell prescriber about any other drugs used. OTC drugs or herbal remedies may contain ephedrine or theophylline salts; excessive CNS stimulation may result.

• If patient smokes, have him inform prescriber if he quits. A dosage reduction may be necessary to prevent toxicity.

43

Expectorants and antitussives

benzonatate
codeine phosphate
  (See Chapter 26, NARCOTIC AND
  OPIOID ANALGESICS.)
codeine sulfate
  (See Chapter 26, NARCOTIC AND
  OPIOID ANALGESICS.)
dextromethorphan
  hydrobromide
diphenhydramine
  hydrochloride
  (See Chapter 41, ANTIHISTAMINES.)
guaifenesin
hydromorphone hydrochloride
  (See Chapter 26, NARCOTIC AND
  OPIOID ANALGESICS.)

COMBINATION PRODUCTS
Preparations are available in the following
combinations:
• Expectorants with decongestants, anti-
histamines, or both
• Antitussives with decongestants, anti-
histamines, or both
• Expectorants and antitussives
• Expectorants and antitussives with de-
congestants, antihistamines, or both

---

benzonatate
Tessalon, Tessalon Perles

Pregnancy risk category C

AVAILABLE FORMS
Capsules: 100 mg, 200 mg

INDICATIONS & DOSAGES
➤ **Symptomatic relief of cough—**
Adults and children older than age 10:
100 to 200 mg P.O. t.i.d.; up to 600 mg
daily may be needed.

ACTION
Chemical relative of tetracaine that suppresses the cough reflex by direct action
on the cough center in the medulla and
through an anesthetic action on stretch

receptors of vagal afferent fibers in the
respiratory passages, lungs, and pleura.

Route	Onset	Peak	Duration
P.O.	15-20 min	Unknown	3-8 hr

ADVERSE REACTIONS
CNS: dizziness, headache, sedation.
EENT: nasal congestion, burning sensa-
tion in eyes.
GI: nausea, constipation, GI upset.
Other: chills, hypersensitivity reactions.

INTERACTIONS
None significant.

EFFECTS ON LAB TEST RESULTS
None reported.

CONTRAINDICATIONS
Contraindicated in patients hypersensitive
to drug or related compounds.

NURSING CONSIDERATIONS
• Use cautiously in patients hypersensitive
to PABA anesthetics (procaine, tetracaine)
because cross-sensitivity reactions may
occur.
• Don't use benzonatate when cough is a
valuable diagnostic sign or is beneficial
(as after thoracic surgery).
• Monitor cough type and frequency.
• Use with percussion and chest vibration.

PATIENT TEACHING
• Warn patient not to chew capsules or
dissolve in mouth. Produces either local
anesthesia that may result in aspiration or
CNS stimulation that may cause restlessness, tremor, and seizures.
• Instruct patient to report adverse reactions.
• Instruct patient to protect drug from
light and moisture.
• *Alert:* Make sure patient understands that
persistent cough may indicate a serious
condition and that he should contact his
prescriber if cough lasts longer than 1

---

*Liquid contains alcohol.   **May contain tartrazine.   †Canada   ‡Australia   §U.K.   ◊OTC

week, recurs frequently, or is accompanied by high fever, rash, or severe headache.

---

dextromethorphan hydrobromide
Balminil DM◇, Benylin DM◇, Broncho-Grippol-DM†, Buckley's DM, Children's Hold◇, Delsym, Hold◇, Koffex DM†, Pertussin CS◇, Pertussin ES◇, Robitussin Pediatric◇, St. Joseph Cough Suppressant for Children◇, Trocal◇, Vicks Formula 44e Pediatric◇

More commonly available in combination products, such as Anti-Tuss DM Expectorant◇, Benylin Expectorant◇, Cheracol D Cough◇, Glycotuss-dM◇, Guiamid D.M. Liquid◇, Guiatuss-DM◇, Halotussin-DM◇, Kolephrin GG/DM◇, Mytussin DM◇, Naldecon Senior DX◇, Pertussin CS◇, Rhinosyn-DMX Expectorant◇, Robitussin-DM◇, Scot-Tussin DM Cough Chasers◇, Tolu-Sed DM◇, Tuss-DM◇, Unproco◇, Vicks Pediatric 44E◇

Pregnancy risk category C

AVAILABLE FORMS
Liquid (extended-release): 30 mg/5 ml ◇
Lozenges: 5 mg◇, 7.5 mg◇
Solution: 3.5 mg/5 ml, 5 mg/5 ml*◇, 7.5 mg/5 ml◇, 10 mg/5 ml*◇, 15 mg/5 ml*◇, 15 mg/15 ml*◇, 12.5 mg/5 ml

INDICATIONS & DOSAGES
➤ **Nonproductive cough—**
Adults and children age 12 and older: 10 to 20 mg P.O. q 4 hours, or 30 mg q 6 to 8 hours. Or, 60 mg extended-release liquid b.i.d. Maximum, 120 mg daily.
Children ages 6 to 11: 5 to 10 mg P.O. q 4 hours, or 15 mg q 6 to 8 hours. Or, 30 mg extended-release liquid b.i.d. Maximum, 60 mg daily.
Children ages 2 to 5: 2.5 to 5 mg P.O. q 4 hours, or 7.5 mg q 6 to 8 hours. Or, 15 mg extended-release liquid b.i.d. Maximum, 30 mg daily.

Children younger than age 2: Dosages must be individualized.

ACTION
Antitussive that suppresses the cough reflex by direct action on the cough center in the medulla.

Route	Onset	Peak	Duration
P.O.	< 0.5 hr	Unknown	3-6 hr

ADVERSE REACTIONS
CNS: drowsiness, dizziness.
GI: nausea, vomiting, stomach pain.

INTERACTIONS
Drug-drug. *MAO inhibitors:* Risk of hypotension, coma, hyperpyrexia, and death. Avoid using together.
Selegiline: Risk of confusion, coma, hyperpyrexia. Avoid using together.
Drug-herb. *Parsley:* May promote or produce serotonin syndrome. Discourage use together.

EFFECTS ON LAB TEST RESULTS
None reported.

CONTRAINDICATIONS
Contraindicated in patients currently taking MAO inhibitors or within 2 weeks of discontinuing MAO inhibitors.

NURSING CONSIDERATIONS
• Use cautiously in atopic children, sedated or debilitated patients, and patients confined to the supine position. Also, use cautiously in patients sensitive to aspirin or tartrazine dyes.
• Don't use dextromethorphan when cough is a valuable diagnostic sign or is beneficial (as after thoracic surgery).
• Dextromethorphan 15 to 30 mg is equivalent to 8 to 15 mg codeine as an antitussive.
• Drug produces no analgesia or addiction and little or no CNS depression.
• Use drug with chest percussion and vibration.
• Monitor cough type and frequency.

PATIENT TEACHING
• Instruct patient to take drug exactly as prescribed.

Reactions may be *common*, uncommon, *life-threatening*, or COMMON AND LIFE-THREATENING.

• Tell patient to report adverse reactions.
• *Alert:* Make sure patient understands that persistent cough may indicate a serious condition and that he should contact his prescriber if cough lasts longer than 1 week, recurs frequently, or is accompanied by high fever, rash, or severe headache.

---

guaifenesin (glyceryl guaiacolate)

Anti-Tuss*◊, Balminil Expectorant†, Breonesin◊, Duratuss-G, Fenesin, Gee-Gee◊, GG-CEN*◊, Glyate*◊, Glycotuss◊, Glytuss◊, Guiatuss*◊, Halotussin, Humibid L.A., Humibid Sprinkle, Hytuss◊, Hytuss 2X◊, Naldecon Senior EX◊, Resyl†, Robitussin*◊, Scot-Tussin Expectorant◊, Uni-tussin*◊

Pregnancy risk category C

AVAILABLE FORMS
Capsules: 200 mg◊
Capsules (extended-release): 300 mg
Solution: 100 mg/5 ml*◊, 200 mg/5 ml
Tablets: 100 mg◊, 200 mg◊
Tablets (extended-release): 600 mg, 1,200 mg

INDICATIONS & DOSAGES
➤ **Expectorant—**
Adults and children age 12 and older: 200 to 400 mg P.O. q 4 hours, or 600 to 1,200 mg extended-release capsules or tablets q 12 hours. Maximum, 2,400 mg daily.
Children ages 6 to 11: 100 to 200 mg P.O. q 4 hours. Maximum, 1,200 mg daily.
Children ages 2 to 5: 50 to 100 mg P.O. q 4 hours. Maximum, 600 mg daily.

ACTION
Increases production of respiratory tract fluids to help liquefy and reduce the viscosity of tenacious secretions.

Route	Onset	Peak	Duration
P.O.	Unknown	Unknown	Unknown

ADVERSE REACTIONS
CNS: dizziness, headache.

GI: vomiting, nausea.
Skin: rash.

INTERACTIONS
None significant.

EFFECTS ON LAB TEST RESULTS
None reported.

CONTRAINDICATIONS
Contraindicated in patients hypersensitive to drug.

NURSING CONSIDERATIONS
• Drug is used to liquefy thick, tenacious sputum. Evidence suggests that guaifenesin is effective as an expectorant, but no evidence exists to support its role as an antitussive.
• Monitor cough type and frequency.
• *Alert:* Don't confuse guaifenesin with guanfacine.

PATIENT TEACHING
• *Alert:* Make sure patient understands that persistent cough may indicate a serious condition and that he should contact his prescriber if cough lasts longer than 1 week, recurs frequently, or is accompanied by high fever, rash, or severe headache.
• Inform patient that drug shouldn't be used for chronic or persistent cough, such as that occurring with smoking, asthma, chronic bronchitis, or emphysema.
• Advise patient to take each dose with one glass of water; increasing fluid intake may prove beneficial.
• Encourage deep-breathing exercises.

44

Miscellaneous respiratory drugs

acetylcysteine
beclomethasone dipropionate
beractant
budesonide
calfactant
cromolyn sodium
dornase alfa
flunisolide
fluticasone propionate
montelukast sodium
palivizumab
triamcinolone acetonide
zafirlukast
zileuton

COMBINATION PRODUCTS
ADVAIR: fluticasone propionate 100 mcg and salmeterol xinafoate 50 mcg.
ADVAIR: fluticasone propionate 250 mcg and salmeterol xinafoate 50 mcg.
ADVAIR: fluticasone propionate 500 mcg and salmeterol xinafoate 50 mcg.

---

acetylcysteine
Mucomyst, Mucomyst-10,
Mucosil-10, Mucosil-20,
Parvolex†‡

Pregnancy risk category B

AVAILABLE FORMS
Injection: 200 mg/ml‡
Solution: 10%, 20%

INDICATIONS & DOSAGES
➤ Adjunct therapy for abnormal viscid or inspissated mucous secretions in patients with pneumonia, bronchitis, bronchiectasis, primary amyloidosis of the lung, tuberculosis, cystic fibrosis, emphysema, atelectasis, pulmonary complications of thoracic surgery, or CV surgery—
Adults and children: 1 to 2 ml 10% or 20% solution by direct instillation into trachea as often as q hour. Or, 1 to 10 ml of 20% solution or 2 to 20 ml of 10% solution by nebulization q 2 to 6 hours, p.r.n.

➤ Acetaminophen toxicity—
P.O.
Adults and children: Initially, 140 mg/kg P.O., then 70 mg/kg P.O. q 4 hours for 17 doses.
I.V.‡
Adults: Dilute initial dose of 150 mg/kg in 200 ml of D_5W and infuse over 15 minutes. Dilute second dose of 50 mg/kg in 500 ml of D_5W and give over 4 hours. Dilute final dose of 100 mg/kg in 1,000 ml of D_5W and infuse over 16 hours.

I.V. ADMINISTRATION
• To prepare I.V. infusion, dilute calculated dose in D_5W.

ACTION
Mucolytic that reduces the viscosity of pulmonary secretions by splitting disulfide linkages between mucoprotein molecular complexes. Also, restores liver stores of glutathione to treat acetaminophen toxicity.

Route	Onset	Peak	Duration
I.V., P.O., inhalation	Unknown	Unknown	Unknown

ADVERSE REACTIONS
CNS: drowsiness.
CV: tachycardia, hypotension, hypertension, chest tightness.
EENT: *rhinorrhea.*
GI: *stomatitis, nausea, vomiting.*
Respiratory: *bronchospasm.*
Skin: rash, clamminess, urticaria.
Other: fever, *angioedema,* chills.

INTERACTIONS
Drug-drug. *Activated charcoal:* Limits acetylcysteine's effectiveness. Don't give activated charcoal before or with acetylcysteine.

EFFECTS ON LAB TEST RESULTS
None reported.

Reactions may be *common,* uncommon, *life-threatening,* or COMMON AND LIFE-THREATENING.

CONTRAINDICATIONS

Contraindicated in patients hypersensitive to drug.

NURSING CONSIDERATIONS

• Use cautiously in elderly or debilitated patients with severe respiratory insufficiency.

• Use plastic, glass, stainless steel, or another nonreactive metal when giving by nebulization. Hand-bulb nebulizers aren't recommended because output is too small and particle size too large.

• Drug is physically or chemically incompatible with tetracyclines, erythromycin lactobionate, amphotericin B, and ampicillin sodium. If given by aerosol inhalation, these drugs should be nebulized separately. Iodized oil, trypsin, and hydrogen peroxide are physically incompatible with acetylcysteine; don't add to nebulizer.

• Drug smells strongly of sulfur. Mixing oral form with juice or cola improves its palatability.

• Monitor cough type and frequency.

• *Alert:* Monitor patient for bronchospasm, especially if he has asthma.

• After opening, store in refrigerator; use within 96 hours.

• *Alert:* Acetylcysteine is given to treat acetaminophen overdose within 24 hours after ingestion. Start treatment immediately as prescribed; don't wait for results of acetaminophen levels.

• When used orally to treat acetaminophen overdose, dilute oral doses with cola, fruit juice, or water before giving. Dilute the 20% solution to 5% (add 3 ml of diluent to each ml of acetylcysteine). If patient vomits within 1 hour of receiving loading or maintenance dose, repeat dose. Diluted solution should be used within 1 hour.

• When acetaminophen levels return to below toxic level according to nomogram, acetylcysteine therapy may be discontinued.

• *Alert:* Don't confuse acetylcysteine with acetylcholine.

PATIENT TEACHING

• Warn patient that drug may have a foul taste or smell that some patients find distressing.

• For maximum effect, instruct patient to clear his airway by coughing before aerosol administration.

---

beclomethasone dipropionate
Beclodisk†, Becloforte Inhaler‡, Beclovent, Beclovent Rotacaps†, Beconase, Beconase AQ, Vancenase, Vancenase AQ, Vanceril

Pregnancy risk category C

AVAILABLE FORMS

Nasal inhalation: 42 mcg/metered spray, 84 mcg/metered spray
Oral inhalation aerosol: 42 mcg/metered spray, 50 mcg/metered spray‡, 84 mcg/metered spray

INDICATIONS & DOSAGES

➤ **Chronic asthma—**
Adults and children age 12 and older: 2 inhalations (84 mcg) t.i.d. or q.i.d. Or, 4 inhalations (168 mcg) b.i.d. Maximum, 20 inhalations (840 mcg) daily.
Children ages 6 to 12: 1 or 2 inhalations (42 to 84 mcg) t.i.d. or q.i.d. Or, 4 inhalations b.i.d. Maximum, 10 inhalations (420 mcg) daily.
➤ **Perennial or seasonal rhinitis; prevention of recurrence of nasal polyps after surgical removal—**
Nasal inhalation
Adults and children older than age 12: 1 spray (42 mcg) in each nostril b.i.d. to q.i.d. Usual total dose is 168 to 336 mcg daily.
Children ages 6 to 12: 1 spray in each nostril t.i.d. (252 mcg daily).
Nasal spray
Adults and children older than age 6: 1 or 2 sprays of single strength (42 to 84 mcg) in each nostril b.i.d. If the double strength preparation is used, 1 or 2 sprays (84 to 168 mcg) into each nostril once daily (168 to 336 mcg). Maintenance dosage: 1 spray (42 mcg) into each nostril t.i.d.

ACTION

Unknown. May decrease inflammation by decreasing the number and activity of inflammatory cells, inhibiting bronchoconstrictor mechanisms producing direct

---

smooth-muscle relaxation, and decreasing airway hyperresponsiveness. In nasal passages it produces anti-inflammatory and vasoconstricting effects.

Route	Onset	Peak	Duration
Inhalation (nasal)	Up to 2 wk	Unknown	Unknown
Inhalation (oral)	1-4 wk	Unknown	Unknown

ADVERSE REACTIONS
EENT: *hoarseness,* fungal infection of throat, *throat irritation, nose irritation.*
GI: dry mouth, *fungal infection of mouth.*
Metabolic: suppression of hypothalamic-pituitary-adrenal function, adrenal insufficiency.
Respiratory: *bronchospasm,* wheezing, cough.
Other: *angioedema,* hypersensitivity reactions, facial edema.

INTERACTIONS
None significant.

EFFECTS ON LAB TEST RESULTS
None reported.

CONTRAINDICATIONS
Contraindicated in patients hypersensitive to drug or its ingredients (fluorocarbons, oleic acid) and in those with status asthmaticus, nonasthmatic bronchial diseases, or asthma controlled by bronchodilators or other noncorticosteroids alone.

NURSING CONSIDERATIONS
● Use with extreme caution, if at all, in patients with tuberculosis, fungal or bacterial infections, ocular herpes simplex, or systemic viral infections.
● Use cautiously in patients receiving systemic corticosteroid therapy.
● A spacer device may help ensure delivery of the proper dose and decrease local (oral) adverse effects.
● Check mucous membranes frequently for signs and symptoms of fungal infection.
● During times of stress (trauma, surgery, or infection), systemic corticosteroids may be needed to prevent adrenal insufficiency in previously corticosteroid-dependent patients.

● Periodic measurement of growth and development may be needed during high-dose or prolonged therapy in children.
● Nasal sprays should be discontinued after 3 weeks if symptomatic improvement isn't evident.
● *Alert:* Taper oral corticosteroid therapy slowly. Acute adrenal insufficiency and death have occurred in patients with asthma who changed abruptly from oral corticosteroids to beclomethasone.
● *Alert:* Don't confuse Vanceril with Vansil.

PATIENT TEACHING
Oral inhaler
● Inform patient that drug doesn't relieve acute asthma attacks.
● Tell patient who needs a bronchodilator to use it several minutes before beclomethasone.
● Instruct patient to carry or wear medical identification indicating his need for supplemental systemic corticosteroids during stress.
● If patient uses a metered-dose inhaler, instruct him to shake canister well before use.
● Advise patient to allow 1 minute to elapse before taking subsequent puffs of drug, and to hold his breath for a few seconds to enhance action of drug.
● Instruct patient to contact prescriber if response to therapy decreases or if signs or symptoms don't improve within 3 weeks; dosage may need to be adjusted. Tell him not to exceed recommended dosage on his own.
● Tell patient to keep inhaler clean and unobstructed, washing it with warm water and drying it thoroughly.
● Advise patient to prevent oral fungal infections by gargling or rinsing his mouth with water after each use. Caution him not to swallow the water.
● Tell patient to report evidence of corticosteroid withdrawal, including fatigue, weakness, arthralgia, orthostatic hypotension, and dyspnea.
● Instruct patient to store drug at 59° to 86° F (15° to 30° C). Advise patient to ensure delivery of proper dose by gently warming canister to room temperature before using.

Nasal inhaler
- It may take 1 to 2 weeks of regular treatment before relief is evident.
- Tell patient to take medication at regular intervals for best results.
- Advise patient to blow nose gently before using nasal spray.
- Tell patient to follow manufacturer's instructions for use and cleaning recommendations.

---

beractant (natural lung surfactant)
Survanta

Pregnancy risk category NR

AVAILABLE FORMS
Suspension for intratracheal instillation: 25 mg/ml

INDICATIONS & DOSAGES
➤ **Prevention of respiratory distress syndrome (RDS), also known as hyaline membrane disease, in premature neonates weighing 1,250 g (2 lb, 12 ounces) or less at birth or having symptoms consistent with surfactant deficiency—**
Neonates: 4 ml/kg intratracheally. Divide each dose into four quarter-doses and give each quarter-dose with infant in a different position to ensure even distribution of drug; between quarter-doses, use a hand-held resuscitation bag at 60 breaths/minute and sufficient oxygen to prevent cyanosis. Give drug as soon as possible, preferably within 15 minutes of birth. Repeat in 6 hours if respiratory distress continues. Give no more than four doses in 48 hours.
➤ **Rescue treatment of RDS in premature infants—**
Neonates: 4 ml/kg intratracheally; before giving, increase ventilator rate to 60 breaths/minute with an inspiratory time of 0.5 second and a fraction of inspired oxygen of 1. Divide each dose into four quarter-doses and give each quarter-dose with infant in a different position to ensure even distribution of drug; between quarter-doses, continue mechanical ventilation for at least 30 seconds or until stable. Give dose as soon as RDS is confirmed by X-ray, preferably within 8 hours of birth. Repeat in 6 hours if respiratory distress con-

tinues. Give no more than four doses in 48 hours.

ACTION
Lowers alveolar surface tension during respiration and stabilizes alveoli against collapse. It's an extract of bovine lung that contains neutral lipids, fatty acids, surfactant-related proteins, and phospholipids that mimics naturally occurring surfactant; palmitic acid, tripalmitin, and colfosceril palmitate are added to standardize the solution's composition.

Route	Onset	Peak	Duration
Intra-tracheal	0.5-2 hr	Unknown	2-3 days

ADVERSE REACTIONS
CV: TRANSIENT BRADYCARDIA, vasoconstriction, hypotension.
Hematologic: decreased oxygen saturation, hypocapnia, hypercapnia.
Respiratory: endotracheal tube reflux or blockage, *apnea.*
Skin: pallor.

INTERACTIONS
None significant.

EFFECTS ON LAB TEST RESULTS
None reported.

CONTRAINDICATIONS
No known contraindications.

NURSING CONSIDERATIONS
- Beractant should be given only by staff experienced in caring for clinically unstable premature neonates, including neonatal intubation and airway management.
- Accurate weight determination is essential to proper measurement of dosage.
- Continuously monitor neonate before, during, and after beractant administration. The endotracheal tube may be suctioned before giving drug; allow neonate to stabilize before proceeding with administration.
- Refrigerate at 36° to 46° F (2° to 8° C). Warm before use by allowing drug to stand at room temperature for at least 20 minutes or by holding in hand for at least 8 minutes. Don't use artificial warming methods. Unopened vials that have been

warmed to room temperature may be returned to the refrigerator within 24 hours; however, warm and return drug to the refrigerator only once. Vials are for single use only; discard unused drug.

• Beractant doesn't need sonication or reconstitution before use. Inspect contents before giving; make sure color is off-white to light brown and that contents are uniform. If settling occurs, swirl vial gently; don't shake. Some foaming is normal.

• Use a large-bore needle (20G or larger) to draw up drug; don't use a filter. Give drug using a #5 French end-hole catheter. Premeasure and shorten catheter before use. Fill catheter with beractant and discard excess drug so that only total dose to be given remains in the syringe. Insert catheter into neonate's endotracheal tube; make sure catheter tip protrudes just beyond end of tube above neonate's carina. Don't instill drug into a mainstream bronchus.

• Even distribution of drug is important. For example, give each dose in four quarter-doses, with each quarter-dose being given over 2 to 3 seconds and with the patient positioned differently after each use. Between giving quarter-doses, remove the catheter and ventilate the patient. Give the first quarter-dose with the patient's head and body inclined slightly downward, and the head turned to the right. Give the second quarter-dose with the head turned to the left. Then, incline the head and body slightly upward with the head turned to the right to give the third quarter-dose. Turn the head to the left for the fourth quarter-dose.

• Immediately after giving, moist breath sounds and crackles can occur. Don't suction the neonate for 1 hour unless other signs or symptoms of airway obstruction are evident.

• Continuous monitoring of ECG and transcutaneous oxygen saturation are essential; frequent arterial blood pressure monitoring and frequent arterial blood gas sampling are highly desirable.

• Transient bradycardia and oxygen desaturation are common after dosing.

• **Alert:** Beractant can rapidly affect oxygenation and lung compliance. Peak ventilator inspiratory pressures may need to be adjusted if chest expansion improves substantially after drug administration. Notify prescriber and adjust immediately as directed because lung overdistention and fatal pulmonary air leakage may result.

• Audiovisual materials that describe dosage and usage procedures are available from the manufacturer.

• **Alert:** Don't confuse Survanta with Sufenta.

PATIENT TEACHING
• Inform parents of neonate's need for drug, and explain drug action and use.
• Encourage parents to ask questions, and address their concerns.

---

budesonide
Pulmicort Turbuhaler

Pregnancy risk category C

AVAILABLE FORMS
Dry powder inhaler: 200 mcg/dose

INDICATIONS & DOSAGES
➤ **Prophylactic therapy in maintenance treatment of asthma—**
In all patients, use lowest effective dose after stabilization of asthma.
Adults previously on bronchodilators alone: Initially, inhaled dose of 200 to 400 mcg b.i.d. to maximum of 400 mcg b.i.d.
Adults previously on inhaled corticosteroids: Initially, inhaled dose of 200 to 400 mcg b.i.d. to maximum of 800 mcg b.i.d.
Adults previously on oral corticosteroids: Initially, inhaled dose of 400 to 800 mcg b.i.d. to maximum of 800 mcg b.i.d.
Children older than age 6 previously on bronchodilators alone or inhaled corticosteroids: Initially, inhaled dose of 200 mcg b.i.d. to maximum of 400 mcg b.i.d.
Children older than age 6 previously on oral corticosteroids: Highest recommended dose is 400 mcg b.i.d.
Children ages 1 to 8: (Respules) 0.25 mg via jet nebulizer with compressor once daily. Increase to 0.5 mg q.d. or 0.25 mg b.i.d. in child not receiving systemic or inhaled corticosteroids or 1 mg daily or 0.5 mg b.i.d. if child is receiving oral corticosteroids.

ACTION

Anti-inflammatory corticosteroid that exhibits potent glucocorticoid activity and weak mineralocorticoid activity. The exact mechanism of the corticosteroids isn't known, but they have a wide range of inhibitory activities against such cell types as mast cells and macrophages and mediators (such as leukotrienes) involved in allergic and nonallergic inflammation.

Route	Onset	Peak	Duration
Inhalation	24 hr	1-2 wk	Unknown

ADVERSE REACTIONS

CNS: *headache,* asthenia, pain, insomnia, syncope, hypertonia.
EENT: *sinusitis, pharyngitis,* rhinitis, voice alteration.
GI: oral candidiasis, dyspepsia, gastroenteritis, nausea, dry mouth, taste perversion, vomiting, abdominal pain.
Metabolic: weight gain.
Musculoskeletal: back pain, fractures, myalgia.
Respiratory: *respiratory tract infections,* increased cough, **bronchospasm.**
Skin: ecchymosis.
Other: flulike symptoms, fever, hypersensitivity reactions.

INTERACTIONS

Drug-drug. *Ketoconazole:* May inhibit metabolism of budesonide and increase plasma levels. Monitor patient.

EFFECTS ON LAB TEST RESULTS

None reported.

CONTRAINDICATIONS

Contraindicated in patients hypersensitive to drug and in those with status asthmaticus or other acute asthma episodes.

NURSING CONSIDERATIONS

● Use cautiously, if at all, in patients with active or quiescent tuberculosis of the respiratory tract, ocular herpes simplex, or untreated systemic fungal, bacterial, viral, or parasitic infections.
● When transferring from systemic corticosteroid to budesonide, use caution and gradually decrease corticosteroid dose to prevent adrenal insufficiency.

● Drug doesn't remove the need for systemic corticosteroid therapy in some situations.
● If bronchospasm occurs after using budesonide, stop therapy and treat with a bronchodilator.
● Improved lung function has been observed within 24 hours of starting budesonide treatment, although maximum benefit may not be achieved for 1 to 2 weeks or longer.
● Watch for *Candida* infections of the mouth or pharynx.
● *Alert:* Corticosteroids may increase risk of developing serious or fatal infections in patients exposed to viral illnesses, such as chickenpox or measles.
● In rare cases, inhaled corticosteroids have been linked to increased intraocular pressure and cataract development. If local irritation occurs, drug should be discontinued.

PATIENT TEACHING

● Tell patient that budesonide inhaler isn't a bronchodilator and isn't intended to treat acute episodes of asthma.
● Instruct patient to use the inhaler at regular intervals as follows because effectiveness depends on twice-daily use on a regular basis:
–Pulmicort Turbuhaler must be kept upright (mouthpiece on top) during loading to provide the correct dose.
–Turbuhaler must be primed when the unit is used for the first time. To prime, hold the unit upright and turn the brown grip fully to the right, then fully to the left until it clicks. Repeat priming.
–When loading the first dose, the unit is held upright and the brown grip turned to the right and then to the left until it clicks.
–Tell patient to turn his head away from the inhaler and breathe out.
–During inhalation, Turbuhaler must be in the upright or horizontal position.
–Tell patient not to shake inhaler.
–Instruct patient to place mouthpiece between lips and to inhale forcefully and deeply.
–Tell patient that he may not taste the drug or sense it entering his lungs, but this doesn't mean it isn't effective.

---

*Liquid contains alcohol.   **May contain tartrazine.   †Canada   ‡Australia   §U.K.   ◇OTC

–Tell patient not to exhale through the Turbuhaler. If more than one dose is required, repeat steps.

–Advise patient to rinse his mouth with water and then spit out the water after each dose to decrease the risk of developing oral candidiasis.

–When 20 doses remain in the Turbuhaler, a red mark appears in the indicator window. When red mark reaches the bottom, it's empty.

–Tell patient not to use Turbuhaler with a spacer device and not to chew or bite the mouthpiece.

–Replace mouthpiece cover after use and always keep it clean and dry.

• Tell patient that improvement in asthma control may be seen within 24 hours, although the maximum benefit may not appear for 1 to 2 weeks. If signs or symptoms worsen during this time, patient should contact prescriber.

• Advise patient to avoid exposure to chickenpox or measles and to contact prescriber if exposure occurs.

• Instruct patient to carry or wear medical identification indicating need for supplementary corticosteroids during periods of stress or an asthma attack.

• Tell patient to read and follow the patient information leaflet contained in the package.

---

calfactant
Infasurf

Pregnancy risk category NR

AVAILABLE FORMS
Intratracheal suspension: 35 mg phospholipids and 0.65 mg proteins/ml; 6-ml vial

INDICATIONS & DOSAGES
➤ **Prevention of respiratory distress syndrome (RDS) in premature infants under 29 weeks' gestational age at high risk for RDS; treatment of infants younger than 72 hours of age in whom RDS develops (confirmed by clinical and radiologic findings) and who need endotracheal intubation—**
Newborns: 3 ml/kg of body weight at birth intratracheally, given in two aliquots

of 1.5 ml/kg each, q 12 hours for total of three doses.

ACTION
Nonpyrogenic lung surfactant that modifies alveolar surface tension, thereby stabilizing the alveoli.

Route	Onset	Peak	Duration
Intra-tracheal	24-48 hr	Unknown	Unknown

ADVERSE REACTIONS
CV: BRADYCARDIA.
Respiratory: AIRWAY OBSTRUCTION, APNEA, *hypoventilation, cyanosis.*
Other: *reflux of drug into endotracheal tube,* dislodgment of endotracheal tube.

INTERACTIONS
None significant.

EFFECTS ON LAB TEST RESULTS
None reported.

CONTRAINDICATIONS
No known contraindications.

NURSING CONSIDERATIONS
• Drug should be given under supervision of medical staff experienced in the acute care of newborn infants with respiratory failure who need intubation.

• Store drug at 36° to 46° F (2° to 8° C). It isn't necessary to warm drug before use.

• Unopened, unused vials that have warmed to room temperature can be re-refrigerated within 24 hours for future use. Avoid repeated warming to room temperature.

• Suspension settles during storage. Gentle swirling or agitation of the vial is commonly needed for redispersion. Don't shake vial. Visible flecks in the suspension and foaming at the surface are normal.

• *Alert:* Drug is intended only for intratracheal use; to prevent RDS, give to infant as soon as possible after birth, preferably within 30 minutes.

• Withdraw dose into a syringe from single-use vial using a 20G or larger needle; avoid excessive foaming.

• Give through a side-port adapter into the endotracheal tube. Two medical staff should be present during dosing. Give

---

dose in two aliquots of 1.5 ml/kg each. Place infant on one side after first aliquot and other side after second aliquot. Give while ventilation is continued over 20 to 30 breaths for each aliquot, with small bursts timed only during the inspiratory cycles. Evaluate respiratory status and reposition infant between each aliquot.

• Monitor patient for reflux of drug into endotracheal tube, cyanosis, bradycardia, or airway obstruction during the dosing procedure. If these occur, stop drug and take appropriate measures to stabilize infant. After infant is stable, resume dosing with appropriate monitoring.

• After giving drug, carefully monitor infant so that oxygen therapy and ventilatory support can be modified in response to improvements in oxygenation and lung compliance.

• Each single-use vial should be entered only once; discard unused material.

PATIENT TEACHING

• Explain to parents the function of drug in preventing and treating RDS.

• Notify parents that, although infant may improve rapidly after treatment, he may continue to need intubation and mechanical ventilation.

• Notify parents of possible adverse effects of drug, including bradycardia, reflux into endotracheal tube, airway obstruction, cyanosis, dislodgment of endotracheal tube, and hypoventilation.

• Reassure parents that infant will be carefully monitored.

---

cromolyn sodium (sodium cromoglycate)
Crolom, Gastrocrom, Intal, Intal Inhaler, Intal Nebulizer Solution, Nasalcrom, Rynacrom†

Pregnancy risk category B

AVAILABLE FORMS
Aerosol: 800 mcg/metered spray
Capsules (for oral solution): 100 mg
Nasal solution: 5.2 mg/metered spray (40 mg/ml)
Ophthalmic solution: 4%
Solution (for nebulization): 20 mg/2 ml

INDICATIONS & DOSAGES
➤**Mild to moderate persistent asthma**—
Adults and children age 5 and older: 2 metered sprays using inhaler q.i.d. at regular intervals. Or, 20 mg via nebulization q.i.d. at regular intervals.
➤**Prevention and treatment of seasonal and perennial allergic rhinitis**—
Adults and children older than age 2: 1 spray in each nostril t.i.d. or q.i.d. Maximum, six times daily.
➤**Prevention of exercise-induced bronchospasm**—
Adults and children age 5 and older: 2 metered sprays inhaled no longer than 1 hour before anticipated exercise.
➤**Conjunctivitis**—
Adults and children age 4 and older: 1 to 2 drops in each eye four to six times daily at regular intervals.
➤**Systemic mastocytosis**—
Adults and children older than age 12: 200 mg P.O. q.i.d. before meals and h.s.
Children ages 2 to 12: 100 mg P.O. q.i.d. 30 minutes before meals or h.s.

ACTION
Inhibits the degranulation of sensitized mast cells that occurs after exposure to specific antigens. Also, inhibits release of histamine and slow-reacting substance of anaphylaxis.

Route	Onset	Peak	Duration
Inhalation, intranasal, ophthalmic, P.O.	Unknown	Unknown	Unknown

ADVERSE REACTIONS
CNS: dizziness, headache.
EENT: *irritated throat and trachea,* lacrimation, nasal congestion, pharyngeal irritation, *sneezing,* nasal burning and irritation, epistaxis.
GI: nausea, esophagitis, abdominal pain, *bad taste.*
GU: dysuria, urinary frequency.
Musculoskeletal: joint swelling and pain.
Respiratory: *bronchospasm* after inhalation of dry powder, *cough,* wheezing, eosinophilic pneumonia.
Skin: rash, urticaria.
Other: swollen parotid gland, *angioedema.*

---

*Liquid contains alcohol.   **May contain tartrazine.   †Canada   ‡Australia   §U.K.   ◇OTC

INTERACTIONS
None significant.

EFFECTS ON LAB TEST RESULTS
None reported.

CONTRAINDICATIONS
Contraindicated in patients hypersensitive to drug and in those experiencing acute asthma attacks and status asthmaticus.

NURSING CONSIDERATIONS
• Use with caution in children. Use of cromolyn oral inhalation solution isn't recommended in children younger than age 2. Cromolyn powder or aerosol for oral inhalation isn't recommended for children younger than age 5. Cromolyn ophthalmic solution isn't recommended for children younger than age 4. Cromolyn nasal solution isn't recommended for children younger than age 6.
• Use inhalation form cautiously in patients with coronary artery disease or a history of arrhythmias.
• Drug (except for ophthalmic solution) should be used only when acute episode of asthma has been controlled, airway is cleared, and patient can breathe independently.
• *Alert:* For full-term neonates and infants, use oral cromolyn sodium only for severe, incapacitating disease when benefits clearly outweigh risks.
• Dissolve powder in capsules for oral dose in hot water, and further dilute with cold water before ingestion. Don't mix with fruit juice, milk, or food.
• Discontinue drug if eosinophilic pneumonia develops, as evidenced by eosinophilia and infiltrates on chest X-ray.
• Watch for recurrence of asthma signs and symptoms when dosage is decreased, especially when corticosteroids are also used.

PATIENT TEACHING
• Teach patient how to use prescribed form of drug.
• Advise patient that full effects of drug may not be noted for 4 weeks.
• Tell patient that esophagitis may be relieved by antacids or a glass of milk.
• Warn patient that nasal solution may cause stinging or sneezing.

dornase alfa
Pulmozyme

Pregnancy risk category B

AVAILABLE FORMS
Inhalation solution: 2.5-mg ampule (1 mg/ml)

INDICATIONS & DOSAGES
➤ **To improve pulmonary function and decrease the frequency of moderate to severe respiratory tract infections in patients with cystic fibrosis—**
Adults and children age 5 and older: 1 ampule or 2.5 mg inhaled once daily. Treatment usually takes 10 to 15 minutes. Use drug only with an approved nebulizer.

ACTION
Hydrolyzes DNA in sputum of cystic fibrosis patients, causing decreased viscosity and elasticity of pulmonary secretions.

Route	Onset	Peak	Duration
Inhalation	3-7 days	9 days	Unknown

ADVERSE REACTIONS
CV: *chest pain.*
EENT: *pharyngitis, voice alteration,* laryngitis, conjunctivitis.
Skin: *rash,* urticaria.

INTERACTIONS
None significant.

EFFECTS ON LAB TEST RESULTS
None reported.

CONTRAINDICATIONS
Contraindicated in patients hypersensitive to drug or to products derived from Chinese hamster ovary cells.

NURSING CONSIDERATIONS
• Drug is used with other standard therapies for cystic fibrosis.
• Patients older than age 21 and those with a forced vital capacity over 85% may benefit from twice-daily use.
• Safety and efficacy haven't been established for use longer than 12 months, for children younger than age 5, and for chil-

---

Reactions may be *common,* uncommon, *life-threatening,* or COMMON AND LIFE-THREATENING.

dren with forced vital capacity below 40% of normal value.

• **Alert:** Give only with the Hudson T Up-draft II disposable jet nebulizer, the Marquest Acorn II disposable jet nebulizer along with Pulmo-Aide compressor, or the PARI LC Jet+ reusable nebulizer along with the PARI PRONEB compressor.

• Discard cloudy or discolored solution.

• Don't mix with other drugs in the nebulizer. Mixing could lead to a physical or chemical reaction that may inactivate dornase alfa.

• Refrigerate drug in its protective foil pouch to protect it from strong light.

• Once opened, the entire ampule must be used or discarded.

PATIENT TEACHING

• Teach patient how to use drug at home.

• Remind patient to breathe only through his mouth when using the nebulizer. If this is difficult, suggest that he use a nose clip.

• Tell patient that if he begins coughing during treatment to turn off nebulizer without spilling drug. To resume, he should turn on nebulizer and continue breathing through the mouthpiece until the nebulizer cup is empty or mist is no longer produced.

---

flunisolide
AeroBid, AeroBid-M, Bronalide†, Nasalide, Nasarel

Pregnancy risk category C

AVAILABLE FORMS
Nasal solution: 25 mcg/metered spray
Oral inhalant: 250 mcg/metered spray (at least 100 metered inhalations/container)

INDICATIONS & DOSAGES
➤ **Chronic asthma—**
Adults and adolescents older than age 15: 2 inhalations (500 mcg) b.i.d. Maximum, 8 inhalations (2,000 mcg) daily.
Children ages 6 to 15: 2 inhalations (500 mcg) b.i.d. Higher dosages haven't been studied. Maximum, 1,000 mcg daily.
➤ **Seasonal or perennial rhinitis—**
Adults and adolescents older than age 14: 2 sprays (50 mcg) in each nostril b.i.d. May be increased to t.i.d. if necessary.

Maximum dose is 8 sprays in each nostril daily (400 mcg).
Children ages 6 to 14: 1 spray (25 mcg) in each nostril t.i.d. or 2 sprays (50 mcg) in each nostril b.i.d. Maximum dose is 4 sprays in each nostril daily (200 mcg).

ACTION
Unknown. May decrease inflammation through inhibitory activities against such cell types as mast cells and macrophages and mediators such as leukotrienes. In nasal passages it produces anti-inflammatory and vasoconstricting effects.

Route	Onset	Peak	Duration
Inhalation (nasal)	Up to 3 wk	Unknown	Unknown
Inhalation (oral)	1-4 wk	Unknown	Unknown

ADVERSE REACTIONS
CNS: dizziness, irritability, nervousness, *headache.*
CV: palpitations, chest pain, edema.
EENT: throat irritation, hoarseness, nasopharyngeal fungal infections, *sore throat, nasal congestion,* nasal irritation, nasal burning or stinging.
GI: *nausea, vomiting,* dry mouth, *unpleasant taste, diarrhea, upset stomach,* abdominal pain, decreased appetite.
Respiratory: *upper respiratory tract infection, cold symptoms.*
Skin: rash, pruritus.
Other: *flu,* fever.

INTERACTIONS
None significant.

EFFECTS ON LAB TEST RESULTS
None reported.

CONTRAINDICATIONS
Contraindicated in patients hypersensitive to drug and in those with status asthmaticus or respiratory tract infections.

NURSING CONSIDERATIONS
• Drug isn't recommended in patients with nonasthmatic bronchial diseases or with asthma controlled by bronchodilators or other noncorticosteroids alone.

• A spacer device may help to ensure proper dosage administration and decrease local (oral) adverse effects.
• Store drug between 59° and 86° F (15° and 30° C).
• Nasal spray should be discontinued after 3 weeks if symptomatic improvement isn't evident.
• *Alert:* Withdraw drug slowly in patients who have received long-term oral corticosteroid therapy.
• After withdrawal of systemic corticosteroids, patient may need supplemental systemic corticosteroids if stress (trauma, surgery, or infection) causes evidence of adrenal insufficiency.
• *Alert:* Don't confuse flunisolide with fluocinonide.
• *Alert:* Nasarel and Nasalide shouldn't be considered the same product.

PATIENT TEACHING
For oral inhalant
• Warn patient that flunisolide doesn't relieve acute asthma attacks.
• Advise patient to ensure delivery of proper dose by gently warming the canister to room temperature before using. Some patients carry the canister in a pocket to keep it warm.
• Tell patient who also is using a bronchodilator to use it several minutes before he uses flunisolide.
• Instruct patient to allow 1 minute to elapse before repeating inhalations and to hold his breath for a few seconds to enhance drug action.
• Teach patient to keep inhaler clean and unobstructed. He should wash it with warm water and dry it thoroughly after use.
• Teach patient to check mucous membranes frequently for signs and symptoms of fungal infection.
• Advise patient to prevent oral fungal infections by gargling or rinsing mouth with water after each inhaler use. Caution him not to swallow the water.
• Advise parents of a child receiving long-term therapy that the child should have periodic growth measurements and be checked for evidence of hypothalamic-pituitary-adrenal axis suppression.

For nasal spray
• The nasal inhaler should be primed (5 to 6 sprays) before initial use and after long periods of no use.
• Advise patient to clear nasal passageways before use.
• Patient should follow manufacturer's instructions for use and cleaning. Open containers should be discarded after 3 months.
• Advise patient that therapeutic results may take several weeks.

---

fluticasone propionate
Flixotide§, Flonase, Flovent, Flovent Rotadisk

Pregnancy risk category C

AVAILABLE FORMS
Nasal spray: 50 mcg/metered spray
Oral inhalation aerosol: 44 mcg, 110 mcg, 220 mcg
Oral inhalation powder: 50 mcg, 100 mcg, 250 mcg, 500 mcg§

INDICATIONS & DOSAGES
➤ **Maintenance treatment of asthma as prophylactic therapy and for patients requiring oral corticosteroid treatment for chronic asthma—**
Flovent
Adults and children age 12 and older: In those previously taking bronchodilators alone, initially, inhaled dose of 88 mcg b.i.d. to maximum of 440 mcg b.i.d.
Patients previously taking inhaled corticosteroids: Initially, inhaled dose of 88 to 220 mcg b.i.d. to maximum of 440 mcg b.i.d.
Patients previously taking oral corticosteroids: Inhaled dose of 880 mcg b.i.d.
Flovent Rotadisk
Adults and adolescents: In patients previously taking bronchodilators alone, initially, inhaled dose of 100 mcg b.i.d. to maximum of 500 mcg b.i.d.
Patients previously taking inhaled corticosteroids: Initially, inhaled dose of 100 to 250 mcg b.i.d. to maximum of 500 mcg b.i.d.
Patients previously taking oral corticosteroids: Inhaled dose of 1,000 mcg b.i.d.

Reactions may be *common*, uncommon, *life-threatening*, or COMMON AND LIFE-THREATENING.

Children ages 4 to 11: For patients previously on bronchodilators alone or on inhaled corticosteroids, initially, inhaled dose of 50 mcg b.i.d. to maximum of 100 mcg b.i.d.

Flonase

➤ **Nasal symptoms of seasonal and perennial and nonallergic rhinitis—**
Adults: Initially, 2 sprays in each nostril daily or b.i.d. Once symptoms are controlled, decrease to 1 spray in each nostril daily.
Adolescents and children older than 4: Initially, 1 spray in each nostril daily. If not responding, increase to 2 sprays in each nostril daily. Once symptoms are controlled, decrease to 1 spray in each nostril daily.

ACTION

Synthetic glucocorticoid with potent anti-inflammatory activity. Inflammation is an important component in the pathogenesis of asthma. Glucocorticoids inhibit many cell types and mediator production or secretion involved in the asthmatic response. These anti-inflammatory actions of fluticasone may contribute to its efficacy in asthma. In nasal passages, it produces anti-inflammatory and vasoconstrictor effects.

Route	Onset	Peak	Duration
Inhalation (nasal)	12 hr	Several days	1-2 wk
Inhalation (oral)	24 hr	Several days	1-2 wk

ADVERSE REACTIONS

CNS: *headache,* dizziness, migraine, nervousness.
EENT: *pharyngitis,* acute nasopharyngitis, nasal congestion, sinusitis, dysphonia, rhinitis, otitis media, tonsillitis, nasal discharge, earache, laryngitis, epistaxis, sneezing, hoarseness, conjunctivitis, eye irritation, dental problems.
GI: mouth irritation, *oral candidiasis,* diarrhea, abdominal pain, viral gastroenteritis, colitis, abdominal discomfort, nausea, vomiting.
GU: dysmenorrhea, candidiasis of vagina, pelvic inflammatory disease, vaginitis, vulvovaginitis, irregular menstrual cycle.
Metabolic: cushingoid features, growth retardation in children, weight gain.
Musculoskeletal: joint pain, aches and pains, disorder or symptoms of neck sprain or strain, muscular soreness.
Respiratory: *upper respiratory tract infection,* bronchitis, chest congestion, dyspnea, irritation from inhalant.
Skin: dermatitis, urticaria.
Other: fever, influenza.

INTERACTIONS

Drug-drug. *Ketoconazole:* Increased mean fluticasone levels. Use care when giving fluticasone with long-term ketoconazole and other known cytochrome P-450 3A4 inhibitors.

EFFECTS ON LAB TEST RESULTS

None reported.

CONTRAINDICATIONS

Contraindicated in patients hypersensitive to ingredients in these preparations. Also contraindicated in primary treatment of patients with status asthmaticus or other acute episodes of asthma in which intensive measures are needed.

NURSING CONSIDERATIONS

● Use cautiously in breast-feeding patients.
● Because of risk of systemic absorption of inhaled corticosteroids, observe patient carefully for evidence of systemic corticosteroid effects.
● Some patients on high doses of fluticasone may have an abnormal response to the 6-hour cosyntropin stimulation test.
● Monitor patient, especially postoperatively or during periods of stress, for evidence of inadequate adrenal response.
● During withdrawal from oral corticosteroids, some patients may experience signs and symptoms of systemically active corticosteroid withdrawal—such as joint or muscle pain, lassitude, and depression—despite maintenance or even improvement of respiratory function.
● For patients starting therapy who are currently receiving oral corticosteroid therapy, reduce dose of prednisone to no more than 2.5 mg/day on a weekly basis, beginning after at least 1 week of therapy with fluticasone.

• *Alert:* As with other inhaled asthma drugs, bronchospasm may occur with an immediate increase in wheezing after dosing. If bronchospasm occurs after dosing with fluticasone inhalation aerosol, it should be treated immediately with a fast-acting inhaled bronchodilator.

PATIENT TEACHING
• Tell patient that drug isn't indicated for the relief of acute bronchospasm.
• For proper use of drug and to attain maximum improvement, tell patient to carefully follow the accompanying patient instructions.
• Advise patient to use drug at regular intervals, as directed.
• Instruct patient not to increase dosage but to contact prescriber if signs or symptoms don't improve or if condition worsens. Or, with nasal spray if signs or symptoms aren't improved after 4 days of treatment.
• Instruct patient to immediately contact prescriber if asthma episodes unresponsive to bronchodilators occur during treatment with fluticasone. During such episodes, patient may need therapy with oral corticosteroids.
• Warn patient to avoid exposure to chickenpox or measles and, if exposed, to consult prescriber immediately.
• Tell patient to carry or wear medical identification indicating that he may need supplementary corticosteroids during stress or a severe asthma attack.
• During periods of stress or a severe asthma attack, instruct patient who has been withdrawn from systemic corticosteroids to resume oral corticosteroids (in prescribed doses) immediately and to contact prescriber for further instruction. Instruct him to rinse his mouth after inhalation.
• Advise patient to avoid spraying inhalation aerosol into eyes.
• Instruct patient to shake canister well before using inhalation aerosol.
• Advise patient to store fluticasone powder in a dry place.
For Flonase nasal spray
• Tell patient to prime the nasal inhaler before initial use or after 1 week or longer of non-use.

• Have patient clear nasal passages before use.
• Advise patient to follow manufacturer's recommendations for use and cleaning.
• Advise patient to use at regular intervals for full benefit.
• Tell patient to contact provider if signs or symptoms don't improve within 4 days or if signs or symptoms worsen.

---

montelukast sodium
Singulair

Pregnancy risk category B

AVAILABLE FORMS
Tablets (chewable): 4 mg, 5 mg
Tablets (film-coated): 10 mg

INDICATIONS & DOSAGES
➤ **Prophylaxis and long-term treatment of asthma—**
Adults and children age 15 and older:
10 mg film-coated tablet P.O. once daily in evening.
Children ages 6 to 14: 5 mg chewable tablet P.O. once daily in evening.
Children ages 2 to 5: 4-mg chewable tablet P.O. once daily in the evening.

ACTION
A selective, competitive leukotriene-receptor antagonist that causes inhibition of airway cysteinyl leukotriene ($CysLT_1$) receptors. Binds with high affinity and selectivity to the $CysLT_1$ receptor and inhibits physiologic action of the cysteinyl leukotriene LTD_4. This receptor inhibition reduces early- and late-phase bronchoconstriction from antigen challenge.

Route	Onset	Peak	Duration
P.O. (chewable)	Unknown	2-2.5 hr	Unknown
P.O. (film-coated)	Unknown	3-4 hr	Unknown

ADVERSE REACTIONS
CNS: *headache,* dizziness, fatigue, asthenia.
EENT: nasal congestion, dental pain.
GI: dyspepsia, infectious gastroenteritis, abdominal pain.
GU: pyuria.

Respiratory: cough.
Skin: rash.
Other: fever, trauma, influenza.

INTERACTIONS
Drug-drug. *Phenobarbital, rifampin:*
May decrease bioavailability of montelukast because of induction of hepatic metabolism. Monitor patient.

EFFECTS ON LAB TEST RESULTS
• May increase ALT and AST levels.

CONTRAINDICATIONS
Contraindicated in patients hypersensitive to drug or its ingredients.

NURSING CONSIDERATIONS
• Use cautiously and with appropriate monitoring in patients whose dosages of systemic corticosteroids are reduced.
• Assess patient's underlying condition, and monitor patient for effectiveness.
• *Alert:* Don't abruptly substitute drug for inhaled or oral corticosteroids. Dose of inhaled corticosteroids may be reduced gradually.
• Drug isn't indicated for use in patients with acute asthmatic attacks, status asthmaticus, or as monotherapy for management of exercise-induced bronchospasm. Appropriate rescue drug should be continued for acute exacerbations.

PATIENT TEACHING
• Advise patient to take drug daily, even if asymptomatic, and to contact his prescriber if asthma isn't well controlled.
• Warn patient not to reduce or stop taking other prescribed antiasthma drugs without prescriber's approval.
• Advise patient to seek medical attention if short-acting inhaled bronchodilators are needed more often than usual during drug therapy.
• Warn patient that drug isn't beneficial in acute asthma attacks or in exercise-induced bronchospasm, and advise him to keep appropriate rescue drugs available.
• Advise patient with known aspirin sensitivity to continue to avoid using aspirin and NSAIDs during drug therapy.
• Advise patient with phenylketonuria that chewable tablet contains phenylalanine.

palivizumab
Synagis

Pregnancy risk category C

AVAILABLE FORMS
Injection: 50 mg, 100-mg vial

INDICATIONS & DOSAGES
➤ **Prevention of serious lower respiratory tract disease caused by respiratory syncytial virus (RSV) in children at high risk—**
Children: 15 mg/kg I.M. monthly throughout RSV season. Give first dose before start of RSV season.

ACTION
Exhibits neutralizing and fusion-inhibitory activity against RSV, which inhibits RSV replication.

Route	Onset	Peak	Duration
I.M.	Unknown	Unknown	Unknown

ADVERSE REACTIONS
CNS: nervousness, pain.
EENT: *otitis media, rhinitis,* pharyngitis, sinusitis, conjunctivitis.
GI: diarrhea, vomiting, gastroenteritis, oral candidiasis.
Hematologic: anemia.
Respiratory: *upper respiratory tract infection,* cough, wheeze, bronchiolitis, *apnea,* pneumonia, bronchitis, asthma, croup, dyspnea.
Skin: *rash,* fungal dermatitis, eczema, seborrhea.
Other: hernia, failure to thrive, injection site reaction, viral infection, flu syndrome.

INTERACTIONS
None significant.

EFFECTS ON LAB TEST RESULTS
• May increase ALT and AST levels.
• May decrease hemoglobin.

CONTRAINDICATIONS
Contraindicated in children hypersensitive to drug or its components.

---

*Liquid contains alcohol.   **May contain tartrazine.   †Canada   ‡Australia   §U.K.   ◇OTC

NURSING CONSIDERATIONS
- Use cautiously in patients with thrombocytopenia or other coagulation disorders.
- Patients should receive monthly doses throughout RSV season, even if RSV infection develops. In the northern hemisphere, RSV season typically lasts from November to April.
- To reconstitute, slowly add 1 ml of sterile water for injection into a 100-mg vial or 0.6 ml of sterile water for injection into a 50-mg vial. Gently swirl the vial for 30 seconds to avoid foaming. Don't shake vial. Let reconstituted solution stand at room temperature for 20 minutes until the solution clears. Give within 6 hours of reconstitution.
- Give drug into anterolateral aspect of thigh. Don't use gluteal muscle routinely as an injection site because of risk of damage to sciatic nerve. Injection volumes over 1 ml should be given as a divided dose.
- *Alert:* Anaphylactoid reactions after use of drug haven't been observed but can occur after use of proteins. If anaphylaxis or severe allergic reaction occurs, give epinephrine (1:1,000), and provide supportive care as needed.

PATIENT TEACHING
- Explain to parent or caregiver that drug is used to prevent RSV and not to treat it.
- Advise parent that monthly injections are recommended throughout RSV season (November to April in the northern hemisphere).
- Tell parent to immediately report adverse reactions or any unusual bruising, bleeding, or weakness.

---

triamcinolone acetonide
Azmacort, Nasacort, Nasacort AQ

Pregnancy risk category C

AVAILABLE FORMS
Inhalation aerosol: 100 mcg/metered spray
Nasal spray: 55 mcg/metered spray

INDICATIONS & DOSAGES
➤ **Persistent asthma—**
Adults and children older than age 12: 2 inhalations t.i.d. to q.i.d. Maximum, 16 inhalations daily. In some patients, maintenance can be accomplished when total daily dose is given b.i.d.
Children ages 6 to 12: 1 to 2 inhalations t.i.d. to q.i.d. Maximum, 12 inhalations daily.
➤ **Nasal treatment of symptoms of seasonal and perennial allergic rhinitis—**
Adults and children older than age 12: 2 sprays in each nostril daily.
Children ages 6 to 12: Initially, 1 spray in each nostril daily. If not responding, increase to 2 sprays in each nostril daily.

ACTION
Unknown. May decrease inflammation through inhibitory activities against such cell types as mast cells and macrophages and mediators such as leukotrienes.

Route	Onset	Peak	Duration
Inhalation (nasal)	12-24 hr	Several days	1-2 weeks
Inhalation (oral)	1-4 wk	Unknown	Unknown

ADVERSE REACTIONS
EENT: dry or irritated nose or throat, hoarseness, *pharyngitis.*
GI: oral candidiasis, dry or irritated tongue or mouth.
Metabolic: hypothalamic-pituitary-adrenal function suppression, adrenal insufficiency.
Respiratory: cough, wheezing.
Other: facial edema.

INTERACTIONS
None significant.

EFFECTS ON LAB TEST RESULTS
None reported.

CONTRAINDICATIONS
Contraindicated in patients hypersensitive to drug or its ingredients and in those with status asthmaticus.

NURSING CONSIDERATIONS
- Use with extreme caution, if at all, in patients with tuberculosis of the respiratory tract, ocular herpes simplex, or untreated fungal, bacterial, or systemic viral infections.

Reactions may be *common,* uncommon, *life-threatening,* or COMMON AND LIFE-THREATENING.

• Unlike other corticosteroids, drug has a spacer built into the drug-delivery device.
• Use cautiously in patients receiving systemic corticosteroids.
• Most adverse reactions to corticosteroids are dose- or duration-dependent.
• Patients who have recently been switched from systemic corticosteroids to oral inhaled corticosteroids may need to resume systemic corticosteroid therapy during periods of stress or severe asthma attacks.
• Taper oral therapy slowly.
• Store drug between 59° and 86° F (15° and 30° C).
• No data exist to demonstrate whether drug appears in breast milk. Because of risk of severe adverse effects, breast-feeding isn't recommended during therapy.
• For nasal spray, if improvement isn't evident after 2 to 3 weeks, the patient should be reevaluated.
• *Alert:* Don't confuse triamcinolone with Triaminicin.

PATIENT TEACHING
For inhalation aerosol
• Inform patient that inhaled corticosteroids don't relieve emergency asthma attacks.
• Advise patient to warm canister to room temperature before using. Some patients carry canister in a pocket to keep it warm.
• If patient needs a bronchodilator, tell him to use it several minutes before triamcinolone. Tell patient to allow 1 minute to elapse before repeat inhalations and to hold his breath for a few seconds to enhance drug action.
• Teach patient to check mucous membranes frequently for evidence of fungal infection. Advise patient to avoid exposure to chickenpox or measles and to contact provider if exposure occurs.
• Tell patient to prevent oral fungal infections by gargling or rinsing mouth with water after each use of the inhaler. Remind him not to swallow the water.
• Tell patient to keep inhaler clean and unobstructed and to wash it with warm water and dry it thoroughly after use.
• Instruct patient to contact prescriber if response to therapy decreases; dosage may need adjustment. Tell him not to exceed recommended dosage on his own.

• Instruct patient to wear or carry medical identification indicating his need for supplemental systemic glucocorticoids during periods of stress.
For nasal spray
• Advise patient to use at regular intervals for full therapeutic effect.
• Advise patient to clear nasal passages before use.
• Have patient follow manufacturer's recommendations for use and cleaning.

zafirlukast
Accolate

Pregnancy risk category B

AVAILABLE FORMS
Tablets: 10 mg, 20 mg

INDICATIONS & DOSAGES
➤ **Prophylaxis and chronic treatment of asthma—**
Adults and children age 12 and older: 20 mg P.O. b.i.d. taken 1 hour before or 2 hours after meals.
Children ages 5 to 11: 10 mg P.O. b.i.d. taken 1 hour before or 2 hours after meals.

ACTION
Selectively competes for leukotriene receptor sites, blocking inflammatory action.

Route	Onset	Peak	Duration
P.O.	Rapid	3 hr	Unknown

ADVERSE REACTIONS
CNS: *headache,* asthenia, dizziness, pain.
GI: nausea, diarrhea, abdominal pain, vomiting, dyspepsia.
Musculoskeletal: myalgia, back pain.
Other: infection, accidental injury, fever.

INTERACTIONS
Drug-drug. *Aspirin:* Increased zafirlukast levels. Monitor patient.
Erythromycin, theophylline: Decreased zafirlukast levels. Monitor patient.
Warfarin: Increased PT. Monitor PT and INR, and adjust anticoagulant dosage.
Drug-food. *Food:* Reduced rate and extent of zafirlukast absorption. Give 1 hour before or 2 hours after a meal.

EFFECTS ON LAB TEST RESULTS
• May increase liver enzyme levels.

CONTRAINDICATIONS
Contraindicated in patients hypersensitive to drug.

NURSING CONSIDERATIONS
• Drug isn't indicated for reversing bronchospasm in acute asthma attacks.
• Give cautiously to elderly patients and those with hepatic impairment.
• Give drug to pregnant patients only if clearly needed. Don't give to breast-feeding women.
• *Alert:* Reduction of oral corticosteroid dose has been followed in rare cases by eosinophilia, vasculitic rash, worsening pulmonary symptoms, cardiac complications, or neuropathy, sometimes presenting as Churg-Strauss syndrome.

PATIENT TEACHING
• Tell patient that drug is used for long-term treatment of asthma and that he should keep taking it even if symptoms resolve.
• Advise patient to continue taking other antiasthma drugs, as prescribed.
• Instruct patient not to take drug with food. Drug should be taken 1 hour before or 2 hours after meals.

zileuton
Zyflo

Pregnancy risk category C

AVAILABLE FORMS
Tablets: 600 mg

INDICATIONS & DOSAGES
➤ **Prophylaxis and chronic treatment of asthma—**
Adults and children age 12 and older: 600 mg P.O. q.i.d.

ACTION
Inhibits enzyme responsible for the formation of leukotrienes, thus reducing inflammatory response.

Route	Onset	Peak	Duration
P.O.	Rapid	2 hr	Unknown

ADVERSE REACTIONS
CNS: *headache,* asthenia, dizziness, pain, insomnia, nervousness, somnolence, malaise.
CV: chest pain.
EENT: conjunctivitis.
GI: dyspepsia, nausea, abdominal pain, constipation, flatulence, vomiting.
GU: urinary tract infection, vaginitis.
Hematologic: *leukopenia.*
Musculoskeletal: myalgia, arthralgia, hypertonia, neck pain, rigidity.
Skin: pruritus.
Other: accidental injury, fever, lymphadenopathy.

INTERACTIONS
Drug-drug. *Propranolol and other beta blockers:* Increased effect of beta blocker. Monitor patient and reduce beta blocker dosage, as directed.
Theophylline: Decreased theophylline clearance. (On average, theophylline levels double.) Reduce theophylline dosage, and monitor serum levels.
Warfarin: Increased PT. Monitor PT and INR, and adjust dosage of anticoagulant.

EFFECTS ON LAB TEST RESULTS
• May increase ALT levels.
• May decrease WBC count.

CONTRAINDICATIONS
Contraindicated in patients hypersensitive to drug and in those with active liver disease or transaminase elevations at least three times the upper limit of normal.

NURSING CONSIDERATIONS
• *Alert:* Drug isn't indicated for reversing bronchospasm in acute asthma attacks.
• Give cautiously to patients with hepatic impairment or history of heavy alcohol use.
• Drug should be used in pregnancy only if benefit to mother outweighs risk to the fetus. Breast-feeding women shouldn't take drug.
• Safety and effectiveness in patients younger than age 12 haven't been established.
• Obtain baseline and periodic liver enzyme levels.

PATIENT TEACHING

● Tell patient that drug is used for long-term treatment of asthma and that he should keep taking drug even if symptoms resolve.

● Caution patient that drug isn't a bronchodilator and shouldn't be used to treat an acute asthma attack.

● Advise patient to continue taking other antiasthma drugs.

● Advise patient that pill may be cut in half if needed.

● Instruct patient to notify prescriber if his short-acting bronchodilator doesn't relieve signs or symptoms.

● Inform patient that he must undergo periodic testing of liver enzyme levels.

● Tell patient to notify prescriber immediately if he develops signs or symptoms of liver dysfunction (right upper quadrant pain, nausea, fatigue, pruritus, jaundice, malaise).

● Tell patient to consult prescriber before taking OTC or new prescription drugs.

● Urge patient to report flu symptoms.

aluminum carbonate
aluminum hydroxide
calcium carbonate
magaldrate
magnesium hydroxide
   (See Chapter 48, LAXATIVES.)
magnesium oxide
simethicone
sodium bicarbonate
   (See Chapter 62, ACIDIFIERS AND
   ALKALINIZERS.)

COMBINATION PRODUCTS
ALKA-SELTZER GOLD ◊ : sodium bicarbonate 958 mg, citric acid 832 mg, and potassium bicarbonate 312 mg.
ALKA-SELTZER ORIGINAL ◊ : aspirin 325 mg, citric acid 1,000 mg, and phenylalanine 9 mg.
ALUDROX ◊ : aluminum hydroxide 307 mg and magnesium hydroxide 103 mg.
DI-GEL: magnesium hydroxide 128 mg and calcium carbonate 280 mg.
EXTRA STRENGTH ALKA-SELTZER ◊ : aspirin 500 mg and citric acid 1,000 mg.
GAVISCON TABLETS ◊ : aluminum hydroxide 80 mg and magnesium trisilicate 20 mg.
GELUSIL ◊ : aluminum hydroxide 200 mg, magnesium hydroxide 200 mg, and simethicone 25 mg.
MAALOX ANTACID PLUS ANTI-GAS EXTRA STRENGTH: aluminum hydroxide 350 mg, magnesium hydroxide 350 mg, and simethicone 30 mg.
MAALOX PLUS ◊ : aluminum hydroxide 200 mg, magnesium hydroxide 200 mg, and simethicone 25 mg.
MAALOX TABLETS ◊ : aluminum hydroxide 200 mg, magnesium hydroxide 200 mg, and simethicone 25 mg.
MAALOX THERAPEUTIC CONCENTRATE SUSPENSION: aluminum hydroxide 600 mg and magnesium hydroxide 300 mg/5 ml.
MYLANTA LIQUID: aluminum hydroxide 200 mg, magnesium hydroxide 200 mg, and simethicone 20 mg/5 ml.
MYLANTA TABLETS ◊ : aluminum hydroxide 200 mg, magnesium hydroxide 200 mg, and simethicone 20 mg.
PEPCID COMPLETE: calcium carbonate 800 mg, magnesium hydroxide 165 mg, and famotidine 10 mg.
RIOPAN PLUS CHEWABLE TABLETS ◊ : magaldrate 480 mg and simethicone 20 mg.
RIOPAN PLUS DOUBLE STRENGTH CHEWABLE TABLETS: magaldrate 1,080 mg and simethicone 20 mg.
RIOPAN PLUS DOUBLE STRENGTH SUSPENSION: magaldrate 1,080 mg and simethicone 40 mg/5 ml.
RIOPAN PLUS SUSPENSION ◊ : magaldrate 540 mg and simethicone 40 mg/5 ml.
TITRALAC PLUS ◊ : calcium carbonate 420 mg and simethicone 21 mg.
UNIVOL† ◊ : aluminum hydroxide and magnesium carbonate co-dried gel 300 mg and magnesium hydroxide 100 mg.

aluminum carbonate
Basaljel ◊

Pregnancy risk category NR

AVAILABLE FORMS
Oral suspension: equivalent to aluminum hydroxide 400 mg/5 ml ◊
Tablets or capsules: equivalent to aluminum hydroxide 500 mg ◊

INDICATIONS & DOSAGES
➤ **Antacid—**
Adults: 5 to 10 ml of suspension P.O. q 2 hours, p.r.n.; or 1 to 2 tablets or capsules P.O. q 2 hours, p.r.n. Maximum, 24 capsules, tablets, or teaspoonfuls per 24 hours.
➤ **To prevent formation of urinary phosphate stones in conjunction with low-phosphate diet—**
Adults: 15 to 30 ml of suspension in water or juice P.O. 1 hour after meals and h.s. Or, 2 to 6 tablets or capsules 1 hour after meals and h.s.

ACTION
Antacid that reduces total acid load in the GI tract, elevates gastric pH to reduce pepsin activity, strengthens the gastric mucosal barrier, and increases esophageal sphincter tone.

Route	Onset	Peak	Duration
P.O.	20 min	Unknown	20-180 min

ADVERSE REACTIONS
CNS: encephalopathy.
GI: *constipation, **intestinal obstruction.***
Metabolic: hypophosphatemia, increased gastrin levels.
Musculoskeletal: osteomalacia.

INTERACTIONS
Drug-drug. *Allopurinol, antibiotics (including quinolones, tetracyclines), corticosteroids, diflunisal, digoxin, ethambutol, H_2-receptor antagonists, iron salts, isoniazid, penicillamine, phenothiazines, thyroid hormones, ticlopidine:* Decreased pharmacologic effect of these drugs because of possible impaired absorption. Separate administration times by 1 to 2 hours.
Enteric-coated drugs: May be released prematurely in stomach. Separate doses by at least 1 hour.

EFFECTS ON LAB TEST RESULTS
• May increase gastrin levels. May decrease phosphate levels.

CONTRAINDICATIONS
No known contraindications.

NURSING CONSIDERATIONS
• Use cautiously in patients with chronic renal disease.
• When giving through nasogastric tube, make sure tube is placed correctly and is patent; after instilling drug, flush tube with water to ensure passage to stomach and to clear tube.
• *Alert:* Monitor long-term, high-dose use in patients on restricted sodium intake. Each tablet, capsule, or 5 ml of suspension contains about 3 mg of sodium.
• Record stool amount and consistency. Manage constipation with laxatives or stool softeners. Alternate with magnesium-

containing antacids (unless patient has renal disease).
• Monitor phosphate levels.
• Watch for evidence of hypophosphatemia (anorexia, malaise, muscle weakness) with prolonged use; also can lead to resorption of calcium and bone demineralization.
• Because drug contains aluminum, it's used in patients with renal failure to help control hyperphosphatemia by binding with phosphate in the GI tract.
• Basaljel liquid contains no sugar.
• Aluminum carbonate may interfere with imaging techniques using sodium pertechnetate Tc99m and thus impair evaluation of Meckel's diverticulum. It may also interfere with reticuloendothelial imaging of liver, spleen, or bone marrow using technetium Tc99m sulfur colloid. It may antagonize effect of pentagastrin during gastric acid secretion tests.

PATIENT TEACHING
• Warn patient not to take aluminum carbonate indiscriminately or to switch antacids without prescriber's advice.
• Tell patient to shake suspension well and to take with small amount of water or fruit juice to facilitate passage.
• Urge patient to notify prescriber about signs and symptoms of bleeding, tarry stools, or coffee-ground vomitus.
• Instruct pregnant patient to seek medical advice before taking drug.

---

aluminum hydroxide
AlternaGEL◇, Alu-Cap§◇, Aluminum Hydroxide Gel◇, Aluminum Hydroxide Gel Concentrated◇, Alu-Tab◇, Amphojel◇, Dialume◇

Pregnancy risk category NR

AVAILABLE FORMS
Capsules: 400 mg◇, 500 mg◇
Oral suspension: 320 mg/5 ml◇, 450 mg/5 ml◇, 600 mg/5 ml◇, 675 mg/ 5 ml◇
Tablets: 300 mg◇, 500 mg◇, 600 mg◇

INDICATIONS & DOSAGES
➤ **Antacid**—
Adults: 500 to 1,500 mg P.O. 1 hour after meals and h.s. Or, 300-mg tablet or 600-mg tablet, chewed before swallowing, taken with milk or water five to six times daily after meals and h.s.

ACTION
Antacid that reduces total acid load in the GI tract, elevates gastric pH to reduce pepsin activity, strengthens the gastric mucosal barrier, and increases esophageal sphincter tone.

Route	Onset	Peak	Duration
P.O.	Variable	Unknown	20-180 min

ADVERSE REACTIONS
CNS: encephalopathy.
GI: *constipation,* ***intestinal obstruction.***
Metabolic: hypophosphatemia.
Musculoskeletal: osteomalacia.

INTERACTIONS
Drug-drug. *Allopurinol, antibiotics (including quinolones, tetracyclines), corticosteroids, diflunisal, digoxin, ethambutol, H_2-receptor antagonists, iron salts, isoniazid, penicillamine, phenothiazines, thyroid hormones, ticlopidine:* Decreased pharmacologic effect of these drugs because of possible impaired absorption. Separate administration times.
Enteric-coated drugs: May be released prematurely in stomach. Separate doses by at least 1 hour.

EFFECTS ON LAB TEST RESULTS
• May increase gastrin levels. May decrease phosphate levels.

CONTRAINDICATIONS
No known contraindications.

NURSING CONSIDERATIONS
• Use cautiously in patients with chronic renal disease.
• When giving through nasogastric tube, make sure tube is placed correctly and is patent; after instilling drug, flush tube with water to ensure passage to stomach and to clear tube.
• **Alert:** Monitor long-term, high-dose use in patient on restricted sodium intake.

Each tablet, capsule, or 5 ml of suspension contains 2 to 3 mg of sodium.
• Record amount and consistency of stools. Manage constipation with laxatives or stool softeners; alternate with magnesium-containing antacids (if patient doesn't have renal disease).
• Monitor phosphate levels.
• Watch for evidence of hypophosphatemia (anorexia, malaise, and muscle weakness) with prolonged use; also can lead to resorption of calcium and bone demineralization.
• Aluminum hydroxide therapy may interfere with imaging techniques using sodium pertechnetate Tc99m and thus impair evaluation of Meckel's diverticulum. It also may interfere with reticuloendothelial imaging of liver, spleen, or bone marrow using technetium Tc99m sulfur colloid. It may antagonize effect of pentagastrin during gastric acid secretion tests.
• Because drug contains aluminum, it's used in patients with renal failure to help control hyperphosphatemia by binding with phosphate in the GI tract.

PATIENT TEACHING
• Instruct patient to shake suspension well and to follow with a small amount of milk or water to facilitate passage.
• Advise patient not to take aluminum hydroxide indiscriminately or to switch antacids without prescriber's advice.
• Urge patient to notify prescriber about signs and symptoms of bleeding, tarry stools, or coffee-ground vomitus.
• Instruct pregnant patient to seek medical advice before taking drug.

---

calcium carbonate
Alka-Mints◇, Amitone◇, Cal-Supp‡, Chooz◇, Dicarbosil◇, Maalox Antacid Caplets◇, Rolaids Calcium Rich◇, Tums◇, Tums E-X◇, Tums Ultra◇

Pregnancy risk category NR

AVAILABLE FORMS
Calcium carbonate contains 40% calcium; 20 mEq calcium per gram.
Chewing gum: 500 mg/piece
Lozenges: 600 mg ◇

Reactions may be *common*, uncommon, ***life-threatening***, or **COMMON AND LIFE-THREATENING**.

Oral suspension: 1,250 mg/5 ml
Tablets: 500 mg ◊, 600 mg ◊, 650 mg ◊,
1,000 mg ◊, 1,250 mg ◊
Tablets (chewable): 350 mg ◊, 420 mg ◊,
500 mg ◊, 750 mg, 850 mg, 1,000 mg,
1,250 mg‡

INDICATIONS & DOSAGES
➤ **Antacid, calcium supplement—**
Adults: 350 mg to 1.5 g P.O. or 2 pieces of
chewing gum 1 hour after meals and h.s.,
p.r.n.

ACTION
Antacid that reduces total acid load in the
GI tract, elevates gastric pH to reduce
pepsin activity, strengthens the gastric
mucosal barrier, and increases esophageal
sphincter tone.

Route	Onset	Peak	Duration
P.O.	20 min	Unknown	20-180 min

ADVERSE REACTIONS
CNS: headache, irritability, weakness.
GI: rebound hyperacidity, *nausea*.
Metabolic: altered phosphate levels.

INTERACTIONS
Drug-drug. *Antibiotics (including quinolones, tetracyclines), hydantoins, iron
salts, isoniazid, salicylates:* Decreased
pharmacologic effect of these drugs because of possible impaired absorption.
Separate administration times by 2 hours.
Enteric-coated drugs: May be released
prematurely in stomach. Separate doses by
at least 1 hour.
Drug-food. *Milk, other foods high in vitamin D:* Possible milk-alkali syndrome
(headache, confusion, distaste for food,
nausea, vomiting, hypercalcemia, hypercalciuria). Avoid using together.

EFFECTS ON LAB TEST RESULTS
● May decrease phosphate levels.

CONTRAINDICATIONS
Contraindicated in patients with ventricular fibrillation or hypercalcemia.

NURSING CONSIDERATIONS
● Use cautiously, if at all, if patient takes a
cardiac glycoside or has sarcoidosis or
renal or cardiac disease.

● Record amount and consistency of
stools. Manage constipation with laxatives
or stool softeners.
● Monitor calcium levels, especially in
patients with mild renal impairment.
● Watch for evidence of hypercalcemia
(nausea, vomiting, headache, confusion,
and anorexia).

PATIENT TEACHING
● Advise patient not to take calcium carbonate indiscriminately or to switch
antacids without prescriber's advice.
● Tell patient who takes chewable tablets
to chew thoroughly before swallowing and
to follow with a glass of water.
● Tell patient who uses suspension form to
shake well and take with a small amount
of water to facilitate passage.
● Urge patient to notify prescriber about
signs and symptoms of bleeding, tarry
stools, or coffee-ground vomitus.

---

magaldrate (aluminum-magnesium complex)
Lowsium ◊, Lowsium Plus,
Riopan ◊

Pregnancy risk category NR

AVAILABLE FORMS
Oral suspension: 540 mg/5 ml ◊

INDICATIONS & DOSAGES
➤ **Antacid—**
Adults: 540 to 1,080 mg (5 to 10 ml) of
suspension P.O. with water between meals
and h.s.

ACTION
Antacid that reduces total acid load in the
GI tract, elevates gastric pH to reduce
pepsin activity, strengthens the gastric mucosal barrier, and increases esophageal
sphincter tone.

Route	Onset	Peak	Duration
P.O.	20 min	Unknown	20-180 min

ADVERSE REACTIONS
GI: mild constipation, diarrhea.
GU: increased urine pH levels.
Metabolic: hypokalemia.

---

*Liquid contains alcohol. **May contain tartrazine. †Canada ‡Australia §U.K. ◊OTC

INTERACTIONS
Drug-drug. *Allopurinol, antibiotics (including quinolones, tetracyclines), diflunisal, digoxin, iron salts, isoniazid, penicillamine, phenothiazines, quinidine, salicylates, ticlopidine:* Decreased pharmacologic effect of these drugs because of possible impaired absorption. Separate administration times by 1 to 2 hours.
Enteric-coated drugs: May be released prematurely in stomach. Separate doses by at least 1 hour.

EFFECTS ON LAB TEST RESULTS
• May increase gastrin levels. May decrease potassium levels.

CONTRAINDICATIONS
Contraindicated in patients with severe renal disease.

NURSING CONSIDERATIONS
• Use cautiously in patients with mild renal impairment.
• When giving drug through nasogastric tube, make sure tube is placed properly and is patent. After instilling drug, flush tube with water to ensure passage to stomach and to clear tube.
• Monitor magnesium level in patients with mild renal impairment. Symptomatic hypermagnesemia usually occurs only in severe renal failure.
• Drug may antagonize effect of pentagastrin during gastric acid secretion tests.
• *Alert:* Drug isn't typically used in patients with renal failure to help control hypophosphatemia because it contains magnesium, which may accumulate.
• Drug has a low sodium content and is good for patients on sodium restriction.

PATIENT TEACHING
• Instruct patient to shake suspension well and to follow dose with water.
• Advise patient not to take magaldrate indiscriminately or to switch antacids without prescriber's advice.
• Urge patient to notify prescriber about signs and symptoms of bleeding, tarry stools, or coffee-ground vomitus.

magnesium oxide
Mag-Ox 400 ◇ , Maox ◇ ,
Uro-Mag ◇

Pregnancy risk category NR

AVAILABLE FORMS
Capsules: 140 mg ◇
Tablets: 400 mg ◇ , 420 mg ◇ , 500 mg

INDICATIONS & DOSAGES
➤ **Antacid—**
Adults: 140 mg P.O. with water or milk after meals and h.s.
➤ **Laxative—**
Adults: 4 g P.O. with water or milk, usually h.s.
➤ **Oral replacement therapy in mild hypomagnesemia—**
Adults: 400 to 840 mg P.O. daily. Monitor magnesium level.

ACTION
Reduces total acid load in the GI tract, elevates gastric pH, strengthens the gastric mucosal barrier, and increases esophageal sphincter tone.

Route	Onset	Peak	Duration
P.O.	20 min	Unknown	20-180 min

ADVERSE REACTIONS
GI: *diarrhea,* nausea, abdominal pain.
Metabolic: hypermagnesemia.

INTERACTIONS
Drug-drug. *Allopurinol, antibiotics, digoxin, iron salts, penicillamine, phenothiazines:* Decreased pharmacologic effect of these drugs because of possible impaired absorption. Separate administration times by 1 to 2 hours.
Enteric-coated drugs: May be released prematurely in stomach. Separate doses by at least 1 hour.

EFFECTS ON LAB TEST RESULTS
• May increase magnesium level.

CONTRAINDICATIONS
Contraindicated in patients with severe renal disease.

NURSING CONSIDERATIONS
- Use cautiously in patients with mild renal impairment.
- When using drug as a laxative, don't give within 1 to 2 hours of other oral drugs.
- *Alert:* Monitor magnesium levels. With prolonged use and renal impairment, watch for evidence of hypermagnesemia (hypotension, nausea, vomiting, depressed reflexes, respiratory depression, and coma).
- If diarrhea occurs, be prepared to suggest alternative preparation.

PATIENT TEACHING
- Advise patient not to take magnesium oxide indiscriminately or to switch antacids without prescriber's advice.
- Urge patient to report bleeding, tarry stools, or coffee-ground vomitus.

---

simethicone
Flatulex◇, Gas Relief◇, Gas-X◇, Gas-X Extra Strength◇, Mylanta Gas◇, Mylanta Anti-Gas Extra Strength◇, Mylicon◇, Ovol†, Ovol-40†, Ovol-80†, Phazyme◇, Phazyme 95◇, Phazyme-125 Maximum Strength◇, Ultra-strength Phazyme-180

Pregnancy risk category NR

AVAILABLE FORMS
Capsules: 125 mg, 180 mg
Drops: 40 mg/0.6 ml◇
Tablets: 40 mg◇, 55 mg†◇, 60 mg◇, 80 mg◇, 95 mg◇, 125 mg◇

INDICATIONS & DOSAGES
➤ **Flatulence, functional gastric bloating—**
Adults and children older than age 12: 40 to 125 mg P.O. after each meal and h.s., up to 500 mg daily. For drops, 40 to 80 mg P.O. after each meal and h.s., up to 500 mg daily.
Children ages 2 to 12: 40 mg after meals and h.s., up to 240 mg daily.
Children younger than age 2: 20 mg after meals and h.s., up to 120 mg daily.

ACTION
By its defoaming action, drug disperses or prevents formation of mucus-surrounded gas pockets in the GI tract.

Route	Onset	Peak	Duration
P.O.	Immediate	Immediate	Unknown

ADVERSE REACTIONS
GI: expulsion of excessive liberated gas as belching, flatus.

INTERACTIONS
None significant.

EFFECTS ON LAB TEST RESULTS
None reported.

CONTRAINDICATIONS
Contraindicated in patients hypersensitive to drug.

NURSING CONSIDERATIONS
- Drug isn't recommended for treating infant colic because information on safety in children is limited.
- Drug doesn't prevent formation of gas.
- *Alert:* Don't confuse simethicone with cimetidine.

PATIENT TEACHING
- Tell patient to chew tablet before swallowing.
- Advise patient to change positions often and to walk to aid passage of flatus.

46

Digestive enzymes and gallstone solubilizers

pancreatin
pancrelipase
ursodiol

COMBINATION PRODUCTS
PANCREASE CAPSULES: lipase 4,000 units, protease 25,000 units, and amylase 20,000 units in enteric-coated microspheres.

---

pancreatin
Donnazyme, Hi-Vegi-Lip Tablets ◇, 4X Pancreatin 600 mg ◇, 8X Pancreatin 900 mg ◇, Pancrezyme 4X Tablets ◇

Pregnancy risk category C

AVAILABLE FORMS
Donnazyme
Tablets: 500 mg pancreatin, 1,000 units lipase, 12,500 units protease, and 12,500 units amylase
Hi-Vegi-Lip Tablets
Tablets (enteric-coated): 2,400 mg pancreatin, 4,800 units lipase, 60,000 units protease, and 60,000 units amylase ◇
4X Pancreatin 600 mg
Tablets (enteric-coated): 2,400 mg pancreatin, 12,000 units lipase, 60,000 units protease, and 60,000 units amylase ◇
8X Pancreatin 900 mg
Tablets (enteric-coated): 7,200 mg pancreatin, 22,500 units lipase, 180,000 units protease, and 180,000 units amylase ◇
Pancrezyme 4X Tablets
Tablets (enteric-coated): 2,400 mg pancreatin, 12,000 units lipase, 60,000 units protease, and 60,000 units amylase ◇

INDICATIONS & DOSAGES
➤ **Exocrine pancreatic secretion insufficiency; digestive aid in diseases related to deficiency of pancreatic enzymes, such as cystic fibrosis—**
Adults and children: Dosage varies with condition being treated. Usual initial dose is 8,000 to 24,000 units of lipase activity P.O. before or with each meal or snack. Total daily dose also may be given in divided doses at 1- to 2-hour intervals throughout day.

ACTION
Replaces endogenous exocrine pancreatic enzymes and aids digestion of starches, fats, and proteins.

Route	Onset	Peak	Duration
P.O.	Unknown	Unknown	1-2 hr

ADVERSE REACTIONS
GI: nausea, diarrhea with high doses.
Skin: perianal irritation.
Other: allergic reactions.

INTERACTIONS
Drug-drug. *Antacids:* May negate pancreatin's beneficial effect. Avoid using together.

EFFECTS ON LAB TEST RESULTS
• May increase uric acid levels.

CONTRAINDICATIONS
Contraindicated in patients hypersensitive to drug, pork protein, or pork enzymes and in those with acute pancreatitis or acute exacerbations of chronic pancreatitis.

NURSING CONSIDERATIONS
• Use with caution in pregnant or breast-feeding women.
• Minimal USP standards dictate that each milligram of bovine or porcine pancreatin contains lipase 2 units, protease 25 units, and amylase 25 units.
• To avoid indigestion, monitor patient's dietary intake to ensure a proper balance of fat, protein, and starch. Dosage varies according to degree of maldigestion and malabsorption, amount of fat in diet, and enzyme activity of individual preparations.
• Fewer bowel movements and improved stool consistency indicate effective therapy.

• Drug isn't effective in GI disorders unrelated to pancreatic enzyme deficiency.
• Enteric coating on some products may reduce available enzyme in upper portion of jejunum.

PATIENT TEACHING
• Instruct patient to take before or with meals and snacks.
• Tell patient not to crush or chew enteric-coated forms. Capsules containing enteric-coated microspheres may be opened and sprinkled on a small quantity of cool, soft food. Stress importance of swallowing immediately, without chewing, and following with a glass of water or juice.
• Warn patient not to inhale powder form or powder from capsules; it may irritate skin or mucous membranes.
• Tell patient to store in airtight container at room temperature.
• Instruct patient not to change brands without consulting prescriber.

---

pancrelipase
Cotazym Capsules, Cotazym S Capsules, Creon 5 Minimicrospheres, Creon 10 Minimicrospheres, Creon 20 Minimicrospheres, Ilozyme Tablets, Ku-Zyme HP Capsules, Pancrease Capsules, Pancrease MT 4, Pancrease MT 10, Pancrease MT 16, Pancrease MT 20, Pancrelipase Capsules, Protilase Capsules, Ultrase MT 12, Ultrase MT 18, Ultrase MT 20, Viokase Powder, Viokase Tablets, Zymase Capsules

Pregnancy risk category C

AVAILABLE FORMS
Cotazym
Capsules: 8,000 units lipase, 30,000 units protease, 30,000 units amylase, and 25 mg calcium carbonate
Cotazym-S
Capsules (enteric-coated spheres): 5,000 units lipase, 20,000 units protease, and 20,000 units amylase

Creon 5
Capsules (delayed-release): 5,000 units lipase, 18,750 units protease, and 16,600 units amylase
Creon 10
Capsules (delayed-release): 10,000 units lipase, 37,500 units protease, and 33,200 units amylase
Creon 20
Capsules (delayed-release): 20,000 units lipase, 75,000 units protease, and 66,400 units amylase
Ilozyme
Tablets: 11,000 units lipase, 30,000 units protease, and 30,000 units amylase
Ku-Zyme HP
Capsules: 8,000 units lipase, 30,000 units protease, and 30,000 units amylase
Pancrease
Capsules (enteric-coated microspheres): 4,000 units lipase, 25,000 units protease, and 20,000 units amylase
Pancrease MT 4
Capsules (enteric-coated microtablets): 4,500 units lipase, 12,000 units protease, and 12,000 units amylase
Pancrease MT 10
Capsules (enteric-coated microtablets): 10,000 units lipase, 30,000 units protease, and 30,000 units amylase
Pancrease MT 16
Capsules (enteric-coated microtablets): 16,000 units lipase, 48,000 units protease, and 48,000 units amylase
Pancrease MT 20
Capsules (enteric-coated microtablets): 20,000 units lipase, 44,000 units protease, and 56,000 units amylase
Pancrelipase
Capsules (enteric-coated pellets): 4,000 units lipase, 25,000 units protease, and 20,000 units amylase
Protilase
Capsules (enteric-coated spheres): 4,000 units lipase, 25,000 units protease, and 20,000 units amylase
Ultrase MT 12
Capsules (delayed-release): 12,000 units lipase, 39,000 units protease, and 39,000 units amylase
Ultrase MT 18
Capsules (delayed-release): 18,000 units lipase, 58,500 units protease, and 58,000 units amylase

---

Ultrase MT 20
Capsules (delayed-release): 20,000 units lipase, 65,000 units protease, and 65,000 units amylase
Viokase
Powder: 16,800 units lipase, 70,000 units protease, and 70,000 units amylase per 0.7 g powder
Tablets: 8,000 units lipase, 30,000 units protease, and 30,000 units amylase
Zymase
Capsules (enteric-coated spheres): 12,000 units lipase, 24,000 units protease, and 24,000 units amylase

INDICATIONS & DOSAGES
➤ **Exocrine pancreatic secretion insufficiency; cystic fibrosis in adults and children; steatorrhea and other disorders of fat metabolism caused by insufficient pancreatic enzymes—**
Adults and children older than age 12: Dosage adjusted to patient's response. Usual initial dose 4,000 to 48,000 units of lipase with each meal.
Children ages 7 to 12: 4,000 to 12,000 units of lipase activity with each meal or snack. More can be taken, if needed.
Children ages 1 to 6: 4,000 to 8,000 units of lipase with each meal and 4,000 units of lipase with each snack.
Children ages 6 months to 11 months: 2,000 units of lipase with each meal.
Children younger than age 6 months: Dosage not established.

ACTION
Replaces endogenous exocrine pancreatic enzymes and aids digestion of starches, fats, and proteins.

Route	Onset	Peak	Duration
P.O.	Variable	Variable	Variable

ADVERSE REACTIONS
GI: *nausea,* cramping, diarrhea with high doses.

INTERACTIONS
Drug-drug. *Antacids:* May destroy enteric coating and enhance degradation of pancrelipase. Avoid using together.
Oral iron: May decrease iron response. Monitor patient for decreased effectiveness.

EFFECTS ON LAB TEST RESULTS
● May increase uric acid levels.

CONTRAINDICATIONS
Contraindicated in patients with severe hypersensitivity to pork and in those with acute pancreatitis or acute exacerbations of chronic pancreatic diseases.

NURSING CONSIDERATIONS
● *Alert:* Use drug only for confirmed exocrine pancreatic insufficiency. It isn't effective in GI disorders unrelated to enzyme deficiency.
● Lipase activity is greater than with other pancreatic enzymes.
● For infants, mix powder with applesauce and give with meals. Avoid contact with or inhalation of powder because it may be highly irritating. Older children may take capsules with food.
● Monitor patient's stools. Adequate replacement decreases number of bowel movements and improves stool consistency.
● Minimal USP standards dictate that each milligram of pancrelipase contains 24 units lipase, 100 units protease, and 100 units amylase.
● Dosage varies with degree of maldigestion and malabsorption, amount of fat in diet, and enzyme activity of individual preparations.
● Enteric coating on some products may reduce available enzyme in upper portion of jejunum.

PATIENT TEACHING
● Instruct patient to take before or with meals and snacks.
● Advise patient not to crush or chew enteric-coated forms. Capsules containing enteric-coated microspheres may be opened and sprinkled on a small quantity of cool, soft food. Stress importance of swallowing immediately, without chewing, and following with glass of water or juice.
● Warn patient not to inhale powder form or powder from capsules; it may irritate skin or mucous membranes.
● Tell patient to store in airtight container at room temperature.
● Instruct patient not to change brands without consulting prescriber.

Reactions may be *common,* uncommon, *life-threatening,* or COMMON AND LIFE-THREATENING.

ursodiol
Actigall, Urso

Pregnancy risk category B

AVAILABLE FORMS
Capsules: 300 mg
Tablets: 250 mg

INDICATIONS & DOSAGES
➤ **Dissolution of gallstones less than 20 mm in diameter when surgery is prohibited—**
Adults: 8 to 10 mg/kg P.O. daily in two or three divided doses.
➤ **Prevention of gallstone formation in obese patients with rapid weight loss—**
Adults: 300 mg P.O. b.i.d.

ACTION
Unknown. Drug is a naturally occurring bile acid that probably suppresses hepatic synthesis and secretion of cholesterol as well as intestinal cholesterol absorption. With long-term use, ursodiol can solubilize cholesterol from gallstones.

Route	Onset	Peak	Duration
P.O.	Unknown	1-3 hr	Unknown

ADVERSE REACTIONS
CNS: *headache,* fatigue, anxiety, depression, *dizziness,* sleep disorders.
EENT: rhinitis.
GI: *nausea, vomiting, dyspepsia,* metallic taste, *abdominal pain,* biliary pain, cholecystitis, *diarrhea, constipation,* stomatitis, flatulence.
GU: *urinary tract infection.*
Musculoskeletal: arthralgia, myalgia, *back pain.*
Respiratory: cough.
Skin: pruritus, rash, dry skin, urticaria, hair thinning, diaphoresis.

INTERACTIONS
Drug-drug. *Aluminum-containing antacids, cholestyramine, colestipol:* Binds ursodiol, preventing its absorption. Avoid using together.
Clofibrate, estrogens, oral contraceptives: Increased hepatic cholesterol secretion; may counteract effects of ursodiol. Avoid using together.

EFFECTS ON LAB TEST RESULTS
None reported.

CONTRAINDICATIONS
Contraindicated in patients hypersensitive to ursodiol or other bile acids and in those with chronic hepatic disease, unremitting acute cholecystitis, cholangitis, biliary obstruction, gallstone-induced pancreatitis, or biliary fistula.

NURSING CONSIDERATIONS
• Drug won't dissolve calcified cholesterol stones, radiolucent bile pigment stones, or radiopaque stones.
• *Alert:* Monitor liver function test results, including AST and ALT, at the start of therapy and after 1 month, 3 months, and then every 6 months during therapy. Abnormal test results may indicate worsening of the disease. A theoretical risk exists that a hepatotoxic metabolite of ursodiol may form in some patients.
• Therapy usually is long-term, with ultrasound images of the gallbladder taken every 6 months. If stones don't partially dissolve within 12 months, eventual success is unlikely. Safety of use for longer than 24 months hasn't been established.

PATIENT TEACHING
• Advise patient about alternative therapies, including watchful waiting (no intervention) and cholecystectomy because the relapse rate may be as high as 50% after 5 years.
• Tell patient to report adverse effects.
• Advise patient that dissolution of gallstones requires months of treatment.

47

Antidiarrheals

attapulgite
bismuth subsalicylate
calcium polycarbophil
  (See Chapter 48, LAXATIVES.)
diphenoxylate hydrochloride and
  atropine sulfate
loperamide
octreotide acetate
opium tincture
opium tincture, camphorated

COMBINATION PRODUCTS
IMODIUM ADVANCED: loperamide 2 mg
and simethicone 125 mg chewable tablets.
KAODENE NON-NARCOTIC ◊: 3.9 g kaolin
and 194.4 mg pectin in 30-ml bismuth
subsalicylate liquid.
KAPECTOLIN: 90 g kaolin and 2 g pectin in
30-ml suspension.
K-C SUSPENSION ◊: 5.2 g kaolin, 260 mg
pectin, 260 mg bismuth subsalicylate in
30-ml suspension.

---

attapulgite
Diasorb, Donnagel, Fowler's†,
Kaopectate Advanced Formula,
Kaopectate Maximum Strength,
K-Pek, Parepectolin, Rheaban
Maximum Strength

Pregnancy risk category NR

AVAILABLE FORMS
Caplets: 750 mg
Oral suspension: 600 mg/15 ml, 750 mg/
5 ml, 750 mg/15 ml†, 900 mg/15 ml†
Tablets: 300 mg, 600 mg†, 630 mg†,
750 mg

INDICATIONS & DOSAGES
➤ **Acute, nonspecific diarrhea—**
Adults and children older than age 12: 1.2
to 1.5 g (up to 3 g if using Diasorb) P.O.
after each loose bowel movement, not to
exceed 9 g in 24 hours.
Children ages 6 to 12: 600 mg suspension or 750 mg tablet P.O. after each loose
bowel movement, not to exceed 4.2 g suspension or 4.5 g tablet in 24 hours.

Children ages 3 to 5: 300 mg P.O. after
each loose bowel movement, not to exceed
2.1 g in 24 hours.

ACTION
Hydrated magnesium aluminum silicate
that's thought to adsorb large numbers of
bacteria and toxins and reduce water loss.

Route	Onset	Peak	Duration
P.O.	Unknown	Unknown	Unknown

ADVERSE REACTIONS
GI: constipation.

INTERACTIONS
Drug-drug. *Oral drugs:* Potential for
impaired absorption of oral drugs. Give
attapulgite not less than 2 hours before or
3 hours after these drugs, and monitor patient for decreased effectiveness.

EFFECTS ON LAB TEST RESULTS
None reported.

CONTRAINDICATIONS
Contraindicated in patients with dysentery
or suspected bowel obstruction.

NURSING CONSIDERATIONS
● Use cautiously in patients with dehydration. Promote adequate fluid intake to
compensate for fluid loss from diarrhea.
● Drug shouldn't be used if diarrhea is
accompanied by fever or blood or mucus
in the stool. If these signs occur during
treatment, withhold drug and notify prescriber.

PATIENT TEACHING
● Tell patient to take drug after each loose
bowel movement until diarrhea is controlled.
● Instruct patient to notify prescriber if
diarrhea isn't controlled within 48 hours
or if fever develops.

---

bismuth subsalicylate
Bismatrol◇, Bismatrol Extra
Strength◇, Pepto-Bismol◇,
Pepto-Bismol Maximum Strength
Liquid◇, Pink Bismuth◇

Pregnancy risk category NR

AVAILABLE FORMS
Oral suspension: 262 mg/15 ml◇,
524 mg/15 ml◇
Tablets (chewable): 262 mg◇

INDICATIONS & DOSAGES
➤ **Mild, nonspecific diarrhea—**
Adults and children older than age 12:
30 ml or 2 tablets P.O. q 30 minutes to 1
hour, up to maximum of eight doses and
for no longer than 2 days.
Children ages 9 to 12: 15 ml or 1 tablet
P.O. q 30 minutes to 1 hour, up to maximum of eight doses and for no longer than
2 days.
Children ages 6 to 9: 10 ml or ⅔ tablet
P.O. q 30 minutes to 1 hour, up to maximum of eight doses and for no longer than
2 days.
Children ages 3 to 6: 5 ml or ⅓ tablet
P.O. q 30 minutes to 1 hour, up to maximum of eight doses and for no longer
than 2 days.

ACTION
Unknown. Has a mild water-binding
capacity. May adsorb toxins and provide
protective coating for mucosa.

Route	Onset	Peak	Duration
P.O.	1 hr	Unknown	Unknown

ADVERSE REACTIONS
GI: temporary darkening of tongue and
stools.
Other: salicylism with high doses.

INTERACTIONS
Drug-drug. *Aspirin, other salicylates:*
Risk of salicylate toxicity. Monitor pa-
tient.
Oral anticoagulants, oral antidiabetics:
Theoretical risk of increased effects of
these drugs after high doses of bismuth
subsalicylate. Monitor patient closely.

Tetracycline: Decreased tetracycline absorption. Separate administration times by
at least 2 hours.

EFFECTS ON LAB TEST RESULTS
None reported.

CONTRAINDICATIONS
Contraindicated in patients hypersensitive
to salicylates.

NURSING CONSIDERATIONS
• Use cautiously in patients taking aspirin.
Discontinue if tinnitus occurs.
• Because bismuth is radiopaque, it may
interfere with radiologic examination of
GI tract.
• Salicylate absorption may occur from
bismuth subsalicylate. Use cautiously in
children and in patients with bleeding disorders or salicylate sensitivity.
• Avoid use before GI radiologic procedures because bismuth is radiopaque and
may interfere with X-rays.

PATIENT TEACHING
• Advise patient that bismuth subsalicylate contains salicylate. Each tablet has
102 mg salicylate. Regular-strength liquid
has 130 mg/15 ml. Extra-strength liquid
has 230 mg/15 ml.
• Instruct patient to chew tablets well before swallowing and to shake liquid before
measuring dose.
• Tell patient to call prescriber if diarrhea
lasts longer than 2 days or is accompanied
by high fever.
• Advise patient to drink plenty of clear
fluids to help prevent dehydration, which
may accompany diarrhea.
• Urge patient to consult with prescriber
before giving bismuth subsalicylate to
children or teenagers during or after recovery from the flu or chickenpox.
• Inform patient that all forms of Pepto-
Bismol are effective against traveler's diarrhea. Tablets and caplets may be more
convenient to carry.

---

diphenoxylate hydrochloride and atropine sulfate
Logen, Lomanate, Lomotil*, Lonox

Pregnancy risk category C
Controlled substance schedule V

AVAILABLE FORMS
Liquid: 2.5 mg/5 ml (with atropine sulfate 0.025 mg/5 ml)*
Tablets: 2.5 mg (with atropine sulfate 0.025 mg)

INDICATIONS & DOSAGES
➤ **Acute, nonspecific diarrhea—**
Adults and children older than age 12:
Initially, 5 mg P.O. q.i.d.; then adjusted, p.r.n.
Children ages 2 to 12: 0.3 to 0.4 mg/kg liquid form P.O. daily in four divided doses. For maintenance, initial dose reduced, p.r.n., up to 75%.

ACTION
Unknown. Probably increases smooth muscle tone in GI tract, inhibits motility and propulsion, and diminishes secretions.

Route	Onset	Peak	Duration
P.O.	45-60 min	3 hr	3-4 hr

ADVERSE REACTIONS
CNS: *sedation, dizziness,* headache, drowsiness, lethargy, restlessness, depression, euphoria, malaise, confusion, numbness in limbs.
CV: tachycardia.
EENT: mydriasis.
GI: *dry mouth,* nausea, vomiting, abdominal discomfort or distention, ***paralytic ileus,*** anorexia, fluid retention in bowel or megacolon, ***pancreatitis,*** swollen gums.
GU: urine retention.
Respiratory: *respiratory depression.*
Skin: pruritus, rash, dry skin.
Other: *angioedema, anaphylaxis,* possible physical dependence with long-term use.

INTERACTIONS
Drug-drug. *Barbiturates, CNS depressants, narcotics, tranquilizers:* Enhanced CNS depression. Monitor patient closely.
MAO inhibitors: May cause hypertensive crisis. Avoid using together.
Drug-lifestyle. *Alcohol use:* Enhanced CNS depression. Discourage use together.

EFFECTS ON LAB TEST RESULTS
None reported.

CONTRAINDICATIONS
Contraindicated in patients hypersensitive to diphenoxylate or atropine, in those with jaundice, and in children younger than age 2. Also contraindicated in those with acute diarrhea resulting from poison (until toxic material is eliminated from GI tract), from organisms that penetrate intestinal mucosa, or from antibiotic-induced pseudomembranous enterocolitis.

NURSING CONSIDERATIONS
• Use cautiously in children age 2 and older; in patients with hepatic disease, narcotic dependence, or acute ulcerative colitis; and in pregnant patients. Stop therapy immediately and notify prescriber if abdominal distention or other signs or symptoms of toxic megacolon develop.
• *Alert:* Monitor fluid and electrolyte balance. Correct fluid and electrolyte disturbances before starting drug. Dehydration, especially in young children, may increase risk of delayed toxicity. Fluid retention in bowel or megacolon may occur with drug use and may mask depletion of extracellular fluid and electrolytes, especially in young children treated for acute gastroenteritis.
• Drug isn't indicated for treating antibiotic-induced diarrhea.
• Drug is unlikely to be effective if no response occurs within 48 hours.
• Risk of physical dependence increases with high dosage and long-term use. Atropine sulfate helps discourage abuse.

PATIENT TEACHING
• Tell patient not to exceed recommended dosage.
• Warn patient not to use drug to treat acute diarrhea for longer than 2 days and

---

to seek medical attention if diarrhea continues.

• Advise patient to avoid hazardous activities, such as driving, until CNS effects of drug are known.

---

loperamide
Imodium, Imodium A-D ◇, Kaopectate II Caplets ◇, Maalox Anti-Diarrheal Caplets ◇, Pepto Diarrhea Control ◇

Pregnancy risk category B

AVAILABLE FORMS
Caplets: 2 mg ◇
Capsules: 2 mg
Oral liquid: 1 mg/5 ml ◇

INDICATIONS & DOSAGES
➤ **Acute, nonspecific diarrhea—**
Adults and children older than age 12:
Initially, 4 mg P.O.; then 2 mg after each unformed stool. Maximum, 8 mg daily.
Children ages 8 to 12: 2 mg t.i.d. P.O. on first day. Subsequent doses of 5 ml or 0.1 mg/kg of body weight may be given after each unformed stool. Maximum, 6 mg daily.
Children ages 6 to 8: 2 mg P.O. b.i.d. on first day. If diarrhea persists, contact prescriber. Don't exceed 4 mg daily.
Children ages 2 to 5: 1 mg P.O. t.i.d. on first day. If diarrhea persists, contact prescriber.
➤ **Chronic diarrhea—**
Adults: Initially, 4 mg P.O.; then 2 mg after each unformed stool until diarrhea subsides. Dosage adjusted to individual response.

ACTION
Inhibits peristaltic activity, prolonging transit of intestinal contents.

Route	Onset	Peak	Duration
P.O.	Unknown	2.5-5 hr	24 hr

ADVERSE REACTIONS
CNS: drowsiness, fatigue, dizziness.
GI: dry mouth; abdominal pain, distention, or discomfort; *constipation;* nausea; vomiting.
Skin: rash, hypersensitivity reactions.

INTERACTIONS
None significant.

EFFECTS ON LAB TEST RESULTS
None reported.

CONTRAINDICATIONS
Contraindicated in patients hypersensitive to drug and when constipation must be avoided. Also contraindicated in children younger than age 2.

NURSING CONSIDERATIONS
• Use cautiously in patients with hepatic disease.
• Drug produces antidiarrheal action similar to diphenoxylate but without as many adverse CNS effects.
• *Alert:* Monitor children closely for CNS effects; they may be more sensitive to them than adults.
• *Alert:* Don't confuse Imodium with Ionamin.

PATIENT TEACHING
• Advise patient not to exceed recommended dosage.
• Tell patient with acute diarrhea to stop drug and seek medical attention if no improvement occurs within 48 hours. In chronic diarrhea, tell him to notify prescriber and to stop drug if no improvement occurs after taking 16 mg daily for at least 10 days.
• Advise patient with acute colitis to stop drug immediately and notify prescriber about abdominal distention.
• Warn patient to avoid activities that require mental alertness until CNS effects of drug are known.
• Tell patient to report nausea, abdominal pain, or abdominal discomfort.
• Advise patient to relieve dry mouth with ice chips or sugarless gum.

---

octreotide acetate
Sandostatin, Sandostatin LAR

Pregnancy risk category B

AVAILABLE FORMS
Injection ampules: 0.05 mg, 0.1 mg, 0.5 mg

Injection (long-acting): 10 mg, 20 mg, 30 mg
Injection-multidose vials: 0.2 mg/ml, 1 mg/ml

INDICATIONS & DOSAGES
➤ **Flushing and diarrhea from carcinoid tumors—**
Adults: 0.1 to 0.6 mg daily S.C. in two to four divided doses for first 2 weeks of therapy. Usual daily dose is 0.3 mg. Subsequent dosage based on individual response.
➤ **Watery diarrhea from vasoactive intestinal polypeptide-secreting tumors (VIPomas)—**
Adults: 0.2 to 0.3 mg daily S.C. in two to four divided doses for first 2 weeks of therapy. Subsequent dosage based on individual response; usually shouldn't exceed 0.45 mg daily.
➤ **Acromegaly—**
Adults: Initially, 50 mcg S.C. t.i.d., then adjusted based on somatomedin C levels q 2 weeks.

ACTION
Mimics action of naturally occurring somatostatin.

Route	Onset	Peak	Duration
S.C.	0.5 hr	0.5 hr	< 12 hr

ADVERSE REACTIONS
CNS: dizziness, light-headedness, fatigue, headache.
CV: *bradycardia,* edema, conduction abnormalities, *arrhythmias.*
EENT: blurred vision.
GI: *nausea, diarrhea, abdominal pain or discomfort, loose stools,* vomiting, fat malabsorption, *gallbladder abnormalities,* flatulence, constipation.
GU: pollakiuria, urinary tract infection.
Metabolic: hyperglycemia; hypoglycemia; hypothyroidism; suppressed secretion of growth hormone and of the gastroenterohepatic peptides gastrin, vasoactive intestinal polypeptide, insulin, glucagon, secretin, motilin, and pancreatic polypeptide.
Musculoskeletal: backache, joint pain.
Skin: flushing, wheal, erythema or pain at injection site, alopecia.

Other: pain or burning at S.C. injection site, cold symptoms, flulike symptoms.

INTERACTIONS
Drug-drug. *Cyclosporine:* May decrease plasma cyclosporine levels. Monitor patient closely.

EFFECTS ON LAB TEST RESULTS
● May increase or decrease glucose levels.

CONTRAINDICATIONS
Contraindicated in patients hypersensitive to drug or its components.

NURSING CONSIDERATIONS
● Monitor baseline thyroid function tests.
● Monitor somatomedin C levels every 2 weeks. Dosage adjustments are based on this level.
● Monitor laboratory tests periodically, such as thyroid function tests, glucose, urine 5-hydroxyindoleacetic acid, plasma serotonin, and plasma substance P (for carcinoid tumors).
● Monitor patient regularly for gallbladder disease. Octreotide therapy may be related to the development of cholelithiasis because of its effect on gallbladder motility or fat absorption.
● Monitor patient closely for signs and symptoms of glucose imbalance. Patients with type 1 diabetes mellitus and patients receiving oral antidiabetics or oral diazoxide may need dosage adjustments during therapy. Monitor glucose levels.
● Octreotide therapy may alter fluid and electrolyte balance and may cause need for adjustment of other drugs used to control symptoms of the disease, such as beta blockers.
● Half-life may be altered in patients with end-stage renal failure who are receiving dialysis.
● *Alert:* Don't confuse Sandostatin with Sandimmune or Sandoglobulin.

PATIENT TEACHING
● Urge patient to report signs and symptoms of abdominal discomfort immediately.
● Stress importance of the need for periodic laboratory testing during octreotide therapy.

Reactions may be *common,* uncommon, *life-threatening,* or **COMMON AND LIFE-THREATENING.**

opium tincture*

Controlled substance schedule II

opium tincture, camphorated* (paregoric)

Pregnancy risk category NR
Controlled substance schedule III

AVAILABLE FORMS
opium tincture
Oral solution: Equivalent to morphine 10 mg/ml*
opium tincture, camphorated
Oral solution: Each 5 ml contains morphine, 2 mg; anise oil, 0.2 ml; benzoic acid, 20 mg; camphor, 20 mg; glycerin, 0.2 ml; and alcohol to make 5 ml*

INDICATIONS & DOSAGES
➤ **Acute, nonspecific diarrhea—**
Opium tincture
Adults: 0.6 ml P.O. q.i.d. Maximum, 6 ml daily.
Opium tincture, camphorated
Adults: 5 to 10 ml P.O. once daily, b.i.d., t.i.d., or q.i.d. until diarrhea subsides.
Children: 0.25 to 0.5 ml/kg P.O. once daily, b.i.d., t.i.d., or q.i.d. until diarrhea subsides.

ACTION
Increases smooth muscle tone in GI tract, inhibits motility and propulsion, and diminishes secretions.

Route	Onset	Peak	Duration
P.O.	Unknown	Unknown	Unknown

ADVERSE REACTIONS
CNS: dizziness, light-headedness.
GI: nausea, vomiting.
Other: physical dependence after long-term use.

INTERACTIONS
None significant.

EFFECTS ON LAB TEST RESULTS
• Increased amylase and lipase levels.

CONTRAINDICATIONS
Contraindicated in patients with acute diarrhea caused by poisoning until toxic material is removed from GI tract. Also contraindicated in patients with diarrhea caused by organisms that penetrate intestinal mucosa.

NURSING CONSIDERATIONS
• Use cautiously in patients with asthma, prostatic hyperplasia, hepatic disease, and history of opioid dependence.
• *Alert:* Opium tincture has 25 times more opium content than camphorated opium tincture. Camphorated opium tincture is more dilute, and teaspoon doses are easier to measure than dropper quantities of opium tincture.
• *Alert:* For overdose, use the narcotic antagonist naloxone, to reverse respiratory depression.
• Mix with sufficient water to ensure passage to stomach.
• Opium tincture and camphorated opium tincture may prevent delivery of Tc99m disofenin to small intestine during hepatobiliary imaging tests; delay test until 24 hours after last dose.
• A milky fluid forms when camphorated opium tincture is added to water.
• Store in tightly capped, light-resistant container.
• *Alert:* Don't confuse opium tincture with camphorated opium tincture.

PATIENT TEACHING
• Advise patient against long-term use of drug; risk of physical dependence increases with long-term use.
• Instruct patient to measure dose carefully to avoid overdose.
• Tell patient to notify prescriber if diarrhea persists.

---

*Liquid contains alcohol.   **May contain tartrazine.   †Canada   ‡Australia   §U.K.   ◇OTC

INTERACTIONS
Drug-drug. *Tetracyclines:* Impaired tetracycline absorption. Avoid using together.

EFFECTS ON LAB TEST RESULTS
None reported.

CONTRAINDICATIONS
Contraindicated in patients with signs or symptoms of GI obstruction or those with swallowing difficulty.

NURSING CONSIDERATIONS
● Before giving drug for constipation, determine whether patient has adequate fluid intake, exercise, and diet.
● In children younger than age 6, use must be directed by prescriber.
● *Alert:* Rectal bleeding or failure to respond to therapy may indicate need for surgery.

PATIENT TEACHING
● Full benefit of drug may take 1 to 3 days to occur.
● Advise patient to chew Equalactin or Mitrolan tablets thoroughly before swallowing and to drink a full (8-ounce) glass of water with each dose. When drug is used as an antidiarrheal, tell patient not to drink a glass of water.
● Advise patient to seek medical attention if he experiences vomiting, chest pain, difficulty breathing or swallowing after taking medication.
● Teach patient about dietary sources of bulk, including bran and other cereals, fresh fruit, and vegetables.
● For severe diarrhea, advise patient to repeat dose every 30 minutes, but not to exceed maximum daily dose. Don't use for longer than 2 days, unless directed by a prescriber.

---

castor oil
Emulsoil ◇ , Purge ◇

Pregnancy risk category X

AVAILABLE FORMS
Capsules: 0.62 ml
Oral liquid: 67%, 95% (Emulsoil ◇ , Purge ◇)

INDICATIONS & DOSAGES
➤ **Preparation for rectal or bowel examination or for surgery—**
Adults and children age 12 and older: 15 to 60 ml P.O. as a single dose about 16 hours before surgery or procedure.
Children ages 2 to 12: 5 to 15 ml P.O. as a single dose about 16 hours before surgery or procedure.
Children younger than age 2: 1 to 5 ml P.O. as a single dose about 16 hours before surgery or procedure.

ACTION
Unknown. Stimulant laxative that increases peristalsis, probably by direct effect on smooth muscle of the intestine. It's thought to either irritate the musculature or stimulate the colonic intramural plexus. Drug also promotes fluid accumulation in colon and small intestine.

Route	Onset	Peak	Duration
P.O.	2-6 hr	Variable	Variable

ADVERSE REACTIONS
GI: *nausea,* vomiting, diarrhea, loss of normal bowel function with excessive use, *abdominal cramps* especially in severe constipation, malabsorption of nutrients, cathartic colon with long-term misuse, protein-losing enteropathy, possible constipation after catharsis.
Metabolic: hypokalemia, other electrolyte imbalances with excessive use.
Other: laxative dependence with long-term or excessive use.

INTERACTIONS
Drug-drug. *Other oral drugs:* Absorption of drugs given together decreased. Separate administration times.

EFFECTS ON LAB TEST RESULTS
● Decreased potassium and electrolyte imbalances.

CONTRAINDICATIONS
Contraindicated during menstruation or pregnancy and in patients with ulcerative bowel lesions, anal or rectal fissures, fecal impaction, intestinal obstruction, intestinal perforation, or symptoms of appendicitis or acute surgical abdomen, such as abdominal pain, nausea, and vomiting.

Reactions may be *common,* uncommon, *life-threatening,* or COMMON AND LIFE-THREATENING.

NURSING CONSIDERATIONS

• Use cautiously in patients with rectal bleeding.

• Give castor oil with juice or carbonated beverage to mask oily taste. Have patient stir mixture and drink it promptly. Ice held in the mouth before taking drug will help reduce taste.

• Shake emulsion well before measuring dose. Emulsion is better tolerated but is more expensive. Store below 40° F (4.4° C). Don't freeze.

• Give on empty stomach for best results.

• Increased dosage produces no greater effect.

• Give drug at times that don't interfere with scheduled activities or sleep.

• Increased intestinal motility reduces absorption of oral drugs given together. Separate administration times.

• *Alert:* Failure of patient to respond to drug may indicate acute condition requiring surgery.

PATIENT TEACHING

• Tell patient not to expect another bowel movement for 1 to 2 days after castor oil has emptied bowel.

• Warn patient about possible adverse reactions.

---

docusate calcium (dioctyl calcium sulfosuccinate)
DC Softgels ◊ , Pro-Cal-Sof ◊ ,
Sulfolax ◊ , Surfak ◊

docusate sodium (dioctyl sodium sulfosuccinate)
Colace ◊ , Coloxyl‡, Coloxyl
Enema Concentrate‡, Diocto ◊ ,
Dioctyl§, Dioeze ◊ , Diosuccin ◊ ,
Di-Sosul ◊ , D.O.S. ◊ , D-S-S ◊ ,
Duosol ◊ , Ex-Lax Stool Softener
Caplets, Fletcher's Enemette§,
Modane Soft ◊ , Norgalax Micro-
enema§, Phillips' Liqui-Gels, Pro-
Sof ◊ , Regulax SS ◊ , Regulex† ◊

Pregnancy risk category C

AVAILABLE FORMS
docusate calcium
Capsules: 50 mg ◊ , 240 mg ◊

docusate sodium
Capsules: 50 mg ◊ , 100 mg ◊ ,
240 mg ◊ , 250 mg ◊
Enema concentrate: 18 g/100 ml (must be diluted)‡
Oral liquid: 150 mg/15 ml ◊
Oral solution: 10 mg/ml ◊ , 50 mg/ml ◊
Syrup: 20 mg/5 ml, 50 mg/15 ml ◊ ,
60 mg/15 ml ◊
Tablets: 50 mg ◊ , 100 mg ◊

INDICATIONS & DOSAGES
➤ **Stool softener—**
Adults and children older than age 12: 50 to 500 mg docusate calcium or sodium P.O. daily until bowel movements are normal. Or, give enema. Dilute 1:24 with sterile water before use, and give 100 to 150 ml retention enema, 300 to 500 ml evacuation enema, or 0.5 to 1.5 L flushing enema P.R.
Children ages 6 to 12: 40 to 120 mg docusate sodium P.O. daily.
Children ages 3 to 6: 20 to 60 mg docusate sodium P.O. daily.
Children younger than age 3: 10 to 40 mg docusate sodium P.O. daily.

Higher dosages used for initial therapy. Dosage adjusted to individual response.

ACTION
Stool softener that reduces surface tension of interfacing liquid contents of the bowel. This detergent activity promotes incorporation of additional liquid into stools, thus forming a softer mass.

Route	Onset	Peak	Duration
P.O.	1-3 days	Unknown	Unknown
P.R.	Unknown	Unknown	Unknown

ADVERSE REACTIONS
GI: bitter taste, mild abdominal cramping, diarrhea.
Other: laxative dependence with long-term or excessive use.

INTERACTIONS
Drug-drug. *Mineral oil:* May increase mineral oil absorption and cause toxicity and lipoid pneumonia. Separate administration times.

EFFECTS ON LAB TEST RESULTS
None reported.

CONTRAINDICATIONS
Contraindicated in patients hypersensitive to drug and in those with intestinal obstruction or signs and symptoms of appendicitis, fecal impaction, or acute surgical abdomen, such as undiagnosed abdominal pain or vomiting.

NURSING CONSIDERATIONS
• Drug isn't for use in treating existing constipation but prevents constipation from developing.
• Before giving drug, determine whether patient has adequate fluid intake, exercise, and diet.
• Give liquid in milk, fruit juice, or infant formula to mask bitter taste.
• Drug is laxative of choice for patients who shouldn't strain during defecation, including patients recovering from MI or rectal surgery, those with rectal or anal disease that makes passage of firm stools difficult, and those with postpartum constipation.
• Store drug at 59° to 86° F (15° to 30° C), and protect liquid from light.

PATIENT TEACHING
• Teach patient about dietary sources of bulk, including bran and other cereals, fresh fruit, and vegetables.
• Instruct patient to use drug only occasionally and not for longer than 1 week without prescriber's knowledge.
• Tell patient to discontinue drug and notify prescriber if severe cramping occurs.
• Notify patient that it may take from 1 to 3 days to soften stools.

---

glycerin
Fleet Babylax ◊, Sani-Supp ◊

Pregnancy risk category NR

AVAILABLE FORMS
Enema (pediatric): 4 ml/applicator ◊
Suppositories: Adult, children, and infant sizes ◊

INDICATIONS & DOSAGES
➤ Constipation—
Adults and children age 6 and older: 2 to 3 g as rectal suppository; or 5 to 15 ml as enema.

Children ages 2 to 5: 1 to 1.7 g as rectal suppository; or 2 to 5 ml as enema.

ACTION
Hyperosmolar laxative that draws water from the tissues into the feces, thus stimulating evacuation.

Route	Onset	Peak	Duration
P.R.	15-30 min	Unknown	Unknown

ADVERSE REACTIONS
GI: *cramping pain,* rectal discomfort, hyperemia of rectal mucosa.

INTERACTIONS
None significant.

EFFECTS ON LAB TEST RESULTS
None reported.

CONTRAINDICATIONS
Contraindicated in patients hypersensitive to drug and in those with intestinal obstruction or signs and symptoms of appendicitis, fecal impaction, or acute surgical abdomen, such as undiagnosed abdominal pain or vomiting.

NURSING CONSIDERATIONS
• Drug is used mainly to reestablish proper toilet habits in laxative-dependent patients.

PATIENT TEACHING
• Tell patient that drug must be retained for at least 15 minutes and that it usually acts within 1 hour. Entire suppository need not melt to be effective.
• Warn patient about adverse GI reactions.

---

lactulose
Cephulac, Cholac, Chronulac, Constilac, Constulose, Duphalac, Enulose, Evalose, Heptalac, Lactulax†

Pregnancy risk category B

AVAILABLE FORMS
Packets: 10 g, 20 g
Syrup: 10 g/15 ml

INDICATIONS & DOSAGES
➤Constipation—
Adults: 10 to 20 g or 15 to 30 ml P.O.
daily, increased to 60 ml/day, if needed.
➤ **To prevent and treat hepatic encephalopathy, including hepatic precoma and coma in patients with severe hepatic disease—**
Adults: Initially, 20 to 30 g or 30 to 45 ml P.O. t.i.d. or q.i.d., until two or three soft stools are produced daily. Usual dose is 60 to 100 g daily in divided doses. Or, 200 g or 300 ml diluted with 700 ml of water or normal saline solution and given as retention enema P.R. q 4 to 6 hours, p.r.n.

ACTION
Produces an osmotic effect in colon; resulting distention promotes peristalsis. Also, decreases ammonia, probably as a result of bacterial degradation, which decreases the pH of colon contents.

Route	Onset	Peak	Duration
P.O.	24-48 hr	Variable	Variable
P.R.	Unknown	Unknown	Unknown

ADVERSE REACTIONS
GI: *abdominal cramps, belching, diarrhea, gaseous distention, flatulence,* nausea, vomiting.

INTERACTIONS
Drug-drug. *Antacids, antibiotics, oral neomycin:* Decreased lactulose effectiveness. Avoid using together.

EFFECTS ON LAB TEST RESULTS
None reported.

CONTRAINDICATIONS
Contraindicated in patients on a low-galactose diet.

NURSING CONSIDERATIONS
• Use cautiously in patients with diabetes mellitus.
• To minimize sweet taste, dilute with water or fruit juice or give with food.
• Prepare enema (not commercially available) by adding 200 g (300 ml) to 700 ml of water or normal saline solution. The diluted solution is given as retention ene-

ma for 30 to 60 minutes. Use a rectal balloon.
• If enema isn't retained for at least 30 minutes, be prepared to repeat dose.
• Monitor sodium level for hypernatremia, especially when giving in higher doses to treat hepatic encephalopathy.
• Monitor mental status when giving to patients with hepatic encephalopathy.
• Be prepared to replace fluid loss.
• *Alert:* Don't confuse lactulose with lactose.

PATIENT TEACHING
• Show home care patient how to mix and use drug.
• Inform patient about adverse reactions and tell him to notify prescriber if reactions become bothersome or if diarrhea occurs.
• Instruct patient not to take other laxatives during lactulose therapy.

---

magnesium citrate (citrate of magnesia)
Citroma◇, Citro-Mag†

magnesium hydroxide (milk of magnesia)
Milk of Magnesia◇, Milk of Magnesia Concentrated◇, Phillips' Milk of Magnesia◇

magnesium sulfate (epsom salts)◇

Pregnancy risk category NR

AVAILABLE FORMS
magnesium citrate
Oral solution: about 168 mEq magnesium/240 ml ◇
magnesium hydroxide
Chewable tablets: 311 mg
Oral suspension: 400 mg/5 ml, 800 mg/5 ml
magnesium sulfate
Granules: about 40 mEq magnesium/5 g◇

INDICATIONS & DOSAGES
➤**Constipation, to evacuate bowel before surgery—**
Adults and children age 12 and older: 11 to 25 g magnesium citrate P.O. daily as a

single dose or divided. Or, 2.4 to 4.8 g or 30 to 60 ml magnesium hydroxide P.O. daily as a single dose or divided. Or, 10 to 30 g magnesium sulfate P.O. daily as a single dose or divided.

Children ages 6 to 11: 5.5 to 12.5 g magnesium citrate P.O. daily as a single dose or divided. Or, 1.2 to 2.4 g or 15 to 30 ml magnesium hydroxide P.O. daily as a single dose or divided. Or, 5 to 10 g magnesium sulfate P.O. daily as a single dose or divided.

Children ages 2 to 5: 2.7 to 6.25 g magnesium citrate P.O. daily as a single dose or divided. Or, 0.4 to 1.2 g or 5 to 15 ml magnesium hydroxide P.O. daily as a single dose or divided. Or, 2.5 to 5 g magnesium sulfate P.O. daily as a single dose or divided.

➤ **Antacid**—
Adults: 5 to 15 ml milk of magnesia P.O. t.i.d. or q.i.d.

ACTION
Saline laxative that produces an osmotic effect in the small intestine by drawing water into the intestinal lumen.

Route	Onset	Peak	Duration
P.O.	0.5-3 hr	Variable	Variable

ADVERSE REACTIONS
GI: *abdominal cramping, nausea, diarrhea.*
Metabolic: fluid and electrolyte disturbances with daily use.
Other: laxative dependence with long-term or excessive use.

INTERACTIONS
Drug-drug. *Oral drugs:* Impaired absorption. Separate administration times.

EFFECTS ON LAB TEST RESULTS
● May alter fluid and electrolyte levels, with prolonged use.

CONTRAINDICATIONS
Contraindicated in pregnant patients about to deliver and in patients with myocardial damage, heart block, fecal impaction, rectal fissures, intestinal obstruction or perforation, renal disease, or signs and symptoms of appendicitis or acute surgical abdomen, such as abdominal pain, nausea, or vomiting.

NURSING CONSIDERATIONS
● Use cautiously in patients with rectal bleeding.
● Give drug at times that don't interfere with scheduled activities or sleep. Drug produces watery stools in 3 to 6 hours.
● Before giving drug for constipation, determine whether patient has adequate fluid intake, exercise, and diet.
● Chill magnesium citrate before use to improve its palatability.
● Shake suspension well; give with a large amount of water when used as laxative. When giving by nasogastric tube, make sure tube is placed properly and is patent. After instilling drug, flush tube with water to ensure passage to stomach and maintain tube patency.
● *Alert:* Monitor electrolyte levels, during prolonged use. Magnesium may accumulate if patient has renal insufficiency.
● Drug is for short-term use.
● Magnesium sulfate is more potent than other saline laxatives.

PATIENT TEACHING
● Teach patient to administer drug.
● Teach patient about dietary sources of bulk, including bran and other cereals, fresh fruit, and vegetables.
● Warn patient that frequent or prolonged use as a laxative may cause dependence.

methylcellulose
Citrucel ◊ , Citrucel Orange Flavor ◊ , Citrucel Sugar-Free Orange Flavor ◊

Pregnancy risk category NR

AVAILABLE FORMS
Powder: 105 mg/g ◊ ; 196 mg/g ◊

INDICATIONS & DOSAGES
➤ **Chronic constipation**—
Adults and children older than age 12: Up to 6 g daily given in divided doses of 0.45 to 3 g per dose.

Reactions may be *common*, uncommon, *life-threatening*, or COMMON AND LIFE-THREATENING.

Children ages 6 to 12: Usual dose 3 g daily given in divided doses of 0.45 to 1.5 g per dose.

ACTION

Bulk-forming laxative that absorbs water and expands to increase bulk and moisture content of stools. The increased bulk encourages peristalsis and bowel movement.

Route	Onset	Peak	Duration
P.O.	12-24 hr	< 3 days	Variable

ADVERSE REACTIONS

GI: *nausea,* vomiting, diarrhea with excessive use; esophageal, gastric, small intestinal, or colonic strictures when drug is chewed or taken in dry form; *abdominal cramps,* especially in severe constipation. **Other:** laxative dependence with long-term or excessive use.

INTERACTIONS

None significant.

EFFECTS ON LAB TEST RESULTS

None reported.

CONTRAINDICATIONS

Contraindicated in patients with intestinal obstruction, intestinal ulceration, disabling adhesions, difficulty swallowing, or signs and symptoms of appendicitis or acute surgical abdomen, such as abdominal pain, nausea, and vomiting.

NURSING CONSIDERATIONS

● Before giving drug for constipation, determine whether patient has adequate fluid intake, exercise, and diet.

● Drug is especially useful in debilitated patients and in those with postpartum constipation, irritable bowel syndrome, diverticulitis, and colostomies. It's also used to treat laxative abuse and to empty colon before barium enema examinations.

● Drug isn't absorbed systemically and is nontoxic.

● **Alert:** Don't confuse Citrucel with Citracal.

PATIENT TEACHING

● Tell patient to take drug with at least 8 ounces (240 ml) of liquid to mask grittiness.

● Teach patient about dietary sources of bulk, including bran and other cereals, fresh fruit, and vegetables.

● Tell patient to increase fluid intake.

polyethylene glycol and electrolyte solution
Co-Lav, Colovage, CoLyte, Glycoprep‡, Go-Evac, GoLYTELY, NuLYTELY, OCL

Pregnancy risk category C

AVAILABLE FORMS

Powder for oral solution: Polyethylene glycol (PEG) 3350 (6 g), anhydrous sodium sulfate (568 mg), NaCl (146 mg), potassium chloride (74.5 mg)/100 ml (Colovage); PEG 3350 (120 g), sodium sulfate (3.36 g), NaCl (2.92 g), potassium chloride (1.49 g)/2 L (CoLyte); PEG 3350 (60 g), NaCl (1.46 g), potassium chloride (0.745 g), sodium bicarbonate (1.68 g), sodium sulfate (5.68 g)/L (Co-Lav); PEG 3350 (60 g), NaCl (1.46 g), potassium chloride (745 mg), sodium bicarbonate (1.68 g), sodium sulfate (5.68 g)/L (Glycoprep‡); PEG 3350 (236 g), sodium sulfate (22.74 g), sodium bicarbonate (6.74 g), NaCl (5.86 g), potassium chloride (2.97 g)/ 4.8 L (GoLYTELY); PEG 3350 (59 g), sodium sulfate (5.685 g), sodium bicarbonate (1.685 g), NaCl (1.465 g), potassium chloride (0.743 g)/L (Go-Evac); PEG 3350 (420 g), sodium bicarbonate (5.72 g), NaCl (11.2 g), potassium chloride (1.48 g)/4 L (NuLYTELY); PEG 3350 (6 g), sodium sulfate decahydrate (1.29 g), NaCl (146 mg), potassium chloride (75 mg), polysorbate-80 (30 mg)/100 ml (OCL)

INDICATIONS & DOSAGES

➤ **Bowel preparation before GI examination—**

Adults: 240 ml P.O. q 10 minutes until 4 L are consumed or until watery stool is clear. Typically, give 4 hours before examination, allowing 3 hours for drinking and 1 hour for bowel evacuation.

ACTION

PEG 3350, a nonabsorbable solution, acts as an osmotic product. Sodium sulfate greatly reduces sodium absorption. The

ACTION

Unknown. Stimulant laxative that increases peristalsis, probably by direct effect on smooth muscle of the intestine. It's thought to either irritate the musculature or stimulate the colonic intramural plexus. Drug also promotes fluid accumulation in colon and small intestine.

Route	Onset	Peak	Duration
P.O.	6-10 hr	Variable	Variable
P.R.	0.5-2 hr	Unknown	Unknown

ADVERSE REACTIONS

GI: *nausea,* vomiting, diarrhea, loss of normal bowel function with excessive use, *abdominal cramps* especially in severe constipation, malabsorption of nutrients, cathartic colon with long-term misuse, possible constipation after catharsis, yellow or yellow-green cast to feces, diarrhea in breast-feeding infants of mothers receiving senna, darkened pigmentation of rectal mucosa with long-term use, protein-losing enteropathy.
GU: red-pink discoloration in alkaline urine, yellow-brown discoloration in acidic urine.
Metabolic: electrolyte imbalance such as hypokalemia.
Other: laxative dependence with long-term or excessive use.

INTERACTIONS

None significant.

EFFECTS ON LAB TEST RESULTS

● May alter fluid and electrolyte levels, with prolonged use.

CONTRAINDICATIONS

Contraindicated in patients with ulcerative bowel lesions, fecal impaction, intestinal obstruction, intestinal perforation, or signs and symptoms of appendicitis or acute surgical abdomen, such as nausea, vomiting, and abdominal pain.

NURSING CONSIDERATIONS

● Before giving drug for constipation, determine whether patient has adequate fluid intake, exercise, and diet.
● In phenolsulfonphthalein excretion test, senna may turn urine pink to red, red to violet, or red to brown.

● Limit diet to clear liquids after X-Prep Liquid is taken.
● Avoid exposing product to excessive heat or light.
● Drug is for short-term use.
● Senna is one of the most effective laxatives for counteracting constipation caused by narcotic analgesics.

PATIENT TEACHING

● Teach patient about dietary sources of bulk, including bran and other cereals, fresh fruit, and vegetables.
● Tell patient to report persistent or severe reactions.

---

sodium phosphates
Fleet Phospho-Soda ◊

Pregnancy risk category NR

AVAILABLE FORMS

Enema: 160 mg/ml sodium phosphate and 60 mg/ml sodium biphosphate ◊
Liquid: 2.4 g/5 ml sodium phosphate and 900 mg sodium biphosphate/5 ml ◊

INDICATIONS & DOSAGES

➤ **Constipation—**
Adults: 20 to 30 ml solution mixed with 120 ml cold water P.O. Or, 60 to 135 ml P.R. as enema.
Children: 5 to 15 ml solution mixed with 120 ml cold water P.O. Or, 67.5 ml P.R. as enema.

ACTION

Saline laxative that produces an osmotic effect in the small intestine by drawing water into the intestinal lumen.

Route	Onset	Peak	Duration
P.O.	0.5-3 hr	Variable	Variable
P.R.	5-10 min	With effect	With effect

ADVERSE REACTIONS

GI: *abdominal cramping.*
Metabolic: fluid and electrolyte disturbances, such as hypernatremia and hyperphosphatemia, with daily use.
Other: laxative dependence with long-term or excessive use.

Reactions may be *common,* uncommon, *life-threatening,* or COMMON AND LIFE-THREATENING.

INTERACTIONS
None significant.

EFFECTS ON LAB TEST RESULTS
• May increase sodium and phosphate levels. May decrease electrolyte levels, with prolonged use.

CONTRAINDICATIONS
Contraindicated in patients on sodium-restricted diets and in patients with intestinal obstruction, intestinal perforation, edema, heart failure, megacolon, impaired renal function, or signs and symptoms of appendicitis or acute surgical abdomen, such as abdominal pain, nausea, or vomiting.

NURSING CONSIDERATIONS
• Use cautiously in patients with large hemorrhoids or anal excoriations.
• Dosages are expressed as sennosides.
• Before giving drug for constipation, determine whether patient has adequate fluid intake, exercise, and diet.
• *Alert:* Up to 10% of sodium content of drug may be absorbed.
• *Alert:* Severe electrolyte imbalances may occur if recommended dosage is exceeded.

PATIENT TEACHING
• Teach patient about dietary sources of bulk, including bran and other cereals, fresh fruit, and vegetables.
• Warn patient about adverse reactions, and stress importance of using drug only for short-term therapy.

chlorpromazine hydrochloride
(See Chapter 31, ANTIPSYCHOTICS.)
dimenhydrinate
dolasetron mesylate
dronabinol
granisetron hydrochloride
meclizine hydrochloride
metoclopramide hydrochloride
ondansetron hydrochloride
perphenazine
(See Chapter 31, ANTIPSYCHOTICS.)
prochlorperazine
prochlorperazine edisylate
prochlorperazine maleate
promethazine hydrochloride
(See Chapter 41, ANTIHISTAMINES.)
scopolamine
(See Chapter 36, ANTICHOLINERGICS.)
thiethylperazine maleate
trimethobenzamide hydrochloride

COMBINATION PRODUCTS
None.

---

dimenhydrinate
Andrumin‡, Apo-Dimenhydrinate†, Calm-X ◇, Children's Dramamine ◇ *, Dimetabs, Dinate, Dramamine ◇ *, Dramamine**, Liquid ◇ *, Dramanate, Dymenate, Gravol†, Gravol L/A†, Hydrate, PMS-Dimenhydrinate†, Triptone Caplets ◇

Pregnancy risk category B

AVAILABLE FORMS
Elixir: 15 mg/5 ml†
Injection: 50 mg/ml
Syrup: 12.5 mg/4 ml* ◇ , 15.62 mg/5 ml
Tablets: 50 mg ◇
Tablets (chewable): 50 mg ◇

INDICATIONS & DOSAGES
➤ **Prevention and treatment of motion sickness—**
Adults and children age 12 and older: 50 to 100 mg P.O. q 4 to 6 hours; 50 mg I.M.,

p.r.n.; or 50 mg I.V. diluted in 10 ml normal saline solution for injection, injected over 2 minutes. Maximum, 400 mg daily. For prevention, take 30 minutes before motion exposure.
Children ages 6 to 11: 25 to 50 mg P.O. q 6 to 8 hours, not to exceed 150 mg in 24 hours. Or, 1.25 mg/kg or 37.5 mg/m^2 I.M. or P.O. q.i.d. Maximum, 300 mg daily.
Children ages 2 to 5: 12.5 to 25 mg P.O. q 6 to 8 hours, not to exceed 75 mg in 24 hours. Or, 1.25 mg/kg or 37.5 mg/m^2 I.M. or P.O. q.i.d. Maximum, 300 mg daily.

I.V. ADMINISTRATION
● Before using, dilute each ml (50 mg) of drug with 10 ml of sterile water for injection, D$_5$W, or normal saline solution for injection. Give by direct injection over at least 2 minutes.
● *Alert:* Most I.V. products contain benzyl alcohol, which has been linked to a fatal gasping syndrome in premature infants and low-birth-weight infants.

ACTION
Unknown. Antihistamine that may affect neural pathways originating in the labyrinth to inhibit nausea and vomiting.

Route	Onset	Peak	Duration
I.M.	20-30 min	Unknown	3-6 hr
I.V.	Immediate	Unknown	3-6 hr
P.O.	15-30 min	Unknown	3-6 hr

ADVERSE REACTIONS
CNS: *drowsiness,* headache, dizziness, confusion, nervousness, vertigo, tingling and weakness of hands, lassitude, excitation, insomnia.
CV: palpitations, hypotension, tachycardia.
EENT: blurred vision, dry respiratory passages, diplopia, nasal congestion.
GI: dry mouth, nausea, vomiting, diarrhea, epigastric distress, constipation, anorexia.
Respiratory: wheezing, thickened bronchial secretions.

Reactions may be *common,* uncommon, *life-threatening,* or COMMON AND LIFE-THREATENING.

Skin: photosensitivity, urticaria, rash.
Other: *anaphylaxis,* tightness of chest.

INTERACTIONS
Drug-drug. *CNS depressants:* Additive CNS depression. Avoid using together.
Ototoxic drugs: Dimenhydrinate may mask symptoms of ototoxicity. Use cautiously.
TCAs, other anticholinergic drugs: Increased anticholinergic activity. Monitor patient.
Drug-lifestyle. *Alcohol use:* Additive CNS depression. Discourage use together.

EFFECTS ON LAB TEST RESULTS
None reported.

CONTRAINDICATIONS
Contraindicated in patients hypersensitive to drug or its components.

NURSING CONSIDERATIONS
• Use cautiously in patients receiving ototoxic drugs and in patients with seizures, acute angle-closure glaucoma, or enlarged prostate gland.
• Elderly patients may be more susceptible to adverse CNS effects.
• Undiluted solution irritates veins and may cause sclerosis.
• Drug may alter or confuse test results for xanthines (caffeine, aminophylline) because of its 8-chlorotheophylline content.
• Because incompatibilities are common, avoid mixing parenteral preparation with other drugs.
• Discontinue drug 4 days before diagnostic skin tests to avoid preventing, reducing, or masking test response.
• *Alert:* Drug may mask symptoms of ototoxicity, brain tumor, or intestinal obstruction.
• *Alert:* Don't confuse dimenhydrinate with diphenhydramine.

PATIENT TEACHING
• Advise patient to avoid activities that require alertness until CNS effects of drug are known.
• Instruct patient to report adverse reactions promptly.

dolasetron mesylate
Anzemet

Pregnancy risk category B

AVAILABLE FORMS
Injection: 20 mg/ml as 12.5/0.625 ml ampule or 100 mg/5 ml vials
Tablets: 50 mg, 100 mg

INDICATIONS & DOSAGES
➤ **Prevention of nausea and vomiting from cancer chemotherapy—**
Adults: 100 mg P.O. given as a single dose 1 hour before chemotherapy. Or, 1.8 mg/kg or a fixed dose of 100 mg as a single I.V. dose given 30 minutes before chemotherapy.
Children ages 2 to 16: 1.8 mg/kg P.O. given 1 hour before chemotherapy. Or, 1.8 mg/kg as a single I.V. dose given 30 minutes before chemotherapy. Injectable formulation can be mixed with apple juice and given P.O. Maximum dose is 100 mg.
➤ **Prevention of postoperative nausea and vomiting—**
Adults: 100 mg P.O. within 2 hours before surgery. Or, 12.5 mg as a single I.V. dose about 15 minutes before cessation of anesthesia or as soon as nausea or vomiting presents.
Children ages 2 to 16: 1.2 mg/kg P.O. given within 2 hours before surgery, to maximum of 100 mg. Or, 0.35 mg/kg, up to 12.5 mg given as a single I.V. dose about 15 minutes before cessation of anesthesia or as soon as nausea or vomiting presents. Injectable formulation can be mixed with apple juice and given P.O.
➤ **Postoperative nausea and vomiting—**
Adults: 12.5 mg as a single I.V. dose as soon as nausea or vomiting occurs.
Children ages 2 to 16: 0.35 mg/kg, to maximum dose of 12.5 mg, given as a single I.V. dose as soon as nausea or vomiting occurs.

I.V. ADMINISTRATION
• Injection can be given as rapidly as 100 mg/30 seconds or diluted in 50 ml compatible solution and infused over 15 minutes.

ACTION
Selective serotonin 5-HT$_3$ receptor antagonist that blocks the action of serotonin. Blocking the activity of the serotonin receptors prevents serotonin from stimulating the vomiting reflex.

Route	Onset	Peak	Duration
I.V.	Rapid	36 min	7 hr
P.O.	Rapid	1 hr	8 hr

ADVERSE REACTIONS
CNS: *headache,* dizziness, drowsiness, fatigue.
CV: *arrhythmias,* ECG changes, hypotension, hypertension, tachycardia.
GI: *diarrhea,* dyspepsia, abdominal pain, constipation, anorexia.
GU: oliguria, urine retention.
Skin: pruritus, rash.
Other: fever, chills, pain at injection site.

INTERACTIONS
Drug-drug. *Drugs that prolong ECG intervals, such as antiarrhythmics:* Increased risk of arrhythmia. Monitor patient closely.
Drugs that inhibit cytochrome P-450 enzymes, such as cimetidine: Increased hydrodolasetron levels. Monitor patient for adverse effects.
Drugs that induce cytochrome P-450 enzymes, such as rifampin: Decreased hydrodolasetron levels. Monitor patient for decreased efficacy of antiemetic.

EFFECTS ON LAB TEST RESULTS
● May increase ALT and AST levels.

CONTRAINDICATIONS
Contraindicated in patients hypersensitive to drug.

NURSING CONSIDERATIONS
● *Alert:* Give with caution in patients who have or may develop prolonged cardiac conduction intervals, such as those with electrolyte abnormalities, history of arrhythmia, and cumulative high-dose anthracycline therapy.
● Drug isn't recommended for use in children younger than age 2. Use cautiously in breast-feeding women.

● Injection for oral use is stable in apple or apple-grape juice for 2 hours at room temperature.
● *Alert:* Don't confuse Anzemet with Aldomet.

PATIENT TEACHING
● Tell patient about possible adverse effects.
● Instruct patient not to mix injection in juice for oral use until just before dosing.
● Tell patient to report nausea or vomiting.

---

dronabinol (delta-9-tetrahydrocannabinol)
Marinol

Pregnancy risk category C
Controlled substance schedule III

AVAILABLE FORMS
Capsules: 2.5 mg, 5 mg, 10 mg

INDICATIONS & DOSAGES
➤ **Nausea and vomiting from cancer chemotherapy—**
Adults: 5 mg/m^2 P.O. 1 to 3 hours before administration of chemotherapy. Then same dose q 2 to 4 hours after chemotherapy for total of four to six doses daily. If needed, dosage increased in 2.5 mg/m^2 increments to maximum of 15 mg/m^2 per dose.
➤ **Anorexia and weight loss in patients with AIDS—**
Adults: 2.5 mg P.O. b.i.d. before lunch and dinner. If patient can't tolerate it, decrease to 2.5 mg P.O. given as a single dose daily in evening or h.s. May gradually increase to maximum of 20 mg daily.

ACTION
Unknown. A derivative of marijuana.

Route	Onset	Peak	Duration
P.O.	0.5-1 hr	2-4 hr	4-6 hr

ADVERSE REACTIONS
CNS: *dizziness, drowsiness, euphoria, ataxia,* depersonalization, hallucinations, somnolence, headache, muddled thinking, asthenia, amnesia, confusion, *paranoia.*

CV: tachycardia, orthostatic hypotension, palpitations, vasodilation.
EENT: visual disturbances.
GI: *dry mouth, nausea, vomiting, abdominal pain,* diarrhea.

INTERACTIONS
Drug-drug. *CNS depressants, psychomimetic substances, sedatives:* Additive CNS depression. Avoid using together.
Drug-lifestyle. *Alcohol use:* Additive CNS depression. Discourage use together.

EFFECTS ON LAB TEST RESULTS
None reported.

CONTRAINDICATIONS
Contraindicated in patients hypersensitive to sesame oil or cannabinoids.

NURSING CONSIDERATIONS
• Use cautiously in elderly, pregnant, or breast-feeding patients and in those with heart disease, psychiatric illness, or history of drug abuse.
• Expect drug to be prescribed only for patients who haven't responded satisfactorily to other antiemetics.
• *Alert:* Dronabinol is the principal active substance in *Cannabis sativa* (marijuana). This substance can produce both physical and psychological dependence and has a high risk of abuse.
• CNS effects are intensified at higher dosages.
• Drug effects may persist for days after treatment ends.
• *Alert:* Don't confuse dronabinol with droperidol.

PATIENT TEACHING
• Tell patient that drug may induce unusual changes in mood or other adverse behavioral effects.
• Advise patient against performing activities that require alertness until CNS effects of drug are known.
• Warn caregivers to supervise patient during and immediately after treatment.
• Advise patient to take drug 1 to 3 hours before chemotherapy use.

granisetron hydrochloride
Kytril

Pregnancy risk category B

AVAILABLE FORMS
Injection: 1 mg/ml
Tablets: 1 mg

INDICATIONS & DOSAGES
➤ **Prevention of nausea and vomiting from emetogenic cancer chemotherapy—**
Adults and children age 2 and older:
10 mcg/kg I.V. infused over 5 minutes. Begin infusion within 30 minutes before use of chemotherapy. Or, 1 mg P.O. up to 1 hour before chemotherapy and repeated 12 hours later. Or, 2 mg P.O. daily given up to 1 hour before chemotherapy.
➤ **Prevention of nausea and vomiting from radiation, including total body irradiation and fractionated abdominal radiation—**
Adults: 2 mg P.O. once daily within 1 hour of radiation.

I.V. ADMINISTRATION
• Dilute drug with normal saline solution for injection or D_5W to a volume of 20 to 50 ml. Infuse over 5 minutes, beginning within 30 minutes before chemotherapy, and only on days chemotherapy is given. Diluted solutions are stable for 24 hours at room temperature.
• For direct I.V. injection, the drug is given undiluted over 30 seconds.

ACTION
Selective antagonist of a specific type of serotonin receptor (5-HT_3) located in the CNS in the chemoreceptor trigger zone and in the peripheral nervous system on nerve terminals of the vagus nerve. Drug's blocking action may occur at both sites.

Route	Onset	Peak	Duration
I.V., P.O.	Unknown	Unknown	Unknown

ADVERSE REACTIONS
CNS: *headache, asthenia,* somnolence, dizziness, anxiety.
CV: hypertension.

CNS depressants: Additive CNS effects. Avoid using together.
Phenothiazines: Increased risk of extrapyramidal effects. Monitor patient closely.
Drug-lifestyle. *Alcohol use:* Additive CNS effects. Discourage use together.

EFFECTS ON LAB TEST RESULTS
● May increase aldosterone and prolactin levels.
● May decrease neutrophil and granulocyte counts.

CONTRAINDICATIONS
Contraindicated in patients hypersensitive to drug and in those with pheochromocytoma or seizure disorders. Also, contraindicated in those for whom stimulation of GI motility might be dangerous (for example, those with hemorrhage, obstruction, or perforation).

NURSING CONSIDERATIONS
● Use cautiously in patients with history of depression, Parkinson's disease, or hypertension.
● Monitor bowel sounds.
● Safety and effectiveness of drug haven't been established for therapy lasting longer than 12 weeks.
● When oral solution is used (10 mg/ml) dilute in pudding, applesauce, juice, or water just before using.
● *Alert:* Use diphenhydramine 25 mg I.V., to counteract extrapyramidal adverse effects from high metoclopramide doses.

PATIENT TEACHING
● Tell patient to avoid activities that require alertness for 2 hours after doses.
● Urge patient to report persistent or serious adverse reactions promptly.
● Advise patient to avoid alcohol ingestion during therapy.

---

ondansetron hydrochloride
Zofran, Zofran ODT

Pregnancy risk category B

AVAILABLE FORMS
Injection: 2 mg/ml
Oral solution: 4 mg/5 ml

Premixed injection: 32 mg/50 ml
Tablets: 4 mg, 8 mg, 24 mg
Tablets (disintegrating): 4 mg, 8 mg

INDICATIONS & DOSAGES
➤ **Prevention of nausea and vomiting from emetogenic chemotherapy—**
Adults and children age 12 and older: 8 mg P.O. 30 minutes before chemotherapy. Then, 8 mg P.O. 8 hours after first dose. Then, 8 mg q 12 hours for 1 to 2 days. Or, a single dose of 32 mg by I.V. infusion over 15 minutes beginning 30 minutes before chemotherapy. Or, three divided doses of 0.15 mg/kg I.V. Give first dose 30 minutes before chemotherapy and subsequent doses 4 and 8 hours after first dose. Infuse drug over 15 minutes.
Children ages 4 to 11: 4 mg P.O. 30 minutes before chemotherapy. Then, 4 mg P.O. 4 and 8 hours after first dose. Then, 4 mg q 8 hours for 1 to 2 days. Or, three doses of 0.15 mg/kg I.V. Give first dose 30 minutes before chemotherapy; use subsequent doses 4 and 8 hours after first dose. Infuse drug over 15 minutes.
➤ **Prevention of postoperative nausea and vomiting—**
Adults: 4 mg I.V. undiluted over 2 to 5 minutes. Or, 16 mg P.O. 1 hour before induction of anesthesia.
Children weighing more than 40 kg (88 lb): 4 mg I.V. as a single dose.
Children weighing 40 kg or less: 0.1 mg/kg I.V. as a single dose.
➤ **Prevention of nausea and vomiting from radiotherapy in patients receiving total body irradiation, single high-dose fraction to abdomen, or daily fractions to abdomen—**
Adults: 8 mg P.O. t.i.d.
Adjust-a-dose: For patients with severe liver failure, total daily dose shouldn't exceed 8 mg.

I.V. ADMINISTRATION
● Dilute drug in 50 ml of D_5W injection or normal saline solution for injection before using.
● Drug is stable for up to 48 hours after dilution in 5% dextrose in normal saline solution for injection, 5% dextrose in half-normal saline solution for injection, and 3% sodium chloride for injection.

Reactions may be *common,* uncommon, *life-threatening,* or **COMMON AND LIFE-THREATENING.**

• *Alert:* Give as I.V. infusion over 15 minutes.

ACTION
Selective antagonist of a specific type of serotonin receptor (5-HT$_3$) located in the CNS at the chemoreceptor trigger zone and in the peripheral nervous system on nerve terminals of the vagus nerve. Drug's blocking action may occur at both sites.

Route	Onset	Peak	Duration
I.V., P.O.	Unknown	Unknown	Unknown

ADVERSE REACTIONS
CNS: *headache, malaise, fatigue, dizziness, sedation.*
CV: *chest pain.*
GI: *diarrhea, constipation,* abdominal pain, xerostomia.
GU: urine retention, gynecologic disorders.
Musculoskeletal: *pain.*
Respiratory: hypoxia.
Skin: rash, pruritus.
Other: chills, injection site reaction, fever.

INTERACTIONS
Drug-drug. *Drugs that alter hepatic drug metabolizing enzymes, such as cimetidine, phenobarbital:* May alter pharmacokinetics of ondansetron. No dosage adjustment appears necessary.
Drug-herb. *Horehound:* May enhance serotoninergic effects. Discourage use together.

EFFECTS ON LAB TEST RESULTS
• May increase ALT and AST levels.

CONTRAINDICATIONS
Contraindicated in patients hypersensitive to drug.

NURSING CONSIDERATIONS
• Use cautiously in patients with hepatic impairment. Monitor liver function test results. Dose shouldn't exceed 8 mg in these patients.
• *Alert:* Don't confuse Zofran with Zosyn, Zantac, or Zoloft.

PATIENT TEACHING
• Instruct patient to immediately report difficulty breathing after drug administration.
• Tell patient receiving drug I.V. to report discomfort at insertion site.
• Instruct patient, when using disintegrating tablets, to open blister just before use by peeling backing off. Don't push through foil blister. Using with a liquid isn't necessary.

prochlorperazine
Compazine, PMS
Prochlorperazine†, Stemetil†

prochlorperazine edisylate
Compazine, Compazine Syrup

prochlorperazine maleate
Compazine, Compazine Spansule,
PMS Prochlorperazine†, Stemetil†

Pregnancy risk category C

AVAILABLE FORMS
prochlorperazine
Injection: 5 mg/ml
Suppositories: 2.5 mg, 5 mg, 25 mg
Tablets: 5 mg, 10 mg
prochlorperazine edisylate
Injection: 5 mg/ml
Syrup: 5 mg/5 ml
prochlorperazine maleate
Capsules (extended-release): 10 mg, 15 mg, 30 mg
Tablets: 5 mg, 10 mg, 25 mg

INDICATIONS & DOSAGES
➤ **Preoperative nausea control—**
Adults: 5 to 10 mg I.M. 1 to 2 hours before induction of anesthesia; repeat once in 30 minutes, if needed. Or, 5 to 10 mg I.V. 15 to 30 minutes before induction of anesthesia; repeat once, if needed.
➤ **Severe nausea and vomiting—**
Adults: 5 to 10 mg P.O., t.i.d. or q.i.d.; 15 mg sustained-release form P.O. on rising; 10 mg sustained-release form P.O. q 12 hours; 25 mg P.R., b.i.d.; or 5 to 10 mg I.M. repeated q 3 to 4 hours, p.r.n. Maximum I.M. dose is 40 mg daily. Or, 2.5 to 10 mg I.V. at no more than 5 mg/minute.

Children weighing 18 to 39 kg (40 to 86 lb): 2.5 mg P.O. or P.R., t.i.d.; or 5 mg P.O. or P.R., b.i.d. Maximum, 15 mg daily. Or, 0.132 mg/kg by deep I.M. injection. Control usually is obtained with one dose.

Children weighing 14 to 17 kg (30 to 37 lb): 2.5 mg P.O. or P.R., b.i.d. or t.i.d. Maximum, 10 mg daily. Or, 0.132 mg/kg by deep I.M. injection. Control usually is obtained with one dose.

Children weighing 9 to 13 kg (20 to 29 lb): 2.5 mg P.O. or P.R. once daily or b.i.d. Maximum, 7.5 mg daily. Or, 0.132 mg/kg by deep I.M. injection. Control usually is obtained with one dose.

➤ **To manage symptoms of psychotic disorders—**
Adults and children age 12 and older: 5 to 10 mg P.O., t.i.d. or q.i.d.
Children ages 2 to 12: 2.5 mg P.O. or P.R., b.i.d. or t.i.d. Don't exceed 10 mg on day 1. Increase dosage gradually to recommended maximum, if needed. In children ages 2 to 5, maximum is 20 mg daily. In children ages 6 to 12, maximum is 25 mg daily.

➤ **To manage symptoms of severe psychosis—**
Adults and children age 12 and older: 10 to 20 mg I.M. repeated in 1 to 4 hours, if needed. Rarely, patients may receive 10 to 20 mg q 4 to 6 hours. Institute oral therapy after symptoms are controlled.
Children ages 2 to 12: 0.13 mg/kg I.M.

➤ **Nonpsychotic anxiety—**
Adults: 5 to 10 mg by deep I.M. injection q 3 to 4 hours. Don't exceed 20 mg daily, and don't give for longer than 12 weeks. Or, 5 to 10 mg P.O., t.i.d. or q.i.d. Or, 15 mg extended-release capsule once daily. Or, 10 mg extended-release capsule q 12 hours.

I.V. ADMINISTRATION

● Add 20 mg prochlorperazine/L D_5W and normal saline solution 15 to 30 minutes before induction. Infusion rate shouldn't exceed 5 mg/minute. Maximum parenteral dose is 40 mg daily. Infuse slowly, never as a bolus.
● Watch for orthostatic hypotension, especially when giving drug I.V.

ACTION

Acts on the chemoreceptor trigger zone to inhibit nausea and vomiting; in larger doses, it partially depresses vomiting center.

Route	Onset	Peak	Duration
I.M.	10-20 min	Unknown	3-4 hr
I.V.	Unknown	Unknown	Unknown
P.O.	30-40 min	Unknown	3-12 hr
P.O. (extended)	30-40 min	Unknown	10-12 hr
P.R.	1 hr	Unknown	3-4 hr

ADVERSE REACTIONS

CNS: *extrapyramidal reactions,* sedation, pseudoparkinsonism, EEG changes, dizziness.
CV: *orthostatic hypotension,* tachycardia, ECG changes.
EENT: *ocular changes, blurred vision.*
GI: *dry mouth, constipation,* increased appetite.
GU: *urine retention,* dark urine, menstrual irregularities, inhibited ejaculation.
Hematologic: *transient leukopenia, agranulocytosis.*
Hepatic: cholestatic jaundice.
Metabolic: weight gain.
Skin: *mild photosensitivity,* allergic reactions, exfoliative dermatitis.
Other: gynecomastia, hyperprolactinemia.

INTERACTIONS

Drug-drug. *Antacids:* Inhibited absorption of oral phenothiazines. Separate antacid and phenothiazine doses by at least 2 hours.
Anticholinergics, including antidepressants and antiparkinsonians: Increased anticholinergic activity and aggravated parkinsonian symptoms. Use together cautiously.
Barbiturates: May decrease phenothiazine effect. Monitor patient for decreased antiemetic effect.
Drug-herb. *Dong quai, St. John's wort:* Increased risk of photosensitivity. Advise patient to avoid prolonged sun exposure.
Kava: Increased risk of dystonic reactions. Discourage use together.
Drug-lifestyle. *Alcohol use:* Increased CNS depression. Discourage use together.

EFFECTS ON LAB TEST RESULTS
• May cause abnormal liver function test result values.
• May decrease WBC and granulocyte counts.

CONTRAINDICATIONS
Contraindicated in patients hypersensitive to phenothiazines and in those with CNS depression, including coma. Also, contraindicated during pediatric surgery, when using spinal or epidural anesthetic or adrenergic blockers, and in children younger than age 2.

NURSING CONSIDERATIONS
• Use cautiously in patients with impaired CV function, glaucoma, seizure disorders, and Parkinson's disease; in those who have been exposed to extreme heat; and in children with acute illness.
• Dilute oral solution with tomato juice, fruit juice, milk, coffee, carbonated beverage, tea, water, or soup. Or, mix with pudding.
• Drug causes false-positive results for urinary porphyrins, urobilinogen, amylase, and 5-hydroxyindoleacetic acid; it also causes false-positive urine pregnancy results in tests using human chorionic gonadotropin.
• For I.M. use, inject deeply into upper outer quadrant of gluteal region.
• Don't give by S.C. route or mix in syringe with another drug.
• To prevent contact dermatitis, avoid getting concentrate or injection solution on hands or clothing.
• Monitor CBC and liver function studies during long-term therapy.
• *Alert:* Use drug only when vomiting can't be controlled by other measures or when only a few doses are needed. If more than four doses are needed in 24 hours, notify prescriber.
• Store in light-resistant container. Slight yellowing doesn't affect potency; discard extremely discolored solutions.

PATIENT TEACHING
• Teach patient what to use to dilute oral solution.
• Advise patient to wear protective clothing when exposed to sunlight.

• Tell patient to call prescriber if more than four doses are needed within 24 hours.

---

thiethylperazine maleate
Torecan**

Pregnancy risk category X

AVAILABLE FORMS
Injection: 5 mg/ml
Tablets: 10 mg

INDICATIONS & DOSAGES
➤ **Nausea and vomiting—**
Adults: 10 mg P.O. or I.M., once daily, b.i.d., or t.i.d.

ACTION
Unknown. Probably acts on the chemoreceptor trigger zone to inhibit nausea and vomiting.

Route	Onset	Peak	Duration
I.M., P.O.	0.5 hr	Unknown	4 hr

ADVERSE REACTIONS
CNS: *extrapyramidal reactions,* sedation, confusion, pseudoparkinsonism, EEG changes, dizziness.
CV: *orthostatic hypotension,* tachycardia, ECG changes.
EENT: *ocular changes, blurred vision.*
GI: *dry mouth, constipation,* increased appetite.
GU: *urine retention,* dark urine, menstrual irregularities, inhibited ejaculation.
Hematologic: *transient leukopenia, agranulocytosis.*
Hepatic: cholestatic jaundice.
Metabolic: weight gain.
Skin: *mild photosensitivity,* allergic reactions.
Other: hyperprolactinemia, gynecomastia.

INTERACTIONS
Drug-drug. *Antacids:* Inhibited absorption of oral phenothiazines. Separate antacid and phenothiazine doses by at least 2 hours.
Anticholinergics, including antidepressants and antiparkinsonians: Increased anticholinergic activity and increased risk

---

of parkinsonian-like symptoms. Use together cautiously.
Barbiturates: May decrease phenothiazine effect. Monitor patient for decreased antiemetic effect.

EFFECTS ON LAB TEST RESULTS
• May increase prolactin levels.
• May decrease WBC and granulocyte counts.

CONTRAINDICATIONS
Contraindicated in patients hypersensitive to phenothiazines and in those with severe CNS depression or hepatic disease; also contraindicated in pregnant and in comatose patients.

NURSING CONSIDERATIONS
• Use cautiously in patients with aspirin or tartrazine hypersensitivity.
• Drug may alter immunologic urine pregnancy test results.
• *Alert:* Don't give I.V. May cause severe hypotension.
• For nausea and vomiting from anesthesia and surgery, give deep I.M. injection shortly before or when terminating anesthesia.
• If drug gets on skin, wash off at once to prevent contact dermatitis.
• Use only when vomiting can't be controlled by other measures or when only a few doses are needed.
• Elderly patients may be more sensitive to therapeutic and adverse effects of drug.

PATIENT TEACHING
• Warn patient about hypotension; suggest that he stay in bed for 1 hour after receiving drug.
• Urge patient to report decreased urine output, visual changes, and CNS effects immediately.

trimethobenzamide hydrochloride
Arrestin, Tebamide, T-Gen, Ticon, Tigan, Triban, Trimazide

Pregnancy risk category C

AVAILABLE FORMS
Capsules: 100 mg, 250 mg

Injection: 100 mg/ml
Suppositories: 100 mg, 200 mg

INDICATIONS & DOSAGES
➤ **Nausea and vomiting—**
Adults: 250 mg P.O. t.i.d. or q.i.d.; or 200 mg I.M. or P.R., t.i.d. or q.i.d.
Children weighing 13 to 40 kg (29 to 88 lb): 100 to 200 mg P.O. or P.R., t.i.d. or q.i.d.
Children weighing less than 13 kg: 100 mg P.R., t.i.d. or q.i.d.

ACTION
Unknown. Probably acts on the chemoreceptor trigger zone to inhibit nausea and vomiting.

Route	Onset	Peak	Duration
I.M.	15-35 min	Unknown	2-3 hr
P.O.	10-20 min	Unknown	3-4 hr
P.R.	Unknown	Unknown	Unknown

ADVERSE REACTIONS
CNS: *drowsiness,* dizziness with large doses, headache, disorientation, depression, parkinsonian-like symptoms, ***coma, seizures.***
CV: hypotension.
EENT: blurred vision.
GI: diarrhea.
Hepatic: jaundice.
Musculoskeletal: muscle cramps.
Other: hypersensitivity reactions.

INTERACTIONS
Drug-drug. *CNS depressants:* Additive CNS depression. Avoid using together.
Drug-lifestyle. *Alcohol use:* Additive CNS depression. Discourage use together.

EFFECTS ON LAB TEST RESULTS
None reported.

CONTRAINDICATIONS
Contraindicated in patients hypersensitive to drug. Suppositories contraindicated in patients hypersensitive to benzocaine hydrochloride or similar local anesthetic.

NURSING CONSIDERATIONS
• Use cautiously in children; drug may be linked to Reye's syndrome.

• For I.M. use, inject deeply into upper outer quadrant of gluteal region to reduce pain and local irritation.

• Drug may mask signs and symptoms of toxic drug overdose, intestinal obstruction, brain tumor, or other conditions.

• Drug may cause pain, stinging, burning, redness, or swelling at I.M. injection site. Withhold drug if skin hypersensitivity reaction occurs.

• *Alert:* Don't confuse Tigan with Ticar.

PATIENT TEACHING

• Tell patient to refrigerate suppositories.

• Advise patient of possible drowsiness and dizziness; caution against performing hazardous activities requiring alertness until CNS effects of drug are known.

cimetidine
cimetidine hydrochloride
esomeprazole magnesium
famotidine
lansoprazole
misoprostol
omeprazole
pantoprazole sodium
rabeprazole sodium
ranitidine hydrochloride
sucralfate

COMBINATION PRODUCTS
ARTHROTEC: 50 mg diclofenac sodium and 200 mcg misoprostol; 75 mg diclofenac sodium and 200 mcg misoprostol.
PEPCID COMPLETE ◊ : 800 mg calcium carbonate, 165 mg magnesium hydroxide, and 10 mg famotidine.
PREVPAK: 4 capsules of amoxicillin 500 mg, 2 capsules of delayed-release lansoprazole 30 mg, and 2 tablets of film-coated clarithromycin 500 mg.

cimetidine
Tagamet, Tagamet HB ◊

cimetidine hydrochloride
Tagamet

Pregnancy risk category B

AVAILABLE FORMS
Injection: 300 mg/2 ml, 300 mg in 50 ml normal saline solution, 300 mg/2 ml ADD-Vantage vial
Oral liquid: 300 mg/5 ml
Tablets: 100 mg ◊ , 200 mg, 300 mg, 400 mg, 800 mg

INDICATIONS & DOSAGES
➤ **Short-term treatment of duodenal ulcer; maintenance therapy—**
Adults and children age 16 and older:
800 mg P.O. h.s. Or, 400 mg P.O. b.i.d. or 300 mg q.i.d. (with meals and h.s.). Or, 200 mg t.i.d. with a 400-mg h.s. dose. Treatment lasts 4 to 6 weeks unless endoscopy shows healing. For maintenance therapy, 400 mg h.s. For parenteral therapy, 300 mg diluted to 20 ml with normal saline solution or other compatible I.V. solution by I.V. push over at least 5 minutes q 6 hours; or 300 mg diluted in 50 ml D_5W or other compatible I.V. solution by I.V. infusion over 15 to 20 minutes q 6 hours; or 300 mg I.M. q 6 hours (no dilution needed). Parenteral dosage increased by giving 300-mg doses more frequently to maximum of 2,400 mg daily, p.r.n. Or, 900 mg/day (37.5 mg/hour) I.V. diluted in 100 to 1,000 ml of compatible solution by continuous I.V. infusion.
➤ **Active benign gastric ulceration—**
Adults: 800 mg P.O. h.s. or 300 mg P.O. q.i.d. (with meals and h.s.) for up to 6 weeks.
➤ **Pathologic hypersecretory conditions, such as Zollinger-Ellison syndrome, systemic mastocytosis, and multiple endocrine adenomas—**
Adults and children age 16 and older:
300 mg P.O. q.i.d. with meals and h.s.; adjusted to patient needs. Maximum oral amount, 2,400 mg daily.
For parenteral therapy, 300 mg diluted to 20 ml with normal saline solution or other compatible I.V. solution by I.V. push over at least 5 minutes q 6 hours; or 300 mg diluted in 50 ml D_5W or other compatible I.V. solution by I.V. infusion over 15 to 20 minutes q 6 hours. Increase parenteral dosage by giving 300-mg doses more frequently to maximum of 2,400 mg daily, p.r.n.
➤ **Gastroesophageal reflux disease—**
Adults: 800 mg P.O. b.i.d. or 400 mg q.i.d. before meals and h.s. for up to 12 weeks.
➤ **Prevention of upper GI bleeding in critically ill patients—**
Adults: 50 mg/hour by continuous I.V. infusion for up to 7 days; 25 mg/hour to patients with creatinine clearance below 30 ml/minute.
➤ **Heartburn—**
Adults: 200 mg (Tagamet HB) P.O. with water as symptoms occur, or as directed, up to b.i.d. Maximum, 400 mg daily. Drug

Nursing2003 Drug Handbook
Photoguide
to tablets and capsules

This photoguide presents nearly 400 pills and capsules, representing the most commonly prescribed generic and trade drugs. These drugs, organized alphabetically by generic name, are shown in actual size and color with cross-references to drug information. Each product is labeled with its trade name and its strength.

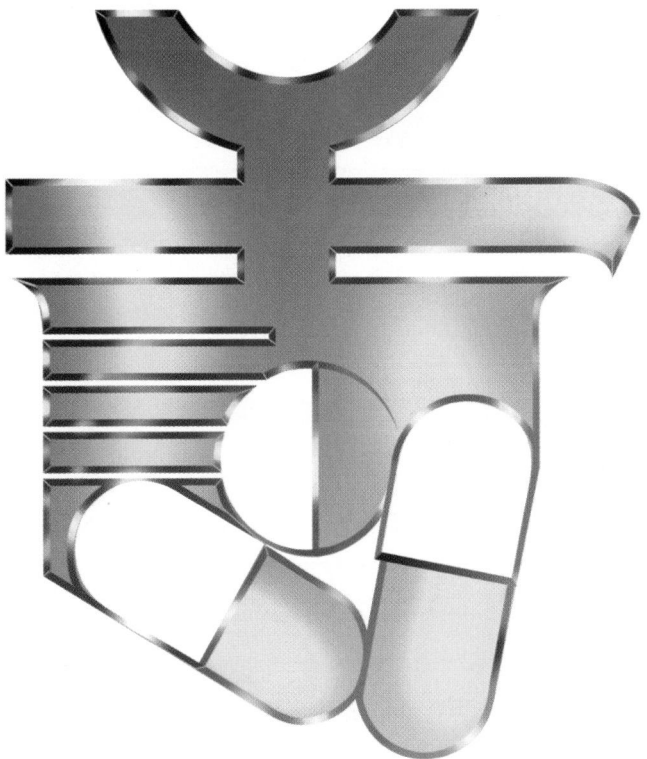

Adapted from Facts and Comparisons, St. Louis, Missouri

ACETAMINOPHEN WITH CODEINE

Tylenol with Codeine #3
(page 373)

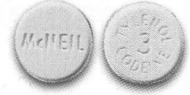

30 mg

ACYCLOVIR

Zovirax
(page 154)

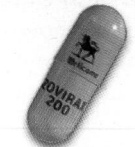

200 mg

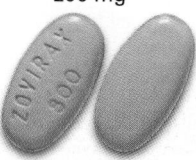

400 mg

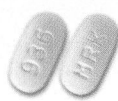

800 mg

ALENDRONATE SODIUM

Fosamax
(page 1241)

 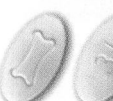

10 mg   40 mg   70 mg

ALPRAZOLAM

Xanax
(page 458)

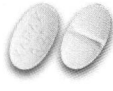 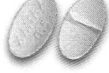 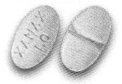

0.25 mg   0.5 mg   1 mg

AMITRIPTYLINE HYDROCHLORIDE

Elavil
(page 432)

10 mg

25 mg

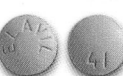

50 mg

75 mg

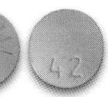 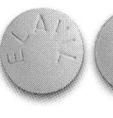 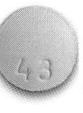

100 mg

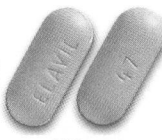

150 mg

AMLODIPINE BESYLATE

Norvasc
(page 248)

2.5 mg

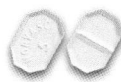

5 mg

AMOXICILLIN/POTASSIUM CLAVULANATE

Augmentin
(page 67)

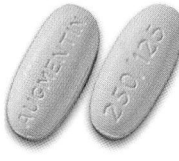

250 mg

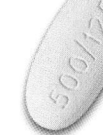

500 mg

Augmentin Chewable
(page 67)

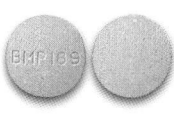

125 mg

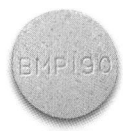

250 mg

AMOXICILLIN TRIHYDRATE

Amoxil
(page 69)

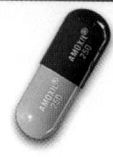 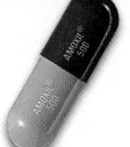

250 mg   500 mg

Amoxil Chewable
(page 69)

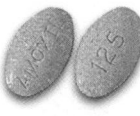 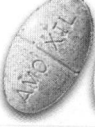

125 mg   250 mg

Trimox
(page 69)

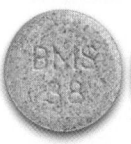

250 mg

ATENOLOL

Tenormin
(page 267)

25 mg   50 mg   100 mg

ATORVASTATIN CALCIUM

Lipitor
(page 312)

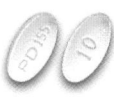 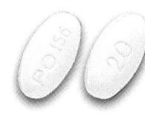

10 mg   20 mg

AZITHROMYCIN

Zithromax
(page 196)

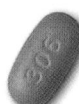

250 mg

BENAZEPRIL HYDROCHLORIDE

Lotensin
(page 269)

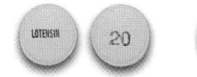 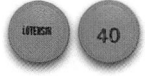

20 mg   40 mg

BUMETANIDE

Bumex
(page 826)

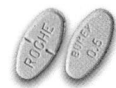 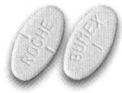 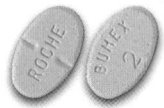

0.5 mg   1 mg   2 mg

BUPROPION HYDROCHLORIDE

Wellbutrin
(page 435)

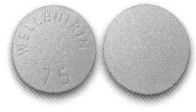 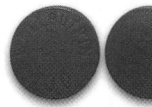

75 mg   100 mg

Wellbutrin SR
(page 435)

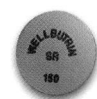

150 mg

Zyban
(page 524)

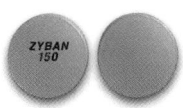

150 mg

BUSPIRONE HYDROCHLORIDE

BuSpar
(page 459)

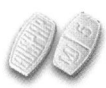 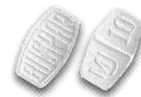

5 mg   10 mg

CAPTOPRIL

Capoten
(page 272)

12.5 mg   25 mg

CARISOPRODOL

Soma
(page 572)

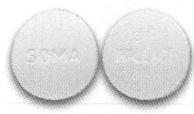

350 mg

CARVEDILOL

Coreg
(page 275)

3.125 mg   6.25 mg   12.5 mg

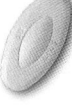

25 mg

CEFPROZIL

Cefzil
(page 112)

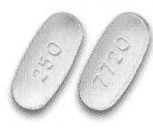 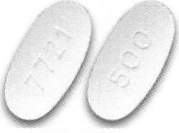

250 mg   500 mg

CEFUROXIME

Ceftin
(page 118)

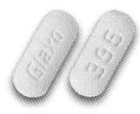 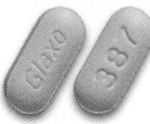 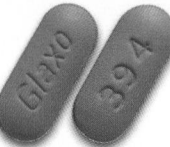

125 mg   250 mg   500mg

CELECOXIB

Celebrex
(page 347)

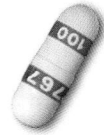 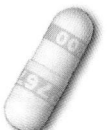

100 mg   200 mg

CETIRIZINE HYDROCHLORIDE

Zyrtec
(page 595)

5 mg   10 mg

CIMETIDINE

Tagamet
(page 690)

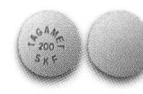 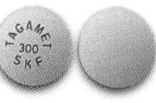 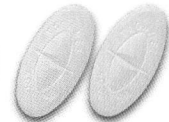

200 mg   300 mg   400 mg

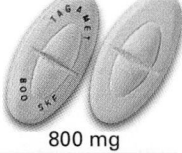

800 mg

CIPROFLOXACIN

Cipro
(page 138)

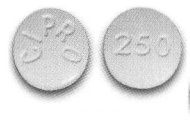 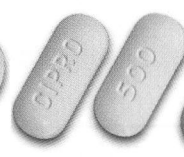 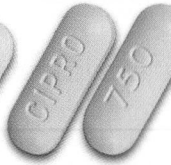

250 mg   500 mg   750 mg

CITALOPRAM HYDROBROMIDE

Celexa
(page 436)

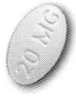 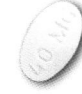

20 mg   40 mg

CLARITHROMYCIN

Biaxin
(page 197)

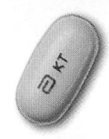 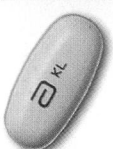

250 mg   500 mg

Biaxin XL
(page 197)

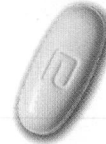

500 mg

CLONAZEPAM

Klonopin
(page 410)

0.5 mg   1 mg   2 mg

CO-TRIMOXAZOLE

Bactrim DS
(page 131)

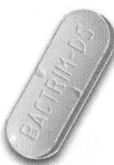

160/800 mg

DIAZEPAM

Valium
(page 463)

2 mg   5 mg   10 mg

DIGOXIN

Lanoxicaps
(page 218)

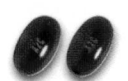 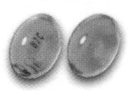 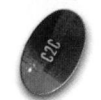

0.05 mg   0.1 mg   0.2 mg

Lanoxin
(page 218)

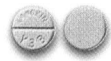 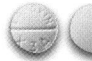

0.125 mg   0.25 mg

DILTIAZEM HYDROCHLORIDE

Cardizem
(page 251)

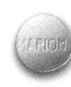 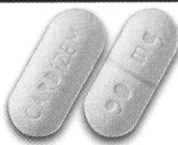

30 mg   90 mg

Cardizem CD
(page 251)

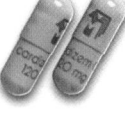 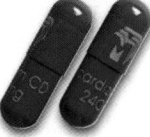 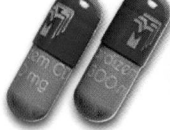

120 mg   240 mg   300 mg

Cardizem SR
(page 251)

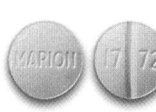 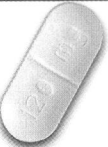

60 mg   120 mg

DOXAZOSIN MESYLATE

Cardura
(page 279)

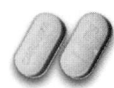 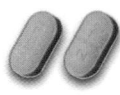 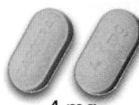

1 mg   2 mg   4 mg

8 mg

ENALAPRIL MALEATE

Vasotec
(page 280)

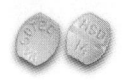

2.5 mg

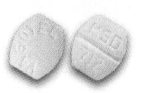

5 mg

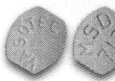

10 mg

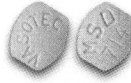

20 mg

ERYTHROMYCIN BASE

E-Mycin
(page 200)

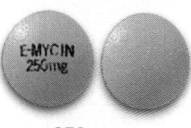

250 mg

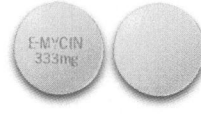

333 mg

Eryc
(page 200)

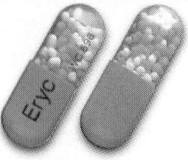

250 mg

Ery-Tab
(page 200)

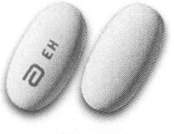

333 mg

ESTRADIOL

Estrace
(page 738)

0.5 mg

1 mg

2 mg

ESTROGENS, CONJUGATED

Premarin
(page 743)

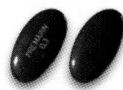

0.3 mg

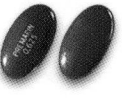

0.625 mg

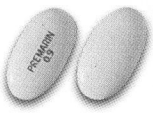

0.9 mg

1.25 mg

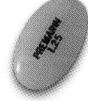

2.5 mg

ETHINYL ESTRADIOL AND ETHYNODIOL DIACETATE

Demulen
(page 749)

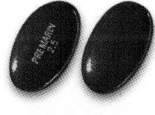

1/35-28

1/50-28

FAMOTIDINE

Pepcid
(page 693)

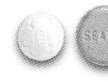

20 mg

40 mg

FEXOFENADINE HYDROCHLORIDE

Allegra
(page 600)

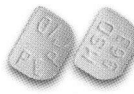

180 mg

FLUCONAZOLE

Diflucan
(page 30)

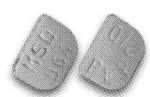

50 mg

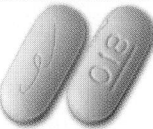

100 mg

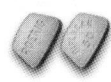

150 mg

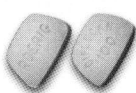

200 mg

FLUOXETINE HYDROCHLORIDE

Prozac
(page 442)

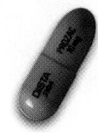

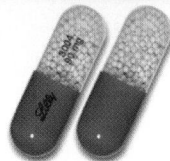

| 10 mg | 20 mg | 90 mg |

Sarafem
(page 442)

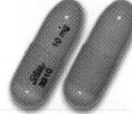

| 10 mg | 20 mg |

FLUVASTATIN SODIUM

Lescol
(page 318)

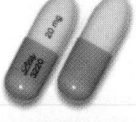

| 20 mg | 40 mg |

FOSINOPRIL SODIUM

Monopril
(page 284)

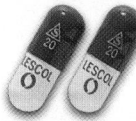

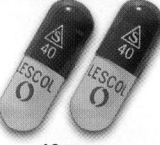

| 10 mg | 20 mg | 40 mg |

FUROSEMIDE

Lasix
(page 831)

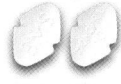

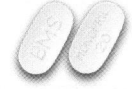

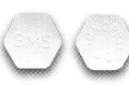

| 20 mg | 40 mg | 80 mg |

GABAPENTIN

Neurontin
(page 413)

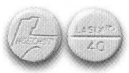

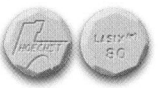

| 100 mg | 300 mg | 400 mg |

GEMFIBROZIL

Lopid
(page 319)

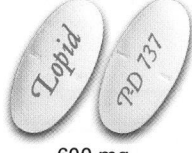

600 mg

GLIPIZIDE

Glucotrol
(page 772)

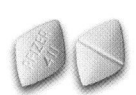 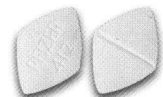

5 mg   10 mg

Glucotrol XL
(page 772)

    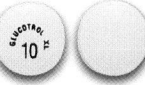

2.5 mg   5 mg   10 mg

GLYBURIDE

DiaBeta
(page 774)

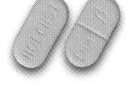 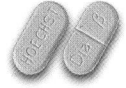 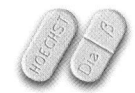

1.25 mg   2.5 mg   5 mg

Micronase
(page 774)

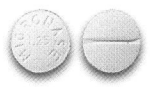  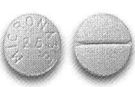 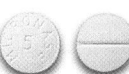

1.25 mg   2.5 mg   5 mg

HYDROCHLOROTHIAZIDE

HydroDIURIL
(page 833)

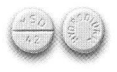 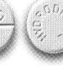

25 mg   50 mg

HYDROCODONE BITARTRATE AND ACETAMINOPHEN

Lortab
(page 372)

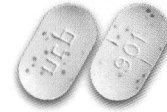 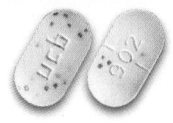 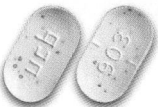

2.5/500 mg   5/500 mg   7.5/500 mg

Vicodin
(page 373)

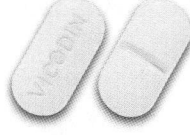

5/500 mg

Vicodin ES
(page 373)

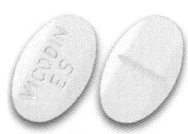

7.5/750 mg

IBUPROFEN

Motrin
(page 355)

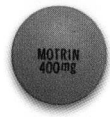

400 mg   600 mg   800 mg

IMATINIB MESYLATE

Gleevec
(page 1254)

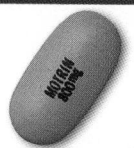

100 mg

LANSOPRAZOLE

Prevacid
(page 694)

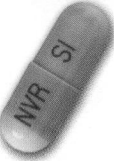 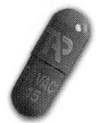 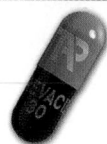

15 mg   30 mg

LEUCOVORIN CALCIUM

Wellcovorin
(page 1179)

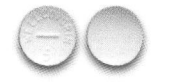 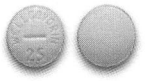

5 mg   25 mg

LEVOFLOXACIN

Levaquin
(page 143)

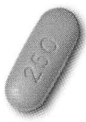 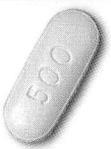

250 mg   500 mg

LEVOTHYROXINE SODIUM

Levothroid
(page 795)

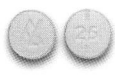 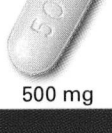

25 mcg   50 mcg   75 mcg

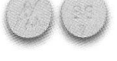 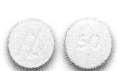

88 mcg   100 mcg   112 mcg

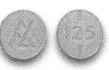 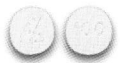 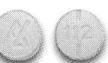

125 mcg   137 mcg   150 mcg

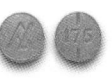 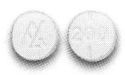 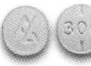

175 mcg   200 mcg   300 mcg

LEVOTHYROXINE SODIUM (CONTINUED)

Levoxyl
(page 795)

25 mcg

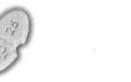

50 mcg

75 mcg

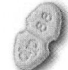

88 mcg

100 mcg

112 mcg

125 mcg

137 mcg

150 mcg

175 mcg

200 mcg

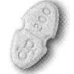

300 mcg

Synthroid
(page 795)

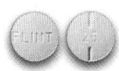

0.025 mg

0.05 mg

0.075 mg

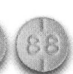

0.088 mg

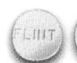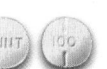

0.1 mg

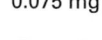

0.112 mg

0.125 mg

0.15 mg

0.175 mg

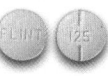

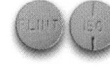

0.2 mg

0.3 mg

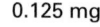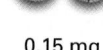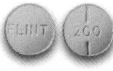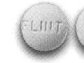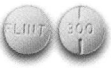

LISINOPRIL

Prinivil
(page 290)

 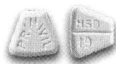

2.5 mg   5 mg   10 mg

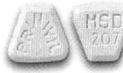

20 mg   40 mg

Zestril
(page 290)

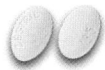 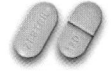

2.5 mg   5 mg   10 mg

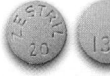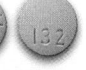 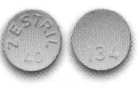

20 mg   40 mg

LORATADINE

Claritin
(page 601)

10 mg

Claritin Reditabs
(page 601)

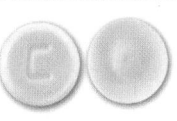

10 mg

LOSARTAN POTASSIUM

Cozaar
(page 291)

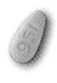

25 mg   50 mg

LOVASTATIN

Mevacor
(page 320)

 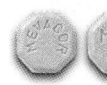

10 mg   20 mg   40 mg

MEDROXYPROGESTERONE ACETATE

Provera
(page 754)

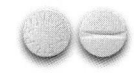 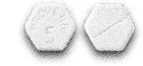 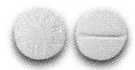

2.5 mg   5 mg   10 mg

MEPERIDINE HYDROCHLORIDE

Demerol
(page 382)

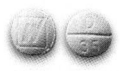 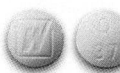

50 mg   100 mg

METFORMIN HYDROCHLORIDE

Glucophage
(page 785)

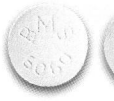 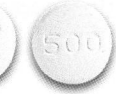 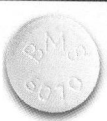 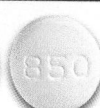

500 mg   850 mg

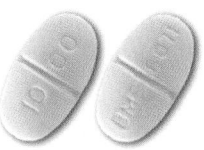

1,000 mg

Glucophage XR
(page 785)

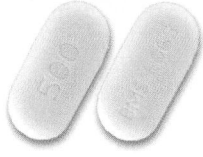

500 mg

METHYLPHENIDATE HYDROCHLORIDE

Concerta
(page 504)

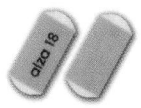 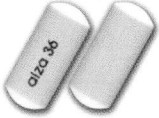 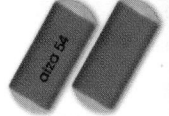

| 18 mg | 36 mg | 54 mg |

Ritalin
(page 504)

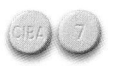 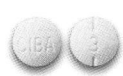 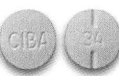

| 5 mg | 10 mg | 20 mg |

Ritalin SR
(page 504)

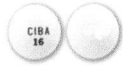

20 mg

METHYLPREDNISOLONE

Medrol
(page 712)

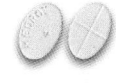 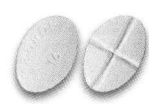

| 4 mg | 16 mg |

METOPROLOL SUCCINATE

Toprol-XL
(page 294)

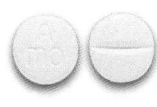 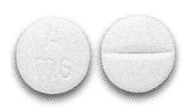 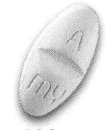

| 50 mg | 100 mg | 200 mg |

MONTELUKAST SODIUM

Singulair
(page 644)

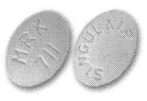

| 4 mg | 5 mg | 10 mg |

NABUMETONE

Relafen
(page 363)

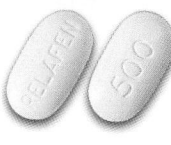 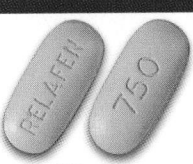

| 500 mg | 750 mg |

NAPROXEN

Naprosyn
(page 364)

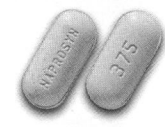 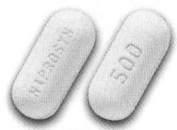

375 mg   500 mg

NEFAZODONE HYDROCHLORIDE

Serzone
(page 446)

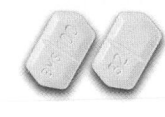 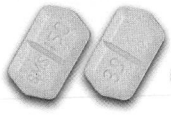 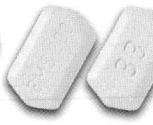

100 mg   150 mg   200 mg

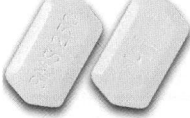

250 mg

NIFEDIPINE

Procardia
(page 256)

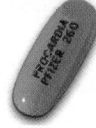 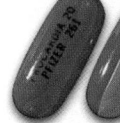

10 mg   20 mg

Procardia XL
(page 256)

  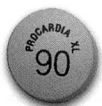

30 mg   60 mg   90 mg

NITROFURANTOIN MACROCRYSTALS

Macrobid
(page 212)

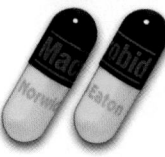

100 mg

NITROGLYCERIN

Nitrostat
(page 257)

0.4 mg

NORTRIPTYLINE HYDROCHLORIDE

Pamelor
(page 447)

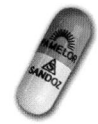
10 mg

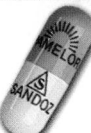
25 mg

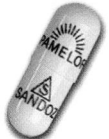
50 mg

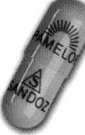
75 mg

OMEPRAZOLE

Prilosec
(page 696)

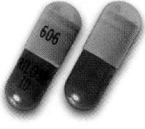
10 mg

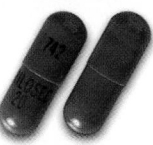
20 mg

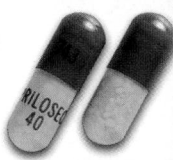
40 mg

OXAPROZIN

Daypro
(page 366)

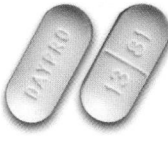

600 mg

OXYCODONE HYDROCHLORIDE

OxyContin
(page 387)

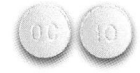 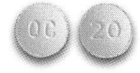 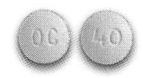

10 mg   20 mg   40 mg

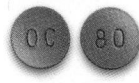

80 mg

PAROXETINE HYDROCHLORIDE

Paxil
(page 448)

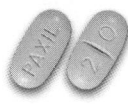 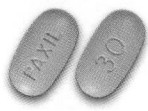

20 mg   30 mg

PENICILLIN V

Pen VK
(page 86)

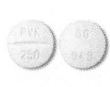 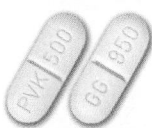

250 mg   500 mg

PENTOXIFYLLINE

Trental
(page 337)

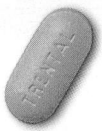

400 mg

PHENYTOIN

Dilantin Infatab
(page 422)

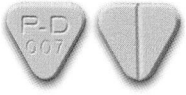

50 mg

PHENYTOIN SODIUM

Dilantin Kapseals
(page 422)

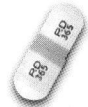 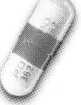

30 mg   100 mg

POTASSIUM CHLORIDE

K-Dur 20
(page 853)

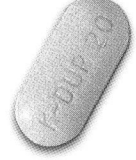

20 mEq

PRAVASTATIN SODIUM

Pravachol
(page 322)

  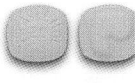 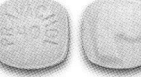

10 mg   20 mg   40 mg

PREDNISONE

Deltasone
(page 717)

   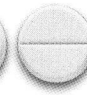

10 mg   50 mg

PROCHLORPERAZINE

Compazine
(page 685)

5 mg   10 mg

PROMETHAZINE HYDROCHLORIDE

Phenergan
(page 602)

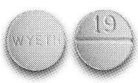 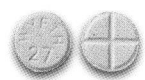

12.5 mg   25 mg   50 mg

PROPRANOLOL HYDROCHLORIDE

Inderal
(page 260)

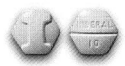

10 mg

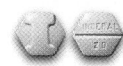

20 mg

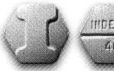

40 mg

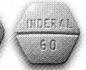

60 mg

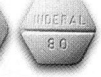

80 mg

Inderal LA
(page 260)

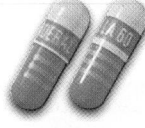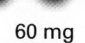

60 mg

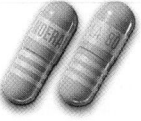

80 mg

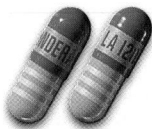

120 mg

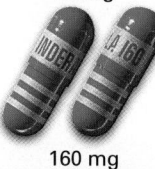

160 mg

QUINAPRIL HYDROCHLORIDE

Accupril
(page 303)

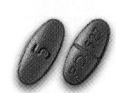

5 mg

10 mg

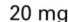

20 mg

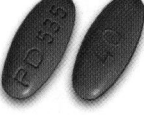

40 mg

RALOXIFENE HYDROCHLORIDE

Evista
(page 1269)

60 mg

RAMIPRIL

Altace
(page 304)

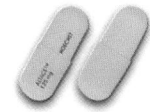 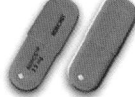 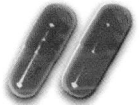

1.25 mg   2.5 mg   5 mg

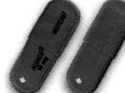

10 mg

RANITIDINE HYDROCHLORIDE

Zantac
(page 699)

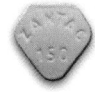 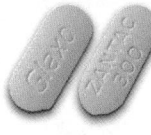

150 mg   300 mg

RISEDRONATE SODIUM

Actonel
(page 1271)

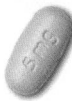

5 mg

RISPERIDONE

Risperdal
(page 488)

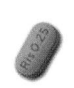  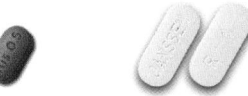

0.25 mg   0.5 mg   1 mg

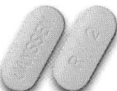 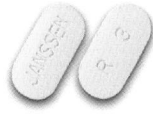 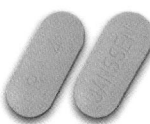

2 mg   3 mg   4 mg

ROFECOXIB

Vioxx
(page 368)

  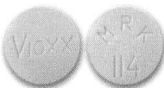

| 12.5 mg | 25 mg | 50 mg |

ROSIGLITAZONE MALEATE

Avandia
(page 792)

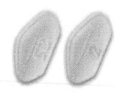 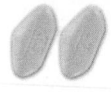 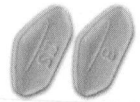

| 2 mg | 4 mg | 8 mg |

SERTRALINE HYDROCHLORIDE

Zoloft
(page 451)

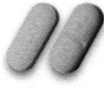 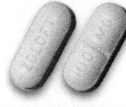

| 50 mg | 100 mg |

SILDENAFIL CITRATE

Viagra
(page 1273)

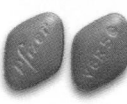 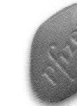 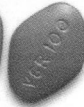

| 50 mg | 100 mg |

SIMVASTATIN

Zocor
(page 323)

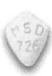 

| 5 mg | 10 mg | 20 mg |

40 mg

SUCRALFATE

Carafate
(page 701)

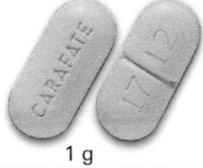

1 g

SUMATRIPTAN SUCCINATE

Imitrex
(page 540)

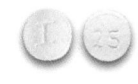　　　　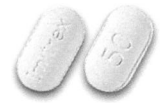

25 mg　　　　50 mg

TAMOXIFEN CITRATE

Nolvadex
(page 960)

　　　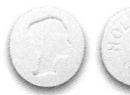

10 mg　　　　20 mg

TEMAZEPAM

Restoril
(page 403)

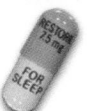　　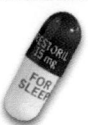　　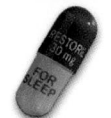

7.5 mg　　　15 mg　　　30 mg

TERAZOSIN HYDROCHLORIDE

Hytrin
(page 307)

　　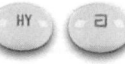　　

1 mg　　　　2 mg　　　　5 mg

10 mg

TICLOPIDINE HYDROCHLORIDE

Ticlid
(page 337)

250 mg

TOLTERODINE TARTRATE

Detrol
(page 1282)

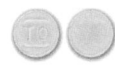 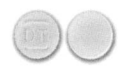

1 mg 2 mg

TRAMADOL HYDROCHLORIDE AND ACETAMINOPHEN

Ultracet
(page 373)

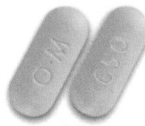

37.5/325 mg

TRAZODONE HYDROCHLORIDE

Desyrel
(page 454)

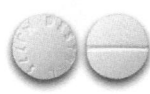 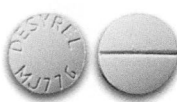

50 mg 100 mg

VALPROIC ACID

Depakote
(page 428)

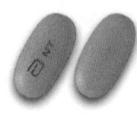 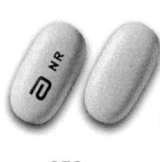 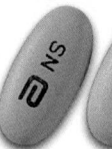

125 mg 250 mg 500 mg

Depakote Sprinkle
(page 428)

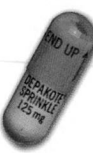

125 mg

VENLAFAXINE HYDROCHLORIDE

Effexor
(page 456)

25 mg

37.5 mg

50 mg

75 mg

100 mg

Effexor XR
(page 456)

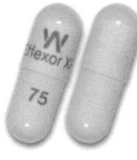

75 mg

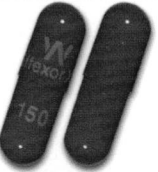

150 mg

VERAPAMIL

Calan
(page 262)

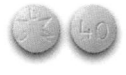

40 mg

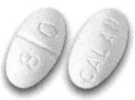

80 mg

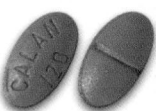

120 mg

VERAPAMIL HYDROCHLORIDE

Isoptin SR
(page 262)

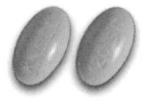

120 mg

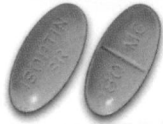

180 mg

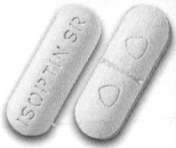

240 mg

Verelan
(page 262)

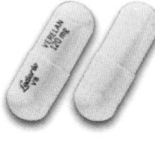

120 mg

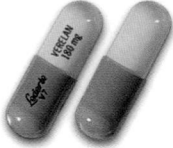

180 mg

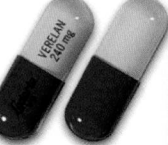

240 mg

WARFARIN SODIUM

Coumadin
(page 880)

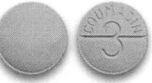

1 mg

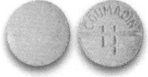

2 mg

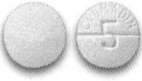

2.5 mg

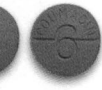

3 mg

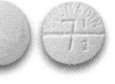

4 mg

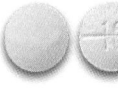

5 mg

6 mg

7.5 mg

10 mg

ZALEPLON

Sonata
(page 404)

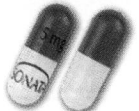 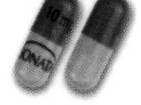

5 mg   10 mg

ZOLPIDEM TARTRATE

Ambien
(page 406)

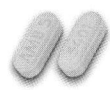 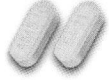

5 mg   10 mg

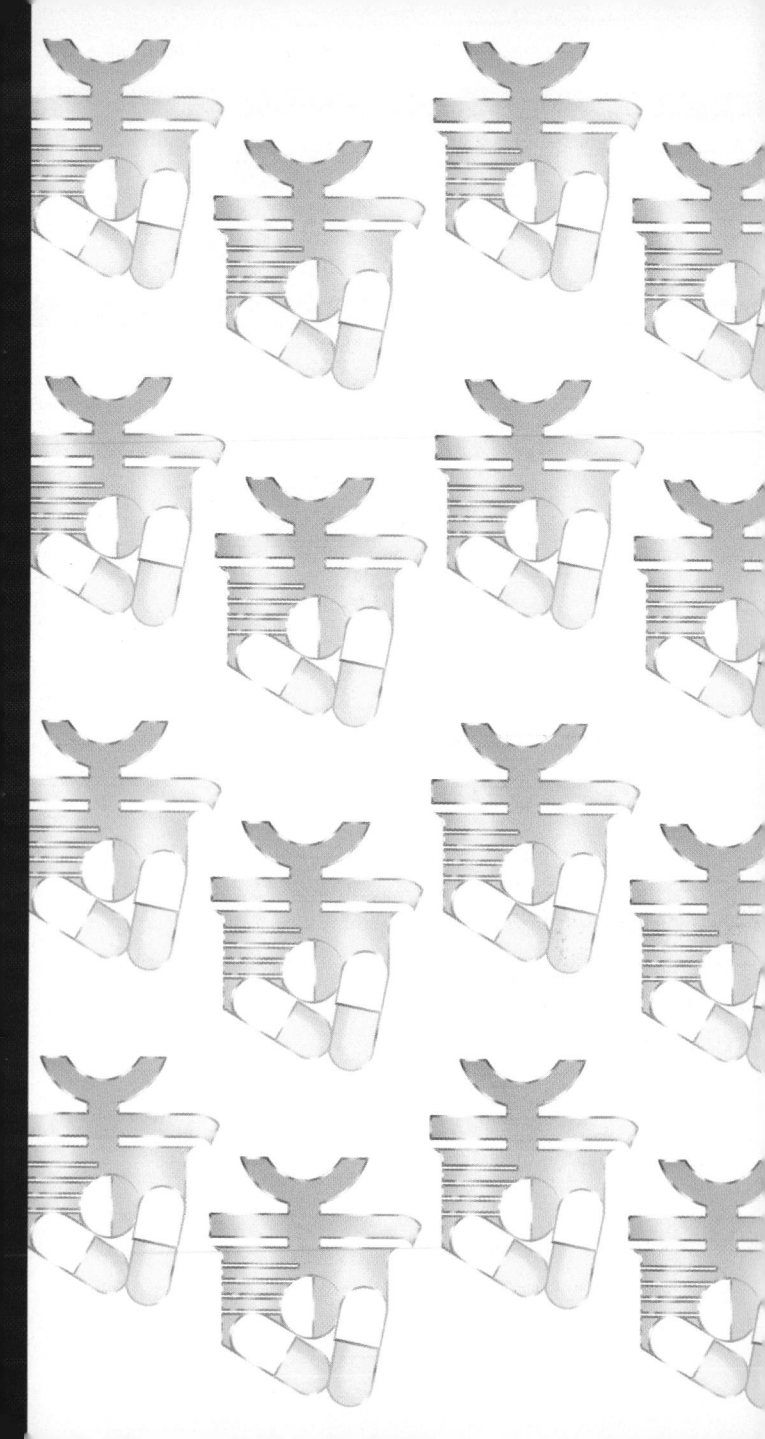

shouldn't be taken daily for longer than 2 weeks.

Adjust-a-dose: For patients with creatinine clearance less than 30 ml/minute, decrease dosage to 300 mg P.O. or I.V. q 12 hours.

I.V. ADMINISTRATION

• *Alert:* Dilute I.V. solutions with normal saline solution, D_5W, dextrose 10% in water (and combinations of these), lactated Ringer's solution, or 5% sodium bicarbonate injection. Don't dilute with sterile water for injection. Cimetidine is also commonly added to total parenteral nutrition solutions with or without fat emulsion.

• Give direct injection over 5 minutes. Rapid I.V. injection may result in arrhythmias and hypotension.

• Infuse drug over at least 30 minutes to minimize risk of adverse cardiac effects. Use infusion pump if cimetidine is given as continuous I.V. infusion in a total volume of 250 ml over 24 hours or less.

ACTION

Competitively inhibits action of histamine on the H_2 at receptor sites of parietal cells, decreasing gastric acid secretion.

Route	Onset	Peak	Duration
I.M.	Unknown	Unknown	Unknown
I.V.	Unknown	Immediate	Unknown
P.O.	Unknown	45-90 min	4-5 hr

ADVERSE REACTIONS

CNS: confusion, dizziness, headache, peripheral neuropathy, somnolence, hallucinations.
GI: mild and transient diarrhea.
GU: impotence.
Musculoskeletal: muscle pain, arthralgia.
Other: mild gynecomastia if used longer than 1 month, hypersensitivity reactions.

INTERACTIONS

Drug-drug. *Antacids:* Interference with cimetidine absorption. Separate administration by at least 1 hour, if possible.
Fosphenytoin, lidocaine, phenytoin, propranolol, some benzodiazepines, theophylline, warfarin: Inhibited hepatic microsomal enzyme metabolism of these drugs. Monitor serum levels.

Ketoconazole and other drugs that depend on gastric pH for absorption: Decreased drug absorption. Separate administration by at least 2 hours.
Drug-herb. *Guarana:* May increase serum caffeine levels or prolong serum caffeine half-life. Monitor patient.
Pennyroyal: May change rate at which toxic metabolites of pennyroyal form. Monitor patient.
Yerba maté: May decrease clearance of yerba maté methylxanthines and cause toxicity. Discourage use together.
Drug-lifestyle. *Alcohol use:* May increase blood alcohol concentration. Discourage use together.

EFFECTS ON LAB TEST RESULTS

• May increase creatinine, alkaline phosphatase, AST, and ALT levels.

CONTRAINDICATIONS

Contraindicated in patients hypersensitive to drug.

NURSING CONSIDERATIONS

• Use cautiously in elderly or debilitated patients because they may be more susceptible to cimetidine-induced confusion.
• Assess patient for abdominal pain. Note blood in emesis, stool, or gastric aspirate.
• Identify tablet strength when obtaining a drug history.
• Schedule cimetidine dose at end of hemodialysis treatment because hemodialysis reduces blood levels of cimetidine. Adjust dosage for patients with renal impairment.
• Drug may antagonize pentagastrin's effect during gastric acid secretion tests; it may cause false-negative results in skin tests using allergen extracts. FD and C blue dye number 2 used in Tagamet tablets may impair interpretation of Hemoccult and Gastroccult tests on gastric content aspirate. Wait at least 15 minutes after giving tablet before drawing sample, and follow test manufacturer's instructions closely.
• I.M. injection may be given undiluted.
• Treatment of gastric ulcer isn't as effective as treatment of duodenal ulcer.
• Up to 10 g overdose can occur without adverse reactions.

ACTION
Competitively inhibits action of histamine on the H$_2$ at receptor sites of parietal cells, decreasing gastric acid secretion.

Route	Onset	Peak	Duration
I.V.	1 hr	1-4 hr	12 hr
P.O.	1 hr	1-3 hr	12 hr

ADVERSE REACTIONS
CNS: *headache,* dizziness, vertigo, malaise, paresthesia.
CV: palpitations, flushing.
EENT: tinnitus, orbital edema.
GI: diarrhea, constipation, anorexia, taste perversion, dry mouth.
Musculoskeletal: bone and muscle pain.
Skin: acne, dry skin.
Other: transient irritation at I.V. site, fever.

INTERACTIONS
None significant.

EFFECTS ON LAB TEST RESULTS
• May increase BUN, creatinine, and liver enzyme levels.

CONTRAINDICATIONS
Contraindicated in patients hypersensitive to drug.

NURSING CONSIDERATIONS
• Assess for abdominal pain. Note blood in emesis, stool, or gastric aspirate.
• Oral suspension must be reconstituted and shaken before use.
• Store reconstituted suspension below 86° F (30° C). Discard after 30 days. Drug may antagonize pentagastrin during gastric acid secretion tests. In skin tests using allergen extracts, drug may cause false-negative results.

PATIENT TEACHING
• Instruct patient on proper use of OTC product (Pepcid AC), if appropriate.
• Tell patient to take prescription drug with a snack, if desired.
• Remind patient that prescription drug is most effective if taken at bedtime. Tell patient taking 20 mg twice daily to take one dose at bedtime.
• Advise patient not to take prescription drug for longer than 8 weeks, unless or-

dered by prescriber, and to limit use of OTC drug to no more than 2 weeks.
• With prescriber's knowledge, allow patient to take antacids together, especially at beginning of therapy when pain is severe.
• Urge patient to avoid cigarette smoking because it may increase gastric acid secretion and worsen disease.
• Advise patient to report abdominal pain and blood in stools or emesis.

lansoprazole
Prevacid, Zoton§

Pregnancy risk category B

AVAILABLE FORMS
Capsules (delayed-release): 15 mg, 30 mg

INDICATIONS & DOSAGES
➤ **Short-term treatment of active duodenal ulcer—**
Adults: 15 mg P.O. daily before eating for 4 weeks.
➤ **Short-term treatment of active benign gastric ulcer—**
Adults: 30 mg P.O. once daily for up to 8 weeks.
➤ **Short-term treatment of erosive esophagitis—**
Adults: 30 mg P.O. daily before eating for up to 8 weeks. If healing doesn't occur, 8 more weeks of therapy may be given. Maintenance dosage for healing is 15 mg P.O. daily.
➤ **Maintenance of healing of erosive esophagitis—**
Adults: 15 mg P.O. once daily.
➤ **Long-term treatment of pathologic hypersecretory conditions, including Zollinger-Ellison syndrome—**
Adults: Initially, 60 mg P.O. once daily. Increase dosage, p.r.n. Daily amounts above 120 mg should be given in evenly divided doses.
➤ **Maintenance of healed duodenal ulcers—**
Adults: 15 mg P.O. daily.
➤ *Helicobacter pylori* **eradication to reduce risk of duodenal ulcer recurrence—**
Adults: For patients receiving dual therapy, 30 mg P.O. lansoprazole with 1 g P.O.

amoxicillin, each given q 8 hours for 14 days. For patients receiving triple therapy, 30 mg P.O. lansoprazole with 1 g P.O. amoxicillin and 500 mg P.O. clarithromycin, all given q 12 hours for 10 to 14 days.
➤ **Short-term treatment of symptomatic gastroesophageal reflux disease—**
Adults: 15 mg P.O. once daily for up to 8 weeks.
✳ *NEW INDICATION:* **Treatment of NSAID-related ulcer in patients who take NSAIDs—**
Adults: 30 mg P.O. daily for 8 weeks.
➤ **Reduction in risk of NSAID-related ulcer in patients who have a history of gastric ulcer but need NSAIDs—**
Adults: 15 mg P.O. daily for up to 12 weeks.

ACTION
Inhibits activity of proton pump and binds to hydrogen-potassium adenosine triphosphatase, located at secretory surface of gastric parietal cells, to block secretion of gastric acid.

Route	Onset	Peak	Duration
P.O.	1-3 hr	Unknown	Unknown

ADVERSE REACTIONS
GI: diarrhea, nausea, abdominal pain.

INTERACTIONS
Drug-drug. *Ampicillin esters, digoxin, iron salts, ketoconazole:* Lansoprazole may inhibit absorption. Monitor patient closely.
Sucralfate: Delayed lansoprazole absorption. Give lansoprazole at least 30 minutes before sucralfate.
Theophylline: Theophylline clearance may increase mildly. Dosage adjustment of theophylline may be needed when lansoprazole is started or stopped. Use together cautiously.
Drug-herb. *Male fern:* Inactivated in alkaline environments. Advise patient to avoid using together.
St. John's wort: Increased risk of sun sensitivity. Advise patient to avoid sun exposure and use sunblock.
Drug-food. *Food:* Decreased rate and extent of GI absorption. Advise patient to take before meals.

EFFECTS ON LAB TEST RESULTS
None reported.

CONTRAINDICATIONS
Contraindicated in patients hypersensitive to drug.

NURSING CONSIDERATIONS
● No dosage adjustment is needed for elderly patients or those with renal insufficiency. Patients with severe liver disease may need dosage adjustment.
● A symptomatic response to lansoprazole therapy doesn't preclude presence of gastric malignancy.
● Safety and efficacy of drug haven't been established in children.
● For patients who have a nasogastric tube in place, capsules can be opened and the intact granules mixed in 40 ml of apple juice and administered through the tube into the stomach. After administering the granules, the tube should be flushed with additional apple juice to clear it.
● Because it's unknown if lansoprazole appears in breast milk, breast-feeding or drug should be discontinued when drug is prescribed for breast-feeding women.

PATIENT TEACHING
● For best effect, instruct patient to take drug no more than 30 minutes before eating.
● If patient has trouble swallowing capsules, tell him to open and sprinkle contents over applesauce, and to swallow immediately. The contents shouldn't be chewed or crushed.

misoprostol
Cytotec

Pregnancy risk category X

AVAILABLE FORMS
Tablets: 100 mcg, 200 mcg

INDICATIONS & DOSAGES
➤ **Prevention of NSAID-induced gastric ulcer in elderly or debilitated patients at high risk for complications**

from gastric ulcer and in patients with history of NSAID-induced ulcer—
Adults: 200 mcg P.O. q.i.d. with food; if not tolerated, decrease to 100 mcg P.O. q.i.d. Dosage should be given for duration of NSAID therapy. Last dose should be given h.s.

ACTION
A synthetic prostaglandin E$_1$ analogue that replaces gastric prostaglandins depleted by NSAID therapy. Also decreases basal and stimulated gastric acid secretion and may increase gastric mucus and bicarbonate production.

Route	Onset	Peak	Duration
P.O.	30 min	60-90 min	3 hr

ADVERSE REACTIONS
CNS: headache.
GI: *diarrhea, abdominal pain,* nausea, flatulence, dyspepsia, vomiting, constipation.
GU: hypermenorrhea, dysmenorrhea, spotting, cramps, menstrual disorders, postmenopausal vaginal bleeding.

INTERACTIONS
Drug-food. *Any food:* May decrease absorption rate of drug. However, manufacturer recommends that patient take drug with food.

EFFECTS ON LAB TEST RESULTS
None reported.

CONTRAINDICATIONS
Contraindicated in patients hypersensitive to misoprostol or any of its components and in pregnant or breast-feeding women.

NURSING CONSIDERATIONS
• Drug shouldn't be routinely given to women of childbearing age unless they have a high risk of ulcers or complications from NSAID-induced ulcers. Use with caution in patients with inflammatory bowel disease.
• *Alert:* Take special precautions to prevent use of drug during pregnancy. Make sure patient understands dangers of drug to fetus and that she receives both oral and written warnings about these dangers.

Also, make sure she can comply with effective contraception and that she has a negative serum pregnancy test within 2 weeks of starting therapy. Patient shouldn't breast-feed during therapy.
• Drug causes modest decrease in basal pepsin secretion.

PATIENT TEACHING
• Instruct patient not to share misoprostol. Remind pregnant patient that drug may cause miscarriage, often with potentially life-threatening bleeding.
• Advise woman not to begin therapy until second or third day of next normal menstrual period.
• Advise patient to take drug as prescribed for duration of NSAID therapy.
• Tell patient that diarrhea usually occurs early in the course of therapy and is usually self-limiting. Taking drug with food helps minimize the diarrhea.

---

omeprazole
Losec†‡, Prilosec

Pregnancy risk category C

AVAILABLE FORMS
Capsules (delayed-release): 10 mg, 20 mg, 40 mg

INDICATIONS & DOSAGES
➤ **Symptomatic gastroesophageal reflux disease (GERD) without esophageal lesions—**
Adults: 20 mg P.O. daily for 4 weeks for patients poorly responsive to customary medical treatment usually including an adequate course of H$_2$-receptor antagonists.
➤ **Erosive esophagitis and accompanying symptoms caused by GERD—**
Adults: 20 mg P.O. daily for 4 to 8 weeks.
➤ **Maintenance of healing erosive esophagitis—**
Adults: 20 mg P.O. daily.
➤ **Pathologic hypersecretory conditions (such as Zollinger-Ellison syndrome)—**
Adults: Initially, 60 mg P.O. daily; adjust dosage based on patient response. If daily dose exceeds 80 mg, administer in divided doses. Doses up to 120 mg t.i.d. have been

---

Reactions may be *common*, uncommon, *life-threatening*, or COMMON AND LIFE-THREATENING.

given. Continue therapy as long as clinically indicated.

➤ **Duodenal ulcer (short-term treatment)**—
Adults: 20 mg P.O. daily for 4 to 8 weeks.
➤ ***Helicobacter pylori* infection and duodenal ulcer disease, to eradicate *H. pylori* with clarithromycin (dual therapy)**—
Adults: 40 mg P.O. every morning with clarithromycin 500 mg P.O. t.i.d. for 14 days. For patients with an ulcer at start of therapy, an additional 14 days of omeprazole 20 mg P.O. once daily is recommended.
➤ ***H. pylori* infection and duodenal ulcer disease, to eradicate *H. pylori* with clarithromycin and amoxicillin (triple therapy)**—
Adults: 20 mg P.O. with clarithromycin 500 mg P.O. and amoxicillin 1,000 mg P.O., each given b.i.d. for 10 days. For patients with an ulcer at start of therapy, another 18 days of omeprazole 20 mg P.O. once daily is recommended.
➤ **Short-term treatment of active benign gastric ulcer**—
Adults: 40 mg P.O. once daily for 4 to 8 weeks.

ACTION
Inhibits activity of acid (proton) pump and binds to hydrogen-potassium adenosine triphosphatase at secretory surface of gastric parietal cells to block formation of gastric acid.

Route	Onset	Peak	Duration
P.O.	1 hr	2 hr	< 3 days

ADVERSE REACTIONS
CNS: headache, dizziness, asthenia.
GI: diarrhea, abdominal pain, nausea, vomiting, constipation, flatulence.
Musculoskeletal: back pain.
Respiratory: cough, upper respiratory tract infection.
Skin: rash.

INTERACTIONS
Drug-drug. *Ampicillin esters, iron derivatives, ketoconazole:* May exhibit poor bioavailability in patients taking omeprazole because these drugs need a low gas-

tric pH for optimal absorption. Avoid using together.
Diazepam, fosphenytoin, phenytoin, warfarin: Decreased hepatic clearance, possibly leading to increased serum levels. Monitor drug levels.
Drug-herb. *Male fern:* Inactivated in alkaline environments. Advise patient to separate administration times.
Pennyroyal: May change rate at which toxic metabolites of pennyroyal form. Ask patient about the use of herbal remedies, and discourage use together.
St. John's wort: Increased risk of sun sensitivity. Advise patient to avoid sun exposure and use sunblock.

EFFECTS ON LAB TEST RESULTS
None reported.

CONTRAINDICATIONS
Contraindicated in patients hypersensitive to drug or its components.

NURSING CONSIDERATIONS
● Dosage adjustments aren't needed for patients with renal or hepatic impairment.
● Omeprazole increases its own bioavailability with repeated doses. Drug is labile in gastric acid; less drug is lost to hydrolysis because drug increases gastric pH.
● *Alert:* Don't confuse Prilosec with Prozac, Prilocaine, or Prinivil.
● Serum gastrin levels rise in most patients during the first 2 weeks of therapy.

PATIENT TEACHING
● Tell patient to swallow capsules whole and not to open, crush, or chew them.
● Instruct patient to take drug 30 minutes before meals.
● Caution patient not to perform hazardous activities if dizziness occurs.

---

pantoprazole sodium
Protonix

Pregnancy risk category B

AVAILABLE FORMS
Injection: 40 mg per vial
Tablet (delayed-release): 40 mg

INDICATIONS & DOSAGES

➤ **Treatment of erosive esophagitis with gastroesophageal reflux disease (GERD)—**
Adults: 40 mg P.O. once daily for up to 8 weeks. For patients who haven't healed after 8 weeks of treatment, another 8-week course may be considered.

➤ **Short-term treatment of GERD, in patients who can't take delayed-release tablets orally—**
Adults: 40 mg I.V. daily for 7 to 10 days.
Treatment with I.V. pantoprazole should be discontinued when P.O. pantoprazole is warranted.

I.V. ADMINISTRATION

● Dilute with D_5W, normal saline, or lactated Ringer's solution to a final concentration of 0.4 mg/ml. Infuse over 15 minutes at a rate not greater than 3 mg/min (7 ml/min). Don't give another infusion simultaneously through the same line. The reconstituted solution may be stored for up to 2 hours at room temperature, and the admixture may be stored for up to 12 hours room temperature.

ACTION

Inhibits proton pump activity by binding to hydrogen-potassium adenosine triphosphatase, located at secretory surface of gastric parietal cells, to suppress gastric acid secretion.

Route	Onset	Peak	Duration
I.V.	15-30 min	Unknown	24 hr
P.O.	Unknown	2.5 hr	> 24 hr

ADVERSE REACTIONS

CNS: headache, insomnia, asthenia, migraine, anxiety, dizziness.
CV: chest pain.
EENT: pharyngitis, rhinitis, sinusitis.
GI: diarrhea, flatulence, abdominal pain, eructation, constipation, dyspepsia, gastroenteritis, GI disorder, nausea, vomiting, rectal disorder.
GU: urinary frequency, urinary tract infection.
Metabolic: hyperglycemia, hyperlipemia.
Musculoskeletal: back pain, neck pain, arthralgia, hypertonia.
Respiratory: bronchitis, increased cough, dyspnea, upper respiratory tract infection.

Skin: rash.
Other: flu syndrome, infection, pain.

INTERACTIONS

Drug-drug. *Ampicillin esters, iron salts, ketoconazole:* May decrease absorption of these drugs. Monitor patient closely.
Proton pump inhibitors: May increase risk of sunburn. Advise patient to use sun protection.
Drug-herb. *St. John's wort:* May increase risk of sunburn. Advise patient to use sun protection.
Drug-food. *Any food:* Delayed absorption of pantoprazole for up to 2 hours; however, the extent of absorption isn't affected. Advise patient to take drug without regard to meals.

EFFECTS ON LAB TEST RESULTS

● May increase glucose, serum lipids, and liver function test result values.

CONTRAINDICATIONS

Contraindicated in patients hypersensitive to any component of the formulation.

NURSING CONSIDERATIONS

Safety and efficacy of using the I.V. formulation to initiate therapy for GERD hasn't been demonstrated.
● *Alert:* Don't confuse with Protonix tablets, Prilosec, Prozac, or Prevacid.
● Drug can be given without regard to meals.
● Drug shouldn't be used for maintenance therapy beyond 16 weeks.
● Symptomatic response to therapy doesn't preclude the presence of gastric malignancy.

PATIENT TEACHING

● Instruct patient to take exactly as prescribed and at about the same time every day.
● Advise patient that drug can be taken without regard to meals.
● Inform patient that tablet should be swallowed whole and not crushed, split, or chewed.
● Tell patient that antacids don't affect pantoprazole absorption.

Reactions may be *common*, uncommon, *life-threatening*, or COMMON AND LIFE-THREATENING.

rabeprazole sodium
Aciphex

Pregnancy risk category B

AVAILABLE FORMS
Tablets (delayed-release): 20 mg

INDICATIONS & DOSAGES
➤ **Healing of erosive or ulcerative gastroesophageal reflux disease (GERD)—**
Adults: 20 mg P.O. daily for 4 to 8 weeks. Additional 8-week course may be considered, if needed.
➤ **Maintenance of healing of erosive or ulcerative GERD—**
Adults: 20 mg P.O. daily.
➤ **Healing of duodenal ulcers—**
Adults: 20 mg P.O. daily after morning meal for up to 4 weeks.
➤ **Pathologic hypersecretory conditions, including Zollinger-Ellison syndrome—**
Adults: 60 mg P.O. daily; may be increased, p.r.n., to 100 mg P.O. daily or 60 mg P.O. b.i.d.

ACTION
Blocks proton pump activity by inhibiting gastric hydrogen-potassium adenosine triphosphatase at secretory surface of gastric parietal cells, thereby blocking gastric acid secretion.

Route	Onset	Peak	Duration
P.O.	< 1 hr	2-5 hr	> 24 hr

ADVERSE REACTIONS
CNS: headache.

INTERACTIONS
Drug-drug. *Cyclosporine:* May inhibit cyclosporine metabolism. Use together cautiously.
Digoxin, ketoconazole, other gastric pH-dependent drugs: Decreased or increased drug absorption at increased pH values. Monitor patient closely.

EFFECTS ON LAB TEST RESULTS
None reported.

CONTRAINDICATIONS
Contraindicated in patients hypersensitive to drug, other benzimidazoles (lansoprazole, omeprazole), or components of these formulations.

NURSING CONSIDERATIONS
• Use cautiously in patients with severe hepatic impairment.
• Consider additional courses of therapy if duodenal ulcer or GERD isn't healed after first course of therapy.
• Symptomatic response to therapy doesn't preclude presence of gastric malignancy.

PATIENT TEACHING
• Explain importance of taking drug exactly as prescribed.
• Advise patient that delayed-release tablets should be swallowed whole and not crushed, chewed, or split.
• Inform patient that drug may be taken without regard to meals.

---

ranitidine hydrochloride
Apo-Ranitidine†, Zantac*, Zantac-C†, Zantac 75 ◊, Zantac 150, Zantac EFFERdose Tablets, Zantac 150 GELdose, Zantac 300, Zantac 300 GELdose

Pregnancy risk category B

AVAILABLE FORMS
Granules (effervescent): 150 mg
Infusion: 0.5 mg/ml in 100-ml containers
Injection: 25 mg/ml
Syrup: 15 mg/ml*
Tablets: 75 mg ◊, 150 mg, 300 mg
Tablets (dispersible): 150 mg‡
Tablets (effervescent): 150 mg

INDICATIONS & DOSAGES
➤ **Duodenal and gastric ulcer (short-term treatment); pathologic hypersecretory conditions, such as Zollinger-Ellison syndrome—**
Adults: 150 mg P.O. b.i.d. or 300 mg daily h.s. Or, 50 mg I.V. or I.M. q 6 to 8 hours. Patients with Zollinger-Ellison syndrome may need doses up to 6 g P.O. daily.

➤ **Maintenance therapy for duodenal or gastric ulcer—**
Adults: 150 mg P.O. h.s.
➤ **Gastroesophageal reflux disease—**
Adults: 150 mg P.O. b.i.d.
Children 1 month to 16 years: 5 to 10 mg/kg daily given as 2 divided doses P.O.
➤ **Erosive esophagitis—**
Adults: 150 mg P.O. q.i.d. Maintenance dosage is 150 mg P.O. b.i.d.
Children 1 month to 16 years: 5 to 10 mg/kg daily given as 2 divided doses P.O.
➤ **Heartburn—**
Adults and children age 12 and older: 75 mg (Zantac 75 only) P.O. as symptoms occur, not to exceed 150 mg daily. Don't exceed 2 weeks of continuous treatment.
Adjust-a-dose: For renally impaired patients with creatinine clearance below 50 ml/minute, 150 mg P.O. q 24 hours or 50 mg I.V. q 18 to 24 hours.

I.V. ADMINISTRATION
● To prepare I.V. injection, dilute 2 ml (50 mg) ranitidine with compatible I.V. solution to a total volume of 20 ml, and inject over at least 5 minutes. Compatible solutions include sterile water for injection, normal saline solution for injection, D_5W or lactated Ringer's injection.
● To give drug by intermittent I.V. infusion, dilute 50 mg (2 ml) ranitidine in 100 ml compatible solution and infuse at a rate of 5 to 7 ml/min. The premixed solution is 50 ml and doesn't need further dilution. Infuse over 15 to 20 minutes. After dilution, solution is stable for 48 hours at room temperature.
● Store I.V. injection in refrigerator at 36° to 46° F (2° to 8° C).

ACTION
Competitively inhibits action of histamine on the H_2 at receptor sites of parietal cells, decreasing gastric acid secretion.

Route	Onset	Peak	Duration
I.V.	Unknown	Unknown	Unknown
P.O.	1 hr	1-3 hr	13 hr

ADVERSE REACTIONS
CNS: vertigo, malaise, headache.
EENT: blurred vision.
Hepatic: jaundice.

Other: burning and itching at injection site, *anaphylaxis, angioedema.*

INTERACTIONS
Drug-drug. *Antacids:* May interfere with ranitidine absorption. Stagger doses, if possible.
Diazepam: Decreased absorption of diazepam. Monitor patient closely.
Glipizide: May increase hypoglycemic effect. Adjust glipizide dosage, as directed.
Procainamide: May decrease renal clearance of procainamide. Monitor patient closely for toxicity.
Warfarin: May interfere with warfarin clearance. Monitor patient closely.
Drug-lifestyle. *Alcohol use:* May increase blood alcohol level. Discourage use together.

EFFECTS ON LAB TEST RESULTS
● May increase creatinine and ALT levels.

CONTRAINDICATIONS
Contraindicated in patients hypersensitive to drug and those with acute porphyria.

NURSING CONSIDERATIONS
● Use cautiously in patients with hepatic dysfunction. Adjust dosage in patients with impaired renal function.
● Assess patient for abdominal pain. Note presence of blood in emesis, stool, or gastric aspirate.
● Drug may cause false-positive results in urine protein tests using Multistix.
● Ranitidine may be added to total parenteral nutrition solutions.
● *Alert:* Don't confuse ranitidine with ritodrine or rimantadine; don't confuse Zantac with Xanax or Zyrtec.

PATIENT TEACHING
● Instruct patient on proper use of OTC preparation, as indicated.
● Remind patient taking prescription drug once daily to take it at bedtime for best results.
● Instruct patient to take without regard to meals because absorption isn't affected by food.

• Tell patient taking EFFERdose to dissolve drug in 6 to 8 ounces of water before taking.

• Urge patient to avoid cigarette smoking because it may increase gastric acid secretion and worsen disease.

• Advise patient to report abdominal pain and blood in stool or emesis.

• Warn patients with phenylketonuria that EFFERdose granules and tablets contain aspartame.

---

sucralfate
Antepsin§, Carafate

Pregnancy risk category B

AVAILABLE FORMS
Suspension: 1 g/10 ml
Tablets: 1 g

INDICATIONS & DOSAGES
➤ **Short-term (up to 8 weeks) treatment of duodenal ulcer—**
Adults: 1 g P.O. q.i.d. 1 hour before meals and h.s.
➤ **Maintenance therapy for duodenal ulcer—**
Adults: 1 g P.O. b.i.d.

ACTION
Unknown. Probably adheres to and protects surface of ulcer by forming a barrier.

Route	Onset	Peak	Duration
P.O.	Unknown	Unknown	6 hr

ADVERSE REACTIONS
CNS: dizziness, sleepiness, headache, vertigo.
GI: *constipation,* nausea, gastric discomfort, diarrhea, bezoar formation, vomiting, flatulence, dry mouth, indigestion.
Musculoskeletal: back pain.
Skin: rash, pruritus.

INTERACTIONS
Drug-drug. *Antacids:* May decrease binding of drug to gastroduodenal mucosa, impairing effectiveness. Separate administration times by 30 minutes.
Cimetidine, digoxin, fluoroquinolones, fosphenytoin, ketoconazole, norfloxacin, phenytoin, quinidine, ranitidine, tetracy-
cline, theophylline: Decreased absorption. Separate administration times by at least 2 hours.

EFFECTS ON LAB TEST RESULTS
None reported.

CONTRAINDICATIONS
No known contraindications.

NURSING CONSIDERATIONS
• Use cautiously in patients with chronic renal failure.
• Reconstitute drug before instillation through a nasogastric tube. Flush tube with water to ensure passage into stomach.
• Drug is minimally absorbed and causes few adverse reactions.
• Monitor patient for severe, persistent constipation.
• Sucralfate is as effective as cimetidine in healing duodenal ulcer.
• Drug contains aluminum but isn't classified as an antacid. Monitor patient with renal insufficiency for aluminum toxicity.

PATIENT TEACHING
• Tell patient to take sucralfate on an empty stomach, 1 hour before each meal and at bedtime.
• Instruct patient to continue prescribed regimen to ensure complete healing. Pain and other ulcer signs and symptoms may subside within first few weeks of therapy.
• Urge patient to avoid cigarette smoking because it may increase gastric acid secretion and worsen disease.
• Antacids may be taken while on sucralfate; however, separate doses by 30 minutes.

---

betamethasone
betamethasone acetate and
  betamethasone sodium
  phosphate
betamethasone sodium
  phosphate
cortisone acetate
dexamethasone
dexamethasone acetate
dexamethasone sodium
  phosphate
fludrocortisone acetate
hydrocortisone
hydrocortisone acetate
hydrocortisone cypionate
hydrocortisone sodium
  phosphate
hydrocortisone sodium
  succinate
methylprednisolone
methylprednisolone acetate
methylprednisolone sodium
  succinate
prednisolone
prednisolone acetate
prednisolone sodium phosphate
prednisolone tebutate
prednisone
triamcinolone
triamcinolone acetonide
triamcinolone diacetate
triamcinolone hexacetonide

COMBINATION PRODUCTS
DECADRON PHOSPHATE WITH XYLO-
CAINE: dexamethasone phosphate 4 mg
and lidocaine hydrochloride 10 mg per ml.

---

betamethasone
Celestone*

betamethasone acetate and
betamethasone sodium
phosphate
Celestone Chronodose‡,
Celestone Soluspan

betamethasone sodium
phosphate
Betnesol§, Celestone Phosphate,
Selestoject

Pregnancy risk category C

AVAILABLE FORMS
betamethasone
Syrup: 600 mcg/5 ml
Tablets: 600 mcg
Tablets (effervescent): 500 mcg†
**betamethasone acetate and betametha-
sone sodium phosphate**
Injection (suspension): betamethasone
acetate 3 mg and betamethasone sodium
phosphate (equivalent to 3-mg base) per ml
betamethasone sodium phosphate
Injection: 4 mg (equivalent to 3-mg base)
per ml in 5-ml vials

INDICATIONS & DOSAGES
➤ **Conditions with severe inflammation,
conditions requiring immunosuppression—**
Adults: 0.6 to 7.2 mg P.O. daily. Or, 0.5 to
9 mg I.M. or into joint or soft tissue daily.
Betamethasone sodium phosphate-acetate
suspension 6 to 12 mg injected into large
joints or 1.5 to 6 mg injected into smaller
joints. Both injections may be given q 1 to
2 weeks, p.r.n.
Children: 0.0175 to 0.25 mg/kg daily or
0.5 to 7.5 mg/m² daily; given in three or
four divided doses. Not recommended for
long-term use; especially likely to inhibit
growth.

ACTION
Not completely defined. Decreases inflammation, mainly by stabilizing leukocyte
lysosomal membranes; suppresses immune response; stimulates bone marrow;
and influences protein, fat, and carbohydrate metabolism.

Route	Onset	Peak	Duration
I.M.	Rapid	1-3 hr	7-14 days
P.O.	Rapid	Unknown	3-25 days

Reactions may be *common*, uncommon, *life-threatening*, or COMMON AND LIFE-THREATENING.

ADVERSE REACTIONS

CNS: *euphoria, insomnia,* psychotic behavior, pseudotumor cerebri, vertigo, headache, paresthesia, *seizures.*

CV: *heart failure,* hypertension, edema, *arrhythmias,* thrombophlebitis, *thromboembolism.*

EENT: cataracts, glaucoma.

GI: *peptic ulceration,* GI irritation, increased appetite, *pancreatitis,* nausea, vomiting.

GU: menstrual irregularities.

Metabolic: hypokalemia, hyperglycemia, carbohydrate intolerance, hypercholesterolemia, hypocalcemia.

Musculoskeletal: muscle weakness, osteoporosis; growth suppression in children.

Skin: hirsutism, delayed wound healing, acne, various skin eruptions.

Other: susceptibility to infections; *acute adrenal insufficiency* after increased stress or abrupt withdrawal after long-term therapy, cushingoid state.

After abrupt withdrawal: rebound inflammation, fatigue, weakness, arthralgia, fever, dizziness, lethargy, depression, fainting, orthostatic hypotension, dyspnea, anorexia, hypoglycemia. *After prolonged use, sudden withdrawal may be fatal.*

INTERACTIONS

Drug-drug. *Antidiabetics, including insulin:* Increased glucose levels. May need dosage adjustment of antidiabetic therapy.

Aspirin, indomethacin, other NSAIDs: Increased risk of GI distress and bleeding. Use together cautiously.

Barbiturates, fosphenytoin, phenytoin, rifampin: Decreased corticosteroid effect. Corticosteroid dosage may need to be increased.

Cardiac glycosides: Increased risk of arrhythmia resulting from hypokalemia. Monitor potassium level.

Oral anticoagulants: Altered dosage requirements. Monitor PT and INR closely.

Potassium-depleting drugs such as thiazide diuretics: Enhanced potassium-wasting effects of betamethasone. Monitor potassium levels.

Salicylates: Reduced salicylate levels with corticosteroids. Monitor patient for lack of salicylate effectiveness.

Skin-test antigens: Decreased response. Defer skin testing until therapy is completed.

Toxoids, vaccines: Decreased antibody response and increased risk of neurologic complications. Avoid using together.

Drug-herb. *Echinacea:* Increased immune-stimulating effects. Discourage use together.

Ginseng: Potentiates immune-modulating response. Discourage use together.

Drug-lifestyle. *Alcohol use:* Increased risk of gastric irritation and GI ulceration. Advise patient to avoid alcohol use.

EFFECTS ON LAB TEST RESULTS

● May increase potassium, glucose, calcium, and cholesterol levels.

CONTRAINDICATIONS

Contraindicated in patients hypersensitive to drug and in those with viral or bacterial infections (except in life-threatening situations) or systemic fungal infections.

NURSING CONSIDERATIONS

● Use with extreme caution and only in life-threatening situations if patient has recent MI or active peptic ulcer.

● Use cautiously in patients with renal disease, hypertension, osteoporosis, diabetes mellitus, hypothyroidism, cirrhosis, diverticulitis, nonspecific ulcerative colitis, recent intestinal anastomoses, thromboembolic disorders, seizures, myasthenia gravis, heart failure, tuberculosis, ocular herpes simplex, emotional instability, or psychotic tendencies. Because some formulations contain sulfite preservatives, also use cautiously in patients hypersensitive to sulfites.

● Check for sensitivity to other corticosteroids.

● Adrenocorticoid therapy suppresses reactions to skin tests, causes false-negative results in the nitroblue tetrazolium tests for systemic bacterial infections, and decreases ^{131}I uptake and protein-bound iodine levels in thyroid function tests.

● Betamethasone sodium phosphate and betamethasone acetate suspension combination product shouldn't be given by I.V. route.

● *Alert:* Don't use drug for alternate-day therapy.

• *Alert:* Avoid using wrong salt formulation of drug; salt formulations aren't interchangeable.
• Obtain baseline weight before starting therapy, and weigh patient daily; report sudden weight gain to prescriber.
• For better results and less toxicity, give once-daily dose in morning.
• Most adverse reactions to corticosteroids are dose- or duration-dependent.
• To reduce GI irritation, give drug with milk or food.
• To prevent muscle atrophy, give I.M. injection deeply. Rotate injection sites.
• Always adjust drug to lowest effective dose.
• Monitor patient for cushingoid symptoms, including moonface, buffalo hump, central obesity, thinning hair, hypertension, and increased susceptibility to infection.
• Monitor glucose level and potassium levels regularly. Diabetic patient may need adjustments in insulin dosage.
• Watch for depression or mood changes, especially in patient receiving long-term therapy.
• A calorie- or sodium-restricted diet with protein supplementation may be needed for patient receiving long-term therapy.
• Elderly patients may be more susceptible to osteoporosis with long-term use.
• Adrenal suppression may last up to 1 year after drug is stopped.
• Gradually reduce drug dosage after long-term therapy.
• Observe patient for evidence of infection, especially after corticosteroid withdrawal.

PATIENT TEACHING
• Tell patient not to stop drug abruptly or without prescriber's consent.
• Instruct patient to take drug with food or milk; tell patient using effervescent tablets to dissolve them in water immediately before ingestion.
• Teach patient about drug's effects. Warn patient on long-term therapy about cushingoid effects (moonface, buffalo hump) and to notify prescriber about sudden weight gain or swelling.
• Instruct patient to report signs and symptoms of corticosteroid withdrawal,

including fatigue, weakness, arthralgia, orthostatic hypotension, and dyspnea.
• Tell patient to contact prescriber if signs and symptoms worsen or drug is no longer effective. Tell him not to increase dosage without prescriber's consent.
• Advise elderly patient receiving long-term therapy to consider exercise or physical therapy. Tell him to ask prescriber about vitamin D or calcium supplement.
• Advise patient receiving prolonged therapy to have periodic ophthalmic examinations.
• Tell patient to report slow healing of wounds.
• Instruct patient to carry or wear medical identification indicating his need for supplemental glucocorticoids during stress. This card should contain prescriber's name, name of drug, and dosage being taken.
• Advise patient to avoid exposure to infections (such as chickenpox or measles) and to notify prescriber if exposure occurs.
• Tell patient to report signs and symptoms of infection (fever, sore throat, dysuria, myalgias) or injuries during therapy and within 12 months after therapy stops.

cortisone acetate
Cortate‡, Cortisyl§, Cortone Acetate

Pregnancy risk category C

AVAILABLE FORMS
Injection (suspension): 50 mg/ml
Tablets: 5 mg, 10 mg, 25 mg

INDICATIONS & DOSAGES
➤ **Adrenal insufficiency, allergy, inflammation—**
Adults: 25 to 300 mg P.O. or 20 to 300 mg I.M. daily. Dosages are highly individualized depending on severity of disease.

ACTION
Not completely defined. Decreases inflammation, mainly by stabilizing leukocyte lysosomal membranes; suppresses immune response; stimulates bone marrow;

and influences protein, fat, and carbohydrate metabolism.

Route	Onset	Peak	Duration
I.M., P.O.	Variable	Variable	Variable

ADVERSE REACTIONS

CNS: *euphoria, insomnia,* psychotic behavior, pseudotumor cerebri, vertigo, headache, paresthesia, *seizures.*
CV: *heart failure,* hypertension, edema, *arrhythmias,* thrombophlebitis, *thromboembolism.*
EENT: cataracts, glaucoma.
GI: *peptic ulceration,* GI irritation, increased appetite, *pancreatitis,* nausea, vomiting.
GU: menstrual irregularities, increased urine glucose levels.
Metabolic: possible hypokalemia, hyperglycemia, and carbohydrate intolerance; hypercholesterolemia; hypocalcemia.
Musculoskeletal: growth suppression in children, muscle weakness, osteoporosis.
Skin: hirsutism, delayed wound healing, acne, various skin eruptions; atrophy at I.M. injection site.
Other: susceptibility to infections; *acute adrenal insufficiency* after increased stress or abrupt withdrawal after long-term therapy, cushingoid state.
After abrupt withdrawal: rebound inflammation, fatigue, weakness, arthralgia, fever, dizziness, lethargy, depression, fainting, orthostatic hypotension, dyspnea, anorexia, hypoglycemia. *After prolonged use, sudden withdrawal may be fatal.*

INTERACTIONS

Drug-drug. *Antidiabetics, including insulin:* Decreased response. May need dosage adjustment.
Aspirin, indomethacin, other NSAIDs: Increased risk of GI distress and bleeding. Use together cautiously.
Barbiturates, fosphenytoin, phenytoin, rifampin: Decreased corticosteroid effect. Increase corticosteroid dosage.
Live attenuated virus vaccines, other toxoids and vaccines: Decreased antibody response and increased risk of neurologic complications. Avoid using together.
Oral anticoagulants: Altered dosage requirements. Monitor PT and INR closely.

Potassium-depleting drugs such as thiazide diuretics: Enhanced potassium-wasting effects of cortisone. Monitor potassium levels.
Salicylates: Decreased salicylate levels with corticosteroids. Watch for lack of salicylate effectiveness.
Skin-test antigens: Decreased response. Defer skin testing until therapy is completed.
Drug-herb. *Echinacea:* Increased immune-stimulating effects. Discourage use together.
Ginseng: Potentiates immune-modulating response. Discourage use together.
Drug-lifestyle. *Alcohol use:* Increased risk of gastric irritation and GI ulceration. Advise patient to avoid alcohol use.

EFFECTS ON LAB TEST RESULTS

● May increase glucose and cholesterol levels. May decrease potassium, calcium, T_3, and T_4 levels.

CONTRAINDICATIONS

Contraindicated in patients hypersensitive to drug or its ingredients and in those with systemic fungal infections.

NURSING CONSIDERATIONS

● Use with extreme caution in patient with recent MI.
● Use cautiously in patients with GI ulcer, renal disease, hypertension, osteoporosis, diabetes mellitus, hypothyroidism, cirrhosis, diverticulitis, nonspecific ulcerative colitis, recent intestinal anastomoses, thromboembolic disorders, seizures, myasthenia gravis, heart failure, tuberculosis, ocular herpes simplex, emotional instability, or psychotic tendencies.
● Check for sensitivity to other corticosteroids.
● Most adverse reactions to corticosteroids are dose- or duration-dependent.
● To reduce GI irritation, give with milk or food. Patient may need adjunctive medication to prevent GI irritation.
● For better results and less toxicity, give a once-daily dose in morning.
● The I.M. route has slow onset of action and shouldn't be used for acute conditions that need rapid effect. This route may be used on a twice-daily schedule matching diurnal variation. Rotate injection sites to

---

*Liquid contains alcohol.   **May contain tartrazine.   †Canada   ‡Australia   §U.K.   ◇OTC

prevent muscle atrophy. The I.M. route is usually reserved for patients unable to take the P.O. form.

● Mixing or diluting parenteral suspension may alter absorption rate and decrease drug effectiveness.

● Cortisone therapy suppresses reactions to skin tests, causes false-negative results in the nitroblue tetrazolium test for systemic bacterial infections, and decreases ^{131}I uptake and protein-bound iodine levels in thyroid function tests.

● **Alert:** Drug isn't for I.V. use.

● Drug should always be adjusted to lowest effective dose.

● Monitor electrolyte and glucose levels. Diabetic patient may need adjustment in insulin dosage.

● Monitor patient for fluid and electrolyte imbalances. Patient may need low-sodium diet and potassium supplements.

● Monitor patient for cushingoid effects, including moonface, buffalo hump, central obesity, thinning hair, hypertension, and increased susceptibility to infection.

● Elderly patients may be more susceptible to osteoporosis with long-term use.

● Gradually reduce dosage after long-term therapy.

● Watch for evidence of infection, especially after corticosteroid withdrawal.

PATIENT TEACHING

● Tell patient not to stop drug abruptly or without prescriber's consent.

● Instruct patient to take drug with milk or food.

● Advise patient receiving long-term therapy to consider exercise or physical therapy. Also, tell him to ask prescriber about vitamin D or calcium supplement.

● Tell patient to report slow healing of wounds.

● Warn patient on long-term therapy about cushingoid effects (moonface, buffalo hump) and the need to notify prescriber about sudden weight gain or swelling.

● Instruct patient to carry or wear medical identification indicating his need for supplemental glucocorticoids during stress. This card should contain prescriber's name, name of drug, and dosage taken.

● Instruct patient to avoid exposure to infections (such as measles and chickenpox) and to notify prescriber if such exposure occurs.

---

dexamethasone
Decadron*, Dexone 0.5, Dexone, 0.75, Dexone 1.5, Dexone 4, Hexadrol

dexamethasone acetate
Cortastat LA, Dalalone D.P., Dalalone L.A., Decadron-LA, Decaject LA, Dexasone L.A., Dexone LA, Solurex LA

dexamethasone sodium phosphate
Cortastat, Dalalone, Decadron Phosphate, Decaject, Dexasone, Hexadrol Phosphate, Solurex

Pregnancy risk category C

AVAILABLE FORMS
dexamethasone
Elixir: 0.5 mg/5 ml*
Oral solution: 0.5 mg/5 ml, 1 mg/ml
Tablets: 0.25 mg, 0.5 mg, 0.75 mg, 1 mg, 1.5 mg, 2 mg, 4 mg, 6 mg
dexamethasone acetate
Injection: 8 mg/ml, 16 mg/ml suspension
dexamethasone sodium phosphate
Injection: 4 mg/ml, 10 mg/ml, 20 mg/ml, 24 mg/ml

INDICATIONS & DOSAGES
➤ **Cerebral edema—**
Adults: Initially, 10 mg (phosphate) I.V.; then 4 to 6 mg I.M. q 6 hours until symptoms subside (usually 2 to 4 days); then tapered over 5 to 7 days.
➤ **Inflammatory conditions, allergic reactions, neoplasias—**
Adults: 0.75 to 9 mg/day P.O. or 0.5 to 9 mg/day (phosphate) I.M. Or, 4 to 16 mg (acetate) I.M. into joint or soft tissue q 1 to 3 weeks. Or, 0.8 to 1.6 mg (acetate) into lesions q 1 to 3 weeks.
➤ **Shock—**
Adults: 20 mg (phosphate) as single initial dose; then 3 mg/kg/24 hours via continuous I.V. infusion. Or, 1 to 6 mg/kg (phosphate) I.V. as single dose. Or, 40 mg I.V. q 2 to 6 hours, p.r.n., continued only until

---

Reactions may be *common*, uncommon, *life-threatening*, or COMMON AND LIFE-THREATENING.

patient is stabilized (usually not longer than 48 to 72 hours).

➤ **Dexamethasone suppression test for Cushing's syndrome—**

Adults: After determining baseline 24-hour urine levels of 17-hydroxycorticosteroids, 0.5 mg P.O. q 6 hours for 48 hours. Twenty-four-hour urine collection made again to determine 17-hydroxycorticosteroid excretion during second 24 hours of dexamethasone administration. Or, 1 mg P.O. as single dose at 11:00 p.m. with determination of plasma cortisol at 8 a.m. the next morning.

➤ **Adrenocortical insufficiency—**

Children: 0.024 to 0.34 mg/kg or 0.66 to 10 mg/m^2 P.O. daily, given in four divided doses.

I.V. ADMINISTRATION

● When giving drug as direct injection, inject undiluted over at least 1 minute.

● When giving as intermittent or continuous infusion, dilute solution according to manufacturer's instructions, and give over prescribed duration. If used for continuous infusion, change solution every 24 hours.

ACTION

Not clearly defined. Decreases inflammation, mainly by stabilizing leukocyte lysosomal membranes; suppresses immune response; stimulates bone marrow; and influences protein, fat, and carbohydrate metabolism.

Route	Onset	Peak	Duration
I.M.	1 hr	1 hr	6 days
I.M. (acetate)	1 hr	8 hr	Unknown
I.V.	1 hr	1 hr	Variable
P.O.	1-2 hr	1-2 hr	2.5 days

ADVERSE REACTIONS

CNS: *euphoria, insomnia,* psychotic behavior, pseudotumor cerebri, vertigo, headache, paresthesia, *seizures.*

CV: *heart failure,* hypertension, edema, *arrhythmias,* thrombophlebitis, *thromboembolism.*

EENT: cataracts, glaucoma.

GI: *peptic ulceration,* GI irritation, increased appetite, *pancreatitis,* nausea, vomiting.

GU: menstrual irregularities, increased urine glucose and calcium levels.

Metabolic: hypokalemia, hyperglycemia, and carbohydrate intolerance; hypercholesterolemia; hypocalcemia.

Musculoskeletal: growth suppression in children, muscle weakness, osteoporosis.

Skin: hirsutism, delayed wound healing, acne, various skin eruptions, atrophy at I.M. injection site.

Other: cushingoid state, susceptibility to infections, *acute adrenal insufficiency* after increased stress or abrupt withdrawal after long-term therapy.

After abrupt withdrawal: rebound inflammation, fatigue, weakness, arthralgia, fever, dizziness, lethargy, depression, fainting, orthostatic hypotension, dyspnea, anorexia, hypoglycemia. *After prolonged use, sudden withdrawal may be fatal.*

INTERACTIONS

Drug-drug. *Aminoglutethimide:* May cause loss of dexamethasone-induced adrenal suppression. Use together cautiously.

Antidiabetics, including insulin: Decreased response. May need dosage adjustment.

Aspirin, indomethacin, other NSAIDs: Increased risk of GI distress and bleeding. Use together cautiously.

Barbiturates, phenytoin, rifampin: Decreased corticosteroid effect. Increase corticosteroid dosage.

Cardiac glycosides: Increased risk of arrhythmia resulting from hypokalemia. May need dosage adjustment.

Ephedrine: A decreased half-life and increased clearance of dexamethasone may occur.

Oral anticoagulants: Altered dosage requirements. Monitor PT and INR closely.

Potassium-depleting drugs such as thiazide diuretics: Enhanced potassium-wasting effects of dexamethasone. Monitor potassium levels.

Salicylates: Decreased salicylate levels. Monitor patient for lack of salicylate effectiveness.

Skin-test antigens: Decreased response. Defer skin testing until therapy is completed.

---

*Liquid contains alcohol.   **May contain tartrazine.   †Canada   ‡Australia   §U.K.   ◇OTC

Toxoids, vaccines: Decreased antibody response and increased risk of neurologic complications. Avoid using together.

Drug-herb. *Echinacea:* Increased immune-stimulating effects. Discourage use together.

Ginseng: Potentiates immune-modulating response. Discourage use together.

Drug-lifestyle. *Alcohol use:* Increased risk of gastric irritation and GI ulceration. Advise patient to avoid alcohol use.

EFFECTS ON LAB TEST RESULTS
● May increase glucose and cholesterol levels. May decrease potassium, calcium, T_3, and T_4 levels.

CONTRAINDICATIONS
Contraindicated in patients hypersensitive to drug or its ingredients and in those with systemic fungal infections.

NURSING CONSIDERATIONS
● Use with extreme caution in patient with recent MI.
● Use cautiously in patients with GI ulcer, renal disease, hypertension, osteoporosis, diabetes mellitus, hypothyroidism, cirrhosis, diverticulitis, nonspecific ulcerative colitis, recent intestinal anastomoses, thromboembolic disorders, seizures, myasthenia gravis, heart failure, tuberculosis, ocular herpes simplex, emotional instability, or psychotic tendencies. Because some formulations contain sulfite preservatives, also use cautiously in patients sensitive to sulfites.
● Determine whether patient is sensitive to other corticosteroids.
● Most adverse reactions to corticosteroids are dose- or duration-dependent.
● For better results and less toxicity, give once-daily dose in morning.
● Give oral dose with food when possible. Patient may need medication to prevent GI irritation.
● Give I.M. injection deeply into gluteal muscle. Rotate injection sites to prevent muscle atrophy. Avoid S.C. injection because atrophy and sterile abscesses may occur.
● Always adjust to lowest effective dose.
● Monitor patient's weight, blood pressure, and electrolyte levels.

● Monitor patient for cushingoid effects, including moonface, buffalo hump, central obesity, thinning hair, hypertension, and increased susceptibility to infection.
● Watch for depression or psychotic episodes, especially in high-dose therapy.
● Diabetic patient may need increased insulin; monitor glucose levels.
● Drug may mask or worsen infections, including latent amebiasis.
● Elderly patients may be more susceptible to osteoporosis with long-term use.
● Inspect patient's skin for petechiae.
● Drug suppresses reactions to skin tests, causes false-negative results in the nitro-blue tetrazolium test for systemic bacterial infections, and decreases ^{131}I uptake and protein-bound iodine levels in thyroid function tests.
● Gradually reduce dosage after long-term therapy.
● **Alert:** Don't confuse dexamethasone with desoximetasone.

PATIENT TEACHING
● Tell patient not to stop drug abruptly or without prescriber's consent.
● Instruct patient to take drug with food or milk.
● Teach patient signs and symptoms of early adrenal insufficiency: fatigue, muscle weakness, joint pain, fever, anorexia, nausea, dyspnea, dizziness, and fainting.
● Instruct patient to carry or wear medical identification indicating his need for supplemental systemic glucocorticoids during stress, especially when dosage is decreased. This card should contain prescriber's name, name of drug, and dosage taken.
● Warn patient on long-term therapy about cushingoid effects (moonface, buffalo hump) and the need to notify prescriber about sudden weight gain or swelling.
● Warn patient about easy bruising.
● Advise patient receiving long-term therapy to consider exercise or physical therapy. Give vitamin D or calcium supplement.
● Instruct patient receiving long-term therapy to have periodic ophthalmic examinations.
● Advise patient to avoid exposure to infections (such as measles and chickenpox) and to notify prescriber if such exposure occurs.

Reactions may be *common*, uncommon, *life-threatening*, or COMMON AND LIFE-THREATENING.

fludrocortisone acetate
Florinef Acetate

Pregnancy risk category C

AVAILABLE FORMS
Tablets: 0.1 mg

INDICATIONS & DOSAGES
➤ **Salt-losing adrenogenital syndrome—**
Adults: 0.1 to 0.2 mg P.O. daily.
➤ **Addison's disease (adrenocortical insufficiency)—**
Adults: 0.1 mg P.O. daily. Usual dosage range is 0.1 mg three times weekly to 0.2 mg daily. Decrease dosage to 0.05 mg daily if transient hypertension develops as a result of drug therapy.

ACTION
Increases sodium reabsorption and potassium and hydrogen secretion at the distal convoluted tubules of nephrons.

Route	Onset	Peak	Duration
P.O.	Variable	2 hr	1-2 days

ADVERSE REACTIONS
CV: hypertension, cardiac hypertrophy, edema, *heart failure.*
Hematologic: bruising.
Metabolic: *sodium and water retention,* hypokalemia.
Skin: diaphoresis, urticaria, allergic rash.

INTERACTIONS
Drug-drug. *Barbiturates, fosphenytoin, phenytoin, rifampin:* Increased clearance of fludrocortisone acetate. Monitor patient for possible diminished effect of corticosteroid. Corticosteroid dosage may need to be increased.
Potassium-depleting drugs such as amphotericin B, thiazide diuretics: Enhanced potassium-wasting effects of fludrocortisone. Monitor potassium levels.
Drug-food. *Sodium-containing drugs or foods:* May increase blood pressure. Sodium intake may need adjustment.

EFFECTS ON LAB TEST RESULTS
● May decrease potassium level.

CONTRAINDICATIONS
Contraindicated in patients hypersensitive to drug and in those with systemic fungal infections.

NURSING CONSIDERATIONS
● Use cautiously in patients with hypothyroidism, recent MI, cirrhosis, ocular herpes simplex, emotional instability, psychotic tendencies, diverticulitis, fresh intestinal anastomoses, active or latent peptic ulcer, renal insufficiency, hypertension, osteoporosis, myasthenia gravis, or nonspecific ulcerative colitis.
● Drug is used with cortisone or hydrocortisone in adrenal insufficiency.
● Glucose tolerance tests should be performed only if needed because addisonian patients tend to develop severe hypoglycemia within 3 hours of the test.
● *Alert:* Monitor patient's blood pressure and electrolyte levels. If hypertension occurs, notify prescriber and expect dosage to be decreased by 50%.
● Weigh patient daily; notify prescriber about sudden weight gain.
● Unless contraindicated, give low-sodium diet that's high in potassium and protein. Potassium supplements may be needed.
● Drug may cause adverse effects similar to those of glucocorticoids.

PATIENT TEACHING
● Tell patient to notify prescriber if hypotension, weakness, cramping, or palpitations worsen or if changes in mental status occur.
● Warn patient that mild peripheral edema is common.

hydrocortisone
Aquacort†, Cortef, Cortenema, Hydrocortone

hydrocortisone acetate
Anucort-HC, Anusol-HC, Cortifoam, Hydrocortone Acetate, Proctocort

hydrocortisone cypionate
Cortef

---

hydrocortisone sodium phosphate
Hydrocortone Phosphate

hydrocortisone sodium succinate
A-hydroCort, Solu-Cortef

Pregnancy risk category C

AVAILABLE FORMS
hydrocortisone
Enema: 100 mg/60 ml
Tablets: 5 mg, 10 mg, 20 mg
hydrocortisone acetate
Injection: 25 mg/ml*, 50 mg/ml* suspension
Rectal aerosol foam: 10% aerosol foam (provides 90 mg/application)
Rectal suppository: 25 mg, 30 mg
hydrocortisone cypionate
Oral suspension: 2 mg/ml
hydrocortisone sodium phosphate
Injection: 50 mg/ml solution
hydrocortisone sodium succinate
Injection: 100-mg vial*, 250-mg vial*, 500-mg vial*, 1,000-mg vial*

INDICATIONS & DOSAGES
➤ **Severe inflammation, adrenal insufficiency—**
Adults: 5 to 30 mg P.O. b.i.d., t.i.d., or q.i.d. (as much as 80 mg q.i.d. may be given in acute situations). Or, initially, 100 to 500 mg succinate I.M. or I.V.; then 50 to 100 mg I.M., as indicated. Or, 15 to 240 mg phosphate I.M., S.C., or I.V. daily in divided doses q 12 hours. Or, 5 to 75 mg acetate into joints or soft tissue repeated at 3 to 5 days for bursae and 1 to 4 weeks for joints. Dosage varies with size of joint. Local anesthetics commonly are injected with dose.
➤ **Shock—**
Adults: Initially, 50 mg/kg succinate I.V., repeated in 4 hours. Repeat dosage q 24 hours, p.r.n. Or, 100 to 500 mg to 2 g q 2 to 6 hours, continued until patient is stabilized (usually not longer than 48 to 72 hours).
Children: Phosphate (I.M.) or succinate (I.M. or I.V.) 0.16 to 1 mg/kg or 6 to 30 mg/m² given once or twice daily.

➤ **Adjunct for ulcerative colitis and proctitis—**
Adults: 1 enema (100 mg) P.R. nightly for 21 days. Or, 1 applicatorful (90-mg foam) P.R. daily or b.i.d. for 14 to 21 days. Or, 25 mg rectal suppository b.i.d. for 2 weeks. For severe proctitis, 25 mg P.R. t.i.d. or 50 mg b.i.d.

I.V. ADMINISTRATION
● Don't use acetate or suspension form for I.V. route. When giving as direct injection, inject directly into vein or an I.V. line containing free-flowing compatible solution over 30 seconds to several minutes. When giving as intermittent or continuous infusion, dilute solution according to manufacturer's instructions, and give over prescribed duration. If used for continuous infusion, change solution every 24 hours.
● Hydrocortisone sodium phosphate may be added directly to D_5W or normal saline solution for I.V. use.
● Reconstitute hydrocortisone sodium succinate with bacteriostatic water or bacteriostatic saline solution before adding to I.V. solutions. When giving by direct I.V. injection, inject over 30 seconds to 10 minutes. For infusion, dilute with D_5W, normal saline solution, or dextrose 5% in normal saline solution to 1 mg/ml or less.

ACTION
Not clearly defined. Decreases inflammation, mainly by stabilizing leukocyte lysosomal membranes; suppresses immune response; stimulates bone marrow; and influences protein, fat, and carbohydrate metabolism.

Route	Onset	Peak	Duration
I.M., I.V., P.O., P.R.	Variable	Variable	Variable

ADVERSE REACTIONS
CNS: *euphoria, insomnia,* psychotic behavior, pseudotumor cerebri, vertigo, headache, paresthesia, *seizures.*
CV: *heart failure,* hypertension, edema, *arrhythmias,* thrombophlebitis, *thromboembolism.*
EENT: cataracts, glaucoma.
GI: *peptic ulceration,* GI irritation, increased appetite, *pancreatitis,* nausea, vomiting.

Reactions may be *common,* uncommon, *life-threatening,* or COMMON AND LIFE-THREATENING.

GU: menstrual irregularities, increased urine calcium levels.

Hematologic: easy bruising.

Metabolic: hypokalemia, hyperglycemia, and carbohydrate intolerance; hypercholesterolemia; hypocalcemia.

Musculoskeletal: growth suppression in children, muscle weakness, osteoporosis.

Skin: hirsutism, delayed wound healing, acne, skin eruptions.

Other: cushingoid state, susceptibility to infections, *acute adrenal insufficiency after increased stress or abrupt withdrawal after long-term therapy.*

After abrupt withdrawal: rebound inflammation, fatigue, weakness, arthralgia, fever, dizziness, lethargy, depression, fainting, orthostatic hypotension, dyspnea, anorexia, hypoglycemia. *After prolonged use, sudden withdrawal may be fatal.*

INTERACTIONS
Drug-drug. *Aspirin, indomethacin, other NSAIDs:* Increased risk of GI distress and bleeding. Use together cautiously.
Barbiturates, fosphenytoin, phenytoin, rifampin: Decreased corticosteroid effect. Increase corticosteroid dosage.
Live attenuated virus vaccines, other toxoids and vaccines: Decreased antibody response and increased risk of neurologic complications. Avoid using together.
Oral anticoagulants: Altered dosage requirements. Monitor PT and INR closely.
Potassium-depleting drugs such as thiazide diuretics: Enhanced potassium-wasting effects of hydrocortisone. Monitor potassium levels.
Skin-test antigens: Decreased response. Defer skin testing until after therapy.
Drug-herb. *Echinacea:* Increased immune-stimulating effects. Discourage use together.
Ginseng: Potentiates immune-modulating response. Discourage use together.

EFFECTS ON LAB TEST RESULTS
• May increase glucose and cholesterol levels. May decrease potassium and calcium levels.

CONTRAINDICATIONS
Contraindicated in patients hypersensitive to drug or its ingredients, in those with systemic fungal infections, and in premature infants (succinate).

NURSING CONSIDERATIONS
• Use with extreme caution in patient with recent MI.
• Use cautiously in patients with GI ulcer, renal disease, hypertension, osteoporosis, diabetes mellitus, hypothyroidism, cirrhosis, diverticulitis, nonspecific ulcerative colitis, recent intestinal anastomoses, thromboembolic disorders, seizures, myasthenia gravis, heart failure, tuberculosis, ocular herpes simplex, emotional instability, and psychotic tendencies.
• Determine whether patient is sensitive to other corticosteroids.
• Most adverse reactions to corticosteroids are dose- or duration-dependent.
• For better results and less toxicity, give a once-daily dose in morning.
• Give oral dose with food when possible. Patient may need medication to prevent GI irritation.
• *Alert:* Salt formulations aren't interchangeable.
• Give I.M. injection deeply into gluteal muscle. Rotate injection sites to prevent muscle atrophy. Avoid S.C. injection because atrophy and sterile abscesses may occur.
• Injectable forms aren't used for alternate-day therapy.
• Enema may produce same systemic effects as other forms of hydrocortisone. If enema therapy must exceed 21 days, discontinue gradually by reducing use to every other night for 2 to 3 weeks.
• High-dose therapy usually isn't continued beyond 48 hours.
• Always adjust to lowest effective dose.
• Monitor patient's weight, blood pressure, and electrolyte levels.
• Monitor patient for cushingoid effects, including moonface, buffalo hump, central obesity, thinning hair, hypertension, and increased susceptibility to infection.
• Unless contraindicated, give a low-sodium diet that's high in potassium and protein. Give potassium supplements.
• Drug may mask or worsen infections, including latent amebiasis.
• Stress (fever, trauma, surgery, and emotional problems) may increase adrenal insufficiency. Increase dosage.

• Watch for depression or psychotic episodes, especially during high-dose therapy.
• Inspect patient's skin for petechiae.
• Diabetic patient may need increased insulin; monitor glucose levels.
• Drug suppresses reactions to skin tests, causes false-negative results in the nitroblue tetrazolium test for systemic bacterial infections, and decreases ^{131}I uptake and protein-bound iodine levels in thyroid function tests.
• Periodic measurement of growth and development may be needed during high-dose or prolonged therapy in children.
• Elderly patients may be more susceptible to osteoporosis with prolonged use.
• Gradually reduce dosage after long-term therapy.
• **Alert:** Don't confuse Solu-Cortef with Solu-Medrol (methylprednisolone sodium succinate), or hydrocortisone with hydroxychloroquine.

PATIENT TEACHING
• Tell patient not to stop drug abruptly or without prescriber's consent.
• Instruct patient to take oral form of drug with milk or food.
• Warn patient on long-term therapy about cushingoid effects (moonface, buffalo hump) and the need to notify prescriber about sudden weight gain or swelling.
• Teach patient signs and symptoms of early adrenal insufficiency: fatigue, muscle weakness, joint pain, fever, anorexia, nausea, dyspnea, dizziness, and fainting.
• Instruct patient to carry or wear medical identification indicating his need for supplemental systemic glucocorticoids during stress. This card should contain prescriber's name, name of drug, and dosage taken.
• Warn patient about easy bruising.
• Urge patient receiving long-term therapy to consider exercise or physical therapy. Also, tell him to ask prescriber about vitamin D or calcium supplement.
• Advise patient receiving long-term therapy to have periodic ophthalmic examinations.
• Caution patient to avoid exposure to infections (such as chickenpox or measles) and to notify prescriber if such exposure occurs.

methylprednisolone
Medrol**, Medrone§

methylprednisolone acetate
depMedalone 40, depMedalone 80, Depoject, Depo-Medrol, Depo-Medrone§, Depopred-40, Depopred-80, Duralone-40, Duralone-80, Medralone-40, Medralone-80, M-Prednisol-40, M-Prednisol-80

methylprednisolone sodium succinate
A-MethaPred, Solu-Medrol

Pregnancy risk category C

AVAILABLE FORMS
methylprednisolone
Tablets: 2 mg, 4 mg, 8 mg, 16 mg, 24 mg, 32 mg
methylprednisolone acetate
Injection (suspension): 20 mg/ml, 40 mg/ml, 80 mg/ml
methylprednisolone sodium succinate
Injection: 40-mg vial, 125-mg vial, 500-mg vial, 1,000-mg vial, 2,000-mg vial

INDICATIONS & DOSAGES
➤ **Severe inflammation or immunosuppression—**
Adults: 2 to 60 mg (base) P.O. usually in four divided doses, 10 to 80 mg acetate I.M. daily, or 10 to 250 mg succinate I.M. or I.V. up to six times daily. Or, 4 to 40 mg acetate into smaller joints or 20 to 80 mg acetate into larger joints. Intralesional use is usually 20 to 60 mg acetate. Intralesional and intra-articular injections may be repeated q 1 to 5 weeks.
Children: 0.03 to 0.2 mg/kg or 1 to 6.25 mg/ m^2 succinate I.M. once daily or b.i.d.
➤ **Shock—**
Adults: 100 to 250 mg succinate I.V. at 2- to 6-hour intervals. Or, 30 mg/kg I.V. initially, repeated q 4 to 6 hours, p.r.n. Give over 3 to 15 minutes. Continue therapy for 2 to 3 days or until patient is stable.

I.V. ADMINISTRATION
• Use only methylprednisolone sodium succinate for I.V. route; never use acetate

---

Reactions may be *common,* uncommon, *life-threatening,* or COMMON AND LIFE-THREATENING.

form. Reconstitute according to manufacturer's directions using supplied diluent, or use bacteriostatic water for injection with benzyl alcohol.

• When giving as direct injection, inject diluted drug into vein or free-flowing compatible I.V. solution over at least 1 minute. For shock, give massive doses over at least 10 minutes to prevent arrhythmias and circulatory collapse. When giving as an intermittent or continuous infusion, dilute solution according to manufacturer's instructions, and give over prescribed duration. If used for continuous infusion, change solution every 24 hours.

• Compatible solutions include D₅W, normal saline solution, and dextrose 5% in normal saline solution.

ACTION

Not clearly defined. Decreases inflammation, mainly by stabilizing leukocyte lysosomal membranes; suppresses immune response; stimulates bone marrow; and influences protein, fat, and carbohydrate metabolism.

Route	Onset	Peak	Duration
I.M.	6-48 hr	4-8 days	4-8 days
Intra-articular	Rapid	7 days	1-5 wk
I.V.	Rapid	Immediate	7 days
P.O.	Rapid	2-3 hr	30-36 hr

ADVERSE REACTIONS

CNS: *euphoria, insomnia,* psychotic behavior, pseudotumor cerebri, vertigo, headache, paresthesia, *seizures.*
CV: *heart failure,* hypertension, edema, *arrhythmias,* thrombophlebitis, *thromboembolism, cardiac arrest, circulatory collapse* after rapid use of large I.V. doses.
EENT: cataracts, glaucoma.
GI: *peptic ulceration,* GI irritation, increased appetite, *pancreatitis,* nausea, vomiting.
GU: menstrual irregularities, increased urine calcium levels.
Metabolic: hypokalemia, hyperglycemia, and carbohydrate intolerance; hypercholesterolemia; hypocalcemia.
Musculoskeletal: growth suppression in children, muscle weakness, osteoporosis.
Skin: hirsutism, delayed wound healing, acne, various skin eruptions.

Other: cushingoid state, susceptibility to infections, *acute adrenal insufficiency after increased stress or abrupt withdrawal after long-term therapy.*
After abrupt withdrawal: rebound inflammation, fatigue, weakness, arthralgia, fever, dizziness, lethargy, depression, fainting, orthostatic hypotension, dyspnea, anorexia, hypoglycemia. *After prolonged use, sudden withdrawal may be fatal.*

INTERACTIONS

Drug-drug. *Aspirin, indomethacin, other NSAIDs:* Increased risk of GI distress and bleeding. Use together cautiously.
Barbiturates, phenytoin, rifampin: Decreased corticosteroid effect. Increase corticosteroid dosage.
Ketoconazole and macrolide antibiotics: Decreased clearance of methylprednisolone. Decreased dose may be required.
Oral anticoagulants: Altered dosage requirements. Monitor PT and INR closely.
Potassium-depleting drugs such as thiazide diuretics: Enhanced potassium-wasting effects of methylprednisolone. Monitor potassium levels.
Salicylates: Decreased salicylate levels. Monitor patient for lack of salicylate effectiveness.
Skin-test antigens: Decreased response. Defer skin testing until after therapy.
Toxoids, vaccines: Decreased antibody response and increased risk of neurologic complications. Avoid using together.
Drug-herb. *Echinacea:* Increased immune-stimulating effects. Discourage use together.
Ginseng: Potentiates immune-modulating response. Discourage use together.

EFFECTS ON LAB TEST RESULTS

• May increase glucose and cholesterol levels. May decrease potassium and calcium levels.

CONTRAINDICATIONS

Contraindicated in patients hypersensitive to drug or its ingredients and in those with systemic fungal infections; also contraindicated in premature infants (acetate and succinate).

NURSING CONSIDERATIONS

• Use cautiously in patients with GI ulceration or renal disease, hypertension, osteoporosis, diabetes mellitus, hypothyroidism, cirrhosis, diverticulitis, nonspecific ulcerative colitis, recent intestinal anastomoses, thromboembolic disorders, seizures, myasthenia gravis, heart failure, tuberculosis, ocular herpes simplex, emotional instability, and psychotic tendencies.

• Determine whether patient is sensitive to other corticosteroids.

• Drug may be used for alternate-day therapy.

• Most adverse reactions to corticosteroids are dose- or duration-dependent.

• For better results and less toxicity, give a once-daily dose in the morning.

• Give oral dose with food when possible. Critically ill patients may need to take drug together with antacid or H_2-receptor antagonist.

• *Alert:* Salt formulations aren't interchangeable.

• *Alert:* Don't give Solu-Medrol intrathecally because severe adverse reactions may occur.

• Give I.M. injection deeply into gluteal muscle. Avoid S.C. injection because atrophy and sterile abscesses may occur.

• Dermal atrophy may occur with large doses of acetate salt. Use several small injections rather than a single large dose, and rotate injection sites.

• Don't use acetate if immediate onset of action is needed.

• Discard reconstituted solution after 48 hours.

• Methylprednisolone suppresses reactions to skin tests, causes false-negative results in the nitroblue tetrazolium test for systemic bacterial infections, and decreases ^{131}I uptake and protein-bound iodine levels in thyroid function tests.

• Always adjust to lowest effective dose.

• Monitor patient's weight, blood pressure, electrolyte levels, and sleep patterns. Euphoria may initially interfere with sleep, but patients typically adjust to therapy in 1 to 3 weeks.

• Monitor patient for cushingoid effects, including moonface, buffalo hump, central obesity, thinning hair, hypertension, and increased susceptibility to infection.

• Drug may mask or worsen infections, including latent amebiasis.

• Watch for depression or psychotic episodes, especially in high-dose therapy.

• Diabetic patient may need increased insulin; monitor glucose levels.

• Watch for an enhanced response to drug in patients with hypothyroidism or cirrhosis.

• Watch for allergic reaction to tartrazine in patients with sensitivity to aspirin.

• Unless contraindicated, give low-sodium diet that's high in potassium and protein. Give potassium supplements, as needed.

• Elderly patients may be more susceptible to osteoporosis with prolonged use.

• Gradually reduce dosage after long-term therapy.

• *Alert:* Don't confuse Solu-Medrol with Solu-Cortef (hydrocortisone sodium succinate) or methylprednisolone with medroxyprogesterone.

PATIENT TEACHING

• Tell patient not to stop drug abruptly or without prescriber's consent.

• Instruct patient to take oral form of drug with milk or food.

• Teach patient signs and symptoms of early adrenal insufficiency: fatigue, muscle weakness, joint pain, fever, anorexia, nausea, dyspnea, dizziness, and fainting.

• Instruct patient to carry or wear medical identification indicating his need for supplemental systemic glucocorticoids during stress. This card should contain prescriber's name, name of drug, and dosage taken.

• Warn patient on long-term therapy about cushingoid effects (moonface, buffalo hump) and the need to notify prescriber about sudden weight gain or swelling.

• Advise patient receiving long-term therapy to consider exercise or physical therapy. Also, tell patient to ask prescriber about vitamin D or calcium supplement.

• Instruct patient to avoid exposure to infections (such as chickenpox or measles) and to contact prescriber if such exposure occurs.

Reactions may be *common*, uncommon, *life-threatening*, or COMMON AND LIFE-THREATENING.

prednisolone
Delta-Cortef, Panafcortelone‡,
Precortisyl Forte§, Predenema§,
Prelone

prednisolone acetate
Cotolone, Key-Pred 25, Key-Pred
50, Predalone

**prednisolone sodium
phosphate**
Hydeltrasol, Key-Pred-SP,
Orapred, Pediapred, Predsol
Retention Enema‡, Predsol
Suppositories‡

prednisolone tebutate
Prednisol TBA

Pregnancy risk category C

AVAILABLE FORMS
prednisolone
Syrup: 5 mg/5 ml, 15 mg/5 ml
Tablets: 1 mg‡, 5 mg, 25 mg‡
prednisolone acetate
Injection (suspension): 25 mg/ml,
50 mg/ml
prednisolone sodium phosphate
Injection: 20 mg/ml
Oral solution: 5 mg/5 ml
Oral solution: 20.2 mg/5 ml
Retention enema: 20 mg/100 ml‡
Suppositories: 5 mg‡
prednisolone tebutate
Injection (suspension): 20 mg/ml

INDICATIONS & DOSAGES
➤ **Severe inflammation, immunosup-
pression—**
Prednisolone
Adults: 2.5 to 15 mg P.O. b.i.d., t.i.d., or
q.i.d.
Children: 0.14 to 2 mg/kg or 4 to
60 mg/m² P.O. daily in divided doses.
Prednisolone acetate
Adults: 4 to 60 mg I.M. q 12 hours.
Children: 0.04 to 0.25 mg/kg or 1.5 to
7.5 mg/m² I.M. once or twice daily.
Prednisolone sodium phosphate
Adults: 5 to 60 mg I.M., I.V., or P.O.
Children: 0.14 to 2 mg/kg or 4 to
60 mg/m² daily in divided doses I.M., I.V.,
or P.O.

Prednisolone tebutate
Adults: 4 to 40 mg into joints and lesions,
p.r.n.
➤ **Asthma and other inflammatory
conditions in children—**
Children: 0.14 to 2 mg/kg or 4 to
60 mg/m² daily in four divided doses.
➤ **Acute exacerbations of multiple
sclerosis—**
Adults: 200 mg/day as single or divided
dose for 7 days; then 80 mg every other
day for 1 month.
➤ **Proctitis‡—**
Adults: 1 suppository b.i.d., preferably in
the morning and h.s.
➤ **Ulcerative colitis‡—**
Adults: 1 retention enema h.s. nightly for
2 to 4 weeks. Contents of enema should
be retained overnight.

I.V. ADMINISTRATION
● Use only prednisolone sodium phosphate. When giving as direct injection,
inject undiluted over at least 1 minute.
When giving as intermittent or continuous
infusion, dilute solution according to manufacturer's instructions, and give over prescribed duration. Use D₅W or normal
saline solution as diluent for I.V. infusion.

ACTION
Not clearly defined. Decreases inflammation, mainly by stabilizing leukocyte lysosomal membranes; suppresses immune
response; stimulates bone marrow; and influences protein, fat, and carbohydrate
metabolism.

Route	Peak	Onset	Duration
I.M.	Rapid	1 hr	4 wk
Intra-articular	1-2 days	Unknown	< 4 wk
I.V.	Rapid	1 hr	Unknown
P.O.	Rapid	1-2 hr	3-36 hr
P.R.	Unknown	Unknown	Unknown

ADVERSE REACTIONS
CNS: *euphoria, insomnia,* psychotic behavior, pseudotumor cerebri, vertigo,
headache, paresthesia, *seizures.*
CV: *heart failure,* hypertension, edema,
arrhythmias, thrombophlebitis, *thromboembolism.*
EENT: cataracts, glaucoma.

GI: *peptic ulceration,* GI irritation, increased appetite, ***pancreatitis,*** nausea, vomiting.
GU: menstrual irregularities, increased urine calcium levels.
Metabolic: hypokalemia, hyperglycemia, and carbohydrate intolerance; hypercholesterolemia; hypokalemia; hypocalcemia.
Musculoskeletal: growth suppression in children, muscle weakness, osteoporosis.
Skin: hirsutism, delayed wound healing, acne, various skin eruptions.
Other: susceptibility to infections, cushingoid state, ***acute adrenal insufficiency*** after increased stress or abrupt withdrawal after long-term therapy.
After abrupt withdrawal: rebound inflammation, fatigue, weakness, arthralgia, fever, dizziness, lethargy, depression, fainting, orthostatic hypotension, dyspnea, anorexia, hypoglycemia. ***After prolonged use, sudden withdrawal may be fatal.***

INTERACTIONS
Drug-drug. *Aspirin, indomethacin, other NSAIDs:* Increased risk of GI distress and bleeding. Use together cautiously.
Barbiturates, fosphenytoin, phenytoin, rifampin: Decreased corticosteroid effect. Increase corticosteroid dosage.
Oral anticoagulants: Altered dosage requirements. Monitor PT and INR closely.
Potassium-depleting drugs such as thiazide diuretics: Enhanced potassium-wasting effects of prednisolone. Monitor potassium levels.
Salicylates: Decreased salicylate levels. Monitor patient for lack of salicylate effectiveness.
Skin-test antigens: Decreased response. Defer skin testing until therapy is completed.
Toxoids, vaccines: Decreased antibody response and increased risk of neurologic complications. Avoid using together.
Drug-herb. *Echinacea:* Increased immune-stimulating effects. Discourage use together.
Ginseng: Potentiates immune-modulating response. Discourage use together.

EFFECTS ON LAB TEST RESULTS
• May increase glucose and cholesterol levels. May decrease potassium and calcium levels.

CONTRAINDICATIONS
Contraindicated in patients hypersensitive to drug or its ingredients and in those with systemic fungal infections.

NURSING CONSIDERATIONS
• Use with extreme caution in patients with recent MI.
• Use cautiously in patients with GI ulcer, renal disease, hypertension, osteoporosis, diabetes mellitus, hypothyroidism, cirrhosis, diverticulitis, nonspecific ulcerative colitis, recent intestinal anastomoses, thromboembolic disorders, seizures, myasthenia gravis, heart failure, tuberculosis, ocular herpes simplex, emotional instability, and psychotic tendencies.
• Determine whether patient is sensitive to other corticosteroids.
• Always adjust to lowest effective dose.
• Prednisolone salts (sodium phosphate and tebutate) are used parenterally less often than other corticosteroids that have more potent anti-inflammatory action.
• Drug may be used for alternate-day therapy.
• Most adverse reactions to corticosteroids are dose- or duration-dependent.
• Give oral dose with food, when possible, to reduce GI irritation. Patient may need medication to prevent GI irritation.
• Give I.M. injection deeply into gluteal muscle. Rotate injection sites to prevent muscle atrophy. Avoid S.C. injection because atrophy and sterile abscesses may occur.
• *Alert:* Prednisolone acetate isn't for I.V. use.
• Monitor patient's weight, blood pressure, and electrolyte levels.
• Monitor patient for cushingoid effects, including moonface, buffalo hump, central obesity, thinning hair, hypertension, and increased susceptibility to infection.
• Watch for depression or psychotic episodes, especially during high-dose therapy.
• Drug suppresses reactions to skin tests, causes false-negative results in the nitro-blue tetrazolium test for systemic bacterial infections, and decreases ^{131}I uptake and protein-bound iodine levels in thyroid function tests.
• Diabetic patient may need increased insulin; monitor glucose levels.

Reactions may be *common*, uncommon, *life-threatening*, or **COMMON AND LIFE-THREATENING**.

• Unless contraindicated, give low-sodium diet that's high in potassium and protein. Give potassium supplements, as needed.

• Drug may mask or worsen infections, including latent amebiasis.

• Elderly patients may be more susceptible to osteoporosis with long-term use.

• Gradually reduce dosage after long-term therapy.

• *Alert:* Don't confuse prednisolone with prednisone.

PATIENT TEACHING

• Tell patient not to stop drug abruptly or without prescriber's consent.

• Instruct patient to take oral form of drug with food or milk.

• Teach patient signs and symptoms of early adrenal insufficiency: fatigue, muscle weakness, joint pain, fever, anorexia, nausea, dyspnea, dizziness, and fainting.

• Instruct patient to carry or wear medical identification indicating his need for supplemental systemic glucocorticoids during stress. It should include prescriber's name, name of drug, and dosage taken.

• Warn patient on long-term therapy about cushingoid effects (moonface, buffalo hump) and the need to notify prescriber about sudden weight gain or swelling.

• Tell patient to report slow healing.

• Advise patient receiving long-term therapy to consider exercise or physical therapy. Also, tell him to ask prescriber about vitamin D or calcium supplement.

• Instruct patient to avoid exposure to infections and to notify prescriber if exposure occurs.

• Tell patient to avoid immunizations while taking drug.

---

prednisone

Apo-Prednisone†, Deltasone, Liquid Pred*, Meticorten, Orasone, Panafcort‡, Panasol-S, Prednicen-M, Prednisone Intensol*, Sterapred, Winpred†

Pregnancy risk category C

AVAILABLE FORMS

Oral solution: 5 mg/5 ml*, 5 mg/ml (concentrate)*
Syrup: 5 mg/5 ml*

Tablet: 1 mg, 2.5 mg, 5 mg, 10 mg, 20 mg, 50 mg
Tablet (film-coated): 5 mg

INDICATIONS & DOSAGES

➤ **Severe inflammation, immunosuppression—**
Adults: 5 to 60 mg P.O. daily in single dose or as two to four divided doses. Maintenance dose given once daily or every other day. Dosage must be individualized.
Children: 0.14 to 2 mg/kg or 4 to 60 mg/m² daily P.O. in four divided doses.
➤ **Acute exacerbations of multiple sclerosis—**
Adults: 200 mg P.O. daily for 7 days; then 80 mg P.O. every other day for 1 month.

ACTION

Not clearly defined. Decreases inflammation, mainly by stabilizing leukocyte lysosomal membranes; suppresses immune response; stimulates bone marrow; and influences protein, fat, and carbohydrate metabolism.

Route	Onset	Peak	Duration
P.O.	Variable	Variable	Variable

ADVERSE REACTIONS

CNS: *euphoria, insomnia,* psychotic behavior, pseudotumor cerebri, vertigo, headache, paresthesia, *seizures.*
CV: *heart failure,* hypertension, edema, *arrhythmias,* thrombophlebitis, *thromboembolism.*
EENT: cataracts, glaucoma.
GI: *peptic ulceration,* GI irritation, increased appetite, *pancreatitis,* nausea, vomiting.
GU: menstrual irregularities, increased urine calcium levels.
Metabolic: hypokalemia, hyperglycemia, and carbohydrate intolerance; hypercholesterolemia; hypocalcemia.
Musculoskeletal: growth suppression in children, muscle weakness, osteoporosis.
Skin: hirsutism, delayed wound healing, acne, various skin eruptions.
Other: cushingoid state, susceptibility to infections, *acute adrenal insufficiency* after increased stress or abrupt withdrawal after long-term therapy.
After abrupt withdrawal: rebound inflammation, fatigue, weakness, arthralgia,

---

*Liquid contains alcohol.   **May contain tartrazine.   †Canada   ‡Australia   §U.K.   ◊OTC

fever, dizziness, lethargy, depression, fainting, orthostatic hypotension, dyspnea, anorexia, hypoglycemia. ***After prolonged use, sudden withdrawal may be fatal.***

INTERACTIONS
Drug-drug. *Aspirin, indomethacin, other NSAIDs:* Increased risk of GI distress and bleeding. Use together cautiously.
Barbiturates, fosphenytoin, phenytoin, rifampin: Decreased corticosteroid effect. Increase corticosteroid dosage.
Oral anticoagulants: Altered dosage requirements. Monitor PT and INR closely.
Potassium-depleting drugs such as thiazide diuretics: Enhanced potassium-wasting effects of prednisone. Monitor potassium levels.
Salicylates: Decreased salicylate levels. Monitor patient for lack of salicylate effectiveness.
Skin-test antigens: Decreased response. Defer skin testing until therapy is completed.
Toxoids, vaccines: Decreased antibody response and increased risk of neurologic complications. Avoid using together.
Drug-herb. *Alfalfa sprouts, astragalus, echinacea, licorice:* May interfere with immunosuppressive effect of the drug. Advise patient to avoid using together.
Echinacea: Increased immune-stimulating effects. Advise patient to avoid using together.
Ginseng: Potentiates immune-modulating response. Advise patient to avoid using together.

EFFECTS ON LAB TEST RESULTS
● May increase glucose and cholesterol levels. May decrease potassium and calcium levels.

CONTRAINDICATIONS
Contraindicated in patients hypersensitive to drug and in those with systemic fungal infections.

NURSING CONSIDERATIONS
● Use cautiously in patients with recent MI, GI ulcer, renal disease, hypertension, osteoporosis, diabetes mellitus, hypothyroidism, cirrhosis, diverticulitis, nonspecific ulcerative colitis, recent intestinal anastomoses, thromboembolic disorders, seizures, myasthenia gravis, heart failure, tuberculosis, ocular herpes simplex, emotional instability, and psychotic tendencies.
● Determine whether patient is sensitive to other corticosteroids.
● Drug may be used for alternate-day therapy.
● Always adjust to lowest effective dose.
● Drug suppresses reactions to skin tests, causes false-negative results in the nitroblue tetrazolium test for systemic bacterial infections, and decreases ^{131}I uptake and protein-bound iodine levels in thyroid function tests.
● Most adverse reactions to corticosteroids are dose- or duration-dependent.
● For better results and less toxicity, give a once-daily dose in the morning.
● Unless contraindicated, give oral dose with food when possible to reduce GI irritation. Patient may need medication to prevent GI irritation.
● The oral solution may be diluted in juice or other flavored diluent or semi-solid food (such as applesauce) before using.
● Monitor patient's blood pressure, sleep patterns, and potassium levels.
● Weigh patient daily; report sudden weight gain to prescriber.
● Monitor patient for cushingoid effects, including moonface, buffalo hump, central obesity, thinning hair, hypertension, and increased susceptibility to infection.
● Watch for depression or psychotic episodes, especially during high-dose therapy.
● Diabetic patient may need increased insulin; monitor glucose levels.
● Elderly patients may be more susceptible to osteoporosis with long-term use.
● Drug may mask or worsen infections, including latent amebiasis.
● Unless contraindicated, give low-sodium diet that's high in potassium and protein. Give potassium supplements, as needed.
● Gradually reduce dosage after long-term therapy.
● ***Alert:*** Don't confuse prednisone with prednisolone, primidone, or prednimustine.

PATIENT TEACHING
● Tell patient not to stop drug abruptly or without prescriber's consent.

Reactions may be *common*, uncommon, ***life-threatening***, or COMMON AND LIFE-THREATENING.

• Instruct patient to take drug with food or milk.
• Teach patient signs and symptoms of early adrenal insufficiency: fatigue, muscle weakness, joint pain, fever, anorexia, nausea, dyspnea, dizziness, and fainting.
• Instruct patient to carry or wear medical identification indicating his need for supplemental systemic glucocorticoids during stress. It should include prescriber's name, name of drug, and dosage taken.
• Warn patient on long-term therapy about cushingoid effects (moonface, buffalo hump) and the need to notify prescriber about sudden weight gain or swelling.
• Advise patient receiving long-term therapy to consider exercise or physical therapy. Also, tell patient to ask prescriber about vitamin D or calcium supplement.
• Tell patient to report slow healing.
• Advise patient receiving long-term therapy to have periodic ophthalmic examinations.
• Instruct patient to avoid exposure to infections and to contact prescriber if exposure occurs.

---

triamcinolone
Aristocort, Aristopak, Atolone, Kenacort**

triamcinolone acetonide
Azmacort, Kenaject-40, Kenalog-10, Kenalog-40, Tac-3, Tac-40, Triam-A, Triamonide 40, Tri-Kort, Trilog

triamcinolone diacetate
Amcort, Aristocort Forte, Aristocort Intralesional, Cinalone, Triam Forte, Trilone, Tristoject

triamcinolone hexacetonide
Aristospan Intra-Articular, Aristospan Intralesional

Pregnancy risk category C

AVAILABLE FORMS
triamcinolone
Tablets: 4 mg, 8 mg
triamcinolone acetonide
Injection (suspension): 3 mg/ml, 10 mg/ml, 40 mg/ml

Metered spray: 100 mcg/spray
triamcinolone diacetate
Injectable suspension: 25 mg/ml, 40 mg/ml
triamcinolone hexacetonide
Injectable suspension: 5 mg/ml (intralesional); 20 mg/ml (intra-articular)

INDICATIONS & DOSAGES
➤ **Severe inflammation, immunosuppression—**
Adults: 4 to 48 mg P.O. daily in single dose or divided doses. Or, 40 to 80 mg I.M. (acetonide) at 4-week intervals. Or, 1 mg (acetonide) into lesions. Or, 2.5 to 15 mg (acetonide) into joints (depending on joint size) or soft tissue. A local anesthetic is commonly injected with triamcinolone into the joint. For triamcinolone hexacetonide, up to 0.5 mg (of 5 mg/ml suspension) intralesional or sublesional injection per square inch of affected skin. Additional injections based on patient's response. Or, 2 to 20 mg (using the 20 mg/ml suspension) via intra-articular injection. Dose may be repeated every 3 to 4 weeks.
➤ **Adrenocortical insufficiency—**
Children: 0.117 to 1.66 mg/kg/day or 3.3 to 50 mg/m²/day P.O. in four divided doses.
➤ **Asthma—**
Adults and children age 12 and older: 2 inhalations t.i.d. or q.i.d. Maximum, 16 inhalations daily.
Children ages 6 to 12: 1 to 2 inhalations t.i.d. or q.i.d. Maximum, 12 inhalations daily.

ACTION
Not clearly defined. Decreases inflammation, mainly by stabilizing leukocyte lysosomal membranes; suppresses immune response; stimulates bone marrow; and influences protein, fat, and carbohydrate metabolism.

Route	Onset	Peak	Duration
I.M., inhalation, intra-articular, intralesional, P.O.	Variable	Variable	Variable

---

ADVERSE REACTIONS

CNS: *euphoria, insomnia,* psychotic behavior, pseudotumor cerebri, vertigo, headache, paresthesia, *seizures.*

CV: *heart failure,* hypertension, edema, *arrhythmias,* thrombophlebitis, *thromboembolism.*

EENT: cataracts, glaucoma.

GI: *peptic ulceration,* GI irritation, increased appetite, *pancreatitis,* nausea, vomiting.

GU: menstrual irregularities, increased urine calcium levels.

Metabolic: hypokalemia, hyperglycemia, and carbohydrate intolerance; hypercholesterolemia; hypokalemia; hypocalcemia.

Musculoskeletal: growth suppression in children, muscle weakness, osteoporosis.

Skin: hirsutism, delayed wound healing, acne, various skin eruptions.

Other: cushingoid state, susceptibility to infections, *acute adrenal insufficiency* after increased stress or abrupt withdrawal after long-term therapy.

After abrupt withdrawal: rebound inflammation, fatigue, weakness, arthralgia, fever, dizziness, lethargy, depression, fainting, orthostatic hypotension, dyspnea, anorexia, hypoglycemia. *After prolonged use, sudden withdrawal may be fatal.*

INTERACTIONS

Drug-drug. *Aspirin, indomethacin, other NSAIDs:* Increased risk of GI distress and bleeding. Use together cautiously.

Barbiturates, fosphenytoin, phenytoin, rifampin: Decreased corticosteroid effect. Increase corticosteroid dosage.

Oral anticoagulants: Altered dosage requirements. Monitor PT and INR closely.

Potassium-depleting drugs such as thiazide diuretics: Enhanced potassium-wasting effects of triamcinolone. Monitor potassium levels.

Salicylates: Decreased salicylate levels. Monitor patient for lack of salicylate effectiveness.

Skin-test antigens: Decreased response. Defer skin testing until after therapy.

Toxoids, vaccines: Decreased antibody response and increased risk of neurologic complications. Avoid using together.

Drug-herb. *Echinacea:* Increased immune-stimulating effects. Discourage use together.

Ginseng: Potentiates immune-modulating response. Discourage use together.

EFFECTS ON LAB TEST RESULTS

• May increase glucose and cholesterol levels. May decrease potassium and calcium levels.

CONTRAINDICATIONS

Contraindicated in patients hypersensitive to drug or its ingredients and in those with systemic fungal infections.

NURSING CONSIDERATIONS

• Use cautiously in patients with recent MI, GI ulcer, renal disease, hypertension, osteoporosis, diabetes mellitus, hypothyroidism, cirrhosis, diverticulitis, nonspecific ulcerative colitis, recent intestinal anastomoses, thromboembolic disorders, seizures, myasthenia gravis, heart failure, tuberculosis, ocular herpes simplex, emotional instability, or psychotic tendencies.

• Determine whether patient is sensitive to other corticosteroids.

• Drug isn't used for alternate-day therapy.

• Always adjust to lowest effective dose.

• Most adverse reactions to corticosteroids are dose- or duration-dependent.

• For better results and less toxicity, give a once-daily oral dose in the morning with food.

• *Alert:* Parenteral form isn't for I.V. use.

• *Alert:* Salt formulations aren't interchangeable.

• Don't use 40 mg/ml strength for intradermal or intralesional use.

• Don't use 10 mg/ml strength for I.M. use.

• Don't use diluents that contain preservatives; flocculation may occur.

• Drug suppresses reactions to skin tests, causes false-negative results in the nitroblue tetrazolium test for systemic bacterial infections, and decreases ^{131}I uptake and protein-bound iodine levels in thyroid function tests.

• Give I.M. injection deeply into gluteal muscle. Rotate injection sites to prevent muscle atrophy.

• Monitor patient's weight, blood pressure, and electrolyte levels.

• Monitor patient for cushingoid effects, including moonface, buffalo hump, cen-

tral obesity, thinning hair, hypertension, and increased susceptibility to infection.
• Watch for allergic reaction to tartrazine in patients with sensitivity to aspirin.
• Watch for depression or psychotic episodes, especially during high-dose therapy.
• Diabetic patient may need increased insulin dosage; monitor glucose levels.
• Drug may mask or worsen infections, including latent amebiasis.
• Elderly patients may be more susceptible to osteoporosis with long-term use.
• Unless contraindicated, give low-sodium diet that's high in potassium and protein. Give potassium supplements, as needed.
• Gradually reduce dosage after long-term therapy. Drug may affect patient's sleep.
• *Alert:* Don't confuse triamcinolone with Triaminicin or Triaminicol.

PATIENT TEACHING
• Tell patient not to stop drug abruptly or without prescriber's consent.
• Instruct patient to take drug with food or milk.
• Teach patient signs and symptoms of early adrenal insufficiency: fatigue, muscle weakness, joint pain, fever, anorexia, nausea, dyspnea, dizziness, and fainting.
• Instruct patient to carry or wear medical identification indicating his need for supplemental systemic glucocorticoids during stress. It should include prescriber's name, name of drug, and dosage taken.
• Warn patient on long-term therapy about cushingoid effects (moonface, buffalo hump) and the need to notify prescriber about sudden weight gain and swelling.
• Tell patient to report slow healing.
• Advise patient receiving long-term therapy to consider exercise or physical therapy. Also, tell patient to ask prescriber about vitamin D or calcium supplement.
• Instruct patient to avoid exposure to infections and to notify prescriber if exposure occurs.

➤ **Male hypogonadism—**
Men: 10 to 50 mg P.O. daily; or 5 to
25 mg buccally daily.
➤ **Postpubertal cryptorchidism—**
Men: 30 mg P.O. daily; or 15 mg buccally
daily.
➤ **Prevention of postpartum breast engorgement—**
Women: 80 mg daily in divided doses for
3 to 5 days.

ACTION

Stimulates target tissues to develop normally in androgen-deficient men. May
have some antiestrogen properties, making
it useful in treating certain estrogen-dependent breast cancers. Action in postpartum breast engorgement isn't known
because testosterone doesn't suppress lactation.

Route	Onset	Peak	Duration
Buccal	Unknown	1 hr	Unknown
P.O.	Unknown	2 hr	Unknown

ADVERSE REACTIONS

CNS: headache, anxiety, depression,
paresthesia.
CV: edema.
GI: irritation of oral mucosa with buccal
administration, nausea.
GU: *hypoestrogenic effects in women,* excessive hormonal effects in men.
Hematologic: *suppression of clotting factors,* polycythemia.
Hepatic: reversible jaundice, *cholestatic hepatitis.*
Metabolic: hypernatremia, hyperkalemia,
hyperphosphatemia, hypercholesterolemia, hypercalcemia.
Musculoskeletal: muscle cramps or
spasms.
Skin: hypersensitivity reactions.
Other: androgenic effects in women.

INTERACTIONS

Drug-drug. *Hepatotoxic drugs:* Increased
risk of hepatotoxicity. Monitor liver function closely.
Imipramine: Dramatic paranoid response.
Monitor patient closely.
Insulin, oral antidiabetics: Decreased glucose may alter dosage requirements. Monitor glucose levels in diabetic patients.

Oral anticoagulants: Increased sensitivity
to oral anticoagulants may alter dosage requirements. Monitor PT and INR.

EFFECTS ON LAB TEST RESULTS

● May increase sodium, potassium, phosphate, cholesterol, liver enzyme, lipid, and
calcium levels. May decrease thyroxine-binding globulin and total T_4 levels.
● May increase resin uptake of T_3 and T_4.
Also may increase RBC count.

CONTRAINDICATIONS

Contraindicated in pregnant or breast-feeding women and in men with breast
cancer or known or suspected prostate
cancer.

NURSING CONSIDERATIONS

● Use cautiously in elderly patients; patients with cardiac, renal, or hepatic disease; or healthy men with delayed puberty.
● Don't give to women of childbearing age
until pregnancy is ruled out.
● In children, obtain X-rays of wrist bones
before therapy begins to establish level of
bone maturation. During treatment, bone
maturation may proceed more rapidly than
linear growth. Periodically review X-ray
results to monitor bone maturation.
● Drug is typically used only for intermittent therapy. Because of potential hepatotoxicity, watch closely for jaundice.
● Promptly report evidence of virilization
in women.
● Watch for hypoestrogenic effects in
women (flushing; diaphoresis; vaginitis,
including itching, dryness, and burning;
vaginal bleeding; nervousness; emotional
lability; menstrual irregularities).
● Watch for excessive hormonal effects in
male patients. If patient is prepubertal,
watch for premature epiphyseal closure,
acne, priapism, growth of body and facial
hair, and phallic enlargement. If postpubertal, watch for testicular atrophy,
oligospermia, decreased ejaculatory volume, impotence, gynecomastia, and epididymitis.
● Unless contraindicated, use with diet
high in calories and protein. Give small,
frequent meals.
● Periodically check hemoglobin level and
hematocrit, cholesterol and calcium levels,
and cardiac and liver function test results.

• Drug may cause abnormal glucose tolerance test results.
• Check weight regularly. Edema can be controlled with sodium restriction or diuretics.
• *Alert:* Therapeutic response in breast cancer is usually apparent within 3 months. Therapy should be stopped if signs of disease progression appear.
• Report signs of hypercalcemia. In metastatic breast cancer, hypercalcemia may indicate progression of bone metastases.
• Semen evaluation is routinely performed every 3 to 4 months, especially in adolescent boys.
• *Alert:* Drug shouldn't be given to enhance athletic performance or physique.
• *Alert:* Testosterone and methyltestosterone aren't interchangeable. Don't confuse methyltestosterone with medroxyprogesterone.

PATIENT TEACHING
• Make sure patient understands importance of using an effective nonhormonal contraceptive during therapy.
• Tell woman to report menstrual irregularities and to stop drug pending examination.
• Instruct patient to stop drug immediately and notify prescriber about suspected pregnancy.
• Buccal tablets are twice as potent as oral tablets. Tell patient to avoid eating, drinking, chewing, or smoking while buccal tablet is in place and not to swallow tablet. Place in upper or lower buccal pouch between cheek and gum; tablet needs 30 to 60 minutes to dissolve.
• Instruct patient to change tablet absorption site with each dose to minimize risk of buccal irritation. Advise patient to rinse mouth after using buccal tablet.
• Tell woman to immediately report evidence of virilization, such as acne, edema, weight gain, hirsutism, hoarseness, clitoral enlargement, decreased breast size, deepening voice, changes in libido, male-pattern baldness, and oily skin or hair.
• Teach patient signs and symptoms of hypoglycemia and method for checking glucose level; drug enhances hypoglycemia. Instruct patient to report hypoglycemia immediately.

• Advise woman to wash after intercourse to decrease risk of vaginitis. Instruct her to wear cotton underwear.

---

nandrolone decanoate
Deca-Durabolin

Pregnancy risk category X
Controlled substance schedule III

AVAILABLE FORMS
Injection (in oil): 100 mg/ml, 200 mg/ml

INDICATIONS & DOSAGES
➤ **Severe debility or disease states, refractory anemias—**
Adults and children older than age 13: 50 to 100 mg decanoate I.M. at 1- to 4-week intervals for women; 50 to 200 mg decanoate I.M. at 1- to 4-week intervals for men. Therapy should be intermittent and discontinued if no improvement in 6 months.
Children ages 2 to 13: 25 to 50 mg decanoate I.M. q 3 to 4 weeks.

ACTION
An anabolic steroid that promotes tissue-building processes, reverses catabolism, and stimulates erythropoiesis.

Route	Onset	Peak	Duration
I.M.	Unknown	3-6 days	Unknown

ADVERSE REACTIONS
CNS: excitation, insomnia, habituation, depression.
CV: edema.
GI: nausea, vomiting, diarrhea.
GU: bladder irritability.
Hematologic: *suppression of clotting factors.*
Hepatic: reversible jaundice, *peliosis hepatis, liver cell tumors.*
Metabolic: hypernatremia, hyperkalemia, hypercalcemia, hyperphosphatemia, hypercholesterolemia.
Skin: pain, induration at injection site, acne.
Other: *hypoestrogenic effects in women,* excessive hormonal effects in men, androgenic effects in women.

INTERACTIONS
Drug-drug. *Hepatotoxic drugs:* Increased risk of hepatotoxicity. Monitor liver function closely.
Insulin, oral antidiabetics: Altered dosage requirements. Monitor glucose levels in diabetic patients.
Oral anticoagulants: Altered dosage requirements. Monitor PT and INR.

EFFECTS ON LAB TEST RESULTS
• May increase creatinine, lipid, sodium, potassium, calcium, phosphate, cholesterol, and liver enzyme levels.
• May decrease thyroid function test result values.

CONTRAINDICATIONS
Contraindicated in patients hypersensitive to anabolic steroids, in those with nephrosis or the nephrotic phase of nephritis, in men with breast cancer or known or suspected prostate cancer, in women with breast cancer and hypercalcemia, and in pregnant or breast-feeding women.

NURSING CONSIDERATIONS
• Use cautiously in patients with diabetes; cardiac, renal, or hepatic disease; epilepsy; or migraine or other conditions that may be aggravated by fluid retention.
• Don't give to women of childbearing age until pregnancy is ruled out.
• Make sure patient understands importance of using an effective nonhormonal contraceptive during therapy.
• Instruct patient to discontinue drug immediately and notify prescriber if she suspects pregnancy.
• In children, obtain X-rays of wrist bones before surgery to establish level of bone maturation. During treatment, bone maturation may proceed more rapidly than linear growth; periodically review X-ray results to monitor bone maturation.
• Inject I.M. drug deeply, preferably into upper outer quadrant of gluteal muscle in adults. Rotate injection sites to prevent muscle atrophy.
• Unless contraindicated, use with diet high in calories and protein. Give small, frequent feedings.
• Watch for signs of virilization, which may be irreversible despite prompt discontinuation of therapy. Androgenic effects in women include acne, edema, weight gain, hirsutism, hoarseness, clitoral enlargement, decreased breast size, changes in libido, male-pattern baldness, and oily skin or hair.
• Watch for hypoestrogenic effects in women, including flushing; diaphoresis; vaginitis, including itching, dryness, and burning; vaginal bleeding; nervousness; emotional lability; menstrual irregularities.
• Watch for excessive hormonal effects in male patients. If patient is prepubertal, watch for premature epiphyseal closure, acne, priapism, growth of body and facial hair, and phallic enlargement. If postpubertal, watch for testicular atrophy, oligospermia, decreased ejaculatory volume, impotence, gynecomastia, and epididymitis.
• Closely observe boys younger than age 7 for precocious development of male sexual characteristics.
• Semen evaluation is routinely performed every 3 to 4 months, especially in adolescent boys.
• *Alert:* Periodically evaluate hepatic function. Watch for jaundice; dosage adjustment may reverse condition. If liver function test results are abnormal, therapy should be stopped.
• Check weight regularly. Edema usually can be controlled with sodium restrictions or diuretics.
• Drug may cause abnormal results of fasting plasma glucose, glucose tolerance, and metyrapone tests.
• Watch for evidence of hypoglycemia in diabetic patients. Check glucose levels. Adjust dosage of antidiabetic.
• Check quantitative urine and serum calcium levels. Hypercalcemia is most likely to occur in patients with breast cancer.
• When used to promote erythropoiesis in patient with refractory anemia, make sure he has adequate daily iron intake.
• Anabolic steroids may alter results of laboratory studies performed during therapy and for 2 to 3 weeks after therapy ends.

PATIENT TEACHING
• Make sure patient understands importance of using an effective nonhormonal contraceptive during therapy.

• Review signs and symptoms of virilization with woman, and instruct her to notify prescriber immediately if they occur.
• Advise woman to wash after intercourse to decrease risk of vaginitis. Instruct her to wear cotton underwear.
• Warn diabetic patient to be alert for hypoglycemia, and tell him to notify prescriber if it occurs.
• Tell patient to report sudden weight gain to prescriber.
• Tell woman to report menstrual irregularities and to stop drug when these occur, pending examination.

testosterone
Histerone 100, Testamone 100, Testaqua, Testopel Pellets

testosterone cypionate
depAndro 100, depAndro 200, Depo-Testosterone, Duratest-100, Duratest-200, T-Cypionate, T-E Cypionate, Virilon IM

testosterone enanthate
Andro LA, Delatestryl, Everone 200

testosterone propionate
Malogen†, Virormone§

Pregnancy risk category X
Controlled substance schedule III

AVAILABLE FORMS
testosterone
Injection (aqueous suspension): 100 mg/ml
Pellets (S.C. implant): 75 mg
testosterone cypionate
Injection (in oil): 100 mg/ml, 200 mg/ml
testosterone enanthate
Injection (in oil): 100 mg/ml, 200 mg/ml
testosterone propionate
Injection (in oil): 50 mg/ml, 100 mg/ml

INDICATIONS & DOSAGES
➤ **Male hypogonadism—**
Men: 10 to 25 mg (testosterone) I.M. two to three times weekly; or 50 to 400 mg (cypionate or enanthate) I.M. q 2 to 4 weeks.

➤ **Metastatic breast cancer in women 1 to 5 years after menopause—**
Women: 50 to 100 mg I.M. three times weekly; or 200 to 400 mg (enanthate) I.M. q 2 to 4 weeks.
➤ **Postpartum breast pain and engorgement—**
Women: 25 to 50 mg I.M. of testosterone or testosterone propionate daily for 3 to 4 days.

ACTION
Stimulates target tissues to develop normally in androgen-deficient men. Testosterone may have some antiestrogen properties, making it useful in treating certain estrogen-dependent breast cancers. Its action in postpartum breast engorgement isn't known because testosterone doesn't suppress lactation.

Route	Onset	Peak	Duration
I.M.	Unknown	10-100 min	Unknown
S.C.	Unknown	Unknown	3-4 mo

ADVERSE REACTIONS
CNS: headache, anxiety, depression, paresthesia, sleep apnea.
CV: edema.
GI: nausea.
Hematologic: polycythemia, *suppression of clotting factors.*
Hepatic: reversible jaundice, *cholestatic hepatitis.*
Metabolic: hypernatremia, hyperkalemia, hypercalcemia, hyperphosphatemia, hypercholesterolemia.
Skin: pain, induration at injection site, local edema, acne.
Other: androgenic effects in women, hypersensitivity reactions, hypoestrogenic effects in women, excessive hormonal effects in men.

INTERACTIONS
Drug-drug. *Hepatotoxic drugs:* Increased risk of hepatotoxicity. Monitor liver function closely.
Insulin, oral antidiabetics: Decreased glucose levels may alter dosage requirements. Monitor glucose levels in diabetic patients.
Oral anticoagulants: Increased sensitivity may alter dosage requirements. Monitor PT and INR.

Oxyphenbutazone: May increase oxyphenbutazone levels. Monitor patient.

EFFECTS ON LAB TEST RESULTS
• May increase sodium, potassium, phosphate, cholesterol, liver enzyme, calcium, and creatinine levels.
• May decrease thyroxine-binding globulin and total T_4 levels.
• May increase resin uptake of T_3 and T_4 and RBC count.

CONTRAINDICATIONS
Contraindicated in patients hypersensitive to drug and in those with hypercalcemia or cardiac, hepatic, or renal decompensation; also contraindicated in men with breast cancer or known or suspected prostate cancer and in pregnant or breast-feeding women.

NURSING CONSIDERATIONS
• Use cautiously in elderly patients.
• Don't give to women of childbearing age until pregnancy is ruled out.
• Store I.M. preparations at room temperature. If crystals appear, warm and shake bottle to disperse them.
• Cypionate and Enanthate are long-acting solutions.
• Inject deep into upper outer quadrant of gluteal muscle. Rotate injection sites. Report soreness at site.
• Unless contraindicated, administer with diet high in calories and protein. Provide small, frequent meals to help avoid nausea.
• Monitor patient's liver function test results.
• Testosterone may cause abnormal glucose tolerance test results.
• In patients with metastatic breast cancer, hypercalcemia usually indicates progression of bone metastases. Report signs and symptoms of hypercalcemia.
• Report evidence of virilization in women. Androgenic effects include acne, edema, weight gain, hirsutism, hoarseness, clitoral enlargement, decreased breast size, changes in libido, male-pattern baldness, and oily skin or hair.
• Watch for hypoestrogenic effects in women (flushing; diaphoresis; vaginitis, including itching, drying, and burning; vaginal bleeding; menstrual irregularities).
• Watch for excessive hormonal effects in male patients. If patient is prepubertal, watch for premature epiphyseal closure, acne, priapism, growth of body and facial hair, and phallic enlargement. If postpubertal, watch for testicular atrophy, oligospermia, decreased ejaculatory volume, impotence, gynecomastia, epididymitis.
• Monitor patient's weight and blood pressure routinely.
• Monitor prepubertal boys by X-ray for rate of bone maturation.
• *Alert:* Therapeutic response in breast cancer is usually apparent within 3 months. Therapy should be stopped if disease progresses.
• Androgens may alter results of laboratory studies during therapy and for 2 to 3 weeks after therapy ends.
• *Alert:* Testosterone and methyltestosterone aren't interchangeable. Don't confuse testosterone with testolactone.
• Testosterone salts aren't interchangeable.

PATIENT TEACHING
• Make sure patient understands importance of using an effective nonhormonal contraceptive during therapy.
• Instruct patient to stop drug immediately and notify prescriber about suspected pregnancy.
• Review signs and symptoms of virilization with woman, and instruct her to notify prescriber if they occur.
• Advise woman to wash after intercourse to decrease risk of vaginitis. Instruct her to wear cotton underwear.
• Instruct man to notify prescriber about priapism, reduced ejaculatory volume, or gynecomastia.
• Warn diabetic patient to be alert for hypoglycemia, and to notify prescriber if it occurs.
• Instruct male patients using testosterone for delayed puberty to have radiographs of hand and wrist taken every 6 months while receiving treatment.
• Tell patient to report sudden weight gain.
• Warn patient that drug shouldn't be used to enhance athletic performance.

Reactions may be *common*, uncommon, *life-threatening*, or COMMON AND LIFE-THREATENING.

testosterone transdermal system
Androderm, Testoderm, Testoderm TTS, Testoderm w/Adhesive

Pregnancy risk category X
Controlled substance schedule III

AVAILABLE FORMS
Transdermal system: 2.5 mg/day, 4 mg/day, 5 mg/day, 6 mg/day

INDICATIONS & DOSAGES
➤ **Primary or hypogonadotropic hypogonadism in men—**
Adult men: Testoderm—One 6-mg/day patch applied to scrotal area daily; or 4 mg/day if scrotal area is small. Patch is worn for 22 to 24 hours daily. *Androderm*—Two systems applied h.s. for total dose of 5 mg/day.

ACTION
Releases testosterone, which stimulates target tissues to develop normally in androgen-deficient men.

Route	Onset	Peak	Duration
Transdermal	Unknown	2-4 hr	2 hr after removal

ADVERSE REACTIONS
CNS: *CVA,* asthenia, depression, headache.
GI: GI bleeding.
GU: prostatitis, prostate abnormalities, urinary tract infection.
Hepatic: reversible jaundice, *cholestatic hepatitis.*
Metabolic: hypernatremia, hyperkalemia, hypercalcemia, hyperphosphatemia, hypercholesterolemia.
Skin: acne irritation, *pruritus, blister under system,* allergic contact dermatitis, burning.
Other: gynecomastia, breast tenderness, flu syndrome.

INTERACTIONS
Drug-drug. *Insulin:* Altered insulin dosage requirements. Monitor glucose levels.
Oral anticoagulants: Altered anticoagulant dosage requirements. Monitor PT and INR.
Oxyphenbutazone: May increase oxyphenbutazone levels. Monitor patient.

EFFECTS ON LAB TEST RESULTS
● May increase sodium, potassium, phosphate, cholesterol, liver enzyme, calcium, and creatinine levels.
● May increase RBC count.

CONTRAINDICATIONS
Contraindicated in patients hypersensitive to drug, in women, and in men with known or suspected breast or prostate cancer.

NURSING CONSIDERATIONS
● Use cautiously in elderly men and in patients with renal, hepatic, or cardiac disease.
● If scrotal area is too small for 6-mg/day Testoderm patch, start therapy with 4-mg/day patch.
● Apply Androderm system to clean, dry skin on back, abdomen, upper arms, or thigh.
● Wear gloves while handling transdermal patches. Fold used patches with adhesive side together; discard so that they can't be handled.
● Periodically assess liver function test results, lipid profiles, hemoglobin level, hematocrit (with long-term use), and prostatic acid phosphatase and prostate-specific antigen levels.
● Monitor for excessive hormonal effects in male patients.
● Monitor for evidence of virilization in women whose sexual partner uses the drug.
● *Alert:* Don't confuse Testoderm with Estraderm.

PATIENT TEACHING
● Teach patient how to apply transdermal system. Warn him that adequate serum levels won't be attained if Testoderm patch isn't applied to genital skin. Scrotal area may be dry-shaved for best contact. Tell patient using Androderm that patch isn't to be applied to scrotum. Application site should be rotated, with an interval of 7

days between applications to same site. Avoid bony prominences.

• Don't interchange patch brands.

• Tell patient not to apply Testoderm TTS to scrotum.

• Tell patient that if patch falls off, it may be reapplied. If patch falls off, can't be reapplied, and has been worn at least 12 hours, a new patch may be applied at the next application time.

• Advise patient to wear underwear briefs to prevent the patch from falling off.

• Instruct patient that system must be changed every 24 hours.

• Warn diabetic patient that testosterone may decrease glucose levels and that he should be alert for hypoglycemia.

• Tell patient that topical testosterone has caused virilization in women partners, who should report acne or changes in body hair distribution.

• Advise patient to report persistent erections, nausea, vomiting, changes in skin color, ankle edema, or sudden weight gain to prescriber.

• Tell patient that Androderm doesn't have to be removed during sexual intercourse or while showering.

17 beta-estradiol/norgestimate
drospirenone and ethinyl
    estradiol
esterified estrogens
estradiol
estradiol cypionate
estradiol valerate
estradiol/norethindrone acetate
    transdermal system
estrogens, conjugated
estropipate
ethinyl estradiol
ethinyl estradiol and desogestrel
ethinyl estradiol and ethynodiol
    diacetate
ethinyl estradiol and
    levonorgestrel
ethinyl estradiol and
    norethindrone
ethinyl estradiol and
    norethindrone acetate
ethinyl estradiol and
    norgestimate
ethinyl estradiol and norgestrel
ethinyl estradiol, norethindrone
    acetate, and ferrous fumarate
levonorgestrel
medroxyprogesterone acetate
medroxyprogesterone acetate
    and estradiol cypionate
mestranol and norethindrone
norethindrone
norethindrone acetate
norgestrel
progesterone

COMBINATION PRODUCTS
ESTRATEST: esterified estrogens 1.25 mg
and methyltestosterone 1.25 mg.
PMB 200: conjugated estrogens 0.45 mg
and meprobamate 200 mg.
PMB 400: conjugated estrogens 0.45 mg
and meprobamate 400 mg.
PREMPHASE: conjugated estrogens
0.625 mg and conjugated estrogens
0.625 mg/medroxyprogesterone acetate
5 mg.
PREMPRO 0.625 mg/2.5 mg: conjugated
estrogens 0.625 mg/medroxyprogesterone
acetate 2.5 mg.

PREMPRO 0.625 mg/5 mg: conjugated estrogens 0.625 mg/medroxyprogesterone
acetate 5 mg.
PREVEN EMERGENCY: ethinyl estradiol
(50 mcg) and levonorgestrel (0.25 mg).

17 beta-estradiol/norgestimate
Ortho-Prefest

Pregnancy risk category X

AVAILABLE FORMS
Tablets: Blister card of 15 pink and 15
white tablets, for a total of 30 tablets
Pink tablets—1 mg estradiol
White tablets—1 mg estradiol and
0.09 mg norgestimate

INDICATIONS & DOSAGES
➤ Treatment of moderate to severe
vasomotor symptoms caused by menopause; treatment of vulvar and vaginal
atrophy; prevention of osteoporosis in
women with an intact uterus—
Women: 1 mg estradiol (pink tablet) P.O.
daily for 3 days; then 1 mg estradiol/
0.09 mg norgestimate (white tablet) P.O.
daily for 3 days. Repeat continuously until
blister card is finished.

ACTION
Circulating estrogens modulate the pituitary secretion of luteinizing hormone and
follicle-stimulating hormone through a
negative feedback mechanism. Estrogen
replacement therapy reduces elevated levels of these hormones in postmenopausal
women. Norgestimate binds to androgen
and progesterone receptors. Progestins
counter the estrogenic effects by decreasing
the number of estradiol receptors and suppressing synthesis of endometrial tissue.

Route	Onset	Peak	Duration
P.O.	Unknown	7 hr (estradiol) 2 hr (norgesti-mate)	Unknown

ADVERSE REACTIONS

CNS: depression, dizziness, fatigue, pain, *headache.*

CV: *venous thromboembolism, MI, pulmonary embolism,* thrombophlebitis, edema.

EENT: steepening of corneal curvature, intolerance to contact lenses.

GI: flatulence, nausea, *abdominal pain,* gallbladder disease.

GU: dysmenorrhea, vaginal bleeding, vaginitis.

Metabolic: weight changes, reduced carbohydrate tolerance, aggravation of porphyria.

Musculoskeletal: arthralgia, myalgia, *back pain.*

Respiratory: cough, pharyngitis, sinusitis, *upper respiratory tract infection.*

Skin: chloasma, melasma, hirsutism, ***erythema multiforme,*** erythema nodosum, hemorrhagic eruption, loss of scalp hair.

Other: changes in libido, *flulike symptoms,* viral infection, tooth disorder, breast pain, galactorrhea.

INTERACTIONS

Drug-herb. *Black cohosh:* Increased side effects of estrogens. Discourage use together.

Saw palmetto: Antiestrogenic effects. Discourage use together.

St. John's wort: Decreased effects of estrogens. Discourage use together.

Drug-lifestyle. *Smoking:* Increased risk of CV effects. Advise patient to avoid smoking.

EFFECTS ON LAB TEST RESULTS

• May increase thyroid-binding globulin; factor II, VII antigen, VIII antigen, VIII coagulant activity, IX, X, XII, VII-X complex, II-VII-X complex; beta-thromboglobulin; HDL; triglyceride; corticosteroid; sex steroid; angiotensin and renin substrate; alpha$_1$-antitrypsin; ceruloplasmin; fibrinogen; and plasminogen antigen levels. May decrease folate, metyrapone, LDL, anti-factor Xa, and antithrombin III levels.

• May increase PT, PTT, platelet aggregation time, and platelet count. May decrease T$_3$ resin uptake and glucose tolerance.

CONTRAINDICATIONS

Ortho-Prefest is contraindicated in patients hypersensitive to any of its components, in postmenopausal women, in women with known or suspected pregnancy, and in patients with breast cancer, estrogen-dependent neoplasia, undiagnosed abnormal genital bleeding, and active or previous thrombophlebitis or thromboembolic disorders.

NURSING CONSIDERATIONS

• Give Ortho-Prefest cautiously to women who have had a hysterectomy, to overweight women, to women with abnormal lipid profiles, and to women with impaired liver function.

• Reassess patient at 6-month intervals to determine whether treatment for symptoms is still necessary.

• Use of estrogens is linked to development of malignant tumors. Giving progestin with estrogen significantly reduces this risk.

• Users of estrogen replacement have an increased risk of venous thromboembolism.

• Hormone replacement therapy may increase the risk of breast cancer in postmenopausal women.

• Estrogens can lead to severe hypercalcemia in patients with breast cancer and bone metastases. If this occurs, stop the drug and take appropriate measures to reduce calcium level.

• Monitor glucose closely in patients with diabetes.

PATIENT TEACHING

• Inform patient about the risks of estrogen therapy, such as breast cancer, cancer of the uterus, abnormal blood clotting, and gallbladder disease.

• Tell patient to immediately report undiagnosed, persistent, or recurring abnormal vaginal bleeding.

• Instruct patient to perform monthly breast self-examinations and to obtain yearly mammograms after age 50.

• Tell patient to report warning signals of blood clots, including pain in the calves or chest, sudden shortness of breath, coughing of blood, severe headaches, vomiting, dizziness, faintness, changes in vision or

---

Reactions may be *common,* uncommon, *life-threatening,* or **COMMON AND LIFE-THREATENING.**

speech, and weakness or numbness in arms or legs.

• Urge patient to report evidence of liver problems, such as yellowing of skin or eyes and upper right quadrant pain.

• Instruct patient to report abdominal pain, swelling, or tenderness, which may suggest gallbladder problems.

• Encourage patient to stop smoking or reduce number of cigarettes because of the risk of CV complications.

• Tell patient to store Ortho-Prefest at room temperature away from excessive heat and moisture. Product will remain stable for 18 months.

✳ NEW DRUG

drospirenone and ethinyl estradiol
Yasmin

Pregnancy risk category X

AVAILABLE FORMS
Tablets: Each tablet contains 3 mg drospirenone (DRSP) and 0.03 mg ethinyl estradiol (EE)

INDICATIONS AND DOSAGES
➤ **Prevention of pregnancy**—
Women and postpubertal female adolescents: Day 1 start—1 yellow tablet P.O. daily beginning on day 1 of menstrual cycle (first day of menstruation). Continue taking 1 yellow tablet P.O. daily for 21 consecutive days, at the same time each day, preferably after the evening meal or at bedtime; then take 1 white inert tablet P.O. daily on days 22 through 28. Begin the next and all subsequent 28-day regimens on the same day of the week that the first regimen began, following the same schedule. Restart taking yellow tablets on the next day after taking the last white tablet.

Sunday start—1 yellow tablet P.O. daily, beginning on the first Sunday after the onset of menstruation. Continue taking 1 yellow tablet P.O. daily for 21 consecutive days, at the same time each day, preferably after the evening meal or at bedtime; then take 1 white inert tablet P.O. daily on days 22 through 28. Begin the next and all subsequent 28-day regimens on the same day of the week that the first regimen began,

following the same schedule. Restart taking yellow tablets on the next day after taking the last white tablet.

ACTION
Drug reduces the opportunity for conception by inhibiting ovulation, inhibiting progression of sperm, and reducing the chance of implantation.

Route	Onset	Peak	Duration
P.O.	Unknown	1-3 hr	Unknown

ADVERSE REACTIONS
CNS: asthenia, *cerebral hemorrhage, cerebral thrombosis,* depression, dizziness, emotional lability, headache, migraine, nervousness.
CV: *arterial thromboembolism,* hypertension, *mesenteric thrombosis, MI, thrombophlebitis.*
EENT: cataracts, change in corneal curvature (steepening), intolerance to contact lenses, pharyngitis, retinal thrombosis, sinusitis.
GI: abdominal pain, abdominal cramping, bloating, changes in appetite, colitis, diarrhea, gastroenteritis, nausea, vomiting.
GU: amenorrhea, breakthrough bleeding, change in cervical erosion and secretion, change in menstrual flow, cystitis, cystitis-like syndrome, dysmenorrhea, *hemolytic-uremic syndrome,* impaired renal function, leukorrhea, menstrual disorder, premenstrual syndrome, spotting, temporary infertility after discontinuing treatment, urinary tract infection, vaginal candidiasis, vaginitis.
Hepatic: *Budd-Chiari syndrome,* cholestatic jaundice, gallbladder disease, *hepatic adenomas,* benign liver tumors.
Metabolic: reduced tolerance to carbohydrates, porphyria, weight change.
Musculoskeletal: back pain.
Respiratory: bronchitis, *pulmonary embolism,* upper respiratory tract infection.
Skin: acne, *erythema multiforme,* erythema nodosum, hemorrhagic eruption, hirsutism, loss of scalp hair, melasma, pruritus, rash.
Other: changes in libido.

INTERACTIONS
Drug-drug. *ACE inhibitors, aldosterone antagonists, angiotensin II receptor antag-*

---

*Liquid contains alcohol.   **May contain tartrazine.   †Canada   ‡Australia   §U.K.   ◇OTC

onists, NSAIDs, potassium-sparing diuretics: Increased risk of hyperkalemia. Monitor potassium levels.

Acetaminophen: Increased plasma concentrations of contraceptive and decreased effectiveness of acetaminophen. Monitor for adverse effects. Adjust acetaminophen dose as needed.

Ampicillin, griseofulvin, tetracycline: Decreased contraceptive effect. Encourage use of additional method of birth control while taking the antibiotic.

Ascorbic acid, atorvastatin: Increased concentrations of contraceptive. Monitor for adverse effects.

Carbamazepine, phenobarbital, phenytoin: Increased metabolism of ethinyl estradiol and decreased contraceptive effectiveness. Encourage use of alternative method of birth control.

Clofibrate, morphine, salicylic acid, temazepam: Decreased plasma concentrations and increased clearance of these drugs. Monitor for effectiveness.

Cyclosporine, prednisolone, theophylline: Increased plasma concentrations of these drugs. Monitor for adverse effects and toxicity.

Phenylbutazone, rifampin: Decreased contraceptive effectiveness and increased menstrual irregularities. Advise patient to use alternative method of birth control.

Drug-herb. *St. John's wort:* Decreased contraceptive effect and breakthrough bleeding. Encourage use of additional method of birth control or discourage use together.

Drug-lifestyle. *Smoking:* Increased risk of CV adverse effects. Tell patient not to smoke.

EFFECTS ON LAB TEST RESULTS
● May increase thyroid-binding globulin, total thyroid hormone, total circulating sex steroids, prothrombin, corticoid, folate, triglyceride, and factor VII, VIII, IX, and X levels. May decrease antithrombin III level.
● May increase norepinephrine-induced platelet aggregability. May decrease free T_3 resin uptake and glucose tolerance.

CONTRAINDICATIONS
Contraindicated in women with hepatic dysfunction, tumor, or disease; renal or adrenal insufficiency; thrombophlebitis, thromboembolic disorders, or history of deep vein thrombosis or thromboembolic disorders; cerebrovascular or coronary artery disease; known or suspected breast cancer, endometrial cancer, or other estrogen-dependent neoplasia; abnormal genital bleeding; or cholestatic jaundice of pregnancy or jaundice with other contraceptive pill use. Also contraindicated in women who are pregnant or suspect they may be pregnant and in women older than age 35 who smoke heavily (15 or more cigarettes daily).

NURSING CONSIDERATIONS
● Use cautiously in patients with risk factors for CV disease, such as hypertension, hyperlipidemias, obesity, and diabetes. Also use cautiously in patients with conditions aggravated by fluid retention.
● The use of contraceptives causes increased risk of MI, thromboembolism, stroke, hepatic neoplasia, gallbladder disease, and hypertension. Risk increases in patients with hypertension, diabetes, hyperlipidemia, and obesity.
● Smoking increases the risk of serious CV adverse effects. The risk increases with age (especially older than 35 years) and with heavy smoking (15 or more cigarettes daily).
● The relationship between the use of oral contraceptives and breast and cervical cancers is unclear. Encourage women to schedule a complete gynecologic examination at least yearly and to perform breast self-examinations monthly.
● In patients scheduled to have elective surgery that may increase the risk of thromboembolism, discontinue contraceptive use from at least 4 weeks before until 2 weeks after surgery. Also discontinue use during and after prolonged immobilization.
● Because of increased risk of thromboembolism in the postpartum period, don't start contraceptive use earlier than 4 to 6 weeks after delivery.
● Discontinue use and evaluate patient if loss of vision, proptosis, diplopia, papilledema, or retinal vascular lesions occur. Recommend that contact lens wearers be evaluated by an ophthalmologist if they have changes in vision or lens intolerance.

Reactions may be *common,* uncommon, *life-threatening,* or COMMON AND LIFE-THREATENING.

• If patient misses two consecutive periods, she should obtain a negative pregnancy test result before continuing contraceptive.

• Immediately discontinue use if pregnancy is confirmed.

• Monitor patient with diabetes closely. Glucose intolerance may occur.

• Monitor patient with hypertension closely. If hypertension occurs, discontinue drug.

• Monitor patient with history of depression. Discontinue use if serious depression recurs.

• In patient taking medications that may increase potassium, check potassium level during the first treatment cycle.

• Discontinue use and evaluate patient if persistent, severe headaches occur or if migraines occur or are exacerbated.

• Evaluate patient who experiences breakthrough bleeding and spotting for malignancy or pregnancy.

• Monitor patient with hyperlipidemias closely.

• Discontinue use if jaundice occurs.

PATIENT TEACHING

• Inform patient that pills are used to prevent pregnancy and don't protect against sexually transmitted diseases, such as HIV.

• Advise patient of the dangers of smoking while taking oral contraceptives. Suggest that she choose a different form of birth control if she is a smoker.

• Tell patient to schedule gynecologic examinations yearly and perform breast self-examination monthly.

• Inform patient that spotting, light bleeding, or stomach upset may occur during the first 1 to 3 packs of pills. Tell her to continue taking the pills and to notify her health care provider if these symptoms persist.

• Tell patient to take the pill at the same time each day.

• Tell patient to immediately report sharp chest pain, coughing of blood, or sudden shortness of breath; pain in the calf; crushing chest pain or chest heaviness; sudden severe headache or vomiting, dizziness or fainting, visual or speech disturbances, weakness, or numbness in an arm or leg; loss of vision; breast lumps; severe stomach pain or tenderness; difficulty sleeping, lack of energy, fatigue, or change in mood; jaundice with fever, fatigue, loss of appetite, dark urine, or light-colored bowel movements.

• Tell patient to notify health care provider if she wears contact lenses and notices a change in vision or has difficulty wearing the lenses.

• Advise patient to use additional method of birth control during the first 7 days of the first cycle of oral contraceptive.

• Tell patient to continue taking drug as directed if spotting or breakthrough bleeding occurs. If bleeding is persistent or prolonged, advise patient to notify health care provider.

• Tell patient that the risk of pregnancy increases with each active yellow tablet she forgets to take.

• If patient misses 1 tablet, tell her to take it as soon as she remembers and to take the next pill at the regular time.

• If patient misses 2 tablets during week 1 or 2 of the pack, tell her to use an additional method of birth control for 7 days. Instruct her to take 2 pills on the day she remembers and 2 pills the next day, and then to resume the normal schedule.

• If patient misses 2 tablets during week 3, tell her to use an additional method of birth control for 7 days. If patient uses the "day 1 start" method, tell her to throw away the rest of the pack and start a new pack the same day. If the patient uses the "Sunday start" method, tell her to keep taking 1 pill each day until Sunday. She should throw away the pack on Sunday and start a new pack that day. Tell patient that she may miss her period this month, but to notify health care provider if she misses it 2 months in a row because it may mean she is pregnant.

• If patient misses 3 or more tablets during the first 3 weeks, tell her to use an additional method of birth control for 7 days. If patient uses the "day 1 start" method, tell her to throw away the rest of the pack and start a new pack the same day. If the patient uses the "Sunday start" method, tell her to keep taking 1 pill each day until Sunday. She should throw away the pack on Sunday and start a new pack that day. Tell patient that she may miss her period this month, but to notify health care provider if she misses it 2 months in a row because it may mean she is pregnant.

• If patient misses any of the white tablets, tell her to throw away the missed pills and keep taking 1 pill each day until the pack is empty. She doesn't need to use an additional method of birth control.

• Tell patient to use an additional method of birth control and notify health care provider if she isn't sure what to do about missed pills.

• Small amounts of oral contraceptives are excreted in breast milk. Jaundice and breast enlargement may occur in breast-feeding infants. Drug may also interfere with lactation by decreasing the quantity and quality of breast milk. Advise use of other forms of contraception until infant is completely weaned.

---

esterified estrogens
Estratab, Menest, Neo-Estrone†

Pregnancy risk category X

AVAILABLE FORMS
Tablets: 0.3 mg, 0.625 mg, 1.25 mg, 2.5 mg
Tablets (film-coated): 0.3 mg, 0.625 mg, 1.25 mg, 2.5 mg

INDICATIONS & DOSAGES
➤ **Inoperable prostate cancer—**
Men: 1.25 to 2.5 mg P.O. t.i.d.
➤ **Breast cancer—**
Men and postmenopausal women: 10 mg P.O. t.i.d. for 3 or more months.
➤ **Female hypogonadism—**
Women: 2.5 to 7.5 mg daily in divided doses in cycles of 20 days on, 10 days off.
➤ **Castration, primary ovarian failure—**
Women: 1.25 mg daily in cycles of 3 weeks on, 1 week off. Adjust for symptoms. Can be given continuously.
➤ **Vasomotor menopausal symptoms—**
Women: Average dosage is 1.25 mg P.O. daily in cycles of 3 weeks on, 1 week off. Dosage may be increased to 2.5 to 3.75 mg P.O. daily if needed.
➤ **Atrophic vaginitis, atrophic urethritis—**
Women: 0.3 to 1.25 mg or more P.O. daily in cycles of 3 weeks on, 1 week off.

➤ **Prevention of osteoporosis (Estratab, Neo-Estrone†)—**
Women: Initially, 0.3 mg P.O. daily; may be increased to maximum of 1.25 mg daily.

ACTION
Increases synthesis of DNA, RNA, and protein in responsive tissues. Also, reduces release of follicle-stimulating and luteinizing hormones from the pituitary gland.

Route	Onset	Peak	Duration
P.O.	Unknown	Unknown	Unknown

ADVERSE REACTIONS
CNS: headache, dizziness, chorea, depression, *CVA, seizures.*
CV: thrombophlebitis, *thromboembolism,* hypertension, *edema, pulmonary embolism, MI.*
EENT: worsening myopia or astigmatism, intolerance of contact lenses.
GI: *nausea,* vomiting, abdominal cramps, bloating, anorexia, increased appetite, *pancreatitis,* increased risk of gallbladder disease.
GU: breakthrough bleeding, altered menstrual flow, dysmenorrhea, amenorrhea, *increased risk of endometrial cancer,* cervical erosion, altered cervical secretions, enlargement of uterine fibromas, vaginal candidiasis, testicular atrophy, impotence.
Hepatic: cholestatic jaundice, *hepatic adenoma.*
Metabolic: hypercalcemia, weight changes.
Skin: melasma, rash, hirsutism or hair loss, erythema nodosum, dermatitis.
Other: *breast tenderness, enlargement, or secretion; gynecomastia; possible increased risk of breast cancer.*

INTERACTIONS
Drug-drug. *Carbamazepine, fosphenytoin, phenobarbital, phenytoin, rifampin:* Decreased effectiveness of estrogen therapy. Monitor patient closely.
Corticosteroids: Possible enhanced effects. Monitor patient closely.
Cyclosporine: Increased risk of toxicity. Use together with caution, and monitor cyclosporine levels frequently.

Reactions may be *common*, uncommon, *life-threatening*, or COMMON AND LIFE-THREATENING.

Dantrolene, hepatotoxic drugs: Increased risk of hepatotoxicity. Monitor liver function closely.

Oral anticoagulants: Effect of anticoagulant may be decreased. Dosage adjustments may be needed. Monitor PT and INR.

Tamoxifen: Estrogens may interfere with tamoxifen effectiveness. Discourage use together.

Drug-herb. *Black cohosh:* Increased side effects of estrogens. Discourage use together.

Saw palmetto: Antiestrogenic effects. Discourage use together.

St. John's wort: Decreased effects of estrogens. Discourage use together.

Drug-food. *Caffeine:* May increase caffeine levels. Advise caution.

Drug-lifestyle. *Smoking:* Increased risk of CV effects. If smoking continues, may need alternative form of therapy.

EFFECTS ON LAB TEST RESULTS
● May increase calcium and clotting factor VII to X levels.
● May increase PT and norepinephrine-induced platelet aggregation.

CONTRAINDICATIONS
Contraindicated in pregnant patients, in patients hypersensitive to drug, and in patients with breast cancer (except metastatic disease), estrogen-dependent neoplasia, active thrombophlebitis, thromboembolic disorders, undiagnosed abnormal genital bleeding, or history of thromboembolic disease.

NURSING CONSIDERATIONS
● Use cautiously in patients with history of hypertension, mental depression, cardiac or renal dysfunction, liver impairment, bone disease, migraine, seizures, or diabetes mellitus.
● When used for vasomotor symptoms in menstruating women, cyclic administration is started on day 5 of bleeding.
● Make sure patient has thorough physical examination before starting estrogen therapy. Patients receiving long-term therapy should have annual examinations. Periodically monitor body weight, blood pressure, lipid levels, and hepatic function.

● Notify pathologist about patient's estrogen therapy when sending specimens to laboratory for evaluation.
● Because of risk of thromboembolism, therapy should be discontinued at least 1 month before procedures that cause prolonged immobilization or increased risk of thromboembolism, such as knee or hip surgery.
● Glucose tolerance may be impaired. Response to metyrapone test may be reduced.
● Monitor glucose closely in patients with diabetes.
● *Alert:* Don't confuse Estratab with Estratest.

PATIENT TEACHING
● Tell patient to read package insert describing estrogen's adverse effects; also, give patient verbal explanation.
● Emphasize importance of regular physical examinations. Postmenopausal women who use estrogen replacement for longer than 5 years to treat menopausal symptoms may be at increased risk for endometrial cancer. This risk is reduced by using cyclic rather than continuous therapy and the lowest possible estrogen dosage. Adding progestins to the regimen decreases risk of endometrial hyperplasia; however, it isn't known if progestins affect risk of endometrial cancer. No increased risk of breast cancer has been reported.
● *Alert:* Warn patient to immediately report abdominal pain; pain, numbness, or stiffness in legs or buttocks; pressure or pain in chest or shortness of breath; severe headaches; visual disturbances, such as blind spots, flashing lights, or blurriness; vaginal bleeding or discharge; breast lumps; swelling of hands or feet; yellow skin or sclera; dark urine; and light-colored stools.
● Tell diabetic patient to report elevated glucose levels so that antidiabetic dosage can be adjusted.
● Explain to patient on cyclic therapy for postmenopausal symptoms that she may experience withdrawal bleeding during week off drug. Tell her to report unusual vaginal bleeding.
● Teach woman to perform routine breast self-examination.

---

peanut oil; estradiol cypionate, as a solution in cottonseed oil; estradiol valerate, as a solution in castor oil or sesame oil.

● To administer I.M. injection, make sure drug is well dispersed by rolling vial between palms. Inject deeply into large muscle. Rotate injection sites to prevent muscle atrophy. Never give drug I.V.

● Apply transdermal patch to clean, dry, hairless, intact skin on abdomen or buttocks. Don't apply it to breasts, waistline, or other areas where clothing can loosen patch. When applying, ensure thorough contact between patch and skin, especially around edges, and hold in place for about 10 seconds. Apply patch immediately after opening and removing protective cover. Rotate application sites.

● In women also taking oral estrogen, treatment with the Estraderm transdermal patch can begin 1 week after withdrawal of oral therapy, sooner if menopausal symptoms appear before the end of the week.

● Transdermal systems are sometimes used on a continuous basis (not cyclic). Other alternatives are 1 to 5 mg (cypionate) I.M. q 3 to 4 weeks; or 10 to 20 mg (valerate) I.M. q 4 weeks, p.r.n.

● Because of risk of thromboembolism, therapy should be discontinued at least 1 month before procedures that cause prolonged immobilization or raise the risk of thromboembolism, such as knee or hip surgery.

● Glucose tolerance may be impaired. Monitor glucose closely in patients with diabetes. Response to metyrapone testing may be reduced.

● Notify pathologist about estrogen therapy when sending specimens to laboratory for evaluation.

PATIENT TEACHING

● Tell patient to read package insert describing estrogen's adverse effects; also, give patient verbal explanation.

● Emphasize importance of regular physical examinations. Postmenopausal women who use estrogen replacement for longer than 5 years may be at increased risk for endometrial cancer. Risk is reduced by using cyclic rather than continuous therapy and the lowest possible dosages of estrogen. Adding progestins to the regimen

decreases risk of endometrial hyperplasia; however, it isn't known if progestins affect risk of endometrial cancer. No increased risk of breast cancer has been reported.

● Teach patient how to use cream. Patient should wash vaginal area with soap and water before applying and take drug at bedtime or lie flat for 30 minutes after instillation to minimize drug loss. Vaginal cream should be inserted high into the vagina (approximately ⅔ the length of the applicator).

● Tell patient to use transdermal system correctly, to rotate sites, to avoid breasts and waistline, and to reapply patch if it falls off.

● *Alert:* Warn patient to immediately report abdominal pain; pain, numbness, or stiffness in legs or buttocks; pressure or pain in chest; shortness of breath; severe headaches; visual disturbances; vaginal bleeding or discharge; breast lumps; swelling of hands or feet; yellow skin or sclera; dark urine; and light-colored stools.

● Explain to patient on cyclic therapy for postmenopausal symptoms that withdrawal bleeding may occur during week off drug. Tell her to report unusual vaginal bleeding.

● Tell diabetic patient to report elevated glucose levels so that antidiabetic dosage can be adjusted.

● Teach woman how to perform routine breast self-examination.

● Teach patient methods to decrease risk of thromboembolism.

● Advise woman not to become pregnant during estrogen therapy.

● Advise woman of childbearing age to consult prescriber before taking drug, and to advise prescriber immediately if she becomes pregnant.

● Encourage patient to stop smoking or reduce number of cigarettes because of the risk of CV complications.

estradiol/norethindrone acetate transdermal system
Combipatch

Pregnancy risk category X

AVAILABLE FORMS
Transdermal: 9-cm² system releasing 0.05 mg estradiol and 0.14 mg norethindrone acetate per day; 16-cm² system releasing 0.05 mg estradiol and 0.25 mg norethindrone acetate per day

INDICATIONS & DOSAGES
➤ Moderate to severe vasomotor symptoms from menopause; vulvar and vaginal atrophy; hypoestrogenemia from hypogonadism, castration, or primary ovarian failure in women with intact uterus—
Women: Continuous combined regimen— 9-cm² patch worn continuously on lower abdomen. Old system should be removed and new system applied twice weekly during a 28-day cycle. May increase to 16-cm² patch.
Continuous sequential regimen— Patch can be applied as a sequential regimen with an estradiol transdermal system (such as Alora, Esclim, Estraderm, Vivelle). A 0.05 mg estradiol transdermal patch is worn for first 14 days of a 28-day cycle; replace system twice weekly. For rest of 28-day cycle, 9-cm² patch system should be worn on lower abdomen. May increase to 16-cm² patch, p.r.n.

ACTION
A matrix transdermal system in which estradiol and norethindrone are released continuously. Estrogen replacement therapy can reduce frequency of menopausal symptoms and release of follicle-stimulating and luteinizing hormones from the pituitary gland in postmenopausal women.

Route	Onset	Peak	Duration
Transdermal	12-24 hr	Unknown	3-4 days

ADVERSE REACTIONS
CNS: *asthenia,* **increased risk of CVA,** depression, insomnia, nervousness, dizziness, *headache.*

CV: ***thromboembolism,*** thrombophlebitis, hypertension, *edema,* **pulmonary embolism, MI.**
EENT: *pharyngitis, rhinitis, sinusitis.*
GI: *abdominal pain, diarrhea,* dyspepsia, flatulence, *nausea,* constipation.
GU: *dysmenorrhea, leukorrhea, menstrual disorder,* suspicious Papanicolaou smears, *vaginitis,* menorrhagia, vaginal hemorrhage.
Musculoskeletal: arthralgia, *back pain.*
Respiratory: *respiratory disorder,* bronchitis.
Skin: application site reactions, acne.
Other: *accidental injury, flu syndrome, pain, breast pain,* tooth disorder, peripheral edema, breast enlargement, infection.

INTERACTIONS
Drug-drug. *Carbamazepine, fosphenytoin, phenobarbital, phenytoin, rifampin:* Decreased effectiveness of estrogen therapy. Monitor patient closely.
Corticosteroids: Possible enhanced effects of corticosteroids. Monitor patient closely.
Cyclosporine: Increased risk of toxicity. Use together with caution, and monitor cyclosporine levels frequently.
Dantrolene, hepatotoxic drugs: Increased risk of hepatotoxicity. Monitor liver function closely.
Oral anticoagulants: Effect of anticoagulant may be decreased. Dosage adjustments may be needed. Monitor PT and INR.
Tamoxifen: Estrogens may interfere with tamoxifen effectiveness. Discourage use together.
Drug-herb. *Black cohosh:* Increased side effects of estrogens. Discourage use together.
Saw palmetto: Antiestrogenic effects. Discourage use together.
St. John's wort: Decreased effects of estrogens. Discourage use together.
Drug-food. *Caffeine:* May increase caffeine levels. Advise patient to avoid caffeine.
Grapefruit juice: Elevated estrogen levels. Advise patient to take with liquid other than grapefruit juice.
Drug-lifestyle. *Smoking:* Increased risk of adverse CV effects. If smoking continues, may need alternative therapy.

---

*Liquid contains alcohol.   **May contain tartrazine.   †Canada   ‡Australia   §U.K.   ◊OTC

EFFECTS ON LAB TEST RESULTS
None reported.

CONTRAINDICATIONS
Contraindicated in women hypersensitive to estrogen, progestin, or any component of the patch; in pregnant patients; and in patients with known or suspected breast cancer, known or suspected estrogen-dependent neoplasia, undiagnosed abnormal genital bleeding, active thrombophlebitis, thromboembolic disorders, or CVA.

NURSING CONSIDERATIONS
• Use cautiously in breast-feeding patients and in patients with impaired liver function, asthma, epilepsy, migraine, or cardiac or renal dysfunction.
• Women not receiving continuous estrogen or estrogen/progestin therapy may start therapy at any time.
• Women receiving continuous hormone replacement therapy should complete the current cycle before starting therapy. Women commonly have withdrawal bleeding at completion of cycle; first day of withdrawal bleeding would be an appropriate time to start therapy.
• Store norethindrone patches in refrigerator before dispensing. Patient may then store patches at room temperature for up to 3 months.
• Advise patient not to store patches where extreme temperatures can occur.
• Reevaluate therapy at 3- to 6-month intervals. Combination estrogen/progestin regimens are indicated for women with intact uterus.
• Progestins taken with estrogen significantly reduce, but don't eliminate, risk of endometrial cancer linked to use of estrogen.
• Blood pressure increases have been linked to estrogen use. Monitor patient's blood pressure regularly.
• Treatment of postmenopausal symptoms usually starts during menopausal stage when vasomotor symptoms occur.
• Apply patch system to a smooth (fold-free), clean, dry, nonirritated area of skin on lower abdomen, avoiding the waistline. Application sites should be rotated, with an interval of at least 1 week between applications to same site.
• Don't apply patch on or near breasts.

• Avoid applying to areas that may get prolonged sun exposure.
• Reapply system, if needed, to another area of lower abdomen. If system fails to adhere, replace with a new one.
• INR, activated PTT, and platelet aggregation times may be altered; platelet count and fibrinogen activity may increase. Increased thyroid-binding globulin may lead to increased T_3 and T_4 levels and decreased T_3 resin uptake. Total cholesterol, high-density lipoprotein cholesterol, low-density lipoprotein cholesterol, and triglyceride levels may also decrease.
• Glucose tolerance test may be impaired. Monitor glucose closely in patients with diabetes.
• Response to metyrapone testing may be reduced.
• **Alert:** Don't interchange CombiPatch with other estrogen patches. Verify therapy before application.

PATIENT TEACHING
• Teach patient how to apply system properly. Only one system should be worn at any time during the dosing intervals. Apply patch immediately after opening protective cover.
• Tell patient an oil-based cream or lotion may help remove adhesive from the skin once system has been removed and the area allowed to dry for 15 minutes.
• Advise patient not to use patch if she's pregnant or plans to become pregnant.
• Urge woman of childbearing age to consult prescriber before taking drug and to advise prescriber immediately if she becomes pregnant.
• Instruct patient that the continuous combined regimen may lead to irregular bleeding, particularly in the first 6 months, but that it usually decreases with time, often to an amenorrheic state.
• Tell patient that, for the continuous sequential regimen, monthly withdrawal bleeding is common.
• Advise patient to alert prescriber and remove patch at first sign of thrombotic disorders (thrombophlebitis, cerebrovascular disorders, and pulmonary embolism).
• Instruct patient to discontinue patch and call prescriber about any loss of vision, sudden onset of proptosis (protrusion of the eyeball), double vision, or migraine.

• Encourage patient to stop smoking or reduce number of cigarettes because of the risk of CV complications.

estrogens, conjugated (estrogenic substances, conjugated; oestrogens, conjugated)
C.E.S.†, Premarin, Premarin Intravenous

Pregnancy risk category X

AVAILABLE FORMS
Injection: 25 mg/5 ml
Tablets: 0.3 mg, 0.625 mg, 0.9 mg, 1.25 mg, 2.5 mg
Vaginal cream: 0.625 mg/g

INDICATIONS & DOSAGES
➤ **Abnormal uterine bleeding (hormonal imbalance)—**
Women: 25 mg I.V. or I.M., repeated in 6 to 12 hours, p.r.n.
➤ **Palliative treatment of breast cancer (at least 5 years after menopause)—**
Men and postmenopausal women: 10 mg P.O. t.i.d. for 3 months or more.
➤ **Female castration, primary ovarian failure—**
Women: 1.25 mg P.O. daily in cycles of 3 weeks on and 1 week off. Can be given continuously.
➤ **Osteoporosis—**
Postmenopausal women: 0.625 mg P.O. daily in cyclic regimen (3 weeks on, 1 week off). Can be given continuously.
➤ **Hypogonadism—**
Women: 2.5 to 7.5 mg daily in divided doses for 20 days followed by 10 days off.
➤ **Vasomotor menopausal symptoms—**
Women: 0.3 to 1.25 mg P.O. daily in cycles of 3 weeks on and 1 week off. Can be given continuously.
➤ **Atrophic vaginitis, kraurosis vulvae—**
Women: 0.5 to 2 g intravaginally once daily on a cyclical basis (3 weeks on and 1 week off).
➤ **Palliative treatment of inoperable prostate cancer—**
Men: 1.25 to 2.5 mg P.O. t.i.d.

I.V. ADMINISTRATION
• Refrigerate before reconstituting. Reconstitute only with diluent provided. Agitate gently after adding diluent. Drug is compatible with normal saline, dextrose, or invert sugar solutions. I.V. solution isn't compatible with protein hydrolysate, ascorbic acid, or solutions with an acid pH.
• Use reconstituted solution within a few hours. Don't use parenteral preparations if darkening or precipitation is noted.
• When giving drug by direct I.V. injection, administer slowly to avoid flushing reaction.

ACTION
Increases synthesis of DNA, RNA, and protein in responsive tissues. Also reduces release of follicle-stimulating and luteinizing hormones from the pituitary gland.

Route	Onset	Peak	Duration
I.M., intra-vaginal, I.V., P.O.	Unknown	Unknown	Unknown

ADVERSE REACTIONS
CNS: headache, dizziness, chorea, depression, *increased risk of CVA, seizures.*
CV: flushing with rapid I.V. administration; thrombophlebitis; *thromboembolism;* hypertension; *edema; pulmonary embolism, MI.*
EENT: worsening myopia or astigmatism, intolerance of contact lenses.
GI: *nausea,* vomiting, abdominal cramps, bloating, anorexia, increased appetite, *pancreatitis,* gallbladder disease.
GU: breakthrough bleeding, altered menstrual flow, dysmenorrhea, amenorrhea, *increased risk of endometrial cancer,* cervical erosion, altered cervical secretions, enlargement of uterine fibromas, vaginal candidiasis, testicular atrophy, impotence.
Hepatic: cholestatic jaundice, *hepatic adenoma.*
Metabolic: weight changes.
Skin: melasma, urticaria, hirsutism or hair loss, erythema nodosum, dermatitis.
Other: *breast tenderness, enlargement, or secretion; gynecomastia; possible increased risk of breast cancer.*

INTERACTIONS
Drug-drug. *Carbamazepine, fosphenytoin, phenobarbital, phenytoin, rifampin:* Decreased effectiveness of estrogen therapy. Monitor patient closely.
Corticosteroids: May enhance corticosteroid effects. Monitor patient closely.
Cyclosporine: Increased risk of toxicity. Use together with caution, and monitor cyclosporine levels frequently.
Dantrolene, other hepatotoxic drugs: Increased risk of hepatotoxicity. Monitor liver function closely.
Oral anticoagulants: Effect of anticoagulant may be decreased. Dosage adjustments may be needed. Monitor PT and INR.
Tamoxifen: Estrogens may interfere with tamoxifen effectiveness. Discourage use together.
Drug-herb. *Black cohosh:* Increased side effects of estrogens. Discourage use together.
Red clover: May interfere with hormonal therapies. Discourage use together.
Saw palmetto: Antiestrogenic effects. Discourage use together.
St. John's wort: Decreased effects of estrogens. Discourage use together.
Drug-food. *Caffeine:* May increase caffeine levels. Advise caution.
Drug-lifestyle. *Smoking:* Increased risk of adverse CV effects. If smoking continues, may need alternative therapy.

EFFECTS ON LAB TEST RESULTS
• May increase clotting factor VII to X, total T_4, thyroid-binding globulin, phospholipid, and triglyceride levels.
• May increase PT and norepinephrine-induced platelet aggregation.

CONTRAINDICATIONS
Contraindicated in pregnant patients and in patients with thrombophlebitis, thromboembolic disorders, estrogen-dependent neoplasia, breast or reproductive cancer (except for palliative treatment), or undiagnosed abnormal genital bleeding.

NURSING CONSIDERATIONS
• Use cautiously in patients with cerebrovascular or coronary artery disease, asthma, bone disease, migraine, seizures, or cardiac, hepatic, or renal dysfunction.

Also, use cautiously in women with family history (mother, grandmother, sister) of breast or genital tract cancer or who have breast nodules, fibrocystic breasts, or abnormal mammogram findings.
• Make sure patient has thorough physical examination before starting estrogen therapy. Patients receiving long-term therapy should have annual examinations. Periodically monitor lipid levels, blood pressure, body weight, and hepatic function.
• Rapid treatment of dysfunctional uterine bleeding or reduction of surgical bleeding usually demands delivery by I.M. or I.V. route.
• When administering by I.M. injection, inject deeply into large muscle. Rotate injection sites to prevent muscle atrophy.
• Notify pathologist about estrogen therapy when sending specimens to laboratory for evaluation.
• Because of risk of thromboembolism, therapy should be discontinued at least 1 month before procedures that cause prolonged immobilization or raise the risk of thromboembolism, such as knee or hip surgery.
• Glucose tolerance may be impaired. Monitor glucose closely in patients with diabetes.
• Response to metyrapone testing may be reduced.
• ***Alert:*** Don't confuse Premarin with Primaxin.

PATIENT TEACHING
• Tell patient to read package insert describing estrogen's adverse effects; also, explain effects verbally.
• Emphasize importance of regular physical examinations. Postmenopausal women who use estrogen replacement for longer than 5 years to treat menopausal symptoms may be at increased risk for endometrial cancer. This risk is reduced by using cyclic rather than continuous therapy and lowest possible estrogen dosage. Adding progestins to the regimen decreases risk of endometrial hyperplasia; however, it isn't known if progestins affect risk of endometrial cancer. No increased risk of breast cancer has been reported.
• Teach patient how to use vaginal cream. Patient should wash the vaginal area with soap and water before applying. Tell her to

use drug at bedtime or to lie flat for 30 minutes after instillation to minimize drug loss. Vaginal cream should be inserted high into the vagina (about ⅔ of the length of the applicator).

• Explain to patient that cyclic therapy for postmenopausal symptoms may cause withdrawal bleeding during week off drug. Tell her to report unusual vaginal bleeding.

• *Alert:* Warn patient to immediately report abdominal pain; pain, numbness, or stiffness in legs or buttocks; pressure or pain in chest; shortness of breath; severe headaches; visual disturbances, such as blind spots, flashing lights, or blurriness; vaginal bleeding or discharge; breast lumps; swelling of hands or feet; yellow skin or sclera; dark urine; and light-colored stools.

• Tell diabetic patient to report elevated glucose levels so that antidiabetic dosage can be adjusted.

• Teach woman how to perform routine breast self-examination.

• Advise patient not to become pregnant during estrogen therapy.

• Advise woman of childbearing age to consult prescriber before taking drug, and to advise prescriber immediately if she becomes pregnant.

• Encourage patient to stop smoking or reduce number of cigarettes because of the risk of CV complications.

---

estropiate (piperazine estrone sulfate)
Harmogen§, Ogen, Ortho-Est

Pregnancy risk category X

AVAILABLE FORMS
Tablets: 0.75 mg, 1.5 mg, 3 mg, 6 mg
Vaginal cream: 1.5 mg/g

INDICATIONS & DOSAGES
➤ **Vulvar and vaginal atrophy—**
Women: 0.75 to 6 mg P.O. daily, 3 weeks on and 1 week off; or 2 to 4 g vaginal cream daily. Typically, drug is given on a cyclic, short-term basis. Can be given continuously.

➤ **Primary ovarian failure, female castration, female hypogonadism—**
Women: Given cyclically, 1.5 to 9 mg P.O. daily for first 3 weeks; then a rest period of 8 to 10 days. If bleeding doesn't occur by end of rest period, cycle is repeated. Can be given continuously.

➤ **Vasomotor menopausal symptoms—**
Women: 0.75 to 6 mg P.O. daily in cyclic method, 3 weeks on and 1 week off. Can be given continuously.

➤ **Prevention of osteoporosis—**
Women: 0.625 mg (0.75 mg estropipate) tablet P.O. daily for 25 days of a 31-day cycle.

ACTION
Increases synthesis of DNA, RNA, and proteins in responsive tissues. Also reduces release of follicle-stimulating and luteinizing hormones from the pituitary gland.

Route	Onset	Peak	Duration
Intravaginal, P.O.	Unknown	Unknown	Unknown

ADVERSE REACTIONS
CNS: depression, headache, dizziness, migraine, *seizures, increased risk of CVA.*
CV: *edema;* thrombophlebitis, *increased risk of pulmonary embolism and MI, thromboembolism.*
GI: nausea, vomiting, gallbladder disease, abdominal cramps, bloating.
GU: increased size of uterine fibromas, *increased risk of endometrial cancer,* vaginal candidiasis, cystitis-like syndrome, dysmenorrhea, amenorrhea, breakthrough bleeding, condition resembling premenstrual syndrome.
Hepatic: cholestatic jaundice, *hepatic adenoma.*
Metabolic: weight changes.
Skin: hemorrhagic eruption, erythema nodosum, *erythema multiforme,* hirsutism or hair loss, melasma.
Other: breast engorgement or enlargement; *possible increased risk of breast cancer.*

INTERACTIONS
Drug-drug. *Carbamazepine, fosphenytoin, phenobarbital, phenytoin, rifampin:*

Decreased effectiveness of estrogen therapy. Monitor patient closely.

Corticosteroids: Possible enhanced effects of corticosteroids. Monitor patient closely.

Cyclosporine: Increased risk of toxicity. Use together with caution and frequently monitor cyclosporine levels.

Dantrolene, other hepatotoxic drugs: Increased risk of hepatotoxicity. Monitor liver function closely.

Oral anticoagulants: Effect of anticoagulant may be decreased. Dosage adjustments may be needed. Monitor PT and INR.

Tamoxifen: Estrogens may interfere with tamoxifen effectiveness. Discourage use together.

Drug-herb. *Black cohosh:* Increased side effects of estrogens. Discourage use together.

Red clover: May interfere with hormonal therapies. Discourage use together.

Saw palmetto: Antiestrogenic effects. Discourage use together.

St. John's wort: Decreased effects of estrogens. Discourage use together.

Drug-food. *Caffeine:* May increase caffeine levels. Advise caution.

Drug-lifestyle. *Smoking:* Increased risk of adverse CV effects. If smoking continues, may need alternative therapy.

EFFECTS ON LAB TEST RESULTS
• May increase clotting factor VII to X, total T_4, thyroid-binding globulin, phospholipid, and triglyceride levels.
• May increase PT and norepinephrine-induced platelet aggregation.

CONTRAINDICATIONS
Contraindicated in pregnant patients and those with active thrombophlebitis, thromboembolic disorders, estrogen-dependent neoplasia, undiagnosed genital bleeding, and breast, reproductive organ, or genital cancer.

NURSING CONSIDERATIONS
• Use cautiously in patients with cerebrovascular or coronary artery disease, asthma, mental depression, bone disease, migraine, seizures, or cardiac, hepatic, or renal dysfunction. Also, use cautiously in women with family history (mother, grandmother, sister) of breast or genital

tract cancer or who have breast nodules, fibrocystic breasts, or abnormal mammogram findings.
• Make sure patient has thorough physical examination before starting estrogen therapy. Patients receiving long-term therapy should have examinations yearly. Periodically monitor lipid levels, blood pressure, body weight, and hepatic function.
• When used to treat hypogonadism, duration of therapy needed to produce withdrawal bleeding depends on patient's endometrial response to drug. If satisfactory withdrawal bleeding doesn't occur, an oral progestin is added to the regimen. Explain to patient that, despite return of withdrawal bleeding, pregnancy can't occur because she doesn't ovulate.
• Estropipate/estrone equivalents are:
0.75 mg estropipate = 0.625 mg estrone
1.5 mg estropipate = 1.25 mg estrone
3 mg estropipate = 2.5 mg estrone
6 mg estropipate = 5 mg estrone.
• May give with meals to minimize GI upset.
• Because of risk of thromboembolism, therapy should be discontinued at least 1 month before procedures that cause prolonged immobilization or raise the risk of thromboembolism, such as knee or hip surgery.
• Glucose tolerance may be impaired. Monitor glucose closely in patients with diabetes.
• Response to metyrapone testing may be reduced.

PATIENT TEACHING
• Tell patient to read package insert describing estrogen's adverse effects; also, explain effects verbally.
• Teach patient how to use vaginal cream. Patient should wash the vaginal area with soap and water before applying. Tell her to use drug at bedtime or to lie flat for 30 minutes after instillation to minimize drug loss. Vaginal cream should be inserted high into the vagina (about ⅔ of the length of the applicator).
• Tell diabetic patient to report elevated glucose levels to prescriber.
• Stress importance of regular physical examinations. Postmenopausal women who use estrogen replacement for longer than 5 years may have increased risk of endome-

trial cancer. Using cyclic therapy and lowest possible estrogen dosage reduces risk. Adding progestins to regimen decreases risk of endometrial hyperplasia; however, it isn't known if progestins affect risk of endometrial cancer. No increased risk of breast cancer has been reported.

• *Alert:* Warn patient to immediately report abdominal pain; pain, stiffness, or numbness in legs or buttocks; pressure or pain in chest; shortness of breath; severe headaches; visual disturbances, such as blind spots or flashing lights; vaginal bleeding or discharge; breast lumps; swelling of hands or feet; yellow skin or sclera; dark urine; and light-colored stools.

• Teach woman how to perform routine breast self-examination.

• Advise patient not to become pregnant while on estrogen therapy.

• Encourage patient to stop smoking or reduce number of cigarettes because of the risk of CV complications.

• Advise woman of childbearing age to consult prescriber before taking drug, and to tell prescriber immediately if she becomes pregnant.

ethinyl estradiol (ethinyloestradiol)
Estinyl**

Pregnancy risk category X

AVAILABLE FORMS
Tablets: 0.02 mg, 0.05 mg, 0.5 mg

INDICATIONS & DOSAGES
➤ **Palliative treatment of metastatic breast cancer (at least 5 years after menopause)—**
Women: 1 mg P.O. t.i.d. for at least 3 months.
➤ **Female hypogonadism—**
Women: 0.05 mg P.O. once daily to t.i.d. 2 weeks per month; then 2 weeks of progesterone therapy. Continued for 3 to 6 monthly dosing cycles; then 2 months off. Can be given continuously.
➤ **Vasomotor menopausal symptoms—**
Women: 0.02 to 0.05 mg P.O. daily for cycles of 3 weeks on and 1 week off. Can be given continuously.

➤ **Palliative treatment of metastatic inoperable prostate cancer—**
Men: 0.15 to 2 mg P.O. daily.

ACTION
Increases synthesis of DNA, RNA, and protein in responsive tissues. Also reduces release of follicle-stimulating and luteinizing hormones from the pituitary gland.

Route	Onset	Peak	Duration
P.O.	Unknown	Unknown	Unknown

ADVERSE REACTIONS
CNS: *increased risk of CVA,* headache, dizziness, chorea, depression, *seizures.*
CV: thrombophlebitis, *thromboembolism,* hypertension, *edema, pulmonary embolism, MI.*
EENT: worsening myopia or astigmatism, intolerance to contact lenses.
GI: *nausea,* vomiting, gallbladder disease, abdominal cramps, bloating, anorexia, increased appetite.
GU: breakthrough bleeding, altered menstrual flow, dysmenorrhea, amenorrhea, cervical erosion, *increased risk of endometrial cancer,* altered cervical secretions, enlargement of uterine fibromas, vaginal candidiasis; testicular atrophy, impotence in men.
Hepatic: cholestatic jaundice, *hepatic adenoma.*
Metabolic: weight changes.
Skin: melasma, urticaria, acne, seborrhea, oily skin, hirsutism or hair loss, erythema nodosum, dermatitis.
Other: *breast tenderness, enlargement, or secretion; possible increased risk of breast cancer;* gynecomastia.

INTERACTIONS
Drug-drug. *Carbamazepine, fosphenytoin, phenobarbital, phenytoin, rifampin:* Decreased effectiveness of estrogen therapy. Monitor patient closely.
Corticosteroids: May enhance effects of corticosteroids. Monitor patient closely.
Cyclosporine: Increased risk of toxicity. Use together cautiously, and monitor cyclosporine levels frequently.
Dantrolene, other hepatotoxic drugs: Increased risk of hepatotoxicity. Monitor liver function closely.

Oral anticoagulants: May decrease effects of anticoagulant. Dosage adjustments may be needed. Monitor PT and INR.

Tamoxifen: Estrogens may interfere with effectiveness of tamoxifen. Avoid using together.

Drug-herb. *Black cohosh:* Increased side effects of estrogens. Discourage use together.

Saw palmetto: Antiestrogenic effects. Discourage use together.

St. John's wort: Decreased effects of estrogens. Discourage use together.

Drug-food. *Caffeine:* May increase caffeine levels. Advise patient to avoid caffeine.

Grapefruit juice: Elevated estrogen levels. Advise patient to take with liquid other than grapefruit juice.

Drug-lifestyle. *Smoking:* Increased risk of adverse CV effects. If smoking continues, may need alternative therapy.

EFFECTS ON LAB TEST RESULTS
● May increase clotting factor VII to X, total T_4, thyroid-binding globulin, phospholipid, and triglyceride levels.
● May increase PT and norepinephrine-induced platelet aggregation. May decrease antithrombin III activity.

CONTRAINDICATIONS
Contraindicated in pregnant patients and in those with thrombophlebitis, thromboembolic disorders, estrogen-dependent neoplasia, breast or reproductive organ cancer (except for palliative treatment), or undiagnosed abnormal genital bleeding.

NURSING CONSIDERATIONS
● Use cautiously in patients with cerebrovascular or coronary artery disease, asthma, depression, bone disease, or cardiac, hepatic, or renal dysfunction. Also, use cautiously in women with family history (mother, grandmother, sister) of breast or genital tract cancer or who have breast nodules, fibrocystic breasts, or abnormal mammogram findings.
● Make sure patient has thorough physical examination before starting estrogen therapy. Patients receiving long-term therapy should have examinations yearly. Periodically monitor lipid levels, blood pressure, body weight, and hepatic function.

● Because of risk of thromboembolism, therapy should be discontinued at least 1 month before procedures that cause prolonged immobilization or raise the risk of thromboembolism, such as knee or hip surgery.
● Notify pathologist about estrogen therapy when sending specimens to laboratory for evaluation.
● Glucose tolerance may be impaired. Monitor glucose closely in patients with diabetes.
● Response to metyrapone testing may be reduced.

PATIENT TEACHING
● Tell patient to read package insert describing estrogen's adverse effects; also, give verbal explanation.
● Emphasize importance of regular physical examinations. Postmenopausal women who use estrogen replacement for longer than 5 years to treat menopausal symptoms may be at increased risk for endometrial cancer. This risk is reduced by using cyclic rather than continuous therapy and the lowest possible dosages of estrogen. Adding progestins to the regimen decreases risk of endometrial hyperplasia; however, it isn't known if progestins affect risk of endometrial cancer. No increased risk of breast cancer has been reported.
● Explain to patient that cyclic therapy for postmenopausal symptoms may cause withdrawal bleeding during week off drug. Tell her to report unusual vaginal bleeding.
● *Alert:* Warn patient to immediately report abdominal pain; pain, numbness, or stiffness in legs or buttocks; pressure or pain in chest; shortness of breath; severe headaches; visual disturbances such as blind spots, flashing lights, or blurriness; vaginal bleeding or discharge; breast lumps; swelling of hands or feet; yellow skin or sclera; dark urine; or light-colored stools.
● Tell diabetic patient to report elevated glucose levels; antidiabetic dosage may be adjusted.
● Teach woman how to perform routine breast self-examination.
● Teach patient methods to decrease risk of thromboembolism.

Reactions may be *common*, uncommon, *life-threatening*, or COMMON AND LIFE-THREATENING.

• Encourage patient to stop smoking or reduce number of cigarettes because of the
risk of CV complications.

___

ethinyl estradiol and desogestrel
monophasic: Desogen, Marvelon§,
Ortho-Cept

biphasic: Mircette

ethinyl estradiol and ethynodiol diacetate
monophasic: Demulen 1/35,
Demulen 1/50, Zovia 1/35E, Zovia
1/50E

ethinyl estradiol and levonorgestrel
monophasic: Alesse-21, Alesse-
28, Aviane, Levlen, Levora-21,
Levora-28, Nordette-21, Nordette-
28

biphasic: Preven Emergency
Contraceptive Kit

triphasic: Microgynon-30§, Ovran-
30§, Ovranette§, Tri-Levlen,
Triphasil, Trivora-28

ethinyl estradiol and norethindrone
monophasic: Brevicon, Genora
0.5/35, ModiCon,
N.E.E. 1/35, Necon 1/35-21,
Necon 1/35-28, Necon 0.5/35-21,
Necon 0.5/35-28, Nelova 0.5/35E,
Nelova 1/35E, Norethin 1/35E,
Norinyl 1 + 35, Ortho-Novum 1/35,
Ovcon-35, Ovcon-50

biphasic: Jenest, Necon 10/11-21,
Necon 10/11-28, Nelova 10/11,
Ortho-Novum 10/11

triphasic: Ortho-Novum 7/7/7, Tri-
Norinyl

ethinyl estradiol and norethindrone acetate
monophasic: Loestrin 1/20,
Loestrin 1.5/30

triphasic: Estrostep 21, Estrostep
Fe

ethinyl estradiol and norgestimate
monophasic: Ortho-Cyclen

triphasic: Ortho Tri-Cyclen

ethinyl estradiol and norgestrel
monophasic: Lo/Ovral, Ovral

ethinyl estradiol, norethindrone acetate, and ferrous fumarate
monophasic: Loestrin Fe 1/20,
Loestrin Fe 1.5/30

mestranol and norethindrone
monophasic: Genora 1/50, Necon
1/50-21, Necon 1/50-28, Nelova
1/50M, Norethin 1/50M, Norinyl
1+50, Ortho-Novum 1/50

Pregnancy risk category X

___

AVAILABLE FORMS
Monophasic oral contraceptives:
ethinyl estradiol and desogestrel
Tablets: ethinyl estradiol 30 mcg and desogestrel 0.15 mg (Desogen, Ortho-Cept)
ethinyl estradiol and ethynodiol diacetate
Tablets: ethinyl estradiol 35 mcg and
ethynodiol diacetate 1 mg (Demulen
1/35); ethinyl estradiol 50 mcg and ethynodiol diacetate 1 mg (Demulen 1/50);
ethinyl estradiol 35 mcg and ethynodiol
diacetate 1 mg (Zovia 1/35E); ethinyl
estradiol 50 mcg and ethynodiol diacetate
1 mg (Zovia 1/50E)
ethinyl estradiol and levonorgestrel
Tablets: ethinyl estradiol 30 mcg and levonorgestrel 0.15 mg (Levlen, Levora,
Microgynon-30, Ovran-30, Ovranette,
Nordette-21, Nordette-28); ethinyl estradiol 20 mg and levonorgestrel 0.1 mg
(Alesse-21, Alesse-28, Aviane); ethinyl
estradiol 50 mcg and levonorgestrel
0.25 mg (Emergency Contraceptive Kit)
ethinyl estradiol and norethindrone
Tablets: ethinyl estradiol 35 mcg and
norethindrone 0.4 mg (Ovcon-35); ethinyl
estradiol 35 mcg and norethindrone
0.5 mg (Brevicon, Genora 0.5/35, Modi-
Con, Necon 0.5/35-21, Necon 0.5/35-28,
Nelova 0.5/35E); ethinyl estradiol 35 mcg

___

and norethindrone 1 mg (Genora 1/35, N.E.E. 1/35, Necon 1/35-21, Necon 1/35-28, Nelova 1/35E, Norethin 1/35E, Norinyl 1/35, Ortho-Novum 1/35); ethinyl estradiol 50 mcg and norethindrone 1 mg (Ovcon-50)

ethinyl estradiol and norethindrone acetate

Tablets: ethinyl estradiol 20 mcg and norethindrone acetate 1 mg (Loestrin 1/20); ethinyl estradiol 30 mcg and norethindrone acetate 1.5 mg (Loestrin 1.5/30)

ethinyl estradiol and norgestimate

Tablets: ethinyl estradiol 35 mcg and norgestimate 0.25 mg (Ortho-Cyclen)

ethinyl estradiol and norgestrel

Tablets: ethinyl estradiol 30 mcg and norgestrel 0.3 mg (Lo/Ovral); ethinyl estradiol 50 mcg and norgestrel 0.5 mg (Ovral)

ethinyl estradiol, norethindrone acetate, and ferrous fumarate

Tablets: ethinyl estradiol 20 mcg, norethindrone acetate 1 mg, and ferrous fumarate 75 mg (Loestrin Fe 1/20); ethinyl estradiol 30 mcg, norethindrone acetate 1.5 mg, and ferrous fumarate 75 mg (Loestrin Fe 1.5/30)

mestranol and norethindrone

Tablets: mestranol 50 mcg and norethindrone 1 mg (Genora 1/50, Nelova 1/50M, Norethin 1/50M, Norinyl 1/50, Ortho-Novum 1/50)

Biphasic oral contraceptives:
ethinyl estradiol and norethindrone

Tablets: ethinyl estradiol 35 mcg and norethindrone 0.5 mg during phase 1 (10 days); ethinyl estradiol 35 mcg and norethindrone 1 mg during phase 2 (11 days) (Jenest, Necon 10/11-21, Necon 10/11-28, Nelova 10/11, Ortho-Novum 10/11)

ethinyl estradiol and desogestrel

Tablets: ethinyl estradiol 50 mcg and desogestrel 0.15 mg during phase 1 (21 days) and ethinyl estradiol 10 mcg during phase 2 (5 days) (Mircette)

Triphasic oral contraceptives
ethinyl estradiol and levonorgestrel

Tablets: (Tri-Levlen, Triphasil, Trivora-28) ethinyl estradiol 30 mcg and levonorgestrel 0.05 mg during phase 1 (6 days); ethinyl estradiol 40 mcg and levonorgestrel 0.075 mg during phase 2 (5 days);

ethinyl estradiol 30 mcg and levonorgestrel 0.125 mg during phase 3 (10 days); ethinyl estradiol 30 mcg and levonorgestrel 0.15 mg (Microgynon-30§, Ovran-30§, Ovranette§)

ethinyl estradiol and norethindrone

Tablets: (Tri-Norinyl) ethinyl estradiol 35 mcg and norethindrone 0.5 mg during phase 1 (7 days); ethinyl estradiol 35 mcg and norethindrone 1 mg during phase 2 (9 days); ethinyl estradiol 35 mcg and norethindrone 0.5 mg during phase 3 (5 days); (Ortho-Novum 7/7/7) ethinyl estradiol 35 mcg and norethindrone 0.5 mg during phase 1 (7 days); ethinyl estradiol 35 mcg and norethindrone 0.75 mg during phase 2 (7 days); ethinyl estradiol 35 mcg and norethindrone 1 mg during phase 3 (7 days)

ethinyl estradiol and norethindrone acetate

Tablets: (Estrostep21, Estrostep Fe) ethinyl estradiol 20 mcg and norethindrone acetate 1 mg during phase 1 (5 days); ethinyl estradiol 30 mcg and norethindrone acetate 1 mg during phase 2 (7 days); and ethinyl estradiol 35 mcg and norethindrone acetate 1 mg during phase 3 (9 days). Estrostep Fe contains 7 brown 75-mg ferrous fumarate tablets

ethinyl estradiol and norgestimate

Tablets: (Ortho Tri-Cyclen) ethinyl estradiol 35 mcg and norgestimate 0.18 mg during phase 1 (7 days); ethinyl estradiol 35 mcg and norgestimate 0.215 mg during phase 2 (7 days); ethinyl estradiol 35 mcg and norgestimate 0.25 mg during phase 3 (7 days)

INDICATIONS & DOSAGES
➤**Contraception**—

Women: Monophasic oral contraceptives—1 tablet P.O. daily beginning on day 5 of menstrual cycle (first day of menstrual flow is day 1). With 20- and 21-tablet packages, new dosing cycle begins 7 days after last tablet taken. With 28-tablet packages, dosage is 1 tablet daily without interruption; extra tablets taken on days 22 to 28 are placebos or contain iron.

Biphasic oral contraceptives—1 color tablet P.O. daily for 10 days; then next color tablet for 11 days. With 21-tablet packages, new dosing cycle begins 7 days after last tablet taken. With 28-tablet packages, dose is 1 tablet daily without interruption. *Triphasic oral contraceptives*—1 tablet P.O. daily in the sequence specified by the brand. With 21-tablet packages, new dosing cycle begins 7 days after last tablet taken. With 28-tablet packages, dose is 1 tablet daily without interruption.

➤ **Prevention of pregnancy**—
Women: Preven Emergency Contraceptive Kit, 2 tablets P.O. within 72 hours of unprotected intercourse; a second dose is taken 12 hours after the first dose.

➤ **Acne vulgaris**—
Women: 1 tablet P.O. daily, using the 28-day package of Ortho Tri-Cyclen. For acne, Ortho Tri-Cyclen dosage should follow the same guidelines as when used for contraception.

ACTION
Oral contraceptives inhibit ovulation through a negative feedback mechanism directed at the hypothalamus. They also may prevent transport of the ovum through the fallopian tubes.

Estrogen suppresses secretion of follicle-stimulating hormone, blocking follicular development and ovulation.

Progestin suppresses secretion of luteinizing hormone so that ovulation can't occur even if the follicle develops. Progestin thickens cervical mucus, which interferes with sperm migration and causes endometrial changes that prevent implantation of the fertilized ovum.

Route	Onset	Peak	Duration
P.O.	Unknown	0.5-4 hr	Unknown

ADVERSE REACTIONS
CNS: *headache, dizziness,* depression, lethargy, migraine, *CVA.*
CV: *thromboembolism,* hypertension, edema, *pulmonary embolism.*
EENT: worsening myopia or astigmatism, intolerance of contact lenses, exophthalmos, diplopia.
GI: *nausea,* vomiting, abdominal cramps, bloating, anorexia, changes in appetite, gallbladder disease, *pancreatitis.*
GU: *breakthrough bleeding, spotting,* granulomatous colitis, dysmenorrhea, amenorrhea, cervical erosion or abnormal secretions, enlargement of uterine fibromas, vaginal candidiasis.
Hepatic: cholestatic jaundice, *liver tumors.*
Metabolic: weight gain.
Skin: rash, acne, *erythema multiforme.*
Other: breast tenderness, enlargement, or secretion.

INTERACTIONS
Drug-drug. *Beta blockers:* Increased levels of beta blockers. Dosage adjustments may be necessary.
Carbamazepine, fosphenytoin, phenobarbital, phenytoin, rifampin: Decreased effectiveness of estrogen therapy. Use cautiously.
Corticosteroids: May enhance effects of corticosteroids. Monitor patient closely.
Griseofulvin, penicillins, sulfonamides, tetracyclines: May decrease effectiveness of oral contraceptives. Avoid using together, if possible.
Insulin, sulfonylureas: Glucose intolerance may decrease effects of antidiabetics. Monitor effects.
Oral anticoagulants: Anticoagulant effect may be decreased. Dosage adjustments may be needed. Monitor PT and INR.
Tamoxifen: Estrogens may interfere with effectiveness of tamoxifen. Discourage use together.
Drug-herb. *Black cohosh:* Increased side effects of estrogens. Discourage use together.
Red clover: May interfere with hormonal therapies. Discourage use together.
Saw palmetto: Antiestrogenic effects. Discourage use together.
St. John's wort: May decrease efficacy of the oral contraceptive because of increased hepatic metabolism. Discourage use together. If such use cannot be avoided, advise patient to use an additional method of contraception.
Drug-food. *Caffeine:* May increase caffeine levels. Advise caution.
Grapefruit juice: Elevated estrogen levels. Advise patient to take with liquid other than grapefruit juice.
Drug-lifestyle. *Smoking:* Increased risk of adverse CV effects. If smoking continues, may need alternative therapy.

EFFECTS ON LAB TEST RESULTS
• May increase fibrinogen, triglyceride, total T_4, thyroid-binding globulin, plasminogen, and clotting factor II, VII to X, and XII levels.
• May increase PT, phospholipid concentrations, and norepinephrine-induced platelet aggregation.

CONTRAINDICATIONS
Contraindicated in patients with thromboembolic disorders, cerebrovascular or coronary artery disease, diplopia or ocular lesions arising from ophthalmic vascular disease, classic migraine, MI, known or suspected breast cancer, known or suspected estrogen-dependent neoplasia, benign or malignant liver tumors, active liver disease or history of cholestatic jaundice with pregnancy or previous use of oral contraceptives, and undiagnosed abnormal vaginal bleeding. Also, contraindicated in known or suspected pregnancy and in breast-feeding women.

NURSING CONSIDERATIONS
• Use cautiously in patients with hyperlipidemia, hypertension, migraines, seizure disorders, asthma, or cardiac, renal, or hepatic insufficiency.
• Estrogen-containing oral contraceptives should be used with caution in patients who smoke.
• Triphasic oral contraceptives may cause fewer adverse reactions, such as breakthrough bleeding and spotting.
• The Centers for Disease Control and Prevention reports that use of oral contraceptives may decrease ovarian and endometrial cancers. Also, oral contraceptives don't appear to increase woman's risk of breast cancer. However, the FDA reports that oral contraceptives may be linked to an increase in cervical cancer.
• Monitor lipid levels, blood pressure, body weight, and hepatic function.
• *Alert:* Many oral contraceptives share similar names. Make sure to check the strengths of the hormones for verification.
• Many laboratory tests are affected by oral contraceptives.
• Estrogens and progestins may alter glucose tolerance, thus changing dosage requirements for antidiabetics. Monitor glucose levels.

• Response to metyrapone testing may be reduced. Nitroblue tetrazolium test may have false-positive result.
• Oral contraceptives should be discontinued for a few weeks before adrenal function tests.
• Discontinue oral contraceptive and notify prescriber if patient develops granulomatous colitis.
• Drug should be discontinued at least 1 week before surgery to decrease risk of thromboembolism. Tell patient to use an alternative method of birth control.

PATIENT TEACHING
• Tell patient to take tablets at same time each day; nighttime dosing may reduce nausea and headaches.
• Advise patient to use an additional method of birth control, such as condoms or a diaphragm with spermicide, for the first week of the first cycle.
• Tell patient that missing doses in midcycle greatly increases likelihood of pregnancy.
• Tell patient that missing a dose may cause spotting or light bleeding.
• Tell patient that oral contraceptives don't protect against HIV or sexually transmitted diseases.
• If 1 tablet is missed, tell patient to take it as soon as she remembers or to take 2 tablets the next day and continue regular schedule. If patient misses 2 consecutive days, instruct her to take 2 tablets daily for 2 days and then resume normal schedule. Also, advise her to use an additional method of birth control for 7 days after two missed doses. If she misses three or more doses, tell her to discard remaining tablets in monthly package and to substitute another contraceptive method. If next menstrual period doesn't begin on schedule, warn patient to rule out pregnancy before starting new dosing cycle. If menstrual period begins, have patient start new dosing cycle 7 days after last tablet was taken.
• Warn patient that headache, nausea, dizziness, breast tenderness, spotting, and breakthrough bleeding are common initially. These effects should diminish after three to six dosing cycles (months).

Reactions may be *common*, uncommon, *life-threatening*, or **COMMON AND LIFE-THREATENING**.

- Instruct patient to weigh herself at least twice a week and to report any sudden weight gain or edema to prescriber.
- Warn patient to avoid exposure to ultraviolet light or prolonged exposure to sunlight.
- *Alert:* Warn patient to immediately report abdominal pain; numbness, stiffness, or pain in legs or buttocks; pressure or pain in chest; shortness of breath; severe headache; visual disturbances such as blind spots, blurriness, or flashing lights; undiagnosed vaginal bleeding or discharge; two consecutive missed menstrual periods; lumps in the breast; swelling of hands or feet; or severe pain in the abdomen (tumor rupture in liver).
- Advise patient of increased risks created by simultaneous use of cigarettes and oral contraceptives.
- If one menstrual period is missed and tablets have been taken on schedule, tell patient to continue taking them. If two consecutive menstrual periods are missed, tell patient to stop drug and have pregnancy test. Progestins may cause birth defects if taken early in pregnancy.
- Advise patient not to take same drug for longer than 12 months without consulting prescriber. Stress importance of Papanicolaou tests and annual gynecologic examinations.
- Advise patient to check with prescriber about how soon pregnancy may be attempted after hormonal therapy is stopped. Many prescribers recommend that women not become pregnant within 2 months after stopping drug.
- Warn patient of possible delay in achieving pregnancy when drug is discontinued.
- Tell patient that many prescribers advise women on long-term therapy (5 years or longer) to stop drug and use other birth control methods. Periodically reassess patient while she is off hormone therapy.
- Teach woman how to perform routine breast self-examination.
- Teach patient methods to decrease risk of thromboembolism.
- Advise patient taking oral contraceptives to use additional form of birth control during concurrent treatment with certain antibiotics.
- Advise patient that oral contraceptives may change the fit of rigid contact lenses.

levonorgestrel
Norplant System

Pregnancy risk category X

AVAILABLE FORMS
Implants: 36 mg per capsule; 6 capsules in each kit

INDICATIONS & DOSAGES
➤ **Prevention of pregnancy—**
Women: 6 capsules implanted subdermally in the midportion of upper arm, about 8 cm above elbow crease, during first 7 days of onset of menses. Capsules are placed in fanlike position, 15 degrees apart (total of 75 degrees). Contraceptive efficacy lasts for 5 years.

ACTION
Slowly releases synthetic progestin levonorgestrel into bloodstream. How progestins prevent contraception isn't fully understood, but they alter the mucus covering the cervix, prevent implantation of the egg and, in some patients, prevent ovulation.

Route	Onset	Peak	Duration
Subdermal	24 hr	24 hr	Unknown

ADVERSE REACTIONS
CNS: headache, nervousness, dizziness.
GI: nausea, *abdominal discomfort,* appetite change.
GU: *amenorrhea, many days of bleeding or prolonged bleeding, spotting,* irregular onset of bleeding, frequent onset of bleeding, scanty bleeding, cervicitis, vaginitis, leukorrhea.
Metabolic: weight gain.
Musculoskeletal: bone and muscle pain.
Skin: dermatitis, acne, hirsutism, hypertrichosis, alopecia, infection, transient pain or itching at implant site.
Other: adnexal enlargement, mastalgia, *removal difficulty,* breast discharge.

INTERACTIONS
Drug-drug. *Carbamazepine, fosphenytoin, phenytoin, rifampin:* May reduce contraceptive efficacy of levonorgestrel implants. Monitor patient closely.

Drug-food. *Caffeine:* May increase caffeine levels. Advise caution.

Drug-lifestyle. *Smoking:* Increased risk of adverse CV effects. If smoking continues, may need alternative therapy.

EFFECTS ON LAB TEST RESULTS
None reported.

CONTRAINDICATIONS
Contraindicated in patients with active thrombophlebitis or thromboembolic disorders, undiagnosed abnormal genital bleeding, acute liver disease, malignant or benign liver tumors, known or suspected breast cancer; also contraindicated in known or suspected pregnancy.

NURSING CONSIDERATIONS
• Use cautiously in patients with history of depression or hyperlipidemia and in diabetic or prediabetic patients.
• Drug can be used 5 days postpartum after lactation has been established.
• Most patients develop variations in menstrual bleeding patterns, including irregular bleeding, prolonged bleeding, spotting, and amenorrhea. In most patients, these irregularities diminish over time, although they may last up to 1 year.
• Irregular bleeding may mask symptoms of cervical or endometrial cancer.
• Closely monitor patient with condition that may be aggravated by fluid retention because corticosteroid hormones may cause fluid retention.
• Implants don't contain estrogen. Levonorgestrel is a synthetic progestin.
• Expect implants to be removed if patient develops active thrombophlebitis or thromboembolic disease or will be immobilized for a significant length of time.
• If jaundice develops, expect implants to be removed because corticosteroid hormone metabolism is impaired in patients with liver failure.
• Although retinal thrombosis has been reported after use of oral contraceptives, no similar incidents have been documented after use of the implant system. However, patients with sudden unexplained vision problems, including users of contact lenses who develop vision changes or changes in lens tolerance, should be immediately evaluated by an ophthalmologist.

PATIENT TEACHING
• *Alert:* Tell patient to notify prescriber immediately (before the skin heals over the implant) if one of the implanted capsules falls out. Contraceptive efficacy may be impaired.
• Urge patient to contact prescriber if implant site becomes infected.
• Warn patient that missed menstrual periods aren't an accurate indicator of early pregnancy because drug may induce amenorrhea. Advise patient that 6 weeks or longer of amenorrhea (after a pattern of regular menstrual periods) could indicate pregnancy. If pregnancy is confirmed, implants must be removed.
• Instruct patient to report changes in vision.
• Teach patient how to perform breast self-examination.
• Encourage regular (at least annual) physical examinations.
• Teach patient methods to decrease risk of thromboembolism.
• Encourage patient to stop smoking or reduce number of cigarettes because of the risk of CV complications.

---

medroxyprogesterone acetate
Amen, Cycrin, Depo-Provera, Provera

Pregnancy risk category X

AVAILABLE FORMS
Tablets: 2.5 mg, 5 mg, 10 mg
Injection (suspension): 150 mg/ml, 400 mg/ml

INDICATIONS & DOSAGES
➤ **Abnormal uterine bleeding caused by hormonal imbalance—**
Women: 5 to 10 mg P.O. daily for 5 to 10 days beginning on day 16 of menstrual cycle. If patient also has received estrogen, give 10 mg P.O. daily for 10 days beginning on day 16 or 21 of cycle.
➤ **Secondary amenorrhea—**
Women: 5 to 10 mg P.O. daily for 5 to 10 days. Start at any time during menstrual cycle (usually during latter half of cycle).

Reactions may be *common*, uncommon, *life-threatening*, or COMMON AND LIFE-THREATENING.

➤ **Endometrial or renal cancer—**
Adults: 400 to 1,000 mg I.M. weekly.
Dose may be decreased to 400 mg/month
when disease has stabilized.
➤ **Contraception—**
Women: 150 mg I.M. once q 3 months.

ACTION
Suppresses ovulation, possibly by inhibiting pituitary gonadotropin secretion, thus preventing follicular maturation and causing endometrial thinning.

Route	Onset	Peak	Duration
I.M., P.O.	Unknown	Unknown	Unknown

ADVERSE REACTIONS
CNS: depression, *CVA.*
CV: thrombophlebitis, *pulmonary embolism,* edema, *thromboembolism.*
EENT: exophthalmos, diplopia.
GI: *bloating, abdominal pain.*
GU: *breakthrough bleeding,* dysmenorrhea, *amenorrhea,* cervical erosion, abnormal secretions.
Hepatic: cholestatic jaundice.
Metabolic: weight changes.
Skin: rash, induration, sterile abscesses, acne, pruritus, melasma, alopecia, hirsutism.
Other: pain; breast tenderness, enlargement, or secretion.

INTERACTIONS
Drug-drug. *Aminoglutethimide, carbamazepine, fosphenytoin, phenobarbital, phenytoin, rifampin:* Decreased progestin effects. Monitor patient for diminished therapeutic response. Tell patient to use a nonhormonal contraceptive during therapy with these drugs.
Drug-food. *Caffeine:* May increase caffeine levels. Advise caution.
Drug-lifestyle. *Smoking:* Increased risk of adverse CV effects. If smoking continues, may need alternative therapy.

EFFECTS ON LAB TEST RESULTS
• May increase liver function test values and cause abnormal thyroid function test results.

CONTRAINDICATIONS
Contraindicated in patients hypersensitive to drug and in those with active thromboembolic disorders or history of thromboembolic disorders, cerebrovascular disease, apoplexy, breast cancer, undiagnosed abnormal vaginal bleeding, missed abortion, or hepatic dysfunction; also contraindicated during pregnancy. Tablets are contraindicated in patients with liver dysfunction or known or suspected malignant disease of genital organs.

NURSING CONSIDERATIONS
• Use cautiously in patients with diabetes mellitus, seizures, migraine, cardiac or renal disease, asthma, and depression.
• Drug shouldn't be used as test for pregnancy; it may cause birth defects and masculinization of female fetus.
• I.M. injection may be painful. Monitor sites for evidence of sterile abscess. Rotate injection sites to prevent muscle atrophy.
• Monitor patient for pain and swelling, warmth, or redness in calves; sudden, severe headaches; visual disturbances; numbness in extremities; signs of depression; signs of liver dysfunction (abdominal pain, dark urine, jaundice).
• Response to metyrapone testing is reduced.

PATIENT TEACHING
• According to FDA regulations, patient must read package insert explaining possible adverse effects of progestins before receiving first dose. Also, give patient verbal explanation.
• Advise patient to take medication with food if GI upset occurs.
• *Alert:* Tell patient to report unusual symptoms immediately and to stop drug and notify prescriber about visual disturbances or migraine.
• Teach woman how to perform routine breast self-examination.
• Advise patient to report breast abnormalities, vaginal bleeding, edema, jaundice, dark urine, clay-colored stools, dyspnea, chest pain, or pregnancy to prescriber immediately.
• Advise patient that injection must be administered every 3 months to maintain adequate contraceptive effects.
• Tell patient to report suspected pregnancy to prescriber immediately.

✳ *NEW DRUG*

medroxyprogesterone acetate and estradiol cypionate
Lunelle

Pregnancy risk category X

AVAILABLE FORMS
Injection: 25 mg medroxyprogesterone acetate and 5 mg estradiol cypionate per 0.5 ml

INDICATIONS & DOSAGES
➤ **Contraception—**
Women older than age 16 who have achieved menarche: 0.5 ml I.M. into deltoid, gluteus maximus, or anterior thigh. Give first injection within first 5 days of onset of a normal menstrual period, within 5 days of a complete first trimester abortion, or at least 4 weeks postpartum if not breast-feeding (at least 6 weeks postpartum if breast-feeding). Give second and subsequent injections monthly (28 to 30 days, not to exceed 33 days) after previous injection.

ACTION
Medroxyprogesterone acetate and estradiol cypionate inhibit secretion of gonadotropins, which prevents follicular maturation and ovulation. Other possible mechanisms of action include thinning of the endometrium and thickening of reduced volume of cervical mucus.

Route	Onset	Peak	Duration
I.M.	1 day	7-10 days	28-30 days

ADVERSE REACTIONS
CNS: emotional lability, depression, headache, nervousness, dizziness, asthenia.
GI: abdominal pain, nausea, enlarged abdomen.
GU: amenorrhea, dysmenorrhea, menorrhagia, metrorrhagia, vaginal candidiasis, vulvovaginal disorder.
Metabolic: weight gain.
Skin: acne, alopecia.
Other: breast tenderness, decreased libido.

INTERACTIONS
Drug-drug. *Acetaminophen:* Decreased plasma levels. Monitor patient.
Aminoglutethimide: May decrease medroxyprogesterone acetate levels. Recommend additional birth control.
Antibiotics (ampicillin, griseofulvin, tetracycline): Decreased contraceptive effectiveness. Recommend additional birth control.
Anticonvulsants (carbamazepine, phenobarbital, phenytoin): Increased metabolism of some synthetic estrogens and progestins, which could result in reduced contraceptive effectiveness. Recommend additional birth control.
Clofibric acid, morphine, salicylic acid, temazepam: Decreased drug levels. Monitor levels, or recommend alternative therapy.
Cyclosporine, prednisolone, theophylline: Increased levels of these drugs. Monitor serum levels, and adjust as needed.
Phenylbutazone: May decrease contraceptive effectiveness and increase menstrual irregularities. Recommend additional birth control.
Rifampin: Increased metabolism of some synthetic estrogens and progestins, resulting in decreased contraceptive effectiveness and more irregular bleeding. Recommend additional birth control.
Drug-herb. *St. John's wort:* May induce hepatic enzymes (cytochrome P-450) and transporter proteins. May reduce the effectiveness of contraceptives and may result in breakthrough bleeding. Discourage use together or advise the use of a second method of contraception.
Drug-lifestyle. *Smoking:* Increased risk of thromboembolic disorders. Discourage smoking.

EFFECTS ON LAB TEST RESULTS
● May increase total circulating sex steroid, corticoid, triglyceride, plasma and urinary steroid, gonadotropin, sulfobromophthalein, folate, prothrombin, and factor VII, VIII, IX, and X levels. May decrease antithrombin III level.
● May increase liver function test values, norepinephrine-induced platelet aggregability, thyroid-binding globulin, and total thyroid hormone. May decrease free T_3

Reactions may be *common*, uncommon, *life-threatening*, or COMMON AND LIFE-THREATENING.

resin uptake, glucose tolerance, and sex hormone-binding globulin concentration.

CONTRAINDICATIONS

Contraindicated in patients with known or suspected pregnancy, thrombophlebitis or thromboembolic disorders, a history of deep vein thrombophlebitis or thromboembolic disorders, and cerebral vascular or coronary artery disease. Also contraindicated in patients with undiagnosed abnormal genital bleeding, and in patients with liver dysfunction or disease, such as history of hepatic adenoma or carcinoma; history of cholestatic jaundice of pregnancy or jaundice with prior hormonal contraceptive use, including severe pruritus of pregnancy. Contraindicated in patients with carcinoma of the endometrium, breast, or other known or suspected estrogen-dependent neoplasia. Also contraindicated in patients hypersensitive to any of the ingredients, those who are heavy smokers (15 or more cigarettes per day) or older than age 35, and those with severe hypertension, diabetes with vascular involvement, headaches with focal neurologic symptoms, or valvular heart disease with complications.

NURSING CONSIDERATIONS

• Use cautiously in patients with hypertension, hyperlipidemia, obesity, diabetes, and liver dysfunction. Also use cautiously in patients who smoke and in those with a history of depression.

• The use of oral contraceptives is linked to increased risk of MI, CVA, hepatic neoplasia, and gallbladder disease.

• Monthly injection is effective for contraception during the first cycle of use when administered as recommended.

• If more than 33 days have elapsed since last injection, pregnancy should be considered and another injection shouldn't be given until pregnancy is ruled out.

• Shortening the injection interval could lead to a change in menstrual pattern.

• Don't use bleeding episodes to guide the injection schedule.

• Shake the aqueous suspension vigorously just before use to ensure a uniform suspension.

• Provide yearly physical examinations. Monitor breast exam closely in women with breast nodules or family history of breast cancer.

• When switching patients from other methods of birth control, drug should be given in a manner that ensures continuous contraceptive coverage based on the mechanism of action from both methods. For example, patients switching from oral contraceptives should have their first injection within 7 days after taking their last active pill.

• Discontinue use at least 4 weeks before and for 2 weeks after elective surgery that may be linked to increased risk of thromboembolism.

• Don't use during periods of prolonged immobilization or within 4 weeks after childbirth.

• Injection should be stored at 59° to 86° F (15° to 30° C).

• Effects of drug in nursing mothers haven't been evaluated and are unknown. However, estrogen administration to nursing mothers has resulted in a decrease in the quantity and quality of breast milk.

• Small amounts of combined hormonal contraceptives have been identified in milk with no deleterious effects to the child. However, breast-feeding women shouldn't begin a combined hormonal contraceptive until 6 weeks postpartum.

PATIENT TEACHING

• *Alert:* Teach patient that this product is intended to prevent pregnancy and won't protect against sexually transmitted diseases such as HIV (AIDS), genital warts, genital herpes, chlamydia, gonorrhea, hepatitis B, and syphilis.

• Advise patient that injection must be given every 28 to 30 days. If more than 33 days have passed since an injection, pregnancy must be ruled out before another injection can be given.

• Tell patient that menstrual bleeding patterns may be disrupted while she is receiving drug. Advise patient to report excessive or prolonged bleeding.

• Tell patient that weight gain may occur while she is taking drug.

• Advise patient who wears contact lenses to have an eye examination if visual changes or changes in lens tolerance develop while she is taking drug.

• Risk of pregnancy increases with each tablet missed. Tell patient who misses 1 tablet to take it as soon as she remembers and then to take the next tablet at the regular time. Advise patient who misses 2 tablets to take one as soon as she remembers. She must then take the next regular dose at the usual time and use a nonhormonal method of contraception in addition to norgestrel until 14 tablets have been taken. Instruct patient who misses 3 or more tablets to discontinue drug and use a nonhormonal method of contraception until after menses. If menstrual period doesn't occur within 45 days, pregnancy testing is needed.

• Tell patient that missing a dose may cause spotting or light bleeding.

• Tell patient that oral contraceptives don't protect against HIV or sexually transmitted diseases.

• Advise patient that oral contraceptives and heavy cigarette smoking (15 or more cigarettes daily) raise the risk of serious adverse CV reactions, especially in women older than age 35.

• Instruct woman to immediately report excessive bleeding, bleeding between menstrual cycles, breast pain or tenderness, vaginal discharge, or swelling of hands or feet.

• **Alert:** Tell patient to report unusual symptoms immediately and to stop drug and notify prescriber about visual disturbances, migraines, or numbness or tingling in limbs.

• Teach woman how to perform routine breast self-examination.

progesterone
Gestone§

Pregnancy risk category X

AVAILABLE FORMS
Injection (in oil): 50 mg/ml

INDICATIONS & DOSAGES
➤ **Amenorrhea—**
Women: 5 to 10 mg I.M. daily for 6 to 10 days, usually beginning 8 to 10 days before anticipated start of menstruation. Or as a single 100- to 150-mg I.M. dose.

➤ **Dysfunctional uterine bleeding—**
Women: 5 to 10 mg I.M. daily for six doses.

ACTION
Suppresses ovulation, possibly by inhibiting pituitary gonadotropin secretion, and forms thick cervical mucus.

Route	Onset	Peak	Duration
I.M.	Unknown	Unknown	Unknown

ADVERSE REACTIONS
CNS: depression, *CVA.*
CV: thrombophlebitis, *thromboembolism, pulmonary embolism, edema,* hypertension.
GU: *breakthrough bleeding,* dysmenorrhea, *amenorrhea,* cervical erosion, abnormal secretions.
Hepatic: cholestatic jaundice.
Skin: melasma, rash, acne, pruritus, *pain at injection site.*
Other: breast tenderness, enlargement, or secretion.

INTERACTIONS
Drug-drug. *Barbiturates, carbamazepine, fosphenytoin, phenytoin, rifampin:* Decreased progestin effects. Monitor patient for diminished therapeutic response.
Drug-herb. *Red clover:* May interfere with hormonal therapies. Discourage use together.

EFFECTS ON LAB TEST RESULTS
• May increase liver function test values and cause abnormal thyroid function test results. May decrease pregnanediol excretion.

CONTRAINDICATIONS
Contraindicated in pregnant patients, patients hypersensitive to drug, and patients with breast cancer, undiagnosed abnormal vaginal bleeding, severe hepatic disease, missed abortion, or current or previous thromboembolic disorders. Because of possible allergic reaction, drug shouldn't be given to patients allergic to peanuts or sesame.

Reactions may be *common*, uncommon, *life-threatening*, or COMMON AND LIFE-THREATENING.

NURSING CONSIDERATIONS
• Use cautiously in patients with diabetes mellitus, seizures, migraine, cardiac or renal disease, asthma, or depression.
• Preliminary estrogen treatment is usually needed in menstrual disorders.
• *Alert:* Ask patient about food allergies (peanuts, sesame seeds).
• Give oil solutions (peanut oil or sesame oil) via deep I.M. injection. Check sites frequently for irritation. Rotate injection sites.
• Advise woman of childbearing age to consult prescriber before taking drug and to advise prescriber immediately if she becomes pregnant.
• Response to metyrapone testing is reduced.

PATIENT TEACHING
• According to FDA regulations, patient must read package insert explaining possible adverse effects of progestins before receiving first dose. Also, give patient verbal explanation.
• *Alert:* Tell patient to report unusual symptoms immediately and to stop drug and notify prescriber about visual disturbances or migraine.
• *Alert:* Tell patient to report increased depression immediately; drug may need to be discontinued.
• Teach woman how to perform routine breast self-examination.
• Tell patient to report suspected pregnancy to prescriber immediately.
• Encourage patient to stop smoking or reduce number of cigarettes because of the risk of CV complications.

Gonadotropins

cetrorelix acetate
histrelin acetate
menotropins

COMBINATION PRODUCTS
None.

✽ *NEW DRUG*

cetrorelix acetate
Cetrotide

Pregnancy risk category X

AVAILABLE FORMS
Powder for injection: 0.25 mg, 3 mg

INDICATIONS & DOSAGES
➤ **Inhibition of premature luteinizing hormone (LH) surges in women undergoing controlled ovarian stimulation—**
Adults: 3 mg S.C. once during early to middle follicular phase, given when estradiol level indicates an appropriate stimulation response, usually on stimulation day 7 (range, days 5 to 9). If human chorionic gonadotropin (hCG) has not been given within 4 days after injection, cetrorelix 0.25 mg should be given S.C. once daily until the day of hCG administration. Or, 0.25-mg S.C. multiple-dose regimen is given on either stimulation day 5 (morning or evening) or day 6 (morning), and is continued once daily until the day of hCG administration.

ACTION
Competes with natural gonadotropin-releasing hormone (GnRH) for binding to membrane receptors on pituitary cells, which controls the release of LH and follicle-stimulating hormone (FSH).

Route	Onset	Peak	Duration
S.C.	1-2 hr	1-2 hr	≥ 4 days

ADVERSE REACTIONS
CNS: headache.

GI: nausea.
GU: ovarian hyperstimulation syndrome.

INTERACTIONS
None reported.

EFFECTS ON LAB TEST RESULTS
● May increase ALT, AST, GGT, and alkaline phophatase levels.

CONTRAINDICATIONS
Contraindicated in patients hypersensitive to cetrorelix acetate, extrinsic peptide hormones, mannitol, GnRH, or any other GnRH analogs. Also contraindicated in women with known or suspected pregnancy and in those who are breast-feeding.

NURSING CONSIDERATIONS
● Pregnancy must be ruled out before treatment is started.
● Prescriber should be experienced in fertility treatment.
● Dose is adjusted according to patient response.
● When ultrasound shows a sufficient number or follicles of adequate size, hCG is given to induce ovulation and maturation of oocytes.
● To reduce the risk of ovarian hyperstimulation syndrome, don't give hCG if ovaries show an excessive response to treatment.
● Drug can be administered by the patient after proper instruction.
● It isn't known if drug appears in breast milk. Avoid use in breast-feeding patients.

PATIENT TEACHING
● Instruct patient to store 3-mg form at room temperature (77° F [25° C]) and to store 0.25-mg form in refrigerator (36° to 46° F [2° to 8° C]). Tell patient to keep this product away from children.
● Instruct patient to report any adverse effect that becomes bothersome.
● Educate patient on the importance of following the regimen exactly as prescribed, to achieve optimal results.

• Instruct patient on the proper administration technique, as follows: Wash hands thoroughly with soap and water. Flip off the plastic cover of the vial and wipe the top with an alcohol swab. Attach the needle with the yellow mark to the prefilled syringe. Push the needle through the rubber stopper of the vial and slowly inject the liquid into the vial. Leave the syringe in place and gently swirl the vial until the solution is clear and without residue. Don't shake. Draw liquid from the vial into the syringe. If necessary, invert the vial and pull the needle back as far as needed to withdraw the entire contents of the vial. Detach the needle with the yellow mark from the syringe and replace it with the needle with the gray mark. Invert the syringe and push the plunger until all air bubbles are gone.

• Tell patient to choose an injection site on the lower abdomen, around the navel. If she receives a multiple-dose (0.25-mg) regimen, tell her to choose a different site each day to minimize local irritation. Instruct her to clean the site with an alcohol swab and gently pinch a skinfold surrounding the site of injection. Instruct her to insert the needle completely into the skin at about a 45-degree angle and, once the needle has been inserted completely, to release her grasp of the skin. Tell her to gently pull back the plunger of the syringe to check for correct positioning of the needle. If no blood appears, tell her to inject the entire solution by slowly pushing the plunger. She should then withdraw the needle and gently press an alcohol swab onto the injection site.

• If blood appears when the patient pulls back on the plunger, tell her to withdraw the needle and gently press an alcohol swab onto the injection site. Explain that she'll need to discard the syringe and the drug vial and to repeat the procedure using a new pack.

• Urge the patient to use a syringe and needle only once and then to dispose of them properly. If available, suggest that she use a medical waste container for disposal.

histrelin acetate
Supprelin

Pregnancy risk category X

AVAILABLE FORMS
Injection: 120 mcg/0.6 ml, 300 mcg/0.6 ml, 600 mcg/0.6 ml

INDICATIONS & DOSAGES
➤ **Centrally mediated (idiopathic or neurogenic) precocious puberty—**
Children (girls ages 2 to 8; boys ages 2 to 9½): 10 mcg/kg S.C. daily.

ACTION
Agonist that mimics effects of gonadotropin-releasing hormone (GnRH; also called luteinizing hormone–releasing hormone) but is more potent. Long-term use desensitizes responsiveness of pituitary gonadotropin, decreasing sex hormone production by testes or ovaries.

Route	Onset	Peak	Duration
S.C.	Unknown	Unknown	Unknown

ADVERSE REACTIONS
CNS: malaise, *mood changes, nervousness, dizziness, depression, headache, insomnia, anxiety,* paresthesia, cognitive changes, syncope, somnolence, lethargy, impaired consciousness, tremor, hyperkinesia, *seizures,* hot flashes, conduct disorder, fatigue.
CV: *vasodilation,* edema, palpitations, pallor, tachycardia, hypertension.
EENT: epistaxis, ear congestion, abnormal pupillary function, otalgia, visual disturbances, hearing loss, polyopia, photophobia, rhinorrhea, sinusitis, nasal infections.
GI: *abdominal pain, nausea, vomiting, diarrhea, flatulence, decreased appetite, dyspepsia,* cramps, constipation, thirst, gastritis, GI distress.
GU: *menstrual changes, vaginal dryness, leukorrhea, hypermenorrhea, vaginal bleeding, vaginitis, dysmenorrhea,* tenderness of female genitalia, polyuria, incontinence, dysuria, hematuria, nocturia, glycosuria.
Hematologic: hyperlipidemia, anemia, purpura.

---

*Liquid contains alcohol.   **May contain tartrazine.   †Canada   ‡Australia   §U.K.   ◇OTC

Metabolic: *weight gain.*
Musculoskeletal: *arthralgia, muscle stiffness, muscle cramps.*
Respiratory: *upper respiratory tract infection, respiratory congestion, cough,* asthma, breathing disorder, bronchitis, hyperventilation.
Skin: *redness, swelling, acne, rash, diaphoresis,* urticaria, pruritus, alopecia.
Other: *libido changes, breast pain or edema,* breast discharge, decreased breast size, *fever, body pains,* chills, **acute hypersensitivity reactions, anaphylaxis, angioedema.**

INTERACTIONS
None significant.

EFFECTS ON LAB TEST RESULTS
● May increase lipid levels.
● May decrease hemoglobin.

CONTRAINDICATIONS
Contraindicated in patients hypersensitive to drug or its ingredients and in pregnant or breast-feeding women.

NURSING CONSIDERATIONS
● Drug is indicated only for patients who will comply with daily schedule. Noncompliance or inadequate dosing may result in inadequate control of pubertal process, possibly allowing recurrence of symptoms, including onset of menses, breast development, or testicular growth; long-term consequences may involve decreased adult height.
● A complete physical and endocrinologic evaluation should be performed before therapy starts; several indices should be reexamined at 3 months and every 6 to 12 months thereafter. Such evaluations should include height and weight, hand and wrist X-rays for bone-age determination, sex steroid (estradiol or testosterone) levels, and GnRH stimulation test. Monitor these tests periodically to determine effectiveness of therapy.
● Further tests to rule out other causes of precocious puberty include beta human chorionic gonadotropin levels (to detect chorionic gonadotropin-secreting tumor); pelvic, adrenal, or testicular ultrasound (to detect corticosteroid-secreting tumor); and computed tomography scan of the head (to detect previously undiagnosed intracranial tumors). Workup also sets baseline of gonad size for serial monitoring.
● Refrigerate drug (36° to 46° F [2° to 8° C]) and protect from light in its original container. Use vials only once because drug doesn't contain preservatives. Allow drug to reach room temperature before use.
● Give by S.C. route and rotate injection sites to minimize local reactions.
● Decreases in follicle-stimulating hormone, luteinizing hormone, and sex corticosteroid levels occur within 3 months.
● Reevaluate patient if prepubertal levels of sex steroids or GnRH test responses aren't achieved within 3 months of therapy.
● Safety and efficacy of drug haven't been established in children younger than age 2.

PATIENT TEACHING
● Before therapy, make sure patient and caregiver understand importance of adhering to daily schedules. Tell parents to give drug at same time each day to aid compliance and ensure adequate dosing.
● Drug is dispensed as a 30-day kit that contains a patient information leaflet. Make sure caregiver reads and understands leaflet.
● Inform patient that, because drug is a peptide, it is destroyed in GI tract and so must be given parenterally.
● Explain importance of rotating injection sites daily. Sites should include upper arms, thighs, and abdomen.
● Warn patient of potential risks and adverse effects of therapy. During first month of treatment, girls commonly experience a slight menstrual flow, which probably is related to decreasing estrogen levels brought on by treatment. As estrogen levels drop, menses begins because estrogens support the endometrium.
● Advise patient to seek medical attention immediately if signs of hypersensitivity reaction occur: sudden rash, difficulty breathing or swallowing, or rapid heartbeat. Also tell patient to notify prescriber about severe or persistent swelling, redness, or irritation at injection site.

Reactions may be *common*, uncommon, *life-threatening*, or **COMMON AND LIFE-THREATENING.**

menotropins
Humegon, Menogon§, Pergonal,
Repronex

Pregnancy risk category X

AVAILABLE FORMS
Injection: 75 IU of luteinizing hormone
(LH) and 75 IU of follicle-stimulating
hormone (FSH) activity per ampule;
150 IU of LH and 150 IU of FSH activity
per ampule

INDICATIONS & DOSAGES
➤ **Anovulation**—
Women: 75 IU each of FSH and LH I.M.
daily for 7 to 12 days; then 5,000 to
10,000 units of human chorionic gonadotropin (hCG) I.M. 1 day after last dose
of menotropins. Repeated for one to
three menstrual cycles until ovulation
occurs.
➤ **Infertility with ovulation**—
Women: 75 IU each of FSH and LH I.M.
daily for 7 to 12 days; then 10,000 units
hCG I.M. 1 day after last dose of menotropins. Repeated for two menstrual cycles. Then 150 IU each of FSH and LH
daily for 7 to 12 days, followed by 10,000
units hCG I.M. 1 day after last dose of
menotropins. Repeated for two menstrual
cycles.
➤ **Infertility in men**—
Men: Prior treatment with hCG of 5,000
units three times a week for 4 to 6 months;
then 75 IU each of FSH and LH I.M. three
times weekly (given with 2,000 units of
hCG twice weekly) for at least 4 months.
If spermatogenesis doesn't improve, increase to 150 IU each of FSH and LH
three times weekly (dose of hCG remains
unchanged).

ACTION
When given to women who haven't had
primary ovarian failure, drug mimics FSH
in inducing follicular growth and LH in
aiding follicular maturation. Drug induces
spermatogenesis in men.

Route	Onset	Peak	Duration
I.M.	9-12 days	Unknown	Unknown

ADVERSE REACTIONS
CNS: headache, malaise, dizziness, *CVA.*
CV: tachycardia, venous thrombophlebitis, *arterial occlusion, pulmonary embolism.*
GI: nausea, vomiting, diarrhea, abdominal
cramps, bloating.
GU: *ovarian enlargement with pain and
abdominal distention,* multiple births,
ovarian hyperstimulation syndrome, ovarian cysts, ectopic pregnancy.
Musculoskeletal: aches, joint pains.
Respiratory: atelectasis, *adult respiratory
distress syndrome, pulmonary infarction,*
dyspnea, tachypnea.
Skin: rash.
Other: *gynecomastia,* fever, hypersensitivity reactions, *anaphylaxis,* chills.

INTERACTIONS
None significant.

EFFECTS ON LAB TEST RESULTS
None reported.

CONTRAINDICATIONS
Contraindicated in patients hypersensitive
to drug and in those with primary ovarian
failure, uncontrolled thyroid or adrenal
dysfunction, pituitary tumor, abnormal
uterine bleeding, uterine fibromas, or ovarian cysts or enlargement; also contraindicated in pregnant women and in men with
normal pituitary function, primary testicular failure, or infertility disorders other
than hypogonadotropic hypogonadism.

NURSING CONSIDERATIONS
● Monitor patient closely to ensure adequate ovarian stimulation without hyperstimulation.
● Watch for ovarian hyperstimulation syndrome, which may progress rapidly to a
serious medical event characterized by
dramatic increase in vascular permeability,
which causes rapid accumulation of fluid
in the peritoneal cavity, thorax, and peri-
cardium. Evidence includes hypovolemia,
hemoconcentration, electrolyte imbalance,
ascites, hemoperitoneum, pleural effusion,
hydrothorax, and thromboembolitic
events. Cases are more common and severe if patient becomes pregnant.

---

*Liquid contains alcohol.   **May contain tartrazine.   †Canada   ‡Australia   §U.K.   ◇OTC

• Reconstitute with 1 to 2 ml of sterile normal saline solution for injection. Use immediately.
• Rotate injection sites.

PATIENT TEACHING
• Tell patient about possibility of multiple births. (It occurs about 20% of the time.)
• For patient with infertility, encourage daily intercourse from day before hCG is given until ovulation occurs.
• Tell patient that pregnancy usually occurs 4 to 6 weeks after therapy.
• Instruct patient to immediately report severe abdominal pain, bloating, swelling of hands or feet, nausea, vomiting, diarrhea, substantial weight gain, or shortness of breath.

acarbose
chlorpropamide
glimepiride
glipizide
glucagon
glyburide
glyburide and metformin
hydrochloride
insulins
insulin aspart (rDNA origin)
injection
insulin glargine (rDNA origin)
injection
metformin hydrochloride
miglitol
nateglinide
pioglitazone hydrochloride
repaglinide
rosiglitazone maleate

COMBINATION PRODUCTS
Humulin 50/50 ◇: isophane insulin suspension (human) 50% and insulin injection (human) 50%, 100 units/ml.
Humulin 70/30 ◇, Novolin 70/30 ◇: isophane insulin suspension (human) 70% and insulin injection (human) 30%, 100 units/ml.

acarbose
Glucobay§, Prandase†, Precose

Pregnancy risk category B

AVAILABLE FORMS
Tablets: 25 mg, 50 mg, 100 mg

INDICATIONS & DOSAGES
➤ **Adjunct to diet to lower glucose levels in patients with type 2 (non–insulin-dependent) diabetes mellitus whose hyperglycemia can't be managed by diet alone or by diet and a sulfonylurea—**
Adults: Individualized. Initially, 25 mg P.O. t.i.d. with first bite of each main meal. Subsequent dosage adjustment made q 4 to 8 weeks, based on 1-hour postprandial glucose level and tolerance. Maintenance dose is 50 to 100 mg P.O. t.i.d.

Adjust-a-dose: For patients weighing less than 60 kg (132 lb), don't exceed 50 mg P.O. t.i.d. For patients weighing more than 60 kg, don't exceed 100 mg P.O. t.i.d.
➤ **Adjunct to insulin or metformin therapy in patients with type 2 (non–insulin-dependent) diabetes mellitus whose hyperglycemia can't be managed by diet, exercise, and insulin or metformin alone—**
Adults: Initially, 25 mg P.O. t.i.d. with first bite of each main meal. Adjust dosage at 4- to 8-week intervals based on 1-hour postprandial glucose levels and tolerance to determine minimum effective dose of each drug. Maintenance dose is 50 to 100 mg P.O. t.i.d. based on patient's weight. Maximum dose for patients weighing 60 kg or less is 50 mg P.O. t.i.d.; for patients weighing more than 60 kg, maximum dose is 100 mg P.O. t.i.d.

ACTION
An alpha-glucosidase inhibitor that delays digestion of carbohydrates, resulting in a smaller rise in glucose level after meals.

Route	Onset	Peak	Duration
P.O.	Unknown	1 hr	2-4 hr

ADVERSE REACTIONS
GI: *abdominal pain, diarrhea, flatulence.*
Metabolic: hypocalcemia.

INTERACTIONS
Drug-drug. *Calcium channel blockers, corticosteroids, estrogens, fosphenytoin, isoniazid, nicotinic acid, oral contraceptives, phenothiazine, phenytoin, sympathomimetics, thiazides and other diuretics, thyroid products:* May cause hyperglycemia when used together or hypoglycemia when withdrawn. Monitor glucose level.
Digestive enzyme preparations containing carbohydrate-splitting enzymes (such as amylase, pancreatin), intestinal adsorbents (such as activated charcoal): May reduce effect of acarbose. Don't administer together.

Digoxin: May reduce digoxin concentration. Monitor digoxin levels.

EFFECTS ON LAB TEST RESULTS
● May increase ALT and AST levels. May decrease calcium and vitamin B$_6$ levels.

CONTRAINDICATIONS
Contraindicated in patients hypersensitive to drug and in those with diabetic ketoacidosis, cirrhosis, inflammatory bowel disease, colonic ulceration, partial intestinal obstruction, predisposition to intestinal obstruction, chronic intestinal disease with marked disorder of digestion or absorption, or conditions that may deteriorate because of increased intestinal gas formation.

NURSING CONSIDERATIONS
● Drug isn't recommended for use in pregnant women, breast-feeding women, or patients with cirrhosis or creatinine levels higher than 2 mg/dl.
● Use cautiously in patients receiving a sulfonylurea or insulin. Drug isn't recommended for renally impaired patients. Acarbose may increase hypoglycemic potential of the sulfonylurea. Monitor patient receiving both drugs closely. If hypoglycemia occurs, treat patient with oral glucose (dextrose). Severe hypoglycemia may need I.V. glucose infusion or glucagon administration. Because dosage adjustments may be needed to prevent further hypoglycemia, report hypoglycemia and treatment required to prescriber. Insulin therapy may be needed during increased stress (infection, fever, surgery, or trauma). Monitor patient closely for hyperglycemia.
● Safety and efficacy of drug haven't been established in children.
● Monitor patient's 1-hour postprandial plasma glucose level to determine therapeutic effectiveness of acarbose and to identify appropriate dose. Report hyperglycemia to prescriber. Thereafter, glycosylated hemoglobin should be measured every 3 months.
● Monitor transaminase level every 3 months in first year of therapy and periodically thereafter in patients receiving doses in excess of 50 mg t.i.d. Report abnormalities; dosage adjustment or drug withdrawal may be needed.

PATIENT TEACHING
● Tell patient to take drug daily with first bite of each of three main meals.
● Explain that therapy relieves symptoms but doesn't cure the disease.
● Stress importance of adhering to specific diet, weight reduction, exercise, and hygiene programs. Show patient how to monitor glucose level and to recognize and treat hyperglycemia.
● Teach patient taking a sulfonylurea how to recognize hypoglycemia. Advise treating symptoms with a form of dextrose rather than with a product containing table sugar.
● Urge patient to wear or carry medical identification at all times.
● Instruct patient about nature of disease and importance of following therapeutic regimen, adhering to specific diet, and losing weight.
● Advise patient that adverse effects usually occur during the first few weeks of therapy, if they develop. Usually, these effects diminish over time.

---

chlorpropamide
Apo-Chlorpropamide†, Diabinese

Pregnancy risk category C

AVAILABLE FORMS
Tablets: 100 mg, 250 mg

INDICATIONS & DOSAGES
➤ **Adjunct to diet to lower glucose level in patients with type 2 (non–insulin-dependent) diabetes mellitus—**
Adults: 250 mg P.O. daily with breakfast. Initial dosage increased after 5 to 7 days because of extended duration of action; then increased q 3 to 5 days by 50 to 125 mg, if needed, to maximum of 750 mg daily. Some patients with mild diabetes respond well to doses of 100 mg or less daily.
Elderly patients: For patients older than age 65, initially 100 to 125 mg P.O. daily; then increase as with adult dose.
Adjust-a-dose: For patients with renal insufficiency, increase dosage as tolerated.

Reactions may be *common,* uncommon, *life-threatening,* or COMMON AND LIFE-THREATENING.

> ► **To change from insulin to oral therapy—**
Adults: If insulin dosage is less than 40 units daily, stop insulin and start oral therapy as above. If insulin dosage is 40 units or more daily, start oral therapy as above with insulin reduced by 50%. Reduce insulin dosage further according to response.

ACTION

Unknown. A sulfonylurea that probably stimulates insulin release from pancreatic beta cells and reduces glucose output by the liver. An extrapancreatic effect increases peripheral sensitivity to insulin. Also exerts an antidiuretic effect in patients with diabetes insipidus.

Route	Onset	Peak	Duration
P.O.	1 hr	2-4 hr	24 hr

ADVERSE REACTIONS

CNS: paresthesia, fatigue, dizziness, vertigo, malaise, headache.
CV: increased risk of cardiovascular mortality.
EENT: tinnitus.
GI: nausea, heartburn, epigastric distress.
GU: tea-colored urine.
Hematologic: *leukopenia, thrombocytopenia, aplastic anemia, agranulocytosis,* hemolytic anemia.
Hepatic: cholestatic jaundice.
Metabolic: *prolonged hypoglycemia,* dilutional hyponatremia.
Skin: rash, pruritus, erythema, urticaria.
Other: *disulfiram-like reactions,* hypersensitivity reactions.

INTERACTIONS

Drug-drug. *Anabolic steroids, chloramphenicol, clofibrate, guanethidine, MAO inhibitors, salicylates, sulfonamides:* Increased hypoglycemic activity. Monitor glucose level.
Beta blockers: Prolonged hypoglycemic effect and masked symptoms of hypoglycemia. Use together cautiously.
Corticosteroids, glucagon, rifampin, thiazide diuretics: Decreased hypoglycemic response. Monitor glucose level.
Hydantoins: Increased hydantoin levels. Monitor levels.

Oral anticoagulants: Increased hypoglycemic activity or enhanced anticoagulant effect. Monitor glucose level, PT, and INR.
Drug-herb. *Bitter melon (karela), burdock, dandelion, eucalyptus, ginkgo biloba, marshmallow:* Increased hypoglycemic effects. Discourage use together.
Drug-lifestyle. *Alcohol use:* Altered glycemic control, most commonly hypoglycemia. May also cause a disulfiram-like reaction. Discourage use together.

EFFECTS ON LAB TEST RESULTS

● May increase BUN, creatinine, alkaline phosphatase, bilirubin, AST, LDH, and cholesterol levels. May decrease glucose and sodium levels.
● May decrease hemoglobin and WBC, platelet, and granulocyte counts.

CONTRAINDICATIONS

Contraindicated in pregnant women, breast-feeding women, patients hypersensitive to drug, and those with type 2 diabetes complicated by ketosis, acidosis, diabetic coma, major surgery, severe infections, or severe trauma; also contraindicated for treating type 1 (insulin-dependent) diabetes or diabetes that can be adequately controlled by diet.

NURSING CONSIDERATIONS

● Use cautiously in patients with porphyria or impaired hepatic or renal function, or in debilitated, malnourished, or elderly patients. Also use cautiously in patients with known allergy to sulfonamides.
● Elderly patients may be more sensitive to therapeutic and adverse effects.
● Drug may accumulate in patients with renal insufficiency. Watch for and report signs of impending renal insufficiency, such as dysuria, anuria, and hematuria.
● *Alert:* Adverse effects of drug, especially hypoglycemia, may be more frequent, prolonged, or severe than with some other sulfonylureas because of drug's long duration of action. If hypoglycemia occurs, monitor patient closely for minimum of 3 to 5 days.
● Patients switching from another oral antidiabetic don't usually need a transition period.

• Patients may need hospitalization during transition from insulin to an oral antidiabetic. Monitor patient's glucose levels at least three times daily before meals.

• **Alert:** Don't confuse chlorpropamide with chlorpromazine.

PATIENT TEACHING

• Instruct patient about nature of disease and importance of following therapeutic regimen, adhering to specific diet, losing weight, getting exercise, following personal hygiene programs, and avoiding infection. Explain how and when to monitor glucose level, and teach recognition of and intervention for hypoglycemia and hyperglycemia.

• Make sure patient understands that therapy relieves symptoms but doesn't cure the disease. He should also understand potential risks and advantages of taking drug and of other treatment methods.

• Advise woman planning pregnancy to consult prescriber before becoming pregnant. Insulin may be needed during pregnancy and breast-feeding.

• Tell patient not to change drug dosage without prescriber's consent and to report abnormal blood or urine glucose test results.

• Teach patient to carry candy or other simple sugars to treat mild hypoglycemic episodes. Patient experiencing severe episode may need hospital treatment.

• Advise patient not to take other drugs, including OTC drugs, without first checking with prescriber.

• Advise patient to avoid alcohol consumption. Signs and symptoms of chlorpropamide-alcohol flush are facial flushing, light-headedness, headache, and occasional breathlessness. Even very small amounts of alcohol can produce this reaction.

• Advise patient to wear or carry medical identification at all times.

• **Alert:** Tell patient to report rash, skin eruptions, and other signs and symptoms of hypersensitivity to prescriber immediately.

---

glimepiride
Amaryl

Pregnancy risk category C

AVAILABLE FORMS
Tablets: 1 mg, 2 mg, 4 mg

INDICATIONS & DOSAGES

➤ **Adjunct to diet and exercise to lower glucose levels in patients with type 2 (non–insulin-dependent) diabetes mellitus whose hyperglycemia can't be managed by diet and exercise alone—**
Adults: Initially, 1 to 2 mg P.O. once daily with first main meal of day; usual maintenance dose is 1 to 4 mg P.O. once daily. After reaching 2 mg, dosage is increased in increments not exceeding 2 mg q 1 to 2 weeks, based on patient's glucose level response. Maximum dosage is 8 mg/day.

➤ **Adjunct to insulin therapy in patients with type 2 diabetes mellitus whose hyperglycemia can't be managed by diet and exercise in conjunction with oral hypoglycemics—**
Adults: 8 mg P.O. once daily with first main meal of day; used with low-dose insulin. Adjust insulin dosage upward weekly, p.r.n., based on patient's glucose level response.

➤ **Adjunct to metformin therapy in patients with type 2 diabetes mellitus whose hyperglycemia can't be managed by diet, exercise, and glimepiride or metformin alone—**
Adults: 8 mg P.O. once daily with first main meal of day with metformin if patient doesn't respond adequately to glimepiride monotherapy. Adjust dosages based on patient's glucose level to determine minimum effective dose of each drug.

Adjust-a-dose: For renally or hepatically impaired patients, initial dose is 1 mg P.O. once daily with first main meal of day; then adjust to appropriate dosage, p.r.n.

ACTION
Unknown. Lowers glucose levels, possibly by stimulating release of insulin from functioning pancreatic beta cells. Drug

---

also can lead to increased sensitivity of peripheral tissues to insulin.

Route	Onset	Peak	Duration
P.O.	1 hr	2-3 hr	> 24 hr

ADVERSE REACTIONS

CNS: dizziness, asthenia, headache.
EENT: changes in accommodation.
GI: nausea.
Hematologic: *leukopenia,* hemolytic anemia, *agranulocytosis, thrombocytopenia, aplastic anemia, pancytopenia.*
Hepatic: cholestatic jaundice.
Metabolic: *hypoglycemia,* dilutional hyponatremia.
Skin: pruritus, erythema, urticaria, morbilliform or maculopapular eruptions, photosensitivity reactions.

INTERACTIONS

Drug-drug. *Beta blockers:* May mask symptoms of hypoglycemia. Monitor glucose level.
Drugs that tend to produce hyperglycemia (such as corticosteroids, estrogens, fosphenytoin, isoniazid, nicotinic acid, oral contraceptives, other diuretics, phenothiazines, phenytoin, sympathomimetic thiazides, thyroid products): May lead to loss of glucose control. Adjust dosage.
Insulin: May increase risk of hypoglycemia. Don't use together.
NSAIDs, other drugs that are highly protein-bound (such as beta blockers, chloramphenicol, coumarin, MAO inhibitors, probenecid, salicylates, sulfonamides): May potentiate hypoglycemic action of sulfonylureas such as glimepiride. Monitor glucose levels carefully.
Drug-herb. *Burdock, dandelion, eucalyptus, marshmallow:* Increased hypoglycemic effects. Discourage use together.
Drug-lifestyle. *Alcohol use:* Altered glycemic control, most commonly hypoglycemia. May also cause disulfiram-like reaction. Discourage use together.

EFFECTS ON LAB TEST RESULTS

• May increase BUN, creatinine, alkaline phosphatase, and AST levels. May decrease glucose and sodium levels.
• May decrease hemoglobin and WBC, RBC, platelet, granulocytes.

CONTRAINDICATIONS

Contraindicated in patients hypersensitive to drug and in those with diabetic ketoacidosis, which should be treated with insulin.

NURSING CONSIDERATIONS

• Use cautiously in debilitated or malnourished patients and in those with adrenal, pituitary, hepatic, or renal insufficiency; these patients are more susceptible to the hypoglycemic action of glucose-lowering drugs. Use of drug isn't recommended in elderly patients. Also use cautiously in patients with known allergy to sulfonamides.
• Glimepiride and insulin may be used together in patients who lose glucose control after initially responding to therapy (secondary failure).
• Monitor fasting glucose level periodically to determine therapeutic response. Also monitor glycosylated hemoglobin, usually every 3 to 6 months, to precisely assess long-term glycemic control.
• Oral hypoglycemics may cause increased risk of CV mortality compared with diet alone or with diet and insulin therapy.
• Safety and effectiveness of drug in children haven't been established.
• No data exist to demonstrate whether drug appears in breast milk. Don't give drug to breast-feeding women because of potential for hypoglycemia in breast-fed infants.
• When changing patient from other hypoglycemics (sulfonylureas) to glimepiride, a transition period isn't needed.
• **Alert:** Don't confuse glimepiride with glyburide or glipizide.

PATIENT TEACHING

• Tell patient to take drug with first meal of the day.
• Make sure patient understands that therapy relieves symptoms but doesn't cure the disease. He should also understand potential risks and advantages of taking drug and of other treatment methods.
• Stress importance of adhering to diet, weight reduction, exercise, and personal hygiene programs. Explain to patient and family how and when to monitor glucose levels, and teach recognition of and inter-

vention for signs and symptoms of hyperglycemia and hypoglycemia.
● Advise patient to wear or carry medical identification at all times.
● Advise woman planning pregnancy to consult prescriber before becoming pregnant. Insulin may be needed during pregnancy and breast-feeding.
● Advise patient to consult prescriber before taking any OTC products.
● Teach patient to carry candy or other simple sugars to treat mild hypoglycemic episodes. Patient experiencing severe episode may need hospital treatment.
● Inform patient that alcohol lowers glucose level and should be avoided.

glipizide
Glibenese§, Glucotrol, Glucotrol XL, Minidiab‡

Pregnancy risk category C

AVAILABLE FORMS
Tablets: 5 mg, 10 mg
Tablets (extended-release): 2.5 mg, 5 mg, 10 mg

INDICATIONS & DOSAGES
➤ **Adjunct to diet to lower glucose level in patients with type 2 (non–insulin-dependent) diabetes mellitus—**
Adults: Initially, 5 mg P.O. daily 30 minutes before breakfast. Maximum once-daily dose is 15 mg. Doses of more than 15 mg should be divided; maximum total daily dose is 40 mg for immediate-release tablets. **Extended-release tablets:** Initially, 5 mg P.O. with breakfast daily. Adjust in 5-mg increments q 3 months depending on level of glycemic control. Maximum daily dose is 20 mg.
Elderly patients: For patients older than age 65, initial dose is 2.5 mg P.O. daily.
Adjust-a-dose: For patients with liver disease, initial dose is 2.5 mg P.O. daily.
➤ **To replace insulin therapy—**
Adults: If insulin dosage is more than 20 units daily, start patient at usual dosage in addition to 50% of insulin. If insulin dosage is less than or equal to 20 units, insulin may be stopped when glipizide starts.

ACTION
Unknown. A sulfonylurea that probably stimulates insulin release from pancreatic beta cells and reduces glucose output by the liver. An extrapancreatic effect increases peripheral sensitivity to insulin.

Route	Onset	Peak	Duration
P.O.	15-30 min	1-3 hr	24 hr
P.O. (extended)	2-3 hr	6-12 hr	24 hr

ADVERSE REACTIONS
CNS: dizziness, drowsiness, headache.
GI: nausea, constipation, diarrhea.
Hematologic: *leukopenia,* hemolytic anemia, *agranulocytosis, thrombocytopenia, aplastic anemia.*
Hepatic: cholestatic jaundice.
Metabolic: *hypoglycemia.*
Skin: rash, pruritus, photosensitivity.

INTERACTIONS
Drug-drug. *Amantadine, anabolic steroids, antifungal antibiotics (miconazole, fluconazole), chloramphenicol, clofibrate, guanethidine, MAO inhibitors, probenecid, salicylates, sulfonamides:* Increased hypoglycemic activity. Monitor glucose level.
Beta blockers: Prolonged hypoglycemic effect and masked symptoms of hypoglycemia. Use together cautiously.
Corticosteroids, glucagon, rifampin, thiazide diuretics: Decreased hypoglycemic response. Monitor glucose level.
Hydantoins: Increased levels of hydantoins. Monitor glucose level.
Oral anticoagulants: Increased hypoglycemic activity or enhanced anticoagulant effect. Monitor glucose levels, PT, and INR.
Drug-herb. *Burdock, dandelion, eucalyptus, marshmallow:* Increased hypoglycemic effects. Discourage use together.
Drug-lifestyle. *Alcohol use:* Altered glycemic control, most commonly hypoglycemia. Also may cause disulfiram-like reaction. Discourage use together.

EFFECTS ON LAB TEST RESULTS
● May increase BUN, creatinine, alkaline phosphatase, AST, and cholesterol levels. May decrease glucose levels.

Reactions may be *common,* uncommon, ***life-threatening,*** or COMMON AND LIFE-THREATENING.

• May decrease WBCs, platelets, hemoglobin, and granulocytes.

CONTRAINDICATIONS
Contraindicated in patients hypersensitive to drug and in those with diabetic ketoacidosis with or without coma; also contraindicated in pregnant or breast-feeding women.

NURSING CONSIDERATIONS
• Use cautiously in patients with renal or hepatic disease; in debilitated, malnourished, or elderly patients; and in those with known allergy to sulfonamides.
• Give immediate-release preparations about 30 minutes before meals.
• Some patients may attain effective control on a once-daily regimen, whereas others respond better with divided dosing.
• Patient may switch from immediate-release dose to extended-release tablets at the nearest equivalent total daily dose.
• Glipizide is a second-generation sulfonylurea. The frequency of adverse reactions appears to be lower than with first-generation drugs such as chlorpropamide.
• During periods of increased stress, patient may need insulin therapy. Monitor patient closely for hyperglycemia in these situations.
• Patient transferring from insulin therapy to an oral antidiabetic needs glucose level monitoring at least t.i.d. before meals. Patient may need hospitalization during transition.
• *Alert:* Don't confuse glipizide with glyburide or glimepiride.

PATIENT TEACHING
• Instruct patient about disease and importance of following therapeutic regimen, adhering to diet, losing weight, getting exercise, following personal hygiene programs, and avoiding infection. Explain how and when to monitor glucose level, and teach recognition of hypoglycemia and hyperglycemia.
• Tell patient to carry candy or other simple sugars to treat mild hypoglycemic episodes. Patient experiencing severe episode may need hospital treatment.
• Instruct patient not to change drug dosage without prescriber's consent and to report abnormal blood or urine glucose test results.
• Tell patient not to take other drugs, including OTC drugs, without first checking with prescriber.
• Advise patient to wear or carry medical identification at all times.
• Advise woman planning pregnancy to consult prescriber before becoming pregnant. Insulin may be needed during pregnancy and breast-feeding.
• Inform patient that alcohol lowers glucose level and should be avoided.

glucagon
GlucaGen Diagnostic Kit,
Glucagon Diagnostic Kit,
Glucagon Emergency Kit

Pregnancy risk category B

AVAILABLE FORMS
Powder for injection: 1-mg (1-unit) vial

ACTION
Raises glucose level by promoting catalytic depolymerization of hepatic glycogen to glucose.

Route	Onset	Peak	Duration
I.M., S.C.	4-10 min	Unknown	12-32 min
I.V. (hyperglycemia)	Immediate	30 min	60-90 min
I.V. (gastric relaxation)	1 min	30 min	9-25 min

INDICATIONS & DOSAGES
➤ **Hypoglycemia—**
Adults and children weighing more than 20 kg (44 lb): 1 mg S.C., I.M., or I.V.
Children weighing 20 kg or less: 0.5 USP units or 20 to 30 mcg/kg S.C., I.M., or I.V.; maximum dose 1 mg. May repeat in 15 minutes, if needed. I.V. glucose must be given if patient fails to respond.
➤ **Diagnostic aid for radiologic examination—**
Adults: 0.25 to 2 mg I.V. or I.M. before radiologic procedure.

I.V. ADMINISTRATION
• Reconstitute drug in 1-unit vial with 1 ml of diluent. Use only diluent supplied

---

by manufacturer when preparing doses of 2 mg or less. For larger doses, dilute with sterile water for injection.
• Unstable hypoglycemic diabetic patients may not respond to glucagon; give dextrose I.V. instead.

ADVERSE REACTIONS
CV: hypotension.
GI: nausea, vomiting.
Metabolic: hypokalemia.
Respiratory: *bronchospasm, respiratory distress.*
Other: hypersensitivity reactions.

INTERACTIONS
Drug-drug. *Anticoagulants:* Enhanced anticoagulant effect. Monitor prothrombin activity and monitor patient for signs of bleeding.
Fosphenytoin, phenytoin: Inhibited glucagon-induced insulin release. Use cautiously.

EFFECTS ON LAB TEST RESULTS
• May decrease potassium levels.

CONTRAINDICATIONS
Contraindicated in patients hypersensitive to drug and in those with pheochromocytoma.

NURSING CONSIDERATIONS
• Use cautiously in those with history of insulinoma or pheochromocytoma.
• Drug should be used only in emergency situations.
• Monitor glucose concentrations before, during, and after administration.
• *Alert:* Arouse patient from coma as quickly as possible and give additional carbohydrates orally to prevent secondary hypoglycemic reactions.
• *Alert:* Don't confuse glucagon with Glaucon.

PATIENT TEACHING
• Instruct patient and caregivers in proper glucagon administration and recognition of hypoglycemia.
• Explain importance of calling prescriber at once in emergencies.

glyburide (glibenclamide)
Daonil§, DiaBeta**, Euglucon†, Glynase PresTab, Micronase, Semi-Daonil§

Pregnancy risk category B

AVAILABLE FORMS
Tablets: 1.25 mg, 2.5 mg, 5 mg
Tablets (micronized): 1.5 mg, 3 mg, 6 mg

INDICATIONS & DOSAGES
➤ **Adjunct to diet to lower glucose level in patients with type 2 (non–insulin-dependent) diabetes mellitus—**
Adults: Initially, 2.5 to 5 mg regular tablets P.O. once daily with breakfast or first main meal. Usual maintenance dosage is 1.25 to 20 mg daily as a single dose or in divided doses. Or, micronized formulation may be used. Initial dosage is 1.5 to 3 mg daily. Usual maintenance dosage of micronized formulation is 0.75 to 12 mg daily. Patients receiving more than 6 mg daily may have better response with b.i.d. dosing.
Adjust-a-dose: For patients who are more sensitive to antidiabetics and for those with adrenal or pituitary insufficiency, start with 1.25 mg daily. When using micronized tablets, patients who are more sensitive to antidiabetics should start with 0.75 mg daily.
➤ **To replace insulin therapy—**
Adults: If insulin dosage is less than 40 units/day, patient may be switched directly to glyburide when insulin is discontinued. If insulin dosage is 40 or more units/day, initially 5-mg regular tablets or 3-mg micronized formulation can be given P.O. once daily in addition to 50% of insulin dosage.

ACTION
Unknown. A sulfonylurea that probably stimulates insulin release from pancreatic beta cells and reduces glucose output by the liver. An extrapancreatic effect increases peripheral sensitivity to insulin and causes a mild diuretic effect.

Route	Onset	Peak	Duration
P.O.	1-4 hr	2-4 hr	24 hr

Reactions may be *common*, uncommon, ***life-threatening***, or COMMON AND LIFE-THREATENING.

ADVERSE REACTIONS

EENT: changes in accommodation or blurred vision.

GI: nausea, epigastric fullness, heartburn.

Hematologic: *leukopenia,* hemolytic anemia, *agranulocytosis, thrombocytopenia, aplastic anemia.*

Hepatic: cholestatic jaundice, *hepatitis.*

Metabolic: *hypoglycemia.*

Musculoskeletal: arthralgia, myalgia.

Skin: rash, pruritus, other allergic reactions.

Other: *angioedema.*

INTERACTIONS

Drug-drug. *Anabolic steroids, chloramphenicol, clofibrate, guanethidine, MAO inhibitors, probenecid, phenylbutazone, salicylates, sulfonamides:* Increased hypoglycemic activity. Monitor glucose level.

Beta blockers: Prolonged hypoglycemic effect and masked symptoms of hypoglycemia. Use together cautiously.

Corticosteroids, glucagon, rifampin, thiazide diuretics: Decreased hypoglycemic response. Monitor glucose level.

Hydantoins: Increased hydantoin levels. Monitor blood levels.

Oral anticoagulants: Increased hypoglycemic activity or enhanced anticoagulant effect. Monitor glucose level, PT, and INR.

Drug-herb. *Burdock, dandelion, eucalyptus, marshmallow:* Increased hypoglycemic effects. Discourage use together.

Drug-lifestyle. *Alcohol use:* Altered glycemic control, most commonly hypoglycemia. Also may cause disulfiram-like reaction. Discourage use together.

EFFECTS ON LAB TEST RESULTS

• May increase BUN, alkaline phosphatase, bilirubin, AST, ALT, and cholesterol levels. May decrease glucose levels.

• May decrease hemoglobin and WBC, platelet, and granulocyte counts.

CONTRAINDICATIONS

Contraindicated in patients hypersensitive to drug and in those with diabetic ketoacidosis with or without coma; also contraindicated in pregnant or breast-feeding women.

NURSING CONSIDERATIONS

• Use cautiously in patients with hepatic or renal impairment; in debilitated, malnourished, or elderly patients; and in patients with known allergy to sulfonamides.

• *Alert:* Micronized glyburide (Glynase PresTab) contains drug in a smaller particle size and isn't bioequivalent to regular glyburide tablets. Patients who have been taking Micronase or DiaBeta need to be readjusted.

• Although most patients may take drug once daily, those taking more than 10 mg daily may achieve better results with b.i.d. dosage.

• Glyburide is a second-generation sulfonylurea. Adverse effects are less common than with first-generation drugs such as chlorpropamide.

• During periods of increased stress, such as infection, fever, surgery, or trauma, patient may need insulin therapy. Monitor patient closely for hyperglycemia in these situations.

• Patient transferring from insulin to an oral antidiabetic needs glucose level monitoring at least three times daily before meals. Patient may need hospitalization during transition.

• *Alert:* Don't confuse glyburide with glimepiride or glipizide.

PATIENT TEACHING

• Instruct patient about nature of disease and importance of following therapeutic regimen, adhering to specific diet, losing weight, getting exercise, following personal hygiene programs, and avoiding infection. Explain how and when to monitor glucose levels, and teach recognition of and intervention for hypoglycemia and hyperglycemia.

• Tell patient not to change drug dosage without prescriber's consent and to report abnormal blood or urine glucose test results.

• Teach patient to carry candy or other simple sugars to treat mild hypoglycemic episodes. Patient experiencing severe episode may need hospital treatment.

• Advise patient not to take other drugs, including OTC drugs, without first checking with prescriber.

• Advise patient to wear or carry medical identification at all times.

• *Alert:* Instruct patient to report episodes of hypoglycemia to prescriber immediately; severe hypoglycemia is sometimes fatal in patients receiving as little as 2.5 to 5 mg glyburide daily.
• Inform patient that alcohol may lower glucose levels and should be avoided.

✳ NEW DRUG

glyburide and metformin hydrochloride
Glucovance

Pregnancy risk category B

AVAILABLE FORMS
Tablets: 1.25 mg glyburide/250 mg metformin hydrochloride, 2.5 mg glyburide/ 500 mg metformin hydrochloride, 5 mg glyburide/500 mg metformin hydrochloride

INDICATIONS & DOSAGES
➤ **Adjunct to diet and exercise to improve glycemic control in patients with type 2 (non–insulin-dependent) diabetes whose hyperglycemia can't be controlled with diet and exercise alone—**
Adults: Initially, 1.25 mg glyburide/ 250 mg metformin hydrochloride P.O. once daily or b.i.d. with meals. In patients with HbA_{1c} greater than 9% or a fasting plasma glucose level greater than 200 mg/dl, start with 1.25 mg glyburide/ 250 mg metformin hydrochloride b.i.d. with morning and evening meals. Daily dose may be increased in increments of 1.25 mg glyburide/250 mg metformin hydrochloride daily q 2 weeks, up to the minimum effective dose needed to achieve adequate control of glucose level. Maximum daily dose is 20 mg glyburide/ 2,000 mg metformin.
➤ **Second-line therapy in patients with type 2 diabetes when diet, exercise, and initial treatment with a sulfonylurea or metformin don't result in adequate glycemic control—**
Adults: Initially, 2.5 mg glyburide/500 mg metformin hydrochloride or 5 mg glyburide/500 mg metformin hydrochloride b.i.d. with meals. Increase in increments of no more than 5 mg glyburide/500 mg metformin hydrochloride, up to the mini-

mum effective dose needed to achieve adequate control of glucose level. Maximum daily dose is 20 mg glyburide/2,000 mg metformin hydrochloride.
Adjust-a-dose: Initial and maintenance dosing should be conservative in elderly patients because of the potential for decreased renal function in this population. Any dosage adjustment requires careful assessment of renal function. The dosage in elderly, debilitated, or malnourished patients shouldn't be adjusted to the maximum, to avoid the risk of hypoglycemia.

ACTION
Unknown. Glyburide appears to lower glucose level by stimulating the release of insulin from the pancreas. Metformin decreases hepatic glucose production and intestinal absorption of glucose and improves insulin sensitivity.

Route	Onset	Peak	Duration
P.O. (glyburide)	1 hr	4 hr	24 hr
P.O. (metformin)	Unknown	Unknown	Unknown

ADVERSE REACTIONS
CNS: headache, dizziness.
GI: *diarrhea,* nausea, vomiting, abdominal pain.
Metabolic: *hypoglycemia, lactic acidosis.*
Respiratory: *upper respiratory tract infection.*

INTERACTIONS
Drug-drug. *Beta blockers, chloramphenicol, ciprofloxacin, coumarins, highly protein-bound drugs, MAO inhibitors, miconazole, NSAIDs, probenecid, salicylates, sulfonamides:* Increases hypoglycemic activity of glyburide. Monitor glucose level.
Calcium channel blockers, corticosteroids, estrogens, isoniazid, nicotinic acid, oral contraceptives, phenothiazines, phenytoin, sympathomimetics, thiazides and other diuretics, thyroid agents: May cause hyperglycemia. Monitor glucose level.
Cationic drugs (such as amiloride, cimetidine, digoxin, morphine, procainamide, quinidine, quinine, ranitidine, triamterene, trimethoprim, vancomycin): May increase

---

Reactions may be *common,* uncommon, *life-threatening,* or COMMON AND LIFE-THREATENING.

metformin plasma levels. Monitor glucose level.

Furosemide: Increases levels of metformin and decreases levels of furosemide. Monitor patient closely.

Nifedipine: Increases metformin levels. Metformin dosage may need to be decreased.

Drug-lifestyle. *Alcohol use:* Alters glycemic control, most commonly hypoglycemia. May cause disulfiram-like reaction with glyburide component. Discourage using together.

EFFECTS ON LAB TEST RESULTS
● May increase lactate levels. May decrease glucose levels.

CONTRAINDICATIONS
Contraindicated in patients hypersensitive to glyburide or metformin and in those with renal disease, renal dysfunction, or metabolic acidosis (including diabetic ketoacidosis). Also contraindicated in patients with heart failure requiring pharmacologic treatment.

NURSING CONSIDERATIONS
● Use cautiously in elderly, hepatically impaired, debilitated, or malnourished patients and in those with adrenal or pituitary insufficiency because of increased risk of hypoglycemia. Monitor renal function regularly in elderly patients.
● Assess glucose level before therapy and regularly thereafter. Monitor glycosylated hemoglobin to assess long-term therapy.
● *Alert:* Obtain baseline renal function studies and don't start drug if creatinine levels are 1.5 mg/dl or greater (in men) or 1.4 mg/dl or greater (in women). Monitor renal function at least once yearly while patient is on long-term therapy and more often if renal dysfunction is anticipated. If renal impairment is detected, stop drug.
● Temporarily stop drug in patients undergoing radiologic studies involving intravascular administration of iodinated contrast materials because products may result in acute alteration of renal function.
● For patients previously treated with glyburide or metformin, the starting dose of drug shouldn't exceed daily dose of the glyburide (or equivalent dose of another

sulfonylurea) and metformin already being taken.
● Monitor patient closely during times of increased stress, such as infection, fever, surgery, or trauma; insulin therapy may be needed. Temporarily suspend drug for any surgical procedure that requires restricted intake of food and fluids, and don't restart until patient's oral intake has resumed.
● Lactic acidosis is a rare but serious (50% fatal) metabolic complication that can result from metformin accumulation. Lactic acidosis occurs primarily in diabetic patients with significant renal insufficiency; multiple medical or surgical problems; and multiple drug regimens. The risk of lactic acidosis increases with the degree of renal impairment and patient age.
● Early symptoms of lactic acidosis may include malaise, myalgias, respiratory distress, increasing somnolence, and nonspecific abdominal distress.
● GI symptoms that occur after patient is stabilized on drug are unlikely to be drug-related, and could be caused by lactic acidosis or other serious disease.
● Suspect lactic acidosis in any diabetic patient with metabolic acidosis lacking evidence of ketoacidosis.
● Monitor patient's hematologic status for megaloblastic anemia. Patients with inadequate vitamin B_{12} or calcium intake or absorption seem predisposed to developing subnormal vitamin B_{12} levels when taking metformin. These patients should have vitamin B_{12} level determinations every 2 to 3 years.
● Discontinue drug if CV collapse, acute heart failure, acute MI, or other conditions characterized by hypoxemia occur because these conditions may be associated with lactic acidosis and may cause prerenal azotemia.
● Watch for ketoacidosis or lactic acidosis in patient who develops laboratory abnormalities or clinical illness by evaluating laboratory values, including electrolyte, ketone, glucose, pH, lactate, pyruvate, and metformin levels. Stop drug if there is evidence of acidosis.
● All patients should have a baseline creatinine that indicates normal renal function before initiation of therapy. Don't start treatment in patients age 80 or older, un-

less creatinine clearance level demonstrates that renal function is normal.

• Drug usually shouldn't be adjusted to maximum dose.

• Drug isn't recommended for breast-feeding women.

PATIENT TEACHING

• Tell patient to take once-daily dose with breakfast and twice-daily dose with breakfast and dinner.

• Teach patient about diabetes and importance of following therapeutic regimen; adhering to diet, weight reduction, regular exercise and hygiene programs; and avoiding infection. Explain how and when to self-monitor glucose level and how to differentiate between symptoms of hypoglycemia and hyperglycemia.

• Instruct patient to stop drug and tell prescriber of unexplained hyperventilation, myalgia, malaise, unusual somnolence, or other symptoms of early lactic acidosis.

• Tell patient that GI symptoms are common with initial drug therapy but that GI symptoms that occur after prolonged therapy may be related to lactic acidosis or other serious disease and should be reported promptly.

• Counsel patient against excessive short-term and long-term alcohol intake.

• Advise patient not to take any other drugs, including OTC drugs, without checking with prescriber.

• Instruct patient to carry medical identification.

---

insulins

insulin injection (regular insulin, crystalline zinc insulin)
Actrapid‡, Actrapid PenFill‡, Humulin-R ◊, Humulin R (concentrated) U-500, Hypurin Neutral‡, Insulin 2 Neutral‡, Novolin R ◊, Novolin R PenFill ◊, Novolin R Prefilled, Regular Iletin I ◊, Regular Iletin II ◊, Regular Purified Pork Insulin ◊, Velosulin Human BR†

insulin (lispro)
Humalog, Humalog 75/25

insulin zinc suspension, prompt (semilente)
Human Monotard§, Hypurin Lente§

isophane insulin suspension (neutral protamine Hagedorn insulin, NPH)
Humulin N ◊, Humulin NPH‡, Hypurin Isophane‡, Iletin II NPH Purified Pork ◊, Novolin N ◊, Novolin N PenFill ◊, Novolin N Prefilled, NPH Insulin ◊, NPH Purified Pork ◊, Protaphane‡, Protaphane PenFill‡

isophane insulin suspension with insulin injection
Humulin 50/50 ◊, Humulin 70/30 ◊, Novolin 70/30, Novolin 70/30 PenFill ◊, Novolin 70/30 Prefilled

insulin zinc suspension (lente)
Humulin L ◊, Lente Iletin I ◊, Lente Iletin II ◊, Lente MC‡, Lente Purified Pork Insulin ◊, Novolin L ◊

insulin zinc suspension, extended (ultralente)
Humulin-U Ultralente Insulin ◊

Pregnancy risk category B

AVAILABLE FORMS
insulin injection
Injection (human): 100 units/ml (Humulin-R ◊, Novolin R ◊, Velosulin Human BR‡); 100 units/ml in 1.5-ml cartridge system ◊ (Novolin R PenFill ◊); 100 units/ml in 1.5-ml prefilled syringes (Novolin R Prefilled ◊)
Injection (pork): 100 units/ml ◊
Injection (purified pork): 100 units/ml (Actrapid‡, Pork Regular Iletin II ◊, Regular Purified Pork Insulin ◊); 100 units/ml in 1.5-ml cartridge system‡ (Actrapid PenFill‡); 100 units/ml in 2-ml cartridge

---

Reactions may be *common*, uncommon, ***life-threatening***, or COMMON AND LIFE-THREATENING.

system‡; 500 units/ml (Regular [Concentrated] Iletin II)
insulin lispro injection
Injection (human): 100 units/ml (Humalog); lispro 25 units/ml with lispro protamine 75 units/ml (Humalog Mix 75/25)
insulin zinc suspension, prompt
Injection (purified pork): 100 units/ml ◊
isophane insulin suspension
Injection (human, recombinant): 100 units/ml (Humulin N ◊, Humulin NPH‡, Novolin N ◊); 100 units/ml in 1.5-ml cartridge system (Novolin N PenFill ◊, Protaphane PenFill‡); 100 units/ml in 1.5-ml prefilled syringes (Novolin N Prefilled ◊)
Injection (purified pork): 100 units/ml (NPH Purified Pork ◊, Purified Pork NPH Iletin II, Protaphane‡)
isophane insulin suspension 50% with insulin injection 50%
Injection (human): 100 units/ml (Humulin 50/50 ◊, Novolin 50/50 ◊)
isophane insulin suspension 70% with insulin injection 30%
Injection (human): 100 units/ml (Humulin 70/30 ◊, Novolin 70/30 ◊); 100 units/ml in 1.5-ml cartridge system (Novolin 70/30 PenFill ◊); 100 units/ml in 1.5-ml prefilled syringes (Novolin 70/30 Prefilled ◊)
insulin zinc suspension
Injection (purified pork): 100 units/ml (Lente Iletin II, Lente L Insulin ◊)
Injection (human): 100 units/ml ◊ (Humulin L ◊, Novolin L ◊)
insulin zinc suspension, extended
Injection (human): 100 units/ml (Humulin-U Ultralente ◊)

INDICATIONS & DOSAGES
➤ **Diabetic ketoacidosis (regular insulin)—**
Adults: 0.33 unit/kg as I.V. bolus; then 0.1 unit/kg/hour by continuous infusion. Continue infusion until glucose level drops to 250 mg/dl; then S.C. insulin is begun with dosage, and dosage interval is adjusted according to patient's glucose level.

Or, 50 to 100 units I.V. and 50 to 100 units S.C. immediately; then additional doses q 2 to 6 hours based on glucose levels.

Children: 0.1 unit/kg as I.V. bolus; then 0.1 unit/kg hourly by continuous infusion until glucose level drops to 250 mg/dl; then S.C. insulin started. Or, 1 to 2 units/kg in two divided doses, one I.V. and the other S.C., followed by 0.5 to 1 unit/kg I.V. q 1 to 2 hours based on glucose levels.
➤ **Type 1 (insulin-dependent) diabetes, adjunct to type 2 (non–insulin-dependent) diabetes inadequately controlled by diet and oral antidiabetics—**
Adults and children: Therapeutic regimen adjusted based on patient's glucose levels.
➤ **Control of hyperglycemia with longer-acting insulin (Humalog) in patients with type 1 diabetes and with sulfonylureas in patients with type 2 diabetes—**
Adults and children older than age 3: Dosage varies and must be determined by a prescriber familiar with patient's metabolic needs, eating habits, and other lifestyle variables. Inject S.C. within 15 minutes before or immediately after a meal.

I.V. ADMINISTRATION
● Administer only regular insulin I.V. Inject directly into vein or into a port close to I.V. access site. Intermittent infusion isn't recommended. If given by continuous infusion, infuse drug diluted in normal saline solution at prescribed rate.
● *Alert:* Regular insulin is used in patients with circulatory collapse, diabetic ketoacidosis, or hyperkalemia. Don't use Humulin R (concentrated) U-500 I.V. Don't use intermediate or long-acting insulins for coma or other emergency requiring rapid drug action. Also, ketosis-prone type 1, severely ill, and newly diagnosed diabetic patients with very high glucose levels may need hospitalization and I.V. treatment with regular fast-acting insulin.

ACTION
Increases glucose transport across muscle and fat cell membranes to reduce glucose level. Promotes conversion of glucose to its storage form, glycogen; triggers amino acid uptake and conversion to protein in muscle cells and inhibits protein degradation; stimulates triglyceride formation and inhibits release of free fatty acids from adipose tissue; and stimulates lipoprotein

---

*Liquid contains alcohol.   **May contain tartrazine.   †Canada   ‡Australia   §U.K.   ◊OTC

lipase activity, which converts circulating lipoproteins to fatty acids.

Route	Onset	Peak	Duration
I.V. (rapid)	10-30 min	15-30 min	0.5-1 hr
S.C. (rapid)	0.5-1.5 hr	2-3 hr	5-7 hr
S.C. (inter-mediate)	1-2.5 hr	4-15 hr	12-24 hr
S.C. (long-acting)	4-8 hr	10-30 hr	36 hr
S.C. (Humalog)	15-30 min	30-90 min	3-6.5 hr

ADVERSE REACTIONS
Metabolic: *hypoglycemia,* hyperglycemia, hypomagnesemia, hypokalemia.
Skin: rash, urticaria, pruritus, swelling, redness, stinging, warmth at injection site.
Other: *lipoatrophy, lipohypertrophy,* hypersensitivity reactions, ***anaphylaxis.***

INTERACTIONS
Drug-drug. *Anabolic steroids, beta blockers, clofibrate, fenfluramine, guanethidine, isoniazid, MAO inhibitors, niacin, phenothiazines, salicylates, tetracycline:* Prolonged hypoglycemic effect. Monitor glucose level carefully.
Corticosteroids, dextrothyroxine, epinephrine, thiazide diuretics, thyroid hormone: Diminished insulin response. Monitor patient for hyperglycemia.
Diazoxide, fosphenytoin, phenytoin (high doses): May inhibit endogenous insulin secretion and cause hypoglycemia in diabetic patients. Carefully adjust insulin dosage when using with these drugs.
Oral contraceptives, estrogens: May decrease glucose tolerance in diabetic patients. Monitor glucose levels and adjust insulin dosage carefully.
Drug-herb. *Basil, bay, bee pollen, burdock, sage:* May affect glycemic control. Advise patient and monitor glucose level closely.
Dandelion, eucalyptus, marshmallow: Increased hypoglycemic effects. Discourage use together.
Garlic, ginseng: May decrease glucose levels. Discourage use together.
Drug-lifestyle. *Alcohol use:* Hypoglycemic effect. Discourage use together.

Marijuana use: May increase glucose levels. Tell patient to avoid marijuana.
Smoking: May increase glucose levels and decrease response to insulin administration. Monitor glucose levels.

EFFECTS ON LAB TEST RESULTS
• May decrease glucose, magnesium, potassium, and inorganic phosphate levels.

CONTRAINDICATIONS
Contraindicated in patients with history of systemic allergic reaction to pork when porcine-derived products are used, or hypersensitivity to any component of preparation.

NURSING CONSIDERATIONS
• Insulin is drug of choice to treat diabetes during pregnancy. Insulin requirements increase in pregnant diabetic women and then decline immediately postpartum. Monitor patient closely.
• Dosage is always expressed in USP units. Remember to use only the syringes calibrated for the particular concentration of insulin administered. U-500 insulin must be administered with a U-100 syringe because no syringes are made for this strength.
• Some patients may develop insulin resistance and need large insulin doses to control symptoms of diabetes. U-500 insulin is available as Humulin R (concentrated) U-500 for such patients. Although not every pharmacy may stock it, it's available. Give the pharmacy sufficient notice before requesting refill prescription. Never store U-500 insulin in same area with other insulin preparations because of danger of severe overdose if given accidentally to other patients.
• To mix insulin suspension, swirl vial gently or rotate between palms or between palm and thigh. Don't shake vigorously—this causes bubbling and air in syringe.
• Lente, semilente, and ultralente insulins may be mixed in any proportion. Regular insulin may be mixed with NPH or lente insulins in any proportion. When mixing regular insulin with intermediate or long-acting insulin, always draw up regular insulin into syringe first.

Reactions may be *common,* uncommon, *life-threatening,* or **COMMON AND LIFE-THREATENING.**

• Switching from separate injections to a prepared mixture may alter patient response. When NPH or lente is mixed with regular insulin in the same syringe, give immediately to avoid loss of potency.

• Lispro insulin may be mixed with Humulin N or Humulin U and should be given within 15 minutes before a meal to prevent a hypoglycemic reaction.

• Don't use insulin that changes color or becomes clumped or granular in appearance.

• Check expiration date on vial before using contents.

• Usual administration route is S.C. For proper S.C. administration, remember to pinch a fold of skin with your fingers at least 3 inches (7.6 cm) apart, and insert needle at a 45- to 90-degree angle.

• Press but don't rub site after injection. Rotate injection sites and keep track to avoid overuse of one area. Diabetic patients may achieve better control if injection site is rotated within same anatomic region.

• Monitor patient for hyperglycemia (rebound, or Somogyi effect).

• Store insulin in cool area. Refrigeration is desirable but not essential, except with Humulin R (concentrated) U-500.

PATIENT TEACHING

• Make sure patient knows that drug relieves symptoms but doesn't cure disease.

• Instruct patient about nature of disease and importance of following therapeutic regimen, adhering to specific diet, losing weight, getting exercise, following personal hygiene program, and avoiding infection. Emphasize importance of timing injections with eating and of not skipping meals.

• Stress that accuracy of measurement is important, especially with concentrated regular insulin. Aids, such as magnifying sleeve or dose magnifier, may improve accuracy. Show patient and caregivers how to measure and administer insulin.

• Advise patient not to change order in which insulins are mixed or model or brand of insulin, syringe, or needle.

• Teach patient that glucose levels and urine ketone tests provide essential guides to dosage and success of therapy. It's important for patient to recognize hyper-

glycemic and hypoglycemic symptoms. Insulin-induced hypoglycemia is hazardous and may cause brain damage if prolonged; most adverse effects are temporary. Instruct patient on insulin peak times and their importance.

• Instruct patient on proper use of equipment for monitoring glucose levels.

• Advise patient not to smoke within 30 minutes after insulin injection. Cigarette smoking decreases amount of insulin absorbed by S.C. route.

• Advise patient to avoid vigorous exercise immediately after insulin injection, especially of the area where injection was administered; it causes increased absorption and increased risk of hyperglycemia.

• Inform patient that marijuana may increase insulin requirements.

• Teach patient that alcohol lowers glucose level, and should be avoided.

• Advise patient to wear or carry medical identification at all times, to carry ample insulin and syringes on trips, to keep carbohydrates (lump of sugar or candy) on hand for emergencies, and to note time zone changes for dosage schedule when traveling.

• Advise woman planning pregnancy to consult prescriber before becoming pregnant.

• Advise patient to store insulin at 36° to 46° F (2° to 8° C). Don't freeze or expose vials to excessive heat or sunlight.

---

insulin aspart (rDNA origin) injection
NovoLog

Pregnancy risk category C

AVAILABLE FORMS
Injection: 100 units/ml

INDICATIONS & DOSAGES
➤ **Control of hyperglycemia in patients with diabetes mellitus—**
Adults and children ages 6 and older:
Dosage is highly individualized. Typical daily insulin requirement is 0.5 to 1 unit/kg/day, divided in a meal-related treatment regimen. About 50% to 70% of dose is provided with NovoLog and the remainder by an intermediate- or long-acting insulin.

➤ **Management of type 2 (non–insulin-dependent) diabetes mellitus in patients previously treated with oral antidiabetics—**
Adults: Dosage is highly individualized and based on glucose levels and the patient's response to therapy. Give dose in the evening.

ACTION

Insulin glargine lowers glucose levels by stimulating peripheral glucose uptake, especially by skeletal muscle and fat, and by inhibiting hepatic glucose production.

Route	Onset	Peak	Duration
S.C.	Unknown	None	10.8-24 hr

ADVERSE REACTIONS
Metabolic: *hypoglycemia.*
Skin: lipodystrophy, pruritus, rash.
Other: allergic reactions, pain at injection site.

INTERACTIONS
Drug-drug. *ACE inhibitors, disopyramide, fibrates, fluoxetine, MAO inhibitors, octreotide, oral antidiabetics, propoxyphene, salicylates, sulfonamide antibiotics:* May cause hypoglycemia and increased insulin effect. Monitor glucose. Dosage adjustments of Lantus may be required.
Beta blockers, clonidine: May mask the signs of hypoglycemia. Avoid using together, if possible. Also, may either potentiate or weaken the glucose-lowering effect of insulin. Monitor glucose carefully.
Corticosteroids, danazol, diuretics, estrogens, isoniazid, phenothiazines (such as compazine, phenergan), progestins (such as oral contraceptives), somatropin, sympathomimetics (such as albuterol, epinephrine, terbutaline), thyroid hormones: May reduce the glucose-lowering effect of insulin. Monitor glucose. Dose adjustments of Lantus may be required.
Guanethidine, reserpine: May mask the signs of hypoglycemia. Avoid using together, if possible. Monitor glucose carefully.
Lithium: May either potentiate or weaken the glucose-lowering effect of insulin. Monitor glucose. Dosage adjustments of Lantus may be required.

Pentamidine: May cause hypoglycemia, which may be followed by hyperglycemia. Avoid using together, if possible.
Drug-herb. *Burdock, dandelion, eucalyptus, marshmallow:* Increased hypoglycemic effects. Discourage use together.
Licorice root: May increase dosage requirements of insulin. Discourage use together.
Drug-lifestyle. *Alcohol use, emotional stress:* May potentiate or weaken the glucose-lowering effect of insulin. Monitor glucose.

EFFECTS ON LAB TEST RESULTS
• May decrease glucose levels.

CONTRAINDICATIONS
Contraindicated in patients who are hypersensitive to insulin glargine or its excipients.

NURSING CONSIDERATIONS
• Use cautiously in patients with renal or hepatic impairment.
• **Alert:** Drug isn't intended for I.V. use. It's only for S.C. use.
• Prolonged duration of activity is dependent on injection into S.C. space.
• Because of prolonged duration, this isn't the insulin of choice for diabetic ketoacidosis.
• Desired glucose levels, as well as the doses and timing of antidiabetic medication, must be determined individually, as with any insulin. Glucose monitoring is recommended for all patients with diabetes.
• The rate of absorption, onset, and duration of action may be affected by exercise and other variables, such as illness and emotional stress.
• **Alert:** Lantus must not be diluted or mixed with any other insulin or solution.
• As with any insulin therapy, lipodystrophy may occur at the site of injection and may delay insulin absorption. Continuously rotate injection sites within a given area to reduce lipodystrophy.
• Hypoglycemia is the most common adverse effect of insulin. Early symptoms may be different or less pronounced in patients with long duration of diabetes, diabetic nerve disease, or intensified diabetes control. Monitor glucose closely in these

patients because severe hypoglycemia may result before the patient develops symptoms.

PATIENT TEACHING
● Teach proper glucose monitoring, injection techniques, and diabetes management.
● *Alert:* Educate diabetic patients about signs and symptoms of hypoglycemia, such as fatigue, weakness, confusion, headache, pallor, and diaphoresis.
● Urge patient to wear or carry medical identification at all times.
● Advise patient to treat mild episodes of hypoglycemia with oral glucose tablets. Encourage patient to always carry glucose tablets in case of a hypoglycemic episode.
● Educate patients on the importance of maintaining a diabetic diet, and explain that adjustments in drug dosage, meal patterns, and exercise may be needed to regulate blood sugar.
● *Alert:* Advise patient not to dilute or mix any other insulin or solution with Lantus. If the solution is cloudy, urge patient to discard the vial. Solution should be used only if clear and colorless.
● *Alert:* Any change of insulin should be made cautiously and only under medical supervision. Changes in insulin type, strength, manufacturer, type (such as regular, NPH, or insulin analogs), species (animal, human), or method of manufacturer (rDNA versus animal source insulin) may result in the need for a change in dosage. Oral antidiabetic treatment taken at the same time may need to be adjusted.
● Tell patient to consult prescriber before using OTC medications.
● Inform patient that alcohol lowers glucose level and should be avoided.
● Advise patient to avoid vigorous exercise immediately after insulin injection, especially of the area where injection was administered; it causes increased absorption and increased risk of hyperglycemia.
● Advise woman planning pregnancy to consult prescriber before becoming pregnant.
● Advise patient to store Lantus vials and cartridges in the refrigerator.

metformin hydrochloride
Glucophage, Glucophage XR

Pregnancy risk category B

AVAILABLE FORMS
Tablets: 500 mg, 850 mg, 1,000 mg
Tablets (extended-release): 500 mg

INDICATIONS & DOSAGES
➤ **Adjunct to diet to lower glucose level in patients with type 2 (non–insulin-dependent) diabetes mellitus—**
Adults: Initially, 500 mg P.O. b.i.d. given with morning and evening meals, or 850 mg P.O. once daily given with morning meal. When 500-mg form is used, increase dosage by 500 mg weekly to maximum dose of 2,500 mg P.O. daily in divided doses, p.r.n. When 850-mg form is used, increase dosage by 850 mg every other week to maximum dose of 2,550 mg P.O. daily in divided doses, p.r.n. If using extended-release formulation, initiate therapy at 500 mg P.O. qd with the evening meal. May increase dose weekly in increments of 500 mg/day, up to a maximum dose of 2,000 mg once daily. If higher doses are required, consider using the regular release formulation up to its maximum dose.
Adjust-a-dose: For debilitated and elderly patients, dosing should be conservative because of potential decrease in renal function.

ACTION
Decreases hepatic glucose production and intestinal absorption of glucose and improves insulin sensitivity (increases peripheral glucose uptake and utilization).

Route	Onset	Peak	Duration
P.O. (conventional)	Unknown	2-4 hr	Unknown
P.O. (extended-release)	Unknown	4-8 hr	Unknown

ADVERSE REACTIONS
GI: diarrhea, nausea, vomiting, abdominal bloating, flatulence, anorexia, unpleasant or metallic taste.

Hematologic: megaloblastic anemia.
Metabolic: *lactic acidosis.*

INTERACTIONS

Drug-drug. *Calcium channel blockers, corticosteroids, estrogens, fosphenytoin, isoniazid, nicotinic acid, oral contraceptives, phenothiazines, phenytoin, sympathomimetics, thiazide and other diuretics, thyroid drugs:* May produce hyperglycemia. Monitor patient's glycemic control. Metformin dosage may need to be increased.
Cationic drugs (such as amiloride, cimetidine, digoxin, morphine, procainamide, quinidine, quinine, ranitidine, triamterene, trimethoprim, vancomycin): Have potential to compete for common renal tubular transport systems, which may increase metformin plasma levels. Monitor glucose level.
Nifedipine: Increased metformin plasma levels. Monitor patient closely. Metformin dosage may need to be decreased.
Radiologic contrast dye: Can result in acute renal failure. Withhold metformin for 24 hours before procedure.
Drug-herb. *Guar gum:* Decreased hypoglycemic effect. Discourage use together.
Drug-lifestyle. *Alcohol use:* Potentiates drug effects. Discourage use together.

EFFECTS ON LAB TEST RESULTS
● May decrease hemoglobin.

CONTRAINDICATIONS
Contraindicated in patients hypersensitive to drug and in those with renal disease or metabolic acidosis. Also contraindicated in patients with congestive heart failure requiring pharmacologic intervention, conditions predisposing to renal dysfunction, CV collapse, MI, and septicemia. Drug should be temporarily withheld in patients undergoing radiologic studies involving parenteral administration of iodinated contrast materials because use of such products may result in acute renal dysfunction. Drug should be promptly discontinued if patient enters a hypoxic state. Avoid use in patients with hepatic disease.

NURSING CONSIDERATIONS
● Use caution when giving drug to elderly, debilitated, or malnourished patients and to those with adrenal or pituitary insufficiency because of increased risk of hypoglycemia.
● Before therapy begins and at least annually thereafter, patient's renal function should be assessed. If renal impairment is detected, expect prescriber to switch patient to a different antidiabetic. This is particularly important in elderly patients.
● Administer with meals; once-daily dosage should be given with breakfast and twice-daily dosage with breakfast and dinner. Maximum doses may be better tolerated if total dose is divided into t.i.d. dosing and given with meals.
● When switching patients from standard oral hypoglycemics (except chlorpropamide) to metformin, no transition period is usually needed. When switching patients from chlorpropamide to metformin, care should be taken during the first 2 weeks of metformin therapy because the prolonged retention of chlorpropamide increases the risk of hypoglycemia during this time.
● Monitor patient's glucose levels regularly to evaluate effectiveness of therapy. Notify prescriber if they become elevated despite therapy.
● If patient hasn't responded to 4 weeks of therapy with maximum dosage, prescriber may add an oral sulfonylurea while keeping metformin at maximum dosage. If patient still doesn't respond after several months of therapy with both drugs at maximum dosage, prescriber may discontinue both and start insulin therapy.
● Monitor patient closely during times of increased stress, such as infection, fever, surgery, or trauma. Insulin therapy may be needed in these situations.
● Risk of drug-induced lactic acidosis is very low. Reported cases have occurred primarily in diabetic patients with significant renal insufficiency; in those with other medical or surgical problems; and in those with other drug regimens. Risk increases with degree of renal impairment and patient age.
● *Alert:* Stop drug immediately and notify prescriber if patient develops a condition related to hypoxemia or dehydration because of risk of lactic acidosis.
● Expect drug therapy to be temporarily suspended for surgical procedures (except

minor procedures that don't restrict intake of food and fluids) and for patients undergoing radiologic studies involving use of contrast media containing iodine. Therapy shouldn't be restarted until patient's oral intake has resumed and renal function has been deemed normal by prescriber.

• Monitor patient's hematologic status for evidence of megaloblastic anemia. Patients with inadequate vitamin B_{12} or calcium intake or absorption appear to be predisposed to developing subnormal vitamin B_{12} levels. These patients should have routine vitamin B_{12} level determinations every 2 to 3 years.

PATIENT TEACHING
• *Alert:* Instruct patient about nature of diabetes and importance of following therapeutic regimen, adhering to specific diet, losing weight, getting exercise, following personal hygiene programs, and avoiding infection. Explain how and when to monitor glucose level. Teach evidence of hypoglycemia and hyperglycemia. Explain emergency measures.
• *Alert:* Instruct patient to stop drug and immediately notify prescriber about unexplained hyperventilation, myalgia, malaise, unusual somnolence, or other nonspecific symptoms of early lactic acidosis.
• Warn patient not to consume excessive alcohol while taking drug.
• Tell patient not to change drug dosage without prescriber's consent. Encourage patient to report abnormal glucose level test results.
• Advise patient not to take other drugs, including OTC drugs, without first checking with prescriber.
• Instruct patient to wear or carry medical identification at all times.

---

miglitol
Glyset

Pregnancy risk category B

AVAILABLE FORMS
Tablets: 25 mg, 50 mg, 100 mg

INDICATIONS & DOSAGES
➤ Adjunct to diet to improve glycemic control in patients with type 2 (non–

insulin-dependent) diabetes mellitus whose hyperglycemia can't be managed with diet alone; with a sulfonylurea when diet plus either miglitol or sulfonylurea doesn't result in adequate glycemic control—
Adults: 25 mg P.O. t.i.d. with first bite of each main meal; dosage may be increased after 4 to 8 weeks to 50 mg P.O. t.i.d. Dosage may then be further increased after 3 months, based on glycosylated hemoglobin level, to maximum of 100 mg P.O. t.i.d.

ACTION
Lowers glucose level by inhibiting the alpha-glucosidases in the small intestine. These enzymes convert carbohydrates to glucose. Inhibition of the enzymes delays the digestion of carbohydrates after a meal, resulting in a smaller rise in postprandial glucose levels.

Route	Onset	Peak	Duration
P.O.	Unknown	2-3 hr	Unknown

ADVERSE REACTIONS
GI: *abdominal pain, diarrhea, flatulence.*
Skin: rash.

INTERACTIONS
Drug-drug. *Digoxin, propranolol, ranitidine:* May decrease bioavailability of these drugs. Watch for loss of efficacy of these drugs, and adjust dosage.
Intestinal absorbents (such as charcoal), digestive enzyme preparations (such as amylase, pancreatin): May reduce effectiveness of miglitol. Discourage use together.

EFFECTS ON LAB TEST RESULTS
• May decrease iron levels.

CONTRAINDICATIONS
Contraindicated in patients hypersensitive to drug or its components and in those with diabetic ketoacidosis, inflammatory bowel disease, colonic ulceration, partial intestinal obstruction, chronic intestinal diseases with marked disorders of digestion or absorption, or conditions that may deteriorate because of increased gas formation in the intestine. Also contraindicated in those predisposed to intestinal ob-

struction. Drug isn't recommended for patients with significant renal dysfunction (creatinine higher than 2 mg/dl).

NURSING CONSIDERATIONS
● Use cautiously in patients also receiving insulin or oral sulfonylureas because drug may increase hypoglycemic potential of insulin or sulfonylureas. Adjustments of these drugs may be needed. Monitor patient for increased frequency of hypoglycemia.
● Management of type 2 diabetes should include diet control, exercise program, and regular testing of urine and glucose levels.
● Monitor glucose level regularly, especially during situations of increased stress, such as infection, fever, surgery, or trauma.
● Besides checking glucose levels regularly, monitor glycosylated hemoglobin level every 3 months to evaluate long-term glycemic control.
● Treat mild to moderate hypoglycemia with a form of dextrose, such as glucose tablets or gel. Severe hypoglycemia may need I.V. glucose or glucagon.
● Drug should be given with the first bite of each main meal.
● Monitor patient for adverse GI effects.

PATIENT TEACHING
● Stress importance of adhering to diet, weight reduction, and exercise instructions. Urge patient to have glucose and glycosylated hemoglobin levels tested regularly.
● Inform patient that drug treatment relieves symptoms but doesn't cure diabetes.
● Teach patient how to recognize hyperglycemia and hypoglycemia.
● Instruct patient to have a source of glucose readily available to treat hypoglycemia when miglitol is taken with a sulfonylurea or with insulin.
● Advise patient to seek medical advice promptly during periods of stress, such as fever, trauma, infection, or surgery, because dosage may have to be adjusted.
● Instruct patient to take drug three times daily with first bite of each main meal.
● Show patient how and when to monitor glucose levels.
● Advise patient that sucrose (table sugar, cane sugar) or fruit juices shouldn't be used

to treat hypoglycemic reactions with miglitol. Oral glucose (dextrose) or glucagon is necessary to increase blood sugar.
● Advise patient that adverse GI effects are most common during first few weeks of therapy and should improve over time.
● Urge patient to wear or carry medical identification at all times.

✳ **NEW DRUG**

nateglinide
Starlix

Pregnancy risk category C

AVAILABLE FORMS
Tablets: 60 mg, 120 mg

INDICATIONS & DOSAGES
➤ **As monotherapy, or with metformin, to lower glucose level in patients with type 2 (non–insulin-dependent) diabetes whose hyperglycemia isn't adequately controlled by diet and exercise and who haven't had long-term treatment with other antidiabetics—**
Adults: 120 mg P.O. t.i.d., 1 to 30 minutes before meals. Patients near goal HbA$_{1c}$ when treatment is initiated may receive 60 mg P.O. t.i.d.

ACTION
Lowers glucose levels by stimulating insulin secretion from pancreatic beta cells.

Route	Onset	Peak	Duration
P.O.	20 min	1 hr	4 hr

ADVERSE REACTIONS
CNS: dizziness.
GI: diarrhea.
Metabolic: *hypoglycemia.*
Musculoskeletal: back pain, arthropathy.
Respiratory: *upper respiratory tract infection,* bronchitis, coughing.
Other: flu symptoms, accidental trauma.

INTERACTIONS
Drug-drug. *Corticosteroids, sympathomimetics, thiazides, thyroid products:* May reduce hypoglycemic action of nateglinide. Monitor glucose level closely.
MAO inhibitors, nonselective beta blockers, NSAIDs, salicylates: May potentiate

---

Reactions may be *common,* uncommon, *life-threatening,* or COMMON AND LIFE-THREATENING.

hypoglycemic action of nateglinide. Monitor glucose level closely.

EFFECTS ON LAB TEST RESULTS
• May decrease glucose levels.

CONTRAINDICATIONS
Contraindicated in patients hypersensitive to drug and in patients with type 1 diabetes or diabetic ketoacidosis.

NURSING CONSIDERATIONS
• Use cautiously in patients with moderate to severe liver dysfunction or adrenal or pituitary insufficiency, and in elderly and malnourished patients.
• Don't use with or as a substitute for glyburide or other oral antidiabetics. May be used with metformin.
• Give drug 1 to 30 minutes before a meal. If patient misses a meal, skip the scheduled dose.
• Monitor glucose levels regularly to evaluate drug's efficacy.
• Observe patient for signs and symptoms of hypoglycemia (sweating, rapid pulse, trembling, confusion, headache, irritability, and nausea). To minimize risk of hypoglycemia, make sure that patient has a meal immediately after dose. If hypoglycemia occurs and patient remains conscious, give him an oral form of glucose. If he is unconscious, treat with I.V. glucose.
• Risk of hypoglycemia increases with strenuous exercise, alcohol ingestion, or insufficient caloric intake.
• Symptoms of hypoglycemia may be masked in patients with autonomic neuropathy and in those who use beta blockers.
• Insulin therapy may be needed for glycemic control in patients with fever, infection, or trauma and in those undergoing surgery.
• Monitor glucose levels closely when other drugs are initiated or discontinued to evaluate for possible drug interactions.
• Periodically monitor HbA$_{1c}$ levels.
• Reduced effectiveness may occur over time.
• No special dosage adjustments are usually necessary in elderly patients. However, greater sensitivity to glucose-lowering effect may occur in some elderly patients.

• It's unknown if drug appears in breast milk. Don't use in breast-feeding women.

PATIENT TEACHING
• Tell patient to take drug 1 to 30 minutes before a meal.
• Advise patient to skip the scheduled dose if he skips a meal, to reduce risk of hypoglycemia.
• Instruct patient on risk of hypoglycemia and its signs and symptoms (sweating, rapid pulse, trembling, confusion, headache, irritability, and nausea). Advise him to treat these symptoms by eating or drinking something containing sugar.
• Teach patient how to monitor and log blood sugar levels to evaluate diabetes control.
• Advise patient to notify prescriber for persistent hypoglycemia or hyperglycemia.
• Instruct patient to adhere to prescribed diet and exercise regimen.
• Explain possible long-term complications of diabetes and importance of regular preventive therapy.
• Encourage patient to wear a medical alert bracelet indicating that he has diabetes.

---

pioglitazone hydrochloride
Actos

Pregnancy risk category C

AVAILABLE FORMS
Tablets: 15 mg, 30 mg, 45 mg

INDICATION & DOSAGES
➤ **Adjunct to diet and exercise to improve glycemic control in patients with type 2 (non–insulin-dependent) diabetes mellitus; or when diet, exercise, and a sulfonylurea, metformin, or insulin fails to yield adequate glycemic control—**
Adults: Initially, 15 or 30 mg P.O. once daily. For patients who respond inadequately to initial dosage, it may be increased incrementally; maximum dosage is 45 mg/day. If used in combination therapy, maximum dosage shouldn't exceed 30 mg/day.

ACTION
Lowers glucose levels by decreasing insulin resistance. Improves sensitivity of insulin in muscle and adipose tissue.

Route	Onset	Peak	Duration
P.O.	Unknown	Within 2 hr	Unknown

ADVERSE REACTIONS
CNS: headache.
CV: *edema.*
EENT: sinusitis, pharyngitis.
Hematologic: anemia.
Metabolic: hypoglycemia with combination therapy, aggravated diabetes mellitus, weight gain.
Musculoskeletal: myalgia.
Respiratory: upper respiratory tract infection.
Other: tooth disorder.

INTERACTIONS
Drug-drug. *Ketoconazole:* May inhibit pioglitazone metabolism. Monitor glucose levels more frequently.
Oral contraceptives: May reduce plasma levels of oral contraceptives, resulting in less effective contraception. Advise patient taking drug and oral contraceptives to consider additional birth control measures.
Drug-herb. *Burdock, dandelion, eucalyptus, marshmallow:* Increased hypoglycemic effects. Discourage use together.
Drug-lifestyle. *Alcohol use:* Altered glycemic control; hypoglycemia. Discourage use together.

EFFECTS ON LAB TEST RESULTS
● May decrease glucose and triglyceride levels. May increase HDL levels.
● May decrease hemoglobin.

CONTRAINDICATIONS
Contraindicated in patients hypersensitive to drug or its components and in those with type 1 (insulin-dependent) diabetes mellitus, clinical evidence of active liver disease, ALT level greater than 2½ times the upper limit of normal, or New York Heart Association class III or IV heart failure. Also contraindicated in patients with diabetic ketoacidosis and in those who experienced jaundice while taking troglitazone.

NURSING CONSIDERATIONS
● Use cautiously in patients with edema or heart failure.
● *Alert:* Measure liver enzyme levels at start of therapy, every 2 months for first year of therapy, and periodically thereafter. Liver function tests also should be done in patients who develop evidence of liver dysfunction, such as nausea, vomiting, abdominal pain, fatigue, anorexia, or dark urine. Discontinue drug if patient develops jaundice or if results of liver function tests show elevations in ALT levels greater than three times the upper limit of normal.
● Because ovulation may resume in premenopausal, anovulatory women with insulin resistance, recommend use of additional contraceptive measures.
● Drug should be used in pregnancy only if the benefit justifies risk to fetus. Insulin is the preferred antidiabetic for use during pregnancy.
● Monitor patients with heart failure for increased edema.
● Hemoglobin level and hematocrit may decrease, usually during first 4 to 12 weeks of therapy.
● Patients with normal liver enzyme levels who are switched from troglitazone therapy should undergo a 1-week washout period before starting pioglitazone.
● Management of type 2 diabetes should include diet control. Because caloric restrictions, weight loss, and exercise help improve insulin sensitivity and help make drug therapy effective, these measures are essential for proper diabetes management.
● Watch for hypoglycemia in patients receiving pioglitazone with insulin or a sulfonylurea. Dosage adjustments of these drugs may be needed.
● Monitor glucose levels regularly, especially during situations of increased stress, such as infection, fever, surgery, and trauma.
● Glucose and glycosylated hemoglobin levels should be checked periodically to evaluate therapeutic response to drug.
● Safety and efficacy of drug in children haven't been evaluated.
● *Alert:* Don't confuse pioglitazone with rosiglitazone.

Reactions may be *common*, uncommon, *life-threatening*, or COMMON AND LIFE-THREATENING.

PATIENT TEACHING
• Instruct patient to adhere to dietary instructions and to have glucose and glycosylated hemoglobin levels tested regularly.
• Teach patient taking pioglitazone with insulin or oral antidiabetics the signs and symptoms of hypoglycemia.
• Advise patient to notify prescriber during periods of stress, such as fever, trauma, infection, or surgery, because dosage may have to be changed.
• Instruct patient how and when to monitor glucose levels.
• Notify patient that blood tests of liver function will be performed before therapy starts, every 2 months for the first year, and periodically thereafter.
• Tell patient to report unexplained nausea, vomiting, abdominal pain, fatigue, anorexia, or dark urine immediately because they may indicate liver problems.
• Inform patient that drug can be taken with or without meals. If a dose is missed, it shouldn't be doubled the following day.
• Advise anovulatory, premenopausal women with insulin resistance that therapy may cause resumption of ovulation; recommend use of contraceptive measures.

---

repaglinide
Prandin

Pregnancy risk category C

AVAILABLE FORMS
Tablets: 0.5 mg, 1 mg, 2 mg

INDICATIONS & DOSAGES
➤ **Adjunct to diet and exercise in lowering glucose levels in patients with type 2 (non–insulin-dependent) diabetes mellitus whose hyperglycemia can't be controlled by diet and exercise alone; with metformin to lower glucose levels in patients whose hyperglycemia can't be controlled by exercise, diet, and either repaglinide or metformin alone—**
Adults: If patient hasn't been treated with glucose-lowering drugs or glycosylated hemoglobin (HbA$_{1c}$) is below 8%, initially give 0.5 mg P.O. up to 30 minutes before each meal. If patient has been treated before with glucose-lowering drugs and

HbA$_{1c}$ is 8% or more, initially 1 to 2 mg P.O. taken immediately to 30 minutes before each meal. Recommended range is 0.5 to 4 mg with meals divided b.i.d., t.i.d., or q.i.d. Maximum, 16 mg daily.

ACTION
Stimulates insulin release from beta cells in the pancreas by closing ATP-dependent potassium channels in beta cell membranes, which causes calcium channels to open. Increased calcium influx induces insulin secretion; the overall effect is to lower glucose level.

Route	Onset	Peak	Duration
P.O.	0.5 hr	1 hr	Unknown

ADVERSE REACTIONS
CNS: *headache,* paresthesia.
CV: angina.
EENT: rhinitis, sinusitis.
GI: constipation, diarrhea, dyspepsia, nausea, vomiting.
GU: urinary tract infection.
Metabolic: HYPOGLYCEMIA, hyperglycemia.
Musculoskeletal: arthralgia, back pain.
Respiratory: bronchitis, *upper respiratory tract infection.*
Other: tooth disorder.

INTERACTIONS
Drug-drug. *Barbiturates, carbamazepine, rifampin:* May increase repaglinide metabolism. Monitor glucose level.
Beta blockers, chloramphenicol, coumarins, MAO inhibitors, NSAIDs, other drugs that are highly protein-bound, probenecid, salicylates, sulfonamides: May potentiate hypoglycemic action of repaglinide. Monitor glucose level.
Calcium channel blockers, corticosteroids, estrogens, fosphenytoin, isoniazid, nicotinic acid, oral contraceptives, phenothiazines, phenytoin, sympathomimetics, thiazides and other diuretics, thyroid products: May produce hyperglycemia, resulting in a loss of glycemic control. Monitor glucose level.
Erythromycin, inhibitors of P-450 cytochrome system 3A4, ketoconazole, miconazole: May inhibit repaglinide metabolism. Monitor glucose levels.

Drug-herb. *Burdock, dandelion, eucalyptus, marshmallow:* Increased hypoglycemic effects. Tell patient to avoid using together.
Drug-food. *Grapefruit juice:* Inhibits metabolism of repaglinide. Tell patient to avoid using together.
Drug-lifestyle. *Alcohol use:* Altered glycemic control; hypoglycemia. Advise patient to avoid alcohol.

EFFECTS ON LAB TEST RESULTS
● May increase or decrease glucose levels.

CONTRAINDICATIONS
Contraindicated in patients hypersensitive to drug or its inactive ingredients and in those with type 1 (insulin-dependent) diabetes mellitus or diabetic ketoacidosis.

NURSING CONSIDERATIONS
● Use cautiously in patients with hepatic insufficiency in whom reduced metabolism could cause hypoglycemia and elevated blood levels of repaglinide.
● Use cautiously in elderly, debilitated, or malnourished patients and in those with adrenal or pituitary insufficiency because these patients are more susceptible to hypoglycemic effect of glucose-lowering drugs.
● Increase dosage carefully in patients with impaired renal function or renal failure requiring dialysis.
● Adjust dosage by glucose level response. May double dosage up to 4 mg with each meal until satisfactory glucose level is achieved. At least 1 week should elapse between dosage adjustments to assess response.
● Metformin may be added if repaglinide monotherapy is inadequate.
● Administration of oral antidiabetics may cause increased CV mortality compared with diet alone or diet plus insulin treatment. This association may also apply to repaglinide.
● Loss of glycemic control can occur during stress, such as fever, trauma, infection, or surgery. Discontinue drug and administer insulin.
● Hypoglycemia may be difficult to recognize in elderly patients and in patients taking beta blockers.

● When switching to another oral hypoglycemic, begin new drug on day after last dose of repaglinide.

PATIENT TEACHING
● Stress importance of diet and exercise with drug therapy.
● Discuss symptoms of hypoglycemia with patient and family.
● Tell patient to monitor glucose level periodically to determine minimum effective dose.
● Encourage patient to keep regular appointments and have his HbA_{1c} levels checked every 3 months to determine long-term glucose control.
● Tell patient to administer drug before meals, usually 15 minutes before start of meal; however, time can vary from immediately preceding meal to up to 30 minutes before meal.
● Tell patient that, if a meal is skipped or an extra meal added, he should skip dose or add an extra dose of drug for that meal, respectively.
● Instruct patient to monitor glucose level carefully and tell him what to do when he's ill, undergoing surgery, or under added stress.
● Advise woman planning pregnancy to consult prescriber before becoming pregnant. Insulin may be needed during pregnancy and breast-feeding.
● Teach patient to carry candy or other simple sugars to treat mild hypoglycemic episodes. Patient experiencing severe episode may need hospital treatment.
● Inform patient that alcohol lowers glucose level and should be avoided.

---

rosiglitazone maleate
Avandia

Pregnancy risk category C

AVAILABLE FORMS
Tablets: 2 mg, 4 mg, 8 mg

INDICATIONS & DOSAGES
➤ **Adjunct to diet and exercise to improve glycemic control in patients with type 2 (non–insulin-dependent) diabetes mellitus; with metformin to lower glucose levels in patients whose hypergly-**

---

cemia can't be controlled by diet, exercise, and either rosiglitazone or metformin alone—
Adults: Initially, 4 mg P.O. daily in the morning or in divided doses b.i.d. in the morning and evening. Dosage may be increased to 8 mg P.O. daily or in divided doses b.i.d. if fasting plasma glucose level doesn't improve after 12 weeks of treatment.

✳ *NEW INDICATION:* Adjunct to sulfonylureas, diet, and exercise in patients with type 2 diabetes mellitus—
Adults: 4 mg P.O. once daily or in two divided doses.

ACTION

Lowers glucose levels by improving insulin sensitivity.

Route	Onset	Peak	Duration
P.O.	Unknown	1 hr	Unknown

ADVERSE REACTIONS

CNS: headache, fatigue.
CV: edema.
EENT: sinusitis.
GI: diarrhea.
Hematologic: anemia.
Metabolic: hyperglycemia.
Musculoskeletal: back pain.
Respiratory: upper respiratory tract infection.
Other: injury.

INTERACTIONS

None significant.

EFFECTS ON LAB TEST RESULTS

• May increase glucose levels.
• May decrease hemoglobin.

CONTRAINDICATIONS

Contraindicated in patients hypersensitive to drug or its components and in those with New York Heart Association class III or IV cardiac status unless expected benefits outweigh risks. Also contraindicated in patients with active liver disease, increased baseline liver enzyme levels (ALT level over 2½ times upper limit of normal), type 1 (insulin-dependent) diabetes, or diabetic ketoacidosis and in those who experienced jaundice while taking troglitazone. Because metformin is contraindicated in patients with renal impairment, combination therapy with rosiglitazone is also contraindicated in patients with renal impairment. Rosiglitazone can be used as monotherapy in patients with renal impairment.

NURSING CONSIDERATIONS

• Use cautiously in patients with edema or heart failure.
• Before starting drug therapy, patient should be treated for secondary causes of poor glycemic control, such as infection.
• *Alert:* Liver enzyme levels should be checked before therapy starts. Don't use drug in patients with increased baseline liver enzyme levels. In patients with normal baseline liver enzyme levels, monitor these levels every 2 months for first 12 months and periodically thereafter. If ALT level is elevated during treatment, recheck levels as soon as possible. Drug should be discontinued if levels remain elevated.
• Because ovulation may resume in premenopausal, anovulatory women with insulin resistance, recommend use of contraceptives.
• Management of type 2 diabetes should include diet control. Because caloric restriction, weight loss, and exercise help improve insulin sensitivity and improve effectiveness of drug therapy, these measures are essential to proper diabetes treatment.
• Glucose and glycosylated hemoglobin levels should be checked periodically to monitor therapeutic response to drug.
• Monitor patient with heart failure for increased edema.
• Hemoglobin level and hematocrit may decrease during therapy, usually during first 4 to 8 weeks. Increases in total cholesterol, low-density lipoprotein, and high-density lipoprotein levels and decreases in free fatty acid levels also may occur.
• Patients with normal hepatic enzyme levels who are switched from troglitazone should undergo a 1-week washout before starting rosiglitazone.
• For patients whose glucose levels are inadequately controlled with metformin, rosiglitazone should be added to—not substituted for—metformin.
• *Alert:* Don't confuse rosiglitazone with pioglitazone.

PATIENT TEACHING

• Advise patient that drug can be taken with or without food.

• Notify patient that blood will be tested to check liver function before therapy starts, every 2 months for first 12 months, and then periodically thereafter.

• Tell patient to immediately notify prescriber about unexplained signs and symptoms, such as nausea, vomiting, abdominal pain, fatigue, anorexia, or dark urine; these may indicate liver problems.

• Recommend use of contraceptives to premenopausal, anovulatory women with insulin resistance because ovulation may resume with therapy.

• Advise patient that management of diabetes should include diet control. Because caloric restriction, weight loss, and exercise help improve insulin sensitivity and improve effectiveness of drug therapy, these measures are essential to proper diabetes treatment.

• Instruct patient to monitor glucose level carefully and tell him what to do when he's ill, undergoing surgery, or under added stress.

---

levothyroxine sodium
liothyronine sodium
liotrix
thyroid desiccated

COMBINATION PRODUCTS
None.

---

levothyroxine sodium (T_4, L-thyroxine sodium)
Eltroxin†, Levo-T, Levotec†, Levothroid, Levoxine, Levoxyl, Oroxine‡, Synthroid**

Pregnancy risk category A

AVAILABLE FORMS
Injection: 200-mcg vial, 500-mcg vial
Tablets: 25 mcg, 50 mcg, 75 mcg, 88 mcg, 100 mcg, 112 mcg, 125 mcg, 137 mcg, 150 mcg, 175 mcg, 200 mcg, 300 mcg

INDICATIONS & DOSAGES
➤ **Myxedema coma—**
Adults: 200 to 500 mcg I.V.; then 100 to 300 mcg on second day, followed by parenteral maintenance dose of 50 to 200 mcg I.V. daily. Switch patient to oral maintenance as soon as possible.
➤ **Thyroid hormone replacement—**
Adults: Initially, 25 to 50 mcg P.O. daily, increased by 25 mcg P.O. q 2 to 4 weeks until desired response occurs. Maintenance dose is 75 to 200 mcg P.O. daily.
Children older than age 12: more than 150 mcg or 2 to 3 mcg/kg P.O. daily.
Children ages 6 to 12: 100 to 150 mcg or 4 to 5 mcg/kg P.O. daily.
Children ages 1 to 5: 75 to 100 mcg or 5 to 6 mcg/kg P.O. daily.
Children ages 6 months to 1 year: 50 to 75 mcg or 6 to 8 mcg/kg P.O. daily.
Children younger than age 6 months: 25 to 50 mcg or 8 to 10 mcg/kg P.O. daily.
Patients older than age 65: 12.5 to 50 mcg P.O. daily, increased by 12.5 to 25 mcg q 3 to 8 weeks, depending on response.

I.V. ADMINISTRATION
● Prepare I.V. dose immediately before injection. Dilute Synthroid Powder for Injection with 5 ml of normal saline solution for injection or bacteriostatic saline solution injection with benzyl alcohol to 200- or 500-mcg vial; don't use other diluents. Resulting solutions contain 40 or 100 mcg/ml, respectively. Don't mix with other I.V. infusion solutions. Inject into vein over 1 to 2 minutes.
● Initial I.V. dose is about half the previously established oral dose of Synthroid tablets.
● Monitor blood pressure and heart rate closely. High initial I.V. dosage is usually well tolerated by patients in myxedema coma. Normal levels of T_4 should occur within 24 hours, followed by a threefold increase in T_3 in 3 days.

ACTION
Not completely defined. Stimulates metabolism of all body tissues by accelerating rate of cellular oxidation.

Route	Onset	Peak	Duration
I.V.	Unknown	Unknown	Unknown
P.O.	24 hr	Unknown	Unknown

ADVERSE REACTIONS
CNS: *nervousness, insomnia, tremor,* headache.
CV: *tachycardia, palpitations,* **arrhythmias,** *angina pectoris,* **cardiac arrest.**
GI: diarrhea, vomiting.
GU: menstrual irregularities.
Metabolic: weight loss.
Musculoskeletal: decreased bone density.
Skin: allergic skin reactions, diaphoresis.
Other: heat intolerance, fever.

INTERACTIONS
Drug-drug. *Beta blockers:* May reduce the effects of beta blockers. Monitor patient.
Cholestyramine, colestipol: Impaired levothyroxine absorption. Separate doses by 4 to 5 hours.

Digoxin: Decreased glycoside effects. Monitor patient for clinical effect.

Estrogens: Decreased free levothyroxines. Monitor patient for decreased effectiveness of thyroid hormone.

Fosphenytoin, phenytoin: Free thyroid released. Monitor patient for tachycardia.

Insulin, oral antidiabetics: Altered glucose levels. Monitor glucose levels. Dosage adjustments may be needed.

Oral anticoagulants: Altered PT. Monitor PT and INR. Dosage adjustments may be needed.

Sympathomimetics such as epinephrine: Increased risk of coronary insufficiency. Monitor patient closely.

Theophylline: Decreased theophylline clearance in hypothyroidism; clearance may return to normal when euthyroid state is achieved. Monitor theophylline levels.

Drug-herb. *Horseradish:* Abnormal thyroid function may occur. Discourage use in patients undergoing thyroid function tests.

Lemon balm: Antithyroid effects; herb inhibits thyroid-stimulating hormone. Discourage use together.

EFFECTS ON LAB TEST RESULTS
None reported.

CONTRAINDICATIONS
Contraindicated in patients hypersensitive to drug and in those with acute MI uncomplicated by hypothyroidism, untreated thyrotoxicosis, or uncorrected adrenal insufficiency.

NURSING CONSIDERATIONS
● Use with extreme caution in elderly patients and in those with angina pectoris, hypertension, other CV disorders, renal insufficiency, or ischemia.
● Use cautiously in patients with diabetes mellitus, diabetes insipidus, or myxedema. Patients with diabetes mellitus may need increased antidiabetic doses when starting thyroid hormone replacement.
● *Alert:* Drug may be given I.V. or I.M. when P.O. ingestion is precluded for long periods. However, dosage adjustment is needed.
● Rapid replacement in patients with arteriosclerosis may cause angina, coronary occlusion, or CVA. Use cautiously in

these patients. In patients with coronary artery disease who must receive thyroid hormone, observe carefully for possible coronary insufficiency.
● Thyroid hormone replacement requirements are about 25% lower in patients older than age 60 than in young adults.
● Patients with adult hypothyroidism are unusually sensitive to thyroid hormone. Start at lowest dosage and adjust to higher dosages according to patient's symptoms and laboratory data until euthyroid state is reached.
● When changing from levothyroxine to liothyronine, levothyroxine should be stopped and liothyronine begun. Dosage should be increased in small increments after residual effects of levothyroxine have disappeared. When changing from liothyronine to levothyroxine, levothyroxine is started several days before withdrawing liothyronine to avoid relapse. Drugs aren't interchangeable.
● Thyroid hormones alter thyroid function test results.
● Patients taking levothyroxine who need to have ^{131}I uptake studies performed must discontinue drug 4 weeks before test.
● Patients taking anticoagulants may need their dosage modified; also, careful monitoring of coagulation status is needed.
● Alterations in radioactive iodine (^{131}I) thyroid uptake, protein-bound iodine levels, and liothyronine uptake may occur.
● *Alert:* Don't confuse levothyroxine with liothyronine or liotrix.

PATIENT TEACHING
● Make sure patient understands importance of compliance. Tell him to take thyroid hormones at same time each day, preferably before breakfast, to maintain constant hormone levels and help prevent insomnia.
● Make sure patient understands that replacement therapy is for a lifetime. The drug should never be discontinued unless directed by prescriber.
● Warn patient (especially elderly patient) to notify prescriber at once about chest pain, palpitations, sweating, nervousness, shortness of breath, or other signals of overdose or aggravated CV disease.
● Advise caregiver that for infant or child who can't swallow tablets, crush tablet and

suspend in small amount of formula, breast milk, or water and give by spoon or dropper. Crushed tablet can be sprinkled over food, but avoid foods containing large amounts of soybean, fiber, or iron.
• Advise patient who has achieved stable response not to change brands.
• Tell patient to report unusual bleeding and bruising.
• Advise patient not to take OTC or other prescription medications without first consulting his prescriber.

liothyronine sodium (T$_3$)
Cytomel, Tertroxin‡, Triostat

Pregnancy risk category A

AVAILABLE FORMS
Injection: 10 mcg/ml
Tablets: 5 mcg, 25 mcg, 50 mcg

INDICATIONS & DOSAGES
➤ **Congenital hypothyroidism—**
Children: 5 mcg P.O. daily with a 5-mcg increase q 3 to 4 days until desired response achieved.
➤ **Myxedema—**
Adults: Initially, 2.5 to 5 mcg P.O. daily, increased by 5 to 10 mcg q 1 to 2 weeks until daily dose reaches 25 mcg. Then, increased by 12.5 to 25 mcg daily q 1 to 2 weeks. Maintenance dose is 50 to 100 mcg daily.
➤ **Myxedema coma, premyxedema coma—**
Adults: Initially, 10 to 20 mcg I.V. for patients with known or suspected CV disease; 25 to 50 mcg I.V. for patients who don't have CV disease. Subsequent dosage adjustments made based on patient's condition and response. Switch patient to oral therapy as soon as possible.
➤ **Simple (nontoxic) goiter—**
Adults: Initially, 5 mcg P.O. daily; may increase by 5 to 10 mcg daily q 1 to 2 weeks, until daily dose reaches 25 mcg. Then, increase by 12.5 to 25 mcg daily q 1 to 2 weeks. Usual maintenance dose is 75 mcg daily.
➤ **Thyroid hormone replacement—**
Adults: Initially, 25 mcg P.O. daily, increased by 12.5 to 25 mcg q 1 to 2 weeks

until satisfactory response occurs. Usual maintenance dose is 25 to 50 mcg daily.
Patients older than age 65: 5 mcg daily, increased in 5-mcg daily increments q 1 to 2 weeks.
➤ **T$_3$ suppression test to differentiate hyperthyroidism from euthyroidism—**
Adults: 75 to 100 mcg P.O. daily for 7 days.

I.V. ADMINISTRATION
• Administer repeat doses more than 4 hours but less than 12 hours apart.

ACTION
Not clearly defined. Enhances oxygen consumption by most tissues of the body; increases the basal metabolic rate and the metabolism of carbohydrates, lipids, and proteins.

Route	Onset	Peak	Duration
I.V.	Unknown	Unknown	Unknown
P.O.	Unknown	2-3 days	3 days

ADVERSE REACTIONS
CNS: *nervousness, insomnia, tremor,* headache.
CV: *tachycardia, arrhythmias,* angina, **cardiac decompensation and collapse.**
GI: diarrhea, vomiting.
GU: menstrual irregularities.
Metabolic: weight loss.
Musculoskeletal: accelerated bone maturation in infants and children.
Skin: skin reactions, diaphoresis.
Other: heat intolerance.

INTERACTIONS
Drug-drug. *Beta blockers:* May reduce the effects of beta blockers. Monitor patient using drugs together.
Cholestyramine, colestipol: Impaired liothyronine absorption. Separate doses by 4 to 5 hours.
Digoxin: Decreased glycoside effects. Monitor patient for clinical effect.
Insulin, oral antidiabetics: Initial thyroid replacement therapy may cause increases in insulin or oral hypoglycemic requirements. Monitor glucose levels. Dosage adjustments may be needed.
Oral anticoagulants: Altered PT. Monitor PT and INR. Dosage adjustments may be needed.

roid hormones at same time each day, preferably before breakfast, to maintain constant hormone levels and help prevent insomnia.
• Tell patient that drug should never be discontinued unless directed by prescriber.
• Warn patient (especially elderly patient) to notify prescriber at once about chest pain, palpitations, sweating, nervousness, or other signs of overdose or aggravated CV disease.
• Tell patient not to switch brands; the two commercially prepared liotrix drugs contain different amounts of each ingredient.
• Tell patient to report unusual bleeding and bruising.
• Advise patient not to take OTC or other prescription medications without first consulting his prescriber.

---

thyroid desiccated
Armour Thyroid, S-P-T

Pregnancy risk category A

AVAILABLE FORMS
Capsules (pork origin): 60 mg, 120 mg, 180 mg, 300 mg
Tablets: 15 mg, 30 mg, 60 mg, 65 mg, 90 mg, 120 mg, 130 mg, 180 mg, 240 mg, 300 mg
Tablets (enteric-coated): 60 mg, 120 mg
Tablets (Thyrar; bovine origin): 30 mg, 60 mg, 120 mg

INDICATIONS & DOSAGES
➤ **Mild hypothyroidism—**
Adults: Initially, 60 mg P.O. daily, increased by 60 mg q 30 days until desired response occurs. Usual maintenance dose is 60 to 120 mg daily as single dose.
➤ **Severe hypothyroidism—**
Adults: Initially, 15 mg P.O. daily, increased by 30 mg daily after 2 weeks, and 2 weeks later increased to 60 mg daily. After 2 months, increase to 120 mg daily if response still inadequate.
Patients older than age 65: 7.5 to 15 mg daily. May double dose q 6 to 8 weeks until desired result is obtained.
➤ **Congenital or severe hypothyroidism in children—**
Children older than age 12: 1.2 to 1.8 mg/kg daily P.O.

Children ages 6 to 12: 2.4 to 3 mg/kg daily P.O.
Children ages 1 to 5: 3 to 3.6 mg/kg daily P.O.
Children ages 6 to 12 months: 3.6 to 4.8 mg/kg daily P.O.
Children younger than 6 months: 4.8 to 6 mg/kg daily P.O.

ACTION
Not clearly defined. Stimulates metabolism of all body tissues by accelerating the rate of cellular oxidation.

Route	Onset	Peak	Duration
P.O.	Unknown	Unknown	Unknown

ADVERSE REACTIONS
CNS: *nervousness, insomnia,* tremor, headache.
CV: *tachycardia, **arrhythmias,*** angina pectoris, ***cardiac decompensation and collapse.***
GI: diarrhea, vomiting.
GU: menstrual irregularities.
Metabolic: weight loss.
Musculoskeletal: accelerated rate of bone maturation in infants and children.
Skin: allergic skin reactions, diaphoresis.
Other: heat intolerance.

INTERACTIONS
Drug-drug. *Beta blockers:* May reduce the effects of beta blockers. Monitor patient.
Cholestyramine: Impaired thyroid absorption. Separate doses by 4 to 5 hours.
Digoxin: Decreased glycoside effects. Monitor patient for clinical effect.
Insulin, oral antidiabetics: Altered glucose levels. Monitor glucose levels and adjust dosage as needed.
Oral anticoagulants: Altered PT. Monitor PT and INR. Adjust dosage as needed.
Sympathomimetics, such as epinephrine: Increased risk of coronary insufficiency. Monitor patient closely.
Theophylline: Decreased theophylline clearance in hypothyroidism; clearance may return to normal when euthyroid state is achieved. Monitor theophylline levels.
Drug-herb. *Lemon balm:* Antithyroid effects; herb inhibits thyroid-stimulating hormone. Discourage use together.

EFFECTS ON LAB TEST RESULTS
None reported.

CONTRAINDICATIONS
Contraindicated in patients hypersensitive
to drug and in those with acute MI uncomplicated by hypothyroidism, untreated
thyrotoxicosis, or uncorrected adrenal insufficiency.

NURSING CONSIDERATIONS
● Use with extreme caution in elderly patients and in those with angina pectoris,
hypertension, other CV disorders, renal
insufficiency, or ischemia.
● Use cautiously in patients with myxedema, diabetes mellitus, or diabetes insipidus.
● In patients with coronary artery disease,
check for coronary insufficiency.
● Thyroid hormone replacement requirements are about 25% lower in patients
older than age 60 than in young adults.
● Monitor pulse and blood pressure.
● In children, sleeping pulse rate and basal
morning temperature guide treatment.
● Thyroid hormones alter thyroid function
test results. Alterations in radioactive iodine (^{131}I) uptake, protein-bound iodine
levels, and liothyronine uptake may occur.
● Patient must discontinue thyroid 7 to 10
days before undergoing ^{131}I studies.
● **Alert:** Don't confuse thyroid with Thyrolar.

PATIENT TEACHING
● Tell patient to take thyroid hormones at
same time each day, preferably before
breakfast, to maintain constant hormone
levels and help prevent insomnia.
● Tell patient the drug should never be discontinued unless directed by prescriber.
● Advise patient who has achieved stable
response not to change brands.
● Warn patient (especially elderly patient)
to notify prescriber at once about chest
pain, palpitations, or other signs of overdose or aggravated CV disease.
● Tell patient to report unusual bleeding
and bruising.
● Advise patient not to take OTC or other
prescription medications without first consulting his prescriber.

methimazole
potassium iodide
potassium iodide, saturated
  solution
propylthiouracil
radioactive iodine
strong iodine solution

COMBINATION PRODUCTS
None.

methimazole
Tapazole

Pregnancy risk category D

AVAILABLE FORMS
Tablets: 5 mg, 10 mg

INDICATIONS & DOSAGES
➤ **Hyperthyroidism—**
Adults: If mild, 15 mg P.O. daily. If moderately severe, 30 to 40 mg daily. If severe, 60 mg daily. Daily amount is divided into three equal doses and given at 8-hour intervals. Maintenance dosage is 5 to 30 mg daily.
Children: 0.4 mg/kg P.O. in three divided doses daily. Maintenance dosage is 0.2 mg/kg in divided doses daily.

ACTION
Inhibits oxidation of iodine in thyroid gland, blocking ability of iodine to combine with tyrosine to form T_4. Also may prevent coupling of monoiodotyrosine and diiodotyrosine to form T_4 and T_3.

Route	Onset	Peak	Duration
P.O.	Rapid	0.5-1 hr	Unknown

ADVERSE REACTIONS
CNS: headache, drowsiness, vertigo, paresthesia, neuritis, neuropathies, CNS stimulation, depression.
GI: diarrhea, nausea, vomiting, salivary gland enlargement, loss of taste, epigastric distress.
GU: nephritis.
Hematologic: *agranulocytosis, leukopenia, thrombocytopenia, aplastic anemia.*
Hepatic: jaundice, hepatic dysfunction, *hepatitis.*
Musculoskeletal: arthralgia, myalgia.
Skin: rash, urticaria, discoloration, pruritus, erythema nodosum, exfoliative dermatitis, lupuslike syndrome, abnormal hair loss.
Other: fever, lymphadenopathy, hypothyroidism.

INTERACTIONS
Drug-drug. *Aminophylline, oxtriphylline, theophylline:* Decreased clearance. May need dosage adjustment.
Amiodarone: May decrease methimazole dosage requirements. May need to decrease methimazole dose.
Anticoagulants: May alter dosage requirements. Monitor PT, PTT, and INR.
Cardiac glycosides: Increased levels. May need to decrease cardiac glycoside dosage.
Potassium iodide: May decrease response to drug. May need to increase methimazole dosage.

EFFECTS ON LAB TEST RESULTS
● May decrease hemoglobin and granulocyte, WBC, and platelet counts.

CONTRAINDICATIONS
Contraindicated in patients hypersensitive to drug and in breast-feeding women.

NURSING CONSIDERATIONS
● Use with extreme caution during pregnancy. Pregnant women may need less drug as pregnancy progresses. Monitor thyroid function studies closely. Thyroid hormone may be added to regimen. Drug may be stopped during last few weeks of pregnancy.
● Monitor CBC periodically to detect impending leukopenia, thrombocytopenia, and agranulocytosis. Also, monitor hepatic function.

Reactions may be *common*, uncommon, *life-threatening*, or COMMON AND LIFE-THREATENING.

• *Alert:* Doses higher than 30 mg/day increase risk of agranulocytosis.

• *Alert:* Patients older than age 40 may have an increased risk of drug-induced agranulocytosis.

• Watch for evidence of hypothyroidism (mental depression; cold intolerance; hard, nonpitting edema); notify prescriber because dosage may need to be adjusted.

• *Alert:* Discontinue drug and notify prescriber if severe rash or enlarged cervical lymph nodes develop.

• Drug therapy alters selenomethionine (^{75}Se) uptake by the pancreas and ^{123}I or ^{131}I uptake by the thyroid.

• *Alert:* Don't confuse methimazole with mebendazole or methazolamide.

PATIENT TEACHING
• Tell patient to take drug with meals to reduce adverse GI reactions.

• Warn patient to report fever, sore throat, mouth sores, skin eruptions, anorexia, pruritus, right upper quadrant pain, yellow skin, or sclera.

• Tell patient to ask prescriber about using iodized salt and eating shellfish. The iodine in these may make the drug less effective.

• Warn patient against OTC cough medicines; many contain iodine.

• Warn patient that drug may cause drowsiness; advise patient to use caution when operating machinery or operating a vehicle.

• Instruct patient to store drug in light-resistant container.

• Teach patient to watch for evidence of hypothyroidism (unexplained weight gain, fatigue, cold intolerance) and to notify prescriber if it arises.

• Tell women not to use drug while breastfeeding.

potassium iodide
Pima, Thyro-Block

potassium iodide, saturated solution (SSKI)

strong iodine solution (Lugol's solution)

Pregnancy risk category D

AVAILABLE FORMS
potassium iodide
Syrup: 325 mg/5 ml
Tablets: 130 mg
potassium iodide, saturated solution
Oral solution: 1 g/ml
strong iodine solution
Oral solution: Iodine 50 mg/ml and potassium iodide 100 mg/ml

INDICATIONS & DOSAGES
➤ **Preparation for thyroidectomy—**
Adults and children: Strong iodine solution (USP), 0.1 to 0.3 ml P.O. t.i.d.; or potassium iodide, saturated solution (SSKI), 1 to 5 drops in water P.O. t.i.d. after meals for 10 to 14 days before surgery.
➤ **Thyrotoxic crisis—**
Adults and children: 500 mg P.O. q 4 hours (about 10 drops of SSKI); or 1 ml of strong iodine solution t.i.d. Give at least 1 hour after the first dose of propylthiouracil or methimazole.
➤ **Radiation protectant for thyroid gland—**
Adults and children age 1 and older: 130 mg P.O. daily for 7 to 14 days after radiation exposure. Start no later than 3 to 4 hours after acute exposure.
Children younger than age 1: 65 mg P.O. daily for 7 to 14 days after exposure. Initiate no later than 3 to 4 hours after acute exposure.

ACTION
Inhibits thyroid hormone formation, limits iodide transport into the thyroid gland, and blocks thyroid hormone release.

Route	Onset	Peak	Duration
P.O.	< 24 hr	10-15 days	Unknown

ADVERSE REACTIONS
EENT: periorbital edema.
GI: diarrhea, inflammation of salivary glands, burning mouth and throat, sore teeth and gums, *metallic taste.*
Metabolic: *potassium toxicity.*
Skin: acneiform rash.
Other: fever, hypersensitivity reactions.

INTERACTIONS
Drug-drug. *ACE inhibitors, potassium-sparing diuretics:* Risk of hyperkalemia. Avoid using together.
Antithyroid drugs: Potassium iodide may potentiate hypothyroid or goitrogenic effects. Monitor patient closely.
Lithium carbonate: Hypothyroidism may occur. Use together cautiously.

EFFECTS ON LAB TEST RESULTS
• May increase potassium levels.
• May alter thyroid function test results.

CONTRAINDICATIONS
Contraindicated in patients with tuberculosis, acute bronchitis, iodide hypersensitivity, or hyperkalemia. Some formulations contain sulfites, which may precipitate allergic reactions in hypersensitive patients.

NURSING CONSIDERATIONS
• Use cautiously in patients with hypocomplementemic vasculitis, goiter, or autoimmune thyroid disease.
• Drug is usually given with other antithyroid drugs.
• Prescriber may avoid prescribing enteric-coated tablets, which have been linked to small-bowel lesions and can lead to serious complications, including perforation, hemorrhage, or obstruction.
• For thyrotoxicosis, first iodine dose is given at least 1 hour after first dose of propylthiouracil and methimazole.
• Dilute oral solution in water, milk, or fruit juice, and give after meals to prevent gastric irritation, hydrate patient, and mask salty taste.
• Give iodides through straw to avoid tooth discoloration.
• *Alert:* Earliest signs of delayed hypersensitivity reactions caused by iodides are irritation and swollen eyelids.

• Monitor patient for iodism, which can cause metallic taste, burning in mouth and throat, sore teeth and gums, increased salivation, coryza, sneezing, eye irritation with swelling of eyelids, severe headache, productive cough, GI irritation, diarrhea, rash, or soreness of the pharynx, larynx, and tonsils.
• Store in light-resistant container.

PATIENT TEACHING
• Show patient how to mask salty taste of oral solution. Tell him to take all forms of drug after meals.
• *Alert:* Warn patient that sudden withdrawal may precipitate thyroid crisis.
• *Alert:* Teach patient signs and symptoms of potassium toxicity, including confusion, irregular heartbeat, numbness, tingling, pain or weakness of hands or feet, and tiredness.
• Tell patient to ask prescriber about using iodized salt and eating shellfish. These foods contain iodine and may alter drug's effectiveness.
• Tell patient to stop drug and notify prescriber if epigastric pain, rash, metallic taste, nausea, or vomiting occurs.

---

propylthiouracil (PTU)
Propyl-Thyracil†

Pregnancy risk category D

AVAILABLE FORMS
Tablets: 50 mg, 100 mg†

INDICATIONS & DOSAGES
➤ **Hyperthyroidism—**
Adults: 300 to 450 mg P.O. daily in three divided doses; up to 1,200 mg daily has been used in severe cases. Maintenance dosage varies but usually ranges from 100 to 150 mg daily.
Children older than age 10: 150 to 300 mg P.O. daily in divided doses t.i.d. Maintenance dosage determined by patient response.
Children ages 6 to 10: 50 to 150 mg P.O. daily in divided doses t.i.d or q.i.d. Maintenance dosage determined by patient response.

➤ **Thyrotoxic crisis—**
Adults and children: 200 mg P.O. q 4 to 6 hours on first day; once symptoms are fully controlled, gradually reduce dosage to usual maintenance levels.

ACTION
Inhibits oxidation of iodine in thyroid gland, blocking ability of iodine to combine with tyrosine to form T_4, and may prevent coupling of monoiodotyrosine and diiodotyrosine to form T_4 and T_3.

Route	Onset	Peak	Duration
P.O.	Unknown	1-1.5 hr	Unknown

ADVERSE REACTIONS
CNS: headache, drowsiness, vertigo, paresthesia, neuritis, neuropathies, CNS stimulation, depression.
CV: vasculitis.
EENT: visual disturbances, loss of taste.
GI: diarrhea, *nausea, vomiting,* epigastric distress, salivary gland enlargement.
GU: nephritis.
Hematologic: *agranulocytosis, leukopenia, thrombocytopenia, aplastic anemia.*
Hepatic: jaundice, *hepatotoxicity.*
Musculoskeletal: arthralgia, myalgia.
Skin: rash, urticaria, skin discoloration, pruritus, erythema nodosum, exfoliative dermatitis, lupus-like syndrome.
Other: fever, lymphadenopathy, dose-related hypothyroidism.

INTERACTIONS
Drug-drug. *Aminophylline, oxtriphylline, theophylline:* Decreased clearance. Dosage may need to be altered.
Anticoagulants: Anticoagulant effects may be increased. Monitor PT and INR.
Cardiac glycosides: Increased levels of glycosides. May need dosage reduction.
Potassium iodide: May decrease response to drug. May need to increase dosage of antithyroid drug.

EFFECTS ON LAB TEST RESULTS
• May decrease hemoglobin and granulocyte, WBC, and platelet counts.

CONTRAINDICATIONS
Contraindicated in patients hypersensitive to drug and in breast-feeding women.

NURSING CONSIDERATIONS
• Use cautiously in pregnant women, who may need less drug as pregnancy progresses. Monitor thyroid function studies closely. Thyroid hormone may be added to regimen. Drug may be stopped during last few weeks of pregnancy.
• *Alert:* Patients older than age 40 may have an increased risk of agranulocytosis.
• Give drug with meals to reduce adverse GI reactions.
• Watch for hypothyroidism (mental depression; cold intolerance; hard, nonpitting edema); adjust dosage.
• Monitor CBC periodically to detect impending leukopenia, thrombocytopenia, and agranulocytosis. PTU therapy alters selenomethionine (^{75}Se) levels and liothyronine uptake.
• *Alert:* Stop drug and notify prescriber if severe rash develops or cervical lymph nodes enlarge.
• Store drug in light-resistant container.

PATIENT TEACHING
• Instruct patient to take drug with meals.
• Warn patient to report fever, sore throat, mouth sores, and skin eruptions.
• Tell patient to report unusual bleeding or bruising.
• Tell patient to ask prescriber about using iodized salt and eating shellfish. These foods contain iodine and may alter effectiveness of drug.
• Warn patient against taking OTC cough medicines; many contain iodine.
• Teach patient to watch for signs and symptoms of hypothyroidism (unexplained weight gain, fatigue, cold intolerance) and to notify prescriber if they occur.

radioactive iodine (sodium iodide ^{131}I)
Iodotope, Sodium Iodide ^{131}I
Therapeutic

Pregnancy risk category X

AVAILABLE FORMS
All radioactivity concentrations are determined at time of calibration.

Iodotope
Capsules: radioactivity range is 1 to
50 millicuries (mCi)/capsule at time of
calibration
Oral solution: radioactivity concentration
is 7.05 mCi/ml at time of calibration; in
vials containing about 7, 14, 28, 70, or
106 mCi at time of calibration
Sodium Iodide ¹³¹I Therapeutic
Capsules: Radioactivity range is 0.8 to
100 mCi/capsule at time of calibration
Oral solution: Radioactivity range is 3.5
to 150 mCi/vial at time of calibration

INDICATIONS & DOSAGES
➤ **Hyperthyroidism—**
Adults: Usual dosage is 4 to 10 mCi P.O.
Dosage is based on estimated weight of
thyroid gland and thyroid uptake. Treatment repeated after 6 weeks, based on T_4
level.
➤ **Thyroid cancer—**
Adults: Initially, 30 to 100 mCi P.O., with
subsequent doses of 100 to 200 mCi.
Dosage is based on estimated malignant
thyroid tissue and metastatic tissue as determined by total body scan. Treatment repeated according to clinical status.

ACTION
Limits thyroid hormone secretion by de-
stroying thyroid tissue. Affinity of thyroid
tissue for radioactive iodine facilitates uptake of drug by cancerous thyroid tissue
that has metastasized to other sites in the
body.

Route	Onset	Peak	Duration
P.O.	Unknown	1-1.5 hr	Unknown

ADVERSE REACTIONS
CV: chest pain, tachycardia.
EENT: *fullness in neck,* pain on swallow-
ing, sore throat.
Hematologic: anemia, blood dyscrasia,
leukopenia, thrombocytopenia.
Respiratory: cough.
Skin: rash, pruritus, urticaria, temporary
thinning of hair.
Other: hypothyroidism, radiation-induced
thyroiditis, radiation sickness, allergic-
type reactions.

INTERACTIONS
Drug-drug. *Lithium carbonate:* Hypothyroidism may occur. Use with caution.
    The following drugs may interfere with
the action of ¹³¹I and should be withheld
for the specified time before the ¹³¹I dose
is administered:
Adrenocorticoids: 1 week.
Benzodiazepines: 1 month.
Cholecystographic drugs: 6 to 9 months.
Contrast media that contain iodine: 1 to 2
months.
*Products containing iodine, including an-
titussives, expectorants, topical drugs, and
vitamins:* 2 weeks.
Salicylates: 1 to 2 weeks.

EFFECTS ON LAB TEST RESULTS
• May decrease hemoglobin and WBC and
platelet counts.

CONTRAINDICATIONS
Contraindicated during pregnancy (except
to treat thyroid cancer) and in breast-
feeding women.

NURSING CONSIDERATIONS
• All antithyroid drugs and thyroid preparations must be stopped 1 week before ¹³¹I
dose. If this isn't possible, patient may receive thyroid-stimulating hormone for 3
days before ¹³¹I dose. When treating
women of childbearing age, give dose during menstruation or within 7 days afterward.
• After therapy for hyperthyroidism, patient shouldn't resume antithyroid drugs
but should continue propranolol or other
drugs used to treat symptoms of hyperthyroidism until onset of full ¹³¹I effect (usually 6 weeks).
• ¹³¹I therapy alters ¹³¹I thyroid uptake and
protein-bound iodine levels.
• Monitor thyroid function by T_4 levels.
• Institute full radiation precautions. Have
patient use proper disposal methods when
coughing and expectorating. After dose
for hyperthyroidism, patient's urine and
saliva are slightly radioactive for 24 hours;
vomitus is highly radioactive for 6 to 8
hours.
• After dose for thyroid cancer, patient's
urine, saliva, and perspiration are radioactive for 3 days. Isolate patient and observe
these precautions: Don't allow pregnant

Reactions may be *common*, uncommon, *life-threatening*, or **COMMON AND LIFE-THREATENING**.

personnel to care for patient; provide disposable eating utensils and linens; instruct patient to save urine in lead container for 24 to 48 hours; limit contact with patient to 30 minutes per shift per person on day 1, and increase time, as needed, to 1 hour on day 2 and longer on day 3.

PATIENT TEACHING

● Tell patient to fast overnight before therapy and to drink as much fluid as possible for 48 hours afterward.

● Instruct patient about appropriate radiation exposure precautions to use after receiving drug.

● Warn patient who is discharged less than 7 days after ^{131}I dose for thyroid cancer to avoid close contact with small children and not to sleep in same room with another person for 7 days after treatment.

● Teach patient the signs and symptoms of hypothyroidism (unexplained weight gain, fatigue, cold intolerance) and instruct him to notify prescriber if they occur.

58
Pituitary hormones

corticotropin
desmopressin acetate
leuprolide acetate
   (See Chapter 70, ANTINEOPLASTICS
   THAT ALTER HORMONE BALANCE.)
repository corticotropin
somatrem
somatropin
vasopressin

COMBINATION PRODUCTS
None.

---

corticotropin (ACTH, adrenocorticotropic hormone)
ACTH, Acthar

repository corticotropin
ACTH 40 Gel Repository, ACTH 80 Gel Repository, H.P. Acthar Gel

Pregnancy risk category C

AVAILABLE FORMS
Aqueous injection: 25-unit vial, 40-unit vial
Repository injection: 40 units/ml, 80 units/ml

INDICATIONS & DOSAGES
➤ **Diagnostic test of adrenocortical function—**
Adults: 40 units I.M. (repository) q 12 hours for 1 to 2 days; or 10 to 25 units aqueous form in 500 ml of D_5W I.V. over 8 hours, between blood samplings.
   Individual dosages vary with sensitivity of adrenal glands to stimulation and with specific disease. Infants and younger children need larger doses per kg than older children and adults.
➤ **For therapeutic use—**
Adults: 20 units aqueous form S.C. or I.M. q.i.d. Or, 40 to 80 units q 24 to 72 hours (repository form). For an acute exacerbation of multiple sclerosis, 80 to 120 units (injection or repository) I.M. daily in divided doses for 2 to 3 weeks.

I.V. ADMINISTRATION
• Use only aqueous form for I.V. administration. Dilute in 500 ml D_5W, and infuse over 8 hours.
• Refrigerate reconstituted solution and use within 24 hours.

ACTION
By replacing the body's own tropic hormone, drug stimulates the adrenal cortex to secrete its entire spectrum of hormones.

Route	Onset	Peak	Duration
I.M., I.V.	Rapid	1 hr	2-4 hr
I.M. (repository)	Unknown	Unknown	3 days
S.C.	Unknown	Unknown	Unknown

ADVERSE REACTIONS
CNS: *seizures, dizziness,* vertigo, *increased intracranial pressure with papilledema,* pseudotumor cerebri.
CV: hypertension, *heart failure,* necrotizing vasculitis, *shock.*
EENT: cataracts, glaucoma.
GI: peptic ulceration with perforation and hemorrhage, *pancreatitis,* abdominal distention, ulcerative esophagitis, nausea, vomiting.
GU: menstrual irregularities.
Metabolic: activation of latent diabetes mellitus, *sodium and fluid retention,* hypokalemic alkalosis.
Musculoskeletal: suppression of growth in children, muscle weakness, steroid myopathy, loss of muscle mass, osteoporosis, vertebral compression fractures.
Respiratory: pneumonia, *bronchospasm.*
Skin: impaired wound healing, thin fragile skin, petechiae, facial erythema, diaphoresis, acne, hyperpigmentation, allergic reactions, hirsutism, ecchymoses.
Other: cushingoid symptoms, abscess and septic infection, hypersensitivity reactions.

INTERACTIONS
Drug-drug. *Amphotericin B, potassium-sparing diuretics:* Increased risk of hypokalemia. Monitor potassium levels.

Anticonvulsants, barbiturates, rifampin: Increased metabolism of corticotropin and decreased effectiveness. Watch for lack of effect.

Antidiabetics: May increase antidiabetic requirements because of intrinsic hyperglycemic activity of corticotropin. Monitor glucose levels closely.

Estrogens: May potentiate effects of cortisol. Dosage adjustments may be needed.

NSAIDs, salicylates: Increased risk of GI bleeding. Avoid using together.

Oral anticoagulants: Altered PT. Monitor PT and INR. Dosage adjustments may be needed.

Vaccines: Risk of neurologic complications and lack of antibody response. Don't give with smallpox vaccine, and use extremely cautiously with other immunizations.

EFFECTS ON LAB TEST RESULTS
• May increase glucose levels. May decrease potassium and calcium levels.

CONTRAINDICATIONS
Contraindicated in patients hypersensitive to pork and pork products and in those with peptic ulcer, scleroderma, osteoporosis, systemic fungal infections, ocular herpes simplex, peptic ulceration, heart failure, hypertension, Cushing's syndrome, and adrenocortical hyperfunction or primary insufficiency. Also contraindicated after recent surgery.

NURSING CONSIDERATIONS
• Use cautiously in pregnant women and women of childbearing age. Also, use cautiously in patients being immunized and in those with latent tuberculosis or tuberculin reactivity, hypothyroidism, cirrhosis, acute gouty arthritis, psychotic tendencies, renal insufficiency, diverticulitis, nonspecific ulcerative colitis, thromboembolic disorders, seizures, uncontrolled hypertension, or myasthenia gravis.
• *Alert:* Check product label to be certain medication is for I.V. use; corticotropin repository injection is for I.M. or S.C. use only, not for I.V. use.
• Corticotropin treatment should be preceded by verification of adrenal responsiveness and testing for hypersensitivity and allergic reactions.

• If administering gel, warm it to room temperature and draw into large needle. Replace needle (using 21G or 22G) and give slowly as deep I.M. injection.
• Corticotropin may mask signs of chronic disease and decrease host resistance and ability to localize infection.
• Note and record weight changes, fluid exchange, and resting blood pressures until minimal effective dosage is achieved.
• Watch neonates of corticotropin-treated mothers for signs of hypoadrenalism.
• In patients with diabetes, monitor glucose more frequently.
• Unusual stress may require additional use of rapid-acting steroids. When possible, gradually reduce corticotropin dosage to lowest effective level to minimize induced adrenocortical insufficiency. Therapy can be reinstituted if stressful situation (trauma, surgery, severe illness) occurs shortly after drug is stopped.
• High plasma cortisol levels may be reported erroneously in patients receiving spironolactone, cortisone, or hydrocortisone when fluorometric analysis is used. This doesn't occur with the radioimmunoassay or competitive protein-binding method. However, therapy can be maintained with prednisone, dexamethasone, or betamethasone because they aren't detectable by the fluorometric method. Drug also may alter protein-bound iodine levels and radioactive iodine (^{131}I) and T_3 uptake.
• Drug may cause suppression of skin test reactions and falsely decreased urinary estradiol levels and estriol levels with Brown method.
• *Alert:* Don't confuse corticotropin with cosyntropin.

PATIENT TEACHING
• Warn patient that injection is painful.
• Stress importance of informing all members of health care team about therapeutic use of drug because unusual stress may require additional use of rapidly acting steroids.
• Instruct patient how to handle troublesome adverse reactions, such as limiting sodium intake to reduce severity of edema and increasing protein intake to combat nitrogen loss.
• Inform patient of need for close follow-up care.

- Advise patient not to discontinue therapy abruptly.
- Instruct patient to avoid people with known or suspected varicella infections.
- Tell patient to avoid alcohol, salicylates, and NSAIDs because of the increased risk of ulcer formation.
- Tell patient to report symptoms of fluid retention, muscle weakness, abdominal pain, seizures, or headache to prescriber.
- Tell patient to avoid vaccinations during therapy.

---

desmopressin acetate
DDAVP, Desmospray§, Minirin‡, Stimate

Pregnancy risk category B

AVAILABLE FORMS
Injection: 4 mcg/ml, 15 mcg/ml
Nasal solution: 0.1 mg/ml, 1.5 mg/ml
Tablets: 0.1 mg, 0.2 mg

INDICATIONS & DOSAGES
➤ **Nonnephrogenic diabetes insipidus, temporary polyuria, and polydipsia related to pituitary trauma—**
Adults and children older than age 12: 0.1 to 0.4 ml intranasally daily in one to three doses. Most adults need 0.2 ml daily in divided doses. Or, give 0.5 to 1 ml I.V. or S.C. of the injectable form daily, usually in two divided doses. Or, give 0.05 mg P.O. b.i.d. of the oral form; adjust dosage to patient response. If patient previously received the drug intranasally, begin oral therapy 12 hours after last intranasal dose.
Children ages 3 months to 12 years: 0.05 to 0.3 ml intranasally daily in one or two doses.
➤ **Hemophilia A and von Willebrand's disease—**
Adults and children: 0.3 mcg/kg diluted in normal saline solution and infused I.V. over 15 to 30 minutes. Repeat dose, if needed, as indicated by laboratory response and patient's condition. Or, 300 mcg (one spray in each nostril) of solution containing 1.5 mcg/ml. Dose of 150 mcg (one spray of solution containing 1.5 mg/ml into a single nostril) may be adequate for patients weighing less than 50 kg (110 lb). Give drug 2 hours before surgery.

➤ **Primary nocturnal enuresis—**
Children age 6 and older: Initially, 20 mcg (0.2 ml) intranasally h.s. (10 mcg in each nostril). Adjust dosage based on response; maximum recommended dosage is 40 mcg daily. Or, initially 0.2 mg P.O. h.s., may adjust dose up to 0.6 mg to achieve desired response. For patients previously on intranasal DDAVP therapy, start tablet 24 hours after last intranasal dose in the nighttime.

I.V. ADMINISTRATION
- For adults and children weighing more than 10 kg (22 lb), dilute with 50 ml sterile physiologic saline solution. For children weighing 10 kg or less, 10 ml of diluent is recommended.
- Inspect for particulate matter and discoloration before infusing drug.
- Monitor blood pressure and pulse during infusion.

ACTION
Increases the permeability of renal tubular epithelium to adenosine monophosphate and water; the epithelium promotes reabsorption of water and produces a concentrated urine. Also increases factor VIII activity by releasing endogenous factor VIII from plasma storage sites.

Route	Onset	Peak	Duration
Intranasal	1 hr	1-5 hr	8-12 hr
I.V.	15-30 min	Unknown	4-12 hr
P.O.	1 hr	1-1.5 hr	8-12 hr

ADVERSE REACTIONS
CNS: headache.
CV: flushing, slight rise in blood pressure.
EENT: rhinitis, epistaxis, sore throat.
GI: nausea, abdominal cramps.
GU: vulvar pain.
Respiratory: cough.
Other: local erythema, swelling, or burning after injection.

INTERACTIONS
Drug-drug. *Carbamazepine, chlorpropamide:* Potentiated ADH; may potentiate effects of desmopressin. Avoid using together.
Clofibrate: Enhanced and prolonged effects of desmopressin. Monitor patient closely.

Reactions may be *common*, uncommon, **life-threatening**, or COMMON AND LIFE-THREATENING.

Demeclocycline, epinephrine, heparin, lithium: Increased risk of adverse effects. Monitor patient closely.
Pressor agents: Enhanced pressor effects with large doses of desmopressin. Monitor patient closely.
Drug-lifestyle. *Alcohol use:* Increased risk of adverse effects. Discourage use together.

EFFECTS ON LAB TEST RESULTS
None reported.

CONTRAINDICATIONS
Contraindicated in patients hypersensitive to drug and in those with type IIB von Willebrand's disease.

NURSING CONSIDERATIONS
● Use cautiously in breast-feeding women; no data exist to demonstrate whether drug appears in breast milk.
● Use cautiously in patients with coronary artery insufficiency, hypertensive CV disease, and conditions linked to fluid and electrolyte imbalances, such as cystic fibrosis, because these patients are prone to hyponatremia.
● Morning and evening doses are adjusted separately for adequate diurnal rhythm of water turnover.
● Desmopressin injection shouldn't be used to treat hemophilia A with factor VIII levels of up to 5% or severe cases of von Willebrand's disease.
● Ensure nasal passages are intact, clean, and free of obstruction before intranasal use.
● Intranasal use can cause changes in the nasal mucosa, resulting in erratic, unreliable absorption. Report worsening condition to prescriber, who may prescribe injectable DDAVP.
● Adjust fluid intake to reduce risk of water intoxication and sodium depletion, especially in children or elderly patients.
● *Alert:* Overdose may cause oxytocic or vasopressor activity. Withhold drug and notify prescriber. Use furosemide if fluid retention is excessive.
● *Alert:* Don't confuse desmopressin with vasopressin.

PATIENT TEACHING
● Instruct patient to clear nasal passages before administering drug.

● Instruct patient to press down four times to prime pump. Tell him to discard the bottle after 25 (150 mcg/spray) or 50 doses (10 mcg/spray), depending on the strength, because the amount left may be less than desired dose.
● Some patients may have trouble measuring and inhaling drug into nostrils. Teach patient and caregivers correct method of administration.
● Advise patient to report nasal congestion, allergic rhinitis, or upper respiratory tract infection to prescriber; dosage adjustment may be needed.
● Teach patient using S.C. desmopressin to rotate injection sites to prevent tissue damage.
● Warn patient to drink only enough water to satisfy thirst.
● Inform patient with hemophilia A or von Willebrand's disease that taking desmopressin may avoid hazards of using blood products.
● Advise patient to carry or wear medical identification indicating use of drug.

---

somatrem
Protropin

Pregnancy risk category C

AVAILABLE FORMS
Injectable lyophilized powder: 5-mg (about 15-IU) vial, 10-mg (about 30-IU) vial

INDICATIONS & DOSAGES
➤ **Long-term treatment of children who have growth failure because of lack of adequate endogenous GH secretion—**
Children (prepubertal): Highly individualized; up to 0.1 mg/kg S.C. (preferred) or I.M. three times weekly. Don't exceed 0.3 mg/kg per week.

ACTION
Purified growth hormone (GH) of recombinant DNA origin that stimulates linear, skeletal muscle, and organ growth.

Route	Onset	Peak	Duration
I.M., S.C.	Unknown	3-5 hr	Unknown

ADVERSE REACTIONS
Metabolic: hypothyroidism, hyperglycemia.
Other: *antibodies to GH.*

INTERACTIONS
Drug-drug. *Glucocorticoids:* May inhibit growth-promoting action of somatrem. Adjust glucocorticoid dosage, as needed.

EFFECTS ON LAB TEST RESULTS
● May increase glucose levels.

CONTRAINDICATIONS
Contraindicated in patients hypersensitive to benzyl alcohol and in those with epiphyseal closure or active neoplasia.

NURSING CONSIDERATIONS
● Use cautiously in patients with hypothyroidism and in those whose GH deficiency is caused by an intracranial lesion.
● Make sure to check product's expiration date.
● To prepare solution, inject supplied bacteriostatic water for injection into vial containing drug. Then swirl vial gently until contents are completely dissolved. Don't shake vial.
● After reconstitution, solution should be clear. Don't inject solution if it's cloudy or contains particles.
● If prepared for other than neonatal use, store reconstituted drug in refrigerator; use within 14 days.
● **Alert:** Toxicity in neonates has occurred from exposure to benzyl alcohol used as a preservative. If drug is given to neonates, reconstitute immediately before use with sterile water for injection (without bacteriostat). Use vial once; then discard.
● Regular checkups are needed, including monitoring of height and blood and radiologic studies.
● Drug therapy alters glucose tolerance test results (reduced tolerance with high doses) and total protein and thyroid function tests. T_4-binding capacity and radioactive uptake may be decreased.
● Observe patient for evidence of glucose intolerance and hyperglycemia.
● Watch for slipped capital femoral epiphysis or progression of scoliosis in patients with rapid growth.

● Monitor periodic thyroid function tests for hypothyroidism; condition may need treatment with a thyroid hormone.
● Funduscopic examination of patient for intracranial hypertension should be done at start of therapy and periodically thereafter.
● **Alert:** Don't confuse somatrem with somatropin, Serostim, or sumatriptan.

PATIENT TEACHING
● Reassure patient and caregivers that somatrem is pure and safe. Drug replaces pituitary-derived human GH, which was removed from the market in 1985 because of its link with a rare but fatal viral infection (Creutzfeldt-Jakob disease).
● Review evidence of hypothyroidism and hyperglycemia. Instruct patient and parents to report such evidence promptly.
● Instruct patient to report limb, hip, or knee pain; headache; weakness; localized muscle pain; or edema to prescriber.

---

somatropin
Genotropin, Humatrope, Norditropin, Nutropin, Nutropin AQ, Saizen, Serostim, Zomacton§

Pregnancy risk category C (B; Serostim)

AVAILABLE FORMS
Genotropin injection: 1.5 mg (about 4 IU/ml), 5.8 mg (about 15 IU/ml), 13.8 mg (about 36 IU/ml)
Injection: 2-mg (about 6-IU [Humatrope]) vial†, 5-mg (about 15-IU [Humatrope]) vial, 10-mg (about 30-IU [Nutropin]) vial
Norditropin injection: 4 mg (about 12 IU/ml), 8 mg (about 24 IU/ml)
Norditropin injection cartridges: 5 mg/1.5 ml, 10 mg/1.5 ml, 15 mg/1.5 ml
Nutropin AQ injection: 10 mg (about 30 IU/vial)
Nutropin injection: 5 mg (about 15 IU/vial), 10 mg (about 30 IU/vial)
Saizen injection: 5 mg (about 15 IU/vial)
Serostim injection: 5 mg (about 15 IU/vial), 6 mg (about 18 IU/ml)

INDICATIONS & DOSAGES
➤ **Long-term treatment of growth failure in children with inadequate secre-**

tion of endogenous growth hormone (GH)—
Children: 0.18 mg/kg S.C. or I.M. weekly, divided equally and given on three alternate days, six times weekly or daily using Humatrope. Or, 0.30 mg/kg S.C. weekly in daily divided doses using Nutropin. Or, 0.06 mg/kg I.M. or S.C. three times weekly using Saizen. Or, 0.024 to 0.034 mg/kg S.C., six to seven times weekly using Norditropin. Or, 0.16 to 0.24 mg/kg S.C. weekly, divided into five to seven doses using Genotropin.

➤ **In children, growth failure from chronic renal insufficiency up to time of renal transplantation (Nutropin and Nutropin AQ)—**
Children: Weekly dosage of up to 0.35 mg/kg S.C. divided into daily doses.
➤ **Long-term treatment of short stature related to Turner's syndrome (Humatrope, Nutropin, Nutropin AQ)—**
Children: Up to 0.375 mg/kg/week (about 1.125 IU/kg/week) S.C. divided into equal doses given three to seven times weekly.
➤ **Long-term treatment of growth failure in children with Prader-Willi Syndrome (PWS) diagnosed by genetic testing (Genotropin):**
Children: 0.24 mg/kg S.C. weekly, divided into five to seven doses.
➤ **Replacement of endogenous GH in adult patients with GH deficiency (Humatrope, Nutropin, Nutropin AQ)—**
Adults: Initially, not more than 0.006 mg/kg S.C. weekly. May be increased to maximum of 0.025 mg/kg daily in patients younger than age 35 or 0.0125 mg/kg daily in patients older than age 35. Or, starting dose isn't more than 0.04 mg/kg S.C. weekly (genotropin), divided into six to seven doses. Dose may be increased at 4- to 8-week intervals to a maximum dose of 0.08 mg/kg S.C. weekly, divided into six to seven doses.
➤ **AIDS wasting or cachexia—**
Adults and children weighing more than 55 kg (121 lb): 6 mg S.C. h.s. (Serostim).
Adults and children weighing 45 to 55 kg (99 to 121 lb): 5 mg S.C. h.s. (Serostim).
Adults and children weighing 35 to 45 kg (77 to 99 lb): 4 mg S.C. h.s. (Serostim).
Adults and children weighing less than 35 kg: 0.1 mg/kg/day S.C. h.s. (Serostim).

✳ *NEW INDICATION:* **Long-term treatment of growth failure in children born small for gestational age (SGA) who don't achieve catch-up growth by 2 years of age (Genotropin):**
Children: 0.48 mg/kg S.C. weekly, divided into five to seven doses.

ACTION
Purified GH of recombinant DNA origin that stimulates skeletal, linear, muscle, and organ growth.

Route	Onset	Peak	Duration
I.M., S.C.	Unknown	3-5 hr	12-48 hr

ADVERSE REACTIONS
CNS: headache, weakness.
CV: mild, transient edema.
Hematologic: *leukemia.*
Metabolic: mild hyperglycemia, hypothyroidism.
Musculoskeletal: localized muscle pain.
Other: injection site pain, antibodies to GH.

INTERACTIONS
Drug-drug. *Corticotropin, corticosteroids:* Long-term use inhibits growth response to GH. Monitor patient for lack of effect.

EFFECTS ON LAB TEST RESULTS
● May increase glucose, inorganic phosphorus, alkaline phosphatase, and parathyroid hormone levels.

CONTRAINDICATIONS
Contraindicated in patients with closed epiphyses or an active underlying intracranial lesion. Humatrope shouldn't be reconstituted with supplied diluent for patients hypersensitive to either Metacresol or glycerin.

NURSING CONSIDERATIONS
● Use cautiously in children with hypothyroidism and in those whose GH deficiency is caused by an intracranial lesion. These children should be examined frequently for progression or recurrence of underlying disease.
● To prepare solution, inject supplied diluent into vial containing drug by aiming stream of liquid against wall of glass vial.

Then swirl vial gently until contents are completely dissolved. Don't shake vial.
• After reconstitution, solution should be clear. Don't inject solution if it's cloudy or contains particles.
• Patients on dialysis need changes in drug administration schedule as follows: For hemodialysis, administer before bedtime or 3 to 4 hours after dialysis. For long-term cycling peritoneal dialysis, administer in the morning after completion of dialysis. For long-term ambulatory peritoneal dialysis, administer in the evening at the time of the overnight exchange.
• Store reconstituted drug in refrigerator; use within 14 days.
• If sensitivity to diluent occurs, drug may be reconstituted with sterile water for injection. When drug is reconstituted in this manner, use only 1 reconstituted dose per vial, refrigerate solution if it isn't used immediately after reconstitution, use reconstituted dose within 24 hours, and discard unused portion.
• Monitor child's height regularly. Regular checkups, including monitoring of blood and radiologic studies, also are needed.
• Monitor patient's glucose levels regularly because GH may induce a state of insulin resistance.
• Excessive glucocorticoid therapy inhibits somatropin's growth-promoting effect. Patients with coexisting corticotropin deficiency should have their glucocorticoid replacement dosage carefully adjusted to avoid growth inhibition.
• Watch for slipped capital femoral epiphysis or progression of scoliosis in patients with rapid growth.
• Monitor results of periodic thyroid function tests for hypothyroidism; condition may need thyroid hormone treatment. Laboratory measurements of thyroid hormone may change.
• Funduscopic examination of patient for intracranial hypertension should be done at onset of, and periodically during, therapy.
• *Alert:* Don't confuse somatropin with somatrem or sumatriptan.

PATIENT TEACHING
• Inform parents that child with endocrine disorders (including GH deficiency) may have an increased risk of slipped capital epiphyses. Tell them to notify prescriber if they notice their child limping.
• Instruct diabetic patients to monitor glucose closely and report changes to prescriber.
• Stress importance of close follow-up care.

vasopressin (ADH)
Pitressin

Pregnancy risk category C

AVAILABLE FORMS
Injection: 0.5-ml and 1-ml ampules, 20 units/ml

INDICATIONS & DOSAGES
➤ **Nonnephrogenic, nonpsychogenic diabetes insipidus—**
Adults: 5 to 10 units I.M. or S.C. b.i.d. to q.i.d., p.r.n. Or, intranasally (aqueous solution used as spray or applied to cotton balls) in individualized dosages, based on response.
Children: 2.5 to 10 units I.M. or S.C. b.i.d. to q.i.d., p.r.n. Or, intranasally (aqueous solution used as spray or applied to cotton balls) in individualized doses.
➤ **Prevention and treatment of abdominal distention—**
Adults: Initially, 5 units I.M.; subsequent injections may be given every 3 to 4 hours, increasing to 10 units if needed. Children may receive reduced dosages. Or, for adults, aqueous vasopressin 5 to 15 units S.C. at 2 hours before and repeated at 30 minutes before abdominal radiography or kidney biopsy.

ACTION
Increases permeability of the renal tubular epithelium to adenosine monophosphate and water; the epithelium promotes reabsorption of water and produces a concentrated urine.

Route	Onset	Peak	Duration
I.M., intranasal, S.C.	2-8 hr	Unknown	Unknown

ADVERSE REACTIONS
CNS: tremor, headache, vertigo.

Reactions may be *common,* uncommon, *life-threatening,* or COMMON AND LIFE-THREATENING.

CV: vasoconstriction, *arrhythmias, cardiac arrest,* myocardial ischemia, circumoral pallor, decreased cardiac output, angina in patients with vascular disease.
GI: abdominal cramps, nausea, vomiting, flatulence.
Skin: diaphoresis, cutaneous gangrene.
Other: water intoxication, *hypersensitivity reactions.*

INTERACTIONS
Drug-drug. *Carbamazepine, chlorpropamide, clofibrate, fludrocortisone, TCAs:* Increased antidiuretic response. Use together cautiously.
Demeclocycline, heparin, lithium, norepinephrine: Reduced antidiuretic activity. Use together cautiously.
Drug-lifestyle. *Alcohol use:* Reduced antidiuretic activity. Discourage use together.

EFFECTS ON LAB TEST RESULTS
None reported.

CONTRAINDICATIONS
Contraindicated in patients with chronic nephritis and nitrogen retention.

NURSING CONSIDERATIONS
• Use cautiously in children, elderly patients, pregnant women, preoperative and postoperative polyuric patients, and those with seizure disorders, migraines, asthma, CV disease, heart failure, renal disease, goiter with cardiac complications, arteriosclerosis, or fluid overload.
• Monitor patient for hypersensitivity reactions, including urticaria, angioedema, bronchoconstriction, and anaphylaxis.
• Synthetic desmopressin is sometimes preferred because of its longer duration of action and less frequent adverse reactions. Desmopressin also is available commercially as a nasal solution.
• Drug may be used for transient polyuria resulting from ADH deficiency related to neurosurgery or head injury.
• Use minimum effective dose to reduce adverse reactions.
• Give with 1 to 2 glasses of water to reduce adverse reactions and improve therapeutic response.
• Warm the vasopressin vial in your hands, and mix until the hormone is distributed throughout the solution before administration.
• Monitor urine specific gravity and fluid intake and output to aid evaluation of drug effectiveness.
• To prevent possible seizures, coma, and death, observe patient closely for early evidence of water intoxication, including drowsiness, listlessness, headache, confusion, and weight gain.
• Monitor blood pressure of patient taking vasopressin twice daily. Watch for excessively elevated blood pressure or lack of response to drug, which may be indicated by hypotension. Also, monitor weight daily.
• *Alert:* Don't confuse vasopressin with desmopressin.

PATIENT TEACHING
• Instruct patient to rotate injection sites to prevent tissue damage.
• Tell patient to report adverse reactions to prescriber promptly.
• Tell patient to report drowsiness, listlessness, and headache to prescriber.
• Tell patient to avoid alcohol and OTC medications unless approved by prescriber.
• Tell patient to restrict water intake.

calcifediol
calcitonin (human)
calcitonin (salmon)
calcitriol
pamidronate disodium
zoledronic acid

COMBINATION PRODUCTS
None.

---

calcifediol
Calderol

Pregnancy risk category C

AVAILABLE FORMS
Capsules: 20 mcg, 50 mcg

INDICATIONS & DOSAGES
➤ **Metabolic bone disease and hypocalcemia caused by chronic renal failure—**
Adults: Initially, 300 to 350 mcg P.O. weekly. Give daily or on alternate days. Dosage may be increased at 4-week intervals, if needed.

ACTION
A vitamin D analogue that stimulates calcium absorption from the GI tract and promotes movement of calcium from bone to blood.

Route	Onset	Peak	Duration
P.O.	Unknown	4 hr	15-20 days

ADVERSE REACTIONS
None reported.

INTERACTIONS
Drug-drug. *Cardiac glycosides:* Increased risk of arrhythmias. Avoid using together.
Cholestyramine, colestipol: Decreased absorption of orally administered vitamin D analogues. Avoid using together.
Corticosteroids: Counteract vitamin D analogue effects. Avoid using together.
Fosphenytoin, phenytoin, phenobarbital: May increase metabolism of vitamin to inactive metabolites. Avoid using together.

Magnesium-containing antacids: Possible hypermagnesemia, especially in patients with chronic renal failure. Avoid using together.
Other vitamin D analogues: Increased toxicity. Avoid using together.
Products containing calcium, thiazide diuretics: Increased risk of hypercalcemia. Use together cautiously.

EFFECTS ON LAB TEST RESULTS
None reported.

CONTRAINDICATIONS
Contraindicated in patients with hypercalcemia or vitamin D toxicity.

NURSING CONSIDERATIONS
• Monitor calcium level; when multiplied by phosphate level, it shouldn't exceed 70. During adjustment, calcium level should be determined at least weekly.
• If hypercalcemia occurs, stop calcifediol and notify prescriber. Drug may be resumed after calcium level returns to normal.
• Vitamin D intoxication causes various adverse effects, including headache, somnolence, weakness, irritability, hypertension, arrhythmias, conjunctivitis, photophobia, rhinorrhea, nausea, vomiting, constipation, polydipsia, pancreatitis, metallic taste, dry mouth, anorexia, nephrocalcinosis, polyuria, nocturia, weight loss, bone and muscle pain, pruritus, hyperthermia, and decreased libido.
• Drug may falsely elevate cholesterol tests using the Zlatkis-Zak reaction.
• *Alert:* Don't confuse calcifediol with calcitonin or calcitriol.

PATIENT TEACHING
• Teach patient to report signs and symptoms of hypercalcemia.
• Instruct patient about importance of consuming adequate daily calcium. Inform patient about foods high in calcium and how much to consume daily.

Reactions may be *common*, uncommon, ***life-threatening***, or **COMMON AND LIFE-THREATENING**.

calcitonin (human)
Cibacalcin

calcitonin (salmon)
Calcimar, Calsynar§, Miacalcin,
Osteocalcin, Salmonine

Pregnancy risk category C

AVAILABLE FORMS
calcitonin (human)
Injection: 0.5 mg/vial
calcitonin (salmon)
Injection: 200 IU/ml, 2-ml ampules
Nasal spray: 200 IU/activation in 2-ml
bottle

INDICATIONS & DOSAGES
➤ **Paget's disease of bone (osteitis de-
formans)**—
Adults: Initially, 100 IU of calcitonin
(salmon) daily S.C. or I.M. Maintenance
dosage is 50 to 100 IU daily S.C. or I.M.,
every other day, or three times weekly. Or,
calcitonin (human) 0.5 mg daily, reduced
to 0.25 mg daily. Some patients may need
up to 0.5 mg b.i.d.
➤ **Hypercalcemia**—
Adults: 4 IU/kg of calcitonin (salmon) q
12 hours S.C. or I.M. If response inadequate after 1 or 2 days, increase dosage to
8 IU/kg I.M. q 12 hours. If response remains unsatisfactory after 2 additional
days, increase dosage to maximum of
8 IU/kg I.M. q 6 hours.
➤ **Postmenopausal osteoporosis**—
Adults: 100 IU of calcitonin (salmon)
daily I.M. or S.C. Or, 200 IU (one activation) of calcitonin (salmon) daily intranasally, alternating nostrils daily. Patient
should receive adequate vitamin D and
calcium supplements (1.5 g calcium carbonate and 400 units of vitamin D) daily.

ACTION
Decreases osteoclastic activity by inhibiting osteocytic osteolysis; decreases mineral release and matrix or collagen breakdown in bone.

Route	Onset	Peak	Duration
I.M., S.C.	15 min	4 hr	8-24 hr
Intranasal	Rapid	0.5 hr	1 hr

ADVERSE REACTIONS
CNS: headache, weakness, dizziness,
paresthesia.
CV: chest pressure, *facial flushing.*
EENT: eye pain, *nasal congestion, rhinitis.*
GI: *transient nausea,* unusual taste, diarrhea, anorexia, *vomiting,* epigastric discomfort, abdominal pain.
GU: *increased urinary frequency,* nocturia.
Respiratory: shortness of breath.
Skin: rash, pruritus of ear lobes, *inflammation at injection site.*
Other: hypersensitivity reactions, **anaphylaxis,** edema of feet, chills, tender
palms and soles.

INTERACTIONS
None significant.

EFFECTS ON LAB TEST RESULTS
None reported.

CONTRAINDICATIONS
Contraindicated in patients hypersensitive
to salmon calcitonin. Human calcitonin
has no contraindications.

NURSING CONSIDERATIONS
• Skin test usually is done before therapy.
• *Alert:* Systemic allergic reactions are
possible because hormone is protein. Keep
epinephrine nearby.
• Calcitonin (human) is especially indicated in patients who have developed resistance to calcitonin (salmon). Calcitonin
(human) is linked to a risk of diminishing
efficacy caused by antibody formation or
hypersensitivity reactions. The two calci-
tonins aren't interchangeable.
• Administer at bedtime, when possible, to
minimize nausea and vomiting.
• I.M. route is preferred if volume of dose
to be administered exceeds 2 ml.
• Use freshly reconstituted solution within
2 hours.
• *Alert:* Observe patient for signs of
hypocalcemic tetany during therapy (muscle twitching, tetanic spasms, and seizures
when hypocalcemia is severe).
• Monitor calcium level closely. Watch for
symptoms of hypercalcemia relapse: bone
pain, renal calculi, polyuria, anorexia,
nausea, vomiting, thirst, constipation,

lethargy, bradycardia, muscle hypotonicity, pathologic fracture, psychosis, and coma.
• Periodic examinations of urine sediment are recommended.
• Monitor periodic alkaline phosphatase and 24-hour urine hydroxyproline levels to evaluate drug effect.
• In Paget's disease, maximum reductions of alkaline phosphatase and urinary hydroxyproline excretion may take 6 to 24 months of continuous treatment.
• In patients with good initial clinical response to calcitonin who have a relapse, expect to evaluate antibody response to the hormone protein.
• If symptoms have been relieved after 6 months, treatment may be discontinued until symptoms or radiologic signs recur.
• Store calcitonin (human) at room temperature (77° F [25° C]) and protect from light; refrigerate calcitonin (salmon) at 36° to 46° F (2° to 8° C).
• **Alert:** Don't confuse calcitonin with calcifediol or calcitriol.

PATIENT TEACHING
• When drug is administered for postmenopausal osteoporosis, remind patient to take adequate calcium and vitamin D supplements.
• Show home care patient and family member how to administer drug. Tell them to do so at bedtime if only one dose is needed daily. If nasal spray is prescribed, tell patient to alternate nostrils daily.
• Advise patient to notify prescriber if significant nasal irritation develops.
• Inform patient that facial flushing and warmth occur in 20% to 30% of patients within minutes of injection and usually last about 1 hour. Reassure patient that this is a transient effect.
• Tell patient that nausea and vomiting may occur at the onset of therapy.
• Tell patient to report signs and symptoms of hypercalcemia promptly. Inform patient that, if calcitonin loses its hypocalcemic activity, other drugs or increased dosages won't help.
• Advise patient to notify prescriber immediately if signs of an allergic response occur.

calcitriol (1,25-dihydroxy-cholecalciferol)
Calcijex, Rocaltrol

Pregnancy risk category C

AVAILABLE FORMS
Capsules: 0.25 mcg, 0.5 mcg
Injection: 1 mcg/ml, 2 mcg/ml
Oral solution: 1 mcg/ml

INDICATIONS & DOSAGES
➤ **Hypocalcemia in patients undergoing long-term dialysis—**
Adults: Initially, 0.25 mcg P.O. daily. May be increased by 0.25 mcg daily at 4- to 8-week intervals. Maintenance dosage is 0.5 to 3 mcg daily. Or, 0.5 mcg I.V. three times weekly about every other day. If response to initial dosage is inadequate, may increase by 0.25 to 0.5 mcg at 2- to 4-week intervals. Maintenance dosage is 0.5 to 3 mcg I.V. three times weekly.
➤ **Hypoparathyroidism, pseudohypoparathyroidism—**
Adults and children age 6 and older: Initially, 0.25 mcg P.O. daily in the morning. Dosage may be increased at 2- to 4-week intervals. Maintenance dosage is 0.25 to 2 mcg P.O. daily.
➤ **Hypoparathyroidism—**
Children ages 1 to 5: 0.25 to 0.75 mcg P.O. daily.
➤ **Management of secondary hyperparathyroidism and resulting metabolic bone disease in predialysis patients (moderate to severe chronic renal failure with creatinine clearance of 15 to 55 ml/minute)—**
Adults and children age 3 and older: Initially, 0.25 mcg P.O. daily. Dosage may be increased to 0.5 mcg/day if needed.
Children younger than age 3: Initially, 10 to 15 ng/kg P.O. daily.

I.V. ADMINISTRATION
• For hypocalcemic patients with chronic renal failure who are undergoing hemodialysis, may give drug by rapid I.V. injection through catheter at end of hemodialysis session.

Reactions may be *common*, uncommon, *life-threatening*, or COMMON AND LIFE-THREATENING.

ACTION

A vitamin D analogue that stimulates calcium absorption from the GI tract and promotes movement of calcium from bone to blood.

Route	Onset	Peak	Duration
I.V.	Immediate	Unknown	3-5 days
P.O.	2-6 hr	3-6 hr	3-5 days

ADVERSE REACTIONS

None reported.

INTERACTIONS

Drug-drug. *Cardiac glycosides:* Increased risk of arrhythmias. Avoid using together.

Cholestyramine, colestipol, excessive use of mineral oil: Decreased absorption of orally administered vitamin D analogues. Avoid using together.

Corticosteroids: Counteract vitamin D analogue effects. Avoid using together.

Magnesium-containing antacids: May induce hypermagnesemia, especially in patients with chronic renal failure. Avoid using together.

Phenytoin, phenobarbital: Inhibited calcitriol synthesis. An increased dose may be necessary.

EFFECTS ON LAB TEST RESULTS

None reported.

CONTRAINDICATIONS

Contraindicated in patients with hypercalcemia or vitamin D toxicity. Withhold all preparations containing vitamin D.

NURSING CONSIDERATIONS

• Use cautiously in patients receiving cardiac glycosides and in those with sarcoidosis or hyperparathyroidism.

• Monitor calcium level; multiplied by phosphate level, it shouldn't exceed 70. During adjustment, determine calcium level twice weekly. Stop and notify prescriber if hypercalcemia occurs, but resume after calcium level returns to normal. Patient should receive adequate daily intake of calcium. Observe for hypocalcemia, bone pain, and weakness before and during therapy.

• Vitamin D intoxication causes various adverse effects, including headache, somnolence, weakness, irritability, hypertension, arrhythmias, conjunctivitis, photophobia, rhinorrhea, nausea, vomiting, constipation, polydipsia, pancreatitis, metallic taste, dry mouth, anorexia, nephrocalcinosis, polyuria, nocturia, weight loss, bone and muscle pain, pruritus, hyperthermia, and decreased libido.

• Drug therapy may falsely elevate cholesterol determinations using the Zlatkis-Zak reaction.

• Protect drug from heat and light.

• *Alert:* Don't confuse calcitriol with calcifediol or calcitonin.

PATIENT TEACHING

• Tell patient to immediately report early symptoms of vitamin D intoxication: weakness, nausea, vomiting, dry mouth, constipation, muscle or bone pain, or metallic taste.

• Instruct patient to adhere to diet and calcium supplementation and to avoid unapproved OTC drugs and magnesium-containing antacids.

• *Alert:* Tell patient that drug mustn't be taken by anyone for whom it wasn't prescribed. It's the most potent form of vitamin D available.

---

pamidronate disodium
Aredia

Pregnancy risk category C

AVAILABLE FORMS

Injection: 30-mg, 90-mg vials

INDICATIONS & DOSAGES

➤ **Moderate to severe hypercalcemia from cancer (with or without bone metastases)—**

Adults: Dosage depends on severity of hypercalcemia. Calcium levels should be corrected for albumin. Corrected calcium (CCa) is calculated using this formula:

$$\underset{\text{(mg/dl)}}{CCa} = \underset{\substack{\text{calcium} \\ \text{(mg/dl)}}}{\text{serum}} + \underset{\substack{\text{albumin)} \\ \text{(g/dl)}}}{0.8\ (4-\text{serum}}$$

Patients with moderate hypercalcemia (CCa levels of 12 to 13.5 mg/dl) may receive 60 to 90 mg by I.V. infusion as a single dose over 2 to 24 hours. Patients with

severe hypercalcemia (CCa levels higher than 13.5 mg/dl) may receive 90 mg by I.V. infusion over 2 to 24 hours. A minimum of 7 days should elapse before retreatment to allow for full response to initial dose.
➤ **Moderate to severe Paget's disease—**
Adults: 30 mg I.V. as a 4-hour infusion on 3 consecutive days for total dose of 90 mg. Cycle repeated, p.r.n.
➤ **Osteolytic bone metastases of breast cancer with standard antineoplastic therapy—**
Adults: 90 mg I.V. infusion over 2 hours q 3 to 4 weeks.
➤ **Osteolytic bone lesions of multiple myeloma—**
Adults: 90 mg I.V. over 4 hours once monthly.

I.V. ADMINISTRATION
● Reconstitute drug with 10 ml of sterile water for injection. After drug is completely dissolved, add to 250 ml (2-hour infusion), 500 ml (4-hour infusion), or 1,000 ml (up to 24-hour infusion) of half-normal or normal saline solution for injection or D_5W.
● Don't mix with infusion solutions that contain calcium, such as Ringer's injection or lactated Ringer's injection. Visually inspect for precipitate before use.
● *Alert:* Give drug only by I.V. infusion. Injecting a bolus may cause nephropathy.

ACTION
An antihypercalcemic that inhibits resorption of bone. Adsorbs to hydroxyapatite crystals in bone and may directly block dissolution of calcium phosphate. Blocks mature osteoclast formation. Apparently doesn't inhibit bone formation or mineralization.

Route	Onset	Peak	Duration
I.V.	Unknown	Unknown	Unknown

ADVERSE REACTIONS
CNS: *seizures, fatigue,* somnolence, syncope.
CV: **atrial fibrillation,** tachycardia, *hypertension.*
GI: *abdominal pain, anorexia, constipation, nausea, vomiting,* **GI hemorrhage.**

Hematologic: *leukopenia, thrombocytopenia,* anemia.
Metabolic: hypophosphatemia, hypokalemia, hypomagnesemia, hypocalcemia.
Other: *infusion-site reaction,* fever.

INTERACTIONS
None significant.

EFFECTS ON LAB TEST RESULTS
● May decrease phosphate, potassium, magnesium, and calcium levels.
● May decrease WBCs, platelets, and hemoglobin.

CONTRAINDICATIONS
Contraindicated in patients hypersensitive to drug or other bisphosphonates, such as etidronate.

NURSING CONSIDERATIONS
● Use with extreme caution, and consider risks versus benefits, in patients with renal impairment.
● Assess hydration status before treatment. Use drug only after patient has been vigorously hydrated with normal saline solution. In patients with mild to moderate hypercalcemia, hydration alone may be sufficient.
● Because drug can cause electrolyte disturbances, carefully monitor electrolyte levels, especially calcium, phosphate, and magnesium. Short-term administration of calcium may be needed in patients with severe hypocalcemia. Also monitor creatinine level, CBC and differential count, and hemoglobin levels and hematocrit.
● Carefully monitor patients with anemia, leukopenia, or thrombocytopenia during first 2 weeks of therapy.
● Monitor patient's temperature. Some patients experience an elevation of $1.8°$ F ($1°$ C) for 24 to 48 hours after therapy.
● Solution is stable for 24 hours at room temperature.
● Store reconstituted drug at 36° to 46° F (2° to 8° C).

PATIENT TEACHING
● Explain use and administration of drug to patient and family.
● Instruct patient to report adverse reactions promptly.

Reactions may be *common,* uncommon, *life-threatening,* or **COMMON AND LIFE-THREATENING.**

✳ NEW DRUG

zoledronic acid
Zometa

Pregnancy risk category C

AVAILABLE FORMS
Injection: 4 mg/vial

INDICATIONS & DOSAGES
➤ **Hypercalcemia related to malignancy—**
Adults: 4 mg by I.V. infusion over at least
15 minutes. If albumin-corrected calcium
level doesn't return to normal, consider retreatment with 4 mg. Allow at least 7 days
to pass before retreatment to allow a full
response to the initial dose.
Adjust-a-dose: The following guidelines
are for patients who received zoledronic
acid, have reduced renal function as a result, and must be retreated with the drug.
If patient had a normal creatinine level before treatment and has an increase in
creatinine level of 0.5 mg/dl within 2 weeks of
the next dose, drug should be withheld until level is within 10% of baseline value.
Likewise, if patient had an abnormal creatinine level before treatment and has an increase of 1 mg/dl within 2 weeks of the
next dose, drug should be withheld until
level is within 10% of baseline value.

I.V. ADMINISTRATION
● Reconstitute by adding 5 ml of sterile
water to each vial. The drug must be completely dissolved.
● Withdraw 4 mg of drug and mix in
100 ml of normal saline solution or D_5W.
● The drug must be given as an I.V. infusion over at least 15 minutes.
● If not used immediately after reconstitution, the solution must be refrigerated. It
must be given within 24 hours.
● Inspect the solution to rule out particulate matter and discoloration before giving
it.
● Give drug as a single I.V. solution in a
line separate from all other drugs.
● *Alert:* Don't mix drug with calcium-
containing solutions (such as lactated
Ringer's solution).

ACTION
Zoledronic acid inhibits bone resorption,
probably by inhibiting osteoclast activity
and osteoclastic resorption of mineralized
bone and cartilage. Decreases calcium release induced by the stimulatory factors
produced by tumors.

Route	Onset	Peak	Duration
I.V.	Unknown	Unknown	7-28 days

ADVERSE REACTIONS
CNS: headache, somnolence, *anxiety,
confusion, agitation, insomnia.*
CV: hypotension.
GI: *nausea, constipation, diarrhea, ab-
dominal pain, vomiting,* anorexia, dyspha-
gia.
GU: decreased creatinine level, *urinary
infection.*
Hematologic: *anemia, granulocytopenia,
thrombocytopenia, pancytopenia.*
Metabolic: dehydration.
Musculoskeletal: *skeletal pain,* arthral-
gia.
Respiratory: *dyspnea, cough,* pleural ef-
fusion.
Other: *fever, progression of cancer, infection.*

INTERACTIONS
Drug-drug. *Aminoglycosides, loop diuretics:* Additive effects to lower calcium levels. Give together cautiously, and monitor
calcium levels.

EFFECTS ON LAB TEST RESULTS
● May increase creatinine levels. May decrease calcium, phosphorus, magnesium,
and potassium levels.
● May decrease hemoglobin, hematocrit,
and RBC, WBC, and platelet counts.

CONTRAINDICATIONS
Contraindicated in patients with clinically
significant hypersensitivity to drug, other
bisphosphonates, or ingredients in formulation.

NURSING CONSIDERATIONS
● Use cautiously in patients with aspirin-
sensitive asthma because other bisphosphonates have been linked to bronchoconstriction in aspirin-sensitive patients with

I.V. ADMINISTRATION
● Reconstitute drug in 500-mg vial with at least 5 ml of sterile water for injection. Use within 24 hours of reconstitution.
● Inject 100 to 500 mg/minute into a large vein using a 21G or 23G needle. Intermittent or continuous infusion isn't recommended.

ACTION
Blocks action of carbonic anhydrase, promoting renal excretion of sodium, potassium, bicarbonate, and water. Also decreases secretion of aqueous humor in the eye, thereby lowering intraocular pressure. As an anticonvulsant, it may decrease abnormal paroxysmal or excessive neuronal discharge. In acute mountain sickness, it produces a respiratory and metabolic acidosis that may stimulate ventilation, increase cerebral blood flow, promote the release of oxygen from hemoglobin, and increase ventilation.

Route	Onset	Peak	Duration
I.V.	2 min	15 min	4-5 hr
P.O.	1-1.5 hr	1-4 hr	8-12 hr
P.O. (extended)	2 hr	3-6 hr	18-24 hr

ADVERSE REACTIONS
CNS: drowsiness, paresthesia, confusion, depression, *seizures,* weakness.
EENT: transient myopia, hearing dysfunction, tinnitus.
GI: nausea, vomiting, anorexia, metallic taste, diarrhea, black tarry stools.
GU: polyuria, hematuria, crystalluria, glycosuria, renal calculus.
Hematologic: *aplastic anemia,* hemolytic anemia, *leukopenia.*
Metabolic: hypokalemia, asymptomatic hyperuricemia, hyperchloremic acidosis.
Skin: rash.
Other: *pain at injection site,* sterile abscesses.

INTERACTIONS
Drug-drug. *Amphetamines, anticholinergics, mecamylamine, procainamide, quinidine:* Decreased renal clearance of these drugs, increasing toxicity. Monitor patient for toxicity.

Cyclosporine: Increased cyclosporine levels, which may cause nephrotoxicity and neurotoxicity. Monitor patient for toxicity.
Diflunisal: Increased risk of adverse effects of acetazolamide; significant decrease in intracranial pressure if used together. Use with caution.
Lithium: Increased excretion of lithium, resulting in decreased effectiveness. Monitor lithium level.
Methenamine: Reduced effectiveness of acetazolamide. Avoid using together.
Primidone: Serum and urine levels of primidone may be decreased. Monitor patient closely.
Salicylates: Accumulation and toxicity of acetazolamide, including CNS depression and metabolic acidosis. Monitor patient for toxicity.
Drug-lifestyle. *Sun exposure:* Increased risk for photosensitivity reactions. Advise patient to avoid excessive sunlight exposure.

EFFECTS ON LAB TEST RESULTS
● May increase uric acid levels. May decrease potassium levels.
● May decrease hemoglobin, WBC count, and thyroid iodine uptake.

CONTRAINDICATIONS
Contraindicated in patients hypersensitive to drug and in those with hyponatremia or hypokalemia, renal or hepatic disease or dysfunction, renal calculi, adrenal gland failure, hyperchloremic acidosis, or severe pulmonary obstruction. Also contraindicated in those receiving long-term treatment for chronic noncongestive angle-closure glaucoma.

NURSING CONSIDERATIONS
● Use cautiously in patients receiving other diuretics and in those with respiratory acidosis, emphysema, or chronic pulmonary disease.
● Cross-sensitivity between antibacterial sulfonamides and sulfonamide-derivative diuretics such as acetazolamide has been reported.
● If patient can't swallow oral form, pharmacist may make a suspension using crushed acetazolamide tablets in a highly flavored syrup, such as cherry, raspberry, or chocolate. Although concentrations up

---

Reactions may be *common,* uncommon, *life-threatening,* or **COMMON AND LIFE-THREATENING.**

to 500 mg/5 ml are feasible, concentrations of 250 mg/5 ml are more palatable. Refrigeration improves palatability but doesn't improve stability. Suspensions are stable for 1 week.

• Monitor fluid intake and output, glucose, and electrolytes, especially potassium, bicarbonate, and chloride. When drug is used in diuretic therapy, consult prescriber and dietitian about providing a high-potassium diet.

• Monitor elderly patients closely because they are especially susceptible to excessive diuresis.

• Weigh patient daily. Rapid or excessive fluid loss causes weight loss and hypotension.

• Diuretic effect decreases when acidosis occurs but can be reestablished by withdrawing drug for several days and then restarting or by using intermittent administration schedules.

• Because bicarbonate ion excretion makes patient's urine alkaline, drug may cause false-positive urine protein tests.

• Monitor patient for signs of hemolytic anemia (pallor, weakness, and palpitations).

• Drug may increase glucose level and cause glycosuria.

• *Alert:* Don't confuse acetazolamide with acetohexamide.

PATIENT TEACHING
• Tell patient to take oral form with food if GI upset occurs.

• Caution patient not to perform hazardous activities if adverse CNS reactions occur.

• Instruct patient to avoid prolonged exposure to sunlight; drug may cause phototoxicity.

• Instruct patient to notify prescriber if unusual bleeding, bruising, tingling, or tremors occur.

---

amiloride hydrochloride
Kaluril‡, Midamor

Pregnancy risk category B

AVAILABLE FORMS
Tablets: 5 mg

INDICATIONS & DOSAGES
➤ **Hypertension; hypokalemia; edema from heart failure, usually in patients also taking thiazide or other potassium-wasting diuretics—**
Adults: 5 mg P.O. daily, increased to 10 mg daily, if needed; then 15 mg. Maximum, 20 mg daily.

ACTION
A potassium-sparing diuretic that inhibits sodium reabsorption and potassium excretion in the distal tubules.

Route	Onset	Peak	Duration
P.O.	2 hr	6-10 hr	24 hr

ADVERSE REACTIONS
CNS: fatigue, *headache,* weakness, dizziness, encephalopathy.
CV: orthostatic hypotension.
GI: *nausea, anorexia, diarrhea, vomiting,* abdominal pain, constipation, appetite changes.
GU: impotence.
Hematologic: *aplastic anemia, neutropenia.*
Metabolic: hyperkalemia, hyponatremia.
Musculoskeletal: muscle cramps.
Respiratory: dyspnea.

INTERACTIONS
Drug-drug. *ACE inhibitors, indomethacin, potassium-sparing diuretics, potassium supplements:* May cause hyperkalemia. Avoid using together.
Lithium: Decreased lithium clearance, increasing risk of lithium toxicity. Monitor lithium level.
NSAIDs: Decreased diuretic effectiveness. Avoid using together.
Drug-herb. *Licorice:* Increased risk of hypokalemia. Discourage use together.
Drug-food. *Foods high in potassium (such as bananas, oranges), salt substitutes containing potassium:* May cause hyperkalemia. Advise patient to choose diet carefully and to use low-potassium salt substitutes.

EFFECTS ON LAB TEST RESULTS
• May increase BUN and potassium levels. May decrease sodium level.
• May decrease hemoglobin, neutrophil count, and liver function test values.

CONTRAINDICATIONS

Contraindicated in patients hypersensitive to drug and in those with elevated potassium level (higher than 5.5 mEq/L), anuria, acute or chronic renal insufficiency, or diabetic nephropathy. Don't give to patients receiving potassium supplementation or other potassium-sparing diuretics, such as spironolactone and triamterene.

NURSING CONSIDERATIONS

• Use cautiously in patients with diabetes mellitus, cardiopulmonary disease, or severe, existing hepatic or renal insufficiency. Also use cautiously in elderly or debilitated patients.
• To prevent nausea, give drug with meals.
• Monitor potassium level because of increased risk of hyperkalemia. Alert prescriber immediately if potassium level exceeds 6.5 mEq/L, and expect drug to be discontinued.
• Drug causes severe hyperkalemia in diabetic patients after glucose tolerance testing; stop drug at least 3 days before testing.
• *Alert:* Don't confuse amiloride with amrinone or amiodarone.

PATIENT TEACHING

• Advise patient to avoid sudden postural changes and to rise slowly to avoid effects of orthostatic hypotension.
• Caution patient not to perform hazardous activities if adverse CNS reactions occur.
• To prevent serious hyperkalemia, warn patient to avoid excessive ingestion of potassium-rich foods, potassium-containing salt substitutes, and potassium supplements.
• Advise patient to report signs of hyperkalemia: paresthesia, muscle weakness, fatigue, paralysis of limbs.
• Instruct patient to check with prescriber or pharmacist before taking new prescription or OTC drugs.
• Tell patient to take drug with food if GI upset occurs.

bumetanide
Bumex, Burinex‡§

Pregnancy risk category C

AVAILABLE FORMS
Injection: 0.25 mg/ml
Tablets: 0.5 mg, 1 mg, 2 mg

INDICATIONS & DOSAGES
➤ **Edema caused by heart failure or hepatic or renal disease—**
Adults: 0.5 to 2 mg P.O. once daily. If diuretic response isn't adequate, a second or third dose may be given at 4- to 5-hour intervals. Maximum dose is 10 mg/day. May be given parenterally if oral route isn't feasible. Usual initial dose is 0.5 to 1 mg given I.V. or I.M. If response isn't adequate, a second or third dose may be given at 2- to 3-hour intervals. Maximum, 10 mg/day.

I.V. ADMINISTRATION
• Give I.V. doses directly using a 21G or 23G needle over 1 to 2 minutes. For intermittent infusion, give diluted drug through an intermittent infusion device or piggyback into an I.V. line containing a free-flowing, compatible solution. Infuse at ordered rate. Continuous infusion isn't recommended.
• In patients with severe chronic renal insufficiency, a continuous infusion of bumetanide (12 mg over 12 hours) may be more effective and less toxic than intermittent bolus therapy.

ACTION
A potent loop diuretic that inhibits sodium and chloride reabsorption at the ascending loop of Henle.

Route	Onset	Peak	Duration
I.M.	40 min	Unknown	5-6 hr
I.V.	Within min	15-30 min	0.5-1 hr
P.O.	0.5-1 hr	1-2 hr	4-6 hr

ADVERSE REACTIONS
CNS: *weakness,* dizziness, headache, vertigo.
CV: orthostatic hypotension, ECG changes, chest pain.
EENT: transient deafness, tinnitus.

Reactions may be *common,* uncommon, *life-threatening,* or COMMON AND LIFE-THREATENING.

GI: nausea, vomiting, upset stomach, dry mouth, diarrhea.
GU: premature ejaculation, difficulty maintaining erection, oliguria.
Hematologic: azotemia, *thrombocytopenia.*
Metabolic: volume depletion and dehydration; hypokalemia; hypochloremic alkalosis; hypomagnesemia; asymptomatic hyperuricemia.
Musculoskeletal: arthritic pain, muscle pain and tenderness.
Skin: rash, pruritus, diaphoresis.
Other: pain.

INTERACTIONS
Drug-drug. *Aminoglycoside antibiotics:* Potentiated ototoxicity. Use together cautiously.
Antihypertensives: Increased risk of hypotension. Use together cautiously.
Cardiac glycosides: Increased risk of digoxin toxicity from bumetanide-induced hypokalemia. Monitor potassium and digoxin levels.
Cisplatin: Increased risk of ototoxicity. Monitor patient closely.
Diuretics: Profound diuresis and potential electrolyte loss. Monitor patient for fluid and electrolyte disorders.
Lithium: Decreased lithium clearance, increasing risk of lithium toxicity. Monitor lithium level.
Neuromuscular blockers: Potentially prolonged neuromuscular blockade. Monitor patient closely.
NSAIDs, probenecid: Inhibited diuretic response. Use together cautiously.
Other potassium-wasting drugs (such as amphotericin B, corticosteroids): Increased risk of hypokalemia. Use together cautiously.
Drug-herb. *Dandelion:* May interfere with diuretic activity. Discourage use together.
Licorice: May cause unexpected rapid potassium loss. Discourage use together.

EFFECTS ON LAB TEST RESULTS
● May increase creatinine, nitrogenous compound (urea), glucose, and cholesterol levels. May decrease potassium, magnesium, sodium, and calcium levels.
● May decrease platelet count.

CONTRAINDICATIONS
Contraindicated in patients hypersensitive to drug or sulfonamides (possible cross-sensitivity) and in patients with anuria, hepatic coma, or severe electrolyte depletion.

NURSING CONSIDERATIONS
● Use cautiously in patients with hepatic cirrhosis and ascites, in elderly patients, and in those with depressed renal function.
● To prevent nocturia, give drug in the morning. If second dose is needed, give in early afternoon.
● Safest and most effective dosage schedule for control of edema is intermittent dosage given on alternate days or 3 to 4 days with 1 or 2 days off between cycles.
● Monitor fluid intake and output, weight, and electrolyte, BUN, creatinine, and carbon dioxide levels frequently.
● Watch for evidence of hypokalemia, such as muscle weakness and cramps. Instruct patient to report these symptoms.
● Consult prescriber and dietitian about a high-potassium diet. Foods rich in potassium include citrus fruits, tomatoes, bananas, dates, and apricots.
● Monitor glucose levels in diabetic patients.
● Monitor uric acid levels, especially in patients with history of gout.
● Monitor blood pressure and pulse rate during rapid diuresis. Bumetanide can lead to profound water and electrolyte depletion.
● If oliguria or azotemia develops or increases, prescriber may stop drug.
● Bumetanide can be safely used in patients allergic to furosemide; 1 mg of bumetanide equals 40 mg of furosemide.
● *Alert:* Don't confuse Bumex with Buprenex.

PATIENT TEACHING
● Tell patient to take drug in morning to prevent nocturia, and if second dose is prescribed, to take it in early afternoon. Also instruct patient to take drug with food or milk if adverse GI reactions occur.
● Instruct patient to notify prescriber about muscle weakness, cramps, nausea, or dizziness.

• Advise patient to stand up slowly to prevent dizziness and to limit alcohol intake and strenuous exercise in hot weather to avoid exacerbating orthostatic hypotension.
• Instruct patient to weigh himself daily to monitor fluid status.

chlorthalidone
Apo-Chlorthalidone†, Hygroton, Novo-Thalidone†, Thalitone, Uridon†

Pregnancy risk category B

AVAILABLE FORMS
Tablets: 15 mg, 25 mg, 50 mg, 100 mg

INDICATIONS & DOSAGES
➤ **Edema, hypertension—**
Adults: Initially, 25 to 100 mg P.O. daily, or up to 200 mg P.O. on alternate days.
Children: 2 mg/kg or 60 mg/m^2 P.O. three times weekly.

ACTION
Increases sodium and water excretion by inhibiting sodium and chloride reabsorption in the distal segment of the nephron.

Route	Onset	Peak	Duration
P.O.	2-3 hr	2-6 hr	2-3 days

ADVERSE REACTIONS
CNS: dizziness, vertigo, headache, paresthesia, weakness, restlessness.
CV: orthostatic hypotension, vasculitis.
GI: anorexia, nausea, *pancreatitis,* vomiting, abdominal pain, diarrhea, constipation.
GU: impotence.
Hematologic: *aplastic anemia, agranulocytosis, leukopenia, thrombocytopenia.*
Hepatic: jaundice.
Metabolic: *hypokalemia;* asymptomatic hyperuricemia; hyperglycemia and impaired glucose tolerance; fluid and electrolyte imbalances, including dilutional hyponatremia and hypochloremia, metabolic alkalosis, hypercalcemia, volume depletion, and dehydration.
Skin: dermatitis, photosensitivity reactions, rash, purpura, urticaria.
Other: hypersensitivity reactions, gout.

INTERACTIONS
Drug-drug. *Amphotericin B:* Increased risk of hypokalemia. Monitor potassium level closely.
Antidiabetics: Decreased effectiveness; dosage adjustments may be needed. Monitor glucose levels.
Barbiturates, opiates: Increased orthostatic hypotensive effect. Monitor blood pressure closely.
Cardiac glycosides: Increased risk of digoxin toxicity from chlorthalidone-induced hypokalemia. Monitor potassium and digoxin levels.
Cholestyramine, colestipol: Decreased intestinal absorption of thiazides. Separate doses.
Corticosteroids: Increased risk of hypokalemia. Monitor potassium level closely.
Diazoxide: Increased antihypertensive, hyperglycemic, and hyperuricemic effects. Use together cautiously.
Lithium: Decreased lithium clearance, increasing risk of lithium toxicity. Monitor lithium level.
NSAIDs: Increased risk of NSAID-induced renal failure. Monitor renal function closely.
Drug-herb. *Licorice:* May cause unexpected rapid potassium loss. Discourage use together.
Drug-lifestyle. *Alcohol use:* Increased orthostatic hypotensive effect. Discourage use together.
Sun exposure: Increased risk for photosensitivity reaction. Advise patient to avoid excessive sunlight exposure.

EFFECTS ON LAB TEST RESULTS
• May increase uric acid, glucose, calcium, cholesterol, and triglyceride levels. May decrease potassium, sodium, and chloride levels.
• May decrease hemoglobin and granulocyte, WBC, and platelet counts.

CONTRAINDICATIONS
Contraindicated in patients with anuria and patients hypersensitive to thiazides or other sulfonamide-derived drugs.

NURSING CONSIDERATIONS
• Use cautiously in patients with severe renal disease and impaired hepatic function.

Reactions may be *common*, uncommon, *life-threatening*, or COMMON AND LIFE-THREATENING.

• To prevent nocturia, give drug in the morning.

• Monitor fluid intake and output, weight, blood pressure, and electrolyte levels.

• Watch for signs of hypokalemia, such as muscle weakness and cramps. Drug may be used with potassium-sparing diuretic to prevent potassium loss.

• Consult prescriber and dietitian about a high-potassium diet. Foods rich in potassium include citrus fruits, tomatoes, bananas, apricots, and dates.

• Monitor creatinine and BUN levels regularly. Cumulative effects of drug may occur with impaired renal function.

• Monitor uric acid levels, especially in patients with history of gout.

• Monitor glucose levels, and check insulin requirements in diabetic patients.

• Monitor elderly patients, who are especially susceptible to excessive diuresis.

• *Alert:* Don't use Hygroton and Thalitone interchangeably; they have different bioavailabilities.

• Stop thiazides and thiazide-like diuretics before parathyroid function tests.

• In hypertensive patients, therapeutic response may be delayed several weeks.

• *Alert:* Don't confuse Uridon tablets (available only in Canada) with the urinary anti-infective Uridon Modified (available in the United States).

PATIENT TEACHING

• Instruct patient to take in morning to prevent nocturia.

• Tell patient to avoid sudden postural changes and to rise slowly to avoid effects of orthostatic hypotension.

• Advise patient to use a sunblock to prevent photosensitivity reactions.

• Tell patient that drug may cause GI upset and should be taken with food or milk.

• Advise patient to report signs of hypotension: increased heart rate or pulse, dizziness, tiredness, or restlessness.

ethacrynate sodium
Edecrin Sodium

ethacrynic acid
Edecril‡, Edecrin

Pregnancy risk category B

AVAILABLE FORMS
ethacrynate sodium
Injection: 50 mg (with 62.5 mg of mannitol and 0.1 mg of thimerosal)
ethacrynic acid
Tablets: 25 mg, 50 mg

INDICATIONS & DOSAGES
➤ **Acute pulmonary edema**—
Adults: 50 mg or 0.5 to 1 mg/kg I.V. Usually only one dose is needed, although a second dose may be needed.
➤ **Edema**—
Adults: 50 to 200 mg P.O. daily. Refractory patients may need up to 200 mg b.i.d.
Children: Initial dose is 25 mg P.O., increased cautiously in 25-mg increments daily until desired effect is achieved.
Adjust-a-dose: If added to an existing diuretic regimen, initial dose is 25 mg and dosage adjustments are made in 25-mg increments.

I.V. ADMINISTRATION
• Add to vial 50 ml of D_5W or normal saline solution. Give slowly through tubing of running infusion over several minutes. Discard unused solution after 24 hours. Don't use cloudy or opalescent solutions.

• If more than one I.V. dose is needed, use a new injection site to avoid thrombophlebitis.

• Don't mix with whole blood or its derivatives.

ACTION
A potent loop diuretic that inhibits sodium and chloride reabsorption at the proximal and distal tubules and the ascending loop of Henle.

Route	Onset	Peak	Duration
I.V.	5 min	15-30 min	2 hr
P.O.	30 min	2 hr	6-8 hr

Sucralfate: May reduce diuretic and antihypertensive effect. Separate administration times by 2 hours.

Drug-herb. *Aloe:* May increase drug effects. Discourage use together.

Dandelion: May interfere with diuretic activity. Discourage use together.

Ginseng: Decreased loop diuretic effect. Discourage use together.

Licorice: May cause unexpected rapid potassium loss. Discourage use together.

Drug-lifestyle. *Sun exposure:* Increased risk for photosensitivity reactions. Advise patient to avoid excessive sunlight exposure.

EFFECTS ON LAB TEST RESULTS
● May increase glucose, cholesterol, and uric acid levels. May decrease potassium, sodium, calcium, and magnesium levels.
● May decrease hemoglobin and granulocyte, WBC, and platelet counts.

CONTRAINDICATIONS
Contraindicated in patients hypersensitive to drug and in those with anuria.

NURSING CONSIDERATIONS
● Use cautiously in patients with hepatic cirrhosis and in those allergic to sulfonamides. Furosemide should be used during pregnancy only if potential benefits to mother clearly outweigh risks to fetus.
● To prevent nocturia, give P.O. and I.M. preparations in the morning. Give second dose in early afternoon.
● *Alert:* Monitor weight, blood pressure, and pulse rate routinely with long-term use and during rapid diuresis. Furosemide can lead to profound water and electrolyte depletion.
● If oliguria or azotemia develops or increases, drug may need to be discontinued.
● Monitor fluid intake and output and electrolyte, BUN, and carbon dioxide levels frequently.
● Watch for signs of hypokalemia, such as muscle weakness and cramps.
● Consult prescriber and dietitian about a high-potassium diet. Foods rich in potassium include citrus fruits, tomatoes, bananas, and dates.
● Monitor glucose levels in diabetic patients.

● Furosemide may not be well absorbed orally in patient with severe heart failure. Drug may need to be given I.V. even if patient is taking other oral drugs.
● Monitor uric acid level, especially in patients with a history of gout.
● Monitor elderly patients, who are especially susceptible to excessive diuresis, because circulatory collapse and thromboembolic complications are possible.
● Store tablets in light-resistant container to prevent discoloration (doesn't affect potency). Don't use discolored (yellow) injectable preparation. Refrigerate oral furosemide solution to ensure drug stability.
● *Alert:* Don't confuse furosemide with torsemide.

PATIENT TEACHING
● Advise patient to take drug with food to prevent GI upset, and to take drug in morning to prevent nocturia. If second dose is needed, tell patient to take it in early afternoon, 6 to 8 hours after morning dose.
● Inform patient of possible need for potassium or magnesium supplements.
● Instruct patient to stand slowly to prevent dizziness and to limit alcohol intake and strenuous exercise in hot weather to avoid worsening orthostatic hypotension.
● Advise patient to immediately report ringing in ears, severe abdominal pain, or sore throat and fever; these symptoms may indicate furosemide toxicity.
● *Alert:* Discourage patient taking furosemide at home from storing different types of drugs in the same container, increasing the risk of drug errors. The most popular strengths of furosemide and digoxin are white tablets about equal in size.
● Tell patient to check with prescriber or pharmacist before taking OTC drugs.
● Teach patient to avoid direct sunlight and to use protective clothing and a sunblock because of risk of photosensitivity reactions.

---

hydrochlorothiazide
Apo-Hydro†, Dichlotride‡, Diuchlor
H†, Esidrix, Ezide, HydroDIURIL,
Hydro-Par, HydroSaluric§,
Microzide, Neo-Codema†, Novo-
Hydrazide†, Oretic, Urozide†

Pregnancy risk category B

AVAILABLE FORMS
Capsules: 12.5 mg
Oral solution: 50 mg/5 ml, 100 mg/ml
Tablets: 25 mg, 50 mg, 100 mg

INDICATIONS & DOSAGES
➤ **Edema—**
Adults: 25 to 100 mg P.O. daily or intermittently; up to 200 mg initially for several days until dry weight is attained.
➤ **Hypertension—**
Adults: 12.5 to 50 mg P.O. once daily.
Daily dose increased or decreased based
on blood pressure.
Children ages 2 to 12 years: 37.5 to
100 mg or 2.2 mg/kg P.O. daily in 2 divided doses.
Children ages 6 months to 2 years: 12.5 to
37.5 mg or 2.2 mg/kg P.O. daily in 2 divided doses.
Children younger than age 6 months: Up
to 3.3 mg/kg P.O. daily in 2 divided doses.

ACTION
A thiazide diuretic that increases sodium
and water excretion by inhibiting sodium
and chloride reabsorption in distal segment of the nephron.

Route	Onset	Peak	Duration
P.O.	2 hr	4-6 hr	6-12 hr

ADVERSE REACTIONS
CNS: dizziness, vertigo, headache, paresthesia, weakness, restlessness.
CV: orthostatic hypotension, allergic myocarditis, vasculitis.
GI: anorexia, nausea, *pancreatitis,* epigastric distress, vomiting, abdominal pain, diarrhea, constipation.
GU: polyuria, frequent urination, *renal
failure,* interstitial nephritis.
Hematologic: *aplastic anemia, agranulocytosis, leukopenia, thrombocytopenia,*
hemolytic anemia.

Hepatic: jaundice.
Metabolic: asymptomatic hyperuricemia;
hypokalemia; hyperglycemia and impaired
glucose tolerance; fluid and electrolyte
imbalances, including dilutional hyponatremia and hypochloremia; metabolic alkalosis; hypercalcemia; volume depletion
and dehydration.
Musculoskeletal: muscle cramps.
Respiratory: *respiratory distress,* pneumonitis.
Skin: dermatitis, photosensitivity reactions, rash, purpura, alopecia.
Other: hypersensitivity reactions, gout,
anaphylactic reactions.

INTERACTIONS
Drug-drug. *Amphotericin B, corticosteroids:* Increased risk of hypokalemia.
Monitor potassium level closely.
Antidiabetics: Decreased effectiveness of
hypoglycemics; dosage adjustments may
be needed. Monitor glucose levels.
Antihypertensives: Additive antihypertensive effect. Use together cautiously.
Barbiturates, opiates: Increased orthostatic hypotensive effect. Monitor patient
closely.
Cardiac glycosides: Increased risk of
digoxin toxicity from hydrochlorothiazide-
induced hypokalemia. Monitor potassium
and digoxin levels.
Cholestyramine, colestipol: Decreased intestinal absorption of thiazides. Separate
doses.
Diazoxide: Increased antihypertensive, hyperglycemic, and hyperuricemic effects.
Use together cautiously.
Lithium: Decreased lithium excretion, increasing risk of lithium toxicity. Monitor
lithium level.
NSAIDs: Increased risk of NSAID-
induced renal failure. Monitor renal function closely.
Drug-herb. *Dandelion:* May interfere
with diuretic activity. Discourage use together.
Licorice: May cause unexpected rapid
potassium loss. Discourage use together.
Drug-lifestyle. *Alcohol use:* Increased orthostatic hypotensive effect. Discourage
use together.

EFFECTS ON LAB TEST RESULTS
• May increase glucose, cholesterol, triglyceride, calcium, and uric acid levels. May decrease potassium, sodium, and chloride levels.
• May decrease hemoglobin and granulocyte, WBC, and platelet counts.

CONTRAINDICATIONS
Contraindicated in patients with anuria and patients hypersensitive to other thiazides or other sulfonamide derivatives.

NURSING CONSIDERATIONS
• Use cautiously in children and in patients with severe renal disease, impaired hepatic function, or progressive hepatic disease.
• To prevent nocturia, give drug in the morning.
• Monitor fluid intake and output, weight, blood pressure, and serum electrolyte levels.
• Watch for signs of hypokalemia, such as muscle weakness and cramps. Drug may be used with potassium-sparing diuretic to prevent potassium loss.
• Consult prescriber and dietitian about a high-potassium diet. Foods rich in potassium include citrus fruits, tomatoes, bananas, apricots, and dates.
• Monitor serum creatinine and BUN levels regularly. Cumulative effects of drug may occur with impaired renal function.
• Monitor uric acid levels, especially in patients with history of gout.
• Monitor glucose levels, especially in diabetic patients.
• Monitor elderly patients, who are especially susceptible to excessive diuresis.
• Discontinue thiazides and thiazide-like diuretics before parathyroid function tests.
• In patients with hypertension, therapeutic response may be delayed several weeks.

PATIENT TEACHING
• Instruct patient to take drug with food to minimize GI upset. Also tell him to take drug in morning to avoid nocturia; if second dose is needed, have him take it in early afternoon.
• Advise patient to avoid sudden posture changes and to rise slowly to avoid orthostatic hypotension.

• Encourage patient to use a sunblock to prevent photosensitivity reactions.
• Tell patient to check with prescriber or pharmacist before using alcohol or OTC drugs.

indapamide
Lozide†, Lozol, Natrilix‡

Pregnancy risk category B

AVAILABLE FORMS
Tablets: 1.25 mg, 2.5 mg

INDICATIONS & DOSAGES
➤ **Edema—**
Adults: Initially, 2.5 mg P.O. daily in the morning. Increased to 5 mg daily after 1 week, if needed.
➤ **Hypertension—**
Adults: Initially, 1.25 mg P.O. daily in the morning. Increased to 2.5 mg daily after 4 weeks, if needed. Increased to 5 mg daily after 4 more weeks, if needed.

ACTION
Unknown. A thiazide-like diuretic that probably inhibits sodium reabsorption in distal segment of nephron. Also has a direct vasodilating effect, possibly resulting from calcium channel–blocking action.

Route	Onset	Peak	Duration
P.O.	Unknown	2-5 hr	18 hr

ADVERSE REACTIONS
CNS: headache, nervousness, dizziness, light-headedness, weakness, vertigo, restlessness, drowsiness, fatigue, anxiety, depression, numbness of limbs, irritability, agitation.
CV: orthostatic hypotension, palpitations, PVCs, irregular heartbeat, vasculitis, flushing.
EENT: rhinorrhea.
GI: anorexia, nausea, epigastric distress, vomiting, abdominal pain, diarrhea, constipation.
GU: nocturia, polyuria, frequent urination, impotence.
Metabolic: asymptomatic hyperuricemia; fluid and electrolyte imbalances, including dilutional hyponatremia, hypochloremia, metabolic alkalosis, and hypokalemia;

Reactions may be *common*, uncommon, *life-threatening*, or **COMMON AND LIFE-THREATENING**.

weight loss; volume depletion and dehydration; hyperglycemia.
Musculoskeletal: muscle cramps and spasms.
Skin: rash, pruritus, urticaria.
Other: gout.

INTERACTIONS
Drug-drug. *Amphotericin B, corticosteroids:* Increased risk of hypokalemia. Monitor potassium level closely.
Cardiac glycosides: Increased risk of digoxin toxicity from indapamide-induced hypokalemia. Monitor potassium and digoxin levels.
Diazoxide: Increased antihypertensive, hyperglycemic, and hyperuricemic effects. Use together cautiously.
Lithium: Decreased lithium clearance that may increase lithium toxicity. Avoid using together.
NSAIDs: Increased risk of NSAID-induced renal failure. Monitor patient for signs of renal failure.
Drug-herb. *Licorice:* May cause unexpected rapid potassium loss. Discourage using together.

EFFECTS ON LAB TEST RESULTS
● May increase glucose, cholesterol, triglyceride, and uric acid levels. May decrease potassium, sodium, and chloride levels.

CONTRAINDICATIONS
Contraindicated in patients hypersensitive to other sulfonamide-derived drugs and in those with anuria.

NURSING CONSIDERATIONS
● Use cautiously in patients with severe renal disease, impaired hepatic function, or progressive hepatic disease.
● To prevent nocturia, give drug in the morning.
● Monitor fluid intake and output, weight, blood pressure, and electrolyte levels.
● Watch for signs of hypokalemia, such as muscle weakness and cramps. Drug may be used with potassium-sparing diuretic to prevent potassium loss.
● Consult prescriber and dietitian about a high-potassium diet. Foods rich in potassium include citrus fruits, tomatoes, bananas, apricots, and dates.

● Monitor creatinine and BUN levels regularly. Cumulative effects of drug may occur with impaired renal function.
● Monitor uric acid levels, especially in patients with history of gout.
● Monitor glucose levels, especially in diabetic patients.
● Monitor elderly patients, who are especially susceptible to excessive diuresis.
● Discontinue thiazides and thiazide-like diuretics before parathyroid function tests.
● Therapeutic response may be delayed several weeks in hypertensive patients. Also, if dose must be increased to 5 mg, concomitant therapy may be considered.

PATIENT TEACHING
● Instruct patient to take drug in morning to prevent nocturia and with food if GI upset occurs.
● Advise patient to avoid sudden posture changes and to rise slowly to avoid orthostatic hypotension.

---

mannitol
Osmitrol

Pregnancy risk category C

AVAILABLE FORMS
Injection: 5%, 10%, 15%, 20%, 25%

INDICATIONS & DOSAGES
➤ **Test dose for marked oliguria or suspected inadequate renal function—**
Adults and children older than age 12: 200 mg/kg or 12.5 g as a 15% to 20% I.V. solution over 3 to 5 minutes. Response is adequate if 30 to 50 ml of urine/hour is excreted over 2 to 3 hours; if response is inadequate, a second test dose is given. If still no response after second dose, mannitol shouldn't be continued.
➤ **Oliguria—**
Adults and children older than age 12: 50 to 100 g I.V. as a 15% to 25% solution over 90 minutes to several hours.
➤ **Prevention of oliguria or acute renal failure—**
Adults and children older than age 12: 50 to 100 g I.V. of a concentrated solution; then a 5% to 10% solution. Exact concentration determined by fluid requirements.

---

*Liquid contains alcohol.   **May contain tartrazine.   †Canada   ‡Australia   §U.K.   ◇OTC

➤ **Reduction of intraocular or intracranial pressure—**
Adults and children older than age 12: 1.5 to 2 g/kg as a 15% to 20% I.V. solution over 30 to 60 minutes.
➤ **Diuresis in drug intoxication—**
Adults and children older than age 12: 5% to 10% solution continuously up to 200 g I.V., while maintaining 100 to 500 ml urine output/hour and a positive fluid balance.
➤ **Irrigating solution during transurethral resection of prostate gland—**
Adults: 2.5% to 5% solution, p.r.n.

I.V. ADMINISTRATION
• Administer as intermittent or continuous infusion at prescribed rate using an in-line filter and an infusion pump. Direct injection isn't recommended. Check I.V. line patency at infusion site before and during administration.
• Monitor patient for signs and symptoms of infiltration; if it occurs, watch for inflammation, edema, and necrosis.

ACTION
An osmotic diuretic that increases the osmotic pressure of glomerular filtrate, inhibiting tubular reabsorption of water and electrolytes. It elevates plasma osmolality, resulting in enhanced water flow into extracellular fluid.

Route	Onset	Peak	Duration
I.V.	1-3 hr	Unknown	3-8 hr

ADVERSE REACTIONS
CNS: *seizures,* dizziness, headache.
CV: edema, thrombophlebitis, hypotension, hypertension, *heart failure,* tachycardia, angina-like chest pain, vascular overload.
EENT: blurred vision, rhinitis.
GI: thirst, dry mouth, nausea, vomiting, *diarrhea.*
GU: urine retention.
Metabolic: dehydration.
Other: local pain, fever, chills, urticaria.

INTERACTIONS
Drug-drug. *Lithium:* Increased urinary excretion of lithium. Monitor lithium level closely.

EFFECTS ON LAB TEST RESULTS
• May cause electrolyte imbalances.

CONTRAINDICATIONS
Contraindicated in patients hypersensitive to drug and in those with anuria, severe pulmonary congestion, frank pulmonary edema, severe heart failure, severe dehydration, metabolic edema, progressive renal disease or dysfunction, or active intracranial bleeding except during craniotomy.

NURSING CONSIDERATIONS
• To redissolve crystallized solution (crystallization occurs at low temperatures or in concentrations higher than 15%), warm bottle in hot water bath and shake vigorously. Cool to body temperature before giving. Don't use solution with undissolved crystals.
• For maximum intraocular pressure reduction before surgery, give 60 to 90 minutes preoperatively.
• Monitor vital signs, including central venous pressure and fluid intake and output hourly. Report increasing oliguria. Check weight, renal function, fluid balance, and serum and urine sodium and potassium levels daily.
• Use urinary catheter in comatose or incontinent patient because therapy is based on strict evaluation of fluid intake and output. If patient has urinary catheter, use an hourly urometer collection bag to facilitate accurate evaluation of output.
• Drug can be used to measure glomerular filtration rate.
• To relieve thirst, give frequent mouth care or fluids.
• When drug is used as an irrigating solution for prostate surgery, concentrations of 3.5% or greater are needed to avoid hemolysis.
• Drug is commonly used in chemotherapy regimens to enhance diuresis of renally toxic drugs.
• Drug may interfere with tests for inorganic phosphorus or ethylene glycol levels.

PATIENT TEACHING
• Tell patient that he may feel thirsty or have a dry mouth, and emphasize impor-

tance of drinking only the amount of fluids ordered.

• Instruct patient to promptly report adverse reactions and discomfort at I.V. site.

metolazone
Metenix-5§, Mykrox, Zaroxolyn**

Pregnancy risk category B

AVAILABLE FORMS
Tablets: 5 mg (Metenix-5§)
Tablets (extended-release): 2.5 mg, 5 mg, 10 mg (Zaroxolyn)
Tablets (prompt-release): 0.5 mg (Mykrox)

INDICATIONS & DOSAGES
➤ **Edema in heart failure or renal disease—**
Adults: 5 to 20 mg (extended-release) P.O. daily.
➤ **Hypertension—**
Adults: 2.5 to 5 mg (extended-release) P.O. daily. Maintenance dosage is based on patient's blood pressure. Or, 0.5 mg (prompt-release) P.O. once daily in morning, increased to 1 mg P.O. daily, p.r.n.

ACTION
Increases sodium and water excretion by inhibiting sodium reabsorption in the cortical diluting site of the ascending loop of Henle.

Route	Onset	Peak	Duration
P.O.	1 hr	2-8 hr	12-24 hr

ADVERSE REACTIONS
CNS: *dizziness,* headache, fatigue, vertigo, paresthesia, weakness, restlessness, drowsiness, anxiety, depression, nervousness, blurred vision.
CV: orthostatic hypotension, palpitations, vasculitis.
GI: anorexia, nausea, *pancreatitis,* epigastric distress, vomiting, abdominal pain, diarrhea, constipation, dry mouth.
GU: nocturia, polyuria, frequent urination, impotence.
Hematologic: *aplastic anemia, agranulocytosis, leukopenia,* purpura.
Hepatic: jaundice, *hepatitis.*

Metabolic: hyperglycemia and impaired glucose tolerance; fluid and electrolyte imbalances, including hypokalemia, hypomagnesemia, dilutional hyponatremia and hypochloremia, metabolic alkalosis, and hypercalcemia; volume depletion and dehydration.
Musculoskeletal: muscle cramps.
Skin: dermatitis, photosensitivity reactions, rash, pruritus, urticaria.

INTERACTIONS
Drug-drug. *Amphotericin B, corticosteroids:* Increased risk of hypokalemia. Monitor potassium level closely.
Anticoagulants: May affect hypoprothrombinemic response. Monitor PT and INR.
Antidiabetics: May alter glucose level requiring dosage adjustment of antidiabetics. Monitor glucose levels.
Barbiturates, opiates: Increased orthostatic hypotensive effect. Monitor patient closely.
Cardiac glycosides: Increased risk of digoxin toxicity from metolazone-induced hypokalemia. Monitor potassium and digoxin levels.
Cholestyramine, colestipol: Decreased intestinal absorption of thiazides. Separate doses.
Diazoxide: Increased antihypertensive, hyperglycemic, and hyperuricemic effects. Use together cautiously.
Lithium: Decreased lithium clearance, increasing risk of lithium toxicity. Monitor lithium level.
NSAIDs: Increased risk of NSAID-induced renal failure. Monitor patient for signs of renal failure.
Other antihypertensives: May have additive effects. Use together cautiously.
Drug-herb. *Licorice:* May cause unexpected rapid potassium loss. Discourage use together.
Drug-lifestyle. *Alcohol use:* Increased orthostatic hypotensive effect. Discourage use together.
Sun exposure: Increased risk for photosensitivity reaction. Advise patient to avoid excessive sunlight exposure.

EFFECTS ON LAB TEST RESULTS
• May increase glucose, calcium, cholesterol, and triglyceride levels. May de-

crease potassium, sodium, magnesium, and chloride levels.
• May decrease hemoglobin and granulocyte and WBC counts.

CONTRAINDICATIONS
Contraindicated in patients hypersensitive to thiazides or other sulfonamide-derived drugs and in those with anuria, hepatic coma, or precoma.

NURSING CONSIDERATIONS
• Use cautiously in patients with impaired renal or hepatic function.
• To prevent nocturia, give drug in the morning.
• Mykrox (prompt-release) tablets are more rapidly and completely absorbed than other brands, mimicking an oral solution.
• *Alert:* Don't interchange Mykrox with Zaroxolyn (extended-release) tablets.
• Monitor fluid intake and output, weight, blood pressure, and electrolyte levels.
• Watch for signs and symptoms of hypokalemia, such as muscle weakness and cramps. Drug may be used with potassium-sparing diuretic to prevent potassium loss.
• Consult prescriber and dietitian about a high-potassium diet. Foods rich in potassium include citrus fruits, tomatoes, bananas, dates, and apricots.
• Monitor glucose levels, especially in diabetic patients.
• Monitor uric acid levels, especially in patients with history of gout.
• Monitor elderly patients, who are especially susceptible to excessive diuresis.
• In hypertensive patients, therapeutic response may be delayed several weeks.
• Monitor blood pressure. If response is inadequate, another antihypertensive may be added.
• Metolazone and furosemide may be used together to enhance diuretic effect.
• Unlike thiazide diuretics, metolazone is effective in patients with decreased renal function.
• Drug is used as an adjunct therapy in furosemide-resistant edema.
• Stop thiazides and thiazide-like diuretics before parathyroid function tests.
• *Alert:* Don't confuse Zaroxolyn with Zarontin.

PATIENT TEACHING
• Tell patient to take drug in morning to prevent nocturia.
• Advise patient to avoid sudden posture changes and to rise slowly to avoid effects of orthostatic hypotension.
• Instruct patient to use a sunblock to prevent photosensitivity reactions.

---

spironolactone
Aldactone, Novospiroton†, Spiractin‡, Spiroctan§

Pregnancy risk category D

AVAILABLE FORMS
Tablets: 25 mg, 50 mg, 100 mg

INDICATIONS & DOSAGES
➤ **Edema—**
Adults: 25 to 200 mg P.O. daily or in two to four divided doses.
Children: 3.3 mg/kg P.O. daily or in divided doses.
➤ **Hypertension—**
Adults: 50 to 100 mg P.O. daily or in divided doses.
➤ **Diuretic-induced hypokalemia—**
Adults: 25 to 100 mg P.O. daily.
➤ **Detection of primary hyperaldosteronism—**
Adults: 400 mg P.O. daily for 4 days (short test) or 3 to 4 weeks (long test). If hypokalemia and hypertension are corrected, a presumptive diagnosis of primary hyperaldosteronism is made.
➤ **Management of primary hyperaldosteronism—**
Adults: 100 to 400 mg P.O. daily. Use lowest effective dose.

ACTION
A potassium-sparing diuretic that antagonizes aldosterone in the distal tubules, increasing sodium and water excretion.

Route	Onset	Peak	Duration
P.O.	1-2 days	2-3 days	2-3 days

ADVERSE REACTIONS
CNS: headache, drowsiness, lethargy, confusion, ataxia.
GI: diarrhea, gastric bleeding, ulceration, cramping, gastritis, vomiting.

Reactions may be *common,* uncommon, **life-threatening**, or COMMON AND LIFE-THREATENING.

GU: inability to maintain erection, menstrual disturbances.
Hematologic: *agranulocytosis.*
Metabolic: hyponatremia, *hyperkalemia,* dehydration, mild acidosis.
Skin: urticaria, hirsutism, maculopapular eruptions.
Other: gynecomastia, breast soreness, drug fever, *anaphylaxis.*

INTERACTIONS
Drug-drug. *ACE inhibitors, indomethacin, other potassium-sparing diuretics, potassium supplements:* Increased risk of hyperkalemia. Use together cautiously, especially in patients with renal impairment.
Aspirin: Possible blocked diuretic effect of spironolactone. Watch for diminished spironolactone response.
Digoxin: May alter digoxin clearance, increasing risk of digoxin toxicity. Monitor digoxin levels.
Drug-herb. *Licorice:* May block ulcer healing and aldosterone-like effects of licorice; increased risk of hypokalemia. Discourage use together.
Drug-food. *Potassium-containing salt substitutes, potassium-rich foods (such as citrus fruits, tomatoes):* Increased risk of hyperkalemia. Tell patient to use low-potassium salt substitutes and to eat high-potassium foods cautiously.

EFFECTS ON LAB TEST RESULTS
● May increase BUN and potassium levels. May decrease sodium level.
● May decrease granulocyte count.

CONTRAINDICATIONS
Contraindicated in patients hypersensitive to drug and in those with anuria, acute or progressive renal insufficiency, or hyperkalemia.

NURSING CONSIDERATIONS
● Use cautiously in patients with fluid or electrolyte imbalances, impaired renal function, or hepatic disease.
● Drug or its metabolites may cross the placental barrier. Use with extreme caution in pregnant women.
● To enhance absorption, give drug with meals.
● Protect drug from light.

● Monitor electrolyte levels, fluid intake and output, weight, and blood pressure.
● Monitor elderly patients, who are more susceptible to excessive diuresis.
● Inform laboratory that patient is taking spironolactone because drug may interfere with tests that measure digoxin levels. Drug therapy alters fluorometric determinations of plasma and urinary 17-hydroxycorticosteroid levels.
● Drug is less potent than thiazide and loop diuretics and is useful as an adjunct to other diuretic therapy. Diuretic effect is delayed 2 to 3 days when used alone.
● Maximum antihypertensive response may be delayed for up to 2 weeks.
● Watch for hyperchloremic metabolic acidosis, which may occur during therapy, especially in patients with hepatic cirrhosis.
● Breast cancer has been reported in some patients taking spironolactone, although a causal relationship hasn't been established.
● *Alert:* Don't confuse Aldactone with Aldactazide.

PATIENT TEACHING
● Instruct patient to take drug in morning to prevent nocturia. If second dose is needed, tell him to take it with food in early afternoon.
● *Alert:* Warn patient to avoid excessive ingestion of potassium-rich foods (such as citrus fruits, tomatoes, bananas, dates, and apricots), potassium-containing salt substitutes, and potassium supplements to prevent serious hyperkalemia.
● Caution patient not to perform hazardous activities if adverse CNS reactions occur.
● Advise men about possible breast tenderness or gynecomastia.

---

torsemide
Demadex, Torem§

Pregnancy risk category B

AVAILABLE FORMS
Injection: 10 mg/ml
Tablets: 5 mg, 10 mg, 20 mg, 100 mg

INDICATIONS & DOSAGES
➤ **Diuresis in patients with heart failure—**
Adults: Initially, 10 to 20 mg P.O. or I.V. once daily. If response is inadequate, dose is doubled until response is obtained. Maximum, 200 mg daily.
➤ **Diuresis in patients with chronic renal failure—**
Adults: Initially, 20 mg P.O. or I.V. once daily. If response is inadequate, dose is doubled until response is obtained. Maximum, 200 mg daily.
➤ **Diuresis in patients with hepatic cirrhosis—**
Adults: Initially, 5 to 10 mg P.O. or I.V. once daily with an aldosterone antagonist or a potassium-sparing diuretic. If response is inadequate, dose is doubled until response is obtained. Maximum, 40 mg daily.
➤ **Hypertension—**
Adults: Initially, 5 mg P.O. daily. Increased to 10 mg if needed and tolerated. If response is still inadequate, another antihypertensive should be added.

I.V. ADMINISTRATION
• Inspect ampules for precipitate or discoloration before use.
• Drug may be given by direct injection over at least 2 minutes. Rapid injection may cause ototoxicity. Don't give more than 200 mg at a time.

ACTION
A loop diuretic that enhances excretion of sodium, chloride, and water by acting on the ascending loop of Henle.

Route	Onset	Peak	Duration
I.V.	10 min	1 hr	6-8 hr
P.O.	1 hr	1-2 hr	6-8 hr

ADVERSE REACTIONS
CNS: asthenia, dizziness, headache, nervousness, insomnia, syncope.
CV: ECG abnormalities, chest pain, edema, orthostatic hypotension.
EENT: rhinitis, sore throat.
GI: *excessive thirst,* diarrhea, constipation, nausea, dyspepsia, ***hemorrhage.***
GU: *excessive urination,* impotence.
Metabolic: *electrolyte imbalances including hypokalemia and hypomagnesemia,*

dehydration, hypochloremic alkalosis, hyperuricemia, hypercholesterolemia.
Musculoskeletal: arthralgia, myalgia.
Respiratory: cough.
Skin: rash.

INTERACTIONS
Drug-drug. *Cholestyramine:* Decreased absorption of torsemide. Separate administration times by at least 3 hours.
Digoxin: Decreased torsemide clearance. No dosage adjustments are needed.
Indomethacin: Decreased diuretic effectiveness in sodium-restricted patients. Avoid using together.
Lithium, ototoxic drugs (such as aminoglycosides, ethacrynic acid): May increase toxicity of these drugs. Avoid using together.
NSAIDs: May potentiate nephrotoxicity of NSAIDs. Use together cautiously.
Probenecid: Decreased diuretic effectiveness. Avoid using together.
Salicylates: Decreased excretion, possibly leading to salicylate toxicity. Avoid using together.
Spironolactone: Decreased renal clearance of spironolactone. No dosage adjustments are needed. Use together cautiously.
Drug-herb. *Dandelion:* May interfere with diuretic activity. Discourage use together.
Licorice: May cause unexpected rapid potassium loss. Discourage use together.

EFFECTS ON LAB TEST RESULTS
• May increase BUN, creatinine, cholesterol, and uric acid levels. May decrease potassium and magnesium levels.

CONTRAINDICATIONS
Contraindicated in patients hypersensitive to drug or other sulfonamide derivatives and in those with anuria.

NURSING CONSIDERATIONS
• Use cautiously in patients with hepatic disease and related cirrhosis and ascites; sudden changes in fluid and electrolyte balance may precipitate hepatic coma in these patients.
• To prevent nocturia, give drug in the morning.
• Monitor fluid intake and output, electrolyte levels, blood pressure, weight, and

---

Reactions may be *common*, uncommon, *life-threatening*, or COMMON AND LIFE-THREATENING.

pulse rate during rapid diuresis and routinely with long-term use. Drug can cause profound diuresis and water and electrolyte depletion.

• Watch for signs of hypokalemia, such as muscle weakness and cramps.

• Consult prescriber and dietitian about providing a high-potassium diet. Foods rich in potassium include citrus fruits, tomatoes, bananas, dates, and apricots.

• Monitor elderly patients, who are especially susceptible to excessive diuresis with potential for circulatory collapse and thromboembolic complications.

• **Alert:** Don't confuse torsemide with furosemide.

PATIENT TEACHING
• Tell patient to take drug in morning to prevent nocturia.

• Advise patient to change positions slowly to prevent dizziness and to limit alcohol intake and strenuous exercise in hot weather to prevent effects of orthostatic hypotension.

• Advise patient to immediately report ringing in ears because it may indicate toxicity.

• Tell patient to check with prescriber or pharmacist before taking OTC drugs.

---

triamterene
Dyrenium, Dytac§

Pregnancy risk category B

AVAILABLE FORMS
Capsules: 50 mg, 100 mg

INDICATIONS & DOSAGES
➤ **Edema—**
Adults: Initially, 100 mg P.O. b.i.d. after meals. Maximum, 300 mg daily.

ACTION
A potassium-sparing diuretic that inhibits sodium reabsorption and potassium and hydrogen excretion by direct action on the distal tubules.

Route	Onset	Peak	Duration
P.O.	2-4 hr	6-8 hr	12-16 hr

ADVERSE REACTIONS
CNS: dizziness, weakness, fatigue, headache.
CV: hypotension.
GI: dry mouth, nausea, vomiting, diarrhea.
GU: interstitial nephritis, nephrolithiasis.
Hematologic: megaloblastic anemia related to low folic acid levels, *thrombocytopenia, agranulocytosis.*
Hepatic: jaundice.
Metabolic: azotemia, *hyperkalemia,* hypokalemia, hyponatremia, hyperglycemia, acidosis.
Musculoskeletal: muscle cramps.
Skin: photosensitivity reactions, rash.
Other: *anaphylaxis.*

INTERACTIONS
Drug-drug. *ACE inhibitors, potassium supplements:* Increased risk of hyperkalemia. Use together as long as potassium level is monitored.
Amantadine: Increased risk of amantadine toxicity. Avoid using together.
Lithium: Decreased lithium clearance, increasing risk of lithium toxicity. Monitor lithium level.
NSAIDs: May enhance risk of nephrotoxicity. Use together cautiously.
Quinidine: May interfere with some laboratory tests that measure quinidine levels. Inform laboratory that patient is taking triamterene.
Drug-herb. *Licorice:* Increased risk of hypokalemia. Discourage use together.
Drug-food. *Potassium-containing salt substitutes, potassium-rich foods:* Increased risk of hyperkalemia. Use cautiously, and monitor potassium levels.
Drug-lifestyle. *Sun exposure:* Increased risk for photosensitivity reactions. Advise patient to avoid excessive sunlight exposure.

EFFECTS ON LAB TEST RESULTS
• May increase BUN, creatinine, glucose, and uric acid levels. May decrease sodium levels. May increase or decrease potassium levels.
• May increase liver function test values. May decrease hemoglobin and granulocyte and platelet counts.

CONTRAINDICATIONS

Contraindicated in patients hypersensitive to drug and in those with anuria, severe or progressive renal disease or dysfunction, severe hepatic disease, or hyperkalemia.

NURSING CONSIDERATIONS

• Use cautiously in elderly or debilitated patients and in those with hepatic impairment or diabetes mellitus.
• To minimize nausea, give drug after meals.
• Monitor blood pressure, uric acid, CBC, and glucose, BUN, and electrolyte levels.
• Watch for blood dyscrasia.
• Drug therapy may interfere with enzyme assays that use fluorometry, such as quinidine determinations.
• To minimize excessive rebound potassium excretion, withdraw drug gradually.
• Drug is less potent than thiazides and loop diuretics and is useful as an adjunct to other diuretic therapy. It's usually used with potassium-wasting diuretics; full effect is delayed 2 to 3 days when used alone.
• **Alert:** Don't confuse triamterene with trimipramine.

PATIENT TEACHING

• Tell patient to take drug after meals to minimize nausea.
• If a single daily dose is prescribed, instruct patient to take it in the morning to prevent nocturia.
• **Alert:** Warn patient to avoid excessive ingestion of potassium-rich foods (such as citrus fruits, tomatoes, bananas, dates, and apricots), potassium-containing salt substitutes, and potassium supplements to prevent serious hyperkalemia.
• Teach patient to avoid direct sunlight, wear protective clothing, and use sunblock to prevent photosensitivity reactions.
• Tell patient that urine may turn blue.

---

urea (carbamide)
Ureaphil

Pregnancy risk category C

AVAILABLE FORMS
Injection: 40 g/150 ml

INDICATIONS & DOSAGES
➤ **Elevated intracranial or intraocular pressure—**
Adults: 1 to 1.5 g/kg as a 30% solution by slow I.V. infusion over 1 to 2½ hours. Rate shouldn't exceed 4 ml/minute. Maximum, 120 g daily.
Children: 0.1 to 1.5 g/kg by slow I.V. infusion (rate not to exceed 4 ml/minute) or 35 g/m² in 24 hours. Children younger than age 2 may receive as little as 0.1 g/kg by slow I.V. infusion.

I.V. ADMINISTRATION
• **Alert:** Avoid rapid I.V. infusion because it may cause hemolysis or increased capillary bleeding. Maximum infusion rate is 4 ml/minute.
• To prepare 135 ml of 30% solution, mix contents of 40-g vial of urea with 105 ml of D_5W, $D_{10}W$, or 10% invert sugar in water. Each milliliter of 30% solution provides 300 mg urea.
• Use only freshly reconstituted urea for I.V. infusion; solution becomes ammonia upon standing. Use within minutes of reconstitution and discard within 24 hours.
• **Alert:** Extravasation may cause reactions ranging from mild irritation to necrosis.

ACTION
An osmotic diuretic that increases the osmotic pressure of glomerular filtrate, inhibiting tubular reabsorption of water and electrolytes. It also elevates plasma osmolality, resulting in enhanced water flow into extracellular fluid.

Route	Onset	Peak	Duration
I.V.	30-45 min	1-2 hr	3-10 hr

ADVERSE REACTIONS
CNS: *headache,* syncope, disorientation.
CV: hypotension, tachycardia, dizziness, ECG changes.
GI: *nausea, vomiting.*
Hematologic: hemolysis with rapid administration.
Metabolic: fluid overload, hyponatremia, hypokalemia; alterations in electrolytes.
Skin: irritation or necrotic sloughing with extravasation.

Reactions may be *common,* uncommon, ***life-threatening****,* or COMMON AND LIFE-THREATENING.

INTERACTIONS

Drug-drug. *Lithium:* Increased lithium clearance and decreased lithium effectiveness. Monitor lithium level.

EFFECTS ON LAB TEST RESULTS

• Decreased potassium and sodium levels.

CONTRAINDICATIONS

Contraindicated in patients with severely impaired renal function, marked dehydration, frank hepatic failure, active intracranial bleeding, or sickle-cell disease with CNS involvement.

NURSING CONSIDERATIONS

• Use cautiously in pregnant women, breast-feeding women, and patients with cardiac disease or hepatic or renal impairment.
• Assess breath sounds for crackles, indicating pulmonary edema.
• Watch for signs and symptoms of hyponatremia (nausea, vomiting, tachycardia) or hypokalemia (muscle weakness, lethargy), which may indicate electrolyte depletion before serum levels are reduced.
• Maintain adequate hydration; monitor blood pressure, fluid intake and output, and electrolyte levels.
• Monitor BUN level in patients with renal disease.
• To ensure bladder emptying in comatose patients, use an indwelling urinary catheter and an hourly urometer collection bag for accurate evaluation of diuresis.
• If satisfactory diuresis doesn't occur in 6 to 12 hours, urea should be discontinued and renal function reevaluated.

PATIENT TEACHING

• Instruct patient to report adverse reactions promptly.
• Tell patient to report discomfort at I.V. insertion site.

61

Electrolytes and replacement solutions

calcium acetate
calcium carbonate
calcium chloride
calcium citrate
calcium glubionate
calcium gluceptate
calcium gluconate
calcium lactate
calcium phosphate, dibasic
calcium phosphate, tribasic
dextran, high-molecular-weight
dextran, low-molecular-weight
hetastarch
magnesium chloride
magnesium sulfate
potassium acetate
potassium bicarbonate
potassium chloride
potassium gluconate
Ringer's injection
Ringer's injection, lactated
sodium chloride

COMBINATION PRODUCTS

CITRACAL +D: calcium 316.5 mg with 200 units cholecalciferol.
DICAL-D; DIOSTATE D: calcium 116.7 mg (as phosphate tribasic) with cholecalciferol 133 units.
DICAL-D WAFERS: calcium 232 mg (as phosphate tribasic) with cholecalciferol 200 units.
KLORVESS*: potassium and chloride 20 mEq each (from potassium chloride, potassium bicarbonate, and L-lysine monohydrochloride).
K-LYTE/CL: potassium 25 mEq, chloride 25 mEq (from potassium chloride, potassium bicarbonate, and lysine hydrochloride).
KOLYUM: potassium 20 mEq, chloride 3.4 mEq per 15 ml (from potassium gluconate and potassium chloride).
NEUTRA-PHOS: phosphorus 250 mg, sodium 164 mg, potassium 278 mg (from dibasic and monobasic sodium and potassium phosphate).
POSTURE-D: calcium 600 mg (as phosphate tribasic) with cholecalciferol 125 units.

TWIN-K: 15 ml supplies 20 mEq of potassium ions as a combination of potassium gluconate and potassium citrate.

calcium acetate
PhosLo

calcium carbonate
Apo-Cal†◊, Cal Carb-HD◊, Calci-Chew◊, Calciday-667◊, Calci-Mix◊, Calcite 500†◊, Calcium 600◊, Calglycine◊, Cal-Plus◊, Calsan†◊, Caltrate 600◊, Chooz◊, Dicarbosil◊, Gencalc 600◊, Mallamint◊, Nephro-Calci◊, Nu-Cal†◊, Os-Cal†◊, Os-Cal 500◊, Os-Cal Chewable†◊, Oysco◊, Oysco 500 Chewable◊, Oyst-Cal 500◊, Oystercal 500◊, Oyster Shell Calcium-500◊, Rolaids Calcium Rich◊, Super Calcium '1200'◊, Titralac◊, Tums◊, Tums E-X◊

calcium chloride ◊
Calciject†

calcium citrate ◊
Citracal◊, Citracal Liquitab†◊

calcium glubionate
Calcium-Sandoz†, Neo-Calglucon

calcium gluceptate ◊

calcium gluconate

calcium lactate ◊

calcium phosphate, dibasic ◊

calcium phosphate, tribasic
Posture ◊

Pregnancy risk category C

AVAILABLE FORMS
calcium acetate
Contains 253 mg or 12.7 mEq of elemental calcium/g

Reactions may be *common*, uncommon, **life-threatening**, or COMMON AND LIFE-THREATENING.

Injection: 0.5 mEq Ca++/ml
Tablets: 250 mg ◊, 500 mg ◊, 667 mg, 668 mg ◊, 1,000 mg ◊
calcium carbonate
Contains 400 mg or 20 mEq of elemental calcium/g
Capsules: 600 mg ◊, 1.25 g ◊
Oral suspension: 1 g/5 ml ◊, 1.25 g/ 5 ml ◊
Powder packets: 6.5 g (2,400 mg calcium) per packet ◊
Tablets: 650 mg ◊, 1.25 g ◊, 1.5 g ◊
Tablets (chewable): 350 mg ◊, 420 mg ◊, 500 mg ◊, 550 mg ◊, 625 mg ◊†, 750 mg ◊, 835 mg ◊, 850 mg ◊, 1 g ◊, 1.25 g ◊
calcium chloride
Contains 270 mg or 13.5 mEq of elemental calcium/g
Injection: 10% solution in 10-ml ampules, vials, and syringes
calcium citrate
Contains 211 mg or 10.6 mEq of elemental calcium/g
Tablets: 950 mg ◊, 1.04 g
Tablets (effervescent): 2.376 g ◊
calcium glubionate
Contains 64 mg or 3.2 mEq elemental calcium/g
Syrup: 1.8 g/5 ml
calcium gluceptate
Contains 82 mg or 4.1 mEq elemental calcium/g
Injection: 1.1 g/5 ml in 5-ml ampules or 10-ml vials
calcium gluconate
Contains 90 mg or 4.5 mEq of elemental calcium/g
Injection: 10% solution in 10-ml ampules and vials, 10-ml or 50-ml vials
Tablets: 500 mg ◊, 650 mg ◊, 1 g ◊
calcium lactate
Contains 130 mg or 6.5 mEq of elemental calcium/g
Tablets: 325 mg, 650 mg
calcium phosphate, dibasic
Contains 230 mg or 11.5 mEq of elemental calcium/g
Tablets: 500 mg ◊
calcium phosphate, tribasic
Contains 400 mg or 20 mEq of elemental calcium/g
Tablets: 300 mg ◊, 600 mg ◊

INDICATIONS & DOSAGES
➤ **Hypocalcemic emergency—**
Adults: 7 to 14 mEq calcium I.V. May be given as a 10% calcium gluconate solution, 2% to 10% calcium chloride solution, or 22% calcium gluceptate solution.
Children: 1 to 7 mEq calcium I.V.
Infants: Up to 1 mEq calcium I.V.
➤ **Hypocalcemic tetany—**
Adults: 4.5 to 16 mEq calcium I.V. Repeated until tetany is controlled.
Children: 0.5 to 0.7 mEq/kg calcium I.V. three to four times a day until tetany is controlled.
Neonates: 2.4 mEq/kg I.V. daily in divided doses.
➤ **Adjunctive treatment of cardiac arrest—**
Adults: 0.027 to 0.054 mEq/kg calcium chloride I.V., 4.5 to 6.3 mEq calcium gluceptate I.V., or 2.3 to 3.7 mEq calcium gluconate I.V.
Children: 0.27 mEq/kg calcium chloride I.V. Repeat in 10 minutes if needed; determine calcium levels before giving more doses.
➤ **Adjunctive treatment of magnesium intoxication—**
Adults: Initially, 7 mEq I.V. Subsequent doses based on patient's response.
➤ **During exchange transfusions—**
Adults: 1.35 mEq I.V. with each 100 ml citrated blood.
Neonates: 0.45 mEq I.V. after each 100 ml citrated blood.
➤ **Hyperphosphatemia—**
Adults: 1,334 to 2,000 mg P.O. calcium acetate or 2 to 5.2 g calcium ion t.i.d. with meals. Most dialysis patients will need 3 to 4 tablets with each meal.
➤ **Dietary supplement—**
Adults: 500 mg to 2 g P.O. daily.

I.V. ADMINISTRATION
● Give calcium chloride only by I.V. route. When adding to parenteral solutions that contain other additives (especially phosphorus or phosphate), watch for precipitate. Use an in-line filter.
● Give calcium gluconate only by I.V. route.
● *Alert:* Calcium salts aren't interchangeable; verify preparation before use.
● Monitor ECG when giving calcium I.V. Stop and notify prescriber if patient com-

plains of discomfort. After I.V. injection, patient should remain recumbent for 15 minutes.
• *Alert:* Severe necrosis and tissue sloughing can occur after extravasation. Calcium gluconate is less irritating to veins and tissues than calcium chloride.

Direct injection
• Warm solution to body temperature before administration.
• Administer slowly through a small needle into a large vein or through an I.V. line containing a free-flowing, compatible solution at 1 ml/minute (1.5 mEq/minute) for calcium chloride, 1.5 to 5 ml/minute for calcium gluconate, or 2 ml/minute for calcium gluceptate. Don't use scalp veins in children.

Intermittent infusion
• Infuse diluted solution through an I.V. line containing a compatible solution. Maximum of 200 mg/minute suggested for calcium gluceptate and calcium gluconate.
• Drug will precipitate if administered I.V. with sodium bicarbonate or other alkaline drugs.

ACTION
Replaces calcium and maintains calcium level.

Route	Onset	Peak	Duration
I.V.	Immediate	Immediate	0.5-2 hr
P.O.	Unknown	Unknown	Unknown

ADVERSE REACTIONS
CNS: tingling sensations, sense of oppression or heat waves with I.V. use; syncope with rapid I.V. injection.
CV: mild drop in blood pressure, vasodilation, *bradycardia, arrhythmias, cardiac arrest with rapid I.V. injection.*
GI: irritation, *constipation,* chalky taste, hemorrhage, nausea, vomiting, thirst, abdominal pain.
GU: polyuria, renal calculi.
Metabolic: hypercalcemia.
Skin: local reactions, including burning, necrosis, tissue sloughing, cellulitis, soft-tissue calcification with I.M. use.
Other: pain, irritation at S.C. injection site; *vein irritation.*

INTERACTIONS
Drug-drug. *Atenolol, fluoroquinolones, tetracyclines:* Decreased bioavailability of these drugs and calcium when oral preparations are taken together. Separate administration times.
Calcium channel blockers: Decreased calcium effectiveness. Avoid using together.
Cardiac glycosides: Increased digoxin toxicity. Give calcium cautiously, if at all, to digitalized patients.
Fosphenytoin, phenytoin: Use together decreases absorption of both drugs. Avoid using together, or monitor levels carefully.
Sodium polystyrene sulfonate: Risk of metabolic acidosis in patients with renal disease. Avoid using together.
Thiazide diuretics: Risk of hypercalcemia. Avoid using together.
Drug-food. *Foods containing oxalic acid (rhubarb, spinach), phytic acid (bran, whole-grain cereals), phosphorus (dairy products, milk):* May interfere with calcium absorption. Discourage use together.

EFFECTS ON LAB TEST RESULTS
• May increase calcium levels.

CONTRAINDICATIONS
Contraindicated in cancer patients with bone metastases and in patients with ventricular fibrillation, hypercalcemia, hypophosphatemia, or renal calculi.

NURSING CONSIDERATIONS
• Use all calcium products with extreme caution in digitalized patients and patients with sarcoidosis and renal or cardiac disease. Use calcium chloride cautiously in patients with cor pulmonale, respiratory acidosis, or respiratory failure.
• Give I.M. injection in the gluteal region in adults, lateral thigh in infants. Use I.M. route only in emergencies when no I.V. route is available because of irritation of tissue by calcium salts.
• *Alert:* Make sure prescriber specifies form of calcium to be given; crash carts usually contain both calcium gluconate and calcium chloride.
• Monitor calcium levels frequently. Hypercalcemia may result after large doses in chronic renal failure. Report abnormalities.

Reactions may be *common*, uncommon, *life-threatening*, or COMMON AND LIFE-THREATENING.

• To avoid constipation and bloating, and to improve absorption, administer calcium carbonate in divided doses.

• I.V. calcium may produce transient elevation of plasma 11-hydroxycorticosteroid levels (Glenn-Nelson technique) and false-negative values for serum and urine magnesium, as measured by the Titan yellow method.

PATIENT TEACHING
• Tell patient to take oral calcium 1 to 1½ hours after meals if GI upset occurs.
• Warn patient to avoid oxalic acid (in rhubarb and spinach), phytic acid (in bran and whole-grain cereals), and phosphorus (in dairy products) in the meal preceding calcium consumption; these substances may interfere with calcium absorption.

---

dextran, high-molecular-weight (dextran 70, dextran 75)
Dextran 75, Gendex 75, Gentran 70, Macrodex

Pregnancy risk category C

AVAILABLE FORMS
Injection: 6% dextran 70 in normal saline solution or D_5W; 6% dextran 75 in normal saline solution or D_5W

INDICATIONS & DOSAGES
➤ **Plasma expander—**
Adults: 30 g (500 ml of 6% solution) I.V. In emergencies, may be given at 1.2 to 2.4 g (20 to 40 ml)/minute. In normovolemic or nearly normovolemic patients, infusion shouldn't exceed 240 mg (4 ml)/minute.

Total dose during first 24 hours not to exceed 1.2 g/kg; actual dose depends on amount of fluid loss and resulting hemoconcentration and must be determined for each patient.

I.V. ADMINISTRATION
• Prescriber may order dextran 1 to protect against dextran-induced anaphylaxis. Give 20 ml of dextran 1 (containing 150 mg/ml) I.V. over 60 seconds, 1 to 2 minutes before I.V. infusion of dextran 70.

• Use D_5W solution instead of normal saline solution for patients with heart failure.

• *Alert:* Observe patient closely during early phase of infusion when most anaphylactic reactions occur.

ACTION
Expands plasma volume via colloidal osmotic effect, drawing fluid from interstitial to intravascular space, providing fluid replacement.

Route	Onset	Peak	Duration
I.V.	Immediate	Immediate	Unknown

ADVERSE REACTIONS
CV: thrombophlebitis.
EENT: nasal congestion.
GI: nausea, vomiting.
GU: increased specific gravity and viscosity of urine, tubular stasis and blocking, oliguria, anuria.
Metabolic: fluid overload.
Musculoskeletal: arthralgia.
Skin: urticaria.
Other: fever, *anaphylaxis,* hypersensitivity reactions.

INTERACTIONS
Drug-drug. *Abciximab, aspirin, heparin, thrombolytics, warfarin:* Increased bleeding if given together. Use together with extreme caution.

EFFECTS ON LAB TEST RESULTS
• May increase ALT and AST levels.
• May increase bleeding time. May decrease hemoglobin and hematocrit.

CONTRAINDICATIONS
Contraindicated in patients hypersensitive to dextran and in those with marked hemostatic defects, cardiac decompensation, renal disease with severe oliguria or anuria, hypervolemic conditions, or severe bleeding disorders.

NURSING CONSIDERATIONS
• Use cautiously in patients undergoing bowel surgery and in patients with active hemorrhage, thrombocytopenia, impaired renal clearance, chronic liver disease, or abdominal conditions.

• Assess hydration before starting therapy; otherwise, use urine or serum osmolality because urine specific gravity is affected by urine dextran level.

• **Alert:** Low- and high-molecular-weight dextrans aren't interchangeable. Verify preparation before use.

• Have blood samples drawn before starting infusion.

• Monitor urine flow rate during administration. If oliguria or anuria occurs or isn't relieved by infusion, stop dextran and give loop diuretic.

• Watch for circulatory overload. Drug provides plasma expansion slightly greater than volume infused.

• Monitor hemoglobin levels and hematocrit; if values fall below 30% by volume, notify prescriber.

• Drug may interfere with analyses of blood grouping, crossmatching, bilirubin, glucose level, and protein.

• Drug may precipitate in storage but can be heated to dissolve, if needed.

• Monitor glucose levels before and during infusion; drug metabolizes to glucose.

PATIENT TEACHING

• Explain use and administration of dextran to patient and family.

• Tell patient to report adverse effects.

---

dextran, low-molecular-weight (dextran 40)
Dextran 40, Gentran 40, LMD 10%, Rheomacrodex

Pregnancy risk category C

AVAILABLE FORMS
Injection: 10% dextran 40 in D_5W or normal saline solution

INDICATIONS & DOSAGES
➤ **Plasma volume expansion—**
Adults: Dosage by I.V. infusion depends on amount of fluid loss. Infuse first 10 ml/kg of dextran rapidly with central venous pressure monitoring; then infuse remaining dose slowly. Total dose not to exceed 20 ml/kg daily. If therapy continues longer than 24 hours, don't exceed 10 ml/kg daily, continued for no longer than 5 days.

➤ **Prophylaxis of venous thrombosis—**
Adults: 10 ml/kg (500 to 1,000 ml) I.V. on day of procedure; 500 ml on days 2 and 3.

➤ **Hemodiluent in extracorporeal circulation—**
Adults: 10 to 20 ml/kg added to the perfusion circuit, not to exceed total dose of 20 ml/kg.

I.V. ADMINISTRATION

• Use D_5W solution instead of normal saline solution for patients with heart failure.

• Prescriber may order dextran 1 to protect against dextran-induced anaphylaxis. Administer 20 ml of dextran 1 (containing 150 mg/ml) I.V. over 60 seconds, 1 to 2 minutes before I.V. infusion of dextran.

• Observe patient closely during early phase of infusion when most anaphylactic reactions occur.

• Store at constant 77° F (25° C). Drug may precipitate in storage but can be heated to dissolve, if needed.

• Discard partially used containers.

ACTION
Expands plasma volume by colloidal osmotic effect, drawing fluid from interstitial to intravascular space, providing fluid replacement.

Route	Onset	Peak	Duration
I.V.	Immediate	Immediate	3 hr

ADVERSE REACTIONS
CV: thrombophlebitis.
GI: nausea, vomiting.
GU: tubular stasis and blocking, increased urine viscosity.
Skin: urticaria.
Other: *anaphylaxis,* hypersensitivity reactions.

INTERACTIONS
None significant.

EFFECTS ON LAB TEST RESULTS
• May increase ALT and AST levels.
• May increase bleeding time. May decrease hemoglobin and hematocrit.

CONTRAINDICATIONS
Contraindicated in patients hypersensitive to drug and in those with marked hemo-

---

Reactions may be common, uncommon, *life-threatening*, or COMMON AND LIFE-THREATENING.

static defects, cardiac decompensation, or renal disease with severe oliguria or anuria.

NURSING CONSIDERATIONS
• Use cautiously in patients with active hemorrhage, thrombocytopenia, or diabetes mellitus.
• Assess hydration before starting therapy; otherwise, use urine or serum osmolality because urine specific gravity is affected by urine dextran level.
• Watch for circulatory overload and a rise in central venous pressure. Drug provides plasma expansion slightly greater than volume infused.
• Monitor urine flow rate during administration. If oliguria or anuria occurs or isn't relieved, stop dextran and give loop diuretic.
• Check hemoglobin levels and hematocrit; if values fall below 30% by volume, notify prescriber.
• Drug may interfere with analyses of blood grouping, crossmatching, bilirubin, glucose levels, and protein.
• Monitor glucose levels before and during infusion; drug metabolizes to glucose.
• *Alert:* Low- and high-molecular-weight dextrans aren't interchangeable. Verify preparation before use.

PATIENT TEACHING
• Explain use and administration of dextran to patient and family.
• Tell patient to report adverse effects.

---

hetastarch
Hespan

Pregnancy risk category C

AVAILABLE FORMS
Injection: 500 ml (6 g/100 ml in normal saline solution)

INDICATIONS & DOSAGES
➤ **Plasma expander—**
Adults: 500 to 1,000 ml I.V., depending on amount of blood lost and resulting hemoconcentration. Total daily dose shouldn't exceed 1,500 ml.

➤ **Continuous-flow centrifugation leukapheresis—**
Adults: 250 ml to 700 ml I.V. infused at a constant fixed ratio (usually 1:8) to venous whole blood.

I.V. ADMINISTRATION
• Up to 20 ml/kg hourly may be used in hemorrhagic shock. Slower rates of administration are typically used in patients with burns or septic shock.
• Discard partially used bottles.

ACTION
Expands plasma volume and provides fluid replacement.

Route	Onset	Peak	Duration
I.V.	Immediate	Immediate	Unknown

ADVERSE REACTIONS
CNS: headache.
CV: peripheral edema of legs.
EENT: periorbital edema.
GI: nausea, vomiting.
Hematologic: dilution of clotting factors.
Metabolic: fluid overload.
Musculoskeletal: muscle pain.
Respiratory: wheezing.
Skin: rash, urticaria.
Other: mild fever, chills, hypersensitivity reactions.

INTERACTIONS
None significant.

EFFECTS ON LAB TEST RESULTS
None reported.

CONTRAINDICATIONS
Contraindicated in patients hypersensitive to drug and in those with severe bleeding disorders, severe heart failure, or renal failure with oliguria and anuria.

NURSING CONSIDERATIONS
• Use cautiously in patients with liver disease.
• Hetastarch isn't a substitute for blood or plasma.
• To avoid circulatory overload, monitor patients with renal impairment carefully.
• When used in continuous-flow centrifugation, leukapheresis ratio is usually one

part hetastarch to eight parts venous whole blood.

• When added to whole blood, hetastarch increases the erythrocyte sedimentation rate.

• Discontinue drug and notify prescriber if allergic or sensitivity reactions occur. If needed, give an antihistamine.

PATIENT TEACHING

• Explain use and administration of drug to patient and family.

• Tell patient to report adverse reactions promptly.

---

magnesium chloride
Slow-Mag ◊

magnesium sulfate

Pregnancy risk category D

AVAILABLE FORMS
magnesium chloride
Tablets (delayed-release): 64 mg
magnesium sulfate
Injectable solutions: 10%, 12.5%, 50% in 2-ml, 5-ml, 10-ml, 20-ml, and 30-ml ampules, vials, and prefilled syringes

INDICATIONS & DOSAGES
➤ **Mild hypomagnesemia—**
Adults: 1 g I.V. by piggyback or I.M. q 6 hours for four doses, depending on magnesium level. Or, 3 g P.O. q 6 hours for four doses.
➤ **Severe hypomagnesemia (serum magnesium 0.8 mEq/L or less, with symptoms)—**
Adults: 2 to 5 g I.V. in 1 L of solution over 3 hours. Subsequent doses depend on magnesium levels.
➤ **Magnesium supplementation—**
Adults: 64 mg (one tablet) P.O. t.i.d.
➤ **Magnesium supplementation in total parenteral nutrition (TPN)—**
Adults and children: 4 to 24 mEq I.V. daily added to TPN solution.
Infants: 2 to 10 mEq I.V. daily added to TPN solution. Each 2 ml of 50% solution contains 1 g, or 8.12 mEq, magnesium sulfate.

I.V. ADMINISTRATION
• Inject I.V. bolus dose slowly, using infusion pump for continuous infusion, if available, to avoid respiratory or cardiac arrest. Maximum infusion rate is 150 mg/minute. Rapid drip causes feeling of heat.
• *Alert:* When giving I.V. for severe hypomagnesemia, watch for respiratory depression and evidence of heart block. Respirations should exceed 16 breaths/minute before dose is given.
• Drug is incompatible with alkalis, including carbonates and bicarbonates. Precipitate may form if mixed with solutions containing alcohol, arsenates, barium, calcium, clindamycin, heavy metals, hydrocortisone sodium succinate, phosphates, polymyxin B sulfate, procaine, salicylates, or tartrates.

ACTION
Replaces magnesium and maintains magnesium level; as an anticonvulsant, reduces muscle contractions by interfering with release of acetylcholine at myoneural junction.

Route	Onset	Peak	Duration
I.M.	1 hr	Unknown	3-4 hr
I.V.	Immediate	Unknown	30 min
P.O.	Unknown	4 hr	4-6 hr

ADVERSE REACTIONS
CNS: toxicity, *weak or absent deep tendon reflexes,* flaccid paralysis, drowsiness, stupor.
CV: slow, weak pulse; *arrhythmias, hypotension, circulatory collapse,* flushing.
GI: diarrhea.
Metabolic: hypocalcemia.
Respiratory: *respiratory paralysis.*
Skin: diaphoresis.
Other: hypothermia.

INTERACTIONS
Drug-drug. *Alendronate, nitrofurantoin, penicillamine, quinolones, sodium polystyrene sulfonate, tetracyclines:* Decreased bioavailability with oral magnesium supplements. Separate administration by 2 to 3 hours.
Cardiac glycosides: May cause serious cardiac conduction changes. Use together with extreme caution.

Reactions may be *common,* uncommon, *life-threatening*, or COMMON AND LIFE-THREATENING.

CNS depressants: May have additive effect. Use together cautiously.
Neuromuscular blockers: May cause increased neuromuscular blockage. Use together cautiously.

EFFECTS ON LAB TEST RESULTS
• May decrease calcium levels.

CONTRAINDICATIONS
Contraindicated in patients with myocardial damage or heart block and in pregnant women in actively progressing labor.

NURSING CONSIDERATIONS
• Use parenteral magnesium with extreme caution in patients with impaired renal function.
• Undiluted 50% solutions may be given by deep I.M. injection to adults. Dilute solutions to 20% or less for use in children.
• Keep I.V. calcium available to reverse magnesium intoxication.
• Test knee-jerk and patellar reflexes before each additional dose. If absent, notify prescriber and give no more magnesium until reflexes return; otherwise, patient may develop temporary respiratory failure and need cardiopulmonary resuscitation or I.V. administration of calcium.
• Check magnesium level after repeated doses.
• Monitor fluid intake and output. Output should be 100 ml or more during 4-hour period before dose.
• Monitor renal function.
• After giving to toxemic pregnant woman within 24 hours before delivery, watch neonate for signs and symptoms of magnesium toxicity, including neuromuscular and respiratory depression.

PATIENT TEACHING
• Explain use and administration of drug to patient and family.
• Tell patient to report adverse effects.

---

potassium acetate

Pregnancy risk category C

AVAILABLE FORMS
Injection: 2 mEq/ml in 20-ml, 30-ml vials; 4 mEq/ml in 50-ml vials

INDICATIONS & DOSAGES
➤ **Hypokalemia—**
Adults: No more than 20 mEq hourly in concentration of 40 mEq/L or less. Total 24-hour dose shouldn't exceed 150 mEq (3 mEq/kg in children).
➤ **Prevention of hypokalemia—**
Adults: Dosage is individualized to patient's needs, not to exceed 150 mEq/day. Administered as an additive to I.V. infusions. Usual dose is 20 mEq/L infused at no more than 20 mEq/hour.
Children: Individualized dose not to exceed 3 mEq/kg/day. Administered as an additive to I.V. infusions.

I.V. ADMINISTRATION
• Give only by I.V. infusion, never I.V. push or I.M. Watch for pain and redness at infusion site. Large-bore needle reduces local irritation.
• *Alert:* Give slowly as diluted solution; potentially fatal hyperkalemia may result from too-rapid infusion.

ACTION
Replaces potassium and maintains potassium level.

Route	Onset	Peak	Duration
I.V.	Immediate	Immediate	Unknown

ADVERSE REACTIONS
CNS: paresthesia of limbs, listlessness, mental confusion, weakness or heaviness of legs, flaccid paralysis.
CV: hypotension, *arrhythmias, heart block,* ECG changes, *cardiac arrest.*
GI: nausea, vomiting, abdominal pain, diarrhea.
Metabolic: hyperkalemia.
Respiratory: *respiratory paralysis.*
Other: pain, redness at infusion site, fever.

INTERACTIONS
Drug-drug. *ACE inhibitors, potassium-sparing diuretics:* Increased risk of hyperkalemia. Use with extreme caution.

EFFECTS ON LAB TEST RESULTS
• May increase potassium levels.

CONTRAINDICATIONS
Contraindicated in patients with severe renal impairment with oliguria, anuria, or

azotemia; untreated Addison's disease; or acute dehydration, heat cramps, hyperkalemia, hyperkalemic form of familial periodic paralysis, or conditions linked to extensive tissue breakdown.

NURSING CONSIDERATIONS
• Use cautiously in patients with cardiac disease or renal impairment.
• During therapy, monitor ECG, renal function, fluid intake and output, and potassium, creatinine, and BUN levels. Never give potassium postoperatively until urine flow is established.
• Potassium replacement should be done with ECG monitoring and frequent potassium determinations. I.V. route should be used only for life-threatening hypokalemia or when oral replacement isn't feasible.
• Many adverse reactions may reflect hyperkalemia.
• *Alert:* Potassium preparations aren't interchangeable; verify preparation before use.

PATIENT TEACHING
• Explain use and administration to patient and family.
• Tell patient to report adverse effects, especially pain at insertion site.

potassium bicarbonate
K+Care ET, Klor-Con/EF, K-Lyte, K-Vescent

Pregnancy risk category C

AVAILABLE FORMS
Tablets (effervescent): 25 mEq

INDICATIONS & DOSAGES
➤ Hypokalemia—
Adults: 25 to 50 mEq dissolved in 4 to 8 oz (120 to 240 ml) of water once daily to q.i.d.

ACTION
Replaces potassium and maintains potassium level.

Route	Onset	Peak	Duration
P.O.	Unknown	4 hr	Unknown

ADVERSE REACTIONS
CNS: paresthesia of limbs, listlessness, confusion, weakness or heaviness of legs, flaccid paralysis.
CV: *arrhythmias,* ECG changes, hypotension, *heart block, cardiac arrest.*
GI: *nausea, vomiting, abdominal pain,* diarrhea.

INTERACTIONS
Drug-drug. *ACE inhibitors, potassium-sparing diuretics:* May cause hyperkalemia. Use with extreme caution.

EFFECTS ON LAB TEST RESULTS
• May increase potassium levels.

CONTRAINDICATIONS
Contraindicated in patients with severe renal impairment with oliguria, anuria, or azotemia; untreated Addison's disease; or acute dehydration, heat cramps, hyperkalemia, hyperkalemic form of familial periodic paralysis, or other conditions linked to extensive tissue breakdown.

NURSING CONSIDERATIONS
• Use cautiously in patients with cardiac disease or renal impairment.
• Dissolve potassium bicarbonate tablets completely in 4 to 8 oz of cold water.
• Ask patient's flavor preference. Available in lime, fruit punch, citrus, and orange flavors.
• Don't administer potassium supplements postoperatively until urine flow has been established.
• *Alert:* Potassium preparations aren't interchangeable; verify preparation before use. Never switch potassium products without prescriber's order. Potassium chloride can't be given instead of potassium bicarbonate.
• Monitor fluid intake and output and BUN, potassium, and creatinine levels.

PATIENT TEACHING
• Tell patient to take drug with meals and sip slowly over 5 to 10 minutes.
• Tell patient to report adverse effects.
• Warn patient not to use salt substitutes at the same time, except with prescriber's permission.

Reactions may be *common,* uncommon, *life-threatening,* or COMMON AND LIFE-THREATENING.

potassium chloride
Cena-K, K + 10, Kaochlor 10%*, Kaochlor S-F 10%*, Kaon-Cl, Kaon-Cl 20%*, Kay-Cee-L§, Kay Ciel*, K + Care, K-Dur, K-Lease, K-Lor, Klor-Con, Klor-Con/25, Klorvess, Klotrix, K-Lyte/Cl, K-Norm, K-Tab, Micro-K Extencaps, Rum-K, Slow-K, Ten-K

Pregnancy risk category C

AVAILABLE FORMS
Capsules (controlled-release): 8 mEq (600 mg), 10 mEq (750 mg)
Injection: 20-mEq, 40-mEq ampules; additive syringes containing 30-mEq or 40-mEq; 10-mEq, 20-mEq, 30-mEq, 40-mEq, 60-mEq, 100-mEq, 200-mEq, 400-mEq, or 1,000-mEq vials
Oral liquid: 10% (20 mEq/15 ml), 15% (30 mEq/15 ml), 20% (40 mEq/15 ml)
Powder for oral use: 15-mEq packet, 20-mEq packet, 25-mEq packet, 25-mEq dose
Tablets (controlled-release): 6.7 mEq (500 mg), 8 mEq (600 mg), 10 mEq (750 mg), 20 mEq (1,500 mg)
Tablets (film-coated): 2.5 mEq (200 mg), 8 mEq (600 mg), 10 mEq (750 mg)

INDICATIONS & DOSAGES
➤ **Hypokalemia—**
Adults: 40 to 100 mEq P.O. daily in three or four divided doses for treatment; 10 to 20 mEq for prevention. Further dosage based on potassium level.
Children: 3 mEq/kg daily. Total daily dose not to exceed 40 mEq/m^2.

Use I.V. route only when oral replacement isn't feasible or when hypokalemia is life-threatening. If potassium level is less than 2 mEq/ml, maximum infusion rate is 40 mEq/hour, maximum infusion concentration is 80 mEq/L, and maximum 24-hour dose is 400 mEq. If potassium level is more than 2 mEq/ml, maximum infusion rate is 10 mEq/hour, maximum infusion concentration is 40 mEq/L, and maximum 24-hour dose is 200 mEq. For routine supplementation, usual dose is 10 to 20 mEq hourly in concentrations of 40 mEq/L or less.

I.V. ADMINISTRATION
● *Alert:* Give by infusion only, never I.V. push or I.M. Give slowly as dilute solution; potentially fatal hyperkalemia may result from too-rapid infusion. Decrease I.V. rate if burning occurs during infusion.

ACTION
Replaces potassium and maintains potassium level.

Route	Onset	Peak	Duration
I.V.	Immediate	Immediate	Unknown
P.O.	Unknown	Unknown	Unknown

ADVERSE REACTIONS
CNS: paresthesia of limbs, listlessness, confusion, weakness or heaviness of limbs, flaccid paralysis.
CV: *arrhythmias, heart block, cardiac arrest,* ECG changes, hypotension, *postinfusion phlebitis.*
GI: nausea, vomiting, abdominal pain, diarrhea.
Metabolic: hyperkalemia.
Respiratory: *respiratory paralysis.*

INTERACTIONS
Drug-drug. *ACE inhibitors, potassium-sparing diuretics:* Risk of hyperkalemia. Use with extreme caution.

EFFECTS ON LAB TEST RESULTS
● May increase potassium levels.

CONTRAINDICATIONS
Contraindicated in patients with severe renal impairment with oliguria, anuria, or azotemia; with untreated Addison's disease; or with acute dehydration, heat cramps, hyperkalemia, hyperkalemic form of familial periodic paralysis, or other conditions linked to extensive tissue breakdown.

NURSING CONSIDERATIONS
● Use cautiously in patients with cardiac disease or renal impairment.
● *Alert:* Give oral potassium supplements with extreme caution because different forms deliver varying amounts of potassium. Never switch products without prescriber's order.
● *Alert:* Potassium preparations aren't interchangeable; verify preparation before use.

---

*Liquid contains alcohol. **May contain tartarzine. †Canada ‡Australia §U.K. ◊OTC

- Make sure powders are completely dissolved before giving.
- Enteric-coated tablets aren't recommended because of increased risk of GI bleeding and small-bowel ulcerations.
- Tablets in wax matrix sometimes lodge in esophagus and cause ulceration in cardiac patients who have esophageal compression from enlarged left atrium. Use liquid form in such patients and in those with esophageal stasis or obstruction.
- Drug is commonly used orally with potassium-wasting diuretics to maintain potassium levels.
- Sugar-free liquid is available (Kaochlor S-F 10%); use if tablet or capsule passage is likely to be delayed, as in GI obstruction. Have patient sip slowly to minimize GI irritation.
- Don't crush sustained-release potassium products.
- Monitor ECG and electrolyte levels during therapy.
- Monitor renal function. Potassium shouldn't be given during immediate postoperative period until urine flow is established.
- Many adverse reactions may reflect hyperkalemia.

PATIENT TEACHING
- Instruct patient how to prepare (powders) and administer drug form prescribed. Tell patient to take with or after meals with full glass of water or fruit juice to lessen GI distress.
- Teach patient signs and symptoms of hyperkalemia, and tell patient to notify prescriber if they occur.
- Tell patient to report discomfort at I.V. insertion site.
- Warn patient not to use salt substitutes concurrently, except with prescriber's permission.

potassium gluconate
Glu-K, Kaon, Kaylixir*, K-G Elixir*

Pregnancy risk category C

AVAILABLE FORMS
Elixir: 4.68 g (20 mEq K+)/15 ml*
Tablets: 500 mg (2 mEq K+)

INDICATIONS & DOSAGES
➤ Hypokalemia—
Adults: 40 to 100 mEq P.O. daily in three or four divided doses for treatment; 10 to 20 mEq daily for prevention. Further dosage adjustments are based on potassium determinations.

ACTION
Replaces potassium and maintains intracellular and extracellular potassium levels.

Route	Onset	Peak	Duration
P.O.	Unknown	Unknown	4 hr

ADVERSE REACTIONS
CNS: paresthesia of limbs, listlessness, confusion, weakness or heaviness of legs, flaccid paralysis.
CV: *arrhythmias,* ECG changes.
GI: *nausea, vomiting, abdominal pain,* diarrhea.

INTERACTIONS
Drug-drug. *ACE inhibitors, potassium-sparing diuretics:* Risk of hyperkalemia. Use with extreme caution.

EFFECTS ON LAB TEST RESULTS
- May increase potassium levels.

CONTRAINDICATIONS
Contraindicated in patients with severe renal impairment with oliguria, anuria, or azotemia; untreated Addison's disease; or acute dehydration, heat cramps, hyperkalemia, hyperkalemic form of familial periodic paralysis, or other conditions linked to extensive tissue breakdown.

NURSING CONSIDERATIONS
- Use cautiously in patients with cardiac disease or renal impairment.
- *Alert:* Give oral potassium supplements with extreme caution because different forms deliver varying amounts of potassium. Never switch products without prescriber's order.
- *Alert:* Potassium preparations aren't interchangeable; verify preparation before use.
- Don't administer potassium supplements postoperatively until urine flow has been established.

Reactions may be *common,* uncommon, *life-threatening,* or COMMON AND LIFE-THREATENING.

• Monitor ECG, fluid intake and output, and BUN, potassium, and creatinine levels.

PATIENT TEACHING
• Advise patient to sip liquid potassium slowly to minimize GI irritation. Also tell him to take drug with or after meals with a full glass of water or fruit juice.
• Warn patient not to use salt substitutes concurrently, except with prescriber's permission.

Ringer's injection

Pregnancy risk category NR

AVAILABLE FORMS
Injection: 250 ml, 500 ml, 1,000 ml

INDICATIONS & DOSAGES
➤ **Fluid and electrolyte replacement—**
Adults and children: Dosage highly individualized, but usually 1.5 to 3 L (2% to 6% body weight), infused I.V. over 18 to 24 hours.

I.V. ADMINISTRATION
• Give at ordered rate, using an infusion device.

ACTION
Replaces fluids and electrolytes.

Route	Onset	Peak	Duration
I.V.	Immediate	Immediate	Unknown

ADVERSE REACTIONS
Metabolic: fluid overload.

INTERACTIONS
None significant.

EFFECTS ON LAB TEST RESULTS
• May cause electrolyte imbalances.

CONTRAINDICATIONS
Contraindicated in patients with renal failure, except as emergency volume expander.

NURSING CONSIDERATIONS
• Use cautiously in patients with heart failure, circulatory insufficiency, renal

dysfunction, hypoproteinemia, or pulmonary edema.
• Ringer's injection contains sodium, 147 mEq/L; potassium, 4 mEq/L; calcium, 4.5 mEq/L; and chloride, 155.5 mEq/L.
• Electrolyte content is insufficient for treating severe electrolyte deficiencies but does provide electrolytes in levels about equal to those in blood.
• *Alert:* Don't confuse Ringer's injection with Ringer's lactate solution.

PATIENT TEACHING
• Explain use and administration of drug to patient and family.
• Tell patient to report unusual signs or symptoms promptly.

Ringer's injection, lactated (Ringer's lactate solution)

Pregnancy risk category NR

AVAILABLE FORMS
Injection: 150 ml, 250 ml, 500 ml, 1,000 ml

INDICATIONS & DOSAGES
➤ **Fluid and electrolyte replacement—**
Adults and children: Dosage highly individualized, but usually 1.5 to 3 L (2% to 6% body weight) infused I.V. over 18 to 24 hours.

I.V. ADMINISTRATION
• Give at ordered rate, using an infusion device.

ACTION
Replaces fluids and electrolytes.

Route	Onset	Peak	Duration
I.V.	Immediate	Immediate	Unknown

ADVERSE REACTIONS
Metabolic: fluid overload.

INTERACTIONS
None significant.

EFFECTS ON LAB TEST RESULTS
• May cause electrolyte imbalance.

CONTRAINDICATIONS
Contraindicated in patients with renal failure, except as emergency volume expander.

NURSING CONSIDERATIONS
• Use cautiously in patients with heart failure, circulatory insufficiency, renal dysfunction, hypoproteinemia, or pulmonary edema.
• Use cautiously in patients with hepatic dysfunction because of possible lactic acid accumulation.
• Lactated Ringer's injection contains sodium, 130 mEq/L; potassium, 4 mEq/L; calcium, 3 mEq/L; chloride, 109.7 mEq/L; and lactate, 28 mEq/L.
• Lactated Ringer's injection more closely approximates electrolyte levels in blood plasma.
• *Alert:* Don't confuse Ringer's injection with Ringer's lactate solution.

PATIENT TEACHING
• Explain use and administration of drug to patient and family.
• Tell patient to report unusual signs or symptoms promptly.

---

sodium chloride
Slow-Sodium§

Pregnancy risk category C

AVAILABLE FORMS
Injection: Half-normal saline solution 25 ml, 50 ml, 150 ml, 250 ml, 500 ml, 1,000 ml; normal saline solution 2 ml, 3 ml, 5 ml, 10 ml, 20 ml, 25 ml, 30 ml, 50 ml, 100 ml, 150 ml, 250 ml, 500 ml, 1,000 ml; 3% sodium chloride solution 500 ml; 5% sodium chloride solution 500 ml; 14.6% sodium chloride solution 20 ml, 40 ml, 200 ml; 23.4% sodium chloride solution 30 ml, 50 ml, 100 ml, and 200 ml
Tablets: 650 mg
Tablets (slow-release): 600 mg, 1 g, 2.25 g

INDICATIONS & DOSAGES
➤ **Fluid and electrolyte replacement in hyponatremia caused by electrolyte loss or in severe salt depletion—**
Adults: Dosage is individualized; 3% or 5% solution used only with frequent elec-

trolyte determination and given only slow I.V. With 0.45% solution: 3% to 8% of body weight, according to deficiencies, over 18 to 24 hours; with 0.9% solution: 2% to 6% of body weight, according to deficiencies, over 18 to 24 hours.
➤ **Management of heat cramp caused by excessive perspiration—**
Adults: 1 g P.O. with each glass of water.

I.V. ADMINISTRATION
• *Alert:* Don't confuse concentrates (14.6%, 23.4%) available to add to parenteral nutrient solutions with normal saline solution for injection, and never give without diluting. Read labels carefully.
• *Alert:* Infuse 3% and 5% solutions slowly and cautiously to avoid pulmonary edema. Use only for critical situations, and observe patient continually.
• Never use bacteriostatic sodium chloride injection with newborns.

ACTION
Replaces sodium and chloride and maintains levels.

Route	Onset	Peak	Duration
I.V.	Immediate	Immediate	Unknown
P.O.	Unknown	Unknown	Unknown

ADVERSE REACTIONS
CV: aggravation of heart failure, thrombophlebitis, edema when given too rapidly or in excess.
Metabolic: hypernatremia, aggravation of existing metabolic acidosis with excessive infusion.
Respiratory: *pulmonary edema.*
Other: local tenderness, abscess, tissue necrosis at injection site.

INTERACTIONS
None significant.

EFFECTS ON LAB TEST RESULTS
• May increase sodium levels. May decrease potassium levels.
• May cause electrolyte imbalance.

CONTRAINDICATIONS
Contraindicated in patients with conditions in which sodium and chloride administration is detrimental. Sodium chlo-

---

ride 3% and 5% injections are contraindicated in patients with increased, normal, or only slightly decreased serum electrolyte levels.

NURSING CONSIDERATIONS
• Use cautiously in elderly or postoperative patients and in patients with heart failure, circulatory insufficiency, renal dysfunction, or hypoproteinemia.
• Monitor electrolyte levels.

PATIENT TEACHING
• Explain use and administration of drug to patient and family.
• Tell patient to report adverse reactions promptly.

62

Acidifiers and alkalinizers

sodium bicarbonate
sodium lactate
tromethamine

COMBINATION PRODUCTS
None.

---

sodium bicarbonate
Arm and Hammer Pure Baking
Soda ◊ , Bell/ans ◊ ,
Citrocarbonate, Soda Mint ◊

Pregnancy risk category C

AVAILABLE FORMS
Injection (powder): 4% (2.4 mEq/5 ml),
4.2% (5 mEq/10 ml), 5% (297.5 mEq/
500 ml), 7.5% (8.92 mEq/10 ml and
44.6 mEq/50 ml), 8.4% (10 mEq/10 ml
and 50 mEq/50 ml)
Tablets ◊ : 325 mg, 650 mg

INDICATIONS & DOSAGES
➤ **Cardiac arrest**—
Adults and children: 1 mEq/kg I.V. of
7.5% or 8.4% solution; then 0.5 mEq/kg
I.V. q 10 minutes, depending on arterial
blood gases (ABGs). Base further dosages
on results of ABG analysis. If ABG results
are unavailable, use 0.5 mEq/kg I.V. q 10
minutes until spontaneous circulation re-
turns.
Infants up to age 2: Not to exceed 8
mEq/kg I.V. of 4.2% solution daily.
➤ **Metabolic acidosis**—
Adults and children: Dosage depends on
blood carbon dioxide content, pH, and patient's condition. Generally, 2 to 5 mEq/kg
I.V. infused over 4- to 8-hour period.
➤ **Systemic or urinary alkalinization**—
Adults: Initially, 4 g P.O.; then 1 to 2 g q 4
hours.
Children: 84 to 840 mg/kg P.O. daily.
➤ **Antacid**—
Adults: 300 mg to 2 g P.O. up to q.i.d. tak-
en with glass of water.

I.V. ADMINISTRATION
● Drug may be added to other I.V. fluids.
Sodium bicarbonate inactivates such catecholamines as norepinephrine and dopamine and forms precipitate with calcium.
Don't mix sodium bicarbonate with I.V.
solutions of these drugs, and flush I.V. line
adequately.
● *Alert:* Sodium bicarbonate isn't routinely
recommended for use in cardiac arrest because it may produce a paradoxical acidosis from carbon dioxide production. It
shouldn't be routinely administered during
the early stages of resuscitation unless acidosis is clearly present.
● Four percent sodium bicarbonate is usually used for neutralizing certain I.V.
drugs, such as erythromycin. Consult
pharmacist before use.

ACTION
Restores buffering capacity of the body
and neutralizes excess acid.

Route	Onset	Peak	Duration
I.V.	Immediate	Immediate	Unknown
P.O.	Unknown	Unknown	Unknown

ADVERSE REACTIONS
GI: gastric distention, belching, flatulence.
Metabolic: hypokalemia, *metabolic alkalosis,* hypernatremia, hyperosmolarity
with overdose.
Other: pain and irritation at injection site.

INTERACTIONS
Drug-drug. *Anorexiants, flecainide,
mecamylamine, methenamine, quinidine,
sympathomimetics:* Urine alkalinization
decreases renal clearance of these drugs
and increases risk of toxicity. Monitor patient closely for toxicity.
*Chlorpropamide, lithium, methotrexate,
salicylates, tetracycline:* Increased urine
alkalinization increases renal clearance of
these drugs and decreases effectiveness.
Monitor patient closely for effectiveness.

Reactions may be *common,* uncommon, *life-threatening,* or COMMON AND LIFE-THREATENING.

Enteric-coated drugs: May be released prematurely in stomach. Avoid using together.
Ketoconazole: Concurrent use may decrease absorption. Use together with caution.

EFFECTS ON LAB TEST RESULTS
• May increase sodium and lactate levels. May decrease potassium levels.

CONTRAINDICATIONS
Contraindicated in patients with metabolic or respiratory alkalosis and in those with hypocalcemia in which alkalosis may produce tetany, hypertension, seizures, or heart failure. Also contraindicated in patients who are losing chlorides because of vomiting or continuous GI suction and in those receiving diuretics known to produce hypochloremic alkalosis. Orally administered sodium bicarbonate is contraindicated for patients with acute ingestion of strong mineral acids.

NURSING CONSIDERATIONS
• Use with extreme caution in patients with renal insufficiency, heart failure, or other edematous or sodium-retaining condition.
• To avoid risk of alkalosis, obtain blood pH, partial pressure of arterial oxygen, partial pressure of arterial carbon dioxide, and electrolyte levels. Keep prescriber informed of laboratory results.

PATIENT TEACHING
• Tell patient not to take drug with milk because doing so may cause hypercalcemia, alkalosis, and renal calculi.

---

sodium lactate

Pregnancy risk category NR

AVAILABLE FORMS
Injection: 1/6 M solution (167 mEq/L)

INDICATIONS & DOSAGES
➤ **Alkalinize urine—**
Adults: 30 ml of 1/6 M solution/kg of body weight I.V., given in divided doses over 24 hours.

➤ **Metabolic acidosis—**
Adults: 1/6 M injection (167 mEq lactate/L I.V.); dosage depends on degree of bicarbonate deficit.

I.V. ADMINISTRATION
• Add sodium lactate to other I.V. solutions, or give as an isotonic 1/6 M solution. Drug is compatible with most common I.V. solutions.
• Don't mix with sodium bicarbonate; drugs are incompatible.

ACTION
Metabolized to sodium bicarbonate, producing buffering effect.

Route	Onset	Peak	Duration
I.V.	Immediate	1-2 hr	Unknown

ADVERSE REACTIONS
CV: thrombophlebitis at injection site.
Metabolic: *metabolic alkalosis,* hypernatremia, hyperosmolarity with overdose.
Other: fever, infection.

INTERACTIONS
None significant.

EFFECTS ON LAB TEST RESULTS
• May increase sodium levels.

CONTRAINDICATIONS
Contraindicated in patients with hypernatremia, severe acidosis, lactic acidosis, or situations in which sodium administration is detrimental, such as during heart failure or corticosteroid administration.

NURSING CONSIDERATIONS
• Use with extreme caution in patients with metabolic or respiratory alkalosis, severe hepatic or renal disease, heart failure, shock, hypoxia, or beriberi.
• Monitor electrolyte levels to avoid alkalosis.

PATIENT TEACHING
• Explain use and administration of drug to patient and family.
• Tell patient to report unusual signs and symptoms.

tromethamine
Tham

Pregnancy risk category C

AVAILABLE FORMS
Injection: 18 g/500 ml

INDICATIONS & DOSAGES
➤ **Metabolic acidosis during cardiac bypass surgery or cardiac arrest—**
Adults: Dosage depends on bicarbonate deficit. Calculate as follows: each milliliter of 0.3 M tromethamine solution needed equals weight in kilograms multiplied by bicarbonate deficit (mEq/L). Base additional therapy on serial determinations of existing bicarbonate deficit. Administer over at least 1 hour; individual doses shouldn't exceed 500 mg/kg.
➤ **Acidosis during bypass surgery—**
Adults: Average dose of 9 ml/kg (2.7 mEq/kg or 0.32 g/kg); total single dose of 500 ml (150 mEq or 18 g) is adequate for most adults; not to exceed 500 mg/kg over a period of less than 1 hour.
➤ **Cardiac arrest—**
Adults: 3.5 to 6 ml/kg (126 to 216 mg/kg) of a 0.3 M solution or 3.6 to 10.8 g (111 to 333 ml) injected into large peripheral vein.

I.V. ADMINISTRATION
● Give slowly either through 18G to 20G needle into largest antecubital vein or through indwelling I.V. catheter.
● If extravasation occurs, infiltrate area with 1% procaine and 150 units hyaluronidase.

ACTION
Combines with hydrogen ions and associated acid anions; resulting salts are excreted. Also has osmotic diuretic effect.

Route	Onset	Peak	Duration
I.V.	Immediate	Immediate	Unknown

ADVERSE REACTIONS
Hepatic: *hemorrhagic hepatic necrosis.*
Metabolic: hypoglycemia, *hyperkalemia with decreased urine output.*
Respiratory: *respiratory depression.*

Other: venospasm, I.V. thrombosis, inflammation, necrosis, sloughing if extravasation occurs, fever.

INTERACTIONS
None significant.

EFFECTS ON LAB TEST RESULTS
● May increase potassium levels. May decrease glucose levels.

CONTRAINDICATIONS
Contraindicated in patients with anuria, uremia, or chronic respiratory acidosis; also contraindicated during pregnancy (except in acute, life-threatening situations).

NURSING CONSIDERATIONS
● Use cautiously in patients with renal disease and poor urine output. Monitor ECG and potassium levels.
● Make these determinations before, during, and after therapy: blood pH, carbon dioxide tension, and bicarbonate, glucose, and electrolyte levels.
● Have mechanical ventilation available for patients with respiratory acidosis.
● To prevent blood pH from rising above normal, be prepared to adjust dosage carefully.

PATIENT TEACHING
● Explain use of drug to patient and family.
● Tell patient to report adverse reactions.

Reactions may be *common,* uncommon, *life-threatening,* or COMMON AND LIFE-THREATENING.

ferrous fumarate
ferrous gluconate
ferrous sulfate
ferrous sulfate, dried
iron dextran
iron sucrose injection
polysaccharide-iron complex
sodium ferric gluconate
    complex

COMBINATION PRODUCTS
FERRO-DSS: ferrous fumarate 150 mg and
docusate sodium 100 mg.
FERRO-SEQUELS ◊: ferrous fumarate
150 mg and docusate sodium 100 mg.

ferrous fumarate
Femiron◊, Feostat◊, Feostat
Drops◊, Fersamal§, Hemocyte◊,
Ircon◊, Nephro-Fer◊,
Novofumar†, Palafer†, Palafer
Pediatric Drops†, Span-FF◊

Pregnancy risk category A

AVAILABLE FORMS
Each 100 mg of ferrous fumarate provides
33 mg of elemental iron.
Drops: 45 mg/0.6 ml ◊
Oral suspension: 100 mg/5 ml ◊
Tablets: 63 mg ◊, 200 mg ◊, 324 mg ◊,
325 mg ◊, 350 mg ◊
Tablets (chewable): 100 mg ◊

INDICATIONS & DOSAGES
➤ **Iron deficiency—**
Adults: 50 to 100 mg P.O. of elemental
iron t.i.d.
Children: 3 to 6 mg/kg/day P.O. of ele-
mental iron in three divided doses.

ACTION
Provides elemental iron, an essential component in the formation of hemoglobin.

Route	Onset	Peak	Duration
P.O.	4 days	7-10 days	2-4 mo

ADVERSE REACTIONS
GI: nausea, epigastric pain, vomiting, constipation, diarrhea, black stools, anorexia.
Other: temporarily stained teeth from suspension and drops.

INTERACTIONS
Drug-drug. *Antacids, cholestyramine
resin, cimetidine, vitamin E:* Decreased
iron absorption. Separate doses by at least
2 hours.
Chloramphenicol: Delayed response to
iron therapy. Monitor patient.
*Fluoroquinolones, penicillamine, tetracy-
clines:* Decreased GI absorption, possibly
resulting in decreased serum levels or efficacy. Separate doses by 2 to 4 hours.
Levodopa, methyldopa: Decreased absorption and efficacy of levodopa and
methyldopa. Watch for decreased effect of
these drugs.
L-Thyroxine: Decreased L-thyroxine absorption. Separate doses by at least 2
hours. Monitor thyroid function.
Vitamin C: May increase iron absorption.
Give together.
Drug-herb. *Black cohosh, chamomile,
feverfew, gossypol, hawthorn, nettle, plantain, St. John's wort:* Decreased iron absorption. Discourage use together.
Oregano: May reduce iron absorption.
Tell patient to separate oregano from iron
supplements or iron-containing foods by
at least 2 hours.
Drug-food. *Cereals, cheese, coffee, eggs,
milk, tea, whole-grain breads, yogurt:*
May impair oral iron absorption. Discourage use together.

EFFECTS ON LAB TEST RESULTS
None reported.

CONTRAINDICATIONS
Contraindicated in patients with primary
hemochromatosis or hemosiderosis, hemolytic anemia (unless iron deficiency
anemia is also present), peptic ulcer disease, regional enteritis, or ulcerative colitis. Also contraindicated in those receiving
repeated blood transfusions.

---

*Liquid contains alcohol.   **May contain tartrazine.   †Canada   ‡Australia   §U.K.   ◊OTC

NURSING CONSIDERATIONS

- Use cautiously on long-term basis.
- GI upset may be related to dose.
- Between-meal doses are preferable, but drug can be given with some foods, although absorption may be decreased.
- Enteric-coated products reduce GI upset but also reduce amount of iron absorbed.
- Check for constipation; record color and amount of stools.
- *Alert:* Oral iron may turn stools black. Although this unabsorbed iron is harmless, it could mask presence of melena. Guaiac test and orthotoluidine tests may yield false-positive results, but benzidine test isn't usually affected.
- Monitor hemoglobin levels, hematocrit, and reticulocyte count during therapy.
- Combination products such as Ferro-Sequels contain stool softeners, which help prevent constipation, a common adverse reaction.
- Iron overload may decrease uptake of technetium 99m and thus interfere with skeletal imaging.

PATIENT TEACHING

- Tell patient to take tablets with juice (preferably orange juice) or water, but not with milk or antacids.
- To avoid staining teeth, tell patient to take suspension with straw and place drops at back of throat.
- Caution patient not to crush tablets or chew extended-release forms.
- Advise patient not to substitute one iron salt for another; the amount of elemental iron may vary.
- *Alert:* Inform parents that as little as 3 or 4 tablets can cause serious poisoning in children.

ferrous gluconate
Fergon* ◊, Fertinic†, Novoferrogluc†

Pregnancy risk category A

AVAILABLE FORMS
Each 100 mg of ferrous gluconate provides 11.6 mg of elemental iron.
Tablets: 300 mg, 320 mg ◊, 325 mg ◊

INDICATIONS & DOSAGES
➤ **Iron deficiency—**
Adults: 50 to 100 mg P.O. of elemental iron t.i.d.
Children: 3 to 6 mg/kg/day P.O. of elemental iron in three divided doses.

ACTION
Provides elemental iron, an essential component in the formation of hemoglobin.

Route	Onset	Peak	Duration
P.O.	4 days	7-10 days	2-4 mo

ADVERSE REACTIONS
GI: *nausea,* epigastric pain, vomiting, *constipation,* diarrhea, *black stools,* anorexia.

INTERACTIONS
Drug-drug. *Antacids, cholestyramine resin, cimetidine, vitamin E:* Decreased iron absorption. Separate doses by at least 2 hours.
Chloramphenicol: Delayed response to iron therapy. Monitor patient.
Fluoroquinolones, penicillamine, tetracyclines: Decreased GI absorption, possibly resulting in decreased serum levels or efficacy. Separate doses by 2 to 4 hours.
Levodopa, methyldopa: Decreased absorption and efficacy of levodopa and methyldopa. Watch for decreased effect of these drugs.
L-Thyroxine: Decreased L-thyroxine absorption. Separate doses by at least 2 hours. Monitor thyroid function.
Vitamin C: May increase iron absorption. Give together.
Drug-herb. *Black cohosh, chamomile, feverfew, gossypol, hawthorn, nettle, plantain, St. John's wort:* Decreased iron absorption. Discourage use together.
Oregano: May reduce iron absorption. Tell patient to separate oregano from iron supplements or iron-containing foods by at least 2 hours.
Drug-food. *Cereals, cheese, coffee, eggs, milk, tea, whole-grain breads, yogurt:* May impair oral iron absorption. Discourage use together.

EFFECTS ON LAB TEST RESULTS
None reported.

CONTRAINDICATIONS
Contraindicated in patients with peptic ulceration, regional enteritis, ulcerative colitis, hemosiderosis, primary hemochromatosis, or hemolytic anemia (unless an iron deficiency anemia is also present) and in those receiving repeated blood transfusions.

NURSING CONSIDERATIONS
• Use cautiously on long-term basis.
• GI upset may be related to dose.
• Between-meal doses are preferable, but drug can be given with some foods, although absorption may be decreased.
• Enteric-coated products reduce GI upset but also reduce amount of iron absorbed.
• Check for constipation; record color and amount of stools.
• *Alert:* Oral iron may turn stools black. Although this unabsorbed iron is harmless, it could mask melena. Guaiac and orthotoluidine test may yield false-positive results, but benzidine test isn't usually affected.
• Monitor hemoglobin levels, hematocrit, and reticulocyte count during therapy.
• Iron overload may decrease uptake of technetium 99m and thus interfere with skeletal imaging.

PATIENT TEACHING
• To promote absorption, tell patient to take tablets with orange juice.
• *Alert:* Inform parents that as few as 3 or 4 tablets can cause serious iron poisoning in children.
• Caution patient not to substitute one iron salt for another because the amounts of elemental iron vary.

---

ferrous sulfate
Apo-Ferrous Sulfate†, Feosol*◊, Fer-Gen-Sol, Fer-In-Sol Drops*◊, Fer-In-Sol Syrup*◊, Fer-Iron Drops◊, Fero-Gradumet, Mol-Iron*◊

ferrous sulfate, dried
Fe⁵⁰, Feosol◊, Feospan§, Feratab, Novoferrosulfa†,

PMS-Ferrous Sulfate†, Slow FE◊

Pregnancy risk category A

AVAILABLE FORMS
Each 100 mg of ferrous sulfate provides 20 mg of elemental iron, about 30 mg of elemental iron in ferrous sulfate dried products.
Caplets (extended-release): 160 mg (dried)
Capsules: 250 mg ◊
Drops: 125 mg/ml
Elixir: 220 mg/5 ml*◊
Tablets: 195 mg, 300 mg 325 mg; 200 mg (dried)
Tablets (extended-release): 160 mg (dried)◊, 525 mg
Solution: 300 mg/5 ml
Syrup: 90 mg/5 ml ◊

INDICATIONS & DOSAGES
➤ **Iron deficiency—**
Adults: 50 to 100 mg P.O. of elemental iron t.i.d.
Children: 3 to 6 mg/kg/day P.O. of elemental iron in three divided doses.

ACTION
Provides elemental iron, an essential component in the formation of hemoglobin.

Route	Onset	Peak	Duration
P.O.	4 days	7-10 days	2-4 mo

ADVERSE REACTIONS
GI: *nausea,* epigastric pain, vomiting, *constipation, black stools,* diarrhea, anorexia.
Other: temporarily stained teeth from liquid forms.

INTERACTIONS
Drug-drug. *Antacids, cholestyramine resin, cimetidine, vitamin E:* Decreased iron absorption. Separate doses if possible.
Chloramphenicol: Delayed response to iron therapy. Monitor patient.
Fluoroquinolones, penicillamine, tetracyclines: Decreased GI absorption, possibly resulting in decreased serum levels or efficacy. Separate doses by 2 to 4 hours.
Levodopa, methyldopa: Decreased absorption and efficacy of levodopa and methyldopa. Watch for decreased effect of these drugs.

---

*Liquid contains alcohol.   **May contain tartrazine.   †Canada   ‡Australia   §U.K.   ◊OTC

L-Thyroxine: Decreased L-thyroxine absorption. Separate doses by at least 2 hours. Monitor thyroid function.

Vitamin C: May increase iron absorption. Give together.

Drug-herb. *Black cohosh, chamomile, feverfew, gossypol, hawthorn, nettle, plantain, St. John's wort:* Decreased iron absorption. Discourage use together.

Oregano: May reduce iron absorption. Tell patient to separate oregano from iron supplements or iron-containing foods by at least 2 hours.

Drug-food. *Cereals, cheese, coffee, eggs, milk, tea, whole-grain breads, yogurt:* May impair oral iron absorption. Discourage use together.

EFFECTS ON LAB TEST RESULTS
None reported.

CONTRAINDICATIONS
Contraindicated in patients with hemosiderosis, primary hemochromatosis, hemolytic anemia (unless iron deficiency anemia is also present), peptic ulceration, ulcerative colitis, or regional enteritis and in those receiving repeated blood transfusions.

NURSING CONSIDERATIONS
- Use cautiously on long-term basis.
- GI upset may be related to dose.
- Between-meal doses are preferable. Drug can be given with some foods, although absorption may be decreased.
- Enteric-coated products reduce GI upset but also reduce amount of iron absorbed.
- *Alert:* Oral iron may turn stools black. Although this unabsorbed iron is harmless, it could mask melena. Guaiac test and orthotoluidine test may yield false-positive results, but benzidine test isn't usually affected.
- Monitor hemoglobin levels, hematocrit, and reticulocyte count during therapy.
- Iron overload may decrease uptake of technetium 99m and thus interfere with skeletal imaging.
- *Alert:* Don't confuse different iron salts; elemental content may vary.

PATIENT TEACHING
- Tell patient to take with juice.

- Instruct patient not to crush or chew extended-release forms.
- *Alert:* Inform parents that as little as 3 to 4 tablets can cause serious iron poisoning in children.
- Caution patient not to substitute one iron salt for another because amounts of elemental iron vary.
- Advise patient to report constipation and change in stool color or consistency.

iron dextran
DexFerrum, InFeD

Pregnancy risk category C

AVAILABLE FORMS
1 ml iron dextran provides 50 mg elemental iron.
Injection: 50 mg elemental iron/ml

INDICATIONS & DOSAGES
➤ **Iron deficiency anemia—**
Adults and children: Total dose is calculated using the following formula:

$$\text{Dose (ml)} = 0.0442 \text{ (desired Hb} - \text{observed Hb)} \times \text{Weight in kg} + (0.26 \times \text{Weight in kg)}.$$

I.M. or I.V. test dose is needed before administration.

I.M. (by Z-track method): Inject 0.5-ml test dose. If no reaction occurs in 1 hour, give remainder of dose. Daily dose should ordinarily not exceed 0.5 ml (25 mg) for infants weighing less than 5 kg (11 lb); 1 ml (50 mg) for those weighing less than 10 kg (22 lb); and 2 ml (100 mg) for heavier children and adults. Don't give iron dextran in the first 4 months of life.

I.V.: Inject 0.5-ml test dose over 30 seconds. If no reaction occurs in 1 hour, give remainder of therapeutic I.V. dose. Repeat therapeutic I.V. dose daily. Single dose shouldn't exceed 100 mg. Give slowly (1 ml/minute).

I.V. ADMINISTRATION
- Check hospital policy before giving I.V. Don't mix with other parenteral drug or nutritional solutions containing liquid emulsions.
- After completing I.V. dose, flush the vein with 10 ml of normal saline solution. Pa-

tient should rest for 15 to 30 minutes after I.V. administration.

ACTION
Provides elemental iron, an essential component in the formation of hemoglobin.

Route	Onset	Peak	Duration
I.M.	72 hr	Unknown	3-4 wk
I.V.	Unknown	Unknown	Unknown

ADVERSE REACTIONS
CNS: headache, transitory paresthesia, dizziness, malaise.
CV: chest pain, tachycardia, *bradycardia, hypotension reaction, peripheral vascular flushing.*
GI: nausea, anorexia.
Musculoskeletal: arthralgia, myalgia.
Respiratory: *bronchospasm,* dyspnea.
Skin: rash; urticaria; *soreness, inflammation, brown skin discoloration at I.M. injection site; local phlebitis at I.V. injection site;* sterile abscess; necrosis; atrophy.
Other: fibrosis, *anaphylaxis, delayed sensitivity reactions,* fever, chills.

INTERACTIONS
None significant.

EFFECTS ON LAB TEST RESULTS
None reported.

CONTRAINDICATIONS
Contraindicated in patients hypersensitive to drug, in those with acute infectious renal disease, and in those with any anemia except iron deficiency anemia.

NURSING CONSIDERATIONS
• Don't administer iron dextran with oral iron preparations.
• Use with extreme caution in patients who have serious hepatic impairment, rheumatoid arthritis, or other inflammatory diseases because these patients may be at higher risk for certain delays and reactions.
• Use cautiously in patients with history of significant allergies or asthma.
• I.M. or I.V. injections of iron are advisable only for patients in whom oral administration is impossible or ineffective.
• For I.M. route, inject deeply into upper outer quadrant of buttock—never into arm or other exposed area—with a 2- to 3-inch

19G or 20G needle. Use Z-track method to avoid leakage into subcutaneous tissue and staining of skin. After drawing up drug, use a new sterile needle to give injection.
• Monitor hemoglobin levels and hematocrit and reticulocyte count.
• Large doses (more than 250 mg iron) may color the serum brown. Iron dextran prevents meaningful measurement of iron level and total iron-binding capacity for up to 3 weeks; I.M. injection may cause dense areas of activity for 1 to 6 days on bone scans using technetium 99m diphosphonate.
• Drug causes false increases of bilirubin and false decreases in calcium.

PATIENT TEACHING
• Teach patient signs and symptoms of hypersensitivity or iron toxicity, and tell him to report them if they occur.
• Inform patient that drug may stain skin.

✳ **NEW DRUG**

iron sucrose injection
Venofer

Pregnancy risk category B

AVAILABLE FORMS
Injection: 20 mg/ml of elemental iron

INDICATIONS & DOSAGES
➤ **Iron deficiency anemia in patients undergoing long-term hemodialysis who are receiving supplemental erythropoietin therapy—**
Adults: 100 mg (5 ml) of elemental iron I.V. directly in the dialysis line, either by slow injection at a rate of 1 ml/minute or by infusion over 15 minutes during the dialysis session one to three times a week to a total of 1,000 mg in 10 doses; repeat p.r.n.

I.V. ADMINISTRATION
• For administration by slow injection, give drug at a rate of 1 ml (20 mg elemental iron) undiluted solution per minute, not exceeding 1 vial (100 mg elemental iron) per injection.
• For administration by infusion, dilute drug to a maximum of 100 ml in normal

---

*Liquid contains alcohol.   **May contain tartrazine.   †Canada   ‡Australia   §U.K.   ◇OTC

saline solution immediately before infusion and infuse at a rate of 100 mg elemental iron over at least 15 minutes.
● Don't mix with other drugs or add to parenteral nutrition solutions of I.V. infusion.
● Inspect drugs for particulate matter and discoloration before administration.

ACTION

Exogenous source of iron that replenishes depleted body iron stores and is essential for hemoglobin synthesis.

Route	Onset	Peak	Duration
I.V.	Unknown	Unknown	Variable

ADVERSE REACTIONS

CNS: headache, asthenia, malaise, dizziness.
CV: *hypotension,* chest pain, hypertension, fluid retention.
GI: nausea, vomiting, diarrhea, abdominal pain.
Musculoskeletal: *leg cramps,* bone and muscle pain.
Respiratory: dyspnea, pneumonia, cough.
Skin: pruritus, application site reaction.
Other: fever, accidental injury, pain.

INTERACTIONS

Drug-drug. *Oral iron preparations:* Reduces absorption of orally administered iron preparations. Avoid using together.

EFFECTS ON LAB TEST RESULTS

● May increase liver enzyme levels.

CONTRAINDICATIONS

Contraindicated in patients with hypersensitivity to drug or its components, evidence of iron overload, or anemia not caused by iron deficiency.

NURSING CONSIDERATIONS

● **Alert:** Rare but fatal hypersensitivity reactions characterized by anaphylactic shock, loss of consciousness, collapse, hypotension, dyspnea, or convulsion have occurred.
● Giving drug by infusion may reduce the risk of hypotension.
● Transferrin saturation levels increase rapidly after I.V. administration of iron su-

crose. Obtain iron levels 48 hours after I.V. administration.
● Monitor hematocrit and hemoglobin, ferritin, and transferrin saturation levels.
● Withhold dose in patient with signs and symptoms of iron overload.
● Dose selection in elderly patients should be conservative because of decreased hepatic, renal, or cardiac function; other disease; and other drug therapy.
● It's unknown if drug appears in breast milk. Use cautiously in breast-feeding women.

PATIENT TEACHING

● Instruct patient to notify prescriber if symptoms of overdose occur, such as headache, nausea, dizziness, joint aches, paresthesia, or abdominal and muscle pain.

polysaccharide-iron complex
Ferrex-150, Fe-Tinic-150, Hytinic, Niferex, Niferex-150, Nu-Iron, Nu-Iron 150

Pregnancy risk category NR

AVAILABLE FORMS

Capsules: 150 mg
Solution: 100 mg/5 ml
Tablets (film-coated): 50 mg

ACTION

Provides elemental iron, an essential component in the formation of hemoglobin.

Route	Onset	Peak	Duration
P.O.	Few days	2-10 days	2 mo

INDICATIONS & DOSAGES

➤ **Uncomplicated iron deficiency anemia—**
Adults: 50 to 100 mg P.O. of elemental iron t.i.d.
Children: 3 to 6 mg/kg/day P.O. of elemental iron in three divided doses.

ADVERSE REACTIONS

GI: *nausea,* epigastric pain, vomiting, *constipation, black stools,* diarrhea, anorexia.
Other: temporarily stained teeth from liquid forms.

INTERACTIONS
Drug-drug. *Antacids, cholestyramine resin, cimetidine, vitamin E:* Decreased iron absorption. Separate doses by 2 to 4 hours.

Chloramphenicol: Delayed response to iron therapy. Monitor patient.

Fluoroquinolones, penicillamine, tetracyclines: Decreased GI absorption, possibly resulting in decreased serum levels or efficacy. Separate doses by 2 to 4 hours.

Levodopa, methyldopa: Decreased absorption and efficacy of levodopa and methyldopa. Watch for decreased effect of these drugs.

Thyroid: May inhibit thyroid hormone absorption. Separate doses by 2 hours.

Vitamin C: May increase iron absorption. Give together.

Drug-herb. *Black cohosh, chamomile, feverfew, gossypol, hawthorn, nettle, plantain, St. John's wort:* Decreased iron absorption. Discourage use together.

Oregano: May reduce iron absorption. Tell patient to separate oregano from iron supplements or iron-containing foods by at least 2 hours.

Drug-food. *Cereals, cheese, coffee, eggs, milk, tea, whole-grain breads, yogurt:* May impair oral iron absorption. Discourage use together.

EFFECTS ON LAB TEST RESULTS
None reported.

CONTRAINDICATIONS
Contraindicated in patients hypersensitive to drug or its ingredients and in those with hemochromatosis or hemosiderosis.

NURSING CONSIDERATIONS
• **Alert:** Oral iron may turn stools black. Although this unabsorbed iron is harmless, it may mask melena. Guaiac and orthotoluidine tests may yield false-positive results, but benzidine test isn't usually affected.

• Monitor hemoglobin levels and hematocrit and reticulocyte count.

• Although nausea, constipation, black stools, and epigastric pain are common adverse reactions to iron therapy, few, if any, occur with polysaccharide iron complex.

• Iron overload may decrease uptake of technetium 99m and thus interfere with skeletal imaging.

PATIENT TEACHING
• Tell patient to take drug with juice.

• **Alert:** Inform parents that as few as 3 tablets can cause serious iron poisoning in children.

• Caution patient not to substitute one iron salt for another because the amounts of elemental iron vary.

---

sodium ferric gluconate complex
Ferrlecit

Pregnancy risk category B

AVAILABLE FORMS
Injection: 62.5 mg elemental iron (12.5 mg/ml) in 5-ml ampules

INDICATIONS & DOSAGES
➤ **Iron deficiency anemia in patients undergoing long-term hemodialysis and receiving supplemental erythropoietin therapy**—
Adults: Before starting therapeutic doses, give test dose of 2 ml sodium ferric gluconate complex (25 mg elemental iron), diluted in 50 ml normal saline solution and given I.V. over 1 hour. If test dose is tolerated, give therapeutic dose of 10 ml (125 mg elemental iron) diluted in 100 ml normal saline solution and given I.V. over 1 hour. Most patients need minimum cumulative dose of 1 g elemental iron administered at more than eight sequential dialysis treatments to achieve a favorable hemoglobin or hematocrit response.

I.V. ADMINISTRATION
• Dilute test dose of sodium ferric gluconate complex in 50 ml normal saline solution and give over 1 hour. Dilute therapeutic doses of drug in 100 ml normal saline solution and give over 1 hour.

• Don't mix sodium ferric gluconate complex with other drugs or add to parenteral nutrition solutions for I.V. infusion. Use immediately after dilution in normal saline solution.

• *Alert:* Profound hypotension with flushing, light-headedness, malaise, fatigue, weakness, or severe chest, back, flank, or groin pain has been reported after rapid I.V. administration of iron. These reactions aren't related to hypersensitivity reactions and may result from too-rapid administration. Don't exceed recommended rate of administration (2.1 mg/minute). Monitor patient closely during infusion.

ACTION

Restores total body iron content, which is critical for normal hemoglobin synthesis and oxygen transport.

Route	Onset	Peak	Duration
I.V.	Unknown	Unknown	Unknown

ADVERSE REACTIONS

CNS: asthenia, headache, fatigue, malaise, dizziness, paresthesia, agitation, insomnia, somnolence, syncope.
CV: hypotension, hypertension, tachycardia, *bradycardia,* angina, chest pain, *MI,* edema, flushing.
EENT: conjunctivitis, abnormal vision, rhinitis.
GI: nausea, vomiting, diarrhea, rectal disorder, dyspepsia, eructation, flatulence, melena, abdominal pain.
GU: urinary tract infection.
Hematologic: abnormal erythrocytes, anemia.
Metabolic: hyperkalemia, hypoglycemia, hypokalemia, hypervolemia.
Musculoskeletal: myalgia, arthralgia, back pain, arm pain, cramps.
Respiratory: dyspnea, coughing, upper respiratory tract infection, pneumonia, pulmonary edema.
Skin: pruritus, increased sweating, rash.
Other: injection site reaction, pain, fever, infection, rigors, chills, flu syndrome, *sepsis, carcinoma,* hypersensitivity reactions, lymphadenopathy.

INTERACTIONS

None significant.

EFFECTS ON LAB TEST RESULTS

• May increase or decrease potassium levels. May decrease glucose levels.
• May decrease hemoglobin.

CONTRAINDICATIONS

Contraindicated in patients hypersensitive to drug or its components (such as benzyl alcohol) and in those with anemias not related to iron deficiency. Don't give to patients with iron overload.

NURSING CONSIDERATIONS

• Use cautiously in elderly patients.
• *Alert:* Dosage is expressed in milligrams of elemental iron.
• Drug shouldn't be given to patients with iron overload, which typically occurs in hemoglobinopathies and other refractory anemias.
• *Alert:* Potentially life-threatening hypersensitivity reactions (characterized by CV collapse, cardiac arrest, bronchospasm, oral or pharyngeal edema, dyspnea, angioedema, urticaria, or pruritus sometimes linked to pain and muscle spasm of chest or back) may occur during infusion. Have adequate supportive measures readily available. Monitor patient closely during infusion.
• Monitor hemoglobin levels, hematocrit, and ferritin and iron saturation levels.
• Some adverse reactions in hemodialysis patients may be related to dialysis itself or to chronic renal failure.
• Check with patient about other potential sources of iron, such as OTC iron preparations and iron-containing multiple vitamins with minerals.

PATIENT TEACHING

• Urge patient to notify prescriber immediately if abdominal pain, diarrhea, vomiting, drowsiness, or hyperventilation occurs. These symptoms may indicate iron poisoning.

Reactions may be *common*, uncommon, *life-threatening*, or COMMON AND LIFE-THREATENING.

64

Anticoagulants

argatroban
bivalirudin
dalteparin sodium
danaparoid sodium
enoxaparin sodium
heparin calcium
heparin sodium
tinzaparin sodium
warfarin sodium

COMBINATION PRODUCTS
None.

✳ *NEW DRUG*

argatroban
Acova

Pregnancy risk category B

AVAILABLE FORMS
Injection: 100 mg/ml

INDICATIONS & DOSAGE
➤ **Prophylaxis or treatment of thrombosis in patients with heparin-induced thrombocytopenia—**
Adults: 2 mcg/kg/minute, given as a continuous I.V. infusion; adjust dose until the steady-state activated partial thromboplastin time (aPTT) is 1.5 to 3 times the initial baseline value, not to exceed 100 seconds; maximum dose 10 mcg/kg/minute.
Adjust-a-dose: For patients with moderate hepatic impairment, the initial dose should be reduced to 0.5 mcg/kg/minute, given as a continuous infusion. The aPTT should be monitored closely and the dosage adjusted as clinically indicated.

I.V. ADMINISTRATION
● Dilute in normal saline solution, D_5W, or lactated Ringer's injection to a final concentration of 1 mg/ml.
● Each 2.5-ml vial should be diluted 100-fold by mixing it with 250 ml of diluent.
● Mix the constituted solution by repeated inversion of the diluent bag for 1 minute.
● Prepared solutions are stable for up to 24 hours at 77° F (25° C).

ACTION
Argatroban reversibly binds to the thrombin-active site and inhibits thrombin-catalyzed or -induced reactions: fibrin formation, coagulation factor V, VIII, and XIII activation, protein C activation, and platelet aggregation. Argatroban can inhibit the action of free and clot-associated thrombin.

Route	Onset	Peak	Duration
I.V.	Rapid	1-3 hr	Duration of infusion

ADVERSE REACTIONS
CNS: *cerebrovascular disorder.*
CV: *atrial fibrillation, cardiac arrest,* hypotension, *ventricular tachycardia.*
GI: abdominal pain, diarrhea, *GI bleeding,* nausea, vomiting.
GU: abnormal renal function, groin bleeding, *hematuria,* urinary tract infection.
Respiratory: cough, dyspnea, pneumonia, hemoptysis.
Other: allergic reactions, brachial bleeding, fever, infection, pain, *sepsis.*

INTERACTIONS
Drug-drug. *Oral anticoagulants:* May prolong PT and INR and may increase the risk of bleeding. Monitor patient closely.
Thrombolytic agents: Increased risk of intracranial bleeding. Avoid using together.

EFFECTS ON LAB TEST RESULTS
● May decrease hemoglobin and hematocrit.

CONTRAINDICATIONS
Contraindicated in patients who have overt major bleeding who are hypersensitive to drug or any of its components.

NURSING CONSIDERATIONS
● Use cautiously in patients with hepatic disease or conditions that increase the risk of hemorrhage, such as severe hypertension.
● Use cautiously in patients who have just had lumbar puncture, spinal anesthesia, or

---

major surgery, especially of the brain, spinal cord, or eye; patients with hematologic conditions associated with increased bleeding tendencies, such as congenital or acquired bleeding disorders; and patients with GI ulcers or other lesions.

• Discontinue all parenteral anticoagulants before giving argatroban. Giving argatroban together with antiplatelets, thrombolytics, and other anticoagulants may increase the risk of bleeding.

• Get results of baseline coagulation tests, platelets, hemoglobin, and hematocrit before starting therapy, and report any abnormalities to the prescriber.

• Check aPTT 2 hours after giving drug; dose adjustments may be required to get a targeted aPTT of 1.5 to 3 times the baseline, no longer than 100 seconds. Steady state is achieved 1 to 3 hours after starting argatroban.

• Hemorrhage in patients receiving argatroban can occur at any site in the body. Any unexplained fall in hematocrit or blood pressure or any other unexplained symptoms may signify a hemorrhagic event.

• To convert to oral anticoagulant therapy, give warfarin P.O. with argatroban at up to 2 mcg/kg/minute until the INR exceeds 4 on combined therapy. After argatroban is discontinued, repeat the INR in 4 to 6 hours. If the repeat INR is below the desired therapeutic range, resume the I.V. argatroban infusion. Repeat the procedure daily until the desired therapeutic range on warfarin alone is reached.

• **Alert:** Don't confuse Acova (argatroban) with Aggrastat (tirofiban).

• It's unknown whether argatroban is excreted in breast milk. A decision should be made to discontinue either breast-feeding or the drug, taking into account the importance of the drug to the mother.

PATIENT TEACHING

• Tell patient that this drug can cause bleeding, and ask him to report any unusual bruising or bleeding (nosebleeds, bleeding gums) or tarry stools to the prescriber immediately.

• Advise patient to avoid activities that carry a risk of injury and to use a soft toothbrush and an electric razor while receiving argatroban.

• Instruct patient to notify prescriber if he has wheezing, trouble breathing, or skin rash.

• Instruct patient to notify prescriber if she is pregnant or breast-feeding or has recently had a baby.

• Tell patient to notify prescriber if he has GI ulcers, hepatic disease, recent surgery, radiation treatment, falling episodes, or injury.

✳ *NEW DRUG*

bivalirudin
Angiomax

Pregnancy risk category B

AVAILABLE FORMS
Injection: 250-mg vial

INDICATIONS & DOSAGES
➤ **Unstable angina in patients undergoing percutaneous transluminal coronary angioplasty (PTCA)—**
Adults: 1 mg/kg I.V. bolus just before PTCA; then begin 4-hour I.V. infusion at 2.5 mg/kg/hour. After initial 4-hour infusion, an additional I.V. infusion at a rate of 0.2 mg/kg/hour for up to 20 hours may be given as needed. Give with 300 to 325 mg aspirin.
Adjust-a-dose: For patients with renal impairment, adjust dose according to creatinine clearance. For moderate renal impairment (creatinine clearance 30 to 59 ml/minute), reduce dose by 20%. For severe renal impairment (creatinine clearance 10 to 29 ml/minute), reduce dose by 60%. For dialysis-dependent patients (off dialysis), reduce dose by 90%.

I.V. ADMINISTRATION
• Reconstitute each 250-mg vial with 5 ml of sterile water for injection. Further dilute each reconstituted vial in 50 ml D_5W or normal saline solution to yield a final concentration of 5 mg/ml.

• To prepare low-rate infusion, further dilute each reconstituted vial in 500 ml D_5W or normal saline solution to yield a final concentration of 0.5 mg/ml.

• Don't mix other drugs with bivalirudin before or during administration.

Reactions may be *common,* uncommon, *life-threatening,* or COMMON AND LIFE-THREATENING.

• The prepared solution is stable for 24 hours at 36° to 46° F (2° to 8° C).
• It's unknown if drug appears in breast milk; use cautiously in breast-feeding women.
• Puncture-site hemorrhage and catheterization site hematoma may occur in more patients age 65 and older than in younger patients.

ACTION
Drug binds specifically and rapidly to thrombin to produce an anticoagulant effect.

Route	Onset	Peak	Duration
I.V.	Rapid	Immediate	Duration of infusion

ADVERSE REACTIONS
CNS: anxiety, *headache,* insomnia, nervousness.
CV: *bradycardia,* hypertension, *hypotension.*
GI: abdominal pain, dyspepsia, *nausea,* vomiting.
GU: urine retention.
Hematologic: *severe, spontaneous bleeding* (cerebral, retroperitoneal, GU, GI).
Musculoskeletal: *back pain,* pelvic pain.
Other: fever, *pain,* pain at injection site.

INTERACTIONS
Drug-drug. *Glycoprotein IIb/IIIa inhibitors:* Safety and effectiveness not yet established. Avoid using together.
Heparin, warfarin, other oral anticoagulants: Increases risk of bleeding. Use together cautiously. Stop heparin at least 8 hours before giving bivalirudin.

EFFECTS ON LAB TEST RESULTS
None reported.

CONTRAINDICATIONS
Contraindicated in patients hypersensitive to drug or its components and in those with active major bleeding. Avoid using in patients with unstable angina who aren't undergoing PTCA or in patients with other acute coronary syndromes.

NURSING CONSIDERATIONS
• Use cautiously in patients with heparin-induced thrombocytopenia or heparin-induced thrombocytopenia-thrombosis syndrome, and in patients with diseases associated with increased risk of bleeding.
• Don't give by I.M. route.
• Hemorrhage can occur at any site in the body in patients receiving bivalirudin. Consider a hemorrhagic event if unexplained drop in hematocrit, fall in blood pressure, or other unexplained symptom occurs.
• Monitor baseline coagulation tests, hemoglobin, and hematocrit before initiation of therapy and periodically throughout therapy.
• Monitor venipuncture sites for bleeding, hematoma, or inflammation.

PATIENT TEACHING
• Advise patient that drug can cause bleeding and tell him to report unusual bruising or bleeding (nosebleeds, bleeding gums) or tarry stools immediately.
• Counsel patient that drug is given with aspirin and caution him to avoid other aspirin-containing drugs or drugs to treat swelling or pain (Motrin, Naprosyn, Aleve) while receiving bivalirudin.
• Advise patient to avoid activities that carry a risk of injury and instruct him to use a soft toothbrush and electric razor while on drug.

dalteparin sodium
Fragmin

Pregnancy risk category B

AVAILABLE FORMS
Syringe: 2,500 antifactor Xa IU/0.2 ml, 5,000 antifactor Xa IU/0.2 ml, 10,000 antifactor Xa IU/ml in 9.5-ml vial

INDICATIONS & DOSAGES
➤ **Prevention of deep vein thrombosis (DVT) in patients undergoing abdominal surgery who are at risk for thromboembolic complications—**
Adults: 2,500 IU S.C. daily, starting 1 to 2 hours before surgery and repeated once daily for 5 to 10 days postoperatively.
➤ **DVT prophylaxis in patients undergoing hip replacement surgery—**
Adults: 2,500 IU S.C. within 2 hours before surgery and second dose 2,500 IU

S.C. in the evening of surgery (at least 6 hours after first dose). If surgery is performed in the evening, omit second dose on day of surgery. Starting on first postoperative day, administer 5,000 IU S.C. once daily for 5 to 10 days. Or, 5,000 IU S.C. on the evening before surgery; then 5,000 IU S.C. once daily starting in the evening of surgery for 5 to 10 days postoperatively.

➤ **Unstable angina and non–Q-wave MI—**

Adults: 120 IU/kg S.C. q 12 hours with aspirin P.O. unless contraindicated. Maximum dose, 10,000 IU. Usual duration of treatment is 5 to 8 days.

ACTION

A low-molecular-weight heparin derivative that enhances inhibition of factor Xa and thrombin by antithrombin.

Route	Onset	Peak	Duration
S.C.	Unknown	4 hr	Unknown

ADVERSE REACTIONS

Hematologic: *thrombocytopenia, hemorrhage,* ecchymoses, bleeding complications.

Skin: pruritus, rash, pain, *hematoma at injection site.*

Other: fever, *anaphylaxis,* injection site pain.

INTERACTIONS

Drug-drug. *Antiplatelet drugs, oral anticoagulants:* May increase risk of bleeding. Use together cautiously.

EFFECTS ON LAB TEST RESULTS

• May increase ALT and AST levels.
• May decrease platelet count.

CONTRAINDICATIONS

Contraindicated in patients hypersensitive to drug, heparin, or pork products; in those with active major bleeding; and in those with thrombocytopenia and antiplatelet antibodies in presence of drug.

NURSING CONSIDERATIONS

• Use with extreme caution in patients with history of heparin-induced thrombocytopenia and in patients at increased risk for hemorrhage, such as those with severe uncontrolled hypertension, bacterial endocarditis, congenital or acquired bleeding disorders, active ulceration, angiodysplastic GI disease, or hemorrhagic CVA; also use with extreme caution shortly after brain, spinal, or ophthalmic surgery. Monitor vital signs.

• **Alert:** Patients receiving low-molecular-weight heparins or heparinoids who have epidural or spinal anesthesia or spinal puncture are at risk for developing epidural or spinal hematoma that can result in long-term paralysis. Risk increases with use of epidural catheters, drugs affecting hemostasis, or traumatic or repeated epidural or spinal punctures. Monitor these patients frequently for signs of neurologic impairment. Urgent treatment is needed.

• Use with caution in patients with bleeding diathesis, thrombocytopenia, platelet defects, severe hepatic or renal insufficiency, hypertension or diabetic retinopathy, or recent GI bleeding.

• DVT is a risk factor in patients who are candidates for therapy, including those older than age 40, those who are obese, those undergoing surgery under general anesthesia lasting longer than 30 minutes, and those who have additional risk factors (such as malignancy or history of DVT or pulmonary embolism).

• Have patient assume a sitting or supine position when administering drug. Give S.C. injection deeply. Injection sites include a U-shaped area around the navel, upper outer side of thigh, and upper outer quadrangle of buttock. Rotate sites daily. When area around the navel or thigh is used, use thumb and forefinger to lift up a fold of skin while giving injection. The entire length of needle should be inserted at a 45- to 90-degree angle.

• Never give drug I.M.

• Don't mix with other injections or infusions unless specific compatibility data support such mixing.

• Multidose vial shouldn't be used in pregnant women.

• **Alert:** Drug isn't interchangeable (unit for unit) with unfractionated heparin or other low-molecular-weight heparin.

• Periodic, routine CBC and fecal occult blood tests are recommended during ther-

apy. Patients don't need regular monitoring of PT or activated PTT.
• Monitor patient closely for thrombocytopenia.
• Drug should be discontinued if a thromboembolic event occurs despite dalteparin prophylaxis.

PATIENT TEACHING
• Instruct patient and family to watch for and report signs of bleeding (bruising and blood in stools).
• Tell patient to avoid OTC drugs containing aspirin or other salicylates unless ordered by prescriber.

---

danaparoid sodium
Orgaran

Pregnancy risk category B

AVAILABLE FORMS
Ampule: 750 anti-Xa units/0.6 ml
Syringe: 750 anti-Xa units/0.6 ml

INDICATIONS & DOSAGES
➤ **Prevention of postoperative deep vein thrombosis (DVT) in patients undergoing elective hip replacement surgery—**
Adults: 750 anti-Xa units S.C. b.i.d. starting 1 to 4 hours preoperatively, and then no sooner than 2 hours after surgery. Treatment continued for 7 to 10 days postoperatively or until risk of DVT has diminished.

ACTION
Prevents fibrin formation by inhibiting generation of thrombin by factor Xa and factor IIa.

Route	Onset	Peak	Duration
S.C.	Unknown	2-5 hr	Unknown

ADVERSE REACTIONS
CNS: insomnia, headache, asthenia, dizziness.
CV: peripheral edema, *hemorrhage.*
GI: *nausea, constipation,* vomiting.
GU: urinary tract infection, urine retention.
Hematologic: anemia.
Musculoskeletal: joint disorder.

Skin: rash, pruritus.
Other: *fever, injection site pain,* infection.

INTERACTIONS
Drug-drug. *Oral anticoagulants, platelet inhibitors:* May increase risk of bleeding. Use together cautiously. Monitor PT and INR.

EFFECTS ON LAB TEST RESULTS
• May decrease hemoglobin.

CONTRAINDICATIONS
Contraindicated in patients hypersensitive to drug or pork products and in those with severe hemorrhagic diathesis (such as hemophilia or idiopathic thrombocytopenic purpura), active major bleeding, or thrombocytopenia and antiplatelet antibodies in presence of drug.

NURSING CONSIDERATIONS
• Use with extreme caution in patients at increased risk for hemorrhage, such as those with severe uncontrolled hypertension, acute bacterial endocarditis, congenital or acquired bleeding disorders, active ulcerative and angiodysplastic GI disease, nonhemorrhagic CVA, or postoperative indwelling epidural catheter; also use with extreme caution shortly after brain, spinal, or ophthalmic surgery. Monitor vital signs.
• *Alert:* Drug contains sodium sulfite, which can cause allergic reactions in some people, especially asthmatics.
• Use with caution in patients with impaired renal function.
• Drug should be used in pregnancy only if clearly needed. Use cautiously in breast-feeding women.
• Safety and effectiveness of drug in children haven't been established.
• Danaparoid should never be given I.M. To give drug, have patient lie down. Give S.C. injection deeply using a 25G to 26G needle. Alternate injection sites between the left and right anterolateral and posterolateral abdominal wall. Gently pull up a skinfold with thumb and forefinger and insert entire length of needle into tissue. Don't rub afterward.
• *Alert:* Drug isn't interchangeable (unit for unit) with heparin or low-molecular-weight heparin.

• *Alert:* Patients receiving low-molecular-weight heparins or heparinoids who have epidural or spinal anesthesia or spinal puncture are at risk for developing epidural or spinal hematoma that can result in long-term paralysis. Risk increases with use of epidural catheters, drugs affecting hemostasis, or traumatic or repeated epidural or spinal punctures. Monitor these patients frequently for signs of neurologic impairment. Urgent treatment is needed.

• Periodic, routine CBC (including platelet count) and fecal occult blood tests are recommended during therapy. Patients don't need regular monitoring of PT and PTT.

• Drug has little effect on PT, PTT, fibrinolytic activity, or bleeding time. Drug may cause unreliable PT and Thrombotest results within 5 hours after administration.

• *Alert:* Monitor patient's hematocrit and blood pressure closely; a decrease in either may signal hemorrhage.

• If serious bleeding occurs, drug should be stopped and blood products transfused. There is no evidence that protamine sulfate is effective in reversing bleeding induced by danaparoid.

• Store ampules at room temperature; syringes should be refrigerated at 36° to 46° F (2° to 8° C). Protect drug from light.

PATIENT TEACHING
• Instruct patient and family to watch for and report signs of bleeding or abnormal bruising.

• Tell patient to avoid OTC drugs containing aspirin or other salicylates unless ordered by prescriber.

---

enoxaparin sodium
Lovenox

Pregnancy risk category B

AVAILABLE FORMS
Injection: 30-mg/0.3 ml, 40-mg/0.4 ml, 60-mg/0.6 ml, 80-mg/0.8 ml, 100-mg/1 ml ampules and syringes

INDICATIONS & DOSAGES
➤ **Prevention of pulmonary embolism and deep vein thrombosis (DVT) after hip or knee replacement surgery—**
Adults: 30 mg S.C. q 12 hours for 7 to 10 days. Give initial dose between 12 and 24 hours postoperatively, provided hemostasis has been established. Treatment should continue during postoperative period until risk of DVT has diminished. Hip replacement patients may receive 40 mg S.C. given 12 hours preoperatively. After initial phase of therapy, hip replacement patients should continue with 40 mg S.C. daily for 3 weeks.
➤ **Prevention of pulmonary embolism and DVT after abdominal surgery—**
Adults: 40 mg S.C. daily with initial dose 2 hours before surgery. Give subsequent dose, provided hemostasis has been established, 24 hours after initial preoperative dose and continue once daily for 7 to 10 days. Continue treatment during postoperative period until risk of DVT has diminished.
➤ **Prevention of ischemic complications of unstable angina and non–Q-wave MI with oral aspirin therapy—**
Adults: 1 mg/kg S.C. q 12 hours until clinical stabilization (minimum 2 days) with aspirin 100 to 325 mg P.O. once daily.
➤ **Inpatient treatment of acute DVT with and without pulmonary embolism when administered with warfarin sodium—**
Adults: 1 mg/kg S.C. q 12 hours; or, 1.5 mg/kg S.C. once daily (at same time daily) for 5 to 7 days until therapeutic oral anticoagulant effect (INR 2 to 3) has been achieved. Warfarin sodium therapy is usually initiated within 72 hours of enoxaparin injection.
➤ **Outpatient treatment of acute DVT without pulmonary embolism when administered with warfarin sodium—**
Adults: 1 mg/kg S.C. q 12 hours for 5 to 7 days until therapeutic oral anticoagulant effect (INR 2 to 3) has been achieved. Warfarin sodium therapy is usually initiated within 72 hours of enoxaparin injection.
Adjust-a-dose: If patient weighs less than 45 kg (99 lb) or has a creatinine clearance of less than 30 ml/minute, decrease dose.

ACTION

A low-molecular-weight heparin derivative that accelerates formation of antithrombin III–thrombin complex and deactivates thrombin, preventing conversion of fibrinogen to fibrin. Has a higher antifactor Xa–to–antifactor IIa activity ratio.

Route	Onset	Peak	Duration
S.C.	Unknown	3-5 hr	24 hr

ADVERSE REACTIONS

CV: edema, peripheral edema.
GI: nausea.
Hematologic: hypochromic anemia, *thrombocytopenia, hemorrhage,* ecchymoses, bleeding complications.
Skin: irritation, pain, hematoma, and erythema at injection site; *rash; urticaria.*
Other: fever, pain, *angioedema, anaphylaxis.*

INTERACTIONS

Drug-drug. *Anticoagulants, antiplatelet drugs, NSAIDs:* Increased risk of bleeding.

EFFECTS ON LAB TEST RESULTS

• May increase ALT and AST levels.
• May decrease hemoglobin.

CONTRAINDICATIONS

Contraindicated in patients hypersensitive to drug, heparin, or pork products; in those with active major bleeding; and in those with thrombocytopenia and antiplatelet antibodies in presence of drug.

NURSING CONSIDERATIONS

• Use with extreme caution in patients with history of heparin-induced thrombocytopenia, aneurysms, cerebrovascular hemorrhage, spinal or epidural punctures (as with anesthesia), uncontrolled hypertension, or threatened abortion.
• The vascular access sheath for instrumentation should remain in place for 6 to 8 hours after a dose, and next dose should be given no sooner than 6 to 8 hours after sheath removal. Monitor vital signs.
• Use cautiously in elderly patients and in those with conditions that place them at increased risk for hemorrhage, such as bacterial endocarditis, congenital or acquired bleeding disorders, ulcer disease, angiodysplastic GI disease, hemorrhagic CVA, or recent spinal, eye, or brain surgery. Also, use cautiously in patients with regional or lumbar block anesthesia, blood dyscrasias, recent childbirth, pericarditis or pericardial effusion, renal insufficiency, or severe CNS trauma.
• *Alert:* Patients receiving low-molecular-weight heparins or heparinoids who have epidural or spinal anesthesia or spinal puncture are at risk for developing epidural or spinal hematoma that can result in long-term paralysis. Risk increases with use of epidural catheters, drugs affecting hemostasis, or traumatic or repeated epidural or spinal punctures. Monitor these patients frequently for signs of neurologic impairment. Urgent treatment is needed.
• Draw blood to establish baseline coagulation parameters before therapy.
• Never give drug I.M.
• *Alert:* Don't try to expel the air bubble from the 30- or 40-mg prefilled syringes. This may lead to loss of drug and an incorrect dosage administration.
• Don't massage after S.C. injection. Watch for signs of bleeding at site. Rotate sites and keep record.
• Avoid excessive I.M. injections of other drugs to prevent or minimize hematomas. If possible, don't give I.M. injections at all.
• Monitor platelet counts regularly. Patients with normal coagulation won't need close monitoring of PT or PTT.
• Regularly inspect patient for bleeding gums, bruises on arms or legs, petechiae, nosebleeds, melena, tarry stools, hematuria, hematemesis.
• To treat severe overdose, give protamine sulfate (a heparin antagonist) by slow I.V. infusion at concentration of 1% to equal dose of drug injected.
• *Alert:* Enoxaparin isn't interchangeable with heparin or other low-molecular-weight heparins.

PATIENT TEACHING

• Instruct patient and family to watch for signs of bleeding or abnormal bruising and to notify prescriber immediately if any occur.

---

*Liquid contains alcohol.   **May contain tartrazine.   †Canada   ‡Australia   §U.K.   ◊OTC

• Tell patient to avoid OTC drugs containing aspirin or other salicylates unless ordered by prescriber.

---

heparin calcium‡
Uniparin-Ca‡

heparin sodium
Hepalean†, Heparin Leo†, Heparin Lock Flush Solution (with Tubex), Heparin Sodium Injection, Hep-Lock, Hep-Pak, Monoparin§, Multiparin§, Pump-Hep§, Unihep§, Uniparin‡

Pregnancy risk category C

AVAILABLE FORMS
Products are derived from beef lung or pork intestinal mucosa.
heparin calcium‡
Ampule: 12,500 units/0.5 ml; 20,000 units/0.8 ml
Syringe: 5,000 units/0.2 ml
heparin sodium
Carpuject: 10,000 units/ml
Disposable syringes: 1,000 units/ml, 2,500 units/ml, 5,000 units/ml, 7,500 units/ml, 10,000 units/ml, 15,000 units/ml, 20,000 units/ml, 40,000 units/ml
Premixed I.V. solutions: 1,000 units in 500 ml of normal saline solution; 2,000 units in 1,000 ml of normal saline solution; 12,500 units in 250 ml of half-normal saline solution; 25,000 units in 250 ml of half-normal saline solution; 25,000 units in 500 ml of half-normal saline solution; 10,000 units in 100 ml of D_5W; 12,500 units in 250 ml of D_5W; 20,000 units in 500 ml of D_5W; 25,000 units in 250 ml D_5W; 25,000 units in 500 ml D_5W
Unit-dose vials: 1,000 units/ml, 5,000 units/ml, 10,000 units/ml, 20,000 units/ml, 40,000 units/ml
Vials: 1,000 units/ml, 2,000 units/ml, 2,500 units/ml, 5,000 units/ml, 7,500 units/ml, 10,000 units/ml, 20,000 units/ml, 40,000 units/ml
heparin sodium flush
Disposable syringes: 10 units/ml, 100 units/ml
Vials: 10 units/ml, 100 units/ml

INDICATIONS & DOSAGES
Dosage is highly individualized depending on disease state, age, and renal and hepatic status.
➤ **Full-dose continuous I.V. infusion therapy for deep vein thrombosis (DVT), MI, pulmonary embolism—**
Adults: Initially, 5,000 units by I.V. bolus; then 750 to 1,500 units/hour by I.V. infusion with pump. Hourly rate titrated based on PTT results (q 4 hours in the early stages of treatment).
Children: Initially, 50 units/kg I.V.; then 25 units/kg/hour or 20,000 U/m² daily by I.V. infusion pump. Dosage titrated based on PTT.
➤ **Full-dose S.C. therapy for DVT, MI, pulmonary embolism—**
Adults: Initially, 5,000 units I.V. bolus and 10,000 to 20,000 units in a concentrated solution S.C.; then 8,000 to 10,000 units S.C. q 8 hours or 15,000 to 20,000 units in a concentrated solution q 12 hours.
➤ **Full-dose intermittent I.V. therapy for DVT, MI, pulmonary embolism—**
Adults: Initially, 10,000 units by I.V. bolus; then titrated according to PTT, and 5,000 to 10,000 units I.V. q 4 to 6 hours.
Children: Initially, 100 units/kg by I.V. bolus; then 50 to 100 units/kg q 4 hours.
➤ **Fixed low-dose therapy for venous thrombosis, pulmonary embolism, atrial fibrillation with embolism, postoperative DVT, and prevention of embolism—**
Adults: 5,000 units S.C. q 12 hours. In surgical patients, first dose given 2 hours before procedure; then 5,000 units S.C. q 8 to 12 hours for 5 to 7 days or until patient can walk.
➤ **Consumptive coagulopathy (such as disseminated intravascular coagulation)—**
Adults: 50 to 100 units/kg by I.V. bolus or continuous I.V. infusion q 4 hours.
Children: 25 to 50 units/kg by I.V. bolus or continuous I.V. infusion q 4 hours. If no improvement within 4 to 8 hours, discontinue heparin.
➤ **Open-heart surgery—**
Adults: (Total body perfusion) 150 to 300 units/kg continuous I.V. infusion.

> **Patency maintenance of I.V. in-dwelling catheters—**
Adults: 10 to 100 units I.V. flush. Use sufficient volume to fill device. Not intended for therapeutic use.

I.V. ADMINISTRATION
• Administer I.V. using infusion pump to provide maximum safety because of long-term effect and irregular absorption when given S.C. Check constant I.V. infusions regularly, even when pumps are in good working order, to prevent overdose or underdose. Place notice above patient's bed to caution I.V. team or laboratory personnel to apply pressure dressings after taking blood.
• During intermittent I.V. therapy, always draw blood 30 minutes before next scheduled dose to avoid falsely elevated PTT. Blood for PTT may be drawn 4 hours after continuous I.V. heparin therapy starts. Blood for PTT should never be drawn from the I.V. tubing of the heparin infusion or from the infused vein. Falsely elevated PTT will result. Always draw blood from the opposite arm.
• Don't skip a dose or "catch up" with an I.V. solution containing heparin. If I.V. solution runs out, restart it as soon as possible, and reschedule bolus dose immediately.
• Concentrated heparin solutions (more than 100 units/ml) can irritate blood vessels.
• Never piggyback other drugs into an infusion line while heparin infusion is running. Never mix another drug and heparin in same syringe when giving a bolus.

ACTION
Accelerates formation of antithrombin III–thrombin complex and deactivates thrombin, preventing conversion of fibrinogen to fibrin.

Route	Onset	Peak	Duration
I.V.	Immediate	Unknown	Variable
S.C.	20-60 min	2-4 hr	Variable

ADVERSE REACTIONS
EENT: rhinitis.
Hematologic: *hemorrhage, overly prolonged clotting time, thrombocytopenia.*

Skin: irritation, mild pain, hematoma, ulceration, cutaneous or S.C. necrosis, pruritus, urticaria.
Other: *white clot syndrome;* hypersensitivity reactions, including chills, fever, *anaphylactoid reactions.*

INTERACTIONS
Drug-drug. *Oral anticoagulants:* Increased additive anticoagulation. Monitor PT, INR, and PTT.
Salicylates, other antiplatelet drugs: Increased anticoagulant effect. Avoid using together.
Thrombolytics: Increased risk of hemorrhage. Monitor patient closely.
Drug-herb. *Garlic, ginkgo, motherwort, red clover, white willow:* May increase risk of bleeding. Discourage using together.

EFFECTS ON LAB TEST RESULTS
• May increase ALT and AST levels.
• May increase INR, PT, and PTT. May decrease platelets.

CONTRAINDICATIONS
Contraindicated in patients hypersensitive to drug. Conditionally contraindicated in patients with active bleeding, blood dyscrasia, or bleeding tendencies, such as hemophilia, thrombocytopenia, or hepatic disease with hypoprothrombinemia; suspected intracranial hemorrhage; suppurative thrombophlebitis; inaccessible ulcerative lesions (especially of GI tract) and open ulcerative wounds; extensive denudation of skin; ascorbic acid deficiency and other conditions that cause increased capillary permeability. Also conditionally contraindicated during or after brain, eye, or spinal cord surgery; during spinal tap or spinal anesthesia; during continuous tube drainage of stomach or small intestine; in subacute bacterial endocarditis, shock, advanced renal disease, threatened abortion, or severe hypertension.

Although heparin use is clearly hazardous in these conditions, its risks and benefits must be evaluated.

NURSING CONSIDERATIONS
• Use cautiously during menses and in patients with mild hepatic or renal disease, alcoholism, occupations with high risk of physical injury, or history of allergies,

---

*Liquid contains alcohol.   **May contain tartrazine.   †Canada   ‡Australia   §U.K.   ◊OTC

asthma, or GI ulcerations; also use cautiously immediately postpartum.
• Draw blood to establish baseline coagulation parameters before therapy.
• Drug may cause false elevations in some tests for thyroxine levels.
• When patient needs anticoagulation during pregnancy, most prescribers use heparin.
• Some commercially available heparin injections contain benzyl alcohol. These products should be avoided in neonates and pregnant women if possible.
• Drug requirements are higher in early phases of thrombogenic diseases and febrile states; they're lower when patient's condition stabilizes.
• Elderly patients should usually start at lower dosage.
• Check order and vial carefully; heparin comes in various concentrations.
• *Alert:* USP units and IU aren't equivalent for heparin.
• *Alert:* Heparin, low-molecular-weight heparins, and danaparoid aren't interchangeable.
• Give low-dose injections sequentially between iliac crests in lower abdomen deep into S.C. fat. Inject drug S.C. slowly into fat pad. Leave needle in place for 10 seconds after injection; then withdraw needle. Don't massage after S.C. injection, and watch for signs of bleeding at injection site. Alternate sites every 12 hours—right for morning, left for evening.
• PTT should be drawn 4 to 6 hours after dose administered by S.C. injection.
• Avoid excessive I.M. injections of other drugs to prevent or minimize hematomas. If possible, don't give I.M. injections at all.
• Measure PTT carefully and regularly. Anticoagulation is present when PTT values are 1½ to 2 times the control values.
• Monitor platelet count regularly. When new thrombosis accompanies thrombocytopenia (white clot syndrome), discontinue heparin.
• Regularly inspect patient for bleeding gums, bruises on arms or legs, petechiae, nosebleeds, melena, tarry stools, hematuria, and hematemesis.
• Monitor vital signs.
• *Alert:* To treat severe heparin calcium or sodium overdose, use protamine sulfate, a heparin antagonist. Dosage is based on the dose of heparin, its route of administration, and the time elapsed since it was given. Generally, 1 to 1.5 mg of protamine/100 units of heparin is given if only a few minutes have elapsed; 0.5 to 0.75 mg protamine/100 units heparin if 30 to 60 minutes have elapsed; 0.25 to 0.375 mg protamine/100 units heparin if 2 hours or more have elapsed. Don't give more than 50 mg protamine in a 10-minute period.
• Abrupt withdrawal may cause increased coagulability; warfarin therapy usually overlaps heparin therapy for continuation of prophylaxis or treatment.

PATIENT TEACHING
• Instruct patient and family to watch for signs of bleeding or bruising and to notify prescriber immediately if any occur.
• Tell patient to avoid OTC drugs containing aspirin, other salicylates, or drugs that may interact with heparin unless ordered by prescriber.

✳ *NEW DRUG*

---

tinzaparin sodium
Innohep

Pregnancy risk category B

AVAILABLE FORMS
Injection: 20,000 anti-Xa IU/ml, in 2-ml vials

INDICATIONS & DOSAGES
➤ **Symptomatic deep vein thrombosis with or without pulmonary embolism with warfarin sodium—**
Adults: 175 anti-Xa IU/kg of body weight S.C. once daily for at least 6 days and until patient is adequately anticoagulated with warfarin sodium (INR of at least 2.0) for 2 consecutive days. Initiate warfarin sodium therapy when appropriate, usually within 1 to 3 days of tinzaparin initiation. Volume of dose to be given may be calculated as follows:
Patient weight in kg $\times$ 0.00875 ml/kg = volume to be administered in ml.

ACTION
A low-molecular-weight heparin that inhibits reactions that lead to blood clotting,

---

Reactions may be *common*, uncommon, *life-threatening*, or COMMON AND LIFE-THREATENING.

including formation of fibrin clots. Also acts as a potent coinhibitor of several activated coagulation factors, especially factors Xa and IIa (thrombin). Drug binds antithrombin, thereby increasing ability to inactivate coagulation enzymes factor Xa and thrombin. Drug also induces release of tissue factor pathway inhibitor, which may contribute to the antithrombotic effect.

Route	Onset	Peak	Duration
S.C.	2-3 hr	4-5 hr	18-24 hr

ADVERSE REACTIONS

CNS: headache, dizziness, insomnia, confusion, *cerebral or intracranial bleeding.*
CV: *arrhythmias,* chest pain, hypotension, hypertension, *pulmonary embolism, MI, thromboembolism,* tachycardia, dependent edema, angina pectoris.
EENT: epistaxis, ocular hemorrhage.
GI: anorectal bleeding, constipation, flatulence, hematemesis, hemarthrosis, *GI hemorrhage,* nausea, vomiting, dyspepsia, retroperitoneal or intra-abdominal bleeding.
GU: dysuria, hematuria, urinary tract infection, urine retention, *vaginal hemorrhage.*
Hematologic: *granulocytopenia, thrombocytopenia,* anemia, *agranulocytosis, pancytopenia, hemorrhage.*
Musculoskeletal: back pain.
Respiratory: pneumonia, respiratory disorder, dyspnea.
Skin: bullous eruption, cellulitis, *injection site hematoma,* pruritus, purpura, rash, melena, skin necrosis, wound hematoma, bullous eruption.
Other: hypersensitivity reaction, *spinal or epidural hematoma,* fever, pain, infection, impaired healing, *allergic reaction,* congenital anomaly, *fetal death,* fetal distress.

INTERACTIONS

Drug-drug. *Oral anticoagulants, platelet inhibitors (such as dextran, dipyridamole, NSAIDs, salicylates, sulfinpyrazone), thrombolytics:* May increase risk of bleeding. Use together cautiously. If drugs must be given together, monitor patient.

EFFECTS ON LAB TEST RESULTS
• May increase AST and ALT levels.

• May decrease hemoglobin and granulocyte, platelet, RBC, and WBC count.

CONTRAINDICATIONS
Contraindicated in patients hypersensitive to tinzaparin sodium, heparin, sulfites, benzyl alcohol, or pork products. Also contraindicated in patients with active major bleeding and in those with history of heparin-induced thrombocytopenia.

NURSING CONSIDERATIONS
• Use cautiously in patients with increased risk of hemorrhage, such as those with bacterial endocarditis; uncontrolled hypertension; diabetic retinopathy; congenital or acquired bleeding disorders, including hepatic failure and amyloidosis; GI ulceration; or hemorrhagic stroke.
• Use cautiously in patients who have recently undergone brain, spinal, or ophthalmologic surgery, and in patients being treated with platelet inhibitors.
• Elderly patients and patients with renal insufficiency may show reduced elimination of drug. Use drug with care in these patients.
• It's unknown if drug appears in breast milk. Use cautiously in breast-feeding patients.
• Drug isn't intended for I.M. or I.V. administration, nor should it be mixed with other injections or infusions.
• Don't interchange drug (unit to unit) with heparin or other low-molecular-weight heparins.
• When giving drug, have patient lie or sit down. Give by deep S.C. injection into abdominal wall. Introduce whole length of needle into skinfold held between thumb and forefinger. Make sure to hold skinfold throughout injection. Rotate injection sites between right and left anterolateral and posterolateral abdominal wall. To minimize bruising, don't rub injection site after administration.
• Use an appropriate calibrated syringe to ensure correct withdrawal of volume of drug from vials.
• Monitor platelet count during therapy. Stop drug if platelet count falls below 100,000/mm³.
• Periodically monitor CBC count and stool tests for occult blood during treatment.

• Drug may affect PT and INR levels. Patient also receiving warfarin should have blood for PT and INR drawn just before next scheduled dose of tinzaparin.

• Drug contains sodium metabisulfite, which may cause allergic reactions in susceptible people.

• *Alert:* When neuraxial anesthesia (epidural or spinal anesthesia) or spinal puncture is used, patient is at risk for developing spinal hematoma, which can result in long-term or permanent paralysis. Watch for signs and symptoms of neurologic impairment. Consider risk versus benefit of neuraxial intervention in patient being anticoagulated with low-molecular-weight heparins or heparinoids.

• If patient becomes pregnant while taking drug, she should be notified of potential hazards to fetus. Cases of gasping syndrome have occurred in premature infants when large amounts of benzyl alcohol have been administered.

• Store drug at room temperature.

PATIENT TEACHING

• Explain to patient importance of laboratory monitoring to ensure effectiveness of drugs while maintaining safety.

• Teach patient warning signs of bleeding and instruct him to report these signs immediately.

• Caution patient to take such safety measures as using soft toothbrush and electric razor to prevent cuts and bruises.

• Instruct patient that warfarin therapy will be started when appropriate, within 1 to 3 days of tinzaparin administration. Explain importance of warfarin therapy and monitoring to ensure safety and efficacy.

---

warfarin sodium
Coumadin, Warfilone†

Pregnancy risk category X

AVAILABLE FORMS
Injection: 2 mg/ml (powder)
Tablets: 1 mg, 2 mg, 2.5 mg, 3 mg, 4 mg, 5 mg, 6 mg, 7.5 mg, 10 mg

INDICATIONS & DOSAGES
➤ **Pulmonary embolism with deep vein thrombosis, MI, rheumatic heart dis-**ease with heart valve damage, prosthetic heart valves, chronic atrial fibrillation—
Adults: 2 to 5 mg P.O. daily for 2 to 4 days; then dosage based on daily PT and INR. Usual maintenance dosage is 2 to 10 mg P.O. daily; I.V. dosage is same as that used P.O.

I.V. ADMINISTRATION
• I.V. form may be ordered in rare instances when oral therapy can't be given. Reconstitute powder with 2.7 ml sterile water, or as instructed in manufacturer guidelines. Give I.V. as a slow bolus injection over 1 to 2 minutes into a peripheral vein.

• Because onset of action is delayed, heparin sodium is often given during first few days of treatment. When heparin is being given simultaneously, blood for PT and INR shouldn't be drawn within 5 hours of intermittent I.V. heparin administration. However, blood for PT and INR may be drawn at any time during continuous heparin infusion.

ACTION
Inhibits vitamin K–dependent activation of clotting factors II, VII, IX, and X, formed in the liver.

Route	Onset	Peak	Duration
I.V.	Unknown	Unknown	Unknown
P.O.	0.5-3 days	Unknown	2-5 days

ADVERSE REACTIONS
CNS: headache.
GI: anorexia, nausea, vomiting, cramps, *diarrhea,* mouth ulcerations, sore mouth, melena.
GU: hematuria, excessive menstrual bleeding.
Hematologic: *hemorrhage.*
Hepatic: *hepatitis,* jaundice.
Skin: dermatitis, urticaria, necrosis, gangrene, alopecia, *rash.*
Other: *fever,* enhanced uric acid excretion.

INTERACTIONS
Drug-drug. *Acetaminophen:* May increase bleeding with long-term therapy (more than 2 weeks) at high doses (more

---

Reactions may be *common,* uncommon, *life-threatening,* or COMMON AND LIFE-THREATENING.

than 2 g/day) of acetaminophen. Monitor patient very carefully.

Allopurinol, amiodarone, anabolic steroids, cephalosporins, chloramphenicol, cimetidine, ciprofloxacin, clofibrate, danazol, diazoxide, diflunisal, disulfiram, erythromycin, ethacrynic acid, fenoprofen calcium, fluconazole, fluoroquinolones, glucagon, heparin, ibuprofen, influenza virus vaccine, isoniazid, itraconazole, ketoprofen, lovastatin, meclofenamate, methimazole, methylthiouracil, metronidazole, miconazole, nalidixic acid, neomycin (oral), norfloxacin, ofloxacin, omeprazole, pentoxifylline, propafenone, propoxyphene, propylthiouracil, quinidine, simvastatin, streptokinase, sulfinpyrazone, sulfonamides, sulindac, tamoxifen, tetracyclines, thiazides, thyroid drugs, TCAs, urokinase, vitamin E: Increased PT and INR. Monitor patient carefully for bleeding. Reduce anticoagulant dosage as directed.

Anticonvulsants: Increased levels of phenytoin and phenobarbital. Monitor drug levels closely.

Barbiturates, carbamazepine, corticosteroids, corticotropin, dicloxacillin, ethchlorvynol, griseofulvin, haloperidol, meprobamate, mercaptopurine, methaqualone, nafcillin, oral contraceptives containing estrogen, rifampin, spironolactone, sucralfate, trazodone: Decreased PT and INR with reduced anticoagulant effect. Monitor patient carefully.

Chloral hydrate, glutethimide, propylthiouracil, sulfinpyrazone: Increased or decreased PT. Avoid using, if possible, and monitor patient carefully.

Cholestyramine: Decreased response when administered too closely together. Give 6 hours after oral anticoagulants.

NSAIDs, salicylates: Increased PT and INR; ulcerogenic effects. Avoid using together.

Sulfonylureas (oral antidiabetics): Increased hypoglycemic response. Monitor glucose levels.

Drug-herb. *Angelica:* Significantly prolonged PT when *Angelica sinensis* is given with warfarin. Discourage using together.

Anise, arnica flower, asafoetida, bromelain, celery, chamomile, clove, Danshen, devil's claw, dong quai, fenugreek, fever- *few, garlic, ginger, ginkgo, horse chestnut, licorice, meadowsweet, motherwort, onion, papain, parsley, passion flower, quassia, red clover, reishi mushroom, rue, sweet clover, turmeric, white willow:* May increase risk of bleeding. Discourage using together.

Coenzyme Q10, ginseng, St. John's wort: May reduce action of drug. Ask patient about use of herbal remedies, and advise caution.

Green tea: Decreased anticoagulant effect caused by vitamin K content of green tea. Advise patient to minimize variable consumption of green tea and other foods or nutritional supplements containing vitamin K.

Drug-food. *Foods, multivitamins, or enteral products containing vitamin K:* May impair anticoagulation. Tell patient to maintain consistent daily intake of leafy green vegetables.

Drug-lifestyle. *Alcohol use:* Enhanced anticoagulant effects may occur. Tell patient to avoid large amounts of alcohol.

EFFECTS ON LAB TEST RESULTS
● May increase ALT and AST levels.
● May increase INR, PT, and PTT.

CONTRAINDICATIONS
Contraindicated in patients hypersensitive to drug and in those with bleeding from the GI, GU, or respiratory tract; aneurysm; cerebrovascular hemorrhage; severe or malignant hypertension; severe renal or hepatic disease; subacute bacterial endocarditis, pericarditis, or pericardial effusion; or blood dyscrasias or hemorrhagic tendencies. Also contraindicated during pregnancy, threatened abortion, eclampsia, or preeclampsia, and after recent surgery involving large open areas, eye, brain, or spinal cord; recent prostatectomy; major regional lumbar block anesthesia, spinal puncture, or diagnostic or therapeutic invasive procedures.

Avoid using in patients with a history of warfarin-induced necrosis; in unsupervised patients with senility, alcoholism, or psychosis; or in situations in which there are inadequate laboratory facilities for coagulation testing.

NURSING CONSIDERATIONS

• Use cautiously in patients with diverticulitis, colitis, mild or moderate hypertension, or mild or moderate hepatic or renal disease; with drainage tubes in any orifice; with regional or lumbar block anesthesia; or in conditions that increase risk of hemorrhage; also use cautiously in breastfeeding women.

• Draw blood to establish baseline coagulation parameters before therapy.

• PT and INR determinations are essential for proper control. Prescribers typically try to maintain PT at 1½ to 2 times normal. There is a high risk of bleeding when PT exceeds 2½ times the control values.

• Give warfarin at same time daily. INR range for chronic atrial fibrillation is 2 to 3.

• I.M. administration isn't recommended.

• Regularly inspect patient for bleeding gums, bruises on arms or legs, petechiae, nosebleeds, melena, tarry stools, hematuria, and hematemesis.

• Observe breast-fed infants of women on drug for unexpected bleeding.

• *Alert:* Withhold drug and call prescriber at once if fever or rash (signs of severe adverse reactions) occurs.

• Half-life of warfarin's anticoagulant effect is 36 to 44 hours. Effect can be neutralized by vitamin K injections or oral vitamin K.

• Drug is best oral anticoagulant for patient taking antacids, phenytoin, or fosphenytoin.

• Elderly patients and patients with renal or hepatic failure are especially sensitive to warfarin effect.

• Warfarin can cause false-negative theophylline levels.

PATIENT TEACHING

• Stress importance of complying with prescribed dosage and follow-up appointments. Tell patient to carry a card that identifies his increased risk of bleeding.

• Tell patient and family to watch for signs of bleeding or abnormal bruising and to call prescriber at once if they occur.

• Warn patient to avoid OTC products containing aspirin, other salicylates, or drugs that may interact with warfarin unless ordered by prescriber.

• Tell patient to consult a prescriber before using miconazole vaginal cream or suppositories. Abnormal bleeding and bruising have occurred.

• Instruct woman to notify prescriber if menses is heavier than usual; she may need dosage adjustment.

• Tell patient to use electric razor when shaving to avoid scratching skin, and to use a soft toothbrush.

• Warn patient to read food labels. Food, nutritional supplements, and multivitamins that contain vitamin K may impair anticoagulation.

• Tell patient to eat a daily, consistent amount of leafy green vegetables containing vitamin K. Eating varied amounts daily may alter anticoagulant effects.

65
Blood derivatives

albumin 5%
albumin 25%
antihemophilic factor
anti-inhibitor coagulant complex
antithrombin III, human
factor IX (human)
factor IX complex
plasma protein fractions

COMBINATION PRODUCTS
None.

albumin 5%
Albumarc, Albuminar-5, Albutein 5%, Buminate 5%, Plasbumin-5

albumin 25%
Albumarc, Albuminar-25, Albutein 25%, Buminate 25%, Plasbumin-25

Pregnancy risk category C

AVAILABLE FORMS
albumin 5%
Injection: 50-ml, 250-ml, 500-ml, 1,000-ml vials
albumin 25%
Injection: 20-ml, 50-ml, 100-ml vials

INDICATIONS & DOSAGES
➤ **Hypovolemic shock—**
Adults: Initially, 500 to 750 ml 5% solution by I.V. infusion, repeated q 30 minutes, p.r.n. As plasma volume approaches normal, rate of infusion of 5% solution shouldn't exceed 2 to 4 ml/minute. Or, 100 to 200 ml I.V. of 25% solution, repeated after 10 to 30 minutes, if needed. Dosage varies with patient's condition and response. As plasma volume approaches normal, rate of infusion of 25% solution shouldn't exceed 1 ml/minute.
Children: 12 to 20 ml 5% solution/kg by I.V. infusion, repeated in 15 to 30 minutes if response is inadequate. Or, 2.5 to 5 ml I.V. of 25% solution/kg, repeated after 10 to 30 minutes, if needed.

➤ **Hypoproteinemia—**
Adults: 200 to 300 ml of 25% albumin. Dosage varies with patient's condition and response. Rate of infusion shouldn't exceed 2 to 3 ml/minute.
➤ **Hyperbilirubinemia—**
Infants: 1 g albumin (4 ml 25%)/kg during or 1 to 2 hours before exchange transfusion.

I.V. ADMINISTRATION
• Make sure patient is properly hydrated before infusion.
• To minimize waste, take care when preparing and administering drug. This product is expensive, and supply shortages frequently occur.
• Avoid rapid I.V. infusion. Specific rate is individualized based on patient's age, condition, and diagnosis. Albumin 5% is infused undiluted; albumin 25% may be infused undiluted or diluted with normal saline solution or D₅W injection. Use solution promptly. Discard unused solution. Don't use cloudy solutions or those containing sediment. Solution should be a clear amber color.
• *Alert:* Don't give more than 250 g in 48 hours.

ACTION
Albumin 5% supplies colloid to the blood and expands plasma volume. Albumin 25% provides intravascular oncotic pressure in a 5:1 ratio, causing a fluid shift from interstitial spaces to the circulation and slightly increasing plasma protein level.

Route	Onset	Peak	Duration
I.V.	< 15 min	< 15 min	Several hr

ADVERSE REACTIONS
CNS: headache.
CV: *vascular overload after rapid infusion,* hypotension, tachycardia.
GI: increased salivation, nausea, vomiting.
Musculoskeletal: back pain.
Respiratory: altered respiration, dyspnea, pulmonary edema.
Skin: urticaria, rash.
Other: chills, fever.

---

*Liquid contains alcohol.   **May contain tartrazine.   †Canada   ‡Australia   §U.K.   ◊OTC

INTERACTIONS
Drug-drug. *ACE inhibitors:* Increased risk of atypical reactions. Withhold ACE inhibitors 24 hours before giving albumin, if possible.

EFFECTS ON LAB TEST RESULTS
• May increase albumin level.

CONTRAINDICATIONS
Contraindicated in patients hypersensitive to drug and in those with severe anemia or cardiac failure.

NURSING CONSIDERATIONS
• Use with extreme caution in patients with hypertension, low cardiac reserve, hypervolemia, pulmonary edema, or hypoalbuminemia with peripheral edema.
• Watch for hemorrhage or shock after surgery or injury. Rapid rise in blood pressure may cause bleeding from sites that aren't apparent at lower pressures.
• Monitor vital signs carefully.
• Watch for signs of vascular overload (heart failure or pulmonary edema).
• Monitor fluid intake and output; hemoglobin, hematocrit, protein, and electrolyte levels during therapy.
• Preparations of albumin derived from placental tissue may increase alkaline phosphatase level.
• Follow storage instructions on bottle. Freezing may cause bottle to break.

PATIENT TEACHING
• Explain use and administration of albumin to patient and family.
• Tell patient to report adverse reactions promptly.

---

antihemophilic factor (AHF)
Human: Alphanate, Hemofil M, Humate-P, Koate-DVI, Monarc-M, Monoclate-P

Recombinant: Bioclate, Helixate, Kogenate, Recombinate

Pregnancy risk category C

AVAILABLE FORMS
Injection: vials, with diluent. Units specified on label

INDICATIONS & DOSAGES
➤ **Spontaneous hemorrhage in patients with hemophilia A (factor VIII deficiency)—**
Adults and children: Calculate dosage using this formula:

$$\text{AHF required (IU)} = \text{body weight (kg)} \times \text{desired factor VIII increase (\% of normal)} \times 0.5$$

Note: Severely bleeding patients may require higher doses.

To prevent spontaneous hemorrhage, the desired level of factor VIII is 5% of normal; for mild hemorrhage, 30% of normal; for moderate hemorrhage and minor surgery, 30% to 50% of normal; for severe hemorrhage, 80% to 100% of normal.
➤ **Bleeding in patients with hemophilia A (factor VIII deficiency)—**
Adults and children: For minor hemorrhage into muscle and joints, 8 IU/kg I.V. (or calculated dose to raise plasma factor VIII levels to 20% to 40% of normal) q 8 to 12 hours for 1 to 3 days, as needed. For overt bleeding, initial dose of 15 to 25 IU/kg I.V.; then 8 to 15 IU/kg q 8 to 12 hours for 3 to 4 days. To treat massive bleeding or hemorrhage involving major organs, initial dose of 40 to 50 IU/kg I.V.; then 20 to 25 IU/kg I.V. q 8 to 12 hours. Refer to manufacturer recommendations regarding specific products.
➤ **Prevention of bleeding in hemophilic patients who need surgery—**
Adults: 25 to 30 IU/kg I.V. 1 hour before surgery; then 50% of initial dose 5 hours later. Dosage titrated to achieve a level of AHF 80% to 100% of normal during surgery and maintained at 30% to 60% of normal for at least 10 to 14 days postoperatively.

I.V. ADMINISTRATION
• Refrigerate concentrate until ready to use. Warm concentrate and diluent bottles to room temperature before reconstituting. To mix drug, gently roll vial between hands.
• Use reconstituted solution within 3 hours. Store away from heat and don't refrigerate. Refrigeration after reconstitution may cause active ingredient to precipitate. Don't shake or mix with other I.V. solu-

tions. Solution should be filtered before administration.

● Administer I.V. preparations at 2 ml/minute; may be given up to 10 ml/minute, depending on the preparation being used.

● Take baseline pulse rate before I.V. administration. Use plastic syringe; drug may interact with glass syringe and bind to its surface. If pulse rate increases significantly, flow rate should be reduced or administration stopped.

ACTION
Directly replaces deficient clotting factor.

Route	Onset	Peak	Duration
I.V.	Immediate	1-2 hr	Unknown

ADVERSE REACTIONS
CV: tightness in chest, *thrombosis.*
GI: nausea.
Hematologic: *hemolytic anemia, thrombocytopenia.*
Respiratory: wheezing.
Skin: *urticaria,* stinging at injection site.
Other: *chills, fever,* hypersensitivity reactions, *anaphylaxis, risk of hepatitis B and HIV.*

INTERACTIONS
None significant.

EFFECTS ON LAB TEST RESULTS
● May decrease hemoglobin and platelet count.

CONTRAINDICATIONS
Monoclonally prepared AHF is contraindicated in patients hypersensitive to drug or murine (mouse) protein.

NURSING CONSIDERATIONS
● Use cautiously in neonates, infants, and patients with hepatic disease because of their susceptibility to hepatitis, which may be transmitted in AHF.
● Monitor coagulation studies before therapy.
● Monitor patients with blood types A, B, and AB for possible hemolysis.
● Change in urine color to an orange or red hue can signify a hemolytic reaction.
● Administer hepatitis B vaccine before administering AHF.
● Don't give drug S.C. or I.M.

● Monitor vital signs regularly.
● Monitor coagulation studies frequently during therapy.
● Monitor patient for allergic reactions.
● Some patients develop inhibitors to factor VIII, resulting in decreased response to drug.
● Risk of hepatitis must be weighed against risk of patient not receiving drug.
● Because of manufacturing process, risk of HIV transmission is extremely low.

PATIENT TEACHING
● Explain use and administration of AHF to patient and family.
● Advise patient to report adverse reactions promptly.
● Advise patient to carry or wear medical identification.
● Tell patient to notify prescriber if drug seems less effective; a change may signify the development of antibodies.

anti-inhibitor coagulant complex
Autoplex T, Feiba VH Immuno

Pregnancy risk category C

AVAILABLE FORMS
Injection: Number of units of factor VIII correctional activity indicated on label of vial

INDICATIONS & DOSAGES
➤ **Prevention and control of hemorrhagic episodes in patients with hemophilia A who have developed inhibitor antibodies to antihemophilic factor; management of bleeding in patients with acquired hemophilia who have spontaneously acquired inhibitors to factor VIII—**
Adults and children: Highly individualized and varies among manufacturers. For Autoplex T, 25 to 100 units/kg I.V., depending on severity of hemorrhage. If no hemostatic improvement occurs within 6 hours after initial administration, dosage repeated. For Feiba VH Immuno, 50 to 100 units/kg I.V. q 6 or 12 hours until clear signs of improvement. Maximum daily dose is 200 units/kg.

I.V. ADMINISTRATION
• Warm drug and diluent to room temperature before reconstitution. Reconstitute according to manufacturer's directions. Use filter needle provided by manufacturer to withdraw reconstituted solution from vial into syringe; filter needle should then be replaced with a sterile injection needle for administration. Administer as soon as possible. If drug is given as an I.V. infusion, administration set must contain a filter. Autoplex T infusions should be completed within 1 hour after reconstitution; Feiba VH Immuno infusions, within 3 hours.
• Dosages of the two available products aren't equivalent.
• Individualize rate of administration based on patient's response. Autoplex T infusions may begin at 2 ml/minute; if well tolerated, infusion rate may be increased gradually to 10 ml/minute. Feiba VH Immuno infusion rate shouldn't exceed 2 units/kg/minute.
• *Alert:* If flushing, lethargy, headache, transient chest discomfort, or changes in blood pressure or pulse rate develop because of a rapid infusion, stop drug and notify prescriber. These symptoms usually disappear when infusion stops. The infusion may then be resumed at a slower rate.

ACTION
Unknown. Efficacy may be related in part to presence of activated factors, which leads to more complete factor X activation with tissue factor, phospholipid, and ionic calcium and allows the coagulation process to proceed beyond those stages in which factor VIII is needed.

Route	Onset	Peak	Duration
I.V.	10-30 min	Unknown	Unknown

ADVERSE REACTIONS
CNS: headache, lethargy.
CV: changes in blood pressure, flushing, *acute MI, thromboembolic events.*
GI: nausea, vomiting.
Hematologic: *disseminated intravascular coagulation.*
Skin: rash, urticaria.

Other: fever, chills, hypersensitivity reactions, *anaphylaxis, risk of hepatitis B and HIV.*

INTERACTIONS
Drug-drug. *Antifibrinolytic drugs:* May alter effects of anti-inhibitor coagulant complex. Avoid using together.

EFFECTS ON LAB TEST RESULTS
None reported.

CONTRAINDICATIONS
Contraindicated in patients with disseminated intravascular coagulation or a normal coagulation mechanism and in those showing signs of fibrinolysis.

NURSING CONSIDERATIONS
• Use cautiously in patients with liver disease.
• Administer hepatitis B vaccine before giving drug.
• Keep epinephrine available to treat anaphylaxis.
• Feiba VH Immuno shouldn't be used with newborns, but Autoplex T can be used with caution.
• Monitor patient closely for hypersensitivity reactions.
• Monitor vital signs regularly, and report significant changes to prescriber.
• Observe patient closely for signs of thromboembolic events.
• Reassure patient that, because of manufacturing process, risk of HIV transmission is extremely low.

PATIENT TEACHING
• Explain use and administration of anti-inhibitor coagulant complex to patient and family.
• Tell patient to report adverse reactions promptly.

---

antithrombin III, human (AT-III, heparin cofactor I)
Thrombate III

Pregnancy risk category B

AVAILABLE FORMS
Injection: 500 IU, 1,000 IU

INDICATIONS & DOSAGES
➤ **Thromboembolism related to hereditary AT-III deficiency—**
Adults and children: Initial dose is individualized to quantity needed to increase AT-III activity to 120% of normal activity as determined 30 minutes after administration. Usual dose is 50 to 100 IU/minute I.V., not to exceed 100 IU/minute. Dose is calculated based on anticipated 1.4 % increase in plasma AT-III activity produced by 1 IU/kg of body weight using the formula:

$$\text{Dose required (IU)} = \frac{(\text{desired activity [\%]} - \text{baseline activity [\%]}) \times \text{weight (kg)}}{1.4}$$

Maintenance dose is individualized to quantity needed to increase AT-III activity to 80% of normal activity and is administered at 24-hour intervals.

To calculate subsequent dosages, multiply desired AT-III activity (as percentage of normal) minus baseline AT-III activity (as percentage of normal) by body weight (in kg). Divide by actual increase in AT-III activity (as percentage) produced by 1 IU/kg as determined 30 minutes after initial dose is given.

I.V. ADMINISTRATION
● Reconstitute using 10 ml of sterile water (provided), normal saline solution, or D_5W. Don't shake vial. Withdraw the dissolved solution using the manufacturer-provided filter needle. Dilute further in same diluent solution if desired. Infuse over 10 to 20 minutes. Give I.V. only. Don't mix with other medication or diluents. Administer within 3 hours after reconstitution.

ACTION
Replaces deficient AT-III in patients with hereditary AT-III deficiency, normalizing coagulation inhibition and inhibiting thromboembolism formation. Also deactivates plasmin (to lesser extent than clotting factor).

Route	Onset	Peak	Duration
I.V.	Immediate	Unknown	4 days

ADVERSE REACTIONS
CNS: dizziness.
CV: vasodilation, lowered blood pressure, chest tightness.
GI: nausea, foul taste.
GU: diuresis.
Other: chills.

INTERACTIONS
Drug-drug. *Heparin:* Increased anticoagulant effect of both drugs. Heparin dosage reduction may be needed.

EFFECTS ON LAB TEST RESULTS
None reported.

CONTRAINDICATIONS
No known contraindications.

NURSING CONSIDERATIONS
● Use with extreme caution in children and neonates because safety and efficacy haven't been established.
● Use cautiously. Prepared from pooled plasma from human donors, drug carries minimal risk of transmission of viruses, including hepatitis and HIV.
● Treatment usually lasts 2 to 8 days but may be prolonged in pregnancy or when used with surgery or immobilization.
● *Alert:* Because of risk of neonatal thromboembolism (sometimes fatal) in children of parents with hereditary AT-III deficiency, anticipate obtaining AT-III levels immediately after birth.
● Bring solution to room temperature before administration. Use solution within 3 hours of preparation.
● Obtain AT-III activity levels b.i.d. until dosage requirement has stabilized, and then daily immediately before dose. Functional assays are preferred because quantitative immunologic test results may be normal despite decreased AT-III activity.
● Watch for dyspnea and increased blood pressure, which may occur if administration rate is too rapid.
● One IU is equivalent to quantity of endogenous AT-III present in 1 ml of normal human plasma.
● Heparin binds to AT-III lysine-binding sites, increasing heparin efficacy.
● Drug isn't recommended for long-term prophylaxis of thrombotic episodes.
● Store drug at 36° to 46° F (2° to 8° C).

PATIENT TEACHING
• Explain use and administration of AT-III to patient and parents.
• Instruct patient to report adverse reactions promptly.

---

factor IX (human)
AlphaNine SD, Mononine

factor IX complex
Bebulin VH, Immuno, Konyne 80, Profilnine SD, Proplex T

Pregnancy risk category C

AVAILABLE FORMS
Injection: Vials, with diluent. Units specified on label.

INDICATIONS & DOSAGES
➤ **Factor IX deficiency (hemophilia B or Christmas disease), anticoagulant overdosage—**
Adults and children: To calculate approximate units of factor IX needed, use the following equations:
Human product: 1 unit/kg × body weight in kilograms × percentage of desired increase of factor IX level.
Recombinant product: 1.2 units/kg × body weight in kilograms × percentage of desired increase of factor IX level.
Proplex T: 0.5 units/kg × body weight in kilograms × percentage of desired increase of factor IX level.
Infusion rates vary with product and patient comfort. Dosage is highly individualized, depending on degree of deficiency, level of factor IX desired, patient weight, and severity of bleeding.

I.V. ADMINISTRATION
• Reconstitute with 20 ml of sterile water for injection for each vial of lyophilized drug. Keep refrigerated until ready to use; warm to room temperature before reconstituting. Factor IX (Human) should be used within 3 hours after reconstitution. Factor IX Complex is stable for 12 hours after reconstitution, although administration should begin within 3 hours of reconstitution. Unstable in solution.
• Don't shake, refrigerate, or mix with other I.V. solutions. Store away from heat.

• Avoid rapid infusion. If tingling sensation, fever, chills, or headache develops, decrease flow rate and notify prescriber.

ACTION
Directly replaces deficient clotting factor.

Route	Onset	Peak	Duration
I.V.	Immediate	10-30 min	Unknown

ADVERSE REACTIONS
CNS: headache.
CV: *thromboembolic reactions, MI, disseminated intravascular coagulation, pulmonary embolism,* changes in blood pressure, *flushing.*
GI: nausea, vomiting.
Skin: urticaria.
Other: *transient fever, chills, tingling.*

INTERACTIONS
Drug-drug. *Aminocaproic acid:* Increased risk of thrombosis. Avoid using together.

EFFECTS ON LAB TEST RESULTS
None reported.

CONTRAINDICATIONS
Contraindicated in patients with hepatic disease in whom intravascular coagulation or fibrinolysis is suspected. Mononine is contraindicated in patients hypersensitive to murine (mouse) protein.

NURSING CONSIDERATIONS
• Use cautiously in neonates and infants because of susceptibility to hepatitis, which may be transmitted with factor IX complex.
• Administer hepatitis B vaccine before giving factor IX complex.
• Observe patient for allergic reactions and monitor vital signs regularly.
• Observe patient closely for signs and symptoms of thromboembolic events.
• Risk of hepatitis must be weighed against risk of not receiving drug.
• Risk of HIV transmission is extremely low because of manufacturing process.

PATIENT TEACHING
• Explain use and administration of factor IX to patient and family.

Reactions may be *common*, uncommon, *life-threatening*, or COMMON AND LIFE-THREATENING.

• Tell patient to report adverse reactions promptly and to discontinue drug if they occur.
• Advise patient to report chest tightness, wheezing, respiratory distress, cough, or hypotension.

---

plasma protein fractions
Plasmanate, Plasma-Plex, Plasmatein, Protenate

Pregnancy risk category C

AVAILABLE FORMS
Injection: 5% solution in 50-ml, 250-ml, 500-ml vials

INDICATIONS & DOSAGES
➤ **Shock—**
Adults: Varies with patient's condition and response, but usual dose is 250 to 500 ml I.V. (12.5 to 25 g protein), usually no faster than 10 ml/minute.
Children: 6.6 to 33 ml/kg (0.33 to 1.65 g/ kg of protein) I.V., 5 to 10 ml/minute.
➤ **Hypoproteinemia—**
Adults: 1,000 to 1,500 ml I.V. daily. Maximum infusion rate is 8 ml/minute.

I.V. ADMINISTRATION
• Check expiration date before using. Don't use solutions that are cloudy, contain sediment, or have been frozen. Discard solutions in containers that have been open for longer than 4 hours because solution contains no preservatives.
• Don't infuse solutions containing amino acids or alcohol through same I.V. line; proteins may precipitate.
• If patient is dehydrated, give additional fluids either P.O. or I.V.
• Don't give more than 250 g or 5,000 ml in 48 hours.

ACTION
Supplies colloid to the blood and expands plasma volume. Primary constituent is albumin.

Route	Onset	Peak	Duration
I.V.	Immediate	Immediate	Unknown

ADVERSE REACTIONS
CNS: headache.

CV: hypotension, *vascular overload,* tachycardia, flushing.
GI: nausea, vomiting, hypersalivation.
Musculoskeletal: back pain.
Respiratory: dyspnea, *pulmonary edema.*
Skin: rash.
Other: chills, fever.

INTERACTIONS
None significant.

EFFECTS ON LAB TEST RESULTS
None reported.

CONTRAINDICATIONS
Contraindicated in patients with severe anemia or heart failure and in those undergoing cardiac bypass.

NURSING CONSIDERATIONS
• Use cautiously in patients with hepatic or renal failure, low cardiac reserve, or restricted sodium intake.
• Hypotension risk is greater when infusion rate exceeds 10 ml/minute.
• Monitor blood pressure. Be prepared to slow or stop infusion if hypotension suddenly occurs. Vital signs should return to normal gradually; assess them hourly.
• Watch for signs of vascular overload (heart failure or pulmonary edema).
• *Alert:* Watch for hemorrhage or shock after surgery or injury. A rapid rise in blood pressure may cause bleeding from sites that isn't apparent at lower pressures.
• Report decreased urine output.
• Drug contains 130 to 160 mEq sodium/L.

PATIENT TEACHING
• Explain use and administration of drug to patient and family.
• Tell patient to report adverse reactions promptly.

---

alteplase
anistreplase
reteplase, recombinant
streptokinase
tenecteplase
urokinase

COMBINATION PRODUCTS
None.

alteplase (tissue plasminogen activator, recombinant; t-PA)
Actilyse‡, Activase, Cathflo Activase

Pregnancy risk category C

AVAILABLE FORMS
Injection: 20-mg (11.6 million–IU), 50-mg (29 million–IU), 100-mg (58 million–IU) vials
Injection (Cathflo Activase): 2-mg single-patient vials (lyophilized powder for intracatheter instillation)

INDICATIONS & DOSAGES
➤ **Lysis of thrombi obstructing coronary arteries in acute MI—**
3-hour infusion
Adults: 100 mg by I.V. infusion over 3 hours, as follows: 60 mg in first hour, of which 6 to 10 mg is given as a bolus over first 1 to 2 minutes. Then 20 mg/hour infused for 2 hours. Adults weighing less than 65 kg (143 lb) should receive 1.25 mg/kg in a similar fashion (60% in first hour, 10% as a bolus; then 20% of total dose per hour for 2 hours).
Accelerated infusion
Adults weighing more than 67 kg: 100 mg total dose. Give 15 mg I.V. bolus over 1 to 2 minutes, followed by 50 mg infused over the next 30 minutes; then 35 mg infused over the next hour.
Adults weighing 67 kg or less: 15 mg I.V. bolus over 1 to 2 minutes, followed by 0.75 mg/kg infused over the next 30 minutes; then 0.5 mg/kg infused over the next hour.

➤ **Management of acute massive pulmonary embolism—**
Adults: 100 mg by I.V. infusion over 2 hours. Heparin begun at end of infusion when PTT or thrombin time returns to twice normal or less. Don't exceed 100-mg dose. Higher doses may increase risk of intracranial bleeding.
➤ **Acute ischemic CVA—**
Adults: 0.9 mg/kg by I.V. infusion over 1 hour with 10% of total dose administered as an initial I.V. bolus over 1 minute. Maximum total dose is 90 mg.
✻ *NEW INDICATION:* **Restoration of function to central venous access devices as assessed by the ability to withdraw blood—**
Adults and children older than age 2: For patients weighing more than 30 kg (66 lb), instill 2 mg in 2 ml sterile water into catheter. For patients weighing 10 kg (22 lb) to 30 kg (66 lb), instill 110% of the internal lumen volume of the catheter, not to exceed 2 mg in 2 ml sterile water. After 30 minutes of dwell time, assess catheter function by aspirating blood. If function is restored, aspirate 4 to 5 ml of blood to remove Cathflo Activase and residual clot, and gently irrigate the catheter with normal saline solution. If catheter function not restored after 120 minutes, instill a second dose.

I.V. ADMINISTRATION
● Give alteplase I.V. only, using a controlled infusion device.
● Reconstitute drug only with unpreserved sterile water for injection. (Check manufacturer's labeling for specific information.) Don't use 50-mg vial if vacuum isn't present; 100-mg vials don't have a vacuum. Reconstitute with large-bore (18G) needle, directing stream of sterile water at lyophilized cake. Don't shake. Slight foaming is common (allow foaming to settle before use), and solution should be clear or pale yellow.
● Drug may be given reconstituted (1 mg/ml) or diluted with an equal volume of normal saline solution or D_5W to

---

Reactions may be common, uncommon, *life-threatening*, or COMMON AND LIFE-THREATENING.

make a 0.5-mg/ml solution. Adding other drugs to the infusion isn't recommended.
• Reconstitute solution immediately before administration; discard any unused portion after 8 hours.

For Cathflo Activase
• Reconstitute Cathflo Activase with 2.2 ml sterile water; dissolve completely into a colorless to pale yellow solution that yields a concentration of 1 mg/ml. Solutions are stable for up to 8 hours at room temperature.
• Assess the cause of catheter dysfunction before using alteplase. Some conditions that have occluded the catheter include catheter malposition, mechanical failure, constriction by a suture, and lipid deposits or drug precipitates within the catheter lumen. Don't try to suction because of the risk of damage to the vascular wall or collapse of soft-walled catheters.
• Don't use excessive pressure while instilling alteplase into the catheter, which could cause catheter rupture or expulsion of the clot into the circulation.

ACTION
Binds to fibrin in a thrombus and locally converts plasminogen to plasmin, which initiates local fibrinolysis.

Route	Onset	Peak	Duration
I.V.	Unknown	Unknown	Unknown

ADVERSE REACTIONS
CNS: *cerebral hemorrhage.*
CV: hypotension, *arrhythmias,* edema.
GI: nausea, vomiting, *GI bleeding* (Cathflo Activase).
Hematologic: *spontaneous bleeding.*
Other: bleeding at puncture sites, *cholesterol embolization,* hypersensitivity reactions, *anaphylaxis,* fever; *venous thrombosis, sepsis* (Cathflo Activase).

INTERACTIONS
Drug-drug. *Aspirin, coumadin anticoagulants, dipyridamole, drugs affecting platelet activity (abciximab), heparin:* Increased risk of bleeding. Monitor patient carefully.

EFFECTS ON LAB TEST RESULTS
None reported.

CONTRAINDICATIONS
Contraindicated in patients with active internal bleeding, intracranial neoplasm, arteriovenous malformation, aneurysm, severe uncontrolled hypertension, or history or current evidence of intracranial hemorrhage, suspicion of subarachnoid hemorrhage, or seizure at onset of CVA when used for acute ischemic CVA. Also contraindicated in patients with history of CVA, intraspinal or intracranial trauma or surgery within 2 months, or known bleeding diathesis.

NURSING CONSIDERATIONS
• Use cautiously in patients with major surgery within 10 days (when bleeding is difficult to control because of its location); organ biopsy; trauma (including cardiopulmonary resuscitation); GI or GU bleeding; cerebrovascular disease; systolic pressure of 180 mm Hg or higher or diastolic pressure of 110 mm Hg or higher; mitral stenosis, atrial fibrillation, or other conditions that may lead to left heart thrombus; acute pericarditis or subacute bacterial endocarditis; hemostatic defects caused by hepatic or renal impairment; septic thrombophlebitis; or diabetic hemorrhagic retinopathy. Also use cautiously in patients receiving anticoagulants, in patients ages 75 and older, and during pregnancy and the first 10 days postpartum.
• *Alert:* When used for acute ischemic CVA, drug should be given within 3 hours after symptoms occur and only when intracranial bleeding has been ruled out.
• Drug may be given to menstruating women.
• To attain recanalization of occluded coronary arteries and improvement of heart function, treatment with alteplase should start as soon as possible after onset of symptoms.
• Anticoagulant and antiplatelet therapy is commonly started during or after treatment, to decrease risk of another thrombosis.
• Monitor vital signs and neurologic status carefully. Keep patient on strict bed rest.
• Have antiarrhythmics readily available, and carefully monitor ECG. Coronary thrombolysis is linked with arrhythmias caused by reperfusion of ischemic my-

ocardium. Such arrhythmias don't differ from those commonly linked with MI.
• Avoid invasive procedures during thrombolytic therapy. Carefully monitor patient for signs of internal bleeding, and frequently check all puncture sites. Bleeding is the most common adverse effect and may occur internally and at external puncture sites.
• If uncontrollable bleeding occurs, stop infusion (and heparin) and notify prescriber.
• Results of coagulation and fibrinolytic tests may be altered. Use of aprotinin (150 to 200 units/ml) in blood sample may attenuate this interference.

PATIENT TEACHING
• Explain use and administration of drug to patient and family.
• Tell patient to report adverse reactions promptly.

---

anistreplase (anisoylated plasminogen-streptokinase activator complex; APSAC)
Eminase

Pregnancy risk category C

AVAILABLE FORMS
Injection: 30-unit vial

INDICATIONS & DOSAGES
➤ **Lysis of coronary artery thrombi after acute MI—**
Adults: 30 units I.V. over 2 to 5 minutes by direct injection.

I.V. ADMINISTRATION
• Unlike other thrombolytics that must be infused, this drug should be given by direct injection into an I.V. line over 2 to 5 minutes.
• Reconstitute drug by slowly adding 5 ml of sterile water for injection. Direct stream against side of vial, not at drug itself. Gently roll vial to mix dry powder and water. To avoid excessive foaming, don't shake vial. Reconstituted solution should be colorless to pale yellow. Inspect for precipitate. If drug isn't administered within 30 minutes of reconstituting, discard vial.

• Don't mix with other drugs; don't dilute solution after reconstitution.

ACTION
Anistreplase, derived from Lys-plasminogen and streptokinase, is formulated into a fibrinolytic enzyme plus activator complex with the activator temporarily blocked by an anisoyl group. It's activated in vivo by a nonenzymatic process that removes the anisoyl group. Active drug converts plasminogen to plasmin, resulting in thrombolysis.

Route	Onset	Peak	Duration
I.V.	Immediate	45 min	6 hr-2 days

ADVERSE REACTIONS
CNS: *intracranial hemorrhage.*
CV: ARRHYTHMIAS, *conduction disorders, hypotension,* flushing.
EENT: gum or mouth hemorrhage.
GI: *hemorrhage.*
GU: hematuria.
Hematologic: *bleeding tendency,* eosinophilia.
Musculoskeletal: arthralgia.
Respiratory: hemoptysis.
Skin: hematoma, urticaria, pruritus, delayed purpuric rash.
Other: bleeding at puncture sites.

INTERACTIONS
Drug-drug. *Drugs that alter platelet function (including aspirin, dipyridamole), heparin, oral anticoagulants:* May increase risk of bleeding. Use together cautiously.

EFFECTS ON LAB TEST RESULTS
• May decrease hemoglobin and hematocrit. May decrease alpha$_2$-antiplasmin, factor V, factor VIII, fibrinogen, and plasminogen activities.
• May increase PT, PTT, INR, and eosinophil count.

CONTRAINDICATIONS
Contraindicated in patients with history of severe allergic reaction to anistreplase or streptokinase, active internal bleeding, CVA, recent (within past 2 months) intraspinal or intracranial surgery or trauma, aneurysm, arteriovenous malformation,

---

intracranial neoplasm, uncontrolled hypertension, or known bleeding diathesis.

NURSING CONSIDERATIONS
● Use cautiously in patients with recent (within 10 days) major surgery (when bleeding is difficult to control because of its location); trauma (including cardiopulmonary resuscitation); GI or GU bleeding; cerebrovascular disease; hypertension (systolic pressure of 180 mm Hg or higher, or diastolic pressure of 110 mm Hg or higher); mitral stenosis, atrial fibrillation, or other conditions that may lead to left heart thrombus; acute pericarditis or subacute bacterial endocarditis; hemostatic defects caused by hepatic or renal impairment; septic thrombophlebitis; or diabetic hemorrhagic retinopathy. Also contraindicated during pregnancy and first 10 days postpartum, in patients receiving anticoagulants, and in those ages 75 and older.
● Drug may be given to menstruating women.
● Carefully monitor ECG during treatment. Be prepared to treat bradycardia or ventricular irritability. Thrombolytic therapy is linked with reperfusion arrhythmias that may signify successful thrombolysis. These arrhythmias are similar to those seen in the course of an acute MI and may include sinus bradycardia, accelerated idioventricular rhythm, ventricular tachycardia, or premature ventricular depolarizations.
● Carefully monitor patient; avoid I.M. injections and nonessential handling or moving of patient. Bleeding is the most common adverse reaction and may occur internally and at external puncture sites.
● Anticoagulant or antiplatelet therapy may be used with drug treatment to decrease risk of another thrombosis.
● Anistreplase is derived from human plasma. No cases of hepatitis or HIV infection have been reported to date. The manufacturing process is designed to purify the plasma used in preparation of drug.
● *Alert:* Drug efficacy may be limited if antistreptokinase antibodies are present. Antibody levels may be elevated if more than 5 days have elapsed since previous treatment with anistreplase or streptoki-

nase, or if patient has had a recent streptococcal infection.
● In vitro coagulation tests will be affected by presence of anistreplase. This can be attenuated if blood samples are collected with aprotinin (150 to 200 units/ml).
● *Alert:* Don't confuse anistreplase with alteplase.

PATIENT TEACHING
● Explain use and administration of drug to patient and family.
● Tell patient to report adverse reactions promptly.

---

reteplase, recombinant
Rapilysin§, Retavase

Pregnancy risk category C

AVAILABLE FORMS
Injection: 10.4 units (18.1 mg)/vial. Supplied in a kit with components for reconstitution for two single-use vials.

INDICATIONS & DOSAGES
➤ **Management of acute MI—**
Adults: Double-bolus injection of 10 + 10 units. Give each bolus I.V. over 2 minutes. If complications, such as serious bleeding or an anaphylactoid reaction, don't occur after first bolus, give second bolus 30 minutes after start of first bolus.

I.V. ADMINISTRATION
● Drug is administered I.V. as a double-bolus injection. If bleeding or anaphylactoid reactions occur after first bolus, notify prescriber; second bolus may be withheld.
● Reconstitute drug according to manufacturer's instructions using items provided in kit. Reconstitute with sterile water for injection, USP (without preservatives). Reconstituted solution should be colorless; resulting concentration will be 1 unit/ml. If foaming occurs, allow vial to stand for several minutes. Inspect for precipitation. Use within 4 hours of reconstitution; discard unused portions.
● Don't administer with other I.V. drugs through same I.V. line. Note that heparin and reteplase are incompatible in solution.

ACTION
Enhances cleavage of plasminogen to generate plasmin, which leads to fibrinolysis.

Route	Onset	Peak	Duration
I.V.	Unknown	Unknown	Unknown

ADVERSE REACTIONS
CNS: *intracranial hemorrhage.*
CV: *arrhythmias, cholesterol embolization, hemorrhage.*
GI: *hemorrhage.*
GU: hematuria.
Hematologic: *bleeding tendency,* anemia.
Other: bleeding at puncture sites.

INTERACTIONS
Drug-drug. *Heparin, oral anticoagulants, platelet inhibitors (abciximab, aspirin, dipyridamole):* May increase risk of bleeding. Use together cautiously.

EFFECTS ON LAB TEST RESULTS
• May increase PT, PTT, and INR. May decrease hemoglobin.

CONTRAINDICATIONS
Contraindicated in patients with active internal bleeding, known bleeding diathesis, history of CVA, recent intracranial or intraspinal surgery or trauma, severe uncontrolled hypertension, intracranial neoplasm, arteriovenous malformation, or aneurysm.

NURSING CONSIDERATIONS
• Use cautiously in patients with previous puncture of noncompressible vessels; in those with recent (within 10 days) major surgery, obstetric delivery, organ biopsy, GI or GU bleeding, or trauma; in those with cerebrovascular disease, hypertension (systolic pressure ≥ 180 mm Hg, diastolic pressure ≥ 110 mm Hg), and conditions that may lead to left heart thrombus, including mitral stenosis, acute pericarditis, subacute bacterial endocarditis, and hemostatic defects; and in those with diabetic hemorrhagic retinopathy, septic thrombophlebitis, and other conditions in which bleeding would be difficult to manage. Also use cautiously in patients ages 75 and older and in breast-feeding women.
• Drug may be given to menstruating women.

• Carefully monitor ECG during treatment. Coronary thrombolysis may result in arrhythmias linked with reperfusion. Be prepared to treat bradycardia or ventricular irritability.
• Carefully monitor patient for bleeding. Avoid I.M. injections, invasive procedures, and nonessential handling of patient. Bleeding is the most common adverse reaction and may occur internally or at external puncture sites. If local measures don't control serious bleeding, discontinue anticoagulation therapy and notify prescriber. Withhold second bolus of reteplase.
• Reteplase may alter coagulation studies; drug remains active in vitro and can lead to degradation of fibrinogen in sample. Collect blood samples in the presence of PPACK (chloromethylketone) at 2-micromolar concentrations.
• Drug should be used in pregnancy only if benefit to mother justifies risk to fetus.
• Safety and efficacy of drug in children haven't been established.
• Potency is expressed in units specific to reteplase and isn't comparable with other thrombolytic drugs.
• Avoid use of noncompressible pressure sites during therapy. If an arterial puncture is needed, use an arm vessel that can be compressed manually. Apply pressure for at least 30 minutes; then apply a pressure dressing. Check site frequently.

PATIENT TEACHING
• Explain use and administration of drug to patient and family.
• Tell patient to report adverse reactions immediately.

streptokinase
Kabikinase§, Streptase

Pregnancy risk category C

AVAILABLE FORMS
Injection: 250,000 IU, 750,000 IU, 1,500,000 IU in vials for reconstitution

INDICATIONS & DOSAGES
➤ **Arteriovenous cannula occlusion—**
Adults: 250,000 IU in 2 ml I.V. solution by I.V. pump infusion into each occluded limb of the cannula over 25 to 35 minutes.

Reactions may be *common,* uncommon, *life-threatening,* or COMMON AND LIFE-THREATENING.

Clamp off cannula for 2 hours. Then aspirate contents of cannula, flush with saline solution, and reconnect.

➤ **Venous thrombosis, pulmonary embolism, arterial thrombosis, and embolism—**

Adults: Loading dose is 250,000 IU by I.V. infusion over 30 minutes. Sustaining dose is 100,000 IU/hour I.V. infusion for 72 hours for deep vein thrombosis and 100,000 IU/hour over 24 to 72 hours by I.V. infusion pump for pulmonary embolism and arterial thrombosis or embolism.

➤ **Lysis of coronary artery thrombi following acute MI—**

Adults: Loading dose is 20,000 IU bolus through coronary catheter; then infuse a maintenance dose of 2,000 IU/minute over 60 minutes. Or, may be administered as an I.V. infusion. Usual adult dose is 1.5 million IU infused I.V. over 60 minutes.

I.V. ADMINISTRATION

• Reconstitute drug in each vial with 5 ml of normal saline solution for injection or D_5W solution. Further dilute to 45 ml (if needed, total volume may be increased to 500 ml in a glass or 50 ml in a plastic container). Don't shake; roll gently to mix. Some flocculation may be present after reconstituting; discard if large amounts are present. Filter solution with 0.8-micron or larger filter. Use within 8 hours. Store powder at room temperature and refrigerate after reconstitution.

• *Alert:* Don't mix with other drugs or give other drugs through the same I.V. line.

• Heparin by continuous infusion is usually started within 1 to 4 hours after stopping streptokinase. Use infusion pump to administer heparin. Initiating heparin 12 hours after intracoronary streptokinase may minimize bleeding risk.

ACTION

Activates plasminogen in two steps: Plasminogen and streptokinase form a complex that exposes the plasminogen-activating site; plasminogen is then converted to plasmin by cleavage of the peptide bond, which leads to fibrinolysis.

Route	Onset	Peak	Duration
I.V.	Immediate	20 min-2 hr	4-24 hr

ADVERSE REACTIONS

CNS: polyradiculoneuropathy, headache.
CV: *reperfusion arrhythmias, hypotension,* vasculitis, flushing.
EENT: periorbital edema.
GI: nausea.
Hematologic: *bleeding;* increased thrombin time, activated PTT, and PT; moderately decreased hematocrit.
Respiratory: minor breathing difficulty, *bronchospasm, pulmonary edema.*
Skin: urticaria, pruritus.
Other: phlebitis at injection site, hypersensitivity reactions, *anaphylaxis,* delayed hypersensitivity reactions, *angioedema, fever.*

INTERACTIONS

Drug-drug. *Anticoagulants:* Increased risk of bleeding. Monitor patient closely.
Antifibrinolytic drugs: Streptokinase activity is inhibited and reversed by antifibrinolytic drugs such as aminocaproic acid. Don't use together.
Aspirin, dipyridamole, drugs affecting platelet activity, indomethacin, phenylbutazone: Increased risk of bleeding. Monitor patient closely.

EFFECTS ON LAB TEST RESULTS

• May increase PT, PTT, and INR. May decrease hematocrit.

CONTRAINDICATIONS

Contraindicated in patients with ulcerative wounds, active internal bleeding, recent CVA, recent trauma with possible internal injuries, visceral or intracranial malignant neoplasms, ulcerative colitis, diverticulitis, severe hypertension, acute or chronic hepatic or renal insufficiency, uncontrolled hypocoagulation, chronic pulmonary disease with cavitation, subacute bacterial endocarditis or rheumatic valvular disease, previous severe allergic reaction to streptokinase, or recent cerebral embolism, thrombosis, or hemorrhage.

Also contraindicated within 10 days after intra-arterial diagnostic procedure or any surgery, including liver or kidney biopsy, lumbar puncture, thoracentesis, paracentesis, or extensive or multiple cutdowns.

---

*Liquid contains alcohol.   **May contain tartrazine.   †Canada   ‡Australia   §U.K.   ◇OTC

I.M. injections and other invasive procedures are contraindicated during streptokinase therapy.

NURSING CONSIDERATIONS

• Use cautiously when treating arterial embolism that originates from left side of heart because of danger of cerebral infarction.

• Drug may be given to menstruating women.

• Only prescribers with wide experience in thrombotic disease management should use streptokinase. Drug should be given only where clinical and laboratory monitoring can be performed.

• Before using streptokinase to clear an occluded arteriovenous cannula, try flushing with heparinized saline solution.

• Keep aminocaproic acid available to treat bleeding, and corticosteroids to treat allergic reactions.

• Before starting therapy, draw blood for coagulation studies, hematocrit, platelet count, and type and crossmatching. Rate of I.V. infusion depends on thrombin time and streptokinase resistance.

• To check for hypersensitivity reactions, give 100 IU intradermally; a wheal-and-flare response within 20 minutes means patient is probably allergic. Monitor vital signs frequently.

• If patient has had either a recent streptococcal infection or recent treatment with streptokinase, a higher loading dose may be needed. Alternative thrombolytics should be considered.

• Combined therapy with low-dose aspirin (162.5 mg) or dipyridamole has improved short- and long-term results.

• Monitor patient for excessive bleeding every 15 minutes for first hour, every 30 minutes for second through eighth hours, and then every 4 hours. If bleeding is evident, stop therapy and notify prescriber. Pretreatment with heparin or drugs that affect platelets causes high risk of bleeding but may improve long-term results.

• Monitor pulse, color, and sensation of limbs every hour.

• Keep involved limb in straight alignment to prevent bleeding from infusion site.

• Avoid unnecessary handling of patient; pad side rails. Bruising is more likely during therapy.

• Keep a laboratory flow sheet on patient's chart to monitor PTT, PT, thrombin time, and hemoglobin level and hematocrit. Monitor vital signs and neurologic status.

• Avoid I.M. injection. Keep venipuncture sites to a minimum; use pressure dressing on puncture sites for at least 15 minutes.

• *Alert:* Watch for signs of hypersensitivity and notify prescriber immediately if any occur. Antihistamines or corticosteroids may be used to treat mild allergic reactions. If a severe reaction occurs, stop infusion immediately and notify prescriber.

• Thrombolytic therapy in patients with acute MI may decrease infarct size, improve ventricular function, and decrease risk of heart failure. For optimal effect, streptokinase must be given within 6 hours after symptoms start.

PATIENT TEACHING

• Explain use and administration of drug to patient and family.

• Tell patient to report adverse reactions promptly.

---

tenecteplase
TNKase

Pregnancy risk category C

AVAILABLE FORMS
Injection: 50 mg

INDICATIONS & DOSAGES
➤ **Reduction of mortality from acute MI—**
Adults weighing 90 kg (198 lb) or more: 50 mg (10 ml) by I.V. bolus over 5 seconds.
Adults weighing 80 to 89 kg (176 to 196 lb): 45 mg (9 ml) by I.V. bolus over 5 seconds.
Adults weighing 70 to 79 kg (154 to 174 lb): 40 mg (8 ml) by I.V. bolus over 5 seconds.
Adults weighing 60 to 69 kg (132 to 152 lb): 35 mg (7 ml) by I.V. bolus over 5 seconds.
Adults weighing less than 60 kg (132 lb): 30 mg (6 ml) by I.V. bolus over 5 seconds. Maximum dose is 50 mg.

Reactions may be *common*, uncommon, *life-threatening*, or COMMON AND LIFE-THREATENING.

I.V. ADMINISTRATION

- Use syringe prefilled with sterile water for injection, and inject the entire contents into drug vial.
- *Alert:* Gently swirl solution once mixed. Don't shake.
- Draw up the appropriate dose needed from the reconstituted vial with the syringe and discard any unused portion.
- Visually inspect product for particulate matter before administration.
- Administer the drug rapidly over 5 seconds.

ACTION

A human tissue plasminogen activator that binds to fibrin and converts plasminogen to plasmin. The specificity to fibrin decreases systemic activation of plasminogen and the resulting breakdown of circulating fibrinogen.

Route	Onset	Peak	Duration
I.V.	Immediate	Immediate	Unknown

ADVERSE REACTIONS

CNS: *CVA, intracranial hemorrhage.*
CV: *arrhythmias.*
EENT: pharyngeal bleed, epistaxis.
GI: *GI bleeding.*
GU: hematuria.
Skin: *hematoma.*
Other: bleeding at puncture site.

INTERACTIONS

Drug-drug. *Anticoagulants (heparin, vitamin K antagonists), drugs that alter platelet function (acetylsalicylic acid, dipyridamole, glycoprotein IIb/IIIa inhibitors):* Increased risk of bleeding when used before, during, or after therapy with tenecteplase. Use cautiously.

EFFECTS ON LAB TEST RESULTS

- May increase PT, PTT, and INR.

CONTRAINDICATIONS

Contraindicated in patients with an active internal bleed; history of CVA; intracranial or intraspinal surgery or trauma during previous 2 months; intracranial neoplasm, aneurysm, or arteriovenous malformation; severe uncontrolled hypertension; or bleeding diathesis.

NURSING CONSIDERATIONS

- Use cautiously in patients who have had recent major surgery (such as coronary artery bypass graft), organ biopsy, obstetric delivery, or previous puncture of noncompressible vessels. Also use cautiously in pregnant women, patients ages 75 and older, and patients with recent trauma, recent GI or GU bleeding, high risk of left ventricular thrombus, acute pericarditis, hypertension (systolic pressure ≥ 180 mm Hg or diastolic pressure ≥ 110 mm Hg), severe hepatic dysfunction, hemostatic defects, subacute bacterial endocarditis, septic thrombophlebitis, diabetic hemorrhagic retinopathy, or cerebrovascular disease. Begin therapy as soon as possible after onset of MI symptoms.
- Minimize arterial and venous punctures during treatment.
- Avoid noncompressible arterial punctures and internal jugular and subclavian venous punctures.
- Give drug immediately once reconstituted, or refrigerate and use within 8 hours.
- Don't give drug in the same I.V. line as dextrose. Flush dextrose-containing lines with normal saline solution before administration.
- Administer tenecteplase by a designated line.
- Give heparin with tenecteplase but not in the same I.V. line.
- Monitor patient for bleeding. If serious bleeding occurs, discontinue heparin and antiplatelet drugs immediately.
- Monitor ECG for reperfusion arrhythmias.
- Cholesterol embolism is rarely related to thrombolytic use, but it may be lethal. Signs and symptoms may include livedo reticularis ("purple toe" syndrome), acute renal failure, gangrenous digits, hypertension, pancreatitis, MI, cerebral infarction, spinal cord infarction, retinal artery occlusion, bowel infarction, and rhabdomyolysis.

PATIENT TEACHING

- Advise patient about proper dental care to avoid excessive gum bleeding.
- Tell patient to report any adverse effects or excess bleeding immediately.
- Explain to patient and family about the use of tenecteplase.

---

urokinase
Abbokinase, Abbokinase Open-Cath, Ukidan‡

Pregnancy risk category B

AVAILABLE FORMS
Injection: 5,000 units (IU) per unit-dose vial; 9,000 units (IU) per unit-dose vial; 250,000-IU vial

INDICATIONS & DOSAGES
➤ **Lysis of acute massive pulmonary embolism and lysis of pulmonary embolism with unstable hemodynamics—**
Adults: For I.V. infusion *only* by constant infusion pump. Priming dose: 4,400 IU/kg of urokinase with normal saline or D₅W solution admixture, given over 10 minutes. Then 4,400 IU/kg/hour for 12 hours. Therapy followed by continuous I.V. infusion of heparin and then oral anticoagulants.
➤ **Coronary artery thrombosis—**
Adults: After bolus dose of heparin ranging from 2,500 to 10,000 units, 6,000 IU/minute of urokinase is infused into occluded artery for up to 2 hours. Average total dose is 500,000 IU. Urokinase therapy should start within 6 hours after symptoms start.
➤ **Venous catheter occlusion—**
Adults: Solution containing 5,000 IU/ml is instilled into occluded line and, after 5 minutes, is aspirated. Repeat aspiration attempts q 5 minutes for 30 minutes. If line isn't patent after 30 minutes, it's capped and urokinase is left to work for 30 to 60 minutes before it is aspirated again. May require second instillation. Flush with 10 ml normal saline solution after patency is restored.

I.V. ADMINISTRATION
• Reconstitute according to manufacturer's directions using sterile water for injection. Gently roll vial; don't shake. Don't use bacteriostatic water for injection to reconstitute; it contains preservatives. Dilute further with normal saline solution or D₅W solution before infusion. Urokinase solutions may be filtered through a 0.45-micron or smaller cellulose-membrane filter before administration. Discard unused solution. Total volume of fluid adminis-tered by I.V. infusion should not exceed 200 ml.
• Don't mix with other drugs. Administer through separate I.V. line.
• Heparin by continuous infusion may be started concurrently or within 3 to 4 hours after urokinase has been stopped to prevent recurrent thrombosis.

ACTION
Activates plasminogen to plasmin by directly cleaving peptide bonds at two different sites, causing fibrinolysis.

Route	Onset	Peak	Duration
I.V.	Immediate	20 min-4 hr	12-24 hr

ADVERSE REACTIONS
CV: *reperfusion arrhythmias,* hypotension.
GI: nausea, vomiting.
Hematologic: *bleeding.*
Respiratory: *bronchospasm,* minor breathing difficulties.
Other: phlebitis at injection site, fever, chills, hypersensitivity reactions.

INTERACTIONS
Drug-drug. *Anticoagulants:* Increased risk of bleeding. Monitor patient closely.
Aspirin, dipyridamole, indomethacin, phenylbutazone, other drugs affecting platelet activity: Increased risk of bleeding. Monitor patient.

EFFECTS ON LAB TEST RESULTS
• May increase PT, PTT, and INR. May decrease hematocrit.

CONTRAINDICATIONS
Contraindicated in patients with active internal bleeding, history of CVA, aneurysm, arteriovenous malformation, known bleeding diathesis, recent trauma with possible internal injuries, visceral or intracranial malignancy, ulcerative colitis, diverticulitis, severe hypertension, hemostatic defects including those secondary to severe hepatic or renal insufficiency, uncontrolled hypocoagulation, chronic pulmonary disease with cavitation, subacute bacterial endocarditis or rheumatic valvular disease, and recent cerebral embolism, thrombosis, or hemorrhage.

Reactions may be *common,* uncommon, *life-threatening,* or **COMMON AND LIFE-THREATENING.**

Also contraindicated within 10 days after intra-arterial diagnostic procedure or surgery (liver or kidney biopsy, lumbar puncture, thoracentesis, paracentesis, or extensive or multiple cutdowns) or within 2 months after intracranial or intraspinal surgery. Don't use during pregnancy or first 10 days postpartum.

I.M. injections and other invasive procedures are contraindicated during urokinase therapy.

NURSING CONSIDERATIONS
• Have typed and crossmatched RBCs, whole blood, plasma expanders (other than dextran), and aminocaproic acid available to treat bleeding. Keep corticosteroids, epinephrine, and antihistamines available to treat allergic reactions.
• Drug may be given to menstruating women.
• Only prescribers with extensive experience in thrombotic disease management should use urokinase and only in facilities where clinical and laboratory monitoring can be performed.
• Monitor patient for excessive bleeding every 15 minutes for first hour; every 30 minutes for second through eighth hours; then once every 4 hours. Pretreatment with drugs affecting platelets places patient at high risk of bleeding.
• Monitor pulse, color, and sensation of limbs every hour.
• Although risk of hypersensitivity reactions is low, monitor patient.
• Keep a laboratory flow sheet on patient's chart to monitor PTT, PT, thrombin time, hemoglobin level, and hematocrit.
• Monitor vital signs and neurologic status. Don't take blood pressure in legs because doing so could dislodge a clot.
• Keep venipuncture sites to a minimum; use pressure dressing on puncture sites for at least 15 minutes.
• Keep involved limb in straight alignment to prevent bleeding from infusion site.
• Because bruising is more likely during therapy, avoid unnecessary handling of patient, and pad side rails.

PATIENT TEACHING
• Explain use and administration of drug to patient and family.

• Instruct patient to report adverse reactions promptly.

---

*Liquid contains alcohol.   **May contain tartrazine.   †Canada   ‡Australia   §U.K.   ◊OTC

67

Alkylating drugs

busulfan
carboplatin
carmustine
chlorambucil
cisplatin
cyclophosphamide
ifosfamide
lomustine
mechlorethamine hydrochloride
melphalan
melphalan hydrochloride
temozolomide
thiotepa

COMBINATION PRODUCTS
None.

busulfan
Busulfex, Myleran

Pregnancy risk category D

AVAILABLE FORMS
Injection: 6 mg/ml
Tablets: 2 mg

INDICATIONS & DOSAGES
➤ **Chronic myelocytic (granulocytic) leukemia—**
Adults: 4 to 8 mg P.O. daily until WBC count falls to 15,000/mm³; drug stopped until WBC count rises to 50,000/mm³, and then resumed as before. Or, 4 to 8 mg P.O. daily until WBC count falls to 10,000 to 20,000/mm³; then reduce daily dose, p.r.n., to maintain WBC count at this level. Dosage is highly variable; range is 2 mg/week to 4 mg/day.
Children: 0.06 to 0.12 mg/kg/day or 1.8 to 4.6 mg/m²/day P.O.; adjust dosage to maintain WBC count at 20,000/mm³, but never below 10,000/mm³.
➤ **Allogenic hematopoietic stem cell transplantation in patients with chronic myelogenous leukemia—**
Adults: 0.8 mg/kg I.V. q 6 hours for 4 days (a total of 16 doses). Give cyclophosphamide 60 mg/kg I.V. over 1 hour daily

for 2 days beginning 6 hours after the 16th dose of busulfan injection.

I.V. ADMINISTRATION
● Dilute drug in either D_5W or normal saline to a final concentration of ≥ 0.5 mg/ml. Use the 5-micron nylon filter to withdraw the calculated volume from the ampule. A new needle should then be used to inject the drug into the I.V. bag or syringe. Invert several times to ensure mixing.
● Infuse over 2 hours through a central venous catheter using a controlled-infusion device. Flush the catheter line with 5 ml of D_5W or normal saline before and after each infusion.
● Busulfan solutions are stable for 8 hours at room temperature, or 12 hours when diluted in normal saline and refrigerated. Infusions must be used and completed during these time frames.

ACTION
Unknown. Thought to cross-link strands of cellular DNA and interfere with RNA transcription, causing an imbalance of growth that leads to cell death. Not specific to cell cycle.

Route	Onset	Peak	Duration
I.V.	Unknown	Unknown	Unknown
P.O.	1-2 wk	Unknown	Unknown

ADVERSE REACTIONS
CNS: unusual tiredness or weakness, fatigue, *seizures.*
EENT: cataracts.
GI: cheilosis, dry mouth, anorexia, *nausea, vomiting.*
GU: amenorrhea, azoospermia.
Hematologic: *leukopenia, thrombocytopenia, anemia, severe pancytopenia.*
Hepatic: jaundice.
Metabolic: profound hyperuricemia.
Respiratory: *irreversible pulmonary fibrosis.*
Skin: alopecia, *transient hyperpigmentation,* rash, urticaria, anhidrosis.

Reactions may be *common*, uncommon, *life-threatening*, or COMMON AND LIFE-THREATENING.

Other: gynecomastia, Addison-like wasting syndrome.

INTERACTIONS
Drug-drug. *Anticoagulants, aspirin:* Increased risk of bleeding. Avoid using together.
Cyclophosphamide: May increase risk of cardiac tamponade in patients with thalassemia. Monitor patient.
Myelosuppressives: May cause increased myelosuppression. Monitor patient.
Phenytoin: May decrease busulfan levels. Monitor busulfan levels.
Thioguanine: May cause hepatotoxicity, esophageal varices, or portal hypertension. Use together cautiously.

EFFECTS ON LAB TEST RESULTS
• May increase uric acid levels.
• May decrease hemoglobin and WBC and platelet counts.

CONTRAINDICATIONS
Contraindicated in patients with chronic myelogenous leukemia that has shown prior resistance to drug. Not useful with chronic lymphocytic or acute leukemia or in the blastic crisis of chronic myelogenous leukemia.

NURSING CONSIDERATIONS
• Use cautiously in patients recently given other myelosuppressives or radiation treatment and in those with depressed neutrophil or platelet count. Because high-dose therapy has been linked to seizures, use cautiously in patients with history of head trauma or seizures and in those receiving other drugs that lower the seizure threshold.
• Manufacturer recommends that patients receiving busulfan injection be premedicated with antiemetics before first dose and then on a fixed schedule during therapy; phenytoin should be used to prevent seizures.
• Follow facility policy when preparing and handling drug. Label as a hazardous drug.
• Therapeutic effects are commonly accompanied by toxicity.
• To prevent bleeding, avoid all I.M. injections when platelet count is less than 50,000/mm³.

• Monitor patient response (increased appetite and sense of well-being, decreased total WBC count, reduced size of spleen), which usually begins in 1 to 2 weeks.
• Monitor uric acid level. To prevent hyperuricemia with resulting uric acid nephropathy, allopurinol may be ordered in addition to keeping patient adequately hydrated.
• Anticipate possible blood transfusion during treatment because of cumulative anemia. Patients may receive injections of RBC colony-stimulating factor to promote RBC production and decrease the need for blood transfusions.
• *Alert:* Pulmonary fibrosis may occur as late as 8 months to 10 years after treatment with busulfan. (Average duration of therapy is 4 years.)

PATIENT TEACHING
• Advise patient to watch for signs of infection (fever, sore throat, fatigue) and bleeding (easy bruising, nosebleeds, bleeding gums, melena). Tell patient to take temperature daily.
• Instruct patient to report signs and symptoms of toxicity so dosage can be adjusted. Persistent cough and progressive dyspnea with alveolar exudate, suggestive of pneumonia, may be result of drug toxicity.
• Instruct patient to avoid OTC products containing aspirin and NSAIDs.
• Inform patient that drug may cause darkening of skin.
• Advise woman of childbearing age to avoid becoming pregnant during therapy. Recommend that she consult prescriber before becoming pregnant.
• Warn breast-feeding woman to discontinue breast-feeding because of risk of toxicity to infant.
• Instruct patient to take drug on empty stomach to decrease nausea and vomiting.
• Because of risk of impotence and male sterility, advise man of childbearing potential about sperm banking before therapy begins.

carboplatin
Paraplatin, Paraplatin-AQ†

Pregnancy risk category D

AVAILABLE FORMS
Injection: 50-mg, 150-mg, 450-mg vials

INDICATIONS & DOSAGES
➤ **Advanced ovarian cancer—**
Adults: 360 mg/m² I.V. on day 1 q 4 weeks or 300 mg/m² when used with other chemotherapy drugs; doses shouldn't be repeated until platelet count exceeds 100,000/mm³ and neutrophil count exceeds 2,000/mm³. Subsequent doses are based on blood counts. Alternatively, refer to Package for Formula Dosing.
Adjust-a-dose: For renally impaired patients with creatinine clearance of 41 to 59 ml/minute, initial dose is 250 mg/m²; if between 16 and 40 ml/minute, initial dose is 200 mg/m². Drug isn't recommended for patients with creatinine clearance of 15 ml/minute or less.

I.V. ADMINISTRATION
● *Alert:* Have epinephrine, corticosteroids, and antihistamines available when administering carboplatin because anaphylactoid reactions may occur within minutes of administration.
● Reconstitute with D₅W, normal saline solution, or sterile water for injection to yield 10 mg/ml. Add 5 ml of diluent to 50 mg vial, 15 ml of diluent to 150-mg vial, or 45 ml of diluent to 450-mg vial. Reconstituted drug can then be further diluted for infusion with normal saline solution or D₅W. A concentration as low as 0.5 mg/ml can be prepared. Give drug by continuous or intermittent infusion over at least 15 minutes.
● Don't use needles or I.V. administration sets containing aluminum to administer carboplatin; precipitation and loss of potency may occur.
● Store unopened vials at room temperature. Once reconstituted and diluted as directed, drug is stable at room temperature for 8 hours. Because drug doesn't contain antibacterial preservatives, discard unused drug after 8 hours.

ACTION
Unknown. Thought to cross-link strands of cellular DNA and interferes with RNA transcription, causing an imbalance of growth that leads to cell death. Not specific to cell cycle.

Route	Onset	Peak	Duration
I.V.	Unknown	Unknown	Unknown

ADVERSE REACTIONS
CNS: *asthenia,* dizziness, confusion, **CVA,** peripheral neuropathy, central neurotoxicity, paresthesia.
CV: *heart failure, embolism.*
EENT: ototoxicity, visual disturbances.
GI: constipation, diarrhea, *nausea, vomiting,* mucositis, change in taste, stomatitis.
Hematologic: THROMBOCYTOPENIA, *leukopenia, neutropenia,* anemia, BONE MARROW SUPPRESSION.
Skin: alopecia.
Other: hypersensitivity reactions, *pain, anaphylaxis.*

INTERACTIONS
Drug-drug. *Aspirin, NSAIDs:* Increased risk of bleeding. Avoid using together.
Bone marrow suppressants, including radiation therapy: Increased hematologic toxicity. Monitor CBC with differential closely.
Myelosuppressives: May cause increased myelosuppression. Monitor patient.
Nephrotoxic drugs, especially aminoglycosides: Enhanced nephrotoxicity of carboplatin. Use together cautiously.

EFFECTS ON LAB TEST RESULTS
● May increase BUN, creatinine, AST, and alkaline phosphatase levels. May decrease electrolyte levels.
● May decrease neutrophils, WBCs, RBCs, and platelet counts. May decrease hemoglobin and hematocrit.

CONTRAINDICATIONS
Contraindicated in patients with severe bone marrow suppression or bleeding or with history of hypersensitivity to cisplatin, platinum-containing compounds, or mannitol.

Reactions may be *common*, uncommon, *life-threatening*, or COMMON AND LIFE-THREATENING.

NURSING CONSIDERATIONS

• Determine electrolyte, creatinine, and BUN levels, CBC, and creatinine clearance before first infusion and before each course of treatment.

• Monitor CBC and platelet count frequently during therapy and, when indicated, until recovery. WBC and platelet count nadirs usually occur by day 21. Levels usually return to baseline by day 28. Dose shouldn't be repeated unless platelet count exceeds 100,000/mm³. Give WBC colony-stimulating factor to promote neutrophil recovery.

• Bone marrow suppression may be more severe in patients with creatinine clearance below 60 ml/minute; dosage adjustments are recommended for such patients.

• Follow facility policy to reduce risks because preparation and administration of parenteral form of drug are linked to mutagenic, teratogenic, and carcinogenic risks for staff.

• *Alert:* Carefully check ordered dose against laboratory test results. Only one increase in dosage is recommended. Subsequent doses shouldn't exceed 125% of starting dose.

• Therapeutic effects are commonly accompanied by toxicity.

• Carboplatin has less nephrotoxicity and neurotoxicity than cisplatin, but it causes more severe myelosuppression.

• To prevent bleeding, avoid all I.M. injections when platelet count is below 50,000/mm³.

• Monitor vital signs during infusion.

• Administer antiemetic therapy. Carboplatin can produce severe vomiting.

• Anticipate blood transfusions during treatment because of cumulative anemia. Patient may receive injections of RBC colony-stimulating factor to promote cell production.

• Hydration or diuresis before or after treatment isn't needed.

• Patients older than age 65 are at greater risk for neurotoxicity.

• *Alert:* Don't confuse carboplatin with cisplatin.

PATIENT TEACHING

• Advise patient of most common adverse reactions: nausea, vomiting, bone marrow suppression, anemia, and thrombocytopenia.

• Advise patient to watch for signs of infection (fever, sore throat, fatigue) and bleeding (easy bruising, nosebleeds, bleeding gums, melena). Tell patient to take temperature daily.

• Instruct patient to avoid OTC products containing aspirin and NSAIDs.

• Advise breast-feeding woman taking drug to discontinue breast-feeding because of risk of toxicity to infant.

• Because of risk of impotence, sterility, and amenorrhea, counsel both men and women of childbearing age before starting therapy. Also recommend that women consult prescriber before becoming pregnant.

---

carmustine (BCNU)
BiCNU, Gliadel Wafer

Pregnancy risk category D

AVAILABLE FORMS
Injection: 100-mg vial (lyophilized), with a 3-ml vial of absolute alcohol supplied as a diluent
Wafer: 7.7 mg, for intracavitary use

INDICATIONS & DOSAGES
➤ **Brain tumors, Hodgkin's disease, malignant lymphoma, multiple myeloma—**
Adults: 150 to 200 mg/ m² I.V. by slow infusion q 6 weeks; may be divided into daily injections of 75 to 100 mg/m² on two successive days; repeat dose q 6 weeks if platelet count is greater than 100,000/mm³ and WBC count is greater than 4,000/mm³.
Adjust-a-dose: Dosage is reduced by 30% when WBC nadir is 2,000 to 2,999/mm³ and platelet nadir is 25,000 to 74,999/mm³. Dosage is reduced by 50% when WBC nadir is less than 2,000/mm³ and platelet nadir is less than 25,000/mm³.
➤ **Adjunct to surgery to prolong survival in patients with recurrent glioblastoma multiforme for whom surgical resection is indicated—**
Adults: 8 wafers placed in the resection cavity if size and shape of cavity allow. If 8 wafers can't be accommodated, use

---

maximum number of wafers allowed. Or, 150 to 200 mg/m^2 I.V. by slow infusion as single dose, repeated q 6 to 8 weeks.

I.V. ADMINISTRATION
● Follow facility policy to reduce risks because preparation and administration of parenteral form of this drug are linked to carcinogenic, mutagenic, and teratogenic risks for staff. Manufacturer recommends wearing gloves when handling either form.
● To reconstitute, dissolve 100 mg of carmustine in 3 ml of absolute alcohol provided by manufacturer. Dilute solution with 27 ml of sterile water for injection. Resulting solution contains 3.3 mg of carmustine/ml in 10% alcohol. Dilute in normal saline solution or D$_5$W for I.V. infusion. Give at least 250 ml over 1 to 2 hours. To reduce pain on infusion, dilute further or slow infusion rate.
● Discard drug if powder liquefies or appears oily (decomposition has occurred).
● Administer only in glass containers. Solution is unstable in plastic I.V. bags.
● Don't mix with other drugs during administration.
● Store reconstituted solution in refrigerator for 24 hours or at room temperature for 8 hours. May decompose at temperatures higher than 80° F (27° C).

ACTION
Inhibits enzymatic reactions involved with DNA synthesis, cross-links strands of cellular DNA, and interferes with RNA transcription, causing an imbalance of growth that leads to cell death. Not specific to cell cycle.

Route	Onset	Peak	Duration
I.V., intra-cavitary	Unknown	Unknown	Unknown

ADVERSE REACTIONS
CNS: ataxia, drowsiness.
EENT: ocular toxicities.
GI: *nausea beginning in 2 to 6 hours, vomiting, stomatitis.*
GU: *nephrotoxicity, renal failure.*
Hematologic: azotemia, *cumulative bone marrow suppression, leukopenia, thrombocytopenia, acute leukemia or bone marrow dysplasia,* anemia.

Hepatic: *hepatotoxicity.*
Respiratory: *pulmonary fibrosis.*
Skin: facial flushing, hyperpigmentation.
Other: *intense pain at infusion site from venous spasm, secondary malignancies.*

INTERACTIONS
Drug-drug. *Anticoagulants, aspirin, NSAIDs:* Increased risk of bleeding. Avoid using together.
Cimetidine: May increase carmustine's bone marrow toxicity. Avoid combination, if possible.
Digoxin, phenytoin: Decreased levels of these drugs. Monitor patient.
Myelosuppressives: May cause increased myelosuppression. Monitor patient.

EFFECTS ON LAB TEST RESULTS
● May increase nitrogenous compound (urea), AST, bilirubin, and alkaline phosphatase levels.
● May decrease hemoglobin and WBC and platelet counts.

CONTRAINDICATIONS
Contraindicated in patients hypersensitive to drug.

NURSING CONSIDERATIONS
● Pulmonary toxicity appears to be dose-related and may occur 9 days to 15 years after treatment. Obtain pulmonary function tests, before and during therapy.
● Bone marrow suppression is delayed with carmustine. Drug shouldn't be given more often than every 6 weeks.
● To reduce nausea, give antiemetic before drug.
● Avoid contact with skin because carmustine causes a brown stain. If drug comes into contact with skin, wash off thoroughly.
● Perform liver, renal function, and pulmonary function tests periodically.
● Monitor CBC with differential. The absolute neutrophil count may be used to better calculate the patient's immunosuppressive state.
● Monitor uric acid level. To prevent hyperuricemia with resulting uric acid nephropathy, allopurinol may be used with adequate hydration.
● Therapeutic effects are commonly accompanied by toxicity.

Reactions may be *common*, uncommon, *life-threatening*, or **COMMON AND LIFE-THREATENING.**

• Acute leukemia or bone marrow dysplasia may occur after long-term use.
• To prevent bleeding, avoid all I.M. injections when platelet count is less than 50,000/mm³.
• Anticipate blood transfusions during treatment because of cumulative anemia. Patient may receive injections of RBC colony-stimulating factor to promote cell production.
• Unopened foil pouches of wafer may be kept at ambient room temperature for a maximum of 6 hours.
• Wafers broken in half may be used; however, wafers broken into more than two pieces should be discarded.

PATIENT TEACHING
• Advise patient about common adverse reactions to drug.
• Tell patient to watch for signs and symptoms of infection (fever, sore throat, fatigue) and bleeding (easy bruising, nosebleeds, bleeding gums, melena). Tell him to take temperature daily.
• Instruct patient to avoid OTC products containing aspirin and NSAIDs.
• Advise breast-feeding woman to discontinue breast-feeding during therapy because of possible risk of toxicity to infant.
• Caution woman of childbearing age to avoid becoming pregnant during therapy. Recommend that she consult prescriber before becoming pregnant.

---

chlorambucil
Leukeran

Pregnancy risk category D

AVAILABLE FORMS
Tablets: 2 mg

INDICATIONS & DOSAGES
➤ **Chronic lymphocytic leukemia; malignant lymphomas, including lymphosarcoma, giant follicular lymphoma, and Hodgkin's disease—**
Adults: 0.1 to 0.2 mg/kg P.O. daily for 3 to 6 weeks, then adjusted for maintenance (usually 4 to 10 mg daily); or, 3 to 6 mg/m² P.O. daily.
Children: 0.1 to 0.2 mg/kg P.O. or 4.5 mg/m² P.O. daily for 3 to 6 weeks.

Adjust-a-dose: Reduce initial dose if given within 4 weeks after a full course of radiation therapy or myelosuppressive drugs, or if pretreatment leukocyte or platelet counts are depressed from bone marrow disease.

ACTION
Cross-links strands of cellular DNA and interferes with RNA transcription, causing an imbalance of growth that leads to cell death. Not specific to cell cycle.

Route	Onset	Peak	Duration
P.O.	Unknown	1 hr	Unknown

ADVERSE REACTIONS
CNS: *seizures,* peripheral neuropathy, tremor, muscle twitching, confusion, agitation, ataxia, flaccid paresis.
GI: *nausea, vomiting,* stomatitis, diarrhea.
GU: *azoospermia, infertility,* sterile cystitis.
Hematologic: *neutropenia, bone marrow suppression, thrombocytopenia,* anemia, *myelosuppression.*
Hepatic: *hepatotoxicity.*
Respiratory: interstitial pneumonitis, *pulmonary fibrosis.*
Skin: rash, *erythema multiforme,* epidermal necrolysis, *Stevens-Johnson syndrome.*
Other: allergic febrile reaction, hypersensitivity reactions, *secondary malignancies.*

INTERACTIONS
Drug-drug. *Anticoagulants, aspirin:* Increased risk of bleeding. Avoid using together.
Myelosuppressives: May cause increased myelosuppression. Monitor patient.

EFFECTS ON LAB TEST RESULTS
• May increase AST and alkaline phosphatase levels. May increase blood and urine uric acid levels.
• May decrease hemoglobin, neutrophil and platelet counts. May decrease WBC, granulocyte, and RBC counts.

CONTRAINDICATIONS
Contraindicated in patients with hypersensitivity or resistance to previous therapy. Patients hypersensitive to other alkylating

---

drugs may also be hypersensitive to chlorambucil.

NURSING CONSIDERATIONS
• Use cautiously in patients with history of head trauma or seizures and in patients receiving other drugs that lower the seizure threshold. Also use cautiously within 4 weeks of a full course of radiation or chemotherapy.
• Monitor CBC with differential.
• Monitor patient for neutropenia, which may not appear until after the third week of treatment. The neutrophil count may continue to decrease for up to 10 days after treatment ends.
• The absolute neutrophil count may be used to better calculate the patient's immunosuppressive state.
• Monitor uric acid level. To prevent hyperuricemia with resulting uric acid nephropathy, allopurinol may be used with adequate hydration.
• If WBC count falls below 2,000/mm³ or granulocyte count falls below 1,000/mm³, follow institutional policy for infection control in immunocompromised patients. Patients may receive injections of WBC colony-stimulating factor to increase WBC count recovery. Severe neutropenia is reversible up to cumulative dose of 6.5 mg/kg in a single course.
• Therapeutic effects are frequently accompanied by toxicity.
• To prevent bleeding, avoid all I.M. injections when platelet count is below 50,000/mm³.
• Anticipate blood transfusions during treatment because of cumulative anemia. Patient may receive injections of RBC colony-stimulating factor to promote RBC production and decrease need for blood transfusions.

PATIENT TEACHING
• Advise patient to watch for signs of infection (fever, sore throat, fatigue) and bleeding (easy bruising, nosebleeds, bleeding gums, melena). Tell patient to take temperature daily.
• Tell patient to take drug with food.
• Instruct patient to avoid OTC products containing aspirin and NSAIDs.

• Tell breast-feeding woman to discontinue breast-feeding during therapy because of risk of toxicity to infant.
• Advise woman of childbearing age to avoid becoming pregnant during therapy and to notify prescriber immediately if pregnancy is suspected.

---

cisplatin (CDDP, cis-platinum†)
Platinol AQ

Pregnancy risk category D

AVAILABLE FORMS
Injection: 0.5 mg/ml†, 1 mg/ml

INDICATIONS & DOSAGES
➤ **Adjunctive therapy in metastatic testicular cancer—**
Adults: 20 mg/m² I.V. daily for 5 days. Repeated q 3 weeks for three cycles or longer.
➤ **Adjunctive therapy in metastatic ovarian cancer—**
Adults: 100 mg/m² I.V.; repeated q 4 weeks. Or, 50 to 100 mg/m² I.V. once q 3 to 4 weeks with cyclophosphamide.
➤ **Advanced bladder cancer—**
Adults: 50 to 70 mg/m² I.V. q 3 to 4 weeks. Patients who have received other antineoplastic drugs or radiation therapy should receive 50 mg/m² q 4 weeks.

I.V. ADMINISTRATION
• Administer mannitol or furosemide boluses or infusions before and during cisplatin infusion to maintain diuresis of 100 to 400 ml/hour during and for 24 hours after therapy.
• Hydrate patient with normal saline solution before giving drug. Maintain urine output of at least 100 ml/hour for 4 consecutive hours before therapy and for 24 hours after therapy.
• Follow facility policy to reduce risks because preparation and administration of parenteral form of drug are linked to carcinogenic, mutagenic, and teratogenic risks for staff.
• Reconstitute powder using sterile water for injection. Add 10 ml to 10-mg vial or 50 ml to 50-mg vial to make a solution containing 1 mg/ml. Further dilute with

---

dextrose 5% in 0.3% sodium chloride injection or dextrose 5% in half-normal saline solution for injection. Solutions are stable for 20 hours at room temperature. Don't refrigerate.

• Infusions are most stable in chloride-containing solutions (such as normal or half-normal saline solution and 0.22% sodium chloride). Don't use D_5W alone.

• The manufacturer recommends giving drug as an I.V. infusion in 2 L of dextrose 5% in half-normal saline solution or dextrose 5% in 0.33% sodium chloride solution with 37.5 g of mannitol over 6 to 8 hours.

• Don't use needles or I.V. administration sets that contain aluminum because they will displace the platinum, causing loss of potency and formation of a black precipitate.

• To prevent hypokalemia, potassium chloride (10 to 20 mEq/L) is commonly added to I.V. fluids before and after cisplatin therapy. Magnesium sulfate may be added to prevent hypomagnesemia.

ACTION
Unknown. Thought to cross-link strands of cellular DNA and interfere with RNA transcription, causing an imbalance of growth that leads to cell death. Not specific to cell cycle.

Route	Onset	Peak	Duration
I.V.	Unknown	Unknown	Several days

ADVERSE REACTIONS
CNS: *peripheral neuritis,* **seizures.**
EENT: *tinnitus, hearing loss, ototoxicity, vestibular toxicity, optic neuritis, papilledema, cerebral blindness, blurred vision.*
GI: loss of taste, *nausea, vomiting beginning 1 to 4 hours after dose and lasting 24 hours or longer.*
GU: **PROLONGED RENAL TOXICITY** with repeated courses of therapy.
Hematologic: MYELOSUPPRESSION, *leukopenia, thrombocytopenia,* anemia.
Metabolic: *hypomagnesemia,* hypokalemia, hypocalcemia, hyponatremia, hypophosphatemia, hyperuricemia.
Other: *anaphylactoid reaction.*

INTERACTIONS
Drug-drug. *Aminoglycoside antibiotics:* Increased nephrotoxicity. Carefully monitor renal function studies.
Aspirin, NSAIDs: Increased risk of bleeding. Avoid using together.
Bumetanide, ethacrynic acid, furosemide: Increased ototoxicity. Avoid using together, if possible.
Fosphenytoin, phenytoin: Decreased phenytoin and fosphenytoin levels. Monitor levels.
Myelosuppressives: May cause increased myelosuppression. Monitor patient.
Sodium bicarbonate, mesna, sodium thiosulfate: Inactivates cisplatin. Don't administer through same I.V. line.

EFFECTS ON LAB TEST RESULTS
• May increase uric acid levels. May decrease magnesium, potassium, calcium, sodium, and phosphate levels.
• May decrease hemoglobin and WBC and platelet levels.

CONTRAINDICATIONS
Contraindicated in patients hypersensitive to drug or other platinum-containing compounds and in those with severe renal disease, hearing impairment, or myelosuppression.

NURSING CONSIDERATIONS
• Use cautiously in patients previously treated with radiation or cytotoxic drugs and in those with peripheral neuropathies; also use cautiously with other ototoxic and nephrotoxic drugs.
• Monitor CBC, electrolyte levels (especially potassium and magnesium), platelet count, and renal function studies before initial and subsequent doses.
• To detect hearing loss, obtain audiometry tests before initial and subsequent doses.
• Prehydration and mannitol diuresis may significantly reduce renal toxicity and ototoxicity.
• Therapeutic effects are frequently accompanied by toxicity.
• Check current protocol. Some prescribers use I.V. sodium thiosulfate or amifostine to minimize toxicity.
• Administer antiemetics. Nausea and vomiting may be severe and protracted;

however, occurrence and severity have been significantly reduced with use of ondansetron and granisetron. Monitor intake and output. Continue I.V. hydration until patient can tolerate adequate oral intake.

• Some prescribers combine metoclopramide with dexamethasone and antihistamines, or ondansetron or granisetron with dexamethasone.

• Delayed-onset vomiting (3 to 5 days after treatment) has been reported; patients may need prolonged antiemetic treatment.

• Renal toxicity is cumulative; renal function must return to normal before next dose can be given.

• Dose shouldn't be repeated unless platelet count is greater than 100,000/mm³, WBC count is greater than 4,000/mm³, creatinine level is less than 1.5 mg/dl, creatine clearance is 50 ml/minute or more, or BUN level is less than 25 mg/dl.

• To prevent bleeding, avoid all I.M. injections when platelet count is less than 50,000/mm³.

• Anticipate blood transfusions during treatment because of cumulative anemia.

• *Alert:* Immediately administer epinephrine, corticosteroids, or antihistamines for anaphylactoid reactions.

• Safety of drug in children hasn't been established.

• *Alert:* Don't confuse cisplatin with carboplatin; they aren't interchangeable.

PATIENT TEACHING
• Advise patient to watch for signs and symptoms of infection (fever, sore throat, fatigue) and bleeding (easy bruising, nosebleeds, bleeding gums, melena). Tell patient to take temperature daily.

• Tell patient to immediately report tinnitus or numbness in hands or feet.

• Instruct patient to avoid OTC products containing aspirin.

• Advise breast-feeding woman taking drug to discontinue breast-feeding because of risk of toxicity to infant.

• Advise woman of childbearing age to avoid becoming pregnant during therapy. Recommend that she consult prescriber before becoming pregnant.

cyclophosphamide
Cycloblastin‡, Cytoxan**, Cytoxan Lyophilized, Endoxan§, Endoxan-Asta‡, Neosar, Procytox†

Pregnancy risk category D

AVAILABLE FORMS
Injection: 100-mg, 200-mg, 500-mg, 1-g, 2-g vials
Tablets: 25 mg, 50 mg

INDICATIONS & DOSAGES
➤ **Breast and ovarian cancers, Hodgkin's disease, chronic lymphocytic leukemia, chronic myelocytic leukemia, acute lymphoblastic leukemia, acute myelocytic and monocytic leukemia, neuroblastoma, retinoblastoma, malignant lymphoma, multiple myeloma, mycosis fungoides, sarcoma—**
Adults: Initially for induction, 40 to 50 mg/kg I.V. in divided doses over 2 to 5 days. Or, 10 to 15 mg/kg I.V. q 7 to 10 days, 3 to 5 mg/kg I.V. twice weekly, or 1 to 5 mg/kg P.O. daily, based on patient tolerance.
Children: Initially for induction, 2 to 8 mg/kg or 60 to 250 mg/m² P.O. or I.V. daily. Maintenance dose is 2 to 5 mg/kg P.O. or 50 to 150 mg/m² P.O. twice weekly.

Adjust subsequent doses according to evidence of antitumor activity or leukopenia.
➤ **Minimal change nephrotic syndrome in children—**
Children: 2 to 3 mg/kg P.O. daily for 60 to 90 days.

I.V. ADMINISTRATION
• Follow facility policy to reduce risks. Preparation and administration of parenteral form of this drug are linked to carcinogenic, mutagenic, and teratogenic risks for staff.

• Reconstitute powder using sterile water for injection or bacteriostatic water for injection containing only parabens. For the nonlyophilized product, add 5 ml to 100-mg vial, 10 ml to 200-mg vial, 25 ml to 500-mg vial, 50 ml to 1-g vial, or 100 ml to 2-g vial to produce a solution containing 20 mg/ml. Shake to dissolve;

Reactions may be *common*, uncommon, **life-threatening**, or COMMON AND LIFE-THREATENING.

this may take up to 6 minutes, and it may be difficult to completely dissolve drug. Lyophilized preparation is much easier to reconstitute; check package insert for quantity of diluent needed to reconstitute drug.

• After reconstitution, administer, by direct I.V. injection or infusion. For I.V. infusion, further dilute with D_5W, dextrose 5% in normal saline solution for injection, dextrose 5% in Ringer's injection, lactated Ringer's injection, sodium lactate injection, or half-normal saline solution for injection.

• Check reconstituted solution for small particles. Filter solution if needed.

• Reconstituted solution is stable for 6 days if refrigerated, or 24 hours at room temperature. However, use stored solutions cautiously because drug contains no preservatives.

ACTION

Cross-links strands of cellular DNA and interferes with RNA transcription, causing an imbalance of growth that leads to cell death. Not specific to cell cycle.

Route	Onset	Peak	Duration
I.V., P.O.	Unknown	Unknown	Unknown

ADVERSE REACTIONS

CV: *cardiotoxicity with very high doses and with doxorubicin,* flushing.
GI: anorexia, *nausea and vomiting beginning within 6 hours,* abdominal pain, stomatitis, mucositis.
GU: HEMORRHAGIC CYSTITIS, impaired fertility.
Hematologic: *leukopenia, thrombocytopenia,* anemia.
Hepatic: *hepatotoxicity.*
Metabolic: hyperuricemia, SIADH.
Respiratory: *pulmonary fibrosis with high doses.*
Skin: *reversible alopecia,* rash, pigmentation, nail changes, itching.
Other: *secondary malignant disease, anaphylaxis,* hypersensitivity reactions.

INTERACTIONS

Drug-drug. *Allopurinol:* Increased myelosuppression. Monitor toxicity.
Aspirin, NSAIDs: Increased risk of bleeding. Avoid using together.

Barbiturates: Increased pharmacologic effect and enhanced cyclophosphamide toxicity from induction of hepatic enzymes. Monitor patient closely.
Cardiotoxic drugs: Increased adverse cardiac effects. Monitor toxicity.
Chloramphenicol, corticosteroids: Reduced activity of cyclophosphamide. Use together cautiously.
Digoxin: May decrease digoxin levels. Monitor levels closely.
Myelosuppressives: May cause increased myelosuppression. Monitor patient.
Succinylcholine: Prolonged neuromuscular blockade. Avoid using together.

EFFECTS ON LAB TEST RESULTS

• May increase uric acid levels. May decrease pseudocholinesterase levels.
• May decrease hemoglobin and WBC, RBC, and platelet counts.

CONTRAINDICATIONS

Contraindicated in patients hypersensitive to drug and in those with severe bone marrow suppression.

NURSING CONSIDERATIONS

• Use cautiously in patients with leukopenia, thrombocytopenia, malignant cell infiltration of bone marrow, or hepatic or renal disease and in those who have recently undergone radiation therapy or chemotherapy.
• Don't give drug at bedtime; infrequent urination during the night may increase possibility of cystitis. If cystitis occurs, discontinue drug and notify prescriber. Cystitis can occur months after therapy ceases. Mesna may be given to lower occurrence and severity of bladder toxicity. Test urine for blood.
• Patients should receive adequate hydration before and after dose to decrease risk of cystitis.
• Use caution to ensure correct dose to decrease risk of cardiac toxicity.
• Monitor CBC and renal and liver function test results.
• Monitor patient closely for leukopenia (nadir between days 8 and 15, recovery in 17 to 28 days).
• Monitor uric acid level. To prevent hyperuricemia with resulting uric acid

nephropathy, allopurinol may be used with adequate hydration.

• Drug may suppress positive reaction to *Candida,* mumps, *Trichophyton,* and tuberculin skin test. A false-positive result for the Papanicolaou test may occur.

• *Alert:* Monitor patient for cyclophosphamide toxicity (leukopenia, thrombocytopenia, cardiotoxicity) if patient's corticosteroid therapy is discontinued.

• To prevent bleeding, avoid all I.M. injections when platelet count is below 50,000/mm^3.

• Anticipate blood transfusions because of cumulative anemia. Patients may receive injections of RBC colony-stimulating factor to promote RBC production and decrease need for blood transfusions.

• Therapeutic effects are commonly accompanied by toxicity.

• Drug has been used to treat nononcologic disorders such as lupus, nephritis, and rheumatoid arthritis.

PATIENT TEACHING

• Warn patient that hair loss is likely to occur but that it's reversible.

• Advise patient to watch for signs and symptoms of infection (fever, sore throat, fatigue) and bleeding (easy bruising, nosebleeds, bleeding gums, melena). Tell patient to take temperature daily.

• Instruct patient to avoid OTC products that contain aspirin.

• To minimize risk of hemorrhagic cystitis, encourage patient to void every 1 to 2 hours while awake and to drink at least 3 L of fluid daily. If patient is taking oral form of drug, instruct him to avoid taking it at bedtime because infrequent urination increases risk of cystitis.

• Advise both men and women to practice contraception during therapy and for 4 months afterward; drug is potentially teratogenic.

• Advise breast-feeding woman taking drug to stop breast-feeding because of risk of toxicity to infant.

• Drug can cause irreversible sterility in both men and women. Counsel patients of childbearing potential before starting therapy. Also recommend that women consult prescriber before becoming pregnant.

---

ifosfamide
Holoxan‡, Ifex, Mitoxana§

Pregnancy risk category D

AVAILABLE FORMS
Injection: 1 g, 2 g†‡, 3 g

INDICATIONS & DOSAGES
➤ **Testicular cancer—**
Adults: 1.2 g/m^2/day I.V. for 5 consecutive days. Treatment is repeated q 3 weeks or after patient recovers from hematologic toxicity.

I.V. ADMINISTRATION

• Follow facility policy to reduce risks. Preparation and administration of parenteral form of drug are linked to carcinogenic, mutagenic, and teratogenic risks for staff.

• Reconstitute each gram of drug with 20 ml of diluent to yield a solution of 50 mg/ml. Use sterile water for injection or bacteriostatic water for injection. Solutions may then be further diluted with sterile water, dextrose 2.5% or 5% in water, half-normal or normal saline solution for injection, dextrose 5% and normal saline solution for injection, or lactated Ringer's injection.

• Infuse each dose over at least 30 minutes.

• Give ifosfamide with a protective drug such as mesna to prevent hemorrhagic cystitis. Obtain urinalysis before each dose. If microscopic hematuria is present, notify prescriber. Mesna is given with or before ifosfamide to prevent cystitis. (Dosage adjustments of mesna given concomitantly may be needed.) Adequate fluid intake (2 L/day, either P.O. or I.V.) is essential before, and 72 hours after, therapy.

• Ifosfamide and mesna are physically compatible and may be mixed in the same I.V. solution.

• Reconstituted solution is stable for 1 week at room temperature, or 6 weeks if refrigerated. However, use solution within 6 hours if drug was reconstituted with sterile water without a preservative (such as benzyl alcohol or parabens).

Reactions may be *common,* uncommon, *life-threatening,* or COMMON AND LIFE-THREATENING.

ACTION
Cross-links strands of cellular DNA and interferes with RNA transcription, causing an imbalance of growth that leads to cell death. Not specific to cell cycle.

Route	Onset	Peak	Duration
I.V.	Unknown	Unknown	Unknown

ADVERSE REACTIONS
CNS: *somnolence, confusion,* **coma, seizures,** ataxia, hallucinations, depressive psychosis, dizziness, disorientation, cranial nerve dysfunction.
GI: *nausea, vomiting.*
GU: *hemorrhagic cystitis, hematuria,* **nephrotoxicity.**
Hematologic: leukopenia, thrombocytopenia, myelosuppression.
Metabolic: *metabolic acidosis.*
Skin: *alopecia.*
Other: infection, phlebitis.

INTERACTIONS
Drug-drug. *Anticoagulants, aspirin, NSAIDs:* Increased risk of bleeding. Avoid using together.
Barbiturates, chloral hydrate, fosphenytoin, phenytoin: May increase ifosfamide toxicity by inducing hepatic enzymes that hasten formation of toxic metabolites. Monitor patient closely.
Corticosteroids: May inhibit hepatic enzymes, reducing ifosfamide's effect. Monitor patient for increased ifosfamide toxicity if corticosteroid dosage is suddenly reduced or discontinued.
Cyclophosphamides: May increase risk of cardiac tamponade in patients with thalassemia. Monitor patient closely during use.
Myelosuppressives: Enhanced hematologic toxicity. Dosage adjustment may be needed.

EFFECTS ON LAB TEST RESULTS
• May increase liver enzyme levels.
• May decrease WBCs and platelets.

CONTRAINDICATIONS
Contraindicated in patients hypersensitive to drug and in those with severe bone marrow suppression.

NURSING CONSIDERATIONS
• Use cautiously in patients with renal impairment or compromised bone marrow reserve as indicated by leukopenia, granulocytopenia, extensive bone marrow metastases, previous radiation therapy, or previous therapy with cytotoxic drugs.
• Administer antiemetics before giving ifosfamide to help decrease nausea.
• Don't give drug at bedtime; infrequent voiding during the night may increase possibility of cystitis. If cystitis develops, discontinue drug and notify prescriber.
• Bladder irrigation with normal saline solution may be done to treat cystitis.
• Monitor CBC and renal and liver function tests.
• To prevent bleeding, avoid all I.M. injections when platelet count is below 50,000/mm³.
• Anticipate blood transfusions because of cumulative anemia. Patients may receive injections of RBC colony-stimulating factor to promote RBC production and decrease need for blood transfusions.
• Assess patient for mental status changes; dosage may have to be decreased.
• *Alert:* Don't confuse ifosfamide with cyclophosphamide.

PATIENT TEACHING
• Remind patient to void frequently to minimize contact of drug and its metabolites with the bladder mucosa.
• Advise patient to watch for signs and symptoms of infection (fever, sore throat, fatigue) and bleeding (easy bruising, nosebleeds, bleeding gums, melena). Tell patient to take temperature daily.
• Instruct patient to avoid OTC products that contain aspirin.
• Advise breast-feeding woman to discontinue breast-feeding during therapy because of possible risk of toxicity to infant.
• Caution woman of childbearing age to avoid becoming pregnant during therapy. Recommend that she consult prescriber before becoming pregnant.

---

*Liquid contains alcohol.   **May contain tartrazine.   †Canada   ‡Australia   §U.K.   ◇OTC

lomustine (CCNU)
CeeNu

Pregnancy risk category D

AVAILABLE FORMS
Capsules: 10 mg, 40 mg, 100 mg, dose pack (two 10-mg, two 40-mg, two 100-mg capsules)

INDICATIONS & DOSAGES
➤ Brain tumor, Hodgkin's disease—
Adults and children: 100 to 130 mg/m² P.O. as single dose q 6 weeks. Repeat doses shouldn't be given until WBC count exceeds 4,000/mm³ and platelet count is over 100,000/mm³.
Adjust-a-dose: Reduce dosage according to degree of bone marrow suppression or when used with other myelosuppressive drugs. Reduce dosage by 30% for WBC count nadir 2,000 to 2,999/mm³; by 50% for WBC count nadir less than 2,000/mm³.

ACTION
Cross-links strands of cellular DNA and interferes with RNA transcription, causing an imbalance of growth that leads to cell death. Not specific to cell cycle.

Route	Onset	Peak	Duration
P.O.	Unknown	Unknown	Unknown

ADVERSE REACTIONS
CNS: disorientation, lethargy, ataxia.
GI: *nausea, vomiting,* stomatitis.
GU: *nephrotoxicity,* progressive azotemia, *renal failure,* amenorrhea, azoospermia.
Hematologic: *anemia, leukopenia, thrombocytopenia, bone marrow suppression.*
Hepatic: *hepatotoxicity.*
Respiratory: *pulmonary fibrosis.*
Skin: alopecia.
Other: *secondary malignant disease.*

INTERACTIONS
Drug-drug. *Anticoagulants, aspirin, NSAIDs:* Increased risk of bleeding. Avoid using together.
Myelosuppressives: May cause increased myelosuppression. Monitor patient.

EFFECTS ON LAB TEST RESULTS
• May increase nitrogenous compound (urea) level.
• May decrease hemoglobin and WBC, RBC, and platelet counts.

CONTRAINDICATIONS
Contraindicated in patients hypersensitive to drug.

NURSING CONSIDERATIONS
• Use cautiously in patients with decreased platelet, WBC, or RBC counts and in those receiving other myelosuppressives.
• To avoid nausea, give antiemetic before drug.
• Give 2 to 4 hours after meals; drug will be more completely absorbed if taken when stomach is empty.
• Monitor CBC weekly. Usually not administered more often than every 6 weeks; bone marrow toxicity is cumulative and delayed, usually occurring 4 to 6 weeks after drug administration.
• Periodically monitor liver function test results.
• To prevent bleeding, avoid all I.M. injections when platelet count is below 50,000/mm³.
• Anticipate blood transfusions because of cumulative anemia. Patients may receive RBC colony-stimulating factor to promote RBC production and decrease need for blood transfusions.
• Therapeutic effects are commonly accompanied by toxicity.
• Store capsules at room temperature. Avoid exposure to moisture, and protect from temperatures above 104° F (40° C).

PATIENT TEACHING
• Advise patient to take capsules on an empty stomach, if possible.
• Advise patient to watch for signs and symptoms of infection (fever, sore throat, fatigue) and bleeding (easy bruising, nosebleeds, bleeding gums, melena). Tell patient to take temperature daily.
• Instruct patient to avoid OTC products that contain aspirin or NSAIDs.
• Advise breast-feeding woman to discontinue breast-feeding during therapy because of possible risk of toxicity to infant.

Reactions may be *common,* uncommon, *life-threatening,* or COMMON AND LIFE-THREATENING.

● Caution woman of childbearing age to avoid becoming pregnant during therapy. Recommend that she consult prescriber before becoming pregnant.

---

mechlorethamine hydrochloride (nitrogen mustard)
Mustargen

Pregnancy risk category D

AVAILABLE FORMS
Injection: 10-mg vials

INDICATIONS & DOSAGES
➤ **Polycythemia vera, chronic lymphocytic leukemia, chronic myelocytic leukemia, malignant effusions (pericardial, peritoneal, pleural), mycosis fungoides, Hodgkin's disease, lymphosarcoma, bronchogenic cancer—**
Adults: 0.4 mg/kg I.V. as single dose or in divided doses of 0.1 to 0.2 mg/kg/day. Given through running I.V. infusion. Subsequent courses of therapy given when patient has recovered hematologically from previous course (usually 3 to 6 weeks).
➤ **Malignant effusions—**
Adults: 0.4 mg/kg intracavitarily, although 0.2 mg/kg has been used intrapericardially.

I.V. ADMINISTRATION
● Follow facility policy to reduce risks. Preparation and administration of parenteral form of drug are linked to carcinogenic, mutagenic, and teratogenic risks for staff.
● Reconstitute drug using 10 ml of sterile water for injection or normal saline solution for injection. Resulting solution contains 1 mg/ml of mechlorethamine. Give by direct injection into a vein or into tubing of a free-flowing I.V. solution.
● Prepare immediately before infusion. Solution is very unstable. Visually inspect before using; use within 15 minutes, and discard unused solution.
● Dispose of equipment used in preparation and administration of mechlorethamine properly and according to institutional policy. Neutralize unused solution with an equal volume of 5% sodium bicarbonate and 5% sodium thiosulfate for 45 minutes.
● *Alert:* Make sure that I.V. solution doesn't infiltrate. Mechlorethamine is a potent vesicant. If extravasation occurs, apply cold compresses for 6 to 12 hours, and infiltrate area with isotonic sodium thiosulfate.

ACTION
Cross-links strands of cellular DNA and interferes with RNA transcription, causing an imbalance of growth that leads to cell death. Not specific to cell cycle.

Route	Onset	Peak	Duration
I.V., intra-cavitary	Few sec–few min	Unknown	Unknown

ADVERSE REACTIONS
CNS: weakness, vertigo, neurotoxicity.
CV: *thrombophlebitis.*
EENT: tinnitus, deafness with high doses.
GI: *nausea, vomiting, anorexia,* diarrhea, metallic taste.
GU: menstrual irregularities, impaired spermatogenesis.
Hematologic: *thrombocytopenia,* lymphocytopenia, *agranulocytosis,* mild anemia beginning in 2 to 3 weeks.
Hepatic: jaundice.
Metabolic: hyperuricemia.
Skin: *alopecia,* rash, sloughing, severe skin irritation with extravasation or contact.
Other: precipitation of herpes zoster, *anaphylaxis, secondary malignant disease.*

INTERACTIONS
Drug-drug. *Anticoagulants, aspirin, NSAIDs:* Increased risk of bleeding. Avoid using together.
Myelosuppressives: May cause increased myelosuppression. Monitor patient.

EFFECTS ON LAB TEST RESULTS
● May increase nitrogenous compound (urea) level.
● May decrease hemoglobin and granulocyte, lymphocyte, RBC, and platelet counts.

CONTRAINDICATIONS
Contraindicated in patients hypersensitive to drug and in those with infectious diseases.

NURSING CONSIDERATIONS
• Use cautiously in patients with severe anemia or depressed neutrophil or platelet count. Also use cautiously in those who have recently undergone radiation therapy or chemotherapy. Monitor CBC.
• When given intracavitarily for sclerosing effect, dilute using up to 100 ml of normal saline solution for injection. Turn patient from side to side every 5 to 10 minutes for 1 hour to distribute drug.
• Monitor uric acid level. To prevent hyperuricemia with resulting uric acid nephropathy, mechlorethamine may be used with adequate hydration.
• Therapeutic effects are commonly accompanied by toxicity.
• Neurotoxicity increases with dosage and patient age.
• To prevent bleeding, avoid all I.M. injections when platelet count is less than 50,000/mm³.
• Monitor patient closely for bone marrow suppression (nadir of myelosuppression occurring between days 4 and 10 and lasting 10 to 21 days).
• Anticipate blood transfusions because of cumulative anemia. Patients may receive RBC colony-stimulating factor to promote RBC cell production and decrease need for blood transfusions.

PATIENT TEACHING
• Advise patient to report any pain or burning at site of injection during or after administration.
• Advise patient to watch for signs and symptoms of infection (fever, sore throat, fatigue) and bleeding (easy bruising, nosebleeds, bleeding gums, melena). Tell patient to take temperature daily.
• Tell patient that severe nausea and vomiting can occur.
• Instruct patient to avoid OTC products that contain aspirin or NSAIDs.
• Caution breast-feeding woman taking drug to discontinue breast-feeding because of risk of toxicity to infant.
• Advise woman of childbearing age to avoid becoming pregnant during therapy.

Suggest that she consult prescriber before becoming pregnant.

---

melphalan (L-phenylalanine mustard)
Alkeran

melphalan hydrochloride
Alkeran

Pregnancy risk category D

AVAILABLE FORMS
Injection: 50 mg
Tablets (scored): 2 mg

INDICATIONS & DOSAGES
➤ **Multiple myeloma—**
Adults: Initially, 6 mg P.O. daily for 2 to 3 weeks; then stop drug for up to 4 weeks or until WBC and platelet counts stop dropping and begin to rise again; maintenance dose is 2 mg daily. Or, 0.15 mg/kg P.O. daily for 7 days, or 0.25 mg/kg for 4 days; repeated q 4 to 6 weeks.

Or, administer I.V. to patients who can't tolerate oral therapy, 16 mg/m² given by infusion over 15 to 20 minutes at 2-week intervals for four doses. After patient has recovered from toxicity, give drug at 4-week intervals.
Adjust-a-dose: For patients with renal insufficiency, dosage is reduced by up to 50%.
➤ **Nonresectable advanced ovarian cancer—**
Adults: 0.2 mg/kg P.O. daily for 5 days. Repeat q 4 to 6 weeks, depending on bone marrow recovery.

I.V. ADMINISTRATION
• Follow facility policy to reduce risks. Preparation and administration of parenteral form of drug are linked to carcinogenic, mutagenic, and teratogenic risks for staff.
• Because drug isn't stable in solution, reconstitute immediately before administering with the 10 ml of sterile diluent supplied by manufacturer. Shake vigorously until solution is clear. The resulting solution will contain 5 mg/ml of melphalan. Immediately dilute required dose in normal saline solution for injection. Final con-

centration shouldn't exceed 0.45 mg/ml. Give infusion over 15 to 20 minutes.

• Promptly dilute and administer; reconstituted product begins to degrade within 30 minutes. After final dilution, nearly 1% of drug degrades every 10 minutes. Don't refrigerate reconstituted product because a precipitate will form. Administration must be completed within 60 minutes of reconstitution.

ACTION

Cross-links strands of cellular DNA and interferes with RNA transcription, causing an imbalance of growth that leads to cell death. Not specific to cell cycle.

Route	Onset	Peak	Duration
I.V., P.O.	Unknown	Unknown	Unknown

ADVERSE REACTIONS

CV: hypotension, tachycardia, edema.
GI: nausea, vomiting, diarrhea, oral ulceration, stomatitis.
Hematologic: *thrombocytopenia, leukopenia, bone marrow suppression,* hemolytic anemia.
Hepatic: *hepatotoxicity.*
Metabolic: hyperuricemia.
Respiratory: *pneumonitis, pulmonary fibrosis,* dyspnea, *bronchospasm.*
Skin: pruritus, alopecia, urticaria, ulceration at injection site.
Other: *anaphylaxis,* hypersensitivity reactions.

INTERACTIONS

Drug-drug. *Anticoagulants, aspirin, NSAIDs:* Increased risk of bleeding. Avoid using together.
Antigout drugs: Decreased effectiveness. Dosage adjustments may be needed.
Bone marrow suppressants: Increased toxicity. Monitor patient for toxicity.
Cyclosporine: Severe renal failure may occur. Monitor renal function closely.
Myelosuppressives: May cause increased myelosuppression. Monitor patient.
Vaccines: Decreased effectiveness of killed virus vaccines and increased risk of toxicity from live virus vaccines. Postpone routine immunization for at least 3 months after last dose of melphalan.

Drug-food. *Any food:* Decreased oral drug absorption. Advise patient to take drug on an empty stomach.

EFFECTS ON LAB TEST RESULTS

• May increase nitrogenous compound (urea) level.
• May decrease hemoglobin and RBC, WBC, and platelet counts.

CONTRAINDICATIONS

Contraindicated in patients hypersensitive to drug and in those whose disease is resistant to drug. Patients hypersensitive to chlorambucil may have cross-sensitivity to melphalan. Drug isn't recommended in patients with severe leukopenia, thrombocytopenia, or anemia or in those with chronic lymphocytic leukemia.

NURSING CONSIDERATIONS

• Use cautiously in patients receiving radiation and chemotherapy.
• Dosage may need to be reduced in patients with renal impairment.
• Melphalan is drug of choice with prednisone in patients with multiple myeloma.
• Give oral form on empty stomach. Food decreases drug absorption.
• Monitor uric acid level and CBC.
• To prevent bleeding, avoid all I.M. injections when platelet count is less than 50,000/mm^3.
• Anticipate blood transfusions because of cumulative anemia. Patients may receive RBC colony-stimulating factor to promote RBC production and decrease need for blood transfusions.
• Anaphylaxis may occur. Keep antihistamines and steroids readily available, and administer.
• *Alert:* Don't confuse melphalan with Mephyton.

PATIENT TEACHING

• Advise patient to take tablets on empty stomach.
• Advise patient to watch for signs and symptoms of infection (fever, sore throat, fatigue) and bleeding (easy bruising, nosebleeds, bleeding gums, melena). Tell patient to take temperature daily.
• Instruct patient to avoid OTC products that contain aspirin or NSAIDs.

• Caution breast-feeding woman taking drug to discontinue breast-feeding because of risk of toxicity to infant.

• Advise woman of childbearing age to avoid becoming pregnant during therapy. Suggest that she consult prescriber before becoming pregnant.

---

temozolomide
Temodar

Pregnancy risk category D

AVAILABLE FORMS
Capsules: 5 mg, 20 mg, 100 mg, 250 mg

INDICATIONS & DOSAGES
➤ **Refractory anaplastic astrocytoma that has relapsed after chemotherapy regimen containing a nitrosourea and procarbazine—**
Adults: Initial cycle: 150 mg/m^2 P.O. once daily for first 5 days of 28-day treatment cycle. Subsequent cycles: 100 to 200 mg/m^2 P.O. once daily for first 5 days of subsequent 28-day treatment cycles. Timing and dosage of subsequent cycles must be adjusted according to absolute neutrophil count (ANC) and platelet count measured on cycle day 22 (expected nadir) and day 29 (start of next cycle).

Dosage adjustments are based on lowest of ANC and platelet results. For ANC below 1,000/mm^3 or platelet count below 50,000/mm^3, hold therapy until ANC is greater than 1,500/mm^3 and platelet count is greater than 100,000/mm^3. Reduce dose by 50 mg/m^2 for subsequent cycle. Minimum dose is 100 mg/m^2.

For ANC of 1,000 to 1,500/mm^3 or platelet count of 50,000 to 100,000/mm^3, hold therapy until ANC exceeds 1,500/mm^3 and platelet count exceeds 100,000/mm^3. Maintain previous dose for subsequent cycle.

For ANC greater than 1,500/mm^3 and platelet count greater than 100,000/mm^3, increase dose to, or maintain at, 200 mg/m^2 for first 5 days of subsequent cycle.

ACTION
Active metabolite of temozolomide is thought to promote alkylation of DNA in rapidly dividing tissues, interfering with DNA replication.

Route	Onset	Peak	Duration
P.O.	Unknown	1 hr	Unknown

ADVERSE REACTIONS
CNS: amnesia, anxiety, asthenia, ataxia, confusion, SEIZURES, coordination abnormality, depression, dizziness, dysphasia, fatigue, gait abnormality, headache, hemiparesis, insomnia, paresis, paresthesia, somnolence.
CV: peripheral edema.
EENT: abnormal vision, diplopia, pharyngitis, sinusitis.
GI: abdominal pain, anorexia, constipation, diarrhea, nausea, vomiting.
GU: increased urinary frequency, urinary incontinence, urinary tract infection.
Hematologic: anemia, LEUKOPENIA, NEUTROPENIA, THROMBOCYTOPENIA.
Metabolic: weight increase.
Musculoskeletal: back pain, myalgia.
Respiratory: coughing, upper respiratory tract infection.
Skin: pruritus, rash.
Other: hyperadrenocorticism, breast pain in women, fever, viral infection.

INTERACTIONS
Drug-drug. *Valproic acid:* Decreases oral clearance of temozolomide by about 5%. Use together cautiously.
Drug-food. *Any food:* Reduces rate and extent of drug absorption; however, there are no dietary restrictions with drug administration. Advise patient to take drug on empty stomach to reduce nausea and vomiting.

EFFECTS ON LAB TEST RESULTS
• May decrease hemoglobin and WBC, platelet, and neutrophil counts.

CONTRAINDICATIONS
Contraindicated in patients hypersensitive to drug or its components and in those allergic to dacarbazine, which is structurally similar to temozolomide.

NURSING CONSIDERATIONS
• Use cautiously in elderly patients and in those with severe hepatic or renal impairment.

• A CBC should be drawn on days 22 and 29 of each treatment cycle. If ANC falls below 1,500/mm³ or platelet count falls below 100,000/mm³, a weekly CBC should be obtained until counts have recovered.

• Women and elderly patients are at higher risk for developing myelosuppression.

• Nausea and vomiting, which may be self-limiting, are the most common side effects. Advise patient to take drug on an empty stomach or at bedtime to lessen these effects. Antiemetics effectively control nausea and vomiting caused by drug use.

• Avoid skin contact with, or inhalation of, capsule contents if capsule is accidentally opened or damaged. Follow procedures for safe handling and disposal of antineoplastics.

• Store capsules at 59° to 86° F (15° to 30° C).

PATIENT TEACHING

• Emphasize importance of taking dose exactly as prescribed, usually on an empty stomach or at bedtime.

• Stress importance of continuing drug despite nausea and vomiting.

• Tell patient to call immediately if vomiting occurs shortly after he takes a dose.

• Tell patient to promptly report sore throat, fever, unusual bruising or bleeding, rash, or seizures.

• Advise patient to avoid exposure to people with infections.

• Advise sexually active patient to use effective birth control measures during treatment because drug may cause birth defects.

• Tell patient to swallow capsules whole and not to break them open.

---

thiotepa (TESPA, triethylenethiophosphoramide, TSPA)
Thioplex

Pregnancy risk category D

AVAILABLE FORMS
Injection: 15-mg vials

INDICATIONS & DOSAGES
➤ **Breast and ovarian cancers, lymphoma, Hodgkin's disease—**
Adults and children older than age 12: 0.3 to 0.4 mg/kg I.V. q 1 to 4 weeks or 0.2 mg/kg for 4 to 5 days at intervals of 2 to 4 weeks.

➤ **Bladder tumor—**
Adults and children older than age 12: 30 to 60 mg in 30 to 60 ml of saline solution instilled in bladder for 2 hours once weekly for 4 weeks.

➤ **Neoplastic effusions—**
Adults and children older than age 12: 0.6 to 0.8 mg/kg intracavitarily q 1 to 4 weeks.

I.V. ADMINISTRATION
• *Alert:* Follow institutional policy to minimize risks. Preparation and administration of parenteral form of drug are linked with mutagenic, teratogenic, and carcinogenic risks to personnel.

• Reconstitute with 1.5 ml of sterile water for injection. Don't reconstitute with other solutions. Further dilute with normal saline solution for injection. If larger volume is desired, may further dilute with sodium chloride, D_5W, dextrose 5% in normal saline solution for injection, Ringer's injection, or lactated Ringer's injection. Use solutions within 8 hours.

• If pain occurs at insertion site, dilute drug further or use a local anesthetic, to reduce pain. Make sure drug doesn't infiltrate.

• Discard if solution appears grossly opaque or has a precipitate. Solutions should be clear to slightly opaque. To eliminate haze, filter solutions through a 0.22-micron filter before use.

ACTION
Cross-links strands of cellular DNA and interferes with RNA transcription, causing an imbalance of growth that leads to cell death. Not specific to cell cycle.

Route	Onset	Peak	Duration
I.V., intra-cavitary	Unknown	Unknown	Unknown

ADVERSE REACTIONS
CNS: headache, dizziness, fatigue, weakness.

EENT: blurred vision, laryngeal edema, conjunctivitis.
GI: *nausea, vomiting,* abdominal pain, anorexia, stomatitis.
GU: amenorrhea, decreased spermatogenesis, dysuria, increased urine levels of uric acid, urine retention, hemorrhagic cystitis (with intravesicle administration).
Hematologic: *leukopenia beginning within 5 to 10 days, thrombocytopenia, neutropenia,* anemia.
Metabolic: hyperuricemia.
Respiratory: asthma.
Skin: urticaria, rash, dermatitis, alopecia, pain at injection site.
Other: fever, *hypersensitivity, anaphylactic shock.*

INTERACTIONS
Drug-drug. *Anticoagulants, aspirin, NSAIDs:* Increased risk of bleeding. Avoid using together.
Myelosuppressives: May cause increased myelosuppression. Monitor patient.
Neuromuscular blockers: May prolong muscular paralysis. Monitor patient.
Other alkylating drugs, irradiation therapy: May intensify toxicity rather than enhance therapeutic response. Avoid using together.
Succinylcholine: Increased apnea when used together. Avoid using together.

EFFECTS ON LAB TEST RESULTS
• May increase uric acid levels. May decrease pseudocholinesterase levels.
• May decrease hemoglobin and lymphocyte, platelet, WBC, RBC, and neutrophil counts.

CONTRAINDICATIONS
Contraindicated in patients hypersensitive to drug and in those with severe bone marrow, hepatic, or renal dysfunction.

NURSING CONSIDERATIONS
• Use in pregnant women isn't recommended except when benefits to mother outweigh risk of teratogenicity.
• Use cautiously in patients with mild bone marrow suppression and renal or hepatic dysfunction.
• For bladder instillation: dehydrate patient 8 to 10 hours before therapy. Instill drug into bladder by catheter; ask patient

to retain solution for 2 hours. Volume may be reduced to 30 ml if discomfort is too great with 60 ml. Reposition patient every 15 minutes for maximum area contact.
• Monitor CBC weekly for at least 3 weeks after last dose.
• Discontinue drug and notify prescriber if patient's WBC count drops below 3,000/mm³ or if platelet count falls below 150,000/mm³. If WBC count falls below 2,000/mm³ or granulocyte count falls below 1,000/mm³, follow institutional policy for infection control in immunocompromised patients.
• Monitor uric acid levels. To prevent hyperuricemia with resulting uric acid nephropathy, allopurinol may be used with adequate hydration.
• Therapeutic effects are commonly accompanied by toxicity.
• To prevent bleeding, avoid all I.M. injections when platelet count is below 50,000/mm³.
• Anticipate blood transfusions because of cumulative anemia. Patient may need injections of RBC colony-stimulating factor to promote RBC production and decrease need for blood transfusions.
• Refrigerate and protect dry powder from direct sunlight to avoid possible drug breakdown.

PATIENT TEACHING
• Advise patient to watch for signs and symptoms of infection (fever, sore throat, fatigue) and bleeding (easy bruising, nosebleeds, bleeding gums, melena). Tell patient to take temperature daily. Tell patient to report even mild infections.
• Instruct patient to avoid OTC products containing aspirin or NSAIDs.
• Advise breast-feeding woman to stop breast-feeding during therapy because of risk of toxicity to infant.
• Caution woman of childbearing age to avoid becoming pregnant during therapy. Suggest that she consult prescriber before becoming pregnant.

Reactions may be common, uncommon, *life-threatening,* or **COMMON AND LIFE-THREATENING.**

68
Antimetabolites

capecitabine
cytarabine
floxuridine
fludarabine phosphate
fluorouracil
hydroxyurea
mercaptopurine
methotrexate
methotrexate sodium
thioguanine

COMBINATION PRODUCTS
None.

---

capecitabine
Xeloda

Pregnancy risk category D

AVAILABLE FORMS
Tablets: 150 mg, 500 mg

INDICATIONS & DOSAGES
➤ **Patients with metastatic breast cancer resistant to both paclitaxel and a chemotherapy regimen containing anthracycline or resistant to paclitaxel and for whom further anthracycline therapy isn't indicated—**
Adults: 2,500 mg/m² P.O. daily in two divided doses (about 12 hours apart) at end of a meal for 2 weeks, followed by a 1-week rest period given in 3-week cycles.
Adjust-a-dose: Follow National Cancer Institute of Canada (NCIC) Common Toxicity Criteria, as directed, when adjusting dosage. Toxicity criteria relate to degrees of severity of diarrhea, nausea, vomiting, stomatitis, and hand-and-foot syndrome. Refer to drug package insert for specific toxicity definitions.

NCIC grade 1: Maintain dose level.

NCIC grade 2: At first appearance, interrupt treatment until resolved to grade 0 to 1; then restart at 100% of starting dose for next cycle. At second appearance, interrupt treatment until resolved to grade

0 to 1 and use 75% of starting dose for next cycle. At third appearance, interrupt treatment until resolved to grade 0 to 1 and use 50% of starting dose for next cycle. At fourth appearance, discontinue treatment permanently.

NCIC grade 3: At first appearance, interrupt treatment until resolved to grade 0 to 1 and use 75% of starting dose for next cycle. At second appearance, interrupt treatment until resolved to grade 0 to 1 and use 50% of starting dose for next cycle. At third appearance, discontinue treatment permanently.

NCIC grade 4: At first appearance, discontinue treatment permanently or interrupt treatment until resolved to grade 0 to 1 and use 50% of starting dose for next cycle.
✹ *NEW INDICATION:* **First-line treatment of patients with metastatic colorectal cancer when treatment with fluoropyrimidine therapy alone is preferred—**
Adults: 2,500 mg/m²/day P.O., in two divided doses, taken about 12 hours apart and after a meal, for 2 weeks; repeated every 3 weeks. Dosage may need to be adjusted, based on toxicity. See manufacturer's insert for details on specific dosage reduction.
Adjust-a-dose: Starting dose for patients with moderate renal impairment (creatinine clearance 30 to 50 ml/min) should be reduced to 75% of the recommended starting dose.

ACTION
Converted to active drug 5-fluorouracil (5-FU), which is metabolized by both normal and tumor cells to metabolites that cause cellular injury by two different mechanisms: interference with DNA synthesis to inhibit cell division and interference with RNA processing and protein synthesis.

Route	Onset	Peak	Duration
P.O.	Unknown	1.5-2 hr	Unknown

ADVERSE REACTIONS
CNS: dizziness, *fatigue,* headache, insomnia, *paresthesia.*
CV: edema.
EENT: eye irritation.
GI: *diarrhea, nausea, vomiting, stomatitis, abdominal pain, constipation, anorexia,* **intestinal obstruction,** *dyspepsia.*
Hematologic: NEUTROPENIA, THROMBO-CYTOPENIA, *anemia, lymphopenia.*
Hepatic: *hyperbilirubinemia.*
Metabolic: dehydration.
Musculoskeletal: myalgia, limb pain.
Skin: *hand-and-foot syndrome, dermatitis,* nail disorder.
Other: *pyrexia.*

INTERACTIONS
Drug-drug. *Leucovorin:* Increased cytotoxic effects of 5-FU with enhanced toxicity. Monitor patient carefully.

EFFECTS ON LAB TEST RESULTS
• May increase bilirubin levels.
• May decrease hemoglobin and WBC, platelet, and neutrophil counts.

CONTRAINDICATIONS
Contraindicated in patients hypersensitive to 5-FU. Contraindicated in patients with severe renal impairment.

NURSING CONSIDERATIONS
• Use cautiously in elderly patients and patients with history of coronary artery disease, mild to moderate hepatic dysfunction from liver metastases, hyperbilirubinemia, and renal insufficiency. Safety and efficacy of drug in patients ages 18 or younger haven't been established.
• Patients older than age 80 may have a greater risk of adverse GI effects.
• Assess patient for severe diarrhea, and notify prescriber if it occurs. Give fluid and electrolyte replacement, if patient becomes dehydrated. Drug may need to be immediately interrupted until diarrhea resolves or decreases in intensity.
• Monitor patient for hand-and-foot syndrome (numbness, paresthesia, tingling, painless or painful swelling, erythema, desquamation, blistering, and severe pain of hands or feet), hyperbilirubinemia, and severe nausea. Drug therapy will need to

be immediately adjusted. Hand-and-foot syndrome is staged from 1 to 4; drug may be discontinued if severe or recurrent episodes occur.
• Hyperbilirubinemia may require stopping drug.
• *Alert:* Monitor patient carefully for toxicity. It may be managed by symptomatic treatment, dose interruptions, and dosage adjustments.

PATIENT TEACHING
• Inform patient and caregiver about expected adverse effects of drug, especially nausea, vomiting, diarrhea, and hand-and-foot syndrome (pain, swelling or redness of hands or feet). Tell him that patient-specific dose adaptations during therapy are expected and needed.
• *Alert:* Instruct patient to stop taking drug and contact prescriber immediately if the following occur: diarrhea (over four bowel movements daily or diarrhea at night), vomiting (two to five episodes in 24 hours), nausea, appetite loss or decrease in amount of food taken each day, stomatitis (pain, redness, swelling or sores in mouth), hand-and-foot syndrome, fever of 100.5° F (38° C) or higher, or other evidence of infection.
• Tell patient that most adverse effects improve within 2 to 3 days after drug is stopped. If improvement doesn't occur, tell him to contact prescriber.
• Tell patient how to take drug. Drug is usually taken for 14 days followed by 7-day rest period (no drug) given as a 21-day cycle. Prescriber determines number of treatment cycles.
• Instruct patient to take drug with water within 30 minutes after end of a meal (breakfast and dinner).
• If a combination of tablets is prescribed, teach patient importance of correctly identifying the tablets to avoid possible misdosing.
• For missed doses, instruct patient not to take the missed dose and not to double the next one. Instead, he should continue with regular dosing schedule and check with prescriber.
• Instruct patient to inform prescriber if he's taking folic acid.
• Advise woman of childbearing age to avoid becoming pregnant during therapy.

Reactions may be *common,* uncommon, *life-threatening,* or COMMON AND LIFE-THREATENING.

• Advise breast-feeding woman to discontinue breast-feeding during therapy.

---

cytarabine (ara-C, cytosine arabinoside)
Cytosar†§, Cytosar-U

Pregnancy risk category D

AVAILABLE FORMS
Injection: 100-mg, 500-mg, 1-g, 2-g vials

INDICATIONS & DOSAGES
➤ **Acute nonlymphocytic leukemia, acute lymphocytic leukemia, blast phase of chronic myelocytic leukemia—**
Adults and children: 100 mg/m² daily by continuous I.V. infusion or 100 mg/m² I.V. q 12 hours. Given for 7 days and repeated q 2 weeks. For maintenance, 1 mg/kg S.C. once or twice weekly.
➤ **Meningeal leukemia—**
Adults and children: Highly variable from 5 to 75 mg/m² intrathecally. Frequency also varies from once daily for 4 days to once q 4 days. The most frequently used dose is 30 mg/m² q 4 days until CSF fluid is normal; then one additional dose.

I.V. ADMINISTRATION
• Follow facility policy to reduce risks. Preparation and administration of parenteral form are linked to carcinogenic, mutagenic, and teratogenic risks for staff.
• To reduce nausea, give antiemetic before administering. Nausea and vomiting are more frequent when large doses are administered rapidly by I.V. push. These reactions are less frequent when given by infusion. Dizziness may occur with rapid infusion.
• Reconstitute drug using the provided diluent, which is bacteriostatic water for injection containing benzyl alcohol. Avoid this diluent when preparing drug for neonates or intrathecal use. Reconstitute drug in 100-mg vial with 5 ml of diluent or 500-mg vial with 10 ml of diluent. Reconstituted solution is stable for 48 hours. Discard cloudy reconstituted solution.
• For I.V. infusion, further dilute using normal saline solution for injection or D₅W.

ACTION
Inhibits DNA synthesis.

Route	Onset	Peak	Duration
I.V., intrathecal	Unknown	Unknown	Unknown
S.C.	Unknown	20-60 min	Unknown

ADVERSE REACTIONS
CNS: neurotoxicity, malaise, dizziness, headache.
CV: *thrombophlebitis,* edema.
EENT: conjunctivitis.
GI: *nausea, vomiting, diarrhea, anorexia, anal ulceration,* abdominal pain, oral ulcers in 5 to 10 days, projectile vomiting, bowel necrosis with high doses given rapid I.V.
GU: urine retention, renal dysfunction.
Hematologic: *leukopenia,* anemia, reticulocytopenia, *thrombocytopenia, megaloblastosis.*
Hepatic: *hepatotoxicity,* jaundice.
Metabolic: hyperuricemia.
Musculoskeletal: myalgia, bone pain.
Skin: *rash,* pruritus, alopecia, freckling.
Other: flu syndrome, infection, *fever, anaphylaxis.*

INTERACTIONS
Drug-drug. *Digoxin:* May decrease digoxin absorption. Monitor digoxin level closely. Digoxin oral liquid and liquid-filled capsules may not be affected.
Flucytosine: Decreased flucytosine activity. Avoid using together.
Gentamicin: Decreased activity against *Klebsiella pneumoniae.* Avoid using together.

EFFECTS ON LAB TEST RESULTS
• May increase uric acid levels.
• May increase megaloblasts. May decrease hemoglobin and WBC, RBC, platelet, and reticulocyte levels.

CONTRAINDICATIONS
Contraindicated in patients hypersensitive to drug.

NURSING CONSIDERATIONS
• Use cautiously in patients with hepatic or renal compromise, gout, or myelosuppression.

• For intrathecal administration, use preservative-free normal saline solution. Add 5 ml to 100-mg vial or 10 ml to 500-mg vial. Use immediately after reconstitution. Discard unused drug.

• Monitor fluid intake and output carefully. Maintain high fluid intake and give allopurinol to avoid urate nephropathy in leukemia-induction therapy. Monitor uric acid level.

• Monitor hepatic and renal function studies and CBC.

• Therapy may be modified or stopped if granulocyte count is below 1,000/mm³ or platelet count is below 50,000/mm³.

• Corticosteroid eyedrops are prescribed to prevent drug-induced conjunctivitis.

• Provide diligent mouth care to help prevent stomatitis.

• *Alert:* Assess patient receiving high doses for neurotoxicity, which may first appear as nystagmus, but can progress to ataxia and cerebellar dysfunction.

• To prevent bleeding, avoid all I.M. injections when platelet count is below 50,000/mm³.

• Anticipate blood transfusions because of cumulative anemia. Patient may receive RBC colony-stimulating factors to promote RBC production and decrease need for blood transfusions.

• Therapeutic effects are frequently accompanied by toxicity.

• In leukopenia, initial WBC count nadir occurs 7 to 9 days after drug is stopped. A second, more severe nadir occurs 15 to 24 days after drug is stopped. In thrombocytopenia, platelet count nadir occurs on days 12 to 15.

PATIENT TEACHING
• Instruct patient to watch for signs and symptoms of infection (fever, sore throat, fatigue) and bleeding (easy bruising, nosebleeds, bleeding gums, melena). Tell patient to take temperature daily.

• Advise patient to report visual changes, blurred vision, or pain in eyes to prescriber.

• Advise breast-feeding woman to discontinue breast-feeding during therapy because of risk of toxicity to infant.

• Caution woman of childbearing age to avoid becoming pregnant during therapy. Recommend that she consult prescriber

before becoming pregnant. Drug may harm fetus.

floxuridine
(fluorodeoxyuridine)
FUDR

Pregnancy risk category D

AVAILABLE FORMS
Powder for injection: 500 mg for reconstitution (5-ml, 10-ml vials)
Preservative-free injection: 100 mg/ml (5-ml vials)

INDICATIONS & DOSAGES
➤ **GI adenocarcinoma metastatic to the liver—**
Adults: 0.1 to 0.6 mg/kg daily by intra-arterial infusion for 14 to 21 days or until toxicity occurs; or 0.4 to 0.6 mg/kg daily into hepatic artery.

I.V. ADMINISTRATION
• Follow facility policy to reduce risks. Preparation and administration of parenteral form of drug are linked to carcinogenic, mutagenic, and teratogenic risks for staff.

• Reconstitute with 5 ml sterile water for injection to yield a solution of 100 mg/ml. To prepare infusion, dilute in D_5W or normal saline solution.

• Refrigerated solution is stable for up to 2 weeks.

• Use an infusion pump with intra-arterial infusions.

ACTION
Inhibits DNA synthesis.

Route	Onset	Peak	Duration
Intra-arterial	Unknown	Unknown	Unknown

ADVERSE REACTIONS
CNS: malaise, weakness, headache, lethargy, disorientation, confusion, euphoria.
CV: thrombophlebitis, *myocardial ischemia*, angina.
EENT: blurred vision, nystagmus, photophobia, epistaxis.

Reactions may be *common*, uncommon, *life-threatening*, or COMMON AND LIFE-THREATENING.

GI: *anorexia, stomatitis, nausea, vomiting, diarrhea, bleeding, abdominal pain, enteritis,* GI ulceration, intrahepatic and extrahepatic biliary sclerosis, acalculous cholecystitis.
Hematologic: *leukopenia, anemia, thrombocytopenia, agranulocytosis.*
Hepatic: *hepatotoxicity.*
Skin: *erythema,* dermatitis, pruritus, rash, alopecia, photosensitivity.
Other: *anaphylaxis,* fever.

INTERACTIONS
Drug-lifestyle. *Sun exposure:* May increase skin reaction. Advise patient to avoid excessive sunlight exposure.

EFFECTS ON LAB TEST RESULTS
● May decrease hemoglobin and WBC, RBC, platelet, and granulocyte counts.

CONTRAINDICATIONS
Contraindicated in patients with poor nutritional state, bone marrow suppression, or serious infection.

NURSING CONSIDERATIONS
● Use cautiously after high-dose pelvic radiation therapy or use of alkylating drugs and in patients with impaired hepatic or renal function.
● Check line for bleeding, blockage, displacement, or leakage.
● Monitor fluid intake and output, CBC, and renal and hepatic function.
● Use of antacid eases but won't prevent GI distress. An H_2 antihistamine is recommended to prevent peptic ulcer disease during drug therapy.
● Provide diligent mouth care to help prevent stomatitis.
● If patient develops severe skin and adverse GI reactions, therapy must stop.
● Discontinue drug and notify prescriber if patient's WBC count drops below 3,500/mm³ or if platelet count falls below 100,000/mm³. If WBC count falls below 2,000/mm³ or granulocyte count falls below 1,000/mm³, follow institutional policy for infection control in immunocompromised patients.
● To prevent bleeding, avoid all I.M. injections when platelet count is below 50,000/mm³.

● Anticipate blood transfusions because of cumulative anemia. Patients may receive injections of RBC colony-stimulating factors to promote RBC production and decrease need for blood transfusions.
● Higher doses (0.4 to 0.6 mg/kg) are used for intra-arterial infusions into the liver. The liver metabolizes the drug before systemic exposure.
● *Alert:* Don't confuse floxuridine with fludarabine, fluorouracil, or flucytosine.

PATIENT TEACHING
● Inform patient that therapeutic effect may be delayed for 1 to 6 weeks.
● Inform patient receiving drug at home to monitor placement of needle into catheter site and to call his infusion provider immediately if needle becomes dislodged.
● Advise patient to watch for signs and symptoms of infection (fever, sore throat, fatigue) and bleeding (easy bruising, nosebleeds, bleeding gums, melena). Tell patient to take temperature daily.
● Tell patient that exposure to sun may cause or intensify skin reaction.
● Advise breast-feeding woman to discontinue breast-feeding during therapy because of risk of toxicity to infant.
● Caution woman of childbearing age to avoid becoming pregnant during therapy. Recommend that she consult prescriber before becoming pregnant.

fludarabine phosphate
Fludara

Pregnancy risk category D

AVAILABLE FORMS
Powder for injection: 50 mg

INDICATIONS & DOSAGES
➤ **B-cell chronic lymphocytic leukemia in patients who either have not responded or have responded inadequately to at least one standard alkylating drug regimen—**
Adults: 25 mg/m² I.V. over 30 minutes for 5 consecutive days. Cycle repeated q 28 days.

I.V. ADMINISTRATION
● Follow facility policy to reduce risks. Preparation and administration of parenteral form of drug are linked to mutagenic, teratogenic, and carcinogenic risks for staff.
● To prepare solution, add 2 ml of sterile water for injection to the solid cake of fludarabine. Dissolution should occur within 15 seconds; each milliliter will contain 25 mg of drug. Dilute further in 100 or 125 ml of D_5W or normal saline solution for injection. Use within 8 hours of reconstitution.

ACTION
Unknown. An antineoplastic antimetabolite that may have multifaceted actions. After conversion to its active metabolite, fludarabine interferes with DNA synthesis by inhibiting DNA polymerase alpha, ribonucleotide reductase, and DNA primase.

Route	Onset	Peak	Duration
I.V.	7-21 wk	Unknown	Unknown

ADVERSE REACTIONS
CNS: *fatigue, malaise, weakness, paresthesia,* peripheral neuropathy, *CVA,* headache, sleep disorder, depression, cerebellar syndrome, transient ischemic attack, agitation, *confusion, coma.*
CV: *edema,* angina, phlebitis, ***arrhythmias, heart failure, MI,*** supraventricular tachycardia, deep vein thrombosis, ***aneurysm, hemorrhage.***
EENT: *visual disturbances,* hearing loss, delayed blindness, sinusitis, pharyngitis, epistaxis.
GI: *nausea, vomiting, diarrhea,* constipation, *anorexia,* stomatitis, ***GI bleeding,*** esophagitis, mucositis.
GU: dysuria, *urinary tract infection,* urinary hesitancy, proteinuria, hematuria, ***renal failure.***
Hematologic: *hemolytic anemia,* MYELOSUPPRESSION.
Hepatic: *liver failure,* cholelithiasis.
Metabolic: hypocalcemia, hyperkalemia, hyperglycemia, dehydration, hyperuricemia, hyperphosphatemia.
Musculoskeletal: *myalgia.*
Respiratory: *cough, pneumonia, dyspnea, upper respiratory tract infection,* allergic pneumonitis, hemoptysis, hypoxia, bronchitis.
Skin: *rash,* pruritus, alopecia, seborrhea, diaphoresis.
Other: *fever, chills, pain,* tumor lysis syndrome, INFECTION, ***anaphylaxis.***

INTERACTIONS
Drug-drug. *Other myelosuppressives:* Increased toxicity. Avoid using together, if possible.
Pentostatin: Increased risk of pulmonary toxicity, which can be fatal. Avoid using together.

EFFECTS ON LAB TEST RESULTS
● May increase uric acid, glucose, and phosphate levels. May decrease calcium levels.
● May decrease hemoglobin and RBC count.

CONTRAINDICATIONS
Contraindicated in patients hypersensitive to drug or its components.

NURSING CONSIDERATIONS
● Use cautiously in patients with renal insufficiency.
● *Alert:* Monitor patient closely and expect modified dosage based on toxicity. Most toxic effects are dose-dependent. Advanced age, renal insufficiency, and bone marrow impairment may predispose patients to increased or excessive toxicity.
● *Alert:* Careful hematologic monitoring is needed, especially of neutrophil and platelet counts. Bone marrow suppression can be severe.
● To prevent bleeding, avoid all I.M. injections when platelet count is below 50,000/mm^3.
● Anticipate blood transfusions because of cumulative anemia. Patients may receive RBC colony-stimulating factors to promote RBC production and decrease need for blood transfusions.
● Take preventive measures before starting drug treatment. Hyperuricemia, hypocalcemia, hyperkalemia, and renal failure may result from rapid lysis of tumor cells.
● Store drug in refrigerator at 36° to 46° F (2° to 8° C).
● *Alert:* Don't confuse fludarabine with floxuridine, fluorouracil, or flucytosine.

Reactions may be *common*, uncommon, ***life-threatening***, or COMMON AND LIFE-THREATENING.

PATIENT TEACHING
• Instruct patient to watch for signs and symptoms of infection (fever, sore throat, fatigue) and bleeding (easy bruising, nosebleeds, bleeding gums, melena). Tell patient to take temperature daily.
• Advise woman of childbearing age to avoid becoming pregnant during therapy. Recommend that she consult prescriber before becoming pregnant.
• Caution breast-feeding woman to discontinue breast-feeding during therapy because of risk of toxicity to infant.

---

fluorouracil (5-fluorouracil, 5-FU)
Adrucil, Efudex, Fluoroplex

Pregnancy risk category D (injection); X (topical form)

AVAILABLE FORMS
Cream: 1%, 5%
Injection: 50 mg/ml
Topical solution: 1%, 2%, 5%

INDICATIONS & DOSAGES
➤ **Colon, rectal, breast, stomach, and pancreatic cancers—**
Adults: Initially, 12 mg/kg I.V. daily for 4 days; if no toxicity, 6 mg/kg given on days 6, 8, 10, and 12; then a single weekly maintenance dose of 10 to 15 mg/kg I.V. begun after toxicity (if any) from initial course has subsided. (Recommended dosages are based on actual body weight unless patient is obese or retaining fluid.) Maximum single recommended dose is 800 mg/day.
➤ **Palliative treatment of advanced colorectal cancer—**
Adults: 425 mg/m² I.V. daily for 5 consecutive days. Give with 20 mg/m² of leucovorin I.V. Repeat at 4-week intervals for two additional courses; then repeat at intervals of 4 to 5 weeks if tolerated.
➤ **Early breast cancer—**
Adults: 600 mg/m² I.V. on days 1 and 8 of each cycle, combined with cyclophosphamide 100 mg/m² on days 1 through 14 of each cycle and methotrexate 40 mg/m² on days 1 and 8 of each cycle. Repeat monthly for 6 to 12 months allowing for a 2-week rest period between cycles. In adults older than age 60, initial fluorouracil dose is 400 mg/m² and methotrexate dose is 30 mg/m².
➤ **Multiple actinic (solar) keratoses, superficial basal cell carcinoma—**
Adults: Apply cream or topical solution once daily or b.i.d. Usual duration of treatment is 2 to 6 weeks.

I.V. ADMINISTRATION
• Follow facility policy to reduce risks. Preparation and administration of parenteral form of drug are linked to carcinogenic, mutagenic, and teratogenic risks for staff.
• Give antiemetic before drug to reduce nausea.
• Drug may be administered by direct injection without dilution. For I.V. infusion, drug may be diluted with D₅W, sterile water for injection, or normal saline solution for injection. Discard unused portion of vial after 1 hour.
• Don't use cloudy solution. If crystals form, redissolve by warming.
• Use plastic I.V. containers for administering continuous infusions. Solution is more stable in plastic I.V. bags than in glass bottles.
• Don't refrigerate fluorouracil. Protect drug from sunlight.

ACTION
Thought to inhibit DNA and RNA synthesis.

Route	Onset	Peak	Duration
I.V., topical	Unknown	Unknown	Unknown

ADVERSE REACTIONS
CNS: acute cerebellar syndrome, confusion, disorientation, euphoria, ataxia, headache, *weakness, malaise.*
CV: *myocardial ischemia,* angina, thrombophlebitis.
EENT: epistaxis, photophobia, lacrimation, lacrimal duct stenosis, nystagmus, visual changes.
GI: *stomatitis, GI ulcer, nausea, vomiting, diarrhea, anorexia,* **GI bleeding.**
Hematologic: *leukopenia, thrombocytopenia, agranulocytosis,* anemia.
Skin: *dermatitis, erythema, scaling, pruritus,* nail changes, pigmented palmar creas-

---

es, erythematous contact dermatitis, desquamative rash of hands and feet, hand-and-foot syndrome with long-term use, photosensitivity, *reversible alopecia.* **Other:** *pain, burning,* soreness, suppuration, swelling with topical use, ***anaphylaxis,*** decreased plasma albumin.

INTERACTIONS
Drug-drug. *Leucovorin calcium:* Increased cytotoxicity and toxicity of fluorouracil. Monitor patient closely when used together.
Drug-lifestyle. *Sun exposure:* May cause photosensitivity reactions. Advise patient to avoid excessive sunlight exposure.

EFFECTS ON LAB TEST RESULTS
• May increase alkaline phosphatase, AST, ALT, bilirubin, and LD levels. May increase 5-hydroxyindoleacetic acid in urine.
• May decrease hemoglobin and WBC, RBC, platelet, and granulocyte counts.

CONTRAINDICATIONS
Contraindicated in patients hypersensitive to drug and in those with bone marrow suppression (WBC counts of 5,000/mm^3 or less or platelet counts of 100,000/mm^3 or less) or potentially serious infections. Also contraindicated in patients in a poor nutritional state and those who have had major surgery within previous month.

NURSING CONSIDERATIONS
• Use cautiously in patients who have received high-dose pelvic radiation or alkylating drugs, and in patients with impaired hepatic or renal function or widespread neoplastic infiltration of bone marrow.
• Apply topical form cautiously near eyes, nose, and mouth.
• Avoid occlusive dressings with topical form because they increase risk of inflammatory reactions in adjacent normal skin.
• Apply topical form with a nonmetal applicator or suitable gloves. Wash hands immediately after handling topical form.
• Expect to use 1% topical concentration on the face. Higher concentrations are used for thicker-skinned areas or resistant lesions.
• Expect to use 5% topical strength for superficial basal cell carcinoma confirmed by biopsy.

• Ingestion and systemic absorption of topical form may cause leukopenia, thrombocytopenia, stomatitis, diarrhea, or GI ulceration, bleeding, and hemorrhage. Application to large ulcerated areas may cause systemic toxicity.
• Watch for stomatitis or diarrhea (signs of toxicity). May use topical oral anesthetic to soothe lesions. Discontinue drug and notify prescriber if diarrhea occurs.
• Encourage diligent oral hygiene to prevent superinfection of denuded mucosa.
• Monitor WBC and platelet counts daily. Watch for ecchymoses, petechiae, easy bruising, and anemia.
• Monitor fluid intake and output, CBC, and renal and hepatic function tests.
• Long-term use of drug may cause erythematous, desquamative rash of the hands and feet. May be treated with pyridoxine (50 to 150 mg P.O. daily) for 5 to 7 days.
• Dermatologic adverse effects are reversible when drug is stopped.
• To prevent bleeding, avoid all I.M. injections when platelet count is below 50,000/mm^3.
• Anticipate blood transfusions because of cumulative anemia. Patient may receive injections of RBC colony-stimulating factors to promote RBC production and decrease need for blood transfusions.
• ***Alert:*** Fluorouracil toxicity may be delayed for 1 to 3 weeks.
• The WBC count nadir occurs 9 to 14 days after first dose; the platelet count nadir occurs in 7 to 14 days.
• ***Alert:*** Drug is sometimes ordered as 5-fluorouracil or 5-FU. The numeral 5 is part of drug name and shouldn't be confused with dosage units.
• ***Alert:*** Don't confuse fluorouracil with floxuridine, fludarabine, or flucytosine.

PATIENT TEACHING
• Warn patient that alopecia may occur, but that it's reversible.
• Caution patient to avoid prolonged exposure to sunlight or ultraviolet light when topical form is used.
• Tell patient to use highly protective sunblock to avoid inflammatory erythematous dermatitis.
• Warn patient that topically treated area may be unsightly during therapy and for

several weeks afterward. Complete healing may take 1 or 2 months.
• Caution woman of childbearing age to avoid becoming pregnant during therapy. Recommend that she consult prescriber before becoming pregnant.
• Advise breast-feeding woman to discontinue breast-feeding during therapy because of risk of toxicity to infant.

hydroxyurea
Droxia, Hydrea**

Pregnancy risk category D

AVAILABLE FORMS
Capsules: 200 mg, 250 mg, 300 mg, 400 mg, 500 mg

INDICATIONS & DOSAGES
➤ **Melanoma; resistant chronic myelocytic leukemia; recurrent, metastatic, or inoperable ovarian cancer; head and neck cancers—**
Adults: 80 mg/kg P.O. as single dose q 3 days; or 20 to 30 mg/kg P.O. as single daily dose.
➤ **To reduce frequency of painful crises and need for blood transfusions in adult patients with sickle-cell anemia with recurrent moderate to severe painful crises—**
Adults: 15 mg/kg P.O. once daily. If blood counts are in acceptable range, dose may be increased by 5 mg/kg/day q 12 weeks until maximum tolerated dose or 35 mg/kg/day has been reached. If blood counts are considered toxic, withhold drug until hematologic recovery occurs. Resume treatment after reducing dose by 2.5 mg/kg/day. Every 12 weeks, drug may then be adjusted up or down in 2.5-mg/kg/day increments until patient is at stable, nontoxic dose for 24 weeks.

ACTION
Unknown. Thought to inhibit DNA synthesis.

Route	Onset	Peak	Duration
P.O.	Unknown	2 hr	24 hr

ADVERSE REACTIONS
CNS: hallucinations, headache, dizziness, disorientation, *seizures,* malaise.
GI: *anorexia, nausea, vomiting, diarrhea,* stomatitis, constipation.
Hematologic: *leukopenia, thrombocytopenia, anemia, megaloblastosis, bone marrow suppression.*
Metabolic: hyperuricemia.
Skin: rash, itching.
Other: fever, chills.

INTERACTIONS
Drug-drug. *Cytotoxic drugs, radiation therapy:* Enhanced toxicity of hydroxyurea. Use together cautiously.

EFFECTS ON LAB TEST RESULTS
• May increase BUN, creatinine, and uric acid levels.
• May decrease hemoglobin and WBC, RBC, and platelet counts.

CONTRAINDICATIONS
Contraindicated in patients hypersensitive to drug and in those with marked bone marrow depression (leukopenia [less than 2,500/mm³ WBCs], thrombocytopenia [less than 100,000/mm³ platelets], or severe anemia).

NURSING CONSIDERATIONS
• Use cautiously in patients with renal dysfunction.
• Routinely measure BUN, uric acid, and creatinine levels; blood counts must be monitored every 2 weeks.
• Acceptable blood counts during dosage adjustment: neutrophils, 2,500 cells/mm³ or more; platelets, 95,000/mm³ or more; hemoglobin, more than 5.3 g/dl; and reticulocytes (if Hg is below 9 g/dl), more than 95,000/mm³. Toxic levels are considered when neutrophil count is below 2,000 cells/mm³, platelets are below 80,000/mm³, hemoglobin is less than 4.5 g/dl, and reticulocytes (if Hg is below 9 g/dl) are below 80,000/mm³.
• Hydroxyurea may dramatically lower the WBC count in 24 to 48 hours.
• Monitor fluid intake and output; keep patient hydrated.
• Allopurinol is used for treatment or prevention of tumor lysis syndrome.

• To prevent bleeding, avoid all I.M. injections when platelet count is below 50,000/mm³.
• Anticipate blood transfusions because of cumulative anemia. Patient may receive injections of RBC colony-stimulating factors to promote RBC production and decrease need for blood transfusions.
• Dosage modification may be needed after chemotherapy or radiation therapy.
• Auditory and visual hallucinations and hematologic toxicity increase when renal function decreases.
• Drug crosses blood-brain barrier.
• Radiation therapy may increase risk or severity of GI distress or stomatitis.

PATIENT TEACHING
• Tell patient who can't swallow capsules that he may empty contents into water and take immediately. Patient should rinse mouth with water after taking drug this way. Inform patient that some inert material may not dissolve.
• Advise patient to watch for signs and symptoms of infection (fever, sore throat, fatigue) and bleeding (easy bruising, nosebleeds, bleeding gums, melena). He also should take his temperature daily.
• Caution woman of childbearing age to avoid becoming pregnant during therapy. Recommend that she consult prescriber before becoming pregnant.

---

mercaptopurine (6-mercaptopurine, 6-MP)
Purinethol

Pregnancy risk category D

AVAILABLE FORMS
Tablets (scored): 50 mg

INDICATIONS & DOSAGES
➤ **Acute myeloblastic leukemia, chronic myelocytic leukemia—**
Adults: 80 to 100 mg/m² (rounded to nearest 25 mg) P.O. daily as single dose, up to 5 mg/kg/day.
Children: 75 mg/m² (rounded to nearest 25 mg) P.O. daily.
➤ **Acute lymphoblastic leukemia—**
Children: 75 mg/m² (rounded to nearest 25 mg) P.O. daily.

After remission is attained, usual maintenance dose for adults and children is 1.5 to 2.5 mg/kg/day.

ACTION
Inhibits RNA and DNA synthesis.

Route	Onset	Peak	Duration
P.O.	Unknown	Unknown	Unknown

ADVERSE REACTIONS
GI: nausea, vomiting, anorexia, painful oral ulcers, diarrhea, *pancreatitis*, GI ulceration.
Hematologic: *leukopenia, thrombocytopenia,* anemia.
Hepatic: *jaundice, hepatotoxicity.*
Metabolic: hyperuricemia.
Skin: rash, hyperpigmentation.

INTERACTIONS
Drug-drug. *Allopurinol:* Slowed inactivation of mercaptopurine. Decrease mercaptopurine to 25% or 33% of normal dose.
Co-trimoxazole: Enhanced bone marrow suppression; monitor CBC with differential carefully.
Hepatotoxic drugs: May enhance hepatotoxicity of mercaptopurine. Monitor patient for hepatotoxicity.
Nondepolarizing neuromuscular blockers: Antagonized muscle relaxant effect. Notify anesthesiologist that patient is receiving mercaptopurine.
Warfarin: Antagonized or potentiated anticoagulant effect. Monitor PT and INR.

EFFECTS ON LAB TEST RESULTS
• May increase uric acid levels.
• May decrease hemoglobin and WBC, RBC, and platelet counts.

CONTRAINDICATIONS
Contraindicated in patients whose disease has shown resistance to drug and in patients hypersensitive to the drug.

NURSING CONSIDERATIONS
• Dosage modifications may be needed after chemotherapy or radiation therapy in patients with depressed neutrophil or platelet counts and in those with impaired hepatic or renal function.

• Drug is sometimes ordered as 6-mercaptopurine or 6-MP. The numeral 6 is part of drug name and doesn't signify number of dosage units.

• Monitor CBC and transaminase, alkaline phosphatase, and bilirubin levels weekly during induction and monthly during maintenance.

• Leukopenia, thrombocytopenia, or anemia may persist for several days after drug is stopped.

• Observe for signs of bleeding and infection.

• Monitor fluid intake and output. Encourage adequate fluid intake (3 L daily).

• *Alert:* Watch for jaundice, clay-colored stools, and frothy, dark urine. Hepatic dysfunction is reversible when drug is stopped. If right-sided abdominal tenderness occurs, drug should be stopped and prescriber notified.

• Monitor uric acid level. If allopurinol is ordered, use cautiously.

• To prevent bleeding, avoid all I.M. injections when platelet count is below 100,000/mm^3.

• Anticipate blood transfusions because of cumulative anemia. Patient may receive injections of RBC colony-stimulating factors to promote RBC production and decrease need for blood transfusions.

• GI adverse reactions are less common in children than in adults.

PATIENT TEACHING
• Instruct patient to watch for signs and symptoms of infection (fever, sore throat, fatigue) and bleeding (easy bruising, nosebleeds, bleeding gums, melena). Tell patient to take temperature daily.

• Caution woman of childbearing age to avoid becoming pregnant during therapy. Recommend that she consult prescriber before becoming pregnant.

• Advise breast-feeding woman to discontinue breast-feeding during therapy because of risk of toxicity to infant.

methotrexate (amethopterin, MTX)

methotrexate sodium
Folex, Folex PFS, Ledertrexate‡, Methoblastin‡, Rheumatrex

Pregnancy risk category X

AVAILABLE FORMS
Injection: 20-mg, 25-mg, 50-mg, 100-mg, 250-mg, 1000-mg vials, lyophilized powder, preservative free; 25-mg/ml vials, preservative-free solution; 2.5-mg/ml, 25-mg/ml vials, lyophilized powder, preserved
Tablets (scored): 2.5 mg, 10 mg‡

INDICATIONS & DOSAGES
➤ **Trophoblastic tumors (choriocarcinoma, hydatidiform mole)—**
Adults: 15 to 30 mg P.O. or I.M. daily for 5 days. Repeated after 1 or more weeks, based on response or toxicity. Number of courses is three to five, not to exceed five.
➤ **Acute lymphocytic leukemia—**
Adults and children: 3.3 mg/m^2/day P.O., I.M., or I.V. for 4 to 6 weeks or until remission occurs; then 20 to 30 mg/m^2 P.O. or I.M. weekly in two divided doses or 2.5 mg/kg I.V. q 14 days.
➤ **Meningeal leukemia—**
Adults and children: 12 mg/m^2 or less (maximum 15 mg) intrathecally q 2 to 5 days until CSF is normal; then one additional dose.
➤ **Burkitt's lymphoma (stage I, II, or III)—**
Adults: 10 to 25 mg P.O. daily for 4 to 8 days with 1-week rest intervals.
➤ **Lymphosarcoma (stage III)—**
Adults: 0.625 to 2.5 mg/kg daily P.O., I.M., or I.V.
➤ **Osteosarcoma—**
Adults: Initially, 12 g/m^2 I.V. as 4-hour infusion. Subsequent doses 12 to 15 g/m^2 I.V. as 4-hour I.V. infusion given at postoperative weeks 4, 5, 6, 7, 11, 12, 15, 16, 29, 30, 44, and 45. Given with leucovorin, 15 mg P.O., I.M., or I.V. q 6 hours for 10 doses, beginning 24 hours after start of methotrexate infusion.

➤ **Breast cancer—**
Adults: 40 mg/m² I.V. on days 1 and 8 of each cycle combined with cyclophosphamide and fluorouracil. In patients older than age 60, 30 mg/m².
➤ **Mycosis fungoides—**
Adults: 2.5 to 10 mg P.O. daily; or 50 mg I.M. weekly; or 25 mg I.M. twice weekly.
➤ **Psoriasis—**
Adults: 10 to 25 mg P.O., I.M., or I.V. as single weekly dose; or 2.5 mg P.O. every 12 hours for three doses. Dosage shouldn't exceed 30 mg/week.
➤ **Rheumatoid arthritis—**
Adults: Initially, 7.5 mg P.O. weekly, either in single dose or divided as 2.5 mg P.O. q 12 hours for three doses once weekly. Dosage may be gradually increased to maximum of 20 mg weekly.

I.V. ADMINISTRATION

• Follow facility policy to reduce risks. Preparation and administration of parenteral form of drug are linked to carcinogenic, mutagenic, and teratogenic risks for staff.
• Dilution of drug depends on product, and infusion guidelines vary, depending on dose.
• Reconstitute solutions without preservatives immediately before use, and discard unused drug.

ACTION

Reversibly binds to dihydrofolate reductase, blocking reduction of folic acid to tetrahydrofolate, a cofactor necessary for purine, protein, and DNA synthesis.

Route	Onset	Peak	Duration
I.M.	Unknown	0.5-1 hr	Unknown
Intrathecal	Unknown	Unknown	Unknown
I.V.	Immediate	Immediate	Unknown
P.O.	Unknown	1-2 hr	Unknown

ADVERSE REACTIONS

CNS: *arachnoiditis within hours of intrathecal use,* subacute neurotoxicity possibly beginning few weeks later, *leukoencephalopathy,* demyelination, malaise, fatigue, dizziness, headache, aphasia, hemiparesis, drowsiness, *seizures.*
EENT: pharyngitis, blurred vision.

GI: gingivitis, *stomatitis, diarrhea,* abdominal distress, anorexia, GI ulceration and bleeding, enteritis, *nausea, vomiting.*
GU: nephropathy, *tubular necrosis, renal failure,* hematuria, menstrual dysfunction, defective spermatogenesis, infertility, abortion, cystitis.
Hematologic: *anemia, leukopenia, thrombocytopenia.*
Hepatic: *acute toxicity, chronic toxicity,* including cirrhosis and *hepatic fibrosis.*
Metabolic: diabetes, hyperuricemia.
Musculoskeletal: arthralgia, myalgia, osteoporosis in children on long-term therapy.
Respiratory: *pulmonary fibrosis; pulmonary interstitial infiltrates;* pneumonitis; dry, nonproductive cough.
Skin: *urticaria,* pruritus, hyperpigmentation, erythematous rashes, ecchymoses, rash, photosensitivity, alopecia, acne, psoriatic lesions aggravated by exposure to sun.
Other: fever, chills, reduced resistance to infection, septicemia, *sudden death.*

INTERACTIONS

Drug-drug. *Acyclovir:* Use with intrathecal MTX may cause neurologic abnormalities. Monitor patient closely.
Digoxin: May decrease digoxin levels. Monitor digoxin levels closely.
Folic acid derivatives: Antagonized methotrexate effect. Avoid using together, except for leucovorin rescue with high-dose methotrexate therapy.
Fosphenytoin, phenytoin: May decrease phenytoin/fosphenytoin levels. Monitor drug levels closely.
Hepatotoxic drugs: May increase risk of hepatotoxicity. Monitor patient closely.
NSAIDs, phenylbutazone, probenecid, salicylates, sulfonamides: Increased methotrexate toxicity. Avoid using together.
Oral antibiotics: May decrease absorption of methotrexate. Monitor patient closely.
Penicillins, sulfonamides: Increased methotrexate levels. Monitor for methotrexate toxicity.
Theophylline: May increase level of theophylline. Monitor theophylline levels closely.
Vaccines: Immunizations may be ineffective; risk of disseminated infection with

---

Reactions may be *common,* uncommon, *life-threatening,* or COMMON AND LIFE-THREATENING.

live virus vaccines. Defer immunization, if possible.

Drug-food. *Any food:* May delay absorption and reduce peak level of methotrexate. Instruct patient to take drug on an empty stomach.

Drug-lifestyle. *Alcohol use:* May increase hepatotoxicity. Discourage alcohol use. *Sun exposure:* May cause photosensitivity reactions. Advise patient to avoid excessive sunlight exposure.

EFFECTS ON LAB TEST RESULTS
● May increase uric acid levels.
● May decrease hemoglobin and WBC, RBC, and platelet counts.

CONTRAINDICATIONS
Contraindicated in patients hypersensitive to drug and in those with psoriasis or rheumatoid arthritis who also have alcoholism, alcoholic liver, chronic liver disease, immunodeficiency syndromes, or blood dyscrasias. Also contraindicated in pregnant or breast-feeding women.

NURSING CONSIDERATIONS
● Use cautiously and at modified dosage in patients with impaired hepatic or renal function, bone marrow suppression, aplasia, leukopenia, thrombocytopenia, or anemia. Also use cautiously in very young, elderly, or debilitated patients and in patients with infection, peptic ulceration, or ulcerative colitis.
● Monitor pulmonary function tests periodically and fluid intake and output daily. Encourage fluid intake of 2 to 3 L daily.
● Monitor uric acid level.
● Methotrexate distributes readily into pleural effusions and other third space compartments, such as ascites, leading to prolonged systemic levels. Drug should be used cautiously in these patients.
● **Alert:** Alkalinize urine, by giving sodium bicarbonate tablets or I.V. fluids containing sodium bicarbonate to prevent precipitation of drug, especially at high doses. Maintain urine pH above 6.5. Reduce dosage, if BUN level is 20 to 30 mg/dl or creatinine level is 1.2 to 2 mg/dl. Stop drug and notify prescriber if BUN level exceeds 30 mg/dl or creatinine level is higher than 2 mg/dl.

● Use preservative-free formulation for intrathecal administration.
● Watch for increases in AST, ALT, and alkaline phosphatase levels, which may signal hepatic dysfunction.
● Drug may alter results of laboratory assay for folate, thus interfering with detection of folic acid deficiency.
● Watch for signs and symptoms of bleeding (especially GI) and infection.
● To prevent bleeding, avoid all I.M. injections when platelet count is below 50,000/mm^3.
● Anticipate blood transfusions because of cumulative anemia. Patient may receive injections of RBC colony-stimulating factors to promote RBC production and decrease need for blood transfusions.
● Leucovorin rescue is needed with high-dose (over 100 mg) protocols and is started 24 hours after methotrexate therapy is begun. Leucovorin therapy is continued until methotrexate levels are less than 10^{-8} M.
● Monitor methotrexate levels and adjust leucovorin dose.
● The WBC and platelet count nadirs usually occur on day 7.

PATIENT TEACHING
● Advise patient to watch for signs and symptoms of infection (fever, sore throat, fatigue) and bleeding (easy bruising, nosebleeds, bleeding gums, melena). Tell patient to take temperature daily.
● Teach and encourage diligent mouth care to reduce risk of superinfection in the mouth.
● Instruct patient how to take leucovorin ordered by prescriber. Stress the importance of taking medication as prescribed until instructed by prescriber to stop medication.
● Tell patient to use highly protective sunblock when exposed to sunlight.
● Warn patient to avoid conception during and immediately after therapy because of possible abortion or congenital anomalies.
● Advise breast-feeding woman to discontinue breast-feeding during therapy because of risk of toxicity to infant.

---

*Liquid contains alcohol. **May contain tartrazine. †Canada ‡Australia §U.K. ◇OTC

thioguanine (6-TG, 6-thioguanine)
Lanvist†

Pregnancy risk category D

AVAILABLE FORMS
Tablets (scored): 40 mg

INDICATIONS & DOSAGES
➤ **Acute nonlymphocytic leukemia, chronic myelogenous leukemia—**
Adults and children: Initially, 2 mg/kg P.O. daily (usually calculated to nearest 20 mg). If after 4 weeks at 2 mg/kg there is no clinical improvement, dose may be cautiously increased to 3 mg/kg/day if not contraindicated.

ACTION
Inhibits DNA and (to a lesser degree) RNA synthesis.

Route	Onset	Peak	Duration
P.O.	Unknown	Unknown	Unknown

ADVERSE REACTIONS
GI: nausea, vomiting, stomatitis, diarrhea, anorexia.
Hematologic: *leukopenia,* anemia, *thrombocytopenia occurring slowly over 2 to 4 weeks.*
Hepatic: *hepatotoxicity,* jaundice, hepatic fibrosis, *toxic hepatitis.*
Metabolic: hyperuricemia.

INTERACTIONS
Drug-drug. *Myelosuppressives:* Increased risk of toxicity, especially myelosuppression, bleeding, and hepatotoxicity. Use together cautiously.

EFFECTS ON LAB TEST RESULTS
● May increase uric acid levels.
● May decrease hemoglobin and WBC, RBC, and platelet counts.

CONTRAINDICATIONS
Contraindicated in patients whose disease has shown resistance to drug and in patients hypersensitive to the drug. There is usually complete cross-resistance between mercaptopurine and thioguanine.

NURSING CONSIDERATIONS
● Use cautiously and with dosage modification in patients with renal or hepatic dysfunction.
● Monitor CBC daily during induction and then weekly during maintenance therapy. Leukocyte or platelet count depression is a contraindication to increasing dosage.
● Monitor uric acid level. Hyperuricemia can be minimized by increased urine alkalization and administration of allopurinol.
● Watch for jaundice; it may be reversible if drug is stopped promptly.
● To prevent bleeding, avoid all I.M. injections when platelet count is below 100,000/mm^3.
● Anticipate blood transfusions because of cumulative anemia. Patient may receive injections of RBC colony-stimulating factors to promote RBC production and decrease need for blood transfusions.
● **Alert:** Drug is sometimes ordered as 6-thioguanine. The numeral 6 is part of drug name and doesn't signify dosage units.

PATIENT TEACHING
● Instruct patient to watch for signs and symptoms of infection (fever, sore throat, fatigue) and bleeding (easy bruising, nosebleeds, bleeding gums, melena). Tell patient to take temperature daily.
● Caution woman of childbearing age to avoid becoming pregnant during therapy. Recommend that she consult prescriber before becoming pregnant.
● Advise breast-feeding woman to discontinue breast-feeding during therapy because of risk of toxicity to infant.

Reactions may be *common*, uncommon, *life-threatening*, or COMMON AND LIFE-THREATENING.

69
Antibiotic antineoplastics

bleomycin sulfate
dactinomycin
daunorubicin citrate liposomal
daunorubicin hydrochloride
doxorubicin hydrochloride
doxorubicin hydrochloride
  liposomal
epirubicin hydrochloride
idarubicin hydrochloride
mitomycin
pentostatin
plicamycin
valrubicin

COMBINATION PRODUCTS
None.

---

bleomycin sulfate
Blenoxane

Pregnancy risk category D

AVAILABLE FORMS
Injection: 15-unit vials, 30-unit vials

INDICATIONS & DOSAGES
Dosages may vary. Check treatment protocol with prescriber.
➤ **Squamous cell carcinoma (head,
neck, skin, penis, cervix, and vulva),
lymphosarcoma, reticulum cell carcinoma, testicular carcinoma**—
Adults: 10 to 20 units/m² I.V., I.M., or
S.C. once or two times weekly to total of
400 units.
➤ **Hodgkin's disease**—
Adults: 10 to 20 units/m² I.V., I.M., or
S.C. one or two times weekly. After 50%
response, maintenance dose is 1 unit I.M.
or I.V. daily or 5 units I.M. or I.V. weekly
to total of 400 units.
➤ **Treatment of malignant pleural effusion, prevention of recurrent pleural effusions**—
Adults: 60 units given as single-dose bolus
intrapleural injection.

I.V. ADMINISTRATION
● Follow facility policy to reduce risks.
Preparation and administration of parenteral form of drug are linked to carcinogenic,
mutagenic, and teratogenic risks for staff.
● Reconstitute drug with 5 or 10 ml of
normal saline solution for injection to
equal 3 unit/ml solution. Drug may be giv-
en at this concentration over 10 minutes.
● Refrigerate unopened vials containing
dry powder. Reconstituted solution should
be used within 24 hours. Bleomycin may
adsorb to plastic I.V. bags. For prolonged
infusions, use glass containers.

ACTION
Unknown. Thought to inhibit DNA synthesis and cause scission of single- and
double-stranded DNA. To a lesser extent,
inhibits RNA and protein synthesis.

Route	Onset	Peak	Duration
I.M.	Unknown	30-60 min	Unknown
I.V., S.C.	Unknown	Unknown	Unknown

ADVERSE REACTIONS
GI: *stomatitis, anorexia, nausea, vomiting,* diarrhea.
Metabolic: weight loss, hyperuricemia.
Respiratory: PNEUMONITIS, *pulmonary
fibrosis.*
Skin: *erythema, hyperpigmentation, acne,
rash, striae, skin tenderness, pruritus, reversible alopecia,* hyperkeratosis, nail
changes.
Other: *chills,* fever, *anaphylactoid reactions.*

INTERACTIONS
Drug-drug. *Anesthesia:* May increase
oxygen requirements. Monitor patient
closely.
Cardiac glycosides: Decreased digoxin
levels. Monitor digoxin levels closely.
Fosphenytoin, phenytoin: Decreased
phenytoin and fosphenytoin levels. Monitor drug levels closely.

EFFECTS ON LAB TEST RESULTS
● May increase uric acid levels.

CONTRAINDICATIONS
Contraindicated in patients hypersensitive to drug.

NURSING CONSIDERATIONS
• Use cautiously in patients with renal or pulmonary impairment.
• Obtain pulmonary function tests. Drug should be stopped if tests show a marked decline.
• *Alert:* Pulmonary toxicity appears to be dose-related, with an increase when total dose is more than 400 units. Give total doses of more than 400 units with caution.
• For intrapleural administration, dilute 60 units of drug in 50 to 100 ml normal saline solution for injection; drug is given through a thoracotomy tube.
• For I.M. use, dilute drug in 1 to 5 ml of sterile water for injection, bacteriostatic water for injection, or normal saline solution for injection.
• Monitor injection site for irritation.
• *Alert:* Adverse pulmonary reactions are more common in patients older than age 70. Pulmonary fibrosis is fatal in 1% of patients, especially when cumulative dosage exceeds 400 units. Also, pulmonary toxic adverse effects may be increased in patients receiving radiation therapy, patients with preexisting lung disease, and patients requiring O_2 therapy.
• Monitor chest X-ray and listen to lungs regularly.
• Pulmonary function tests and chest X-rays should be obtained before each course of therapy.
• If patient's condition requires sclerosis, drug may be instilled when chest tube drainage is 100 to 300 ml/24 hours before therapy; ideally, drainage should be less than 100 ml. After instillation, thoracotomy tube is clamped and patient is moved alternately from the supine to left and right lateral positions for the next 4 hours. The clamp is then removed and suction reestablished. Amount of time chest tube is left in place after sclerosis depends on patient's condition.
• Watch for fever, which may be treated with antipyretics. Fever usually occurs within 3 to 6 hours of administration.
• Watch for hypersensitivity reactions, which may be delayed for several hours, especially in patients with lymphoma.

(Test dose of 1 to 2 units should be given before first two doses in these patients. If no reaction occurs, follow regular dosage.)
• Don't use adhesive dressings on skin.

PATIENT TEACHING
• Warn patient that alopecia may occur, but that it's usually reversible.
• Tell patient to report adverse reactions promptly and to take infection-control and bleeding precautions.
• Instruct patient that, if he's to receive anesthesia, he must inform anesthesiologist of previous treatment with bleomycin. Pulmonary toxicity of drug may be enhanced by high oxygen levels inhaled during surgery.

---

dactinomycin (actinomycin D)
Cosmegen

Pregnancy risk category C

AVAILABLE FORMS
Injection: 500-mcg vial

INDICATIONS & DOSAGES
Dosages vary. Check treatment protocol with prescriber.
➤ **Sarcoma, trophoblastic tumors in women, testicular cancer—**
Adults: 500 mcg (0.5 mg) I.V. daily for 5 days. Maximum, 15 mcg/kg or 400 to 600 mcg/m²/day for 5 days. After bone marrow recovery, and at least 3 weeks, course may be repeated.
➤ **Wilms' tumor, rhabdomyosarcoma, Ewing's sarcoma—**
Children: 10 to 15 mcg/kg or 400 to 500 mcg/m²/day I.V. for 5 days. Maximum, 500 mcg/day. Or, 2.5 mg/m² I.V. in equally divided daily doses over 7 days. After bone marrow recovery, course may be repeated. Not recommended for infants younger than age 6 months.

I.V. ADMINISTRATION
• Follow facility policy to reduce risks. Preparation and administration of parenteral form of drug are linked to carcinogenic, mutagenic, and teratogenic risks for staff.
• Use only sterile water (without preservatives) as diluent for reconstitution. Add 1.1 ml to vial to yield gold-colored solu-

---

Reactions may be *common*, uncommon, *life-threatening*, or COMMON AND LIFE-THREATENING.

tion containing 0.5 mg/ml. Give by direct injection into a vein or through tubing of a free-flowing I.V. solution of normal saline solution for injection or D_5W. An in-line cellulose ester membrane filter shouldn't be used during dactinomycin administration.

• For I.V. infusion, dilute with up to 50 ml of D_5W or normal saline solution for injection; infuse over 15 minutes.

• Give through a running I.V. line with good blood return. Drug is a vesicant; if extravasation occurs, severe tissue necrosis may result. If infiltration occurs, apply cold compresses to area and notify prescriber.

• Discard unused solutions.

ACTION

May interfere with DNA-dependent RNA synthesis by intercalation. Protein and DNA synthesis are inhibited to a lesser extent.

Route	Onset	Peak	Duration
I.V.	Unknown	Unknown	Unknown

ADVERSE REACTIONS

CNS: malaise, fatigue, lethargy.
GI: *anorexia, nausea, vomiting,* abdominal pain, diarrhea, *stomatitis,* ulceration, proctitis.
GU: increased urine levels of uric acid.
Hematologic: *anemia, leukopenia, thrombocytopenia, pancytopenia, aplastic anemia, agranulocytosis.*
Hepatic: *hepatotoxicity.*
Metabolic: hyperuricemia, hypocalcemia.
Musculoskeletal: myalgia.
Skin: *erythema;* desquamation; reversible alopecia; *hyperpigmentation of skin, especially in previously irradiated areas, acnelike eruptions,* radiation recall effect.
Other: phlebitis and severe damage to soft tissue at injection site, fever, *anaphylactoid reaction.*

INTERACTIONS

Drug-drug. *Bone marrow suppressants:* Additive toxicity. Monitor CBC with differential.

EFFECTS ON LAB TEST RESULTS

• May increase uric acid levels. May decrease calcium levels.

• May decrease WBCs, RBCs, granulocytes, platelets, and hemoglobin.

CONTRAINDICATIONS

Contraindicated in patients with chickenpox or herpes zoster. Contraindicated in patients hypersensitive to the drug.

NURSING CONSIDERATIONS

• If skin contact occurs, irrigate with water for at least 15 minutes.

• *Alert:* Use caution when interpreting orders for dactinomycin as some regimens use milligrams per m^2 or milligrams per kilogram, and others use micrograms per m^2 or micrograms per kilogram.

• *Alert:* Dosage must be reduced in patients who have recently been treated with or who will also receive treatment with radiation therapy or other chemotherapy drugs.

• In the event of a spill, use a solution of trisodium phosphate 5% to inactivate drug.

• Monitor CBC with differential and platelet counts and renal and hepatic functions.

• If WBC count falls below 2,000/mm³ or granulocyte count falls below 1,000/mm³, follow institutional policy for infection control in immunocompromised patients.

• Watch for stomatitis, diarrhea, leukopenia, or thrombocytopenia. Implement preventive mouth care.

• *Alert:* If patient has previously received radiation therapy, he's susceptible to radiation recall effect, which is a reactivation of adverse effects, such as erythema at the site of irradiation, followed by hyperpigmentation, edema, desquamation, vesiculation, and necrosis.

• To reduce nausea, give antiemetic before drug.

• Drug may interfere with determination of antibiotic drug levels (peak and trough).

PATIENT TEACHING

• Advise patient to report any pain or burning at site of injection during or after administration.

• Advise patient to watch for evidence of infection (fever, sore throat, fatigue) and bleeding (easy bruising, nosebleeds,

---

bleeding gums, melena), and to take temperature daily.
• Tell patient that alopecia may occur, but that it's usually reversible.
• Inform patient who received a course of radiation therapy that he may experience radiation recall effect.

daunorubicin citrate liposomal
DaunoXome

Pregnancy risk category D

AVAILABLE FORMS
Injection: 2 mg/ml (equivalent to 50 mg daunorubicin base)

INDICATIONS & DOSAGES
➤ **First-line cytotoxic therapy for advanced HIV-related Kaposi's sarcoma—**
Adults: 40 mg/m² I.V. over 60 minutes once q 2 weeks. Treatment should be continued until there is evidence of progressive disease or until other complications of HIV preclude continuation of therapy.
Adjust-a-dose: For patients with impaired hepatic and renal function, reduce dosage as follows: if bilirubin level is 1.2 to 3 mg/dl, give three-fourths normal dose; if bilirubin or creatinine level exceeds 3 mg/dl, give one-half normal dose.

I.V. ADMINISTRATION
• Dilute drug with D₅W before use. Withdraw calculated volume of drug from vial and transfer into an equivalent amount of D₅W. Recommended concentration after dilution is 1 mg/ml.
• Don't mix daunorubicin citrate liposomal with bacteriostatic or other drugs, saline solution, or other solutions.
• After dilution, immediately give I.V. over 60 minutes. If unable to use immediately, refrigerate at 36° to 46° F (2° to 8° C) for up to 6 hours.
• Don't use in-line filters for I.V. infusion.
• *Alert:* A triad of back pain, flushing, and chest tightness may occur within first 5 minutes of infusion. These symptoms subside after infusion is stopped and usually don't recur when infusion is given at a slower rate.

• Because local tissue necrosis is possible, monitor I.V. site closely to avoid extravasation.
• Follow procedures for proper handling and disposal of antineoplastics.

ACTION
Maximizes selectivity of daunorubicin for solid tumors in situ. After penetrating tumor, drug is released over time to exert antineoplastic activity by inhibiting DNA synthesis and DNA-dependent RNA synthesis through intercalation.

Route	Onset	Peak	Duration
I.V.	Unknown	Unknown	Unknown

ADVERSE REACTIONS
CNS: *headache, neuropathy,* depression, dizziness, syncope, insomnia, amnesia, anxiety, ataxia, confusion, *seizures,* hallucination, tremor, hypertonia, meningitis, *fatigue,* malaise, emotional lability, abnormal gait, hyperkinesia, somnolence, abnormal thinking.
CV: *dose-related cardiomyopathy,* chest pain, hypertension, palpitations, *arrhythmias, pericardial effusion, pericardial tamponade, cardiac arrest,* angina pectoris, *pulmonary hypertension,* flushing, edema, tachycardia, *MI.*
EENT: *rhinitis,* stomatitis, sinusitis, abnormal vision, conjunctivitis, tinnitus, eye pain, deafness, earache.
GI: taste disturbances, dry mouth, gingival bleeding, *nausea, diarrhea, abdominal pain, vomiting, anorexia,* constipation, thirst, *GI hemorrhage,* gastritis, dysphagia, stomatitis, increased appetite, melena, hemorrhoids, tenesmus.
GU: dysuria, nocturia, polyuria.
Hematologic: NEUTROPENIA, THROMBOCYTOPENIA.
Hepatic: hepatomegaly.
Metabolic: dehydration.
Musculoskeletal: *rigors, back pain,* arthralgia, myalgia.
Respiratory: *cough, dyspnea,* hemoptysis, hiccups, pulmonary infiltration, increased sputum.
Skin: alopecia, pruritus, *increased sweating,* dry skin, seborrhea, folliculitis.
Other: *fever,* splenomegaly, lymphadenopathy, tooth caries, *opportunistic infec-*

tions, allergic reactions, flu symptoms, injection site inflammation.

INTERACTIONS
None significant.

EFFECTS ON LAB TEST RESULTS
• May decrease neutrophils and platelet count.

CONTRAINDICATIONS
Contraindicated in patients who have experienced severe hypersensitivity reaction to drug or its components.

NURSING CONSIDERATIONS
• Use cautiously in patients with myelosuppression, cardiac disease, previous radiotherapy encompassing the heart, previous anthracycline use (doxorubicin is 300 mg/m² or above), or hepatic or renal dysfunction.
• Liposomal daunorubicin is associated with less nausea, vomiting, alopecia, neutropenia, thrombocytopenia, and potentially less cardiotoxicity than conventional daunorubicin.
• Give only under supervision of prescriber specializing in cancer chemotherapy.
• Monitor cardiac function regularly. Assess patient before giving each dose because of risk of cardiac toxicity and heart failure. Determine left ventricular ejection fraction at total cumulative doses of 320 mg/m² and every 160 mg/m² thereafter. Total cumulative doses generally shouldn't exceed 550 mg/m².
• Careful hematologic monitoring is needed because severe myelosuppression may occur. Repeat blood counts and evaluate before giving each dose. Withhold treatment if absolute granulocyte count is below 750 cells/mm³.
• Monitor patient closely for signs and symptoms of opportunistic infection, especially because patients with HIV infection are immunocompromised.

PATIENT TEACHING
• Inform patient that alopecia may occur, but that it's usually reversible.
• Instruct patient to call prescriber if sore throat, fever, or other signs or symptoms

of infection occur. Tell patient to avoid exposure to people with infections.
• Advise woman to report suspected or confirmed pregnancy during therapy.
• Tell patient to report back pain, flushing, and chest tightness during infusion.

---

daunorubicin hydrochloride
Cerubidine

Pregnancy risk category D

AVAILABLE FORMS
Injection: 20-mg vial

INDICATIONS & DOSAGES
Dosages vary. Check treatment protocol with prescriber.
➤ **Remission induction in acute non-lymphocytic (myelogenous, monocytic, erythroid) leukemia—**
Adults: In combination, 30 to 45 mg/m²/day I.V. on days 1, 2, and 3 of first course and on days 1 and 2 of subsequent courses with cytarabine infusions.
➤ **Remission induction in acute lymphocytic leukemia—**
Adults: In combination, 45 mg/m²/day I.V. on days 1, 2, and 3 of first course.
Children age 2 and older: 25 mg/m² I.V. on day 1 q week, for up to 6 weeks, if needed.
Children younger than age 2 or body surface area less than 0.5 m²: Dose based on body weight (1 mg/kg), not surface area.
Adjust-a-dose: For patients with impaired hepatic and renal function, reduce dosage as follows: if bilirubin level is 1.2 to 3 mg/dl, give three-fourths normal dose; if bilirubin or creatinine level exceeds 3 mg/dl, give one-half normal dose.

I.V. ADMINISTRATION
• *Alert:* Follow facility policy to reduce risks. Preparation and administration of parenteral form of drug are linked to carcinogenic, mutagenic, and teratogenic risks for staff.
• Reconstitute drug using 4 ml of sterile water for injection to produce a 5 mg/ml solution.
• Withdraw desired dose into syringe containing 10 to 15 ml of normal saline solution for injection. Inject into tubing of a

---

*Liquid contains alcohol.   **May contain tartrazine.   †Canada   ‡Australia   §U.K.   ◊OTC

free-flowing I.V. solution of D_5W or normal saline solution for injection as a slow I.V. push.
• If extravasation occurs, stop I.V. infusion immediately, apply ice to area for 24 to 48 hours, and notify prescriber. Because drug is a vesicant, extravasation could cause severe tissue necrosis.
• *Alert:* Dexamethasone and heparin may form a precipitate. Don't mix together.

ACTION
May interfere with DNA-dependent RNA synthesis by intercalation.

Route	Onset	Peak	Duration
I.V.	Unknown	Unknown	Unknown

ADVERSE REACTIONS
CV: IRREVERSIBLE CARDIOMYOPATHY, ECG changes.
GI: *nausea, vomiting,* diarrhea, stomatitis.
GU: red urine.
Hematologic: *bone marrow suppression.*
Hepatic: *hepatotoxicity.*
Metabolic: hyperuricemia.
Skin: rash, *reversible alopecia,* darkening or redness of previously irradiated areas.
Other: *severe cellulitis, tissue sloughing with drug extravasation, anaphylactoid reaction,* fever, chills.

INTERACTIONS
Drug-drug. *Doxorubicin:* Additive cardiotoxicity. Monitor patient for toxicity.
Hepatotoxic drugs: Increased risk of additive hepatotoxicity. Monitor hepatic function closely.

EFFECTS ON LAB TEST RESULTS
• May increase uric acid levels.

CONTRAINDICATIONS
Contraindicated in patients hypersensitive to the drug.

NURSING CONSIDERATIONS
• Use cautiously in patients with myelosuppression or impaired cardiac, renal, or hepatic function.
• Take preventive measures (including adequate hydration) before starting treatment. Hyperuricemia may result from rapid lysis of leukemic cells. Allopurinol may be ordered.

• Cardiac function studies, including ECG and ejection fraction, should be performed before treatment and then periodically throughout therapy.
• Never give drug I.M. or S.C.
• Cumulative adult dosage is limited to 400 to 550 mg/m² (450 mg/m² when patient is also receiving or has received cyclophosphamide or radiation therapy to cardiac area).
• Therapeutic effects are commonly accompanied by toxicity.
• Monitor CBC and hepatic function tests; monitor ECG every month during therapy.
• Monitor pulse rate closely. Notify prescriber if light resting pulse rate (a sign of cardiac adverse reactions) occurs.
• *Alert:* Stop drug immediately and notify prescriber if signs of heart failure, cardiomyopathy, or arrhythmia develop.
• Watch for nausea and vomiting, which may last 24 to 48 hours.
• Anticipate the need for blood transfusions to combat anemia. Patient may receive injected RBC colony-stimulating factor to promote RBC production and decrease need for blood transfusions.
• *Alert:* Reddish color of drug is similar to that of doxorubicin; don't confuse the two.
• Optimally, use within 8 hours of preparation. Reconstituted solution is stable for 24 hours at room temperature, or 48 hours if refrigerated.
• Lowest blood counts occur 10 to 14 days after administration.

PATIENT TEACHING
• Advise patient to report any pain or burning at site of injection during or after administration.
• Advise patient to watch for signs and symptoms of infection (fever, sore throat, fatigue) and bleeding (easy bruising, nosebleeds, bleeding gums, melena) and to take temperature daily.
• Inform patient that red urine for 1 to 2 days is normal and doesn't indicate the presence of blood in urine.
• Advise patient that alopecia may occur, but that it's usually reversible.
• Caution woman of childbearing age to avoid becoming pregnant during therapy. Recommend that she consult prescriber before becoming pregnant.

Reactions may be *common,* uncommon, *life-threatening,* or COMMON AND LIFE-THREATENING.

doxorubicin hydrochloride
Adriamycin‡, Adriamycin PFS,
Adriamycin RDF, Rubex

Pregnancy risk category D

AVAILABLE FORMS
Injection (preservative-free): 2 mg/ml
Powder for injection: 10-mg, 20-mg,
50-mg, 100-mg, 150-mg vials

INDICATIONS & DOSAGES
Dosages vary. Check treatment protocol
with prescriber.
➤ **Bladder, breast, lung, ovarian, stomach, and thyroid cancers; Hodgkin's disease; acute lymphoblastic and myeloblastic leukemia; Wilms' tumor; neuroblastoma; lymphoma; sarcoma**—
Adults: 60 to 75 mg/m² I.V. as single dose
q 3 weeks; or 30 mg/m² I.V. in single daily
dose, days 1 to 3 of 4-week cycle. Or,
20 mg/m² I.V. once weekly. Maximum
cumulative dose is 550 mg/m².
Elderly patients: May need reduced
dosages.
Adjust-a-dose: For patients with myelosuppression or impaired cardiac or liver
function, dosage may be reduced. Be prepared to decrease dosage if bilirubin level
rises: give 50% of dose when bilirubin
level is 1.2 to 3 mg/100 ml; 25% when it's
3.1 to 5 mg/100 ml.

I.V. ADMINISTRATION
● Follow facility policy to reduce risks.
Preparation and administration of parenteral form of drug are linked to carcinogenic, mutagenic, and teratogenic risks for
staff.
● Reconstitute drug using preservative-free normal saline solution for injection.
Add 5 ml to 10-mg vial, 10 ml to 20-mg
vial, or 25 ml to 50-mg vial. Shake vial
and allow drug to dissolve; final concentration will be 2 mg/ml. Give by direct injection into the tubing of a free-flowing
I.V. solution containing D₅W or normal
saline solution for injection. Administration rate shouldn't be less than 3 minutes.
Drug is a severe vesicant; if extravasation
occurs, tissue necrosis may result.
● Don't place I.V. line over joints or in
limbs with poor venous or lymphatic

drainage. If extravasation occurs, stop I.V.
infusion immediately, apply ice to area for
24 to 48 hours, and notify prescriber.
Monitor area closely because extravasation may be progressive. Early consultation with a plastic surgeon may be advisable.
● If vein streaking occurs, slow administration rate. However, if welts occur, stop
administration and notify prescriber.
● Some protocols give doxorubicin as a
prolonged infusion. This requires central
venous access.
● Refrigerated, reconstituted solution is
stable for 48 hours; at room temperature,
it's stable for 24 hours.

ACTION
May interfere with DNA-dependent RNA
synthesis by intercalation.

Route	Onset	Peak	Duration
I.V.	Unknown	Unknown	Unknown

ADVERSE REACTIONS
CV: cardiac depression, *arrhythmias,
acute left ventricular failure, irreversible
cardiomyopathy.*
EENT: conjunctivitis.
GI: *nausea, vomiting,* diarrhea, *stomatitis,*
esophagitis, anorexia.
GU: transient red urine.
Hematologic: *leukopenia, thrombocytopenia,* MYELOSUPPRESSION.
Metabolic: hyperuricemia.
Skin: *severe cellulitis, tissue sloughing
with drug extravasation,* urticaria, facial
flushing, *complete alopecia within 3 to 4
weeks,* hyperpigmentation of nail beds and
dermal creases, radiation recall effect.
Other: fever, chills, *anaphylaxis.*

INTERACTIONS
Drug-drug. *Aminophylline, cephalothin,
dexamethasone, fluorouracil, heparin, hydrocortisone:* May form a precipitate.
Don't mix together.
Calcium channel blockers: May potentiate
cardiotoxic effects. Monitor patient's ECG
closely.
Digoxin: May decrease digoxin levels.
Monitor digoxin levels closely.
Fosphenytoin, phenytoin: Decreased levels
of phenytoin or fosphenytoin. Check levels.

Streptozocin: Increased and prolonged blood levels. Dosage may have to be adjusted.

EFFECTS ON LAB TEST RESULTS
● May increase uric acid levels.
● May decrease WBCs and platelet count.

CONTRAINDICATIONS
Contraindicated in patients with marked myelosuppression induced by previous treatment with other antitumor drugs or radiotherapy and in patients who have received a lifetime cumulative dose of 550 mg/m^3 of doxorubicin or daunorubicin.

NURSING CONSIDERATIONS
● Cardiac function studies, including ECG and ejection fraction, should be performed before treatment and then periodically throughout therapy. Dexrazoxane may be given within 30 minutes of doxorubicin if the accumulated dose of doxorubicin has reached 300 mg/m^2.
● Take preventive measures, including adequate hydration, before starting treatment. Hyperuricemia may result from rapid lysis of leukemic cells. Allopurinol may be ordered.
● Premedicate with antiemetic to reduce nausea.
● If skin or mucosal contact occurs, immediately wash with soap and water.
● If drug leaks or spills, inactivate it with 5% sodium hypochlorite solution (household bleach).
● Never give drug I.M. or S.C.
● Dosage modification may be needed in patients with myelosuppression or impaired cardiac or hepatic function, and in elderly patients.
● Monitor CBC with differential and hepatic function tests; monitor ECG monthly during therapy. If WBC count falls below 2,000/mm^3 or granulocyte count falls below 1,000/mm^3, follow institutional policy for infection control in immunocompromised patients.
● Monitor ECG for changes such as sinus tachycardia, T-wave flattening, ST-segment depression, and voltage reduction.
● Leukopenia may occur during days 10 to 15, with recovery by day 21.

● Be prepared to stop drug or slow rate of infusion, and notify prescriber if tachycardia develops.
● *Alert:* If signs of heart failure develop, stop drug and notify prescriber. Heart failure can often be prevented by limiting cumulative dose to 550 mg/m^2 (400 mg/m^2 when patient is also receiving or has received cyclophosphamide or radiation therapy to cardiac area).
● Reddish color of drug is similar to that of daunorubicin; don't confuse the two drugs.
● Esophagitis is common in patients who also have received radiation therapy.
● *Alert:* If patient has previously received radiation therapy, he is susceptible to radiation recall effect.

PATIENT TEACHING
● Advise patient to report any pain or burning at site of injection during or after administration.
● Advise patient to watch for signs and symptoms of infection (fever, sore throat, fatigue) and bleeding (easy bruising, nosebleeds, bleeding gums, melena) and to take temperature daily.
● Advise patient that orange to red urine for 1 to 2 days is normal and doesn't indicate presence of blood.
● Inform patient that alopecia may occur, but it's usually reversible. Hair may regrow 2 to 5 months after drug is stopped.

---

doxorubicin hydrochloride liposomal
Doxil

Pregnancy risk category D

AVAILABLE FORMS
Injection: 2 mg/ml

INDICATIONS & DOSAGES
➤ **Metastatic carcinoma of ovary in patients with disease that's refractory to both paclitaxel- and platinum-based chemotherapy regimen—**
Women: 50 mg/m^2 (doxorubicin hydrochloride equivalent) I.V. at initial infusion rate of 1 mg/minute once every 4 weeks for minimum of 4 courses. Continue as long as condition doesn't progress, patient

---

shows no evidence of cardiotoxicity, and patient continues to tolerate treatment. If no infusion-related adverse reactions are observed, increase infusion rate to complete administration over 1 hour.

➤ **AIDS-related Kaposi's sarcoma in patients with disease that has progressed on previous combination chemotherapy and in patients intolerant to such therapy—**
Adults: 20 mg/m² (doxorubicin hydrochloride equivalent) I.V. over 30 minutes once every 3 weeks. Continue as long as patient responds satisfactorily and tolerates treatment.
Adjust-a-dose: For patients with impaired hepatic function, reduce dosage as follows: If bilirubin level is 1.2 to 3 mg/dl, give one-half normal dose; if bilirubin level is more than 3 mg/dl, give one-quarter normal dose.

I.V. ADMINISTRATION
● Follow procedures for proper handling and disposal of antineoplastics.
● Dilute appropriate dose (to maximum of 90 mg) in 250 ml D₅W using aseptic technique. Refrigerate diluted solution at 36° to 46° F (2° to 8° C) and give within 24 hours.
● Carefully check label on I.V. bag before giving. Accidental substitution of doxorubicin hydrochloride liposomal for conventional doxorubicin hydrochloride has resulted in severe adverse reactions. The two products cannot be substituted on a mg-per-mg basis.
● *Alert:* Don't use with in-line filters.
● Infuse over 30 to 60 minutes depending on dose. Monitor patient carefully during infusion. Acute infusion-related reactions (flushing, shortness of breath, facial swelling, headache, chills, back pain, tightness in chest or throat, and hypotension) may occur. Reactions resolve over several hours to a day once infusion is stopped, and may resolve when infusion rate is slowed.
● If signs or symptoms of extravasation occur, stop infusion immediately and restart in another vein. Applying ice over site of extravasation for about 30 minutes may help alleviate local reaction.

ACTION
Consists of doxorubicin hydrochloride encapsulated in liposomes. Action possibly related to drug's ability to bind DNA and inhibit nucleic acid synthesis.

Route	Onset	Peak	Duration
I.V.	Unknown	Unknown	Unknown

ADVERSE REACTIONS
CNS: *asthenia,* paresthesia, headache, somnolence, dizziness, depression, insomnia, anxiety, malaise, emotional lability, fatigue.
CV: chest pain, hypotension, tachycardia, peripheral edema, ***cardiomyopathy, heart failure, arrhythmias,*** pericardial effusion.
EENT: *stomatitis,* pharyngitis, rhinitis, conjunctivitis, retinitis, optic neuritis.
GI: *nausea, vomiting, constipation, anorexia, diarrhea,* abdominal pain, dyspepsia, oral candidiasis, enlarged abdomen, esophagitis, dysphagia, *stomatitis,* taste perversion, glossitis.
GU: albuminuria.
Hematologic: LEUKOPENIA, NEUTROPENIA, THROMBOCYTOPENIA, *anemia.*
Hepatic: hyperbilirubinemia.
Metabolic: dehydration, weight loss, hypocalcemia, hyperglycemia.
Musculoskeletal: myalgia, back pain.
Respiratory: dyspnea, increased cough, pneumonia.
Skin: *rash, alopecia,* dry skin, pruritus, skin discoloration, skin disorder, exfoliative dermatitis, sweating, *palmar-plantar erythrodysesthesia,* alopecia.
Other: fever, allergic reaction, chills, *herpes zoster,* infection, infusion-related reactions.

INTERACTIONS
None reported. However, doxorubicin hydrochloride liposomal may interact with drugs known to affect the conventional formulation of doxorubicin hydrochloride.

EFFECTS ON LAB TEST RESULTS
● May increase PT, bilirubin, and glucose levels. May decrease calcium levels.
● May decrease WBCs, neutrophils, hemoglobin, and platelet count.

CONTRAINDICATIONS

Contraindicated in patients hypersensitive to conventional formulation of doxorubicin hydrochloride or any component in the liposomal formulation. Also contraindicated in patients with marked myelosuppression and those who have received a lifetime cumulative dose of 550 mg/m^2 (400 mg/m^2 in patients who have received radiotherapy to the mediastinal area or therapy with other cardiotoxic drugs such as cyclophosphamide).

NURSING CONSIDERATIONS

● Don't give I.M. or S.C.
● Use cautiously in patients who have received other anthracyclines. Previous or current therapy with related compounds such as daunorubicin should be considered when total dose of drug to be given is calculated. Heart failure and cardiomyopathy may occur after discontinuation of therapy.
● Give drug to patient with history of CV disease only when benefit outweighs risk to patient.
● *Alert:* Monitor patient for signs and symptoms of palmar-plantar erythrodysesthesia, hematologic toxicity, or stomatitis. These adverse reactions may be managed with dosage delays and adjustments.
● Evaluate patient's hepatic function before therapy, and adjust dosage accordingly.
● Drug exhibits unique pharmacokinetic properties compared to conventional doxorubicin hydrochloride and shouldn't be substituted on a mg-per-mg basis.
● Drug may potentiate toxicity of other antineoplastic therapies.
● Closely monitor cardiac function by endomyocardial biopsy, echocardiography, or gated radionuclide scans. If results indicate possible cardiac injury, the benefit of continued therapy must be weighed against the risk of myocardial injury.
● Monitor CBC, including platelets, before each dose and frequently throughout therapy. Leukopenia is usually transient. Persistent severe myelosuppression may result in superinfection or hemorrhage. Patient may need G-CSF (or GM-CSF) to support blood counts.

PATIENT TEACHING

● Tell patient to notify prescriber if he experiences signs and symptoms of hand-foot syndrome (such as tingling or burning, redness, flaking, bothersome swelling, small blisters, or small sores on palms of hands or soles of feet).
● Advise patient to report signs and symptoms of stomatitis (such as painful redness, swelling, or sores in mouth).
● Warn patient to avoid exposure to people with infections. Tell patient to report temperature of 100.5° F (38° C) or higher.
● Tell patient to report nausea, vomiting, tiredness, weakness, rash, or mild hair loss.
● Advise woman of childbearing age to avoid pregnancy during therapy.

epirubicin hydrochloride
Ellence

Pregnancy risk category D

AVAILABLE FORMS
Injection: 2 mg/ml

INDICATIONS & DOSAGES
➤ **Adjuvant therapy in patients with evidence of axillary node tumor involvement after resection of primary breast cancer—**
Adults: 100 to 120 mg/m^2 I.V. infusion over 3 to 5 minutes through a free-flowing I.V. solution on day 1 of each cycle, or divided equally in two doses on days 1 and 8 of each cycle; cycle repeated q 3 to 4 weeks for six cycles; used with regimens containing cyclophosphamide and fluorouracil.

Dosage modification after first cycle is based on toxicity. For patients with platelet count nadir below 50,000/mm^3, absolute neutrophil count (ANC) below 250/mm^3, neutropenic fever, or grade 3 or 4 nonhematologic toxicity, reduce day 1 dose in subsequent cycles to 75% of day 1 dose given in current cycle. Delay day 1 therapy in subsequent cycles until platelet count is at least 100,000/mm^3, ANC is at least 1,500/mm^3, and nonhematologic toxicities recover to grade 1.

For patients receiving divided doses (days 1 and 8), day 8 dose should be 75% of day 1 dose if platelet count is 75,000 to 100,000/mm^3 and ANC is 1,000 to 1,499/mm^3. If day 8 platelet count is below 75,000/mm³, ANC is below 1,000/mm³, or grade 3 or 4 nonhematologic toxicity has occurred, omit day 8 dose.

Adjust-a-dose: For patients with bone marrow dysfunction (heavily pretreated patients, patients with bone marrow depression, or those with neoplastic bone marrow infiltration), start at lower doses of 75 to 90 mg/m². For patients with hepatic dysfunction, if bilirubin is 1.2 to 3 mg/dl or AST is two to four times upper limit of normal, give one-half recommended starting dose. If bilirubin level is above 3 mg/dl or AST is more than four times upper limit of normal, give one-quarter recommended starting dose. For patients with severe renal dysfunction (creatinine level over 5 mg/dl), consider lower doses.

I.V. ADMINISTRATION
● *Alert:* Drug is a vesicant. Never give I.M. or S.C. Always give through free-flowing I.V. solution of normal saline solution or D₅W over 3 to 5 minutes.
● Facial flushing and local erythematous streaking along vein may indicate excessively rapid administration.
● Avoid veins over joints or in limbs with compromised venous or lymphatic drainage.
● Immediately stop infusion if burning or stinging occurs, and restart in another vein.
● Don't mix drug with heparin or fluorouracil because precipitation may result.
● Don't mix in same syringe with other drugs.
● Discard unused solution left in vial 24 hours after vial has been penetrated.

ACTION
Exact mechanism unknown. Thought to form a complex with DNA by intercalation between nucleotide base pairs, thereby inhibiting DNA, RNA, and protein synthesis; DNA cleavage occurs, resulting in cytocidal activity. Drug may also interfere with replication and transcription of DNA and may generate cytotoxic free radicals.

Route	Onset	Peak	Duration
I.V.	Unknown	Unknown	Unknown

ADVERSE REACTIONS
CNS: *lethargy.*
CV: *cardiomyopathy, heart failure.*
EENT: *conjunctivitis, keratitis.*
GI: *nausea, vomiting, diarrhea,* anorexia, *mucositis.*
GU: *amenorrhea,* red urine.
Hematologic: LEUKOPENIA, NEUTROPENIA, *febrile neutropenia, anemia,* THROMBOCYTOPENIA.
Skin: *alopecia,* rash, itch, skin changes.
Other: *infection,* fever, hot flashes, local toxicity.

INTERACTIONS
Drug-drug. *Calcium channel blockers, other cardioactive compounds:* May increase risk of heart failure. Monitor cardiac function closely.
Cimetidine: Increased epirubicin levels by 50%. Avoid using together.
Cytotoxic drugs: Additive toxicities (especially hematologic and GI) may occur. Monitor patient closely.
Radiation therapy: Effects may be enhanced. Monitor patient closely.

EFFECTS ON LAB TEST RESULTS
● May decrease hemoglobin and WBC, neutrophil, and platelet counts.

CONTRAINDICATIONS
Contraindicated in patients hypersensitive to drug, other anthracyclines, or anthracenediones, and in patients with baseline neutrophil counts below 1,500 cells/mm³, severe myocardial insufficiency, recent MI, or severe hepatic dysfunction. Also contraindicated in patients who have had previous treatment with anthracyclines to total cumulative doses.

NURSING CONSIDERATIONS
● Use cautiously in patients with active or dormant cardiac disease, previous or current radiotherapy to mediastinal and pericardial areas, or previous therapy with other anthracyclines or anthracenediones; also use cautiously in patients receiving other cardiotoxic drugs.
● Patients receiving 120 mg/m² of epirubicin should also receive prophylactic antibiotic therapy with co-trimoxazole or a fluoroquinolone.

---

*Liquid contains alcohol.   **May contain tartrazine.   †Canada   ‡Australia   §U.K.   ◇OTC

• Antiemetics may be needed before epirubicin to reduce nausea and vomiting.
• Obtain the following measurements before therapy begins: total bilirubin, AST, and creatinine levels; CBC including ANC; and left ventricular ejection fraction (LVEF).
• Monitor LVEF regularly during therapy. Discontinue drug at first sign of impaired cardiac function. Early signs of cardiac toxicity include sinus tachycardia, ECG abnormalities, tachyarrhythmias, bradycardia, AV block, and bundle-branch block.
• Delayed cardiac toxicity may occur 2 to 3 months after treatment ends; indications include reduced LVEF and signs and symptoms of heart failure (tachycardia, dyspnea, pulmonary edema, dependent edema, hepatomegaly, ascites, pleural effusion, and gallop rhythm). Delayed cardiac toxicity depends on cumulative dose of epirubicin. Don't exceed cumulative dose of 900 mg/m².
• Obtain total and differential WBC, CBC, platelet counts, and liver function tests before and during each cycle of therapy.
• WBC nadir is usually reached 10 to 14 days after drug administration, and returns to normal by day 21.
• Monitor uric acid, potassium, calcium phosphate, and creatinine levels immediately after initial chemotherapy administration in patients susceptible to tumor lysis syndrome. Hydration, urine alkalinization, and prophylaxis with allopurinol may prevent hyperuricemia and minimize potential complications of tumor lysis syndrome.
• Administration of drug after previous radiation therapy may induce an inflammatory cell reaction at irradiation site.
• Give drug under supervision of prescriber experienced in cancer chemotherapy. Pregnant nurses shouldn't handle drug.
• Wear protective clothing (goggles, gown, disposable gloves) when handling drug.

PATIENT TEACHING
• Advise patient to report any pain or burning at site of injection during or after administration.
• Advise patient to report nausea, vomiting, stomatitis, dehydration, fever, evidence of infection, or symptoms of heart failure (tachycardia, dyspnea, edema).
• Tell patient that urine will be reddish-pink for 1 to 2 days after treatment.
• Inform patient of risk of cardiac damage and treatment-related leukemia with use of drug.
• Advise men to use effective contraception during treatment.
• Advise women that irreversible amenorrhea or premature menopause may occur.
• Tell patient that hair usually regrows within 2 to 3 months after therapy stops.

---

idarubicin hydrochloride
Idamycin, Zavedos§

Pregnancy risk category D

AVAILABLE FORMS
Powder for injection: 5 mg, 10 mg, 20 mg

INDICATIONS & DOSAGES
Dosages vary. Check treatment protocol with prescriber.
➤ **Acute myeloid leukemia, including FAB (French-American-British) classifications M1 through M7, with other approved antileukemic drugs—**
Adults: 12 mg/m²/day for 3 days by slow I.V. injection (over 10 to 15 minutes) with 100 mg/m²/day of cytarabine for 7 days by continuous I.V. infusion. Or, as a 25-mg/m² bolus (cytarabine); then 200 mg/m²/day (cytarabine) for 5 days by continuous infusion. A second course may be given, if needed.
Adjust-a-dose: If patient experiences severe mucositis, delay therapy until recovery is complete and reduce dosage by 25%. Reduce dosage in patients with hepatic or renal impairment. Don't give idarubicin if bilirubin level exceeds 5 mg/dl.

I.V. ADMINISTRATION
• Follow facility policy to reduce risks. Preparation and administration of parenteral form of drug are linked to carcinogenic, mutagenic, and teratogenic risks for staff.
• Reconstitute to final concentration of 1 mg/ml using normal saline solution for injection without preservatives. Add 5 ml

---

to 5-mg vial, 10 ml to 10-mg vial, or 20 ml to 20-mg vial. Don't use bacteriostatic saline solution. Vial is under negative pressure.

• Give drug over 10 to 15 minutes into a free-flowing I.V. infusion of normal saline or D_5W solution running into a large vein.

• Drug is a vesicant; tissue necrosis may result. If extravasation occurs, stop infusion immediately and notify prescriber. Treat with intermittent ice packs—for one-half hour immediately, and then for one-half hour q.i.d. for 4 days.

• Reconstituted solutions are stable for 72 hours at 59° to 86° F (15° to 30° C); 7 days if refrigerated. Label unused solutions with chemotherapy hazard label.

ACTION
Unknown. Probably inhibits nucleic acid synthesis by intercalation and interacts with the enzyme topoisomerase II. It's highly lipophilic, which results in an increased rate of cellular uptake.

Route	Onset	Peak	Duration
I.V.	Unknown	Few min	Unknown

ADVERSE REACTIONS
CNS: *headache, changed mental status,* peripheral neuropathy, *seizures.*
CV: *heart failure,* atrial fibrillation, chest pain, *MI,* asymptomatic decline in left ventricular ejection fraction, *myocardial insufficiency, arrhythmias,* HEMORRHAGE, *myocardial toxicity.*
GI: *nausea, vomiting, cramps, diarrhea, mucositis.*
GU: decreased renal function, red urine.
Hematologic: *myelosuppression.*
Hepatic: changes in hepatic function.
Metabolic: hyperuricemia.
Skin: *alopecia, rash, urticaria, bullous erythrodermatous rash on palms and soles,* urticaria at injection site, erythema at previously irradiated sites, tissue necrosis at injection site if extravasation occurs.
Other: INFECTION, *fever, hypersensitivity reactions.*

INTERACTIONS
Drug-drug. *Alkaline solutions, heparin:* Incompatible. Don't mix idarubicin with other drugs unless specific compatibility data are available.

EFFECTS ON LAB TEST RESULTS
• May increase uric acid levels.

CONTRAINDICATIONS
No known contraindications.

NURSING CONSIDERATIONS
• Use with extreme caution in patients with bone marrow suppression induced by previous drug therapy or radiotherapy, impaired hepatic or renal function, previous treatment with anthracyclines or cardiotoxic drugs, or a cardiac condition.
• Cardiotoxicity is the dose-limiting toxicity of drug.
• Take preventive measures, including adequate hydration, before starting treatment. Hyperuricemia may result from rapid lysis of leukemic cells. Allopurinol may be ordered.
• Assess patient for systemic infection and ensure that it's controlled before therapy begins.
• Give antiemetics to prevent or treat nausea and vomiting.
• Drug must never be given I.M. or S.C.
• Monitor hepatic and renal function tests and CBC frequently.
• To prevent bleeding, avoid all I.M. injections when platelet count is below 50,000/mm³.
• Anticipate need for blood transfusions to combat anemia. Patient may receive injections of RBC colony-stimulating factor to promote RBC production and decrease need for blood transfusions.
• Notify prescriber if signs or symptoms of heart failure occur.
• *Alert:* Don't confuse idarubicin with daunorubicin or doxorubicin.

PATIENT TEACHING
• Teach patient to recognize signs and symptoms of extravasation, and tell him to report them if they occur.
• Warn patient to watch for signs and symptoms of infection (fever, sore throat, fatigue) and bleeding (easy bruising, nosebleeds, bleeding gums, melena).
• Advise patient that red urine for several days is normal and doesn't indicate presence of blood.
• Caution woman of childbearing age to avoid becoming pregnant during therapy.

---

*Liquid contains alcohol. **May contain tartrazine. †Canada ‡Australia §U.K. ◇OTC

Recommend that she consult prescriber before becoming pregnant.

mitomycin (mitomycin-C)
Mutamycin

Pregnancy risk category NR

AVAILABLE FORMS
Injection: 5-mg, 20-mg, 40-mg vials

INDICATIONS & DOSAGES
Dosage and indications vary. Check treatment protocol with prescriber.
➤ **Disseminated adenocarcinoma of stomach or pancreas—**
Adults: 10 to 20 mg/m^2 as an I.V. single dose. Repeat cycle after 6 to 8 weeks when WBC and platelet counts have returned to normal.

I.V. ADMINISTRATION
• Follow facility policy to reduce risks. Preparation and administration of parenteral form of drug are linked to mutagenic, teratogenic, and carcinogenic risks to staff.
• Using sterile water for injection, reconstitute drug in 5-mg vials with 10 ml, 20-mg vials with 40 ml, and 40-mg vials with 80 ml. When reconstituted with sterile water, the solution is stable for 14 days under refrigeration and 7 days at room temperature.
• Give drug into the side arm of a free-flowing I.V.
• Avoid extravasation. Stop infusion immediately and notify prescriber if extravasation occurs because of potential for severe ulceration and necrosis.

ACTION
Similar to an alkylating drug, cross-linking strands of DNA and causing an imbalance of cell growth, leading to cell death.

Route	Onset	Peak	Duration
I.V.	Unknown	Unknown	Unknown

ADVERSE REACTIONS
CNS: headache, neurologic abnormalities, confusion, drowsiness, fatigue.
EENT: blurred vision.

GI: mucositis, *nausea, vomiting, anorexia, diarrhea.*
GU: *renal toxicity.*
Hematologic: THROMBOCYTOPENIA, LEUKOPENIA, *microangiopathic hemolytic anemia.*
Respiratory: *interstitial pneumonitis,* pulmonary edema, dyspnea, nonproductive cough, *adult respiratory distress syndrome.*
Skin: cellulitis, induration, desquamation, pruritus, *pain at injection site, reversible alopecia,* purple bands on nails, rash, sloughing with extravasation.
Other: *septicemia,* ulceration, *fever,* pain.

INTERACTIONS
Drug-drug. *Vinca alkaloids:* May cause acute respiratory distress when given together. Monitor patient closely.

EFFECTS ON LAB TEST RESULTS
• May decrease platelet count and hemoglobin.

CONTRAINDICATIONS
Contraindicated in patients hypersensitive to drug and in those with thrombocytopenia, coagulation disorders, or an increased bleeding tendency from other causes.

NURSING CONSIDERATIONS
• Never give drug I.M. or S.C.
• Continue CBC and blood studies at least 8 weeks after therapy stops. Leukopenia and thrombocytopenia are cumulative. If WBC count falls below 2,000/mm^3 or granulocyte count falls below 1,000/mm^3, follow institutional policy for infection control in immunocompromised patients.
• To prevent bleeding, avoid all I.M. injections when platelet count is below 100,000/mm^3.
• Anticipate need for blood transfusions to combat anemia. Patients may receive injections of RBC colony-stimulating factor to promote RBC production and decrease need for blood transfusions.
• Monitor patient for dyspnea with nonproductive cough; chest X-ray may show infiltrates.
• Monitor renal function tests.
• Leukopenia may occur up to 8 weeks after therapy and may be cumulative with successive doses.

Reactions may be *common*, uncommon, *life-threatening*, or COMMON AND LIFE-THREATENING.

• Microangiopathic hemolytic anemia is characterized by thrombocytopenia, renal failure, and hypertension.
• *Alert:* Don't confuse mitomycin with mithramycin.

PATIENT TEACHING
• Advise patient to report any pain or burning at site of injection during or after administration.
• Warn patient to watch for signs and symptoms of infection (fever, sore throat, fatigue) and bleeding (easy bruising, nosebleeds, bleeding gums, melena). Tell patient to take temperature daily.
• Inform patient that alopecia may occur, but that it's usually reversible.

---

pentostatin (2-deoxycoformycin)
Nipent

Pregnancy risk category D

AVAILABLE FORMS
Powder for injection: 10-mg vial

INDICATIONS & DOSAGES
➤ **Alpha interferon–refractory hairy cell leukemia—**
Adults: 4 mg/m² I.V. every other week.

I.V. ADMINISTRATION
• Make sure patient is adequately hydrated before therapy. Give 500 to 1,000 ml of dextrose 5% in half-normal saline solution for hydration. Ensure at least 2 L of urine output daily during therapy.
• Follow facility policy to reduce risks. Preparation and administration of parenteral form of drug are linked to mutagenic, teratogenic, and carcinogenic risks to staff.
• Add 5 ml of sterile water for injection to vial containing pentostatin powder for injection. Mix thoroughly to make a solution of 2 mg/ml. Drug may be given by I.V. bolus injection or diluted further in 25 or 50 ml of D₅W or normal saline solution for injection and infused over 20 to 30 minutes. Avoid extravasation; drug is a vesicant.
• Use reconstituted solution within 8 hours; it contains no preservatives.

• Give an additional 500 ml of D₅W for hydration after drug is administered.

ACTION
Inhibits the enzyme adenosine deaminase (ADA), causing an increase in intracellular levels of deoxyadenosine triphosphate, which leads to cell damage and death. Because the greatest activity of ADA is in cells of the lymphoid system (especially malignant T cells), pentostatin is useful in treating leukemias. The exact antitumor effect for leukemia is unknown.

Route	Onset	Peak	Duration
I.V.	Unknown	Unknown	Unknown

ADVERSE REACTIONS
CNS: *headache, neurologic symptoms,* malaise, anxiety, confusion, depression, dizziness, insomnia, nervousness, paresthesia, somnolence, abnormal thinking, *fatigue, asthenia.*
CV: *arrhythmias,* abnormal ECG, *MI,* angina, ***heart failure,*** thrombophlebitis, peripheral edema, ***hemorrhage.***
EENT: abnormal vision, conjunctivitis, ear pain, eye pain, *epistaxis, pharyngitis, rhinitis,* sinusitis.
GI: *abdominal pain, nausea, vomiting, anorexia, diarrhea,* constipation, flatulence, *stomatitis.*
GU: hematuria, dysuria.
Hematologic: *myelosuppression,* LEUKOPENIA, *anemia,* THROMBOCYTOPENIA, lymphadenopathy.
Metabolic: hyperuricemia, weight loss.
Musculoskeletal: chest pain, back pain, *myalgia,* arthralgia.
Respiratory: *cough, bronchitis, dyspnea,* ***pulmonary edema,*** pneumonia, *upper respiratory tract infection.*
Skin: *petechiae, rash,* eczema, dry skin, maculopapular rash, vesiculobullous rash, *pruritus, seborrhea, discoloration, diaphoresis.*
Other: *ecchymosis, fever,* INFECTION, *pain,* HYPERSENSITIVITY REACTIONS, *chills,* ***sepsis,*** herpes simplex or zoster, ***neoplasm,*** flu syndrome.

INTERACTIONS
Drug-drug. *Cytarabine, vidarabine:* Increased risk or severity of adverse effects from either drug. Avoid using together.

Fludarabine: Risk of severe or fatal pulmonary toxicity. Avoid using together.

EFFECTS ON LAB TEST RESULTS
• May increase BUN, creatinine, liver enzymes, and uric acid levels.
• May decrease hemoglobin, platelets, and granulocytes.

CONTRAINDICATIONS
Contraindicated in patients hypersensitive to drug.

NURSING CONSIDERATIONS
• Use cautiously and only under supervision of prescriber qualified in and experienced with chemotherapeutic drugs. Adverse reactions after pentostatin therapy are common.
• Avoid use in patients with renal insufficiency (creatinine clearance of 60 ml/minute or less) unless the potential benefit outweighs the risk.
• Treat all spills and waste products with 5% sodium hypochlorite (household bleach).
• Optimal duration of therapy is unknown. Current recommendations suggest two additional courses of therapy after a complete response. If a partial response isn't evident after 6 months of therapy, discontinue drug. If partial response occurs, continue drug for another 6 months.
• *Alert:* Withhold or discontinue drug and notify prescriber if there is evidence of CNS toxicity, severe rash, or active infection. Drug may be resumed when the infection clears.
• Obtain baseline neurologic and mental function before starting therapy; mental status changes may progress to neurotoxicity very rapidly.
• Therapy together with psychotropic medications may worsen signs and symptoms of neurotoxicity.
• Temporarily withhold drug and notify prescriber if absolute neutrophil count falls below 200/mm³ and pretreatment level was over 500/mm³. No recommendations exist regarding dosage adjustments in patients with anemia, neutropenia, or thrombocytopenia.
• If WBC count falls below 2,000/mm³ or granulocyte count falls below 1,000/mm³,

follow institutional policy for infection control in immunocompromised patients.
• Anticipate possible blood transfusion during treatment because of cumulative anemia. Patient may receive injections of RBC colony-stimulating factor to promote RBC production and decrease need for blood transfusions.
• Drug should be used only in patients with hairy cell leukemia refractory to alpha interferon. This is defined as disease that progresses after minimum of 3 months of treatment with alpha interferon or disease that doesn't exhibit response after 6 months of therapy.
• Monitor renal function.
• *Alert:* Don't confuse pentostatin with pentosan.

PATIENT TEACHING
• Advise patient to report any pain or burning at site of injection during or after administration.
• Advise patient to watch for signs and symptoms of infection (fever, sore throat, fatigue) and bleeding (easy bruising, nosebleeds, bleeding gums, melena), and to take temperature daily.
• Caution woman of childbearing age to avoid becoming pregnant during therapy. Recommend that she consult prescriber before becoming pregnant.

---

plicamycin (mithramycin)
Mithracin

Pregnancy risk category X

AVAILABLE FORMS
Injection: 2.5-mg vials (contains mannitol 100 mg)

INDICATIONS & DOSAGES
Dosages vary. Check treatment protocol with prescriber.
➤ **Hypercalcemia and hypercalciuria with advanced malignant disease—**
Adults: 25 mcg/kg/day I.V. over 4 to 6 hours for 3 to 4 days. Dosage repeated at weekly intervals until desired response occurs.
➤ **Testicular cancer—**
Adults: 25 to 30 mcg/kg/day I.V. for 8 to 10 days or until toxicity occurs. Don't use

more than 10 daily doses, or 30 mcg/kg individual daily doses.

I.V. ADMINISTRATION
● Follow facility policy to reduce risks. Preparation and administration of parenteral form of drug are linked to carcinogenic, mutagenic, and teratogenic risks for staff.
● To prepare solution, add 4.9 ml of sterile water for injection to vial and shake to dissolve. Then dilute for I.V. infusion in 1,000 ml of D_5W or normal saline solution. Give drug by infusion over 4 to 6 hours. Discard unused drug.
● Slow infusion reduces nausea that develops with I.V. push.
● Avoid extravasation. Plicamycin is a vesicant, and tissue necrosis may result. If I.V. solution infiltrates, stop infusion immediately, notify prescriber, and use ice packs. Restart I.V. line.
● Store lyophilized powder in refrigerator and protect from light.

ACTION
Unknown. Thought to form a complex with DNA, thus inhibiting RNA synthesis. Drug also inhibits parathyroid effects on osteoclasts and inhibits the hypercalcemic effects of vitamin D, leading to lowered calcium concentrations.

Route	Onset	Peak	Duration
I.V.	1-2 days	3 days	3-15 days

ADVERSE REACTIONS
CNS: drowsiness, weakness, lethargy, depression, headache, malaise.
CV: facial flushing.
GI: *nausea, vomiting,* anorexia, diarrhea, stomatitis.
Hematologic: *leukopenia, thrombocytopenia,* bleeding syndrome.
Hepatic: *hepatotoxicity.*
Metabolic: hypocalcemia, hypokalemia, hypophosphatemia.
Skin: rash; pain, redness, swelling at injection site; cellulitis with extravasation; phlebitis.
Other: fever.

INTERACTIONS
None significant.

EFFECTS ON LAB TEST RESULTS
● May increase BUN, creatinine, and liver enzyme levels. May decrease calcium, potassium, and phosphate levels.
● May decrease WBC and platelet counts.

CONTRAINDICATIONS
Contraindicated in women who are or may become pregnant and in patients with thrombocytopenia, bone marrow suppression, or coagulation and bleeding disorders.

NURSING CONSIDERATIONS
● Use with extreme caution in patients with significant renal or hepatic impairment.
● Obtain baseline platelet count and PT before therapy.
● To reduce nausea, give antiemetic before drug.
● Use ideal body weight to calculate dose if patient has edema or fluid retention.
● Avoid contact with skin or mucous membranes.
● Monitor platelet count and PT during therapy. Discontinue drug and notify prescriber if patient's WBC count falls below 4,000/mm³, if platelet count falls below 150,000/mm³, or if PT is prolonged more than 4 seconds longer than control.
● *Alert:* Facial flushing is an early indicator of bleeding. The first evidence of a bleeding syndrome may range from epistaxis (nosebleed) to generalized hemorrhage.
● *Alert:* Hemorrhagic diathesis is dose-related and more likely if plicamycin dose is more than 30 mcg/kg/day or the patient has received more than 10 doses. It's also more common in patients with advanced disease.
● To prevent bleeding, avoid all I.M. injections when platelet count is below 50,000/mm³.
● Anticipate need for blood transfusions to combat anemia. Patient may receive injections of RBC colony-stimulating factor to promote RBC production and decrease need for blood transfusions.
● Monitor LD, AST, ALT, alkaline phosphatase, BUN, creatinine, potassium, calcium, and phosphorus levels.
● Monitor patient for tetany, carpopedal spasm, Chvostek's sign, and muscle

---

*Liquid contains alcohol.   **May contain tartrazine.   †Canada   ‡Australia   §U.K.   ◇OTC

cramps; check calcium level. Precipitous drop in calcium level is possible. Rebound hypercalcemia after administration has also been reported.
● Patients receiving drug for treatment of testicular cancer may need calcium supplementation.

PATIENT TEACHING
● Advise patient to report any pain or burning at site of injection during or after administration.
● Advise patient to watch for signs and symptoms of infection (fever, sore throat, fatigue) and bleeding (easy bruising, nosebleeds, bleeding gums, melena), and to take temperature daily.
● Caution woman of childbearing age to avoid becoming pregnant during therapy. Recommend that she consult prescriber before becoming pregnant.

---

valrubicin
Valstar

Pregnancy risk category C

AVAILABLE FORMS
Solution for intravesical instillation: 200 mg/5 ml

INDICATIONS & DOSAGES
➤ **Intravesical therapy of bacillus Calmette-Guérin–refractory carcinoma in situ of urinary bladder in patients for whom immediate cystectomy would risk unacceptable morbidity or mortality—**
Adults: 800 mg intravesically once weekly for 6 weeks.

ACTION
An anthracycline that exerts its cytotoxic activity by penetrating into cells, where it inhibits the incorporation of nucleosides into nucleic acids, causes extensive chromosomal damage, and stops the cell cycle. Also interferes with the normal DNA breaking-resealing, thereby inhibiting DNA synthesis.

Route	Onset	Peak	Duration
Intravesical	Unknown	Unknown	Unknown

ADVERSE REACTIONS
CNS: asthenia, headache, malaise, dizziness.
CV: vasodilation, chest pain, peripheral edema.
GI: diarrhea, flatulence, nausea, vomiting, abdominal pain.
GU: urine retention, *urinary tract infection,* urinary frequency, dysuria, urinary urgency, bladder spasm, hematuria, *bladder pain, urinary incontinence,* pelvic pain, urethral pain, nocturia, *cystitis,* local burning symptoms.
Hematologic: anemia.
Metabolic: hyperglycemia.
Musculoskeletal: myalgia, back pain.
Respiratory: pneumonia.
Skin: rash.
Other: fever.

INTERACTIONS
None significant.

EFFECTS ON LAB TEST RESULTS
● May increase glucose level.
● May decrease hemoglobin.

CONTRAINDICATIONS
Contraindicated in patients hypersensitive to drug, other anthracyclines, or Cremophor EL (polyoxyethyleneglycol triricinoleate) and in those with concurrent urinary tract infections, small bladder capacity (unable to tolerate a 75-ml instillation), or perforated bladder. Also contraindicated in those in whom the integrity of the bladder mucosa has been compromised.

NURSING CONSIDERATIONS
● Use cautiously in patients with severe irritable bladder symptoms. Bladder spasm and spontaneous discharge of intravesical instillate may occur. Don't clamp the urinary catheter; if absolutely necessary, perform under medical supervision.
● For patients undergoing transurethral resection of the bladder, evaluate status of bladder before intravesical instillation of drug to avoid dangerous systemic exposure. If bladder perforation occurs, delay administration until bladder integrity has been restored.
● If there isn't a complete response of carcinoma in situ to drug treatment after 3

months, or if disorder recurs, cystectomy must be reconsidered because delaying cystectomy could lead to development of metastatic bladder cancer.

• Myelosuppression is possible if drug is inadvertently given systemically or if significant systemic exposure occurs after intravesical administration, such as in patients with bladder rupture or perforation. If drug is given when bladder rupture or perforation is suspected, monitor CBC weekly for 3 weeks. Myelosuppression begins during first week, with nadir by second week, and recovery by third week.

• Monitor patient closely for disease recurrence or progression by cystoscopy, biopsy, and urine cytology every 3 months.

• Drug should be given intravesically only under supervision of prescriber experienced in use of intravesical antineoplastics. Don't give drug I.V. or I.M.

• *Alert:* Use caution when handling and preparing solution. Wear gloves during dose preparation and administration. Prepare and store solution in glass, polypropylene, or polyolefin containers and tubing. Use polyethylene-lined administration sets. Don't use with products containing polyvinyl chloride.

• To prepare, warm four vials containing drug slowly to room temperature. Withdraw total of 20 ml from the four vials (200 mg valrubicin in each 5-ml vial), and dilute with 55 ml of normal saline solution, providing 75 ml of diluted valrubicin solution.

• Use aseptic technique during administration to avoid introducing contaminants into urinary tract or traumatizing urinary mucosa.

• To give drug, first drain bladder by inserting a urinary catheter into patient's bladder under aseptic conditions. Then, instill solution slowly by gravity flow over several minutes. Withdraw catheter. Patient should retain drug for 2 hours before voiding. (Some patients are unable to retain drug for 2 hours.)

• Use procedures for proper handling and disposal of antineoplastics.

• Refrigerate unopened vials at 36° to 46° F (2° to 8° C). Diluted valrubicin is stable for 12 hours at temperatures up to 77° F (25° C).

PATIENT TEACHING
• Inform patient that drug has been shown to induce complete response in only about one in five patients with refractory carcinoma in situ. If it doesn't respond completely after 3 months of treatment or if it recurs, tell patient to discuss with prescriber risks of cystectomy versus risks of metastatic bladder cancer.

• Advise patient to retain drug for 2 hours before voiding, if possible, and to void at end of 2 hours.

• Instruct patient to maintain adequate hydration after treatment.

• Inform patient about irritable bladder symptoms, such as bladder spasm and urinary urgency, frequency, and pain that may occur during instillation and retention of drug and for a limited period after voiding. For first 24 hours after administration, red-tinged urine is common. Tell patient to immediately report prolonged irritable bladder symptoms or prolonged passage of red urine.

• Advise women of childbearing age and their partners to avoid pregnancy during treatment. Recommend use of effective contraception during therapy.

70

Antineoplastics that alter hormone balance

anastrozole
estramustine phosphate sodium
exemestane
flutamide
goserelin acetate
letrozole
leuprolide acetate
megestrol acetate
nilutamide
tamoxifen citrate
testolactone
toremifene citrate

COMBINATION PRODUCTS
None.

---

anastrozole
Arimidex

Pregnancy risk category D

AVAILABLE FORMS
Tablets: 1 mg

INDICATIONS & DOSAGES
➤ **Advanced breast cancer in post-menopausal women with disease progression after tamoxifen therapy—**
Adults: 1 mg P.O. daily.
✷ *NEW INDICATION:* **Treatment of locally advanced or metastatic breast cancer in postmenopausal women—**
Adults: 1 mg P.O. daily until tumor progression is evident.

ACTION
A selective nonsteroidal aromatase inhibitor that significantly lowers estradiol levels, thereby inhibiting stimulation of breast cancer cell growth in postmenopausal women.

Route	Onset	Peak	Duration
P.O.	< 24 hr	Unknown	< 6 days

ADVERSE REACTIONS
CNS: *headache, asthenia,* dizziness, depression, paresthesia.

CV: chest pain, edema, thromboembolic disease, peripheral edema.
EENT: pharyngitis.
GI: *nausea,* vomiting, diarrhea, constipation, abdominal pain, anorexia, dry mouth.
GU: vaginal hemorrhage, vaginal dryness, pelvic pain.
Metabolic: weight gain.
Musculoskeletal: bone pain, *back pain.*
Respiratory: dyspnea, increased cough.
Skin: alopecia, rash, sweating.
Other: *pain, hot flashes.*

INTERACTIONS
None significant.

EFFECTS ON LAB TEST RESULTS
● May increase liver enzyme levels.

CONTRAINDICATIONS
No known contraindications.

NURSING CONSIDERATIONS
● Use cautiously in breast-feeding women.
● Pregnancy must be ruled out before treatment begins.
● Drug should be administered under supervision of a prescriber experienced in use of anticancer drugs.

PATIENT TEACHING
● Instruct patient to report adverse reactions, especially difficulty breathing or chest pain.
● Tell patient to take medication at the same time each day.
● Stress need for follow-up care.
● Counsel woman of childbearing age about risks to pregnancy during therapy.

---

estramustine phosphate sodium
Emcyt, Estracyt‡ , Estracyt§

Pregnancy risk category NR

AVAILABLE FORMS
Capsules: 140 mg

Reactions may be *common,* uncommon, *life-threatening,* or COMMON AND LIFE-THREATENING.

INDICATIONS & DOSAGES
➤ **Palliative treatment of metastatic or progressive prostate cancer—**
Adults: 10 to 16 mg/kg/day P.O. in three or four divided doses. Usual dose is 14 mg/kg daily. Continue therapy for up to 3 months and, if successful, maintain it as long as patient responds.

ACTION
Unknown. A combination of estradiol and a nornitrogen mustard. This drug's uptake into prostate cancer cells is facilitated by the estrogen component. Once intracellular, it may have weak alkylating activity.

Route	Onset	Peak	Duration
P.O.	Unknown	Unknown	Unknown

ADVERSE REACTIONS
CNS: lethargy, insomnia, headache, anxiety, *CVA.*
CV: *MI, edema,* chest pain, thrombophlebitis, *heart failure, edema,* hypertension, flushing.
GI: *nausea, vomiting,* diarrhea, anorexia, flatulence, GI bleeding, thirst.
Hematologic: *leukopenia, thrombocytopenia, thrombosis.*
Metabolic: sodium and fluid retention.
Musculoskeletal: leg cramps.
Respiratory: *pulmonary embolism,* dyspnea.
Skin: rash, pruritus, dry skin, thinning of hair.
Other: decreased libido, *breast tenderness, painful gynecomastia.*

INTERACTIONS
Drug-drug. *Calcium-containing drugs such as antacids:* Impaired absorption of estramustine. Avoid using together.
Drug-food. *Calcium-rich foods, such as dairy products:* Impaired absorption of estramustine. Tell patient to avoid using together.

EFFECTS ON LAB TEST RESULTS
• May increase AST, ALT, LDH, triglyceride, ceruloplasmin, cortisol, phospholipid, and prolactin levels. May decrease folate, pregnanediol, pyroxidine, and phosphate levels.

• May increase PT. May decrease glucose tolerance and WBC and platelet counts.

CONTRAINDICATIONS
Contraindicated in patients hypersensitive to estradiol or nitrogen mustard and in those with active thrombophlebitis or thromboembolic disorders, except when actual tumor mass is cause of thromboembolic phenomenon.

NURSING CONSIDERATIONS
• Use cautiously in patients with history of thrombophlebitis, thromboembolic disorders, or cerebrovascular or coronary artery disease. Monitor weight regularly in these patients. Drug may exaggerate peripheral edema or heart failure.
• Also use cautiously in patients with impaired liver function. Monitor liver function periodically throughout therapy.
• Each 140-mg capsule contains 12.5 mg of sodium.
• Drug may increase blood pressure and decrease glucose level. Monitor periodically throughout therapy.
• Drug is a combination of estrogen estradiol and a nitrogen mustard and may be effective in patients refractory to estrogen therapy alone.
• Patient may continue therapy as long as response is favorable. Some patients have taken drug for more than 3 years.
• Drug may increase norepinephrine-induced platelet aggregation and decrease response to the metyrapone test.
• Store capsules in refrigerator.

PATIENT TEACHING
• Tell patient to take drug on an empty stomach (1 hour before or 2 hours after meals) and to avoid taking within 2 hours of dairy products.
• Because of risk of mutagenic effects, advise patient and partner to use contraception if woman is of childbearing age.
• Instruct patient to store tablets in the refrigerator.

exemestane
Aromasin

Pregnancy risk category D

AVAILABLE FORMS
Tablets: 25 mg

INDICATIONS & DOSAGES
➤ **Advanced breast cancer in post-menopausal women whose disease has progressed after treatment with tamoxifen—**
Adults: 25 mg P.O. once daily after food.

ACTION
A highly protein-bound, irreversible, steroidal aromatase inactivator that leads to reduced levels of circulating estrogens, thereby decreasing cell growth in estrogen-dependent breast cancer.

Route	Onset	Peak	Duration
P.O.	Unknown	1.2 hr	24 hr

ADVERSE REACTIONS
CNS: *depression, insomnia, anxiety, fatigue, pain,* dizziness, headache, paresthesia, generalized weakness, asthenia, confusion, hypoesthesia.
CV: hypertension, edema, chest pain.
EENT: sinusitis, rhinitis, pharyngitis.
GI: *nausea,* vomiting, abdominal pain, anorexia, constipation, diarrhea, increased appetite, dyspepsia.
GU: urinary tract infection.
Musculoskeletal: pathologic fractures, arthritis, back pain, skeletal pain.
Respiratory: *dyspnea,* bronchitis, cough, upper respiratory tract infection.
Skin: rash, increased sweating, alopecia, itching.
Other: fever, infection, flu syndrome, lymphedema, *hot flashes.*

INTERACTIONS
Drug-drug. *Drugs that induce CYP 3A4, estrogenic agents:* May decrease exemestane plasma levels. Monitor patient closely.

EFFECTS ON LAB TEST RESULTS
None reported.

CONTRAINDICATIONS
Contraindicated in patients hypersensitive to drug or its components.

NURSING CONSIDERATIONS
• Use drug only in postmenopausal women.
• Continue treatment until tumor progression is apparent.

PATIENT TEACHING
• Direct patient to take drug after a meal.
• Tell patient that she may need to take drug for a long time.
• Advise patient to report adverse effects, especially fever or swelling of arms or legs.

flutamide
Drogenil§, Euflex†, Eulexin

Pregnancy risk category D

AVAILABLE FORMS
Capsules: 125 mg, 250 mg†

INDICATIONS & DOSAGES
➤ **Metastatic locally confined prostate cancer (stages B_2, C, D_2) with luteinizing hormone–releasing hormone analogues such as leuprolide acetate—**
Adults: 250 mg P.O. q 8 hours.

ACTION
Inhibits androgen uptake or prevents binding of androgens in nucleus of cells in target tissues.

Route	Onset	Peak	Duration
P.O.	Unknown	2 hr	Unknown

ADVERSE REACTIONS
CNS: drowsiness, confusion, depression, anxiety, nervousness, paresthesia.
CV: peripheral edema, hypertension.
GI: *diarrhea, nausea, vomiting,* anorexia.
GU: *impotence.*
Hematologic: anemia, *leukopenia, thrombocytopenia,* hemolytic anemia.
Hepatic: *hepatitis,* encephalopathy.
Skin: rash, photosensitivity reactions.
Other: *hot flashes,* loss of libido, gynecomastia.

Reactions may be *common,* uncommon, *life-threatening,* or **COMMON AND LIFE-THREATENING.**

INTERACTIONS
Drug-drug. *Warfarin:* May increase PT. Monitor PT and INR.
Drug-lifestyle. *Sun exposure:* May cause photosensitivity reactions. Advise patient to avoid excessive sunlight exposure.

EFFECTS ON LAB TEST RESULTS
• May increase BUN, creatinine, and liver enzyme levels.
• May decrease hemoglobin and WBC and platelet levels.

CONTRAINDICATIONS
Contraindicated in patients hypersensitive to drug.

NURSING CONSIDERATIONS
• Monitor liver function tests and CBC periodically.
• Flutamide must be taken continuously with drug used for medical castration (such as leuprolide) to allow full benefit of therapy. Leuprolide suppresses testosterone production, whereas flutamide inhibits testosterone action at cellular level; together, they can impair growth of androgen-responsive tumors.

PATIENT TEACHING
• Advise patient not to stop drug therapy without consulting prescriber.
• Instruct patient to report adverse reactions promptly, especially dark yellow or brown urine, vomiting, or yellowing of the eyes or skin.

---

goserelin acetate
Zoladex

Pregnancy risk category X (endometriosis and endometrial thinning); D (breast cancer)

AVAILABLE FORMS
Implants: 3.6 mg, 10.8 mg

ACTION
A luteinizing hormone–releasing hormone (LH-RH) analogue that acts on the pituitary gland to decrease the release of follicle-stimulating hormone and luteinizing hormone, resulting in dramatically lowered levels of sex hormones (estrogen in women and testosterone in men).

Route	Onset	Peak	Duration
S.C.	Rapid	0.5-1 hr	Throughout therapy

INDICATIONS & DOSAGES
➤ **Endometriosis, palliative treatment of advanced prostate cancer—**
Adults: 3.6 mg S.C. q 28 days into upper abdominal wall. For endometriosis, maximum duration of therapy is 6 months. For prostate cancer, 10.8 mg S.C. into upper abdominal wall q 12 weeks.
➤ **Palliative treatment of advanced breast cancer in premenopausal and perimenopausal women—**
Adults: 3.6 mg S.C. q 28 days into upper abdominal wall.
➤ **For endometrial thinning before endometrial ablation—**
Adults: 3.6 mg S.C. into upper abdominal wall. One or two depots are recommended, given 4 weeks apart.

ADVERSE REACTIONS
CNS: lethargy, pain, dizziness, *insomnia,* anxiety, *depression, headache,* chills, *emotional lability,* **CVA,** *asthenia.*
CV: edema, **heart failure, arrhythmias,** *peripheral edema,* hypertension, **MI,** peripheral vascular disorder, chest pain, *vasodilation.*
GI: nausea, vomiting, diarrhea, constipation, ulcer, anorexia, abdominal pain.
GU: *sexual dysfunction, impotence, lower urinary tract symptoms,* renal insufficiency, urinary obstruction, *vaginitis,* urinary tract infection, *amenorrhea.*
Hematologic: anemia.
Metabolic: hypercalcemia, hyperglycemia, weight increase.
Musculoskeletal: back pain.
Respiratory: COPD, upper respiratory tract infection.
Skin: rash, *diaphoresis, acne, seborrhea,* hirsutism.
Other: *hot flashes,* gout, breast swelling and tenderness, *changes in breast size,* breast pain, *changes in libido,* infection.

INTERACTIONS
None significant.

---

*Liquid contains alcohol.   **May contain tartrazine.   †Canada   ‡Australia   §U.K.   ◊OTC

EFFECTS ON LAB TEST RESULTS
- May increase calcium and glucose levels.
- May decrease hemoglobin.

CONTRAINDICATIONS
Contraindicated in patients hypersensitive to LH-RH, LH-RH agonist analogues, or goserelin acetate. Also contraindicated in pregnant or breast-feeding women and in patients with obstructive uropathy or vertebral metastases. The 10.8-mg implant is contraindicated in women because data are insufficient to support reliable suppression of estradiol.

NURSING CONSIDERATIONS
- Because use of drug is related to loss of bone mineral density in women, use cautiously in patients with risk factors for osteoporosis, such as family history of osteoporosis, chronic alcohol or tobacco abuse, or use of drugs, such as corticosteroids or anticonvulsants, that affect bone density.
- Before administering to women, rule out pregnancy.
- Never administer by I.V. injection.
- Administer drug into upper abdominal wall using aseptic technique. After cleaning area with an alcohol swab and injecting a local anesthetic, stretch patient's skin with one hand while grasping barrel of syringe with the other. Insert needle into the subcutaneous fat; then change direction of needle so that it parallels the abdominal wall. Push needle in until hub touches patient's skin; withdraw about 1 cm (this creates a gap for drug to be injected) before depressing plunger completely.
- To avoid need for a new syringe and injection site, don't aspirate after inserting needle. If needle penetrates a blood vessel, blood will appear in the syringe chamber. Withdraw needle, and inject elsewhere with a new syringe.
- *Alert:* Implant comes in a preloaded syringe. If package is damaged, don't use the syringe. Make sure drug is visible in the translucent chamber of the syringe.
- When used for prostate cancer, LH-RH analogues such as goserelin may initially worsen symptoms because drug initially increases testosterone levels. Some pa-

tients may experience increased bone pain. Rarely, disease exacerbation (either spinal cord compression or ureteral obstruction) has occurred.
- When drug is used for endometrial thinning, surgery should be performed at 4 weeks if one depot is administered. When two depots are given, surgery should be performed within 2 to 4 weeks after administration of second depot.

PATIENT TEACHING
- Advise patient to report every 28 days for a new implant. A delay of a couple of days is permissible.
- Tell patient that pain may worsen for first 30 days of treatment.
- Tell woman to use a nonhormonal form of contraception during treatment. Caution patient about significant risks to fetus.
- Urge woman to call prescriber if menstruation persists or if breakthrough bleeding occurs. Menstruation should stop during treatment.
- Inform woman that a delayed return of menses may occur after therapy ends. Persistent amenorrhea is rare.

---

letrozole
Femara

Pregnancy risk category D

AVAILABLE FORMS
Tablets: 2.5 mg

INDICATIONS & DOSAGES
➤ **Metastatic breast cancer in postmenopausal women with disease progression after antiestrogen therapy (such as tamoxifen)—**
Adults: 2.5 mg P.O. as single daily dose.
✱ **NEW INDICATION: First-line treatment of hormone receptor–positive or hormone receptor–unknown, locally advanced or metastatic breast cancer in postmenopausal women—**
Adults: 2.5 mg P.O. once daily until tumor progression is evident.

ACTION
A nonsteroidal competitive inhibitor of the aromatase enzyme system, which inhibits conversion of androgens to estrogens. De-

creased estrogens lead to decreased tumor mass or delayed progression of tumor growth in some women.

Route	Onset	Peak	Duration
P.O.	Unknown	2 days	Unknown

ADVERSE REACTIONS
CNS: headache, somnolence, dizziness, fatigue, mood changes.
CV: hypertension, *thromboembolism*, chest pain, edema.
GI: *nausea,* vomiting, constipation, diarrhea, abdominal pain, anorexia.
Metabolic: hypercholesterolemia, weight gain.
Musculoskeletal: *bone pain, limb pain, back pain,* arthralgia.
Respiratory: dyspnea, cough.
Skin: rash, pruritus.
Other: viral infections, hot flashes.

INTERACTIONS
None significant.

EFFECTS ON LAB TEST RESULTS
• May increase cholesterol levels.

CONTRAINDICATIONS
Contraindicated in patients hypersensitive to drug or its components.

NURSING CONSIDERATIONS
• Dosage adjustment isn't needed in renally impaired patients with creatinine clearance of 10 ml/minute or more.
• Use cautiously in patients with severe liver impairment; dosage adjustment isn't needed for mild to moderate liver dysfunction.
• Food doesn't affect drug absorption.

PATIENT TEACHING
• Instruct patient to take drug exactly as prescribed.
• Tell patient that drug can be taken with or without food.
• Inform patient about potential adverse reactions.

leuprolide acetate
Lucrin‡, Lupron, Lupron Depot, Lupron Depot-Ped, Lupron Depot-3 Month, Lupron Depot-4 Month, Lupron for Pediatric Use

Pregnancy risk category X

AVAILABLE FORMS
Depot injection: 3.75 mg, 7.5 mg, 11.25 mg, 15 mg, 22.5 mg, 30 mg
Injection: 1 mg/0.2 ml (5 mg/ml) in 2.8-ml multiple-dose vials

INDICATIONS & DOSAGES
➤ **Advanced prostate cancer—**
Adults: 1 mg S.C. daily. Or, 7.5 mg I.M. (depot injection) monthly. Or, 22.5 mg I.M. q 3 months (depot injection). Or, 30 mg I.M. q 4 months (depot injection).
➤ **Endometriosis—**
Adults: 3.75 mg I.M. (depot injection only) as single injection once monthly for up to 6 months. Or, 11.25 mg I.M. q 3 months for up to 6 months.
➤ **Central precocious puberty—**
Children: Initially, 0.3 mg/kg (minimum 7.5 mg) I.M. (depot injection only) as single injection q 4 weeks. Dosage may be increased in increments of 3.75 mg q 4 weeks, if needed. Therapy should be discontinued before girl reaches age 11 and before boy reaches age 12.
➤ **Correction of anemia related to uterine fibroids—**
Adults: 3.75 mg I.M. once monthly for up to 3 consecutive months in combination with iron therapy.

ACTION
Initially stimulates but then inhibits release of follicle-stimulating hormone and luteinizing hormone, resulting in testosterone and estrogen suppression.

Route	Onset	Peak	Duration
I.M., S.C.	< 2-4 wk	1-2 mo	60-90 days

ADVERSE REACTIONS
CNS: *dizziness, depression, headache, pain,* insomnia, paresthesia, *asthenia.*
CV: *arrhythmias,* angina, *MI, peripheral edema, ECG changes,* hypotension, hypertension, murmur.

GI: *nausea, vomiting,* anorexia, constipation.

GU: *impotence, vaginitis,* urinary frequency, hematuria, urinary tract infection, *amenorrhea.*

Hematologic: anemia.

Metabolic: *weight gain or loss.*

Musculoskeletal: transient bone pain during first week of treatment, joint disorder, myalgia, neuromuscular disorder.

Respiratory: dyspnea, sinus congestion, *pulmonary fibrosis.*

Skin: reactions at injection site, dermatitis.

Other: gynecomastia, *hot flashes,* androgen-like effects.

INTERACTIONS
None significant.

EFFECTS ON LAB TEST RESULTS
• May increase BUN, creatinine, bilirubin, alkaline phosphatase, LDH, glucose, uric acid, albumin, calcium, and phosphorus levels.
• May decrease hemoglobin.

CONTRAINDICATIONS
Contraindicated in patients hypersensitive to drug or other gonadotropin-releasing hormone analogues, in women with undiagnosed vaginal bleeding, and in pregnant or breast-feeding women. The 30-mg depot injection is contraindicated in women.

NURSING CONSIDERATIONS
• Use cautiously in patients hypersensitive to benzyl alcohol.
• Never give by I.V. injection.
• Depot injections should be given under medical supervision. Use supplied diluent to reconstitute drug (extra diluent is provided and remainder should be discarded). Draw 1 ml into a syringe with a 22G needle. (When preparing Lupron Depot-3 Month 22.5 mg, use a 23G or larger needle.) Withdraw 1.5 ml from ampule for the 3-month formulation. Inject into vial; then shake well. Suspension will appear milky. Although suspension is stable for 24 hours after reconstitution, it contains no bacteriostatic product. Use immediately.
• When using prefilled dual-chamber syringes, prepare for injection by screwing white plunger into end stopper until stop-

per begins to turn. Remove and discard tab around base of needle. Hold syringe upright and release diluent by slowly pushing plunger until first stopper is at blue line in middle of barrel. Gently shake syringe to form a uniform milky suspension. If particles adhere to stopper, tap syringe against your finger. Remove needle guard and advance plunger to expel air from syringe. Inject entire contents I.M. as with a normal injection.
• A fractional dose of drug formulated to give every 3 months isn't equivalent to same dose of once-a-month formulation.
• After the start of treatment for central precocious puberty, patient response should be monitored every 1 to 2 months with a gonadotropin-releasing hormone stimulation test and sex corticosteroid level determinations. Measurement of bone age for advancement should be performed every 6 to 12 months.
• During first few weeks of therapy, drug may increase signs and symptoms being treated (flare).

PATIENT TEACHING
• Before starting child on treatment for central precocious puberty, make sure parents understand importance of continuous therapy.
• Carefully instruct patient who will self-administer S.C. injection about proper administration techniques and advise her to use only the syringes provided by manufacturer.
• Advise patient that, if another syringe must be substituted, a low-dose insulin syringe (U-100, 0.5 ml) may be an appropriate choice but that needle gauge should be no smaller than 22G (except when using Lupron Depot-3 Month 22.5 mg).
• Instruct patient to store leuprolide acetate powder (depot) and diluent at room temperature. Unopened vials of leuprolide acetate injection should be refrigerated; vial in use may be stored at room temperature for several months. Protect leuprolide acetate injection from heat and light.
• Inform patient with history of undesirable effects from other endocrine therapies that leuprolide is easier to tolerate.
• Reassure patient that adverse effects disappear after about 1 week. Explain that

symptoms of prostate cancer or central precocious puberty may worsen initially.
• Advise woman of childbearing age to use a nonhormonal form of contraception during treatment.

megestrol acetate
Megace, Megace OS†, Megostat‡

Pregnancy risk category D

AVAILABLE FORMS
Oral suspension: 40 mg/ml
Tablets: 20 mg, 40 mg

INDICATIONS & DOSAGES
➤ **Breast cancer—**
Adults: 40 mg P.O. q.i.d.
➤ **Endometrial cancer—**
Adults: 40 to 320 mg P.O. daily in divided doses.
➤ **Anorexia, cachexia, or unexplained significant weight loss in patients with AIDS—**
Adults: 800 mg P.O. (oral suspension) daily.

ACTION
A progestin that inhibits hormone-dependent tumor growth by inhibiting pituitary and adrenal steroidogenesis. Drug may also have direct cytotoxicity.

Route	Onset	Peak	Duration
P.O.	Unknown	Unknown	Unknown

ADVERSE REACTIONS
CV: thrombophlebitis, *heart failure,* hypertension, *thromboembolism.*
GI: nausea, vomiting, diarrhea, flatulence, constipation, dry mouth, increased appetite.
GU: breakthrough menstrual bleeding, impotence, vaginal bleeding or discharge, urinary tract infection.
Metabolic: hyperglycemia, *weight gain.*
Musculoskeletal: carpal tunnel syndrome.
Respiratory: *pulmonary embolism,* dyspnea.
Skin: alopecia, rash.
Other: gynecomastia, tumor flare.

INTERACTIONS
None significant.

EFFECTS ON LAB TEST RESULTS
• May increase glucose levels.

CONTRAINDICATIONS
Contraindicated in patients hypersensitive to drug. Also contraindicated as a diagnostic test for pregnancy.

NURSING CONSIDERATIONS
• Use cautiously in patients with history of thrombophlebitis or thromboembolism.
• Glucose levels may increase in diabetic patients.
• Drug is relatively nontoxic with a low risk of adverse effects.
• In patients with cancer, 2 months is an adequate trial period.

PATIENT TEACHING
• Inform patient that therapeutic response isn't immediate.
• Advise breast-feeding woman to stop breast-feeding during therapy because of risk of toxicity to infant.
• Advise woman of childbearing age to use an effective form of contraception while receiving drug.

nilutamide
Anandron†, Nilandron

Pregnancy risk category C

AVAILABLE FORMS
Tablets: 50 mg, 100 mg†

INDICATIONS & DOSAGES
➤ **Adjunct therapy with surgical castration for treatment of metastatic prostate cancer—**
Adults: 300 mg P.O. daily for 30 days; then 150 mg P.O. daily thereafter.

ACTION
A nonsteroidal antiandrogen that interacts with the androgen receptor and prevents normal androgenic response.

Route	Onset	Peak	Duration
P.O.	Unknown	Unknown	Unknown

ADVERSE REACTIONS

CNS: dizziness.
CV: hypertension.
EENT: *impaired adaptation to darkness,* photophobia, abnormal vision.
GI: nausea, constipation, diarrhea.
GU: urinary tract infection, impotence.
Hepatic: *hepatitis.*
Respiratory: dyspnea, interstitial pneumonitis.
Other: *hot flashes, decreased libido.*

INTERACTIONS

Drug-drug. *Phenytoin, theophylline, vitamin K antagonists:* Possible delayed elimination and toxicity. Modify doses accordingly.
Drug-lifestyle. *Alcohol use:* Possible disulfiram-like reaction as evidenced by facial flushing, malaise, and hypotension. Discourage alcohol use.

EFFECTS ON LAB TEST RESULTS
• May increase AST and ALT levels.

CONTRAINDICATIONS
Contraindicated in patients hypersensitive to drug and in those with severe hepatic or respiratory disease.

NURSING CONSIDERATIONS
• Drug is used with surgical castration and should begin on same day as, or on day after, surgery for maximum benefit.
• Safety and efficacy of drug in children haven't been determined.
• Obtain baseline liver enzyme levels, and repeat at 3-month intervals. Drug should be discontinued if transaminase level exceeds three times upper limit of normal.
• Obtain a baseline chest X-ray before therapy begins. Monitor patient (especially if Asian) for signs and symptoms of interstitial pneumonitis, and notify prescriber if they occur.

PATIENT TEACHING
• Explain purpose of drug, how it's given, and importance of not stopping treatment without consulting prescriber.
• Tell patient to immediately report dyspnea or aggravation of dyspnea.
• Inform patient about risk of developing hepatitis. Tell him to report nausea, vomiting, abdominal pain, or jaundice. Tell patient to avoid alcohol during therapy.
• Warn patient that visual disturbances, such as a delay in adaptation to darkness, may affect driving at night and in tunnels.

---

tamoxifen citrate
Nolvadex, Nolvadex-D†‡, Novo-Tamoxifen†, Tamofen†, Tamonet†

Pregnancy risk category D

AVAILABLE FORMS
Tablets: 10 mg, 20 mg
Tablets (enteric-coated)†: 10 mg, 20 mg

INDICATIONS & DOSAGES
➤ **Advanced breast cancer in women and men—**
Adults: 20 mg to 40 mg P.O. daily; doses greater than 20 mg per day should be divided b.i.d.
➤ **Adjunct treatment of breast cancer in women—**
Adults: 20 mg to 40 mg P.O. daily for 5 years; doses greater than 20 mg per day should be divided b.i.d.
➤ **Reduction of breast cancer occurrence in high-risk women—**
Adults: 20 mg P.O. daily for 5 years.
✳ *NEW INDICATION:* **To reduce risk of invasive breast cancer in patients with ductal carcinoma in situ after breast surgery and radiation—**
Adults: 20 mg P.O. daily for 5 years.

ACTION
Exact neoplastic action unknown. Acts as an estrogen antagonist.

Route	Onset	Peak	Duration
P.O.	1-several mo	Unknown	Several wk

ADVERSE REACTIONS
CNS: confusion, weakness, sleepiness, headache.
CV: *fluid retention, thromboembolism.*
EENT: corneal changes, cataracts, retinopathy.
GI: *nausea, vomiting, diarrhea.*
GU: *vaginal discharge,* vaginal bleeding, *irregular menses, amenorrhea.*

Reactions may be *common*, uncommon, *life-threatening*, or COMMON AND LIFE-THREATENING.

Hematologic: *leukopenia, thrombocy-topenia.*
Hepatic: fatty liver, cholestasis, *hepatic necrosis.*
Metabolic: *hypercalcemia, weight gain or loss.*
Musculoskeletal: brief worsening of pain from osseous metastases.
Skin: *skin changes,* rash.
Other: temporary bone or tumor pain, *hot flashes.*

INTERACTIONS
Drug-drug. *Antacids:* May affect absorption of enteric-coated tablet. Don't use within 2 hours.
Bromocriptine: May elevate tamoxifen levels. Monitor patient closely.
Coumadin-type anticoagulants: May cause significant increase in anticoagulant effect. Monitor patient, PT, and INR closely.

EFFECTS ON LAB TEST RESULTS
• May increase BUN, calcium, and liver enzyme levels.
• May decrease WBC and platelet counts.

CONTRAINDICATIONS
Contraindicated in patients hypersensitive to drug. Also contraindicated as therapy to reduce risk of breast cancer in high-risk women who also need coumarin-type anticoagulant therapy or in women with history of deep vein thrombosis or pulmonary embolism.

NURSING CONSIDERATIONS
• Use cautiously in patients with leukopenia or thrombocytopenia. Monitor CBC closely.
• Monitor lipid levels during long-term therapy in patients with hyperlipidemia.
• Monitor calcium levels. At start of therapy, drug may compound hypercalcemia related to bone metastases.
• Patient should have a baseline and periodic gynecologic exams because of the small increased risk of endometrial cancer.
• Drug acts as an antiestrogen. Best results have been reported in patients with positive estrogen receptors.
• Patient may initially experience worsening symptoms (disease flare).

• Adverse reactions are usually minor and well tolerated.
• Variations on karyopyknotic index in vaginal smears and various degrees of estrogen effect on Papanicolaou smears have been seen infrequently in postmenopausal patients.

PATIENT TEACHING
• Tell patient taking enteric-coated tablets (Nolvadex-D) to swallow them whole without crushing or chewing. Tell her not to take antacids within 2 hours of dose.
• Reassure patient that acute exacerbation of bone pain during therapy usually indicates drug will produce good response. Recommend analgesics to relieve pain.
• Strongly encourage woman who is taking or has taken tamoxifen to have regular gynecologic examinations because of increased risk of uterine cancer related to therapy.
• Encourage woman to have annual mammograms and breast examinations.
• Advise patient to use barrier form of contraception because short-term therapy induces ovulation in premenopausal patients.
• Instruct patient to report vaginal bleeding or changes in menstrual cycle.
• Caution woman of childbearing age to avoid becoming pregnant during therapy and first 2 months after stopping drug. Recommend that she consult prescriber before becoming pregnant.
• Advise patient that breast cancer risk assessment tools are available and that she should discuss her concerns with her prescriber.

testolactone
Teslac

Pregnancy risk category C
Controlled substance schedule III

AVAILABLE FORMS
Tablets: 50 mg

INDICATIONS & DOSAGES
➤ **Advanced premenopausal breast cancer in women whose ovarian func-**

tion has been terminated; advanced postmenopausal breast cancer—
Adults: 250 mg P.O. q.i.d.

ACTION
Exact antineoplastic action unknown. Appears to inhibit steroid aromatase activity and decrease estrone synthesis.

Route	Onset	Peak	Duration
P.O.	6-12 wk	Unknown	Unknown

ADVERSE REACTIONS
CNS: paresthesia, peripheral neuropathy.
CV: increased blood pressure, edema.
GI: nausea, vomiting, diarrhea, anorexia, glossitis.
Skin: alopecia, erythema, nail changes.

INTERACTIONS
Drug-drug. *Oral anticoagulants:* Increased pharmacologic effects. Monitor patient, PT, and INR carefully.

EFFECTS ON LAB TEST RESULTS
None reported.

CONTRAINDICATIONS
Contraindicated in patients hypersensitive to drug and in men with breast cancer.

NURSING CONSIDERATIONS
● Monitor fluid and electrolyte levels, especially calcium level.
● Force fluids to aid calcium excretion and encourage exercise to prevent hypercalcemia. Immobilized patients are prone to hypercalcemia.
● Higher-than-recommended doses may increase risk of remission in patients with visceral metastases.
● Estradiol levels measured by radioimmunoassay may be decreased.

PATIENT TEACHING
● Inform patient that therapeutic response isn't immediate; 3 months is an adequate trial for drug.
● Tell patient to notify prescriber if numbness or tingling occurs in fingers, toes, or face.

toremifene citrate
Fareston

Pregnancy risk category D

AVAILABLE FORMS
Tablets: 60 mg

INDICATIONS & DOSAGES
➤ **Metastatic breast cancer in postmenopausal women with estrogen receptor–positive or unknown tumors—**
Adults: 60 mg P.O. as single daily dose. Treatment usually continues until disease progression is observed.

ACTION
A nonsteroidal triphenylethylene that exerts its antitumor effect by competing with estrogen for binding sites in the tumor. This blocks the growth-stimulating effects of endogenous estrogen in the tumor, causing an antiestrogenic effect.

Route	Onset	Peak	Duration
P.O.	Unknown	3 hr	Unknown

ADVERSE REACTIONS
CNS: dizziness, fatigue, depression.
CV: edema, *thromboembolism, heart failure, MI, pulmonary embolism.*
EENT: visual disturbances, glaucoma, dry eyes, *cataracts.*
GI: *nausea,* vomiting.
GU: *vaginal discharge,* vaginal bleeding.
Metabolic: hypercalcemia.
Skin: *sweating.*
Other: *hot flashes.*

INTERACTIONS
Drug-drug. *Calcium-elevating drugs such as hydrochlorothiazide:* Increased risk of hypercalcemia. Monitor calcium levels closely.
Coumadin-like anticoagulants such as warfarin: Prolonged PT and INR. Monitor PT and INR closely.
Cytochrome P-450 3A4 enzyme inducers, such as carbamazepine, phenobarbital, phenytoin: Increased rate of toremifene metabolism. Monitor patient closely.
Cytochrome P-450 3A4-6 enzyme inhibitors, such as erythromycin, ketocona-

zole: Decreased toremifene metabolism. Clinical relevance is uncertain.

EFFECTS ON LAB TEST RESULTS
● May increase calcium and liver enzyme levels.

CONTRAINDICATIONS
Contraindicated in patients hypersensitive to drug. Also contraindicated in patients with a history of thromboembolic disease.

NURSING CONSIDERATIONS
● Obtain periodic CBC, calcium levels, and liver function tests.
● Monitor calcium levels closely during first weeks of treatment in patients with bone metastases because of increased risk of hypercalcemia.

PATIENT TEACHING
● Instruct patient to take drug exactly as prescribed.
● Advise patient that doses may be taken without regard to meals.
● Warn patient not to stop therapy without consulting prescriber.
● Inform patient about vaginal bleeding and other adverse effects; tell her to notify prescriber if bleeding occurs.
● Warn patient that disease flare-up may occur during first weeks of therapy. Reassure her that this doesn't indicate treatment failure.
● Advise patient to report leg or chest pain, severe headache, visual changes, or dyspnea.

alemtuzumab
arsenic trioxide
asparaginase
bacillus Calmette-Guérin (BCG),
  live intravesical
bexarotene
dacarbazine
docetaxel
etoposide
etoposide phosphate
gemcitabine hydrochloride
gemtuzumab ozogamicin
irinotecan hydrochloride
mitotane
mitoxantrone hydrochloride
paclitaxel
pegaspargase
porfimer sodium
procarbazine hydrochloride
rituximab
teniposide
topotecan hydrochloride
trastuzumab
tretinoin
vinblastine sulfate
vincristine sulfate
vinorelbine tartrate

COMBINATION PRODUCTS
None.

✳ *NEW DRUG*

alemtuzumab
Campath

Pregnancy risk category C

AVAILABLE FORMS
Ampules: 10 mg/ml, 3-ml ampules

INDICATIONS & DOSAGES
➤ **B-cell chronic lymphocytic leukemia**
in patients treated with alkylating
drugs, in whom fludarabine therapy has
failed—
Adults: Initially, 3 mg I.V. infusion over 2
hours daily; if tolerated (infusion-related
toxicities are grade 2 or less), increase

dose to 10 mg daily and continue, as tolerated; then increase to 30 mg daily. As
maintenance, give 30 mg I.V. three times
weekly on nonconsecutive days (such as
Monday, Wednesday, Friday) for up to 12
weeks. Don't give single doses of more
than 30 mg or weekly doses of more than
90 mg.
Adjust-a-dose: For patients with hematologic toxicity, see table.

Hematologic toxicity	Dose modification and reinitiation
First occurrence of absolute neutrophil count (ANC) ≤ 250/mm³ or platelets ≤ 25,000/mm³	Withhold therapy; resume at same dose when ANC ≥ 500/mm³ or platelets ≥ 50,000/mm³. If delay between doses is ≥ 7 days, start therapy at 3 mg; escalate to 10 mg, then 30 mg as tolerated.
Second occurrence of ANC ≤ 250/mm³ or platelets ≤ 25,000/mm³	Withhold therapy; when ANC ≥ 500/mm³ or platelets ≥ 50,000/mm³, resume at 10 mg. If delay between doses is ≥ 7 days, start therapy at 3 mg; escalate to 10 mg only.
Third occurrence of ANC ≤ 250/mm³ or platelets ≤ 25,000/mm³	Discontinue therapy.
For a decrease of ANC or platelet count ≤ 50% of the baseline value in patients starting therapy with ANC ≤ 500/mm³ or platelet count ≤ 25,000/mm³	Withhold therapy; when ANC or platelet count returns to baseline, resume therapy. If delay between dosing is ≥ 7 days, start therapy at 3 mg and escalate to 10 mg, then 30 mg as tolerated.

I.V. ADMINISTRATION
● Don't give as I.V. push or bolus.
● Premedicate with diphenhydramine
50 mg and acetaminophen 650 mg 30 minutes before infusion; give hydrocortisone
200 mg to decrease severe infusion-related
events. Give anti-infective prophylaxis
while patient is on therapy. TMP-sulfa DS
b.i.d. three times a week and famciclovir

(or equivalent) 250 mg b.i.d. have been used at beginning of alemtuzumab therapy. Continue for 2 months, or until CD4+ count is 200 cells/mm³ or more, whichever occurs later.

• Don't shake ampule before use. Withdraw the necessary amount of drug from the ampule and filter with a sterile, low-protein binding, 5-micron filter before dilution. Add to 100 ml normal saline or D₅W. Gently invert bag to mix solution. Infuse over 2 hours.

• Discard any unused portion of drug. Solutions may be stored at room temperature or refrigerated; protect solution from light. Diluted solutions must be used within 8 hours of preparation.

ACTION

Proposed mechanism of action is antibody-dependent lysis of leukemic cells following cell-surface binding.

Route	Onset	Peak	Duration
I.V.	Unknown	Unknown	Unknown

ADVERSE REACTIONS

CNS: *insomnia,* depression, somnolence, *asthenia, headache, dysthenias, dizziness, fatigue,* malaise, tremor.
CV: *edema, peripheral edema, chest pain, hypotension, hypertension, tachycardia, supraventricular tachycardia.*
EENT: epistaxis, rhinitis, *pharyngitis.*
GI: *anorexia, nausea, vomiting, diarrhea, stomatitis, ulcerative stomatitis, mucositis, abdominal pain, dyspepsia,* constipation.
Hematologic: NEUTROPENIA, *anemia,* **pancytopenia,** THROMBOCYTOPENIA, **purpura.**
Musculoskeletal: *pain, skeletal pain, back pain, myalgias.*
Respiratory: *dyspnea, cough, bronchitis, pneumonitis,* **bronchospasm.**
Skin: *rash, urticaria, pruritus, increased sweating.*
Other: INFECTION, SEPSIS, *herpes simplex, rigors, fever,* temperature change sensation, candidiasis.

INTERACTIONS

None reported.

EFFECTS ON LAB TEST RESULTS

• May decrease hemoglobin, hematocrit, and WBC, RBC, CD4+, platelet, neutrophil, and lymphocyte counts.

CONTRAINDICATIONS

Contraindicated in patients with active systemic infections, underlying immunodeficiency (such as HIV), or known type I hypersensitivity or anaphylactic reactions to alemtuzumab or its components.

NURSING CONSIDERATIONS

• Initiate drug at low dose; escalate as tolerated.

• Monitor blood pressure and hypotensive symptoms during administration.

• Irradiate blood if transfusions are necessary to protect against graft vs. host disease. Monitor hematologic studies carefully.

• Don't exceed recommended doses.

• Don't give drug if patient has systemic infection at scheduled dose time.

• Don't immunize with live viral vaccines.

• Obtain CBC and platelet counts weekly during therapy and more frequently if worsening anemia, neutropenia, or thrombocytopenia occurs.

• Obtain CD4+ counts after treatment until CD4+ count is 200 cells/mm³or higher.

• If therapy is interrupted for 7 days or longer, restart with gradual dose escalation.

PATIENT TEACHING

• Tell patient to report immediately any infusion reactions, such as rigors, chills, fever, nausea, or vomiting.

• Advise patient that blood tests will be done during therapy to monitor for adverse effects.

• Advise patient to report immediately any signs or symptoms of infection.

• Safety and efficacy in children are unknown.

• It's unknown whether drug is excreted in breast milk. Advise patient to stop breast-feeding during treatment and for at least 3 months after taking last dose of drug.

---

*Liquid contains alcohol.   **May contain tartrazine.   †Canada   ‡Australia   §U.K.   ◊OTC

✳ *NEW DRUG*

arsenic trioxide
Trisenox

Pregnancy risk category D

AVAILABLE FORMS
Injection: 1 mg/ml

INDICATIONS & DOSAGES
➤ **Acute promyelocytic leukemia (APL) in patients who have relapsed or who are refractory to retinoid and anthracycline chemotherapy—**
Adults and children age 5 and older: For induction phase, 0.15 mg/kg I.V. daily until bone marrow remission. Maximum 60 doses. For consolidation phase, 0.15 mg/kg I.V. daily for 25 doses over a period up to 5 weeks, beginning 3 to 6 weeks after completion of induction therapy.

I.V. ADMINISTRATION
● Follow facility policy regarding preparation and handling of antineoplastic drugs. The active ingredient is a human carcinogen.
● Dilute with 100 to 250 ml of D_5W or normal saline solution. After dilution, drug is stable for 24 hours at room temperature and for 48 hours if refrigerated.
● Administer I.V. over 1 to 2 hours. Infusion time may be extended up to 4 hours if vasomotor reactions occur.
● Discard any remaining drug in the ampule. Don't mix arsenic trioxide with any other medications.

ACTION
Causes morphological changes and DNA fragmentation, resulting in death of promyelocytic leukemic cells.

Route	Onset	Peak	Duration
I.V.	Unknown	Unknown	Unknown

ADVERSE REACTIONS
CNS: *headache, insomnia, paresthesia, dizziness,* tremor, **seizures,** somnolence, **coma,** anxiety, depression, agitation, confusion, *fatigue, weakness.*
CV: tachycardia, PROLONGED QT INTERVAL, *palpitations, edema, chest pain,* ECG abnormalities, *hypotension, flushing, hypertension.*
EENT: *eye irritation, epistaxis, blurred vision,* dry eye, earache, tinnitus, *sore throat, post nasal drip,* eyelid edema, *sinusitis,* nasopharyngitis, painful red eye.
GI: *nausea, vomiting, diarrhea, anorexia, abdominal pain, constipation, loose stools, dyspepsia,* oral blistering, fecal incontinence, **GI hemorrhage,** dry mouth, abdominal tenderness or distention, bloody diarrhea, oral candidiasis.
GU: *renal failure,* renal impairment, oliguria, incontinence, **vaginal hemorrhage,** intermenstrual bleeding.
Hematologic: leukocytosis, anemia, THROMBOCYTOPENIA, NEUTROPENIA, **disseminated intravascular coagulation, hemorrhage,** lymphadenopathy.
Metabolic: *hypokalemia, hypomagnesemia, hyperglycemia, hypocalcemia,* hypoglycemia, acidosis, *weight gain,* weight loss, **hyperkalemia.**
Musculoskeletal: *arthralgia, myalgia, bone pain, back pain, neck pain, limb pain.*
Respiratory: *cough, dyspnea, hypoxia, pleural effusion, wheezing, decreased breath sounds, crepitations, rales,* hemoptysis, tachypnea, rhonchi, *upper respiratory tract infection.*
Skin: *dermatitis, pruritus, ecchymosis, dry skin, erythema, increased sweating,* night sweats, petechiae, hyperpigmentation, urticaria, skin lesions, local exfoliation, *pallor.*
Other: *fever,* **drug hypersensitivity,** *rigors,* lymphadenopathy, facial edema, *herpes simplex infection,* bacterial infection, herpes zoster, **sepsis,** pain, erythema, or edema at injection site.

INTERACTIONS
Drug-drug. *Drugs that can lead to electrolyte abnormalities (diuretics or amphotericin B):* Increases risk of electrolyte abnormalities. Use together cautiously.
Drugs that can prolong the QT interval (antiarrhythmics or thioridazine): May further prolong QT interval. Use together cautiously.

EFFECTS ON LAB TEST RESULTS
● May increase ALT, AST, magnesium, and calcium levels. May increase or decrease glucose and potassium levels.

• May decrease hemoglobin and neutrophil and platelet counts. May increase WBC counts.

CONTRAINDICATIONS
Contraindicated in patients hypersensitive to arsenic.

NURSING CONSIDERATIONS
• Use cautiously in patients with heart failure, renal failure, prolonged QT interval, conditions that result in hypokalemia or hypomagnesemia, or a history of torsades de pointes.
• Before starting drug, perform ECG; obtain potassium, calcium, magnesium, and creatinine levels; and correct electrolyte abnormalities.
• *Alert:* Arsenic trioxide can cause fatal arrhythmias and complete AV block.
• *Alert:* Arsenic trioxide has been linked to APL differentiation syndrome, characterized by fever, dyspnea, weight gain, pulmonary infiltrates, and pleural or pericardial effusions, with or without leukocytosis. This syndrome can be fatal and requires treatment with high-dose steroids
• Monitor electrolytes and hematologic and coagulation profiles at least twice weekly during treatment. Keep potassium levels above 4 mEq/dl and magnesium levels above 1.8 mg/dl.
• Monitor patient for syncope and rapid or irregular heart rate. If these occur, discontinue drug, hospitalize patient, and monitor electrolytes and QTc interval. Drug may be restarted when electrolyte abnormalities are corrected and QTc interval falls below 460 msec.
• Monitor ECG at least weekly during therapy. Prolonged QTc interval commonly occurs between 1 and 5 weeks after infusion, and returns to baseline about 8 weeks after infusion. If QTc interval is higher than 500 msec at any time during therapy, assess patient closely and consider stopping drug.
• Caution woman of childbearing age to avoid becoming pregnant during therapy or to consult prescriber before becoming pregnant.
• Instruct patient to notify prescriber of all medications he is currently taking and to check with prescriber before starting any new medication.

• Arsenic appears in breast milk. Because of the potential for serious adverse reactions in nursing infants, patient should stop breast-feeding during therapy.

PATIENT TEACHING
• Tell patient to report fever, shortness of breath, or weight gain immediately.
• Instruct patient to tell prescriber about all drugs currently being taken and to check with prescriber before staring any new drug.
• Inform diabetic patient that drug may cause hyperglycemia or hypoglycemia, and instruct him to monitor glucose level closely.

asparaginase
Elspar, Kidrolase†

Pregnancy risk category C

AVAILABLE FORMS
Injection: 10,000-IU vial

INDICATIONS & DOSAGES
➤ **Acute lymphocytic leukemia (ALL) (with other drugs)—**
Adults and children: 1,000 IU/kg I.V. daily for 10 days, injected over 30 minutes. Or, 6,000 IU/m² I.M. at intervals specified in protocol.
➤ **Sole induction drug for acute lymphocytic leukemia—**
Adults and children: 200 IU/kg I.V. daily for 28 days.

I.V. ADMINISTRATION
• Follow facility policy to reduce risks. Preparation and administration of parenteral form of drug are linked to carcinogenic, mutagenic, and teratogenic risks for staff.
• Reconstitute drug with 5 ml of either sterile water for injection or saline solution for injection.
• Don't shake vial vigorously because foaming may occur.
• Give I.V. injection over 30 minutes through a running infusion of normal saline solution or D₅W solution.
• Refrigerate unopened dry powder. Reconstituted solution is stable for 8 hours if refrigerated. Use only clear solutions.

ACTION
Destroys the essential amino acid asparagine, which is needed for protein synthesis in acute lymphocytic leukemia, leading to death of the leukemic cell.

Route	Onset	Peak	Duration
I.M.	Unknown	14-24 hr	23-33 days
I.V.	Immediate	Immediate	23-33 days

ADVERSE REACTIONS
CNS: confusion, drowsiness, depression, hallucinations, fatigue, agitation, headache, lethargy, somnolence.
GI: *vomiting, anorexia, nausea,* cramps, stomatitis, **HEMORRHAGIC PANCREATITIS.**
GU: azotemia, *renal failure,* glycosuria, polyuria, uric acid nephropathy.
Hematologic: *anemia, hypofibrinogenemia,* depression of clotting factor synthesis, *leukopenia.*
Hepatic: *hepatotoxicity.*
Metabolic: weight loss, *hyperglycemia,* hyperuricemia, hyperammonemia, hypocalcemia.
Skin: *rash, urticaria.*
Other: ANAPHYLAXIS, chills, fever, hypersensitivity reactions.

INTERACTIONS
Drug-drug. *Methotrexate:* Decreased methotrexate effectiveness. Avoid using together or administer asparaginase after methotrexate.
Prednisone: Hyperglycemia. Monitor glucose levels.
Vincristine: Increased neuropathy. Monitor patient closely; give asparaginase after vincristine.

EFFECTS ON LAB TEST RESULTS
● May increase BUN, AST, ALT, glucose, uric acid, and ammonia levels. May decrease calcium levels.
● May decrease hemoglobin, thyroid function test values, and WBC count.

CONTRAINDICATIONS
Contraindicated in patients hypersensitive to drug (unless desensitized) and in those with pancreatitis or history of pancreatitis.

NURSING CONSIDERATIONS
● Use cautiously in patients with hepatic dysfunction. Drug should initially be given in hospital setting with close supervision.
● Monitor blood and urine glucose levels before and during therapy. Watch for signs and symptoms of hyperglycemia.
● Allopurinol should be started before therapy begins to help prevent uric acid nephropathy.
● *Alert:* Risk of hypersensitivity increases with repeated doses. An intradermal skin test should be performed before initial dose and when drug is given after an interval of 1 week or more between doses. Give 2 IU asparaginase as I.D. injection. Observe site for at least 1 hour for erythema or a wheal, which indicates a positive response. Patient with negative skin test may still develop allergic reaction to drug. Desensitization may be needed before first treatment dose is given and with retreatment. One IU of drug may be ordered I.V. Dose is then doubled every 10 minutes, provided no reaction has occurred, until total amount given equals patient's total dose for that day.
● Drug shouldn't be used alone to induce remission unless combination therapy is inappropriate. Drug isn't recommended for maintenance therapy.
● For I.M. injection, reconstitute with 2 ml normal saline solution to the 10,000-IU vial. Refrigerate and use within 8 hours.
● Don't give more than 2 ml at one injection site.
● Don't use cloudy solutions.
● If drug contacts skin or mucous membranes, wash with a generous amount of water for at least 15 minutes.
● Keep epinephrine, diphenhydramine, and I.V. corticosteroids available for treating anaphylaxis.
● Monitor CBC and bone marrow function tests.
● Obtain amylase levels to check pancreatic status. If levels are elevated, discontinue asparaginase.
● Help prevent occurrence of tumor lysis (which can result in uric acid nephropathy) by increasing fluid intake.
● Drug may affect clotting factor synthesis and cause hypofibrinogenemia, leading to thrombosis or, more commonly, severe bleeding. Monitor patient and bleeding studies closely.

Reactions may be *common,* uncommon, *life-threatening,* or **COMMON AND LIFE-THREATENING.**

• Because of vomiting, administer fluids parenterally for 24 hours or until oral fluids are tolerated.

• Some patients may become hypersensitive to asparaginase derived from cultures of *Escherichia coli. Erwinia asparaginase,* derived from cultures of *Erwinia carotovora,* has been used in these patients without cross-sensitivity.

• Drug toxicity is more likely in adults than in children.

• There are several protocols for use of this drug.

PATIENT TEACHING

• Tell patient to watch for signs of infection (fever, sore throat, fatigue) and bleeding (easy bruising, nosebleeds, bleeding gums, melena). Tell patient to take temperature daily.

• Stress importance of maintaining adequate fluid intake to help prevent hyperuricemia. If adverse GI reactions prevent patient from drinking fluids, tell patient to notify prescriber.

• Urge patient to immediately report severe headache, stomach pain with nausea or vomiting, or inability to move a limb.

• Advise patient to report signs of a hypersensitivity reaction, including rash, pruritus, chills, dizziness, chest tightness, or difficulty breathing.

---

bacillus Calmette-Guérin (BCG), live intravesical
PACIS, TheraCys, TICE BCG

Pregnancy risk category C

AVAILABLE FORMS
PACIS
Injection: 120 mg/ampule
TheraCys
Suspension (freeze-dried) for bladder instillation: 81 mg/vial
TICE BCG
Suspension (freeze-dried) for bladder instillation: About 50 mg/ampule

INDICATIONS & DOSAGES
➤ **In situ carcinoma of the urinary bladder (primary and relapsed)—**
Adults: One reconstituted and diluted vial, 81 mg, given intravesically once weekly

for 6 weeks (induction); then additional treatments at 3, 6, 12, 18, and 24 months (TheraCys). Or, one bladder instillation (one ampule suspended in 50 ml of sterile, preservative-free saline solution) once weekly for 6 weeks; then once monthly for 6 to 12 months (TICE BCG). Or, instill 120 mg or 1 ampule intravesically into the bladder slowly by gravity flow, by catheter once weekly for 6 weeks. Schedule may be repeated if tumor remission isn't achieved and if clinical circumstances warrant (PACIS).

ACTION
Unknown. Instillation of the live bacterial suspension causes a local inflammatory response. Local infiltration of histiocytes and leukocytes is followed by a decrease in superficial tumors in the bladder.

Route	Onset	Peak	Duration
Intravesical	Unknown	Unknown	Unknown

ADVERSE REACTIONS
CNS: *malaise.*
GI: nausea, vomiting, anorexia, diarrhea, abdominal pain.
GU: *bladder irritability, dysuria, urinary frequency, hematuria, cystitis, urinary urgency, nocturia,* urinary incontinence, urinary tract infection, urine retention, local pain.
Musculoskeletal: arthralgia, myalgia.
Other: hypersensitivity reactions, *fever,* chills, *flu syndrome.*

INTERACTIONS
Drug-drug. *Antitubercular agents:* May attenuate response to BCG intravesical. Avoid using together.
Bone marrow suppressants, immunosuppressants, radiation therapy: May impair response to BCG intravesical by decreasing the immune response; may also increase the risk of osteomyelitis or disseminated BCG infection. Avoid using together.

EFFECTS ON LAB TEST RESULTS
None reported.

CONTRAINDICATIONS
Contraindicated in immunocompromised patients, in those receiving immunosuppressive therapy, in asymptomatic carriers

---

*Liquid contains alcohol.   **May contain tartrazine.   †Canada   ‡Australia   §U.K.   ◇OTC

with a positive HIV serology, and in those with urinary tract infection, gross hematuria, or fever of unknown origin.

NURSING CONSIDERATIONS

• Determine patient's reactivity to tuberculin before therapy. Tuberculin sensitivity may be rendered positive by BCG intravesical treatment.

• Drug shouldn't be handled by caregiver with immune deficiency.

• BCG intravesical shouldn't be administered within 7 to 14 days of transurethral resection or biopsy. Fatal disseminated BCG infection has occurred after traumatic catheterization.

• Prepare product using sterile technique in a biocontainment hood. If preparation can't be performed in a biocontainment hood, person responsible for mixing the product should wear gloves, mask, and gown to avoid inhaling BCG organisms or contacting broken skin.

• To avoid cross-contamination, parenteral drugs shouldn't be prepared in areas where BCG has been in use.

• To prepare PACIS, add 1 ml of sterile diluent (preservative-free normal saline solution for injection) to 1 ampule of BCG to resuspend. Leave drug and diluent in contact for 1 minute. Then mix suspension by withdrawing it into syringe and expelling it gently back into ampule two or three times. Avoid creating foam; don't shake. Dilute the reconstituted product in another 49 ml of saline solution diluent, bringing the total volume to 50 ml.

• Use suspension immediately after preparation. Discard any prepared suspension after 2 hours.

• To give TheraCys, reconstitute only with 3 ml of provided diluent per vial just before use. Don't remove rubber stopper to prepare solution. Use immediately. Add contents of 3 reconstituted vials to 50 ml of sterile, preservative-free saline solution (final volume, 53 ml). Insert a urethral catheter into bladder under aseptic conditions, drain bladder, and infuse 53 ml of prepared solution by gravity feed. Remove catheter and properly dispose of unused drug.

• To give TICE BCG, use thermosetting plastic or sterile glass containers and syringes. Draw 1 ml of sterile, preservative-

free saline solution into a 3-ml syringe. Add to 1 ampule of drug; gently expel back into ampule three times to ensure thorough mixing. Use immediately. Dispense cloudy suspension into top end of a catheter-tipped syringe that contains 49 ml of saline solution. Gently rotate syringe. Properly dispose of unused drug.

• Don't use reconstituted product if it has clumps that can't be dispersed with gentle shaking.

• Protect drug from exposure to direct or indirect sunlight.

• Handle drug and material used for instillation as infectious material because it contains live, attenuated mycobacteria. Dispose of equipment (syringes, catheters, and containers) as biohazardous waste.

• Use strict aseptic technique to administer drug to minimize trauma to GU tract and to prevent introduction of other contaminants.

• If there's evidence of traumatic catheterization, don't administer drug; notify prescriber. Subsequent treatment may resume after 1 week as if no interruption occurred.

• Carefully monitor patient's urinary status because drug causes an inflammatory response in the bladder.

• Closely monitor patient for evidence of systemic BCG infection. BCG infections are rarely detected by positive cultures. Withhold therapy if systemic infection is suspected (short-term high temperature over 103° F [39° C] or persistent temperature over 101° F [38° C] for longer than 2 days or with severe malaise). Contact an infectious disease specialist for initiation of fast-acting antituberculosis therapy.

• If fever is caused by infection, drug should be withheld until patient recovers.

• Drug isn't used as an immunizing product to prevent cancer or tuberculosis.

• Drug may cause hypersensitivity. Manage symptomatically.

• Patients with a small bladder capacity may experience increased local irritation with usual dose of BCG intravesical.

• Treat bladder irritation symptomatically with phenazopyridine, acetaminophen, and propantheline. Systemic hypersensitivity can be treated with diphenhydramine. To minimize risk of systemic infection, some prescribers give isoniazid for 3 days starting on first day of treatment.

Reactions may be *common*, uncommon, *life-threatening*, or COMMON AND LIFE-THREATENING.

• *Alert:* Don't confuse BCG intravesical with BCG vaccine.

PATIENT TEACHING

• Tell patient to retain drug in bladder for 2 hours after instillation, if possible. For first hour, have patient lie 15 minutes prone, 15 minutes supine, and 15 minutes on each side; patient may spend second hour in sitting position.

• Advise patient to sit when voiding.

• Instruct patient to disinfect urine for 6 hours after instillation of drug. Tell him to pour undiluted household bleach (5% sodium hypochlorite solution) in equal volume to voided urine into the toilet and wait 15 minutes before flushing.

• Tell patient to notify prescriber if symptoms worsen or if the following symptoms develop: blood in urine, fever and chills, frequent urge to urinate, painful urination, nausea, vomiting, joint pain, or rash.

• *Alert:* Warn patient that a cough that develops after therapy could indicate a life-threatening BCG infection. Tell him to report it immediately.

• Caution woman of childbearing age to avoid becoming pregnant or breast-feeding during therapy.

---

bexarotene
Targretin

Pregnancy risk category X

AVAILABLE FORMS
Capsules: 75 mg
Topical gel: 1%

INDICATIONS & DOSAGES
➤ **Cutaneous T-cell lymphoma in patients refractory to at least one previous systemic therapy—**
Adults: 300 mg/m²/day P.O. as a single dose with a meal. If no response after 8 weeks, increase to 400 mg/m²/day if initial dose was tolerated.
Adjust-a-dose: Patients with hepatic insufficiency may need lower doses. If toxicity occurs, adjust dose to 200 mg/m²/day and then to 100 mg/m²/day; or temporarily suspend drug. When toxicity is controlled, doses may be carefully readjusted upward.

➤ **Refractory cutaneous lesions in patients with cutaneous T-cell lymphoma (stage IA and IB)—**
Adults: Initially, apply generously to affected areas every other day for first week; increase at weekly intervals to once daily, then b.i.d., then t.i.d., and finally q.i.d.

ACTION
The exact mechanism of action in the treatment of cutaneous T-cell lymphoma is unknown. Bexarotene selectively binds and activates retinoid X receptor (RXR) subtypes. Once activated, these receptors function as transcription factors that regulate the expression of genes that control cellular differentiation and proliferation. Bexarotene inhibits the in vitro growth of some tumor cell lines of hematopoietic and squamous cell origin, and it induces in vivo tumor cell regression in some animal models.

Route	Onset	Peak	Duration
P.O., topical	Unknown	Unknown	Unknown

ADVERSE REACTIONS
CNS: *headache,* insomnia, *asthenia,* fatigue, syncope, depression, agitation, ataxia, *CVA,* confusion, dizziness, hyperesthesia, hypoesthesia, neuropathy.
CV: *peripheral edema,* chest pain, hypertension, angina, **heart failure,** tachycardia.
EENT: cataracts, pharyngitis, rhinitis, dry eyes, conjunctivitis, ear pain, blepharitis, corneal lesion, keratitis, otitis externa, visual field defect.
GI: *nausea,* diarrhea, vomiting, anorexia, **pancreatitis,** *abdominal pain,* constipation, dry mouth, flatulence, colitis, dyspepsia, cheilitis, gastroenteritis, gingivitis, melena.
GU: albuminuria, hematuria, incontinence, urinary tract infection, urinary urgency, dysuria, abnormal kidney function.
Hematologic: *leukopenia,* anemia, eosinophilia, **hemorrhage,** thrombocythemia, lymphocytosis, **thrombocytopenia.**
Hepatic: bilirubinemia, **liver failure.**
Metabolic: *hyperlipemia, hypercholesterolemia, hypothyroidism,* hyperglycemia, hypoproteinemia, hypocalcemia, hyponatremia, weight change.

Musculoskeletal: arthralgia, myalgia, back pain, bone pain, myasthenia, arthrosis.

Respiratory: pneumonia, dyspnea, hemoptysis, pleural effusion, bronchitis, cough, *pulmonary edema,* hypoxia.

Skin: *rash, dry skin,* exfoliative dermatitis, *alopecia, photosensitivity reaction,* pruritus, cellulitis, acne, skin ulcer, skin nodule; *contact dermatitis and skin disorder* (topical).

Other: *infection,* chills, fever, flu syndrome, breast pain, *sepsis.*

INTERACTIONS

Drug-drug. *Erythromycin, gemfibrozil, itraconazole, ketoconazole, other inhibitors of cytochrome P-450 3A4:* Increased plasma bexarotene levels. Avoid using together.

Insulin, sulfonylureas: May enhance hypoglycemic action of these drugs, resulting in hypoglycemia in patients with diabetes mellitus. Use together cautiously.

Phenobarbital, phenytoin, rifampin, other inducers of cytochrome P-450 3A4: Decreased plasma bexarotene levels. Avoid using together.

Products containing DEET: Increased DEET toxicity with topical gel preparation. Avoid using together.

Vitamin A preparations: Increased risk of vitamin A toxicity. Avoid vitamin A supplements.

Drug-food. *Any food:* Increased bexarotene absorption. Give drug with food.

Grapefruit juice: May inhibit cytochrome P-450 3A4. Tell patient to avoid grapefruit juice during therapy.

Drug-lifestyle. *Sun exposure:* May cause photosensitivity reaction. Advise patient to avoid excessive sunlight exposure.

EFFECTS ON LAB TEST RESULTS

• May increase creatinine, LDH, AST, ALT, bilirubin, amylase lipid, cholesterol, and glucose levels. May decrease protein, calcium, and sodium levels.

• May increase eosinophil count. May decrease hemoglobin and WBC and lymphocyte counts. May increase or decrease platelet count.

CONTRAINDICATIONS

Contraindicated in patients hypersensitive to drug or its components and in pregnant women. Drug isn't recommended for patients with risk factors for pancreatitis, such as previous pancreatitis, uncontrolled hyperlipidemia, excessive alcohol consumption, uncontrolled diabetes mellitus, or biliary tract disease. Also not recommended for patients taking drugs that increase triglyceride levels or have pancreatic toxicity.

NURSING CONSIDERATIONS

• Use cautiously in women of childbearing age, patients with hepatic insufficiency, and patients hypersensitive to retinoids.

• *Alert:* Woman of childbearing age should use effective contraception for at least 1 month before start of therapy, during therapy, and for at least 1 month after therapy ends. During therapy, she should use two reliable forms of contraception unless abstinence is the chosen method. A negative pregnancy test should be obtained within 1 week before starting therapy and monthly during therapy.

• Start therapy on the second or third day of a normal menstrual period.

• Men who are receiving therapy must wear condoms during sexual intercourse throughout and for at least 1 month after therapy if their sexual partners are pregnant or could become pregnant.

• No more than a 1-month supply of bexarotene should be given to a woman of childbearing potential, so the results of pregnancy testing can be assessed regularly and so the patient can be reminded of the danger of birth defects if she becomes pregnant during therapy.

• Obtain total cholesterol, HDL cholesterol, and triglyceride levels at start of drug therapy, weekly until lipid response is established (2 to 4 weeks), and at 8-week intervals thereafter. Elevated triglyceride levels during therapy should be treated with antilipemic therapy and, if necessary, the dose of bexarotene reduced or suspended.

• Obtain baseline thyroid function tests, and monitor them during treatment.

• Monitor WBC with differential at baseline and periodically during treatment.

● Monitor liver function test results at baseline and after 1, 2, and 4 weeks of treatment. If stable, monitor them every 8 weeks during treatment. Consider suspending treatment if results are three times the upper limit of normal.

● Obtain ophthalmologic evaluation for cataracts if patient has visual difficulties.

● Bexarotene therapy may increase CA 125 assay values in patients with ovarian cancer.

For topical gel:

● A response may be seen within 4 weeks; most patients require longer treatment.

PATIENT TEACHING

● Advise patient to minimize exposure to sunlight and artificial ultraviolet light and to take appropriate precautions.

● Teach patient that it may take several capsules to make the necessary dose and that these capsules should be taken at the same time and with a meal.

● Teach women of childbearing potential the dangers of becoming pregnant while taking bexarotene and the need for monthly pregnancy tests.

● Explain the need for obtaining baseline laboratory tests and for periodic monitoring of these tests.

● Tell patient to report any visual changes.

For topical gel:

● Instruct patient to allow gel to dry before putting clothes on.

● Instruct patient to avoid the use of occlusive dressings.

● Tell patient not to apply drug to unaffected areas or mucosal areas.

---

dacarbazine (DTIC)
DTIC†, DTIC-Dome

Pregnancy risk category C

AVAILABLE FORMS
Injection: 100-mg, 200-mg vials

INDICATIONS & DOSAGES
➤ **Metastatic malignant melanoma—**
Adults: 2 to 4.5 mg/kg I.V. daily for 10 days; repeated q 4 weeks, as tolerated. Or 250 mg/m² I.V. daily for 5 days; repeated at 3-week intervals.

➤ **Hodgkin's disease—**
Adults: 150 mg/m² I.V. daily (with other drugs) for 5 days; repeated q 4 weeks. Or 375 mg/m² on first day of combination regimen; repeated q 15 days.

I.V. ADMINISTRATION

● Administer antiemetics before giving dacarbazine. Nausea and vomiting may subside after several doses.

● Follow institutional policy to reduce risks. Preparation and administration of parenteral form of drug are linked to carcinogenic, mutagenic, and teratogenic risks for personnel.

● Reconstitute drug using sterile water for injection. Add 9.9 ml to 100-mg vial or 19.7 ml to 200-mg vial; resulting solution will be colorless to clear yellow. For infusion, further dilute by using up to 250 ml of normal saline solution or D₅W; infuse over at least 15 to 30 minutes.

● Drug may be diluted further or given at a slower infusion rate to decrease pain at insertion site.

● Avoid extravasation during infusion. If I.V. solution infiltrates, stop immediately, apply ice to area for 24 to 48 hours, and notify prescriber. Extravasation may cause severe pain and tissue damage.

● Reconstituted solutions in the vial are stable for 8 hours at room temperature and normal lighting conditions, or up to 3 days if refrigerated. Further diluted solutions are stable for 8 hours at normal room temperature and light, or up to 24 hours if refrigerated. If solutions turn pink, discard drug because it has decomposed.

ACTION
Unknown. Probably cross-links strands of cellular DNA and interferes with RNA and protein synthesis. Not specific to cell cycle.

Route	Onset	Peak	Duration
I.V.	Unknown	Unknown	Unknown

ADVERSE REACTIONS
CNS: facial paresthesia.
GI: *severe nausea and vomiting, anorexia,* stomatitis.
Hematologic: *leukopenia, thrombocytopenia.*

Skin: phototoxicity, alopecia, rash, facial flushing.
Other: tissue damage, *flu syndrome, anaphylaxis,* severe pain with infiltration or a too-concentrated solution.

INTERACTIONS
Drug-lifestyle. *Sun exposure:* May cause photosensitivity reaction, especially during first 2 days of therapy. Advise patient to avoid excessive sunlight exposure.

EFFECTS ON LAB TEST RESULTS
● May increase BUN and liver enzyme levels.
● May decrease WBC, RBC, and platelet counts.

CONTRAINDICATIONS
Contraindicated in patients hypersensitive to drug.

NURSING CONSIDERATIONS
● Use cautiously in patients with impaired bone marrow function and those with severe renal or hepatic dysfunction.
● To prevent bleeding, avoid all I.M. injections when platelet count is below 50,000/mm³.
● Anticipate need for blood transfusions to combat anemia. Patient may receive injections of RBC colony-stimulating factors to promote RBC production and decrease need for blood transfusions.
● Therapeutic effects are commonly accompanied by toxicity. Monitor CBC and platelet count.
● For Hodgkin's disease, drug is usually given with bleomycin, vinblastine, and doxorubicin.
● *Alert:* Don't confuse dacarbazine with Dicarbosil or procarbazine.

PATIENT TEACHING
● Tell patient to watch for evidence of infection (fever, sore throat, fatigue) and bleeding (easy bruising, nosebleeds, bleeding gums, melena). Tell patient to take temperature daily.
● Tell patient to avoid people with upper respiratory tract infections.
● Instruct patient to avoid OTC products that contain aspirin or NSAIDs.
● Advise patient to avoid sunlight and sunlamps for first 2 days after treatment.

● Reassure patient that flu syndrome (fever, malaise, myalgia beginning 7 days after treatment ends and possibly lasting 7 to 21 days) may be treated with mild antipyretics such as acetaminophen.
● Counsel woman to avoid pregnancy and breast-feeding during therapy.

docetaxel
Taxotere

Pregnancy risk category D

AVAILABLE FORMS
Injection: 20 mg, 80 mg, in single-dose vials

INDICATIONS & DOSAGES
➤ **Locally advanced or metastatic breast cancer after failure of previous chemotherapy—**
Adults: 60 to 100 mg/m² I.V. over 1 hour q 3 weeks.
Adjust-a-dose: In patients receiving 100 mg/m² who experience febrile neutropenia, neutrophil count of less than 500/mm³ for longer than 1 week, severe or cumulative cutaneous reactions, or severe peripheral neuropathy, reduce subsequent dose by 25%, to 75 mg/m². In patients who continue to experience reactions with decreased dose, either decrease it further to 55 mg/m² or discontinue drug.
➤ **Locally advanced or metastatic non–small-cell lung cancer after failure of previous cisplatin-based chemotherapy—**
Adults: 75 mg/m² I.V. over 1 hour every 3 weeks.
Adjust-a-dose: In patients who experience febrile neutropenia, neutrophil count of less than 500/mm³ for longer than 1 week, severe or cumulative cutaneous reactions, or severe peripheral neuropathy, withhold drug until toxicity resolves; then restart at 55 mg/m². In patients who develop grade 3 peripheral neuropathy or above, discontinue drug.

I.V. ADMINISTRATION
● Wear gloves during drug preparation and administration. If solution contacts skin, wash immediately and thoroughly with soap and water. If drug contacts mucous

membranes, flush thoroughly with water. Mark all waste materials with CHEMO-THERAPY HAZARD labels.

• Prepare and store infusion solutions in bottles (glass or polypropylene) or plastic bags, and administer through polyethylene-lined administration sets. Administer drug as 1-hour infusion; store unopened vials in refrigerator.

• Before administration, dilute drug using diluent supplied. Allow drug and diluent to stand at room temperature for 5 minutes before mixing. After adding all the diluent to drug vial, gently rotate vial for about 15 seconds. Allow solution to stand for a few minutes to enable foam to dissipate. All foam need not fully dissipate before proceeding to the next step.

• Prepare drug infusion solution by withdrawing the needed amount of premixed solution from the vial and injecting it into 250 ml normal saline solution or D_5W to yield 0.3 to 0.9 mg/ml. Doses exceeding 240 mg need a larger volume of infusion solution to stay below 0.9 mg/ml of docetaxel. Mix infusion thoroughly by manual rotation.

• Discard solution if it isn't clear or it contains precipitates. Infusion solution should be used within 4 hours.

ACTION

Promotes formation and stabilization of nonfunctional microtubules. This prevents mitosis and leads to cell death.

Route	Onset	Peak	Duration
I.V.	Rapid	Unknown	Unknown

ADVERSE REACTIONS

CNS: *asthenia,* paresthesia, peripheral neuropathy.
CV: *fluid retention, peripheral edema,* hypotension, flushing, chest tightness.
GI: *stomatitis, nausea, vomiting, diarrhea.*
Hematologic: *anemia,* NEUTROPENIA, FEBRILE NEUTROPENIA, MYELOSUPPRESSION, LEUKOPENIA, THROMBOCYTOPENIA.
Musculoskeletal: *myalgia,* arthralgia, back pain.
Respiratory: dyspnea, *pulmonary edema.*

Skin: *alopecia,* skin eruptions, desquamation, nail pigmentation alterations, nail pain, rash, reaction at injection site.
Other: hypersensitivity reactions, *infection,* drug fever, chills.

INTERACTIONS

Drug-drug. *Compounds that induce, inhibit, or are metabolized by cytochrome P-450 3A4, such as cyclosporine, erythromycin, ketoconazole, troleandomycin:* Metabolism of docetaxel may be modified. Use together cautiously.

EFFECTS ON LAB TEST RESULTS

• May increase ALT, AST, bilirubin, and alkaline phosphatase levels.
• May decrease hemoglobin and WBC and platelet counts.

CONTRAINDICATIONS

Contraindicated in patients severely hypersensitive to drug or to other formulations containing polysorbate 80 and in those with neutrophil counts below 1,500 cells/mm³.

NURSING CONSIDERATIONS

• Don't give drug to patients with bilirubin levels exceeding upper limit of normal. Also, avoid use of drug in patients with ALT or AST levels above 1.5 times upper limit of normal and alkaline phosphatase levels over 2.5 times upper limit of normal or in patients with baseline neutrophil count less than 1,500/mm³.
• Give oral corticosteroid such as dexamethasone 16 mg P.O. (8 mg b.i.d.) daily for 3 days starting 1 day before docetaxel administration, to reduce risk and severity of fluid retention and hypersensitivity reactions.
• Bone marrow toxicity is the most frequent and dose-limiting toxicity. Frequent blood count monitoring is needed during therapy.
• Monitor patient closely for hypersensitivity reactions, especially during first and second infusions.
• Safety and efficacy of drug in children haven't been established.
• Contact between undiluted docetaxel concentrate and polyvinyl chloride equipment or devices isn't recommended.

• Fluid retention is dose-related and may be severe. Monitor patient closely.
• *Alert:* Don't confuse Taxotere with Taxol.

PATIENT TEACHING
• Caution woman of childbearing age to avoid pregnancy or breast-feeding during therapy.
• Advise patient to report any pain or burning at site of injection during or after administration.
• Warn patient that alopecia occurs in almost 80% of patients, but is reversible with drug discontinuation.
• Tell patient to promptly report sore throat, fever, or unusual bruising or bleeding, as well as signs and symptoms of fluid retention, such as swelling or dyspnea.

---

etoposide (VP-16, VP-16-213)
VePesid

etoposide phosphate
Etopophos

Pregnancy risk category D

AVAILABLE FORMS
etoposide
Capsules: 50 mg
Injection: 20 mg/ml in 5-ml vials
etoposide phosphate
Injection: 119.3-mg vials equivalent to 100 mg etoposide

INDICATIONS & DOSAGES
➤ **Testicular cancer—**
Adults: 50 to 100 mg/m² I.V. on 5 consecutive days q 3 to 4 weeks. Or, 100 mg/m² on days 1, 3, and 5 q 3 to 4 weeks.
➤ **Small-cell carcinoma of the lung—**
Adults: 35 mg/m²/day I.V. for 4 days. Or, 50 mg/m²/day I.V. for 5 days. P.O. dose is two times I.V. dose, rounded to nearest 50 mg.
Adjust-a-dose: For patients with creatine clearance of 15 to 50 mL/minute, reduce dose by 25%.

I.V. ADMINISTRATION
• Dilute etoposide for infusion in either D₅W or normal saline solution to 0.2 or 0.4 mg/ml. Higher concentrations may crystallize. Etoposide phosphate may be given without further dilution or may be diluted to as low as 0.1 mg/ml in either D₅W or normal saline solution.
• Etoposide diluted to 0.2 mg/ml is stable for 96 hours at room temperature in plastic or glass unprotected from light; solutions diluted to 0.4 mg/ml are stable for 48 hours under same conditions. Diluted solutions of etoposide phosphate are stable at room temperature or under refrigeration for 24 hours.
• Give etoposide by slow I.V. infusion (over at least 30 minutes) to prevent severe hypotension. Etoposide phosphate may be given over 5 to 210 minutes.
• *Alert:* Monitor blood pressure every 15 minutes during infusion. Hypotension can occur with too rapid an infusion. If systolic pressure falls below 90 mm Hg, stop infusion and notify prescriber.
• Follow institutional policy to reduce risks. Preparation and administration of parenteral form of drug are linked to carcinogenic, mutagenic, and teratogenic risks for personnel.
• *Alert:* Don't confuse VePesid with Versed.

ACTION
Unknown. Inhibits topoisomerase II enzyme, which leads to inability to repair DNA strand breaks. This ultimately leads to cell death. Cell cycle specific to G₂ portion of cell cycle.

Route	Onset	Peak	Duration
I.V., P.O.	Unknown	Unknown	Unknown

ADVERSE REACTIONS
CNS: peripheral neuropathy.
CV: hypotension.
GI: *nausea and vomiting, anorexia, diarrhea,* abdominal pain, stomatitis.
Hematologic: *anemia, myelosuppression,* LEUKOPENIA, THROMBOCYTOPENIA, NEUTROPENIA.
Hepatic: *hepatotoxicity.*
Skin: *reversible alopecia,* rash.

INTERACTIONS
Drug-drug. *Warfarin:* May further prolong PT. Monitor PT and INR closely.

---

*Reactions may be common, uncommon, **life-threatening**, or COMMON AND LIFE-THREATENING.*

EFFECTS ON LAB TEST RESULTS
• May decrease hemoglobin and WBC, RBC, platelet, and neutrophil counts.

CONTRAINDICATIONS
Contraindicated in patients hypersensitive to drug.

NURSING CONSIDERATIONS
• Use cautiously in patients who have had cytotoxic or radiation therapy. Use cautiously in patients with hepatic impairment.
• Obtain baseline blood pressure before starting therapy.
• Anticipate need for antiemetics.
• Have diphenhydramine, hydrocortisone, epinephrine, and emergency equipment available to establish an airway in case anaphylaxis occurs.
• Store capsules in refrigerator.
• Monitor CBC. Watch for evidence of bone marrow suppression.
• Observe mouth for signs of ulceration.
• To prevent bleeding, avoid all I.M. injections when platelet count is below 50,000/mm³.
• Anticipate need for blood transfusions to combat anemia. Patient may receive injections of RBC colony-stimulating factors to promote RBC production and decrease need for blood transfusions.
• Dose of etoposide phosphate is expressed as etoposide equivalents; 119.3 mg of etoposide phosphate is equivalent to 100 mg of etoposide.

PATIENT TEACHING
• Tell patient to watch for signs and symptoms of infection (fever, sore throat, fatigue) and bleeding (easy bruising, nosebleeds, bleeding gums, melena). Tell patient to take temperature daily.
• Inform patient of need for frequent blood pressure readings during I.V. administration.
• Caution woman of childbearing age to avoid pregnancy or breast-feeding during therapy.

gemcitabine hydrochloride
Gemzar

Pregnancy risk category D

AVAILABLE FORMS
Powder for injection: 200-mg, 1-g vials

INDICATIONS & DOSAGES
➤ **Locally advanced or metastatic adenocarcinoma of pancreas and patients treated previously with fluorouracil—**
Adults: 1,000 mg/m² I.V. over 30 minutes once weekly for up to 7 weeks, unless toxicity occurs. Monitor CBC with differential and platelet count before giving each dose. If bone marrow suppression is detected, adjust therapy. Give full dose if absolute granulocyte count (AGC) is 1,000/mm³ or more and platelet count is 100,000/mm³ or more. If AGC is 500 to 999/mm³ or platelet count is 50,000 to 99,999/mm³, give 75% of dose. Withhold dose if AGC is below 500/mm³ or platelet count is below 50,000/mm³. Treatment course of 7 weeks is followed by 1 week of rest. Subsequent dosage cycles consist of 1 infusion weekly for 3 of 4 consecutive weeks. Dosage adjustments for subsequent cycles are based on AGC and platelet count nadirs and degree of nonhematologic toxicity.
➤ **With cisplatin as first-line treatment of inoperable, locally advanced, or metastatic non–small-cell lung cancer—**
Adults: For 4-week schedule, 1,000 mg/m² I.V. over 30 minutes on days 1, 8, and 15 of each 28-day cycle. Cisplatin 100 mg/m² on day 1 after gemcitabine infusion.

For 3-week schedule, 1,250 mg/m² I.V. over 30 minutes on days 1 and 8 of each 21-day cycle. Cisplatin 100 mg/m² on day 1 after gemcitabine infusion.

I.V. ADMINISTRATION
• Follow institutional policy to reduce risks. Preparation and administration of parenteral form of drug are linked to mutagenic, teratogenic, and carcinogenic risks for personnel.
• To prepare solution, add 5 ml of unpreserved normal saline solution for injection to 200-mg vial or 25 ml of diluent to a 1-g vial. Shake to dissolve. Resulting concen-

---

tration is 40 mg/ml; reconstitution at higher concentrations isn't recommended. May be further diluted with normal saline solution for injection to a concentration as low as 0.1 mg/ml, if needed. Solution should be clear to light straw-colored and free of particulates. It's stable for 24 hours at room temperature. Don't refrigerate reconstituted drug because crystallization may occur.

• Prolonging infusion time beyond 60 minutes or administering drug more frequently than once weekly may increase toxicity.

ACTION

Cytotoxic and cell cycle–specific; inhibits DNA synthesis and blocks progression of cells through G_1/S-phase boundary.

Route	Onset	Peak	Duration
I.V.	Unknown	Unknown	Unknown

ADVERSE REACTIONS

CNS: *somnolence, paresthesia.*
CV: *edema, peripheral edema.*
GI: *stomatitis, nausea, vomiting, constipation, diarrhea.*
GU: *proteinuria, hematuria.*
Hematologic: *anemia,* **leukopenia, neutropenia, thrombocytopenia.**
Respiratory: *dyspnea,* **bronchospasm.**
Skin: *alopecia, rash.*
Other: *pain, fever, flu syndrome, infection, pain at injection site.*

INTERACTIONS
None significant.

EFFECTS ON LAB TEST RESULTS
• May increase BUN, creatinine, ALT, and AST levels.
• May decrease hemoglobin and WBC, neutrophil, and platelet counts.

CONTRAINDICATIONS
Contraindicated in patients hypersensitive to drug.

NURSING CONSIDERATIONS
• Use cautiously in patients with renal or hepatic impairment.
• Drug isn't recommended for pregnant or breast-feeding women.

• Monitor patient closely. Expect dosage modification according to toxicity and degree of myelosuppression. Age, sex, and presence of renal impairment may predispose patient to toxicity.
• Careful hematologic monitoring, especially of neutrophil and platelet counts, is needed.
• Obtain baseline and periodic renal and hepatic laboratory tests.
• Safety and effectiveness of drug in children haven't been determined.

PATIENT TEACHING
• Advise patient to watch for evidence of infection (fever, sore throat, fatigue) and bleeding (easy bruising, nosebleeds, bleeding gums, melena). Tell patient to take temperature daily.
• Tell patient that adverse effects may continue after treatment ends.
• Caution woman of childbearing age to avoid pregnancy or breast-feeding during therapy.

gemtuzumab ozogamicin
Mylotarg

Pregnancy risk category D

AVAILABLE FORMS
Powder for injection: 5 mg

INDICATIONS & DOSAGES
➤ **Treatment of patients with CD33-positive acute myeloid leukemia in first relapse and who aren't considered candidates for cytotoxic chemotherapy—**
Adults age 60 and older: 9 mg/m² I.V. over 2 hours every 14 days for a total of two doses. Premedicate with diphenhydramine 50 mg P.O. and acetaminophen 650 to 1,000 mg P.O. 1 hour before infusion.

I.V. ADMINISTRATION
• Drug is light sensitive; protect from direct and indirect sunlight and unshielded fluorescent light during infusion preparation and administration.
• Administer in 100 ml of normal saline solution for injection. Place the 100-ml I.V. bag into an ultraviolet protectant bag.

Reactions may be *common,* uncommon, *life-threatening,* or COMMON AND LIFE-THREATENING.

Use the resulting drug solution in the I.V. bag immediately.

• A separate I.V. line equipped with a low–protein binding 1.2-micron terminal filter must be used for drug administration. May be infused by central or peripheral line.

• **Alert:** Don't administer as a push or bolus.

• Reconstituted drug is stable for 8 hours if refrigerated.

ACTION
Binds to the CD33 antigen on the surface of leukemic blasts, resulting in the formation of a complex that's internalized by the cell. The cytotoxic antibiotic is then released inside the cell, causing DNA double strand breaks and cell death.

Route	Onset	Peak	Duration
I.V.	Unknown	Unknown	Unknown

ADVERSE REACTIONS
CNS: *asthenia,* depression, *dizziness, headache, insomnia, pain.*
CV: *hypertension, hypotension, tachycardia, peripheral edema.*
EENT: *epistaxis, pharyngitis, rhinitis.*
GI: enlarged abdomen, *abdominal pain, anorexia, constipation, diarrhea, dyspepsia, nausea, stomatitis, vomiting.*
GU: *hematuria, vaginal hemorrhage.*
Hematologic: *anemia,* HEMORRHAGE, LEUKOPENIA, NEUTROPENIA, NEUTROPENIC FEVER, THROMBOCYTOPENIA.
Hepatic: *hepatotoxicity.*
Metabolic: hyperglycemia, *hypokalemia, hypomagnesemia.*
Musculoskeletal: arthralgia, *back pain.*
Respiratory: *cough, dyspnea,* **hypoxia,** *pneumonia.*
Skin: ecchymoses, local reaction, petechiae, rash.
Other: *chills, fever,* herpes simplex, SEPSIS.

INTERACTIONS
None known.

EFFECTS ON LAB TEST RESULTS
• May increase ALT, AST, LDH, and glucose levels.
• May decrease hemoglobin and WBC, neutrophil, and platelet counts.

CONTRAINDICATIONS
Contraindicated in patients hypersensitive to drug or any of its components.

NURSING CONSIDERATIONS
• Use cautiously in patients with hepatic impairment.
• Drug should be used only under the supervision of a clinician experienced in the use of cancer chemotherapeutics.
• Premedicate with diphenhydramine and acetaminophen. Additional doses of acetaminophen 650 to 1,000 mg P.O. can be given every 4 hours, as needed.
• Monitor vital signs during infusion and for 4 hours after infusion.
• Monitor postinfusion symptom complex of chills, fever, hypotension, hypertension, hyperglycemia, hypoxia, and dyspnea that may occur during the first 24 hours after administration.
• **Alert:** Severe myelosuppression will occur in all patients given the recommended dose of this drug. Careful hematologic monitoring is required.
• Monitor electrolytes, hepatic function, CBC, and platelet counts during therapy.
• Tumor lysis syndrome may occur. Provide adequate hydration and treat with allopurinol to prevent hyperuricemia.

PATIENT TEACHING
• Advise patient about postinfusion symptoms and instruct him to continue to take acetaminophen 650 to 1,000 mg every 4 hours, as needed.
• Urge patient to watch for signs of infection (fever, sore throat, fatigue) and bleeding (easy bruising, nosebleeds, bleeding gums, melena). Tell patient to take temperature daily.
• Tell patient to avoid OTC products that contain aspirin.

---

irinotecan hydrochloride
Campto§, Camptosar

Pregnancy risk category D

AVAILABLE FORMS
Injection: 100 mg/5-ml vial

INDICATIONS & DOSAGES

➤ **Metastatic carcinoma of the colon or rectum that has recurred or progressed after fluorouracil (5-FU) therapy—**

Adults: Initially, 125 mg/m² by I.V. infusion over 90 minutes. Recommended treatment is 125 mg/m² I.V. once weekly for 4 weeks; then 2-week rest period. Thereafter, additional courses of treatment may be repeated q 6 weeks with 4 weeks on and 2 weeks off. Subsequent doses may be adjusted to low of 50 mg/m² or to maximum of 150 mg/m² in 25- to 50-mg/m² increments based on patient's tolerance. Additional courses may continue indefinitely in patients who respond favorably and in those whose disease remains stable, provided intolerable toxicity doesn't occur.

➤ **First-line therapy for metastatic colorectal cancer with 5-fluorouracil (5-FU) and leucovorin—**

Regimen 1

Adults: 125 mg/m² I.V. over 90 minutes on days 1, 8, 15, and 22; then leucovorin 20 mg/m² I.V. bolus on days 1, 8, 15, and 22 and 5-FU 500 mg/m² I.V. bolus on days 1, 8, 15, and 22. Courses are repeated q 6 weeks.

Adjust-a-dose: During a course of therapy, for patients with absolute neutrophil count (ANC) of 1,000 to 1,499/mm³ or four to six stools per day over baseline, decrease irinotecan dose to 100 mg/m² and 5-FU dose to 400 mg/m² and continue leucovorin at 20 mg/m².

For patients with ANC of 500 to 999/mm³ or seven to nine stools per day over baseline, omit one dose; then decrease irinotecan dose to 100 mg/m² and 5-FU dose to 400 mg/m² and continue leucovorin at 20 mg/m² once ANC increases to 1,000/mm³ or more and stools decrease to fewer than seven per day.

For patients with ANC less than 500/mm³ or 10 or more stools per day over baseline, omit one dose; then decrease irinotecan dose to 75 mg/m² and 5-FU dose to 300 mg/m² and continue leucovorin at 20 mg/m² once ANC increases to 1,000/mm³ or more and stools decrease to fewer than seven per day.

For patients with neutropenic fever, omit one dose; then decrease irinotecan dose to 75 mg/m² and 5-FU dose to 300 mg/m² and continue leucovorin at 20 mg/m² once neutropenic fever is resolved.

At the start of subsequent courses of therapy, for patients with ANC of 500 to 999/mm³ or seven to nine stools per day over baseline, decrease irinotecan dose to 100 mg/m² and 5-FU dose to 400 mg/m² and continue leucovorin at 20 mg/m². For patients with ANC less than 500/mm³, neutropenic fever, or 10 or more stools per day over baseline, decrease irinotecan dose to 75 mg/m² and 5-FU dose to 300 mg/m² and continue leucovorin at 20 mg/m².

Regimen 2

Adults: 180 mg/m² I.V. over 90 minutes on days 1, 15, and 29; then leucovorin 200 mg/m² I.V. over 2 hours on days 1, 2, 15, 16, 29, and 30; then 5-FU 400 mg/m² I.V. bolus on days 1, 2, 15, 16, 29, and 30 and 5-FU 600 mg/m² I.V. infusion over 22 hours on days 1, 2, 15, 16, 29, and 30.

Adjust-a-dose: During a course of therapy, for patients with ANC of 1,000 to 1,499/mm³ or four to six stools per day over baseline, decrease irinotecan dose to 150 mg/m², 5-FU bolus dose to 320 mg/m², and 5-FU infusion dose to 480 mg/m², and continue leucovorin at 200 mg/m².

For patients with ANC of 500 to 999/mm³ or seven to nine stools per day over baseline, omit one dose; then decrease irinotecan dose to 150 mg/m², 5-FU bolus dose to 320 mg/m², and 5-FU infusion to 480 mg/m², and continue leucovorin at 200 mg/m² once ANC increases to 1,000/mm³ or more and stools decrease to fewer than seven per day.

For patients with ANC less than 500/mm³ or 10 or more stools per day over baseline, omit one dose; then decrease irinotecan dose to 120 mg/m², 5-FU bolus dose to 240 mg/m², and 5-FU infusion to 360 mg/m², and continue leucovorin at 200 mg/m² once ANC increases to 1,000/mm³ or more and stools decrease to fewer than seven per day.

For patients with neutropenic fever, omit one dose; then decrease irinotecan dose to 120 mg/m², 5-FU bolus to 240 mg/m², 5-FU infusion to 360 mg/m², and continue leucovorin at 200 mg/m^2 once neutropenic fever is resolved.

At the start of subsequent courses of therapy, for patients with ANC of 500 to 999/mm^3 or seven to nine stools per day over baseline, decrease irinotecan dose to 150 mg/m^2, 5-FU bolus dose to 320 mg/m^2, and 5-FU infusion to 480 mg/m^2, and continue leucovorin at 200 mg/m^2. For patients with ANC less than 500/mm^3, neutropenic fever, or 10 or more stools per day over baseline, decrease irinotecan dose to 120 mg/m^2, 5-FU bolus dose to 240 mg/m^2, and 5-FU infusion to 360 mg/m^2, and continue leucovorin at 200 mg/m^2.

I.V. ADMINISTRATION
● Premedicate patient with antiemetic drugs on day of treatment starting at least 30 minutes before giving irinotecan.
● Wear gloves while handling and preparing infusion solutions. If drug contacts skin, wash thoroughly with soap and water. If drug contacts mucous membranes, flush thoroughly with water.
● Irinotecan must be diluted in D$_5$W injection (preferred) or normal saline solution for injection before infusion. Final concentration range is 0.12 to 1.1 mg/ml.
● Irinotecan solution is stable for up to 24 hours at 77° F (25° C) and in ambient fluorescent lighting. Solutions diluted in D$_5$W, stored at 36° to 46° F (2° to 8° C), and protected from light are stable for 48 hours. However, because of possible microbial contamination during dilution, use admixture within 24 hours if refrigerated or 6 hours if kept at room temperature. Refrigerating admixtures using normal saline solution isn't recommended because of low and sporadic risk of visible particulate. Don't freeze admixture because drug may precipitate.
● Don't add other drugs to irinotecan infusion.
● Avoid extravasation. If it occurs, flush site with sterile water and apply ice. Notify prescriber.

ACTION
A derivative of camptothecin. Camptothecins interact specifically with the enzyme topoisomerase I, which relieves torsional strain in DNA by inducing reversible single-strand breaks. Irinotecan and its active metabolite SN-38 bind to the topoisomerase I–DNA complex and prevent relegation of these single-strand breaks.

Route	Onset	Peak	Duration
I.V.	Unknown	1 hr	Unknown

ADVERSE REACTIONS
CNS: *insomnia, dizziness, asthenia, headache,* akathisia.
CV: *vasodilation, edema,* orthostatic hypotension.
EENT: *rhinitis.*
GI: *diarrhea, nausea, vomiting, anorexia, stomatitis, constipation, flatulence, dyspepsia, abdominal cramping and pain, abdominal enlargement.*
Hematologic: *leukopenia, anemia, neutropenia, thrombocytopenia.*
Metabolic: *weight loss, dehydration.*
Musculoskeletal: *back pain.*
Respiratory: *dyspnea, increased cough.*
Skin: *alopecia, sweating, rash.*
Other: *fever, pain, chills, minor infection.*

INTERACTIONS
Drug-drug. *Dexamethasone:* Increased risk of irinotecan-induced lymphocytopenia. Monitor patient closely.
Diuretics: Increased risk of dehydration and electrolyte imbalance. Consider discontinuing diuretic during active periods of nausea and vomiting.
Laxative use: Increased risk of diarrhea. Avoid using together.
Other antineoplastics: May cause additive adverse effects, such as myelosuppression and diarrhea. Monitor patient closely.
Pelvic or abdominal irradiation: Increased risk of severe myelosuppression. Avoid use of drug with irradiation.
Prochlorperazine: Increased risk of akathisia. Monitor patient closely.

EFFECTS ON LAB TEST RESULTS
● May increase alkaline phosphatase and AST levels.
● May decrease hemoglobin and WBC and neutrophil counts.

CONTRAINDICATIONS
Contraindicated in patients hypersensitive to drug.

NURSING CONSIDERATIONS
• Use cautiously in elderly patients.
• Drug is packaged in a plastic blister to protect against inadvertent breakage and leakage. Inspect vial for damage and signs of leakage before removing blister.
• Store vial at 59° to 86° F (15° to 30° C). Protect from light.
• Diuretic may be withheld during therapy and periods of active vomiting or diarrhea to decrease risk of dehydration.
• Drug can induce severe diarrhea. Diarrhea occurring within 24 hours of administration may be preceded by diaphoresis and abdominal cramping and may be relieved by 0.25 to 1 mg atropine I.V., unless contraindicated. Diarrhea occurring more than 24 hours after drug administration may be prolonged, leading to dehydration and electrolyte imbalances; it may be life-threatening. Diarrhea occurring after 24 hours should be treated with loperamide. Monitor patient's fluid status and electrolyte levels.
• Temporarily discontinue therapy if neutropenic fever occurs or if absolute neutrophil count drops below 500/mm³. Dosage should be reduced, especially if WBC count is below 2,000/mm³, neutrophil count is below 1,000/mm³, hemoglobin level is below 8 g/dl, or platelet count is below 100,000/mm³.
• Routine administration of a colony-stimulating factor isn't needed but may be helpful in patients with significant neutropenia.
• Monitor WBC count with differential, hemoglobin level, and platelet count before each dose of irinotecan.
• Safety and effectiveness of drug in children haven't been established.

PATIENT TEACHING
• Inform patient about risk of diarrhea and methods to treat it; tell him to avoid laxatives.
• Tell patient to notify prescriber if vomiting, fever, signs and symptoms of infection, or symptoms of dehydration (fainting, light-headedness, or dizziness) occur after drug administration.

• Warn patient that alopecia may occur.
• Caution woman of childbearing age to avoid pregnancy or breast-feeding during therapy.

---

mitotane (o,p'-DDD)
Lysodren

Pregnancy risk category C

AVAILABLE FORMS
Tablets (scored): 500 mg

INDICATIONS & DOSAGES
➤ **Inoperable adrenocortical cancer—**
Adults: Initially, 2 to 6 g P.O. daily in divided doses t.i.d. or q.i.d.; increased to 9 to 10 g P.O. daily in divided doses t.i.d. or q.i.d. Adjust dosage until maximum tolerated dose is achieved (varies from 2 to 16 g/day but is usually 9 to 10 g/day).

ACTION
Unknown. May suppress function of adrenocortical tissue and hinder extra-adrenal metabolism of cortisol.

Route	Onset	Peak	Duration
P.O.	Unknown	3-5 hr	Unknown

ADVERSE REACTIONS
CNS: *depression, somnolence, lethargy, vertigo.*
CV: hypertension, orthostatic hypotension, flushing.
EENT: visual disturbances, diplopia, lens opacity, toxic retinopathy.
GI: *severe nausea, vomiting, diarrhea, anorexia.*
GU: hemorrhagic cystitis.
Metabolic: adrenal insufficiency, hyperuricemia.
Musculoskeletal: myalgia.
Skin: dermatitis, *maculopapular rash,* muscle twitching.
Other: fever.

INTERACTIONS
Drug-drug. *Corticosteroids:* Increased metabolism of corticosteroids requiring higher corticosteroid doses. Adjust corticosteroid dosage as directed.

Reactions may be *common*, uncommon, *life-threatening*, or COMMON AND LIFE-THREATENING.

Phenytoin, phenobarbital: Increased metabolism of these agents. Monitor levels closely.
Warfarin: Increased metabolism, which may require higher warfarin doses. Monitor PT and INR closely.

EFFECTS ON LAB TEST RESULTS
● May increase plasma cortisol, protein-bound iodine, and uric acid levels.

CONTRAINDICATIONS
Contraindicated in patients hypersensitive to drug, patients in shock, and patients who have suffered trauma.

NURSING CONSIDERATIONS
● Use cautiously in patients with hepatic disease.
● To reduce nausea, give antiemetic before mitotane.
● Monitor effectiveness by reduction in pain, weakness, and anorexia.
● Assess and record behavioral and neurologic signs daily. Prolonged therapy has been linked to significant neurologic impairment.
● Both glucocorticoid and mineralocorticoid therapy are required to avoid acute adrenocortical insufficiency. Glucocorticoid dosage should be increased during periods of physiologic stress, such as infection or trauma.
● Because drug is distributed mostly to body fat, obese patients may need higher dosage and may have longer-lasting adverse reactions.
● An adequate therapeutic trial lasts at least 3 months, but treatment can continue if clinical benefits are observed.

PATIENT TEACHING
● Warn ambulatory patient to avoid activities that require alertness and good motor coordination until CNS effects of drug are known.
● Instruct patient to notify prescriber if severe adverse GI or skin reactions occur because dosage adjustment may be needed.
● Counsel woman of childbearing age to avoid pregnancy or breast-feeding during therapy.

mitoxantrone hydrochloride
Novantrone

Pregnancy risk category D

AVAILABLE FORMS
Injection: 2 mg/ml in 10-ml, 12.5-ml, 15-ml vials

INDICATIONS & DOSAGES
➤ **Combination initial therapy for acute nonlymphocytic leukemia—**
Adults: Induction begins with 12 mg/m^2 I.V. daily on days 1 to 3, with 100 mg/m^2 daily of cytarabine on days 1 to 7. A second induction may be given if response isn't adequate. Maintenance therapy is 12 mg/m^2 on days 1 and 2, with cytarabine on days 1 to 5.

I.V. ADMINISTRATION
● Follow facility policy to minimize risks. Preparation and administration of parenteral form are linked to mutagenic, teratogenic, and carcinogenic risks to staff.
● Dilute dose (available as an aqueous solution of 2 mg/ml in volumes of 10, 12.5, and 15 ml) in at least 50 ml of normal saline solution for injection or D$_5$W injection. Administer by direct injection into free-flowing I.V. line of normal saline solution or D$_5$W injection over at least 3 minutes, usually 15 to 30 minutes. Don't mix with other drugs.
● If extravasation occurs, stop infusion immediately and notify prescriber.
● Once vial is penetrated, undiluted solution may be stored at room temperature for 7 days, or 14 days in refrigerator. Don't freeze.
● Drug is physically incompatible with heparin. Don't mix.

ACTION
Exact mechanism is unknown. Probably not specific to cell cycle. Reacts with DNA, producing cytotoxic effect.

Route	Onset	Peak	Duration
I.V.	Unknown	Unknown	Unknown

ADVERSE REACTIONS
CNS: *seizures,* headache.

CV: *heart failure, arrhythmias,* tachycardia.
EENT: conjunctivitis.
GI: *bleeding, abdominal pain, diarrhea, nausea, mucositis, vomiting, stomatitis.*
GU: *renal failure.*
Hematologic: *myelosuppression.*
Hepatic: jaundice.
Metabolic: hyperuricemia.
Respiratory: *dyspnea, cough.*
Skin: *alopecia,* petechiae, ecchymoses, local irritation or phlebitis.
Other: *fungal infections, fever, sepsis.*

INTERACTIONS
None significant.

EFFECTS ON LAB TEST RESULTS
• May increase ALT, AST, bilirubin, and uric acid levels.

CONTRAINDICATIONS
Contraindicated in patients hypersensitive to drug.

NURSING CONSIDERATIONS
• Use cautiously in patients with previous exposure to anthracyclines or other cardiotoxic drugs, previous radiation therapy to mediastinal area, or heart disease.
• Patients with significant myelosuppression shouldn't receive drug unless benefits outweigh risks.
• Administer allopurinol. Uric acid nephropathy can be avoided by hydrating patient before and during therapy.
• Closely monitor hematologic and laboratory chemistry parameters.
• To prevent bleeding, avoid all I.M. injections if platelet count falls below 50,000/mm³.
• Anticipate need for blood transfusion to combat anemia. Patients may receive injections of RBC colony-stimulating factors to promote RBC production and decrease need for blood transfusions.
• Monitor left ventricular ejection fraction.
• Treat infections with antibiotics. Patients may receive injections of WBC colony-stimulating factors to promote cell growth and decrease risk of infection.
• If severe nonhematologic toxicity occurs during first course, delay second course until patient recovers.

PATIENT TEACHING
• Advise patient to report any pain or burning at site of injection during or after administration.
• Tell patient that urine may appear blue-green within 24 hours after administration and that some bluish discoloration of the sclera may occur. These effects aren't harmful and may persist during therapy.
• Advise patient to watch for signs and symptoms of bleeding and infection.
• Caution woman of childbearing age to avoid pregnancy during therapy. Recommend that she consult prescriber before becoming pregnant.

---

paclitaxel
Taxol

Pregnancy risk category D

AVAILABLE FORMS
Injection: 30 mg/5 ml, 100 mg/16.7 ml

INDICATIONS & DOSAGES
➤ **Metastatic ovarian cancer after failure of first-line or subsequent chemotherapy—**
Adults: 135 mg/m² or 175 mg/m² I.V. over 3 hours q 3 weeks.
✳ **NEW INDICATION: First-line therapy in advanced ovarian cancer—**
Adults: 175 mg/m² I.V. over 3 hours q 3 weeks, followed by cisplatin 75 mg/m² I.V.; or, 135 mg/m² I.V. over 24 hours q 3 weeks, followed by cisplatin 75 mg/m².
➤ **Breast cancer after failure of combination chemotherapy for metastatic disease or relapse within 6 months of adjuvant chemotherapy—**
Adults: 175 mg/m² I.V. over 3 hours q 3 weeks.
➤ **Second-line therapy in AIDS-related Kaposi's sarcoma—**
Adults: 135 mg/m² I.V. over 3 hours q 3 weeks, or 100 mg/m² I.V. over 3 hours q 2 weeks.
➤ **Non–small-cell lung cancer in combination with cisplatin—**
Adults: 135 mg/m² I.V. infusion over 24 hours, followed by cisplatin 75 mg/m² I.V., with cycles repeated q 3 weeks. Or, 175 mg/m² I.V. infusion over 3 hours, fol-

lowed by cisplatin 80 mg/m² I.V., with cycles repeated q 3 weeks.

➤ **Adjuvant treatment of node-positive breast cancer—**

Adults: 175 mg/m² I.V. over 3 hours q 3 weeks for four courses, administered sequentially to doxorubicin-containing combination chemotherapy.

Adjust-a-dose: For patients with severe neutropenia (neutrophil count below 500 cells/mm³ for 1 week or longer) or severe peripheral neuropathy, reduce subsequent courses of drug by 20%.

I.V. ADMINISTRATION

• Follow institutional protocol for safe handling, preparation, and administration of chemotherapeutic drugs. Preparation and administration of parenteral form of drug are linked to carcinogenic, mutagenic, and teratogenic risks for personnel. Mark all waste materials with CHEMO-THERAPY HAZARD labels.

• Dilute concentrate before infusion. Compatible solutions include normal saline solution for injection, D₅W, 5% dextrose in normal saline solution for injection, and 5% dextrose in Ringer's lactate injection. Dilute to a final concentration of 0.3 to 1.2 mg/ml. Diluted solutions are stable for 24 hours at room temperature.

• Prepare and store infusion solutions in glass containers. Undiluted concentrate shouldn't contact polyvinyl chloride I.V. bags or tubing. Prepared solution may appear hazy. Store diluted solution in glass or polypropylene bottles, or use polypropylene or polyolefin bags. Administer through polyethylene-lined administration sets, and use an in-line 0.22-micron filter.

• Avoid extravasation.

• Continuously monitor patient for 30 minutes after starting infusion. Continue close monitoring throughout infusion.

ACTION

Prevents depolymerization of cellular microtubules, thus inhibiting normal reorganization of microtubule network needed for mitosis and other vital cellular functions.

Route	Onset	Peak	Duration
I.V.	Unknown	Unknown	Unknown

ADVERSE REACTIONS

CNS: *peripheral neuropathy, asthenia.*
CV: **bradycardia,** *hypotension, abnormal ECG.*
GI: *nausea, vomiting, diarrhea, mucositis.*
Hematologic: NEUTROPENIA, LEUKOPENIA, THROMBOCYTOPENIA, *anemia, bleeding.*
Musculoskeletal: *myalgia, arthralgia.*
Skin: *alopecia.*
Other: hypersensitivity reactions, **anaphylaxis,** *cellulitis and phlebitis at injection site, infections.*

INTERACTIONS

Drug-drug. *Cisplatin:* Possible additive myelosuppressive effects. When given together, paclitaxel should be given before cisplatin.
Doxorubicin: Plasma levels of doxorubicin and its active metabolite, doxorubicinol, may be increased when coadministered. Use together cautiously.
Drugs that inhibit cytochrome P-450, such as cyclosporine, dexamethasone, diazepam, etoposide, ketoconazole, quinidine, retinoic acid, teniposide, testosterone, verapamil, vincristine: May increase paclitaxel levels. Monitor patient for toxicity.
Ketoconazole: Inhibited paclitaxel metabolism. Use together cautiously.

EFFECTS ON LAB TEST RESULTS

• May increase alkaline phosphatase, AST, and triglyceride levels.
• May decrease hemoglobin and neutrophil, WBC, and platelet counts.

CONTRAINDICATIONS

Contraindicated in patients hypersensitive to drug or polyoxyethylated castor oil (a vehicle used in drug solution) and in those with baseline neutrophil counts below 1,500/mm³ or AIDS-related Kaposi's sarcoma with baseline neutrophil counts below 1,000/mm³.

NURSING CONSIDERATIONS

• Use cautiously in patients with hepatic impairment.
• Some patients experience peripheral neuropathies, which may be cumulative and dose-related. Patients with severe symptoms may need dosage reduction.

• I.M. route is preferred because it has the lowest risk of hepatotoxicity, coagulopathy, and GI and renal disorders.

• When administering I.M., limit volume administered at a single injection site to 2 ml. If volume to be administered exceeds 2 ml, use multiple injection sites.

• **Alert:** Monitor patient closely for hypersensitivity (including life-threatening anaphylaxis), especially those hypersensitive to other forms of L-asparaginase. As a routine precaution, keep patient under observation for 1 hour and have resuscitation equipment and other drugs needed to treat anaphylaxis (such as epinephrine, oxygen, and I.V. corticosteroids) readily available. Moderate to life-threatening hypersensitivity requires stopping L-asparaginase.

• To assess effects of therapy, monitor patient's peripheral blood count and bone marrow. A drop in circulating lymphoblasts is often noted after therapy starts, sometimes accompanied by a marked rise in uric acid levels.

• Obtain frequent amylase determinations to detect pancreatitis. Monitor patient's glucose level during therapy to detect hyperglycemia.

• Monitor patient for liver dysfunction when drug is used with hepatotoxic chemotherapeutic drugs.

• Drug may affect several plasma proteins; monitoring of fibrinogen, PT, INR, and PTT may be indicated.

PATIENT TEACHING
• Inform patient of risk of hypersensitivity reactions and importance of reporting them immediately.

• Tell patient not to take other drugs, including OTC preparations, until approved by prescriber because risk of bleeding is higher when pegaspargase is given with drugs such as aspirin. Pegaspargase may also increase toxicity of other drugs.

• Urge patient to report signs and symptoms of infection (fever, chills, and malaise); drug may have immunosuppressant effect.

• Caution woman of childbearing age to avoid pregnancy and breast-feeding during therapy.

porfimer sodium
Photofrin

Pregnancy risk category C

AVAILABLE FORMS
Injection: 75 mg/vial

INDICATIONS & DOSAGES
➤ **Palliative treatment for patients with completely obstructive esophageal cancer or for those with partially obstructive esophageal cancer who can't be satisfactorily treated with Nd:YAG laser therapy—**
Adults: 2 mg/kg I.V. for 3 to 5 minutes (first stage of therapy); then illumination with laser light 40 to 50 hours later (second stage). A second laser-light application may be given 96 to 120 hours after injection. Total of three courses (each course consisting of both stages) may be given, separated by at least 30 days.
➤ **Microinvasive endobronchial non–small-cell lung cancer in patients for whom surgery and radiotherapy aren't indicated—**
Adults: 2 mg/kg I.V. for 3 to 5 minutes (first stage of therapy); then illumination with laser light 40 to 50 hours later (second stage). A second laser-light application may be given 96 to 120 hours after injection. Total of three courses (each course consisting of both stages) may be given, separated by at least 30 days.

I.V. ADMINISTRATION
• Reconstitute each vial of porfimer with 31.8 ml of D_5W solution or normal saline solution for injection, resulting in final concentration of 2.5 mg/ml. Shake until dissolved. Don't mix porfimer with other drugs in same solution. Reconstituted drug is opaque. Inspect carefully for particulate and discoloration before use. Protect reconstituted drug from bright light, and use immediately.

• Administer drug as a single slow I.V. injection over 3 to 5 minutes.

• Take precautions to prevent extravasation at injection site. If it occurs, protect area from light.

ACTION

Photosensitizing drug that damages cancer cells through propagation of radical reactions. Tumor death occurs through ischemic necrosis secondary to vascular occlusion that appears to be partly mediated by release of thromboxane A_2. Cytotoxic and antitumor actions of porfimer depend on availability of light and oxygen.

Route	Onset	Peak	Duration
I.V.	Unknown	Unknown	Unknown

ADVERSE REACTIONS

CNS: anxiety, confusion, *insomnia,* asthenia.
CV: hypotension, hypertension, ***heart failure,*** atrial fibrillation, *chest pain,* tachycardia, edema.
EENT: *pharyngitis,* diplopia, photophobia.
GI: *constipation, abdominal pain, nausea, vomiting,* diarrhea, dyspepsia, dysphagia, eructation, esophageal edema, esophageal tumor bleeding, esophageal stricture, esophagitis, hematemesis, melena, anorexia.
GU: urinary tract infection, candidiasis.
Hematologic: *anemia.*
Metabolic: dehydration, weight loss.
Respiratory: cough, *dyspnea, pleural effusion, pneumonia,* respiratory insufficiency, tracheoesophageal fistula.
Skin: *photosensitivity reaction.*
Other: *back pain,* substantial or general pain, *fever,* surgical complication.

INTERACTIONS

Drug-drug. *Other photosensitizing drugs (griseofulvin, phenothiazines, sulfonamides, sulfonylurea hypoglycemics, tetracyclines, thiazide diuretics):* May increase photosensitivity reaction. Use together cautiously.
Drug-lifestyle. *Sun exposure:* May cause photosensitivity reaction. Advise patient to avoid excessive sunlight exposure.

EFFECTS ON LAB TEST RESULTS

• May decrease hemoglobin.

CONTRAINDICATIONS

Contraindicated in patients hypersensitive to porphyrins and in those with porphyria, tracheoesophageal or bronchoesophageal fistula, or tumor eroding into major blood vessel.

NURSING CONSIDERATIONS

• Breast-feeding isn't recommended during therapy because no data exist to demonstrate whether drug appears in breast milk.
• Safety and efficacy of drug in children haven't been established.
• Before each course of treatment, patient should be evaluated for a tracheoesophageal or bronchoesophageal fistula.
• Don't allow drug to contact eyes or skin during preparation or administration. Protect an exposed person from bright light.
• Patient must receive 630-nm wavelength laser-light therapy 40 to 50 hours after porfimer injection for drug to be effective. A second laser-light treatment (but not a second injection) may be given as early as 96 hours or as late as 120 hours after injection. Before a second treatment, residual tumor should be debrided; vigorous debridement may cause tumor bleeding. Monitor patient closely.
• Inflammation of treatment area may cause substernal chest pain. Notify prescriber if this occurs; pain may be sufficiently intense to warrant short-term use of opiate analgesics.
• Monitor CBC regularly to detect anemia. Drug and laser therapy may cause tumor bleeding.

PATIENT TEACHING

• Tell patient to avoid direct sunlight and bright indoor light for 30 days after injection, but tell him to expose skin to ambient indoor light. After 30 days, he should expose a small area of skin (not face) to sunlight for 10 minutes. If he doesn't develop a photosensitivity reaction (erythema, edema, blistering) within 24 hours, he can gradually and cautiously resume outdoor activities. If photosensitivity reaction occurs, he should avoid sunlight and bright indoor light for 2 weeks before retesting.
• Urge patient traveling to an area with stronger sun to retest his photosensitivity level.
• Warn patient that ultraviolet sunscreens don't protect against photosensitivity reaction.

• Advise patient to wear dark sunglasses with an average white light transmittance of less than 4% when outdoors.
• Caution woman of childbearing age to use an effective contraceptive method, avoid pregnancy, and notify prescriber of suspected pregnancy.

---

procarbazine hydrochloride
Matulane, Natulan†

Pregnancy risk category D

AVAILABLE FORMS
Capsules: 50 mg

INDICATIONS & DOSAGES
Dosages and indications vary. Check treatment protocol with prescriber.
➤ Adjunct treatment of Hodgkin's disease (stages III and IV), other cancers using MOPP (nitrogen mustard, vincristine, procarbazine, prednisone) regimen—
Adults: 2 to 4 mg/kg P.O. daily in single dose or divided doses for first week. Then, 4 to 6 mg/kg/day until WBC count falls below 4,000/mm^3, platelet count falls below 100,000/mm^3, or maximum response is obtained. Maintenance dose is 1 to 2 mg/kg/day after bone marrow recovery. For MOPP regimen, 100 mg/m^2/day P.O. for 14 days.
Children: 50 mg/m^2 P.O. daily for first week; then 100 mg/m^2 until response or toxicity occurs. Maintenance dose is 50 mg/m^2 P.O. daily after bone marrow recovery.

ACTION
Unknown. Thought to inhibit DNA, RNA, and protein synthesis.

Route	Onset	Peak	Duration
P.O.	Unknown	Unknown	Unknown

ADVERSE REACTIONS
CNS: nervousness, depression, headache, dizziness, *coma*, insomnia, nightmares, paresthesia, neuropathy, *hallucinations,* confusion, syncope.
CV: hypotension, tachycardia, flushing.
EENT: retinal hemorrhage, nystagmus, photophobia.

GI: *nausea, vomiting,* abdominal pain, hematemesis, melena, anorexia, stomatitis, dry mouth, dysphagia, diarrhea, constipation.
GU: hematuria, urinary frequency, nocturia.
Hematologic: *bleeding tendency, thrombocytopenia, leukopenia, anemia,* hemolytic anemia, *pancytopenia,* eosinophilia.
Hepatic: *hepatotoxicity.*
Respiratory: *pleural effusion,* cough, pneumonitis.
Skin: reversible alopecia, dermatitis, pruritus, rash, hyperpigmentation.
Other: gynecomastia, allergic reaction, herpes outbreak.

INTERACTIONS
Drug-drug. *CNS depressants:* Additive depressant effects. Avoid using together.
Digoxin: May decrease digoxin levels. Monitor digoxin levels closely.
Drugs high in tyramine, local anesthetics, MAO inhibitors, sympathomimetics, TCAs: May cause tremor, palpitations, increased blood pressure. Monitor patient closely.
Levodopa: Sudden hypertensive crisis may occur. Don't administer within 2 to 4 weeks of procarbazine.
Drug-food. *Caffeine:* May result in arrhythmias, severe hypertension. Discourage caffeine intake.
Foods high in tyramine (cheese, Chianti wine): May cause tremor, palpitations, increased blood pressure. Monitor patient closely; advise him to avoid or limit intake.
Drug-lifestyle. *Alcohol use:* Mild disulfiram-like reaction may cause flushing, headache, nausea, and hypotension. Warn patient to avoid alcoholic beverages.

EFFECTS ON LAB TEST RESULTS
• May increase eosinophil count. May decrease hemoglobin and platelet, WBC, and RBC counts.

CONTRAINDICATIONS
Contraindicated in patients hypersensitive to drug and in those with inadequate bone marrow reserve as shown by bone marrow aspiration.

Reactions may be *common*, uncommon, *life-threatening*, or **COMMON AND LIFE-THREATENING**.

NURSING CONSIDERATIONS

• Use cautiously in patients with impaired hepatic or renal function.
• Monitor CBC and platelet counts.
• To prevent bleeding, avoid all I.M. injections when platelet count is below 50,000/mm³.
• Anticipate need for blood transfusions to combat anemia. Patients may receive injections of RBC colony-stimulating factors to promote RBC production and decrease need for blood transfusions.
• Discontinue drug if patient becomes confused or if paresthesia or other neuropathies develop. Notify prescriber.

PATIENT TEACHING

• To decrease nausea and vomiting, advise patient to take drug at bedtime and in divided doses.
• Tell patient to watch for signs of infection (fever, sore throat, fatigue) and bleeding (easy bruising, nosebleeds, bleeding gums, melena). Tell patient to take temperature daily.
• Warn patient to avoid alcohol during therapy. Urge him to stop drug and check with prescriber immediately if he experiences a disulfiram-like reaction (chest pains, rapid or irregular heartbeat, severe headache, stiff neck).
• Instruct patient to avoid OTC medications that contain sympathomimetics. Also, tell him to avoid foods and drinks high in tyramine, such as wine, tea, coffee, cola, cheese, and bananas.
• Warn patient to avoid hazardous activities that require alertness and good motor coordination until CNS effects of drug are known.
• Caution woman of childbearing age to avoid becoming pregnant during therapy and to consult prescriber before becoming pregnant.

rituximab
Rituxan

Pregnancy risk category C

AVAILABLE FORMS

Injection: 10 mg/ml; 10-ml, 50-ml single-use, sterile vials

INDICATIONS & DOSAGES

➤ **Relapsed or refractory, low-grade or follicular, CD20-positive, B-cell non-Hodgkin's lymphoma—**
Adults: 375 mg/m² given as I.V. infusion once weekly for four doses (days 1, 8, 15, 22). Initial infusion should be started at 50 mg/hour. If hypersensitivity or infusion-related events don't occur, increase rate 50 mg/hour q 30 minutes, to maximum of 400 mg/hour. Subsequent infusions can be administered at 100 mg/hour initially and increased by increments of 100 mg/hour at 30-minute intervals, to maximum of 400 mg/hour, as tolerated.

I.V. ADMINISTRATION

• *Alert:* Drug must be given as I.V. infusion; don't give as I.V. push or bolus.
• Dilute to a final concentration of 1 to 4 mg/ml in bag of D_5W or normal saline solution. Gently invert bag to mix solution. Discard unused portion left in vial. Diluted solutions are stable for 24 hours if refrigerated and for 12 hours at room temperature.
• Monitor patient's blood pressure closely during infusion. If hypotension, bronchospasm, or angioedema occurs, stop infusion and restart at a 50% rate reduction when symptoms resolve.
• Stop infusion if serious or life-threatening arrhythmias occur. Patients who develop clinically significant arrhythmias should undergo cardiac monitoring during and after subsequent infusions of rituximab.

ACTION

A murine and human monoclonal antibody directed against CD20 antigen found on the surface of normal and malignant B lymphocytes. Binding to this antigen mediates the lysis of the B cells.

Route	Onset	Peak	Duration
I.V.	Variable	Variable	6-12 mo

ADVERSE REACTIONS

CNS: dizziness, *asthenia, headache,* fatigue, paresthesia, malaise, agitation, insomnia, hypesthesia, hypertonia, nervousness.

CV: *hypotension,* **arrhythmias,** hypertension, peripheral edema, chest pain, tachycardia, **bradycardia,** flushing.
EENT: sore throat, rhinitis, sinusitis, lacrimation disorder, conjunctivitis.
GI: *nausea,* vomiting, abdominal pain or enlargement, diarrhea, dyspepsia, anorexia, taste perversion.
Hematologic: LEUKOPENIA, *thrombocytopenia, neutropenia,* anemia.
Metabolic: hyperglycemia, hypocalcemia.
Musculoskeletal: myalgia, back pain.
Respiratory: *bronchospasm,* dyspnea, cough increase, bronchitis.
Skin: *pruritus, rash,* urticaria.
Other: ANGIOEDEMA, *fever, chills, rigors,* pain, pain at injection site, tumor pain.

INTERACTIONS
None significant.

EFFECTS ON LAB TEST RESULTS
• May increase glucose and LDH levels. May decrease calcium levels.
• May decrease hemoglobin and WBC, platelet, and neutrophil counts.

CONTRAINDICATIONS
Contraindicated in patients with type I hypersensitivity or anaphylactic reactions to murine proteins or components of rituximab.

NURSING CONSIDERATIONS
• Monitor patient closely for signs and symptoms of hypersensitivity. Have drugs, such as epinephrine, antihistamines, and corticosteroids, available to immediately treat such a reaction. Premedicate with acetaminophen and diphenhydramine before each infusion.
• Infusion-related reactions are most severe with the first infusion. Subsequent infusions are generally well tolerated.
• Obtain CBC at regular intervals and more frequently in patients who develop cytopenias.
• Protect vials from direct sunlight.

PATIENT TEACHING
• Tell patient to report symptoms of hypersensitivity, such as itching, rash, chills, or rigors, during and after infusion.
• Urge patient to watch for signs and symptoms of infection (fever, sore throat,

fatigue) and bleeding (easy bruising, nosebleeds, bleeding gums, melena). Tell patient to take temperature daily.

---

teniposide (VM-26)
Vumon

Pregnancy risk category D

AVAILABLE FORMS
Injection: 10 mg/ml

INDICATIONS & DOSAGES
➤ **Refractory childhood acute lymphoblastic leukemia—**
Children: Optimum dosage hasn't been established. Dosages ranging from 165 to 250 mg/m² I.V. once or twice weekly for 4 to 6 weeks have been used. Usually given with other drugs.
Adjust-a-dose: Patients with both Down syndrome and leukemia are at higher risk for myelosuppression. Administer first course of treatment at half the recommended dosage.

I.V. ADMINISTRATION
• Dilute drug in either D_5W or normal saline solution for injection to 0.1, 0.2, 0.4, or 1 mg/ml. Don't agitate vigorously; precipitation may occur. Discard cloudy solutions. Prepare and store drug in glass containers. Infuse over at least 30 to 60 minutes to prevent hypotension.
• Don't mix with other drugs or solutions. Heparin solution can cause precipitation. Flush administration apparatus and catheters with D_5W or normal saline solution before and after infusion of drug.
• Ensure careful placement of I.V. catheter. Extravasation can result in local tissue necrosis or sloughing.
• Occlusion of catheters, including those centrally placed, can occur, particularly during 24-hour infusions at 0.1 to 0.2 mg/ml. Monitor catheters carefully.
• Don't use a membrane-type in-line filter because diluent may dissolve it.
• Monitor blood pressure every 30 minutes during infusion. If systolic blood pressure falls below 90 mm Hg, stop infusion and notify prescriber.
• In normal saline solution or D_5W, concentrations of 0.1 to 0.4 mg/ml in glass

---

Reactions may be *common*, uncommon, *life-threatening*, or COMMON AND LIFE-THREATENING.

containers are chemically stable for at least 24 hours at room temperature or refrigerated.

• Follow institutional policy to reduce risks. Preparation and administration of parenteral form of drug are linked to carcinogenic, mutagenic, and teratogenic risks for personnel.

• Use non-DEHP (di[2-ethylhexyl] phthalate) containers and tubing for administration.

ACTION

A phase-specific cytotoxic drug that acts in the late S or early G_2 phase of the cell cycle, thus preventing cells from entering mitosis.

Route	Onset	Peak	Duration
I.V.	Unknown	Unknown	Unknown

ADVERSE REACTIONS

CV: hypotension.
GI: *nausea, vomiting, mucositis, diarrhea.*
Hematologic: MYELOSUPPRESSION, LEUKOPENIA, NEUTROPENIA, THROMBOCYTOPENIA, *anemia.*
Metabolic: hyperuricemia.
Skin: rash.
Other: *infection,* bleeding, hypersensitivity reactions, *phlebitis, extravasation at injection site.*

INTERACTIONS

Drug-drug. *Methotrexate:* May increase clearance and intracellular levels of methotrexate. Avoid using together.
Sodium salicylate, sulfamethizole, tolbutamide: May displace teniposide from protein-binding sites and increase toxicity. Avoid using together.

EFFECTS ON LAB TEST RESULTS

• May increase uric acid levels.
• May decrease hemoglobin and WBC, platelet, and neutrophil levels.

CONTRAINDICATIONS

Contraindicated in patients hypersensitive to drug or to polyoxyethylated castor oil, an injection vehicle.

NURSING CONSIDERATIONS

• Drug may be prescribed despite patient's history of hypersensitivity because therapeutic benefits outweigh risks. Treat such patients with antihistamines and corticosteroids before infusion begins, and observe continuously for first hour of infusion and at frequent intervals thereafter.

• Obtain baseline blood counts and renal and hepatic function tests.

• Monitor blood pressure before and during therapy. Hypotension can occur from rapid infusion.

• Have on hand diphenhydramine, hydrocortisone, epinephrine, and emergency equipment to establish an airway in case of anaphylaxis. Signs of hypersensitivity include chills, fever, urticaria, tachycardia, bronchospasm, dyspnea, hypotension, and flushing.

• Monitor blood counts and renal and hepatic function tests.

PATIENT TEACHING

• Advise patient to report any pain or burning at site of injection during or after administration.

• Tell patient to report signs and symptoms of infection (fever, sore throat, fatigue) and bleeding (easy bruising, nosebleeds, bleeding gums, melena). Tell patient to take temperature daily.

• Caution woman of childbearing age to avoid becoming pregnant during therapy and to consult prescriber before becoming pregnant.

topotecan hydrochloride
Hycamtin

Pregnancy risk category D

AVAILABLE FORMS

Injection: 4-mg single-dose vial

INDICATIONS & DOSAGES

➤ **Metastatic carcinoma of the ovary after failure of initial or subsequent chemotherapy—**
Adults: 1.5 mg/m² I.V. infusion given over 30 minutes daily for 5 consecutive days, starting on day 1 of a 21-day cycle. Minimum of four cycles should be given.

Skin: acne, *rash.*
Other: allergic reaction, herpes simplex, *chills, fever, flu syndrome, infection, pain.*

INTERACTIONS
Drug-drug. *Anthracyclines, cyclophosphamide:* Increased cardiotoxicity. Use together very cautiously.

EFFECTS ON LAB TEST RESULTS
● May decrease hemoglobin and WBC count.

CONTRAINDICATIONS
Contraindicated in patients with known hypersensitivity to the drug.

NURSING CONSIDERATIONS
● Use cautiously in elderly patients, in patients hypersensitive to drug or its components, and in those with cardiac dysfunction.
● Safety and effectiveness of drug in children haven't been established.
● Before beginning therapy, patient should undergo thorough baseline cardiac assessment, including history and physical examination and methods to identify risk of cardiotoxicity.
● Assess patient for signs and symptoms of cardiac dysfunction, especially if patient is receiving drug with anthracyclines and cyclophosphamide.
● Check for dyspnea, increased cough, paroxysmal nocturnal dyspnea, peripheral edema, or S_3 gallop. Treatment may be stopped in patients who develop a significant decrease in left ventricular function.
● Monitor patient receiving both drug and chemotherapy closely for cardiac dysfunction or failure, anemia, leukopenia, diarrhea, and infection.
● Drug should be used only in patients with metastatic breast cancer whose tumors have HER2 protein overexpression.
● Check for first-infusion symptom complex, commonly consisting of chills or fever. Treat with acetaminophen, diphenhydramine, and meperidine (with or without reducing rate of infusion). Other signs or symptoms include nausea, vomiting, pain, rigors, dizziness, dyspnea, hypotension, rash, and asthenia. These symptoms occur infrequently with subsequent infusions.

PATIENT TEACHING
● Tell patient about risk of first-dose infusion-related adverse reactions.
● Urge patient to notify prescriber immediately if signs or symptoms of cardiac dysfunction occur, such as shortness of breath, increased cough, or peripheral edema. Tell patient that these effects can occur after infusion is complete.
● Instruct patient to report adverse effects to prescriber.
● Advise breast-feeding woman to discontinue breast-feeding during drug therapy and for 6 months after last dose of drug.

---

tretinoin
Vesanoid

Pregnancy risk category D

AVAILABLE FORMS
Capsules: 10 mg

INDICATIONS & DOSAGES
➤ **Induction of remission in patients with acute promyelocytic leukemia (APL), French-American-British (FAB) classification M³ (including M³ variant), when anthracycline chemotherapy is contraindicated or unsuccessful—**
Adults and children age 1 and older: 45 mg/m²/day P.O. in two even doses. Therapy should be stopped 30 days after complete remission is documented or after 90 days of treatment, whichever occurs first.

ACTION
Unknown. Thought to induce differentiation of promyelocytic leukemic blasts, leading to apoptosis and remission induction.

Route	Onset	Peak	Duration
P.O.	Unknown	1-2 hr	Unknown

ADVERSE REACTIONS
CNS: dizziness, *paresthesia, anxiety, insomnia, depression, confusion,* **cerebral hemorrhage, CVA,** intracranial hypertension, agitation, hallucination, abnormal gait, agnosia, aphasia, asterixis, cerebellar edema, cerebellar disorders, *seizures,* **coma,** CNS depression, dysarthria, en-

cephalopathy, facial paralysis, hemiplegia, hyporeflexia, hypotaxia, lack of light reflex, neurologic reaction, spinal cord disorder, tremor, dementia, somnolence, slow speech, *fatigue, malaise, weakness.*

CV: *chest discomfort,* ARRHYTHMIAS, *hypotension, hypertension, phlebitis, edema,* **heart failure, MI,** *pericardial effusions, peripheral edema,* impaired myocardial contractility, progressive hypoxemia, enlarged heart, heart murmur, ischemia, myocarditis, pericarditis, secondary cardiomyopathy, *flushing.*

EENT: *earache, ear fullness,* hearing loss, *visual disturbances,* changed visual acuity, visual field defects, *ocular disorders.*

GI: mucositis, *GI hemorrhage, nausea, vomiting, anorexia, abdominal pain, GI disorders, diarrhea, constipation, dyspepsia, abdominal distention,* hepatosplenomegaly, ulcer.

GU: *renal insufficiency,* dysuria, **acute renal failure,** urinary frequency, renal tubular necrosis, enlarged prostate.

Hematologic: *leukocytosis,* HEMORRHAGE, **disseminated intravascular coagulation.**

Hepatic: **hepatitis,** *hypercholesterolemia, hypertriglyceridemia.*

Metabolic: fluid imbalance, acidosis, *weight gain or loss.*

Musculoskeletal: *myalgia, bone pain,* bone inflammation, flank pain.

Respiratory: *pneumonia, upper respiratory tract disorders, dyspnea, respiratory insufficiency, pleural effusion, rales, expiratory wheezing,* lower respiratory tract disorders, pulmonary infiltrates, bronchial asthma, pulmonary edema, laryngeal edema, pulmonary hypertension.

Skin: *rash, dry skin and mucous membranes, pruritus, alopecia, increased sweating, skin changes,* pallor.

Other: **retinoic acid–APL syndrome, septicemia, multiorgan failure,** *fever, infections, shivering,* cellulitis, facial edema, lymph disorder, hypothermia, ascites, *pain.*

INTERACTIONS
Drug-drug. *Ketoconazole:* May enhance tretinoin activity when taken together. Use together cautiously.

Drug-food. *Any food:* May enhance absorption of tretinoin. Advise patient to take drug with food.

EFFECTS ON LAB TEST RESULTS
● May increase cholesterol and triglyceride levels.
● May increase liver function test values and WBC count.

CONTRAINDICATIONS
Contraindicated in patients hypersensitive to retinoids or parabens, which is used as a preservative in gelatin capsule.

NURSING CONSIDERATIONS
● Drug isn't recommended for pregnant or breast-feeding women.
● Because patient with APL is at high risk of severe reactions, give drug under supervision of clinician with experience managing such patients and in a facility able to monitor drug tolerance and protect and maintain patient compromised by toxicity.
● Some patients receiving drug have experienced retinoic acid–APL syndrome, characterized by fever, dyspnea, weight gain, radiographic pulmonary infiltrates, and pleural or pericardial effusions. Notify prescriber immediately if these occur because the syndrome has occasionally been accompanied by impaired myocardial contractility and episodic hypotension with or without leukocytosis. Some patients have died from progressive hypoxemia and multiorgan failure. The syndrome typically occurs during first month of therapy. Prompt treatment with high-dose corticosteroids may reduce morbidity and mortality.
● Monitor CBC and platelet counts regularly. Patients with high WBC counts at diagnosis are at increased risk for further, rapid elevations. Rapidly evolving leukocytosis is linked to higher risk of life-threatening complications.
● Administer drug only to induce remission. Patients should receive standard consolidation or maintenance regimen after induction therapy.
● Monitor patient (especially child) for pseudotumor cerebri. Early evidence includes papilledema, headache, nausea, vomiting, and visual disturbances. Notify prescriber immediately if these occur.

• Monitor cholesterol and triglyceride levels and liver function studies, and report abnormalities.

• Maintain infection control and bleeding precautions, and provide prompt treatment.

• Make sure that pregnancy testing and contraception counseling are repeated monthly throughout therapy and for 1 month after therapy ends.

• **Alert:** Don't confuse tretinoin with trientine or Retin-A.

PATIENT TEACHING

• Explain infection control and bleeding precautions. Tell patient to notify prescriber about signs and symptoms of infection (fever, sore throat, fatigue) or bleeding (easy bruising, nosebleeds, bleeding gums, melena). Tell patient to take temperature daily.

• Inform woman that pregnancy test is needed 1 week before therapy begins and that therapy will be delayed, if possible, until a negative result is obtained.

• Instruct woman to use contraception during therapy and for 1 month after therapy ends, despite history of infertility or menopause, unless a hysterectomy has been performed. Recommend that she use two methods of contraception simultaneously, unless abstinence is the chosen method, and that she notify prescriber if pregnancy is suspected.

---

vinblastine sulfate (VLB)
Velban, Velbe†‡

Pregnancy risk category D

AVAILABLE FORMS
Injection: 10-mg vials (lyophilized powder), 1 mg/ml in 10-ml vials

INDICATIONS & DOSAGES
➤ **Breast or testicular cancer, Hodgkin's disease and malignant lymphoma, choriocarcinoma, lymphosarcoma, mycosis fungoides, Kaposi's sarcoma, histiocytosis—**
Adults: 3.7 mg/m² I.V. weekly. May increase to maximum dose of 18.5 mg/m² I.V. weekly based on response. Don't repeat dose if WBC count is below

4,000/mm³. Increase dosage at weekly intervals in increments of 1.8 mg/m² until desired therapeutic response is obtained, leukocyte count decreases to 3,000/mm³, or maximum weekly dose of 18.5 mg/m² is reached.
Children: Initial dose is 2.5 mg/m² I.V. weekly. Increase dosage by 1.25 mg/m² weekly until WBC count is below 3,000/mm³ or tumor response is seen. Maximum dose is 12.5 mg/m² I.V. weekly.
Adjust-a-dose: For patients with direct bilirubin over 3 mg/dl, reduce dose by 50%. For patients with recent exposure to radiation therapy or chemotherapy, single doses usually don't exceed 5.5 mg/m².

I.V. ADMINISTRATION
• Follow institutional policy to reduce risks. Preparation and administration of parenteral form of drug are linked to carcinogenic, mutagenic, and teratogenic risks for personnel.
• **Alert:** Drug is fatal if given intrathecally; it's for I.V. use only.
• Inject drug directly into vein or tubing of running I.V. line over 1 minute. Drug is a vesicant; if extravasation occurs, stop infusion immediately and notify prescriber. The manufacturer recommends that moderate heat be applied to area of leakage. Local injection of hyaluronidase may help disperse drug. Moderate heat may be applied on and off every 2 hours for 24 hours, with local injection of hydrocortisone or normal saline solution.
• Reconstitute drug in 10-mg vial with 10 ml of saline solution for injection. This yields 1 mg/ml. Refrigerate reconstituted solution. Protect solution from light and discard after 28 days.

ACTION
Arrests mitosis in metaphase, blocking cell division.

Route	Onset	Peak	Duration
I.V.	Unknown	Unknown	Unknown

ADVERSE REACTIONS
CNS: depression, *paresthesia, peripheral neuropathy and neuritis, numbness, loss of deep tendon reflexes, muscle pain and weakness,* headache, *CVA.*
CV: hypertension, *MI.*

Reactions may be *common*, uncommon, *life-threatening*, or COMMON AND LIFE-THREATENING.

EENT: pharyngitis.
GI: *nausea, vomiting,* bleeding ulcer, *constipation, ileus, anorexia,* diarrhea, abdominal pain, *stomatitis.*
Hematologic: *anemia,* **leukopenia, thrombocytopenia.**
Metabolic: hyperuricemia, *weight loss.*
Respiratory: **acute bronchospasm,** shortness of breath.
Skin: reversible alopecia, vesiculation.
Other: *irritation, phlebitis,* cellulitis, necrosis with extravasation.

INTERACTIONS
Drug-drug. *Erythromycin, other drugs that inhibit cytochrome P-450 pathway:* May increase toxicity of vinblastine. Monitor patient closely for toxicity.
Mitomycin: Increased risk of bronchospasm and shortness of breath. Monitor patient's respiratory status.
Phenytoin: Decreased plasma phenytoin levels. Monitor phenytoin levels closely.

EFFECTS ON LAB TEST RESULTS
● May increase uric acid levels.
● May decrease hemoglobin and WBC and platelet counts.

CONTRAINDICATIONS
Contraindicated in patients with severe leukopenia or bacterial infection or in patients hypersensitive to the drug.

NURSING CONSIDERATIONS
● Use cautiously in patients with hepatic dysfunction.
● To reduce nausea, give antiemetic before drug.
● Don't administer drug into a limb with compromised circulation.
● *Alert:* After administering drug, check for development of life-threatening acute bronchospasm. If this occurs, notify prescriber immediately. Reaction is most likely to occur in patients who are also receiving mitomycin.
● Monitor patient for stomatitis. Stop drug if stomatitis occurs and notify prescriber.
● Assess bowel activity. Give laxatives as needed and ordered. Stool softeners may be used prophylactically.
● Dosage shouldn't be repeated more frequently than every 7 days or severe leukopenia will occur. Nadir occurs on

days 4 to 10 and lasts another 7 to 14 days.
● Assess patient for numbness and tingling in hands and feet. Assess gait for early evidence of footdrop.
● Drug is less neurotoxic than vincristine.
● Anticipate a decrease in dosage by 50% if bilirubin levels exceed 3 mg/100 ml.
● Discontinue drugs known to cause urine retention for first few days after vinblastine therapy, particularly in elderly patients.
● *Alert:* Don't confuse vinblastine with vincristine, vindesine, or vinorelbine.

PATIENT TEACHING
● Tell patient to report evidence of infection (fever, sore throat, fatigue) and bleeding (easy bruising, nosebleeds, bleeding gums, melena). Tell patient to take temperature daily.
● Urge patient to report pain, swelling, burning, or any unusual feeling at injection site during infusion.
● Warn patient that alopecia may occur, but explain that it's usually reversible.
● Caution woman of childbearing age to avoid pregnancy during therapy.
● Tell patient that pain may occur in jaw and in organ containing tumor.

---

vincristine sulfate (VCR)
Oncovin, Vincasar PFS

Pregnancy risk category D

AVAILABLE FORMS
Injection: 1 mg/ml in 1-ml, 2-ml, 5-ml multidose vials; 1 mg/ml in 1-ml, 2-ml, 5-ml preservative-free vials

INDICATIONS & DOSAGES
➤ **Acute lymphoblastic and other leukemias, Hodgkin's disease, malignant lymphoma, neuroblastoma, rhabdomyosarcoma, Wilms' tumor—**
Adults: 0.4 to 1.4 mg/m^2 I.V. weekly. Maximum weekly dose is 2 mg.
Children weighing more than 10 kg (22 lb): 1.5 to 2 mg/m^2 I.V. weekly.
Children weighing 10 kg and less or with body surface area less than 1 m^2: Initially, 0.05 mg/kg I.V. weekly.

Adjust-a-dose: For patients with direct bilirubin over 3 mg/dl, reduce dose by 50%.

I.V. ADMINISTRATION

• Follow facility policy to reduce risks. Preparation and administration of parenteral form of drug are linked to carcinogenic, mutagenic, and teratogenic risks for staff.

• Inject directly into vein or tubing of running I.V. line slowly over 1 minute. Vincristine is a vesicant; if it extravasates, stop infusion immediately and notify prescriber. Apply heat on and off every 2 hours for 24 hours. Administer 150 units hyaluronidase to area of infiltrate.

• If protocol requires a continuous infusion of vincristine, a central line must be used.

ACTION

Arrests mitosis in metaphase, blocking cell division.

Route	Onset	Peak	Duration
I.V.	Unknown	Unknown	Unknown

ADVERSE REACTIONS

CNS: *peripheral neuropathy,* sensory loss, *loss of deep tendon reflexes, paresthesia, wristdrop and footdrop,* **seizures, coma,** headache, ataxia, cranial nerve palsies.
CV: hypotension, hypertension.
EENT: visual disturbances, blindness, diplopia, optic and extraocular neuropathy, ptosis, hoarseness, vocal cord paralysis, photophobia.
GI: diarrhea, *constipation, cramps,* ileus that mimics surgical abdomen, paralytic ileus, *nausea, vomiting,* anorexia, dysphagia, **intestinal necrosis,** *stomatitis.*
GU: urine retention, SIADH, dysuria, polyuria.
Hematologic: anemia, **leukopenia, thrombocytopenia.**
Metabolic: weight loss, hyponatremia.
Musculoskeletal: *jaw pain, muscle weakness and cramps.*
Respiratory: *acute bronchospasm,* dyspnea.
Skin: rash, reversible alopecia.
Other: fever, severe local reaction following extravasation, *phlebitis,* cellulitis at injection site.

INTERACTIONS

Drug-drug. *Asparaginase:* Decreased hepatic clearance of vincristine. Use together also may result in additive neurotoxicity. Check for toxicity.
Digoxin: Decreased digoxin effects. Monitor digoxin level.
Mitomycin: May increase frequency of bronchospasm and acute pulmonary reactions. Monitor patient's respiratory status.
Ototoxic drugs: May potentiate loss of hearing. Use together with extreme caution.
Phenytoin: May reduce phenytoin levels. Monitor phenytoin levels closely.

EFFECTS ON LAB TEST RESULTS

• May decrease sodium levels.
• May decrease hemoglobin and WBC and platelet counts.

CONTRAINDICATIONS

Contraindicated in patients hypersensitive to drug and in those with demyelinating form of Charcot-Marie-Tooth syndrome. Don't give to patients who are receiving radiation therapy through ports that include the liver.

NURSING CONSIDERATIONS

• Use cautiously in patients with hepatic dysfunction, neuromuscular disease, or infection.
• Don't administer 5-mg vial as a single dose. The 5-mg vials are for multiple-dose use.
• **Alert:** After administering drug, check for life-threatening acute bronchospasm. If this occurs, notify prescriber immediately. This reaction is most likely to occur in those also receiving mitomycin.
• Check for hyperuricemia, especially in patients with leukemia or lymphoma. Maintain hydration and administer allopurinol to prevent uric acid nephropathy. Check for toxicity.
• Monitor fluid intake and output. Fluid restriction may be needed if SIADH develops.
• Because of risk of neurotoxicity, drug shouldn't be given more often than once weekly. Children are more resistant to neurotoxicity than adults. Neurotoxicity is dose-related and usually reversible. Some neurotoxicities may be permanent.

Reactions may be *common,* uncommon, *life-threatening,* or **COMMON AND LIFE-THREATENING.**

• Check for depression of Achilles tendon reflex, numbness, tingling, footdrop or wristdrop, difficulty in walking, ataxia, and slapping gait. Also check ability to walk on heels. Support patient when walking.
• Monitor bowel function. Give stool softener or laxative or water before giving dose. Constipation may be an early sign of neurotoxicity.
• All vials (1-mg, 2-mg, 5-mg) contain 1-mg/ml solution and should be refrigerated.
• Discontinue drugs known to cause urine retention, particularly in elderly patients, for first few days after vincristine therapy.
• *Alert:* Drug is fatal if given intrathecally; it's for I.V. use only.
• *Alert:* Don't confuse vincristine with vinblastine or vindesine.

PATIENT TEACHING
• Advise patient to report any pain or burning at site of injection during or after administration.
• Tell patient to report evidence of infection (fever, sore throat, fatigue) and bleeding (easy bruising, nosebleeds, bleeding gums, melena). Tell patient to take temperature daily.
• Warn patient that alopecia may occur, but explain that it's usually reversible.
• Caution woman of childbearing age to avoid becoming pregnant during therapy and to consult prescriber before becoming pregnant.

---

vinorelbine tartrate
Navelbine

Pregnancy risk category D

AVAILABLE FORMS
Injection: 10 mg/ml, 50 mg/5 ml

INDICATIONS & DOSAGES
➤ Alone or as adjunct therapy with cisplatin for first-line treatment of ambulatory patients with nonresectable advanced non–small-cell lung cancer (NSCLC); alone or with cisplatin in stage IV of NSCLC; with cisplatin in stage III of NSCLC—
Adults: 30 mg/m^2 I.V. weekly. In combination treatment, same dosage with

120 mg/m^2 of cisplatin given on days 1 and 29, then q 6 weeks.
Adjust-a-dose: If granulocyte count is 1,000 to 1,499 cells/mm^3, give 50% of dose. If less than 1,000 cells/mm^3, dose is withheld. If total bilirubin is 2.1 to 3.0 mg/dl, reduce dose by 50%; if more than 3.0, give 25% of dose.

I.V. ADMINISTRATION
• Dilute drug before use to 1.5 to 3 mg/ml with D$_5$W or normal saline solution in a syringe. Or, dilute to 0.5 to 2 mg/ml in an I.V. bag. Administer drug I.V. over 6 to 10 minutes into side port of a free-flowing I.V. line that is closest to I.V. bag; then flush with 75 to 125 ml or more of D$_5$W or normal saline solution.
• Drug may be stored for up to 24 hours at room temperature.
• Avoid extravasation when administering vinorelbine because drug can cause considerable irritation, localized tissue necrosis, and thrombophlebitis. If extravasation occurs, stop drug immediately and inject remaining dose into a different vein; notify prescriber.

ACTION
A semisynthetic vinca alkaloid that exerts its primary antineoplastic effect by disrupting microtubule assembly, which in turn disrupts spindle formation and prevents mitosis.

Route	Onset	Peak	Duration
I.V.	Unknown	Unknown	Unknown

ADVERSE REACTIONS
CNS: *peripheral neuropathy, asthenia, fatigue.*
CV: chest pain.
GI: *nausea, vomiting, anorexia, diarrhea, constipation, stomatitis.*
Hematologic: **bone marrow suppression, agranulocytosis,** LEUKOPENIA, **thrombocytopenia,** anemia, **granulocytopenia.**
Hepatic: hyperbilirubinemia.
Musculoskeletal: myalgia, arthralgia, jaw pain, loss of deep tendon reflexes.
Respiratory: dyspnea.
Skin: *alopecia,* rash.
Other: *injection pain or reaction.*

• Protect drug from light.
• No adequate, well-controlled studies in pregnant women exist. Use anakinra in pregnant women only if clearly needed.
• It isn't known whether drug appears in milk. Use cautiously in breast-feeding women.
• Safety and efficacy in patients with juvenile rheumatoid arthritis haven't been established.
• Use drug cautiously in elderly patients because they have a greater risk of infection and are more likely to have renal impairment.

PATIENT TEACHING

• Tell patient to store drug in refrigerator and not to freeze or expose to excessive heat. Advise letting drug come to room temperature before giving a dose.
• Teach patient the proper dosage and administration.
• Urge patient to rotate injection sites.
• Teach proper disposal of syringes in a puncture-resistant container. Also, caution patient not to reuse needles.
• Review the signs and symptoms of allergic and other adverse reactions, especially signs of serious infections. Urge patient to contact the prescriber if they arise.
• Inform patient that injection site reactions are common, are usually mild, and typically last 14 to 28 days.
• Tell patient to avoid live-virus vaccines while taking anakinra.

azathioprine
Imuran, Thioprine‡

Pregnancy risk category D

AVAILABLE FORMS
Powder for injection: 100 mg
Tablets: 50 mg

INDICATIONS & DOSAGES
➤ **Immunosuppression in kidney transplantation—**
Adults: Initially, 3 to 5 mg/kg P.O. or I.V. daily, usually beginning on day of transplantation. Maintained at 1 to 3 mg/kg daily based on patient response and tolerance.

Adjust-a-dose: Give drug in lower doses to patients with oliguria in the posttransplant period and for those with impaired renal function.
➤ **Severe, refractory rheumatoid arthritis—**
Adults: Initially, 1 mg/kg P.O. as single dose or divided into two doses. Usual dose is 50 to 100 mg. If patient response isn't satisfactory after 6 to 8 weeks, dosage may be increased by 0.5 mg/kg daily to maximum of 2.5 mg/kg daily at 4-week intervals.

I.V. ADMINISTRATION
• Reconstitute drug in 100-mg vial with 10 ml of sterile water for injection. Inspect for particles before use.
• Drug may be given by direct I.V. injection or further diluted in normal saline solution for injection or D$_5$W solution and infused over 30 to 60 minutes.
• Use only in patients who can't tolerate oral drugs.

ACTION
Unknown, but thought to cause variable alterations in antibody production.

Route	Onset	Peak	Duration
I.V., P.O.	Unknown	Unknown	Unknown

ADVERSE REACTIONS
GI: *nausea, vomiting, **pancreatitis**,* steatorrhea, diarrhea, abdominal pain.
Hematologic: LEUKOPENIA, *myelosuppression,* anemia, *pancytopenia,* THROMBOCYTOPENIA, *immunosuppression.*
Hepatic: *hepatotoxicity,* jaundice.
Musculoskeletal: arthralgia, myalgia.
Skin: rash, alopecia.
Other: *infections,* fever, *increased risk of neoplasia.*

INTERACTIONS
Drug-drug. *ACE inhibitors:* Combination may cause severe leukopenia. Monitor patient closely.
Allopurinol: Impaired inactivation of azathioprine. Decrease azathioprine to one-third to one-quarter normal dose.
Cyclosporine: Plasma cyclosporine levels may be increased. Monitor cyclosporine levels closely.

Methotrexate: May increase plasma levels of methotrexate metabolite. Monitor patient closely.

Nondepolarizing neuromuscular blockers: Azathioprine may reverse the neuromuscular blockade. Monitor patient closely.

Other myelopoiesis drugs: Exaggerated leukopenia, especially in renal transplant patients. Monitor patient closely.

Warfarin: Azathioprine may decrease action of warfarin. Monitor patient closely.

EFFECTS ON LAB TEST RESULTS
● May increase AST, ALT, alkaline phosphatase, and bilirubin levels. May decrease uric acid levels.
● May decrease hemoglobin and WBC, RBC, and platelet counts.

CONTRAINDICATIONS
Contraindicated in patients hypersensitive to drug or its components.

NURSING CONSIDERATIONS
● Use cautiously in patients with hepatic or renal dysfunction.
● Give drug after meals to minimize adverse GI effects.
● To prevent bleeding, avoid all I.M. injections when platelet count is below 100,000/mm³.
● Monitor CBC and platelet counts weekly for 1 month; then twice monthly. Notify prescriber if counts drop suddenly or become dangerously low. Drug may need to be temporarily withheld.
● Watch for early signs and symptoms of hepatotoxicity, such as clay-colored stools, dark urine, pruritus, and yellow skin and sclera; and for increased alkaline phosphatase, bilirubin, AST, and ALT levels.
● Therapeutic response usually occurs within 8 weeks.
● Benefits must be weighed against risk when giving to patient with systemic viral infection, such as chickenpox or herpes zoster.
● Patients with rheumatoid arthritis previously treated with alkylating drugs, such as cyclophosphamide, chlorambucil, or melphalan, may have a prohibitive risk of neoplasia if treated with azathioprine.
● Drug shouldn't be used for treating rheumatoid arthritis in pregnant women.

● **Alert:** Don't confuse azathioprine with azidothymidine, Azulfidine, or azatadine; don't confuse Imuran with Inderal.

PATIENT TEACHING
● Warn patient to report even mild infections (colds, fever, sore throat, malaise) because drug is a potent immunosuppressant.
● Instruct patient to avoid conception during therapy and for 4 months after therapy stops.
● Warn patient that some thinning of hair is possible.
● Tell patient taking drug for refractory rheumatoid arthritis that it may take up to 12 weeks to be effective.
● Advise patient to report unusual bleeding or bruising.
● Tell patient that drug may be taken with food to decrease nausea.
● Advise patient to use soft toothbrush and perform oral care cautiously.

basiliximab
Simulect

Pregnancy risk category B

AVAILABLE FORMS
Injection: 20-mg vials

INDICATIONS & DOSAGES
➤ **Prophylaxis of acute organ rejection in patients receiving renal transplantation when used as part of an immunosuppressive regimen that includes cyclosporine and corticosteroids—**
Adults and children weighing 35 kg (77 lb) or more: 20 mg I.V. given within 2 hours before transplant surgery and 20 mg I.V. given 4 days after transplantation.
Children weighing less than 35 kg: 10 mg I.V. given within 2 hours before transplant surgery and 10 mg I.V. given 4 days after transplantation.
NOTE: The second dose of basiliximab should be withheld if hypersensitivity reactions occur.

I.V. ADMINISTRATION
● Reconstitute with 5 ml sterile water for injection. Shake vial gently to dissolve powder. Dilute reconstituted solution to

volume of 50 ml with normal saline solution or D5W for infusion. When mixing solution, gently invert bag to avoid foaming. Don't shake.

• Infuse over 20 to 30 minutes via a central or peripheral vein. Don't add or infuse other drugs simultaneously through same I.V. line.

• Drug may be given as a bolus injection; however, this method of administration is associated with nausea, vomiting and local reactions, including pain.

• Use reconstituted solution immediately; may be refrigerated at 36° to 46° F (2° to 8° C) for up to 24 hours or kept at room temperature for 4 hours.

ACTION

Binds specifically to and blocks the interleukin (IL)-2 receptor alpha chain on the surface of activated T lymphocytes, inhibiting IL-2-mediated activation of lymphocytes, a critical pathway in the cellular immune response involved in allograft rejection.

Route	Onset	Peak	Duration
I.V.	Unknown	Immediate	Unknown

ADVERSE REACTIONS

CNS: agitation, anxiety, *asthenia,* depression, *dizziness, headache,* hypoesthesia, *insomnia,* neuropathy, paresthesia, *tremor,* fatigue.
CV: angina pectoris, **arrhythmias,** atrial fibrillation, **heart failure,** chest pain, abnormal heart sounds, aggravated hypertension, *hypertension,* hypotension, tachycardia, *leg or peripheral edema,* generalized edema.
EENT: abnormal vision, cataract, conjunctivitis, *rhinitis, pharyngitis,* sinusitis.
GI: *abdominal pain, candidiasis, constipation, diarrhea, dyspepsia,* esophagitis, enlarged abdomen, flatulence, gastroenteritis, GI disorder, **GI hemorrhage,** gum hyperplasia, melena, *nausea,* ulcerative stomatitis, *vomiting.*
GU: abnormal renal function, albuminuria, bladder disorder, *dysuria,* frequent micturition, genital edema, hematuria, *increased nonprotein nitrogen,* oliguria, renal tubular necrosis, ureteral disorder, *urinary tract infection,* urinary retention, impotence.

Hematologic: *anemia,* hematoma, **hemorrhage,** polycythemia, purpura, **thrombocytopenia,** thrombosis.
Metabolic: *acidosis,* dehydration, diabetes mellitus, fluid overload, hypercalcemia, *hypercholesterolemia, hyperglycemia, hyperkalemia,* hyperlipemia, *hyperuricemia, hypocalcemia, hypokalemia, hypomagnesemia, hypophosphatemia, hypoproteinemia, weight gain.*
Musculoskeletal: arthralgia, arthropathy, *back pain,* bone fracture, cramps, hernia, *leg pain,* myalgia.
Respiratory: abnormal chest sounds, bronchitis, **bronchospasm,** *cough, dyspnea,* pneumonia, pulmonary disorder, **pulmonary edema,** upper respiratory tract infection.
Skin: *acne,* cyst, hypertrichosis, pruritus, rash, skin disorder or ulceration.
Other: accidental trauma, *viral infection,* infection, **sepsis,** *fever, surgical wound complications,* herpes zoster, herpes simplex, **hypersensitivity reactions.**

INTERACTIONS
None significant.

EFFECTS ON LAB TEST RESULTS
• May increase calcium, cholesterol, glucose, lipids, and uric acid levels. May decrease magnesium, phosphorus, and protein levels. May increase or decrease potassium levels.
• May increase RBC count. May decrease hemoglobin and platelet count.

CONTRAINDICATIONS
Contraindicated in patients hypersensitive to drug or its components.

NURSING CONSIDERATIONS
• Use cautiously and only under supervision of prescriber qualified and experienced in immunosuppressive therapy and managing organ transplantation.
• Use cautiously in elderly patients.
• Severe acute hypersensitivity reactions can occur within 24 hours after initial exposure or reexposure to basiliximab. Drugs for treating hypersensitivity reactions should be available for immediate use and the second dose of basiliximab should be withheld if hypersensitivity reactions occur.

Reactions may be *common,* uncommon, **life-threatening,** or COMMON AND LIFE-THREATENING.

• Check for electrolyte imbalances and acidosis during drug therapy.
• Monitor patient's intake and output, vital signs, hemoglobin level, and hematocrit during therapy.
• Be alert for signs and symptoms of opportunistic infections during drug therapy.

PATIENT TEACHING
• Inform patient of potential benefits of and risks related to immunosuppressive therapy, including decreased risk of graft loss or acute rejection. Advise patient that immunosuppressive therapy increases risks of developing lymphoproliferative disorders and opportunistic infections. Tell him to report signs and symptoms of infection promptly.
• Inform woman of childbearing age to use effective contraception before therapy starts and for 2 months after therapy ends.
• Instruct patient to report adverse effects immediately.
• Explain that drug is used with cyclosporine and corticosteroids.

---

cyclosporine
Neoral, Sandimmune, Sandimmun‡

cyclosporine, modified
Gengraf

Pregnancy risk category C

AVAILABLE FORMS
Capsules: 25 mg, 50 mg, 100 mg
Capsules for microemulsion: 25 mg, 50 mg
Injection: 50 mg/ml
Oral solution: 100 mg/ml

INDICATIONS & DOSAGES
➤ **Prophylaxis of organ rejection in kidney, liver, or heart transplantation—**
Adults and children: 15 mg/kg P.O. 4 to 12 hours before transplantation and continued daily for 1 to 2 weeks postoperatively. Then reduce dosage by 5% each week to maintenance level of 5 to 10 mg/kg/day. Or, 5 to 6 mg/kg I.V. concentrate 4 to 12 hours before transplantation given as a continuous infusion. Postoperatively, repeat dose daily until patient can tolerate P.O. forms.

For conversion from Sandimmune to Gengraf, use same daily dose as previously used for Sandimmune. Monitor blood levels every 4 to 7 days after conversion along with blood pressure and creatinine level every 2 weeks during the first 2 months.
➤ **Severe, active rheumatoid arthritis that hasn't adequately responded to methotrexate (Gengraf and Neoral only)—**
Adults: 2.5 mg/kg/day P.O., taken b.i.d. as divided dose. Dosage may be increased by 0.5 to 0.75 mg/kg/day after 8 weeks and again after 12 weeks to a maximum of 4 mg/kg/day. If no response is seen after 16 weeks, discontinue therapy.
➤ **Psoriasis (Gengraf and Neoral only)—**
Adults: 1.25 mg/kg P.O. b.i.d. for at least 4 weeks. Dosage may be increased by 0.5 mg/kg/day once every 2 weeks p.r.n. to a maximum dose of 4 mg/kg/day.
Adjust-a-dose: For patients with such adverse effects as hypertension, elevated creatinine level (30% above pretreatment level), or abnormal CBC and liver function test results, decrease dosage by 25% to 50%.

I.V. ADMINISTRATION
• Give cyclosporine I.V. concentrate at one-third oral dose, and dilute before use.
• Dilute each ml of concentrate in 20 to 100 ml of D_5W or normal saline solution for injection. Dilute immediately before use; infuse over 2 to 6 hours.
• I.V. administration is usually reserved for patients who can't tolerate oral drugs.
• Protect I.V. solution from light.

ACTION
Unknown. Thought to inhibit proliferation and function of T lymphocytes and inhibit production and release of lymphokines.

Route	Onset	Peak	Duration
I.V.	Unknown	Unknown	Unknown
P.O.	Unknown	1.5-3.5 hr	Unknown

ADVERSE REACTIONS
CNS: *tremor, headache,* confusion, paresthesia.

CV: *hypertension,* flushing.
EENT: *gum hyperplasia,* oral thrush, sinusitis.
GI: *nausea, vomiting,* diarrhea, abdominal discomfort.
GU: NEPHROTOXICITY.
Hematologic: anemia, *leukopenia, thrombocytopenia.*
Hepatic: *hepatotoxicity.*
Metabolic: increased low-density lipoprotein levels, hyperglycemia.
Skin: *hirsutism,* acne.
Other: *infections, anaphylaxis,* gynecomastia.

INTERACTIONS
Drug-drug. *Acyclovir, aminoglycosides, amphotericin B, cimetidine, co-trimoxazole, diclofenac, gentamycin, ketoconazole, melphalan, NSAIDs, ranitidine, sulfamethoxazole/trimethoprim, tacrolimus, tobramycin, vancomycin:* Increased risk of nephrotoxicity. Avoid using together.
Allopurinol, bromocriptine, cimetidine, clarithromycin, danazol, diltiazem, erythromycin, fluconazole, imipenem-cilastatin, itraconazole, ketoconazole, methylprednisolone, metoclopramide, nicardipine, prednisolone, verapamil: May increase blood levels of cyclosporine. Monitor patient for increased toxicity.
Azathioprine, corticosteroids, cyclophosphamide, verapamil: Increased immunosuppression. Monitor patient closely.
Carbamazepine, isoniazid, nafcillin, octreotide, phenobarbital, phenytoin, rifabutin, rifampin, ticlopidine: Decreased immunosuppressant effect from low cyclosporine levels. Cyclosporine dosage may need to be increased.
Digoxin, lovastatin, prednisolone: Decreased clearance of these drugs. Use together cautiously.
Potassium-sparing diuretics: Cyclosporine may induce hyperkalemia. Monitor patient closely.
Vaccines: Decreased immune response. Postpone routine immunization.
Drug-herb. *Alfalfa sprouts, astragulus, echinacea, licorice:* May interfere with immunosuppressive effect. Discourage use together.
St. John's wort: May reduce cyclosporine levels, resulting in decrease in efficacy. Discourage use together.

Drug-food. *Grapefruit and grapefruit juices:* Decreased metabolism and increased blood levels of cyclosporine. Discourage patient from taking together.
High-fat meals: Neoral absorption may be decreased by a high-fat meal. Urge patient to take on empty stomach.

EFFECTS ON LAB TEST RESULTS
• May increase BUN, creatinine, LDL, bilirubin, AST, ALT, and glucose levels.
• May decrease hemoglobin and WBC and platelet counts.

CONTRAINDICATIONS
Contraindicated in patients hypersensitive to drug or polyoxyethylated castor oil (found in injectable form). Contraindicated in patients with rheumatoid arthritis or psoriasis with abnormal renal function, uncontrolled hypertension or malignancies (Neoral or Gengraf). Psoriasis patients shouldn't receive PUVA or UVB therapy, methotrexate, other immunosuppressants, coal tar, or radiation (Neoral or Gengraf).

NURSING CONSIDERATIONS
• Cyclosporine can cause nephrotoxicity and hepatotoxicity.
• Drug typically is given once or twice daily.
• Neoral has greater bioavailability than Sandimmune. Less Neoral may be needed to provide blood level derived from Sandimmune. Monitor blood levels when switching patients between these two brands.
• Gengraf and Sandimmune aren't bioequivalent and can't be interchanged without prescriber supervision. Conversion of Gengraf to Sandimmune should be done with increased monitoring to prevent underdosing.
• Gengraf is bioequivalent to and interchangeable with Neoral capsules.
• Always give cyclosporine with adrenal corticosteroids.
• For treatment of rheumatoid arthritis or psoriasis, use Neoral or Gengraf.
• Before starting treatment in patients with rheumatoid arthritis, obtain blood pressure measurements (on at least two occasions) and two creatinine levels to estimate baseline. Evaluate blood pressure and creatinine every 2 weeks during initial 3

Reactions may be *common,* uncommon, *life-threatening,* or COMMON AND LIFE-THREATENING.

months, then monthly if the patient is stable. Monitor blood pressure and creatinine level after an increase in NSAID dosage or introduction of a new NSAID. Monitor CBC and liver function tests monthly if patient also receives methotrexate. If hypertension occurs, decrease dosage of Gengraf or Neoral by 25% to 50%. If hypertension persists, decrease dosage further or control blood pressure with antihypertensives.

• Psoriasis patients previously treated with PUVA, methotrexate, immunosuppressants, UVB, coal tar, or radiation therapy are at increased risk for developing skin malignancies when taking Gengraf and Neoral.

• Initially for psoriasis patients, obtain blood pressure measurements on at least two occasions. Evaluate patient for occult infection and tumors initially and throughout treatment. Obtain baseline creatinine level (on two occasions), CBC, and BUN, magnesium, uric acid, potassium, and lipid levels. Evaluate creatinine and BUN levels every 2 weeks during initial 3 months and then monthly thereafter if patient is stable. If creatinine level is 25% above pretreatment levels, repeat creatinine measurement within 2 weeks. If creatinine level stays 25% to 50% above baseline, dosage is reduced by 25% to 50%. If at any time the creatinine level is 50% above baseline, dosage should be reduced by 25% to 50%. Discontinue if creatinine level isn't reversed after two dosage modifications. Monitor creatinine level after increasing NSAID dose or after starting a new NSAID. Evaluate blood pressure, CBC, and uric acid, potassium, lipid, and magnesium levels every 2 weeks for the first 3 months, then monthly if patient is stable, or more frequently when dosage adjustments are made. Dosage should be reduced by 25% to 50% for an abnormality of clinical concern.

• Improvement in psoriasis may not be evident until after 12 to 16 weeks of therapy.

• Measure oral solution doses carefully in an oral syringe. To increase palatability, conventional oral solution may be mixed with milk, chocolate milk, or orange juice. Oral cyclosporine solution for emulsion may be mixed with orange or apple juice (avoid grapefruit juice). Solution for emulsion is less palatable when mixed with milk. Use a glass container to mix, and have patient drink at once. Don't rinse dosing syringe with water. If syringe needs cleaning, it must be completely dry before reuse.

• Monitor elderly patient for renal impairment and hypertension.

• Monitor blood pressure every 2 weeks for the first 3 months of therapy, then monthly if stable.

• Monitor cyclosporine blood levels at regular intervals. Absorption of cyclosporine oral solution can be erratic.

• Monitor BUN and creatinine levels. Nephrotoxicity may develop 2 to 3 months after transplant surgery, possibly requiring dosage reduction. Notify prescriber about signs or symptoms of nephrotoxicity. Prescriber must differentiate between transplanted kidney rejection and cyclosporine-induced nephrotoxicity.

• **Alert:** Don't confuse cyclosporine with cyclophosphamide or cycloserine; don't confuse Sandimmune with Sandoglobulin or Sandostatin.

PATIENT TEACHING
• Encourage patient to take drug at same time each day, and teach him how to measure dosage and mask taste of oral solution, if prescribed. Tell him not to take cyclosporine with grapefruit juice.

• Instruct patient to fill glass with water after dose and drink it to make sure he consumes all of drug.

• Advise patient to take drug with meals if nausea occurs.

• Advise patient to take Neoral or Gengraf on an empty stomach.

• Tell patient being treated for psoriasis that improvement may not occur until after 12 to 16 weeks of therapy.

• Stress that drug shouldn't be stopped without prescriber's approval.

• Explain to patient the importance of frequent laboratory monitoring while receiving therapy.

• Tell patient to avoid people with infections because drug lowers resistance to infection.

• Warn patient that during the use of cyclosporine, vaccination may be less effective.

GI: *nausea, vomiting, diarrhea,* hiccups, epigastric pain, abdominal distention, stomatitis.
GU: renal ARTERY stenosis.
Hematologic: LEUKOPENIA, THROMBO-CYTOPENIA, hemolysis, *aplastic anemia.*
Metabolic: hyperglycemia.
Musculoskeletal: *arthralgia, myalgia.*
Respiratory: *dyspnea, **pulmonary edema.***
Skin: *rash, pruritus, urticaria.*
Other: febrile reactions, hypersensitivity reactions, serum sickness, *anaphylaxis,* infections, night sweats, lymphadenopathy, chills.

INTERACTIONS
None significant.

EFFECTS ON LAB TEST RESULTS
• May increase liver enzyme and glucose levels.
• May decrease hemoglobin and WBC and platelet counts.

CONTRAINDICATIONS
Contraindicated in patients hypersensitive to drug.

NURSING CONSIDERATIONS
• Use cautiously in patients receiving additional immunosuppressive therapy (such as corticosteroids or azathioprine) because of increased risk of infection.
• An intradermal skin test is recommended at least 1 hour before first dose. Marked local swelling or erythema larger than 10 mm indicates increased risk of severe systemic reaction such as anaphylaxis. Severe reactions to skin test, such as hypotension, tachycardia, dyspnea, generalized rash, or anaphylaxis, usually preclude further use of drug.
• Monitor patient for hypotension, respiratory distress, and chest, flank, or back pain, which may indicate anaphylaxis or hemolysis.
• Keep airway adjuncts and anaphylaxis drugs at bedside during administration.
• Watch for signs and symptoms of infection, such as fever, sore throat, malaise.

PATIENT TEACHING
• Instruct patient to report adverse drug reactions promptly, especially signs and symptoms of infection (fever, sore throat, fatigue).
• Tell patient to immediately report discomfort at I.V. insertion site because drug can cause a chemical phlebitis.
• Advise woman of childbearing age to avoid pregnancy during therapy.

muromonab-CD3
Orthoclone OKT3

Pregnancy risk category C

AVAILABLE FORMS
Injection: 1 mg/1 ml in 5-ml ampules

INDICATIONS & DOSAGES
➤ **Acute allograft rejection in renal transplant patients; in corticosteroid-resistant hepatic or cardiac allograft rejection—**
Adults: 5 mg I.V. bolus once daily for 10 to 14 days.

I.V. ADMINISTRATION
• Draw solution into syringe through low protein-binding 0.2- or 0.22-micron filter. Discard filter and attach needle for I.V. bolus injection.
• Give bolus in less than 1 minute.

ACTION
A murine monoclonal antibody that reacts in the T-lymphocyte membrane with a molecule (CD3) needed for antigen recognition. Depletes the blood of CD3+ T cells, which leads to restoration of allograft function and reversal of rejection.

Route	Onset	Peak	Duration
I.V.	Immediate	Unknown	1 wk

ADVERSE REACTIONS
CNS: *tremor, headache, **seizures, encephalopathy, cerebral edema, aseptic meningitis.***
CV: *chest pain, tachycardia,* hypertension, ***cardiac arrest,*** hypotension, ***shock, heart failure.***
EENT: *blindness, blurred vision, tinnitus, otitis media, conjunctivitis.*
GI: *nausea, vomiting, diarrhea.*
GU: oliguria, anuria.

Reactions may be *common*, uncommon, *life-threatening*, or COMMON AND LIFE-THREATENING.

Respiratory: *severe pulmonary edema, dyspnea, wheezing,* **adult respiratory distress syndrome.**
Other: *fever, chills, tremors,* **INFECTION, anaphylaxis, cytokine release syndrome, risk of neoplasia.**

INTERACTIONS

Drug-drug. *Immunosuppressants:* Increased risk of infection. Use cautiously; consider reduced immunosuppressant dosage.
Indomethacin: Increased muromonab-CD3 levels with encephalopathy and other CNS effects. Monitor patient closely.
Live-virus vaccines: May increase replication and effects. Use with extreme caution.

EFFECTS ON LAB TEST RESULTS
● May increase BUN and creatinine levels.

CONTRAINDICATIONS
Contraindicated in patients hypersensitive to drug or other products of murine (mouse) origin and in those who have history of seizures or are predisposed to seizures. Also contraindicated in those who have antimurine antibody titers of 1:1,000 or more or fluid overload, as evidenced by chest X-ray or weight gain greater than 3% within the week before treatment. Don't use in pregnant or breast-feeding women.

NURSING CONSIDERATIONS
● Obtain chest X-ray within 24 hours before starting drug treatment.
● Assess patient for signs and symptoms of fluid overload before treatment.
● Treatment should begin in facility equipped and staffed for cardiopulmonary resuscitation and where patient can be monitored closely.
● Most adverse reactions develop within 30 minutes to 6 hours after first dose.
● Before administering drug, give an antipyretic to help lower risk of expected pyrexia and chills. Treat temperature exceeding 100° F (38° C) with antipyretics before drug administration, and evaluate risk of infection.
● Give corticosteroids before first injection to help decrease risk of adverse reactions. Methylprednisolone sodium succinate (1 mg/kg) before injection, then hydrocorti-

sone sodium succinate (100 mg) 30 minutes after injection, have been recommended to alleviate severity of first-dose reaction.
● Patients develop antibodies to muromonab-CD3 that can lead to loss of effectiveness and more severe adverse reactions if a second course of therapy is attempted. Therefore, some prescribers believe that drug should be used for only a single course of treatment.
● Drug may cause abnormal urine cytologic study results.

PATIENT TEACHING
● Inform patient of expected adverse reactions.
● Reassure patient that reactions will diminish as treatment progresses.
● Tell patient to avoid people with infections because drug lowers resistance to infection.
● Advise woman to avoid pregnancy during therapy.

---

mycophenolate mofetil
CellCept

mycophenolate mofetil hydrochloride
CellCept Intravenous

Pregnancy risk category C

AVAILABLE FORMS
mycophenolate mofetil
Capsules: 250 mg
Tablets: 500 mg
mycophenolate mofetil hydrochloride
Injection: 500 mg/vial

INDICATIONS & DOSAGES
➤ **Prophylaxis of organ rejection in patients receiving allogenic renal transplants—**
Adults: 1 g P.O. or I.V. b.i.d. with corticosteroids and cyclosporine.
Adjust-a-dose: For patients with severe chronic renal impairment outside of immediate posttransplant period, avoid doses above 1 g b.i.d. If neutropenia develops, interrupt or reduce dosing.

➤ **Prophylaxis of organ rejection in patients receiving allogenic cardiac transplant**—
Adults: 1.5 g P.O. or I.V. b.i.d. with cyclosporine and corticosteroids.
✱ *NEW INDICATION:* **Prophylaxis of organ rejection, with cyclosporine and corticosteroids, in patients receiving allogenic hepatic transplants**—
Adults: 1 g I.V. b.i.d. over no less than 2 hours or 1.5 g P.O. b.i.d.

I.V. ADMINISTRATION
• CellCept Intravenous must be reconstituted and diluted to 6 mg/ml using 14 ml of D_5W.
• Never give drug by rapid or bolus I.V. injection. Infuse drug over at least 2 hours.
• Use within 4 hours of reconstitution and dilution.
• Drug is incompatible with other I.V. solutions.

ACTION
Inhibits proliferative response of T and B lymphocytes, suppresses antibody formation by B lymphocytes, and may inhibit recruitment of leukocytes into sites of inflammation and graft rejection.

Route	Onset	Peak	Duration
I.V.	Unknown	Unknown	10-17 hr
P.O.	Unknown	0.5-1.25 hr	7.5-18 hr

ADVERSE REACTIONS
CNS: *tremor,* insomnia, dizziness, *headache,* asthenia.
CV: *chest pain, hypertension, edema.*
EENT: pharyngitis.
GI: *diarrhea, constipation, nausea, dyspepsia, vomiting, oral candidiasis, abdominal pain,* **hemorrhage.**
GU: *urinary tract infection, hematuria,* renal tubular necrosis.
Hematologic: *anemia,* LEUKOPENIA, THROMBOCYTOPENIA, hypochromic anemia, leukocytosis.
Metabolic: *hypercholesterolemia, hypophosphatemia, hypokalemia, hyperkalemia, hyperglycemia.*
Musculoskeletal: *back pain.*
Respiratory: *dyspnea, cough, infection,* bronchitis, pneumonia.
Skin: *acne,* rash.

Other: *pain, fever, infection,* **sepsis,** *peripheral edema.*

INTERACTIONS
Drug-drug. *Acyclovir, ganciclovir, other drugs that undergo renal tubular secretion:* Increased risk of toxicity for both drugs. Monitor patient closely.
Antacids with magnesium and aluminum hydroxides: Decreased mycophenolate absorption. Separate administration times.
Azathioprine: Hasn't been clinically studied. Monitor patient closely when used together.
Cholestyramine: May interfere with enterohepatic recirculation, reducing mycophenolate bioavailability. Avoid use together.
Phenytoin, theophylline: May increase both drug levels. Monitor drug levels closely.
Probenecid, salicylates: May increase mycophenolate levels. Monitor patient closely.

EFFECTS ON LAB TEST RESULTS
• May increase cholesterol and glucose levels. May decrease phosphorous level. May increase or decrease potassium level.
• May decrease hemoglobin and platelet counts. May increase or decrease WBC count.

CONTRAINDICATIONS
Contraindicated in patients hypersensitive to drug, its ingredients, or mycophenolic acid and in patients sensitive to polysorbate 80.

NURSING CONSIDERATIONS
• Drug isn't recommended for use in pregnant women (unless benefits to mother outweigh risks to fetus) or breast-feeding women.
• Use cautiously in patients with GI disorders.
• Safety and effectiveness of drug in children haven't been established.
• Start drug therapy within 24 hours after transplantation. I.V. form is recommended for patients unable to take oral forms.
• I.V. form can be given for up to 14 days; switch patient to capsules or tablets as soon as oral drugs can be tolerated.

Reactions may be *common,* uncommon, *life-threatening,* or COMMON AND LIFE-THREATENING.

• Avoid doses above 1 g b.i.d. after immediate posttransplant period in patients with severe chronic renal impairment.
• Because of potential teratogenic effects, don't open or crush capsule. Avoid inhaling powder in capsule or having it contact skin or mucous membranes. If such contact occurs, wash thoroughly with soap and water, and rinse eyes with water.

PATIENT TEACHING
• Warn patient not to open or crush capsules, but to swallow them whole on an empty stomach.
• Stress importance of not interrupting or stopping therapy without first consulting prescriber.
• Inform woman that pregnancy test is needed 1 week before therapy begins.
• Instruct woman of childbearing age to use two forms of contraception during therapy and for 6 weeks afterward, even with a history of infertility, unless a hysterectomy has been performed or abstinence is the chosen method. Tell her to notify prescriber immediately if she suspects pregnancy.
• Warn patient of the increased risk of lymphoma and other malignancies.

---

sirolimus
Rapamune

Pregnancy risk category C

AVAILABLE FORMS
Oral solution: 1 mg/ml
Tablet: 1 mg

INDICATIONS & DOSAGES
➤ **Prophylaxis of organ rejection in patients receiving renal transplants with cyclosporine and corticosteroids—**
Adults and adolescents: Initially, 6 mg P.O. as one-time dose as soon as possible after transplantation; then maintenance dose of 2 mg P.O. once daily.
Children age 13 and older weighing less than 40 kg (88 lb): Initial dose is 3 mg/m^2 P.O. as one-time dose after transplantation; then 1 mg/m^2 P.O. once daily.
Adjust-a-dose: For patients with mild to moderate hepatic impairment, reduce

maintenance dose by about one-third. It isn't necessary to reduce loading dose.

ACTION
An immunosuppressant that inhibits T-lymphocyte activation and proliferation that occurs in response to antigenic and cytokine stimulation. Also inhibits antibody formation.

Route	Onset	Peak	Duration
P.O.	Unknown	1-3 hr	Unknown

ADVERSE REACTIONS
CNS: *headache, insomnia, tremor, anxiety, depression, asthenia,* malaise, syncope, confusion, dizziness, emotional lability, hypertonia, hypesthesia, hypotonia, neuropathy, paresthesia, somnolence.
CV: *hypertension,* **heart failure, atrial fibrillation,** tachycardia, hypotension, *chest pain, edema,* **hemorrhage,** palpitations, peripheral vascular disorder, thrombophlebitis, thrombosis, vasodilatation, *peripheral edema.*
EENT: facial edema, *pharyngitis,* epistaxis, rhinitis, sinusitis, abnormal vision, cataract, conjunctivitis, deafness, ear pain, otitis media, tinnitus.
GI: *diarrhea, nausea, vomiting, constipation, abdominal pain, dyspepsia,* hernia, enlarged abdomen, ascites, peritonitis, anorexia, dysphagia, eructation, esophagitis, flatulence, gastritis, gastroenteritis, gingivitis, gum hyperplasia, ileus, mouth ulceration, oral candidiasis, stomatitis.
GU: dysuria, hematuria, albuminuria, *kidney tubular necrosis,* urinary tract infection, pelvic pain, glycosuria, bladder pain, hydronephrosis, impotence, kidney pain, nocturia, oliguria, pyuria, scrotal edema, testis disorder, *toxic nephropathy,* urinary frequency, urinary incontinence, urinary retention.
Hematologic: *anemia,* THROMBOCYTO-PENIA, *leukopenia, thrombotic thrombocytopenia purpura,* ecchymosis, leukocytosis, polycythemia.
Metabolic: *hypercholesteremia, hyperlipidemia, hypokalemia, weight gain, hypophosphatemia, hyperkalemia,* hypervolemia, Cushing's syndrome, diabetes mellitus, acidosis, dehydration, hypercalcemia, hyperglycemia, hyperphosphate-

---

mia, hypocalcemia, hypoglycemia, hypomagnesemia, hyponatremia, weight loss.
Musculoskeletal: *back pain, arthralgia,* myalgia, arthrosis, bone necrosis, leg cramps, osteoporosis, tetany.
Respiratory: *dyspnea, cough, atelectasis, upper respiratory tract infection,* asthma, bronchitis, hypoxia, lung edema, pleural effusion, pneumonia.
Skin: *rash, acne,* hirsutism, fungal dermatitis, pruritus, skin hypertrophy, skin ulcer, sweating.
Other: *fever, pain,* abscess, cellulitis, chills, flu syndrome, infection, ***sepsis,*** lymphadenopathy, abnormal healing.

INTERACTIONS
Drug-drug. *Aminoglycosides, amphotericin B, other nephrotoxic drugs:* Increased risk of nephrotoxicity. Use with caution.
Bromocriptine, cimetidine, clarithromycin, clotrimazole, danazol, erythromycin, fluconazole, indinavir, itraconazole, metoclopramide, nicardipine, ritonavir, verapamil, other drugs that inhibit CYP 3A4: May increase blood levels of sirolimus. Monitor sirolimus levels closely.
Carbamazepine, phenobarbital, phenytoin, rifabutin, rifapentine, other drugs that induce CYP 3A4: May decrease blood levels of sirolimus. Monitor patient closely.
Cyclosporine (oral solution and capsules): Increased sirolimus levels. Give sirolimus 4 hours after cyclosporine. After long-term administration, sirolimus may reduce cyclosporine clearance, requiring reduction in cyclosporine dosage.
Diltiazem: Increased sirolimus levels. Monitor sirolimus levels, as needed.
Ketoconazole: Increased rate and extent of sirolimus absorption. Avoid using together.
Live-virus vaccines (BCG; measles; mumps, rubella; oral polio; yellow fever; varicella; TY21a typhoid): Reduced vaccine effectiveness. Avoid using together.
Rifampin: Decreased sirolimus levels. Alternative therapy to rifampin may be prescribed.
Drug-food. *Grapefruit juice:* Decreased metabolism of sirolimus. Discourage patient from taking together.

EFFECTS ON LAB TEST RESULTS
• May increase BUN, creatinine, liver enzyme, cholesterol, and lipid levels. May decrease sodium and magnesium levels. May increase or decrease phosphate, potassium, glucose, and calcium levels.
• May increase RBC count. May decrease hemoglobin and platelet count. May increase or decrease WBC count.

CONTRAINDICATIONS
Contraindicated in patients hypersensitive to active drug, its derivatives, or components of product.

NURSING CONSIDERATIONS
• Use cautiously in patients with hyperlipidemia and impaired liver or renal function.
• Drug should be prescribed only by prescribers experienced in immunosuppressive therapy and management of renal transplant patients.
• Drug should be used in regimen with cyclosporine and corticosteroids; it should be taken 4 hours after cyclosporine dose.
• Drug should be taken consistently either with or without food.
• Dilute drug before use. After dilution, use immediately and discard syringe.
• When diluting oral solution, empty correct amount into glass or plastic (not Styrofoam) container holding at least ¼ cup (60 ml) of either water or orange juice. Don't use grapefruit juice or other liquids. Stir vigorously and have patient drink immediately. Refill container with at least ½ cup (120 ml) of water or orange juice, stir again, and have patient drink all contents.
• After transplantation, antimicrobial prophylaxis for *Pneumocystis carinii* and cytomegalovirus should be given for 1 year and 3 months, respectively.
• ***Alert:*** Patients taking drug are more susceptible to infection and lymphoma.
• Monitor renal function tests, because use with cyclosporine may cause creatinine levels to increase. Adjustment of immunosuppressive regimen may be needed.
• Monitor cholesterol and triglyceride levels. Treatment with lipid-lowering drugs during therapy isn't uncommon. If hyperlipidemia is detected, additional interventions, such as diet and exercise, should begin.

Reactions may be *common*, uncommon, ***life-threatening***, or **COMMON AND LIFE-THREATENING**.

• Check for rhabdomyolysis.

• Monitor drug levels in patients age 13 and older who weigh less than 40 kg, patients with hepatic impairment, patients also receiving drugs that induce or inhibit CYP 3A4, and patients in whom cyclosporine dosing is markedly reduced or discontinued.

• A slight haze may develop during refrigeration. This doesn't affect potency of drug. If haze develops, bring to room temperature and shake until haze disappears.

• Store away from light, and refrigerate at 36° to 46° F (2° to 8° C). After opening bottle, use contents within 1 month. If needed, store bottles and pouches at room temperature (up to 77° F [25° C]) for several days. Drug may be kept in oral dosing syringe for 24 hours at room temperature.

PATIENT TEACHING

• Tell patient how to properly store, dilute, and give drug.

• Advise woman of childbearing age about risks during pregnancy. Tell her to use effective contraception before and during therapy, and for 12 weeks after stopping therapy.

• Tell patient to take drug consistently with or without food to minimize absorption variability.

• Tell patient to take drug 4 hours after cyclosporine to avoid drug interactions.

• Advise patient to wash area with soap and water if drug solution touches skin or mucous membranes.

tacrolimus (FK506)
Prograf

Pregnancy risk category C

AVAILABLE FORMS
Capsules: 1 mg, 5 mg
Injection: 5 mg/ml

INDICATIONS & DOSAGES
➤ **Prophylaxis of organ rejection in allogenic liver or kidney transplants—**
Adults: 0.03 to 0.05 mg/kg/day I.V. as continuous infusion given no sooner than 6 hours after transplantation. Substitute P.O. therapy as soon as possible, with first oral dose given 8 to 12 hours after discontinuing I.V. infusion. Or, give P.O. dose within 24 hours of transplantation after renal function has recovered. Recommended initial P.O. dose for allogenic liver transplants is 0.1 to 0.15 mg/kg/day P.O. in two divided doses q 12 hours. Recommended initial P.O. dose for allogenic kidney transplants is 0.2 mg/kg/day in two divided doses q 12 hours. Adjust dosages based on clinical response.
Children: Initially, 0.03 to 0.05 mg/kg/day I.V.; then 0.15 to 0.2 mg/kg/day P.O. on schedule similar to adults, adjusted p.r.n.
Adjust-a-dose: Give lowest recommended I.V. and P.O. dosages to patients with renal or hepatic impairment.

I.V. ADMINISTRATION

• Dilute drug with normal saline solution for injection or D₅W injection to 0.004 to 0.02 mg/ml before use. Store diluted infusion solution for up to 24 hours in glass or polyethylene containers. Don't store drug in a polyvinyl chloride container because of decreased stability and potential for extraction of phthalates.

• Monitor patient continuously during first 30 minutes of I.V. administration and frequently thereafter for signs and symptoms of anaphylaxis.

ACTION
Exact mechanism unknown. Inhibits T-lymphocyte activation, which results in immunosuppression.

Route	Onset	Peak	Duration
I.V., P.O.	Unknown	1.5-3.5 hr	Unknown

ADVERSE REACTIONS
CNS: *headache, tremor, insomnia, paresthesia, delirium,* **coma,** *asthenia.*
CV: hypertension, *peripheral edema.*
GI: *diarrhea, nausea, vomiting, constipation, anorexia, abdominal pain, ascites.*
GU: *abnormal renal function, urinary tract infection, oliguria.*
Hematologic: *anemia, leukocytosis,* THROMBOCYTOPENIA.
Metabolic: *hyperkalemia, hypokalemia, hyperglycemia, hypomagnesemia.*
Musculoskeletal: *back pain.*
Respiratory: *pleural effusion, atelectasis, dyspnea.*

promotes active immunity to tuberculosis (TB).

Route	Onset	Peak	Duration
Percutaneous	Unknown	Unknown	Unknown

ADVERSE REACTIONS
Musculoskeletal: osteomyelitis.
Other: lymphadenopathy, allergic reaction, *anaphylaxis.*

INTERACTIONS
Drug-drug. *Immunosuppressants:* May reduce response to BCG vaccine. Avoid using together.
Isoniazid, rifampin, streptomycin: Inhibited multiplication of BCG. Avoid using together.

EFFECTS ON LAB TEST RESULTS
None reported.

CONTRAINDICATIONS
Contraindicated in patients hypersensitive to vaccine. Also contraindicated in patients with hypogammaglobulinemia, patients with immunosuppression and a positive tuberculin reaction (when meant for use as immunoprophylactic after exposure to TB), patients with fresh smallpox vaccinations, patients with burns, and patients receiving corticosteroid therapy. Avoid use in pregnant women.

NURSING CONSIDERATIONS
• Don't inject vaccine I.V., S.C., or I.D.
• Use cautiously in patients with chronic skin disease. Inject only into healthy skin.
• Obtain history of allergies and reaction to immunization.
• Keep epinephrine 1:1,000 available to treat anaphylaxis.
• Don't shake vial after reconstitution. Use within 2 hours.
• Don't give to febrile patients unless cause is known.
• Expect lesions in 7 to 14 days. Papules reach maximum diameter of 3 mm, then fade.
• Allow at least 6 to 8 weeks between BCG and live-virus vaccines; give killed-virus vaccines 7 days before or 10 days after BCG.

• Vaccine is of no value as immunoprophylactic in patients with positive tuberculin test.
   Tuberculin sensitivity may be rendered positive by BCG intravesical treatment. Determine patient's reactivity to tuberculin before therapy.
• Destroy live vaccine by autoclaving or treating with formaldehyde solution before disposal.

PATIENT TEACHING
• Advise patient to have tuberculin skin test 2 to 3 months after BCG vaccination.
• Tell patient to report unusual signs and symptoms after vaccination, or signs of allergic reaction, including difficulty breathing, enlarged lymph nodes, or skin ulcer or lesion at injection site.
• Urge patient to keep site dry for 24 hours and not to expose area to others because live vaccine may infect them.

cholera vaccine

Pregnancy risk category C

AVAILABLE FORMS
Injection: Suspension of killed *Vibrio cholerae* (each ml contains 8 units of Inaba and Ogawa serotypes) in 1.5-ml and 20-ml vials

INDICATIONS & DOSAGES
➤ **Primary immunization for persons traveling to areas where cholera is endemic or epidemic—**
I.M. or S.C. route
Adults and children older than age 10: Two doses of 0.5 ml I.M. or S.C., 1 week to 1 month apart, before traveling in cholera area. Booster is 0.5 ml q 6 months, p.r.n.
Children ages 5 to 10: 0.3 ml I.M. or S.C. Boosters of same dose should be given q 6 months, p.r.n.
Children ages 6 months to 4 years: 0.2 ml I.M. or S.C. Boosters of same dose should be given q 6 months, p.r.n.
I.D. route
Adults and children age 5 and older: Two doses of 0.2 ml I.D., 1 week to 1 month apart, and q 6 months, p.r.n.

ACTION

Promotes active immunity to cholera.

Route	Onset	Peak	Duration
I.D., I.M., S.C.	After second dose	Unknown	3-6 mo

ADVERSE REACTIONS

CNS: headache, malaise.
Skin: *erythema, swelling, pain, induration at injection site.*
Other: fever, *anaphylaxis.*

INTERACTIONS

Drug-drug. *Plague, typhoid, other vaccines with systemic adverse reactions:* Increased toxicity. Don't use together.
Yellow fever vaccine: Simultaneous use may interfere with immune response to both vaccines. Give 3 weeks apart.

EFFECTS ON LAB TEST RESULTS

None reported.

CONTRAINDICATIONS

Contraindicated in those with acute illness or history of severe systemic reaction or allergic response to vaccine.

NURSING CONSIDERATIONS

• Obtain history of allergies and reaction to immunization.
• Keep epinephrine 1:1,000 available to treat anaphylaxis.
• Shake vial vigorously before withdrawing each dose.
• Give vaccine I.M. in deltoid muscle in adults and children older than age 3.
• Don't give vaccine I.M. to patients with thrombocytopenia or other coagulation disorders that contraindicate I.M. injection.
• I.M. and S.C. routes give higher levels of protection in children younger than age 5.
• Vaccine is about 50% effective in reducing clinical illness risk for 3 to 6 months.

PATIENT TEACHING

• Advise patient that pain, induration, and swelling at injection site are common for 24 to 48 hours.

• Tell traveler to avoid food and water that may be contaminated.
• Advise patient that malaise, headache, and mild to moderate fever may persist for 1 to 2 days.

---

diphtheria and tetanus toxoids and acellular pertussis vaccine adsorbed (DTaP)

Certiva, Infanrix, Tripedia

Pregnancy risk category C

AVAILABLE FORMS

Injection: 6.7 Lf units diphtheria, 5 Lf units tetanus, and 46.8 mcg pertussis antigens per 0.5 ml in single-dose and 7.5-ml vials; 15 Lf units of diphtheria toxoid, 6 Lf units tetanus toxoid, and 40 mcg pertussis toxoid per 0.5 ml in 7.5-ml vials; 25 Lf units of diphtheria toxoid, 10 Lf units tetanus toxoid, 25 mcg pertussis toxin, 25 mcg FHA, 8 mcg peractin per 0.5 ml in 0.5-ml vials

INDICATIONS & DOSAGES

➤ **Primary immunization—**
Children ages 6 weeks to 7 years: Give 0.5 ml I.M. 4 to 8 weeks apart for three doses and a fourth dose at least 6 months after the third dose.
➤ **Booster immunization—**
If Tripedia was used for the first four doses, a fifth dose is recommended at 4 to 6 years of age before entering school. If the fourth dose was given after age 4, a fifth dose isn't needed.

Certiva as a fourth dose is recommended at 15 to 20 months of age in children who received their first three doses as whole-cell DTP vaccine. A fifth dose is recommended at 4 to 6 years of age in children who received four doses of whole-cell DTP vaccine or three doses of whole-cell vaccine followed by one dose of DTaP, unless the fourth dose was given after the fourth birthday.

Infanrix is recommended as a fifth dose in children 4 to 6 years of age before entering school in those who received one dose or more of whole-cell DTP unless

---

the fourth dose was given after the fourth birthday.

ACTION
Promotes active immunity to diphtheria, tetanus, and pertussis (DTP) by inducing production of antitoxins and antibodies.

Route	Onset	Peak	Duration
I.M.	2 wk after last dose	Unknown	10 yr

ADVERSE REACTIONS
CNS: *seizures, encephalopathy,* peripheral neuropathy, *drowsiness.*
GI: *vomiting, anorexia.*
Skin: *soreness at injection site, redness,* nodule remaining several weeks at injection site, urticaria.
Other: *anaphylaxis, shock,* thrombocytopenic purpura, *fever,* hypersensitivity reactions.

INTERACTIONS
Drug-drug. *Immunosuppressants:* May reduce response to DTP vaccine. Avoid using together.

EFFECTS ON LAB TEST RESULTS
None reported.

CONTRAINDICATIONS
Contraindicated in immunosuppressed patients and in those on corticosteroid therapy or with history of seizures. Children whose seizures are well controlled or those with an explained single-episode seizure may receive the acellular vaccine. Defer vaccination in patients with acute febrile illness. Children with preexisting neurologic disorders shouldn't receive pertussis component. Also, children who exhibit neurologic signs after injection shouldn't receive pertussis component in any succeeding injections. Give diphtheria and tetanus toxoids (called DT) instead. Not recommended for adults or children older than age 7.

NURSING CONSIDERATIONS
• *Alert:* Vaccine isn't routinely given to individuals age 7 and older; it may only be used in special circumstances.

• Obtain history of allergies and reaction to immunization, especially to pertussis vaccine.
• Keep epinephrine 1:1,000 available to treat anaphylaxis.
• Give only by deep I.M. injection, preferably in thigh or deltoid muscle. Don't give S.C.
• In infants, give I.M. injection in the anterolateral thigh.
• Vaccine may be given at same time as trivalent oral polio vaccine and, if indicated, when the patient receives vaccines against *Haemophilus influenzae* type b, measles, mumps, and rubella.
• Acellular vaccine may be linked to a lower risk of local pain and fever.
• *Alert:* DTaP preparations are generally not interchangeable. It's recommended to use the vaccine from the same manufacturer, if possible, for at least the first three doses.

PATIENT TEACHING
• Explain risks and benefits of vaccine to parents before it's given.
• Tell parents to report systemic reactions promptly; remind them that local reactions are common. Acetaminophen in age-appropriate dosing will decrease occurrence of postvaccination fever in children prone to febrile seizure activity.
• Stress importance of keeping scheduled appointments for subsequent doses. Full immunization requires a series of injections.

Haemophilus b conjugate vaccines

Haemophilus b conjugate vaccine, diphtheria CRM$_{197}$ protein conjugate (HbOC)
HibTITER

Haemophilus b conjugate vaccine, diphtheria toxoid conjugate (PRP-D)
Prohibit

Haemophilus b conjugate vaccine, meningococcal protein conjugate (PRP-OMP)
Pedvaxhib

Pregnancy risk category C

AVAILABLE FORMS
***Haemophilus* b conjugate vaccine, diphtheria CRM$_{197}$ protein conjugate**
Injection: 10 mcg of purified *Haemophilus* b saccharide and about 25 mcg CRM$_{197}$ protein per 0.5 ml
***Haemophilus* b conjugate vaccine, diphtheria toxoid conjugate**
Injection: 25 mcg of *Haemophilus influenzae* type B (HIB) capsular polysaccharide and 18 mcg of diphtheria toxoid protein per 0.5 ml
***Haemophilus* b conjugate vaccine, meningococcal protein conjugate**
Injection: 7.5 mcg of *Haemophilus* b PRP and 125 mcg *Neisseria meningitidis* OMPC per 0.5 ml
Powder for injection: 15 mcg of *Haemophilus* b PRP, 250 mcg *N. meningitidis* OMPC per dose

INDICATIONS & DOSAGES
➤ **Immunization against HIB infection—**
Conjugate vaccine, diphtheria CRM$_{197}$ protein conjugate
Infants: 0.5 ml I.M. at age 2 months. Repeated at 4 months and 6 months. Booster dose given at age 15 months.
Previously unvaccinated infants ages 2 to 6 months: 0.5 ml I.M. Repeated in 2 months and again in 4 months for total of three doses. Booster dose given at age 15 months.
Previously unvaccinated infants ages 7 to 11 months: 0.5 ml I.M. Repeated in 2 months, for a total of two doses. Booster dose given at age 15 months (but no sooner than 2 months after last vaccination).
Previously unvaccinated infants ages 12 to 14 months: 0.5 ml I.M. Booster dose given at age 15 months (but no sooner than 2 months after first vaccination).
Previously unvaccinated children ages 15 to 71 months: 0.5 ml I.M. Booster dose isn't needed.

Conjugate vaccine, diphtheria toxoid conjugate
Previously unvaccinated children ages 15 to 71 months: 0.5 ml I.M. Booster dose isn't needed. Not recommended for use in children younger than age 15 months.
Conjugate vaccine, meningococcal protein conjugate
Infants: 0.5 ml I.M. at age 2 months. Repeated at 4 months. Booster dose given at age 12 months.
Previously unvaccinated infants ages 2 to 6 months: 0.5 ml I.M. Repeated in 2 months. Booster dose given at age 12 months.
Previously unvaccinated infants ages 7 to 11 months: 0.5 ml I.M. Repeated in 2 months. Booster dose given at age 15 months (but no sooner than 2 months after last vaccination).
Previously unvaccinated infants ages 12 to 14 months: 0.5 ml I.M. Booster dose given at age 15 months (but no sooner than 2 months after first vaccination).
Previously unvaccinated children ages 15 to 71 months: 0.5 ml I.M. Booster dose isn't needed.

Premature infants follow same schedule as full-term infants.

ACTION
Promotes active immunity to HIB; is a polymer of ribose, ribitol, and phosphate (PRP); and is linked by covalent bonds to highly antigenic substances, enabling the vaccine to promote an immune response in infants.

Route	Onset	Peak	Duration
I.M.	2 wk after last dose	Unknown	Several yr

ADVERSE REACTIONS
GI: diarrhea, vomiting.
Skin: *erythema, pain at injection site.*
Other: *anaphylaxis,* fever, crying.

INTERACTIONS
Drug-drug. *Immunosuppressants:* May suppress antibody response to HIB vaccine. Defer immunization.

EFFECTS ON LAB TEST RESULTS
None reported.

CONTRAINDICATIONS

Contraindicated in patients hypersensitive to vaccine or its components and in those with acute illness.

NURSING CONSIDERATIONS

• HIB is an important cause of meningitis in infants and preschool children.
• Immunization against HIB infection is recommended for children with HIV infections. Follow usual immunization schedule.
• Vaccine and DTP may be given simultaneously. A combination product is commercially available.
• Diphtheria toxoid conjugate vaccine (Prohibit) isn't recommended in children younger than age 15 months.
• Vaccine isn't routinely given to adults or children older than age 5 unless they're at high risk for infection (including patients with chronic conditions, such as functional asplenia, splenectomy, Hodgkin's disease, or sickle cell anemia).
• Keep epinephrine 1:1,000 available to treat anaphylaxis.
• Don't give vaccine I.D. or I.V.; give it I.M.
• *Alert:* Don't give to febrile children.
• Give vaccine into anterolateral aspect of upper thigh in small children. Injections may be made into deltoid muscle of larger children if sufficient muscle is present.
• Drug may interfere with interpretation of antigen detection tests used to diagnose systemic HIB disease.

PATIENT TEACHING

• Warn patient or parents that pain may occur at injection site.
• Tell patient or parents to notify prescriber if adverse reactions persist or become severe.

---

hepatitis A vaccine, inactivated
Havrix, Vaqta

Pregnancy risk category C

AVAILABLE FORMS
Havrix
Injection: 360 ELISA units (EL. units)/ 0.5 ml, 720 EL. units/0.5 ml; 1,440 EL. units/ml

Vaqta
Injection: 25 units/0.5 ml, 50 units/ml

INDICATIONS & DOSAGES
➤ **Active immunization against hepatitis A virus—**
Adults: 1,440 EL. units (Havrix) or 50 units (Vaqta) I.M. as single dose. For booster dose, 1,440 EL. units (Havrix) or 50 units (Vaqta) given 6 to 12 months after initial dose. A booster dose is recommended if prolonged immunity is desired.
Children ages 2 to 18: 720 EL. units (Havrix) or 25 units (Vaqta) I.M. as single dose; then booster dose of 720 EL. units (Havrix) or 25 units (Vaqta) I.M. given 6 to 12 months after initial dose, or 360 EL. units I.M. given 1 month apart and 360 EL. units I.M. 6 to 12 months after primary course. Booster recommended for prolonged immunity.
➤ **Prevention of hepatitis A in patients with chronic liver disease or clotting factor disorders, and in food handlers—**
Adults: 1,440 EL. units (Havrix) I.M. as single dose. For booster dose, 1,440 EL. units (Havrix) I.M. given 6 to 12 months after initial dose. Booster dose is recommended if prolonged immunity is desired.
Children ages 2 to 18: 720 EL. units (Havrix) I.M. as single dose; then booster dose of 720 EL. units (Havrix) I.M. given 6 to 12 months after initial dose; or two doses of 360 EL. units I.M. given 1 month apart and 360 EL. units I.M. 6 to 12 months after primary course. Booster dose is recommended if prolonged immunity is desired.

ACTION
Promotes active immunity to hepatitis A virus.

Route	Onset	Peak	Duration
I.M.	1-15 days	Unknown	6 mo

ADVERSE REACTIONS
CNS: hypertonia, insomnia, vertigo, *headache, fatigue, malaise, seizures,* encephalopathy, dizziness.
EENT: pharyngitis, photophobia.
GI: *anorexia, nausea,* abdominal pain, diarrhea, dysgeusia, vomiting.
GU: menstrual disorders.
Musculoskeletal: arthralgia, myalgia.

Reactions may be *common*, uncommon, *life-threatening*, or **COMMON AND LIFE-THREATENING**.

Respiratory: other upper respiratory tract infections.
Skin: pruritus, rash, urticaria, *induration, redness, swelling,* hematoma, *injection site soreness,* jaundice.
Other: *fever,* lymphadenopathy, ***anaphylaxis.***

INTERACTIONS
Drug-drug. *Anticoagulants:* Increased risk of bleeding. Give I.M. injections cautiously.

EFFECTS ON LAB TEST RESULTS
● May increase CPK level.

CONTRAINDICATIONS
Contraindicated in patients hypersensitive to vaccine's components.

NURSING CONSIDERATIONS
● Use cautiously in patients with thrombocytopenia or bleeding disorders and in those who are taking an anticoagulant because bleeding may occur after an I.M. injection.
● As with other vaccines, administration of hepatitis A vaccine should be delayed, if possible, in patient with febrile illness.
● Keep epinephrine 1:1,000 available to treat anaphylaxis.
● If vaccine is given to immunosuppressed persons or persons receiving immunosuppressants, expected immune response may not occur.
● Persons who should receive vaccine include people traveling to or living in areas of high endemicity for hepatitis A (Africa, Asia [except Japan], the Mediterranean basin, Eastern Europe, the Middle East, Central and South America, Mexico, and parts of the Caribbean), military personnel, native peoples of Alaska and the Americas, persons engaging in high-risk sexual activity, and users of illegal injectable drugs. Certain institutional workers, employees of child day-care centers, laboratory workers who handle live hepatitis A virus, and handlers of primate animals also may benefit.
● For I.M. use, shake vial or syringe well before withdrawal. After it has been agitated thoroughly, vaccine is an opaque white suspension. Discard if it appears

otherwise. No dilution or reconstitution is needed.
● Give as I.M. injection into the deltoid region in adults. It shouldn't be given in the gluteal region; such injections may result in suboptimal response. Never inject I.V., S.C., or I.D.

PATIENT TEACHING
● Inform patient that vaccine won't prevent hepatitis caused by other drugs or pathogens known to infect the liver.
● Warn patient about local adverse reactions. Tell him to report persistent or severe reactions promptly.
● Alert travelers to dangers of eating raw or undercooked shellfish or consuming food or drink in countries with poor hygienic conditions.
● Remind patient to return for second injection 6 to 12 months after the first.

hepatitis B vaccine, recombinant
Engerix-B, Recombivax HB

Pregnancy risk category C

AVAILABLE FORMS
Injection: 5 mcg HBsAg/0.5 ml (Recombivax HB, pediatric/adolescent formulation with or without preservative); 10 mcg HBsAg/0.5 ml (Engerix-B, adolescent/pediatric formulation); 10 mcg HBsAg/ml (Recombivax HB, adult formulation); 20 mcg HBsAg/ml (Engerix-B, adult formulation); 40 mcg HBsAg/ml (Recombivax HB dialysis formulation)

INDICATIONS & DOSAGES
➤ **Immunization against infection from all known subtypes of hepatitis B virus (HBV), primary preexposure prophylaxis against HBV, postexposure prophylaxis (when given with hepatitis B immune globulin)—**
Engerix-B
Adults age 20 and older: Initially, 20 mcg I.M.; then second dose of 20 mcg I.M. after 30 days. A third dose of 20 mcg I.M. is given 6 months after the initial dose.
Adjust-a-dose: For adults undergoing dialysis or receiving immunosuppressants, initially, 40 mcg I.M. (divided into two

Theophylline, warfarin: Clearance may be impaired, causing increased levels of these drugs. Monitor patient closely.

EFFECTS ON LAB TEST RESULTS
None reported.

CONTRAINDICATIONS
Contraindicated in patients hypersensitive to eggs or components of vaccine, including thimerosal. Defer vaccination in patients with acute respiratory or other active infection and in those with active neurologic disorders.

NURSING CONSIDERATIONS
• Use cautiously in patients with history of sulfite allergy.
• Fever and malaise occur most often in children and in others not exposed to influenza viruses. Severe reactions in adults are rare.
• Obtain history of allergies, especially to eggs, and reactions to immunizations.
• Keep epinephrine 1:1,000 available to treat anaphylaxis.
• Thoroughly agitate vial just before administration to restore suspension.
• Give injections for adults and older children in deltoid muscle; for infants and children younger than age 3, give in anterolateral aspect of thigh.
• Ideally, give vaccinations from October to mid-November because outbreaks of influenza typically don't occur until December. Don't give vaccine too early in season because antibody titers may begin to decline before flu season.
• Children age 12 and younger should be given their second dose before December, if possible.
• Give vaccines to both children and adults throughout flu season, even as late as April.
• The American Academy of Pediatrics states that influenza vaccine can be given simultaneously (but at a different site and with a different syringe) with other routine vaccinations in children.
• *Alert:* Don't give influenza vaccine with, or within 3 days after administration of, whole-cell pertussis vaccine or combined diphtheria/tetanus toxoid/whole cell pertussis vaccine, adsorbed.

• Vaccine is considered safe in pregnant women. Vaccination shouldn't be postponed, regardless of stage of pregnancy, in patients who have high-risk conditions and who will be in first trimester of pregnancy when flu season begins.
• Immunodeficient patients may receive two doses 1 month apart; however, there is little evidence that booster doses improve immunogenic response to vaccine. Chemoprophylaxis with amantadine may be helpful.
• Vaccine is strongly recommended for anyone older than 6 months; for patients with chronic disease, metabolic disorders, or medical conditions that put them at risk for complications from influenza; for health care workers, especially doctors, nurses, employees of nursing homes, volunteer workers, and other personnel in both hospital and outpatient settings; and for household members who may contact persons at high risk for medical complications of influenza. Also recommended for anyone who wishes to reduce chance of infection.
• Allergic reactions, which usually occur immediately, are extremely rare. Paralysis related to Guillain-Barré syndrome is rare and has been linked only to the 1976 vaccine.
• Vaccine prepared for a previous influenza season shouldn't be used to provide protection for current season.
• Although there's little information regarding influenza in persons with HIV, it's recommended that these patients receive vaccine. Patients with advanced disease may have a low response; there's no evidence that booster dose will improve immune response.
• *Alert:* No whole virus vaccine (Fluzone) was distributed in the United States during the 2001-2002 influenza season.

PATIENT TEACHING
• Advise patient about risks of vaccination compared with risks of influenza and its complications.
• Make sure patient understands that annual vaccination with current vaccine is needed because immunity to influenza decreases in year after injection.
• Explain that vaccine can't cause influenza. Fever, malaise, and myalgia may begin

---

Reactions may be *common*, uncommon, ***life-threatening***, or **COMMON AND LIFE-THREATENING**.

6 to 12 hours after vaccination and last 1 to 2 days. Such systemic reactions aren't common.

• Instruct patient to take appropriate acetaminophen dose for fever and apply ice compresses to injection site to minimize discomfort.

Japanese encephalitis virus vaccine, inactivated
JE-VAX

Pregnancy risk category C

AVAILABLE FORMS
Injection: 1-ml, 10-ml vials

INDICATIONS & DOSAGES
➤ **Active immunization against Japanese encephalitis (JE)—**
Primary immunization schedule
Adults and children older than age 3: 1 ml S.C. on days 0, 7, and 30.
Children ages 1 to 3: 0.5 ml S.C. on days 0, 7, and 30.
Booster doses
Adults and children older than age 3: 1 ml S.C., 2 years after last dose.
Children ages 1 to 3: 0.5 ml S.C., 2 years after last dose.

ACTION
Provides active immunity against JE, a mosquito-borne arboviral flavivirus infection that's the main cause of viral encephalitis in Asia.

Route	Onset	Peak	Duration
S.C.	Unknown	Unknown	2 yr

ADVERSE REACTIONS
CNS: *headache, dizziness, malaise.*
GI: *nausea, vomiting, abdominal pain.*
Musculoskeletal: *myalgia.*
Respiratory: *respiratory distress.*
Skin: rash, *local tenderness and swelling at injection site,* generalized urticaria.
Other: *anaphylaxis; fever; chills; angioedema of the face, oropharynx, limbs, or lips.*

INTERACTIONS
None significant.

EFFECTS ON LAB TEST RESULTS
None reported.

CONTRAINDICATIONS
Contraindicated in patients hypersensitive to drug or thimerosal (a preservative) and in those who exhibited severe adverse reactions, such as generalized urticaria or angioedema, to previous dose of vaccine. Because vaccine is derived from mouse brain, its use is contraindicated in patients hypersensitive to substances of murine or neural origin.

NURSING CONSIDERATIONS
• Use cautiously in pregnant or breast-feeding women, elderly patients, and those with history of urticaria after vaccines, drugs, or insect bites. Advanced age may be a risk factor for developing symptomatic illness after JE infection. JE acquired during pregnancy can cause intrauterine infection and fetal death.
• Use vaccine to provide protection against JE in persons who reside in areas where virus is endemic and in persons planning to travel 1 month or longer to those areas. It isn't indicated for all persons traveling to or residing in Asia. For most travelers to Asia, the risk of acquiring JE is extremely low. Contact the Centers for Disease Control and Prevention at 877-FYI-TRIP (394-8747) for current travel advisories.
• Keep epinephrine 1:1,000 and other resuscitation equipment and drugs available to treat anaphylaxis and other adverse reactions.
• To prepare vaccine for injection, use supplied diluent (sterile water for injection). Add 1.3 ml of diluent to single-dose vial and 11 ml of diluent to 10-dose vial. Shake vial thoroughly to ensure dissolution of vaccine. After reconstitution, refrigerate vaccine (36° to 46° F [2° to 8° C]) for up to 8 hours. Discard unused vaccine after 8 hours.
• Follow recommended three-dose schedule for best results. When time constraints prohibit use of schedule, an abbreviated schedule with injections on days 0, 7, and 14 may be used.
• When it isn't possible to follow usual dose schedule, a two-dose regimen with injections on days 0 and 7 may be used.

Antibodies will be induced in about 80% of patients with this schedule. A two-dose regimen shouldn't be used unless circumstances are unusual.

• Monitor patient closely for 30 minutes after injection.

• Reactions to first dose have occurred a median of 12 hours after injection (88% occurred within 3 days). The delay between second dose and adverse effects was usually longer, with median of 3 days, and some effects weren't seen for 2 weeks. Some patients exhibited adverse reactions to second or third dose, even when first or second dose was well tolerated.

PATIENT TEACHING

• Warn patient about possibility of delayed generalized urticaria or delayed angioedema of the limbs, face, oropharynx, or (especially) lips. Generalized urticaria or angioedema may occur within minutes of vaccination. Most reactions occur within 48 hours. However, reactions that may be related to vaccine have occurred as late as 17 days after injection.

• Because of risk of delayed reactions, advise patient to remain in areas where medical care is available for 10 days after injection. Caution against international travel during this time. Advise patient to seek medical assistance as soon as a reaction appears.

• Encourage patient and parents to report adverse effects after vaccination. Health care providers should report these adverse effects to the Vaccine Adverse Event Reporting System at (800) 822-7967.

• Teach patient about precautions that may limit exposure to mosquito bites, such as using insect repellents, wearing protective clothing, and avoiding outdoor activities, especially in the evening.

Lyme disease vaccine (recombinant OspA)
LYMErix

Pregnancy risk category C

AVAILABLE FORMS
Injection: 30 mcg/0.5 ml single-dose vials and prefilled syringes

INDICATIONS & DOSAGES
➤ **Active immunization against Lyme disease**—
Adults and adolescents ages 15 to 70:
30 mcg I.M. in deltoid region; repeat dose at 1 and 12 months after first dose. Administration of second and third doses should take place several weeks before onset of *Borrelia burgdorferi* transmission season (varies according to geographic area).

ACTION
Stimulates formation of anti-OspA antibodies, which have demonstrated bactericidal activity against *B. burgdorferi*, the bacterial spirochete that causes Lyme disease.

Route	Onset	Peak	Duration
I.M.	Unknown	Unknown	Unknown

ADVERSE REACTIONS
CNS: *headache, fatigue,* dizziness, depression, hypoesthesia, paresthesia.
EENT: pharyngitis, rhinitis, sinusitis.
GI: diarrhea, nausea.
Musculoskeletal: *arthralgia,* back pain, aches, myalgia, arthritis, arthrosis, stiffness, tendinitis.
Respiratory: bronchitis, coughing, upper respiratory tract infection.
Skin: *rash,* injection site reaction, contact dermatitis, *injection site pain, redness, soreness, swelling.*
Other: chills or rigors, fever, viral infection, flu syndrome.

INTERACTIONS
Drug-drug. *Immunosuppressants:* Expected immune response may not occur. Consider deferring vaccination for 3 months after therapy ends.

EFFECTS ON LAB TEST RESULTS
None reported.

CONTRAINDICATIONS
Contraindicated in patients hypersensitive to vaccine or its components. Don't give vaccine to patients outside indicated age range or to those with treatment-resistant Lyme arthritis (antibiotic refractory) or moderate to severe febrile illness.

Reactions may be *common*, uncommon, *__life-threatening__*, or COMMON AND LIFE-THREATENING.

NURSING CONSIDERATIONS

• Use cautiously in patients who may be allergic to the natural rubber packaging for the prefilled syringe. Packaging for vial doesn't contain rubber.

• Use with caution in breast-feeding women because it's unknown whether vaccine appears in breast milk.

• Vaccine is a preventive measure, not a treatment for Lyme disease.

• Before immunization, review patient's history for possible vaccine sensitivity, allergies, previous vaccination-related adverse reactions, and occurrence of adverse event-related signs and symptoms. Epinephrine injection and other drugs appropriate for controlling immediate allergic reactions must be readily available.

• Immunization against Lyme disease is appropriate in persons who live or work in, travel to, or pursue recreational activities in *B. burgdorferi*-infected grassy or wooded areas.

• Patients with a history of Lyme disease may benefit from vaccination because previous infection with *B. burgdorferi* may not provide protective immunity.

• As with other vaccines, Lyme disease vaccine may not protect everyone.

• Refrigerate vaccine between 36° and 46° F (2° and 8° C). Don't freeze; discard if product has been frozen.

• Shake well before use. Inspect for particulates or discoloration before giving. With thorough agitation, Lyme disease vaccine is a turbid, white suspension. Discard if it appears otherwise.

• Use vaccine as supplied, without diluting or reconstituting it. Use the full, recommended dose of the vaccine. Discard vaccine remaining in single-dose vial.

• Lyme disease vaccine should be given I.M. in deltoid region. Don't give I.V., I.D., or S.C.

• As with other I.M. injections, vaccine shouldn't be given to persons taking anticoagulants or who have clotting disorders, unless potential benefit clearly outweighs risk.

• No information is available on immune response to Lyme disease vaccine when given with other vaccines. When vaccine must be given with other vaccines, each should be given with a different syringe and at a different injection site.

• Register pregnant women who receive Lyme disease vaccine by calling GlaxoSmithKline Pharmaceuticals at (800) 366-8900, ext. 5231.

• Immunization with Lyme disease vaccine may cause a false-positive enzyme-linked immunosorbent assay (ELISA) result for *B. burgdorferi* in the absence of infection. Therefore, it's important to perform Western blot testing if ELISA test is positive or equivocal in vaccinated persons being evaluated for suspected Lyme disease.

PATIENT TEACHING

• Inform patient that vaccine prevents but doesn't treat Lyme disease.

• Inform patient that, like other vaccines, Lyme disease vaccine may not protect everyone.

• Inform patient of benefits and risks of immunization with vaccine and of importance of completing all three vaccinations several weeks before start of *B. burgdorferi* season in his geographic area.

• Tell patient to report adverse effects.

• Advise patient to take standard preventive measures, such as wearing long-sleeved shirts and long pants, tucking pants into socks, treating clothing with tick repellent, and checking for and removing ticks when in endemic areas.

• Show patient the appropriate way to remove ticks, such as using fine-pointed tweezers and not squeezing the tick before withdrawal.

• Advise patient to notify prescriber of immunization with vaccine because it may interfere with laboratory diagnosis of Lyme disease.

---

measles, mumps, and rubella virus vaccine, live
M-M-R II

Pregnancy risk category C

AVAILABLE FORMS

Injection: Single-dose vial containing not less than 1,000 tissue culture infective doses (TCID$_{50}$) of attenuated measles virus derived from Enders' attenuated Edmonston strain (grown in chick embryo

---

culture), 20,000 TCID$_{50}$ of the Jeryl Lynn (B level) mumps strain (grown in chick embryo culture), and 1,000 TCID$_{50}$ of the Wistar RA 27/3 strain of rubella virus (propagated in human diploid cell culture) per 0.5-ml dose. Multidose vial available to institutions or government agencies.

INDICATIONS & DOSAGES
➤ **Routine immunization—**
Adults: One vial S.C. Patients born after 1957 should receive two doses at least 1 month apart.
Children: One vial S.C. A two-dose schedule is recommended, with first dose given at 15 months (12 months in high-risk areas) and second dose given either at ages 4 to 6 or 11 to 12.

ACTION
Promotes immunity to measles, mumps, and rubella virus by inducing production of antibodies.

Route	Onset	Peak	Duration
S.C.	Unknown	Unknown	< 11 yr

ADVERSE REACTIONS
GI: diarrhea.
Musculoskeletal: arthritis, arthralgia.
Skin: rash, erythema at injection site, urticaria.
Other: fever, regional lymphadenopathy, *anaphylaxis.*

INTERACTIONS
Drug-drug. *Immune serum globulin, plasma, whole blood:* Antibodies in serum may interfere with immune response. Don't use vaccine within 3 to 11 months of these products, depending on dose of antibody or blood given.
Immunosuppressants: May decrease immune response to vaccine. Defer immunization until immunosuppressant is discontinued.

EFFECTS ON LAB TEST RESULTS
None reported.

CONTRAINDICATIONS
Contraindicated in immunosuppressed patients; in those with cancer, blood dyscrasia, gamma globulin disorders, fever,

active untreated tuberculosis, or anaphylactic or anaphylactoid reactions to neomycin or eggs; in those receiving corticosteroid or radiation therapy; and in pregnant women.

NURSING CONSIDERATIONS
• Obtain history of allergies, especially anaphylactic reactions to antibiotics, or reaction to immunization.
• Keep epinephrine 1:1,000 available to treat anaphylaxis.
• If skin test is needed, give it either before or simultaneously with vaccine.
• Use only diluent supplied. Discard vaccine 8 hours after reconstituting.
• Inject into outer aspect of upper arm with a 25G ⅝-inch needle. Don't give I.V.
• Refrigerate vaccine; protect from light. Solution may be used if red, pink, or yellow, but must be clear.
• Risk of adverse effects is low (0.5% to 4%).
• Treat fever with antipyretics such as acetaminophen.
• Presence of maternal antibodies may prevent response in children younger than age 12 months.
• The Immunization Practices Advisory Committee recommends that colleges, other post-high school educational institutions, and medical institutions employing prescriber obtain documentation of receipt of two doses of vaccine after age 1 (or other evidence of immunity, such as infection, documented by prescriber). Combined measles, mumps, and rubella vaccine is preferred.
• *Alert:* The Centers for Disease Control and Prevention recommend that, during a measles outbreak in a health care facility, susceptible personnel exposed to measles virus (whether or not they received measles vaccine or immunoglobulin) avoid patient contact for days 5 through 21 after such exposure. If personnel become ill, they should avoid patient contact for at least 7 days after developing rash.
• Vaccine may temporarily decrease response to tuberculin skin testing.

PATIENT TEACHING
• Warn patient or parents about adverse reactions linked to vaccine.

Reactions may be *common*, uncommon, *life-threatening*, or COMMON AND LIFE-THREATENING.

• Review immunization schedule with parents, and stress importance of receiving second injection at the appropriate time to maintain immunization.
• Tell woman of childbearing age to use contraceptive measures until 3 months after immunization.
• Febrile seizures have rarely occurred in children after vaccination. Tell parents to treat and promptly report fever, especially in patient with family history of seizures.

measles and rubella virus vaccine, live attenuated
M-R-Vax II

Pregnancy risk category C

AVAILABLE FORMS
Injection: Single-dose vial containing not less than 1,000 tissue culture infective doses ($TCID_{50}$) per 0.5 ml of attenuated measles virus derived from Enders' attenuated Edmonston strain (grown in chick embryo culture); 1,000 $TCID_{50}$ of the Wistar RA 27/3 strain of rubella virus

INDICATIONS & DOSAGES
➤ **Immunization—**
Adults and children age 15 months and older: 0.5 ml (1,000 units) S.C.

ACTION
Promotes immunity to measles and rubella virus by inducing production of antibodies.

Route	Onset	Peak	Duration
S.C.	Unknown	Unknown	< 11 yr

ADVERSE REACTIONS
Musculoskeletal: arthralgia.
Skin: rash, *burning and stinging at injection site.*
Other: fever, lymphadenopathy, ***anaphylaxis.***

INTERACTIONS
Drug-drug. *Immune serum globulin, plasma, whole blood:* Antibodies in serum may interfere with immune response. Don't use vaccine within 3 months of transfusion.

Immunosuppressants: May reduce immune response to vaccine. Defer immunization until immunosuppressant is discontinued.

EFFECTS ON LAB TEST RESULTS
None reported.

CONTRAINDICATIONS
Contraindicated in immunosuppressed patients; in those with cancer, blood dyscrasia, gamma globulin disorders, fever, active untreated tuberculosis, or anaphylactic or anaphylactoid reactions to eggs or neomycin; in those receiving corticosteroid or radiation therapy; and in pregnant women.

NURSING CONSIDERATIONS
• Obtain history of allergies, especially anaphylactic reactions to antibiotics.
• Keep epinephrine 1:1,000 available to treat anaphylaxis.
• If skin test is needed, give it either before or simultaneously with vaccine.
• Use only diluent supplied. Discard vaccine 8 hours after reconstituting.
• Inject into outer upper arm. Don't inject I.V.
• Store in refrigerator and protect from light. Reconstituted solution should be clear yellow.
• *Alert:* Vaccine shouldn't be given within 1 month of other live virus vaccines, except oral poliovirus vaccine. Immunization should be deferred in patients with acute illness.
• Allow at least 3 weeks between BCG and rubella vaccines.
• Vaccine may temporarily decrease response to tuberculin skin testing.

PATIENT TEACHING
• Warn patient or parents about adverse reactions linked to vaccine.
• Caution woman of childbearing age to avoid pregnancy until 3 months after immunization.
• Advise use of antipyretics to control fever.

measles virus vaccine, live attenuated
Attenuvax

Pregnancy risk category C

AVAILABLE FORMS
Injection: Single-dose vial containing not less than 1,000 tissue culture infective doses ($TCID_{50}$) of measles virus derived from the more attenuated line of Enders' attenuated Edmonston strain (grown in chick embryo culture); available in 10- and 50-dose vials

INDICATIONS & DOSAGES
➤ **Immunization**—
Adults and children age 15 months and older: 0.5 ml (1,000 units) S.C. A two-dose schedule is recommended, with first dose given at 15 months (12 months in high-risk areas) and second dose given at ages 4 to 6 or 11 to 12.
➤ **Measles outbreak control**—
Adults: School personnel born in or after 1957 should be revaccinated if they lack evidence of measles immunity. If outbreak is in a medical facility, all workers born in or after 1957 should be revaccinated if they lack evidence of immunity.
Children: If cases occur in children younger than age 1, children should be vaccinated as young as age 6 months. All students and siblings should be revaccinated if they lack documentation of measles immunity.

ACTION
Promotes immunity to measles virus by inducing production of antibodies.

Route	Onset	Peak	Duration
S.C.	Few days	Unknown	≥ 13 yr

ADVERSE REACTIONS
CNS: *febrile seizures in susceptible children.*
GI: anorexia.
Hematologic: *leukopenia, thrombocytopenia.*
Skin: rash, erythema, swelling, tenderness at injection site.
Other: fever, lymphadenopathy, *anaphylaxis.*

INTERACTIONS
Drug-drug. *Immune serum globulin, plasma, whole blood:* Antibodies in serum may interfere with immune response. Don't use vaccine for at least 3 months after administration of these products.

EFFECTS ON LAB TEST RESULTS
• May decrease WBC and platelet counts.

CONTRAINDICATIONS
Contraindicated in pregnant women; in immunosuppressed patients; in patients with cancer, blood dyscrasia, gamma globulin disorders, fever, active untreated tuberculosis, or anaphylactic or anaphylactoid reactions to neomycin or eggs; and in patients receiving corticosteroid or radiation therapy.

NURSING CONSIDERATIONS
• Obtain history of allergies, especially anaphylactic reactions to antibiotics, or reaction to immunization. Immunization should be deferred in patients with acute illness or after administration of blood or plasma.
• Keep epinephrine 1:1,000 available to treat anaphylaxis.
• If skin test is needed, give it either before or simultaneously with vaccine.
• Use only diluent supplied. Discard vaccine 8 hours after reconstituting.
• Don't give vaccine I.V.
• Vaccine may be given with oral poliovirus vaccine.
• The Immunization Practices Advisory Committee recommends that colleges, other post–high school educational institutions, and medical institutions employing health care providers obtain documentation of receipt of two doses of vaccine after age 1 (or other evidence of immunity, such as infection, documented by prescriber). Combined measles, mumps, and rubella vaccine is preferred.
• Don't give vaccine within 3 months of receiving blood or plasma transfusion or human immune serum globulin.
• *Alert:* The Centers for Disease Control and Prevention recommends that during a measles outbreak in a health care facility, susceptible personnel exposed to the measles virus (whether or not they received measles vaccine or immune globu-

---

Reactions may be *common*, uncommon, *life-threatening*, or COMMON AND LIFE-THREATENING.

lin) avoid patient contact for days 5 through 21 after such exposure. If personnel become ill, they should avoid patient contact for at least 7 days after developing rash.

• If attenuated measles vaccine is given immediately after exposure to the disease, some protection may be provided. This level of protection is significantly increased if vaccine is given even a few days before exposure.

• Vaccine may temporarily decrease response to tuberculin skin test.

PATIENT TEACHING
• Warn patient or parents about adverse reactions linked to vaccine.

• Review immunization schedule with patient or parents and stress importance of receiving second injection at appropriate time.

• Stress importance of avoiding pregnancy for 3 months after vaccination. Provide contraception information, if needed.

meningococcal polysaccharide vaccine
Menomune-A/C/Y/W-135

Pregnancy risk category C

AVAILABLE FORMS
Injection: 1-dose, 10-dose, and 50-dose vials with vial of diluent

INDICATIONS & DOSAGES
➤ **Meningococcal meningitis prophylaxis—**
Adults and children age 2 and older:
0.5 ml S.C.

ACTION
Promotes active immunity to meningitis.

Route	Onset	Peak	Duration
S.C.	Unknown	Unknown	3 yr

ADVERSE REACTIONS
CNS: headache, malaise.
Musculoskeletal: muscle cramps.
Skin: *pain, tenderness, erythema, induration at injection site.*
Other: chills, fever, ***anaphylaxis,*** mild lymphadenopathy.

INTERACTIONS
Drug-drug. *Immunosuppressants:* May reduce immune response to vaccine. Defer immunization until three months after immunosuppressant therapy is discontinued.

EFFECTS ON LAB TEST RESULTS
None reported.

CONTRAINDICATIONS
Contraindicated in patients hypersensitive to thimerosal or other vaccine components; also contraindicated in pregnant women. Defer vaccination in patients with acute illness. Vaccine isn't contraindicated in immunocompromised patients.

NURSING CONSIDERATIONS
• Obtain history of allergies and reaction to immunization.

• Keep epinephrine 1:1,000 available to treat anaphylaxis.

• Don't give I.V., I.M., or I.D.

• Vaccine may be given with other immunizations.

• Routine vaccination isn't recommended. Vaccine should be reserved for persons at risk, such as those who live in or are traveling to epidemic or highly endemic areas, household or institutional contacts of meningococcal disease as an adjunct to appropriate antibiotic chemoprophylaxis, medical and laboratory personnel at risk for exposure to meningococcal disease, patients with terminal complement component deficiency, and those with anatomic or functional asplenia.

• Reconstitute vaccine only with supplied diluent.

• Some prescribers will revaccinate children if they are at high risk and if they previously received vaccine before age 4.

• Don't give vaccine within 3 months of receiving blood or plasma transfusion or human immune serum globulin administration.

PATIENT TEACHING
• Warn patient or parents about adverse reactions linked to vaccine.

• Stress importance of avoiding pregnancy for 3 months after vaccination. Provide contraception information, if needed.

• Instruct patient to take correct acetaminophen dose to control fever.

mumps virus vaccine, live
Mumpsvax

Pregnancy risk category C

AVAILABLE FORMS
Injection: Single-dose vial containing not less than 20,000 tissue culture infective doses ($TCID_{50}$) of attenuated mumps virus derived from Jeryl Lynn mumps strain (grown in chick embryo culture) per 0.5 ml and vial of diluent; single-dose vial containing not less than 5,000 $TCID_{50}$ of the U.S. Reference Mumps Virus in each 0.5 ml†

INDICATIONS & DOSAGES
➤ **Immunization—**
Adults and children age 1 and older:
0.5 ml (20,000 units) S.C.

Not recommended in children younger than age 12 months; children vaccinated at younger than 12 months should be revaccinated.

ACTION
Promotes active immunity to mumps.

Route	Onset	Peak	Duration
S.C.	Unknown	Unknown	> 15 yr

ADVERSE REACTIONS
CNS: malaise.
GI: diarrhea.
Skin: rash, injection site reaction.
Other: *anaphylaxis,* slight fever, mild allergic reactions, mild lymphadenopathy.

INTERACTIONS
Drug-drug. *Immune serum globulin, plasma, whole blood:* Antibodies in serum may interfere with immune response. Don't use vaccine for at least 3 months after administration of these products.

EFFECTS ON LAB TEST RESULTS
None reported.

CONTRAINDICATIONS
Contraindicated in immunosuppressed patients; in those with cancer, blood dyscrasia, gamma globulin disorders, fever, untreated active tuberculosis, or anaphylactic or anaphylactoid reactions to neomycin or eggs; in those receiving corticosteroid or radiation therapy; and in pregnant women.

NURSING CONSIDERATIONS
• Obtain history of allergies, especially anaphylactic reactions to antibiotics, and reaction to immunization. Defer use in patients with acute or febrile illness and for at least 3 months after transfusions or treatment with immune serum globulin.
• Keep epinephrine 1:1,000 available to treat anaphylaxis.
• If skin test is needed, give it either before or simultaneously with vaccine.
• Use only diluent supplied. Discard vaccine 8 hours after reconstituting.
• Use a 25G ⅝-inch needle to inject.
• Don't give vaccine I.V.
• Refrigerate and protect from light. Reconstituted solution is clear yellow; don't use if discolored.
• Don't give vaccine less than 1 month before or after immunization with other live virus vaccines; however, trivalent live, oral poliovirus vaccine may be given simultaneously.
• Give to asymptomatic HIV-infected children.
• Vaccine isn't recommended for infants younger than age 12 months because retained maternal mumps antibodies may interfere with immune response.
• Don't use for delayed hypersensitivity (allergy) skin testing. Use mumps skin-test antigen, a killed viral product.
• Vaccine may temporarily decrease response to tuberculin skin test.

PATIENT TEACHING
• Warn patient or parents about adverse reactions linked to vaccine.
• Stress importance of avoiding pregnancy for 3 months after vaccination. Provide contraception information, if needed.
• Tell patient to treat fever with antipyretics.

---

plague vaccine

Pregnancy risk category C

AVAILABLE FORMS
Injection: 1.8 to 2.2 billion killed plague bacilli (*Yersinia pestis*)/ml in 20-ml vials

---

Reactions may be *common,* uncommon, **life-threatening,** or **COMMON AND LIFE-THREATENING.**

INDICATIONS & DOSAGES
➤ Primary immunization and booster—
Adults: 1 ml I.M.; then 0.2 ml in 4 to 12 weeks, and then 0.2 ml 5 to 6 months after second dose. Booster is 0.1 to 0.2 ml q 6 months while in plague area. After 3 boosters, use 1- to 2-year booster cycle.

ACTION
Promotes active immunity to plague caused by *Y. pestis.*

Route	Onset	Peak	Duration
I.M.	Unknown	Unknown	6-12 mo

ADVERSE REACTIONS
CNS: headache, malaise.
GI: nausea, vomiting.
Hematologic: leukocytosis.
Musculoskeletal: arthralgia, myalgia.
Other: *slight fever, lymphadenopathy,* **anaphylaxis,** swelling, *induration, erythema, tenderness at injection site.*

INTERACTIONS
Drug-drug. *Anticoagulants:* Increased risk of bleeding. Give with caution.
Cholera, typhoid vaccine: Increased risk of adverse effects. Don't give at same time.

EFFECTS ON LAB TEST RESULTS
● May increase WBC count.

CONTRAINDICATIONS
Contraindicated in immunosuppressed patients; in those hypersensitive to beef, soy, casein, phenol, sulfite, or formaldehyde; and in pregnant women. Patients who have had severe local or systemic reactions to plague vaccine shouldn't be revaccinated. Also contraindicated in patients with severe thrombocytopenia or other coagulation disorders that would contraindicate I.M. injections.

NURSING CONSIDERATIONS
● The Centers for Disease Control and Prevention doesn't recommend vaccination in persons younger than age 18 because data are insufficient.
● Obtain history of allergies and reaction to immunization. Immunization should be deferred in patients with respiratory infection.
● Keep epinephrine 1:1,000 available to treat anaphylaxis.
● Inject into the deltoid area.
● Vaccination is recommended for all laboratory and field personnel working with *Y. pestis.*

PATIENT TEACHING
● Warn patient about adverse reactions linked to vaccine.
● Caution woman of childbearing age to report suspected pregnancy before administration.
● Tell patient to treat fever with appropriate acetaminophen dose.

pneumococcal 7-valent conjugate vaccine (diphtheria CRM$_{197}$ protein)
Prevnar

Pregnancy risk category C

AVAILABLE FORMS
Suspension for I.M. injection: 0.5-ml vials

INDICATIONS & DOSAGES
➤ Active immunization of infants and toddlers against invasive disease caused by *Streptococcus pneumoniae* capsular serotypes 4, 6B, 9V, 14, 18C, 19F, and 23F—
Infants and toddlers: A total of four 0.5-ml doses, given I.M. at ages 2, 4, 6, and 12 to 15 months.
Previously unvaccinated older infants and children: 0.5 ml I.M. according to the following schedules based on the age at the first dose.
Ages 7 to 11 months: Two doses at least 4 weeks apart, followed by a third dose given after the 1-year birthday and at least 2 months after the second dose.
Ages 12 to 23 months: Two doses at least 2 months apart.
Ages 24 months through 9 years: One dose.

ACTION
Promotes active immunity against invasive pneumococcal disease, including sepsis and meningitis, caused by the seven pneu-

mococcal capsular serotypes included in the vaccine.

Route	Onset	Peak	Duration
I.M.	Unknown	Unknown	Unknown

ADVERSE REACTIONS
CNS: *drowsiness, irritability, restless sleep.*
GI: *diarrhea, vomiting, decreased appetite.*
Musculoskeletal: interference with limb movement.
Skin: rash or urticaria, *injection site reactions including edema, erythema, induration, inflammation, skin discoloration, and tenderness.*
Other: *fever,* hypersensitivity reactions.

INTERACTIONS
Drug-drug. *Immunosuppressive drugs (antineoplastic drugs, corticosteroids):* May result in suboptimal active immunity. Monitor patient closely.

EFFECTS ON LAB TEST RESULTS
None reported.

CONTRAINDICATIONS
Contraindicated in children who are allergic to any component of the vaccine, including diphtheria toxoid.

NURSING CONSIDERATIONS
• Use with caution in patients with a history of latex allergy; product packaging contains dry natural rubber. Use cautiously in patients with thrombocytopenia or coagulation disorders; I.M. injection may produce bleeding.
• A reduced antibody response may occur in immunocompromised patients.
• Obtain a thorough allergy history, including any reactions to immunizations.
• Epinephrine solution 1:1,000 and other necessary treatments should be available to treat allergic reactions.
• If different sites and separate syringes are used, pneumococcal 7-valent conjugate vaccine may be administered simultaneously with influenza, DTP, poliovirus, or *Haemophilus* b polysaccharide vaccines.
• Pneumococcal 7-valent conjugate vaccine isn't a substitute for routine diphthe-

ria immunization or for 23-valent pneumococcal vaccine, when indicated.
• Shake well to produce a uniform suspension. A nodule may form at injection site if vaccine isn't shaken.
• *Alert:* Don't inject I.V. Give by I.M. injection only, using the deltoid muscle or, in infants, only the anterolateral thigh. Don't inject into or near a nerve or blood vessel.
• Administration should be delayed if the patient or parents report current or recent moderate to severe febrile illness because immunity may be impaired.
• Refrigerate at 36° to 46° F (2° to 8° C). Don't freeze. Reconstitution or dilution is unnecessary.

PATIENT TEACHING
• Provide patient or family with thorough information on the benefits and risks of immunization.
• Inform parent of the immunization schedule.
• Advise parent that the most common adverse effects occur within the first three days and include a mild fever, nausea, vomiting, diarrhea, irritability, decreased appetite, rash, and hives. Adverse effects at the injection site include pain, tenderness, redness, swelling, and inflammation.
• Tell parent to report any bothersome or persistent side effects.

pneumococcal vaccine, polyvalent
Pneumovax 23, Pnu-Imune 23

Pregnancy risk category C

AVAILABLE FORMS
Injection: 25 mcg each of 23 polysaccharide isolates/0.5 ml

INDICATIONS & DOSAGES
➤ **Pneumococcal immunization—**
Adults and children age 2 and older:
0.5 ml I.M. or S.C.

ACTION
Promotes active immunity to infections caused by *Streptococcus pneumoniae.*

Route	Onset	Peak	Duration
I.M., S.C.	2-3 wk	Unknown	5 yr

ADVERSE REACTIONS
Musculoskeletal: myalgia, arthralgia.
Skin: injection site rash, *injection site soreness,* severe local reaction caused by revaccination within 3 years.
Other: *anaphylaxis,* slight fever.

INTERACTIONS
Drug-drug. *Immunosuppressants:* May reduce immune response to vaccine. Defer immunization until three months after immunosuppressant therapy is discontinued.

EFFECTS ON LAB TEST RESULTS
None reported.

CONTRAINDICATIONS
Contraindicated in patients hypersensitive to drug or its components (phenol) and in those with Hodgkin's disease who have received extensive chemotherapy or nodal irradiation. Defer use in patients with acute respiratory distress syndrome.

NURSING CONSIDERATIONS
• Vaccine isn't recommended for children younger than age 2.
• Check immunization history to avoid revaccination within 3 years.
• Obtain history of allergies and reaction to immunization. Eggs and egg protein aren't used during the manufacture of vaccine; contains phenol as a preservative.
• Keep epinephrine 1:1,000 available to treat anaphylaxis.
• Inject in deltoid or midlateral thigh. Don't inject I.V or I.D.
• When splenectomy is being considered, vaccine should be given at least 2 weeks before procedure to ensure adequate antibody response. Vaccine may be less effective in splenectomized patients.
• Vaccine protects against 23 pneumococcal types, accounting for 90% of pneumococcal disease.
• Vaccine may be given to children age 2 and older to prevent pneumococcal otitis media, although the Centers for Disease Control and Prevention doesn't recommend otitis media as an indication for vaccine.
• Vaccine is recommended for all adults older than age 65.

• Administration with influenza virus vaccine is safe and effective.

PATIENT TEACHING
• Warn patient about adverse reactions linked to vaccine.
• Tell patient to treat fever with mild antipyretics and local site reaction with cold compresses.
• Warn patient with idiopathic thrombocytopenic purpura that there is a possibility of relapse 2 to 14 days after vaccination.

---

poliovirus vaccine, inactivated (IPV)
IPOL

poliovirus vaccine, live, oral, trivalent (TOPV)
Orimune

Pregnancy risk category C

AVAILABLE FORMS
Inactivated virus vaccine injection: Mixture of three types of poliovirus (types 1, 2, and 3) grown in tissue culture. IPOL uses monkey kidney cultures and comes in 0.5-ml prefilled syringes
Oral vaccine: Mixture of three live viruses (types 1, 2, and 3), grown in monkey kidney tissue culture; in 0.5-ml single-dose Dispettes

INDICATIONS & DOSAGES
➤ **Poliovirus immunization (IPV)—**
Adults: 0.5 ml S.C.; then second dose in 4 to 8 weeks. A third dose is given in 6 to 12 months.
Children: 0.5 ml S.C. at 2 and 4 months. A third dose is given at 15 to 18 months. A reinforcing dose of 0.5 ml S.C. should be given before entry into school at ages 4 to 6.

ACTION
Promotes immunity to poliomyelitis by inducing humoral antibodies and antibodies in the lymphatic tissue.

Route	Onset	Peak	Duration
P.O.	7-10 days	21 days	Yrs
S.C.	Unknown	Unknown	Yrs

ADVERSE REACTIONS
CNS: sleepiness.
GI: decreased appetite.
Skin: injection site erythema, induration, *pain*.
Other: *poliomyelitis (TOPV only),* fever, crying, hypersensitivity reaction.

INTERACTIONS
Drug-drug. *Immune serum globulin, plasma, whole blood:* Antibodies in serum may interfere with immune response. Don't use vaccine within 3 months of transfusion.
Immunosuppressants: May reduce immune response to vaccine. Defer immunization until immunosuppressant is discontinued.

EFFECTS ON LAB TEST RESULTS
None reported.

CONTRAINDICATIONS
Oral vaccine is contraindicated in immunosuppressed patients; in those with cancer or immunoglobulin abnormalities; in those receiving radiation, antimetabolite, alkylating drug, or corticosteroid therapy; and in those who have a household contact who fits one of these preceding categories. These patients should receive IPV. Injectable vaccine is contraindicated in patients hypersensitive to neomycin, streptomycin, or polymyxin B.

NURSING CONSIDERATIONS
● TOPV is no longer recommended for routine immunization schedule. Special circumstances when oral vaccine would be appropriate include: imminent travel to a polio-endemic area, "catch-up" immunization, or when a parent objects to number of injections a child will receive.
● Don't use TOPV in siblings of child with known immunodeficiency syndrome; IPV is preferred.
● Obtain history of allergies and reaction to immunization.
● If skin test is needed, give it either before or with vaccine.
● Keep TOPV frozen until used. Once thawed, if unopened, may refrigerate up to 30 days; if opened, up to 7 days. Thaw before administration.

● Color change of TOPV from pink to yellow doesn't indicate change in efficacy of vaccine. Yellow color is caused by storage at low temperatures.
● **Alert:** Parenteral form should be given to immunodeficient patients or those with altered immune status because they may be at risk for developing the disease if live virus vaccine is given.
● Keep epinephrine 1:1,000 available to treat anaphylaxis.
● Oral vaccine should be deferred in patients with vomiting or diarrhea. Both forms of vaccine should be deferred in patients with acute illness.
● Don't give to neonates less than 6 weeks old.
● Highest risk of poliovirus infection occurs after first dose of oral vaccine.
● Adults at high risk for exposure who have completed a primary course may receive another dose.
● Vaccine isn't effective in modifying or preventing existing or incubating poliomyelitis.
● Document manufacturer, lot number, date given, and name, address, and title of person giving vaccine on patient's record or log.
● Vaccine may temporarily decrease response to tuberculin skin test.

PATIENT TEACHING
● Inform patient or parents about risks and benefits of vaccine before administration.
● Warn patient or parents about adverse reactions linked to vaccine.

---

rabies vaccine, adsorbed

Pregnancy risk category C

AVAILABLE FORMS
Injection: Single-dose 1-ml vial

INDICATIONS & DOSAGES
➤ **Preexposure prophylaxis rabies immunization for persons in high-risk groups—**
Adults and children: 1 ml I.M. at 0, 7, and 21 or 28 days for total of three injections. Patients at increased risk for rabies should be checked q 6 months and given booster

---

vaccination, 1 ml I.M., p.r.n., to maintain adequate serum titer.

➤ **Postexposure rabies prophylaxis—**
Adults and children not previously vaccinated against rabies: 20 IU/kg doses of human rabies immune globulin (HRIG) I.M. and five 1-ml injections of rabies vaccine, adsorbed I.M. given on days 0, 3, 7, 14, and 28.

Adults and children previously vaccinated against rabies: Two 1-ml injections of rabies vaccine, adsorbed I.M. given on days 0 and 3. HRIG shouldn't be given.

ACTION

Promotes active immunity to rabies.

Route	Onset	Peak	Duration
I.M.	Unknown	2 wk after 3 doses	Unknown

ADVERSE REACTIONS

CNS: *headache, dizziness, fatigue.*
GI: *abdominal pain, nausea.*
Musculoskeletal: *myalgia, aching of injected muscle.*
Skin: *transient pain, erythema, swelling, itching,* mild inflammatory reaction at injection site.
Other: *slight fever,* reaction resembling serum sickness, ***anaphylaxis.***

INTERACTIONS

Drug-drug. *Antimalarials, corticosteroids, immunosuppressants:* Decreased response to rabies vaccine. Avoid using together.

EFFECTS ON LAB TEST RESULTS

None reported.

CONTRAINDICATIONS

Contraindicated in patients who have experienced life-threatening allergic reactions to previous injections of vaccine or to components of vaccine, including thimerosal.

NURSING CONSIDERATIONS

• Use cautiously in patients hypersensitive to monkey-derived proteins, in those with history of non–life-threatening allergic reactions to previous injections of vaccine, and in children.

• Keep epinephrine 1:1,000 available to treat anaphylaxis.
• Give as I.M. injection into deltoid region in adults and older children. For younger children, the midanterolateral aspect of the thigh also is acceptable. Don't use I.D. route. Avoid injecting vaccine near a peripheral nerve or into adipose or S.C. tissue.
• Vaccine is normally a light pink color because of presence of phenol red in suspension.
• **Alert:** If patient experiences serious adverse reaction to vaccine, report reaction promptly to local public health officials.
• **Alert:** Don't confuse vaccine with rabies immune globulin. Both drugs may be given in some situations.

PATIENT TEACHING

• Inform patient about adverse reactions linked to vaccine and importance of reporting serious adverse reactions.
• Warn patient not to perform hazardous activities if dizziness occurs.
• Advise proper antipyretic dose for fever.
• Teach proper wound care and signs and symptoms of infection.

---

rabies vaccine, human diploid cell (HDCV)
Imovax Rabies, Imovax Rabies I.D. Vaccine

Pregnancy risk category C

AVAILABLE FORMS

I.D. injection: 0.25 IU rabies antigen/dose
I.M. injection: 2.5 IU rabies antigen/ml, in single-dose vial with diluent

INDICATIONS & DOSAGES

➤ **Postexposure antirabies immunization—**
Adults and children: Five 1-ml doses of HDCV I.M. First dose given as soon as possible after exposure; an additional dose given on each of days 3, 7, 14, and 28 after first dose. If no antibody response occurs after this primary series, booster dose is recommended.

➤ **Preexposure prophylaxis immunization for persons in high-risk groups—**
Adults and children: Three 1-ml injections
given I.M. First dose given on day 0 (first
day of therapy), second dose on day 7, and
third dose on day 21 or 28. Or, 0.1 ml I.D.
on same dosage schedule.

ACTION
Promotes active immunity to rabies.

Route	Onset	Peak	Duration
I.D., I.M.	1 wk	1-2 mo	> 2 yr

ADVERSE REACTIONS
CNS: *headache,* dizziness, *fatigue.*
GI: *nausea,* abdominal pain, diarrhea.
Musculoskeletal: muscle aches.
Skin: *injection site pain, erythema,
swelling, itching.*
Other: *fever,* **anaphylaxis,** serum sick-
ness.

INTERACTIONS
Drug-drug. *Antimalarials, corticosteroids, immunosuppressants:* Decreased response to rabies vaccine. Avoid using together.

EFFECTS ON LAB TEST RESULTS
None reported.

CONTRAINDICATIONS
No contraindications reported for persons
after exposure. An acute febrile illness
contraindicates use of vaccine for persons
previously exposed.

NURSING CONSIDERATIONS
• Use cautiously in hypersensitive patients.
• Keep epinephrine 1:1,000 available to
treat anaphylaxis.
• Use vaccine immediately after reconstitution.
• *Alert:* Don't use I.D. route for postexposure rabies vaccination.
• Alternative regimen of 0.1-ml doses is
only for preexposure prophylaxis. For
postexposure prophylaxis, only use 1-ml
doses.
• Stop corticosteroid therapy during immunizing period unless therapy is essential for treatment of other conditions.

• Some patients who receive booster doses
experience serum sickness-like hypersensitivity. These reactions usually respond to
antihistamines.
• All serious reactions should be reported
to the State Department of Health.
• *Alert:* Don't confuse vaccine with rabies
immune globulin. Both drugs may be giv-
en in some situations.

PATIENT TEACHING
• Inform patient about adverse reactions
linked to vaccine. Tell patient to report
persistent or severe reactions.
• Stress importance of receiving booster,
if appropriate for patient.
• Tell patient to treat mild reaction with
anti-inflammatory or antipyretic at appropriate doses.

rubella and mumps virus
vaccine, live
Biavax II

Pregnancy risk category C

AVAILABLE FORMS
Injection: Single-dose vial containing not
less than 1,000 tissue culture infective
doses (TCID$_{50}$) of Wistar RA 27/3 rubella
virus (propagated in human diploid cell
culture) and not less than 20,000 TCID$_{50}$
of Jeryl Lynn mumps strain (grown in
chick embryo cell culture)

INDICATIONS & DOSAGES
➤ **Rubella and mumps immunization—**
Adults and children age 1 and older:
0.5 ml S.C.

ACTION
Promotes immunity to rubella and mumps
by inducing antibody production.

Route	Onset	Peak	Duration
S.C.	Unknown	Unknown	10.5 yr

ADVERSE REACTIONS
CNS: polyneuritis.
GI: diarrhea.
Musculoskeletal: *arthritis, arthralgia.*
Skin: rash, pain, erythema, and indura-
tion at injection site; ***thrombocytopenic purpu-
ra;*** urticaria.

Other: fever, *anaphylaxis,* lymphadenopathy.

INTERACTIONS
Drug-drug. *Immune serum globulin, plasma, whole blood:* Antibodies in serum may interfere with immune response. Don't give vaccine for at least 3 months after use of these products.
Immunosuppressants: May reduce immune response to vaccine. Defer immunization until immunosuppressant is discontinued.

EFFECTS ON LAB TEST RESULTS
None reported.

CONTRAINDICATIONS
Contraindicated in immunosuppressed patients; in those with cancer, blood dyscrasia, gamma globulin disorders, fever, active untreated tuberculosis, or history of anaphylaxis or anaphylactoid reactions to neomycin or eggs; in those receiving corticosteroid (except those receiving corticosteroids as replacement therapy) or radiation therapy; and in pregnant women.

NURSING CONSIDERATIONS
• Obtain history of allergies, especially anaphylactic reaction to antibiotics, and reaction to immunization.
• Keep epinephrine 1:1,000 available to treat anaphylaxis.
• If skin test is needed, give it either before or with vaccine.
• Vaccination should be deferred in patients with acute illness and after administration of immune serum globulin, blood, or plasma.
• Use only diluent supplied. Discard vaccine 8 hours after reconstituting.
• Inject into outer upper arm. Don't inject I.V.
• Allow an interval of at least 3 weeks between BCG and rubella vaccines.
• Vaccine may temporarily decrease response to tuberculin skin test.
• Document drug manufacturer, lot number, date, and name, address, and title of person giving dose on patient record or log.
• Patients born before 1956 are believed to have acquired natural immunity.

PATIENT TEACHING
• Inform patient about adverse reactions linked to vaccine.
• Stress importance of avoiding pregnancy for 3 months after vaccination. Provide contraception information, if needed.
• Inform women and girls older than age 12 about risk of self-limited arthralgia or arthritis 2 to 4 weeks after vaccination.

---

rubella virus vaccine, live attenuated (RA 27/3)
Meruvax II

Pregnancy risk category C

AVAILABLE FORMS
Injection: Single-dose vial containing not less than 1,000 tissue culture infective doses ($TCID_{50}$) of Wistar RA 27/3 strain of rubella virus (propagated in human diploid cell culture)

INDICATIONS & DOSAGES
➤ **Rubella immunization—**
Adults and children age 1 and older:
0.5 ml or 1,000 units S.C.

ACTION
Promotes immunity to rubella by inducing production of antibodies.

Route	Onset	Peak	Duration
S.C.	2-6 wk	Unknown	> 10 yr

ADVERSE REACTIONS
CNS: headache, malaise, polyneuritis.
EENT: sore throat.
Musculoskeletal: arthralgia, arthritis.
Skin: rash, pain, erythema, and induration at injection site; ***thrombocytopenic purpura;*** urticaria.
Other: fever, *anaphylaxis,* lymphadenopathy.

INTERACTIONS
Drug-drug. *Immune serum globulin, plasma, whole blood:* Antibodies in serum may interfere with immune response. Don't give vaccine for at least 3 months after use of these products.
Immunosuppressants, interferon: May reduce immune response to vaccine. Defer

---

immunization until immunosuppressant is discontinued.

EFFECTS ON LAB TEST RESULTS
None reported.

CONTRAINDICATIONS
Contraindicated in immunosuppressed patients; in patients with cancer, blood dyscrasia, gamma globulin disorders, fever, or active untreated tuberculosis; in patients hypersensitive to neomycin; in patients receiving corticosteroids (except those receiving corticosteroids as replacement therapy) or radiation therapy; and in pregnant women. Don't vaccinate patients who have AIDS or symptomatic HIV.

NURSING CONSIDERATIONS
• Obtain history of allergies and reaction to immunization.
• Keep epinephrine 1:1,000 available to treat anaphylaxis.
• If skin test is needed, give it either before or with vaccine.
• Immunization should be deferred in patients with acute illness and after administration of human immune serum globulin, blood, or plasma.
• Use only diluent supplied. Discard vaccine 8 hours after reconstituting. Protect from light.
• Inject into outer upper arm. Don't inject vaccine I.V.
• Document drug manufacturer, lot number, date, and name, address, and title of person giving dose on patient record or log.
• Allow at least 3 weeks between BCG and rubella vaccinations.
• Vaccine may temporarily decrease response to tuberculin skin test.

PATIENT TEACHING
• Inform patient about adverse reactions linked to vaccine.
• Stress importance of avoiding pregnancy for 3 months after vaccination. Provide contraception information, if needed.
• Tell patient to use correct dose of antipyretic for treating fever.

tetanus toxoid, adsorbed

tetanus toxoid, fluid

Pregnancy risk category C

AVAILABLE FORMS
tetanus toxoid, adsorbed
Injection: 5 to 10 limit flocculation (Lf) units inactivated tetanus/0.5-ml dose, in 0.5-ml syringes and 5-ml vials
tetanus toxoid, fluid
Injection: 4 to 5 Lf units inactivated tetanus/0.5-ml dose, in 0.5-ml syringes and 7.5-ml vials

INDICATIONS & DOSAGES
➤ **Primary immunization—**
Adults and children age 7 and older: 0.5 ml (adsorbed) I.M. 4 to 8 weeks apart for two doses; then third dose given 6 to 12 months after second. Or, 0.5 ml (fluid) I.M. or S.C. 4 to 8 weeks apart for three doses; then fourth dose of 0.5 ml 6 to 12 months after third dose.
Children ages 6 weeks to 6 years: 0.5 ml (adsorbed) I.M. at ages 2, 4, and 6 months. Give fourth dose at 15 to 18 months. Give fifth dose at ages 4 to 6, just before entry into school, if indicated.
➤ **Booster doses—**
Adults: 0.5 ml I.M. at 10-year intervals.

ACTION
Promotes immunity to tetanus by inducing antitoxin production.

Route	Onset	Peak	Duration
I.M., S.C.	After 2 doses	Unknown	> 10 yr

ADVERSE REACTIONS
CNS: headache, *seizures,* malaise, encephalopathy.
CV: tachycardia, hypotension, flushing.
Musculoskeletal: aches, pains.
Skin: erythema, induration, nodule at injection site; urticaria; pruritus.
Other: slight fever, chills, *anaphylaxis.*

INTERACTIONS
Drug-drug. *Chloramphenicol:* May interfere with response to tetanus toxoid. Watch patient for effect.

Immunosuppressants, tetanus immune globulin: May reduce immune response to vaccine. Defer immunization until 1 month after immunosuppressant is discontinued.

EFFECTS ON LAB TEST RESULTS
None reported.

CONTRAINDICATIONS
Contraindicated in immunosuppressed patients, in those with immunoglobulin abnormalities, and in those with severe hypersensitivity or neurologic reactions to toxoid or its ingredients. Also contraindicated in patients with thrombocytopenia or other coagulation disorders that would contraindicate I.M. injection unless potential benefits outweigh risks. Defer vaccination in patients with acute illness and during polio outbreaks, except in emergencies.

NURSING CONSIDERATIONS
• Use cautiously (adsorbed form) in infants or children with cerebral damage, neurologic disorders, or history of febrile seizures.
• Obtain history of allergies and reaction to immunization.
• Determine date of last tetanus immunization.
• Keep epinephrine 1:1,000 available to treat anaphylaxis.
• Adsorbed form produces longer duration of immunity. Fluid form provides quicker booster effect in patients actively immunized previously.
• Document manufacturer, lot number, date, and name, address, and title of person giving dose on patient record or log.
• *Alert:* Don't confuse drug with tetanus immune globulin, human. Both drugs may be given in some situations.

PATIENT TEACHING
• Advise patient to avoid using hot or cold compresses at injection site; this may increase severity of local reaction.
• Instruct patient to report persistent or severe adverse reactions.
• Advise patient of proper antipyretic dose for fever reaction.
• Tell patient that nodule at injection site may be present for a few weeks.

typhoid vaccine, oral
Vivotif Berna Vaccine

typhoid vaccine, parenteral

Pregnancy risk category C

AVAILABLE FORMS
Capsules (enteric-coated): 2 to 6×10^9 colony-forming units of viable *Salmonella typhi* Ty21a and 5 to 50×10^9 bacterial cells of nonviable Ty21a2 (four doses of vaccine in a single package)
Injection: suspension of killed Ty-2 strain of *S. typhi;* 8 units/ml in 5- and 10-ml vials

INDICATIONS & DOSAGES
➤ **Primary immunization—**
P.O.
Adults: One capsule P.O. on alternate days 1 hour before meals for four doses. Protocol repeated as booster q 5 years.
S.C.
Adults and children older than age 10: 0.5 ml S.C.; repeated in 4 weeks. Protocol repeated as booster q 3 years with either 0.5 ml S.C. or 0.1 ml I.D.
Children ages 6 months to 10 years: 0.25 ml S.C.; repeated in 4 weeks. Protocol repeated as booster q 3 years with either 0.25 ml S.C. or 0.1 ml I.D.

ACTION
Provides active immunity to typhoid fever.

Route	Onset	Peak	Duration
I.D., P.O., S.C.	After last dose	Unknown	3-5 yr

ADVERSE REACTIONS
CNS: headache, malaise.
GI: nausea, abdominal cramps, vomiting.
Musculoskeletal: myalgia.
Skin: rash; urticaria; swelling, pain, inflammation at injection site; induration.
Other: fever, *anaphylaxis.*

INTERACTIONS
Drug-drug. *Immunosuppressants, phenytoin, sulfonamides:* May impair antibody response. Don't use together.
Other vaccines (cholera, plague): May increase adverse effects. Don't give together.

EFFECTS ON LAB TEST RESULTS
None reported.

CONTRAINDICATIONS
Contraindicated in patients hypersensitive to vaccine or its components and in immunosuppressed patients. Defer vaccination in patients with acute illness. Use parenteral, inactivated vaccine in HIV-positive patients.

NURSING CONSIDERATIONS
• Obtain history of allergies and reaction to immunization. Keep epinephrine 1:1,000 available to treat anaphylaxis.
• Treat fever with antipyretics.
• Shake thoroughly before withdrawing from vial.
• Refrigerate vaccine at 36° to 46° F (2° to 8° C).

PATIENT TEACHING
• When giving oral vaccine, make sure patient understands importance of taking all four doses and following alternate-day regimen.
• Tell patient to take oral vaccine with cold or lukewarm water and not to chew or crush enteric-coated capsules. Capsules should be swallowed immediately.
• Tell patient to take oral vaccine 1 hour before meals.
• Inform patient about adverse reactions linked to vaccine; reactions usually appear within 24 hours and last 1 to 2 days.

---

typhoid Vi polysaccharide vaccine
Typhim Vi

Pregnancy risk category C

AVAILABLE FORMS
Injection: 0.5-ml syringe, 20-dose vial, 50-dose vial

INDICATIONS & DOSAGES
➤ **Active immunization against typhoid fever—**
Adults and children age 2 and older: 0.5 ml I.M. as single dose. Reimmunize q 2 years with 0.5 ml I.M. as single dose, if needed.

ACTION
Promotes active immunity to typhoid fever.

Route	Onset	Peak	Duration
I.M.	2 wk	Unknown	2 yr

ADVERSE REACTIONS
CNS: *headache,* malaise.
GI: nausea, vomiting, abdominal cramps.
Musculoskeletal: myalgia.
Skin: *pain, tenderness, induration, erythema at injection site;* rash; urticaria.
Other: *anaphylaxis,* fever.

INTERACTIONS
Drug-drug. *Anticoagulants:* Increased effect of anticoagulants. Check patient for bleeding.

EFFECTS ON LAB TEST RESULTS
None reported.

CONTRAINDICATIONS
Contraindicated in patients hypersensitive to vaccine's components. Don't use vaccine to treat patients with typhoid fever; don't give to those who are chronic typhoid carriers.

NURSING CONSIDERATIONS
• Use cautiously in patients with thrombocytopenia or bleeding disorder and in those taking an anticoagulant; bleeding may occur after an I.M. injection in these patients.
• As with other vaccines, administration should be delayed, if possible, in patients with febrile illness.
• Although anaphylaxis is rare, keep epinephrine available to treat an anaphylactoid reaction.
• Give as an I.M. injection into deltoid region in adults and into deltoid or vastus lateralis in children. Don't give in gluteal region or areas where there may be a nerve trunk. Never inject vaccine I.V.
• Record drug manufacturer, lot number, date, and name, address, and title of person giving dose on patient record or log.

PATIENT TEACHING
• Advise patient to take all precautions needed to avoid contact with or ingestion of contaminated food and water.

• Inform patient that immunization should be given at least 2 weeks before expected exposure. Although an optimal reimmunization schedule hasn't been established, recommended reimmunization consists of single dose for U.S. travelers every 2 years if exposure to typhoid fever is possible.
• Inform patient about adverse reactions linked to vaccine.

---

varicella virus vaccine
Varivax

Pregnancy risk category C

AVAILABLE FORMS
Injection: Single-dose vial containing 1,350 plague-forming units of Oka/Merck varicella virus (live)

INDICATIONS & DOSAGES
➤ **Prevention of varicella-zoster (chickenpox) infections—**
Adults and children age 13 and older: 0.5 ml S.C.; then second 0.5-ml dose 4 to 8 weeks later.
Children ages 1 to 12: 0.5 ml S.C.

ACTION
Prevents chickenpox by inducing production of antibodies to varicella-zoster virus.

Route	Onset	Peak	Duration
S.C.	4-6 wk	Unknown	> 2 yr

ADVERSE REACTIONS
Skin: swelling, redness, pain, rash, varicella-like rash at injection site.
Other: *anaphylaxis, fever,* herpes zoster, stiffness.

INTERACTIONS
Drug-drug. *Blood products, immune globulin:* May inactivate vaccine. Defer vaccination for at least 5 months after blood or plasma transfusions or administration of immune globulin or varicella-zoster immune globulin.
Immunosuppressants: Risk of severe reactions to live virus vaccines. Postpone routine vaccination.
Salicylates: Reye's syndrome has been reported after natural varicella infection.

Avoid use of salicylates for 6 weeks after varicella immunization.

EFFECTS ON LAB TEST RESULTS
None reported.

CONTRAINDICATIONS
Contraindicated in patients hypersensitive to drug; in those with history of anaphylactoid reaction to neomycin; in those with blood dyscrasia, leukemia, lymphomas, neoplasms affecting bone marrow or lymphatic system, primary and acquired immunosuppressive states, active untreated tuberculosis, or any febrile respiratory illness or other active febrile infection; and in pregnant women.

NURSING CONSIDERATIONS
• Vaccine must be stored frozen. Diluent should be stored separately at room temperature or refrigerated.
• To reconstitute vaccine, first withdraw 0.7 ml of diluent into syringe to be used for reconstitution. Inject all diluent in syringe into vial of lyophilized vaccine, and gently agitate to mix thoroughly. Give immediately after reconstitution. Discard if not used within 30 minutes.
• Keep epinephrine available to treat anaphylaxis.
• Vaccine has been used safely and effectively with measles, mumps, and rubella vaccine.
• Document manufacturer, lot number, date, and name, address, and title of person giving dose on patient record or log.
• *Alert:* Vaccine contains live, attenuated virus. Vaccinated patients who develop rash may be able to transmit virus.

PATIENT TEACHING
• Inform patient or parents about adverse reactions linked to vaccine.
• Caution woman of childbearing age to report suspected pregnancy before administration.
• Instruct patient to avoid salicylates for 6 weeks after vaccination to prevent Reye's syndrome.
• Tell patient to avoid pregnancy for 3 months after vaccination.
• Inform patient to avoid postinjection close contact with susceptible high-risk

---

*Liquid contains alcohol. **May contain tartrazine. †Canada ‡Australia §U.K. ◇OTC

individuals (such as pregnant women or immunocompromised persons).

---

yellow fever vaccine
YF-Vax

Pregnancy risk category C

AVAILABLE FORMS
Injection: Live, attenuated 17D yellow fever virus in 1-, 5-, and 20-dose vials, with diluent; supplied only to centers authorized to issue yellow fever vaccination certificates

ACTION
Provides active immunity to yellow fever.

Route	Onset	Peak	Duration
S.C.	7-10 days	28 days	> 10 yr

INDICATIONS & DOSAGES
➤ **Primary vaccination—**
Adults and children age 9 months and older: 0.5 ml deep S.C.; booster is 0.5 ml S.C. q 10 years.
Children ages 6 to 9 months: Same dose as above if they are traveling to areas of epidemic yellow fever.

ADVERSE REACTIONS
CNS: headache, *malaise.*
Musculoskeletal: myalgia.
Skin: mild swelling, pain at injection site.
Other: *anaphylaxis, fever.*

INTERACTIONS
Drug-drug. *Cholera vaccine:* Administration together may interfere with immune response to both yellow fever and cholera vaccines. Give 3 weeks apart.
Immunosuppressants: May increase viral replication and development of infection with yellow fever virus. Defer immunization until immunosuppressant is stopped.

EFFECTS ON LAB TEST RESULTS
None reported.

CONTRAINDICATIONS
Contraindicated in immunosuppressed patients; in those with cancer, gamma globulin deficiency, or those hypersensitive to eggs; and in those receiving corticosteroid

or radiation therapy. Also contraindicated in pregnant women and in infants younger than age 6 months, except in high-risk areas.

NURSING CONSIDERATIONS
● Obtain history of allergies, especially to eggs, and reactions to immunizations.
● Keep epinephrine 1:1,000 available to treat anaphylaxis.
● In patients who have received blood or plasma transfusions, 8 weeks should pass before you give vaccine.
● Reconstitute with unpreserved saline solution for injection (preservatives inactivate the yellow fever viruses).
● Keep vaccine frozen. Don't use unless shipping case contains some dry ice on arrival. Avoid vigorous shaking; carefully swirl mixture until suspension is uniform. Use within 1 hour after reconstituting. Discard remainder.
● Yellow fever vaccine shouldn't be given within 1 month of other live-virus vaccines; may be given with hepatitis B vaccine.

PATIENT TEACHING
● Inform patient about adverse reactions linked to vaccine.
● Caution woman of childbearing age to report suspected pregnancy before administration.
● Advise patient to avoid bites by using sprays, repellents, protective clothing, and screens.

Reactions may be *common*, uncommon, *life-threatening*, or **COMMON AND LIFE-THREATENING.**

74

Antitoxins and antivenins

**black widow spider antivenin
Crotalidae antivenom,
     polyvalent
diphtheria antitoxin, equine
Micrurus fulvius antivenin**

COMBINATION PRODUCTS
None.

---

black widow spider antivenin
Antivenin (*Latrodectus mactans*)

Pregnancy risk category C

AVAILABLE FORMS
Injection: Combination package—one vial of antivenin (6,000-unit vial), one 2.5-ml vial of diluent (sterile water for injection), and one 1-ml vial of normal equine serum (1:10 dilution) for sensitivity testing

INDICATIONS & DOSAGES
➤ **Black widow spider bite—**
Adults and children: 2.5 ml I.M. in antero-lateral thigh. Second dose may be needed. In severe cases, antivenin may be given I.V.

Test for sensitivity before giving drug with 0.02 ml of 1:10 antivenin in normal saline solution. Evaluate result in 10 minutes.

For desensitization, use 1:10 and 1:100 dilutions of antivenin in normal saline solution for injection.

I.V. ADMINISTRATION
• I.V. route is preferred in severe cases, in patients in shock, and in patients younger than age 12.
• Reconstitute antivenin with 2.5 ml of diluent. Further dilute reconstituted solution in 10 to 50 ml normal saline solution for injection and infuse over 15 minutes.
• Reconstituted solutions should be used within 48 hours; diluted solutions, within 12 hours.

ACTION
Unknown.

Route	Onset	Peak	Duration
I.M.	Unknown	2-3 days	Unknown
I.V.	Immediate	Unknown	Unknown

ADVERSE REACTIONS
CNS: *neurotoxicity.*
Other: hypersensitivity reactions, *anaphylaxis, serum sickness.*

INTERACTIONS
Drug-drug. *Antihistamines:* May interfere with sensitivity tests. Avoid using together.

EFFECTS ON LAB TEST RESULTS
None reported.

CONTRAINDICATIONS
Contraindicated in patients hypersensitive to drug or its components (horse serum) when desensitization isn't feasible.

NURSING CONSIDERATIONS
• Immobilize patient; splint the bitten limb to prevent spread of venom.
• Obtain history of allergies, especially to horses, and reaction to immunization. Have epinephrine 1:1,000 available to treat anaphylaxis.
• For best results, give antivenin as soon as possible.
• Perform a skin or conjunctival test before administration.
• *Alert:* Give I.M. injection in anterolateral thigh so that a tourniquet may be applied if a systemic reaction occurs.
• Watch patient for 2 to 3 days. Venom is neurotoxic and may cause respiratory paralysis and seizures.
• Signs and symptoms usually subside in 1 to 3 hours.
• Refrigerate at 36° to 46° F (2° to 8° C).
• Discard if injection is frozen.

PATIENT TEACHING
• Explain to patient and family how drug will be given.

---

*Liquid contains alcohol.   **May contain tartrazine.   †Canada   ‡Australia   §U.K.   ◊OTC

• Instruct patient to report adverse reactions promptly.

• Tell patient that serum sickness can occur 8 to 12 days after administration.

Crotalidae antivenom, polyvalent

Pregnancy risk category C

AVAILABLE FORMS
Injection: Combination package—one vial of lyophilized serum, one vial of diluent (10 ml of bacteriostatic water for injection), and one 1-ml vial of normal horse serum (diluted 1:10) for sensitivity testing

INDICATIONS & DOSAGES
➤ **Crotalid (rattlesnake) bites—**
Adults and children: Initially, 20 to 150 ml I.V., depending on severity of bite and patient response. For minimal envenomation: 20 to 40 ml I.V.; for moderate envenomation: 50 to 90 ml I.V.; for severe envenomation: 100 to 150 ml I.V. For a large amount of venom, more than 150 ml may be given I.V. directly into superficial vein. Subsequent doses are based on patient's response; may need another 10 to 50 ml if swelling progresses, systemic symptoms increase, or new signs and symptoms appear.

Test for sensitivity before giving drug. Give 0.02 to 0.03 ml of 1:10 dilution in normal saline solution I.D. Read results after 5 to 10 minutes. Watch carefully for delayed allergic reaction or relapse.

If sensitivity test is positive, desensitize; prepare 1:10 and 1:100 dilutions of antivenom in normal saline solution for injection.
Adjust-a-dose: Children, who have less resistance and less body fluid to dilute venom, may need twice adult dose.

I.V. ADMINISTRATION
• Reconstitute drug by adding 10 ml of supplied diluent. Further dilute to make a 1:1 to 1:10 solution using normal saline solution or D₅W. To avoid foaming, don't shake while mixing. Start by infusing 5 to 10 ml of diluted antivenom over 3 to 5 minutes; observe patient carefully. If no signs or symptoms of immediate systemic reaction occur, continue infusion.

• Use reconstituted solution within 48 hours and dilutions within 12 hours.

ACTION
Neutralizes and binds venom of crotalids (pit vipers), including rattlesnakes, water moccasins, and copperheads.

Route	Onset	Peak	Duration
I.V.	Immediate	Unknown	Unknown

ADVERSE REACTIONS
Musculoskeletal: arthralgia.
Skin: erythema, urticaria.
Other: pain, hypersensitivity reactions, *anaphylaxis, serum sickness,* lymphadenopathy, fever.

INTERACTIONS
Drug-drug. *Antihistamines:* Increased toxicity of crotalid venoms. Don't use together.

EFFECTS ON LAB TEST RESULTS
None reported.

CONTRAINDICATIONS
Contraindicated in patients hypersensitive to drug or its components.

NURSING CONSIDERATIONS
• Use drug cautiously. About 60% of patients treated with antivenom develop hypersensitivity.

• Immobilize patient immediately. Splint bitten limb.

• Obtain history of allergies, especially to horses, and reactions to immunizations. Have epinephrine 1:1,000 available in case of hypersensitivity reaction.

• *Alert:* Type and crossmatch blood as soon as possible; hemolysis from venom prevents accurate crossmatching.

• For best results, give antivenom as soon as possible, preferably within 4 hours of bite. In severe cases, may be given within 24 hours of bite.

• Give corticosteroids, as prescribed. If a large number of vials is given, serum sickness may result 5 to 24 days after infusion.

• Antivenom may be stored without refrigeration for 60 days, but it shouldn't be exposed to temperatures over 98.6° F (37° C).

PATIENT TEACHING
• Explain to patient and family that test dose will be given first to check for sensitivity to drug.
• Instruct patient to report adverse reactions promptly.

---

diphtheria antitoxin, equine

Pregnancy risk category C

AVAILABLE FORMS
Injection: Not less than 500 units/ml in 10,000-unit and 20,000-unit vials

INDICATIONS & DOSAGES
➤ **Diphtheria prevention—**
Adults and children: 5,000 to 10,000 units I.M.
➤ **Pharyngeal or laryngeal diphtheria of 48 hours' duration—**
Adults and children: 20,000 to 40,000 units I.M. or slow I.V. infusion.
➤ **Nasopharyngeal lesions—**
Adults and children: 40,000 to 60,000 units I.M. or slow I.V. infusion.
➤ **Extensive disease of 3 or more days' duration or disease with neck swelling—**
Adults and children: 80,000 to 120,000 units by slow I.V. infusion.

I.V. ADMINISTRATION
• Dilute appropriate dose in D_5W or normal saline solution to achieve a 1:20 dilution.
• Give solution by direct infusion at no more than 1 ml/minute.

ACTION
Binds with circulating toxin and prevents disease progression.

Route	Onset	Peak	Duration
I.M.	Unknown	2 days	Unknown
I.V.	Immediate	Unknown	Unknown

ADVERSE REACTIONS
Skin: erythema, urticaria.
Other: pain, hypersensitivity reactions, *anaphylaxis,* serum sickness.

INTERACTIONS
None significant.

EFFECTS ON LAB TEST RESULTS
None reported.

CONTRAINDICATIONS
Contraindicated in patients hypersensitive to drug or its components.

NURSING CONSIDERATIONS
• Obtain history of allergies, especially to horses, and reactions to immunizations. Have epinephrine 1:1,000 available in case of anaphylaxis. Antitoxin should be used with extreme caution in patients with history of allergic disorders.
• Test for sensitivity before giving drug.
• *Alert:* If patient has signs or symptoms of diphtheria (sore throat, fever, tonsillar membrane), start therapy immediately, without waiting for culture reports.
• For storage, refrigerate antitoxin at 36° to 50° F (2° to 10° C). Before giving, warm to 90° to 95° F (32° to 35° C), never higher.
• Begin appropriate antimicrobial therapy.
• Monitor patient for serum sickness (urticaria, pruritus, fever, malaise, arthralgia), which may occur in 7 to 12 days.

PATIENT TEACHING
• Explain to patient and family that test dose will be given first to check for sensitivity to drug.
• Tell patient to report adverse reactions promptly.

Micrurus fulvius antivenin

Pregnancy risk category C

AVAILABLE FORMS
Injection: Combination package with 10 ml of diluent

INDICATIONS & DOSAGES
➤ **Eastern and Texas coral snake bite—**
Adults and children: 30 to 50 ml or 3 to 5 vials slow I.V. through running I.V. of normal saline solution. Give 1 to 2 ml over 3 to 5 minutes; monitor patient closely for allergic reaction. If no signs or symptoms

---

of allergic reaction develop, continue injection; 100 ml or more may be needed.

Test for sensitivity before giving drug. If sensitivity test is positive, prepare to desensitize; prepare 1:10 and 1:100 dilutions of antivenin in saline solution for injection.

I.V. ADMINISTRATION
• Reconstitute antivenin powder with diluent. Further dilute in normal saline solution to achieve a 1:1 to 1:10 dilution. Gently swirl solution to avoid foaming.
• Infuse initial 1 to 2 ml over 3 to 5 minutes while closely monitoring patient. If no immediate systemic response occurs, continue infusion at maximum safe rate for I.V. fluid administration.
• Use reconstituted solution within 48 hours and dilutions within 12 hours.

ACTION
Neutralizes and binds coral snake venom.

Route	Onset	Peak	Duration
I.V.	Immediate	Unknown	Unknown

ADVERSE REACTIONS
Musculoskeletal: arthralgia.
Skin: erythema, urticaria.
Other: pain, hypersensitivity reactions, *anaphylaxis,* fever, lymphadenopathy.

INTERACTIONS
None significant.

EFFECTS ON LAB TEST RESULTS
None reported.

CONTRAINDICATIONS
Contraindicated in patients hypersensitive to drug or its components.

NURSING CONSIDERATIONS
• *Alert:* Drug isn't effective for Sonoran or Arizona coral snake bites.
• Immobilize patient and splint bitten limb to prevent spread of venom.
• Obtain accurate patient history of allergies, especially to horses, and reactions to immunizations. Keep epinephrine 1:1,000 available to treat anaphylaxis.
• Antivenin should be given as soon as possible (before onset of neurotoxic signs), preferably within 4 hours of bite;

asymptomatic patients should be treated because systemic symptoms usually develop later.
• Watch patient carefully for 24 hours. Venom is neurotoxic and may cause respiratory paralysis.
• Antivenin can be stored at room temperature for 10 days.

PATIENT TEACHING
• Explain to patient and family that test dose will be given first to check for sensitivity to drug.
• Tell patient to report adverse reactions promptly.

Reactions may be *common,* uncommon, *life-threatening,* or COMMON AND LIFE-THREATENING.

cytomegalovirus immune
  globulin, intravenous
hepatitis B immune globulin,
  human
immune globulin intramuscular
immune globulin intravenous
rabies immune globulin, human
respiratory syncytial virus
  immune globulin intravenous,
  human
Rh$_o$(D) immune globulin, human
Rh$_o$(D) immune globulin
  intravenous, human
tetanus immune globulin,
  human
varicella-zoster immune
  globulin

COMBINATION PRODUCTS
None.

---

cytomegalovirus immune globulin (human), intravenous (CMV-IGIV)
CytoGam

Pregnancy risk category C

AVAILABLE FORMS
Injection: 2.5 g/50 ml†; 1 g/20 ml

INDICATIONS & DOSAGES
➤ **To attenuate primary CMV disease in seronegative kidney transplant recipients who receive a kidney from a CMV seropositive donor—**
Adults: Give I.V. based on time after transplantation: within 72 hours, 150 mg/kg; 2 weeks after, 100 mg/kg; 4 weeks after, 100 mg/kg; 6 weeks after, 100 mg/kg; 8 weeks after, 100 mg/kg; 12 weeks after, 50 mg/kg; 16 weeks after, 50 mg/kg.

Give initial dose at 15 mg/kg/hour. Increase to 30 mg/kg/hour after 30 minutes if no adverse reactions occur, and then to 60 mg/kg/hour after another 30 minutes if no reactions occur. Volume shouldn't exceed 75 ml/hour. Subsequent doses may be given at 15 mg/kg/hour for 15 minutes,

increasing q 15 minutes in a stepwise fashion to 60 mg/kg/hour.
➤ **Prophylaxis of CMV disease linked with lung, liver, pancreas, and heart transplants—**
Adults: Used with ganciclovir in organ transplants from CMV seropositive donors into seronegative recipients. Maximum total dose per infusion is 150 mg/kg I.V. given as follows based on time after transplantation: within 72 hours, 150 mg/kg; 2 weeks after, 150 mg/kg; 4 weeks after, 150 mg/kg; 6 weeks after, 150 mg/kg; 8 weeks after, 150 mg/kg; 12 weeks after, 100 mg/kg; 16 weeks after, 100 mg/kg.

Give initial dose at 15 mg/kg/hour. If no adverse reactions occur after 30 minutes, increase rate to 30 mg/kg/hour. If no adverse reactions occur after another 30 minutes, infusion may be increased to 60 mg/kg/hour (volume shouldn't exceed 75 ml/hour). Subsequent doses may be given at 15 mg/kg/hour for 15 minutes, increasing every 15 minutes in a stepwise fashion to maximum rate of 60 mg/kg/hour (volume shouldn't exceed 75 ml/hour). Monitor patient closely during and after each rate change.

I.V. ADMINISTRATION
● Remove tab portion of vial cap and clean rubber stopper with 70% alcohol or equivalent. To avoid foaming, don't shake vial. Inspect vial for clarity and particles.
● If possible, give through a separate I.V. line, using an infusion pump. Filters aren't needed. If unable to give through separate line, piggyback into line of saline solution for injection or into 5%, 10%, 20%, or 25% dextrose in water, with or without sodium chloride. Don't dilute more than 1:2 with any of these solutions.
● Begin infusion within 6 hours of entering vial; finish within 12 hours.

ACTION
Provides passive immunity by supplying a relatively high level of immunoglobulin G

(IgG) antibodies against CMV. Increasing these antibody levels in CMV-exposed patients may attenuate or reduce risk of serious CMV disease.

Route	Onset	Peak	Duration
I.V.	Unknown	Unknown	Unknown

ADVERSE REACTIONS
CNS: aseptic meningitis syndrome.
CV: hypotension, *flushing.*
GI: *nausea, vomiting.*
Musculoskeletal: muscle cramps, *back pain.*
Respiratory: *wheezing.*
Other: *anaphylaxis, chills,* fever.

INTERACTIONS
Drug-drug. *Live-virus vaccines:* May interfere with immune response to live-virus vaccines. Defer vaccination for at least 3 months.

EFFECTS ON LAB TEST RESULTS
None reported.

CONTRAINDICATIONS
Contraindicated in patients sensitive to other human immunoglobulin preparations or with selective IgA deficiency.

NURSING CONSIDERATIONS
• Monitor patient's vital signs closely before, during, and after infusion, and before and after increases in infusion rate.
• *Alert:* If anaphylaxis occurs or blood pressure drops, stop infusion, notify prescriber, and be prepared to give cardiopulmonary resuscitation and such drugs as diphenhydramine and epinephrine.
• Refrigerate drug at 36° to 46° F (2° to 8° C).

PATIENT TEACHING
• Review drug therapy regimen with patient, and stress importance of compliance in follow-up visits.
• Instruct patient to report adverse reactions promptly.

hepatitis B immune globulin, human
BayHep, HyperHep

Pregnancy risk category C

AVAILABLE FORMS
Injection: 1-ml, 4-ml, 5-ml vials; 0.5-ml neonatal single-dose syringe

INDICATIONS & DOSAGES
➤ **Hepatitis B exposure in high-risk patients—**
Adults and children: 0.06 ml/kg (usual dose is 3 ml to 5 ml) I.M. within 7 days after exposure. Dose repeated 28 days after exposure if patient refuses hepatitis B vaccine.
Neonates born to patients who test positive for hepatitis B surface antigen (HBsAg): 0.5 ml I.M. within 12 hours of birth.

ACTION
Provides passive immunity to hepatitis B.

Route	Onset	Peak	Duration
I.M.	1-6 days	3-11 days	2 mo

ADVERSE REACTIONS
Skin: urticaria, *pain and tenderness at injection site.*
Other: *anaphylaxis, angioedema.*

INTERACTIONS
Drug-drug. *Live-virus vaccines:* May interfere with response to live-virus vaccines. Defer routine immunization for 3 months.

EFFECTS ON LAB TEST RESULTS
None reported.

CONTRAINDICATIONS
Contraindicated in patients with history of anaphylactic reactions to immune serum. Give to patients with coagulation disorders or thrombocytopenia only if benefit outweighs risk.

NURSING CONSIDERATIONS
• Obtain history of allergies and reactions to immunizations. Keep epinephrine 1:1,000 available.

• Inspect for discoloration or particulates. Drug is clear, slightly amber, and moderately viscous.

• Inject into anterolateral thigh or deltoid muscle in older children and adults; inject into anterolateral thigh in neonates and children younger than age 3.

• For postexposure prophylaxis (for example, needlestick, direct contact), drug is usually given with hepatitis B vaccine.

• *Alert:* This immune globulin provides passive immunity; don't confuse with hepatitis B vaccine. Both drugs may be given at same time. Don't mix in the same syringe.

• *Alert:* Don't confuse HyperHep with Hyperstat or Hyper-Tet.

PATIENT TEACHING
• Inform patient that pain and tenderness may occur at injection site.
• Tell patient to report signs and symptoms of hypersensitivity immediately.

immune globulin intramuscular (gamma globulin, IG, IGIM)

immune globulin intravenous (IGIV)
Gamimune N, Gammagard S/D, Gammar-P I.V., Iveegam, Polygam S/D, Sandoglobulin, Venoglobulin-I, Venoglobulin-S

Pregnancy risk category C

AVAILABLE FORMS
immune globulin intramuscular
Injection: 2-ml, 10-ml vials
immune globulin intravenous
Injection: 5% and 10% in 10-ml, 50-ml, 100-ml, 250-ml vials (Gamimune N) 5% in 2.5-g, 5-g, 10-g vials; 5%, 10% in 5-g, 10-g, 20-g vials (Venoglobulin-S)
Powder for injection: 50 mg protein/ml in 2.5-g, 5-g, 10-g vials (Gammagard S/D); 2.5-g, 1-g, 5-g vials (Gammar-P I.V.); 500-mg, 1-g, 2.5-g, 5-g vials (Iveegam); 2.5-g, 5-g, 10-g vials (Polygam S/D); 1-g, 3-g, 6-g, 12-g vials (Sandoglobulin); 500-mg, 2.5-g, 5-g, 10-g vials (Venoglobulin-I)

INDICATIONS & DOSAGES
➤ **Primary humoral immunodeficiency (IGIV)—**
Adults and children: Gamimune N—100 to 200 mg/kg I.V. monthly, at 0.01 to 0.02 ml/kg/minute for 30 minutes. If no problems, rate can be slowly increased to maximum of 0.08 ml/kg/minute.

Gammagard S/D—200 to 400 mg/kg I.V.; then monthly doses of 100 mg/kg. Initiate infusion at 0.5 ml/kg/hour and increase to maximum of 4 ml/kg/hour. Dose related to patient response.

Gammar-P I.V.—200 to 400 mg/kg infused I.V. at 0.01 ml/kg/minute and increased to 0.02 ml/kg/minute after 15 to 30 minutes if no problems, given q 3 to 4 weeks. Maximum infusion rate is 0.06 ml/kg/minute.

✳ *NEW INDICATION:* Treatment of primary defective antibody synthesis such as agammaglobulinemia or hypogammaglobulinemia in patients who are at increased risk of infection—
Adolescents and children: Gammar-P I.V. () I.V. every three to four weeks. Adjust dosage according to clinical effect and to maintain IgG at desired level.

Iveegam—200 mg/kg I.V. monthly. May increase dose to maximum of 800 mg/kg or give more frequently to produce desired effect. Infusion rate is 1 to 2 ml/minute for 5% solution.

Polygam S/D—Initially, 200 to 400 mg/kg I.V. at 0.5 ml/kg/hour, increasing to maximum of 4 ml/kg/hour. Subsequent dose is 100 mg/kg I.V. monthly.

Sandoglobulin—200 mg/kg I.V. monthly. Start with 0.5 to 1 ml/minute of 3% solution; gradually increase dose to 2.5 ml/minute after 15 to 30 minutes.

Venoglobulin-I—Initially, 200 mg/kg I.V. monthly at 0.01 to 0.02 ml/kg/minute for 30 minutes; then increase to 0.04 ml/kg/minute or more if no adverse reaction. Dose may be increased to 300 to 400 mg/kg and given more often than once monthly if needed and tolerated.

Venoglobulin-S—200 mg/kg I.V. monthly. Dose may be increased to 300 to 400 mg/kg and given more often than once monthly if adequate IgG levels haven't occurred. Begin infusion at 0.01 to 0.02 ml/kg/minute for 30 minutes; then increase 5% solutions to 0.04 ml/kg/minute

---

and 10% solutions to 0.05 ml/kg/minute, if tolerated.

➤ **Idiopathic thrombocytopenic purpura (IGIV)—**

Adults and children: Gamimune N— 400 mg/kg 5% solution I.V. for 5 days; or 1,000 mg/kg 10% solution I.V. for 1 to 2 days with maintenance dose of 10% solution at 400 to 1,000 mg/kg I.V. single infusion to maintain 30,000/mm³ platelet count.

*Sandoglobulin—*0.4 g/kg I.V. for 2 to 5 consecutive days.

➤ **Bone marrow transplant (IGIV)—**

Adults older than age 20: Gamimune N— 500 mg/kg 5% or 10% solution I.V. on days 7 and 2 before transplantation; then weekly until 90 days after transplantation.

➤ **B-cell chronic lymphocytic leukemia (IGIV)—**

Adults: 400 mg/kg Gammagard S/D or Polygam S/D I.V. q 3 to 4 weeks.

➤ **Hepatitis A exposure (IGIM)—**

Adults and children: 0.02 ml/kg I.M. as soon as possible after exposure. Up to 0.1 ml/kg may be given if prolonged or intense exposure.

➤ **Measles exposure (IGIM)—**

Adults and children: 0.25 ml/kg I.M. within 6 days after exposure.

➤ **Postexposure prophylaxis of measles (IGIM)—**

Children: 0.5 ml/kg I.M. within 6 days after exposure (maximum 15 ml).

➤ **Chickenpox exposure (IGIM)—**

Adults and children: 0.6 to 1.2 ml/kg I.M. as soon as exposed.

➤ **Rubella exposure in first trimester pregnancy (IGIM)—**

Women: 0.55 ml/kg I.M. as soon as possible after exposure (within 72 hours).

➤ **Pediatric HIV infection (IGIV)—**

Children: 400 mg/kg Gamimune N I.V. q 28 days, at 0.01 to 0.02 ml/kg/minute for 30 minutes; increase to maximum of 0.08 ml/kg/minute.

I.V. ADMINISTRATION

• When giving Polygam S/D, Gammagard S/D, or Iveegam, use a 15-micron in-line filter.

• Gamimune N 5% and 10% are incompatible with saline solutions; they may be diluted with D₅W, if needed.

• Reconstitute Gammagard S/D and Polygam S/D according to package directions using sterile water for injection as diluent and the transfer device provided to prepare a solution containing 50 mg of protein per ml for 5% immune globulin solution or 100 mg of protein per ml for 10% immune globulin solution. Warm powder and sterile water for injection to room temperature before reconstitution. Give no more than 2 hours after reconstitution. Infuse with administration set provided or with an adequate filter.

• Reconstitute Gammar-P I.V. with sterile water for injection diluent provided. Warm powder and diluent to room temperature before reconstitution. After adding diluent, keep vial in upright position and undisturbed for 5 minutes. Gently swirl vial after 5 minutes. Don't shake. Dissolution may take up to 20 minutes.

• Reconstitute Iveegam with sterile water for injection diluent provided. Agitate or rotate vial gently. Don't shake.

• Reconstitute Sandoglobulin with normal saline solution diluent provided. Or, reconstitute with sterile water for injection or D₅W. Consider patient's fluid, electrolyte, and calorie requirements when choosing diluent.

• When preparing Sandoglobulin, don't shake vial. Swirl gently to dissolve drug. Dissolution may take up to 20 minutes. Solution should be clear and at room temperature before use. If large doses are to be given, several reconstituted vials of same concentration and diluent may be pooled into an empty sterile glass or plastic I.V. infusion container using aseptic technique. Filtering isn't needed. If filtering, use a filter with pore size of 15 microns or larger to prevent slowing of infusion. Antibacterial filters may be used. If drug is reconstituted outside of sterile laminar airflow conditions, use promptly. Drug reconstituted in a sterile laminar flow hood and stored under refrigeration is stable for up to 24 hours.

• Don't mix with other drugs or I.V. fluids.

• Most adverse reactions are related to a rapid infusion rate. If adverse reactions occur, decrease infusion rate or discontinue infusion until reaction subsides. Resume infusion at a rate that patient can tolerate.

Reactions may be *common*, uncommon, *life-threatening*, or COMMON AND LIFE-THREATENING.

ACTION

Provides passive immunity by increasing antibody titer. The primary component is immunoglobulin G (IgG). The mechanism for treating idiopathic thrombocytopenic purpura is unknown.

Route	Onset	Peak	Duration
I.M.	Unknown	2-5 hr	Unknown
I.V.	Immediate	Immediate	Unknown

ADVERSE REACTIONS

CNS: headache, faintness, malaise.
GI: nausea, vomiting.
Musculoskeletal: hip pain, chest pain, chest tightness, muscle stiffness at injection site.
Respiratory: dyspnea.
Skin: urticaria; pain, erythema.
Other: fever, *anaphylaxis,* chills.

INTERACTIONS

Drug-drug. *Live-virus vaccines:* Length of time to wait before giving live-virus vaccinations varies with dose of immune globulin given. Refer to recommendations by American Academy of Pediatrics.

EFFECTS ON LAB TEST RESULTS

None reported.

CONTRAINDICATIONS

Contraindicated in patients hypersensitive to drug or its components.

NURSING CONSIDERATIONS

● Obtain history of allergies and reactions to immunizations. Keep epinephrine 1:1,000 available to treat anaphylaxis.
● When giving I.M., use gluteal region. Divide doses larger than 10 ml and inject into several muscle sites to reduce pain and discomfort.
● Give drug soon after reconstitution.
● Immune globulin shouldn't be given for prophylaxis against hepatitis A if 6 weeks or more have elapsed since exposure or onset of clinical illness.
● *Alert:* Don't confuse Sandoglobulin with Sandostatin or Sandimmune.

PATIENT TEACHING

● Explain to patient and family how drug will be given.

● Tell patient that local reactions may occur at injection site. Instruct him to notify prescriber promptly if adverse reactions persist or become severe.
● Inform patient of possible need to have therapy more than once monthly to maintain appropriate IgG levels.

---

rabies immune globulin, human
Hyperab, Imogam Rabies-HT

Pregnancy risk category C

AVAILABLE FORMS

Injection: 150 IU/ml in 2-ml, 10-ml vials

INDICATIONS & DOSAGES

➤ **Rabies exposure—**
Adults and children: 20 IU/kg I.M. at time of first dose of rabies vaccine. Half of dose is used to infiltrate wound area; remainder is given I.M. in a different site.

ACTION

Provides passive immunity to rabies.

Route	Onset	Peak	Duration
I.M.	24 hr	Unknown	Unknown

ADVERSE REACTIONS

GU: *nephrotic syndrome.*
Skin: *rash;* pain, redness, and induration at injection site.
Other: slight fever, *anaphylaxis, angioedema.*

INTERACTIONS

Drug-drug. *Live-virus vaccines (measles, mumps, polio, or rubella):* Interferes with response to vaccine. Delay immunization, if possible.

EFFECTS ON LAB TEST RESULTS

None reported.

CONTRAINDICATIONS

No known contraindications.

NURSING CONSIDERATIONS

● Use with caution in patients hypersensitive to thimerosal or history of systemic allergic reactions to human immunoglobu-

lin preparations; also use cautiously in those with IgA deficiency.
• Obtain history of animal bites, allergies, and reactions to immunizations. Have epinephrine 1:1,000 ready to treat anaphylaxis.
• Ask patient when last tetanus immunization was received; many prescribers order a booster at this time.
• Use only with rabies vaccine and immediate local treatment of wound. Don't give rabies vaccine and rabies immune globulin in same syringe or at same site. Give as soon as possible after exposure or through day 7. After day 8, antibody response to culture vaccine has occurred.
• Don't give live-virus vaccines within 3 months of rabies immune globulin.
• Don't give more than 5 ml I.M. at one injection site; divide I.M. doses over 5 ml; give at different sites.
• Give large volumes (5 ml) in adults only. Use upper outer quadrant of gluteal area.
• *Alert:* This immune serum provides passive immunity. Don't confuse with rabies vaccine, a suspension of killed microorganisms that confers active immunity. The two drugs are often used together prophylactically after exposure to rabid animals.
• Clean wound thoroughly with soap and water; this is the best prophylaxis against rabies.

PATIENT TEACHING
• Inform patient that local reactions may occur at injection site. Instruct him to notify prescriber promptly if reactions persist or become severe.
• Tell patient that a tetanus shot also may be needed.
• Instruct patient in wound care.

respiratory syncytial virus immune globulin intravenous, human (RSV-IGIV)
RespiGam

Pregnancy risk category C

AVAILABLE FORMS
Injection: 50 mg ± 10 mg/ml in 20-ml, 50-ml single-use vial

INDICATIONS & DOSAGES
➤ **Prevention of serious lower respiratory tract infections from RSV in children with bronchopulmonary dysplasia (BPD) or history of premature birth (35 weeks' gestation or less)—**
Premature infants and children younger than age 2: Single infusion monthly. Give 1.5 ml/kg/hour I.V. for 15 minutes; then, if clinical condition allows higher rate, increase to 3 ml/kg/hour for 15 minutes and then to maximum of 6 ml/kg/hour until infusion ends. Maximum recommended total dose per monthly infusion is 750 mg/kg.

I.V. ADMINISTRATION
• Drug doesn't contain a preservative. Enter single-use vial only once; don't shake; avoid foaming. Begin infusion within 6 hours and end within 12 hours after vial is entered. Don't use if solution is turbid. Give through I.V. line using a constant infusion pump. Don't predilute drug before infusion. Although filters aren't needed for infusion, an in-line filter with pore size larger than 15 microns may be used. Give drug separately from other drugs.
• Adhere to infusion rate guidelines; most adverse reactions may be related to rate used. In especially ill children with BPD, slower rates may be indicated.
• Assess cardiopulmonary status and vital signs before beginning infusion, before each rate increase, and every 30 minutes thereafter until 30 minutes after completion of infusion.
• *Alert:* If patient develops hypotension, anaphylaxis, or severe allergic reaction, stop infusion and give epinephrine (1:1,000). Patients with selective IgA deficiency can develop antibodies to IgA and have anaphylactic or allergic reactions to subsequent administration of blood products containing IgA, including RSV-IGIV.

ACTION
Provides passive immunity to RSV.

Route	Onset	Peak	Duration
I.V.	Unknown	Unknown	≥ 1 mo

ADVERSE REACTIONS
CNS: dizziness, anxiety.

Reactions may be *common*, uncommon, *life-threatening*, or COMMON AND LIFE-THREATENING.

CV: tachycardia, hypertension, palpitations, chest tightness, flushing.
GI: vomiting, diarrhea, gastroenteritis, abdominal cramps.
Metabolic: fluid overload.
Musculoskeletal: myalgia, arthralgia.
Respiratory: respiratory distress, wheezing, crackles, hypoxia, tachypnea, dyspnea.
Skin: rash, pruritus, inflammation at injection site.
Other: fever; overdose effect; hypersensitivity reactions including *anaphylaxis, angioneurotic edema.*

INTERACTIONS
Drug-drug. *Live-virus vaccines (such as mumps, rubella, and especially measles):* May interfere with response. If such vaccines are given during or within 10 months after RSV-IGIV, reimmunization is recommended, if appropriate.

EFFECTS ON LAB TEST RESULTS
None reported.

CONTRAINDICATIONS
Contraindicated in patients severely hypersensitive to drug or other human immunoglobulin and selective immunoglobulin A (IgA) deficiency.

NURSING CONSIDERATIONS
• Children with fluid overload shouldn't receive drug.
• First dose should be given before RSV season (November to April) begins; subsequent doses should be given monthly throughout RSV season to maintain protection. Children with RSV should continue to receive monthly doses for duration of RSV season.
• Watch patient closely for signs and symptoms of fluid overload. Children with BPD may be more prone to this condition. Report increases in heart rate, respiratory rate, retractions, or crackles. Keep a loop diuretic, such as furosemide or bumetanide, available.

PATIENT TEACHING
• Explain to parents importance of child receiving drug monthly throughout RSV season, even if child is already infected.

• Teach parents how drug is given and which adverse reactions are related to administration. Tell parents to report all adverse reactions promptly.

$Rh_o(D)$ immune globulin, human
Gamulin Rh, HypRho-D,
HypRho-D Mini-Dose,
MICRhoGAM, RhoGAM

$Rh_o(D)$ immune globulin intravenous, human

Pregnancy risk category C

AVAILABLE FORMS
$Rh_o(D)$ immune globulin, human
Injection: 300 mcg of $Rh_o(D)$ immune globulin/vial (standard dose); 50 mcg of $Rh_o(D)$ immune globulin/vial (microdose)
$Rh_o(D)$ immune globulin I.V., human
Injection: 120 mcg, 300 mcg

INDICATIONS & DOSAGES
➤ **$Rh_o(D)$ immune globulin, human Rh exposure after abortion, miscarriage, ectopic pregnancy; or postpartum—**
Adults: Transfusion unit or blood bank determines fetal packed RBC volume entering patient's blood; one vial is given I.M. if fetal packed RBC volume is less than 15 ml. More than one vial I.M. may be needed if severe fetomaternal hemorrhage occurs; must be given within 72 hours after delivery or miscarriage.
➤ **After abortion or miscarriage to prevent Rh antibody formation—**
Adults: Consult transfusion unit or blood bank. One microdose vial I.M. will suppress immune reaction to 2.5 ml $Rh_o(D)$-positive RBCs. Ideally, should be given within 3 hours, but may be given up to 72 hours after abortion or miscarriage.
➤ **$Rh_o(D)$ immune globulin I.V., human Rh exposure after abortion, amniocentesis after 34 weeks' gestation, or other manipulations after 34 weeks' gestation with increased risk of Rh isoimmunization—**
Adults: 120 mcg I.M. or I.V.; must be given within 72 hours after delivery, miscarriage, or manipulation.

---

*Liquid contains alcohol.   **May contain tartrazine.   †Canada   ‡Australia   §U.K.   ◊OTC

➤ **Pregnancy—**

Adults: 300 mcg I.M. or I.V. at 28 weeks' gestation. If given early in pregnancy, additional doses should be given at 12-week intervals to maintain adequate levels of passively acquired anti-Rh antibodies. Then, within 72 hours of delivery, 120 mcg should be given I.M. or I.V. If 72 hours have elapsed, drug should be given as soon as possible, up to 28 days.

➤ **Transfusion accidents—**

Adults: 600 mcg I.V. q 8 hours or 1,200 mcg I.M. q 12 hours until total dose given. Total dose depends on volume of packed RBCs or whole blood infused. Consult blood bank or transfusion unit at once; must be given within 72 hours.

➤ **Idiopathic thrombocytopenic purpura in adults who are Rh$_o$(D) antigen-positive—**

Adults: Initially, 50 mcg/kg I.V. If hemoglobin is less than 10 g/dl, reduce initial dose to 25 to 40 mcg/kg. Initial dose may be given as single dose or divided into two doses and given on separate days. Then, 25 to 60 mcg/kg I.V. may be given, p.r.n., to elevate platelet counts with specific dosage that's determined individually.

I.V. ADMINISTRATION

● Reconstitute only with normal saline solution.

● Reconstitute drug in vials containing 600 or 1,500 units with 2.5 ml of normal saline solution and vials containing 5,000 units with 8.5 ml of normal saline solution.

● Slowly inject diluent onto the outside wall of vial and gently swirl vial until lyophilized pellet is dissolved. Don't shake vial.

● Give injection over 3 to 5 minutes.

● Don't give with other products.

ACTION

Suppresses the active antibody response and formation of anti-Rh$_o$(D) antibodies in Rh$_o$(D)-negative, Du-negative persons exposed to Rh-positive blood. Rh$_o$(D) immune globulin I.V. may form complexes with RBCs, blocking platelet destruction in adults who are Rh$_o$(D) antigen-positive.

However, mechanism of action isn't completely known.

Route	Onset	Peak	Duration
I.M., I.V.	Unknown	Unknown	Unknown

ADVERSE REACTIONS

Skin: discomfort at injection site.
Other: *anaphylaxis,* slight fever.

INTERACTIONS

Drug-drug. *Live-virus vaccines:* May interfere with response. Delay immunization for 3 months, if possible.

EFFECTS ON LAB TEST RESULTS

None reported.

CONTRAINDICATIONS

Contraindicated in Rh$_o$(D)-positive or D^u-positive patients and in those previously immunized to Rh$_o$(D) blood factor. Also contraindicated in patients with anaphylactic or severe systemic reaction to human globulin.

NURSING CONSIDERATIONS

● Use extreme caution when giving drug to patients with immunoglobulin A (IgA) deficiency. Because of risk of patient developing IgA antibodies and having an anaphylactic reaction, prescriber must weigh potential benefits of treatment against risk of hypersensitivity reactions.

● Obtain history of allergies and reactions to immunizations. Keep epinephrine 1:1,000 ready to treat anaphylaxis.

● *Alert:* Immediately after delivery, send a sample of neonate's cord blood to laboratory for typing and crossmatching. Confirm if mother is Rh$_o$(D)-negative and D^u-negative. Give drug to mother, only if infant is Rh$_o$(D)-positive or D^u-positive. Administration must occur within 72 hours of delivery.

● This immune serum provides passive immunity to patient exposed to Rh$_o$(D)-positive fetal blood during pregnancy and prevents formation of maternal antibodies (active immunity), which would endanger future Rh$_o$(D)-positive pregnancies.

● Defer vaccination with live-virus vaccines for 3 months after administration of Rh$_o$(D) immune globulin.

• Minidose preparations are recommended for patient undergoing abortion or miscarriage up to 12 weeks' gestation unless she is Rh₀(D)-positive or Dᵘ-positive or has Rh antibodies, or unless the father or fetus is Rh-negative.

PATIENT TEACHING
• Explain how drug protects future Rh₀(D)-positive fetuses if used because of pregnancy, or explain other use, if indicated.
• Warn patient about adverse reactions related to drug.
• Assure patient receiving this drug that there's no risk of HIV transmission.

---

tetanus immune globulin, human
Hyper-Tet

Pregnancy risk category C

AVAILABLE FORMS
Injection: 250-unit vial or syringe

INDICATIONS & DOSAGES
➤ **Postexposure tetanus prophylaxis following injury in those persons whose immunization is incomplete or unknown—**
Adults and children: 250 units deep I.M. injection.
➤ **Tetanus treatment—**
Adults and children: Single doses of 3,000 to 6,000 units I.M. have been used. Optimal dosage schedules haven't been established.

ACTION
Provides passive immunity to tetanus.

Route	Onset	Peak	Duration
I.M.	Unknown	2-3 days	4 wk

ADVERSE REACTIONS
GU: *nephrotic syndrome.*
Musculoskeletal: stiffness.
Skin: erythema at injection site.
Other: pain, slight fever, hypersensitivity reactions, *anaphylaxis, angioedema.*

INTERACTIONS
Drug-drug. *Live-virus vaccines:* May interfere with response. Defer administration of live-virus vaccines for 3 months after administration of tetanus immune globulin.

EFFECTS ON LAB TEST RESULTS
None reported.

CONTRAINDICATIONS
Contraindicated in patients with thrombocytopenia or other coagulation disorders that would contraindicate I.M. injection unless potential benefits outweigh risks.

NURSING CONSIDERATIONS
• Use cautiously in patients with history of previous systemic allergic reactions after administration of human immunoglobulin preparations and in those allergic to thimerosal.
• Obtain history of injury, tetanus immunizations, last tetanus toxoid injection, allergies, and reactions to immunizations. Keep epinephrine 1:1,000 available to treat hypersensitivity reaction.
• Don't give I.V. or I.D. Don't give in gluteal area.
• Tetanus immune globulin is used only if wound is more than 24 hours old or patient has had fewer than two tetanus toxoid injections.
• Thoroughly clean wound and remove all foreign matter.
• *Alert:* Don't confuse drug with tetanus toxoid. Tetanus immune globulin isn't a substitute for tetanus toxoid, which should be given at same time to produce active immunization. Don't give at same site as toxoid.
• Antibodies remain at effective levels for about 4 weeks, which is several times the duration of equine antitetanus antibodies, therefore protecting patients for incubation period of most tetanus cases.
• Don't give live-virus vaccines for 3 months after giving tetanus immune globulin.
• *Alert:* Don't confuse Hyper-Tet with HyperHep or Hyperstat.

PATIENT TEACHING
• Warn patient about local adverse reactions related to drug.

• Instruct patient to report serious adverse reactions promptly.
• Advise patient to complete full series of tetanus immunizations.
• Instruct patient to take acetaminophen for fever reduction and apply cool compresses at injection site for comfort.

varicella-zoster immune globulin (VZIG)

Pregnancy risk category C

AVAILABLE FORMS
Injection: 10% to 18% solution of the globulin fraction of human plasma containing 125 units of varicella-zoster virus antibody (volume is about 2.5 ml or less)

INDICATIONS & DOSAGES
➤ **Passive immunization of susceptible immunodeficient patients after exposure to varicella (chickenpox or herpes zoster)—**
Adults and children weighing more than 40 kg (88 lb): 625 units I.M.
Children weighing 29.9 to 40 kg (66 to 88 lb): 500 units I.M.
Children weighing 19.9 to 30 kg (44 to 66 lb): 375 units I.M.
Children weighing 10 to 20 kg (22 to 44 lb): 250 units I.M.
Children weighing up to 10 kg (22 lb): 125 units I.M.

ACTION
Provides passive immunity to varicella-zoster virus in immunodeficient patients.

Route	Onset	Peak	Duration
I.M.	Unknown	Unknown	1 mo

ADVERSE REACTIONS
CNS: headache, malaise.
GI: GI distress.
Respiratory: respiratory distress.
Skin: discomfort at injection site, rash.
Other: *anaphylaxis.*

INTERACTIONS
Drug-drug. *Live-virus vaccines:* May interfere with response. Defer vaccination for 3 months after administration of VZIG.

EFFECTS ON LAB TEST RESULTS
None reported.

CONTRAINDICATIONS
Contraindicated in patients with thrombocytopenia or history of severe reaction to human immune serum globulin or thimerosal; also contraindicated during pregnancy.

NURSING CONSIDERATIONS
• Obtain accurate patient history of allergies and reactions to immunizations. Keep epinephrine 1:1,000 ready to treat anaphylaxis.
• For maximum benefit, give as soon as possible after presumed exposure. Drug may be of benefit when given as late as 96 hours after exposure.
• Give only by deep I.M. injection into a large muscle such as gluteal muscle. Never give I.V.
• Don't give in divided doses.
• Although usually restricted to children younger than age 15, VZIG may be given to adolescents and adults, if needed.
• VZIG isn't recommended for nonimmunosuppressed patients.
• *Alert:* VZIG provides passive immunity; don't confuse with varicella vaccine. Don't use these two drugs together.
• Drug isn't commercially distributed and is available only from 20 regional United States distribution centers. These centers will distribute to Canada and overseas. Contact the Massachusetts Public Health Biologic Laboratories or the Centers for Disease Control and Prevention at (800) 232-2522 for more information.

PATIENT TEACHING
• Warn patient about local adverse reactions related to drug.
• Instruct patient to report serious adverse reactions to prescriber promptly.
• Suggest use of acetaminophen for fever reduction and cool compresses at injection site for comfort.

Reactions may be *common,* uncommon, *life-threatening,* or COMMON AND LIFE-THREATENING.

darbepoetin alpha
epoetin alfa
filgrastim
glatiramer acetate for injection
interferon alfacon-1
interferon alfa-2a, recombinant
  (rIFN-A)
interferon alfa-2b, recombinant
  (IFN-alpha 2)
interferon beta-1a
interferon beta-1b,
  recombinant
interferon gamma-1b
levamisole hydrochloride
oprelvekin
peginterferon alfa-2b
sargostim

COMBINATION PRODUCTS
None.

✳ *NEW DRUG*

___

darbepoetin alpha
Aranesp

Pregnancy risk category C

AVAILABLE FORMS
Injection: 25 mcg/ml, 40 mcg/ml,
60 mcg/ml, and 100 mcg/ml single-dose
vials, polysorbate solution; 25 mcg/ml,
40 mcg/ml, 60 mcg/ml, and 100 mcg/ml
single-dose vials, albumin solution

INDICATIONS & DOSAGES
➤ **Anemia from chronic renal failure—**
Adults: 0.45 mcg/kg I.V. or S.C. once
weekly. Adjust doses so that hemoglobin
doesn't exceed 12 g/dl. Dose shouldn't be
increased more frequently than once a
month. In patients being converted
from epoetin alpha, starting dose should
be based on the previous epoetin alpha
dose (see table).

Previous weekly epoetin alpha dose (units/wk)	Weekly Aranesp dose (mcg/wk)
< 2,500	6.25
2,500-4,999	12.5
5,000-10,999	25
11,000-17,999	40
18,000-33,999	60
34,000-89,999	100
≥ 90,000	200

Aranesp should be given less frequently
than epoetin alpha. If patient was receiving epoetin alpha 2 to 3 times weekly, give
Aranesp once weekly. If patient was receiving epoetin alpha once weekly, give
Aranesp once every 2 weeks.
Adjust-a-dose: If increasing hemoglobin
approaches 12 g/dl, the dose should be reduced by 25%. If hemoglobin continues to
increase, the dose should be withheld until hemoglobin begins to decrease; then,
restart at a dose 25% below the previous
dose. If hemoglobin increases by more
than 1 g/dl over 2 weeks, decrease the
dose by 25%. If increase in hemoglobin is
less than 1 g/dl over 4 weeks and iron
stores are adequate, increase the dose by
25% of previous dose. Further increases
can be made at 4-week intervals until target hemoglobin is reached.
  Patients who don't need dialysis may
need lower maintenance doses.

I.V. ADMINISTRATION
● Give undiluted by I.V. injection.
● Don't shake. Shaking can denature the
drug.
● Don't mix with other drugs or solutions.
● Single-dose vials contain no preserva-
tives; don't pool unused portions.
● Don't use if drug contains particles or is
discolored.

ACTION
Mimics effects of erythropoietin, a naturally occurring hormone produced by the
kidneys. Helps to control RBC production. Acts on erythroid tissues in bone

___

marrow, stimulating mitotic activity of erythroid progenitor cells and early precursor cells. Functions as a growth factor and as a differentiating factor, enhancing RBC production.

Route	Onset	Peak	Duration
I.V.	Unknown	Unknown	21 hr
S.C.	Unknown	34 hr	49 hr

ADVERSE REACTIONS
CNS: *headache,* dizziness, fatigue, asthenia.
CV: *hypertension, hypotension,* **CARDIAC ARRHYTHMIA, CARDIAC ARREST,** angina, ***heart failure,*** thrombosis, *edema,* chest pain, ***acute MI.***
GI: *diarrhea, vomiting, nausea, abdominal pain,* constipation.
Musculoskeletal: *myalgia, arthralgia, limb pain,* back pain.
Respiratory: *upper respiratory tract infection, dyspnea, cough,* bronchitis.
Skin: *pruritus.*
Other: *infection,* fever, fluid overload, flu-like symptoms, access site hemorrhage.

INTERACTIONS
None reported.

EFFECTS ON LAB TEST RESULTS
None reported.

CONTRAINDICATIONS
Aranesp is contraindicated in patients hypersensitive to the drug or its components and in patients with uncontrolled hypertension.

NURSING CONSIDERATIONS
• Safety and effectiveness haven't been established in patients with underlying hematologic disease, such as hemolytic anemia, sickle cell anemia, thalassemia or porphyria. Use with caution.
• Safety and efficacy of drug haven't been established in pediatric patients.
• Some patients have been treated successfully with a S.C. dose given once every 2 weeks.
• Hemoglobin may not increase until 2 to 6 weeks after starting therapy.
• Aranesp may increase the risk of CV events. Blood pressure should be carefully monitored and controlled.

• Patient may experience seizures. Monitor patients closely, especially during the first several months of therapy.
• ***Alert:*** Monitor hemoglobin weekly until stabilized. Don't exceed the target of 12 g/dl.
• Monitor renal function and electrolytes in predialysis patients.
• Monitor iron status before and during treatment. Provide supplemental iron in patients whose ferritin is less than 100 mcg/L and transferrin saturation is less than 20%.
• Patients who are marginally dialyzed may need adjustments in dialysis prescriptions.
• There is a potential for serious allergic reactions, including skin rash and urticaria. If an anaphylactic reaction occurs, the drug should be stopped and appropriate therapy given.
• Safety and efficacy are no different in elderly patients, but they might have greater sensitivity to the drug.
• It isn't known whether the drug appears in breast milk. Caution should be used in breast-feeding women.
• Store drug in the refrigerator; don't freeze. Protect drug from light.
• ***Alert:*** Decrease dosage if the hemoglobin increases 1g/dl in any 2-week period.

PATIENT TEACHING
• Instruct patients on proper administration and use and disposal of needles.
• Advise patient of possible side effects and allergic reactions.
• Inform patient of the need for frequent monitoring of blood pressure and hemoglobin; stress compliance with his antihypertensive therapy.
• Instruct patient how to take drug correctly at home, including how to dispose of supplies properly.

---

epoetin alfa (erythropoietin)
Epogen, Eprex§, Procrit

Pregnancy risk category C

AVAILABLE FORMS
Injection: 2,000 units/ml, 3,000 units/ml, 4,000 units/ml, 10,000 units/ml; multidose vials of 10,000 units/ml, 20,000 units/ml

---

Reactions may be *common,* uncommon, ***life-threatening,*** or COMMON AND LIFE-THREATENING.

INDICATIONS & DOSAGES

➤ **Anemia from reduced production of endogenous erythropoietin caused by end-stage renal disease—**
Adults: Dosage is individualized. Starting dose is 50 to 100 units/kg I.V. three times weekly. Nondialysis patients with chronic renal failure or patients receiving continuous peritoneal dialysis may receive drug by S.C. injection or I.V. Maintenance dosage is highly individualized.
Adjust-a-dose: Dosage is reduced when target hematocrit is reached or if hematocrit rises more than 4 points in a 2-week period. Dosage is increased if hematocrit doesn't increase by 5 to 6 points after 8 weeks of therapy.

➤ **Adjunctive treatment of HIV-infected patients with anemia caused by zidovudine therapy—**
Adults: 100 units/kg I.V. or S.C. three times weekly for 8 weeks or until target hemoglobin level is reached. If response isn't satisfactory after 8 weeks, dosage may be increased by 50 to 100 units/kg I.V. or S.C. three times weekly. After 4 to 8 weeks, dosage may be further increased in increments of 50 to 100 units/kg three times weekly, up to maximum of 300 units/kg I.V. or S.C. three times weekly.

➤ **Anemia caused by cancer chemotherapy—**
Adults: 150 units/kg S.C. three times weekly for 8 weeks or until target hemoglobin level is reached. If response isn't satisfactory after 8 weeks, dosage may be increased up to 300 units/kg S.C. three times weekly.
Adjust-a-dose: If hematocrit exceeds 40%, drug should be withheld until hematocrit falls to 36%.

➤ **Reduction of need for allogenic blood transfusion in anemic patients scheduled to have elective, noncardiac, nonvascular surgery—**
Adults: 300 units/kg/day S.C. daily for 10 days before surgery, on day of surgery, and for 4 days after surgery. Or, 600 units/kg S.C. in once-weekly doses (21, 14, and 7 days before surgery), plus one-quarter dose on day of surgery.

➤ **Anemia in pediatric patients with chronic renal failure who are having dialysis—**
Infants and children ages 1 month to 16 years: 50 units/kg I.V. or S.C. three times weekly. Maintenance dosage is highly individualized to maintain hematocrit level within target range.
Adjust-a-dose: Reduce dosage when target hematocrit level is reached or if hematocrit level rises more than 4 points within a 2-week period. Increase dosage if hematocrit level doesn't rise by 5 to 6 points after 8 weeks of therapy and is below target range.

I.V. ADMINISTRATION

• Give by direct injection without dilution. Solution contains no preservatives. Discard unused portion. Don't mix with other drugs. Don't shake.
• Drug may be given via the venous return line of dialysis tubing after dialysis to eliminate need for additional I.V. access.
• To prevent adherence to tubing, inject drug while blood is still in I.V. line, and follow with a normal saline solution flush.

ACTION

Mimics effects of erythropoietin, a naturally occurring hormone produced by the kidneys. Helps to control RBC production. Acts on erythroid tissues in bone marrow, stimulating mitotic activity of erythroid progenitor cells and early precursor cells. Functions as a growth factor and as a differentiating factor, enhancing RBC production.

Route	Onset	Peak	Duration
I.V.	Immediate	Immediate	Unknown
S.C.	Unknown	5-24 hr	Unknown

ADVERSE REACTIONS

CNS: *headache,* **seizures,** *paresthesia, fatigue,* dizziness, *asthenia.*
CV: *hypertension, edema,* increased clotting of arteriovenous grafts.
GI: *nausea, vomiting, diarrhea.*
Metabolic: hyperuricemia, hyperkalemia, hyperphosphatemia.
Musculoskeletal: *arthralgia.*
Respiratory: *cough, shortness of breath.*
Skin: *rash, injection site reactions,* urticaria.
Other: *pyrexia.*

INTERACTIONS
None significant.

EFFECTS ON LAB TEST RESULTS
• May increase BUN, creatinine, uric acid, potassium, and phosphate levels.

CONTRAINDICATIONS
Contraindicated in patients hypersensitive to products derived from mammal cells or albumin (human) and in those with uncontrolled hypertension.

NURSING CONSIDERATIONS
• Use cautiously in breast-feeding women.
• Monitor blood pressure before therapy. Up to 80% of patients with chronic renal failure have hypertension. Blood pressure may rise, especially when hematocrit is increasing in the early part of therapy.
• If hematocrit is increasing and approaching 36%, reduce dosage to maintain target hematocrit range. If hematocrit remains unchanged after reducing dosage, withhold dose temporarily until hematocrit decreases.
• When used in HIV-infected patients, be prepared to individualize dosage based on response. Dosage recommendations are for patients with endogenous erythropoietin levels of 500 units/L or less and cumulative zidovudine doses of 4.2 g/week or less.
• Patient treated with epoetin alfa may need additional heparin to prevent clotting during dialysis treatments.
• Monitor blood count. Hematocrit may rise and cause excessive clotting. Renal function, uric acid, and potassium levels may rise.
• Institute diet restrictions or drug therapy to control blood pressure. Reduce dosage in patients who exhibit rapid rise in hematocrit (more than 4 points in a 2-week period), to prevent hypertension.
• Patient's response to epoetin alfa depends on amount of endogenous erythropoietin in the plasma. Patients with levels of 500 units/L or more usually have transfusion-dependent anemia and probably won't respond to drug. Those with levels below 500 units/L usually respond well.
• Patient should receive adequate iron supplementation beginning no later than

when epoetin alfa treatment starts and continuing throughout therapy. Patient also may need vitamin B_{12} and folic acid.
• *Alert:* Don't confuse Epogen with Neupogen.

PATIENT TEACHING
• Inform patient that pain or discomfort in limbs (long bones) and pelvis, and coldness and sweating aren't uncommon after injection (usually occurring within 2 hours). Symptoms may last for 12 hours and then disappear.
• Advise patient that blood specimens will be drawn weekly for blood counts and that dosage adjustments may be made based on results.
• Advise patient to avoid driving or operating heavy machinery at start of therapy. There may be a relationship between excessively rapid hematocrit rise and seizures.
• Tell patient to monitor blood pressure at home and to adhere to dietary restrictions.
• Instruct patient to check that syringes used to give drug are in tenths-of-milliliter increments.

---

filgrastim (G-CSF; granulocyte-colony stimulating factor)
Neupogen

Pregnancy risk category C

AVAILABLE FORMS
Injection: 300 mcg/ml

INDICATIONS & DOSAGES
➤ **To decrease risk of infection in patients with nonmyeloid malignant disease receiving myelosuppressive antineoplastics—**
Adults and children: 5 mcg/kg/day I.V. or S.C. as single dose given no sooner than 24 hours after cytotoxic chemotherapy. Doses may be increased in increments of 5 mcg/kg for each chemotherapy cycle depending on duration and severity of the nadir of absolute neutrophil count (ANC).
➤ **To decrease risk of infection in patients with nonmyeloid malignant disease receiving myelosuppressive anti-**

neoplastics followed by bone marrow transplantation—
Adults and children: 10 mcg/kg/day I.V. infusion of 4 or 24 hours or as continuous 24-hour S.C. infusion at least 24 hours after cytotoxic chemotherapy and bone marrow infusion. Adjust subsequent dosages based on neutrophil response.
Adjust-a-dose: For patients with ANC over 1,000/mm³ for 3 consecutive days, reduce dosage to 5 mcg/kg/day; if ANC remains over 1,000/mm³ for 3 more consecutive days, discontinue drug. If ANC decreases to below 1,000/mm³, resume therapy at 5 mcg/kg/day.
➤ **Congenital neutropenia**—
Adults: 6 mcg/kg S.C. b.i.d. Adjust dosage based on patient response.
Adjust-a-dose: For patients with a persistently elevated ANC (above 10,000/mm³), reduce dosage, as directed.
➤ **Idiopathic or cyclic neutropenia**—
Adults: 5 mcg/kg S.C. daily. Adjust dosage based on patient response.
➤ **Peripheral blood progenitor cell collection and therapy in cancer patients**—
Adults: 10 mcg/kg/day S.C. Give 4 days before leukapheresis and continue until last leukapheresis.
Adjust-a-dose: Patients with WBC count over 100,000/mm³ may need dosage adjustment.

I.V. ADMINISTRATION
● Dilute in 50 to 100 ml of D₅W and give by intermittent infusion over 15 to 60 minutes or continuous infusion over 24 hours.
● Don't dilute with normal saline solution. Dilution to final concentration of less than 5 mcg/ml isn't recommended.
● If final concentration of drug is 5 to 15 mcg/ml, add albumin at a concentration of 2 mg/ml (0.2%) to minimize binding of drug to plastic containers or tubing.

ACTION
A glycoprotein that stimulates proliferation and differentiation of hematopoietic cells. Is specific for neutrophils.

Route	Onset	Peak	Duration
I.V.	5-60 min	24 hr	1-7 days
S.C.	5-60 min	2-8 hr	1-7 days

ADVERSE REACTIONS
CNS: headache, weakness, *fatigue.*
CV: *MI, arrhythmias,* chest pain, hypotension.
GI: *nausea, vomiting, diarrhea, mucositis,* stomatitis, constipation.
Hematologic: *thrombocytopenia,* leukocytosis.
Metabolic: hyperuricemia.
Musculoskeletal: *bone pain.*
Respiratory: dyspnea, cough.
Skin: *alopecia,* rash, cutaneous vasculitis.
Other: *fever,* hypersensitivity reactions.

INTERACTIONS
Drug-drug. *Chemotherapeutic drugs:* Rapidly dividing myeloid cells are potentially sensitive to cytotoxic drugs. Don't use within 24 hours before or after a dose of one of these drugs. Use with caution in patients taking lithium.

EFFECTS ON LAB TEST RESULTS
● May increase creatinine, uric acid, alkaline phosphatase, and LDH levels.
● May increase WBC count and decrease platelet counts.

CONTRAINDICATIONS
Contraindicated in patients hypersensitive to drug or its components or to proteins derived from *Escherichia coli.*

NURSING CONSIDERATIONS
● Use cautiously in breast-feeding women.
● Obtain baseline CBC and platelet count before therapy.
● Once a dose is withdrawn, don't reenter vial. Discard unused portion. Vials are for single-dose use and contain no preservatives.
● Obtain CBC and platelet count two to three times weekly during therapy. Patients who receive drug may potentially receive high doses of chemotherapy, which may increase risk of toxicities.
● A transiently increased neutrophil count is common 1 or 2 days after therapy starts. Give daily for up to 2 weeks or until ANC has returned to 10,000/mm³ after the expected chemotherapy-induced neutrophil nadir.
● *Alert:* Don't confuse Neupogen with Epogen.

PATIENT TEACHING

• If patient will give drug, teach him how to do so and how to dispose of used needles, syringes, drug containers, and unused medicine.

• Instruct patient to report persistent or serious adverse reactions promptly.

---

glatiramer acetate for injection (formerly copolymer 1)
Copaxone

Pregnancy risk category B

AVAILABLE FORMS
Injection: 20 mg lyophilized glatiramer acetate and 40 mg mannitol, USP, in a single-use 2-ml vial; 1-ml vial of sterile water for injection is included for reconstitution

INDICATIONS & DOSAGES
➤ **To reduce frequency of relapse in patients with relapsing-remitting multiple sclerosis—**
Adults: 20 mg S.C. daily.

ACTION
Unknown. Thought to act by modifying immune processes responsible for the pathogenesis of multiple sclerosis.

Route	Onset	Peak	Duration
S.C.	Unknown	Unknown	Unknown

ADVERSE REACTIONS
CNS: abnormal dreams, agitation, *anxiety, asthenia,* confusion, emotional lability, migraine, nervousness, speech disorder, stupor, tremor, vertigo, syncope.
CV: *chest pain,* hypertension, *palpitations, vasodilation,* tachycardia.
EENT: ear pain, eye disorder, laryngismus, *rhinitis,* nystagmus.
GI: anorexia, bowel urgency, *diarrhea,* gastroenteritis, GI disorder, *nausea,* oral candidiasis, salivary gland enlargement, ulcerative stomatitis, vomiting.
GU: amenorrhea, dysmenorrhea, hematuria, impotence, menorrhagia, abnormal Papanicolaou smear, *urinary urgency,* vaginal candidiasis, vaginal hemorrhage.
Hematologic: ecchymosis, *lymphadenopathy.*

Metabolic: weight gain.
Musculoskeletal: *arthralgia, back pain,* neck pain, foot drop, *hypertonia.*
Respiratory: bronchitis, *dyspnea,* hyperventilation.
Skin: eczema; erythema; *pruritus, rash, injection site reaction* or hemorrhage; skin atrophy; skin nodule; *diaphoresis;* urticaria; warts.
Other: bacterial infection, herpes simplex and zoster; chills, cyst, dental caries, peripheral and facial edema, fever, *flu syndrome, infection, pain.*

INTERACTIONS
None significant.

EFFECTS ON LAB TEST RESULTS
None reported.

CONTRAINDICATIONS
Contraindicated in patients hypersensitive to drug or mannitol.

NURSING CONSIDERATIONS
• Give drug only by S.C. injection.
• Store drug in refrigerator (36° to 46° F [2° to 8° C]); diluent can be kept at room temperature.
• Swirl lyophilized material and diluent gently and let stand at room temperature until completely dissolved, about 5 minutes.
• Use immediately after reconstitution because drug doesn't contain preservatives; discard unused drug. Use diluent provided for reconstitution.
• Immediate postinjection reactions have occurred in 10% of patients with multiple sclerosis; symptoms include flushing, chest pain, palpitations, anxiety, dyspnea, constriction of the throat, and urticaria. They typically are transient and self-limiting and don't need specific treatment. Onset of postinjection reaction may occur several months after treatment starts, and patients may have more than one episode.
• About 26% of patients have experienced at least one episode of transient chest pain, which usually begins at least 1 month after treatment starts; it isn't accompanied by other signs or symptoms and doesn't appear to be clinically important.
• Because drug can modify immune response, it could interfere with normal im-

---

Reactions may be *common,* uncommon, **life-threatening,** or COMMON AND LIFE-THREATENING.

mune function. Although evidence is lacking, there has been no evaluation of this risk.

• Drug is antigenic and may lead to induction of unwanted host responses. Systemic study of these effects hasn't been done.

• It isn't known if drug appears in breast milk.

• *Alert:* Don't confuse Copaxone with Compazine.

PATIENT TEACHING

• Instruct patient how to reconstitute and self-inject drug. Supervise first injection.

• Explain need for aseptic self-injection techniques and warn patient against reuse of needles and syringes. Periodically review proper disposal of needles, syringes, drug containers, and unused drug.

• Tell patient to notify prescriber about planned, suspected, or known pregnancy.

• Tell woman to notify prescriber if she is breast-feeding.

• Advise patient not to change drug or dosing schedule or to stop drug without medical approval.

• Tell patient to notify prescriber immediately if dizziness, urticaria, diaphoresis, chest pain, difficulty breathing, or if severe pain occurs after drug injection.

interferon alfacon-1
Infergen

Pregnancy risk category C

AVAILABLE FORMS
Injection: 9 mcg/0.3-ml, 15 mcg/0.5-ml vials

INDICATIONS & DOSAGES
➤ **Chronic hepatitis C viral infection—**
Adults: 9 mcg S.C. three times weekly for 24 weeks; for patients who don't respond or who relapse, 15 mcg S.C. three times weekly for 6 months.
Adjust-a-dose: For patients intolerant to higher doses, dose may be reduced to 7.5 mcg. Don't give doses below 7.5 mcg because decreased efficacy may result.

ACTION
Type-I interferons induce genetic-mediated biological responses that include antiviral, antiproliferative, and immunomodulatory effects and regulation of cytokine expression.

Route	Onset	Peak	Duration
S.C.	Unknown	24-36 hr	Unknown

ADVERSE REACTIONS
CNS: *headache, insomnia, dizziness, paresthesia, amnesia, nervousness, depression, anxiety, emotional lability,* confusion, agitation, **suicidal ideation,** *malaise.*
CV: hypertension, tachycardia, palpitations.
EENT: *retinal hemorrhages,* loss of visual acuity or visual field, conjunctivitis, tinnitus, ear pain, *pharyngitis, sinusitis, rhinitis,* epistaxis.
GI: *abdominal pain, nausea, diarrhea,* taste perversion, *anorexia, dyspepsia, vomiting,* constipation, flatulence, hemorrhoids, decreased saliva.
GU: dysmenorrhea, vaginitis.
Hematologic: *granulocytopenia,* **leukopenia, thrombocytopenia,** ecchymosis, lymphadenopathy, lymphocytosis.
Metabolic: hypothyroidism.
Respiratory: *infection, cough, congestion,* dyspnea, bronchitis.
Skin: *alopecia, pruritus, rash,* dry skin, *pain, erythema* at injection site.
Other: toothache, decreased libido, **hypersensitivity reactions,** body pain, *flulike symptoms.*

INTERACTIONS
Drug-drug. *Drugs metabolized by cytochrome P-450:* May alter drug levels. Monitor changes in levels of these drugs.
Myelosuppressives: No studies have been conducted; however, use cautiously with interferon alfacon-1. Monitor CBC and therapeutic or toxic levels of drugs taken together with interferon alfacon-1.

EFFECTS ON LAB TEST RESULTS
• May increase triglyceride levels.
• May increase PT and INR. May decrease granulocyte, WBC, and platelet counts.

CONTRAINDICATIONS
Contraindicated in patients hypersensitive to alpha interferons, to *Escherichia coli*–derived products, or to any component of product. Also contraindicated in patients with history of severe psychiatric disorders, autoimmune hepatitis, or decompensated hepatic disease.

NURSING CONSIDERATIONS
• Use with caution in patients with history of cardiac disease and other autoimmune or endocrine disorders, in those with abnormally low peripheral blood cell counts, and in those receiving drugs known to cause myelosuppression.
• Depression and suicidal behavior have been linked to drug.
• The following laboratory tests should be performed before therapy, 2 weeks after it starts, and periodically during therapy: CBC with platelets, creatinine, albumin, bilirubin, thyroid-stimulating hormone, and T_4.
• *Alert:* If hypersensitivity reaction occurs, stop drug immediately and treat. Premedication with acetaminophen or ibuprofen may decrease adverse effects.
• Allow at least 48 hours to elapse between doses.
• Dosages and adverse reactions vary among different subtypes of drug. Don't use different subtypes in a single treatment regimen.
• Store drug in refrigerator at 36° to 46° F (2° to 8° C); don't freeze. Injection may be allowed to reach room temperature just before use. Avoid vigorous shaking. Discard unused portion.

PATIENT TEACHING
• If drug is to be used at home, instruct patient on appropriate use, dosage, and administration. A patient information leaflet is available from the manufacturer and should be given to the patient. Also teach patient proper disposal procedures for needles, syringes, drug containers, and unused drug.
• Instruct patient not to reuse needles or syringes or reenter vial.
• Tell patient to discard all syringes and needles in a puncture-resistant container.

• Urge patient to inspect vial for discoloration and particulates before use; don't use if either appear.
• Tell patient that nonnarcotic analgesics and bedtime administration may be used to prevent or lessen flulike symptoms (headache, fever, malaise, myalgia) related to therapy.
• Instruct patient to immediately report symptoms of depression.

interferon alfa-2a, recombinant (rIFN-A)
Roferon-A

Pregnancy risk category C

AVAILABLE FORMS
Injection: 3, 6, 9, 36 million IU/single-use vial; 9, 18 million IU/multidose vial
Sterile powder for injection: 18 million IU/vial with diluent

INDICATIONS & DOSAGES
➤ **Chronic hepatitis C—**
Adults: 3 million IU 3 times a week S.C. or I.M. for 12 months (48 to 52 weeks). Alternatively, induction dose of 6 million IU 3 times weekly for the first 3 months (12 weeks) followed by 3 million IU 3 times weekly for 9 months (36 weeks). If no response after 3 months, discontinue therapy. Retreatment with either 3 or 6 million IU 3 times weekly for 6 to 12 months may be considered.
➤ **Hairy cell leukemia—**
Adults: For induction, 3 million IU S.C. or I.M. daily for 16 to 24 weeks. For maintenance, 3 million IU S.C. or I.M. 3 times weekly.
➤ **AIDS-related Kaposi's sarcoma—**
Adults: For induction, 36 million IU S.C. or I.M. daily for 10 to 12 weeks. For maintenance, 36 million IU S.C. or I.M. 3 times weekly. Doses may begin at 3 million IU and escalated upward every 3 days until patient is given 36 million IU daily; in order to decrease toxicity.
➤ **Philadelphia chromosome–positive chronic myelogenous leukemia—**
Adults: Initially, 3 million IU S.C. or I.M. daily for 3 days; then 6 million IU for 3 days; then 9 million IU for duration of treatment.

Children: 2.5 to 5 million IU/m² I.M. daily.

ACTION
Unknown. Appears to involve direct antiproliferative action against tumor or viral cells to inhibit replication and modulation of host immune response by enhancing phagocytic activity of macrophages and augmenting specific cytotoxicity of lymphocytes for target cells.

Route	Onset	Peak	Duration
I.M.	Unknown	2-12 hr	Unknown
S.C.	Unknown	3-12 hr	Unknown

ADVERSE REACTIONS
CNS: *dizziness, confusion,* paresthesia, numbness, lethargy, *depression, decreased mental status,* forgetfulness, **coma,** nervousness, insomnia, sedation, apathy, anxiety, irritability, fatigue, vertigo, gait disturbances, incoordination, syncope.
CV: hypotension, chest pain, **arrhythmias,** palpitations, **heart failure,** hypertension, edema, **MI,** flushing.
EENT: *dryness or inflammation of the oropharynx,* rhinorrhea, sinusitis, conjunctivitis, earache, eye irritation.
GI: *anorexia, nausea, diarrhea, vomiting,* abdominal fullness, *abdominal pain,* flatulence, constipation, hypermotility, gastric distress, excessive salivation, *change in taste.*
GU: transient impotence.
Hematologic: *leukopenia, mild thrombocytopenia.*
Hepatic: *hepatitis.*
Metabolic: *weight loss,* hypercalcemia, hyperphosphatemia.
Respiratory: cyanosis, cough, dyspnea.
Skin: *rash,* dryness, pruritus, *partial alopecia,* urticaria, diaphoresis, *inflammation at injection site.*
Other: *flu syndrome,* night sweats, hot flashes.

INTERACTIONS
Drug-drug. *Aminophylline, theophylline:* May reduce theophylline clearance. Monitor serum levels.
Aspirin: Increased risk of GI bleeding. Avoid using together.
CNS depressants: Increased CNS effects. Avoid using together.

Live-virus vaccines: Increased risk of adverse reactions and decreased antibody response. Avoid using together.
Drug-lifestyle. *Alcohol use:* Increased risk of GI bleeding. Discourage patient from use during therapy.

EFFECTS ON LAB TEST RESULTS
● May increase calcium, phosphate, AST, ALT, alkaline phosphatase, LDH, and fasting glucose levels.
● May increase PT, INR, and PTT. May decrease WBC and platelet counts.

CONTRAINDICATIONS
Contraindicated in patients hypersensitive to drug, murine (mouse) immunoglobulin, or other drug components.

NURSING CONSIDERATIONS
● Use cautiously in patients with severe hepatic or renal function impairment, seizure disorders, compromised CNS function, cardiac disease, or myelosuppression.
● Depression and suicidal behavior have been linked to treatment.
● Obtain allergy history. Drug contains phenol as a preservative and albumin as a stabilizer.
● Use S.C. administration route in patients whose platelet count is below 50,000/mm³.
● Give drug at bedtime to minimize daytime drowsiness.
● Ensure patient is well hydrated, especially during initial stages of treatment.
● At beginning of therapy, assess patient for flulike signs and symptoms, which tend to diminish with continued therapy. Premedicate patient with acetaminophen to minimize signs and symptoms.
● Monitor patient for CNS adverse reactions, such as decreased mental status and dizziness, during therapy.
● Monitor CBC with differential, platelet count, blood chemistry and electrolyte studies, and liver function tests. If patient has cardiac disorder or advanced stages of cancer, monitor ECG.
● For patients who develop thrombocytopenia, exercise extreme care in performing invasive procedures; inspect injection site and skin frequently for bruising; limit frequency of I.M. injections; test urine,

emesis fluid, stool, and secretions for occult blood.
- *Alert:* Different brands of interferon may not be equivalent and may need different dosages.
- Severe adverse reactions may need dosage reduction to one-half or discontinuation of drug until reactions subside.
- *Alert:* Neurotoxicity and cardiotoxicity are more common in elderly patients, especially those with underlying CNS or cardiac impairment.
- Use with blood dyscrasia-causing drugs, bone marrow suppressant, or radiation therapy may increase bone marrow suppression. Dosage may need to be reduced.
- Keep drug refrigerated. Don't freeze.

PATIENT TEACHING
- Advise patient that laboratory tests will be performed before and periodically during therapy.
- Teach patient proper oral hygiene during treatment because the bone marrow suppressant effects of interferon may lead to microbial infection, delayed healing, and gingival bleeding. Drug also may decrease salivary flow.
- Stress need to follow prescriber's instructions about taking and recording temperature and how and when to take acetaminophen.
- Advise patient to check with prescriber for instructions after missing dose.
- Tell patient that drug may cause temporary partial hair loss; hair should return when drug is withdrawn.
- If patient will be giving drug to himself, teach him how to prepare and give it and how to dispose of used needles, syringes, containers, and unused drug.
- Instruct patient not to take aspirin or alcohol because use together increases risk of GI bleeding.
- Instruct patient not to change brands of interferon without medical consultation.
- Warn patient against performing tasks that require mental alertness.
- Advise patient to immediately report signs and symptoms of depression.

interferon alfa-2b, recombinant (IFN-alpha 2)
Intron A

Pregnancy risk category C

AVAILABLE FORMS
Injection: 3, 5 million IU/0.5-ml vial; 1, 10 million IU/1-ml vial; 18 million IU/3.8-ml vial; 25 million IU/3.2-ml vial
Powder for injection: 3, 5, 10, 18, 25, 50 million IU/vial with diluent

INDICATIONS & DOSAGES
➤ **Hairy cell leukemia—**
Adults: 2 million IU/m² I.M. or S.C., 3 times weekly for 6 months or more.
➤ **Condylomata acuminata (genital or venereal warts)—**
Adults: 1 million IU for each lesion intralesionally 3 times weekly for 3 weeks.
➤ **AIDS-related Kaposi's sarcoma—**
Adults: 30 million IU/m² S.C. or I.M. 3 times weekly. Maintain dose unless disease progresses rapidly or intolerance occurs.
➤ **Chronic hepatitis B—**
Adults: 30 to 35 million IU weekly I.M. or S.C., given as 5 million IU daily or 10 million IU 3 times weekly for 16 weeks.
Children ages 1 to 17 years: 3 million IU/m² S.C. 3 times weekly for first week; then increase to 6 million IU/m² S.C. 3 times weekly (maximum is 10 million IU 3 times weekly) for total of 16 to 24 weeks.
➤ **Chronic hepatitis C—**
Adults: 3 million IU I.M. or S.C. 3 times weekly. In patients tolerating therapy with normalization of ALT at 16 weeks of therapy, continue for 18 to 24 months. In patients who have not normalized the ALT, consider discontinuing therapy.
➤ **Adjunct to surgical treatment in patients with malignant melanoma who are asymptomatic after surgery but at high risk for systemic recurrence for up to 8 weeks after surgery—**
Adults: Initially, 20 million IU/m² by I.V. infusion five consecutive days weekly for 4 weeks; then maintenance dose of 10

million IU/m² S.C. 3 times weekly for 48 weeks. If adverse effects occur, discontinue therapy until they abate, then resume therapy at 50% of the previous dose. If intolerance persists, stop therapy.

➤ **Initial treatment of clinically aggressive follicular non-Hodgkin's lymphoma in conjunction with chemotherapy containing anthracycline—**
Adults: 5 million IU S.C. 3 times weekly for up to 18 months.

I.V. ADMINISTRATION
● Prepare infusion solution immediately before use.
● Based on desired dose, reconstitute appropriate vial strength of drug with diluent provided. Withdraw dose and inject into a 100-ml bag of normal saline solution. Final concentration of drug shouldn't be less than 10 million IU/100 ml.
● Infuse over 20 minutes.

ACTION
Unknown. Appears to involve direct antiproliferative action against tumor or viral cells to inhibit replication and modulation of host immune response by enhancing phagocytic activity of macrophages and augmenting specific cytotoxicity of lymphocytes for target cells.

Route	Onset	Peak	Duration
I.M., S.C.	Unknown	3-12 hr	16 hr
I.V.	Unknown	15-60 min	4 hr

ADVERSE REACTIONS
CNS: *dizziness, confusion, paresthesia,* lethargy, *depression, difficulty in thinking or concentrating, insomnia,* anxiety, *fatigue, hypoesthesia, amnesia,* nervousness, *somnolence,* weakness, *malaise, asthenia.*
CV: hypotension, *chest pain,* flushing.
EENT: visual disturbances, hearing disorders, pharyngitis, *nasal congestion, sinusitis,* rhinitis, stye.
GI: *anorexia, nausea, diarrhea, vomiting,* abdominal pain, *dyspepsia,* constipation, loose stools, eructation, *dry mouth,* dysgeusia, stomatitis, gingivitis.
GU: transient impotence.
Hematologic: *leukopenia; thrombocytopenia;* anemia.
Metabolic: hypercalcemia, hyperphosphatemia.
Musculoskeletal: *arthralgia, back pain.*
Respiratory: *dyspnea, coughing.*
Skin: *rash, dryness, pruritus, alopecia,* candidiasis, dermatitis, *increased diaphoresis.*
Other: *flu syndrome, rigors,* gynecomastia.

INTERACTIONS
Drug-drug. *Aminophylline, theophylline:* May reduce theophylline clearance. Monitor serum levels.
CNS depressants: Increased CNS effects. Avoid using together.
Live-virus vaccines: Risk of increased adverse reactions to vaccine or decreased antibody response. Postpone immunization.
Zidovudine: Synergistic adverse effects (higher risk of neutropenia) may occur. Carefully monitor WBC count.

EFFECTS ON LAB TEST RESULTS
● May increase calcium, phosphate, AST, ALT, LDH, alkaline phosphatase, and fasting glucose levels.
● May increase PT, INR, and PTT. May decrease hemoglobin and WBC and platelet counts.

CONTRAINDICATIONS
Contraindicated in patients hypersensitive to drug or its components.

NURSING CONSIDERATIONS
● Use cautiously in patients with history of CV disease, pulmonary disease, diabetes mellitus, coagulation disorders, and severe myelosuppression.
● Use S.C. administration route in patients whose platelet count is below 50,000/mm³.
● Depression and suicidal behavior have been linked to drug use; patients with psychotic disorders, especially depression, shouldn't continue drug treatment.
● Give drug at bedtime to minimize daytime drowsiness.
● When giving interferon for condylomata acuminata, use only 10 million-IU vial because dilution of other strengths needed for intralesional use results in a hypertonic solution. Don't reconstitute drug in 10 million-IU vial with more than 1 ml of diluent. Use tuberculin or similar syringe and 25G to 30G needle. Don't inject too

deeply beneath lesion or too superficially. As many as five lesions can be treated at one time. To ease discomfort, give in evening with acetaminophen.
• Ensure patient is well hydrated, especially during initial treatment.
• At beginning of treatment, monitor patient for flulike signs and symptoms, which tend to diminish with continued therapy. Premedicate patient with acetaminophen to minimize these symptoms.
• Periodically check for adverse CNS reactions, such as decreased mental status and dizziness, during therapy.
• Monitor CBC with differential, platelet count, blood chemistry and electrolyte studies, and liver function tests. If patient has cardiac disorder or advanced stages of cancer, monitor ECG.
• For patients who develop thrombocytopenia, exercise extreme care in performing invasive procedures; inspect injection site and skin frequently for signs and symptoms of bruising; limit frequency of I.M. injections; test urine, emesis fluid, stool, and secretions for occult blood.
• Severe adverse reactions may need dosage reduction to one-half or discontinuation of drug until reactions subside.
• *Alert:* Neurotoxicity and cardiotoxicity are more common in elderly patients, especially those with underlying CNS or cardiac impairment.
• Use with blood dyscrasia-causing drugs, bone marrow suppressants, or radiation therapy may increase bone marrow suppression. Dosage reduction may be needed.
• In treatment of condylomata acuminata, maximum response usually occurs 4 to 8 weeks after therapy starts. If results aren't satisfactory after 12 to 16 weeks, a second course may be instituted. Patients with 6 to 10 condylomata may receive a second course of treatment; patients with more than 10 condylomata may receive additional courses.

PATIENT TEACHING
• Advise patient to avoid contact with persons with viral illness; patient is at increased risk for infection during therapy.
• Advise patient that laboratory tests will be performed before and periodically during therapy.

• Teach patient proper oral hygiene during treatment because bone marrow suppressant effects of interferon may lead to microbial infection, delayed healing, and gingival bleeding. Drug also may decrease salivary flow.
• Advise patient to check with prescriber for instructions after missing a dose.
• Stress need to follow prescriber's instructions about taking and recording temperature and how and when to take acetaminophen.
• If patient will give drug to himself, teach him how to prepare injection and how to use disposable syringe. Give him information on drug stability.
• Tell patient that drug may cause temporary partial hair loss; hair should return after drug is withdrawn.
• Advise patient to notify prescriber if signs or symptoms of depression occur.

---

interferon beta-1a
Avonex

Pregnancy risk category C

AVAILABLE FORMS
Lyophilized powder for injection: 33 mcg (6.6 million IU)

INDICATIONS & DOSAGES
➤ **Relapsing forms of multiple sclerosis to slow accumulation of physical disability and decrease frequency of clinical exacerbation—**
Adults age 18 and older: 30 mcg I.M. once weekly.

ACTION
Exact mechanism unknown. Its biological response-modifying properties are mediated through its interactions with specific cell receptors found on the surface of human cells. Binding of these receptors induces the expression of a number of interferon-induced gene products believed to mediate the biological actions of interferon beta-1a.

Route	Onset	Peak	Duration
I.M.	Unknown	3-15 hr	Unknown

ADVERSE REACTIONS
CNS: *headache, sleep difficulty, dizziness,* syncope, ***suicidal tendency, seizures,*** speech disorder, ataxia, *asthenia,* malaise.
CV: chest pain, vasodilation.
EENT: otitis media, decreased hearing, *sinusitis.*
GI: *nausea, diarrhea, dyspepsia,* anorexia, abdominal pain.
GU: ovarian cyst, vaginitis.
Hematologic: anemia.
Musculoskeletal: *muscle ache,* muscle spasm, arthralgia.
Respiratory: *upper respiratory tract infection,* dyspnea.
Skin: ecchymosis at injection site, injection site reaction, urticaria, alopecia, nevus.
Other: *flu syndrome, pain, fever, chills, infection,* herpes zoster, herpes simplex, hypersensitivity reactions.

INTERACTIONS
Drug-lifestyle. *Sun exposure:* Photosensitivity reactions may occur. Advise patient to take precautions against sun exposure.

EFFECTS ON LAB TEST RESULTS
• May increase AST levels.
• May increase eosinophil count. May decrease hemoglobin and hematocrit.

CONTRAINDICATIONS
Contraindicated in patients hypersensitive to natural or recombinant interferon beta, human albumin, or other components of drug.

NURSING CONSIDERATIONS
• Use cautiously in patients with depression, seizure disorders, or severe cardiac conditions.
• Safety and efficacy of drug in chronic progressive multiple sclerosis or in children younger than age 18 haven't been established.
• Monitor patient closely for depression and suicidal ideation. It isn't known if these symptoms are related to the underlying neurologic basis of multiple sclerosis or to interferon beta-1a.
• Monitor WBC count, platelet count, and blood chemistries, including liver function tests.

• To reconstitute drug, inject 1.1 ml of supplied diluent (sterile water for injection) into vial and gently swirl to dissolve drug. Don't shake.
• Drug should be used as soon as possible but may be used within 6 hours after being reconstituted if stored at 36° to 46° F (2° to 8° C).
• It isn't known if drug appears in breast milk. Because of potential for serious adverse reactions in breast-fed infants, the patient must decide whether to discontinue breast-feeding or drug therapy.

PATIENT TEACHING
• Teach patient and family member how to reconstitute drug and give I.M.
• Caution patient not to change dosage or schedule of administration. If a dose is missed, tell him to take it as soon as he remembers. The regular schedule may then be resumed. Two injections shouldn't be given within 2 days of each other.
• Show patient how to store drug.
• Inform patient that flulike signs and symptoms, such as fever, fatigue, myalgia, headache, chills, and arthralgia, aren't uncommon at start of therapy. Acetaminophen 650 mg P.O. may be taken immediately before injection and for another 24 hours after each injection, to lessen severity of flulike signs and symptoms.
• Advise patient to report depression, suicidal ideation, or other adverse reactions.
• Instruct patient to keep syringes and needles away from children. Also, instruct him not to reuse needles or syringes and to discard them in a syringe-disposal unit.
• Caution woman of childbearing age not to become pregnant during therapy because of potential of drug to cause spontaneous abortion. If pregnancy occurs, instruct patient to notify prescriber immediately and to discontinue drug.
• Advise patient to use sunscreen and avoid sun exposure while taking drug because photosensitivity may occur.

---

interferon beta-1b, recombinant
Betaferon§, Betaseron

Pregnancy risk category C

AVAILABLE FORMS
Powder for injection: 9.6 million IU (0.3 mg)

INDICATIONS & DOSAGES
➤ **To reduce frequency of exacerbations in patients with relapsing-remitting multiple sclerosis—**
Adults: 8 million IU (0.25 mg) S.C. every other day.

ACTION
A naturally occurring antiviral and immunoregulatory drug derived from human fibroblasts. Attaches to membrane receptors and causes cellular changes, including increased protein synthesis.

Route	Onset	Peak	Duration
S.C.	Unknown	1-8 hr	Unknown

ADVERSE REACTIONS
CNS: depression, anxiety, emotional lability, depersonalization, *suicidal tendencies,* confusion, somnolence, *hypertonia, asthenia, migraine, seizures,* headache, dizziness.
CV: palpitations, hypertension, tachycardia, peripheral vascular disorder, ***hemorrhage.***
EENT: laryngitis, *sinusitis, conjunctivitis,* abnormal vision.
GI: *diarrhea, constipation, abdominal pain, vomiting.*
GU: *menstrual bleeding or spotting, early or delayed menses, fewer days of menstrual flow, menorrhagia.*
Musculoskeletal: *myasthenia.*
Respiratory: dyspnea.
Skin: *inflammation, pain, necrosis at injection site, diaphoresis, alopecia.*
Other: breast pain, *flu syndrome, pelvic pain, lymphadenopathy, pain,* generalized edema.

INTERACTIONS
None significant.

EFFECTS ON LAB TEST RESULTS
● May increase ALT and bilirubin levels.
● May decrease WBC and neutrophil counts.

CONTRAINDICATIONS
Contraindicated in patients hypersensitive to interferon beta, human albumin, or components of drug.

NURSING CONSIDERATIONS
● Use cautiously in women of childbearing age. Evidence is inconclusive about teratogenic effects, but drug may be an abortifacient.
● To reconstitute, inject 1.2 ml of supplied diluent (half normal saline solution for injection) into vial and gently swirl to dissolve drug. Don't shake. Reconstituted solution will contain 8 million IU (0.25 mg)/ml. Discard vial that contains particulates or discolored solution.
● Inject immediately after preparation.
● Rotate injection sites to minimize local reactions and observe site for necrosis.
● Monitor patient for signs of depression.

PATIENT TEACHING
● Warn woman of childbearing age about dangers to fetus. If pregnancy occurs during therapy, tell her to notify prescriber and stop taking drug.
● Teach patient how to perform S.C. injections, including solution preparation, use of aseptic technique, rotation of injection sites, and equipment disposal. Periodically reevaluate patient's technique.
● Tell patient to take drug at bedtime to minimize mild flulike signs and symptoms that commonly occur.
● Advise patient to report suicidal ideation or depression.
● Urge patient to immediately report signs or symptoms of necrosis at injection site.

interferon gamma-1b
Actimmune

Pregnancy risk category C

AVAILABLE FORMS
Injection: 100 mcg (3 million IU)/0.5-ml vial

Reactions may be *common,* uncommon, *life-threatening,* or **COMMON AND LIFE-THREATENING.**

INDICATIONS & DOSAGES

➤ **Chronic granulomatous disease—**
Adults with body surface area (BSA) over 0.5 m^2: 50 mcg/m^2 (1 million IU/m^2) S.C. 3 times weekly, preferably h.s., in deltoid or anterior thigh muscle.
Adults with a BSA 0.5 m^2 or below: 1.5 mcg/kg S.C. 3 times weekly.

➤ **To delay disease progression in patients with severe, malignant osteopetrosis—**
Patients with body surface area greater than 0.5 m^2: 50 mcg/m^2 (1 million IU/m^2) S.C. 3 times weekly in the deltoid or anterior thigh muscle.
Patients with body surface area 0.5 m^2 or less: 1.5 mcg/kg/dose S.C. 3 times weekly in the deltoid or anterior thigh muscle.

ACTION

Acts as an interleukin-type lymphokine. Has potent phagocyte-activating properties and increases the oxidative metabolism of tissue macrophages.

Route	Onset	Peak	Duration
S.C.	Unknown	7 hr	Unknown

ADVERSE REACTIONS

CNS: *fatigue,* decreased mental status, gait disturbance, dizziness.
GI: *nausea, vomiting, diarrhea,* abdominal pain.
GU: proteinuria.
Hematologic: *neutropenia, thrombocytopenia.*
Metabolic: weight loss.
Musculoskeletal: back pain.
Skin: *erythema and tenderness at injection site, rash.*
Other: *flu syndrome.*

INTERACTIONS

Drug-drug. *Myelosuppressives:* May increase myelosuppression. Monitor patient closely.
Zidovudine: Increased plasma levels of zidovudine. Dosage adjustments are needed when used together.

EFFECTS ON LAB TEST RESULTS

• May increase liver enzyme levels.
• May decrease neutrophil and platelet counts.

CONTRAINDICATIONS

Contraindicated in patients hypersensitive to drug or to genetically engineered products derived from *Escherichia coli.*

NURSING CONSIDERATIONS

• Use cautiously in patients with cardiac disease, including arrhythmias, ischemia, or heart failure. The flu syndrome commonly seen with high doses of drug can worsen these conditions.
• Use cautiously in patients with compromised CNS function or seizure disorders. CNS adverse reactions that may occur at high doses of drug can worsen these conditions.
• Use myelosuppressives together with caution.
• Premedicate patient with acetaminophen to minimize signs and symptoms at start of therapy; these tend to diminish with continued therapy.
• Before beginning therapy and at 3-month intervals, monitor CBC, platelets, renal and hepatic function tests, and urinalysis.
• Discard unused drug. Each vial is for single-dose use only and doesn't contain a preservative.

PATIENT TEACHING

• If patient will give drug to himself, teach him how to give it and how to dispose of used needles, syringes, containers, and unused drug.
• Instruct patient how to manage flulike signs and symptoms (fever, fatigue, myalgia, headache, chills, arthralgia) that commonly occur.
• Advise use of acetaminophen.

levamisole hydrochloride
Ergamisol

Pregnancy risk category C

AVAILABLE FORMS
Tablets: 50 mg (base)

INDICATIONS & DOSAGES
➤ **Adjuvant treatment of Dukes' stage C colon cancer (with fluorouracil) after surgical resection—**
Adults: 50 mg P.O. q 8 hours for 3 days, beginning no earlier than 7 days and no

later than 30 days after surgery, provided patient is out of the hospital, ambulatory, and maintaining normal oral nutrition; has well-healed wounds; and has recovered from postoperative complications. Fluorouracil (450 mg/m²/day I.V.) is given for 5 days with a 3-day course of levamisole starting 21 to 34 days after surgery.

Maintenance dosage is 50 mg P.O. q 8 hours for 3 days q 2 weeks for 1 year. Given with fluorouracil maintenance therapy (450 mg/m²/day by rapid I.V. push once weekly, beginning 28 days after initial 5-day course) for 1 year.

Adjust-a-dose: Dosage modifications are based on hematologic values. If WBC count is 2,500 to 3,500/mm³, don't give fluorouracil, until WBC count is above 3,500/mm³. When fluorouracil is restarted, reduce dosage by 20%. If WBC count stays below 2,500/mm³ for over 10 days after fluorouracil is withdrawn, discontinue levamisole. If platelet count is below 100,000/mm³, therapy with both fluorouracil and levamisole should be discontinued.

ACTION
Unknown. Appears to restore depressed immune function, increase the actions of monocytes and macrophages, and increase T-cell responses. Also inhibits alkaline phosphatase and cholinergic activity.

Route	Onset	Peak	Duration
P.O.	Unknown	1.5-2 hr	Unknown

ADVERSE REACTIONS
CNS: *dizziness, headache, paresthesia, somnolence, depression, nervousness, insomnia, anxiety, fatigue.*
CV: chest pain, edema.
EENT: blurred vision, conjunctivitis, *stomatitis, dysgeusia, altered sense of smell.*
GI: *nausea, diarrhea, vomiting,* anorexia, abdominal pain, constipation, flatulence, dyspepsia.
GU: hyperbilirubinemia.
Hematologic: ***agranulocytosis, leukopenia, thrombocytopenia,*** anemia.
Musculoskeletal: arthralgia, myalgia.
Skin: dermatitis, exfoliative dermatitis, pruritus, urticaria, *alopecia.*
Other: rigors, *infection, fever.*

INTERACTIONS
Drug-drug. *Phenytoin:* Plasma phenytoin levels may be elevated when drug is given with levamisole and fluorouracil. Monitor plasma phenytoin levels.
Warfarin: May prolong coagulation times if taken together. May need dosage adjustment.
Drug-lifestyle. *Alcohol use:* May precipitate a disulfiram-like reaction. Urge patient to avoid using together.

EFFECTS ON LAB TEST RESULTS
• May increase bilirubin levels.
• May decrease hemoglobin and granulocyte, WBC, and platelet counts.

CONTRAINDICATIONS
Contraindicated in patients hypersensitive to drug or its components.

NURSING CONSIDERATIONS
• *Alert:* Use cautiously and with close hematologic monitoring because agranulocytosis, which is sometimes fatal, may occur. Neutropenia is usually reversible when therapy is discontinued.
• If levamisole therapy begins 7 to 20 days after surgery, fluorouracil should be started with second course of levamisole therapy. It should begin no earlier than 21 days and no later than 34 days after surgery. If levamisole is deferred until 21 to 30 days after surgery, fluorouracil therapy should begin with first course of levamisole.
• Don't exceed recommended doses. Higher doses may cause greater risk of agranulocytosis.
• Obtain CBC with differential and platelet count at weekly intervals, before treatment with fluorouracil. Obtain electrolyte levels and liver function studies every 3 months for 1 year.

PATIENT TEACHING
• Tell patient to promptly report development of stomatitis or diarrhea. If either of these reactions occurs during initial course of fluorouracil therapy, drug is discontinued and then weekly fluorouracil therapy is begun 28 days after start of initial course. If stomatitis or diarrhea develops during weekly doses of fluorouracil, fluorouracil therapy is deferred until these

---

symptoms subside. Then fluorouracil therapy is started at dosage reduced by 20%.
• Urge patient to immediately report flu-like signs and symptoms, such as fever, malaise, headache, chills, arthralgia, and fatigue.
• Advise breast-feeding woman to discontinue nursing during drug therapy.

oprelvekin
Neumega

Pregnancy risk category C

AVAILABLE FORMS
Injection: 5 mg single-dose vial with diluent

INDICATIONS & DOSAGES
➤ **Prevention of severe thrombocytopenia and reduction of need for platelet transfusions following myelosuppressive chemotherapy with nonmyeloid malignancies—**
Adults: 50 mcg/kg as single daily S.C. injection.

ACTION
A thrombopoietic growth factor that directly stimulates proliferation of hematopoietic stem cells and megakaryocyte progenitor cells. Also induces megakaryocyte maturation, resulting in increased platelet production.

Route	Onset	Peak	Duration
S.C.	Unknown	3-5 hr	Unknown

ADVERSE REACTIONS
CNS: *asthenia, headache, insomnia, dizziness,* paresthesia, *syncope.*
CV: *tachycardia, palpitations,* **ATRIAL FLUTTER OR FIBRILLATION,** *edema.*
EENT: blurred vision, *conjunctival injection,* eye hemorrhage, pharyngitis.
GI: *oral candidiasis, nausea, vomiting, diarrhea.*
Hematologic: anemia.
Metabolic: dehydration, hypocalcemia.
Respiratory: dyspnea, cough, pleural effusions.
Skin: *rash,* skin discoloration, exfoliative dermatitis.

INTERACTIONS
Drug-drug. *Diuretics, ifosfamide:* Severe hypokalemia resulting in death has occurred in patients receiving these drugs together with oprelvekin. Use with extreme caution.

EFFECTS ON LAB TEST RESULTS
• May decrease calcium level.
• May decrease hemoglobin.

CONTRAINDICATIONS
Contraindicated in patients hypersensitive to drug or its components.

NURSING CONSIDERATIONS
• *Alert:* Administration to children, especially those younger than age 12, should be restricted to controlled clinical trial settings. Papilledema may be a dose-limiting reaction in this population.
• Give S.C. in the abdomen, thigh, hip, or upper arm. Don't inject I.D. or intravascularly.
• Dosing should begin 6 to 24 hours after completion of chemotherapy and end at least 2 days before starting next planned cycle of chemotherapy.
• Each single-dose vial should be reconstituted with 1 ml of supplied diluent. Avoid excessive or vigorous agitation. Discard unused portions.
• Use reconstituted drug within 3 hours.
• Store drug and diluent in refrigerator until ready to use. Don't freeze.
• Use drug cautiously in patients with heart failure because of fluid retention.
• Closely monitor fluid and electrolyte status in patients receiving long-term diuretic therapy.
• Obtain a CBC before chemotherapy and at regular intervals during drug therapy.
• Fluid retention can be severe; monitor patient closely.

PATIENT TEACHING
• Instruct patient about appropriate preparation and administration of drug if he is to self-administer at home.
• Warn patient about potential adverse reactions. Tell him to report any occurrence.
• Tell patient to keep drug refrigerated and not to reconstitute until just before use.

• Urge patient to call prescriber immediately if swelling, rapid heart beat, or difficulty breathing occurs.
• Tell patient to report signs and symptoms of increased bleeding or bruising.

❊ NEW DRUG

peginterferon alfa-2b
PEG-Intron

Pregnancy risk category C

AVAILABLE FORMS
Injection: 100 mcg/ml, 160 mcg/ml, 240 mcg/ml, 300 mcg/ml

INDICATIONS & DOSAGES
Chronic hepatitis C in patients not previously treated with interferon alpha—
Give S.C. once weekly for 48 weeks on same day each week, initial dose based on weight:
Adults weighing 37 to 45 kg (82 to 99 lb): 40 mcg (0.4 ml) of 100-mcg/ml strength.
Adults weighing 46 to 56 kg (101 to 123 lb): 50 mcg (0.5 ml) of 100-mcg/ml strength.
Adults weighing 57 to 72 kg (126 to 159 lb): 64 mcg (0.4 ml) of 160-mcg/ml strength.
Adults weighing 73 to 88 kg (161 to 194 lb): 80 mcg (0.5 ml) of 160-mcg/ml strength.
Adults weighing 89 to 106 kg (196 to 234 lb): 96 mcg (0.4 ml) of 240-mcg/ml strength.
Adults weighing 107 to 136 kg (236 to 300 lb): 120 mcg (0.5 ml) of 240-mcg/ml strength.
Adults weighing 137 to 160 kg (302 to 353 lb): 150 mcg (0.5 ml) of 300-mcg/ml strength.
Adjust-a-dose: For patients who develop a serious adverse reaction, discontinue drug or decrease dose to one-half starting dose. For patients with neutrophil count < 0.75 × 10⁹/L, reduce dose. If neutrophil count is < 0.5 × 10⁹/L, discontinue drug. For patients with platelet count < 80 × 10⁹/L, reduce dose. If platelet count is < 50 × 10⁹/L, discontinue drug.

ACTION
Binds to specific membrane receptors on the cell surface, initiating induction of certain enzymes, suppression of cell proliferation, and immunomodulating activities and inhibition of virus replication in virus-infected cells. Increases levels of effector proteins and body temperature, and decreases leukocyte and platelet counts.

Route	Onset	Peak	Duration
S.C.	Unknown	15-44 hr	Unknown

ADVERSE REACTIONS
CNS: *dizziness,* hypertonia, *depression, insomnia, anxiety, emotional lability, irritability, headache, fatigue,* malaise, **suicidal behavior.**
CV: flushing.
EENT: *pharyngitis,* sinusitis.
GI: *nausea, anorexia, diarrhea, abdominal pain,* vomiting, dyspepsia, right upper quadrant pain.
Hematologic: *neutropenia, thrombocytopenia.*
Hepatic: hepatomegaly.
Metabolic: hypothyroidism, hyperthyroidism, *weight decrease.*
Musculoskeletal: *musculoskeletal pain.*
Respiratory: cough.
Skin: *alopecia, pruritus, dry skin, rash, injection site inflammation or reaction, increased sweating,* injection site pain.
Other: *viral infection, fever, flulike symptoms, rigors.*

INTERACTIONS
None reported.

EFFECTS ON LAB TEST RESULTS
• May increase ALT levels. May increase or decrease TSH levels.
• May decrease neutrophil and platelet counts.

CONTRAINDICATIONS
Contraindicated in patients hypersensitive to drug or any of its components. Also contraindicated in patients with autoimmune hepatitis or decompensated liver disease.

NURSING CONSIDERATIONS
• Use cautiously in patients with psychiatric disorders, diabetes mellitus, CV disease, renal impairment (creatinine clearance < 50 ml/minute), pulmonary infiltrates, or pulmonary function impairment. Also use cautiously in patients with autoimmune, ischemic, and infectious disorders.
• Don't use drug in patients with diabetes or thyroid disorders that can't be controlled with medication. Drug may cause or aggravate hypothyroidism, hyperthyroidism, or diabetes.
• Don't use drug in patients who have failed other alpha interferon treatment or received liver or other organ transplants, or in patients with HIV or hepatitis B virus (HBV).
• Perform ECG on patient with cardiac history before starting drug.
• Initiate treatment in patient who is well hydrated.
• Monitor patient with history of MI or arrhythmias closely for hypotension, arrhythmias, tachycardia, cardiomyopathy, and MI.
• Monitor patient for depression and other mental health disorders. If symptoms are severe, stop drug and refer patient for psychiatric care.
• Monitor patient for signs and symptoms of colitis, such as abdominal pain, bloody diarrhea, and fever. Stop drug if colitis occurs. Symptoms should resolve within 1 to 3 weeks after discontinuing drug.
• Monitor patient for signs and symptoms of pancreatitis or hypersensitivity reactions and stop drug if these occur.
• Monitor patient with pulmonary disease for dyspnea, pulmonary infiltrates, pneumonitis, and pneumonia.
• Eye examination should be done in patient with diabetes or hypertension before starting drug. Retinal hemorrhages, cotton-wool spots, and retinal artery or vein obstruction may occur.
• Monitor patient with renal disease for signs and symptoms of toxicity.
• Monitor CBC count, platelets, and AST, ALT, bilirubin, and thyroid-stimulating hormone (TSH) levels before starting drug and periodically during treatment.
• Stop drug if severe neutropenia or thrombocytopenia occurs.

• It's unknown if drug appears in breast milk. Because of the potential for adverse reactions in breast-feeding infants, the patient must decide whether to stop breast-feeding or stop drug.

PATIENT TEACHING
• Advise patient on the appropriate use of drug and the benefits and risks associated with treatment. Tell patient that adverse reactions may continue for several months after treatment is stopped.
• Advise patient to immediately report symptoms of depression or suicidal ideation.
• Instruct patient on importance of proper disposal of needles and syringes and caution him against reuse of old needles and syringes.
• Tell patient that drug isn't known to prevent transmission of hepatitis C virus (HCV) to others and that it's also unknown if drug will cure hepatitis C or prevent cirrhosis, liver failure, or liver cancer that may result from HCV infection.
• Advise patient that laboratory tests are needed before starting therapy and periodically thereafter.
• Tell patient to take drug at bedtime and to use antipyretics to decrease incidence of flulike signs and symptoms.

---

sargostim (GM-CSF; granulocyte macrophage-colony stimulating factor)
Leukine

Pregnancy risk category C

AVAILABLE FORMS
Powder for injection: 250 mcg, 500 mcg
Solution: 500 mcg/ml

INDICATIONS & DOSAGES
➤ **Acceleration of hematopoietic reconstitution after autologous bone marrow transplantation in patients with malignant lymphoma or acute lymphoblastic leukemia or during autologous bone marrow transplantation in patients with Hodgkin's disease—**
Adults: 250 mcg/m² daily for 21 consecutive days given as 2-hour I.V. infusion be-

ginning 2 to 4 hours after bone marrow transplantation.

➤ **Bone marrow transplantation failure or engraftment delay—**
Adults: 250 mcg/m²/day for 14 days as 2-hour I.V. infusion. Dose may be repeated after 7 days of no therapy. If engraftment still hasn't occurred, a third course of 500 mcg/m²/day I.V. for 14 days may be attempted after another therapy-free 7 days.

Adjust-a-dose: Stimulation of marrow precursors may result in rapid rise of WBC count. If blast cells appear or increase to 10% or more of WBC count or if the underlying disease progresses, discontinue therapy. If absolute neutrophil count is above 20,000/mm³ or if platelet count is above 50,000/mm³, temporarily discontinue drug or reduce dose by 50%.

I.V. ADMINISTRATION
● Reconstitute with 1 ml of sterile water for injection. Direct stream of sterile water against side of vial and gently swirl contents to minimize foaming. Avoid excessive or vigorous agitation or shaking. Dilute in normal saline solution. If final concentration is below 10 mcg/ml, add human albumin at final concentration of 0.1% to saline solution before adding sargostim to prevent adsorption to components of the delivery system. For a final concentration of 0.1% human albumin, add 1 mg human albumin/1 ml saline solution (dilute 1 ml of 5% human albumin in 50 ml of saline solution). Give as soon as possible after mixing and no later than 6 hours after reconstituting.
● Don't add other drugs to infusion solution because no data exist regarding solution compatibility and stability.
● Don't use in-line filter for I.V. administration.

ACTION
A glycoprotein containing 127 amino acids manufactured by recombinant DNA technology in a yeast expression system. It differs from the natural human granulocyte-macrophage colony-stimulating factor by substitution of leucine for arginine at position 23. The carbohydrate moiety also may be different. Drug induces cellular re-

sponses by binding to specific receptors on cell surfaces of target cells.

Route	Onset	Peak	Duration
I.V., S.C.	15 min	2-4 hr	Unknown

ADVERSE REACTIONS
CNS: *malaise, CNS disorders, asthenia.*
CV: *blood dyscrasias, edema,* **supraventricular arrhythmias,** *pericardial effusion.*
GI: *nausea, vomiting, diarrhea, anorexia,* **hemorrhage,** *GI disorders, stomatitis.*
GU: *urinary tract disorder,* abnormal kidney function.
Hepatic: *liver damage.*
Respiratory: *dyspnea, lung disorders,* pleural effusion.
Skin: *alopecia, rash.*
Other: *fever, mucous membrane disorder, peripheral edema,* SEPSIS.

INTERACTIONS
Drug-drug. *Corticosteroids, lithium:* May increase myeloproliferative effects of sargostim. Use cautiously together.

EFFECTS ON LAB TEST RESULTS
● May increase BUN, creatinine, AST, ALT, and bilirubin levels.

CONTRAINDICATIONS
Contraindicated in patients hypersensitive to drug or its components or to yeast-derived products and in those with excessive leukemic myeloid blasts in bone marrow or peripheral blood.

NURSING CONSIDERATIONS
● Use cautiously in patients with cardiac disease, hypoxia, fluid retention, pulmonary infiltrates, heart failure, or impaired renal or hepatic function because these conditions may be exacerbated.
● Anticipate reducing dose by 50% or temporarily discontinuing drug if severe adverse reactions occur; notify prescriber. Therapy may be resumed when reactions abate. Transient rash and local reactions at injection site may occur; no serious allergic or anaphylactic reactions have been reported.
● Don't give within 24 hours of last dose of chemotherapy or within 12 hours of last dose of radiotherapy because rapidly dividing progenitor cells may be sensitive to

these cytotoxic therapies and drug would be ineffective.
• Monitor CBC with differential, including examination for presence of blast cells, biweekly.
• Drug is effective in accelerating myeloid recovery in patients receiving bone marrow that is either unpurged or purged by anti-B cell monoclonal antibodies compared with patients who receive bone marrow that is chemically purged.
• Drug may produce a limited response in transplant patients who have received extensive radiotherapy or in patients who have received other myelotoxic drugs.
• Drug can act as a growth factor for any tumor type, particularly myeloid malignant disease.

PATIENT TEACHING
• Review administration schedule with patient and caregivers, and address their concerns.
• Urge patient to report adverse reactions promptly.

77

Ophthalmic anti-infectives

bacitracin
chloramphenicol
ciprofloxacin hydrochloride
erythromycin
gentamicin sulfate
ofloxacin 0.3%
polymyxin B sulfate
sulfacetamide sodium 10%
sulfacetamide sodium 15%
sulfacetamide sodium 30%
tobramycin
vidarabine

COMBINATION PRODUCTS

AK-POLY-BAC: polymyxin B sulfate 10,000 units and bacitracin zinc 500 units.
BLEPHAMIDE STERILE OPHTHALMIC OINTMENT: sulfacetamide sodium 10% and prednisolone acetate 0.2%.
CETAPRED OINTMENT: sulfacetamide sodium 10% and prednisolone acetate 0.25%.
CORTISPORIN OPHTHALMIC OINTMENT: polymyxin B sulfate 10,000 units, bacitracin zinc 400 units, neomycin sulfate 0.35%, and hydrocortisone 1%.
CORTISPORIN OPHTHALMIC SUSPENSION: polymyxin B sulfate 10,000 units, neomycin sulfate 0.35%, and hydrocortisone 1%.
ISOPTO CETAPRED: sulfacetamide sodium 10% and prednisolone acetate 0.25%.
MAXITROL OINTMENT/OPHTHALMIC SUSPENSION: dexamethasone 0.1%, neomycin sulfate 0.35%, and polymyxin B sulfate 10,000 units.
METIMYD OPHTHALMIC OINTMENT/SUSPENSION: sulfacetamide sodium 10% and prednisolone acetate 0.5%.
NEOSPORIN OPHTHALMIC OINTMENT: polymyxin B sulfate 10,000 units, neomycin sulfate 3.5 mg, and bacitracin zinc 400 units/g.
NEOSPORIN OPHTHALMIC SOLUTION: polymyxin B sulfate 10,000 units, neomycin sulfate 1.75 mg, and gicidin 0.025 mg.
POLYSPORIN OPHTHALMIC OINTMENT: polymyxin B sulfate 10,000 units and bacitracin zinc 500 units.
POLYTRIM OPHTHALMIC: trimethoprim sulfate 1 mg and polymyxin B sulfate 10,000 units/ml.

PRED-G S.O.P.: prednisolone acetate 0.6% and gentamicin sulfate equivalent to gentamicin base 0.3%.
TOBRADEX: dexamethasone 0.1% and tobramycin 0.3%.
VASOCIDIN OPHTHALMIC OINTMENT: sulfacetamide sodium 10% and prednisolone acetate 0.5%.
VASOCIDIN OPHTHALMIC SOLUTION: sulfacetamide sodium 10% and prednisolone phosphate 0.25%.
VASOSULF: sulfacetamide sodium 15% and phenylephrine hydrochloride 0.125%.

---

bacitracin
AK-Tracin

Pregnancy risk category C

AVAILABLE FORMS
Ophthalmic ointment: 500 units/g

INDICATIONS & DOSAGES
➤ **Surface bacterial infections involving conjunctiva and cornea—**
Adults and children: Apply small amount of ointment into conjunctival sac one or more times daily or p.r.n. until favorable response is observed.

ACTION
Inhibits bacterial cell-wall synthesis; may be bactericidal or bacteriostatic, depending on concentration and infection.

Route	Onset	Peak	Duration
Ophthalmic	Unknown	Unknown	Unknown

ADVERSE REACTIONS
EENT: slowed corneal wound healing, temporary visual haze.
Other: overgrowth of nonsusceptible organisms.

INTERACTIONS
Drug-drug. *Heavy metals such as silver nitrate:* Inactivation of bacitracin. Don't use together.

Reactions may be *common*, uncommon, *life-threatening*, or COMMON AND LIFE-THREATENING.

EFFECTS ON LAB TEST RESULTS
None reported.

CONTRAINDICATIONS
Contraindicated in patients hypersensitive to drug and in those with atopy.

NURSING CONSIDERATIONS
• Ophthalmic ointment may be stored at room temperature.
• For external use only.
• Clean eye area of excessive exudate before application.
• Watch for signs and symptoms of superinfection.
Urine sediment tests may show increased protein and cast excretion.
• *Alert:* Don't confuse bacitracin with Bactrim or Bactroban.

PATIENT TEACHING
• Teach patient how to apply drug; tell him that only small amount of ointment is needed and that it may cause blurred vision. Advise him to wash hands before and after administering and not to touch tip of tube to eye or surrounding tissue.
• Instruct patient to stop drug and notify prescriber of signs and symptoms of sensitivity (itching lids, swelling, constant burning, or failure to heal).
• Tell patient not to share drug, washcloths, or towels with family members and to notify prescriber if anyone develops same symptoms.
• Stress importance of compliance with recommended therapy.

---

chloramphenicol
AK-Chlor, Chloromycetin Ophthalmic, Chloroptic, Chloroptic S.O.P., Chlorsig‡, Pentamycetin†, Sno Phenicol§, Sopamycetin†

Pregnancy risk category C

AVAILABLE FORMS
Ophthalmic ointment: 1%
Ophthalmic solution: 0.5%
Powder for ophthalmic solution: 25 mg/vial

INDICATIONS & DOSAGES
➤ **Surface bacterial infection involving conjunctiva or cornea—**
Adults and children: 1 or 2 drops of solution in eye q 3 to 6 hours or more often, if needed. Or, apply small amount of ointment to lower conjunctival sac q 3 to 6 hours or more often, if needed. Continue for at least 48 hours after eye appears normal.

ACTION
Inhibits protein synthesis; may be bacteriostatic or bactericidal, depending on concentration.

Route	Onset	Peak	Duration
Ophthalmic	Unknown	Unknown	Unknown

ADVERSE REACTIONS
EENT: optic atrophy in children, stinging or burning of eye after instillation, blurred vision (with ointment).
Skin: dermatitis.

INTERACTIONS
None significant.

EFFECTS ON LAB TEST RESULTS
None reported.

CONTRAINDICATIONS
Contraindicated in patients hypersensitive to drug.

NURSING CONSIDERATIONS
• If chloramphenicol drops are to be given hourly and then tapered, follow order closely to ensure adequate anterior chamber levels.
• Reconstitute powder for ophthalmic solution with supplied diluent. Use 5 ml of diluent to make 0.5% solution, 10 ml of diluent to make 0.25% solution, or 15 ml to make 0.16% solution.
• Store drug in tightly closed, light-resistant container.
• If patient has more than a superficial infection, anticipate using systemic therapy as well.
• Drug may cause a false elevation of urinary PABA levels if drug is administered during a bentiromide test for pancreatic function. Drug therapy causes false-

---

positive results on tests for urine glucose level using cupric sulfate (Clinitest).

PATIENT TEACHING
• Teach patient how to instill drops or apply ointment. Advise him to wash hands before and after administering ointment or solution, and warn him not to touch tip of applicator to eye or surrounding tissue.
• Tell patient to clean eye area of excessive exudate before application.
• Instruct patient to apply light finger pressure on lacrimal sac for 1 minute after drops are instilled.
• Tell patient that vision may be blurred for a few minutes after applying ointment.
• Tell patient not to share drug, washcloths, or towels with family members and to notify prescriber if anyone develops same signs or symptoms.
• Instruct patient to stop drug and notify prescriber of sensitivity (itching lids, swelling, or constant burning).
• Tell patient to notify prescriber if improvement doesn't occur within 3 days.
• Stress importance of compliance with recommended therapy.
• Instruct patient to watch for signs and symptoms of superinfection, such as redness, drainage, soreness, or failure to heal.

---

ciprofloxacin hydrochloride
Ciloxan

Pregnancy risk category C

AVAILABLE FORMS
Ophthalmic solution: 0.3% (base) in 2.5- and 5-ml containers

INDICATIONS & DOSAGES
➤ **Corneal ulcers caused by *Pseudomonas aeruginosa, Staphylococcus aureus, Staphylococcus epidermidis, Streptococcus pneumoniae,* and possibly *Serratia marcescens* and *Streptococcus viridans*—**
Adults and children older than age 12: 2 drops in affected eye q 15 minutes for first 6 hours; then 2 drops q 30 minutes for remainder of first day. On day 2, 2 drops hourly. On days 3 to 14, 2 drops q 4 hours.
➤ **Bacterial conjunctivitis caused by *Haemophilus influenzae, S. aureus,***

***S. epidermidis,* and possibly *S. pneumoniae*—**
Adults and children older than age 12: 1 or 2 drops into conjunctival sac of affected eye q 2 hours while awake for first 2 days. Then, 1 or 2 drops q 4 hours while awake for next 5 days.

ACTION
Inhibits bacterial DNA gyrase, an enzyme needed for bacterial replication. May be bacteriostatic or bactericidal, depending on concentration.

Route	Onset	Peak	Duration
Ophthalmic	Unknown	Unknown	Unknown

ADVERSE REACTIONS
EENT: *local burning or discomfort, white crystalline precipitate in superficial portion of corneal defect in patients with corneal ulcers, margin crusting, crystals or scales, foreign body sensation, itching, conjunctival hyperemia,* corneal staining, allergic reactions, keratopathy, lid edema, tearing, photophobia, decreased vision.
GI: bad or bitter taste in mouth.

INTERACTIONS
None significant.

EFFECTS ON LAB TEST RESULTS
None reported.

CONTRAINDICATIONS
Contraindicated in patients hypersensitive to ciprofloxacin or other fluoroquinolone antibiotics.

NURSING CONSIDERATIONS
• It's unknown if drug appears in breast milk after application to eye; however, systemically administered ciprofloxacin has appeared in breast milk. Use with caution in breast-feeding women.
• *Alert:* Discontinue drug at first sign of hypersensitivity, such as rash, and notify prescriber. Serious hypersensitivity reactions, including anaphylaxis, may occur in patients receiving systemic fluoroquinolone therapy.
• A topical overdose may be flushed from eyes with warm tap water.

● If corneal epithelium is still compromised after 14 days of treatment, continue therapy.

● Institute appropriate therapy if superinfection occurs. Prolonged use may result in overgrowth of nonsusceptible organisms, including fungi.

● *Alert:* Don't confuse Ciloxan with Cytoxan or cinoxacin.

PATIENT TEACHING
● Tell patient to clean eye area of excessive exudate before instilling.

● Teach patient how to instill drops. Advise him to wash hands before and after administering solution and not to touch tip of dropper to eye or surrounding tissues.

● Instruct patient to apply light finger pressure on lacrimal sac for 1 minute after drops are instilled.

● Tell patient not to share drug, washcloths, or towels with family members and to notify prescriber if anyone develops same signs or symptoms.

● Stress importance of compliance with recommended therapy.

---

erythromycin
Ilotycin

Pregnancy risk category B

AVAILABLE FORMS
Ophthalmic ointment: 0.5%

INDICATIONS & DOSAGES
➤ **Acute and chronic conjunctivitis, other eye infections—**
Adults and children: Apply a ribbon of ointment about 1 cm long directly to infected eye up to six times daily, depending on severity of infection.
➤ **Chlamydial ophthalmic infections (trachoma)—**
Adults and children: Apply small amount to each eye b.i.d. for 2 months or b.i.d. on first 5 days of each month for 6 months.
➤ **Prophylaxis of ophthalmia neonatorum caused by** *Neisseria gonorrhoeae* **or** *Chlamydia trachomatis—*
Neonates: Apply a ribbon of ointment about 1 cm long in lower conjunctival sac of each eye shortly after birth.

ACTION
Inhibits protein synthesis; usually bacteriostatic, but may be bactericidal in high concentrations or against highly susceptible organisms.

Route	Onset	Peak	Duration
Ophthalmic	Unknown	Unknown	Unknown

ADVERSE REACTIONS
EENT: slowed corneal wound healing, blurred vision, itching and burning eyes.
Skin: urticaria, dermatitis.
Other: overgrowth of nonsusceptible organisms with long-term use.

INTERACTIONS
None significant.

EFFECTS ON LAB TEST RESULTS
None reported.

CONTRAINDICATIONS
Contraindicated in patients hypersensitive to drug.

NURSING CONSIDERATIONS
● For prophylaxis of ophthalmia neonatorum, apply ointment no later than 1 hour after birth. Drug is used in neonates born by either vaginal delivery or cesarean section. Gently massage eyelids for 1 minute to spread ointment.

● Drug should be used only when sensitivity studies show it's effective against infecting organisms; it shouldn't be used in infections of unknown etiology.

● Use cautiously in breast-feeding women.

● Drug may interfere with fluorometric determinations of urinary catecholamines.

● Store drug at room temperature in tightly closed, light-resistant container.

PATIENT TEACHING
● Tell patient to clean eye area of excessive exudate before application.

● Teach patient how to apply drug. Advise him to wash hands before and after applying ointment, and warn him not to touch tip of applicator to eye or surrounding tissue.

● Tell patient that vision may be blurred for a few minutes after applying ointment.

• Advise patient to watch for and report signs and symptoms of sensitivity (itching lids, redness, swelling, or constant burning).
• Tell patient not to share drug, washcloths, or towels with family members and to notify prescriber if anyone develops same signs or symptoms.
• Stress importance of compliance with recommended therapy.

---

gentamicin sulfate
Cidomycin§, Garamycin, Genoptic, Gentacidin, Gentak, Genticin§

Pregnancy risk category C

AVAILABLE FORMS
Ophthalmic ointment: 0.3% (base)
Ophthalmic solution: 0.3% (base)

INDICATIONS & DOSAGES
➤ External ocular infections (conjunctivitis, keratoconjunctivitis, corneal ulcers, blepharitis, blepharoconjunctivitis, meibomianitis, and dacryocystitis) caused by susceptible organisms, especially *Pseudomonas aeruginosa, Proteus, Klebsiella pneumoniae, Escherichia coli,* and other g-negative organisms—
Adults and children: 1 to 2 drops in eye q 4 hours. In severe infections, up to 2 drops q hour. Or, apply ointment to lower conjunctival sac b.i.d. or t.i.d.

ACTION
Unknown. Thought to inhibit protein synthesis and is usually bactericidal.

Route	Onset	Peak	Duration
Ophthalmic	Unknown	Unknown	Unknown

ADVERSE REACTIONS
EENT: burning, stinging, or blurred vision with ointment, transient irritation from solution, conjunctival hyperemia.
Other: overgrowth of nonsusceptible organisms with long-term use.

INTERACTIONS
None significant.

EFFECTS ON LAB TEST RESULTS
None reported.

CONTRAINDICATIONS
Contraindicated in patients hypersensitive to drug.

NURSING CONSIDERATIONS
• Use cautiously in patients with history of sensitivity to aminoglycosides because cross-sensitivity may occur.
• Have culture taken before giving drug. Therapy may begin before culture results are known.
• If ophthalmic gentamicin is given together with systemic gentamicin, monitor gentamicin levels.
• Systemic absorption from excessive use may cause systemic toxicities.
• Solution isn't for injection into conjunctiva or anterior chamber of eye.
• Store drug away from heat.

PATIENT TEACHING
• Tell patient to clean eye area of excessive exudate before administering drug.
• Teach patient how to instill drops or apply ointment. Advise him to wash hands before and after administering ointment or solution and not to touch tip of dropper or tube to eye or surrounding tissues.
• Instruct patient to apply light finger pressure on lacrimal sac for 1 minute after drops are instilled.
• Instruct patient to stop drug and notify prescriber if signs and symptoms of sensitivity (itching lids, swelling, or constant burning) occur.
• Advise patient not to share drug, washcloths, or towels with family members and to notify prescriber if anyone develops same signs or symptoms.
• Tell patient that vision may be blurred for few minutes after application of ointment.
• *Alert:* Stress importance of following recommended therapy. *Pseudomonas* infections can cause complete vision loss within 24 hours if infection isn't controlled.

Reactions may be *common,* uncommon, *life-threatening,* or COMMON AND LIFE-THREATENING.

ofloxacin 0.3%
Exocin§, Ocuflox

Pregnancy risk category C

AVAILABLE FORMS
Ophthalmic solution: 0.3% in 1-ml and 5-ml solution

INDICATIONS & DOSAGES
➤ **Conjunctivitis caused by *Staphylococcus aureus, Staphylococcus epidermidis, Streptococcus pneumoniae, Enterobacter cloacae, Haemophilus influenzae, Proteus mirabilis, Pseudomonas aeruginosa,* and *Propionibacterium acnes*—**
Adults and children older than age 1: 1 to 2 drops in conjunctival sac q 2 to 4 hours daily, while awake, for first 2 days; then q.i.d. for up to 5 additional days.
➤ **Bacterial corneal ulcer caused by *S. aureus, S. epidermidis, S. pneumoniae, E. cloacae, H. influenzae, P. mirabilis, P. aeruginosa, Serratia marcescens,* and *P. acnes*—**
Adults and children older than age 1: 1 to 2 drops q 30 minutes while awake and 1 to 2 drops 4 to 6 hours after retiring on days 1 and 2. Days 3 to 7, 1 to 2 drops hourly while awake. Days 7 to 9, 1 to 2 drops q.i.d.

ACTION
Bactericidal. Inhibits bacterial DNA gyrase, an enzyme needed for bacterial replication.

Route	Onset	Peak	Duration
Ophthalmic	Unknown	Unknown	Unknown

ADVERSE REACTIONS
EENT: *transient ocular burning or discomfort,* stinging, redness, itching, photophobia, lacrimation, eye dryness.
Metabolic: hyperglycemia.

INTERACTIONS
None significant.

EFFECTS ON LAB TEST RESULTS
• May increase glucose levels.

CONTRAINDICATIONS
Contraindicated in patients hypersensitive to ofloxacin, other fluoroquinolones, or other components of drug; also contraindicated in breast-feeding women.

NURSING CONSIDERATIONS
• *Alert:* Don't inject drug into conjunctiva or introduce directly into anterior chamber of eye.
• Discontinue drug if improvement doesn't occur within 7 days. Prolonged use may result in overgrowth of nonsusceptible organisms, including fungi.
• *Alert:* Don't confuse Ocuflox with Ocufen.

PATIENT TEACHING
• If an allergic reaction occurs, tell patient to discontinue drug and call prescriber. Serious acute hypersensitivity reactions may need emergency treatment.
• Teach patient how to instill drops. Advise him to wash hands before and after instilling solution, and warn him not to touch tip of dropper to eye or surrounding tissue.
• Advise patient to apply light finger pressure on lacrimal sac for 1 minute after drug instillation.
• Tell patient not to share drug, washcloths, or towels with family members and to notify prescriber if anyone develops same signs or symptoms.
• Stress importance of compliance with recommended therapy.
• Warn patient not to use leftover drug for new eye infection.
• Remind patient to discard drug when no longer needed.

polymyxin B sulfate
Polyfax§

Pregnancy risk category C

AVAILABLE FORMS
Ophthalmic sterile powder for solution: 500,000-unit vials to be reconstituted to 20 to 50 ml

INDICATIONS & DOSAGES
➤ **Alone or with other drugs to treat superficial eye infections involving con-**

junctiva and cornea resulting from infection with *Pseudomonas* or other g-negative organisms—
Adults and children: 1 to 3 drops of 0.1% to 0.25% (10,000 to 25,000 units/ml) hourly. Increase interval based on patient response; or up to 10,000 units daily, injected subconjunctivally.

ACTION
Bactericidal. Alters osmotic barrier of bacteria cell membrane.

Route	Onset	Peak	Duration
Ophthalmic	Unknown	Unknown	Unknown

ADVERSE REACTIONS
EENT: eye irritation, conjunctivitis.
Other: overgrowth of nonsusceptible organisms.

INTERACTIONS
None significant.

EFFECTS ON LAB TEST RESULTS
None reported.

CONTRAINDICATIONS
Contraindicated in patients hypersensitive to drug. Drug shouldn't be injected into eye or anterior chamber of eye.

NURSING CONSIDERATIONS
● Reconstitute carefully to ensure correct drug concentration in solution.
● Drug is often used with neomycin sulfate.
● Drug is one of the most effective antibiotics against g-negative organisms, especially *Pseudomonas.*
● In severe, life-threatening *Pseudomonas* infections, polymyxin B may be used as an ocular irrigant.

PATIENT TEACHING
● Tell patient to clean excessive exudate from eye area before application.
● Teach patient how to instill drops. Advise him to wash hands before and after administering solution, and warn him not to touch tip of dropper to eye or surrounding tissue.

● Instruct patient to apply light finger pressure on lacrimal sac for 1 minute after drops are instilled.
● Advise patient to watch for and report signs and symptoms of sensitivity (itching lids, swelling, or constant burning).
● Tell patient not to share drug, washcloths, or towels with family members and to notify prescriber if anyone develops same signs or symptoms.
● Stress importance of compliance with recommended therapy.

---

sulfacetamide sodium 10%
AK-Sulf, Bleph-10, Cetamide, OcuSulf-10, Sodium Sulamyd Ophthalmic, Sulf-10 Ophthalmic

sulfacetamide sodium 15%
Isopto-Cetamide Ophthalmic

sulfacetamide sodium 30%
Sodium Sulamyd Ophthalmic

Pregnancy risk category C

AVAILABLE FORMS
Ophthalmic ointment: 10%
Ophthalmic solution: 10%, 15%, 30%

INDICATIONS & DOSAGES
➤ **Inclusion conjunctivitis, corneal ulcers, chlamydial infection—**
Adults and children: 1 to 2 drops of 10% solution into lower conjunctival sac q 2 to 3 hours during day, less often at night. Or, 1 to 2 drops of 15% solution instilled into lower conjunctival sac q 1 to 2 hours initially. Increase interval as condition responds. Or, instill 1 drop of 30% solution into lower conjunctival sac q 2 hours. Apply 1.25 to 2.5 cm of 10% ointment into conjunctival sac q.i.d. and h.s. Ointment may be used at night along with drops during the day.
➤ **Trachoma—**
Adults and children: 2 drops of 30% solution into lower conjunctival sac q 2 hours with systemic sulfonamide or tetracycline.

ACTION
Bacteriostatic, although may be bactericidal in high concentrations. Prevents up-

---

take of PABA, a metabolite of bacterial folic acid synthesis.

Route	Onset	Peak	Duration
Ophthalmic	Unknown	Unknown	Unknown

ADVERSE REACTIONS
EENT: slowed corneal wound healing with ointment, pain on instillation of eyedrops, headache or brow pain, photophobia, periorbital edema, eye itching, burning.
Other: overgrowth of nonsusceptible organisms.

INTERACTIONS
Drug-drug. *Gentamicin (ophthalmic):* In vitro antagonism. Avoid using together.
Local anesthetics (procaine, tetracaine), PABA derivatives: Decreased sulfacetamide sodium action. Wait ½ to 1 hour after instilling anesthetic or PABA derivative before instilling sulfacetamide.
Silver preparations: Precipitate formation. Avoid using together.
Drug-lifestyle. *Sun exposure:* Photophobia may occur. Urge patient to take precautions against sun exposure.

EFFECTS ON LAB TEST RESULTS
None reported.

CONTRAINDICATIONS
Contraindicated in patients hypersensitive to sulfonamides. Drug isn't recommended for children younger than age 2 months.

NURSING CONSIDERATIONS
• Drug is often used with oral tetracycline in treating trachoma and inclusion conjunctivitis.
• Store drug away from heat in tightly closed, light-resistant container.

PATIENT TEACHING
• Tell patient to clean excessive exudates from eye area before using drug.
• Teach patient how to instill drops or apply ointment. Advise him to wash hands before and after administering ointment or solution and not to touch tip of dropper to eye or surrounding tissues.

• Instruct patient to apply light finger pressure on lacrimal sac for 1 minute after drops are instilled.
• Warn patient that eyedrops burn slightly.
• Advise patient to watch for and report signs and symptoms of sensitivity (itching lids, swelling, or constant burning).
• Tell patient to wait at least 5 minutes before instilling other eyedrops.
• Warn patient that solution may stain clothing.
• Tell patient to minimize photophobia by wearing sunglasses and avoiding prolonged exposure to sunlight.
• Advise patient not to use discolored solution.
• Tell patient not to share drug, washcloths, or towels with family members and to notify prescriber if anyone develops same signs or symptoms.
• Stress importance of compliance with recommended therapy.

tobramycin
AKTob, Tobrex

Pregnancy risk category B

AVAILABLE FORMS
Ophthalmic ointment: 0.3%
Ophthalmic solution: 0.3%

INDICATIONS & DOSAGES
➤ **External ocular infections by susceptible bacteria—**
Adults and children: In mild to moderate infections, instill 1 or 2 drops into affected eye q 4 hours, or apply thin strip (1 cm long) of ointment q 8 to 12 hours. In severe infections, instill 2 drops into infected eye q 30 to 60 minutes until condition improves; then reduce frequency. Or, apply thin strip (1 cm long) of ointment q 3 to 4 hours until improvement; then reduce frequency.

ACTION
Unknown. Thought to inhibit protein synthesis; usually bactericidal.

Route	Onset	Peak	Duration
Ophthalmic	Unknown	Unknown	Unknown

ADVERSE REACTIONS
EENT: burning or stinging on instillation, lid itching or swelling, conjunctival erythema, blurred vision with ointment, increased lacrimation.

INTERACTIONS
None significant.

EFFECTS ON LAB TEST RESULTS
None reported.

CONTRAINDICATIONS
Contraindicated in patients hypersensitive to drug or other aminoglycosides.

NURSING CONSIDERATIONS
• When two different ophthalmic solutions are used, allow at least 5 minutes between instillations.
• *Alert:* Tobramycin ophthalmic solution isn't for injection.
• If topical ocular tobramycin is administered with systemic tobramycin, carefully monitor levels.
• Prolonged use may result in overgrowth of nonsusceptible organisms, including fungi.
• *Alert:* Don't confuse tobramycin with Trobicin, or Tobrex with Tobradex.

PATIENT TEACHING
• Tell patient to clean excessive exudate from eye area before administering drug.
• Teach patient how to instill drops or apply ointment. Advise him to wash hands before and after administering and to avoid touching tip of dropper to eye or surrounding tissue.
• Instruct patient to apply light finger pressure on lacrimal sac for 1 minute after drops are instilled.
• Advise patient to watch for itching lids, swelling, or constant burning. Tell him to discontinue drug and notify prescriber if these signs and symptoms develop.
• Tell patient not to share drug, washcloths, or towels with family members and to notify prescriber if anyone develops same signs or symptoms.
• Stress importance of compliance with recommended therapy.

vidarabine
Vira-A

Pregnancy risk category C

AVAILABLE FORMS
Ophthalmic ointment: 3% in 3.5-g tube (equivalent to 2.8% vidarabine)

INDICATIONS & DOSAGES
➤ **Acute keratoconjunctivitis, superficial keratitis, and recurrent epithelial keratitis caused by herpes simplex I and II—**
Adults and children: 1 cm of ointment into lower conjunctival sac five times daily at 3-hour intervals. If there are no signs or symptoms of improvement after 7 days, or if complete reepithelialization hasn't occurred in 21 days, consider other forms of therapy. Some cases may need longer treatment if severe. After reepithelialization has occurred, treat for an additional 5 to 7 days at reduced dosage (such as b.i.d.) to prevent recurrence.

ACTION
Unknown. Thought to interfere with DNA synthesis.

Route	Onset	Peak	Duration
Ophthalmic	Unknown	Unknown	Unknown

ADVERSE REACTIONS
EENT: temporary burning, itching, mild irritation, pain, lacrimation, foreign body sensation, conjunctival injection, punctal occlusion, sensitivity, superficial punctate keratitis, photophobia.

INTERACTIONS
None significant.

EFFECTS ON LAB TEST RESULTS
None reported.

CONTRAINDICATIONS
Contraindicated in patients hypersensitive to drug.

NURSING CONSIDERATIONS
• Use corticosteroids cautiously and monitor patient closely. Drug therapy should be

continued for several days after corticosteroid therapy.

● Drug isn't effective against RNA virus, adenoviral ocular infections, or bacterial, fungal, or chlamydial infections.

● Store drug in tightly closed, light-resistant container.

● **Alert:** Don't confuse vidarabine with cytarabine.

PATIENT TEACHING

● Tell patient to clean excessive exudate from eye area before application.

● Teach patient how to apply. Advise him to wash hands before and after applying ointment and to avoid touching tip of tube to eye or surrounding tissue.

● Instruct patient to apply light finger pressure on lacrimal sac for 1 minute after drops are instilled.

● Explain that ointment may produce a temporary visual haze.

● Advise patient to watch for signs of sensitivity, such as itching lids, swelling, or constant burning. Tell patient who develops such signs and symptoms to stop drug and notify prescriber immediately.

● Tell patient to minimize photophobia by wearing sunglasses and avoiding prolonged exposure to sunlight.

● Tell patient not to share drug, washcloths, or towels with family members and to notify prescriber if anyone develops same signs or symptoms.

● Stress importance of compliance with recommended therapy.

78

Ophthalmic anti-inflammatories

dexamethasone
dexamethasone sodium
   phosphate
diclofenac sodium
fluorometholone
flurbiprofen sodium
ketorolac tromethamine
prednisolone acetate
   (suspension)
prednisolone sodium phosphate
   (solution)

COMBINATION PRODUCTS
Corticosteroids for ophthalmic use are commonly used with antibiotics and sulfonamides. See Chapter 77, Ophthalmic anti-infectives.

---

dexamethasone
Maxidex

dexamethasone sodium
phosphate
AK-Dex, Decadron Phosphate,
Maxidex

Pregnancy risk category C

AVAILABLE FORMS
dexamethasone
Ophthalmic suspension: 0.1%
dexamethasone sodium phosphate
Ophthalmic ointment: 0.05%
Ophthalmic solution: 0.1%

INDICATIONS & DOSAGES
➤ **Uveitis; iridocyclitis; inflammatory conditions of eyelids, conjunctiva, cornea, anterior segment of globe; corneal injury from chemical or thermal burns, or penetration of foreign bodies; allergic conjunctivitis; suppression of graft rejection after keratoplasty—**
Adults and children: 1 to 2 drops of suspension or solution or 1.25 to 2.5 cm of ointment into conjunctival sac. In severe disease, drops may be used every 1 to 2 hours, tapering to discontinuation as con-

dition improves. In mild conditions, drops may be used up to four to six times daily or ointment applied t.i.d. or q.i.d. As condition improves, taper dosage to b.i.d.; then once daily. Treatment may extend from a few days to several weeks.

ACTION
Exerts anti-inflammatory action. Edema, fibrin deposition, capillary dilation, leukocyte migration, capillary proliferation, and collagen deposition are suppressed.

Route	Onset	Peak	Duration
Ophthalmic	Unknown	Unknown	Unknown

ADVERSE REACTIONS
EENT: increased intraocular pressure; thinning of cornea; interference with corneal wound healing; increased susceptibility to viral or fungal corneal infection; corneal ulceration; glaucoma exacerbation, cataracts, defects in visual acuity and visual field, optic nerve damage with excessive or long-term use; mild blurred vision; burning, stinging, or redness of eyes; watery eyes; discharge; discomfort; ocular pain; foreign body sensation.
Other: systemic effects, adrenal suppression with excessive or long-term use.

INTERACTIONS
None significant.

EFFECTS ON LAB TEST RESULTS
None reported.

CONTRAINDICATIONS
Contraindicated in patients hypersensitive to any component of drug; in those with ocular tuberculosis or acute superficial herpes simplex (dendritic keratitis), vaccinia, varicella, or other fungal or viral diseases of cornea and conjunctiva; in patients with acute, purulent, untreated infections of eye; and in those who have had uncomplicated removal of superficial corneal foreign body.

Reactions may be *common*, uncommon, *life-threatening*, or COMMON AND LIFE-THREATENING.

NURSING CONSIDERATIONS

• Use cautiously in patients with corneal abrasions that may be infected (especially with herpes).

• Use cautiously in patients with glaucoma (any form) because intraocular pressure may increase. Dosage of glaucoma drugs may need to be increased to compensate.

• Drug isn't for long-term use.

• Watch for corneal ulceration; may require stopping drug.

• Corneal viral and fungal infections may be worsened by corticosteroid application.

• Safe use in pregnant and breast-feeding women hasn't been established.

• *Alert:* Don't confuse dexamethasone with desoximetasone, or Maxidex with Maxzide.

PATIENT TEACHING

• Tell patient to shake suspension well before use.

• Teach patient how to instill drops or apply ointment. Advise him to wash hands before and after applying ointment or solution, and warn him not to touch tip of dropper to eye or surrounding tissue.

• Tell patient to apply light finger pressure on lacrimal sac for 1 minute after instillation.

• Advise patient that he may use eye pad with ointment.

• Warn patient not to use leftover drug for new eye inflammation; doing so may cause serious problems.

• *Alert:* Warn patient to call prescriber immediately and to stop drug if visual acuity changes or visual field diminishes.

• Tell patient not to share drug, washcloths, or towels with family members and to notify prescriber if anyone develops same signs or symptoms.

• Stress importance of compliance with recommended therapy.

• Tell patient who wears contact lenses to check with prescriber before using lenses again.

diclofenac sodium
Voltaren Ophthalmic, Voltarol§

Pregnancy risk category B

AVAILABLE FORMS
Ophthalmic solution: 0.1%

INDICATIONS & DOSAGES

➤ **Postoperative inflammation following removal of cataract—**
Adults: 1 drop in conjunctival sac q.i.d., beginning 24 hours after surgery and continuing throughout first 2 weeks of postoperative period.

➤ **Photophobia in incisional refractive surgery—**
Adults: 1 to 2 drops to operative eye 1 hour before surgery. Within 15 minutes after surgery, instill 1 to 2 drops into operative eye. Then 1 drop q.i.d. beginning 4 to 6 hours after surgery up to 3 days, p.r.n.

ACTION
Unknown. Thought to inhibit the enzyme cyclooxygenase, which is essential in biosynthesis of prostaglandins. Prostaglandins may be mediators of certain kinds of intraocular inflammation.

Route	Onset	Peak	Duration
Ophthalmic	Unknown	Unknown	Unknown

ADVERSE REACTIONS
EENT: *transient stinging and burning, increased intraocular pressure, keratitis,* anterior chamber reaction, ocular allergy, increased bleeding of ocular tissues, including hyphemas with ocular surgery.
GI: nausea, vomiting.
Other: viral infection.

INTERACTIONS
None significant.

EFFECTS ON LAB TEST RESULTS
None reported.

CONTRAINDICATIONS
Contraindicated in patients hypersensitive to any component of drug and in those wearing soft contact lenses. Because of known effects of prostaglandin-inhibiting drugs on fetal CV system (closure of duc-

tus arteriosus), avoid use of drug during late pregnancy.

NURSING CONSIDERATIONS
• Use cautiously in patients hypersensitive to acetylsalicylic acid, phenylacetic acid derivatives, and other NSAIDs; potential for cross-sensitivity exists. Also use cautiously in surgical patients with known bleeding tendencies and in those receiving drugs that may prolong bleeding time.
• Drug may slow or delay healing.
• Most cases of increased intraocular pressure have occurred postoperatively and before drug administration.
• *Alert:* Don't confuse diclofenac with Diflucan or Duphalac; don't confuse Voltaren with Verelan.

PATIENT TEACHING
• Teach patient how to instill drops. Advise him to wash hands before and after instilling solution, and warn him not to touch tip of dropper to eye or surrounding tissue.
• Advise patient to apply light finger pressure on lacrimal sac for 1 minute after instilling drops.
• Stress importance of compliance with recommended therapy.
• Warn patient not to use leftover drug for new eye inflammation.
• Remind patient to discard drug when no longer needed.

---

fluorometholone
Flarex, Fluor-Op, FML Forte, FML Liquifilm Ophthalmic, FML S.O.P.

Pregnancy risk category C

AVAILABLE FORMS
Ophthalmic ointment: 0.1%
Ophthalmic suspension: 0.1%, 0.25%

INDICATIONS & DOSAGES
➤ **Inflammatory and allergic conditions of cornea, conjunctiva, sclera, anterior uvea—**
Adults and children: 1 to 2 drops in conjunctival sac b.i.d. to q.i.d. May be given q 2 hours during first 1 to 2 days, if needed. Or, apply 1.25-cm ribbon of ointment to conjunctival sac q 4 hours, decreased to

once daily to t.i.d. as inflammation subsides.

ACTION
Exerts anti-inflammatory action. Edema, fibrin deposition, capillary dilation, leukocyte migration, capillary proliferation, and collagen deposition are suppressed.

Route	Onset	Peak	Duration
Ophthalmic	Unknown	Unknown	Unknown

ADVERSE REACTIONS
EENT: increased intraocular pressure, thinning of cornea, interference with corneal wound healing, corneal ulceration, increased susceptibility to viral or fungal corneal infections, glaucoma exacerbation, discharge, discomfort, ocular pain, foreign body sensation, cataracts, decreased visual acuity, diminished visual field, optic nerve damage with excessive or long-term use.
Other: systemic effects, adrenal suppression with excessive or long-term use.

INTERACTIONS
None significant.

EFFECTS ON LAB TEST RESULTS
None reported.

CONTRAINDICATIONS
Contraindicated in patients with vaccinia, varicella, acute superficial herpes simplex (dendritic keratitis), other fungal or viral eye diseases, ocular tuberculosis, or acute, purulent, untreated eye infections.

NURSING CONSIDERATIONS
• Use cautiously in patients with corneal abrasions that may be contaminated (especially with herpes).
• Safety and efficacy of drug in children younger than age 2 haven't been established.
• Duration of treatment may range from a few days to several weeks; however, long-term use should be avoided. Monitor intraocular pressure.
• Drug is less likely to cause increased intraocular pressure with extended use than other ophthalmic anti-inflammatory drugs (except medrysone).

Reactions may be *common*, uncommon, *life-threatening*, or COMMON AND LIFE-THREATENING.

• Consult prescriber if no improvement after 2 days. Don't discontinue treatment prematurely.

• In chronic conditions, withdraw treatment by gradually decreasing frequency of applications.

• Shake well before use.

• Store drug in tightly covered, light-resistant container.

PATIENT TEACHING
• Teach patient how to instill drops or apply ointment. Advise him to wash hands before and after administering ointment or solution, and warn him not to touch tip of dropper to eye or surrounding tissue.

• Advise patient to apply light finger pressure on lacrimal sac for 1 minute after instillation.

• Urge patient to call prescriber immediately and to stop drug if visual acuity decreases or visual field diminishes.

• Tell patient not to share drug, washcloths, or towels with family members and to notify prescriber if anyone develops same signs or symptoms.

• Warn patient not to use leftover drug for new eye inflammation; it may cause serious problems.

---

flurbiprofen sodium
Ocufen

Pregnancy risk category C

AVAILABLE FORMS
Ophthalmic solution: 0.03%

INDICATIONS & DOSAGES
➤ **Inhibition of intraoperative miosis—**
Adults: Instill 1 drop into affected eye about q 30 minutes, beginning 2 hours before surgery; give total of 4 drops.

ACTION
Unknown. An NSAID thought to inhibit the cyclooxygenase enzyme essential in biosynthesis of prostaglandins.

Route	Onset	Peak	Duration
Ophthalmic	Unknown	Unknown	Unknown

ADVERSE REACTIONS
EENT: transient burning and stinging on instillation, ocular irritation.

INTERACTIONS
Drug-drug. *Acetylcholine, carbachol:* May be rendered ineffective. Avoid using together.
Anticoagulants: Increased risk of bleeding if significant systemic absorption occurs. Monitor patient closely for bleeding.

EFFECTS ON LAB TEST RESULTS
None reported.

CONTRAINDICATIONS
Contraindicated in patients hypersensitive to drug. Safe use in pregnant and breast-feeding women hasn't been established.

NURSING CONSIDERATIONS
• Use cautiously in patients who may be allergic to aspirin and other NSAIDs.
• Use cautiously in patients with bleeding tendencies and in those receiving drugs that may prolong clotting times.
• Wound healing may be delayed with drug use.
• *Alert:* Don't confuse Ocufen with Ocuflox.

PATIENT TEACHING
• Advise patient to alert prescriber immediately if visual acuity decreases or visual field diminishes.
• Urge patient to take drug as prescribed.
• Tell patient to report excessive bleeding or bruising.

---

ketorolac tromethamine
Acular

Pregnancy risk category C

AVAILABLE FORMS
Ophthalmic solution: 0.5%

INDICATIONS & DOSAGES
➤ **Relief from ocular itching caused by seasonal allergic conjunctivitis—**
Adults: 1 drop into conjunctival sac in each eye q.i.d.

➤ **Postoperative inflammation in patients who have undergone cataract extraction—**
Adults: 1 drop to operative eye or eyes q.i.d. beginning 24 hours after cataract surgery and continuing through first 2 weeks of postoperative period.

ACTION
Unknown. An NSAID thought to inhibit the action of cyclooxygenase, an enzyme responsible for prostaglandin synthesis. Prostaglandins mediate the inflammatory response and also cause miosis.

Route	Onset	Peak	Duration
Ophthalmic	Unknown	Unknown	Unknown

ADVERSE REACTIONS
EENT: *transient stinging and burning on instillation,* superficial keratitis, superficial ocular infections, ocular irritation.

INTERACTIONS
None significant.

EFFECTS ON LAB TEST RESULTS
None reported.

CONTRAINDICATIONS
Contraindicated in patients hypersensitive to components of drug and in those wearing soft contact lenses.

NURSING CONSIDERATIONS
• Use cautiously in patients with bleeding disorders or those hypersensitive to other NSAIDs or aspirin.
• Use cautiously in breast-feeding women.
• Store drug away from heat in a dark, tightly closed container and protect from freezing.
• *Alert:* Don't confuse Acular with Acthar.

PATIENT TEACHING
• Teach patient how to instill drops. Advise him to wash hands before and after instilling solution, and warn him not to touch tip of dropper to eye or surrounding tissue.
• Advise patient to apply light finger pressure on lacrimal sac for 1 minute after instillation.
• Stress importance of compliance with recommended therapy.

• Tell patient not to instill drops while wearing contact lenses.
• Advise patient to report excessive bleeding or bruising to prescriber.
• Remind patient to discard drug when it's no longer needed.

---

prednisolone acetate (suspension)
Econopred Ophthalmic, Econopred Plus Ophthalmic, Pred Forte, Pred Mild Ophthalmic

prednisolone sodium phosphate (solution)
AK-Pred, Inflamase Forte, Inflamase Mild, Predsol Eye Drops‡

Pregnancy risk category C

AVAILABLE FORMS
prednisolone acetate
Ophthalmic suspension: 0.12%, 0.125%, 1%
prednisolone sodium phosphate
Ophthalmic solution: 0.125%, 1%

INDICATIONS & DOSAGES
➤ **Inflammation of palpebral and bulbar conjunctiva, cornea, and anterior segment of globe—**
Adults and children: Instill 1 to 2 drops into eye. In severe conditions, may be used hourly, tapering to discontinuation as inflammation subsides. In mild conditions, may be used b.i.d. to q.i.d.

ACTION
Exerts anti-inflammatory action. Edema, fibrin deposition, capillary dilation, leukocyte migration, capillary proliferation, and collagen deposition are suppressed.

Route	Onset	Peak	Duration
Ophthalmic	Unknown	Unknown	Unknown

ADVERSE REACTIONS
EENT: increased intraocular pressure, thinning of cornea, interference with corneal wound healing, increased susceptibility to viral or fungal corneal infection, corneal ulceration, discharge, discomfort, foreign body sensation, glaucoma exacer-

bation, cataracts, visual acuity and visual field defects, optic nerve damage with excessive or long-term use.
Other: systemic effects, adrenal suppression with excessive or long-term use.

INTERACTIONS
None significant.

EFFECTS ON LAB TEST RESULTS
None reported.

CONTRAINDICATIONS
Contraindicated in patients with acute, untreated, purulent ocular infections; acute superficial herpes simplex (dendritic keratitis); vaccinia, varicella, or other viral or fungal eye diseases; or ocular tuberculosis.

NURSING CONSIDERATIONS
• Use cautiously in patients with corneal abrasions that may be contaminated (especially with herpes).
• Shake suspension and check dosage before administering to ensure correct strength. Store in tightly covered container.
• *Alert:* Don't confuse prednisolone with prednisone.

PATIENT TEACHING
• Teach patient how to instill drops. Advise him to wash hands before and after instillation, and warn him not to touch tip of dropper to eye or surrounding area.
• Advise patient to apply light finger pressure on lacrimal sac for 1 minute after instillation.
• Tell patient on long-term therapy to have frequent tests of intraocular pressure.
• Tell patient not to share drug, washcloths, or towels with family members and to notify prescriber if anyone develops same signs or symptoms.
• Stress importance of compliance with recommended therapy.
• Tell patient to notify prescriber if improvement doesn't occur within several days or if pain, itching, or swelling of eye occurs.
• Warn patient not to use leftover drug for new eye inflammation because serious problems may occur.

---

*Liquid contains alcohol.   **May contain tartrazine.   †Canada   ‡Australia   §U.K.   ◊OTC

acetylcholine chloride
carbachol (intraocular)
carbachol (topical)
echothiophate iodide
pilocarpine
pilocarpine hydrochloride
pilocarpine nitrate

COMBINATION PRODUCTS
E-PILO: epinephrine bitartrate 1% and pilocarpine hydrochloride 1%, 2%, 3%, 4%, or 6%.

---

acetylcholine chloride
Miochol-E

Pregnancy risk category NR

AVAILABLE FORMS
Ophthalmic injection: 1%

INDICATIONS & DOSAGES
➤ **Anterior segment surgery—**
Adults and children: Before or after securing sutures, prescriber gently instills 0.5 to 2 ml into anterior chamber.

ACTION
A cholinergic that causes contraction of the sphincter muscles of the iris, resulting in miosis, and that produces ciliary spasm, deepening of the anterior chamber, and vasodilation of conjunctival vessels of the outflow tract.

Route	Onset	Peak	Duration
Ophthalmic	Immediate	Unknown	10 min

ADVERSE REACTIONS
EENT: corneal edema, clouding, decompensation.

INTERACTIONS
None significant.

EFFECTS ON LAB TEST RESULTS
None reported.

CONTRAINDICATIONS
Contraindicated in patients hypersensitive to drug or its components.

NURSING CONSIDERATIONS
● Reconstitute immediately before using, shaking vial gently until clear solution is obtained.
● Discard unused solution.
● Don't gas-sterilize vial. Ethylene oxide may produce formic acid. Watch for signs and symptoms of hypotension and bradycardia if this occurs.
● *Alert:* Don't confuse acetylcholine with acetylcysteine.

PATIENT TEACHING
● Inform patient about need for drug during surgical procedure, and answer questions and address concerns.
● Instruct patient to immediately report breathing difficulties.

---

carbachol (intraocular)
Miostat

carbachol (topical)
Carboptic, Isopto Carbachol

Pregnancy risk category C

AVAILABLE FORMS
Intraocular injection: 0.01%
Topical ophthalmic solution: 0.75%, 1.5%, 2.25%, 3%

INDICATIONS & DOSAGES
➤ **To produce pupillary miosis in ocular surgery—**
Adults: Before or after securing sutures, prescriber gently instills 0.5 ml (intraocular form) into anterior chamber.
➤ **Glaucoma—**
Adults: 1 to 2 drops (topical form) instilled up to t.i.d.

ACTION
A cholinergic that causes contraction of the sphincter muscles of the iris, resulting

---

Reactions may be *common*, uncommon, *life-threatening*, or COMMON AND LIFE-THREATENING.

in miosis, and that produces ciliary spasm, deepening of the anterior chamber, and vasodilation of conjunctival vessels of the outflow tract.

Route	Onset	Peak	Duration
Intraocular	Unknown	2-5 min	24 hr
Ophthalmic (topical)	10-20 min	4 hr	4-8 hr

ADVERSE REACTIONS
EENT: spasm of eye accommodation, conjunctival vasodilation, eye and brow pain, *transient stinging and burning,* corneal clouding, bullous keratopathy, salivation.

INTERACTIONS
Drug-drug. *Pilocarpine:* Additive effect. Use together cautiously.

EFFECTS ON LAB TEST RESULTS
None reported.

CONTRAINDICATIONS
Contraindicated in patients hypersensitive to drug and in patients with conditions in which cholinergic effects such as constriction are undesirable (for example, acute iritis, some forms of secondary glaucoma, pupillary block glaucoma, or acute inflammatory disease of the anterior chamber).

NURSING CONSIDERATIONS
● Use cautiously in patients with acute heart failure, bronchial asthma, peptic ulcer, hyperthyroidism, GI spasm, Parkinson's disease, and urinary tract obstruction.
● In case of toxicity, give atropine parenterally.
● Drug is used in open-angle glaucoma, especially when patients are resistant or allergic to pilocarpine hydrochloride or nitrate.
● *Alert:* Patients with dark eyes (hazel or brown irises) may need stronger solutions or more frequent instillation because eye pigment may absorb drug.
● If tolerance to drug develops, prescriber may switch to another miotic for a short time.

PATIENT TEACHING
● Teach patient how to instill drug. Advise him to wash hands before and after instillation and to apply light finger pressure on lacrimal sac for 1 minute after drops are instilled. Warn him not to exceed recommended dosage.
● Warn patient to avoid hazardous activities, such as operating machinery or driving, until temporary blurring subsides. Reassure patient that blurred vision usually diminishes with prolonged use.
● Tell glaucoma patient that long-term use may be needed. Stress compliance. Tell him to remain under medical supervision for periodic tests of intraocular pressure.
● Warn patient to use caution during night driving and while performing other hazardous activities in reduced light.

---

echothiophate iodide
(ecotiophate iodide)
Phospholine Iodide

Pregnancy risk category C

AVAILABLE FORMS
Ophthalmic powder for solution: For reconstitution to make 0.03%, 0.06%, 0.125%, and 0.25% solutions

INDICATIONS & DOSAGES
➤ **Primary open-angle glaucoma, conditions obstructing aqueous outflow—**
Adults and children: Instill 1 drop of 0.03% to 0.125% solution into conjunctival sac daily. Maximum dose is 1 drop b.i.d. Use lowest possible dose for continuous control of intraocular pressure.
➤ **Diagnosis of convergent strabismus—**
Adults: Instill 1 drop of 0.125% solution into each eye daily h.s. for 2 to 3 weeks.
➤ **Treatment of convergent strabismus—**
Adults: Initially, instill 1 drop of 0.125% solution into each eye daily h.s. for 2 to 3 weeks. Decrease dosage to 1 drop of 0.125% solution every other day or 1 drop of 0.06% solution daily. The 0.03% solution may be effective for some patients.

ACTION

An anticholinesterase that inhibits the enzymatic destruction of acetylcholine by inactivating cholinesterase, leaving acetylcholine free to act on the effector cells of the iridic sphincter and ciliary muscles, causing pupillary constriction and spasm of accommodation.

Route	Onset	Peak	Duration
Ophthalmic	10 min-8 hr	0.5-24 hr	1-4 wk

ADVERSE REACTIONS

EENT: ciliary spasm or spasm of eye accommodation, ciliary or circumcorneal injection, nonreversible cataract formation (time- and dose-related), reversible iris cysts, pupillary block, blurred or dimmed vision, eye or brow pain, twitching of eyelids, hyperemia, photophobia, lens opacities, lacrimation, retinal detachment.

INTERACTIONS

Drug-drug. *Anticholinergics, cyclopentolate, ophthalmic belladonna alkaloids such as atropine:* Antagonized miotic effects. Avoid using together.
Cholinesterase inhibitors: Possible additive effect causing systemic effects. Monitor patient closely.
Local anesthetics, ophthalmic tetracaine: Increased systemic toxicity and prolonged ocular anesthesia. Monitor patient closely.
Ophthalmic adrenocorticoids: Increased intraocular pressure and decreased antiglaucoma effectiveness. Avoid using together.
Succinylcholine: Respiratory and CV collapse. Don't use together.
Systemic anticholinesterases for myasthenia gravis, pilocarpine: Effects may be additive. Watch for signs and symptoms of toxicity.
Drug-lifestyle. *Cocaine use:* Increased risk of cocaine toxicity. Inform patient of this interaction.
Organophosphate insecticides such as malathion, parathion: May cause systemic effects. Encorage at-risk patient to protect himself from exposure.

EFFECTS ON LAB TEST RESULTS

None reported.

CONTRAINDICATIONS

Contraindicated in patients hypersensitive to drug or iodine and in those with uveal inflammation, acute angle-closure glaucoma before iridectomy, or other forms of glaucoma (except for primary open-angle glaucoma).

NURSING CONSIDERATIONS

• Use with extreme caution, if at all, in patients with seizure disorders, vasomotor instability, parkinsonism, bronchial asthma, spastic GI conditions, urinary tract obstruction, peptic ulcer, severe bradycardia or hypotension, vascular hypertension, MI, or history or risk of retinal detachment.
• Use with caution in patients with corneal abrasion.
• Reconstitute powder, using only diluent provided to avoid contamination. Discard refrigerated, reconstituted solution after 6 months; discard solution stored at room temperature after 1 month.
• Stop drug, at least 2 weeks preoperatively if succinylcholine will be used in surgery.
• Toxicity is cumulative; toxic systemic signs and symptoms may not appear for weeks or months after start of therapy. Atropine sulfate S.C., I.M., or I.V. is antidote of choice.

PATIENT TEACHING

• Teach patient how to instill drug. Advise him to wash hands before and after instillation, to avoid touching applicator tip to any surface, and to apply light finger pressure on lacrimal sac for 1 minute after instillation.
• Tell patient to instill drug at bedtime because it causes transient blurred vision. Warn him that transient brow pain or dimmed or blurred vision is common at first but usually disappears in 5 to 10 days.
• Warn patient to notify prescriber if salivation, diarrhea, profuse diaphoresis, urinary incontinence, or muscle weakness occurs.
• Tell patient to remain under constant medical supervision and not to exceed recommended dosage.

Reactions may be *common*, uncommon, *life-threatening*, or COMMON AND LIFE-THREATENING.

• Advise patient to avoid driving if visual blurring occurs, particularly at night.
• Advise patient to wear or carry medical identification at all times during therapy. Drug is potent, long-acting, and irreversible.

---

pilocarpine
Ocusert Pilo Ocular System

pilocarpine hydrochloride
Adsorbocarpine, Akarpine, Isopto Carpine, Miocarpine†, Pilocar, Pilogel§, Pilopine HS, Pilopt‡, Pilostat, Sno Pilo§

pilocarpine nitrate
Pilagan Liquifilm

Pregnancy risk category C

AVAILABLE FORMS
pilocarpine
Extended-release insert: 20 mcg/hour for 7 days, 40 mcg/hour for 7 days
pilocarpine hydrochloride
Ophthalmic gel: 4%
Ophthalmic solution: 0.25%, 0.5%, 1%, 2%, 3%, 4%, 5%, 6%, 8%, 10%
pilocarpine nitrate
Ophthalmic solution: 1%, 2%, 4%

INDICATIONS & DOSAGES
➤ **Primary open-angle glaucoma—**
Adults and children: Instill 1 to 2 drops up to q.i.d. or apply 1-cm ribbon of 4% gel h.s. Or, apply one Ocusert Pilo system (20 or 40 mcg/hour) q 7 days.
➤ **Emergency treatment of acute angle-closure glaucoma—**
Adults and children: Instill 1 drop of 2% solution q 5 to 10 minutes for three to six doses; then 1 drop q 1 to 3 hours until pressure is controlled.
➤ **Mydriasis caused by mydriatic or cycloplegic drugs—**
Adults and children: 1 drop of 1% solution.

ACTION
A cholinergic that causes contraction of iris sphincter muscles, resulting in miosis, and that produces ciliary spasm, deepen-

ing of the anterior chamber, and vasodilation of conjunctival vessels of the outflow tract.

Route	Onset	Peak	Duration
Ophthalmic	10-30 min	30-85 min	4-8 hr

ADVERSE REACTIONS
EENT: periorbital or supraorbital headache, *myopia,* ciliary spasm, *blurred vision,* conjunctival irritation, transient stinging and burning, keratitis, lens opacity, retinal detachment, lacrimation, changes in visual field, *brow pain.*

INTERACTIONS
Drug-drug. *Carbachol, echothiophate:* Additive effect. Don't use together.
Cyclopentolate, ophthalmic belladonna alkaloids such as atropine, scopolamine: Decreased pilocarpine antiglaucoma effectiveness and blocked mydriatic effects of these drugs. Avoid using together.
Phenylephrine: Decreased dilation by phenylephrine. Don't use together.

EFFECTS ON LAB TEST RESULTS
None reported.

CONTRAINDICATIONS
Contraindicated in patients hypersensitive to drug and in conditions in which cholinergic effects such as constriction are undesirable (for example, acute iritis, some forms of secondary glaucoma, pupillary block glaucoma, acute inflammatory disease of the anterior chamber).

NURSING CONSIDERATIONS
• Use cautiously in patients with acute cardiac failure, bronchial asthma, peptic ulcer, hyperthyroidism, GI spasm, urinary tract obstruction, and Parkinson's disease.
• Monitor vital signs.
• *Alert:* Patients with dark eyes (hazel or brown irises) may need stronger solutions or more frequent instillation because eye pigment may absorb drug.

PATIENT TEACHING
• Instruct patient to apply gel at bedtime because it will blur vision. Warn him to avoid hazardous activities, such as operat-

---

ing machinery or driving, until temporary blurring subsides.

• Teach patient how to instill drug. Advise him to wash hands before and after instillation and to apply light finger pressure on lacrimal sac for 1 minute after drops are instilled. Warn patient not to touch applicator tip to eye or surrounding tissue.

• If Ocusert Pilo system falls out of eye during sleep, tell patient to wash hands, rinse insert in cool tap water, and reposition in eye. Tell him not to use a deformed insert.

• Warn patient that transient brow pain and myopia are common at first but usually disappear in 10 to 14 days.

• Advise patient to wear or carry medical identification at all times during therapy.

atropine sulfate
cyclopentolate hydrochloride
epinephrine hydrochloride
epinephryl borate
homatropine hydrobromide
phenylephrine hydrochloride
scopolamine hydrobromide

COMBINATION PRODUCTS

CYCLOMYDRIL OPHTHALMIC: cyclopentolate hydrochloride 0.2% and phenylephrine hydrochloride 1%.
MUROCOLL-2: scopolamine hydrobromide 0.3% and phenylephrine hydrochloride 10%.
ZINCFRIN ◊: phenylephrine hydrochloride 0.12% and zinc sulfate 0.25%.

---

atropine sulfate
Atropine 1, Atropisol, Atropt‡,
Isopto Atropine

Pregnancy risk category C

AVAILABLE FORMS
Ophthalmic ointment: 1%
Ophthalmic solution: 0.5%, 1%, 2%

INDICATIONS & DOSAGES
➤ **Acute iritis, uveitis—**
Adults: Instill 1 to 2 drops up to q.i.d. or apply small strip of ointment to conjunctival sac up to t.i.d.
Children: 1 to 2 drops of 0.5% solution up to t.i.d. or small strip of ointment applied to conjunctival sac up to t.i.d.
➤ **Cycloplegic refraction—**
Adults: 1 to 2 drops of 1% solution 1 hour before refraction.
Children: 1 to 2 drops of 0.5% solution in each eye b.i.d. for 1 to 3 days before eye examination and 1 hour before refraction.

ACTION
A potent mydriatic and cycloplegic whose anticholinergic action leaves the pupil un-der unopposed adrenergic influence, causing it to dilate.

Route	Onset	Peak	Duration
Ophthalmic	Unknown	0.5-3 hr	7-10 days

ADVERSE REACTIONS
CNS: confusion, somnolence, headache.
CV: tachycardia.
EENT: ocular congestion with long-term use, conjunctivitis, contact dermatitis of eye, ocular edema, *blurred vision,* eye dryness, photophobia, increased intraocular pressure (IOP), transient stinging and burning, irritation, hyperemia.
GI: dry mouth, abdominal distention in infants.
Skin: dryness.

INTERACTIONS
Drug-lifestyle. *Sun exposure:* Photophobia may occur. Advise patient to avoid excessive sun exposure.

EFFECTS ON LAB TEST RESULTS
None reported.

CONTRAINDICATIONS
Contraindicated in patients hypersensitive to drug or belladonna alkaloids and in those with glaucoma or adhesions between the iris and lens. Atropine shouldn't be used in infants age 3 months or younger because of possible link between cyclo plegia produced and development of amblyopia.

NURSING CONSIDERATIONS
● Use cautiously in elderly patients and in others who may have increased IOP. Excessive use in children or in certain susceptible patients, including those with spastic paralysis, brain damage, or Down syndrome, may produce systemic symptoms of atropine poisoning.
● *Alert:* Treat drops and ointment as poison (not for internal use); signs of poisoning are disorientation and confusion. Antidote of choice is physostigmine salicylate I.V. or I.M.

• Watch patient for signs and symptoms of glaucoma, including increased IOP, ocular pain, headache, and progressive blurring of vision; notify prescriber if they occur.
• *Alert:* Don't confuse Atropisol with Aplisol.

PATIENT TEACHING
• Teach patient how to instill atropine. Advise him to wash hands before and after instillation and to apply light finger pressure on lacrimal sac for 1 minute after instillation. Warn patient not to touch tip of dropper or tube to eye or surrounding tissue.
• Warn patient to avoid hazardous activities, such as operating machinery or driving, until temporary blurring subsides.
• Advise patient to ease photophobia by wearing dark glasses or staying out of bright light.

cyclopentolate hydrochloride
AK-Pentolate, Cyclogyl, Mydrilate§, Pentolair

Pregnancy risk category C

AVAILABLE FORMS
Ophthalmic solution: 0.5%, 1%, 2%

INDICATIONS & DOSAGES
➤ **Diagnostic procedures requiring mydriasis and cycloplegia—**
Adults: 1 or 2 drops of 0.5%, 1%, or 2% solution into each eye; then 1 or 2 drops in 5 to 10 minutes, if needed.
Children: 1 drop of 0.5%, 1%, or 2% solution into each eye; then 1 drop of 0.5% or 1% solution in 5 to 10 minutes, if needed.

ACTION
A potent mydriatic and cycloplegic whose anticholinergic action leaves the pupil under unopposed adrenergic influence, causing it to dilate.

Route	Onset	Peak	Duration
Ophthalmic	Rapid	0.5-1.25 hr	6-24 hr

ADVERSE REACTIONS
CNS: irritability, confusion, somnolence, hallucinations, ataxia, *seizures,* behavioral disturbances in children.
CV: tachycardia.
EENT: eye burning on instillation, blurred vision, eye dryness, *photophobia,* ocular congestion, contact dermatitis in eye, conjunctivitis, increased intraocular pressure (IOP), transient stinging and burning, irritation, hyperemia.
GU: urine retention.
Skin: dryness.

INTERACTIONS
Drug-drug. *Carbachol, pilocarpine:* May counteract mydriatic effect. Avoid using together.
Long-acting cholinergic antiglaucoma drugs: Miotic actions may be inhibited. Avoid using together.
Drug-lifestyle. *Sun exposure:* Photophobia may occur. Advise patient to avoid excessive sun exposure.

EFFECTS ON LAB TEST RESULTS
None reported.

CONTRAINDICATIONS
Contraindicated in patients hypersensitive to drug or belladonna alkaloids and in those with glaucoma or adhesions between the iris and lens.

NURSING CONSIDERATIONS
• Use with extreme caution in infants and young children.
• The combination product containing 1% phenylephrine hydrochloride shouldn't be used in infants younger than age 1 because of risk of severe hypertension.
• Use cautiously in elderly patients and in those who may have increased IOP.
• Drug is superior to homatropine hydrobromide and has a shorter duration of action. Physostigmine is antidote of choice.

PATIENT TEACHING
• Teach patient how to instill drug. Advise him to wash hands before and after instillation and to apply light finger pressure on lacrimal sac for 1 minute after instillation. Warn him not to touch tip of dropper to eye or surrounding tissue and that drug will burn when instilled.

• Warn patient to avoid hazardous activities, such as operating machinery or driving, until temporary blurring subsides.
• Advise patient to ease photophobia by wearing dark glasses.

---

epinephrine hydrochloride
Epifrin, Eppy§, Glaucon

epinephryl borate
Epinal

Pregnancy risk category C

AVAILABLE FORMS
epinephrine hydrochloride
Ophthalmic solution: 0.1%, 0.5%, 1%, 2%
epinephryl borate
Ophthalmic solution: 0.5%, 1%

INDICATIONS & DOSAGES
➤ **Open-angle glaucoma—**
Adults: 1 or 2 drops of 1% or 2% solution once daily or b.i.d. Adjust dosage based on tonometric readings.

ACTION
An adrenergic that dilates the pupil by contracting the dilator muscle.

Route	Onset	Peak	Duration
Ophthalmic	1 hr	4-8 hr	24 hr

ADVERSE REACTIONS
CNS: brow ache, headache, lightheadedness.
CV: palpitations, tachycardia, ***arrhythmias,*** hypertension.
EENT: corneal or conjunctival pigmentation; corneal edema with long-term use; follicular hypertrophy; chemosis; conjunctivitis; iritis; hyperemic conjunctiva; eye stinging, burning, tearing on instillation; eye pain; allergic lid reaction; ocular irritation.
Metabolic: hyperglycemia.
Skin: maculopapular rash.

INTERACTIONS
Drug-drug. *Antihistamines (dexchlorpheniramine, diphenhydramine), TCAs:* Increased cardiac effects of epinephrine. Monitor patient closely.

Beta blockers, osmotic drugs, systemic carbonic anhydrase inhibitors, topical miotics: Additive lowering of intraocular pressure. Use together cautiously.
Cardiac glycosides: Increased risk of arrhythmias. Monitor patient closely.
Cyclopropane, halogenated hydrocarbons: Arrhythmias, tachycardia. Use together cautiously, if at all.
Local or systemic sympathomimetics: Additive toxic effects. Avoid using together.
MAO inhibitors: Exaggerated adrenergic effects. Adjust dosage of epinephrine carefully.

EFFECTS ON LAB TEST RESULTS
• May increase BUN and glucose levels.

CONTRAINDICATIONS
Contraindicated in patients hypersensitive to drug or sulfites and in those with hypertensive CV disease or coronary artery disease. Also contraindicated in patients with angle-closure glaucoma or when nature of glaucoma hasn't been established.

NURSING CONSIDERATIONS
• Use cautiously in elderly patients and in those with diabetes mellitus, hypertension, Parkinson's disease, hyperthyroidism, aphakia (eye without lens), cardiac disease, cerebral arteriosclerosis, or bronchial asthma.
• Drug can be injected into anterior chamber to produce rapid mydriasis during cataract removal or can be used to control local bleeding during surgery.
• ***Alert:*** Don't substitute one salt if another one is ordered; drugs aren't interchangeable.
• Monitor blood pressure and other vital signs.
Drug therapy interferes with tests for urinary catecholamines.
• ***Alert:*** Don't confuse epinephrine with ephedrine, or Glaucon with glucagon.

PATIENT TEACHING
• Teach patient how to instill drug. Advise him to wash hands before and after instillation and to apply light finger pressure on lacrimal sac for 1 minute after drops are instilled. Warn him not to touch tip of dropper to eye or surrounding tissue.

• Urge patient to immediately report any decrease in visual acuity.

• Advise patient not to use drug while wearing soft contact lenses because lenses may discolor.

• Tell patient not to use darkened solution.

homatropine hydrobromide
Isopto Homatropine, Minims Homatropine†

Pregnancy risk category C

AVAILABLE FORMS
Ophthalmic solution: 2%, 5%

INDICATIONS & DOSAGES
➤ **Cycloplegic refraction—**
Adults and children: 1 to 2 drops into each eye; if needed, repeat in 5 to 10 minutes for two or three doses.
➤ **Uveitis—**
Adults and children: 1 to 2 drops into each eye q 3 to 4 hours.

ACTION
An anticholinergic that leaves the pupil under unopposed adrenergic influence, causing it to dilate.

Route	Onset	Peak	Duration
Ophthalmic	Rapid	40-60 min	1-3 days

ADVERSE REACTIONS
CNS: confusion, headache, somnolence, edema.
CV: tachycardia.
EENT: eye irritation, *blurred vision, photophobia,* increased intraocular pressure (IOP), transient stinging and burning, conjunctivitis, vascular congestion.
GI: dry mouth.
Skin: dryness, rash.

INTERACTIONS
Drug-lifestyle. *Sun exposure:* Photophobia may occur. Advise patient to avoid excessive sun exposure.

EFFECTS ON LAB TEST RESULTS
None reported.

CONTRAINDICATIONS
Contraindicated in patients hypersensitive to drug or other belladonna alkaloids such as atropine and in those with glaucoma or adhesions between the iris and lens.

NURSING CONSIDERATIONS
• Use cautiously in elderly patients, in those in whom increased IOP may be encountered, and in those with cardiac disease or hypertension.

• Use only 2% solution with children.

• In patients with heavily pigmented irises, larger doses may be needed.

• Monitor vital signs.

• *Alert:* Homatropine is similar to atropine but weaker, with a shorter duration of action. Drug may produce signs or symptoms of atropine poisoning, such as severe mouth dryness or tachycardia.

PATIENT TEACHING
• Teach patient how to instill drug. Advise him to wash hands before and after instillation and to apply light finger pressure on lacrimal sac for 1 minute after drops are instilled.

• Warn patient not to touch tip of dropper to eye or surrounding tissue.

• Caution patient to avoid hazardous activities, such as operating machinery or driving, until temporary blurring subsides.

• Instruct patient to ease photophobia by wearing dark glasses.

• Advise patient to wear or carry medical identification during therapy.

phenylephrine hydrochloride
AK-Dilate, AK-Nefrin Ophthalmic ◇, Isopto Frin ◇, Mydfrin, Phenoptic, Prefrin Liquifilm ◇, Relief ◇

Pregnancy risk category C

AVAILABLE FORMS
Ophthalmic solution: 0.12%, 2.5%, 10%

INDICATIONS & DOSAGES
➤ **Mydriasis without cycloplegia—**
Adults and children: Instill 1 drop of 2.5% or 10% solution before examination. May be repeated in 1 hour, if needed.

➤ **Mydriasis and vasoconstriction—**
Adults and adolescents: 1 drop of 2.5% or 10% solution.
Children: 1 drop of 2.5% solution.
➤ **Chronic mydriasis—**
Adults and adolescents: 1 drop of 2.5% or 10% solution b.i.d. or t.i.d.
Children: Instill 1 drop of 2.5% solution b.i.d. or t.i.d.
➤ **Posterior synechia (adhesion of iris)—**
Adults and children: Instill 1 drop of 2.5% or 10% solution. Don't use 10% concentration in infants.

ACTION

An adrenergic that dilates the pupil by contracting the dilator muscle.

Route	Onset	Peak	Duration
Ophthalmic	Rapid	10-90 min	3-7 hr

ADVERSE REACTIONS

CNS: brow ache, headache.
CV: *hypertension* with 10% solution, tachycardia, palpitations, *PVCs, MI.*
EENT: transient eye burning or stinging on instillation, blurred vision, increased intraocular pressure, keratitis, lacrimation, reactive hyperemia of eye, allergic conjunctivitis, rebound miosis.
Skin: pallor, dermatitis, diaphoresis.
Other: trembling.

INTERACTIONS

Drug-drug. *Atropine (topical), cyclopentolate, homatropine, scopolamine:* May increase dilation of pupil. Use together cautiously.
Beta blockers, MAO inhibitors: May cause arrhythmias because of increased pressor effect. Use together cautiously.
Guanethidine: Increased mydriatic and pressor effects of phenylephrine. Use together cautiously.
Levodopa: Reduced mydriatic effect of phenylephrine. Use together cautiously.
TCAs: Increased cardiac effects of epinephrine. Use together cautiously.
Drug-lifestyle. *Sun exposure:* Photophobia may occur. Advise patient to avoid excessive sun exposure.

EFFECTS ON LAB TEST RESULTS
None reported.

CONTRAINDICATIONS

Contraindicated in patients hypersensitive to drug; also contraindicated in those with angle-closure glaucoma and in patients who wear soft contact lenses.

NURSING CONSIDERATIONS

• Use cautiously in patients with marked hypertension, cardiac disorders, advanced arteriosclerotic changes, type 1 diabetes, or hyperthyroidism; in children with low body weight; and in elderly patients.
• Systemic adverse reactions are least likely with 2.5% solution and most likely with 10% solution.
Drug may lower intraocular pressure in normal eyes or in open-angle glaucoma; it also may cause false-normal tonometry readings.
• *Alert:* Don't confuse Mydfrin with Midrin.

PATIENT TEACHING

• Teach patient how to instill drug. Advise him to wash hands before and after instillation and to apply light finger pressure on lacrimal sac for 1 minute after drops are instilled. Warn him not to touch tip of dropper to eye or surrounding tissue.
• Warn patient not to exceed recommended dosage because systemic effects can result. Monitor blood pressure and pulse rate.
• Tell patient not to use brown solution or solution that contains precipitate.
• Warn patient to avoid hazardous activities, such as operating machinery or driving, until temporary blurring subsides.
• Advise patient to contact prescriber if condition persists longer than 12 hours after discontinuation of drug.
• Advise patient to ease photophobia by wearing dark glasses.

---

*Liquid contains alcohol.   **May contain tartrazine.   †Canada   ‡Australia   §U.K.   ◇OTC

scopolamine hydrobromide
Isopto Hyoscine

Pregnancy risk category NR

AVAILABLE FORMS
Ophthalmic solution: 0.25%

INDICATIONS & DOSAGES
➤ **Cycloplegic refraction—**
Adults: Instill 1 to 2 drops of 0.25% solution 1 hour before refraction.
Children: Instill 1 drop of 0.25% solution b.i.d. for 2 days before refraction.
➤ **Iritis, uveitis—**
Adults: Instill 1 to 2 drops of 0.25% solution once daily to q.i.d.
Children: Instill 1 drop of 0.25% solution once daily to q.i.d.

ACTION
An anticholinergic that leaves the pupil under unopposed adrenergic influence, causing it to dilate.

Route	Onset	Peak	Duration
Ophthalmic	Rapid	15-45 min	< 1 wk

ADVERSE REACTIONS
CNS: confusion, delirium, somnolence, acute psychotic reactions, headache, hallucinations.
CV: tachycardia, edema.
EENT: ocular congestion with prolonged use, conjunctivitis, *blurred vision,* eye dryness, increased intraocular pressure, *photophobia,* transient stinging and burning.
GI: dry mouth.
Skin: dryness, contact dermatitis.

INTERACTIONS
Drug-lifestyle. *Sun exposure:* Photophobia may occur. Advise patient to avoid excessive sun exposure.

EFFECTS ON LAB TEST RESULTS
None reported.

CONTRAINDICATIONS
Contraindicated in patients hypersensitive to drug and in those with shallow anterior chamber, angle-closure glaucoma, or adhesions between the iris and lens; also contraindicated in children with previous severe systemic reaction to atropine.

NURSING CONSIDERATIONS
● *Alert:* If you must use this drug in infants and small children, use it with extreme caution.
● Use cautiously in patients with cardiac disease and in elderly patients.
● Observe patients closely for adverse CNS effects (such as disorientation and delirium).
● Drug may be used in patients sensitive to atropine because it's faster acting and has a shorter duration of action and fewer adverse reactions.

PATIENT TEACHING
● Teach patient how to instill drug. Advise him to wash hands before and after instillation and to apply light finger pressure on lacrimal sac for 1 minute after drops are instilled. Warn him to avoid touching tip of dropper to eye or surrounding tissue.
● Warn patient to avoid hazardous activities, such as operating machinery or driving, until temporary blurring subsides.
● Advise patient to ease photophobia by wearing dark glasses.
● Instruct patient to wear or carry medical identification at all times during therapy.

Ophthalmic vasoconstrictors

naphazoline hydrochloride
oxymetazoline hydrochloride
tetrahydrozoline hydrochloride

COMBINATION PRODUCTS
OPCON-A OPHTHALMIC SOLUTION ◇:
naphazoline hydrochloride 0.027% and
pheniramine maleate 0.315%.

---

naphazoline hydrochloride
AK-Con, Albalon Liquifilm,
Allerest ◇, Clear Eyes ◇, Comfort
Eye Drops ◇, Degest 2, Nafazair,
Naphcon ◇, Naphcon Forte,
Optazine‡, Vasocon Regular

Pregnancy risk category C

AVAILABLE FORMS
Ophthalmic solution: 0.012% ◇,
0.02% ◇, 0.03% ◇, 0.1%

INDICATIONS & DOSAGES
➤ **Ocular congestion, irritation,
itching—**
Adults— Instill 1 drop of 0.1% solution q 3
to 4 hours or 1 drop of 0.012% to 0.03%
solution up to q.i.d.

ACTION
Unknown. Thought to cause vasoconstriction by local adrenergic action on the
blood vessels of the conjunctiva.

Route	Onset	Peak	Duration
Ophthalmic	10 min	Unknown	2-6 hr

ADVERSE REACTIONS
CNS: headache, dizziness, nervousness,
weakness.
EENT: transient eye stinging, pupillary
dilation, eye irritation, photophobia,
blurred vision, increased intraocular pressure, keratitis, lacrimation.
GI: nausea.
Skin: diaphoresis.

INTERACTIONS
Drug-drug. *MAO inhibitors, maprotiline,
tricyclic antidepressants:* Hypertensive
crisis if naphazoline is systemically absorbed. Use together cautiously.

EFFECTS ON LAB TEST RESULTS
None reported.

CONTRAINDICATIONS
Contraindicated in patients hypersensitive
to drug's ingredients and in those with
acute angle-closure glaucoma. Use of
0.1% solution is contraindicated in infants
and small children.

NURSING CONSIDERATIONS
• Use cautiously in patients with hyperthyroidism, cardiac disease, hypertension, or
diabetes mellitus.
• Drug is most widely used ocular decongestant.
• Store drug in tightly closed container.

PATIENT TEACHING
• Teach patient how to instill drug. Advise him to wash hands before and after
instillation and to apply light finger pressure on lacrimal sac for 1 minute after
drops are instilled. Warn him not to touch
tip of dropper to eye or surrounding tissue.
• Warn patient not to exceed recommended dosage. Rebound congestion and conjunctivitis may occur with frequent or prolonged use.
• Tell patient to notify prescriber if photophobia, blurred vision, pain, or lid edema
develops.
• Instruct patient not to use OTC preparations longer than 72 hours without consulting prescriber.

---

oxymetazoline hydrochloride
OcuClear◇, Visine L.R.◇

Pregnancy risk category C

AVAILABLE FORMS
Ophthalmic solution: 0.025%

INDICATIONS & DOSAGES
➤ **Relief from eye redness caused by minor eye irritations—**
Adults and children age 6 and older: Instill 1 to 2 drops into conjunctival sac b.i.d. to q.i.d. (at least 6 hours apart).

ACTION
A direct-acting sympathomimetic amine that acts on alpha-adrenergic receptors in the arterioles of the conjunctiva to produce vasoconstriction, resulting in decreased conjunctival congestion.

Route	Onset	Peak	Duration
Ophthalmic	5 min	Unknown	6 hr

ADVERSE REACTIONS
CNS: headache, light-headedness, nervousness, insomnia.
CV: palpitations, tachycardia, irregular heartbeat.
EENT: *transient stinging on initial instillation,* blurred vision, keratitis, lacrimation, increased intraocular pressure, reactive hyperemia with excessive doses or prolonged use.
Other: trembling.

INTERACTIONS
Drug-drug. *MAO inhibitors, maprotiline, tricyclic antidepressants:* If significant systemic absorption of oxymetazoline occurs, use together may increase pressor effect of oxymetazoline. Avoid using together.

EFFECTS ON LAB TEST RESULTS
None reported.

CONTRAINDICATIONS
Contraindicated in patients hypersensitive to drug or its components and in those with angle-closure glaucoma.

NURSING CONSIDERATIONS
• Use cautiously in patients with hyperthyroidism, cardiac disease, hypertension, and eye disease, infection, or injury.
• Don't use if solution has become cloudy or changes color.
• *Alert:* Don't confuse Visine with Visken.

PATIENT TEACHING
• Teach patient how to instill drops. Advise him to wash hands before and after instillation, and warn him not to touch tip of dropper to eye or surrounding tissue.
• Instruct patient to apply light finger pressure on lacrimal sac for 1 minute after drug instillation.
• Advise patient to stop drug and consult prescriber if eye pain occurs, if vision changes, or if redness or irritation continues, worsens, or lasts for longer than 72 hours.

tetrahydrozoline hydrochloride
Collyrium Fresh◇, Eyesine◇, Geneye◇, Murine Plus◇, Optigene 3◇, Tetrasine◇

Pregnancy risk category C

AVAILABLE FORMS
Ophthalmic solution: 0.05%◇

INDICATIONS & DOSAGES
➤ **Conjunctival congestion, irritation, and allergic conditions—**
Adults and children older than age 2: Instill 1 to 2 drops of 0.05% solution up to q.i.d. or as directed by prescriber.

ACTION
Unknown. Thought to cause vasoconstriction by local adrenergic action on the blood vessels of the conjunctiva.

Route	Onset	Peak	Duration
Ophthalmic	Few min	Unknown	1-4 hr

ADVERSE REACTIONS
CNS: headache, drowsiness, insomnia, dizziness, tremor.
CV: *arrhythmias.*

Reactions may be *common,* uncommon, *life-threatening,* or **COMMON AND LIFE-THREATENING.**

EENT: transient eye stinging, pupillary dilation, increased intraocular pressure, keratitis, lacrimation, eye irritation.

INTERACTIONS
Drug-drug. *Guanethidine, MAO inhibitors, tricyclic antidepressants:* Hypertensive crisis if tetrahydrozoline is systemically absorbed. Don't use together.

EFFECTS ON LAB TEST RESULTS
None reported.

CONTRAINDICATIONS
Contraindicated in patients hypersensitive to drug or its components and in those with angle-closure glaucoma or other serious eye diseases.

NURSING CONSIDERATIONS
• Use cautiously in patients with hyperthyroidism, heart disease, hypertension, or diabetes mellitus.
• Rebound congestion may occur with frequent or prolonged use.
• *Alert:* Don't confuse Visine with Visken.

PATIENT TEACHING
• Teach patient how to instill drug. Advise him to wash hands before and after instillation and to apply light finger pressure on lacrimal sac for 1 minute after drops are instilled. Warn him not to touch tip of dropper to eye or surrounding tissue.
• Warn patient not to exceed recommended dosage.
• Tell patient to stop drug and notify prescriber if redness or irritation persists or increases or if no relief occurs within 2 days.
• Warn patient not to share ophthalmic drugs.

azelastine hydrochloride
betaxolol hydrochloride
bimatoprost
brimonidine tartrate
carteolol hydrochloride
dorzolamide hydrochloride
emedastine difumarate
ketotifen fumarate
latanoprost
levobunolol hydrochloride
metipranolol hydrochloride
sodium chloride, hypertonic
timolol maleate
travoprost
unoprostone isopropyl

COMBINATION PRODUCTS
None.

---

azelastine hydrochloride
Optivar

Pregnancy risk category C

AVAILABLE FORMS
Ophthalmic solution: 0.05%

INDICATIONS & DOSAGES
➤ **Itching of the eye with allergic conjunctivitis—**
Adults and children age 3 and older: Instill 1 drop into affected eye b.i.d.

ACTION
Inhibits the release of histamine and other mediators from cells involved in the allergic response.

Route	Onset	Peak	Duration
Ophthalmic	3 min	Unknown	8 hr

ADVERSE REACTIONS
CNS: fatigue, *headaches.*
EENT: *transient eye burning or stinging,* bitter taste, conjunctivitis, eye pain, pharyngitis, rhinitis, temporary blurring.
Respiratory: asthma, dyspnea.
Skin: pruritus.
Other: flulike symptoms.

INTERACTIONS
None reported.

EFFECTS ON LAB TEST RESULTS
None reported.

CONTRAINDICATIONS
Contraindicated in patients hypersensitive to any of drug's components.

NURSING CONSIDERATIONS
• Indicated only for ocular use.
• Don't use to treat contact lens-related irritation.
• The preservative benzalkonium may be absorbed by soft contact lenses.

PATIENT TEACHING
• Instruct patient not to touch any surface, eyelid, or surrounding areas with tip of dropper bottle.
• Tell patient to keep bottle tightly closed when not in use.
• Advise patient not to wear contact lens if eye is red.
• Warn patient that the preservative benzalkonium may be absorbed by soft contact lenses.
• Instruct patient who wears soft contact lenses and whose eyes aren't red to wait at least 10 minutes after instilling drug before inserting contact lenses.

---

betaxolol hydrochloride
Betoptic, Betoptic S

Pregnancy risk category C

AVAILABLE FORMS
Ophthalmic solution: 0.5%
Ophthalmic suspension: 0.25%

INDICATIONS & DOSAGES
➤ **Chronic open-angle glaucoma, ocular hypertension—**
Adults: Instill 1 or 2 drops of 0.5% solution or 0.25% suspension b.i.d.

Reactions may be *common*, uncommon, *life-threatening*, or COMMON AND LIFE-THREATENING.

ACTION
Unknown. A cardioselective beta blocker that reduces aqueous formation and possibly increases outflow of aqueous humor.

Route	Onset	Peak	Duration
Ophthalmic	0.5-1 hr	2 hr	> 12 hr

ADVERSE REACTIONS
CNS: insomnia, *CVA,* depressive neurosis.
CV: *arrhythmias, heart block, heart failure,* palpitations.
EENT: *eye stinging on instillation causing brief discomfort,* photophobia, erythema, itching, keratitis, occasional tearing.
Respiratory: asthma, *bronchospasm.*

INTERACTIONS
Drug-drug. *Calcium channel blockers:* AV conduction disturbances, ventricular failure, and hypotension if significant systemic absorption occurs. Monitor patient closely.
Cardiac glycosides: Risk of excessive bradycardia. Patient may need ECG monitoring if significant systemic absorption occurs.
Dipivefrin, ophthalmic epinephrine: May produce mydriasis. Use together cautiously.
Inhaled hydrocarbon anesthetics: Prolonged severe hypotension if significant systemic absorption occurs. Tell anesthesiologist that patient is receiving ophthalmic betaxolol.
Insulin, oral antidiabetics: Risk of hypoglycemia or hyperglycemia if significant systemic absorption occurs. May need to adjust dosage of antidiabetics.
Phenothiazines: Additive hypotensive effects; increased risk of adverse effects if significant systemic absorption occurs. Monitor patient closely.
Reserpine: Excessive beta blockade. Monitor patient closely.
Systemic beta blockers: Additive effects. Monitor patient closely.
Drug-lifestyle. *Cocaine use:* May inhibit betaxolol's effects. Inform patient of this interaction.
Sun exposure: Photophobia may occur. Advise patient to avoid excessive sun exposure.

EFFECTS ON LAB TEST RESULTS
None reported.

CONTRAINDICATIONS
Contraindicated in patients hypersensitive to drug and in those with sinus bradycardia, greater-than-first-degree AV block, cardiogenic shock, or overt heart failure.

NURSING CONSIDERATIONS
• Use cautiously in patients with restricted pulmonary function, diabetes mellitus, hyperthyroidism, or history of heart failure.
• Some patients may need a few weeks' treatment to stabilize intraocular pressure (IOP)-lowering response. Determine IOP after 4 weeks of treatment.

PATIENT TEACHING
• Teach patient how to instill drug. Advise him to wash hands before and after instillation and to apply light finger pressure on lacrimal sac for 1 minute after instilling drug. Warn him not to touch tip of dropper to eye or surrounding tissue. Tell him to shake suspension well before instilling.
• Encourage patient to comply with b.i.d. regimen.
• Tell patient to remove contact lenses before instilling drug. Lenses may be reinserted about 15 minutes after using drops.
• Advise patient to ease photophobia by wearing dark glasses.
• Tell patient to avoid using other eye products with drug.

✹ *NEW DRUG*

bimatoprost
Lumigan

Pregnancy risk category C

AVAILABLE FORMS
Ophthalmic solution: 0.03%

INDICATIONS & DOSAGES
➤ **Increased intraocular pressure (IOP) in patients with open-angle glaucoma or ocular hypertension who can't tolerate or are unresponsive to other IOP-lowering drugs—**
Adults: Instill 1 drop in conjunctival sac of affected eye once daily in the evening.

ACTION
Drug is a prostamide, which is a synthetic analogue of prostaglandin with ocular hypotensive activity. It selectively mimics the effects of naturally occurring prostaglandins. Drug is believed to lower IOP by increasing outflow of aqueous humor through both the trabecular meshwork and uveoscleral routes.

Route	Onset	Peak	Duration
Ophthalmic	Unknown	10 min	1.5 hr

ADVERSE REACTIONS
CNS: headache, asthenia.
EENT: *conjunctival hyperemia, growth of eyelashes, ocular pruritus,* ocular dryness, visual disturbance, ocular burning, foreign body sensation, eye pain, pigmentation of the periocular skin, blepharitis, cataract, superficial punctate keratitis, eyelid erythema, ocular irritation, eyelash darkening, eye discharge, tearing, photophobia, allergic conjunctivitis, asthenopia, increase in iris pigmentation, conjunctival edema.
Respiratory: *upper respiratory tract infection.*
Skin: hirsutism.
Other: *infection.*

INTERACTIONS
Drug-herb. *Area, jaborandi:* May have additive IOP-lowering effects. Discourage use together.

EFFECTS ON LAB TEST RESULTS
• May cause abnormal liver function test values.

CONTRAINDICATIONS
Contraindicated in patients hypersensitive to bimatoprost, benzalkonium chloride, or other ingredients in product. Also contraindicated in patients with angle-closure glaucoma or inflammatory or neovascular glaucoma.

NURSING CONSIDERATIONS
• Use cautiously in patients with renal or hepatic impairment.
• Use cautiously in patients with active intraocular inflammation (iritis, uveitis), aphakic patients, pseudophakic patients with torn posterior lens capsule, and in patients at risk for macular edema.
• Temporary or permanent increased pigmentation of iris and eyelid, as well as increased pigmentation and growth of eyelashes, may occur.
• Patient should remove contact lenses before using solution. Lenses may be reinserted 15 minutes after administration.
• If more than one ophthalmic drug is being used, give drugs at least 5 minutes apart.
• Store drug in original container between 59° and 77° F (15° and 25° C).

PATIENT TEACHING
• Tell patient receiving treatment in only one eye about potential for increased brown pigmentation of iris, eyelid skin darkening, and increased length, thickness, pigmentation, or number of lashes in treated eye.
• Teach patient to instill drops, and advise him to wash hands before and after instilling solution. Warn him not to touch dropper or tip to eye or surrounding tissue.
• If eye trauma or infection occurs or if eye surgery is needed, tell patient to seek medical advice before continuing to use multidose container.
• Advise patient to immediately report conjunctivitis or lid reactions.
• Advise patient to apply light pressure on lacrimal sac for 1 minute after instillation to minimize systemic absorption of drug.
• Tell patient to remove contact lenses before using solution and that lenses may be reinserted 15 minutes after administration.
• Advise patient that, if more than one ophthalmic drug is being used, drugs should be given at least 5 minutes apart.
• Stress importance of compliance with recommended therapy.

brimonidine tartrate
Alphagan

Pregnancy risk category B

AVAILABLE FORMS
Ophthalmic solution: 0.2%; 5 ml, 10 ml

INDICATIONS & DOSAGES
➤ **Intraocular pressure (IOP) reduction in open-angle glaucoma or ocular hypertension—**
Adults: 1 drop in affected eye t.i.d., about 8 hours apart.

ACTION
A selective alpha$_2$-adrenergic agonist that reduces aqueous humor production and increases uveoscleral outflow.

Route	Onset	Peak	Duration
Ophthalmic	Unknown	1-4 hr	Unknown

ADVERSE REACTIONS
CNS: anxiety, asthenia, depression, dizziness, *drowsiness, fatigue, headache,* insomnia, syncope.
CV: hypertension, palpitations.
EENT: abnormal vision or taste; blepharitis; *blurred vision; burning, stinging eyes;* runny or stuffy nose; sneezing; conjunctival blanching, edema, hemorrhage, or discharge; *conjunctival follicles;* corneal staining or erosion; eyelid erythema or eyelid edema; *foreign body sensation;* lid crusting; nasal dryness; *ocular hyperemia,* ache, pain, *dryness,* tearing, or irritation; photophobia.
GI: nausea, vomiting, *dry mouth.*
Musculoskeletal: muscle pain.
Skin: *pruritus.*
Other: *allergic reactions.*

INTERACTIONS
Drug-drug. *Antihypertensives, beta blockers, cardiac glycosides:* May further decrease blood pressure or pulse. Use cautiously.
CNS depressants: May increase effects. Use cautiously.
TCAs: May interfere with brimonidine's IOP-lowering effects. Use cautiously.
Drug-lifestyle. *Alcohol use:* May increase CNS depressant effect. Urge patient to avoid alcohol.

EFFECTS ON LAB TEST RESULTS
None reported.

CONTRAINDICATIONS
Contraindicated in patients hypersensitive to drug or benzalkonium chloride

and in those receiving MAO inhibitor therapy.

NURSING CONSIDERATIONS
• Use cautiously in patients with CV disease, cerebral or coronary insufficiency, hepatic or renal impairment, depression, Raynaud's phenomenon, orthostatic hypotension, or thromboangiitis obliterans.
• Monitor IOP because effect may reverse after first month of therapy.
• It's unknown if drug appears in breast milk. Use with caution in breast-feeding women.

PATIENT TEACHING
• Tell patient to wait at least 15 minutes after instilling drug before wearing soft contact lenses.
• Caution patient to avoid hazardous activities because of risk of decreased mental alertness, fatigue, or drowsiness.
• Advise patient to avoid alcohol.

---

carteolol hydrochloride
Ocupress, Teoptic§

Pregnancy risk category C

AVAILABLE FORMS
Ophthalmic solution: 1%

INDICATIONS & DOSAGES
➤ **Chronic open-angle glaucoma, intraocular hypertension—**
Adults: 1 drop into conjunctival sac of affected eye b.i.d.

ACTION
Exact mechanism unknown. A nonselective beta blocker that reduces intraocular pressure (IOP) by decreasing aqueous humor production.

Route	Onset	Peak	Duration
Ophthalmic	Unknown	2 hr	12 hr

ADVERSE REACTIONS
CNS: headache, dizziness, insomnia, asthenia.
CV: *bradycardia,* hypotension, *arrhythmias,* palpitations.
EENT: *transient eye irritation, burning, tearing, conjunctival hyperemia, ocular*

edema, blurred and cloudy vision, photophobia, decreased night vision, ptosis, blepharoconjunctivitis, abnormal corneal staining, corneal sensitivity, sinusitis.
GI: taste perversion.
Respiratory: dyspnea.

INTERACTIONS
Drug-drug. *Catecholamine-depleting drugs such as reserpine, oral beta blockers:* May cause additive effects and development of hypotension or bradycardia. Monitor patient closely.
Drug-lifestyle. *Sun exposure:* Photophobia may occur. Advise patient to avoid excessive sun exposure.

EFFECTS ON LAB TEST RESULTS
None reported.

CONTRAINDICATIONS
Contraindicated in patients hypersensitive to drug or its components and in those with bronchial asthma, severe COPD, sinus bradycardia, second- or third-degree AV block, overt cardiac failure, or cardiogenic shock.

NURSING CONSIDERATIONS
• Use cautiously in patients hypersensitive to other beta blockers; in those with nonallergic bronchospastic disease, diabetes mellitus, hyperthyroidism, or decreased pulmonary function; and in breast-feeding women.
• Monitor vital signs.
• *Alert:* Discontinue drug at first sign of cardiac failure, and notify prescriber.
• When used to reduce elevated IOP in angle-closure glaucoma, drug should be given with a miotic and never alone.

PATIENT TEACHING
• Tell patient that, if more than one topical ophthalmic drug is being used, drugs should be given at least 10 minutes apart.
• Teach patient how to instill drops. Advise him to wash hands before and after instillation, and warn him not to touch tip of dropper to eye or surrounding tissue.
• Advise patient to apply light finger pressure on lacrimal sac for 1 minute after drug instillation to minimize systemic absorption.

• Tell patient to remove contact lenses before instilling drug.
• Instruct patient to keep bottle tightly closed when not in use and to protect it from light.
• Tell patient that drug is a beta blocker and, although it's given topically, it has the potential to be absorbed systemically.
• Inform patient that adverse reactions that can result from beta blockers can occur with topical administration. Tell him to discontinue drug and notify prescriber immediately if signs or symptoms of serious adverse reactions or hypersensitivity occur.
• Advise patient to monitor heart rate and blood pressure closely and to report slow heart rate to prescriber.
• Stress importance of compliance with recommended therapy.
• Advise patient to ease photophobia by wearing dark glasses.

---

dorzolamide hydrochloride
Trusopt

Pregnancy risk category C

AVAILABLE FORMS
Ophthalmic solution: 2%

INDICATIONS & DOSAGES
➤ **Increased intraocular pressure (IOP) in patients with ocular hypertension or open-angle glaucoma—**
Adults: 1 drop into conjunctival sac of affected eye t.i.d.

ACTION
Inhibits carbonic anhydrase in the ciliary processes of the eye, which decreases aqueous humor secretion, presumably by slowing the formation of bicarbonate ions, thereby reducing sodium and fluid transport, resulting in a reduction in IOP.

Route	Onset	Peak	Duration
Ophthalmic	Unknown	Unknown	Unknown

ADVERSE REACTIONS
CNS: headache, asthenia, fatigue.
EENT: *ocular burning, stinging, and discomfort; superficial punctate keratitis; ocular allergic reaction; blurred vision;*

---

lacrimation; dryness; photophobia; irido-cyclitis.
GI: nausea, *bitter taste.*
GU: urolithiasis.
Skin: rash.

INTERACTIONS
Drug-drug. *Oral carbonic anhydrase inhibitors:* May cause additive effects. Don't give together.

EFFECTS ON LAB TEST RESULTS
None reported.

CONTRAINDICATIONS
Contraindicated in patients hypersensitive to drug or its components.

NURSING CONSIDERATIONS
• Use cautiously in patients with hepatic or renal impairment.
• If more than one topical ophthalmic drug is being used, drugs should be given at least 10 minutes apart.

PATIENT TEACHING
• Teach patient how to instill drops. Advise him to wash hands before and after instillation, and warn him not to touch tip of dropper to eye or surrounding tissue.
• Tell patient that drug is a sulfonamide and, although it's given topically, it can be absorbed systemically. Advise patient to apply light finger pressure on lacrimal sac for 1 minute after drug instillation to minimize systemic absorption.
• Tell patient that adverse reactions that can result from sulfonamides may occur with topical administration. Tell him to discontinue drug and notify prescriber immediately if signs or symptoms of serious adverse reactions or hypersensitivity occur.
• Advise patient to discontinue drug and notify prescriber if ocular reactions occur, particularly conjunctivitis and eyelid reactions.
• Tell patient not to wear soft contact lenses during therapy.
• Stress importance of compliance with recommended therapy.

emedastine difumarate
Emadine

Pregnancy risk category B

AVAILABLE FORMS
Ophthalmic solution: 0.05%

INDICATIONS & DOSAGES
➤ **Temporary relief from signs and symptoms of allergic conjunctivitis—**
Adults and children age 3 and older: Instill 1 drop into affected eyes up to q.i.d.

ACTION
A selective H_1 receptor antagonist that inhibits histamine-stimulated vascular permeability in the conjunctiva.

Route	Onset	Peak	Duration
Ophthalmic, topical	Unknown	Unknown	Unknown

ADVERSE REACTIONS
CNS: *headache,* abnormal dreams, asthenia.
EENT: blurred vision, burning or stinging, corneal infiltrates, corneal staining, discomfort, dry eye, foreign body sensation, hyperemia, keratitis, tearing, sinusitis, rhinitis.
GI: bad taste.
Skin: pruritus.

INTERACTIONS
None significant.

EFFECTS ON LAB TEST RESULTS
None reported.

CONTRAINDICATIONS
Contraindicated in patients hypersensitive to drug or its components.

NURSING CONSIDERATIONS
• Drug is only for topical use and not for injection or oral use.
• Avoid touching eyelids or surrounding areas with dropper tip of bottle.
• Keep bottle tightly closed when not in use.
• Don't use if solution is discolored.

• Safety and effectiveness of drug in children younger than age 3 haven't been established.

PATIENT TEACHING
• Teach patient how to instill drops. Advise him to wash hands before and after instillation. To prevent contaminating dropper tip and solution, tell patient to use care not to touch eyelids or surrounding areas with dropper tip of bottle.
• Tell patient not to wear contact lens if eye is red.
• Instruct patient not to use drug for contact lens-related irritation.
• Tell patient that solution contains a preservative (benzalkonium chloride) that may be absorbed by soft contact lenses. If patient wears soft contact lenses and his eyes aren't red, instruct him to wait at least 10 minutes after instilling drug before inserting contact lenses.

---

ketotifen fumarate
Zaditor

Pregnancy risk category C

AVAILABLE FORMS
Ophthalmic solution: 0.025%

INDICATIONS & DOSAGES
➤ **Temporary prevention of eye itching caused by allergic conjunctivitis**—
Adults and children age 4 and older: Instill 1 drop in affected eyes q 8 to 12 hours.

ACTION
Stabilizes mast cells to inhibit release of mediators involved in hypersensitivity reactions and blocks action of histamine at the H_1 receptor, temporarily preventing itching of the eye.

Route	Onset	Peak	Duration
Ophthalmic	Within min	Unknown	Unknown

ADVERSE REACTIONS
CNS: headache.
EENT: *conjunctival infection, rhinitis,* ocular allergic reactions, burning or stinging of eyes, conjunctivitis, eye discharge, dry eyes, eye pain, eyelid disorder, itching

of eyes, keratitis, lacrimation disorder, mydriasis, photophobia, ocular rash, pharyngitis.
Other: flu syndrome.

INTERACTIONS
None significant.

EFFECTS ON LAB TEST RESULTS
None reported.

CONTRAINDICATIONS
Contraindicated in patients hypersensitive to components of drug.

NURSING CONSIDERATIONS
• Drug is only for ophthalmic use and not for injection or oral use.
• Drug isn't indicated for irritation related to contact lenses.
• Preservative in drug may be absorbed by soft contact lenses. Contact lenses shouldn't be inserted until 10 minutes after drug is instilled.
• To prevent contaminating dropper tip and solution, don't touch eyelids or surrounding areas with dropper tip of bottle.

PATIENT TEACHING
• Teach patient the proper technique for giving drops.
• Advise patient not to wear contact lens if eye is red. Warn patient not to use drug to treat contact lens-related irritation.
• Instruct patient who wears soft contact lenses and whose eyes aren't red to wait at least 10 minutes after instilling drug before inserting contact lenses.
• Advise patient to report adverse reactions.
• Advise patient to keep bottle tightly closed when not in use.

---

latanoprost
Xalatan

Pregnancy risk category C

AVAILABLE FORMS
Ophthalmic solution: 0.005%
(50 mcg/ml)

Reactions may be *common*, uncommon, *life-threatening*, or COMMON AND LIFE-THREATENING.

INDICATIONS & DOSAGES
➤ **Increased intraocular pressure (IOP) in patients with open-angle glaucoma or ocular hypertension who can't tolerate or who respond inadequately to other IOP-lowering drugs—**
Adults: 1 drop in conjunctival sac of affected eye once daily in the evening.

ACTION
Exact mechanism unknown. Believed to increase outflow of aqueous humor, thereby lowering IOP.

Route	Onset	Peak	Duration
Ophthalmic	2-4 hr	8-12 hr	Unknown

ADVERSE REACTIONS
CV: angina pectoris.
EENT: *blurred vision, burning, stinging,* conjunctival hyperemia, foreign body sensation, itching, increased brown pigmentation of the iris, dry eye, punctate epithelial keratopathy, lid crusting or edema, lid discomfort, excessive tearing, eye pain, photophobia.
Musculoskeletal: muscle, joint, or back pain.
Respiratory: upper respiratory tract infection.
Skin: rash, allergic skin reaction.
Other: cold or flu.

INTERACTIONS
Drug-drug. *Eyedrops that contain thimerosal:* Precipitation occurs when mixed with latanoprost. If used together, administer at least 5 minutes apart.

EFFECTS ON LAB TEST RESULTS
None reported.

CONTRAINDICATIONS
Contraindicated in patients hypersensitive to drug, benzalkonium chloride, or other components of drug.

NURSING CONSIDERATIONS
● Use cautiously when giving to patients with impaired renal or hepatic function.
● Drug shouldn't be given while patient is wearing contact lenses.
● Administering drug more frequently than recommended may decrease its IOP-lowering effects.

● Drug may gradually change eye color, increasing amount of brown pigment in iris. This change in iris color occurs slowly and may not be noticeable for months or years. Increased pigmentation may be permanent.
● To avoid ocular infections, don't allow tip of dispenser to contact eye or surrounding structures. Serious damage to eye and subsequent loss of vision may result from using contaminated solutions.
● Safety and efficacy of drug in children haven't been established.
● It isn't known if drug appears in breast milk; use caution when giving drug to breast-feeding women.

PATIENT TEACHING
● Inform patient of risk that iris color may change. Patients should be told about risk of increased brown pigmentation in treated eye.
● Teach patient how to instill drops. Advise him to wash his hands before and after instillation, and warn him not to touch dropper or its tip to eye or surrounding tissue.
● Advise patient to apply light finger pressure on lacrimal sac for 1 minute after instillation to minimize systemic absorption.
● Instruct patient to report ocular reactions, especially conjunctivitis and lid reactions.
● Tell patient who wears contact lenses to remove them before giving solution and not to reinsert the lenses until 15 minutes have elapsed.
● Advise patient that, if more than one topical ophthalmic drug is being used, drugs should be given at least 5 minutes apart.
● If patient develops another ocular condition (such as trauma or infection) or needs ocular surgery, advise him to contact prescriber about continued use of multidose container.
● Stress importance of compliance with recommended therapy.

levobunolol hydrochloride
AKBeta, Betagan

Pregnancy risk category C

AVAILABLE FORMS
Ophthalmic solution: 0.25%, 0.5%

INDICATIONS & DOSAGES
➤ **Chronic open-angle glaucoma, ocular hypertension—**
Adults: 1 to 2 drops once daily (0.5%) or b.i.d. (0.25%).

ACTION
Unknown. A nonselective beta blocker thought to reduce aqueous formation and possibly increase outflow of aqueous humor.

Route	Onset	Peak	Duration
Ophthalmic	1 hr	2-6 hr	24 hr

ADVERSE REACTIONS
CNS: headache, depression, insomnia, *syncope.*
CV: slight reduction in resting heart rate, *hypotension,* **bradycardia, heart failure.**
EENT: *transient eye stinging and burning,* tearing, erythema, itching, keratitis, corneal punctate staining, photophobia, decreased corneal sensitivity.
GI: nausea.
Respiratory: *asthmatic attacks in patients with history of asthma.*
Skin: urticaria.

INTERACTIONS
Drug-drug. *Dipivefrin, epinephrine, systemically administered carbonic anhydrase inhibitors, topical miotics:* Additive lowered intraocular pressure. Use together cautiously.
Metoprolol, propranolol, other oral beta blockers: Increased ocular and systemic effects. Use together cautiously.
Reserpine, other catecholamine-depleting drugs: Increased hypotensive and bradycardic effects. Monitor blood pressure and heart rate closely.
Drug-lifestyle. *Sun exposure:* Photophobia may occur. Advise patient to avoid excessive sun exposure.

EFFECTS ON LAB TEST RESULTS
None reported.

CONTRAINDICATIONS
Contraindicated in patients hypersensitive to drug and in those with bronchial asthma, sinus bradycardia, second- or third-degree AV block, cardiac failure, cardiogenic shock, or history of bronchial asthma or severe COPD.

NURSING CONSIDERATIONS
● Use cautiously in patients with chronic bronchitis and emphysema, diabetes mellitus, hyperthyroidism, and myasthenia gravis.
● Avoid letting dropper touch patient's eye or surrounding tissue.
● Safe use in pregnant or breast-feeding women hasn't been established.

PATIENT TEACHING
● Teach patient how to instill drug. Advise him to wash hands before and after instillation and to apply light finger pressure on lacrimal sac for 1 minute after drops are instilled.
● Warn patient not to touch dropper to eye or surrounding tissue.
● Advise elderly patient to report dyspnea, chest pain, or heart irregularities to prescriber. Drug may be absorbed systemically and produce signs and symptoms of beta blockade.
● Advise patient to wear or carry medical identification at all times during therapy.

metipranolol hydrochloride
OptiPranolol

Pregnancy risk category C

AVAILABLE FORMS
Ophthalmic solution: 0.3% in 5-ml, 10-ml, or 15-ml dropper bottles

INDICATIONS & DOSAGES
➤ **Increased intraocular pressure (IOP) in ocular conditions, including ocular hypertension and chronic open-angle glaucoma—**
Adults: 1 drop into affected eye b.i.d. If IOP isn't at satisfactory level, therapy together to lower it may be instituted.

ACTION

Unknown. A noncardioselective beta blocker that appears to reduce aqueous production and reduce elevated and normal IOP, with or without glaucoma, with little or no effect on pupil size or accommodation. IOP above 24 mm Hg is usually reduced about 20% to 26%.

Route	Onset	Peak	Duration
Ophthalmic	0.5 hr	2 hr	24 hr

ADVERSE REACTIONS

CNS: headache, anxiety, dizziness, depression, somnolence, nervousness, asthenia, brow ache.
CV: hypertension, *MI,* atrial fibrillation, angina, palpitations, ***bradycardia.***
EENT: transient local eye discomfort, tearing, conjunctivitis, eyelid dermatitis, blurred vision, blepharitis, abnormal vision, photophobia, eye edema, rhinitis, epistaxis.
GI: nausea.
Musculoskeletal: myalgia.
Respiratory: dyspnea, bronchitis, cough.
Skin: rash.
Other: hypersensitivity reactions.

INTERACTIONS

Drug-drug. *Calcium channel blockers, cardiac glycosides, quinidine:* Increased risk of adverse cardiac effects if significant amount of drug is systemically absorbed. Use together cautiously.
Fentanyl, general anesthetics: Excessive hypotension. Monitor blood pressure closely.
Metoprolol tartrate, propranolol, other oral beta blockers: Increased ocular and systemic effects. Use together cautiously.
Reserpine, other catecholamine-depleting drugs: Increased hypotensive and bradycardia-induced effects. Avoid using together.

EFFECTS ON LAB TEST RESULTS

None reported.

CONTRAINDICATIONS

Contraindicated in patients hypersensitive to drug or its components and in those with bronchial asthma, sinus bradycardia, second- or third-degree AV block, cardiac failure, cardiogenic shock, or history of bronchial asthma or severe COPD.

NURSING CONSIDERATIONS

● Use cautiously in patients with nonallergic bronchospasm, chronic bronchitis, emphysema, diabetes mellitus (especially in those subject to spontaneous hypoglycemia), hyperthyroidism, or cerebrovascular insufficiency.
● Anticipate using pilocarpine, other miotics, or systemic carbonic anhydrase inhibitors together if IOP isn't adequately controlled.
● Check expiration date on bottle before use. Don't use if drops have changed color.
● A slight increase in outflow facility has been demonstrated with metipranolol. Like other noncardioselective beta blockers, metipranolol doesn't have significant local anesthetic (membrane-stabilizing) actions or intrinsic sympathomimetic activity.
● *Alert:* Don't confuse metipranolol with metaproterenol.

PATIENT TEACHING

● Teach patient how to instill drug. Instruct him to first wash hands thoroughly and then tilt head back or lie down and gaze upward. Tell patient to gently grasp lower eyelid below eyelashes and pull eyelid away from eye to form a pouch. Then have him place dropper directly over eye, avoiding contact with eye or any surface; look up just before applying drop; and look down for several seconds after instillation and slowly release eyelid.
● Tell patient to close eyes gently for 1 to 2 minutes and to apply gentle pressure to inside corner of eye at bridge of nose to retard draining of solution from intended area. Warn him not to rub eye or rinse dropper.
● Advise patient to report dyspnea, bradycardia, or chest pain.

sodium chloride, hypertonic
Adsorbonac, Ak-NaCl, Muro 128, Muroptic-5

Pregnancy risk category NR

AVAILABLE FORMS
Ophthalmic ointment: 5%
Ophthalmic solution: 2%, 5%

INDICATIONS & DOSAGES
➤ **Temporary relief from corneal edema—**
Adults and children: Apply 1 to 2 drops q 3 to 4 hours, or ¼-inch (6 mm) of ointment q 3 to 4 hours.

ACTION
An osmotic drug that removes excess fluid from cornea.

Route	Onset	Peak	Duration
Ophthalmic	Unknown	Unknown	Unknown

ADVERSE REACTIONS
EENT: slight eye stinging.
Other: hypersensitivity reactions.

INTERACTIONS
None significant.

EFFECTS ON LAB TEST RESULTS
None reported.

CONTRAINDICATIONS
Contraindicated in patients hypersensitive to drug or its components.

NURSING CONSIDERATIONS
• Ophthalmic solution is only for topical use; never inject.
• Check expiration date before use.

PATIENT TEACHING
• Teach patient how to instill drug. Advise him to wash hands before and after instillation and to apply light finger pressure on lacrimal sac for 1 minute after drops are instilled. Warn patient not to touch dropper to eye or surrounding tissue.
• Tell patient to prevent caking on dropper bottle tip by putting a few drops of sterile irrigation solution inside bottle cap.

• Warn patient that ointment may cause blurred vision.
• If patient experiences severe headache, pain, rapid change in vision, acute redness of eyes, sudden appearance of floating spots, pain on exposure to light, or double vision, tell him to discontinue drug and notify prescriber.
• Advise patient to store drug in tightly closed container.

timolol maleate
Betimol, Timoptic, Timoptic-XE

Pregnancy risk category C

AVAILABLE FORMS
Ophthalmic gel: 0.25%, 0.5%
Ophthalmic solution: 0.25%, 0.5%

INDICATIONS & DOSAGES
➤ **Increased intraocular pressure (IOP) in ocular hypertension or open-angle glaucoma—**
Adults: Initially, 1 drop of 0.25% solution in each affected eye b.i.d.; maintenance dosage is 1 drop daily. If no response, 1 drop of 0.5% solution in each affected eye b.i.d. If IOP is controlled, reduce dosage to 1 drop daily. Or, 1 drop of gel in each affected eye once daily.

ACTION
Unknown. A beta blocker thought to reduce aqueous formation and possibly increase aqueous outflow.

Route	Onset	Peak	Duration
Ophthalmic	0.5 hr	1-2 hr	12-24 hr

ADVERSE REACTIONS
CNS: *CVA*, depression, fatigue, dizziness, lethargy, hallucinations, confusion, *syncope.*
CV: slight reduction in resting heart rate, *arrhythmia, cardiac arrest, heart block,* palpitations, *hypotension, bradycardia, heart failure.*
EENT: minor eye irritation, conjunctivitis, blepharitis, keratitis, visual disturbances, diplopia, ptosis, decreased corneal sensitivity with long-term use.
Hematologic: anemia.

Reactions may be *common*, uncommon, *life-threatening*, or COMMON AND LIFE-THREATENING.

Metabolic: hyperkalemia, hyperglycemia, hyperuricemia.
Respiratory: *asthmatic attacks in patients with history of asthma.*

INTERACTIONS
Drug-drug. *Calcium channel blockers, cardiac glycosides, quinidine:* Increased risk of adverse cardiac effects if significant amounts of timolol are systemically absorbed. Use together cautiously.
Fentanyl, general anesthetics: Excessive hypotension. Monitor blood pressure closely.
Metoprolol propranolol, other oral beta blockers: Increased ocular and systemic effects. Use together cautiously.
Reserpine, other catecholamine-depleting drugs: Increased hypotensive and bradycardia-induced effects. Avoid using together.

EFFECTS ON LAB TEST RESULTS
● May increase BUN, potassium, glucose, and uric acid levels.

CONTRAINDICATIONS
Contraindicated in patients hypersensitive to drug and in those with bronchial asthma, sinus bradycardia, second- or third-degree AV block, cardiac failure, cardiogenic shock, or history of bronchial asthma or severe COPD.

NURSING CONSIDERATIONS
● Use cautiously in patients with nonallergic bronchospasm, chronic bronchitis, emphysema, diabetes mellitus, hyperthyroidism, or cerebrovascular insufficiency.
● Give other ophthalmic drugs at least 10 minutes before giving gel form of drug.
● Monitor diabetic patients carefully. Systemic beta-blocking effects can mask some signs and symptoms of hypoglycemia.
● Some patients may need a few weeks of treatment to stabilize pressure-lowering response. Determine IOP after 4 weeks of treatment.
● Drug can be used safely in patients with glaucoma who wear conventional polymethylmethacrylate (PMMA) hard contact lenses.
● *Alert:* Don't confuse timolol with atenolol, or Timoptic with Viroptic.

PATIENT TEACHING
● Teach patient how to instill drops. Advise him to wash hands before and after instillation and to apply light finger pressure on lacrimal sac for 1 minute after drops are instilled. Warn patient not to touch dropper to eye or surrounding tissue.
● Instruct patient using gel to invert container and shake once before each use. Also tell him to give other ophthalmic drugs at least 10 minutes before giving gel.
● Tell patient to instill drug without contact lenses in place. Lenses may be reinserted about 15 minutes after drug use.
● Advise patient to monitor pulse rate and report slow rate to prescriber. Drug may be absorbed systemically and produce signs and symptoms of beta blockade.
● Tell patient to report difficulty breathing or chest pain to prescriber.

✸ *NEW DRUG*

travoprost
Travatan

Pregnancy risk category C

AVAILABLE FORMS
Ophthalmic solution: 0.004%

INDICATIONS & DOSAGES
➤ **Increased intraocular pressure (IOP) in patients with open-angle glaucoma or ocular hypertension who can't tolerate or who respond inadequately to other IOP-lowering drugs—**
Adults: 1 drop in conjunctival sac of affected eye once daily in evening.

ACTION
Unknown. Thought to reduce IOP by increasing uveoscleral outflow.

Route	Onset	Peak	Duration
Ophthalmic	2 hr	30 min-12 hr	12 hr

ADVERSE REACTIONS
CNS: anxiety, depression, headache, pain.
CV: angina pectoris, *bradycardia,* chest pain, hypertension, hypotension.

EENT: *ocular hyperemia, decreased visual acuity, eye discomfort, foreign body sensation, eye pain, eye pruritus,* conjunctival hyperemia, abnormal vision, blepharitis, blurred vision, cataract, conjunctivitis, dry eye, eye disorder, iris discoloration, keratitis, lid margin crusting, photophobia, subconjunctival hemorrhage, tearing, sinusitis.
GI: dyspepsia, GI disorder.
GU: prostate disorder, urinary incontinence, urinary tract infection.
Metabolic: hypercholesterolemia.
Musculoskeletal: arthritis, back pain.
Respiratory: bronchitis.
Other: accidental injury, cold syndrome, infection.

INTERACTIONS
Drug-herb. *Areca, jaborandi:* May increase effects. Discourage use together.

EFFECTS ON LAB TEST RESULTS
• May increase cholesterol level.

CONTRAINDICATIONS
Contraindicated in patients hypersensitive to travoprost, benzalkonium chloride, or other components. Not recommended for pregnant women or in women trying to become pregnant.

NURSING CONSIDERATIONS
• Use cautiously in patients with renal or hepatic impairment, active intraocular inflammation (iritis, uveitis), or risk factors for macular edema. Also use cautiously in aphakic patients and pseudophakic patients with a torn posterior lens capsule.
• Don't use in patients with angle-closure glaucoma or inflammatory or neovascular glaucoma.
• Temporary or permanent increased pigmentation of the iris and eyelid may occur as well as increased pigmentation and growth of eyelashes.
• Patient should remove contact lenses before instilling drug. Lenses may be reinserted 15 minutes after administration.
• If more than one ophthalmic drug is being used, give the drugs at least 5 minutes apart.
• Store drug between 36° and 77° F (2° and 25° C).

• If a pregnant woman or a woman attempting to become pregnant accidentally comes in contact with drug, thoroughly cleanse the exposed area with soap and water immediately.

PATIENT TEACHING
• Teach patient to instill drops, and advise him to wash hands before and after instilling solution. Warn him not to touch dropper or tip to eye or surrounding tissue.
• Tell patient receiving treatment in only one eye about potential for increased brown pigmentation of the iris, eyelid skin darkening, and increased length, thickness, pigmentation, or number of lashes in the treated eye.
• Tell patient that, if eye trauma or infection occur or if eye surgery is needed, he should seek medical advice before continuing to use the multidose container.
• Advise patient to immediately report conjunctivitis or lid reactions.
• Advise patient to apply light finger pressure on lacrimal sac for 1 minute after instillation to minimize systemic absorption of drug.
• Tell patient to remove contact lenses before administration and explain that he can reinsert them 15 minutes afterward.
• Advise patient that, if more than one ophthalmic drug is being used, they should be given at least 5 minutes apart.
• Stress importance of compliance with recommended therapy.
• Tell patient to discard container within 6 weeks of removing it from the sealed pouch.
• If a pregnant woman or a woman attempting to become pregnant accidentally comes in contact with drug, tell her to thoroughly cleanse the exposed area with soap and water immediately.

✳ *NEW DRUG*

unoprostone isopropyl
Rescula

Pregnancy risk category C

AVAILABLE FORMS
Ophthalmic solution: 0.15% (1.5 mg/ml)

INDICATIONS & DOSAGES

➤Increased intraocular pressure (IOP) in patients with open-angle glaucoma or ocular hypertension who can't tolerate or who respond inadequately to other IOP-lowering drugs—
Adults: Instill 1 drop in affected eye b.i.d.

ACTION

Unknown. Thought to reduce elevated IOP by increasing outflow of aqueous humor.

Route	Onset	Peak	Duration
Ophthalmic	Unknown	Unknown	Unknown

ADVERSE REACTIONS

CNS: dizziness, headache, insomnia.
CV: hypertension.
EENT: abnormal vision, blepharitis, cataracts, conjunctivitis, corneal lesion, *dry eyes,* eye discharge, *eye burning or stinging, eye burning or stinging upon instillation, eye itching, eye redness,* eye discomfort, eye irritation, eye hemorrhage, decreased length of eyelashes, *increased length of eyelashes,* eyelid disorder, foreign body sensation, keratitis, lacrimal disorder, pharyngitis, photophobia, rhinitis, sinusitis, vitreous disorder.
Metabolic: diabetes mellitus.
Musculoskeletal: back pain.
Respiratory: bronchitis, increased cough.
Other: accidental injury, *allergic reaction,* flu syndrome, pain.

INTERACTIONS

None reported.

EFFECTS ON LAB TEST RESULTS

None reported.

CONTRAINDICATIONS

Contraindicated in patients hypersensitive to unoprostone isopropyl, benzalkonium chloride, or other components of product.

NURSING CONSIDERATIONS

• Use cautiously in patients with active intraocular inflammation (uveitis) or angle-closure, inflammatory, or neovascular glaucoma.
• Use cautiously in patients with renal or hepatic impairment.
• Don't give to patient wearing contact lenses because product contains benzalkonium chloride, which may be absorbed by the contact lenses. Patient should remove contact lenses before instilling and wait 15 minutes after instilling before reinserting them.
• Avoid touching tip of container to eye to avoid infection.
• Serious eye damage and blindness may result from using contaminated solutions.
• When giving another ophthalmic drug, separate administration times by 5 minutes.
• Effects of drug in breast-feeding infants is unknown. Therefore, consider risk-benefit ratio before giving drug to breast-feeding women.
• Store at 36° to 77° F (2° to 25° C).

PATIENT TEACHING

• Instruct patient to report side effects, especially conjunctivitis or eyelid reactions.
• Inform patient not to instill drops while wearing contact lenses. Tell him to remove contact lenses before instilling and then wait 15 minutes before reinserting them.
• Instruct patient to avoid touching tip of container to eye because tip could become contaminated, possibly causing an eye infection. Tell him that serious eye damage and blindness may result from using contaminated solutions.
• Before continuing to use multidose container, tell patient to notify prescriber if eye trauma or infection occurs or if ocular surgery was performed.
• Tell patient that drug can be used with other eye medications but that it's important to separate administration times by 5 minutes.
• Tell patient that drug may permanently change eye color. Change may be gradual, over months to years.
• Warn patient not to use drug if he's allergic to it, benzalkonium chloride, or other ingredients in this product.
• Instruct a woman to notify prescriber if she is breast-feeding or becomes pregnant while taking drug.

boric acid
chloramphenicol
triethanolamine polypeptide oleate-condensate

COMBINATION PRODUCTS
None.

---

boric acid
Auro-Dri◇, Dri/Ear◇, Ear-Dry◇

Pregnancy risk category NR

AVAILABLE FORMS
Otic solution: 2.75% boric acid in isopropyl alcohol

INDICATIONS & DOSAGES
➤ **External ear canal infection—**
Adults and children: 3 to 8 drops into ear canal; plug with cotton. Repeat t.i.d. or q.i.d.

ACTION
A weak bacteriostatic that inhibits or destroys bacteria in the ear canal. Is also fungistatic.

Route	Onset	Peak	Duration
Otic	Unknown	Unknown	Unknown

ADVERSE REACTIONS
EENT: ear irritation or itching.
Skin: urticaria.
Other: overgrowth of nonsusceptible organisms.

INTERACTIONS
None significant.

EFFECTS ON LAB TEST RESULTS
None reported.

CONTRAINDICATIONS
Contraindicated in patients with a perforated eardrum or excoriated membranes.

NURSING CONSIDERATIONS
• Monitor patient for signs and symptoms of superinfection.

PATIENT TEACHING
• Show patient or caregiver how to give drug.
• To prevent reinfection, warn patient to avoid touching ear with dropper.
• Tell patient using cotton plug to always moisten with drug.

---

chloramphenicol
Chloromycetin Otic

Pregnancy risk category NR

AVAILABLE FORMS
Otic solution: 0.5%

INDICATIONS & DOSAGES
➤ **External ear canal infection—**
Adults and children: 2 to 3 drops into ear canal t.i.d.

ACTION
Inhibits or destroys bacteria in ear canal.

Route	Onset	Peak	Duration
Otic	Unknown	Unknown	Unknown

ADVERSE REACTIONS
EENT: ear itching or burning.
GU: hemoglobinuria.
Hematologic: *bone marrow depression,* bone marrow hypoplasia, *aplastic anemia.*
Metabolic: lactic acidosis.
Skin: pruritus, urticaria.
Other: overgrowth of nonsusceptible organisms.

INTERACTIONS
None significant.

EFFECTS ON LAB TEST RESULTS
• May decrease hemoglobin.

Reactions may be *common*, uncommon, *life-threatening*, or COMMON AND LIFE-THREATENING.

CONTRAINDICATIONS

Contraindicated in patients hypersensitive to drug or its components and in those with perforated eardrum.

NURSING CONSIDERATIONS

• Obtain history of drug use and reactions.
• Monitor patient for signs and symptoms of superinfection. Avoid prolonged use.
• Reculture persistent drainage.
• Monitor patient for sore throat (early sign of toxicity).
• *Alert:* Don't confuse Chloromycetin with chlorambucil.

PATIENT TEACHING

• Show patient or caregiver how to give drug.
• To avoid reinfection, warn patient to avoid touching ear with dropper.

---

triethanolamine polypeptide oleate-condensate
Cerumenex

Pregnancy risk category NR

AVAILABLE FORMS

Otic solution: 10% in 6-ml, 12-ml bottles with droppers

INDICATIONS & DOSAGES

➤ **Impacted cerumen—**
Adults and children: Fill ear canal with solution and insert cotton plug. After 15 to 30 minutes, flush with warm water.

ACTION

A ceruminolytic that emulsifies and disperses accumulated cerumen.

Route	Onset	Peak	Duration
Otic	Unknown	Unknown	15-30 min

ADVERSE REACTIONS

EENT: ear erythema or itching.
Skin: severe eczema.

INTERACTIONS

None significant.

EFFECTS ON LAB TEST RESULTS

None reported.

CONTRAINDICATIONS

Contraindicated in patients with perforated eardrum, otitis media, or otitis externa.

NURSING CONSIDERATIONS

• *Alert:* If hypersensitivity is suspected, anticipate patch test. Place 1 drop of drug on inner forearm; cover with bandage. Read results in 24 hours. If reaction occurs, drug shouldn't be used.
• *Alert:* Ototoxicity may occur if drug enters middle ear.

PATIENT TEACHING

• Teach patient to moisten cotton plug with drug before insertion, leave cotton in place for a maximum of 30 minutes, and flush ear gently with warm water using a rubber bulb syringe.
• Tell patient not to use drops more often than prescribed.
• Warn patient that drug is for use only in the ears.
• Advise patient to discontinue drug and to contact prescriber immediately if adverse reactions occur.
• Tell patient to keep container tightly closed and away from moisture.

beclomethasone dipropionate
budesonide
epinephrine hydrochloride
flunisolide
fluticasone propionate
naphazoline hydrochloride
oxymetazoline hydrochloride
phenylephrine hydrochloride
tetrahydrozoline hydrochloride
triamcinolone acetonide

COMBINATION PRODUCTS
4-WAY FAST ACTING ORIGINAL ◊:
phenylephrine hydrochloride 0.5%, napha-zoline hydrochloride 0.05%, and pyril-amine maleate 0.2%.

---

beclomethasone dipropionate
Beconase, Beconase AQ, Vancenase, Vancenase AQ

Pregnancy risk category C

AVAILABLE FORMS
Nasal aerosol: 42 mcg/metered spray, 50 mcg/metered spray‡
Nasal spray: 42 mcg/metered spray, 50 mcg/metered spray‡, 84 mcg/metered spray

INDICATIONS & DOSAGES
➤ Relief from symptoms of seasonal or perennial rhinitis, prevention of recurrence of nasal polyps after surgical removal—
Adults and children older than age 12: Usual dosage is 1 or 2 sprays in each nostril, b.i.d., t.i.d., or q.i.d.
Children ages 6 to 12: 1 spray into each nostril t.i.d.

ACTION
A corticosteroid that decreases nasal in-flammation, mainly by stabilizing leuko-cyte lysosomal membranes.

Route	Onset	Peak	Duration
Nasal	5-7 days	3 wk	Unknown

ADVERSE REACTIONS
CNS: headache.
EENT: *mild transient nasal burning and stinging,* nasal congestion, sneezing, burn-ing, stinging, dryness, epistaxis, nasopha-ryngeal fungal infections.

INTERACTIONS
None significant.

EFFECTS ON LAB TEST RESULTS
None reported.

CONTRAINDICATIONS
Contraindicated in patients hypersensitive to drug and in those with untreated local-ized infection involving the nasal mucosa.

NURSING CONSIDERATIONS
• Use cautiously, if at all, in patients with active or quiescent respiratory tract tuber-culous infections or untreated fungal, bac-terial, or systemic viral or ocular herpes simplex infections. Also use cautiously in patients who have recently had nasal sep-tal ulcers, nasal surgery, or trauma.
• Observe patient for fungal infections.
• Drug isn't effective for acute exacerba-tions of rhinitis. Decongestants or antihist-amines may be needed.
• *Alert:* Don't confuse Vancenase with Vanceril.

PATIENT TEACHING
• To instill, instruct patient to shake con-tainer before use, blow nose to clear nasal passages, and tilt head slightly forward and insert nozzle into nostril, pointing away from septum. Tell him to hold other nostril closed and inhale gently while spraying. Next, have him shake container and repeat in other nostril.
• Advise patient to pump nasal spray three or four times before first use and once or twice before first use each day. The cap and nosepiece of the activator should be cleaned in warm water every day, then al-lowed to air-dry.

Reactions may be common, uncommon, *life-threatening,* or COMMON AND LIFE-THREATENING.

• Advise patient to use drug regularly, as prescribed, because its effectiveness depends on regular use.

• Explain that drug's therapeutic effects, unlike those of decongestants, aren't immediate. Most patients achieve benefit within a few days, but some may need 2 to 3 weeks.

• Warn patient not to exceed recommended dosage because of risk of hypothalamic-pituitary-adrenal axis suppression.

• Tell patient to notify prescriber if signs and symptoms don't improve within 3 weeks or if nasal irritation persists.

• Teach patient good nasal and oral hygiene.

---

budesonide
Rhinocort

Pregnancy risk category C

AVAILABLE FORMS
Nasal spray: 32 mcg/metered spray (7-g canister)

INDICATIONS & DOSAGES
➤ **Symptoms of seasonal or perennial allergic rhinitis—**
Adults and children age 6 and older:
2 sprays in each nostril in the morning and evening or 4 sprays in each nostril in the morning. Maintenance dosage should be the fewest number of sprays needed to control symptoms.

ACTION
Unknown. A corticosteroid that probably decreases nasal inflammation, mainly by inhibiting the activities of specific cells and the mediators involved in the allergic response.

Route	Onset	Peak	Duration
Nasal	10 hr	Unknown	Unknown

ADVERSE REACTIONS
CNS: nervousness.
EENT: *nasal irritation, epistaxis, pharyngitis,* reduced sense of smell, nasal pain, hoarseness.
GI: bad taste, dry mouth, dyspepsia, nausea.
Musculoskeletal: myalgia.

Respiratory: *cough,* candidiasis, wheezing, dyspnea.
Skin: facial edema, rash, pruritus, contact dermatitis.
Other: hypersensitivity reactions.

INTERACTIONS
None significant.

EFFECTS ON LAB TEST RESULTS
None reported.

CONTRAINDICATIONS
Contraindicated in patients hypersensitive to drug or its components and in those who have had recent septal ulcers, nasal surgery, or nasal trauma until total healing has occurred.

NURSING CONSIDERATIONS
• Use cautiously in patients with tuberculous infections; untreated fungal, bacterial, or systemic viral infections; or ocular herpes simplex.

• Systemic effects of corticosteroid therapy may occur if recommended daily dose is exceeded.

PATIENT TEACHING
• Tell patient to avoid exposure to chickenpox or measles.

• To instill drug, instruct patient to shake container before use, blow nose to clear nasal passages, and tilt head slightly forward and insert nozzle into nostril, pointing away from septum. Tell him to hold other nostril closed and inhale gently while spraying. Next, have him shake container and repeat in other nostril.

• Advise patient not to break, incinerate, or store canister in extreme heat; contents are under pressure.

• Advise patient to store canister with valve upward.

• Warn patient not to exceed prescribed dosage or use for long periods of time because of risk of hypothalamic-pituitary-adrenal axis suppression.

• Tell patient to contact prescriber if signs or symptoms don't improve in 3 weeks or if condition worsens.

• Teach patient good nasal and oral hygiene.

• Tell patient to use drug within 6 months of opening the protective aluminum pouch.
• Instruct patient not to share product to prevent spread of infection.

epinephrine hydrochloride
Adrenalin Chloride

Pregnancy risk category NR

AVAILABLE FORMS
Nasal solution: 0.1%

INDICATIONS & DOSAGES
➤ **Nasal congestion, local superficial bleeding—**
Adults and children age 6 and older: Instill 1 or 2 drops of solution into each nostril.

ACTION
Causes local vasoconstriction of dilated arterioles, reducing blood flow and nasal congestion.

Route	Onset	Peak	Duration
Nasal	1 min	Unknown	Unknown

ADVERSE REACTIONS
CNS: nervousness, excitation.
CV: *tachycardia.*
EENT: rebound nasal congestion, slight stinging on application.
Metabolic: hyperglycemia, lactic acidosis.

INTERACTIONS
None significant.

EFFECTS ON LAB TEST RESULTS
• May increase BUN and glucose levels.

CONTRAINDICATIONS
Contraindicated in patients hypersensitive to drug.

NURSING CONSIDERATIONS
• Use cautiously in patients with hyperthyroidism, coronary artery disease, hypertension, or diabetes mellitus.
• Monitor heart rate.
• Drug therapy may interfere with tests for urinary catecholamines.

• *Alert:* Don't confuse epinephrine with ephedrine.

PATIENT TEACHING
• Teach patient how to instill nose drops.
• Caution patient not to share product to prevent spread of infection.
• Tell patient not to exceed recommended dosage and to use only when needed.

flunisolide
Nasalide, Nasarel, Rhinalar†, Syntaris§

Pregnancy risk category C

AVAILABLE FORMS
Nasal inhalant: 25 mcg/metered spray, 200 doses/bottle‡
Nasal solution: 0.25 mg/ml in pump spray bottle (25 mcg/spray)

INDICATIONS & DOSAGES
➤ **Symptoms of seasonal or perennial rhinitis—**
Adults: Starting dose is 2 sprays (50 mcg) in each nostril b.i.d. Total daily dose is 200 mcg. If needed, dosage may be increased to 2 sprays in each nostril t.i.d. Maximum total daily dose is 8 sprays in each nostril (400 mcg daily).
Children ages 6 to 14: Starting dose is 1 spray (25 mcg) in each nostril t.i.d. or 2 sprays (50 mcg) in each nostril b.i.d. Total daily dose is 150 to 200 mcg. Maximum total daily dose is 4 sprays in each nostril (200 mcg daily).

ACTION
Exact mechanism unknown. Decreases nasal inflammation, mainly by stabilizing leukocyte lysosomal membranes.

Route	Onset	Peak	Duration
Nasal	Unknown	Unknown	Unknown

ADVERSE REACTIONS
CNS: headache.
EENT: *mild, transient nasal burning and stinging;* nasal congestion; nasopharyngeal fungal infection; burning; stinging; dryness; sneezing; epistaxis; watery eyes.
GI: nausea, vomiting.

Reactions may be *common,* uncommon, *life-threatening,* or COMMON AND LIFE-THREATENING.

INTERACTIONS
None significant.

EFFECTS ON LAB TEST RESULTS
None reported.

CONTRAINDICATIONS
Contraindicated in patients hypersensitive to drug and in those with untreated localized infection involving nasal mucosa.

NURSING CONSIDERATIONS
• Use cautiously, if at all, in patients with active or quiescent respiratory tract tuberculous infections or untreated fungal, bacterial, or systemic viral or ocular herpes simplex infections. Also use cautiously in patients who have recently had nasal septal ulcers, nasal surgery, or nasal trauma.
• Drug isn't effective for acute exacerbations of rhinitis. Decongestants or antihistamines may be needed.
• *Alert:* Don't confuse flunisolide with fluocinonide or Flumadine.

PATIENT TEACHING
• Tell patient to avoid exposure to chickenpox or measles.
• To instill drug, instruct patient to shake container before use, blow nose to clear nasal passages, and tilt head slightly forward and insert nozzle into nostril, pointing away from septum. Tell him to hold other nostril closed and inhale gently while spraying. Have him repeat procedure in other nostril. Tell him to clean nosepiece with warm water if it becomes clogged.
• Explain that drug's therapeutic effects aren't immediate. Most patients achieve benefit within few days, but some may need 2 to 3 weeks.
• Advise patient to use drug regularly, as prescribed.
• Warn patient not to exceed recommended dosage to avoid hypothalamic-pituitary-adrenal axis suppression.
• Tell patient to stop drug and notify prescriber if signs and symptoms don't diminish in 3 weeks or if nasal irritation persists.

fluticasone propionate
Flixonase§, Flonase

Pregnancy risk category C

AVAILABLE FORMS
Nasal spray: 50 mcg/metered spray (9-g, 16-g bottles)

INDICATIONS & DOSAGES
➤ **Seasonal and perennial allergic rhinitis—**
Adults: Initially, 2 sprays (100 mcg) in each nostril once daily. Or, 1 spray in each nostril b.i.d. After few days, dose may be reduced to 1 spray in each nostril daily. Maximum daily dose is 2 sprays in each nostril.
Children age 4 and older: Initially, 1 spray (50 mcg) in each nostril once daily. If patient doesn't respond or signs or symptoms are severe, increase to 2 sprays in each nostril daily. Depending on patient's response, may decrease dose to 1 spray in each nostril daily. Maximum daily dose is 2 sprays in each nostril (200 mcg/day).

ACTION
Exact mechanism unknown. Decreases nasal inflammation.

Route	Onset	Peak	Duration
Nasal	Unknown	Unknown	Unknown

ADVERSE REACTIONS
CNS: headache.
EENT: epistaxis, nasal burning, blood in nasal mucus, pharyngitis, nasal irritation.

INTERACTIONS
None significant.

EFFECTS ON LAB TEST RESULTS
None reported.

CONTRAINDICATIONS
Contraindicated in patients hypersensitive to drug or its components. Don't use drug in patients with recent nasal septal ulcers, nasal surgery, or nasal trauma until healing is complete.

NURSING CONSIDERATIONS
• Use cautiously, if at all, in patients with active or quiescent tuberculous infections;

glaucoma; untreated fungal, bacterial, or systemic viral infections; or ocular herpes simplex. Also use cautiously in patients already receiving systemic corticosteroids and in breast-feeding women.

• Although rare, immediate hypersensitivity or contact dermatitis may occur after intranasal administration.

PATIENT TEACHING
• Urge patient to read instruction sheet before using drug for first time.
• To instill drug, tell patient to shake container gently before use, blow nose to clear nasal passages, and tilt head slightly forward and insert nozzle into nostril, pointing away from septum. Tell him to hold other nostril closed and inhale gently while spraying. Next, have patient shake container and repeat procedure in other nostril.
• Stress importance of adhering to a schedule for instillation because drug effectiveness depends on regular use. Caution patient not to exceed recommended dosage; doing so may lead to hyperadrenocorticism, hypothalamic-pituitary-adrenal axis suppression, or suppression of growth in children or teenagers.
• Tell patient to notify prescriber if signs and symptoms don't improve or condition worsens.
• Warn patient to avoid exposure to chickenpox and measles and, if exposed, to obtain medical advice.
• Instruct patient to watch for and report signs and symptoms of nasal infection.
• Tell patient that sugarless gum, hard candy, and water will help to relieve dry mouth.

naphazoline hydrochloride
Privine ◇

Pregnancy risk category NR

AVAILABLE FORMS
Nasal spray: 0.05% solution
Nose drops: 0.05% solution

INDICATIONS & DOSAGES
➤ **Nasal congestion—**
Adults and children age 12 and older: 1 or 2 drops in each nostril at least 6 hours

apart. Or, 1 or 2 sprays in each nostril at least 6 hours apart.

ACTION
Causes local vasoconstriction of dilated arterioles, reducing blood flow and nasal congestion.

Route	Onset	Peak	Duration
Nasal	10 min	Unknown	2-6 hr

ADVERSE REACTIONS
CNS: restlessness, anxiety, headache.
EENT: rebound nasal congestion, sneezing, stinging, dryness of mucosa.
Other: systemic effects in children.

INTERACTIONS
None significant.

EFFECTS ON LAB TEST RESULTS
None reported.

CONTRAINDICATIONS
Contraindicated in patients hypersensitive to drug.

NURSING CONSIDERATIONS
• Use cautiously in patients with hyperthyroidism, heart disease, hypertension, or diabetes mellitus and in those who have difficulty urinating because of enlargement of prostate gland.
• Don't give to children younger than age 12 unless directed by prescriber.

PATIENT TEACHING
• Teach patient how to use drug. For nose drops, instruct patient to tilt head back as far as possible, instill drops, then lean head forward while inhaling; then repeat procedure for other nostril. For nasal spray, instruct him to hold spray container and head upright. Tell patient not to shake container.
• Caution patient not to share product to prevent spread of infection.
• Warn patient not to exceed recommended dosage.
• Tell patient not to use drug for longer than 2 to 3 days because rebound congestion may develop.
• Instruct patient to call prescriber if nasal congestion persists after 5 days.

Reactions may be *common*, uncommon, *life-threatening*, or COMMON AND LIFE-THREATENING.

oxymetazoline hydrochloride
Afrin ◇, Allerest 12 Hour Nasal Spray ◇, Chlorphed-LA ◇, Dristan 12 Hour Nasal ◇, Drixine Nasal‡, Duramist Plus ◇, Duration ◇, Genasal ◇, Neo-Synephrine 12 Hour Spray ◇, Nostrilla ◇, NTZ Long Acting Nasal ◇, Sinarest 12 Hour ◇

Pregnancy risk category NR

AVAILABLE FORMS
Nasal solution: 0.025% ◇, 0.05% ◇

INDICATIONS & DOSAGES
➤ Nasal congestion—
Adults and children age 6 and older: 2 to 3 drops or sprays of 0.05% solution in each nostril b.i.d.
Children ages 2 to 5: 2 to 3 drops of 0.025% solution in each nostril b.i.d. Use no longer than 3 to 5 days.

ACTION
Unknown. Thought to cause local vasoconstriction of dilated arterioles, reducing blood flow and nasal congestion.

Route	Onset	Peak	Duration
Nasal	5-10 min	6 hr	< 12 hr

ADVERSE REACTIONS
CNS: headache, anxiety, restlessness, dizziness, insomnia.
CV: palpitations, *CV collapse,* hypertension.
EENT: rebound nasal congestion or irritation, dryness of nose and throat, increased nasal discharge, stinging, sneezing.
Other: systemic effects in children.

INTERACTIONS
None significant.

EFFECTS ON LAB TEST RESULTS
None reported.

CONTRAINDICATIONS
Contraindicated in patients hypersensitive to drug.

NURSING CONSIDERATIONS
● Use cautiously in patients with hyperthyroidism, cardiac disease, hypertension, or diabetes mellitus.

PATIENT TEACHING
● Teach patient how to use drug. Tell him to hold head upright to minimize swallowing of drug and to sniff spray briskly.
● Caution patient not to share drug to prevent spread of infection.
● Tell patient not to exceed recommended dosage and to use only when needed.
● Inform patient that prolonged use may result in rebound congestion.
● *Alert:* Warn patient that excessive use may cause bradycardia, hypotension, dizziness, and weakness.

phenylephrine hydrochloride
Alconefrin Nasal Drops 12 ◇, Alconefrin Nasal Drops 25 ◇, Alconefrin Nasal Drops 50 ◇, Doktors ◇, Duration ◇, Neo-Synephrine ◇, Nostril ◇, Rhinall ◇, Rhinall-10 Children's Flavored Nose Drops ◇, Sinex ◇

Pregnancy risk category NR

AVAILABLE FORMS
Nasal solution: 0.125%, 0.16%, 0.25%, 0.5%, 1%

INDICATIONS & DOSAGES
➤ Nasal congestion—
Adults and children age 12 and older: 2 to 3 drops or 1 to 2 sprays in each nostril q 4 hours, p.r.n. Don't use for longer than 3 to 5 days.
Children ages 6 to 12: 2 to 3 drops or 1 to 2 sprays of 0.25% solution in each nostril q 4 hours, p.r.n.
Children younger than age 6: 2 to 3 drops of 0.125% solution q 4 hours, p.r.n.

ACTION
Causes local vasoconstriction of dilated arterioles, reducing blood flow and nasal congestion.

Route	Onset	Peak	Duration
Nasal	Rapid	Unknown	0.5-4 hr

ADVERSE REACTIONS
CNS: headache, tremor, dizziness, nervousness.
CV: *palpitations, tachycardia, **PVCs**,* hypertension, pallor.
EENT: transient burning or stinging, dryness of nasal mucosa; rebound nasal congestion.
GI: nausea.

INTERACTIONS
None significant.

EFFECTS ON LAB TEST RESULTS
None reported.

CONTRAINDICATIONS
Contraindicated in patients hypersensitive to drug.

NURSING CONSIDERATIONS
• Use cautiously in patients with hyperthyroidism, marked hypertension, type 1 diabetes mellitus, cardiac disease, or advanced arteriosclerotic changes; in children with low body weight; and in elderly patients.
• Drug may lower intraocular pressure in normal eyes or in open-angle glaucoma. It also may cause false-normal tonometry readings.

PATIENT TEACHING
• Teach patient how to use drug. Tell him to hold head upright to minimize swallowing of drug, then to sniff spray briskly.
• Caution patient not to share drug to prevent spread of infection.
• Tell patient not to exceed recommended dosage and to use only when needed.
• Advise patient to contact prescriber if signs and symptoms persist longer than 3 days.
• Inform patient that prolonged use may result in rebound congestion.

tetrahydrozoline hydrochloride
Tyzine, Tyzine Pediatric

Pregnancy risk category C

AVAILABLE FORMS
Nasal solution: 0.05%, 0.1%

INDICATIONS & DOSAGES
➤**Nasal congestion—**
Adults and children older than age 6: 2 to 4 drops of 0.1% solution or spray into each nostril q 4 to 6 hours, p.r.n.
Children ages 2 to 6: 2 to 3 drops of 0.05% solution into each nostril q 4 to 6 hours, p.r.n.

ACTION
Unknown. Thought to cause local vasoconstriction of dilated arterioles, reducing blood flow and nasal congestion.

Route	Onset	Peak	Duration
Nasal	Few min	Unknown	4-8 hr

ADVERSE REACTIONS
EENT: transient burning, stinging; sneezing; rebound nasal congestion.

INTERACTIONS
None significant.

EFFECTS ON LAB TEST RESULTS
None reported.

CONTRAINDICATIONS
Contraindicated in patients hypersensitive to drug, in those with angle-closure glaucoma or other serious eye diseases, and in children younger than age 2. The 0.1% solution is contraindicated in children younger than age 6.

NURSING CONSIDERATIONS
• Use cautiously in patients with hyperthyroidism, hypertension, and diabetes mellitus.

PATIENT TEACHING
• Teach patient how to use drug. Tell him to hold head upright to minimize swallowing of drug, then to sniff spray briskly.
• Caution patient not to share product to prevent spread of infection.
• Tell patient not to exceed recommended dosage and to use only as needed for 3 to 5 days.

Reactions may be *common*, uncommon, *life-threatening*, or COMMON AND LIFE-THREATENING.

triamcinolone acetonide
Nasacort, Nasacort AQ

Pregnancy risk category C

AVAILABLE FORMS
Nasal aerosol: 55 mcg/metered spray
Nasal spray pump: 55 mcg/spray

INDICATIONS & DOSAGES
➤ **Rhinitis, allergic disorders, inflammatory conditions, nasal polyps—**
Adults: 2 sprays (Nasacort) in each nostril daily; may increase dose to maximum of 4 sprays per nostril daily, if needed. Or 2 sprays (Nasacort AQ) in each nostril daily; may decrease to 1 spray in each nostril daily for allergic disorders.
Children ages 6 to 12: 2 sprays (Nasacort) in each nostril daily. Or, 1 spray (Nasacort AQ) in each nostril daily. Maximum 2 sprays in each nostril daily.

ACTION
Unknown. A glucocorticoid with anti-inflammatory properties.

Route	Onset	Peak	Duration
Nasal	12 hr	3-4 days	Unknown

ADVERSE REACTIONS
CNS: *headache.*
EENT: *nasal irritation,* dry mucous membranes, nasal and sinus congestion, irritation, burning, stinging, throat discomfort, sneezing, epistaxis.

INTERACTIONS
None significant.

EFFECTS ON LAB TEST RESULTS
None reported.

CONTRAINDICATIONS
Contraindicated in patients hypersensitive to drug or its components.

NURSING CONSIDERATIONS
• Use with extreme caution, if at all, in patients with active or quiescent tuberculosis infection of respiratory tract and in patients with untreated fungal, bacterial, or systemic viral infection or ocular herpes simplex.
• Use cautiously in patients already receiving systemic corticosteroids because of increased likelihood of hypothalamic-pituitary-adrenal axis suppression compared with therapeutic dosage of either one alone; in those with recent nasal septal ulcers, nasal surgery, or trauma because of inhibitory effect on wound healing; and in breast-feeding women.
• **Alert:** When excessive doses are used, signs and symptoms of hyperadrenocorticism and adrenal axis suppression may occur; drug should be discontinued slowly.
• **Alert:** Don't confuse triamcinolone with Triaminicin.

PATIENT TEACHING
• Urge patient to read patient instruction sheet contained in each package before using drug for first time.
• To instill, instruct patient to shake container before use, blow nose to clear nasal passages, and tilt head slightly forward and insert nozzle into nostril, pointing away from septum. Tell him to hold other nostril closed and inhale gently while spraying. Next, have patient shake container and repeat procedure in other nostril.
• Instruct patient to avoid getting aerosol in eyes. If this occurs, rinse with copious amounts of cool tap water.
• Tell patient to discard canister after 100 actuations.
• Stress importance of using drug on a regular schedule because its effectiveness depends on regular use. However, caution patient not to exceed dosage prescribed because serious adverse reactions can occur.
• Tell patient to notify prescriber if signs and symptoms don't diminish in 2 to 3 weeks or if condition worsens.
• Warn patient to avoid exposure to chickenpox or measles and, if exposed, to obtain medical advice.
• Instruct patient to watch for and report signs and symptoms of nasal infection. Drug may need to be discontinued and appropriate local therapy given.
• Advise patient not to break or incinerate canister or store it in extreme heat; contents are under pressure and may explode.

---

acyclovir
amphotericin B
azelaic acid cream
bacitracin
clindamycin phosphate
clotrimazole
docosanol
econazole nitrate
erythromycin
gentamicin sulfate
ketoconazole
metronidazole
miconazole nitrate
mupirocin
neomycin sulfate
nitrofurazone
nystatin
silver sulfadiazine
terbinafine hydrochloride
terconazole
tolnaftate

COMBINATION PRODUCTS
BENZAMYCIN: erythromycin 3% and benzoyl peroxide 5%.
LANABIOTIC ◇: polymyxin B sulfate 10,000 units, neomycin sulfate 3.5 mg, bacitracin 500 units, and lidocaine 40 mg/g.
LOTRISONE: clotrimazole 1% and betamethasone dipropionate 0.05%.
MYCITRACIN ◇: polymyxin B sulfate 5,000 units, bacitracin 500 units, and neomycin sulfate 3.5 mg/g.
MYCOLOG-II: triamcinolone acetonide 0.1% and nystatin 100,000 units/g.
NEOSPORIN CREAM ◇: polymyxin B sulfate 10,000 units and neomycin sulfate 3.5 mg/g.
NEOSPORIN OINTMENT ◇: polymyxin B sulfate 5,000 units, bacitracin zinc 400 units, and neomycin sulfate 3.5 mg/g.
POLYSPORIN OPHTHALMIC OINTMENT ◇: polymyxin B sulfate 10,000 units and bacitracin zinc 500 units/g.

acyclovir
Acyclo-V‡, Avirax†, Zovirax

Pregnancy risk category C

AVAILABLE FORMS
Ointment: 5%

INDICATIONS & DOSAGES
➤ Initial herpes genitalis; limited, non–life-threatening mucocutaneous herpes simplex virus infections in immunocompromised patients—
Adults: Cover all lesions q 3 hours six times daily for 7 days. Although dose varies depending on total lesion area, use about ½-inch (1.3-cm) ribbon of ointment on each 4-inch (10-cm) square of surface area.

ACTION
Inhibits herpes simplex and varicella-zoster viral DNA synthesis by inhibiting viral DNA polymerase action.

Route	Onset	Peak	Duration
Topical	Unknown	Unknown	Unknown

ADVERSE REACTIONS
GU: vulvitis.
Skin: *transient burning and stinging,* rash, pruritus.
Other: edema, pain at application site.

INTERACTIONS
None significant.

EFFECTS ON LAB TEST RESULTS
None reported.

CONTRAINDICATIONS
Contraindicated in patients hypersensitive to drug and patients with chemical intolerance to drug.

NURSING CONSIDERATIONS
● Start therapy as early as possible after signs or symptoms begin.
● Apply drug with a finger cot or rubber glove to prevent autoinoculation of other

body sites and transmission of infection to other persons.
• All lesions must be thoroughly covered.
• Drug is for cutaneous use only; don't apply to eye.
• Drug isn't a cure, but it will help with signs and symptoms.

PATIENT TEACHING
• Teach patient that virus transmission can occur during treatment.
• Tell patient that there may be some discomfort with application.
• Stress importance of compliance for successful therapy.
• Teach patient that therapy should begin as soon as signs and symptoms appear.
• Tell patient to notify prescriber if adverse reactions occur.
• Instruct patient to store drug in a dry place at 59° to 77° F (15° to 25° C).

---

amphotericin B
Fungizone

Pregnancy risk category B

AVAILABLE FORMS
Cream: 3%
Lotion: 3%
Ointment: 3%

INDICATIONS & DOSAGES
➤ **Cutaneous or mucocutaneous candidal infections—**
Adults and children: Apply liberally, rubbing in gently b.i.d. to q.i.d. for 1 to 3 weeks. Interdigital lesions and paronychias are treated for 2 to 4 weeks, and onychomycosis for several months because relapses are common.

ACTION
Usually fungistatic; binds to sterols in the fungal cell membrane, resulting in increased membrane permeability and subsequent cell leakage.

Route	Onset	Peak	Duration
Topical	Unknown	Unknown	Unknown

ADVERSE REACTIONS
Skin: possible dryness, contact sensitivity, erythema, burning, pruritus.

INTERACTIONS
None significant.

EFFECTS ON LAB TEST RESULTS
None reported.

CONTRAINDICATIONS
Contraindicated in patients hypersensitive to drug or its components.

NURSING CONSIDERATIONS
• Clean area before applying drug.
• Report local irritation. Cream may dry skin; ointment may irritate if applied to moist, hairy areas.
• Avoid using occlusive dressings.
• Cream or lotion is preferred for such areas as groin folds, armpits, and neck creases.
• Stop drug if irritation or hypersensitivity occurs, and notify prescriber.

PATIENT TEACHING
• Tell patient to use drug for full treatment period, even if condition has improved.
• Inform patient that skin may become discolored if amphotericin B isn't rubbed in thoroughly; nail lesions may become stained.
• Caution patient against application to eyes.
• Tell patient that fabric discoloration caused by cream or lotion can be removed by washing; discoloration by ointment can be removed with cleaning fluid.
• Instruct patient not to apply occlusive dressing.

---

azelaic acid cream
Azelex, Finevin, Skinoren§

Pregnancy risk category B

AVAILABLE FORMS
Cream: 20%

INDICATIONS & DOSAGES
➤ **Mild to moderate inflammatory acne vulgaris—**
Adults: Apply thin film and gently but thoroughly massage into affected areas b.i.d., in morning and evening.

---

*Liquid contains alcohol.   **May contain tartrazine.   †Canada   ‡Australia   §U.K.   ◇OTC

ACTION
Unknown. May inhibit microbial cellular protein synthesis.

Route	Onset	Peak	Duration
Topical	Unknown	Unknown	Unknown

ADVERSE REACTIONS
Skin: pruritus, burning, stinging, tingling.

INTERACTIONS
None significant.

EFFECTS ON LAB TEST RESULTS
None reported.

CONTRAINDICATIONS
Contraindicated in patients hypersensitive to drug or its components.

NURSING CONSIDERATIONS
• Use cautiously in pregnant and breast-feeding women.
• Monitor patient for early signs and symptoms of hypopigmentation, especially patient with dark complexion.
• If sensitivity or severe irritation occurs, notify prescriber, who may discontinue drug and order appropriate treatment.
• Avoid using occlusive dressings.

PATIENT TEACHING
• Instruct patient to wash and pat dry affected areas before applying drug and to wash hands well after application. Warn him not to apply occlusive dressings or wrappings to affected areas.
• Warn patient that skin irritation may occur, usually at start of therapy, when drug is applied to broken or inflamed skin. Tell him to notify prescriber if irritation persists.
• Advise patient to keep drug away from mouth, eyes, and other mucous membranes. If contact occurs, tell him to rinse thoroughly with water and to notify prescriber if irritation persists.
• Advise patient to report abnormal changes in skin color.
• Urge patient to use drug for full treatment period. In most patients with inflammatory lesions, improvement occurs in 1 to 2 months.
• Instruct patient to store drug at 59° to 86° F (15° to 30° C) and protect it from freezing.

bacitracin
Baciguent ◇

Pregnancy risk category C

AVAILABLE FORMS
Ointment: 500 units/g

INDICATIONS & DOSAGES
➤ **Topical infections, abrasions, cuts, minor burns or wounds—**
Adults and children: Apply thin film daily to t.i.d., based on severity of condition. Drug shouldn't be used for longer than 1 week.

ACTION
Bactericidal or bacteriostatic, depending on organism and concentration of drug; inhibits bacterial cell-wall synthesis. Effective against gram-positive organisms.

Route	Onset	Peak	Duration
Topical	Unknown	Unknown	Unknown

ADVERSE REACTIONS
Skin: stinging, rash, other allergic reactions, allergic contact dermatitis, pruritus, burning, swelling of lips or face.
Other: *anaphylaxis.*

INTERACTIONS
None significant.

EFFECTS ON LAB TEST RESULTS
None reported.

CONTRAINDICATIONS
Contraindicated in patients hypersensitive to drug and in patients with atopy.

NURSING CONSIDERATIONS
• Clean skin before applying drug, especially if skin is crusted or suppurative.
• Anticipate alternative treatment for burns that cover over 20% of body surface area, especially if patient has impaired renal function.
• Prolonged use may result in overgrowth of nonsusceptible organisms, particularly *Candida* species.
• Patients allergic to neomycin may also be sensitive to bacitracin.

Reactions may be *common,* uncommon, *life-threatening,* or COMMON AND LIFE-THREATENING.

• Before applying drug, obtain culture and sensitivity tests.
• *Alert:* Don't confuse bacitracin with Bactroban.

PATIENT TEACHING
• Tell patient to stop using drug and notify prescriber if improvement doesn't occur or if condition worsens.
• Instruct patient to report persistent or severe adverse reactions.
• Tell patient not to use drug for longer than 1 week, except on prescriber's advice.

---

clindamycin phosphate
Cleocin, Cleocin T, Clinda-Derm, Clindets

Pregnancy risk category B

AVAILABLE FORMS
Gel: 1%
Lotion: 1%
Pledget: 1%
Topical solution: 1%
Vaginal cream: 2%

INDICATIONS & DOSAGES
➤ **Inflammatory acne vulgaris—**
Adults and adolescents: Apply to skin b.i.d., morning and evening.
➤ **Bacterial vaginosis—**
Adults: 1 applicatorful intravaginally h.s. for 7 consecutive days.

ACTION
Bacteriostatic or bactericidal based on drug level and susceptibility of organism; suppresses growth of susceptible organisms in sebaceous glands by blocking protein synthesis.

Route	Onset	Peak	Duration
Intravaginal, topical	Unknown	Unknown	Unknown

ADVERSE REACTIONS
GI: GI upset, diarrhea, bloody diarrhea, abdominal pain, colitis including pseudomembranous colitis.
GU: *cervicitis, vaginitis, Candida albicans* overgrowth, *vulvar irritation.*

Skin: *dryness,* rash, *redness,* pruritus, swelling, irritation, contact dermatitis, burning.

INTERACTIONS
Drug-drug. *Erythromycin:* May antagonize clindamycin's effect. Separate administration times.
Isotretinoin: Potential cumulative dryness, resulting in excessive skin irritation. Use cautiously.
Neuromuscular blockers: May increase action of neuromuscular blocker. Use cautiously together.
Drug-lifestyle. *Abrasive or medicated soaps or cleansers, acne products or other preparations containing peeling drugs (benzoyl peroxide, resorcinol, salicylic acid, sulfur, tretinoin), alcohol-containing products (aftershave, cosmetics, perfumed toiletries, shaving creams or lotions), astringent soaps or cosmetics, medicated cosmetics or cover-ups:* Potential cumulative dryness, resulting in excessive skin irritation. Urge caution.

EFFECTS ON LAB TEST RESULTS
• May increase liver enzyme levels.

CONTRAINDICATIONS
Contraindicated in patients hypersensitive to drug and in those with history of ulcerative colitis, regional enteritis, or antibiotic-related colitis.

NURSING CONSIDERATIONS
• For treating acne, drug may be used with tretinoin or benzoyl peroxide as well as systemic antibiotics.
• Drug can cause excessive dryness.
• Monitor elderly patients for systemic effects.

PATIENT TEACHING
• Tell patient to wash area with warm water and soap, rinse, pat dry, and wait 30 minutes after washing or shaving to apply.
• Warn patient to avoid excessive washing of area. Tell patient to cover entire affected area but to avoid contact with eyes, nose, mouth, and other areas bearing mucous membranes.
• Instruct patient to use other prescribed acne medicines at a different time.
• Tell patient to use only as prescribed.

- Instruct patient to dab, not roll, applicator-tipped bottle. If tip becomes dry, patient should invert bottle and depress tip several times to moisten.
- Warn patient not to smoke while applying topical solution.
- For intravaginal application, make sure patient knows how to use applicators that come with drug.
- Advise patient to avoid sexual intercourse during intravaginal treatment.
- Instruct patient to notify prescriber immediately if abdominal pain or diarrhea occurs. Inform him that antidiarrheal drug may worsen condition and should only be used as directed by prescriber.
- Tell patient to remove pledgets from foil before use.
- Advise patients that pledgets should be used only once, then discarded. Also, more than 1 pledget may be used per application.
- Advise patient to complete the entire course of therapy.

---

clotrimazole
Canesten†, Fungoid Crème,
Gyne-Lotrimin ◇, Lotrimin,
Lotrimin AF, Mycelex,
Mycelex-7 ◇, Mycelex-G

Pregnancy risk category B (C for troches)

AVAILABLE FORMS
Combination pack: Vaginal tablets 100 mg and vulvar cream 1% ◇; vaginal tablets 200 mg and vulvar cream 1% ◇
Topical cream: 1%
Topical lotion: 1%
Topical solution: 1%
Troches: 10 mg
Vaginal cream: 1% ◇
Vaginal tablets: 100 mg ◇, 200 mg ◇

INDICATIONS & DOSAGES
➤ **Superficial fungal infections (tinea corporis, tinea cruris, tinea pedis, tinea versicolor, candidiasis)—**
Adults and children: Apply thinly and massage into affected and surrounding area, morning and evening, for 2 to 4 weeks. If improvement doesn't occur after 4 weeks, patient should be reevaluated.

➤ **Vulvovaginal candidiasis—**
Adults: One 100-mg vaginal tablet inserted daily h.s. for 7 consecutive days. Or, one 500-mg vaginal tablet daily h.s. for 1 day. Or, 1 applicatorful of vaginal cream daily h.s. for 7 days.
➤ **Oropharyngeal candidiasis—**
Adults and children age 3 and older: Dissolve troche over 15 to 30 minutes in mouth five times daily for 14 consecutive days.
➤ **Prevention of oropharyngeal candidiasis in patients immunocompromised by such conditions as chemotherapy, radiotherapy, or corticosteroid therapy in the treatment of leukemia, solid tumors, or renal transplantation—**
Adults and children: Dissolve troche over 15 to 30 minutes in mouth t.i.d. for duration of chemotherapy or until corticosteroid is reduced to maintenance levels.

ACTION
Fungistatic but may be fungicidal depending on level. Alters fungal cell-wall permeability and produces osmotic instability.

Route	Onset	Peak	Duration
Intravaginal, topical	Unknown	Unknown	Unknown
P.O.	Unknown	Unknown	3 hr

ADVERSE REACTIONS
GI: lower abdominal cramps, nausea and vomiting with lozenges.
GU: *mild vaginal burning or irritation,* cramping, urinary frequency.
Skin: blistering, *erythema,* edema, pruritus, burning, stinging, peeling, urticaria, skin fissures, general irritation.

INTERACTIONS
None significant.

EFFECTS ON LAB TEST RESULTS
- May increase liver enzyme levels.

CONTRAINDICATIONS
Contraindicated in patients hypersensitive to drug. Also contraindicated for ophthalmic use.

NURSING CONSIDERATIONS
- Clean area before applying drug.

• Watch for and report irritation or sensitivity; discontinue if irritation occurs, and notify prescriber.

• Improvement usually occurs within 1 week; if no improvement is seen within 4 weeks, diagnosis should be reviewed.

• *Alert:* Don't confuse clotrimazole with co-trimoxazole.

PATIENT TEACHING

• Reassure patient that hypopigmentation from tinea versicolor will resolve gradually.

• Warn patient not to use occlusive wrappings or dressings.

• Warn patient to avoid drug contact with eyes.

• Caution patient that frequent or persistent yeast infections may suggest a more serious medical problem.

• Tell patient to refrain from sexual intercourse during intravaginal treatment.

• Warn patient that topical preparation may stain clothing.

• Tell patient that use of a sanitary napkin will protect clothing when using vaginal preparation.

• Emphasize continued use of vaginal preparations, as prescribed, even if menses begins.

• Tell patient with tinea pedis to change shoes and cotton socks daily.

• Tell patient to allow troches to dissolve in mouth; for maximum benefit, advise against chewing.

• Emphasize need to continue treatment for full course and to notify prescriber if no improvement occurs after 4 weeks.

✳ *NEW DRUG*

docosanol
Abreva ◇

Pregnancy risk category B

AVAILABLE FORMS
Cream: 10% ◇

INDICATIONS & DOSAGES
➤ **Recurrent oral and facial herpes simplex—**

Adults and children age 12 and older: Applied topically five times daily, starting with first indication of an episode and continuing until lesion is healed. Rub in gently but completely.

ACTION
Main mechanism appears to be inhibition of fusion between the cell's plasma membrane and the herpes simplex virus envelope, which blocks the entry and subsequent replication of the virus.

Route	Onset	Peak	Duration
Topical	Unknown	Unknown	Unknown

ADVERSE REACTIONS
CNS: *headache.*
Skin: reaction at application site.

INTERACTIONS
None reported.

EFFECTS ON LAB TEST RESULTS
None reported.

CONTRAINDICATIONS
Contraindicated in patients hypersensitive to drug or any of its components.

NURSING CONSIDERATIONS
• Use drug only to treat oral and facial herpes simplex lesions.

• Start treatment as early as possible after signs or symptoms begin.

• Continue treatment until the lesion has healed.

• Avoid application in or near the patient's eyes.

• It isn't known if docosanol appears in breast milk. Use cautiously in breast-feeding patients.

PATIENT TEACHING
• Advise patient to start treatment as soon as signs or symptoms appear.

• Tell patient to use cream only on lips or face.

• Caution patient not to apply drug in or near the eyes because it may cause irritation.

• Tell patient to continue treatment until the lesion has healed.

• Notify patient that lesions are considered contagious until completely healed.

• Urge patient to notify prescriber if the condition gets worse.

• Caution patient that drug should be used during pregnancy only if clearly needed.
• Advise patient to store drug at room temperature and not to freeze it.

econazole nitrate
Ecostatin†, Prevaryl§, Spectazole

Pregnancy risk category C

AVAILABLE FORMS
Cream: 1%

INDICATIONS & DOSAGES
➤ **Tinea corporis, tinea cruris, tinea pedis, tinea versicolor, cutaneous candidiasis—**
Adults and children: Rub into affected areas daily for at least 2 weeks.
➤ **Cutaneous candidiasis—**
Adults and children: Rub into affected areas b.i.d.

ACTION
Fungistatic but may be fungicidal depending on level. Alters fungal cell-wall permeability and produces osmotic instability.

Route	Onset	Peak	Duration
Topical	Unknown	Unknown	Unknown

ADVERSE REACTIONS
Skin: burning, pruritus, stinging, erythema.

INTERACTIONS
None significant.

EFFECTS ON LAB TEST RESULTS
None reported.

CONTRAINDICATIONS
Contraindicated in patients hypersensitive to drug or its components.

NURSING CONSIDERATIONS
• Clean affected area before applying.
• Don't use occlusive dressings.

PATIENT TEACHING
• Tell patient to use drug for entire treatment period, even if signs and symptoms improve. Instruct him to notify prescriber if no improvement occurs after 2 weeks

(tinea corporis, tinea cruris, and tinea versicolor) or 4 weeks (tinea pedis).
• Reassure patient that hypopigmentation from tinea versicolor will resolve gradually.
• Tell patient to stop drug and call prescriber if condition persists or worsens or if irritation occurs.
• Warn patient that drug may stain clothing.
• Tell patient with tinea pedis to change shoes and cotton socks daily.
• Tell patient to keep drug out of eyes.

erythromycin
Akne-mycin, A/T/S, Del-Mycin, Erycette, EryDerm, Erygel, Erymax, Erysol†, ETS†, Sans-Acne†, Staticin, T-Stat†

Pregnancy risk category C (B for EryDerm, Erygel)

AVAILABLE FORMS
Ointment: 2%
Pledgets: 2%
Topical gel: 2%
Topical solution: 1.5%*, 2%*

INDICATIONS & DOSAGES
➤ **Inflammatory acne vulgaris—**
Adults and children: Apply to affected areas b.i.d. morning and evening.

ACTION
Usually bacteriostatic but may be bactericidal in high concentrations or against highly susceptible organisms. Disrupts protein synthesis in susceptible bacteria.

Route	Onset	Peak	Duration
Topical	Unknown	Unknown	Unknown

ADVERSE REACTIONS
Skin: sensitivity reactions, erythema, *burning, dryness, pruritus,* irritation, peeling, oily skin.

INTERACTIONS
Drug-drug. *Clindamycin:* May antagonize clindamycin's effect. Separate administration times.

Reactions may be *common*, uncommon, *life-threatening*, or COMMON AND LIFE-THREATENING.

Isotretinoin: May cause cumulative dryness, resulting in excessive skin irritation. Use cautiously.

Drug-lifestyle. *Abrasive or medicated soaps or cleansers, acne products or other preparations containing peeling drugs (benzoyl peroxide, resorcinol, salicylic acid, sulfur, tretinoin), alcohol-containing products (aftershave, cosmetics, perfumed toiletries, shaving creams or lotions), astringent soaps or cosmetics, medicated cosmetics or cover-ups:* May cause cumulative dryness, resulting in excessive skin irritation. Urge caution.

EFFECTS ON LAB TEST RESULTS
None reported.

CONTRAINDICATIONS
Contraindicated in patients hypersensitive to drug or its components.

NURSING CONSIDERATIONS
● Obtain cultures before beginning therapy.
● Before reconstitution, store drug at room temperature. After reconstitution, refrigerate drug; don't freeze. Expiration date is up to 4 months from date of reconstitution.
● Wash, rinse, and dry affected areas before application.
● Prolonged use may be needed when treating acne vulgaris, which may result in overgrowth of nonsusceptible organisms.
● Drug may interfere with fluorometric determinations of urinary catecholamines.

PATIENT TEACHING
● Advise patient to wash, rinse, and dry face thoroughly before each use.
● Advise patient to avoid use near eyes, nose, mouth, or other areas bearing mucous membranes.
● Tell patient to wash hands after each application.
● Tell patient to stop using drug and notify prescriber if no improvement occurs or if condition worsens.
● Advise patient not to share towels or washcloths.
● Instruct patient to use each pledget once, then discard.

● Caution patient to keep drug away from heat and open flame.

---

gentamicin sulfate
Garamycin, G-Myticin

Pregnancy risk category C

AVAILABLE FORMS
Cream: 0.1%
Ointment: 0.1%

INDICATIONS & DOSAGES
➤ **Treatment and prophylaxis of superficial infections and superficial burns of the skin caused by susceptible bacteria—**
Adults and children older than age 1: Rub in small amount gently t.i.d. or q.i.d., with or without gauze dressing.

ACTION
Exact mechanism unknown. A bactericidal drug that disrupts bacterial protein synthesis by binding to ribosomes.

Route	Onset	Peak	Duration
Topical	Unknown	Unknown	Unknown

ADVERSE REACTIONS
Skin: minor skin irritation, possible photosensitivity, allergic contact dermatitis.

INTERACTIONS
None significant.

EFFECTS ON LAB TEST RESULTS
None reported.

CONTRAINDICATIONS
Contraindicated in patients hypersensitive to drug and its components and in those who may have cross-sensitivity with other aminoglycosides such as neomycin.

NURSING CONSIDERATIONS
● *Alert:* Avoid use on large skin lesions or over a wide area because of possible systemic toxic effects.
● Restrict use of drug to selected patients; widespread use may lead to resistant organisms.
● Prolonged use may result in overgrowth of nonsusceptible organisms.

PATIENT TEACHING
• Tell patient to clean affected area before applying drug and, to increase absorption, have him remove crusts for impetigo before applying drug.
• Instruct patient to store drug in cool place.
• Tell patient to stop drug and notify prescriber immediately if no improvement occurs or if condition worsens.

---

ketoconazole
Nizoral, Nizoral A-D ◇

Pregnancy risk category C

AVAILABLE FORMS
Cream: 2%
Shampoo: 1% ◇, 2%

INDICATIONS & DOSAGES
➤ **Tinea corporis, tinea cruris, tinea pedis, tinea versicolor from susceptible organisms; seborrheic dermatitis; cutaneous candidiasis—**
Adults: Cover affected and immediate surrounding area daily for at least 2 weeks. For seborrheic dermatitis, apply b.i.d. for 4 weeks. Patients with tinea pedis need 6 weeks of treatment. When using shampoo, wet hair, lather, and massage for 1 minute. Rinse and repeat, but leave drug on scalp for 3 minutes before rinsing. Shampoo twice weekly for 4 weeks, with at least 3 days between shampoos and then intermittently, p.r.n., to maintain control.

ACTION
Unknown. An imidazole that probably inhibits yeast growth by altering the permeability of the cell membrane.

Route	Onset	Peak	Duration
Topical	Unknown	Unknown	Unknown

ADVERSE REACTIONS
Skin: severe irritation, pruritus, and stinging with cream; increase in normal hair loss; irritation; abnormal hair texture; scalp pustules; pruritus, oiliness, or dryness of hair and scalp with shampoo use.

INTERACTIONS
Drug-drug. *Topical corticosteroids:* May cause increased absorption of corticosteroid. Avoid using together.

EFFECTS ON LAB TEST RESULTS
None reported.

CONTRAINDICATIONS
Contraindicated in patients hypersensitive to drug or its components.

NURSING CONSIDERATIONS
• Use cautiously in breast-feeding women.
• Most patients show improvement soon after treatment begins.
• Treatment of tinea corporis or tinea cruris should continue for at least 2 weeks to reduce possibility of recurrence.
• *Alert:* Product contains sodium sulfite anhydrous, which may cause severe or life-threatening allergic reactions, including anaphylaxis, in patients with asthma.

PATIENT TEACHING
• Tell patient to stop drug and notify prescriber if hypersensitivity reaction occurs.
• Advise patient to check with prescriber if condition worsens; drug may have to be discontinued and diagnosis reevaluated.
• Warn patient that shampoo applied to permanent-waved hair removes curl.
• Warn patient to avoid contact of drug with eyes.
• Tell patient to continue drug for intended duration of therapy, even if signs and symptoms improve soon after starting treatment.
• Tell patient not to store drug above room temperature (77° F [25° C]) and to protect from light.

---

metronidazole
MetroCream, MetroGel, MetroGel Vaginal, MetroLotion, Noritate

Pregnancy risk category B

AVAILABLE FORMS
Topical cream: 0.75%, 1%
Topical gel: 0.75%
Topical lotion: 0.75%
Vaginal gel: 0.75%

INDICATIONS & DOSAGES
➤ **Inflammatory papules and pustules of acne rosacea—**
Adults: Apply thin film to affected area b.i.d., morning and evening. Frequency and duration of therapy adjusted after response is seen. Results usually noticed within 3 weeks.
➤ **Bacterial vaginosis—**
Adults: 1 applicatorful intravaginally daily or b.i.d. for 5 days. For once-daily dosing, give h.s.

ACTION
Unknown. May cause bactericidal effect by interacting with bacterial DNA. It's active against many anaerobic gram-negative bacilli, anaerobic gram-positive cocci, *Gardnerella vaginalis,* and *Campylobacter fetus.*

Route	Onset	Peak	Duration
Intravaginal	Unknown	6-12 hr	Unknown
Topical	Unknown	Unknown	Unknown

ADVERSE REACTIONS
Topical cream or gel
EENT: lacrimation if applied around eyes.
Skin: rash, *transient redness, dryness, mild burning, stinging.*
Vaginal form
CNS: dizziness, headache.
GI: cramps, pain, nausea, diarrhea, constipation, metallic or bad taste in mouth, decreased appetite.
GU: *cervicitis, vaginitis,* perineal and vulvovaginal itching.
Skin: rash, *transient redness, dryness, mild burning, stinging.*
Other: overgrowth of nonsusceptible organisms.

INTERACTIONS
Drug-drug. *Disulfiram:* Disulfiram-like reaction may occur. Avoid using together and wait 2 weeks after stopping disulfiram before starting metronidazole vaginal therapy.
Oral anticoagulants: May increase anticoagulant effect. Monitor patient for adverse reactions.
Drug-lifestyle. *Alcohol use:* Disulfiram-like reaction may occur. Discourage patient from use together.

EFFECTS ON LAB TEST RESULTS
● May increase or decrease WBC count.

CONTRAINDICATIONS
Contraindicated in patients hypersensitive to drug or its ingredients, such as parabens, and other nitroimidazole derivatives.

NURSING CONSIDERATIONS
● Use cautiously in patients with history or evidence of blood dyscrasia and in those with severe hepatic disease.
● Use vaginal gel cautiously in patients with history of CNS diseases. Oral form may cause seizures and peripheral neuropathy.
● Topical therapy hasn't been linked to adverse effects observed with parenteral or oral therapy; however, some drug may be absorbed after topical use.
● Don't use vaginal gel in patients who have taken disulfiram within past 2 weeks.
● Oral form has been linked to psychotic reaction.

PATIENT TEACHING
● Instruct patient to avoid use of topical gel around eyes.
● Advise patient to clean area thoroughly before use and to wait 15 to 20 minutes after cleaning skin before applying drug to minimize risk of local irritation. Cosmetics may be used after applying drug.
● If local reactions occur, advise patient to apply drug less frequently or discontinue its use and contact prescriber.
● Advise patient to avoid sexual intercourse while using vaginal preparation.
● Caution patient not to drink alcohol while being treated with vaginal preparation.

---

miconazole nitrate
Daktarin§, Femizol-M, Gyno-Daktarin§, Lotrimin AF◇, Micatin◇, Monistat Derm, Monistat 3, Monistat 7◇

Pregnancy risk category C

AVAILABLE FORMS
Cream: 2%
Powder: 2%

Spray: 2%
Topical ointment: 2%
Topical solution: 2%
Vaginal cream: 2%
Vaginal suppositories: 100 mg, 200 mg

INDICATIONS & DOSAGES
➤ **Tinea corporis, tinea cruris, tinea pedis; cutaneous candidiasis; common dermatophyte infections—**
Adults and children older than age 1: Apply sparingly b.i.d. for 2 to 4 weeks. Powder or spray can be used liberally over affected area.
➤ **Tinea versicolor—**
Adults and children older than age 1: Apply sparingly daily for 2 weeks.
➤ **Vulvovaginal candidiasis—**
Adults: 1 applicatorful or 100-mg suppository (Monistat 7) intravaginally h.s. for 7 days; course repeated, if needed. Or, 200-mg suppository (Monistat 3) intravaginally h.s. for 3 days. Apply topical cream sparingly to affected area b.i.d. for 7 days.

ACTION
A fungicidal imidazole that disrupts fungal cell membrane permeability.

Route	Onset	Peak	Duration
Intravaginal, topical	Unknown	Unknown	Unknown

ADVERSE REACTIONS
CNS: headache.
GU: pelvic cramps; vulvovaginal burning, pruritus, and irritation with vaginal cream.
Skin: irritation, burning, maceration, allergic contact dermatitis.

INTERACTIONS
None significant.

EFFECTS ON LAB TEST RESULTS
None reported.

CONTRAINDICATIONS
Contraindicated in patients hypersensitive to drug or its components.

NURSING CONSIDERATIONS
• Use together (within 72 hours) of intravaginal forms and certain latex products, such as condoms or vaginal contraceptive diaphragms, isn't recommended because of possible interaction.
• Don't use occlusive dressings.
• Lotion should be used in intertriginous areas.

PATIENT TEACHING
• Advise patient that vaginal form of drug is for perineal or intravaginal use only and to keep drug out of eyes.
• Caution patient that frequent or persistent yeast infections may suggest a more serious medical problem.
• Tell patient to cautiously insert intravaginal form high into the vagina with applicator provided.
• *Alert:* Vaginal preparation shouldn't be used during first trimester of pregnancy. Vaginal preparation should only be used during pregnancy if recommended by prescriber.
• Tell patient that drug may stain clothing.
• Warn patient to discontinue drug if sensitivity or chemical irritation occurs.
• Tell patient to use drug for full treatment period prescribed and to notify prescriber if signs and symptoms persist or worsen at end of therapy.
• Advise patient to avoid tampons and sexual intercourse during vaginal treatment.
• Instruct patient to apply sparingly in skin-fold areas and rub in well to prevent maceration.
• Tell patient to store vaginal product between 59° and 86° F (15° and 30° C).

mupirocin
Bactroban, Bactroban Cream, Bactroban Nasal

Pregnancy risk category B

AVAILABLE FORMS
Intranasal ointment: 2%
Topical cream: 2%
Topical ointment: 2%

INDICATIONS & DOSAGES
➤ **Impetigo—**
Adults and children: Apply to affected areas t.i.d. for 1 to 2 weeks. Reevaluate pa-

tient in 3 to 5 days; may cover affected area with dressing.

➤ **Secondarily infected traumatic skin lesions caused by *Staphylococcus aureus* or *Streptococcus pyogenes*—**
Adults and children: Apply thin film t.i.d. for 10 days; may cover with gauze dressing, if needed. Reevaluate patient if improvement doesn't occur in 3 to 5 days.

➤ **Eradication of nasal colonization by methicillin-resistant *S. aureus* in adult patients and health care workers—**
Adults and children age 12 and older: Divide ointment in single-use tube between nostrils (¼ tube per nostril) b.i.d. for 5 days. After application, close nostrils by pressing together and releasing sides of nose repeatedly for 1 minute to spread ointment throughout nares.

ACTION
Unknown. Thought to inhibit bacterial protein and RNA synthesis.

Route	Onset	Peak	Duration
Topical	Unknown	Unknown	Unknown

ADVERSE REACTIONS
CNS: headache.
EENT: rhinitis, pharyngitis, burning or stinging with intranasal use.
GI: taste perversion.
Respiratory: upper respiratory tract congestion, cough with intranasal use.
Skin: burning, pruritus, stinging, rash, pain, erythema with topical use.

INTERACTIONS
None significant.

EFFECTS ON LAB TEST RESULTS
None reported.

CONTRAINDICATIONS
Contraindicated in patients hypersensitive to drug or its components.

NURSING CONSIDERATIONS
● Use cautiously in patients with burns or impaired renal function because serious renal toxicity may occur.
● Drug isn't for ophthalmic or internal use.

● Prolonged use may cause overgrowth of nonsusceptible bacteria and fungi.
● Local reactions appear to be caused by polyethylene glycol vehicle.
● Patient shouldn't use other nasal products with intranasal ointment.
● *Alert:* Don't confuse Bactroban with bacitracin.

PATIENT TEACHING
● Tell patient to notify prescriber immediately if no improvement occurs in 3 to 5 days or if condition worsens.
● Tell patient not to use other nasal products with mupirocin.
● Warn patient about local adverse reactions related to drug use.
● Caution patient not to use cosmetics or other skin products on treated area.

---

neomycin sulfate
Myciguent ◇

Pregnancy risk category C

AVAILABLE FORMS
Cream: 0.5% ◇
Ointment: 0.5% ◇

INDICATIONS & DOSAGES
➤ **Prevention or treatment of superficial bacterial infections—**
Adults and children: Rub fingertip-size dose into affected area daily to t.i.d.

ACTION
Unknown. Thought to disrupt bacterial protein synthesis by binding to bacterial ribosomes.

Route	Onset	Peak	Duration
Topical	Unknown	Unknown	Unknown

ADVERSE REACTIONS
CNS: *neuromuscular blockade.*
EENT: *ototoxicity.*
GU: *nephrotoxicity.*
Skin: *rash, contact dermatitis,* urticaria.

INTERACTIONS
None significant.

EFFECTS ON LAB TEST RESULTS
None reported.

CONTRAINDICATIONS
Contraindicated in patients hypersensitive to drug or its components.

NURSING CONSIDERATIONS
• Don't use more than once daily on burns covering more than 20% of body surface area.
• Prolonged use may result in overgrowth of nonsusceptible organisms.
• In products containing corticosteroids, use of occlusive dressings increases corticosteroid absorption and likelihood of systemic effects.
• Enhanced systemic absorption occurs on denuded or abraded areas.
• Watch for signs and symptoms of hypersensitivity and contact dermatitis.
• *Alert:* Watch for signs of ototoxicity with prolonged use.

PATIENT TEACHING
• Tell patient to discontinue drug and notify prescriber if no improvement occurs or if condition worsens.
• Tell patient to report adverse reactions, especially systemic reactions.
• Instruct patient not to use drug for longer than 1 week unless otherwise directed.

nitrofurazone
Furacin

Pregnancy risk category C

AVAILABLE FORMS
Cream: 0.2%
Ointment: 0.2% (soluble dressing)
Topical solution: 0.2%

INDICATIONS & DOSAGES
➤ **Adjunctive treatment of second- and third-degree burns (especially when resistance to other antibiotics and sulfonamides occurs), prevention of skin allograft rejection—**
Adults and children: Apply directly to lesion daily or q few days, depending on severity of burn. Drug may also be ap-

plied to dressings used to cover affected area.

ACTION
Unknown. A broad-spectrum antibiotic that probably inhibits bacterial enzymes involved in carbohydrate metabolism.

Route	Onset	Peak	Duration
Topical	Unknown	Unknown	Unknown

ADVERSE REACTIONS
Skin: erythema, pruritus, burning, local edema, allergic contact dermatitis.

INTERACTIONS
None significant.

EFFECTS ON LAB TEST RESULTS
None reported.

CONTRAINDICATIONS
Contraindicated in patients hypersensitive to drug.

NURSING CONSIDERATIONS
• Use cautiously in patients with known or suspected renal impairment. Monitor creatinine levels regularly.
• Flushing dressing with sterile normal saline solution facilitates removal.
• Clean wound, as indicated by prescriber, before reapplying dressings.
• Use sterile application technique to prevent further wound contamination.
• When using wet dressing, protect skin around wound with zinc oxide ointment.
• Dressings impregnated with drug shouldn't be stored for longer than 24 hours.
• Drug may discolor in light but still retains its potency.
• Discard cloudy solutions if warming to 131° to 140° F (55° to 60° C) doesn't restore clarity.
• Store solution in tight, light-resistant container (brown bottle). Avoid exposure to direct light, prolonged heat, and alkaline materials.

PATIENT TEACHING
• Tell patient to report irritation, sensitization, or infection.
• Explain all procedures to patient.

Reactions may be *common*, uncommon, *life-threatening*, or COMMON AND LIFE-THREATENING.

● Tell patient to notify prescriber if condition worsens.
● Tell patient to avoid contact with eyes.

nystatin
Mycostatin, Nilstat, Nystaform§,
Nystan§, Nystex

Pregnancy risk category NR

AVAILABLE FORMS
Cream: 100,000 units/g
Lozenges: 200,000 units
Ointment: 100,000 units/g
Oral suspension: 100,000 units/ml
Powder: 100,000 units/g
Vaginal tablets: 100,000 units

INDICATIONS & DOSAGES
➤ **Cutaneous and mucocutaneous infections caused by *Candida albicans*—**
Adults and children: Apply to affected area up to several times daily until healing is complete. Apply cream b.i.d. or as indicated; powder, b.i.d. or t.i.d.; lozenges, 1 or 2 four to five times daily until 48 hours after oral symptoms subside, but not longer than 14 days; suspension, 4 to 6 ml q.i.d. (one-half of dose in each side of mouth); retain dose as long as possible before swallowing.
➤ **Vulvovaginal candidiasis—**
Adults: 1 vaginal tablet daily for 14 days.

ACTION
Disrupts integrity of fungal cell wall, promoting osmotic instability.

Route	Onset	Peak	Duration
Intravaginal, P.O., topical	Unknown	Unknown	Unknown

ADVERSE REACTIONS
GI: vomiting with vaginal tablet.
Skin: occasional contact dermatitis from preservatives in some forms.

INTERACTIONS
None significant.

EFFECTS ON LAB TEST RESULTS
None reported.

CONTRAINDICATIONS
Contraindicated in patients hypersensitive to drug or its components.

NURSING CONSIDERATIONS
● Don't use occlusive dressings.
● Preparation doesn't stain skin or mucous membranes.
● Cream is recommended for intertriginous areas; powder, for moist areas; ointment, for dry areas.
● Immunosuppressed patients may tolerate vaginal tablets orally for longer exposure to mucous membrane.
● ***Alert:*** Don't confuse nystatin with Nitrostat.

PATIENT TEACHING
● Show woman how to give vaginal tablets and tell her to continue using vaginal tablets during menstrual period.
● Tell patient to insert drug high in vagina (except during pregnancy) and to refrain from sexual intercourse during vaginal treatment.
● Instruct patient to refrigerate tablets.
● Tell patient to use drug for full prescribed period even if condition improves and to continue use at least 2 days after symptoms subside (for oral therapy). Immunosuppressed patients may use drug on long-term basis.
● Warn patient to keep drug away from eyes.
● Instruct patient not to use occlusive dressings with skin application.
● Tell patient to dissolve oral lozenges slowly in mouth.
● Demonstrate and stress importance of proper oral hygiene, especially for denture wearers.

silver sulfadiazine
Flamazine†, Silvadene, SSD,
SSD AF, Thermazene

Pregnancy risk category B

AVAILABLE FORMS
Cream: 1%

INDICATIONS & DOSAGES
➤ **Prevention and treatment of wound infection in second- and third-degree burns—**
Adults: Apply ¹⁄₁₆-inch thickness to clean debrided wound daily or b.i.d.

ACTION
A broad-spectrum sulfonamide that acts on cell membrane and cell wall; it's bactericidal for many gram-positive and gram-negative organisms.

Route	Onset	Peak	Duration
Topical	Unknown	Unknown	Unknown

ADVERSE REACTIONS
Hematologic: *leukopenia.*
Metabolic: altered serum osmolarity.
Skin: pain, burning, rash, pruritus, skin necrosis, *erythema multiforme,* skin discoloration.

INTERACTIONS
Drug-drug. *Topical proteolytic enzymes:* Inactivation of enzymes. Don't use together.
Drug-lifestyle. *Sun exposure:* Photosensitivity reactions may occur. Urge patient to take precautions against sun exposure.

EFFECTS ON LAB TEST RESULTS
• May decrease WBC count.

CONTRAINDICATIONS
Contraindicated in patients hypersensitive to drug and in those with G6PD deficiency. Also contraindicated in pregnant women at or near term and in premature or full-term neonates during first 2 months after birth. Drug may increase possibility of kernicterus.

NURSING CONSIDERATIONS
• **Alert:** Use cautiously in patients hypersensitive to sulfonamides.
• Use sterile application technique to prevent wound contamination.
• Use drug only on affected areas. Keep these areas medicated at all times.
• Bathe patient daily, if possible.

• Inspect patient's skin daily, and note any changes. Notify prescriber if burning or excessive pain develops.
• Monitor sulfadiazine levels and renal function, and check urine for sulfa crystals in patients with extensive burns.
• Tell prescriber if hepatic or renal dysfunction occurs; drug may need to be stopped.
• Absorption of propylene glycol (contained in the cream) can interfere with serum osmolality.
• Discard darkened cream because drug is ineffective.

PATIENT TEACHING
• Instruct patient to promptly report adverse reactions, especially burning or excessive pain with application.
• Inform patient of need for frequent blood and urine tests to watch for adverse effects.
• Tell patient that he may develop photosensitivity.
• Tell patient to continue treatment until satisfactory healing occurs or until site is ready for grafting.

terbinafine hydrochloride
Lamisil

Pregnancy risk category B

AVAILABLE FORMS
Cream: 1%
Gel: 1%

INDICATIONS & DOSAGES
➤ **Interdigital tinea corporis, tinea cruris, tinea pedis; plantar tinea pedis—**
Adults and children age 12 and older: Cover affected area and immediate surrounding area b.i.d. for at least 1 week; use for 2 weeks for plantar tinea pedis. Treatment shouldn't exceed 4 weeks.
✳ *NEW INDICATION:* **Onychomycosis of fingernails or toenails caused by dermatophytes (tinea unguium)—**
Adults and children older than age 12: For fingernails, 250 mg P.O. daily for 6 weeks. For toenails, 250 mg P.O. daily for 12 weeks.

ACTION
A fungicidal that selectively inhibits an early step in synthesis of sterols used by fungi for cell-wall synthesis.

Route	Onset	Peak	Duration
Topical	Unknown	Unknown	Unknown

ADVERSE REACTIONS
Skin: irritation, burning, pruritus, dryness.

INTERACTIONS
None significant.

EFFECTS ON LAB TEST RESULTS
None reported.

CONTRAINDICATIONS
Contraindicated in patients hypersensitive to drug or its components.

NURSING CONSIDERATIONS
• Before starting treatment, appropriate nail specimens for laboratory testing (KOH preparation, fungal culture, or nail biopsy) should be obtained to confirm the diagnosis of onychomycosis.
• Observe patient for 2 to 6 weeks after therapy is complete to determine whether treatment was successful; review diagnosis if condition persists.
• **Alert:** Rare cases of liver failure, some leading to death or liver transplant, have occurred with the use of tablets in individuals with and without preexisting liver disease.
• Drug isn't intended for oral, ophthalmic, or vaginal use.
• Tablets aren't recommended for patients with chronic or active liver disease. Pretreatment transaminase (ALT, AST) tests are advised for all patients.
• Drug isn't for use in breast-feeding women.
• **Alert:** Don't confuse terbinafine with terfenadine or terbutaline. Don't confuse Lamisil with Lamictal.

PATIENT TEACHING
• Teach patient proper use of drug. Tell him to use only as directed for full recommended course, even if signs and symptoms disappear, and not to apply near eyes, mouth, or mucous membranes or to use occlusive dressings unless so directed.
• Tell patient to report signs and symptoms of persistent nausea, anorexia, fatigue, vomiting, right upper abdominal pain or jaundice, dark urine or pale stools. Discontinue therapy with tablets and have liver tests evaluated.
• Tell patient to discontinue drug and contact prescriber if irritation or sensitivity develops.
• Tell patient to store drug between 41° and 86° F (5° and 30° C).

---

terconazole
Terazol 3, Terazol 7

Pregnancy risk category C

AVAILABLE FORMS
Vaginal cream: 0.4%, 0.8%
Vaginal suppositories: 80 mg

INDICATIONS & DOSAGES
➤ **Vulvovaginal candidiasis—**
Adults: 1 applicatorful of cream or 1 suppository inserted into vagina h.s.; 0.4% cream used for 7 consecutive days; 0.8% cream or 80-mg suppository for 3 consecutive days. Course repeated, if needed, after reconfirmation by smear or culture.

ACTION
Unknown. May increase fungal cell membrane permeability (*Candida* species only).

Route	Onset	Peak	Duration
Intravaginal	Unknown	Unknown	Unknown

ADVERSE REACTIONS
CNS: *headache.*
GI: abdominal pain.
GU: dysmenorrhea, genitalia pain, vulvovaginal burning.
Skin: irritation, *pruritus,* photosensitivity.
Other: fever, chills, body aches.

INTERACTIONS
None significant.

EFFECTS ON LAB TEST RESULTS
None reported.

CONTRAINDICATIONS
Contraindicated in patients hypersensitive to drug or its inactive ingredients.

NURSING CONSIDERATIONS
• Therapeutic effect of drug is unaffected by menstruation or oral contraceptive use.
• *Alert:* Don't confuse terconazole with tioconazole.

PATIENT TEACHING
• Advise patient to continue treatment during menstrual period. However, tell her not to use tampons.
• Instruct patient to insert drug high in vagina (except during pregnancy).
• Tell patient to use for full treatment period prescribed. Explain how to prevent reinfection.
• Instruct patient to notify prescriber and discontinue drug if fever, chills, other flu-like signs and symptoms, or sensitivity develops.
• Caution patient to refrain from sexual intercourse during treatment.
• Tell patient that drug base may react with latex, causing decreased effectiveness of condoms and diaphragms (for up to 72 hours after treatment is completed).
• Instruct patient to store drug at room temperature.

---

tolnaftate
Absorbine Footcare, Aftate for Athlete's Foot ◇, Aftate for Jock Itch ◇, Genaspor ◇, Quinsana Plus, Tinactin ◇, Ting ◇

Pregnancy risk category C

AVAILABLE FORMS
Aerosol liquid: 1% (36% alcohol) ◇
Aerosol powder: 1% (14% alcohol) ◇
Cream: 1% ◇
Gel: 1% ◇
Powder: 1% ◇
Pump spray liquid: 1% (36% alcohol) ◇
Topical solution: 1% ◇

INDICATIONS & DOSAGES
➤ **Superficial fungal infections of the skin; infections caused by common pathogenic fungi; tinea pedis, tinea cruris, tinea corporis, tinea versi-color—**
Adults and children: Apply ¼-inch to ½-inch (6-mm to 1.3-cm) ribbon of cream or 2 to 3 drops of solution to cover area; same amount of cream or solution to cover toes and interdigital webs of one foot; or gel, powder, or spray to cover affected area. Apply drug and massage gently into skin b.i.d. for 2 to 6 weeks.

ACTION
Unknown, although has been shown to distort the hyphae and stunt mycelial growth in susceptible fungi.

Route	Onset	Peak	Duration
Topical	Unknown	Unknown	Unknown

ADVERSE REACTIONS
Skin: may cause irritation.

INTERACTIONS
None significant.

EFFECTS ON LAB TEST RESULTS
None reported.

CONTRAINDICATIONS
Contraindicated in patients hypersensitive to drug or its components.

NURSING CONSIDERATIONS
• Drug isn't used to treat fungal infections of hair or nails; tolnaftate is ineffective against these fungi.
• Drug is odorless and greaseless; it won't stain or discolor skin, hair, nails, or clothing.
• Powder or aerosol may be used inside socks and shoes of persons susceptible to tinea infections.
• Ointments, creams, and liquid are primarily used for treatment; powder and aerosol are adjuncts unless infection is very mild.
• *Alert:* Don't confuse tolnaftate with Tornalate.

PATIENT TEACHING
• Teach patient to clean area and dry thoroughly before applying drug.
• Tell patient to use drug for full treatment period prescribed, even if condition has improved. Treatment should continue for

---

at least 2 weeks after signs and symptoms have resolved.
● Advise patient to use only small quantity of cream or lotion; treated area shouldn't be wet with solution.
● Tell patient to call prescriber if no improvement occurs after 10 days.
● Tell patient to discontinue drug and notify prescriber if condition worsens.
● Advise patient to wear shoes and cotton socks that fit well, and to change footwear daily.
● Tell patient to keep drug away from eyes.

86

Scabicides and pediculicides

crotamiton
lindane
permethrin
pyrethrins

COMBINATION PRODUCTS
None.

---

crotamiton
Eurax

Pregnancy risk category C

AVAILABLE FORMS
Cream: 10%
Lotion: 10%

INDICATIONS & DOSAGES
➤ **Parasitic infestation (scabies)—**
Adults: Scrub entire body with soap and water. Remove scales or crusts. Then apply thin layer of cream over entire body, from chin down (with special attention to skin folds, creases, interdigital spaces, and genital area). Apply second coat in 24 hours. Wait another 48 hours; then wash off. Treatment is repeated in 7 to 10 days if mites reappear or if new lesions develop.
➤ **Itching—**
Adults: Apply locally, massaging gently into affected area until completely absorbed; repeat, p.r.n.

ACTION
Unknown.

Route	Onset	Peak	Duration
Topical	Unknown	Unknown	Unknown

ADVERSE REACTIONS
Skin: *irritation,* allergic skin sensitivity.

INTERACTIONS
None significant.

EFFECTS ON LAB TEST RESULTS
None reported.

CONTRAINDICATIONS
Contraindicated in patients hypersensitive to drug or its components and in those whose skin is raw or inflamed.

NURSING CONSIDERATIONS
● Estimate amount of cream needed per application; most patients tend to overuse scabicides. For most adults, a single tube of cream provides enough for two applications.
● Don't apply drug to acutely inflamed or raw, weeping areas.
● Apply topical corticosteroids, as prescribed, if dermatitis develops from scratching.
● Make sure hospitalized patients are placed in isolation, with special linen-handling precautions, until treatment is completed.
● Monthly maintenance treatments may be needed in long-term care facilities where infestation is a problem.
● *Alert:* Don't confuse Eurax with Serax or Urex.

PATIENT TEACHING
● Tell patient or family member to shake product well before each use.
● Teach patient or family member how to apply drug. Tell patient not to apply to face, eyes, mucous membranes, or urethral meatus. If accidental contact with eyes occurs, tell patient to flush with water and notify prescriber.
● Tell patient to discontinue drug, wash it off skin, and notify prescriber immediately if skin irritation or hypersensitivity develops.
● Instruct patient to change all clothing and bed linens and launder them in hot cycle of washing machine or dry clean after drug is washed off body.
● Instruct patient to reapply drug if it's washed off during treatment time.
● Tell patient to warn other family members and sexual contacts about infestation. Sexual contacts should be treated simultaneously.

Reactions may be *common*, uncommon, *life-threatening*, or COMMON AND LIFE-THREATENING.

● Reassure patient that, although itching may continue for several weeks, it will stop; continued itching doesn't indicate that therapy is ineffective.

---

lindane
GBH†, G-well, Kwellada†

Pregnancy risk category B

AVAILABLE FORMS
Cream: 1%†
Lotion: 1%
Shampoo: 1%

INDICATIONS & DOSAGES
➤ **Parasitic infestation (scabies, pediculosis)—**
Adults and children: Centers for Disease Control and Prevention recommends avoiding bathing before application on skin. If patient does bathe, let skin dry and cool thoroughly before using. For scabies, apply thin layer of cream or lotion over entire skin surface from the neck down (with special attention to skin folds, creases, interdigital spaces, and genital area) and rub in thoroughly; for pediculosis, apply thin layer of cream or lotion to hairy areas. After 8 to 12 hours, wash drug off. Repeat process in 1 week if mites appear or new lesions develop.

Apply shampoo undiluted to dry hair and work into lather for 4 to 5 minutes; small amounts of water may increase lathering. Apply 30 ml of shampoo for short hair, 45 ml for medium-length hair, or 60 ml for long hair. Rinse thoroughly and rub dry with towel. Comb with a fine-tooth comb.
Elderly patients: May need to reduce dosage because of increased skin absorption.

ACTION
Unclear. Appears to inhibit neuronal membrane function in arthropods, causing neuronal hyperactivity, seizures, and death after penetrating the parasite's exoskeleton.

Route	Onset	Peak	Duration
Topical	190 min	Unknown	Unknown

ADVERSE REACTIONS
CNS: *dizziness, seizures.*
Skin: *irritation.*

INTERACTIONS
Drug-lifestyle. *Oils:* May increase absorption of drug; if oil-based hair products are used, urge patient to wash and dry hair before using lindane.

EFFECTS ON LAB TEST RESULTS
None reported.

CONTRAINDICATIONS
Contraindicated in patients hypersensitive to drug or its components, in those with seizure disorders, and in those with inflamed skin. Lotion form is contraindicated in premature neonates.

NURSING CONSIDERATIONS
● Use cautiously in infants, young children, and elderly patients; all are at greater risk for CNS toxicity.
● Apply topical corticosteroids or give oral antihistamines, as prescribed, for pruritus.
● Make sure that hospitalized patients are placed in isolation, with special linen-handling precautions, until treatment is completed.
● Modest amounts (6% to 13%) are absorbed through intact skin. Absorption is increased if applied to face, scalp, axillae, neck, scrotum, or irritated or broken skin.
● Avoid contact of drug with eyes.

PATIENT TEACHING
● Teach patient or family member how to give drug. Apply thin layer to cover body only once: 1 ounce is used for children younger than age 6 and 1 to 2 ounces for older children and adults. Drug shouldn't be left on for longer than 12 hours and should be removed thoroughly by washing.
● If patient bathes before application, tell him to let skin dry thoroughly and cool before applying drug.
● Inform patient that drug can be poisonous when misused. Warn patient not to apply to open areas, acutely inflamed skin, or to face, eyes, mucous membranes, or urethral meatus. If accidental contact with eyes occurs, advise patient to flush with water and notify prescriber.
● Tell patient to avoid inhaling vapors.

• Advise patient to wear gloves if applying to another person.

• Tell patient to wash drug off skin and to notify prescriber immediately if skin irritation or hypersensitivity develops.

• Discourage repeated use, which can lead to skin irritation, systemic toxicity, or seizures. Advise patient to repeat use only if live lice or nits are found after 1 week.

• Warn patient not to use other creams or oils during treatment because of potential for increased absorption.

• Instruct patient to change all clothing and bed linens and launder them in hot water or dry clean after drug is washed off body.

• After application for lice infestation, tell patient to use fine-tooth comb or tweezers to remove nits from hairy areas.

• Advise patient to use lindane shampoo to clean combs or brushes and to wash them thoroughly afterward. Warn patient not to use lindane routinely.

• Warn patient that itching may continue for several weeks after effective treatment, especially for scabies.

• Instruct patient to reapply drug if it's washed off during treatment time.

• Tell patient to warn other family members and sexual contacts about infestation. Sexual contacts should be treated simultaneously.

---

permethrin
Acticin, Elimite, Lyclear§, Nix

Pregnancy risk category B

AVAILABLE FORMS
Cream: 5%
Topical liquid (cream rinse): 1%

INDICATIONS & DOSAGES
➤ **Infestation with *Pediculus humanus capitis* (head lice) and its nits—**
Adults and children age 2 and older: Use after hair has been washed with shampoo, rinsed with water, and towel-dried. Apply 25 to 50 ml of liquid to saturate the hair and scalp. Allow drug to remain on hair for 10 minutes before rinsing off with water. Usually only one application is needed.

➤ **Treatment of *Sarcoptes scabiei*—**
Adults and children age 2 months and older: Thoroughly massage into the skin from the head to the soles. Infants should be treated on the hairline, neck, scalp, temple, and forehead. Cream should be removed after 8 to 14 hours by washing. Usually only one application is needed.

ACTION
Acts on parasites' nerve cells to disrupt the sodium channel current, causing parasitic paralysis.

Route	Onset	Peak	Duration
Topical	10-15 min	Unknown	10 days

ADVERSE REACTIONS
Skin: pruritus, *burning, stinging,* edema, tingling, scalp numbness or discomfort, mild erythema, scalp rash.

INTERACTIONS
None significant.

EFFECTS ON LAB TEST RESULTS
None reported.

CONTRAINDICATIONS
Contraindicated in patients hypersensitive to pyrethrins, chrysanthemums, or components of drug.

NURSING CONSIDERATIONS
• A single treatment is usually needed. Combing of nits isn't needed for effectiveness, but drug package supplies a fine-tooth comb for cosmetic use, as desired.

• Retreat for lice, as prescribed, if lice are observed 7 days after initial application.

PATIENT TEACHING
• Explain that treatment may temporarily worsen signs and symptoms of head lice infestation, such as pruritus, erythema, and edema.

• Tell patient that headgear, comb and brush, scarves, coats, and bed linens should be disinfected by machine washing with hot water and machine drying for at least 20 minutes, using hot cycle. Nonwashable items should be sealed in plastic bag for 2 weeks, or sprayed with product designed to eliminate lice and their nits.

Reactions may be *common*, uncommon, *life-threatening*, or COMMON AND LIFE-THREATENING.

• Warn patient not to use drug on eyelashes or eyebrows. Tell patient to avoid use in eyes, nose, mouth, and mucous membranes.

• Tell patient to warn other family members and sexual contacts about infestation. Sexual contacts should be treated simultaneously.

---

pyrethrins
A-200, Barc◇, Blue, End Lice, Pronto, Pyrinyl◇, R & C, RID◇, Tegrin-LT, Tisit◇, Triple X

Pregnancy risk category C

AVAILABLE FORMS
Shampoo: Pyrethrins 0.2% and piperonyl butoxide 2%; pyrethrins 0.3% and piperonyl butoxide 3%; pyrethrins 0.33% and piperonyl butoxide 4%
Shampoo and conditioner: Pyrethrins 0.33%; piperonyl butoxide technical 3.15%
Topical gel: Pyrethrins 0.3% and piperonyl butoxide 3%
Topical solution: Pyrethrins 0.18% and piperonyl butoxide 2%; pyrethrins 0.2%, piperonyl butoxide 2%, and deodorized kerosene 0.8%; pyrethrins 0.3% and piperonyl butoxide 3%; pyrethrins 0.3% and piperonyl butoxide 2%

INDICATIONS & DOSAGES
➤ **Infestations of head, body, and pubic (crab) lice and their eggs—**
Adults and children: Apply to hair, scalp, or other infested areas until entirely wet. Allow to remain for 10 minutes but no longer. Wash thoroughly with warm water and soap or shampoo. Remove dead lice and eggs with fine-tooth comb. Repeat treatment, if needed, in 7 to 10 days to kill newly hatched lice; not to exceed two applications within 24 hours.

ACTION
Acts as contact poison that disrupts parasites' nervous systems, causing paralysis and death of parasites.

Route	Onset	Peak	Duration
Topical	Unknown	Unknown	Unknown

ADVERSE REACTIONS
Skin: *irritation with repeated use.*

INTERACTIONS
None significant.

EFFECTS ON LAB TEST RESULTS
None reported.

CONTRAINDICATIONS
Contraindicated in patients hypersensitive to drug, ragweed, or chrysanthemums.

NURSING CONSIDERATIONS
• Use cautiously in infants and small children.

• Apply topical corticosteroids or oral antihistamines, as prescribed, if dermatitis develops from scratching.

• Discard container by wrapping in several layers of newspaper.

• Inspect all family members daily for at least 2 weeks for infestation.

• Drug isn't effective against scabies.

PATIENT TEACHING
• Instruct patient not to apply to open areas, acutely inflamed skin, eyebrows or eyelashes, or face, eyes, mucous membranes, or urethral meatus. If accidental contact with eyes occurs, advise patient to flush with water and notify prescriber.

• Warn patient not to swallow or inhale vapors from the drug.

• Tell patient to discontinue drug, wash it off skin, and notify prescriber immediately if skin irritation develops. All preparations contain petroleum distillates.

• Instruct patient to change and sterilize all clothing and bed linens after drug is washed off body. Washable items should be disinfected by machine washing in hot water and drying on hot cycle for at least 20 minutes. Other items can be dry cleaned and sealed in plastic bags for 2 weeks, or treated with products made for this purpose.

• Teach patient to remove dead parasites with a fine-tooth comb.

• Urge patient to warn other family members and sexual contacts about infestation. Sexual contacts should be treated simultaneously.

87

Topical corticosteroids

betamethasone dipropionate
betamethasone valerate
clobetasol propionate
desoximetasone
dexamethasone
dexamethasone sodium
  phosphate
diflorasone diacetate
fluocinolone acetonide
fluocinonide
flurandrenolide
fluticasone propionate
halcinonide
hydrocortisone
hydrocortisone acetate
hydrocortisone butyrate
hydrocortisone valerate
mometasone furoate
triamcinolone acetonide

COMBINATION PRODUCTS
Corticosteroids for topical use are commonly combined with antibiotics and antifungals. (See Chapter 85, LOCAL ANTI-INFECTIVES.)

betamethasone dipropionate
Alphatrex, Diprolene, Diprolene AF, Diprosone, Maxivate, Teladar

betamethasone valerate
Betatrex, Beta-Val, Betnovate†‡, Luxiq, Valisone

Pregnancy risk category C

AVAILABLE FORMS
betamethasone dipropionate
Aerosol: 0.1%
Cream: 0.05%
Gel: 0.05%
Lotion: 0.05%
Ointment: 0.05%
betamethasone valerate
Cream: 0.01%, 0.1%
Foam: 0.12%
Lotion: 0.1%
Ointment: 0.1%

INDICATIONS & DOSAGES
➤ **Inflammation and pruritus from corticosteroid-responsive dermatoses—**
Adults and children older than age 12:
Clean area; apply cream, ointment, lotion, aerosol spray, or gel sparingly. Dipropionate products are given once daily to b.i.d.; valerate products are given once daily to q.i.d. Maximum dose is 45 g/week for Diprolene cream and 50 ml/week for Diprolene lotion.
➤ **Inflammation and pruritus from corticosteroid-responsive dermatoses of scalp (valerate only)—**
Adults: Gently massage small amounts of foam into affected scalp areas b.i.d., morning and evening, until control is achieved. If no improvement is seen in 2 weeks, reassess diagnosis.

ACTION
Unclear. Diffuses across cell membranes to form complexes with specific cytoplasmic receptors. Exhibits anti-inflammatory, antipruritic, vasoconstrictive, and antiproliferative activity. Considered a group III (medium-potency) drug, according to vasoconstrictive properties.

Route	Onset	Peak	Duration
Topical	Unknown	Unknown	Unknown

ADVERSE REACTIONS
GU: glycosuria with dipropionate.
Metabolic: hyperglycemia.
Skin: burning, pruritus, irritation, dryness, erythema, folliculitis, striae, acneiform eruptions, perioral dermatitis, hypopigmentation, hypertrichosis, allergic contact dermatitis, secondary infection, maceration, atrophy, miliaria with occlusive dressings.
Other: *hypothalamic-pituitary-adrenal axis suppression,* Cushing's syndrome.

INTERACTIONS
None significant.

EFFECTS ON LAB TEST RESULTS
• May increase glucose level.

Reactions may be *common*, uncommon, *life-threatening*, or COMMON AND LIFE-THREATENING.

CONTRAINDICATIONS
Contraindicated in patients hypersensitive to corticosteroids.

NURSING CONSIDERATIONS
- Gently wash skin before applying. To prevent skin damage, rub in gently, leaving a thin coat. When treating hairy sites, part hair and apply directly to lesions.
- Avoid applying near eyes or mucous membranes or in ear canal, groin area, or axillae.
- Don't dispense foam directly into warm hands because foam will begin to melt upon contact.
- Because of alcohol content of vehicle, gel products may cause mild, transient stinging, especially when used on or near excoriated skin.
- For patients with eczematous dermatitis whose skin may be irritated by adhesive material, hold dressing in place with gauze, elastic bandages, stockings, or stockinette.
- *Alert:* Don't use occlusive dressings.
- If antifungals or antibiotics are used together without prompt improvement, stop corticosteroid until infection is controlled.
- Systemic absorption is likely with prolonged or extensive body surface treatment. Watch for symptoms.
- Avoid using plastic pants or tight-fitting diapers on treated areas in young children. Children may absorb larger amounts of drug and be more prone to systemic toxicity.
- Continue drug for a few days after lesions clear.
- *Alert:* Diprolene and Diprolene AF may not be replaced with generics because other products have different potencies.

PATIENT TEACHING
- Teach patient how to apply drug.
- Emphasize that drug is for external use only.
- Tell patient to stop drug and report signs of systemic absorption, skin irritation or ulceration, hypersensitivity, or infection.
- Instruct patient not to use occlusive dressings.
- Discuss personal hygiene measures to reduce chance of infection.

clobetasol propionate
Cormax, Dermovate†, Embeline E, Temovate

Pregnancy risk category C

AVAILABLE FORMS
Cream: 0.05%
Gel: 0.05%
Solution: 0.05%
Ointment: 0.05%

INDICATIONS & DOSAGES
➤ **Inflammation and pruritus from corticosteroid-responsive dermatoses—**
Adults and children age 12 and older: Apply thin layer to affected skin areas b.i.d., morning and evening, for maximum of 14 days. Total dose shouldn't exceed 50 g or 50 ml of solution weekly.

ACTION
Unclear. Diffuses across cell membranes to form complexes with specific cytoplasmic receptors. Exhibits anti-inflammatory, antipruritic, vasoconstrictive, and antiproliferative activity. Considered a group I (very high-potency) drug, according to vasoconstrictive properties.

Route	Onset	Peak	Duration
Topical	Unknown	Unknown	Unknown

ADVERSE REACTIONS
GU: glycosuria.
Metabolic: hyperglycemia.
Skin: burning, pruritus, irritation, dryness, erythema, folliculitis, perioral dermatitis, allergic contact dermatitis, hypopigmentation, hypertrichosis, acneiform eruptions.
Other: *hypothalamic-pituitary-adrenal axis suppression,* Cushing's syndrome.

INTERACTIONS
None significant.

EFFECTS ON LAB TEST RESULTS
- May increase glucose level.

CONTRAINDICATIONS
Contraindicated in patients hypersensitive to corticosteroids and in those with primary scalp infections.

---

*Liquid contains alcohol.   **May contain tartrazine.   †Canada   ‡Australia   §U.K.   ◊OTC

NURSING CONSIDERATIONS
• Gently wash skin before applying. To prevent skin damage, rub medication in gently and completely. When treating hairy sites, part hair and apply directly to lesions.
• Avoid applying near eyes or mucous membranes or in ear canal.
• *Alert:* Don't use occlusive dressings or bandages. Don't cover or wrap treated areas unless directed by prescriber.
• If antifungals or antibiotics are used together and there isn't prompt improvement, stop corticosteroid until infection is controlled.
• Discontinue drug and notify prescriber if skin infection, striae, or atrophy occurs.
• HPA axis suppression occurs at doses as low as 2 g/day.

PATIENT TEACHING
• Teach patient how to apply drug and to avoid contact with eyes.
• Tell patient to stop drug and report signs of systemic absorption, skin irritation or ulceration, hypersensitivity, or infection.
• Warn patient to use drug for no more than 14 consecutive days.

---

desoximetasone
Topicort, Topicort LP

Pregnancy risk category C

AVAILABLE FORMS
Cream: 0.05%, 0.25%
Gel: 0.05%
Ointment: 0.25%

INDICATIONS & DOSAGES
➤ **Inflammation from corticosteroid-responsive dermatoses—**
Adults and children: Clean area; apply sparingly b.i.d.

ACTION
Unclear. Diffuses across cell membranes to form complexes with specific cytoplasmic receptors. Exhibits anti-inflammatory, antipruritic, vasoconstrictive, and antiproliferative activity. Considered a group III (medium-potency) drug, according to vasoconstrictive properties.

Route	Onset	Peak	Duration
Topical	Unknown	Unknown	Unknown

ADVERSE REACTIONS
GU: glycosuria.
Metabolic: hyperglycemia.
Skin: burning, pruritus, irritation, dryness, erythema, folliculitis, hypertrichosis, acneiform eruptions, perioral dermatitis, hypopigmentation, allergic contact dermatitis, *maceration, secondary infection, atrophy, striae, miliaria with occlusive dressings.*
Other: *hypothalamic-pituitary-adrenal axis suppression,* Cushing's syndrome.

INTERACTIONS
None significant.

EFFECTS ON LAB TEST RESULTS
• May increase glucose level.

CONTRAINDICATIONS
Contraindicated in patients hypersensitive to drug or its components.

NURSING CONSIDERATIONS
• Gently wash skin before applying. To prevent skin damage, rub in gently, leaving thin coat. When treating hairy sites, part hair and apply directly to lesions.
• Avoid applying near eyes or mucous membranes, or in ear canal.
• For patients with eczematous dermatitis whose skin may be irritated by adhesive material, hold dressing in place with gauze, elastic bandages, stockings, or stockinette.
• Change dressing as prescribed. Stop drug and notify prescriber if skin infection, striae, or atrophy occurs.
• If fever develops and occlusive dressing is in place, notify prescriber and remove occlusive dressing.
• If antifungals or antibiotics are used together, stop corticosteroid until infection is controlled.
• Systemic absorption is likely with use of occlusive dressings, prolonged treatment, or extensive body surface treatment. Watch for symptoms.

Reactions may be *common*, uncommon, *life-threatening*, or COMMON AND LIFE-THREATENING.

• Avoid using plastic pants or tight-fitting diapers on treated areas in young children. Children may absorb larger amounts of drug and be more prone to systemic toxicity.
• Continue drug for a few days after lesions clear.
• Gel contains alcohol and may cause burning or irritation in open lesions.
• *Alert:* Don't confuse desoximetasone with dexamethasone.

PATIENT TEACHING
• Teach patient how to apply drug.
• If an occlusive dressing is ordered, advise patient to leave it in place for no longer than 12 hours each day and not to use the dressing on infected or exudative lesions.
• Tell patient to stop drug and report signs of systemic absorption, skin irritation or ulceration, hypersensitivity, or infection.

---

dexamethasone
Aeroseb-Dex, Decaspray

dexamethasone sodium phosphate
Decadron Phosphate

Pregnancy risk category C

AVAILABLE FORMS
dexamethasone
Aerosol: 0.01%, 0.04%
dexamethasone sodium phosphate
Cream: 0.1%

INDICATIONS & DOSAGES
➤ **Inflammation from corticosteroid-responsive dermatoses—**
Adults and children: Clean area; apply cream or aerosol sparingly t.i.d. or q.i.d. For aerosol use on scalp, shake can well but gently, and apply to dry scalp after shampooing. Hold can upright or inverted and 6 inches away from area. Spray while moving container to all affected areas, which should take about 2 seconds. Don't massage drug into scalp or spray forehead or near eyes. When result is obtained, reduce dose gradually; then discontinue.

ACTION
Unclear. Diffuses across cell membranes to form complexes with specific cytoplasmic receptors. Exhibits anti-inflammatory, antipruritic, vasoconstrictive, and antiproliferative activity. Considered a group IV (low-potency) drug, according to vasoconstrictive properties.

Route	Onset	Peak	Duration
Topical	Unknown	Unknown	Unknown

ADVERSE REACTIONS
GU: glycosuria.
Metabolic: hyperglycemia.
Skin: burning, pruritus, irritation, dryness, erythema, folliculitis, hypertrichosis, acneiform eruptions, perioral dermatitis, hypopigmentation, allergic contact dermatitis, *maceration, secondary infection, atrophy, striae, miliaria with occlusive dressings.*
Other: *hypothalamic-pituitary-adrenal axis suppression,* Cushing's syndrome, altered growth and development in children.

INTERACTIONS
None significant.

EFFECTS ON LAB TEST RESULTS
• May increase glucose level.

CONTRAINDICATIONS
Contraindicated in patients hypersensitive to drug or its components.

NURSING CONSIDERATIONS
• Gently wash skin before applying. To prevent skin damage, rub cream in gently, leaving a thin coat. When treating hairy sites, part hair and apply directly to lesions.
• Avoid applying near eyes or mucous membranes or in ear canal, groin, or axillae.
• For patients with eczematous dermatitis whose skin may be irritated by adhesive material, hold dressing in place with gauze, stockings, or stockinette.
• Change dressing as prescribed. Stop drug and tell prescriber if skin infection, striae, or atrophy occurs.
• If an occlusive dressing has been applied and a fever develops, notify prescriber and remove dressing.

• When using aerosol around face, cover patient's eyes and warn against inhalation of spray. Aerosol preparation contains alcohol and may cause irritation or burning when used on open lesions. To avoid freezing tissues, don't spray longer than 1 to 2 seconds or from less than 6 inches (15 cm) away.

• If antifungals or antibiotics are used together, stop corticosteroid until infection is controlled.

• Systemic absorption is likely with use of occlusive dressings, prolonged treatment, or extensive body surface treatment. Watch for symptoms.

• Avoid using plastic pants or tight-fitting diapers on treated areas in young children. Children may absorb larger amounts of drug and be more prone to systemic toxicity.

• Continue treatment for a few days after lesions clear.

• *Alert:* Don't confuse dexamethasone with desoximetasone.

PATIENT TEACHING
• Teach patient and family how to apply drug.

• If an occlusive dressing is ordered, advise patient to leave it in place for no longer than 12 hours each day and not to use the dressing on infected or exudative lesions.

• Tell patient to stop drug and report signs of systemic absorption, skin irritation or ulceration, hypersensitivity, or infection.

• Tell patient to avoid scratching.

diflorasone diacetate
Florone, Florone E, Maxiflor, Psorcon

Pregnancy risk category C

AVAILABLE FORMS
Cream: 0.05%
Ointment: 0.05%

INDICATIONS & DOSAGES
➤ **Inflammation and pruritus from corticosteroid-responsive dermatoses—**
Adults and children: Clean area; apply sparingly in thin film. Apply cream b.i.d. to q.i.d. and emollient cream and ointment once daily to t.i.d. In children, use lowest dosage that promotes healing.

ACTION
Unclear. Diffuses across cell membranes to form complexes with specific cytoplasmic receptors. Exhibits anti-inflammatory, antipruritic, vasoconstrictive, and antiproliferative activity. Considered a group I or II (very high- or high-potency) drug, according to vasoconstrictive properties.

Route	Onset	Peak	Duration
Topical	Unknown	Unknown	Unknown

ADVERSE REACTIONS
CV: hypertension.
GU: glycosuria.
Metabolic: hyperglycemia.
Musculoskeletal: osteoporosis.
Skin: burning, pruritus, irritation, dryness, erythema, folliculitis, perioral dermatitis, hypertrichosis, hypopigmentation, acneiform eruptions, *maceration, secondary infection, atrophy, striae, miliaria with occlusive dressings.*
Other: *hypothalamic-pituitary-adrenal axis suppression,* Cushing's syndrome.

INTERACTIONS
None significant.

EFFECTS ON LAB TEST RESULTS
• May increase glucose level.

CONTRAINDICATIONS
Contraindicated in patients hypersensitive to drug or its components.

NURSING CONSIDERATIONS
• Before applying, gently wash skin. To prevent skin damage, rub in gently, leaving a thin coat. When treating hairy sites, part hair and apply directly to lesions. Wear gloves to apply drug.

• Avoid applying near eyes, mucous membranes, or rectum or in ear canal, groin, or axillae.

• For patients with eczematous dermatitis whose skin may be irritated by adhesive material, hold dressing in place with gauze, elastic bandages, stockings, or stockinette.

Reactions may be *common,* uncommon, *life-threatening,* or COMMON AND LIFE-THREATENING.

• Change dressing as prescribed. Stop drug and notify prescriber if skin infection, striae, or atrophy occurs.
• If occlusive dressing has been applied and a fever develops, notify prescriber and remove dressing.
• If antifungals or antibiotics are used together, stop corticosteroid until infection is controlled.
• Systemic absorption is likely with use of occlusive dressings, prolonged treatment, or extensive body surface treatment. Watch for symptoms.
• Avoid using plastic pants or tight-fitting diapers on treated areas in young children. Children may absorb larger amounts of drug and be more prone to systemic toxicity.

PATIENT TEACHING
• Teach patient how to apply drug.
• Tell patient to wash hands after drug application.
• If an occlusive dressing is ordered, advise patient to leave it in place for no longer than 12 hours each day and not to use the dressing on infected or exudative lesions.
• Tell patient to stop drug and report signs of systemic absorption, skin irritation or ulceration, hypersensitivity, or infection.

fluocinolone acetonide
Derma-Smoothe/FS, Fluonid, Flurosyn, FS Shampoo, Synalar

Pregnancy risk category C

AVAILABLE FORMS
Cream: 0.01%, 0.025%, 0.2%
Oil: 0.01%
Ointment: 0.025%
Shampoo: 0.01%
Topical solution: 0.01%

INDICATIONS & DOSAGES
➤ **Inflammation from corticosteroid-responsive dermatoses—**
Adults and children: Clean area; apply cream, ointment, or topical solution sparingly b.i.d. to q.i.d.

ACTION
Unclear. Diffuses across cell membranes to form complexes with specific cytoplasmic receptors. Exhibits anti-inflammatory, antipruritic, vasoconstrictive, and antiproliferative activity. Considered a group IV to VI (low-potency) drug, according to vasoconstrictive properties.

Route	Onset	Peak	Duration
Topical	Unknown	Unknown	Unknown

ADVERSE REACTIONS
GU: glycosuria.
Metabolic: hyperglycemia.
Skin: burning, pruritus, irritation, dryness, erythema, folliculitis, hypertrichosis, hypopigmentation, acneiform eruptions, perioral dermatitis, allergic contact dermatitis, *maceration, secondary infection, atrophy, striae, miliaria with occlusive dressings.*
Other: *hypothalamic-pituitary-adrenal axis suppression,* Cushing's syndrome.

INTERACTIONS
None significant.

EFFECTS ON LAB TEST RESULTS
• May increase glucose level.

CONTRAINDICATIONS
Contraindicated in patients hypersensitive to drug or its components.

NURSING CONSIDERATIONS
• Gently wash skin before applying. To prevent skin damage, rub in gently, leaving a thin coat. When treating hairy sites, part hair and apply directly to lesions.
• Avoid application near eyes or mucous membranes; in axillae, groin, or rectal area; or in ear canal if ear drum is perforated.
• For patients with eczematous dermatitis whose skin may be irritated by adhesive material, hold dressing in place with gauze, elastic bandages, stockings, or stockinette.
• Change dressing as prescribed. Stop drug and notify prescriber if skin infection, striae, or atrophy occurs.
• If an occlusive dressing has been applied and a fever develops, notify prescriber and remove dressing.

- If antifungals or antibiotics are used together, stop corticosteroid until infection is controlled.
- Systemic absorption is likely with use of occlusive dressings, prolonged treatment, or extensive body surface treatment. Watch for symptoms.
- Avoid using plastic pants or tight-fitting diapers on treated areas in young children. Children may absorb larger amounts of drug and be more prone to systemic toxicity.
- Fluonid solution on dry lesions may increase dryness, scaling, or pruritus; on denuded or fissured areas, it may cause burning or stinging. If these signs and symptoms persist and dermatitis hasn't improved, discontinue solution and notify prescriber.
- *Alert:* Don't confuse fluocinolone with fluocinonide.

PATIENT TEACHING
- Teach patient or family how to apply drug using gloves or sterile applicator.
- If an occlusive dressing is ordered, advise patient to leave it in place for no longer than 12 hours each day and not to use the dressing on infected or exudative lesions.
- Tell patient to stop drug and report signs of systemic absorption, skin irritation or ulceration, hypersensitivity, or infection.

---

fluocinonide
Lidex, Lidex-E

Pregnancy risk category C

AVAILABLE FORMS
Cream: 0.05%
Gel: 0.05%
Ointment: 0.05%
Topical solution: 0.05%

INDICATIONS & DOSAGES
➤ **Inflammation from corticosteroid-responsive dermatoses—**
Adults and children: Clean area; apply cream, gel, ointment, or topical solution sparingly t.i.d. or q.i.d. In children, use lowest dosage that promotes healing.

ACTION
Unclear. Diffuses across cell membranes to form complexes with specific cytoplasmic receptors. Exhibits anti-inflammatory, antipruritic, vasoconstrictive, and antiproliferative activity. Considered a group II (high-potency) drug, according to vasoconstrictive properties.

Route	Onset	Peak	Duration
Topical	Unknown	Unknown	Unknown

ADVERSE REACTIONS
GU: glycosuria.
Metabolic: hyperglycemia.
Skin: burning, pruritus, irritation, dryness, erythema, folliculitis, hypertrichosis, hypopigmentation, acneiform eruptions, perioral dermatitis, allergic contact dermatitis, *maceration, secondary infection, atrophy, striae, miliaria with occlusive dressings.*
Other: *hypothalamic-pituitary-adrenal axis suppression,* Cushing's syndrome.

INTERACTIONS
None significant.

EFFECTS ON LAB TEST RESULTS
- May increase glucose level.

CONTRAINDICATIONS
Contraindicated in patients hypersensitive to drug or its components.

NURSING CONSIDERATIONS
- Gently wash skin before applying. To prevent skin damage, rub in gently, leaving a thin coat. When treating hairy sites, part hair and apply directly to lesion.
- Avoid applying near eyes or mucous membranes, or in ear canal.
- For patients with eczematous dermatitis whose skin may be irritated by adhesive material, hold dressing in place with gauze, elastic bandages, stockings, or stockinette.
- Change dressing as prescribed. Stop drug and notify prescriber if skin infection, striae, or atrophy occurs.
- If an occlusive dressing has been applied and a fever develops, notify prescriber and remove dressing.
- If antifungals or antibiotics are used together, stop drug until infection is controlled.

Reactions may be *common,* uncommon, *life-threatening,* or **COMMON AND LIFE-THREATENING.**

• Systemic absorption is likely with use of occlusive dressings, prolonged treatment, or extensive body surface treatment. Watch for symptoms.

• Avoid using plastic pants or tight-fitting diapers on treated areas in young children. Children may absorb larger amounts of drug and be more prone to systemic toxicity.

• Continue treatment for a few days after lesions clear.

• *Alert:* Don't confuse fluocinolone with fluocinonide.

PATIENT TEACHING

• Teach patient and family how to apply drug using gloves, sterile applicator, or careful hand washing.

• If an occlusive dressing is ordered, advise patient to leave it in place no more than 12 hours each day and not to use the dressing on infected or exudative lesions.

• Tell patient to stop drug and report signs of systemic absorption, skin irritation or ulceration, hypersensitivity, or infection.

---

flurandrenolide
Cordran, Cordran SP, Drenison Tape†

Pregnancy risk category C

AVAILABLE FORMS
Cream: 0.025%, 0.05%
Lotion: 0.05%
Ointment: 0.025%, 0.05%
Tape: 4 mcg/cm^2

INDICATIONS & DOSAGES
➤ **Inflammation and pruritus from corticosteroid-responsive dermatoses—**
Adults and children: Clean area; apply cream, lotion, or ointment sparingly b.i.d. or t.i.d.

Before applying Cordran tape, clean skin carefully, removing scales, crust, and dried exudate. Apply tape q 12 hours. Let skin dry for 1 hour before applying new tape. Shave or clip hair to allow good contact with skin and comfortable removal. If tape ends loosen prematurely, trim off and replace with fresh tape.

ACTION
Unclear. Diffuses across cell membranes to form complexes with specific cytoplasmic receptors. Exhibits anti-inflammatory, antipruritic, vasoconstrictive, and antiproliferative activity. Considered a group III (medium-potency) drug, according to vasoconstrictive properties.

Route	Onset	Peak	Duration
Topical	Unknown	Unknown	Unknown

ADVERSE REACTIONS
GU: glycosuria.
Metabolic: hyperglycemia.
Skin: burning, pruritus, irritation, dryness, erythema, folliculitis, hypertrichosis, hypopigmentation, acneiform eruptions, allergic contact dermatitis, *maceration, secondary infection, atrophy, striae, miliaria with occlusive dressings,* purpura, stripping of epidermis, furunculosis with tape.
Other: *hypothalamic-pituitary-adrenal axis suppression,* Cushing's syndrome.

INTERACTIONS
None significant.

EFFECTS ON LAB TEST RESULTS
• May increase glucose level.

CONTRAINDICATIONS
Contraindicated in patients hypersensitive to drug or its components.

NURSING CONSIDERATIONS
• Gently wash skin before applying. To prevent skin damage, rub in gently, leaving a thin coat. When treating hairy sites, part hair and apply directly to lesions.

• Avoid applying near eyes or mucous membranes, or in ear canal.

• *Alert:* Don't use tape for exudative lesions or lesions in intertriginous areas.

• Don't tear Cordran tape; cut it with scissors. Make sure skin is dry for 1 hour before applying tape.

• For patients with eczematous dermatitis whose skin may be irritated by adhesive material, hold dressing in place with gauze, elastic bandages, stockings, or stockinette.

• Stop drug and tell prescriber if skin infection, striae, or atrophy occurs.

• Notify prescriber and remove occlusive dressing if fever develops.
• If antifungals or antibiotics are used together, stop drug until infection is controlled.
• Systemic absorption is likely with use of occlusive dressings, prolonged treatment, or extensive body surface treatment. Watch for symptoms.
• Avoid using plastic pants or tight-fitting diapers on treated areas in young children. Children may absorb larger amounts of drug and be more prone to systemic toxicity.
• Continue treatment for a few days after lesions clear.

PATIENT TEACHING
• Teach patient or family how to apply drug.
• If an occlusive dressing is ordered, advise patient to leave it in place for no longer than 12 hours each day and not to use the dressing on infected or exudative lesions.
• Tell patient to stop drug and report signs of systemic absorption, skin irritation or ulceration, hypersensitivity, or infection.

---

fluticasone propionate
Cutivate

Pregnancy risk category C

AVAILABLE FORMS
Cream: 0.05%
Ointment: 0.005%

INDICATIONS & DOSAGES
➤ **Inflammation and pruritus from corticosteroid-responsive dermatoses—**
Adults: Apply sparingly to affected area b.i.d.; rub in gently and completely.
✷ *NEW INDICATION:* **Inflammation and pruritus from atopic dermatitis—**
Children age 3 months and older: Apply thin film (0.05%) to affected areas once daily or b.i.d. Rub in gently. Don't use for longer than 4 weeks.
✷ *NEW INDICATION:* **Inflammation and pruritus from other corticosteroid-responsive dermatoses—**
Children age 3 months and older: Apply a thin film (0.05%) to affected areas b.i.d.

Rub in gently. Don't use for longer than 4 weeks.

ACTION
Unclear. Diffuses across cell membranes to form complexes with specific cytoplasmic receptors. Exhibits anti-inflammatory, antipruritic, vasoconstrictive, and antiproliferative activity. Considered a group III (medium-potency) drug, according to vasoconstrictive properties.

Route	Onset	Peak	Duration
Topical	Rapid	Unknown	10 hr

ADVERSE REACTIONS
CNS: light-headedness.
GU: glycosuria.
Metabolic: hyperglycemia.
Skin: urticaria, burning, hypertrichosis, pruritus, irritation, erythema.
Other: *hypothalamic-pituitary-adrenal axis suppression,* Cushing's syndrome.

INTERACTIONS
None significant.

EFFECTS ON LAB TEST RESULTS
• May increase glucose level.

CONTRAINDICATIONS
Contraindicated in patients hypersensitive to drug or its components and in those with viral, fungal, herpetic, or tubercular skin lesions.

NURSING CONSIDERATIONS
• Don't mix drug with other bases or vehicles because doing so may affect potency.
• If adverse reactions occur, prescriber may order less potent drug.
• Discontinue drug if local irritation or systemic infection, absorption, or hypersensitivity occurs.
• Absorption of corticosteroid is increased when drug is applied to inflamed or damaged skin, eyelids, or scrotal area; it's lowest when applied to intact normal skin, palms of hands, or soles of feet.
• Don't use drug with an occlusive dressing or in diaper area.
• *Alert:* Don't confuse fluticasone with fluconazole.

Reactions may be *common,* uncommon, *life-threatening,* or COMMON AND LIFE-THREATENING.

PATIENT TEACHING
• Teach patient or family member how to apply drug using gloves, sterile applicator, or careful hand washing.
• Tell patient to avoid prolonged use and contact with eyes. Warn him not to apply on face, in skin creases, or around eyes, genitals, axillae, or rectum.
• Instruct patient to notify prescriber if condition persists or worsens or if burning or irritation develops.

halcinonide
Halog, Halog-E

Pregnancy risk category C

AVAILABLE FORMS
Cream: 0.025%, 0.1%
Ointment: 0.1%
Topical solution: 0.1%

INDICATIONS & DOSAGES
➤ **Inflammation from corticosteroid-responsive dermatoses—**
Adults and children: Clean area; apply cream, ointment, or topical solution sparingly b.i.d. or t.i.d. Rub cream in gently.

ACTION
Unclear. Diffuses across cell membranes to form complexes with cytoplasmic receptors. Exhibits anti-inflammatory, antipruritic, vasoconstrictive, and antiproliferative activity. Considered a group II (high-potency) drug, according to vasoconstrictive properties.

Route	Onset	Peak	Duration
Topical	Unknown	Unknown	Unknown

ADVERSE REACTIONS
GU: glycosuria.
Metabolic: hyperglycemia.
Skin: burning, pruritus, irritation, dryness, erythema, folliculitis, hypertrichosis, hypopigmentation, acneiform eruptions, allergic contact dermatitis, *maceration, secondary infection, atrophy, striae, miliaria with occlusive dressings.*
Other: *hypothalamic-pituitary-adrenal axis suppression,* Cushing's syndrome.

INTERACTIONS
None significant.

EFFECTS ON LAB TEST RESULTS
• May increase glucose level.

CONTRAINDICATIONS
Contraindicated in patients hypersensitive to drug or its components.

NURSING CONSIDERATIONS
• Gently wash skin before applying. To prevent skin damage, rub in gently, leaving a thin coat. When treating hairy sites, part hair and apply directly to lesions.
• Avoid applying near eyes or mucous membranes or in ear canal, axillae, groin, or rectal area.
• Gently rub small amount of cream into lesion until it disappears. Reapply, leaving a thin coating on lesion, and cover with occlusive dressing, if ordered. Don't leave dressing in place for longer than 12 hours each day.
• Don't use occlusive dressings on infected or exudative lesions.
• For patients with eczematous dermatitis whose skin may be irritated by adhesive material, hold dressing in place with gauze, stockings, or stockinette.
• Stop drug and tell prescriber if skin infection, striae, or atrophy occurs.
• Good results have been obtained by applying occlusive dressings in the evening and removing them in the morning, providing 12-hour occlusion. Then reapply drug; don't apply occlusive dressings during the day.
• If an occlusive dressing has been applied and a fever develops, notify prescriber and remove dressing.
• If antifungals or antibiotics are used together, stop corticosteroid until infection is controlled.
• Systemic absorption is especially likely with use of occlusive dressings, prolonged treatment, or extensive body surface treatment. Watch for symptoms.
• Avoid using plastic pants or tight-fitting diapers on treated areas in young children. Children may absorb larger amounts of drug and be more prone to systemic toxicity.
• Continue treatment for a few days after lesions clear.

PATIENT TEACHING
• Teach patient how to apply drug.
• If an occlusive dressing is ordered, advise patient to leave it in place for no longer than 12 hours each day and not to use the dressing on infected or exudative lesions.
• Tell patient to stop drug and report signs of systemic absorption, skin irritation or ulceration, hypersensitivity, or infection.

hydrocortisone
Acticort 100, Aeroseb-HC, Ala-Cort, Ala-Scalp, Anusol-HC, Bactine Hydrocortisone ◇, Cetacort, Cort-Dome, Cortizone-5 ◇, Delcort, Dermolate Anti-Itch ◇, Dermtex HC ◇, Efcortelan§, Hi-Cor 2.5, Hycort, Hydro-Tex, Hytone, LactiCare-HC, Penecort, Proctocort ◇, Scalpicin ◇, Synacort, Tegrin-HC ◇, Texacort, T/Scalp

hydrocortisone acetate
Anu-Med HC, Anusol HC-1 ◇, Caldecort (Maximum Strength), Cortaid ◇, Cortamed†, Cortef Feminine Itch ◇, Corticaine ◇, Dermol HC, Gynecort ◇, Hemril-HC Uniserts, Lanacort-5 ◇, Lanacort 10 ◇, ProctoCream-HC, ProctoFoam-HC

hydrocortisone butyrate
Locoid

hydrocortisone valerate
Westcort

Pregnancy risk category C

AVAILABLE FORMS
hydrocortisone
Cream: 0.5% ◇, 1% ◇, 2.5%
Gel: 1%
Lotion: 0.25%, 0.5% ◇, 1% ◇, 1%, 2%, 2.5%
Ointment: 0.5% ◇, 1% ◇, 2.5%
Rectal cream: 1% ◇
Rectal ointment: 1%
Spray: 1% ◇
Stick roll-on: 1%
Topical solution: 1%

hydrocortisone acetate
Cream: 0.5% ◇, 1% ◇, 1%
Ointment: 0.5% ◇, 1% ◇
Rectal foam: 90 mg per application
Suppositories: 25 mg, 30 mg
hydrocortisone butyrate
Cream: 0.1%
Ointment: 0.1%
Solution: 0.1%
hydrocortisone valerate
Cream: 0.2%
Ointment: 0.2%

INDICATIONS & DOSAGES
➤ **Inflammation and pruritus from corticosteroid-responsive dermatoses, adjunctive topical management of seborrheic dermatitis of scalp—**
Adults and children: Clean area; apply cream, gel, lotion, ointment, or topical solution sparingly daily to q.i.d. Spray aerosol onto affected area daily to q.i.d. until acute phase is controlled; then reduce dosage to one to three times weekly, p.r.n. Children should receive lowest dose that provides positive results.
➤ **Inflammation from proctitis—**
Adults: 1 applicatorful of rectal foam P.R. daily or b.i.d. for 2 to 3 weeks; then every other day, p.r.n. Enema is given once nightly for 21 days or until patient improves; may be used for 2 to 3 months if used every other night. Suppositories are inserted b.i.d. for 2 weeks.

ACTION
Unclear. Diffuses across cell membranes to form complexes with specific cytoplasmic receptors. Exhibits anti-inflammatory, antipruritic, vasoconstrictive, and antiproliferative activity.

Route	Onset	Peak	Duration
P.R., topical	Unknown	Unknown	Unknown

ADVERSE REACTIONS
Topical use
GU: glycosuria.
Metabolic: hyperglycemia.
Skin: burning, pruritus, irritation, dryness, erythema, folliculitis, hypertrichosis, hypopigmentation, acneiform eruptions, allergic contact dermatitis, *maceration,*

secondary infection, atrophy, striae, miliaria with occlusive dressings.
Other: *hypothalamic-pituitary-adrenal axis suppression,* Cushing's syndrome.
Rectal use
CNS: *seizures, increased intracranial pressure,* vertigo, headache.
CV: hypertension.
EENT: cataracts, glaucoma.
GI: peptic ulcer, *pancreatitis,* abdominal distention.
GU: menstrual irregularities.
Metabolic: fluid or electrolyte disturbances, decreased carbohydrate tolerance.
Musculoskeletal: muscle weakness, osteoporosis, necrosis and fractures in bone.
Skin: impaired wound healing, fragile skin, petechiae, erythema, sweating.

INTERACTIONS
None significant.

EFFECTS ON LAB TEST RESULTS
● May increase glucose level.

CONTRAINDICATIONS
Contraindicated in patients hypersensitive to drug or its components.

NURSING CONSIDERATIONS
● Gently wash skin before applying. To prevent skin damage, rub in gently, leaving a thin coat. When treating hairy sites, part hair and apply directly to lesions.
● Avoid applying near eyes or mucous membranes or in ear canal; may be safely used on face, groin, and armpits and under breasts.
● If an occlusive dressing is applied and a fever develops, notify prescriber and remove dressing.
● Change dressing as prescribed. Stop drug and tell prescriber if skin infection, striae, or atrophy occurs.
● When using aerosol near the face, cover patient's eyes and warn against inhalation of spray. Aerosol contains alcohol and may cause irritation or burning when used on open lesions. Don't spray longer than 3 seconds or from closer than 6 inches (15 cm) to avoid freezing tissues. If spray is applied to dry scalp after shampooing, drug need not be massaged into scalp.

● If antifungals or antibiotics are used together, stop corticosteroid drug until infection is controlled.
● Systemic absorption is likely with use of occlusive dressings, prolonged treatment, or extensive body surface treatment. Watch for symptoms.
● Avoid using plastic pants or tight-fitting diapers on treated areas in young children. Children may absorb larger amounts of drug and be more prone to systemic toxicity.
● Continue treatment for a few days after lesions clear.
● Monitor patient for fluid or electrolyte disturbances (sodium and fluid retention, potassium loss, hypokalemic alkalosis, negative nitrogen balance from catabolism of protein).
● Drug may suppress skin reaction testing.
● *Alert:* Don't confuse hydrocortisone with hydroxychloroquine.

PATIENT TEACHING
● Teach patient or family member how to apply drug.
● If an occlusive dressing is ordered, advise patient to leave it in place for no longer than 12 hours each day and not to use the dressing on infected or exudative lesions.
● Tell patient to stop drug and report signs of systemic absorption, skin irritation or ulceration, hypersensitivity, infection, or lack of improvement.
● Instruct patient to insert suppositories blunt end first after removing foil wrapper.
● For perianal application, instruct patient to place small amount of drug on a tissue and gently rub in.
● Tell patient to disassemble applicator or aerosol cap and clean with warm water after each use.

---

mometasone furoate
Elocon

Pregnancy risk category C

AVAILABLE FORMS
Cream: 0.1%
Ointment: 0.1%
Lotion: 0.1%

INDICATIONS & DOSAGES
➤ **Inflammation and pruritus from corticosteroid-responsive dermatoses—**
Adults: Apply thin film of cream or ointment to affected areas once daily or apply a few drops of lotion to affected area once daily.
Children age 2 and older: Apply thin film to affected areas once daily for no longer than 3 weeks.

ACTION
Unclear. Diffuses across cell membranes to form complexes with specific cytoplasmic receptors. Exhibits anti-inflammatory, antipruritic, vasoconstrictive, and antiproliferative activity. Considered a group III (medium-potency) drug, according to vasoconstrictive properties.

Route	Onset	Peak	Duration
Topical	Unknown	Unknown	Unknown

ADVERSE REACTIONS
GU: glycosuria.
Metabolic: hyperglycemia.
Skin: burning, erythema, pruritus, atrophy, irritation, acneiform eruptions, hypopigmentation, allergic contact dermatitis.
Other: *hypothalamic-pituitary-adrenal axis suppression,* Cushing's syndrome.

INTERACTIONS
None significant.

EFFECTS ON LAB TEST RESULTS
• May increase glucose level.

CONTRAINDICATIONS
Contraindicated in patients hypersensitive to drug, its components, or other corticosteroids.

NURSING CONSIDERATIONS
• Use cautiously in children age 2 and older.
• Gently wash skin before applying. To prevent skin damage, rub in gently, leaving a thin coat. When treating hairy sites, part hair and apply directly to lesions.
• Don't apply near eyes or mucous membranes or in ear canal, axillae, groin, or rectal area.
• *Alert:* Don't use occlusive dressings.

• Systemic absorption is likely with use of occlusive dressings, prolonged treatment, or extensive body surface treatment.
• If antimicrobials are used together, stop corticosteroid drug until infection is controlled.
• Avoid using plastic pants or tight-fitting diapers on treated areas in young children. Children may absorb larger amounts of drug and be more prone to systemic toxicity.

PATIENT TEACHING
• Teach patient or family member how to apply drug.
• Tell patient to stop drug and report signs of systemic absorption, skin irritation or ulceration, hypersensitivity, infection, or lack of improvement after 2 weeks.

---

triamcinolone acetonide
Aristocort, Delta-Tritex, Flutex, Kenalog, Kenalog in Orabase, Kenalone‡, Triacet, Triderm

Pregnancy risk category C

AVAILABLE FORMS
Aerosol: 0.2 mg/2-second spray
Cream: 0.02%‡, 0.025%, 0.1%, 0.5%
Lotion: 0.025%, 0.1%
Ointment: 0.02%‡, 0.025%, 0.1%, 0.5%
Paste: 0.1%

INDICATIONS & DOSAGES
➤ **Inflammation and pruritus from corticosteroid-responsive dermatoses—**
Adults and children: Clean area; apply aerosol, cream, lotion, or ointment sparingly b.i.d. to q.i.d. Rub in lightly.
➤ **Inflammation from oral lesions—**
Adults and children: Apply paste h.s. and, if needed, b.i.d. or t.i.d., preferably after meals. Apply small amount without rubbing; press to lesion in mouth until thin film develops.

ACTION
Unclear. Diffuses across cell membranes to form complexes with specific cytoplasmic receptors. Exhibits anti-inflammatory, antipruritic, vasoconstrictive, and antiproliferative activity. Considered a group III

Reactions may be *common*, uncommon, *life-threatening*, or COMMON AND LIFE-THREATENING.

(medium-potency) drug, according to vasoconstrictive properties.

Route	Onset	Peak	Duration
Topical	Several hr	Unknown	≥ 1 wk

ADVERSE REACTIONS
CV: syncope.
GU: glycosuria.
Metabolic: hyperglycemia.
Skin: burning, pruritus, irritation, dryness, erythema, folliculitis, hypertrichosis, hypopigmentation, acneiform eruptions, perioral dermatitis, allergic contact dermatitis, *maceration, secondary infection, atrophy, striae, miliaria with occlusive dressings.*
Other: *hypothalamic-pituitary-adrenal axis suppression,* Cushing's syndrome.

INTERACTIONS
None significant.

EFFECTS ON LAB TEST RESULTS
• May increase glucose level.

CONTRAINDICATIONS
Contraindicated in patients hypersensitive to drug or its components.

NURSING CONSIDERATIONS
• Gently wash skin before applying. To avoid skin damage, rub in gently, leaving a thin coat. When treating hairy sites, part hair and apply directly to lesions.
• Don't apply near eyes or in ear canal.
• Stop drug and tell prescriber if skin infection, striae, or atrophy occurs.
• When using aerosol near the face, cover patient's eyes and warn against inhalation of spray. Aerosol contains alcohol and may cause irritation or burning when used on open lesions. Don't spray longer than 3 seconds or from closer than 6 inches (15 cm) to avoid freezing tissues.
• If antifungals or antibiotics are used together, stop corticosteroid until infection is controlled.
• Systemic absorption is likely with the use of occlusive dressings, prolonged treatment, or extensive body surface treatment. Watch for symptoms.
• Avoid using plastic pants or tight-fitting diapers on treated areas in young children. Children may absorb larger amounts of

drug and be more prone to systemic toxicity.
• *Alert:* Don't confuse triamcinolone with Triaminicin or Triaminicol.

PATIENT TEACHING
• Teach patient or family member how to apply drug.
• If an occlusive dressing is ordered, advise patient to leave it in place for no longer than 12 hours each day and not to use the dressing on infected or exudative lesions.
• Tell patient to stop drug and report signs of systemic absorption, skin irritation or ulceration, hypersensitivity, infection, or lack of improvement.

88

Vitamins and minerals

vitamin A
vitamin B complex
   cyanocobalamin,
      hydroxocobalamin
   folic acid
   leucovorin calcium
   niacin
   niacinamide
   pyridoxine hydrochloride
   riboflavin
   thiamine hydrochloride
vitamin C
vitamin D
   cholecalciferol
   ergocalciferol
vitamin D analogue
   doxercalciferol
   paricalcitol
vitamin E
vitamin K analogue
   phytonadione
sodium fluoride
sodium fluoride, topical
trace elements
   chromium
   copper
   iodine
   manganese
   selenium
   zinc

VITAMIN COMBINATION PRODUCTS
B complex vitamins ◊
B complex vitamins with iron ◊
B complex with vitamin C ◊
B vitamin combinations ◊
Calcium and vitamin products ◊
Fluoride with vitamins ◊
Geriatric supplements with multivitamins
and minerals ◊
Miscellaneous vitamins and minerals ◊
Multivitamins ◊
Multivitamins and minerals with hormones ◊
Multivitamins with B_{12} ◊
Vitamin A and D combinations ◊

TRACE ELEMENT COMBINATION PRODUCTS
MULTIPLE TRACE ELEMENT NEONATAL: zinc sulfate 1.5 mg, copper sulfate 0.1 mg, manganese sulfate 0.025 mg, chromium chloride 0.85 mcg per ml.
MULTIPLE TRACE ELEMENT PEDIATRIC: zinc sulfate 0.5 mg, copper sulfate 0.1 mg, manganese sulfate 0.03 mg, and chromium chloride 1 mcg per ml.
MULTIPLE TRACE ELEMENT WITH SELENIUM: zinc sulfate 1 mg, copper sulfate 0.4 mg, manganese sulfate 0.1 mg, chromium chloride 4 mcg, and selenious acid 20 mcg per ml.
NEOTRACE-4: zinc sulfate 1.5 mg, copper sulfate 0.1 mg, manganese sulfate 0.025 mg, and chromium chloride 0.85 mcg per ml.
PEDTRACE-4: zinc sulfate 0.5 mg, copper sulfate 0.1 mg, manganese sulfate 0.025 mg, and chromium chloride 0.85 mcg per ml.
PTE-4: zinc sulfate 1 mg, copper sulfate 0.1 mg, manganese sulfate 0.025 mg, and chromium chloride 1 mcg per ml.
PTE-5: zinc sulfate 1 mg, copper sulfate 0.1 mg, manganese sulfate 0.025 mg, chromium chloride 1 mcg, and selenium (as selenious acid) 15 mcg per ml.
TRACE METALS ADDITIVE: zinc chloride 0.8 mg, copper chloride 0.2 mg, manganese chloride 0.16 mg, and chromium chloride 2 mcg per ml.

---

vitamin A (retinol)
Aquasol A, Del-Vi-A, Palmitate-A-5000

Pregnancy risk category C (in doses more than 800 mcg retinol equivalents); A (in doses less than 800 mcg retinol equivalents); X (in Aquasol)

AVAILABLE FORMS
Capsules: 10,000 IU ◊, 15,000 IU ◊, 25,000 IU

Reactions may be *common*, uncommon, **_life-threatening_**, or **COMMON AND LIFE-THREATENING.**

Drops: 30 ml with dropper (5,000 IU/0.1 ml, 50,000 IU/1 ml)
Injection: 2-ml vials (50,000 IU/ml with 0.5% chlorobutanol, polysorbate 80, butylated hydroxyanisole, and butylated hydroxytoluene)
Tablets: 5,000 IU ◇, 10,000 IU

INDICATIONS & DOSAGES
➤ **Dietary supplement—**
Men and boys older than age 11:
1,000 mcg retinol equivalent (RE) or 3,330 IU.
Women and girls older than age 11:
800 mcg RE or 2,665 IU.
Children ages 7 to 10: 700 mcg RE or 2,330 IU.
Children ages 4 to 6: 500 mcg RE or 1,665 IU.
Children ages 1 to 3: 400 mcg RE or 1,330 IU.
Neonates and infants younger than age 1: 375 mcg RE or 1,500 IU.
Pregnant women: 800 mcg RE or 2,665 IU.
Breast-feeding women (first 6 months): 1,300 mcg RE or 4,330 IU.
Breast-feeding women (second 6 months): 1,200 mcg RE or 4,000 IU.
➤ **Severe vitamin A deficiency—**
Adults and children older than age 8:
100,000 IU I.M. or 100,000 to 500,000 IU P.O. for 3 days; then 50,000 IU I.M. or P.O. for 2 weeks, followed by 10,000 to 20,000 IU P.O. for 2 months. Follow with adequate dietary nutrition and RE vitamin A supplements.
Children age 8 and younger: 5,000 to 15,000 IU I.M. daily for 10 days.
➤ **Maintenance dose to prevent recurrence of vitamin A deficiency—**
Children ages 1 to 8: 5,000 to 10,000 IU P.O. daily for 2 months; then adequate dietary nutrition and RE vitamin A supplements.

ACTION
A coenzyme that stimulates retinal function, bone growth, reproduction, and integrity of epithelial and mucosal tissues.

Route	Onset	Peak	Duration
I.M.	Unknown	Unknown	Unknown
P.O.	Unknown	3-5 hr	Unknown

ADVERSE REACTIONS
Adverse reactions usually occur only with doses that exceed physiologic requirement.
CNS: irritability, headache, ***increased intracranial pressure,*** fatigue, lethargy, malaise.
EENT: papilledema, exophthalmos.
GI: anorexia, epigastric pain, vomiting, polydipsia.
GU: hypomenorrhea, polyuria.
Hepatic: jaundice, hepatomegaly, ***cirrhosis.***
Metabolic: slow growth, hypercalcemia, weight loss.
Musculoskeletal: decalcification, periostitis, premature closure of epiphyses, migratory arthralgia, cortical thickening over the radius and tibia.
Skin: alopecia; dry, cracked, scaly skin; pruritus; lip fissures; erythema; inflamed tongue, lips, and gums; massive desquamation; increased pigmentation; night sweats.
Other: splenomegaly, ***anaphylactic shock.***

INTERACTIONS
Drug-drug. *Cholestyramine resin, mineral oil:* Reduced GI absorption of fat-soluble vitamins. Avoid using together.
Isotretinoin, multivitamins containing vitamin A: Increased risk of toxicity. Avoid using together.
Neomycin (oral): Decreased vitamin A absorption. Avoid using together.
Oral contraceptives: May increase plasma vitamin A levels. Monitor patient closely.
Orlistat: Decreased absorption of fat soluble vitamins. Separate administration time by 2 hours.
Warfarin: Increased risk of bleeding with large doses of vitamin A. Monitor PT and INR closely.

EFFECTS ON LAB TEST RESULTS
● May increase liver enzyme levels.

CONTRAINDICATIONS
Contraindicated orally in patients with malabsorption syndrome; if malabsorption is from inadequate bile secretion, oral route may be used together with bile salts (dehydrocholic acid). Also contraindicated in patients hypersensitive to any ingredi-

---

ent in product and in those with hypervitaminosis A. I.V. route contraindicated except for special water-miscible forms intended for infusion with large parenteral volumes. I.V. push of vitamin A of any type is also contraindicated (anaphylaxis or anaphylactoid reactions and death have resulted).

NURSING CONSIDERATIONS
• RDAs have been converted to REs. One RE has the activity of 1 mcg all-*trans* retinol, 6 mcg beta carotene.
• *Alert:* Give parenteral form by I.M. route or continuous I.V. infusion (that is, in total parenteral nutrition infusion). Never give as I.V. bolus.
• Use cautiously in pregnant patients, avoiding doses exceeding RE.
• Assess patient's vitamin A intake from all sources. Consider dietary intake.
• Liquid products are available for nasogastric route. Preparation may be mixed with cereal or fruit juice.
• Vitamin may be given I.M. for malabsorption syndrome or when oral administration isn't feasible.
• Adequate vitamin A absorption needs suitable dietary protein, fat, vitamin E, and zinc intake and bile secretion; give supplemental salts. Zinc supplements may be needed in patients receiving long-term total parenteral nutrition.
• Watch for adverse reactions if dosage is high. Monitor patient taking more than 25,000 units daily for adverse effects.
• Acute toxicity has resulted from single doses of 25,000 IU/kg of body weight; 350,000 IU in infants and over 2 million IU in adults have also caused acute toxicity. Doses that don't exceed RE are usually nontoxic.
• Chronic toxicity in infants (ages 3 to 6 months) has resulted from doses of 18,500 IU daily for 1 to 3 months. In adults, chronic toxicity has resulted from doses of 50,000 IU daily for over 18 months, 500,000 IU daily for 2 months, and 1 million IU daily for 3 days.
• Watch for skin disorders; high dosages may induce chronic toxicity.
• Vitamin A therapy may falsely increase cholesterol and bilirubin levels.
• *Alert:* Don't confuse Aquasol A with AquaMEPHYTON.

PATIENT TEACHING
• To avoid toxicity, tell patient not to take megadoses of vitamins without specific indications.
• Stress that prescribed vitamins shouldn't be shared with others.
• Instruct patient to protect drug from light.
• Teach patient about good food sources of vitamin A, such as green and yellow vegetables, cantaloupe, and liver (note that liver is also high in saturated fat).
• Advise patient that liquid product can be mixed with food, if desired.
• Tell patient to notify prescriber of signs of overdose (nausea, vomiting, anorexia, malaise, dry and cracking skin and lips, irritability, hair loss, headache, visual disturbances, vertigo, bulging fontanelles in infants).

---

cyanocobalamin (vitamin B$_{12}$)
Crystamine, Crysti-12, Crysti 1000, Cyanocobalamin, Cyanoject, Cyomin, Rubramin PC

hydroxocobalamin (vitamin B$_{12}$)
Hydro-Cobex, Hydro-Crysti-12, LA-12

Pregnancy risk category C (in doses exceeding RDA)

AVAILABLE FORMS
cyanocobalamin
Injection: 100 mcg/ml, 1,000 mcg/ml
Tablets: 25 mcg ◇, 50 mcg ◇, 100 mcg ◇, 250 mcg ◇, 500 mcg ◇, 1,000 mcg ◇
hydroxocobalamin
Injection: 1,000 mcg/ml

INDICATIONS & DOSAGES
➤ **RDA for cyanocobalamin—**
Adults and children age 11 and older: 2.4 mcg.
Children ages 7 to 10: 1.8 mcg.
Children ages 4 to 6: 1.2 mcg.
Children ages 1 to 3: 0.9 mcg.
Infants ages 6 months to 1 year: 0.5 mcg.
Neonates and infants younger than age 6 months: 0.4 mcg.
Pregnant women: 2.4 mcg.
Breast-feeding women: 2.8 mcg.

➤ **Vitamin B$_{12}$ deficiency from inadequate diet, subtotal gastrectomy, or other condition, disorder, or disease, except malabsorption, related to pernicious anemia or other GI disease—**
Adults: 30 mcg hydroxocobalamin I.M. daily for 5 to 10 days, depending on severity of deficiency. Maintenance dose is 100 to 200 mcg I.M. once monthly. For subsequent prophylaxis, advise adequate nutrition and daily RDA vitamin B$_{12}$ supplements.
Children: 1 to 5 mg hydroxocobalamin given over 2 or more weeks in doses of 100 mcg I.M., depending on severity of deficiency. Maintenance dose is 60 mcg/month I.M. For subsequent prophylaxis, advise adequate nutrition and daily RDA vitamin B$_{12}$ supplements.
➤ **Pernicious anemia or vitamin B$_{12}$ malabsorption—**
Adults: Initially, 100 mcg cyanocobalamin I.M. or S.C. daily for 6 to 7 days; then 100 mcg I.M. or S.C. once monthly.
Children: 30 to 50 mcg I.M. or S.C. daily over 2 or more weeks; then 100 mcg I.M. or S.C. monthly for life.
➤ **Methylmalonicaciduria—**
Neonates: 1,000 mcg cyanocobalamin I.M. daily.
➤ **Schilling test flushing dose—**
Adults and children: 1,000 mcg hydroxocobalamin I.M. as single dose.

ACTION

A coenzyme that stimulates metabolic function and is needed for cell replication, hematopoiesis, and nucleoprotein and myelin synthesis.

Route	Onset	Peak	Duration
I.M., S.C.	Unknown	1 hr	Unknown
P.O.	Unknown	8-12 hr	Unknown

ADVERSE REACTIONS

CV: peripheral vascular thrombosis, *heart failure.*
GI: transient diarrhea.
Respiratory: pulmonary edema.
Skin: itching, transitory exanthema, urticaria.
Other: *anaphylaxis, anaphylactoid reactions with parenteral administration,* pain or burning at S.C. or I.M. injection sites.

INTERACTIONS

Drug-drug. *Aminoglycosides, anticonvulsants, colchicine, extended-release potassium products, aminosalicylic acid, and salts:* Malabsorption of vitamin B$_{12}$ from GI tract. Avoid using together.
Ascorbic acid: Large doses may destroy vitamin B$_{12}$ in GI tract. Separate administration times by 1 hour.
Chloramphenicol: Decreased hematopoietic response to vitamin B$_{12}$. Monitor hematologic response and consider alternative anti-infectives.
Drug-lifestyle. *Alcohol use:* Malabsorption of vitamin B$_{12}$. Discourage use together.

CONTRAINDICATIONS

Contraindicated in patients hypersensitive to vitamin B$_{12}$ or cobalt and in those with early Leber's disease.

EFFECTS ON LAB TEST RESULTS

None reported.

NURSING CONSIDERATIONS

● Use cautiously in anemic patients with coexisting cardiac, pulmonary, or hypertensive disease.
● Use cautiously in premature infants; product may contain benzyl alcohol, which may cause "gasping syndrome."
● Determine reticulocyte count, hematocrit, vitamin B$_{12}$, iron, and folate levels before beginning therapy.
● A sensitivity test history should be obtained before administration. An intradermal test dose is recommended in patients with possible sensitivity.
● Vitamin B$_{12}$ may cause false-positive results for intrinsic factor antibodies, which are present in the blood of half of all patients with pernicious anemia. Methotrexate, pyrimethamine, and most anti-infectives invalidate diagnostic blood assays for vitamin B$_{12}$.
● *Alert:* Avoid I.V. administration because of more rapid systemic elimination with resulting decreased utilization.
● Don't mix parenteral preparations in same syringe with other drugs.
● Drug is physically incompatible with dextrose solutions, alkaline or strongly acidic solutions, oxidizing or reducing agents, heavy metals, chlorpromazine,

phytonadione, prochlorperazine, and other drugs.

• Hydroxocobalamin is approved for I.M. or deep S.C. use only. Its only advantage over cyanocobalamin is its longer duration.

• Don't give large oral doses of B_{12} routinely; drug is lost through excretion.

• Closely monitor potassium levels for first 48 hours. Give potassium supplement, if ordered.

• Infection, tumors, or renal, hepatic, and other debilitating diseases may reduce therapeutic response.

• Deficiencies are more common in patients who are strict vegetarians and in their breast-fed infants.

• Vitamin B_{12} deficiency may suppress symptoms of polycythemia vera.

• Protect vitamin B_{12} from light. Don't refrigerate or freeze.

PATIENT TEACHING

• Stress need for patient with pernicious anemia to return for monthly injections. Although total body stores may last 3 to 6 years, anemia will recur if not treated monthly.

• Stress importance of follow-up visits and laboratory studies.

• Teach patient healthy dietary habits.

• Instruct patient not to take folic acid as a replacement for vitamin B_{12}; folic acid may alleviate hematologic manifestations of pernicious anemia, but neurologic complications will progress.

---

folic acid (vitamin B_9)
Folvite, Novo-Folacid†

Pregnancy risk category A

AVAILABLE FORMS
Injection: 10-ml vials (5 mg/ml with 1.5% benzyl alcohol, 5 mg/ml with 1.5% benzyl alcohol and 0.2% ethylenediaminetetraacetic acid)
Tablets: 0.4 mg, 0.8 mg, 1 mg

INDICATIONS & DOSAGES
➤ **RDA—**
Adults and children age 14 and older: 400 mcg.
Children ages 9 to 13: 100 mcg.

Children ages 4 to 8: 200 mcg.
Children ages 1 to 3: 150 mcg.
Infants ages 6 months to 1 year: 80 mcg.
Neonates and infants younger than age 6 months: 65 mcg.
Pregnant women: 600 mcg.
Breast-feeding women: 500 mcg.
➤ **Megaloblastic or macrocytic anemia secondary to folic acid or other nutritional deficiency, hepatic disease, alcoholism, intestinal obstruction, excessive hemolysis—**
Adults and children older than age 4: 0.4 to 1 mg P.O., S.C., or I.M. daily. After anemia caused by folic acid deficiency is corrected, proper diet and RDA supplements are needed to prevent recurrence.
Children younger than age 4: Up to 0.3 mg P.O., S.C., or I.M. daily.
Pregnant and breast-feeding women: 0.8 mg P.O., S.C., or I.M. daily.
➤ **Prevention of megaloblastic anemia during pregnancy to prevent fetal damage—**
Adults: Up to 1 mg P.O., S.C., or I.M. daily throughout pregnancy.
➤ **Test for folic acid deficiency in patients with megaloblastic anemia without masking pernicious anemia—**
Adults and children: 0.1 to 0.2 mg P.O. or I.M. for 10 days while maintaining a diet low in folate and vitamin B_{12}.
➤ **Tropical sprue—**
Adults: 3 to 15 mg P.O. daily.

ACTION
Stimulates normal erythropoiesis and nucleoprotein synthesis.

Route	Onset	Peak	Duration
I.M., P.O., S.C.	Unknown	30-60 min	Unknown

ADVERSE REACTIONS
CNS: altered sleep pattern, general malaise, difficulty concentrating, confusion, impaired judgment, irritability, overactivity.
GI: anorexia, nausea, flatulence, bitter taste.
Respiratory: *bronchospasm.*
Skin: allergic reactions including rash, pruritus, and erythema.

Reactions may be *common*, uncommon, *life-threatening*, or COMMON AND LIFE-THREATENING.

INTERACTIONS

Drug-drug. *Aminosalicylic acid, chloramphenicol, methotrexate, oral contraceptives, sulfasalazine, trimethoprim:* Antagonism of folic acid. Watch for decreased folic acid effect. Use together cautiously.

Phenytoin: Increased anticonvulsant metabolism causing decreased blood levels of the anticonvulsant. Monitor phenytoin levels closely.

EFFECTS ON LAB TEST RESULTS
• May decrease serum and RBC folate levels.

CONTRAINDICATIONS
Contraindicated in patients with undiagnosed anemia (it may mask pernicious anemia) and in those with B_{12} deficiency.

NURSING CONSIDERATIONS
• The U.S. Public Health Service recommends use of folic acid during pregnancy to decrease neural tube defects. In patients with a history of neural tube defects in pregnancy, increased folic acid intake 1 month before and 3 months after conception is recommended.
• Patients with small-bowel resections and intestinal malabsorption may need parenteral administration.
• Most CNS and GI adverse reactions occur at higher doses, such as 15 mg daily for 1 month.
• Don't mix with other drugs in same syringe for I.M. injections.
• Protect drug from light and heat; store at room temperature.
• *Alert:* Don't confuse folic acid with folinic acid.

PATIENT TEACHING
• Teach patient about proper nutrition to prevent recurrence of anemia.
• Stress importance of follow-up visits and laboratory studies.
• Teach patient about foods that contain folic acid: liver, oranges, whole wheat, broccoli, Brussels sprouts.

leucovorin calcium (citrovorum factor, folinic acid)
Wellcovorin

Pregnancy risk category C

AVAILABLE FORMS
Injection: 10 mg/ml
Powder for injection: 50-mg vial, 100-mg vial, 200-mg vial, 350-mg vial, 500-mg vial
Tablets: 5 mg, 10 mg, 15 mg, 25 mg

INDICATIONS & DOSAGES
➤ **Overdose of folic acid antagonist (methotrexate, trimethoprim, or pyrimethamine)—**
Adults and children: I.M. or I.V. dose equivalent to weight of antagonist given. For methotrexate overdose, up to 75 mg I.V. infusion within 12 hours, followed by 12 mg I.M. q 6 hours for four doses. For adverse effects following average doses of methotrexate, 6 to 12 mg I.M. q 6 hours for four doses.
➤ **Leucovorin rescue after high methotrexate dose in treatment of malignant disease—**
Adults and children: 10 mg/m² P.O., I.M., or I.V. q 6 hours until methotrexate levels fall below 5×10^{-8} M.
➤ **Megaloblastic anemia from congenital enzyme deficiency—**
Adults and children: 3 to 6 mg I.M. daily.
➤ **Folate-deficient megaloblastic anemia—**
Adults and children: Up to 1 mg leucovorin I.M. daily. Duration of treatment depends on hematologic response.
➤ **Prevention of hematologic toxicity from pyrimethamine or trimethoprim therapy—**
Adults and children: 400 mcg to 5 mg I.M. with each dose of folic acid antagonist. Oral dosages of 10 to 35 mg once daily or 25 mg once weekly have also been used.
➤ **Hematologic toxicity from pyrimethamine or trimethoprim therapy—**
Adults and children: 5 to 15 mg I.M. daily.

---

*Liquid contains alcohol.   **May contain tartrazine.   †Canada   ‡Australia   §U.K.   ◇OTC

➤ **Palliative treatment of advanced colorectal cancer—**
Adults: 20 mg/m^2 I.V.; then fluorouracil 425 mg/m^2 I.V. or 200 mg/m^2 I.V. (over 3 minutes or longer) followed by fluorouracil 370 mg/m^2 daily for 5 consecutive days. Repeated at 4-week intervals for two additional courses; then at intervals of 4 to 5 weeks, if tolerated.

I.V. ADMINISTRATION

• When using powder for injection, reconstitute 50-mg vial with 5 ml, 100-mg vial with 10 ml, or 350-mg vial with 17 ml of sterile or bacteriostatic water for injection. When doses exceed 10 mg/m^2, don't use diluents containing benzyl alcohol.
• *Alert:* Don't exceed 160 mg/minute when giving by I.V. infusion.

ACTION

A reduced form of folic acid that is readily converted to other tetrahydrofolic acid derivatives.

Route	Onset	Peak	Duration
I.M.	10-20 min	< 1 hr	3-6 hr
I.V.	5 min	10 min	3-6 hr
P.O.	20-30 min	2-3 hr	3-6 hr

ADVERSE REACTIONS

Skin: urticaria.
Other: hypersensitivity reactions, *anaphylactoid reactions.*

INTERACTIONS

Drug-drug. *Anticonvulsants:* May decrease effectiveness of these drugs. Monitor patient.
Fluorouracil: May increase fluorouracil toxicity. Fluorouracil dose may need to be reduced.
Methotrexate: High doses of leucovorin may decrease efficacy of intrathecal methotrexate. Monitor effects.

EFFECTS ON LAB TEST RESULTS

None reported.

CONTRAINDICATIONS

Contraindicated in patients with pernicious anemia and other megaloblastic anemias secondary to lack of vitamin B$_{12}$. Don't give leucovorin calcium intrathecally.

NURSING CONSIDERATIONS

• I.V. route is preferred in patients with GI toxicity when doses exceed 25 mg.
• Drug may mask diagnosis of pernicious anemia.
• Follow leucovorin rescue schedule and protocol closely.
• Combined leucovorin and fluorouracil therapy should be used with extreme caution in elderly or debilitated patients because of increased risk of severe GI toxicity.
• Don't give leucovorin with systemic methotrexate.
• Protect from light and heat; maintain protection and immediately give reconstituted parenteral drug.
• *Alert:* Don't confuse leucovorin (folinic acid) with folic acid.

PATIENT TEACHING

• Explain need for drug to patient and family, and answer any questions or concerns.
• Tell patient to report symptoms of hypersensitivity promptly.

niacin (nicotinic acid, vitamin B$_3$)

Nia-Bid ◇ , Niacor ◇ , Niaspan, Nico-400, Nicobid ◇ , Nicolar** , Nicotinex, Slo-Niacin ◇

niacinamide (nicotinamide) ◇

Pregnancy risk category C

AVAILABLE FORMS

niacin
Capsules (timed-release): 125 mg ◇ , 250 mg ◇ , 300 mg ◇ , 400 mg ◇ , 500 mg
Elixir: 50 mg/5 ml* ◇
Tablets: 25 mg ◇ , 50 mg ◇ , 100 mg ◇ , 250 mg ◇ , 500 mg
Tablets (timed-release): 250 mg ◇ , 375 mg ◇ , 500 mg ◇ , 750 mg ◇ , 1,000 mg ◇
niacinamide
Tablets: 50 mg ◇ , 100 mg ◇ , 125 mg ◇ , 250 mg ◇ , 500 mg ◇

INDICATIONS & DOSAGES

➤ **RDA—**
Healthy adult men and boys ages 14 to 18: 16 mg.

Healthy adult women and girls ages 14 to 18: 14 mg.
Children ages 9 to 13: 12 mg.
Children ages 4 to 8: 8 mg.
Children ages 1 to 3: 6 mg.
Infants ages 6 months to 1 year: 4 mg.
Neonates and infants younger than age 6 months: 2 mg.
Pregnant women: 18 mg.
Breast-feeding women: 17 mg.
➤ **Pellagra—**
Adults: 300 to 500 mg P.O. daily in divided doses.
Children: 100 to 300 mg P.O. daily in divided doses.
➤ **Hartnup disease—**
Adults: 50 to 200 mg P.O. daily.
➤ **Niacin deficiency—**
Adults: Up to 100 mg P.O. daily.
➤ **Hyperlipidemias, especially with hypercholesterolemia—**
Adults: 1 to 2 g P.O. divided b.i.d. to q.i.d. with or after meals, increased at intervals to 6 g daily; or 1 to 2 g extended-release tablets P.O. daily h.s.

ACTION
Stimulates lipid metabolism, tissue respiration, and glycogenolysis; niacin decreases synthesis of LDL and inhibits lipolysis in adipose tissue.

Route	Onset	Peak	Duration
P.O.	Unknown	45 min	Unknown

ADVERSE REACTIONS
CV: *excessive peripheral vasodilation, especially with niacin;* hypotension; atrial fibrillation; *arrhythmias; flushing.*
EENT: toxic amblyopia.
GI: *nausea, vomiting, diarrhea,* possible activation of peptic ulceration, epigastric or substernal pain.
Hepatic: *hepatic dysfunction.*
Metabolic: hyperglycemia, hyperuricemia.
Skin: pruritus, dryness, tingling, rash, hyperpigmentation.

INTERACTIONS
Drug-drug. *Antihypertensives (ganglionic or sympathetic blockers):* May increase vasodilating effect, causing orthostatic hypotension. Use together cautiously and

warn patient about orthostatic hypotension.
Cholestyramine, colestipol: May decrease bioavailability of extended release products. Separate administration time by 4 to 6 hours.
Lovastatin (statin class): May lead to rhabdomyolysis. Use together cautiously.
Sulfinpyrazone: Uricosuric effects may be decreased by niacin. Avoid using together.
Drug-food. *Hot drinks:* May increase flushing and pruritus. Urge patient not to take with hot liquids.
Drug-lifestyle. *Alcohol:* May increase flushing and pruritus. Urge patient to avoid use together.

EFFECTS ON LAB TEST RESULTS
● May increase glucose, AST, ALT, and uric acid levels.

CONTRAINDICATIONS
Contraindicated in patients hypersensitive to drug and in those with hepatic dysfunction, active peptic ulcers, severe hypotension, or arterial hemorrhage.

NURSING CONSIDERATIONS
● After symptoms of niacin deficiency subside, advise adequate nutrition and RDA supplements to prevent recurrence.
● Use cautiously in patients with gallbladder disease, diabetes mellitus, or unstable angina and in patients with history of liver disease, peptic ulcer, allergy, gout, or large alcohol intake.
● Most reactions are dose-dependent.
● Drug may cause dose-related rise in glucose intolerance; carefully monitor glucose level in diabetic patients. Glycosuria may occur.
● Give niacin with meals to minimize adverse GI effects.
● Give aspirin (325 mg P.O. 30 minutes before niacin dose) to help reduce flushing response to niacin.
● Timed-release niacin or niacinamide may prevent excessive flushing that occurs with large doses. However, timed-release niacin is linked to hepatic dysfunction, even at very low doses.
● Monitor hepatic function and glucose level early in therapy.

● *Alert:* Don't confuse Nicobid and Nicotinex with nicotine (Nicoderm, Nicotrol, Nicorette).

PATIENT TEACHING
● Stress that niacin is a potent drug, not just a vitamin, and may cause serious adverse effects. Explain importance of adhering to therapy.
● Explain harmlessness of flushing syndrome.
● Tell patient that flushing and warmth may subside with continued use and that concurrent use of alcohol may increase flushing.
● Tell patient to take with food to minimize stomach upset.

---

pyridoxine hydrochloride (vitamin B$_6$)
Nestrex ◇ , Rodex

Pregnancy risk category C (in doses exceeding RDA)

AVAILABLE FORMS
Injection: 100 mg/ml
Tablets: 10 mg ◇ , 25 mg ◇ , 50 mg ◇ , 100 mg ◇ , 200 mg ◇ , 250 mg ◇ , 500 mg ◇

INDICATIONS & DOSAGES
➤ **RDA—**
Men age 51 and older: 1.7 mg.
Women age 51 and older: 1.5 mg.
Healthy adults ages 19 to 50: 1.3 mg.
Boys ages 14 to 19: 1.3 mg.
Girls ages 14 to 19: 1.2 mg.
Children ages 9 to 13: 1.0 mg.
Children ages 4 to 8: 0.6 mg.
Children ages 1 to 3: 0.5 mg.
Infants ages 6 months to 1 year: 0.3 mg.
Neonates and infants younger than age 6 months: 0.1 mg.
Pregnant women: 1.9 mg.
Breast-feeding women: 2.0 mg.
➤ **Dietary vitamin B$_6$ deficiency—**
Adults: 10 to 20 mg P.O., I.M., or I.V. daily for 3 weeks; then 2 to 5 mg daily as supplement to proper diet.
➤ **Seizures related to vitamin B$_6$ deficiency or dependency—**
Adults and children: 100 mg I.M. or I.V. in single dose.

➤ **Vitamin B$_6$–responsive anemias or dependency syndrome (inborn errors of metabolism)—**
Adults: Up to 500 mg P.O., I.M., or I.V. daily until symptoms subside; then 30 mg daily for life.
➤ **Prevention of vitamin B$_6$ deficiency during drug therapy with isoniazid or penicillamine—**
Adults: 10 to 50 mg P.O. daily.
➤ **Prevention of seizures during cycloserine therapy—**
Adults: 100 to 300 mg P.O. daily.
➤ **Antidote for isoniazid poisoning—**
Adults: 4 g I.V.; then 1 g I.M. q 30 minutes until amount of pyridoxine given equals amount of isoniazid ingested.

I.V. ADMINISTRATION
● Drug isn't for I.V. use in patients with heart disease.
● *Alert:* Seizures have occurred after giving large I.V. doses.
● Protect from light. Don't use solution if it contains a precipitate, although slight darkening is acceptable.
● Inject undiluted drug into I.V. line of free-flowing compatible solution. Or, infuse diluted drug over prescribed duration for intermittent infusion. Don't use for continuous infusion.

ACTION
Acts as a coenzyme that stimulates various metabolic functions, including amino acid metabolism.

Route	Onset	Peak	Duration
I.M., I.V., P.O.	Unknown	Unknown	Unknown

ADVERSE REACTIONS
CNS: paresthesia, unsteady gait, numbness, somnolence, *seizures,* headache.
Skin: photoallergic reaction.

INTERACTIONS
Drug-drug. *Levodopa:* Decreased levodopa effect. Pyridoxine doses should not exceed 5 mg/day in patients receiving levodopa.
Phenobarbital, phenytoin: Decreased anticonvulsant levels, increasing risk of seizures. Avoid using together.

Reactions may be *common,* uncommon, *life-threatening,* or COMMON AND LIFE-THREATENING.

Drug-lifestyle. *Alcohol use:* No conclusive evidence, but delirium and lactic acidosis have been reported after drinking alcohol. Discourage patient from use together.

EFFECTS ON LAB TEST RESULTS
• May increase AST level. May decrease folic acid level.

CONTRAINDICATIONS
Contraindicated in patients hypersensitive to drug.

NURSING CONSIDERATIONS
• When used to treat isoniazid toxicity, expect to also give anticonvulsants.
• If sodium bicarbonate is needed to control acidosis in isoniazid toxicity, don't mix in same syringe with pyridoxine.
• Patients taking high doses (2 to 6 g/day) may experience difficulty walking because of diminished proprioceptive and sensory function.
• Carefully monitor patient's diet. Excessive protein intake increases daily pyridoxine requirements.
• Long-term use of large doses may cause neurotoxicity.
• *Alert:* Don't confuse pyridoxine with pralidoxime or pyridium.

PATIENT TEACHING
• Stress importance of compliance and of good nutrition if drug is prescribed for maintenance therapy to prevent recurrence of deficiency. Explain that pyridoxine with isoniazid has a specific therapeutic purpose and isn't just a vitamin.
• Advise patient taking levodopa alone to avoid multivitamins containing pyridoxine because of decreased levodopa effect.
• Warn patient that there may be burning at the injection site.

---

riboflavin (vitamin B₂) ◇

Pregnancy risk category A (C in doses exceeding the RDA)

AVAILABLE FORMS
Tablets: 25 mg ◇, 50 mg ◇, 100 mg ◇
Tablets (sugar-free): 50 mg ◇, 100 mg ◇

INDICATIONS & DOSAGES
➤ **RDA—**
Adult men: 1.3 mg.
Adult women: 1.1 mg.
Boys ages 14 to 19: 1.3 mg.
Girls ages 14 to 19: 1 mg.
Children ages 9 to 13: 0.9 mg.
Children ages 4 to 8: 0.6 mg.
Children ages 1 to 3: 0.5 mg.
Infants ages 6 months to 1 year: 0.4 mg.
Neonates and infants younger than age 6 months: 0.3 mg.
Pregnant women: 1.4 mg.
Breast-feeding women: 1.6 mg.
➤ **Riboflavin deficiency or adjunct to thiamine treatment for polyneuritis or cheilosis secondary to pellagra—**
Adults and children older than age 12: 5 to 30 mg P.O. daily, depending on severity.
Children younger than age 12: 3 to 10 mg P.O. daily, depending on severity.
  For maintenance, increase nutritional intake and supplement with vitamin B complex.

ACTION
Converts to two other coenzymes needed for normal tissue respiration. Drug is necessary for activation of pyridoxine.

Route	Onset	Peak	Duration
P.O.	Unknown	Unknown	Unknown

ADVERSE REACTIONS
GU: bright yellow urine.

INTERACTIONS
Drug-drug. *Probenecid:* Reduced urinary excretion of riboflavin. Avoid using together.
Propantheline, other anticholinergics: Decreased rate and extent of absorption of riboflavin. Avoid using together.

EFFECTS ON LAB TEST RESULTS
None reported.

CONTRAINDICATIONS
No known contraindications.

NURSING CONSIDERATIONS
• Drug may be given I.M. or I.V. as a component of multiple vitamins.

• Riboflavin deficiency usually accompanies other vitamin B complex deficiencies; patient may need multivitamin therapy.
• Protect drug from air and light.
• *Alert:* Don't confuse riboflavin with ribavirin.

PATIENT TEACHING
• Tell patient to take drug with meals; food increases its absorption.
• Stress proper nutritional habits to prevent recurrence of deficiency.
• Inform patient that riboflavin usually causes bright yellow or orange discoloration of urine.

---

thiamine hydrochloride (vitamin B₁)
Betamin‡, Beta-Sol‡

Pregnancy risk category C (in doses exceeding the RDA)

AVAILABLE FORMS
Elixir†: 250 mcg/5 ml
Injection: 100 mg/ml
Tablets: 25 mg ◊, 50 mg ◊, 100 mg ◊, 250 mg ◊, 500 mg
Tablet (enteric-coated): 20 mg

INDICATIONS & DOSAGES
➤ RDA—
Adult men: 1.2 mg.
Adult women: 1.1 mg.
Boys ages 14 to 18: 1.2 mg.
Girls ages 14 to 18: 1 mg.
Children ages 9 to 13: 0.9 mg.
Children ages 4 to 8: 0.6 mg.
Children ages 1 to 3: 0.5 mg.
Infants ages 6 months to 1 year: 0.3 mg.
Neonates and infants younger than age 6 months: 0.2 mg.
Pregnant women: 1.4 mg.
Breast-feeding women: 1.5 mg.
➤ Beriberi—
Adults: Depending on severity, 5 to 30 mg I.M. t.i.d. for 2 weeks; then dietary correction and multivitamin supplement containing 5 to 30 mg thiamine daily for 1 month.
Children: Depending on severity, 10 to 25 mg I.M. or I.V. daily. For noncritically ill children 10 to 50 mg P.O. daily in divid-

ed doses for several weeks with adequate diet.
➤ **Wet beriberi with myocardial failure**—
Adults and children: 10 to 30 mg I.V. t.i.d.
➤ **Wernicke's encephalopathy**—
Adults: Initially, 100 mg I.V.; then 50 to 100 mg I.V. or I.M. daily until patient is consuming a regular balanced diet.

I.V. ADMINISTRATION
• Dilute drug before use.
• *Alert:* Give large I.V. doses cautiously; give patient a skin test before therapy if he has history of hypersensitivity reactions. Have epinephrine available to treat anaphylaxis.
• Don't use drug with materials that yield alkaline solutions. Thiamine is unstable in alkaline solutions.

ACTION
Combines with adenosine triphosphate to form a coenzyme needed for carbohydrate metabolism.

Route	Onset	Peak	Duration
I.M., I.V., P.O.	Unknown	Unknown	Unknown

ADVERSE REACTIONS
CNS: restlessness, weakness.
CV: cyanosis, *CV collapse (with repeated I.V. injections).*
EENT: tightness of throat.
GI: nausea, *hemorrhage.*
Respiratory: pulmonary edema.
Skin: feeling of warmth, pruritus, urticaria, diaphoresis.
Other: *angioedema,* tenderness, induration after I.M. administration.

INTERACTIONS
Drug-drug. *Neuromuscular blockers:* Increased effects of these drugs. Monitor patient closely.

EFFECTS ON LAB TEST RESULTS
None reported.

CONTRAINDICATIONS
Contraindicated in patients hypersensitive to thiamine products.

Reactions may be *common*, uncommon, *life-threatening*, or COMMON AND LIFE-THREATENING.

NURSING CONSIDERATIONS
• Use parenteral route only when P.O. route isn't feasible.
• Thiamine malabsorption is most likely in alcoholism, cirrhosis, and GI disease.
• Clinically significant deficiency can occur after about 3 weeks of totally thiamine-free diet.
• Thiamine deficiency usually requires concurrent treatment for multiple deficiencies.
• Dosages over 30 mg t.i.d. may not be fully used. After tissue saturation with thiamine, drug is excreted in urine as pyrimidine.
• In Wernicke's encephalopathy, give thiamine before dextrose because dextrose increases thiamine requirement.
• **Alert:** Don't confuse thiamine with Thorazine.

PATIENT TEACHING
• Inform breast-feeding woman that, if beriberi occurs in infant, both she and her child should be treated with thiamine.
• Stress proper nutritional habits to prevent recurrence of deficiency.
• Instruct patient to protect oral doses from light.

---

vitamin C (ascorbic acid)
Cebid Timecelles ◊ , Cecon ◊ ,
Cenolate ◊ , Cevi-Bid, Ce-Vi-Sol*,
Dull-C ◊ , Flavorcee ◊ , N'ice
w/Vitamin C Drops ◊ , Vicks
Vitamin C drops

Pregnancy risk category A (C in doses exceeding the RDA)

AVAILABLE FORMS
Capsules (timed-release): 250 mg, 500 mg ◊
Crystals: 100 g (4 g/tsp) ◊ , 500 g (4 g/tsp) ◊
Injection: 100 mg/ml, 222 mg/ml, 250 mg/ml, 500 mg/ml
Lozenges: 60 mg ◊
Oral liquid: 50 ml (35 mg/0.6 ml)* ◊
Oral solution: 100 mg/ml ◊
Powder: 100 g (4 g/tsp) ◊ , 500 g (4 g/tsp) ◊
Syrup: 500 mg/5 ml ◊

Tablets: 25 mg ◊ , 50 mg ◊ , 100 mg ◊ , 250 mg ◊ , 500 mg ◊ , 1,000 mg ◊
Tablets (chewable): 100 mg ◊ , 250 mg ◊ , 500 mg ◊ , 1,000 mg ◊
Tablets (timed-release): 500 mg ◊ , 1,000 mg ◊ , 1,500 mg

INDICATIONS & DOSAGES
➤ **RDA—**
Men age 19 and older: 90 mg.
Women age 19 and older: 75 mg.
Boys ages 14 to 18: 75 mg.
Girls ages 14 to 18: 65 mg.
Children ages 9 to 13: 45 mg.
Children ages 4 to 8: 25 mg.
Children ages 1 to 3: 15 mg.
Infants ages 7 months to 1 year: 50 mg.
Neonates and infants up to age 6 months: 40 mg.
Pregnant women: 80 to 85 mg.
Breast-feeding women: 115 to 120 mg.
➤ **Frank and subclinical scurvy—**
Adults: Depending on severity, 100 to 250 mg P.O., S.C., I.M., or I.V. daily; then 70 to 150 mg daily for maintenance.
Children: Depending on severity, 100 to 300 mg P.O., S.C., I.M., or I.V. daily; then at least 30 mg daily for maintenance.
➤ **Extensive burns, delayed fracture or wound healing, postoperative wound healing, severe febrile or chronic disease states—**
Adults: 300 to 500 mg S.C., I.M., or I.V. daily for 7 to 10 days. 1 to 2 g daily for extensive burns.
Children: 100 to 200 mg P.O., S.C., I.M., or I.V. daily.
➤ **Prevention of vitamin C deficiency in patients with poor nutritional habits or increased requirements—**
Adults: 70 to 150 mg P.O., S.C., I.M., or I.V. daily.
Children: At least 40 mg P.O., S.C., I.M., or I.V. daily.
Infants: At least 35 mg P.O., S.C., I.M., or I.V. daily.
Pregnant and breast-feeding women: At least 70 to 150 mg P.O., S.C., I.M., or I.V. daily.

I.V. ADMINISTRATION
• Infuse cautiously in patients with renal insufficiency.

---

*Liquid contains alcohol.   **May contain tartrazine.   †Canada   ‡Australia   §U.K.   ◊OTC

• *Alert:* Rapid infusion may cause faintness or dizziness.

ACTION
Stimulates collagen formation and tissue repair; involved in oxidation-reduction reactions.

Route	Onset	Peak	Duration
I.M., I.V., S.C.	Unknown	Unknown	Unknown
P.O.	Unknown	2-3 hr	Unknown

ADVERSE REACTIONS
CNS: faintness, dizziness.
GI: diarrhea, heartburn, nausea, vomiting.
GU: acid urine, oxaluria, renal calculi.
Other: discomfort at injection site.

INTERACTIONS
Drug-drug. *Aspirin (high doses):* Increased risk of salicylate toxicity. Monitor patient closely.
Contraceptives, estrogen: Increased levels of estrogen. Watch for adverse reactions.
Oral iron supplements: Increased iron absorption. Give together.
Drug-herb. *Bearberry:* Inactivation of bearberry in urine. Tell patient to watch for effect.
Drug-lifestyle. *Smoking:* Increased metabolism of vitamin C. Tell patient to increase RDA by 35 mg daily.

EFFECTS ON LAB TEST RESULTS
None reported.

CONTRAINDICATIONS
Contraindicated in patients with an allergy to tartrazine or sulfites. Large doses are contraindicated during pregnancy.

NURSING CONSIDERATIONS
• When giving for urine acidification, check urine pH to ensure efficacy.
• Protect solution from light, and refrigerate ampules.

PATIENT TEACHING
• For patient receiving vitamin C I.M., explain that I.M. route may promote better utilization.
• Stress proper nutritional habits to prevent recurrence of deficiency.

• Inform patient that vitamin C is readily absorbed from citrus fruits, tomatoes, potatoes, and leafy vegetables.
• Advise smokers to increase intake of Vitamin C.

vitamin D

cholecalciferol (vitamin D₃)
Delta-D ◊

ergocalciferol (vitamin D₂)
Calciferol, Drisdol, Radiostol†, Vitamin D

Pregnancy risk category A (C in doses exceeding the RDA)

AVAILABLE FORMS
Capsules: 1.25 mg (50,000 IU)
Injection: 12.5 mg (500,000 IU)/ml
Oral liquid: 8,000 IU/ml in 60-ml dropper bottle ◊
Tablets: 1.25 mg (50,000 IU)

INDICATIONS & DOSAGES
➤ **RDA for cholecalciferol—**
Children and adults up to age 70: 200 IU.
Adults older than age 70: 400 IU.
Pregnant or breast-feeding women: 200 IU.
➤ **Rickets and other vitamin D deficiency diseases, renal osteodystrophy—**
Adults: Initially, 10,000 IU P.O. or I.M. daily; usually increased, based on response, to maximum of 500,000 IU daily.
Children: 1,500 to 5,000 IU P.O. or I.M. daily for 2 to 4 weeks; repeated after 2 weeks, if needed. Or, give single dose of 600,000 IU. After correction of deficiency, maintenance includes adequate diet and RDA supplements.
➤ **Hypoparathyroidism—**
Adults and children: 25,000 to 200,000 IU P.O. or I.M. daily, with calcium supplement.
➤ **Familial hypophosphatemia—**
Adults: 250 mcg to 1.5 mg P.O. daily with phosphate supplements.
Children: 1 to 2 mg P.O. daily with phosphorus supplement, increased in 250- to 500-mcg increments at 3- to 4-month intervals.

ACTION
Promotes absorption and utilization of calcium and phosphate, helping to regulate calcium homeostasis.

Route	Onset	Peak	Duration
I.M., P.O.	2-14 hr	4-12 hr	2 days-6 mo

ADVERSE REACTIONS
Adverse reactions usually occur only in vitamin D toxicity.
CNS: headache, weakness, somnolence, overt psychosis, irritability.
CV: *calcification of soft tissues, including the heart;* hypertension; ***arrhythmias.***
EENT: rhinorrhea, conjunctivitis (calcific), photophobia.
GI: anorexia, nausea, vomiting, constipation, dry mouth, metallic taste, polydipsia.
GU: polyuria, albuminuria, hypercalciuria, nocturia, *impaired renal function,* reversible azotemia.
Metabolic: hypercalcemia, hyperthermia.
Musculoskeletal: bone and muscle pain, bone demineralization, weight loss.
Skin: pruritus.
Other: decreased libido.

INTERACTIONS
Drug-drug. *Cardiac glycosides:* Increased risk of arrhythmias. Monitor calcium levels.
Cholestyramine, colestipol, mineral oil: Inhibited GI absorption of oral vitamin D. Space doses. Use together cautiously.
Corticosteroids: Antagonized effect of vitamin D. Monitor vitamin D levels closely.
Magnesium-containing antacids: May cause hypermagnesemia, especially in patients with chronic renal failure. Monitor magnesium levels.
Orlistat: Decreased GI absorption of vitamin D. Separate dosing by 2 hours.
Phenobarbital, phenytoin: Increased vitamin D metabolism and decreased effectiveness. Monitor patient closely.
Thiazide diuretics: May cause hypercalcemia in patients with hypoparathyroidism. Monitor calcium levels closely.
Verapamil: Atrial fibrillation has occurred as a result of increased calcium. Monitor calcium levels closely.

EFFECTS ON LAB TEST RESULTS
• May increase BUN, creatinine, AST, ALT, nitrogenous compound (urea), calcium, and cholesterol levels.

CONTRAINDICATIONS
Contraindicated in patients with hypercalcemia, hypervitaminosis D, malabsorption syndrome, decreased renal function, or renal osteodystrophy with hyperphosphatemia.

NURSING CONSIDERATIONS
• Use ergocalciferol with extreme caution, if at all, in patients with heart disease, renal stones, or arteriosclerosis.
• Use cautiously in cardiac patients, especially those taking cardiac glycosides, and in patients with increased sensitivity to these drugs.
• Use I.M. injection of vitamin D dispersed in oil for patients unable to absorb oral form.
• *Alert:* Monitor patient's eating and bowel habits; dry mouth, nausea, vomiting, metallic taste, and constipation may be early signs of toxicity.
• Monitor serum and urine calcium, phosphorus, potassium, and urea levels when high therapeutic dosages are used.
• Doses of 60,000 IU/day can cause hypercalcemia. Hypercalcemia may require I.V. hydration and aggressive diuresis.
• Malabsorption from inadequate bile or hepatic dysfunction may require addition of exogenous bile salts to oral form.
• Patients with hyperphosphatemia need dietary phosphate restrictions and binding drugs to avoid metastatic calcifications and renal calculi.
• Mineral oil interferes with absorption of fat-soluble vitamins.

PATIENT TEACHING
• Teach patient that vitamin D is needed to absorb calcium. Instruct patient to read labels for vitamin D content.
• Advise patient that vitamin D is fat soluble and that mineral oil will interfere with absorption.
• Instruct patient to take only as directed, and stress the dangers of excessive doses of fat-soluble vitamins.

• Instruct patient taking vitamin D to restrict intake of magnesium-containing antacids.

• Instruct patient to notify prescriber if signs of toxicity occur, such as weakness, lethargy, headache, anorexia, weight loss, nausea, vomiting, abdominal cramps, diarrhea, constipation, vertigo, polydipsia, polyuria, dry mouth, or muscle or bone pain.

doxercalciferol
Hectorol

Pregnancy risk category B

AVAILABLE FORMS
Capsules: 2.5 mcg

INDICATION & DOSAGES
➤ **Reduction of elevated intact parathyroid hormone (PTH) levels in management of secondary hyperparathyroidism in patients undergoing long-term renal dialysis—**
Adults: Initially, 10 mcg P.O. three times weekly at dialysis. Dosage adjusted p.r.n. to lower intact PTH levels to 150 to 300 pg/ml. Dosage may be increased by 2.5 mcg at 8-week intervals if intact PTH level isn't decreased by 50% and fails to reach target range. Maximum dose is 20 mcg P.O. three times weekly. If intact PTH levels fall below 100 pg/ml, drug should be suspended for 1 week, then resumed at dose that is at least 2.5 mcg lower than last given dose.

ACTION
A vitamin D analogue that acts directly on the parathyroid glands to suppress PTH synthesis and secretion.

Route	Onset	Peak	Duration
P.O.	Unknown	11-12 hr	Unknown

ADVERSE REACTIONS
CNS: *dizziness, headache, malaise, sleep disorder.*
CV: *bradycardia,* edema.
GI: anorexia, dyspepsia, *nausea, vomiting,* constipation.
Metabolic: weight loss.
Musculoskeletal: arthralgia.

Respiratory: *dyspnea.*
Skin: pruritus.
Other: abscess.

INTERACTIONS
Drug-drug. *Calcium-containing or non–aluminum-containing phosphate binders:* May cause hypercalcemia or hyperphosphatemia and decrease effectiveness of doxercalciferol. Use together cautiously and adjust dosage of phosphate binders, as appropriate.
Cholestyramine, mineral oil: Reduced intestinal absorption of doxercalciferol. Avoid using together.
Glutethimide, phenobarbital, other enzyme inducers; phenytoin and other enzyme inhibitors: May affect metabolism of doxercalciferol. Adjust dosage, as appropriate.
Magnesium-containing antacids: May cause hypermagnesemia. Avoid using together.
Vitamin D supplements: May cause additive effects and hypercalcemia. Avoid using together.

EFFECTS ON LAB TEST RESULTS
None reported.

CONTRAINDICATIONS
Contraindicated in patients with recent history of hypercalcemia, hyperphosphatemia, or vitamin D toxicity.

NURSING CONSIDERATIONS
• Use cautiously in patients with hepatic insufficiency.
• Monitor calcium, phosphorus, and intact PTH levels.
• Doxercalciferol is given with dialysis (about every other day). Dosing must be individualized and based on intact PTH levels, with monitoring of calcium and phosphorus levels before doxercalciferol therapy and weekly thereafter in the early phase of treatment.
• Management of secondary hyperparathyroidism may prevent bone disease in patients with renal failure.
• Calcium-based or non–aluminum-containing phosphate binders and a low-phosphate diet are used to control phosphorus levels in patients undergoing dialysis. Expect adjustments in dosages of

Reactions may be *common,* uncommon, *life-threatening,* or COMMON AND LIFE-THREATENING.

doxercalciferol and concurrent therapies such as dietary phosphate binders in order to sustain PTH suppression and maintain calcium and phosphorus levels within acceptable ranges.

• Progressive hypercalcemia secondary to vitamin D overdose may require emergency attention. Acute hypercalcemia may worsen arrhythmias and seizures, and affects action of digoxin. Chronic hypercalcemia can lead to vascular and soft-tissue calcification.

• If hypercalcemia or hyperphosphatemia occur or if the calcium-phosphorus product (Ca × P) is > 70, immediately suspend administration until these values return to normal.

PATIENT TEACHING

• Inform patient that dosage must be adjusted over several months to achieve satisfactory PTH suppression.

• Tell patient to follow instructions regarding calcium supplementation and to adhere to a low-phosphorus diet.

• Tell patient to obtain prescriber's approval before using OTC drugs, including antacids and vitamin products containing calcium or vitamin D.

• Inform patient that early signs and symptoms of hypercalcemia include weakness, headache, somnolence, nausea, vomiting, dry mouth, constipation, muscle pain, bone pain, and metallic taste. Late signs and symptoms include polyuria, polydipsia, anorexia, weight loss, nocturia, conjunctivitis, pancreatitis, photophobia, rhinorrhea, pruritus, hyperthermia, decreased libido, hypertension, and arrhythmias.

paricalcitol
Zemplar

Pregnancy risk category C

AVAILABLE FORMS
Injection: 5 mcg/ml

INDICATIONS & DOSAGES
➤ **Prevention and treatment of secondary hyperparathyroidism and chronic renal failure—**
Adults: 0.04 to 0.1 mcg/kg (2.8 to 7 mcg) I.V. no more frequently than every other

day during dialysis. Doses as high as 0.24 mcg/kg (16.8 mcg) have been safely given. If satisfactory response isn't observed, dosage may be increased by 2 to 4 mcg at 2- to 4-week intervals.

I.V. ADMINISTRATION
• Give drug only as an I.V. bolus. Discard unused portion.
• Inspect drug for particulates and discoloration before use.

ACTION
A synthetic vitamin D analogue that reduces parathyroid hormone (PTH) levels.

Route	Onset	Peak	Duration
I.V.	Immediate	Unknown	15 hr

ADVERSE REACTIONS
CNS: light-headedness, malaise.
CV: palpitations, edema.
GI: dry mouth, *GI bleeding, nausea,* vomiting.
Respiratory: pneumonia.
Other: chills, fever, flulike syndrome, *sepsis.*

INTERACTIONS
None significant.

EFFECTS ON LAB TEST RESULTS
• May decrease total alkaline phosphatase level.

CONTRAINDICATIONS
Contraindicated in patients hypersensitive to drug or its ingredients and in those with evidence of vitamin D toxicity or hypercalcemia.

NURSING CONSIDERATIONS
• Use cautiously in patients taking digitalis compounds. Patients taking digoxin are at greater risk for digitalis toxicity during drug therapy secondary to potential for hypercalcemia.
• Watch for ECG abnormalities.
• Monitor patient for symptoms of hypercalcemia, such as fatigue, muscle weakness, anorexia, depression, nausea, and constipation. Immediately notify prescriber if hypercalcemia is suspected.
• Monitor calcium and phosphorus levels twice weekly when dosage is being adjust-

ed, and then monitor monthly. Measure PTH level every 3 months during therapy.
• As PTH level decreases, paricalcitol dose may need to be decreased. Acute overdose of paricalcitol may cause hypercalcemia, which may require emergency attention.
• In patients with chronic renal failure, appropriate types of phosphate-binding compounds may be needed to control phosphorus levels, but excessive use of aluminum-containing compounds should be avoided.
• Store drug at a controlled room temperature (59° to 86° F [15° to 30° C]).

PATIENT TEACHING
• Stress importance of adhering to a dietary regimen of calcium supplementation and phosphorus restriction during drug therapy.
• Caution against use of phosphate or vitamin D–related compounds during drug therapy.
• Explain need for frequent laboratory tests.
• Instruct patient with chronic renal failure to take phosphate-binding compounds as prescribed but to avoid excessive use of aluminum-containing compounds. Alert patient to early symptoms of hypercalcemia and vitamin D intoxication, such as weakness, headache, somnolence, nausea, vomiting, dry mouth, constipation, muscle and bone pain, and metallic taste.
• Instruct patient to promptly report adverse reactions.
• Remind patient taking digoxin to watch for signs and symptoms of digitalis toxicity.

---

vitamin E (tocopherols)
Aquasol E ◇, Aquavit-E ◇, d'Alpha E, Dry E, Vita-Plus E ◇

Pregnancy risk category A

AVAILABLE FORMS
Capsules: 100 IU ◇, 200 IU ◇, 400 IU ◇, 600 IU ◇, 1,000 IU ◇
Oral solution: 50 mg/ml ◇
Tablets: 100 IU ◇, 200 IU ◇, 400 IU ◇, 500 IU ◇, 600 IU ◇, 1,000 IU ◇

INDICATIONS & DOSAGES
Note: RDAs for vitamin E have been converted to α-tocopherol equivalents (α-TE). One α-TE equals 1 mg of D-α tocopherol, or 1.49 IU.
Healthy adults and children ages 14 to 18: 15 mg.
Children ages 9 to 13: 11 mg.
Children ages 4 to 8: 7 mg.
Children ages 1 to 3: 6 mg.
Infants ages 6 months to 1 year: 5 mg.
Neonates and infants younger than age 6 months: 4 mg.
Pregnant women: 15 mg.
Breast-feeding women: 19 mg.
➤ **Vitamin E deficiency in premature neonates and in patients with impaired fat absorption—**
Adults: Depending on severity, 60 to 75 IU P.O. daily.
Children: 1 IU/kg daily.

ACTION
Unknown. Thought to act as an antioxidant and protect RBC membranes against hemolysis.

Route	Onset	Peak	Duration
P.O.	Unknown	Unknown	Unknown

ADVERSE REACTIONS
None reported with recommended dosages.

INTERACTIONS
Drug-drug. *Anticoagulants (oral):* Hypoprothrombinemic effects may be increased, possibly causing bleeding. Monitor patient closely.
Cholestyramine, colestipol, mineral oil, orlistat: Inhibited GI absorption of oral vitamin E. Separate administration times. Use together cautiously.
Iron: Vitamin E may reduce hematologic response to iron therapy in children with iron-deficiency anemia. Monitor child's response to iron therapy.
Vitamin K: Antagonized effects of vitamin K possible with large doses of vitamin E. Avoid using together.

EFFECTS ON LAB TEST RESULTS
None reported.

CONTRAINDICATIONS
No known contraindications.

Reactions may be *common*, uncommon, **life-threatening**, or COMMON AND LIFE-THREATENING.

NURSING CONSIDERATIONS
• Monitor patient with liver or gallbladder disease for response to therapy. Adequate bile is essential for vitamin E absorption.
• Water-miscible forms are more completely absorbed in GI tract.
• Requirements increase with rise in dietary polyunsaturated acids.
• Don't give drug I.V. (death is possible).
• Hypervitaminosis E symptoms include fatigue, weakness, nausea, headache, blurred vision, flatulence, diarrhea.

PATIENT TEACHING
• Tell patient not to crush tablets or open capsules. An oral solution and chewable tablets are commercially available.
• Warn patient against taking megadoses, which can cause thrombophlebitis. Vitamin is fat soluble and may accumulate.
• Tell patient to store in dry, airtight container.

---

phytonadione (vitamin K₁)
AquaMEPHYTON, Konakion, Mephyton

Pregnancy risk category C

AVAILABLE FORMS
Injection (aqueous colloidal solution):
2 mg/ml, 10 mg/ml
Injection (aqueous dispersion): 2 mg/ml,
10 mg/ml
Tablets: 5 mg

INDICATIONS & DOSAGES
➤ **RDA—**
Women age 25 and older: 65 mcg.
Women ages 19 to 24: 60 mcg.
Girls ages 15 to 18: 55 mcg.
Men age 25 and older: 80 mcg.
Men ages 19 to 24: 70 mcg.
Boys ages 15 to 18: 65 mcg.
Children ages 11 to 14: 45 mcg.
Children ages 7 to 10: 30 mcg.
Children ages 4 to 6: 20 mcg.
Children ages 1 to 3: 15 mcg.
Infants ages 6 months to 1 year: 10 mcg.
Neonates and infants younger than age 6 months: 5 mcg.
Pregnant and breast-feeding women:
65 mcg.

➤ **Hypoprothrombinemia secondary to vitamin K malabsorption, drug therapy, or excessive vitamin A dosage—**
Adults: Depending on severity, 2.5 to 10 mg P.O., S.C., or I.M., repeated and increased up to 50 mg, if needed.
Children: 5 to 10 mg P.O. or parenterally.
Infants: 2 mg P.O. or parenterally.
➤ **Hypoprothrombinemia secondary to effect of oral anticoagulants—**
Adults: 2.5 to 10 mg P.O., S.C., or I.M. based on PT, repeated if needed within 12 to 48 hours after oral dose or within 6 to 8 hours after parenteral dose. In emergency, 10 to 50 mg slow I.V., rate not to exceed 1 mg/minute, repeated q 4 hours, p.r.n.
➤ **Prevention of hemorrhagic disease of newborn—**
Neonates: 0.5 to 1 mg I.M. within 1 hour after birth.
➤ **Hemorrhagic disease of newborn—**
Neonates: 1 mg S.C. or I.M. Higher doses may be needed if mother has been receiving oral anticoagulants.
➤ **Prevention of hypoprothrombinemia related to vitamin K deficiency in long-term parenteral nutrition—**
Adults: 5 to 10 mg I.M. or P.O. weekly.
Children: 2 to 5 mg I.M. or P.O. weekly.
➤ **Prevention of hypoprothrombinemia in infants receiving less than 0.1 mg/L vitamin K in breast milk or milk substitutes—**
Infants: 1 mg I.M. monthly.

I.V. ADMINISTRATION
• Dilute with normal saline solution for injection, D₅W, or 5% dextrose in normal saline solution for injection. Give I.V. by slow infusion over 2 to 3 hours. Don't exceed 1 mg/minute.
• Protect parenteral products from light. Wrap infusion container with aluminum foil or other dark cover.

ACTION
An antihemorrhagic factor that promotes hepatic formation of active coagulation factors.

Route	Onset	Peak	Duration
I.M., I.V., S.C.	1-2 hr	Unknown	Unknown
P.O.	6-12 hr	Unknown	Unknown

ADVERSE REACTIONS
CNS: dizziness.
CV: flushing, transient hypotension after I.V. administration, rapid and weak pulse.
Skin: diaphoresis, erythema.
Other: *anaphylaxis or anaphylactoid reactions, usually after too-rapid I.V. administration;* pain, swelling, and hematoma at injection site.

INTERACTIONS
Drug-drug. *Anticoagulants:* Temporary resistance to prothrombin-depressing anticoagulants may result, especially when larger doses of phytonadione are used. Monitor closely.
Cholestyramine, mineral oil: Inhibited GI absorption of oral vitamin K. Space doses. Use together cautiously.

EFFECTS ON LAB TEST RESULTS
None reported.

CONTRAINDICATIONS
Contraindicated in patients hypersensitive to drug.

NURSING CONSIDERATIONS
● Check brand name labels for administration route restrictions.
● Effects of I.V. injection are more rapid but shorter-lived than S.C. or I.M. injections.
● **Alert:** I.V. use has resulted in fatalities; use only when other routes of administration aren't feasible.
● For I.M. administration in adults and older children, give in upper outer quadrant of buttocks; for infants, give in anterolateral aspect of thigh or deltoid region. S.C. route is preferred to avoid hematoma formation.
● Allergic reactions may also occur after I.M. or S.C. use.
● Anticipate order for weekly addition of 5 to 10 mg of phytonadione to total parenteral nutrition solutions.
● Monitor PT or INR to determine dosage effectiveness.
● If severe bleeding occurs, don't delay other measures, such as administration of fresh frozen plasma or whole blood.
● Vitamin K doesn't reverse the anticoagulant effects of heparin.

● **Alert:** Watch for flushing, weakness, tachycardia, and hypotension; condition may progress to shock.
● Phytonadione therapy for hemorrhagic disease in infants causes fewer adverse reactions than other vitamin K analogues.
● **Alert:** Don't confuse AquaMEPHYTON with Aquasol A.

PATIENT TEACHING
● Explain purpose of drug.
● Tell patient to avoid hazardous activities if dizziness occurs.
● Inform patient that drug is fat soluble; it should be taken only as prescribed to avoid accumulation.
● Teach patient that foods that provide vitamin K include cabbage, cauliflower, kale, spinach, fish, liver, eggs, meats, and dairy products.

sodium fluoride
Fluor-A-Day†, Fluoritab, Fluorodex, Flura, Flura-Drops, Flura-Loz, Karidium, Luride, Luride Lozi-Tabs, Luride-SF Lozi-Tabs, Pediaflor, Pedi-Dent†, Pharmaflur, Pharmaflur df, Pharmaflur 1.1, Phos-Flur

sodium fluoride, topical
ACT◇, Fluorigard◇, Fluorinse, Gel-Kam, Gel-Tin◇, Karigel, Karigel-N, Minute-Gel, Point-Two, Prevident, Stop Gel◇, Thera-Flur, Thera-Flur-N

Pregnancy risk category NR

AVAILABLE FORMS
sodium fluoride
Drops: 0.125 mg/drop, 0.25 mg/drop, 0.2 mg/ml, 0.5 mg/ml
Lozenges: 1 mg
Tablets: 1 mg
Tablets (chewable): 0.25 mg, 0.5 mg, 1 mg
sodium fluoride, topical
Gel: 0.1%, 0.5%, 1.2%, 1.23%
Gel drops: 0.5%
Rinse: 0.02%◇, 0.04%◇, 0.09%, 0.2%

Reactions may be *common*, uncommon, *life-threatening*, or COMMON AND LIFE-THREATENING.

INDICATIONS & DOSAGES
➤ **Prevention of dental caries—**
Adults and children older than age 6: 5 to 10 ml of rinse or thin ribbon of gel applied to teeth with toothbrush or mouth trays for at least 1 minute h.s.
If fluoride ion level in drinking water is below 0.3 parts per million (ppm)
Infants and children ages 6 months to 3 years: 0.25 mg P.O. daily.
Children ages 3 to 6: 0.5 mg P.O. daily.
Children ages 6 to 16: 1 mg P.O. daily.
If fluoride ion level in drinking water is 0.3 to 0.6 ppm
Children ages 3 to 6: 0.25 mg P.O. daily.
Children ages 6 to 16: 0.5 mg P.O. daily.

ACTION
Stabilizes the apatite crystal of bone and teeth. Increases tooth resistance to acid breakdown.

Route	Onset	Peak	Duration
P.O.	Unknown	30-60 min	Unknown

ADVERSE REACTIONS
CNS: headache, weakness.
EENT: staining of teeth.
GI: gastric distress.
Other: hypersensitivity reactions.

INTERACTIONS
Drug-drug. *Aluminum hydroxide, calcium, iron, magnesium:* May decrease absorption. Separate administration times.
Drug-food. *Dairy products:* Incompatibility may occur as a result of formation of calcium fluoride, which is poorly absorbed. Urge patient not to use together.

EFFECTS ON LAB TEST RESULTS
None reported.

CONTRAINDICATIONS
Contraindicated in patients hypersensitive to fluoride and in those whose intake from drinking water exceeds 0.6 ppm.

NURSING CONSIDERATIONS
• Give oral drops undiluted or mixed with fluids or food. Avoid simultaneous ingestion of dairy products.
• *Alert:* Chronic toxicity (fluorosis) may result from prolonged use of higher-than-recommended doses.

PATIENT TEACHING
• Tell patient that tablets may be dissolved in mouth, chewed, or swallowed whole.
• Advise patient that topical rinses and gels shouldn't be swallowed by children younger than age 3 or used if water supply is fluorinated. Drug is most effective when used right after brushing teeth and just before bedtime. Tell patient to rinse around and between teeth for 1 minute; then spit out.
• Tell patient not to eat, drink, or rinse mouth for 30 minutes after application.
• Tell patient to dilute drops or rinses in plastic, not glass, containers.
• Advise patient to notify dentist if tooth mottling occurs.
• Instruct patient not to exceed recommended dosage.

---

trace elements

chromium (chromic chloride)
Chroma-Pak, Chromic Chloride

copper (cupric sulfate)
Cupric Sulfate

iodine (sodium iodide)
Iodopen

manganese (manganese chloride, manganese sulfate)

selenium (selenious acid)
Sele-Pak, Selepen

zinc (zinc sulfate)
Zinca-Pak

Pregnancy risk category C

AVAILABLE FORMS
chromium
Injection: 4 mcg/ml, 20 mcg/ml
copper
Injection: 0.4 mg/ml, 2 mg/ml
iodine
Injection: 100 mcg/ml
manganese
Injection: 0.1 mg/ml
selenium
Injection: 40 mcg/ml

---

*Liquid contains alcohol.   **May contain tartrazine.   †Canada   ‡Australia   §U.K.   ◇OTC

zinc
Injection: 1 mg/ml, 5 mg/ml

INDICATIONS & DOSAGES
➤ **Prevention of individual trace element deficiencies in patients receiving long-term total parenteral nutrition (TPN)—**
chromium
Adults: 10 to 15 mcg I.V. daily.
Children: 0.14 to 0.20 mcg/kg I.V. daily.
copper
Adults: 0.5 to 1.5 mg I.V. daily.
Children: 20 mcg/kg I.V. daily.
iodine
Adults: 1 to 2 mcg/kg I.V. daily.
Children: 2 to 3 mcg/kg I.V. daily.
manganese
Adults: 0.15 to 0.8 mg I.V. daily.
Children: 2 to 10 mcg/kg I.V. daily.
selenium
Adults: 20 to 40 mcg I.V. daily.
Children: 3 mcg/kg I.V. daily.
zinc
Adults: 2.5 to 4 mg I.V. daily.
Full-term infants and children younger than age 5: 100 mcg/kg/day.
Premature infants weighing less than 1.5 to 3 kg (3.3 to 7 lb): 300 mcg/kg/day.

I.V. ADMINISTRATION
● Cautiously infuse diluted solution through patent I.V. line over prescribed duration.
● Don't give undiluted because of potential for phlebitis.

ACTION
Participate in synthesis and stabilization of proteins and nucleic acids in subcellular and membrane transport systems.

Route	Onset	Peak	Duration
I.V.	Immediate	Immediate	Unknown

ADVERSE REACTIONS
Other: hypersensitivity reactions to iodides.

INTERACTIONS
None significant.

EFFECTS ON LAB TEST RESULTS
None reported.

CONTRAINDICATIONS
Contraindicated in patients hypersensitive to iodine.

NURSING CONSIDERATIONS
● Check serum levels of trace elements in patients who have received TPN for 2 months or longer. Give supplement, if ordered. Report low levels of these elements.
● Normal serum levels are 1 to 5 mcg/L chromium; 80 to 163 mcg/dl copper; 6 to 12 mcg/dl manganese; 0.1 to 0.19 mcg/ml selenium; and 88 to 112 mcg/dl zinc.
● Solutions of trace elements are compounded by pharmacist for addition to TPN solutions according to various formulas.

PATIENT TEACHING
● Explain need for zinc administration to patient and family.
● Tell patient to report signs of hypersensitivity promptly.
● Inform patient and family that trace elements are normally received from dietary intake and that, when patient begins eating well, supplements won't be needed.

amino acid infusions, crystalline
amino acid infusions in dextrose
amino acid infusions with
  electrolytes
amino acid infusions with
  electrolytes in dextrose
amino acid infusions for hepatic
  failure
amino acid infusions for high
  metabolic stress
amino acid infusions for renal
  failure
dextrose
fat emulsions
medium chain triglycerides

COMBINATION PRODUCTS
Various products contain dextrose or invert sugar in combination with electrolytes.

---

amino acid infusions,
crystalline
Aminosyn, Aminosyn II,
Aminosyn-PF, Aminosyn-RF,
FreAmine III, Novamine, Travasol,
TrophAmine

amino acid infusions in
dextrose
Aminosyn II with Dextrose,
Travasol in Dextrose

amino acid infusions with
electrolytes
Aminosyn with Electrolytes,
Aminosyn II with Electrolytes,
FreAmine III with Electrolytes,
ProcalAmine with Electrolytes,
Travasol with Electrolytes

amino acid infusions with
electrolytes in dextrose
Aminosyn II with Electrolytes in
Dextrose, Travasol with
Electrolytes in Dextrose

amino acid infusions for
hepatic failure
HepatAmine

amino acid infusions for high
metabolic stress
Aminosyn-HBC, BranchAmin,
FreAmine HBC

amino acid infusions for renal
failure
Aminess, Aminosyn-RF,
NephrAmine, RenAmin

Pregnancy risk category C

AVAILABLE FORMS
Injection: 250 ml, 500 ml, 1,000 ml,
2,000 ml containing amino acids in various concentrations
amino acid infusions, crystalline
Aminosyn: 3.5%, 5%, 7%, 8.5%, 10%
Aminosyn II: 3.5%, 5%, 7%, 8.5%, 10%,
15%
Aminosyn-PF: 7%, 10%
Aminosyn-RF: 5.2%
FreAmine III: 8.5%, 10%
Novamine: 11.4%, 15%
Travasol: 5.5%, 8.5%, 10%
TrophAmine: 6%, 10%
amino acid infusions in dextrose
Aminosyn II: 3.5% in 5% dextrose, 3.5%
in 25% dextrose, 4.25% in 10% dextrose,
4.25% in 20% dextrose, 4.25% in 25%
dextrose, 5% in 25% dextrose
Travasol: 2.75% in 5% dextrose, 2.75% in
10% dextrose, 2.75% in 25% dextrose,
4.25% in 5% dextrose, 4.25% in 10% dextrose, 4.25% in 25% dextrose
amino acid infusions with electrolytes
Aminosyn: 3.5%, 7%, 8.5%
Aminosyn II: 3.5%, 7%, 8.5%, 10%
FreAmine III: 3%, 8.5%
ProcalAmine: 3%
Travasol: 3.5%, 5.5%, 8.5%
**amino acid infusions with electrolytes in
dextrose**
Aminosyn II: 3.5% with electrolytes in 5%
dextrose, 3.5% with electrolytes in 25%
dextrose, 4.25% with electrolytes in 10%

---

dextrose, 4.25% with electrolytes in 20% dextrose, 4.25% with electrolytes in 25% dextrose
Travasol: 2.75% with electrolytes in 5% dextrose, 2.75% with electrolytes in dextrose, 4.25% with electrolytes in 5% dextrose, 4.25% with electrolytes in 10% dextrose, 4.25% with electrolytes in 25% dextrose
amino acid infusions for hepatic failure
HepatAmine: 8%
amino acid infusions for high metabolic stress
Aminosyn-HBC: 7%
BranchAmin: 4%
FreAmine HBC: 6.9%
amino acid infusions for renal failure
Aminess: 5.2%
Aminosyn-RF: 5.2%
NephrAmine: 5.4%
RenAmin: 6.5%

INDICATIONS & DOSAGES
➤ **Total parenteral nutrition (TPN) in patients who can't or won't eat—**
Adults: 1 to 1.7 g/kg I.V. daily.
Children weighing more than 10 kg (22 lb): 20 to 25 g I.V. daily for first 10 kg; then 1 to 1.25 g/kg I.V. daily for each kg over 10 kg.
Children weighing less than 10 kg: 2 to 4 g/kg I.V. daily.
➤ **Nutritional support in patients with cirrhosis, hepatitis, or hepatic encephalopathy—**
Adults: 80 to 120 g of amino acids (12 to 18 g of nitrogen) I.V. daily of formulation for hepatic failure.
➤ **Nutritional support in patients with high metabolic stress—**
Adults: 1.5 g/kg I.V. daily of formulation for high metabolic stress.
➤ **Nutritional support in patients with renal failure—**
Adults: 0.3 to 0.5 g/kg I.V. daily (to total of 26 g daily). Patients on dialysis may need 1 to 1.2 g/kg daily.

I.V. ADMINISTRATION
● Control infusion rate carefully with infusion pump. If infusion rate falls behind, notify prescriber; don't increase rate to catch up.

ACTION
Provides a substrate for protein synthesis or increases conservation of existing body protein.

Route	Onset	Peak	Duration
I.V.	Immediate	Immediate	Unknown

ADVERSE REACTIONS
CV: thrombophlebitis, edema, thrombosis, flushing.
GI: nausea.
GU: glycosuria, osmotic diuresis.
Metabolic: *rebound hypoglycemia when long-term infusions are abruptly stopped,* hyperglycemia, metabolic acidosis, alkalosis, hypophosphatemia, ***hyperosmolar hyperglycemic nonketotic syndrome,*** hyperammonemia, electrolyte imbalances, weight gain.
Musculoskeletal: osteoporosis.
Other: fever, hypersensitivity reactions, tissue sloughing at infusion site from extravasation, *catheter sepsis.*

INTERACTIONS
Drug-drug. *Tetracycline:* May reduce protein-sparing effects of infused amino acids because of its antianabolic activity. Monitor patient.

EFFECTS ON LAB TEST RESULTS
● May increase ammonia and liver enzyme levels. May decrease phosphate, magnesium, and potassium levels. May increase or decrease glucose levels.

CONTRAINDICATIONS
Contraindicated in patients with anuria and in those with inborn errors of amino acid metabolism, such as maple syrup urine disease and isovaleric acidemia. Standard amino acid formulations are contraindicated in patients with severe renal failure or liver disease.

NURSING CONSIDERATIONS
● Use with extreme caution in children and neonates, especially those with low birth weight.
● Use cautiously in patients with renal insufficiency or failure, cardiac disease, or hepatic impairment.
● Give cautiously to diabetic patients; insulin may be needed to prevent hyper-

glycemia. Also give cautiously to patients with cardiac insufficiency; may cause circulatory overload. Patients with fluid restriction may tolerate only 1 to 2 L.

● Some products contain sulfites. Check contents before giving to patients with known sulfite sensitivity.

● Obtain baseline electrolyte, glucose, BUN, calcium, and phosphorus levels before therapy; monitor these levels periodically throughout therapy.

● *Alert:* Infuse amino acids only in I.V. fluids or TPN solution.

● Safe and effective use of parenteral nutrition requires knowledge of nutrition as well as clinical expertise in recognizing and treating complications. Frequent evaluations of patient and laboratory studies are needed.

● Limit peripheral infusions to 2.5% amino acids and dextrose 10%. Check infusion site frequently for erythema, inflammation, irritation, tissue sloughing, necrosis, and phlebitis. Change peripheral I.V. sites routinely to prevent irritation and infection. If subclavian catheter is used, give solution into midsuperior vena cava.

● Check fractional urine every 6 hours for glycosuria initially, then every 12 to 24 hours in stable patients. Abrupt onset of glycosuria may be an early sign of impending sepsis.

● Assess body temperature every 4 hours; elevation may indicate sepsis or infection.

● Watch for extraordinary electrolyte losses that may occur during nasogastric suction, vomiting, diarrhea, or drainage from GI fistula.

● Be prepared to individualize dosage to metabolic and clinical response as determined by nitrogen balance and body weight corrected for fluid balance.

● If patient has chills, fever, or other signs of sepsis, replace I.V. tubing and bottle and send tubing and bottle to the laboratory to be cultured.

● *Alert:* Don't confuse Aminosyn with Amikacin.

PATIENT TEACHING
● Explain need for use to patient and family, and answer any questions.
● Tell patient to report adverse reactions promptly.

dextrose (d-glucose)

Pregnancy risk category C

AVAILABLE FORMS
Injection: 3-ml ampule (10%); 10 ml (25%); 25 ml (5%); 50 ml (5% and 50% available in vial, ampule, and Bristoject); 70-ml pin-top vial (70% for additive use only); 100 ml (5%); 150 ml (5%); 250 ml (5%, 10%); 500 ml (5%, 10%, 20%, 30%, 40%, 50%, 60%, 70%); 650 ml (38.5%); 1,000 ml (2.5%, 5%, 10%, 20%, 30%, 40%, 50%, 60%, 70%); 2,000 ml (50%, 70%)

INDICATIONS & DOSAGES
➤ **Fluid replacement and caloric supplementation in patients who can't maintain adequate oral intake or who are restricted from doing so—**
Adults and children: Dosage depends on fluid and caloric requirements. Peripheral I.V. infusion of 2.5%, 5%, or 10% solution or central I.V. infusion of 20% solution is used for minimal fluid needs. A 10% to 25% solution is used to treat acute hypoglycemia in neonate or older infant (2 ml/kg). A 50% solution is used to treat insulin-induced hypoglycemia (20 to 50 ml). Solutions of 10%, 20%, 30%, 40%, 50%, 60%, and 70% are diluted in admixtures, usually amino acid solutions, for total parenteral nutrition (TPN) given through a central vein.

I.V. ADMINISTRATION
● Control infusion rate carefully; maximum rate is 0.8 g/kg/hour. Use infusion pump when giving with amino acids for TPN.

● *Alert:* Never infuse concentrated solutions rapidly. Rapid infusion may cause hyperglycemia and fluid shift.

● *Alert:* Use central veins to infuse dextrose solutions with concentrations above 10%.

● Check injection site frequently to prevent irritation, tissue sloughing, necrosis, and phlebitis.

ACTION
A simple water-soluble sugar that minimizes glyconeogenesis and promotes an-

abolism in patients whose oral caloric intake is limited.

Route	Onset	Peak	Duration
I.V.	Immediate	Immediate	Unknown

ADVERSE REACTIONS
CNS: confusion, *unconsciousness in hyperosmolar hyperglycemic nonketotic syndrome.*
CV: *exacerbated hypertension and heart failure with fluid overload in susceptible patients;* phlebitis, venous sclerosis, and tissue necrosis with prolonged or concentrated infusions, especially when given peripherally.
GU: glycosuria, osmotic diuresis.
Metabolic: hyperglycemia, dehydration, and hyperosmolarity with rapid infusion of concentrated solution or prolonged infusion; hypoglycemia from rebound hyperinsulinemia with rapid termination of long-term infusions; hypervolemia; hypovolemia.
Respiratory: *pulmonary edema.*
Skin: sloughing and tissue necrosis if extravasation occurs with concentrated solutions.
Other: fever.

INTERACTIONS
Drug-drug. *Corticosteroids:* May cause salt and water retention and increased potassium excretion. Monitor glucose, sodium, and potassium levels.

EFFECTS ON LAB TEST RESULTS
● May increase or decrease glucose level.

CONTRAINDICATIONS
Contraindicated in patients in diabetic coma while glucose level remains excessively high. Use of concentrated solutions contraindicated in patients with intracranial or intraspinal hemorrhage; in dehydrated patients with delirium tremens; and in patients with severe dehydration, anuria, diabetic coma, or glucose-galactose malabsorption syndrome. Also contraindicated in patients with known allergy to corn or corn products.

NURSING CONSIDERATIONS
● Use cautiously in patients with cardiac or pulmonary disease, hypertension, renal insufficiency, urinary obstruction, or hypovolemia.
● *Alert:* Never stop hypertonic solutions abruptly. If needed, have dextrose 10% in water available to treat hypoglycemia if rebound hyperinsulinemia occurs.
● Don't give concentrated solutions S.C. or I.M.
● Monitor glucose levels carefully. Prolonged therapy with D_5W can cause reduction of pancreatic insulin production and secretion.
● Check vital signs frequently. Report adverse reactions promptly.
● Monitor fluid intake and output and weight carefully, especially in patients with renal function impairment.
● Watch closely for signs and symptoms of fluid overload, especially if fluid intake is restricted.
● Monitor for signs of mental confusion.

PATIENT TEACHING
● Explain need for drug to patient and family, and answer any questions.
● Tell patient to report adverse reactions promptly.

fat emulsions
Intralipid 10%, Intralipid 20%, Liposyn II 10%, Liposyn II 20%, Liposyn III 10%, Liposyn III 20%

Pregnancy risk category C

AVAILABLE FORMS
Injection: 50 ml (10%, 20%), 100 ml (10%, 20%), 200 ml (10%, 20%), 250 ml (10%, 20%), 500 ml (10%, 20%)

INDICATIONS & DOSAGES
Intralipid
➤ **Source of calories as adjunct to total parenteral nutrition (TPN)—**
Adults: 1 ml/minute I.V. for 15 to 30 minutes (10% emulsion); 0.5 ml/minute I.V. for 15 to 30 minutes (20% emulsion). If no adverse reactions occur, rate increased to deliver 500 ml over 4 to 8 hours; total daily dose shouldn't exceed 3 g/kg.
Children: 0.1 ml/minute for 10 to 15 minutes (10% emulsion), 0.05 ml/minute I.V. for 10 to 15 minutes (20% emulsion). If no adverse reactions occur, rate increased

to deliver 1 g/kg over 4 hours; daily dose shouldn't exceed 3 g/kg. Equals up to 60% of daily caloric intake; protein-carbohydrate TPN should supply remaining 40%.

➤ **Fatty acid deficiency—**
Adults and children: 8% to 10% of total caloric intake I.V.

Liposyn
➤ **Prevention of fatty acid deficiency—**
Adults: 500 ml (10% emulsion) I.V. twice weekly. Infused initially at rate of 1 ml/minute for 30 minutes. Rate may be increased to, but shouldn't exceed, 500 ml over 4 to 6 hours.
Children: 5 to 10 ml/kg (10% emulsion) I.V. daily. Initially infused at rate of 0.1 ml/minute for 30 minutes. Rate may be increased to, but shouldn't exceed, 100 ml/hour.

I.V. ADMINISTRATION
● *Alert:* Avoid rapid infusion, and use an infusion pump to regulate rate. Rapid infusion may cause fluid or fat overloading.
● Because lipids support bacterial growth, change all I.V. tubing before each infusion. Check injection site daily. Report signs and symptoms of inflammation or infection promptly.
● Drug may be mixed with amino acid solution, dextrose, electrolytes, and vitamins in same I.V. container. Check with pharmacist for acceptable proportions and compatibility information.

ACTION
Provides neutral triglycerides, predominantly unsaturated fatty acids; acts as a source of calories and prevents fatty acid deficiency. When substituted for dextrose as a source of calories, fat emulsions decrease carbon dioxide production.

Route	Onset	Peak	Duration
I.V.	Immediate	Immediate	Unknown

ADVERSE REACTIONS
Early reactions
CNS: headache, sleepiness, dizziness.
CV: chest and back pains, flushing.
EENT: pressure over eyes.
GI: nausea, vomiting.
Hematologic: hypercoagulability.
Respiratory: dyspnea, cyanosis.

Skin: diaphoresis.
Other: hypersensitivity reactions, irritation at infusion site, fever.
Delayed reactions
CNS: *focal seizures.*
Hematologic: *thrombocytopenia, leukopenia,* leukocytosis.
Hepatic: hepatomegaly.
Other: fever, splenomegaly.

INTERACTIONS
None significant.

EFFECTS ON LAB TEST RESULTS
● May increase lipid, bilirubin, and liver enzyme levels.
● May decrease platelet count. May increase or decrease WBC count.

CONTRAINDICATIONS
Contraindicated in patients with severe egg allergies, hyperlipidemia, lipid nephrosis, or acute pancreatitis accompanied by hyperlipidemia.

NURSING CONSIDERATIONS
● Use cautiously in patients with severe hepatic or pulmonary disease, anemia, or blood coagulation disorders including thrombocytopenia, and in patients at risk for fat embolism.
● Use cautiously in jaundiced or premature infants.
● Don't use fat emulsion if it separates or becomes oily.
● Watch for adverse reactions, especially during first half of infusion.
● Monitor lipid levels closely when patient is receiving fat emulsion therapy. Lipemia must clear between doses.
● Monitor hepatic function carefully in long-term therapy.
● Check platelet count frequently in neonates receiving fat emulsions I.V.
● Carefully monitor triglyceride levels and free fatty acids in infants, especially premature and jaundiced infants.
● Refrigeration of fat emulsions isn't needed unless part of an admixture.
● Intralipid and Liposyn differ mainly by their fatty acid components.

PATIENT TEACHING
● Explain need for fat emulsion therapy, and answer any questions.

• Tell patient to report adverse reactions promptly.

---

medium-chain triglycerides
MCT ◇

Pregnancy risk category NR

AVAILABLE FORMS
Oil: 960 ml (115 calories/15 ml) ◇

INDICATIONS & DOSAGES
➤ **Inadequate digestion or absorption of food fats—**
Adults: 15 ml P.O. t.i.d. or q.i.d.

ACTION
A source of rapidly hydrolyzable lipid.

Route	Onset	Peak	Duration
P.O.	Unknown	Unknown	Unknown

ADVERSE REACTIONS
CNS: *reversible coma in susceptible patients.*
GI: *nausea, vomiting, diarrhea, abdominal distention, cramps.*

INTERACTIONS
None significant.

EFFECTS ON LAB TEST RESULTS
None reported.

CONTRAINDICATIONS
No known contraindications.

NURSING CONSIDERATIONS
• Use cautiously in patients with hepatic cirrhosis, portacaval shunts, or tendency to encephalopathy.
• To minimize GI adverse reactions, give smaller, more frequent doses with meals (mixed with salad dressing, chilled fruit juice, or sauces).
• Drug is more easily absorbed than long-chain fats; not dependent on bile salts for emulsification.
• Drug's rapid metabolism provides quick energy.
• Drug provides 7.7 calories/ml and no essential fatty acids.

PATIENT TEACHING
• Instruct patient when and how to take drug to minimize GI adverse reactions.
• Tell patient to report persistent or severe adverse reactions promptly.
• Caution patient not to use plastic containers or utensils with drug.

---

allopurinol
colchicine
probenecid
sulfinpyrazone

COMBINATION PRODUCTS
COLBENEMID, PROBEN-C, PROBENECID WITH COLCHICINE: probenecid 500 mg and colchicine 0.5 mg.

---

allopurinol
Aloprim, Apo-Allopurinol†, Capurate‡, Purinol†, Zyloprim

Pregnancy risk category C

AVAILABLE FORMS
Capsules: 100 mg‡, 300 mg‡
Injection: 500 mg/30 ml vial
Tablets (scored): 100 mg, 200 mg†, 300 mg

INDICATIONS & DOSAGES
➤ **Gout caused by hyperuricemia or by diseases such as acute or chronic leukemia, polycythemia vera, multiple myeloma, psoriasis—**
Dosage varies with severity of disease; can be given as single dose or divided, but doses greater than 300 mg should be divided.
Adults: Mild gout, 200 to 300 mg P.O. daily; severe gout with large tophi, 400 to 600 mg P.O. daily. Same dosage for maintenance in secondary hyperuricemia. Maximum dose is 800 mg/day. Or, give 200 to 400 mg/m²/day I.V. as a single infusion or equally divided dose q 6, 8, or 12 hours.
Children: Initially, 200 mg/m²/day I.V. as single infusion or equally divided dose q 6, 8, or 12 hours. Then titrate according to uric acid levels.
➤ **Hyperuricemia caused by malignancies—**
Children ages 6 to 10: 300 mg P.O. daily or divided t.i.d.
Children younger than age 6: 50 mg P.O. t.i.d.

➤ **Prevention of acute gout attacks—**
Adults: 100 mg P.O. daily; increase at weekly intervals by 100 mg without exceeding maximum dose (800 mg) until uric acid falls to 6 mg/dl or less.
➤ **Prevention of uric acid nephropathy during cancer chemotherapy—**
Adults: 600 to 800 mg P.O. daily for 2 to 3 days, with high fluid intake.
➤ **Recurrent calcium oxalate calculi—**
Adults: 200 to 300 mg P.O. daily in single or divided doses.
Adjust-a-dose: For renally impaired patients, 200 mg P.O. or I.V. daily if creatinine clearance is 10 to 20 ml/minute; 100 mg P.O. or I.V. daily if clearance is less than 10 ml/minute; and 100 mg P.O. or I.V. at extended intervals if clearance is less than 3 ml/minute.

I.V. ADMINISTRATION
● Preparation of allopurinol includes reconstitution and dilution. Dissolve contents of each 30-ml vial in 25 ml of sterile water for injection. Solution should be diluted to desired concentration (no greater than 6 mg/ml) with normal saline solution for injection or D_5W. Don't use solutions containing sodium bicarbonate.
● Store solution at 68° to 77° F (20° to 25° C) and use within 10 hours. Don't use if particulates or discoloration are present.
● Refer to package insert for full list of drugs that are incompatible with allopurinol in solution.

ACTION
Reduces uric acid production by inhibiting xanthine oxidase.

Route	Onset	Peak	Duration
I.V.	Unknown	0.5 hr	Unknown
P.O.	Unknown	0.5-2 hr	1-2 wk

ADVERSE REACTIONS
CNS: drowsiness, headache, paresthesia, peripheral neuropathy, neuritis.
CV: hypersensitivity vasculitis, necrotizing angiitis.
EENT: epistaxis.

---

*Liquid contains alcohol.   **May contain tartrazine.   †Canada   ‡Australia   §U.K.   ◊OTC

GI: nausea, vomiting, diarrhea, abdominal pain, gastritis, taste loss or perversion, dyspepsia.
GU: *renal failure,* uremia.
Hematologic: *agranulocytosis,* anemia, *aplastic anemia, thrombocytopenia, leukopenia,* leukocytosis, eosinophilia.
Hepatic: *hepatitis, hepatic necrosis,* hepatomegaly, cholestatic jaundice.
Musculoskeletal: arthralgia, myopathy.
Skin: *rash;* exfoliative, urticarial, and purpuric lesions; *erythema multiforme;* severe furunculosis of nose; ichthyosis; alopecia; *toxic epidermal necrolysis.*
Other: ecchymoses, fever, chills.

INTERACTIONS

Drug-drug. *Amoxicillin, ampicillin, bacampicillin:* Increased possibility of rash. Avoid using together.
Anticoagulants except warfarin: Increased anticoagulant effect. Dosage adjustments may be needed.
Antineoplastics: Increased potential for bone marrow suppression. Monitor patient carefully.
Chlorpropamide: May increase hypoglycemic effect. Avoid using together.
Diazoxide, diuretics, mecamylamine, pyrazinamide: Increased uric acid level. Adjust dosage of allopurinol.
Ethacrynic acid, thiazide diuretics: Increased risk of allopurinol toxicity. Reduce dosage of allopurinol, and monitor renal function closely.
Uricosurics: Additive effect. May be used to therapeutic advantage.
Urine-acidifying drugs (ammonium chloride, ascorbic acid, potassium or sodium phosphate): May increase possibility of kidney stone formation. Monitor patient carefully.
Xanthines: Increased theophylline levels. Adjust dosage of theophylline, as needed.
Drug-lifestyle. *Alcohol use:* Increased uric acid levels. Discourage patient from alcohol use.

EFFECTS ON LAB TEST RESULTS
● May increase alkaline phosphatase, AST, and ALT levels.
● May increase eosinophil count. May decrease hemoglobin and granulocyte and platelet counts. May increase or decrease WBC count.

CONTRAINDICATIONS
Contraindicated in patients hypersensitive to drug and in those with idiopathic hemochromatosis.

NURSING CONSIDERATIONS
● Monitor uric acid levels to evaluate drug's effectiveness.
● Monitor fluid intake and output; daily urine output of at least 2 L and maintenance of neutral or slightly alkaline urine are desirable.
● Periodically monitor CBC and hepatic and renal function, especially at start of therapy.
● Optimal benefits may need 2 to 6 weeks of therapy. Because acute gout attacks may occur during this time, concurrent use of colchicine may be prescribed prophylactically.
● Don't restart drug in patients who experience a severe reaction.
● *Alert:* Don't confuse Zyloprim with ZORprin.

PATIENT TEACHING
● To minimize GI adverse reactions, tell patient to take drug with or immediately after meals.
● Encourage patient to drink plenty of fluids while taking drug unless otherwise contraindicated.
● Drug may cause drowsiness; tell patient not to drive or perform hazardous tasks requiring mental alertness until CNS effects of drug are known.
● If patient is taking allopurinol for recurrent calcium oxalate stones, advise him also to reduce his dietary intake of animal protein, sodium, refined sugars, oxalate-rich foods, and calcium.
● Tell patient to stop drug at first sign of rash, which may precede severe hypersensitivity or other adverse reactions. Rash is more common in patients taking diuretics and in those with renal disorders. Tell patient to report all adverse reactions.
● Advise patient to avoid alcohol during therapy.
● Teach patient importance of continuing drug even if asymptomatic.

Reactions may be *common,* uncommon, *life-threatening*, or COMMON AND LIFE-THREATENING.

colchicine
Colgout‡

*Pregnancy risk category C (P.O.),
D (I.V.)*

AVAILABLE FORMS
Injection: 1 mg (1/60 grain)/2 ml
Tablets: 0.5 mg (1/120 grain), 0.6 mg
(1/100 grain) as sugar-coated granules

INDICATIONS & DOSAGES
➤ **Prevention of acute gout attacks as
prophylactic or maintenance therapy—**
Adults: 0.5 or 0.6 mg P.O. daily. Patients
who normally have one attack per year or
fewer should receive drug only 3 to 4 days
weekly; patients who have more than one
attack per year should receive drug daily.
In severe cases, 1.0 to 1.8 mg P.O. daily.
➤ **Prevention of gout attacks in patients
undergoing surgery—**
Adults: 0.5 to 0.6 mg P.O. t.i.d. 3 days before and 3 days after surgery.
➤ **Acute gout, acute gouty arthritis—**
Adults: Initially, 0.5 to 1.2 mg P.O.; then
0.5 to 1.2 mg q 1 to 2 hours until pain is
relieved; nausea, vomiting, or diarrhea
ensues; or maximum dose of 8 mg is
reached. Or, 2 mg I.V.; then 0.5 mg I.V. q
6 hours if needed. Wait 3 days before a
second course to reduce cumulative toxicity. (Note that some prescribers prefer to
give a single I.V. injection of 3 mg.) Total
I.V. dose over 24 hours (one course of
treatment) shouldn't exceed 4 mg.

I.V. ADMINISTRATION
● Give by slow I.V. push over 2 to 5 minutes.
● Monitor patient for extravasation because colchicine irritates tissues.
● Don't dilute colchicine injection with
D_5W injection or other fluids that might
change pH of colchicine solution. If lower
concentration of colchicine injection is
needed, dilute with normal saline solution
or sterile water for injection and give
over 2 to 5 minutes by direct injection.
Preferably, inject into the tubing of a free-
flowing I.V. solution. Don't inject if diluted solution becomes turbid.

ACTION
Unknown. As an antigout drug, probably
decreases WBC motility, phagocytosis,
and lactic acid production, decreasing
urate crystal deposits and reducing inflammation. As antiosteolytic drug, probably
inhibits mitosis of osteoprogenitor cells
and decreases osteoclast activity.

Route	Onset	Peak	Duration
I.V.	6-12 hr	Unknown	Unknown
P.O.	12 hr	0.5-2 hr	Unknown

ADVERSE REACTIONS
CNS: peripheral neuritis.
GI: *nausea, vomiting, abdominal pain, di-
arrhea.*
GU: reversible azoospermia.
Hematologic: *aplastic anemia, thrombo-
cytopenia, agranulocytosis with long-
term use,* nonthrombocytopenic purpura.
Musculoskeletal: myopathy.
Skin: alopecia, urticaria, dermatitis.
Other: severe local irritation if extravasa-
tion occurs, hypersensitivity reactions.

INTERACTIONS
Drug-drug. *Vitamin B_{12}:* Impaired absorption of oral vitamin B_{12}. Avoid using
together.
Drug-lifestyle. *Alcohol use:* May impair
efficacy of colchicine prophylaxis. Discourage patient from use together.

EFFECTS ON LAB TEST RESULTS
● May increase alkaline phosphatase, AST,
and ALT levels. May decrease carotene
and cholesterol levels.
● May decrease hemoglobin and platelet
and granulocyte counts.

CONTRAINDICATIONS
Contraindicated in patients hypersensitive
to drug and in those with blood dyscrasias, serious CV disease, renal disease, or
GI disorders.

NURSING CONSIDERATIONS
● Use cautiously in elderly or debilitated
patients and in those with early signs of
CV, renal, or GI disease.
● Obtain baseline laboratory test results,
including CBC, before therapy and periodically throughout therapy.

• **Alert:** Don't give I.M. or S.C.; severe local irritation occurs.
• As maintenance therapy, give drug with meals to reduce GI effects. Drug may be used with uricosurics.
• Monitor fluid intake and output; keep output at 2 L daily.
• **Alert:** After full course of I.V. colchicine (4 mg), don't give colchicine by any route for at least 7 days. Colchicine is a toxic drug and death has resulted from overdose.
• First sign of acute overdose may be GI symptoms, followed by vascular damage, muscle weakness, and ascending paralysis. Delirium and seizures may occur without patient losing consciousness.
• Discontinue drug as soon as gout pain is relieved or at first sign of GI symptoms.

PATIENT TEACHING
• Teach patient how to take drug, and tell him to drink extra fluids.
• Tell patient to report adverse reactions, especially signs of acute overdose (nausea, vomiting, abdominal pain, diarrhea, unusual bleeding, bruising, tiredness, weakness, numbness, or tingling).
• Advise patient to avoid using alcohol while taking drug.
• Tell patient with gout to limit intake of foods high in purine, such as anchovies, liver, sardines, kidneys, sweetbreads, peas, and lentils.

---

probenecid
Benuryl†

Pregnancy risk category B

AVAILABLE FORMS
Tablets: 500 mg

INDICATIONS & DOSAGES
➤ **Adjunct to penicillin therapy—**
Adults and children weighing more than 50 kg (111 lb): 500 mg P.O. q.i.d.
Children ages 2 to 14 or weighing 50 kg or less: Initially, 25 mg/kg P.O.; then 40 mg/kg/day in divided doses q.i.d.
➤ **Gonorrhea—**
Adults: 3.5 g ampicillin P.O. with 1 g probenecid P.O. given together. Or, 1 g probenecid P.O. 30 minutes before dose of

4.8 million units of aqueous penicillin G procaine I.M., injected at two different sites.
➤ **Hyperuricemia of gout, gouty arthritis—**
Adults: 250 mg P.O. b.i.d. for first week; then 500 mg b.i.d., to maximum of 2 to 3 g daily. Maintenance dose should be reviewed q 6 months and reduced by increments of 500 mg, if indicated.

ACTION
Blocks renal tubular reabsorption of uric acid, increasing excretion, and inhibits active renal tubular secretion of many weak organic acids, such as penicillins and cephalosporins.

Route	Onset	Peak	Duration
P.O.	Unknown	2-4 hr	Unknown

ADVERSE REACTIONS
CNS: *headache,* dizziness.
CV: flushing.
GI: anorexia, nausea, vomiting, sore gums.
GU: urinary frequency, renal colic, nephrotic syndrome, costovertebral pain.
Hematologic: *hemolytic anemia,* anemia, *aplastic anemia.*
Hepatic: *hepatic necrosis.*
Skin: dermatitis, pruritus.
Other: fever, exacerbation of gout, hypersensitivity reactions including *anaphylaxis.*

INTERACTIONS
Drug-drug. *Acetaminophen, acyclovir, cephalosporins, ketamine, lorazepam, meclofenamate, penicillin, rifampin, thiopental:* May increase levels of these drugs. Use together cautiously.
Allopurinol: Giving together increases uric acid–lowering effects. May be used to therapeutic advantage.
Methotrexate: Decreased methotrexate excretion. Determine serum levels and reduce methotrexate dosage, if needed.
Nitrofurantoin: Increased toxicity and reduced effectiveness. Reduce probenecid dose.
NSAIDs: May increase toxicity. Avoid using together.

Salicylates: Inhibited uricosuric effect of probenecid, causing urate retention. Avoid using together.

Sulfonylureas: Increased hypoglycemic effect. Monitor blood glucose levels closely. Dosage adjustment may be needed.

Zidovudine: May increase zidovudine levels and toxicity symptoms. Monitor patient.

Drug-lifestyle. *Alcohol use:* Increased urate levels. Discourage patient from use together.

EFFECTS ON LAB TEST RESULTS
• May decrease hemoglobin.

CONTRAINDICATIONS
Contraindicated in patients hypersensitive to drug and in those with uric acid kidney stones or blood dyscrasias; also contraindicated in patients with an acute gout attack and in children younger than age 2.

NURSING CONSIDERATIONS
• Use cautiously in patients with peptic ulcer or renal impairment.
• Use cautiously in patients with sulfa allergy because probenecid is a sulfonamide derivative.
• To minimize GI distress, give drug with milk, food, or antacids. Continued disturbances might indicate need to reduce dosage.
• Force fluids to maintain minimum daily output of 2 to 3 L. Alkalinize urine with sodium bicarbonate or potassium citrate. These measures will prevent hematuria, renal colic, urate stone development, and costovertebral pain.
• Treatment of gout doesn't start until acute attack subsides. Drug doesn't contain an analgesic or anti-inflammatory, and it's of no value during acute gout attacks.
• Monitor BUN level and renal function test results periodically in long-term therapy.
• Drug is suitable for long-term use; no cumulative effects or tolerance have been reported.
• Drug is ineffective in patients with chronic renal insufficiency (glomerular filtration rate below 30 ml/minute).
• Drug may increase frequency, severity, and length of acute gout attacks during first

6 to 12 months of therapy. Prophylactic colchicine or another anti-inflammatory is given during first 3 to 6 months.
• Drug may falsely elevate theophylline levels.
• **Alert:** Don't confuse probenecid with Procanbid.

PATIENT TEACHING
• Instruct patient and family that, when prescribed as treatment for gout, drug must be taken regularly, or gout attacks might occur.
• Tell patient to visit prescriber regularly so that uric acid can be monitored and dosage adjusted, if needed. Lifelong therapy may be needed in patients with hyperuricemia.
• Advise patient with gout to avoid all drugs that contain aspirin, which may precipitate gout. Acetaminophen may be used for pain.
• Instruct patient to drink at least 6 to 8 glasses of water per day.
• Urge patient with gout to avoid alcohol; it increases urate level.
• Tell patient with gout to limit intake of foods high in purine, such as anchovies, liver, sardines, kidneys, sweetbreads, peas, and lentils. Also tell him to identify and avoid other foods that may trigger gout attacks.
• Instruct patient to take all medicine as prescribed when given with penicillin.

sulfinpyrazone
Anturan†, Anturane

Pregnancy risk category NR

AVAILABLE FORMS
Capsules: 200 mg
Tablets: 100 mg

INDICATIONS & DOSAGES
➤ **Intermittent or chronic gouty arthritis—**
Adults: 200 to 400 mg P.O. b.i.d. first week; then 400 mg P.O. b.i.d. Maximum dose is 800 mg daily.

ACTION
A pyrazolone derivative that blocks renal tubular reabsorption of uric acid, increas-

ing excretion, and inhibits platelet aggregation.

Route	Onset	Peak	Duration
P.O.	Unknown	1-2 hr	4-6 hr

ADVERSE REACTIONS

GI: *nausea, dyspepsia,* epigastric pain, reactivation of peptic ulcerations.
GU: altered renal function test results.
Hematologic: anemia, *leukopenia, agranulocytosis, thrombocytopenia, aplastic anemia.*
Respiratory: *bronchoconstriction in patients with aspirin-induced asthma.*
Skin: rash.

INTERACTIONS

Drug-drug. *Aspirin, salicylates:* Inhibited uricosuric effect of sulfinpyrazone. Avoid using together.
Oral anticoagulants: Increased anticoagulant effect and risk of bleeding. Use together cautiously.
Oral antidiabetics: Increased effects. Monitor glucose levels.
Probenecid: Inhibited renal excretion of sulfinpyrazone. Use together cautiously.
Theophylline, verapamil: Increased clearance. Use together cautiously.
Drug-lifestyle. *Alcohol use:* Decreased effectiveness. Discourage patient from use together.

EFFECTS ON LAB TEST RESULTS

• May increase BUN and creatinine levels.
• May decrease hemoglobin and WBC, granulocyte, and platelet counts.

CONTRAINDICATIONS

Contraindicated in patients hypersensitive to pyrazole derivatives (including oxyphenbutazone and phenylbutazone) and in those with blood dyscrasias, active peptic ulcer, or symptoms of GI inflammation or ulceration.

NURSING CONSIDERATIONS

• Use cautiously in patients with healed peptic ulcer and in pregnant women.
• Monitor BUN level, CBC, and renal function studies periodically during long-term use.
• Monitor fluid intake and output closely. Therapy, especially at start, may lead to renal colic and formation of uric acid stones until acid levels are normal (about 6 mg/dl).
• Force fluids to maintain minimum daily output of 2 to 3 L. Alkalinize urine with sodium bicarbonate or other drug.
• Drug doesn't contain an analgesic or anti-inflammatory, and it's of no value during acute gout attacks.
• Drug may increase frequency, severity, and length of acute gout attacks during first 6 to 12 months of therapy. Prophylactic colchicine or another anti-inflammatory is given during first 3 to 6 months.
• Lifelong therapy may be needed in patients with hyperuricemia.
• *Alert:* Don't confuse Anturane with Accutane, Artane, or Antabuse.

PATIENT TEACHING

• Instruct patient and family that drug must be taken regularly, even during acute exacerbations.
• Tell patient to visit prescriber regularly so blood levels can be monitored and dosage adjusted, if needed.
• Warn patient with gout not to take aspirin-containing drugs because these may precipitate gout. Acetaminophen may be used for pain.
• Tell patient with gout to avoid foods high in purine, such as anchovies, liver, sardines, kidneys, sweetbreads, peas, and lentils, and to identify and avoid any other foods that may trigger gout attacks.
• Instruct patient to drink at least 10 to 12 glasses of fluid daily.
• Advise patient to avoid alcohol during therapy.
• Instruct patient to report unusual bleeding or bruising or flulike symptoms.

Reactions may be *common,* uncommon, *life-threatening,* or COMMON AND LIFE-THREATENING.

chymopapain
hyaluronidase

COMBINATION PRODUCTS
None.

---

chymopapain
Chymodiactin

Pregnancy risk category C

AVAILABLE FORMS
Powder for injection: 4,000 units/vial;
each unit of chymopapain is also known
as 1 nanoKatal (nKat)

INDICATIONS & DOSAGES
➤ **Herniated lumbar disk—**
Adults: 2,000 to 4,000 units (nKat)/disk
injected intradiskally. Maximum dose for
multiple disk herniation is 8,000 units.

ACTION
A refined proteolytic enzyme that hydrolyzes noncollagenous proteins in the
chondromucoprotein of the nucleus pulpo-
sus, lowering pressure within the disk.

Route	Onset	Peak	Duration
Intradisk	30 min	Unknown	1 wk

ADVERSE REACTIONS
CNS: *subarachnoid and intracerebral
hemorrhage, seizures,* headache, paresthesia, dizziness.
EENT: conjunctivitis, vasomotor rhinitis.
GI: nausea.
Musculoskeletal: leg weakness, numbness of legs and toes, *back pain, stiffness,
back spasm, soreness,* paraplegia, acute
transverse myelitis.
Skin: erythema, rash, pruritic urticaria.
Other: *anaphylaxis, anaphylactoid reaction, angioedema.*

INTERACTIONS
Drug-drug. *Radiographic contrast media:*
May cause adverse reactions (increased

risk of neurotoxicity) when injected with
chymopapain. Avoid using together.

EFFECTS ON LAB TEST RESULTS
None reported.

CONTRAINDICATIONS
Contraindicated in patients with history of
allergy to drug, papaya, or papaya derivatives such as meat tenderizers; in those
who have previously received an injection
of chymopapain; and in those with severe
spondylolisthesis in addition to spinal
stenosis, severe progressing paralysis, or
evidence of spinal cord tumor or cauda
equina lesion.

NURSING CONSIDERATIONS
• A ChymoFAST test can detect hypersensitivity to drug. To lessen the severity of
anaphylactoid reactions, give histamine-
receptor antagonists before drug (such as
cimetidine 300 mg P.O. q 6 hours and diphenhydramine 50 mg P.O. q 6 hours for 24
hours before chymopapain administration).
• *Alert:* Drug should be used only by prescribers qualified and experienced to perform laminectomy, diskectomy, or other
spinal procedures, and who have received
specialized training in chemonucleolysis.
It shouldn't be injected in regions other
than the lumbar spine; extremely toxic if
injected into subarachnoid space.
• Use sterile water, not bacteriostatic water for injection, to reconstitute drug. Add
2 ml of sterile water for injection to vial
containing 4,000 units (nKat) to make a
solution containing 2,000 units/ml. Use
within 1 hour after reconstitution. Discard
unused drug.
• After wiping stopper with alcohol, allow
to dry before drawing up drug because alcohol inactivates the enzyme.
• Watch very closely for anaphylactoid reaction (0.5% of patients). Reaction may be
immediate or delayed up to 1 hour after
injection and may last for minutes to several hours. Watch for hypotension and
bronchospasm, possibly leading to laryngeal edema, arrhythmias, cardiac arrest,

---

coma, and death. Other signs of allergic response include erythema, pilomotor erection, rash, pruritic urticaria, conjunctivitis, vasomotor rhinitis, angioedema, and various GI disturbances.
• Keep an I.V. line open to manage anaphylaxis quickly, if needed. Keep epinephrine and corticosteroids available.

PATIENT TEACHING
• Instruct patient to anticipate delayed allergic reactions, such as rash, urticaria, or pruritus, which may occur up to 15 days after injection. Tell him to report these at once.
• Warn patient that he may experience back pain or involuntary muscle spasm in the lower back for several days after injection. Reassure him that this is common and temporary.

hyaluronidase
Hyalase§, Wydase

Pregnancy risk category C

AVAILABLE FORMS
Injection: 150 units/ml in 1-ml, 10-ml vials

INDICATIONS & DOSAGES
➤ **Adjunct to increase absorption and dispersion of other injected drugs—**
Adults and children: 150 USP units added to solution containing other drug.
➤ **Hypodermoclysis—**
Adults and children older than age 3: 150 USP units injected S.C. before clysis or injected into clysis tubing near needle for each 1,000-ml clysis solution.
➤ **Excretory urography when contrast medium is given S.C.—**
Adults and children: With patient in a prone position, 75 USP units S.C. over each scapula; then injection of contrast medium at same sites.

ACTION
Hydrolyzes hyaluronic acid, promoting diffusion of fluids in tissues.

Route	Onset	Peak	Duration
S.C.	Immediate	Unknown	1-2 days

ADVERSE REACTIONS
None significant.

INTERACTIONS
Drug-drug. *Local anesthetics:* Increased potential for toxic local reaction. Use together cautiously.

EFFECTS ON LAB TEST RESULTS
None reported.

CONTRAINDICATIONS
Contraindicated in patients hypersensitive to drug.

NURSING CONSIDERATIONS
• Perform a skin test (0.02 ml of solution) for sensitivity. Don't inject into diseased areas. Watch for local reactions (wheal and pseudopods within 5 minutes and persisting, with itching, for 20 to 30 minutes). Erythema alone isn't considered a positive reaction.
• Drug may be given as the commercially available solution or prepared from powder for injection. Prepare a solution of 150 units/ml by adding 1 or 10 ml of normal saline solution to a vial labeled 150 or 1,500 USP units of hyaluronidase, respectively.
• Don't inject into acutely inflamed or cancerous areas.
• *Alert:* Drug isn't recommended for I.V. use but may be given S.C., I.D., or I.M.
• For children, add 15 units to each 100 ml of solution. Drip rate shouldn't exceed 2 ml/minute.
• In children younger than age 3, the volume of a single clysis shouldn't exceed 200 ml.
• Don't add to solutions containing epinephrine or heparin.
• For hypodermoclysis, adjust dosage, rate of injection, and type of solution per patient's response.
• If solution gets in eyes, flush with water.
• Protect from heat. Don't use cloudy or discolored solution. Store reconstituted solution below 86° F (30° C), and use within 14 days.

PATIENT TEACHING
• Explain need for drug to patient and family and describe how drug is given.
• Inform patient about possible adverse skin reactions.

Reactions may be *common*, uncommon, *life-threatening*, or COMMON AND LIFE-THREATENING.

carboprost tromethamine
dinoprostone
methylergonovine maleate
mifepristone
oxytocin, synthetic injection

COMBINATION PRODUCTS
None.

---

carboprost tromethamine
Hemabate

Pregnancy risk category C

AVAILABLE FORMS
Injection: 250 mcg/ml

INDICATIONS & DOSAGES
➤ **To terminate pregnancy between weeks 13 and 20 of gestation—**
Adults: Initially, 250 mcg deep I.M. Subsequent doses of 250 mcg given at intervals of 1½ to 3½ hours, depending on uterine response. Dosage may be increased in increments to 500 mcg if contractility is inadequate after several 250-mcg doses. Total dose shouldn't exceed 12 mg on continuous administration for more than 2 days.
➤ **Postpartum hemorrhage from uterine atony not managed by conventional methods—**
Adults: 250 mcg by deep I.M. injection. Repeat doses given at 15- to 90-minute intervals, p.r.n. Maximum total dose is 2 mg.

ACTION
A prostaglandin that produces strong, prompt contractions of uterine smooth muscle, possibly mediated by calcium and cAMP.

Route	Onset	Peak	Duration
I.M.	Unknown	15-60 min	24 hr

ADVERSE REACTIONS
CNS: headache, anxiety, paresthesia, syncope, weakness.

CV: chest pain, *arrhythmias,* flushing.
EENT: blurred vision, eye pain.
GI: *vomiting, diarrhea, nausea.*
GU: endometritis, *uterine rupture,* uterine or vaginal pain.
Musculoskeletal: backache, leg cramps.
Respiratory: coughing, wheezing.
Skin: rash, diaphoresis.
Other: breast tenderness, *fever,* chills, hot flashes.

INTERACTIONS
Drug-drug. *Other oxytocics:* May increase action. Avoid using together.

EFFECTS ON LAB TEST RESULTS
None reported.

CONTRAINDICATIONS
Contraindicated in patients hypersensitive to drug and in those with acute pelvic inflammatory disease or active cardiac, pulmonary, renal, or hepatic disease.

NURSING CONSIDERATIONS
• Use cautiously in patients with history of asthma, hypotension, hypertension, anemia, jaundice, diabetes; seizure disorders; previous uterine surgery, or CV, adrenal, renal, or hepatic disease.
• Unlike other prostaglandin abortifacients, drug is given by I.M. injection. Injectable form avoids risk of expelling vaginal suppositories if patient has profuse vaginal bleeding.
• Drug should be used only by trained personnel in a hospital setting.

PATIENT TEACHING
• Explain use and administration of drug to patient and family.
• Instruct patient to report adverse reactions promptly.

---

dinoprostone
Cervidil, Prepidil, Prostin E2

Pregnancy risk category C

AVAILABLE FORMS
Endocervical gel: 0.5 mg per application (2.5-ml syringe)
Vaginal insert: 10 mg
Vaginal suppositories: 20 mg

INDICATIONS & DOSAGES
➤ **To terminate second-trimester pregnancy; to evacuate uterus in missed abortion, intrauterine fetal death up to 28 weeks' gestation, or benign hydatidiform mole (suppository)—**
Adults: 20-mg suppository inserted high into posterior vaginal fornix; repeated q 3 to 5 hours until abortion is complete.
➤ **To ripen an unfavorable cervix in pregnant patients at or near term (gel or vaginal insert)—**
Adults: Contents of one syringe given intravaginally; if cervix remains unfavorable after 6 hours, dosage repeated. No more than 1.5 mg (three applications) should be given within 24-hour period.
➤ **Vaginal insert—**
Adults: 10-mg vaginal insert placed transversely in posterior fornix of vagina immediately after removal from foil.

ACTION
A prostaglandin that produces strong, prompt contractions of uterine smooth muscle, possibly mediated by calcium and cAMP.

Route	Onset	Peak	Duration
Intravaginal (gel)	15-30 min	Unknown	Unknown
Intravaginal (insert)	Unknown	Unknown	Unknown
Intravaginal (suppository)	10 min	Unknown	2-6 hr

ADVERSE REACTIONS
CNS: *headache, dizziness,* anxiety, paresthesia, weakness, syncope.
CV: chest pain, *arrhythmias.*
EENT: blurred vision, eye pain.
GI: *nausea, vomiting, diarrhea.*

GU: vaginal pain, vaginitis, endometritis, uterine rupture.
Musculoskeletal: *nocturnal leg cramps,* backache, muscle cramps.
Respiratory: coughing, dyspnea.
Skin: rash, diaphoresis.
Other: breast tenderness, *fever, shivering, chills,* hot flashes.

INTERACTIONS
Drug-drug. *Other oxytocics:* May increase action. Avoid using together.
Drug-lifestyle. *Alcohol use:* Inhibited effectiveness of dinoprostone with high doses. Discourage use together.

EFFECTS ON LAB TEST RESULTS
None reported.

CONTRAINDICATIONS
Gel form is contraindicated in patients hypersensitive to prostaglandins or constituents of gel. Also contraindicated when prolonged contractions of the uterus are considered inappropriate. Also contraindicated in patients with placenta previa or unexplained vaginal bleeding during pregnancy and in whom vaginal delivery isn't indicated (because of vasa previa or active herpes genitalia).

Suppository form is contraindicated in patients hypersensitive to drug, in those with acute pelvic inflammatory disease, and in those with active cardiac, pulmonary, renal, or hepatic disease.

Insert form is contraindicated in patients hypersensitive to drug. Also contraindicated when there's clinical suspicion or evidence of fetal distress when delivery isn't imminent, when patient has unexplained vaginal bleeding during pregnancy, when there's evidence or strong suspicion of marked cephalopelvic disproportion, when oxytocic drugs are contraindicated, when prolonged contraction of the uterus may be detrimental to fetal safety or uterine integrity, when membranes have ruptured, when patient is already receiving oxytocic drugs, and when patient is multipara with 6 or more previous term pregnancies.

NURSING CONSIDERATIONS
• Use suppository form cautiously in patients with asthma, seizure disorders, ane-

mia, diabetes, hypertension or hypotension, jaundice, scarred uterus, cervicitis, acute vaginitis, or CV, renal, or hepatic disease.

• Use gel form and insert forms cautiously in patients with asthma and in those with a history of asthma, glaucoma, or intraocular pressure; renal or hepatic dysfunction; or ruptured membranes.

• Give only when critical care facilities are available.

• When using drug as an abortifacient, be prepared to pretreat patient with an antiemetic and antidiarrheal.

• For cervical ripening, have patient lie on her back; the cervix is examined using a speculum. Assist with insertion of gel, using aseptic technique: A catheter provided with drug is used to give gel into cervical canal just below level of the internal os.

• When using gel, warm to room temperature.

• After administration of gel, patient should remain supine for 10 minutes.

• When gel form is used, contents of syringe are used for one patient only. Discard syringe, catheter, and unused drug after administration; don't attempt to give small amount of drug remaining in catheter.

• It isn't necessary to warm vaginal insert before giving. A minimal amount of water-soluble jelly may be used to aid insertion.

• Have patient remain supine for 2 hours following insertion of vaginal insert; thereafter, she may be ambulatory. Remove insert on onset of active labor or 12 hours after insertion.

• Treat dinoprostone-induced fever (self-limiting and transient and occurs in about 50% of patients) with water sponging and increased fluid intake, not with aspirin.

• Check vaginal discharge regularly.

• Abortion should be complete within 30 hours when suppository form is used.

• Freeze suppositories and inserts at –4° F (–20° C). Store gel in refrigerator at 36° to 46° F (2° to 8° C).

PATIENT TEACHING

• Explain use and administration of drug to patient and family.

• Instruct patient to report adverse reactions promptly.

methylergonovine maleate
Methergine

Pregnancy risk category C

AVAILABLE FORMS
Injection: 0.2 mg/ml
Tablets: 0.2 mg

INDICATIONS & DOSAGES
➤ **Prevention and treatment of postpartum hemorrhage caused by uterine atony or subinvolution—**
Adults: 0.2 mg I.M. q 2 to 4 hours. For excessive uterine bleeding or other emergencies, 0.2 mg I.V. over 1 minute while monitoring blood pressure and uterine contractions. After initial I.M. or I.V. dose, 0.2 mg P.O. q 6 to 8 hours for 2 to 7 days. Decrease dosage if severe cramping occurs.

I.V. ADMINISTRATION
• *Alert:* Don't routinely give drug I.V. because of risk of severe hypertension and CVA. If it must be given I.V., give slowly over at least 1 minute, while carefully monitoring blood pressure. I.V. dose may be diluted to 5 ml with normal saline solution before use. Contractions begin immediately after I.V. use and continue for up to 45 minutes.

• Store I.V. solution below 46° F (8° C). Daily stock may be kept at room temperature for 60 to 90 days.

ACTION
Increases motor activity of the uterus by direct stimulation of the smooth muscle, shortening the third stage of labor and reducing blood loss.

Route	Onset	Peak	Duration
I.M.	2-5 min	Unknown	3 hr
I.V.	Immediate	Unknown	45 min
P.O.	5-10 min	30 min	3 hr

ADVERSE REACTIONS
CNS: dizziness, headache, *seizures,* hallucinations, *CVA with I.V. use.*
CV: hypertension, transient chest pain, palpitations, hypotension, thrombophlebitis.
EENT: tinnitus, nasal congestion.

GI: *nausea, vomiting,* diarrhea, foul taste.
GU: hematuria.
Musculoskeletal: leg cramps.
Respiratory: dyspnea.
Skin: diaphoresis.

INTERACTIONS
Drug-drug. *Dopamine, I.V. oxytocin, regional anesthetics, vasoconstrictors:* Excessive vasoconstriction. Use together cautiously.

EFFECTS ON LAB TEST RESULTS
• May decrease prolactin level.

CONTRAINDICATIONS
Contraindicated in pregnant patients, in patients sensitive to ergot preparations, and in patients with hypertension or toxemia.

NURSING CONSIDERATIONS
• Use cautiously in patients with sepsis, obliterative vascular disease, or hepatic or renal disease. Also use cautiously during last stage of labor.
• Monitor and record blood pressure, pulse rate, and uterine response; report sudden change in vital signs, frequent periods of uterine relaxation, and character and amount of vaginal bleeding.
• Monitor contractions, which may continue 3 hours or more after P.O. or I.M. administration.
• Store tablets in tightly closed, light-resistant container. Discard if discolored.

PATIENT TEACHING
• Explain use and administration of drug to patient and family.
• Instruct patient to report adverse reactions promptly.

✳ *NEW DRUG*

mifepristone
Mifeprex

Pregnancy risk category NR

AVAILABLE FORMS
Tablets: 200 mg

INDICATIONS & DOSAGES
➤ **Termination of intrauterine pregnancy during first 7 weeks—**
Adults: 600 mg (three 200-mg tablets) P.O. as a single dose (considered day 1). On day 3, unless abortion is confirmed by clinical examination or ultrasonographic scan, give 400 mcg (two 200-mcg tablets) of misoprostol P.O.

ACTION
Competitively interacts with progesterone at progesterone-receptor sites. Drug inhibits activity of endogenous and exogenous progesterone, resulting in termination of pregnancy.

Route	Onset	Peak	Duration
P.O.	Rapid	90 min	11 days

ADVERSE REACTIONS
CNS: *headache, dizziness, fatigue,* insomnia, asthenia, anxiety, syncope, fainting.
EENT: sinusitis.
GI: *abdominal cramping, nausea, vomiting, diarrhea,* dyspepsia.
GU: vaginitis, *uterine cramping,* pelvic pain, ***uterine hemorrhage.***
Hematologic: anemia, leukorrhea, decrease in hemoglobin of more than 2 g/dl.
Musculoskeletal: back pain, leg pain.
Other: fever, rigors, viral infections.

INTERACTIONS
Drug-drug. *Carbamazepine, dexamethasone, phenobarbital, phenytoin, rifampin:* May stimulate metabolism, reducing mifepristone levels. Use together cautiously.
Drugs that are CYP 3A4 substrates and have narrow therapeutic ranges (general anesthetics): Increases levels and prolongs elimination of these drugs. Use together cautiously.
Erythromycin, itraconazole, ketoconazole: May inhibit metabolism and increase mifepristone levels. Use together cautiously.
Drug-herb. *St. John's wort:* May stimulate metabolism, reducing mifepristone levels. Discourage use together.
Drug-food. *Grapefruit juice:* May inhibit metabolism and increase mifepristone level. Advise patient to avoid taking drug with grapefruit juice.

Reactions may be *common,* uncommon, *life-threatening,* or COMMON AND LIFE-THREATENING.

EFFECTS ON LAB TEST RESULTS
• May decrease hemoglobin more than 2 g/dl.

CONTRAINDICATIONS
Contraindicated in patients allergic to mifepristone, misoprostol, or other prostaglandins; in those with confirmed or suspected ectopic pregnancy or undiagnosed adnexal mass; and in patients with an intrauterine device (IUD) in place. Also contraindicated in patients with chronic adrenal failure, inherited porphyrias, or hemorrhagic disorders, and in those on long-term corticosteroid therapy or taking anticoagulants.

Don't use in patients without access to a medical facility equipped to provide emergency treatment of incomplete abortion, blood transfusions, and emergency resuscitation from the first visit until discharged by the prescriber.

Don't give to patient who may be unable to understand effects of procedure or to comply with its regimen.

NURSING CONSIDERATIONS
• Use cautiously in patients with CV disease; hypertension; respiratory, renal, or hepatic disease; type 1 diabetes; or severe anemia, and in those who are heavy smokers. Also use cautiously in women older than age 35 who smoke 10 or more cigarettes per day because drug's effects in these patients aren't known.
• Drug is supplied only to health care providers who sign and return a Prescriber's Agreement. It's not available through pharmacies.
• For purposes of this treatment, pregnancy is dated from the first day of the last menstrual period in a presumed 28-day cycle with ovulation occurring at midcycle. Duration of pregnancy may be determined from menstrual history and clinical examination. Ultrasonographic scan should be used if duration of pregnancy is uncertain or if ectopic pregnancy is suspected.
• Patient must read the medication guide and sign the Patient Agreement before drug is given.
• *Alert:* If patient has an IUD in place, make sure that it is removed before treatment begins.

• For proper administration of mifepristone and misoprostol to terminate pregnancy, the patient must visit the prescriber three times. This treatment may be given only in a clinic, medical office, or hospital by or under the supervision of a health care provider able to assess the gestational age of an embryo and to diagnose ectopic pregnancies. The prescriber must also be able to provide surgical intervention in case of incomplete abortion or severe bleeding, or have made plans to provide such care through others, and be able to ensure patient access to medical facilities equipped to provide blood transfusions and resuscitation, if needed.
• After taking misoprostol, patient may need medication for cramps or GI symptoms.
• Patient must return for a follow-up visit about 14 days after taking mifepristone to determine by clinical examination or ultrasound that a complete termination of pregnancy has occurred and to assess the degree of bleeding. If the patient is still pregnant at this visit, the fetus is at risk for malformation resulting from the treatment. Surgical termination is recommended.
• Vaginal bleeding and uterine or abdominal cramping are expected effects of the drug. Vaginal bleeding or spotting occurs for about 9 to 16 days. Excessive bleeding may need treatment with vasoconstrictors, curettage, saline infusions, or blood transfusions. Persistence of heavy or moderate bleeding at the 14-day follow-up visit may indicate incomplete abortion.
• It's unknown if drug appears in breast milk. A breast-feeding woman should consult her prescriber to decide whether to discard her breast milk for a few days after taking drug.
• Store drug at controlled room temperature.
• *Alert:* Don't confuse mifepristone and misoprostol.

PATIENT TEACHING
• Give patient a copy of the medication guide and Patient Agreement. Review these with patient and allow her the chance to ask questions.
• Inform patient of importance of completing the treatment schedule and stress the necessity of returning for a follow-up

---

visit about 14 days after taking mifepristone.
- Advise patient that vaginal bleeding, which may be heavy at times and accompanied by uterine cramping, will probably occur.
- Inform patient that vaginal bleeding isn't proof of a complete abortion and that she must return for follow-up visit to confirm the abortion.
- Tell patient that, if treatment fails, there is a risk of fetal harm and that surgical intervention may be needed.
- Supply patient with a name and telephone number to contact in case of emergency.
- Advise patient that she may become pregnant again as soon as termination of pregnancy is complete and before normal menses has returned.
- Instruct patient on various forms of contraception.

---

oxytocin, synthetic injection
Oxytocin, Pitocin, Syntocinon

Pregnancy risk category C

AVAILABLE FORMS
Injection: 10 units/ml ampule, vial, or tubex

INDICATIONS & DOSAGES
➤ **Induction or stimulation of labor—**
Adults: Initially, 1-ml (10-unit) ampule in 1,000 ml of D₅W injection, lactated Ringer's, or normal saline solution I.V. infused at 1 to 2 milliunits/minute. Rate increased in increments of 1 to 2 milliunits/minute at 15- to 30-minute intervals until normal contraction pattern is established. Rate decreased when labor is firmly established.
➤ **Reduction of postpartum bleeding after expulsion of placenta—**
Adults: 10 to 40 units added to 1,000 ml of D₅W injection, lactated Ringer's, or normal saline solution infused at rate needed to control bleeding, usually 20 to 40 milliunits/minute. Also, 1 ml (10 units) can be given I.M. after delivery of placenta.
➤ **Incomplete or inevitable abortion—**
Adults: 10 units oxytocin I.V. in 500 ml of normal saline solution, lactated Ringer's,

or dextrose 5% in normal saline solution. Infuse at rate of 10 to 20 milliunits (20 to 40 gtt)/minute.

I.V. ADMINISTRATION
- Dilute drug by adding 10 units to 1 L of normal saline, lactated Ringer's, or D₅W solution for induction or stimulation of labor, or by adding 10 units to 500 ml of normal saline, lactated Ringer's, or D₅W solution to produce intense uterine contractions and reduce postpartum bleeding.
- Don't give drug by I.V. bolus injection. Give by infusion only; give by piggyback infusion so drug may be discontinued without interrupting I.V. line. Use an infusion pump.

ACTION
Hormone that causes potent and selective stimulation of uterine and mammary gland smooth muscle.

Route	Onset	Peak	Duration
I.M.	3-5 min	Unknown	2-3 hr
I.V.	Immediate	Unknown	1 hr

ADVERSE REACTIONS
Maternal
CNS: *subarachnoid hemorrhage, seizures, coma.*
CV: hypertension; increased heart rate, systemic venous return, and cardiac output; *arrhythmias.*
GI: nausea, vomiting.
GU: tetanic uterine contractions, *abruptio placentae,* impaired uterine blood flow, pelvic hematoma, increased uterine motility, *uterine rupture, postpartum hemorrhage.*
Hematologic: *afibrinogenemia possibly related to postpartum bleeding.*
Other: hypersensitivity reactions, *anaphylaxis, death from oxytocin-induced water intoxication.*
Fetal
CNS: *infant brain damage.*
CV: *bradycardia,* PVCs, *arrhythmias.*
EENT: neonatal retinal hemorrhage.
Hepatic: neonatal jaundice.
Respiratory: *anoxia, asphyxia.*
Other: *low Apgar scores at 5 minutes.*

Reactions may be *common*, uncommon, *life-threatening*, or COMMON AND LIFE-THREATENING.

INTERACTIONS
Drug-drug. *Cyclopropane anesthetics:*
Less pronounced bradycardia and hypotension. Use together cautiously.
Thiopental anesthetics: May delay induction. Use together cautiously.
Vasoconstrictors: Severe hypertension if oxytocin is given within 3 to 4 hours of vasoconstrictor in patient receiving caudal block anesthetic. Avoid using together.

EFFECTS ON LAB TEST RESULTS
None reported.

CONTRAINDICATIONS
Contraindicated in patients hypersensitive to drug. Also contraindicated when vaginal delivery isn't advised (placenta previa, vasa previa, invasive cervical carcinoma, genital herpes), when cephalopelvic disproportion is present, or when delivery requires conversion, as in transverse lie. Also contraindicated in fetal distress when delivery isn't imminent, in prematurity, in other obstetric emergencies, and in patients with severe toxemia or hypertonic uterine patterns.

NURSING CONSIDERATIONS
• Use with extreme caution during first and second stages of labor because cervical laceration, uterine rupture, and maternal and fetal death have been reported.
• Use with extreme caution, if at all, in patients with invasive cervical cancer and in those with previous cervical or uterine surgery (including cesarean section), grand multiparity, uterine sepsis, traumatic delivery, or overdistended uterus.
• Drug isn't recommended for routine I.M. use. However, 10 units may be given I.M. after delivery of placenta to control postpartum uterine bleeding.
• Never give oxytocin simultaneously by more than one route.
• Drug is used to induce or reinforce labor only when pelvis is known to be adequate, when vaginal delivery is indicated, when fetal maturity is assured, and when fetal position is favorable. It should be used only in hospital where critical care facilities and prescriber are immediately available.
• Monitor fluid intake and output. Antidiuretic effect may lead to fluid overload, seizures, and coma from water intoxication.
• Monitor and record uterine contractions, heart rate, blood pressure, intrauterine pressure, fetal heart rate, and character of blood loss every 15 minutes.
• Have magnesium sulfate (20% solution) available for relaxation of the myometrium.
• If contractions occur less than 2 minutes apart and if contractions over 50 mm Hg are recorded, or if contractions last 90 seconds or longer, stop infusion, turn patient on her side, and notify prescriber.
• Drug isn't known to cause fetal abnormalities when used as indicated.
• *Alert:* Don't confuse Pitocin with Pitressin.

PATIENT TEACHING
• Explain use and administration of drug to patient and family.
• Instruct patient to report adverse reactions promptly.

Spasmolytics

flavoxate hydrochloride
oxybutynin chloride
phenazopyridine hydrochloride

COMBINATION PRODUCTS
None.

---

flavoxate hydrochloride
Urispas

Pregnancy risk category NR

AVAILABLE FORMS
Tablets: 100 mg

INDICATIONS & DOSAGES
➤ **Symptomatic relief of dysuria, urinary frequency and urgency, nocturia, incontinence, and suprapubic pain from urologic disorders—**
Adults and children older than age 12: 100 to 200 mg P.O. t.i.d. to q.i.d. Dosage may be reduced with improvement of symptoms.

ACTION
Produces a direct spasmolytic effect on urinary tract smooth muscles and provides some local anesthesia and analgesia.

Route	Onset	Peak	Duration
P.O.	Unknown	2 hr	Unknown

ADVERSE REACTIONS
CNS: *confusion,* nervousness, dizziness, headache, drowsiness.
CV: tachycardia, palpitations.
EENT: *blurred vision,* disturbed eye accommodation, increased ocular tension.
GI: dry mouth, nausea, vomiting.
GU: dysuria.
Hematologic: eosinophilia, *leukopenia.*
Skin: urticaria, dermatoses.
Other: fever.

INTERACTIONS
Drug-lifestyle. *Exercise, hot weather:* May precipitate heatstroke. Urge patient to use caution in hot weather.

EFFECTS ON LAB TEST RESULTS
● May increase eosinophil count. May decrease WBC count.

CONTRAINDICATIONS
Contraindicated in patients with pyloric or duodenal obstruction, obstructive intestinal lesions or ileus, achalasia, GI hemorrhage, or obstructive uropathies of lower urinary tract.

NURSING CONSIDERATIONS
● Use cautiously in patients suspected of having glaucoma and in pregnant or breast-feeding women.
● Safety and effectiveness of drug in children age 12 and younger are unknown.
● Check patient history for other drug use before giving drugs with anticholinergic adverse reactions. Such reactions may be intensified by flavoxate.
● *Alert:* Don't confuse Urispas with Urised.

PATIENT TEACHING
● Warn patient to avoid hazardous activities, such as operating machinery or driving, until CNS effects of drug are known.
● Tell patient to contact prescriber if adverse reactions occur or if symptoms aren't diminished.
● Caution patient that using drug during very hot weather may precipitate fever or heatstroke because it suppresses diaphoresis.
● Tell patient drug may cause dry mouth.

---

oxybutynin chloride
Cystrin§, Ditropan, Ditropan XL

Pregnancy risk category B

AVAILABLE FORMS
Syrup: 5 g/5 ml
Tablets: 5 mg
Tablets (extended-release): 5 mg, 10 mg

INDICATIONS & DOSAGES
➤ **Antispasmodic for uninhibited or reflex neurogenic bladder—**
Adults: 5 mg P.O. b.i.d. to t.i.d., to maximum of 5 mg q.i.d.
Children older than age 5: 5 mg P.O. b.i.d., to maximum of 5 mg t.i.d.
➤ **Overactive bladder—**
Adults: Initially, 5 mg P.O. (Ditropan XL) once daily. Dosage adjustments may be made weekly in 5-mg increments, p.r.n., to maximum dose of 30 mg P.O. daily.

ACTION
Produces a direct spasmolytic effect and an antimuscarinic (atropine-like) effect on urinary tract smooth muscles, increasing urinary bladder capacity, and provides some local anesthesia and analgesia.

Route	Onset	Peak	Duration
P.O.	30-60 min	3-4 hr	6-10 hr
P.O. (extended)	Unknown	4-6 hr	24 hr

ADVERSE REACTIONS
CNS: dizziness, insomnia, restlessness, hallucinations, asthenia.
CV: *palpitations, tachycardia,* vasodilation.
EENT: mydriasis, cycloplegia, decreased lacrimation, amblyopia.
GI: nausea, vomiting, *dry mouth, constipation,* decreased GI motility.
GU: impotence, *urinary hesitancy, urine retention.*
Skin: rash, decreased diaphoresis.
Other: suppression of lactation, fever.

INTERACTIONS
Drug-drug. *Anticholinergics:* Increased anticholinergic effects. Use together cautiously.
Atenolol, digoxin: Increased levels of these drugs. Monitor drug levels closely.
CNS depressants: Increased CNS effects. Use together cautiously.
Haloperidol, levodopa: Decreased levels of these drugs. Monitor drug levels closely.
Drug-lifestyle. *Alcohol use:* Increased CNS effects. Discourage use together.
Exercise, hot weather: May precipitate heatstroke. Urge patient to use caution in hot weather.

EFFECTS ON LAB TEST RESULTS
None reported.

CONTRAINDICATIONS
Contraindicated in patients hypersensitive to drug and in those with myasthenia gravis, GI obstruction, untreated narrow-angle glaucoma, adynamic ileus, megacolon, severe colitis, ulcerative colitis when megacolon is present, or obstructive uropathy. Also contraindicated in elderly or debilitated patients with intestinal atony and in hemorrhaging patients with unstable CV status.

NURSING CONSIDERATIONS
● Use cautiously in elderly patients and in patients with autonomic neuropathy, reflux esophagitis, or hepatic or renal disease.
● Before giving drug, anticipate confirmation of neurogenic bladder by cystometry and rule out partial intestinal obstruction in patients with diarrhea, especially those with colostomy or ileostomy.
● If patient has urinary tract infection, give antibiotics.
● Drug may aggravate symptoms of hyperthyroidism, coronary artery disease, heart failure, arrhythmias, tachycardia, hypertension, or prostatic hyperplasia.
● Obtain periodic cystometry as directed to evaluate response to therapy.
● *Alert:* Don't confuse Ditropan with diazepam or Dithranol.

PATIENT TEACHING
● Warn patient to avoid hazardous activities, such as operating machinery or driving, until CNS effects of drug are known.
● Caution patient that using drug during very hot weather may precipitate fever or heatstroke because it suppresses diaphoresis.
● Tell patient that Ditropan XL should be swallowed whole and not chewed or crushed.
● Instruct patient to measure syrup with a teaspoon.
● Advise patient to store drug in tightly closed container at 59° to 86° F (15° to 30° C).
● Advise patient to avoid alcohol while taking drug.
● Tell patient that drug may cause dry mouth.

---

phenazopyridine hydrochloride (phenylazo diamino pyridine hydrochloride)
Azo-Standard ◇, Baridium ◇, Geridium, Phenazot†, Prodium ◇, Pyridiate, Pyridium, Urodine, Urogesic, UTI-Relief

Pregnancy risk category B

AVAILABLE FORMS
Tablets: 95 mg ◇, 97.2 mg, 100 mg, 150 mg, 200 mg

INDICATIONS & DOSAGES
➤ **Pain with urinary tract irritation or infection—**
Adults: 200 mg P.O. t.i.d. after meals for 2 days.
Children: 12 mg/kg P.O. daily in three equally divided doses after meals for 2 days.

ACTION
Exerts local anesthetic action on urinary mucosa through unknown mechanism.

Route	Onset	Peak	Duration
P.O.	Unknown	Unknown	Unknown

ADVERSE REACTIONS
CNS: headache.
EENT: staining of contact lenses.
GI: nausea, GI disturbances.
Hematologic: hemolytic anemia, methemoglobinemia.
Skin: rash, pruritus.
Other: *anaphylactoid reactions.*

INTERACTIONS
None significant.

EFFECTS ON LAB TEST RESULTS
• May decrease hemoglobin.

CONTRAINDICATIONS
Contraindicated in patients hypersensitive to drug and in those with glomerulonephritis, severe hepatitis, uremia, renal insufficiency, or pyelonephritis during pregnancy.

NURSING CONSIDERATIONS
• When drug is used with an antibacterial, therapy shouldn't extend beyond 2 days.
• *Alert:* Don't confuse Pyridium with pyridoxine.

PATIENT TEACHING
• Advise patient that taking drug with meals may minimize GI distress.
• Caution patient to stop drug and notify prescriber immediately if skin or sclera becomes yellow-tinged, which may indicate drug accumulation from impaired renal excretion.
• Inform patient that drug colors urine red or orange and may stain fabrics. Contact lenses may also become stained.
• Tell diabetic patient that drug may alter Diastix or Chemstrip uG results. He should use Clinitest for accurate urine glucose test results. Also tell patient that drug may interfere with urinary ketone tests (Acetest or Ketostix).
• Advise patient to notify prescriber if urinary tract pain persists. Tell him that drug shouldn't be used for long-term treatment.

auranofin
aurothioglucose
gold sodium thiomalate

COMBINATION PRODUCTS
None.

auranofin
Ridaura

Pregnancy risk category C

AVAILABLE FORMS
Capsules: 3 mg

INDICATIONS & DOSAGES
➤ **Rheumatoid arthritis—**
Adults: 6 mg P.O. daily, either as 3 mg b.i.d. or 6 mg once daily. After 6 months, may be increased to 9 mg daily.
Children: Initially, 0.1 mg/kg/day. Maintenance dose is 0.15 mg/kg/day; maximum dose is 0.2 mg/kg/day.

ACTION
Unknown. Anti-inflammatory effects probably result from inhibition of sulfhydryl systems, which alters cellular metabolism. May also alter enzyme function and immune response and suppress phagocytic activity.

Route	Onset	Peak	Duration
P.O.	Unknown	2 hr	Unknown

ADVERSE REACTIONS
CNS: confusion, hallucinations, *seizures.*
EENT: conjunctivitis.
GI: *diarrhea, abdominal pain, nausea, stomatitis,* glossitis, anorexia, metallic taste, dyspepsia, flatulence, constipation, dysgeusia, ulcerative colitis.
GU: proteinuria, hematuria, nephrotic syndrome, glomerulonephritis, *acute renal failure.*
Hematologic: *thrombocytopenia, aplastic anemia, agranulocytosis, leukopenia,* eosinophilia, anemia.
Hepatic: jaundice.

Skin: *rash, pruritus, dermatitis,* exfoliative dermatitis, urticaria, erythema, alopecia.

INTERACTIONS
Drug-drug. *Phenytoin:* May increase phenytoin blood levels. Watch for toxicity.

EFFECTS ON LAB TEST RESULTS
• May increase ALT, AST, and alkaline phosphatase levels.
• May increase eosinophils. May decrease hemoglobin and platelet, granulocyte, and WBC counts.

CONTRAINDICATIONS
Contraindicated in patients with history of severe gold toxicity or toxicity from previous exposure to other heavy metals and in those with necrotizing enterocolitis, pulmonary fibrosis, exfoliative dermatitis, bone marrow aplasia, or severe hematologic disorders. Also contraindicated in patients with urticaria, eczema, colitis, severe debilitation, hemorrhagic conditions, or systemic lupus erythematosus, and in patients who have recently received radiation therapy. The manufacturer recommends avoiding use during pregnancy.

NURSING CONSIDERATIONS
• Use cautiously with other drugs that cause blood dyscrasias. Also use cautiously in patients with rash, history of bone marrow depression, or renal, hepatic, or inflammatory bowel disease.
• Monitor patient's platelet count monthly. Drug should be stopped if platelet count falls below 100,000/mm³, if hemoglobin drops suddenly, if granulocytes are less than 1,500/mm³, or if leukopenia (WBC count less than 4,000/mm³) or eosinophilia over 5% exists.
• *Alert:* Monitor patient's urinalysis results monthly. If proteinuria or hematuria is detected, stop drug because it can cause nephrotic syndrome or glomerulonephritis, and notify prescriber.
• Monitor liver function test results.

• Warn women of childbearing potential about risks of drug therapy during pregnancy.

PATIENT TEACHING
• Encourage patient to take drug as prescribed.
• Tell patient to continue concomitant drug therapy if prescribed.
• Remind patient to see prescriber for monthly platelet counts.
• Suggest that patient have regular urinalysis.
• Tell patient to keep taking drug if mild diarrhea occurs but to immediately report blood in stool. Diarrhea is most common adverse reaction.
• Advise patient to report rash or other skin problems and to stop drug until reaction subsides. Pruritus may precede dermatitis; pruritic skin eruptions during drug therapy should be considered a reaction until proven otherwise.
• Inform patient that stomatitis may be preceded by a metallic taste; tell him to notify prescriber if this occurs. Promote careful oral hygiene during therapy.
• Advise patient to report unusual bleeding or bruising.
• Inform patient that beneficial effect may be delayed as long as 3 months. If response is inadequate and maximum dose has been reached, expect prescriber to discontinue drug.
• Warn patient not to give drug to others. Auranofin should be prescribed only for selected patients with rheumatoid arthritis.

aurothioglucose
Gold-50‡, Solganal

gold sodium thiomalate
Aurolate

Pregnancy risk category C

AVAILABLE FORMS
aurothioglucose
Injection (suspension): 50 mg/ml in sesame oil in 10-ml vial
gold sodium thiomalate
Injection: 50 mg/ml with benzyl alcohol

INDICATIONS & DOSAGES
➤ **Rheumatoid arthritis—**
aurothioglucose
Adults: Initially, 10 mg I.M., followed by 25 mg for second and third doses at weekly intervals. Then, 50 mg weekly until 800 mg to 1 g has been given. If improvement occurs without toxicity, 25 to 50 mg is continued at 3- to 4-week intervals indefinitely.
Children ages 6 to 12: One-quarter usual adult dose. Don't exceed 25 mg per dose.
gold sodium thiomalate
Adults: Initially, 10 mg I.M., followed by 25 mg in 1 week. Then, 25 to 50 mg weekly to total dose of 1 g. If improvement occurs without toxicity, 25 to 50 mg q 2 weeks for 2 to 20 weeks; then, 25 to 50 mg q 3 to 4 weeks as maintenance therapy. If relapse occurs, injections resumed at weekly intervals.
Children: Initially, a test dose of 10 mg I.M.; then, 1 mg/kg I.M. weekly, not to exceed 50 mg for a single injection. Follow adult spacing of doses.

ACTION
Unknown. Anti-inflammatory effects probably result from inhibition of sulfhydryl systems, which alters cellular metabolism. May also alter enzyme function and immune response and suppress phagocytic activity.

Route	Onset	Peak	Duration
I.M.	Unknown	3-6 hr	Unknown

ADVERSE REACTIONS
CNS: confusion, hallucinations, *seizures.*
CV: *bradycardia,* hypotension.
EENT: corneal gold deposition, corneal ulcers.
GI: *diarrhea,* anorexia, abdominal cramps, nausea, vomiting, ulcerative enterocolitis, *metallic taste, stomatitis.*
GU: albuminuria, proteinuria, nephrotic syndrome, nephritis, acute tubular necrosis, hematuria, *acute renal failure.*
Hematologic: *thrombocytopenia, aplastic anemia, agranulocytosis, leukopenia,* eosinophilia, anemia.
Hepatic: *hepatitis,* jaundice.
Skin: photosensitivity reaction, *rash, dermatitis,* erythema, exfoliative dermatitis, diaphoresis.

Reactions may be *common,* uncommon, *life-threatening,* or COMMON AND LIFE-THREATENING.

Other: *anaphylaxis, angioedema.*

INTERACTIONS
Drug-lifestyle. *Sun or ultraviolet light exposure:* May cause photosensitivity reaction. Advise patient to avoid excessive sunlight exposure.

EFFECTS ON LAB TEST RESULTS
• May increase ALT, AST, and alkaline phosphatase levels.
• May increase eosinophils. May decrease hemoglobin and platelet, granulocyte, and WBC counts.

CONTRAINDICATIONS
Contraindicated in patients hypersensitive to drug and in those with history of severe toxicity from previous exposure to gold or other heavy metals. Also contraindicated in those who have recently received radiation therapy and in those with hepatitis, exfoliative dermatitis, severe uncontrollable diabetes, renal disease, hepatic dysfunction, uncontrolled heart failure, systemic lupus erythematosus, colitis, Sjögren's syndrome, urticaria, eczema, hemorrhagic conditions, or severe hematologic disorders.

NURSING CONSIDERATIONS
• Use with extreme caution, if at all, in patients with rash, marked hypertension, compromised cerebral or CV circulation, or history of renal or hepatic disease, drug allergies, or blood dyscrasias.
• Warn women of childbearing potential about risks of gold therapy during pregnancy.
• *Alert:* Give drug I.M. only.
• Give drug only under constant supervision of prescriber thoroughly familiar with drug's toxicities and benefits.
• Immerse aurothioglucose vial in warm water; shake vigorously before injecting.
• Give I.M., preferably intragluteally. Drug is pale yellow; don't use if it darkens.
• When injecting gold sodium thiomalate, have patient lie down for 10 to 20 minutes to minimize hypotension.
• Watch for anaphylactoid reaction for 30 minutes after administration.
• *Alert:* Keep dimercaprol available to treat acute toxicity.

• Analyze urine for protein and sediment changes before each injection.
• Monitor CBC, including platelet count, before every second injection.
• Monitor platelet counts if patient develops purpura or ecchymoses.
• If adverse reactions are mild, some rheumatologists resume gold therapy after 2 to 3 weeks' rest.

PATIENT TEACHING
• Inform patient that increased joint pain may occur for 1 to 2 days after injection but usually subsides.
• Advise patient to report rash or skin problems immediately and to stop drug until reaction subsides. Pruritus may precede dermatitis; pruritic skin eruptions during gold therapy should be considered a reaction until proven otherwise.
• Advise patient to report unusual bleeding or bruising.
• Instruct patient to report a metallic taste. Promote careful oral hygiene.
• Urge patient to avoid sunlight and artificial ultraviolet light.
• Tell patient that benefits may not appear for 3 to 4 months.
• Stress need for medical follow-up.

Miscellaneous antagonists and antidotes

activated charcoal
aminocaproic acid
ammonia spirit, aromatic
digoxin immune Fab
dimercaprol
disulfiram
d-penicillamine
edetate calcium disodium
edetate disodium
flumazenil
ipecac syrup
naloxone hydrochloride
naltrexone hydrochloride
pralidoxime chloride
protamine sulfate
sodium polystyrene sulfonate
succimer

(See also Chapter 38, ANTICHOLINER-GICS.)

(See also Chapter 40, ADRENERGIC BLOCKERS [SYMPATHOLYTICS].)

COMBINATION PRODUCTS
None.

---

activated charcoal
Actidose ◊, Actidose-Aqua ◊,
CharcoAid ◊, CharcoCaps ◊,
Liqui-Char ◊

Pregnancy risk category C

AVAILABLE FORMS
Capsules: 260 mg ◊
Granules: 15 g
Oral suspension: 15 g ◊, 30 g ◊, 50 g ◊
Powder: 15 g ◊, 30 g ◊, 40 g ◊, 120 g ◊, 240 g ◊
Tablets: 250 mg ◊

INDICATIONS & DOSAGES
➤ **Flatulence, dyspepsia—**
Adults: 600 mg to 5 g P.O. as single dose or 0.975 to 3.9 g P.O. t.i.d. after meals.
➤ **Poisoning—**
Adults and children: Initially, 1 to 2 g/kg (30 to 100 g) P.O. or 10 times the amount of poison ingested as a suspension in 120 to 240 ml (4 to 8 ounces) of water.

ACTION
An adsorbent that adheres to many drugs and chemicals, inhibiting their absorption from the GI tract.

Route	Onset	Peak	Duration
P.O.	Immediate	Unknown	Unknown

ADVERSE REACTIONS
GI: *black stools,* nausea, constipation, *intestinal obstruction.*

INTERACTIONS
Drug-drug. *Acetylcysteine, ipecac:* Drugs are inactivated by charcoal. Give charcoal after vomiting has been induced by ipecac; remove charcoal by nasogastric tube before giving acetylcysteine.
Acetaminophen, barbiturates, carbamazepine, digitoxin, digoxin, furosemide, glutethimide, hydantoins, methotrexate, nizatidine, phenothiazines, phenylbutazones, propoxyphene, salicylates, sulfonamides, sulfonylureas, tetracyclines, theophyllines, tricyclic antidepressants, valproic acid: Charcoal may reduce absorption of these drugs. Give charcoal at least 2 hours before or 1 hour after other drugs.
Drug-food. *Milk, ice cream, sherbet:* Decreased adsorptive capacity of charcoal. Discourage use together.

EFFECTS ON LAB TEST RESULTS
None reported.

CONTRAINDICATIONS
No known contraindications.

NURSING CONSIDERATIONS
• Although there are no known contraindications, drug isn't effective for treating all acute poisonings.
• *Alert:* Drug is commonly used for treating poisoning or overdose with acetaminophen, aspirin, atropine, barbiturates, dextropropoxyphene, digoxin, poisonous mushrooms, oxalic acid, parathion, phenol, phenytoin, propantheline, propoxyphene, strychnine, or TCAs. Check with

poison control center for use in other types of poisonings or overdoses.
• Give after emesis is complete because activated charcoal absorbs and inactivates ipecac syrup.
• Mix powder (most effective form) with tap water to consistency of thick syrup. Adding a small amount of fruit juice or flavoring will make mix more palatable. Don't mix with ice cream, milk, or sherbet because these will decrease absorptive capacity of activated charcoal.
• *Alert:* Don't aspirate or allow patient to aspirate charcoal powder; this has resulted in fatalities.
• Give by large-bore nasogastric tube after lavage, if needed.
• If patient vomits shortly after administration, be prepared to repeat dose.
• Space doses at least 1 hour apart from other drugs if treatment is for indications other than poisoning.
• Follow treatment with stool softener or laxative to prevent constipation unless sorbitol is part of product ingredients.
• Preparations made with sorbitol have a laxative effect that lessens risk of severe constipation or fecal impaction.
• Don't use charcoal with sorbitol in fructose-intolerant patients or in children younger than age 1.
• *Alert:* Drug is ineffective for poisoning or overdose of cyanide, mineral acids, caustic alkalis, and organic solvents; not very effective with ethanol, lithium, methanol, and iron salts.
• *Alert:* Don't confuse Actidose with Actos.

PATIENT TEACHING
• Explain use and administration of drug to patient (if awake) and family.
• Warn patient that stools will be black until all the charcoal has passed through the body.
• Instruct patient to drink 6 to 8 glasses of liquid per day, as charcoal can cause constipation.

aminocaproic acid
Amicar

Pregnancy risk category C

AVAILABLE FORMS
Injection: 250 mg/ml
Syrup: 250 mg/ml
Tablets: 500 mg

INDICATIONS & DOSAGES
➤ **Excessive bleeding resulting from hyperfibrinolysis—**
Adults: Initially, 5 g P.O. or slow I.V. infusion; then 1 to 1.25 g hourly until bleeding is controlled. Maximum dose is 30 g daily.

I.V. ADMINISTRATION
• Dilute solution with sterile water for injection, normal saline solution for injection, D_5W, or Ringer's injection.
• Infuse slowly. Arrhythmias may be precipitated by too-rapid infusion.
• Don't give by direct or intermittent injection.

ACTION
Inhibits plasminogen activator substances and, to a lesser degree, blocks antiplasmin activity by inhibiting fibrinolysis.

Route	Onset	Peak	Duration
I.V.	1 hr	Unknown	3 hr
P.O.	1 hr	2 hr	Unknown

ADVERSE REACTIONS
CNS: dizziness, malaise, headache, delirium, *seizures,* hallucinations, weakness.
CV: hypotension, *bradycardia, arrhythmias.*
EENT: tinnitus, nasal congestion, conjunctival suffusion.
GI: nausea, cramps, diarrhea.
GU: *acute renal failure.*
Hematologic: generalized thrombosis.
Musculoskeletal: myopathy.
Skin: rash.

INTERACTIONS
Drug-drug. *Estrogens, oral contraceptives:* Increased probability of hypercoagulability. Use together cautiously.

EFFECTS ON LAB TEST RESULTS
● May increase BUN, creatinine, CK, AST, and ALT levels.

CONTRAINDICATIONS
Contraindicated in patients with hematuria, active intravascular clotting, or disseminated intravascular coagulation, unless heparin is used together. Injectable form is contraindicated in newborns.

NURSING CONSIDERATIONS
● Use cautiously in patients with cardiac, hepatic, or renal disease.
● *Alert:* Don't give by bolus injection because of risk of hypotension, bradycardia, and arrhythmias.
● *Alert:* Monitor coagulation studies, along with heart rhythm and blood pressure. Notify prescriber of changes immediately.
● *Alert:* Don't confuse Amicar with Amikin.

PATIENT TEACHING
● Explain use and administration of drug to patient and family.
● Instruct patient to report adverse reactions promptly.

---

ammonia spirit, aromatic ◇

Pregnancy risk category NR

AVAILABLE FORMS
Inhalant: 0.33 ml ◇, 0.4 ml ◇
Solution: 30 ml ◇, 60 ml ◇, 120 ml ◇

INDICATIONS & DOSAGES
➤ **Treatment or prevention of fainting**—
Adults and children: 1 broken capsule inhaled until awake or no longer faint; or 2 to 4 ml P.O. diluted in at least 30 ml of water.

ACTION
Irritates the sensory receptors in the nasal membranes, producing reflex stimulation of the respiratory centers.

Route	Onset	Peak	Duration
P.O., inhalation	Immediate	Unknown	Unknown

ADVERSE REACTIONS
EENT: irritation.
Respiratory: coughing.

INTERACTIONS
None significant.

EFFECTS ON LAB TEST RESULTS
None reported.

CONTRAINDICATIONS
No known contraindications.

NURSING CONSIDERATIONS
● Avoid inhaling vapors when giving drug.
● Monitor patient closely for response.

PATIENT TEACHING
● Instruct patient how to use drug.
● Tell patient to store drug in refrigerator.

---

digoxin immune Fab (ovine)
Digibind

Pregnancy risk category C

AVAILABLE FORMS
Injection: 38-mg vial

INDICATIONS & DOSAGES
➤ **Potentially life-threatening digoxin or digitoxin intoxication**—
Adults and children: I.V. dosage varies according to amount of digoxin or digitoxin to be neutralized. Each vial binds about 0.5 mg of digoxin or digitoxin. Average adult dosage is 6 vials (228 mg). However, if toxicity resulted from acute digoxin ingestion and neither a digoxin level nor an estimated ingestion amount is known, 20 vials (760 mg) may be needed. For children who weigh less than 20 kg (44 lb), a single vial is usually sufficient. See package insert for complete, specific dosage instructions.

I.V. ADMINISTRATION
● Reconstitute drug in 38-mg vial with 4 ml of sterile water for injection. Gently roll vial to dissolve powder. Reconstituted solution contains 9.5 mg/ml.
● Drug may be given by direct injection if cardiac arrest seems imminent. Or, dilute

---

Reactions may be *common*, uncommon, *life-threatening*, or COMMON AND LIFE-THREATENING.

with normal saline solution for injection to an appropriate volume and give by intermittent infusion over 30 minutes.
● Infuse drug through a 0.22-micron membrane filter.
● Refrigerate powder for injection. Reconstitute drug immediately before use. Reconstituted solutions may be refrigerated for 4 hours.

ACTION
Binds molecules of unbound digoxin and digitoxin, making them unavailable for binding at site of action on cells.

Route	Onset	Peak	Duration
I.V.	30 min	End of infusion	15-20 hr

ADVERSE REACTIONS
CV: *heart failure,* rapid ventricular rate, worsening low cardiac output.
Metabolic: hypokalemia.
Other: hypersensitivity reactions, *anaphylaxis.*

INTERACTIONS
None significant.

EFFECTS ON LAB TEST RESULTS
● May decrease potassium levels.

CONTRAINDICATIONS
No known contraindications.

NURSING CONSIDERATIONS
● Use cautiously in patients known to be allergic to ovine (sheep) proteins and in those who have previously received antibodies. In these high-risk patients, skin testing is recommended because drug is derived from digoxin-specific antibody fragments obtained from immunized sheep.
● Drug is used for life-threatening overdose in patients with anaphylaxis, severe hypotension, or cardiac arrest and in those with ventricular arrhythmias (such as ventricular tachycardia or fibrillation), progressive bradycardia (such as severe sinus bradycardia), or second- or third-degree AV block not responsive to atropine.
● Heart failure and rapid ventricular rate may result by reversal of cardiac glycoside's therapeutic effects.

● Monitor potassium level closely.
● In most patients, signs of digitalis toxicity disappear within a few hours.
● Because drug interferes with digitalis immunoassay measurements, standard digoxin levels are misleading until drug is cleared from body (about 2 days).

PATIENT TEACHING
● Explain use and administration of drug to patient and family.
● Instruct patient to report adverse reactions promptly.

dimercaprol
BAL in Oil

Pregnancy risk category C

AVAILABLE FORMS
Injection: 100 mg/ml

INDICATIONS & DOSAGES
➤ **Severe arsenic or gold poisoning—**
Adults and children: 3 mg/kg deep I.M. q 4 hours for 2 days; then q.i.d. on third day; then b.i.d. for 10 days.
➤ **Mild arsenic or gold poisoning—**
Adults and children: 2.5 mg/kg deep I.M. q.i.d. for 2 days; then b.i.d. on third day; then once daily for 10 days.
➤ **Mercury poisoning—**
Adults and children: Initially, 5 mg/kg deep I.M.; then 2.5 mg/kg daily or b.i.d. for 10 days.
➤ **Acute lead encephalopathy or lead level greater than 100 mcg/ml—**
Adults and children: 4 mg/kg deep I.M.; then q 4 hours with edetate calcium disodium for 2 to 7 days. Use separate sites. For less severe poisoning, doses may be reduced to 3 mg/kg after the initial dose.

ACTION
Forms complexes with heavy metals to create chelates that are renally excreted.

Route	Onset	Peak	Duration
I.M.	Unknown	30-60 min	4 hr

ADVERSE REACTIONS
CNS: headache, paresthesia, muscle pain or weakness, anxiety.

CV: *transient increase in blood pressure, tachycardia.*
EENT: blepharospasm, conjunctivitis, lacrimation, rhinorrhea.
GI: *nausea, vomiting,* excessive salivation, *abdominal pain, burning sensation in lips, mouth, and throat.*
Other: *fever,* pain or tightness in throat, chest, or hands.

INTERACTIONS
Drug-drug. *Iron:* Toxic metal complex formed; concurrent therapy contraindicated. Wait 24 hours after last dimercaprol dose.

EFFECTS ON LAB TEST RESULTS
None reported.

CONTRAINDICATIONS
Contraindicated in patients with hepatic dysfunction (except postarsenical jaundice) or iron, cadmium, or selenium poisoning; also contraindicated in those allergic to peanuts.

NURSING CONSIDERATIONS
• Use cautiously in patients with hypertension, G6PD deficiency, or oliguria.
• Safe use in pregnancy hasn't been established; drug shouldn't be used unless judged by prescriber to be needed to treat life-threatening acute poisoning.
• **Alert:** Don't give drug I.V.; give by deep I.M. route only.
• Don't let drug come in contact with skin because it may cause a skin reaction.
• Drug has an unpleasant, garliclike odor.
• Solution with slight sediment is usable.
• Use antihistamine to prevent or relieve mild adverse reactions.
• Keep urine alkaline to prevent renal damage.
• Drug therapy blocks thyroid uptake of ^{131}I, causing decreased values.

PATIENT TEACHING
• Explain use and administration of drug to patient and family.
• Instruct patient to report adverse reactions promptly.

---

disulfiram
Antabuse

Pregnancy risk category NR

AVAILABLE FORMS
Tablets: 250 mg, 500 mg

INDICATIONS & DOSAGES
➤ **Adjunct in management of chronic alcoholism—**
Adults: 250 to 500 mg P.O. as single dose in morning for 1 to 2 weeks or in evening if drowsiness occurs. Maintenance dose is 125 to 500 mg P.O. daily (average dosage 250 mg) until permanent self-control is established. Treatment may continue for months or years.

ACTION
Blocks oxidation of alcohol at the acetaldehyde stage. Excess acetaldehyde produces a highly unpleasant reaction in the presence of even small amounts of alcohol.

Route	Onset	Peak	Duration
P.O.	1-2 hr	Unknown	14 days

ADVERSE REACTIONS
CNS: drowsiness, headache, fatigue, delirium, depression, neuritis, peripheral neuritis, polyneuritis, restlessness, psychotic reactions.
EENT: optic neuritis.
GI: metallic or garliclike aftertaste.
GU: impotence.
Skin: acneiform or allergic dermatitis, occasional eruptions.
Other: *disulfiram-like reaction precipitated by alcohol use.*

INTERACTIONS
Drug-drug. *Barbiturates:* Prolonged duration of effect. Closely monitor patient.
CNS depressants: Increased CNS depression. Use together cautiously.
Coumarin anticoagulants: Increased anticoagulant effect. Adjust dosage of anticoagulant.
Isoniazid: Ataxia or marked change in behavior. Avoid using together.
Metronidazole: Psychotic reaction. Avoid using together.

Reactions may be *common,* uncommon, *life-threatening,* or COMMON AND LIFE-THREATENING.

Midazolam: Increased plasma levels of midazolam. Use together cautiously.
Paraldehyde: Toxic levels of acetaldehyde. Avoid using together.
Phenytoin: Increased blood levels of phenytoin. Monitor phenytoin blood levels, and expect prescriber to adjust phenytoin dosages.
Tricyclic antidepressants, especially amitriptyline: Transient delirium. Closely monitor patient.
Drug-herb. *Herbal preparations containing alcohol:* May cause disulfiram-like reaction. Warn patient against using together. Alcohol reaction may occur as long as 2 weeks after single disulfiram dose.
Drug-food. *Caffeine:* Increased elimination half-life of caffeine. Tell patient to watch for effects.
Drug-lifestyle. *Alcohol use (all sources, including back-rub preparations, cough syrups, liniments, shaving lotion):* May cause disulfiram-like reaction. Discourage use together. Alcohol reaction may occur as long as 2 weeks after single disulfiram dose.

EFFECTS ON LAB TEST RESULTS
● May increase cholesterol level.

CONTRAINDICATIONS
Contraindicated in patients hypersensitive to disulfiram or other thiram derivatives used in pesticides and rubber vulcanization; in those with psychoses, myocardial disease, or coronary occlusion; in those receiving metronidazole, paraldehyde, alcohol, or alcohol-containing products; and in those experiencing alcohol intoxication or who have ingested alcohol within 12 hours.

NURSING CONSIDERATIONS
● Don't give drug during pregnancy.
● Use with extreme caution in patients receiving concurrent phenytoin therapy and in those with diabetes mellitus, hypothyroidism, seizure disorder, cerebral damage, nephritis, or hepatic cirrhosis or insufficiency.
● Never give until patient has abstained from alcohol for at least 12 hours. He should clearly understand consequences of disulfiram therapy and give permission for its use. Use drug only in patients who are

cooperative, well motivated, and receiving supportive psychiatric therapy.
● Complete physical examination and laboratory studies, including CBC, SMA-12, and transaminase level, should precede therapy and be repeated regularly.
● Disulfiram-like reaction may result from alcohol use, with flushing, throbbing headache, dyspnea, nausea, copious vomiting, diaphoresis, thirst, chest pain, palpitations, hyperventilation, hypotension, syncope, anxiety, weakness, blurred vision, confusion, and arthropathy.
● *Alert:* A severe disulfiram-like reaction can cause respiratory depression, CV collapse, arrhythmias, MI, acute heart failure, seizures, unconsciousness, and death.
● The longer patient remains on drug, the more sensitive he becomes to alcohol.
● *Alert:* Don't confuse Antabuse with Anturane.

PATIENT TEACHING
● *Alert:* Caution patient's family that disulfiram should never be given to patient without his knowledge; severe reaction or death could result if patient ingests alcohol.
● Tell patient to wear or carry medical identification that identifies him as a disulfiram user.
● Mild reactions may occur in sensitive patient with blood alcohol levels of 5 to 10 mg/100 ml; symptoms are fully developed at 50 mg/100 ml; unconsciousness typically occurs at 125 to 150 mg/100 ml level. Reaction may last from 30 minutes to several hours or as long as alcohol remains in blood.
● Reassure patient that disulfiram-induced adverse reactions (unrelated to concomitant alcohol use), such as drowsiness, fatigue, impotence, headache, peripheral neuritis, and metallic or garlic taste, subside after about 2 weeks of therapy.
● Advise patient not to drink alcoholic beverages or use products containing alcohol, including topical preparations and mouthwash.
● Have patient verify content of OTC products with pharmacist before use.

D-penicillamine
Cuprimine, Depen, D-Penamine‡

Pregnancy risk category NR

AVAILABLE FORMS
Capsules: 125 mg, 250 mg
Tablets: 125 mg‡, 250 mg

INDICATIONS & DOSAGES
➤ **Wilson's disease—**
Adults and children: 250 mg P.O. q.i.d.
30 to 60 minutes before meals. Dosage
adjusted to achieve urinary copper excretion of 0.5 to 1 mg daily.
➤ **Cystinuria—**
Adults: 250 mg to 1 g P.O. q.i.d. before
meals. Dosage adjusted to achieve urinary
cystine excretion of less than 100 mg daily
when renal calculi exist, or 100 to 200 mg
daily when calculi don't exist. Maximum
dose is 4 g daily.
Children: 30 mg/kg P.O. daily, divided
q.i.d. before meals. Dosage adjusted to
achieve urinary cystine excretion of less
than 100 mg daily when renal calculi exist, or 100 to 200 mg daily when calculi
don't exist.
➤ **Rheumatoid arthritis—**
Adults: Initially, 125 to 250 mg P.O. daily,
with increases of 125 to 250 mg q 1 to 3
months, p.r.n. Maximum dose is 1.5 g
daily.

ACTION
Chelates heavy metals and may inhibit
collagen formation. Mechanism unknown
for rheumatoid arthritis.

Route	Onset	Peak	Duration
P.O.	Unknown	1 hr	Unknown

ADVERSE REACTIONS
EENT: tinnitus, *optic neuritis.*
GI: *anorexia, epigastric pain, nausea,
vomiting, diarrhea, loss of or altered taste
perception, stomatitis.*
GU: nephrotic syndrome, glomerulonephritis, proteinuria, hematuria.
Hematologic: *leukopenia, eosinophilia,
thrombocytopenia, monocytosis, agranulocytosis, aplastic anemia,* lupus-like syndrome.
Hepatic: *hepatotoxicity.*

Metabolic: hypoglycemia.
Musculoskeletal: *arthralgia.*
Respiratory: *pneumonitis.*
Skin: alopecia; friability, especially at
pressure spots; wrinkling; erythema; urticaria.
Other: myasthenia gravis syndrome with
long-term use, allergic reactions, *lymphadenopathy,* ecchymoses.

INTERACTIONS
Drug-drug. *Antacids, oral iron:* Decreased effectiveness of D-penicillamine.
Give at least 2 hours apart.
*Antimalarials, cytotoxic drugs, gold ther-
apy, phenylbutazone:* Linked to serious
hematologic and renal reactions. Avoid using together.
Drug-food. *Any food:* Delayed and decreased absorption of drug. Tell patient to
take drug 1 hour before or 3 hours after
meals.

EFFECTS ON LAB TEST RESULTS
● May decrease glucose levels.
● May increase eosinophil count. May decrease hemoglobin and WBC, platelet, and
granulocyte counts.

CONTRAINDICATIONS
Contraindicated in breast-feeding women,
in pregnant women who have cystinuria,
in patients with penicillamine-related
aplastic anemia or granulocytosis, and in
those with rheumatoid arthritis or renal insufficiency.

NURSING CONSIDERATIONS
● Use with extreme caution, if at all, in patients hypersensitive to penicillin.
● Patients who have had a major toxic reaction to gold salt therapy may be at
greater risk for serious adverse reactions.
● Patient should receive supplemental
pyridoxine daily.
● If patient has a skin reaction, give antihistamines. Handle patient carefully to
avoid skin damage.
● Monitor CBC and renal and hepatic
function every 2 weeks for first 6 months;
then monthly.
● Monitor urinalysis regularly for protein
loss.

Reactions may be *common*, uncommon, *life-threatening*, or COMMON AND LIFE-THREATENING.

• *Alert:* Report rash and fever (important signs of toxicity) to prescriber immediately.

• Withhold drug and notify prescriber if WBC count falls below 3,500/mm³ or platelet count falls below 100,000/mm³. A progressive decline in platelet or WBC count in three successive blood tests may necessitate temporary cessation of therapy, even if such counts are within normal limits.

• Drug may cause positive test results for antinuclear antibody with or without clinical systemic lupus-like syndrome.

• *Alert:* Don't confuse D-penicillamine with penicillin, or Depen with Endep.

PATIENT TEACHING

• Tell patient that therapeutic effect may be delayed up to 3 months in treatment of rheumatoid arthritis.

• Tell patient to take drug on an empty stomach, at least 1 hour before or 2 hours after meals, and to maintain adequate fluid intake, especially at night.

• Advise patient to report early signs of granulocytopenia: fever, sore throat, chills, bruising, and prolonged bleeding time.

• Reassure patient that taste impairment usually resolves in 6 weeks without changes in dosage.

---

edetate calcium disodium
Calcium Disodium Versenate,
Calcium EDTA

Pregnancy risk category B

AVAILABLE FORMS
Injection: 200 mg/ml

INDICATIONS & DOSAGES
➤ **Acute lead encephalopathy or lead levels greater than 70 mcg/dl—**
Adults and children: 1 to 1.5 g/m² I.V. or I.M. daily in divided doses at 8- to 12-hour intervals for 5 days, usually with dimercaprol. A second course may be given after at least 2-day drug-free interval.

➤ **Lead poisoning without encephalopathy or asymptomatic with lead levels less than 70 mcg/dl—**
Children: 1 g/m² I.V. or I.M. daily in divided doses for 5 days.

I.V. ADMINISTRATION
• Dilute the 5-ml ampule with 500 ml or 250 ml of D_5W or normal saline solution for injection to 2 to 4 mg/ml, respectively.
• Infuse half of daily dose over 1 hour. Give rest of infusion at least 12 hours later. Or, give by slow infusion over at least 8 hours.

ACTION
Forms stable, soluble complexes with metals, particularly lead.

Route	Onset	Peak	Duration
I.M., I.V.	1 hr	24-48 hr	Unknown

ADVERSE REACTIONS
CNS: tremors, headache, numbness, tingling, malaise, fatigue.
CV: hypotension, rhythm irregularities.
EENT: histamine-like reactions including sneezing, congestion, and lacrimation.
GI: cheilosis, nausea, vomiting, anorexia, excessive thirst.
GU: proteinuria, hematuria, *nephrotoxicity with renal tubular necrosis leading to fatal nephrosis.*
Hematologic: *transient bone marrow suppression,* anemia.
Metabolic: zinc deficiency, hypercalcemia.
Musculoskeletal: myalgia, arthralgia.
Skin: rash.
Other: pain at I.M. injection site, fever, chills.

INTERACTIONS
Drug-drug. *Insulin:* Interferes with action of insulin by binding with zinc. Adjust insulin dosage as directed.

EFFECTS ON LAB TEST RESULTS
• May increase AST, ALT, and calcium levels.
• May decrease hemoglobin.

CONTRAINDICATIONS
Contraindicated in patients with anuria, hepatitis, or acute renal disease.

NURSING CONSIDERATIONS

- Use with extreme caution in patients with mild renal disease. Expect dosages to be reduced.
- Add procaine hydrochloride to I.M. solution to minimize pain. Watch for local reactions.
- *Alert:* Because rapid I.V. use may increase intracranial pressure, I.M. route may be preferred for treating lead encephalopathy.
- Although I.M. route may be preferred for children and patients with lead encephalopathy, most experts recommend I.V. infusion whenever possible.
- Monitor fluid intake and output, urinalysis, BUN level, and ECG daily.
- To avoid toxicity, use with dimercaprol; don't mix in same syringe.
- *Alert:* Don't confuse edetate calcium disodium with edetate disodium.

PATIENT TEACHING

- Explain use and administration of drug to patient and family.
- Tell patients with lead encephalopathy to avoid excess fluids.

edetate disodium
Disodium EDTA, Endrate

Pregnancy risk category C

AVAILABLE FORMS
Injection: 150 mg/ml

INDICATIONS & DOSAGES
➤ **Hypercalcemic crisis—**
Adults: 50 mg/kg/day by slow I.V. infusion over at least 3 hours. Maximum dose is 3 g/day.
Children: 40 mg/kg/day by slow I.V. infusion over at least 3 hours. Maximum dose is 70 mg/kg/day.

I.V. ADMINISTRATION
- Dilute drug in 500 ml of D_5W or normal saline solution and infuse over 3 or more hours.
- *Alert:* Avoid rapid I.V. infusion; profound hypocalcemia may occur, leading to tetany, seizures, arrhythmias, and respiratory arrest. Drug isn't recommended for

direct or intermittent injection. Avoid extravasation.
- Record I.V. site used, and avoid repeated use of same site because doing so increases likelihood of thrombophlebitis.

ACTION
Chelates with metals such as calcium to form a stable, soluble complex.

Route	Onset	Peak	Duration
I.V.	Unknown	Unknown	Unknown

ADVERSE REACTIONS
CNS: circumoral paresthesia, numbness, headache.
CV: hypotension, thrombophlebitis.
EENT: erythema.
GI: nausea, vomiting, diarrhea.
GU: *nephrotoxicity with urinary urgency,* nocturia, dysuria, polyuria, proteinuria, renal insufficiency, *renal failure, tubular necrosis.*
Metabolic: severe hypocalcemia.
Skin: exfoliative dermatitis.
Other: pain at infusion site.

INTERACTIONS
None significant.

EFFECTS ON LAB TEST RESULTS
- May decrease calcium and magnesium levels.

CONTRAINDICATIONS
Contraindicated in patients hypersensitive to drug and in those with anuria, known or suspected hypocalcemia, significant renal disease, active or healed tubercular lesions, or history of seizures or intracranial lesions.

NURSING CONSIDERATIONS
- Use cautiously in patients with limited cardiac reserve, heart failure, or hypokalemia.
- Keep I.V. calcium available to treat hypocalcemia.
- Keep patients in bed for 15 minutes after infusion to avoid effects of orthostatic hypotension. Monitor blood pressure closely.
- Monitor ECG and renal function tests frequently.
- Obtain calcium level after each dose.

Reactions may be *common,* uncommon, *life-threatening*, or **COMMON AND LIFE-THREATENING**.

• Don't use to treat lead toxicity; edetate calcium disodium should be used instead.
• **Alert:** Don't confuse edetate disodium with edetate calcium disodium.

PATIENT TEACHING
• Explain use and administration of drug to patient and family.
• Instruct patient to report adverse reactions promptly.

flumazenil
Anexate§, Romazicon

Pregnancy risk category C

AVAILABLE FORMS
Injection: 0.1 mg/ml in 5- and 10-ml multiple-dose vials

INDICATIONS & DOSAGES
➤ **Complete or partial reversal of sedative effects of benzodiazepines after anesthesia or short diagnostic procedures (conscious sedation)—**
Adults: Initially, 0.2 mg I.V. over 15 seconds. If patient doesn't reach desired level of consciousness after 45 seconds, dose is repeated. Repeated at 1-minute intervals until cumulative dose of 1 mg has been given (initial dose plus four more doses), if needed. Most patients respond after 0.6 to 1 mg of drug. For resedation, dosage may be repeated after 20 minutes; however, no more than 1 mg should be given at any one time and no more than 3 mg/hour.
➤ **Suspected benzodiazepine overdose—**
Adults: Initially, 0.2 mg I.V. over 30 seconds. If patient doesn't reach desired level of consciousness after 30 seconds, 0.3 mg is given over 30 seconds. If patient still doesn't respond adequately, 0.5 mg is given over 30 seconds; 0.5-mg doses are repeated, p.r.n., at 1-minute intervals until cumulative dose of 3 mg has been given. Most patients with benzodiazepine overdose respond to cumulative doses between 1 and 3 mg; rarely, patients who respond partially after 3 mg may need additional doses, up to 5 mg total. If patient doesn't respond in 5 minutes after receiving 5 mg, sedation is unlikely to be caused by benzodiazepines. In case of resedation,

dosage may be repeated after 20 minutes; however, no more than 1 mg should be given at any one time and no more than 3 mg/hour.

I.V. ADMINISTRATION
• Make sure airway is secure and patent.
• Give drug into I.V. line in large vein with free-flowing I.V. solution over 15 to 30 seconds to minimize pain at injection site. Compatible solutions include D_5W, lactated Ringer's injection, and normal saline solution.
• Store drug in vial until time of use. Drug is stable in a syringe for maximum of 24 hours.
• Monitor patient for signs of extravasation into perivascular tissues.

ACTION
A benzodiazepine antagonist that competitively inhibits the actions of benzodiazepines on the gamma-aminobutyric acid-benzodiazepine receptor complex.

Route	Onset	Peak	Duration
I.V.	1-2 min	6-10 min	Variable

ADVERSE REACTIONS
CNS: *dizziness, abnormal or blurred vision, headache, seizures,* agitation, emotional lability, tremor, insomnia.
CV: *arrhythmias,* cutaneous vasodilation, palpitations.
GI: *nausea, vomiting.*
Respiratory: dyspnea, hyperventilation.
Skin: *diaphoresis.*
Other: *pain at injection site.*

INTERACTIONS
Drug-drug. *Antidepressants, drugs that can cause seizures or arrhythmias:*
Seizures or arrhythmias can develop after effect of benzodiazepine overdose is removed. Flumazenil shouldn't be used in mixed overdose, especially in cases in which seizures (from any cause) are likely to occur.

EFFECTS ON LAB TEST RESULTS
None reported.

CONTRAINDICATIONS
Contraindicated in patients hypersensitive to flumazenil or benzodiazepines, in those

who show evidence of serious TCA overdose, and in those who have received benzodiazepines to treat a potentially life-threatening condition, such as status epilepticus.

NURSING CONSIDERATIONS
• Use cautiously in patients with head injury, psychiatric disorders, or alcohol dependency. Also use cautiously in patients at high risk for developing seizures, those who have recently received multiple doses of a parenteral benzodiazepine, those who display signs of seizure activity, and those who may be at risk for unrecognized benzodiazepine dependence, such as intensive care unit patients.
• Safety and efficacy of drug in children haven't been established.
• Monitor patient closely for resedation that may occur after reversal of benzodiazepine effects because flumazenil's duration of action is shorter than that of all benzodiazepines. Duration of monitoring period depends on specific drug being reversed. Monitor patient closely after doses of long-acting benzodiazepines, such as diazepam, or after high doses of short-acting benzodiazepines, such as 10 mg of midazolam. In most cases, severe resedation is unlikely in patients who fail to show signs of resedation 2 hours after a 1-mg dose of flumazenil.

PATIENT TEACHING
• Warn patient not to perform hazardous activities within 24 hours of procedure because of resedation risk.
• Tell patient to avoid alcohol, CNS depressants, and OTC drugs for 24 hours.
• Give family necessary instructions or provide patient with written instructions. Patient won't recall information given after the procedure; drug doesn't reverse amnesic effects of benzodiazepines.

---

ipecac syrup

Pregnancy risk category C

AVAILABLE FORMS
Syrup*: 70 mg powdered ipecac/ml (contains glycerin 10% and alcohol 1.5% to 2%) ◊

INDICATIONS & DOSAGES
➤ **To induce vomiting in poisoning—**
Adults and children older than age 12: 15 to 30 ml P.O.; then 3 to 4 glasses of water. Repeat dose if vomiting doesn't occur within 20 to 30 minutes. If no vomiting occurs within 30 to 45 minutes after second dose, gastric lavage should be performed.
Children ages 1 to 12: 15 ml P.O.; then 240 to 480 ml (8 to 16 ounces) of water. Repeat dose if vomiting doesn't occur within 20 to 30 minutes. If no vomiting occurs within 30 to 45 minutes after second dose, gastric lavage should be performed.
Infants and children ages 6 months to 1 year: 5 to 10 ml P.O.; then 120 to 240 ml (4 to 8 ounces) of water.

ACTION
Induces vomiting by acting locally on the gastric mucosa and centrally on the chemoreceptor trigger zone.

Route	Onset	Peak	Duration
P.O.	20-30 min	Unknown	20-25 min

ADVERSE REACTIONS
CNS: depression, *drowsiness.*
CV: *arrhythmias, bradycardia,* hypotension, atrial fibrillation, *fatal myocarditis.*
GI: *diarrhea.*

INTERACTIONS
Drug-drug. *Activated charcoal:* Neutralized emetic effect. Don't give together; may give activated charcoal after vomiting.

EFFECTS ON LAB TEST RESULTS
None reported.

CONTRAINDICATIONS
Contraindicated in semicomatose or unconscious patients and in those with severe inebriation, seizures, anaphylaxis, severe hypotension, or loss of gag reflex.

NURSING CONSIDERATIONS
• *Alert:* Don't give after ingestion of petroleum products or volatile oils because of potential for dangerous or lethal aspiration. Don't give after ingestion of caustic substances such as lye because of poten-

---

tial for additional injury to the esophagus and mediastinum.
• Ipecac syrup usually induces vomiting within 20 to 30 minutes.
• Stomach is usually emptied completely; vomitus also may contain some intestinal material.
• If two doses don't induce vomiting, prepare for gastric lavage.
• In antiemetic toxicity, ipecac syrup is usually effective if less than 1 hour has elapsed since ingestion of antiemetic.
• No systemic toxicity occurs with doses of 1 ounce (30 ml) or less.
• Cardiotoxicity occurs with ipecac abuse.
• Ipecac syrup is commonly abused by bulimics who binge, then purge. Watch for abuse in adolescents and adults.

PATIENT TEACHING
• Advise patient or parent to consult prescriber or poison control center in case of accidental ingestion.
• Recommend to parents that 1 ounce (30 ml) of syrup be available in the home for use in case of emergency.
• *Alert:* Advise parents that drug should only be given with a doctor's or poison control center's direction unless these professionals are not immediately available.
• Show parents how to give drug and tell them what to do in case of accidental poisoning.
• Advise patient or parent to give drug with 200 to 300 ml of water or clear liquid.
• Warn parents not to let child sleep on his back after taking drug. Use a pillow to prop child on his side.

naloxone hydrochloride
Narcan

Pregnancy risk category B

AVAILABLE FORMS
Injection: 0.02 mg/ml, 0.4 mg/ml, 1 mg/ml

INDICATIONS & DOSAGES
➤ **Known or suspected narcotic-induced respiratory depression, includ-**
ing that caused by pentazocine and propoxyphene—
Adults: 0.4 to 2 mg I.V., S.C., or I.M. repeated q 2 to 3 minutes, p.r.n. If no response is observed after 10 mg have been given, diagnosis of narcotic-induced toxicity should be questioned.
Children: 0.01 mg/kg I.V.; then second dose of 0.1 mg/kg I.V., if needed. If I.V. route isn't available, drug may be given I.M. or S.C. in divided doses.
Neonates: 0.01 mg/kg I.V., I.M., or S.C. Repeat dose q 2 to 3 minutes, p.r.n.
➤ **Postoperative narcotic depression—**
Adults: 0.1 to 0.2 mg I.V. q 2 to 3 minutes, p.r.n. Repeat dose within 1 to 2 hours, if needed.
Children: 0.005 to 0.01 mg I.V. repeated q 2 to 3 minutes, p.r.n.
Neonates (asphyxia neonatorum):
0.01 mg/kg I.V. into umbilical vein. May be repeated q 2 to 3 minutes.

I.V. ADMINISTRATION
• Be prepared to give continuous I.V. infusion (needed in many instances to control adverse effects of epidurally given morphine). If 0.02 mg/ml isn't available, adult concentration (0.4 mg) may be diluted by mixing 0.5 ml with 9.5 ml of sterile water for injection to make neonatal concentration (0.02 mg/ml).
• Don't mix with drugs containing bisulfite, metabisulfite, long-chain or high molecular weight anions, or any solution with an alkaline pH.

ACTION
Unknown. Thought to displace previously given narcotic analgesics from their receptors (competitive antagonism); it has no pharmacologic activity of its own.

Route	Onset	Peak	Duration
I.M., S.C.	2-5 min	5-15 min	Variable
I.V.	1-2 min	5-15 min	Variable

ADVERSE REACTIONS
CNS: tremors, *seizures.*
CV: tachycardia, hypertension with higher-than-recommended doses, hypotension, *ventricular fibrillation.*
GI: nausea, vomiting.
Respiratory: pulmonary edema.
Skin: diaphoresis.

Other: withdrawal symptoms in narcotic-dependent patients with higher-than-recommended doses.

INTERACTIONS
None significant.

EFFECTS ON LAB TEST RESULTS
None reported.

CONTRAINDICATIONS
Contraindicated in patients hypersensitive to drug.

NURSING CONSIDERATIONS
• Use cautiously in patients with cardiac irritability and opiate addiction. Abrupt reversal of opiate-induced CNS depression may result in nausea, vomiting, diaphoresis, tachycardia, CNS excitement, and increased blood pressure.
• Duration of action of the narcotic may exceed that of naloxone, and patients may relapse into respiratory depression.
• Respiratory rate increases within 1 to 2 minutes.
• *Alert:* Drug is effective only in reversing respiratory depression caused by opiates, not against other drug-induced respiratory depression, including that caused by benzodiazepines.
• Patients who receive naloxone to reverse opioid-induced respiratory depression may exhibit tachypnea.
• Monitor respiratory depth and rate. Be prepared to provide oxygen, ventilation, and other resuscitation measures.
• *Alert:* Don't confuse naloxone with naltrexone.

PATIENT TEACHING
• Inform family about use and administration of drug.
• Reassure family that patient will be monitored closely until effects of narcotic resolve.

---

naltrexone hydrochloride
ReVia, Trexan

Pregnancy risk category C

AVAILABLE FORMS
Tablets: 50 mg

INDICATIONS & DOSAGES
➤ **Adjunct for maintenance of opioid-free state in detoxified individuals—**
Adults: Initially, 25 mg P.O. If no withdrawal signs occur within 1 hour, an additional 25 mg is given. Once patient has been started on 50 mg q 24 hours, flexible maintenance schedule may be used. From 50 to 150 mg may be given daily, depending on schedule prescribed.
➤ **Alcohol dependence—**
Adults: 50 mg P.O. once daily.

ACTION
Unknown. Probably reversibly blocks the subjective effects of opioids given I.V. by competitively occupying opiate receptors in the brain.

Route	Onset	Peak	Duration
P.O.	15-30 min	1 hr	24 hr

ADVERSE REACTIONS
CNS: *insomnia, anxiety, nervousness, headache,* depression, dizziness, fatigue, somnolence, *suicidal ideation.*
GI: *nausea, vomiting,* anorexia, *abdominal pain,* constipation, increased thirst.
GU: delayed ejaculation, decreased potency.
Hepatic: *hepatotoxicity.*
Musculoskeletal: *muscle and joint pain.*
Skin: rash.
Other: chills.

INTERACTIONS
Drug-drug. *Opioid-containing products:* Decreased effect of opioid. Avoid using together.
Thioridazine: Increased somnolence and lethargy. Monitor patient closely.

EFFECTS ON LAB TEST RESULTS
• May increase AST, ALT, and LDH levels.
• May increase lymphocyte count.

CONTRAINDICATIONS
Contraindicated in patients hypersensitive to drug, in those receiving opioid analgesics, in opioid-dependent patients, in patients in acute opioid withdrawal, and in those with positive urine screen for opioids or acute hepatitis or liver failure.

Reactions may be *common*, uncommon, *life-threatening*, or **COMMON AND LIFE-THREATENING**.

NURSING CONSIDERATIONS

• Use cautiously in patients with mild hepatic disease or history of recent hepatic disease.

• Treatment for opioid dependency shouldn't begin until patients receive naloxone challenge, a provocative test of opioid dependency. If signs and symptoms of opioid withdrawal persist after naloxone challenge, don't give drug.

• Patient must be completely free from opioids before taking drug or severe withdrawal symptoms may occur. Patients who have been addicted to short-acting opioids, such as heroin and meperidine, must wait at least 7 days after last opioid dose before starting drug. Patients who have been addicted to longer-acting opioids such as methadone should wait at least 10 days.

• In an emergency, anticipate that patient receiving naltrexone may be given an opioid analgesic, but dose must be higher than usual to surmount naltrexone's effect. Watch for respiratory depression from the opioid; it may be longer and deeper.

• For patients being treated because of history of opioid dependency and who are expected to be noncompliant, be prepared to try a flexible maintenance dose regimen of 100 mg on Monday and Wednesday and 150 mg on Friday.

• Drug should be used only as part of a comprehensive rehabilitation program.

• **Alert:** Don't confuse naltrexone with naloxone.

PATIENT TEACHING

• Advise patient to wear or carry medical identification and to tell medical personnel that he takes naltrexone.

• Give patient names of nonopioid drugs that he can continue to take for pain, diarrhea, or cough.

• Tell patient to report adverse effects to prescriber immediately.

pralidoxime chloride (2-PAM chloride; 2-pyridine-aldoxime methochloride)
Protopam Chloride

Pregnancy risk category C

AVAILABLE FORMS
Injection: 1 g/20 ml in 20-ml vial without diluent or syringe; 600 mg/2 ml autoinjector, parenteral

INDICATIONS & DOSAGES
➤ **Antidote for organophosphate poisoning—**
Adults: 1 to 2 g in 100 ml of normal saline solution by I.V. infusion over 15 to 30 minutes. Repeated in 1 hour if muscle weakness persists. Additional doses may be given cautiously. I.M. or S.C. injection may be used if I.V. isn't feasible.
Children: 20 to 40 mg/kg I.V., given as for adults.
➤ **Cholinergic crisis in myasthenia gravis—**
Adults: 1 to 2 g I.V.; then 250 mg I.V. q 5 minutes, p.r.n.

I.V. ADMINISTRATION
• Reconstitute by adding 20 ml of sterile water for injection to vial containing 1 g of drug. Further dilute by adding 100 ml of normal saline solution. Infuse over 15 to 30 minutes.

• If patient has pulmonary edema, give drug by slow I.V. push over 5 minutes. Don't exceed 200 mg/minute.

• **Alert:** If drug is infused too rapidly, tachycardia, laryngospasm, and muscle rigidity may result.

ACTION
Reactivates cholinesterase inactivated by organophosphorus pesticides and related compounds, permitting degradation of accumulated acetylcholine and facilitating normal functioning of neuromuscular junctions.

Route	Onset	Peak	Duration
I.M.	Unknown	10-20 min	Unknown
I.V.	Unknown	5-15 min	Unknown
S.C.	Unknown	Unknown	Unknown

ADVERSE REACTIONS
CNS: dizziness, headache, drowsiness.
CV: tachycardia.
EENT: blurred vision, diplopia, impaired accommodation.
GI: nausea.
Musculoskeletal: muscular weakness.
Respiratory: hyperventilation.
Other: mild to moderate pain at injection site.

INTERACTIONS
Drug-drug. *Barbiturates:* Increased by anticholinesterases. Use together cautiously to treat seizures.

EFFECTS ON LAB TEST RESULTS
• May increase liver enzyme levels.

CONTRAINDICATIONS
Contraindicated in patients hypersensitive to drug.

NURSING CONSIDERATIONS
• Use with extreme caution in patients with myasthenia gravis (overdose may trigger myasthenic crisis).
• Initially, remove secretions, maintain patent airway, and institute mechanical ventilation, if needed. After dermal exposure to organophosphate, remove patient's clothing and wash his skin and hair with sodium bicarbonate, soap, water, and alcohol as soon as possible. A second washing may be needed. When washing patient, wear protective gloves and clothes to avoid exposure.
• Draw blood for cholinesterase levels before giving drug.
• Drug should be used in hospitalized patients only; have respiratory and other supportive measures available. If possible, obtain accurate medical history and chronology of poisoning. Drug should be given as soon as possible after poisoning; treatment is most effective if initiated within 24 hours after exposure.
• To ameliorate muscarinic effects and block accumulation of acetylcholine associated with organophosphate poisoning, give atropine 2 to 4 mg I.V. with pralidoxime if cyanosis isn't present; if cyanosis is present, give atropine I.M. Give atropine every 5 to 10 minutes until signs of atropine toxicity (flushing, tachycardia, dry mouth, blurred vision, excitement, delirium, and hallucinations) appear; atropinization should be maintained for at least 48 hours.
• Observe patient for 48 to 72 hours if poison was ingested. Delayed absorption may occur from lower bowel. It's difficult to distinguish between toxic effects produced by atropine or organophosphate compounds and those resulting from pralidoxime.
• Watch patient with myasthenia gravis who is being treated for overdose of cholinergic drugs for signs of rapid weakening. He can pass quickly from cholinergic crisis to myasthenic crisis and needs more cholinergic drugs to treat myasthenia. Keep edrophonium available for establishing differential diagnosis.
• Avoid use of aminophylline, morphine, phenothiazine-like tranquilizers, reserpine, succinylcholine, and theophylline in patients with organophosphate poisoning.
• Drug isn't effective against poisoning caused by phosphorus, inorganic phosphates, or organophosphates with no anticholinesterase activity.
• *Alert:* Don't confuse pralidoxime with pramoxine or pyridoxine.

PATIENT TEACHING
• Explain use and administration of drug to patient and family.
• Tell patient to report adverse effects.
• Caution patient treated for organophosphate poisoning to avoid contact with insecticides for several weeks.

---

protamine sulfate

Pregnancy risk category C

AVAILABLE FORMS
Injection: 10 mg/ml

INDICATIONS & DOSAGES
➤ **Heparin overdose—**
Adults: Dosage based on venous blood coagulation studies, usually 1 mg for each 90 to 115 units of heparin. Give by slow I.V. injection over 10 minutes in doses not to exceed 50 mg.

I.V. ADMINISTRATION
• Give slowly by direct I.V. injection. Have emergency equipment available to treat anaphylaxis or severe hypotension.
• **Alert:** Excessively rapid I.V. administration may cause acute hypotension, bradycardia, pulmonary hypertension, dyspnea, transient flushing, and feeling of warmth.

ACTION
A heparin antagonist that forms a physiologically inert complex with heparin sodium.

Route	Onset	Peak	Duration
I.V.	30-60 sec	Unknown	2 hr

ADVERSE REACTIONS
CNS: lassitude.
CV: fall in blood pressure, *bradycardia, circulatory collapse,* transitory flushing.
GI: nausea, vomiting.
Respiratory: dyspnea, pulmonary edema, *acute pulmonary hypertension.*
Other: feeling of warmth, *anaphylaxis, anaphylactoid reactions.*

INTERACTIONS
None significant.

EFFECTS ON LAB TEST RESULTS
None reported.

CONTRAINDICATIONS
Contraindicated in patients hypersensitive to drug.

NURSING CONSIDERATIONS
• Postoperative dose is based on coagulation studies, and a repeat PT 15 minutes after administration is advised.
• Calculate dosage carefully. One milligram of protamine neutralizes 90 to 115 units of heparin depending on salt (heparin calcium or heparin sodium) and source of heparin (beef or pork).
• Risk of hypersensitivity reaction increases in patients hypersensitive to fish; in vasectomized or infertile men; and in patients taking protamine-insulin products.
• Monitor patient continually.
• Watch for spontaneous bleeding (heparin rebound), especially in dialysis patients and in those who have undergone cardiac surgery.

• Protamine may act as an anticoagulant in very high doses.
• **Alert:** Don't confuse protamine with Protopam or protropin.

PATIENT TEACHING
• Explain use and administration of drug to patient and family.
• Tell patient to report adverse effects.

sodium polystyrene sulfonate
Kayexalate, SPS

Pregnancy risk category C

AVAILABLE FORMS
Powder: 1-lb jar (3.5 g/tsp)
Suspension: 15 g/60 ml*

INDICATIONS & DOSAGES
➤ **Hyperkalemia—**
Adults: 15 g P.O. daily to q.i.d. in water or sorbitol (3 to 4 ml/g of resin). Or, mix powder with appropriate medium—aqueous suspension or diet appropriate for renal failure—and instill through a nasogastric tube. Or, 30 to 50 g/100 ml of sorbitol q 6 hours as warm emulsion deep into sigmoid colon (20 cm).
Children: 1 g/kg of body weight/dose P.O. or P.R., p.r.n., to correct hyperkalemia.

ACTION
A potassium-removing resin that exchanges sodium ions for potassium ions in the intestine: 1 g of sodium polystyrene sulfonate is exchanged for 0.5 to 1 mEq of potassium. The resin is then eliminated. Much of the exchange capacity is used for cations other than potassium (calcium and magnesium) and possibly for fats and proteins.

Route	Onset	Peak	Duration
P.O., P.R.	2-12 hr	Unknown	Unknown

ADVERSE REACTIONS
GI: *constipation,* fecal impaction, anorexia, gastric irritation, nausea, vomiting, *diarrhea with sorbitol emulsions.*
Metabolic: hypokalemia, hypocalcemia, hypomagnesemia, sodium retention.

INTERACTIONS
Drug-drug. *Antacids and laxatives (nonabsorbable cation-donating types, including magnesium hydroxide):* Systemic alkalosis and reduced potassium exchange capability. Avoid using together.

EFFECTS ON LAB TEST RESULTS
• May increase sodium level. May decrease potassium, calcium, and magnesium levels.

CONTRAINDICATIONS
Contraindicated in patients hypersensitive to drug and in those with hypokalemia.

NURSING CONSIDERATIONS
• Use cautiously in patients with severe heart failure, severe hypertension, or marked edema. Drug provides 100 mg of sodium per gram.
• Don't heat resin; this impairs drug's effect. Mix resin only with water or sorbitol for P.O. administration. Never mix with orange juice (high potassium content) to disguise taste.
• Chill oral suspension for greater palatability.
• Oral administration is preferred because drug should remain in intestine for at least 30 minutes.
• If sorbitol is given, mix with resin suspension.
• Consider giving in solid form. Resin cookie and candy recipes are available; ask pharmacist or dietitian to supply.
• Premixed forms are available (SPS and others). If preparing manually, mix polystyrene resin only with water and sorbitol for rectal use. Don't use mineral oil for P.R. administration to prevent impaction; ion exchange needs aqueous medium. Sorbitol content prevents impaction.
• Prepare P.R. dose at room temperature. Stir emulsion gently during administration.
• Use #28 French rubber tube for rectal dose; insert 20 cm into sigmoid colon. Tape tube in place. Or, consider an indwelling urinary catheter with a 30-ml balloon inflated distal to anal sphincter to aid in retention. This is especially helpful for patients with poor sphincter control. Use gravity flow. Drain returns constantly through Y-tube connection. Place patient in knee-chest position or with hips on pillow for a while if back-leakage occurs.
• After P.R. administration, flush tubing with 50 to 100 ml of nonsodium fluid to ensure delivery of all drug. Flush rectum to remove resin.
• Prevent fecal impaction in elderly patients by giving resin P.R. Give cleansing enema before P.R. administration. Have patient retain enema for 6 to 10 hours if possible, but 30 to 60 minutes is acceptable.
• Watch for constipation in oral or nasogastric administration. Use sorbitol (10 to 20 ml of 70% syrup every 2 hours, as needed) to produce one or two watery stools daily.
• Monitor potassium levels at least once daily. Treatment may result in potassium deficiency and is usually stopped when potassium is reduced to 4 or 5 mEq/L.
• Watch for signs of hypokalemia: irritability, confusion, arrhythmias, ECG changes, severe muscle weakness, and sometimes paralysis, and digitalis toxicity in digitalized patients.
• When hyperkalemia is severe, polystyrene resin alone isn't adequate for lowering potassium. Dextrose 50% with regular insulin I.V. push may also be given.
• Watch for symptoms of other electrolyte deficiencies (magnesium, calcium) because drug is nonselective. Monitor calcium in patients receiving sodium polystyrene therapy for more than 3 days. Supplementary calcium may be needed.
• Watch for sodium overload. Drug contains about 100 mg sodium per gram About one-third of resin's sodium is retained.

PATIENT TEACHING
• Explain use and administration of drug to patient.
• Advise patient to report adverse reactions promptly.
• Teach patient about low-potassium diet.

succimer
Chemet

Pregnancy risk category C

AVAILABLE FORMS
Capsules: 100 mg

INDICATIONS & DOSAGES
➤ **Lead poisoning in children with lead levels greater than 45 mcg/dl—**
Children: Initially, 10 mg/kg or 350 mg/m² q 8 hours for 5 days. Because capsules come only in 100 mg, round dose to nearest 100 mg, as appropriate (see table). Then, reduce frequency of administration to q 12 hours for an additional 2 weeks.

Weight in kg (lb)	Dose (mg)
> 45 (> 100)	500
35-44 (78-98)	400
24-34 (53-76)	300
16-23 (36-51)	200
8-15 (18-33)	100

ACTION
A chelating drug that forms water-soluble complexes with lead and increases its excretion in urine.

Route	Onset	Peak	Duration
P.O.	Unknown	1-2 hr	Unknown

ADVERSE REACTIONS
CNS: *drowsiness, dizziness, sensorimotor neuropathy, sleepiness, paresthesia, headache.*
CV: *arrhythmias.*
EENT: plugged ears, cloudy film in eyes, otitis media, watery eyes, sore throat, rhinorrhea, nasal congestion.
GI: *nausea, vomiting, diarrhea, loss of appetite, abdominal cramps, hemorrhoidal symptoms, metallic taste in mouth, loose stools.*
GU: decreased urination, difficult urination, proteinuria.
Hematologic: increased platelet count, intermittent eosinophilia, *neutropenia.*
Musculoskeletal: *leg, kneecap, back, stomach, rib, or flank pain.*
Respiratory: cough, head cold.

Skin: papular rash, herpetic rash, mucocutaneous eruptions, pruritus.
Other: *flulike syndrome,* candidiasis.

INTERACTIONS
Drug-drug. *Other chelation therapy (such as CaNa₂ EDTA):* Unknown adverse effects. Separate administration by 4 weeks.

EFFECTS ON LAB TEST RESULTS
• May increase AST, ALT, alkaline phosphatase, and cholesterol levels.
• May increase eosinophil and platelet counts.

CONTRAINDICATIONS
Contraindicated in patients hypersensitive to drug.

NURSING CONSIDERATIONS
• Use cautiously in patients with compromised renal function.
• Measure severity of poisoning by initial lead level and by rate and degree of rebound of lead level. Severity should be used as a guide for more frequent lead monitoring.
• Monitor transaminase level before and at least weekly during therapy. Transient mild elevations of transaminase levels have been observed. Monitor patients with history of hepatic disease.
• Monitor patient at least once weekly for rebound lead levels. Elevated levels and associated symptoms may return rapidly after drug is stopped because of redistribution of lead from bone to soft tissues and blood.
• Course of treatment lasts 19 days. Repeated courses may be needed if indicated by weekly monitoring of lead levels.
• Minimum of 2 weeks between courses is recommended unless high lead levels indicate need for immediate therapy.
• Concurrent administration with other chelating drugs isn't recommended. Patient who has received edetate calcium disodium with or without dimercaprol may use succimer as subsequent therapy after a 4-week interval.
• Discontinue treatment if absolute neutrophil count is less than 1,200.

PATIENT TEACHING

• Explain use and administration of drug to parents and child. Stress importance of complying with frequently ordered blood tests.

• Tell parents of young child who can't swallow capsules that capsule can be opened and its contents sprinkled on a small amount of soft food. Or, beads from capsule may be poured on a spoon; follow with flavored beverage.

• Tell patient to maintain adequate fluid intake.

• Assist parents with identifying and removing sources of lead in child's environment. Chelation therapy isn't a substitute for preventing further exposure and shouldn't be used to permit continued exposure.

• Tell patient to notify prescriber if rash occurs. Consider possibility of allergic or other mucocutaneous reactions each time drug is used.

alendronate sodium
alprostadil
amifostine
anagrelide hydrochloride
aprotinin
balsalazide disodium
becaplermin
capsaicin
clomiphene citrate
eflornithine hydrochloride
etanercept
finasteride
imatinib mesylate
imiquimod
infliximab
isotretinoin
leflunomide
levocarnitine
mesalamine
mesna
minoxidil (topical)
nimodipine
olsalazine sodium
orlistat
pilocarpine hydrochloride
raloxifene hydrochloride
riluzole
risedronate sodium
sevelamer hydrochloride
sildenafil citrate
sulfasalazine
tacrolimus
tacrolimus (topical)
tamsulosin hydrochloride
thalidomide
tolterodine tartrate
tretinoin

COMBINATION PRODUCTS
None.

alendronate sodium
Fosamax

Pregnancy risk category C

AVAILABLE FORMS
Tablets: 5 mg, 10 mg, 35 mg, 40 mg, 70 mg

INDICATIONS & DOSAGES
➤ **Treatment of osteoporosis in post-menopausal women, to increase bone mass in men with osteoporosis—**
Adults: 10 mg P.O. daily or 70 mg P.O. once weekly taken with water only, at least 30 minutes before first food, beverage, or medication of day.
➤ **Paget's disease of bone—**
Adults: 40 mg P.O. daily for 6 months, taken with water only, at least 30 minutes before first food, beverage, or medication of day.
➤ **Prevention of osteoporosis in post-menopausal women—**
Adults: 5 mg P.O. daily or 35 mg P.O. once weekly taken with water only, at least 30 minutes before first food, beverage, or medication of day.
➤ **Glucocorticoid-induced osteoporosis in men and women receiving glucocorticoids in a daily dose equivalent to 7.5 mg or more of prednisone and who have low bone mineral density—**
Adults: 5 mg P.O. daily, taken with water only, at least 30 minutes before first food, beverage, or medication of day. For postmenopausal women not receiving estrogen, recommended dose is 10 mg P.O. daily taken with water only, at least 30 minutes before first food, beverage, or medication of day.

ACTION
Suppresses osteoclast activity on newly formed resorption surfaces, which reduces bone turnover. Bone formation exceeds resorption at remodeling sites, leading to progressive gains in bone mass.

Route	Onset	Peak	Duration
P.O.	Unknown	Unknown	Unknown

ADVERSE REACTIONS
CNS: headache.
GI: abdominal pain, nausea, dyspepsia, constipation, diarrhea, flatulence, acid regurgitation, esophageal ulcer, vomiting,

dysphagia, abdominal distention, gastritis, taste perversion.
Musculoskeletal: musculoskeletal pain.

INTERACTIONS
Drug-drug. *Antacids, calcium supplements:* May interfere with drug absorption. Separate administration times by at least 30 minutes.
Aspirin, NSAIDs: Increased risk of upper GI adverse reactions with drug doses above 10 mg/day. Monitor patient closely.
Hormone replacement therapy: Not recommended for use with alendronate in treating osteoporosis; evidence of effectiveness is lacking. Avoid using together.
Ranitidine: Increased availability of alendronate. Reduce dosage, as needed.
Drug-food. *Any food:* Decreased absorption of drug. Advise patient to take with full glass of water at least 30 minutes before he eats, drinks, or ingests other drugs.

EFFECTS ON LAB TEST RESULTS
None reported.

CONTRAINDICATIONS
Contraindicated in patients hypersensitive to drug and in those with hypocalcemia, severe renal insufficiency, or abnormalities of the esophagus that delay esophageal emptying.

NURSING CONSIDERATIONS
• Use cautiously in patients with active upper GI problems (dysphagia, symptomatic esophageal diseases, gastritis, duodenitis, ulcers) or mild to moderate renal insufficiency.
• Hypocalcemia and other disturbances of mineral metabolism (such as vitamin D deficiency) should be corrected before therapy begins.
• When used to treat osteoporosis in postmenopausal women, disease may be confirmed by findings of low bone mass on diagnostic studies or by history of osteoporotic fracture.
• When used to treat Paget's disease, drug is indicated for patients with alkaline phosphatase level at least two times upper limit of normal, for those who are symptomatic, and for those at risk for future complications from the disease.

• *Alert:* Make sure patient doesn't lie down for at least 30 minutes after taking drug to facilitate delivery to stomach and to reduce risk of esophageal irritation.
• Monitor patient's calcium and phosphate levels throughout therapy.
• *Alert:* Don't confuse Fosamax with Flomax.

PATIENT TEACHING
• Stress importance of taking tablet only with a glass (6 to 8 ounces) of plain water at least 30 minutes before ingesting anything else, including food, beverages, and other drugs. Tell patient that waiting longer than 30 minutes will improve absorption.
• Warn patient not to lie down for at least 30 minutes after taking drug to facilitate delivery to stomach and to reduce risk of esophageal irritation.
• Advise patient to report adverse effects immediately, especially chest pain or difficulty swallowing.
• Advise patient to take supplemental calcium and vitamin D if dietary intake is inadequate.
• Tell patient about benefits of weight-bearing exercises in increasing bone mass. If applicable, explain importance of reducing or eliminating cigarette smoking and alcohol use.

alprostadil
Caverject, Edex, Muse

Pregnancy risk category X

AVAILABLE FORMS
Injection: 5 mcg/ml, 10 mcg/ml, 20 mcg/ml, 40 mcg/ml after reconstitution
Urogenital suppository: 125 mcg, 250 mcg, 500 mcg, 1,000 mcg

INDICATIONS & DOSAGES
➤ **Erectile dysfunction of vasculogenic, psychogenic, or mixed etiology—**
Adults: Dosages are highly individualized, with initial dose of 2.5 mcg intracavernously. If partial response occurs, second dose of 2.5 mcg is given; then increased further in increments of 5 to 10 mcg until patient achieves erection (one suitable for intercourse and not ex-

ceeding 1 hour's duration). If no response to initial dose occurs, second dose may be increased to 7.5 mcg within 1 hour; then increased further in increments of 5 to 10 mcg until patient achieves suitable erection. Patient must remain in prescriber's office until complete detumescence occurs. Procedure shouldn't be repeated for at least 24 hours.

➤ **For urogenital suppository—**
Adults: Initial dose (125 to 250 mcg) given under supervision of prescriber. Adjust dosage p.r.n. until response is sufficient for sexual intercourse. Maximum of two administrations in 24 hours; maximum dose is 1,000 mcg.

➤ **Erectile dysfunction of neurogenic etiology (spinal cord injury)—**
Adults: Dosages are highly individualized, with initial dose of 1.25 mcg intracavernously. If partial response occurs, second dose of 1.25 mcg is given, followed by an increment of 2.5 mcg, to dose of 5 mcg; then in increments of 5 mcg until patient achieves erection (one suitable for intercourse and not exceeding 1 hour's duration). If no response to initial dose occurs, next higher dose may be given within 1 hour. Patient must remain in prescriber's office until complete detumescence occurs. If there is a response, procedure shouldn't be repeated for at least 24 hours.

➤ **For urogenital suppository—**
Adults: Initial dose (125 to 250 mcg) given under supervision of prescriber. Adjust dosage p.r.n. until response is sufficient for sexual intercourse. Maximum of two administrations in 24 hours; maximum dose is 1,000 mcg.

ACTION
A prostaglandin derivative that induces erection by relaxing trabecular smooth muscle and dilating cavernosal arteries. This leads to expansion of lacunar spaces and entrapment of blood by compressing venules against the tunica albuginea, a process referred to as the corporal venoocclusive mechanism.

Route	Onset	Peak	Duration
Intra-cavernous	5-20 min	5-20 min	1-6 hr
Urogenital	10 min	16 min	1 hr

ADVERSE REACTIONS
CNS: headache, dizziness.
CV: hypertension.
EENT: sinusitis, nasal congestion.
GU: *penile pain;* prolonged erection; penile fibrosis, rash, or edema; penile disorder; prostatic disorder.
Musculoskeletal: back pain.
Respiratory: upper respiratory tract infection, flu syndrome, cough.
Other: injection site hematoma or ecchymosis, localized trauma or pain.

INTERACTIONS
Drug-drug. *Anticoagulants:* Increased risk of bleeding from intracavernosal injection site. Monitor patient closely.
Cyclosporine: Decreased cyclosporine levels. Monitor cyclosporine levels closely.
Vasoactive drugs: Safety and efficacy of concomitant use haven't been studied. Avoid using together.

EFFECTS ON LAB TEST RESULTS
None reported.

CONTRAINDICATIONS
Contraindicated in patients hypersensitive to drug and in those with conditions predisposing them to priapism (sickle cell anemia or trait, multiple myeloma, leukemia) or penile deformation (angulation, cavernosal fibrosis, Peyronie's disease). Don't use drug in men with penile implants or for whom sexual activity is inadvisable or contraindicated. Also, drug shouldn't be used by sexual partners of pregnant women unless condoms are used. Drug isn't given to women or children.

NURSING CONSIDERATIONS
● Regular follow-up care, with thorough examination of the penis, is strongly recommended to detect signs of penile fibrosis. Drug should be discontinued in patients who develop penile angulation, cavernosal fibrosis, or Peyronie's disease.

PATIENT TEACHING
● Teach patient how to prepare and give drug before he begins treatment at home. Stress importance of reading and following patient instructions in each package

insert. Tell him to store unopened suppositories in refrigerator (36° to 46° F [2° to 8° C]) and store injection at or below room temperature (77° F [25° C]).

• Tell patient not to shake contents of reconstituted vial, and remind him that vial is designed for a single use. Tell him to discard vial if solution is discolored or contains precipitate.

• Instruct patient to urinate before inserting suppository because moisture makes it easier to put medicine in penis and will aid in dissolving it.

• Review administration and aseptic technique.

• Inform patient that he can expect an erection 5 to 20 minutes after administration, with a preferable duration of no more than 1 hour. If his erection lasts more than 6 hours, tell him to seek medical attention immediately.

• Remind patient to take drug as instructed (generally, no more than three times weekly, with at least 24 hours between each use). Warn him not to change dosage without consulting prescriber.

• Caution patient to use a condom if his sexual partner could be pregnant.

• Review possible adverse reactions. Tell patient to inspect his penis daily and to report redness, swelling, tenderness, curvature, priapism, unusual pain, nodules, or hard tissue.

• Urge patient not to reuse or share needles, syringes, or drug.

• Warn patient that drug doesn't protect against sexually transmitted diseases. Also, caution him that bleeding at injection site can increase risk of transmitting blood-borne diseases to his partner.

• Remind patient to keep regular follow-up appointments so prescriber can evaluate drug effectiveness and safety.

amifostine
Ethyol

Pregnancy risk category C

AVAILABLE FORMS
Injection: 500 mg anhydrous base and 500 mg mannitol in 10-ml vial

INDICATIONS & DOSAGES
➤ **Reduction of cumulative renal toxicity linked to repeated administration of cisplatin in patients with advanced ovarian cancer or non–small-cell lung cancer—**
Adults: 910 mg/m^2 daily as a 15-minute I.V. infusion, starting 30 minutes before chemotherapy. If hypotension occurs and blood pressure doesn't return to normal within 5 minutes after stopping treatment, subsequent cycles should use dose of 740 mg/m^2.

➤ **Reduction of moderate to severe xerostomia in patients undergoing postoperative radiation treatment for head and neck cancer—**
Adults: 200 mg/m^2 daily as 3-minute I.V. infusion, starting 15 to 30 minutes before standard fraction radiation therapy.

I.V. ADMINISTRATION
• Inspect vial for particulates and discoloration before use; discard drug if it's cloudy or precipitated.

• Reconstitute each single-dose vial with 9.7 ml of sterile normal saline injection. Using other solutions to reconstitute drug isn't recommended. Reconstituted solution (500 mg amifostine/10 ml) is chemically stable for 5 hours at room temperature (about 77° F [25° C]) or 24 hours if refrigerated (35° to 46° F [2° to 8° C]).

• Drug can be prepared in polyvinyl chloride bags in concentrations of 5 to 40 mg/ml and has same stability as when drug is reconstituted in single-use vial.

• Keep patient supine during infusion. Monitor blood pressure every 5 minutes. If hypotension occurs and requires interrupting therapy, notify prescriber and keep patient supine with legs elevated. Then give infusion of normal saline solution, using a separate I.V. line. If blood pressure returns to normal within 5 minutes and patient is asymptomatic, infusion may be restarted so full dose of drug can be given. If full dose can't be given, limit subsequent doses to 740 mg/m^2.

• Don't infuse for longer than 15 minutes; longer infusion has been linked to higher risk of adverse reactions.

ACTION

Dephosphorylated by alkaline phosphatase in tissue to a pharmacologically active free thiol metabolite. Free thiol in normal tissues binds and detoxifies reactive metabolites of cisplatin, reducing the toxic effects of cisplatin on renal tissue. Free thiol can also act as a scavenger of free radicals that may be generated in tissues exposed to cisplatin.

Route	Onset	Peak	Duration
I.V.	5-8 min	Unknown	Unknown

ADVERSE REACTIONS

CNS: dizziness, somnolence.
CV: *hypotension.*
GI: *nausea, vomiting.*
Metabolic: hypocalcemia.
Respiratory: hiccups, sneezing.
Other: flushing or feeling of warmth, chills or feeling of coldness, ***allergic reactions ranging from rash to rigors.***

INTERACTIONS

Drug-drug. *Antihypertensives, other drugs that could increase hypotension:* May cause profound hypotension. Monitor patient closely.

EFFECTS ON LAB TEST RESULTS

• May decrease calcium levels.

CONTRAINDICATIONS

Contraindicated in patients hypersensitive to aminothiol compounds or mannitol. Drug shouldn't be used in patients receiving chemotherapy for potentially curable malignancies (including certain malignancies of germ-cell origin), except for patients involved in clinical studies. Also contraindicated in hypotensive or dehydrated patients and in those receiving antihypertensives that can't be stopped during 24 hours preceding amifostine administration.

NURSING CONSIDERATIONS

• Use cautiously in elderly patients and in patients with ischemic heart disease, arrhythmias, heart failure, or history of CVA or transient ischemic attacks.
• Use cautiously in patients for whom common adverse effects of nausea, vomit-

ing, and hypotension are likely to have serious consequences.
• If possible and if ordered, stop antihypertensive therapy 24 hours preceding amifostine administration.
• Patients receiving drug should be adequately hydrated before administration. Monitor patient's blood pressure before and immediately after infusion, and periodically thereafter as clinically indicated.
• Antiemetics, including dexamethasone 20 mg I.V. and a serotonin 5HT₃-receptor antagonist, should be given before and with amifostine. Additional antiemetics may be needed, based on chemotherapeutic drugs given.
• Monitor patient's fluid balance if drug is used with highly emetogenic chemotherapy.
• Monitor calcium level in patients at risk for hypocalcemia, such as those with nephrotic syndrome. If needed, give calcium supplements.
• Safety and effectiveness of drug in children haven't been established.

PATIENT TEACHING

• Instruct patient to remain in a supine position throughout infusion.
• Advise patient not to breast-feed; it's unknown if drug or its metabolites appear in breast milk.

---

anagrelide hydrochloride
Agrylin

Pregnancy risk category C

AVAILABLE FORMS

Capsules: 0.5 mg, 1 mg

INDICATIONS & DOSAGES

➤ **Essential thrombocythemia to reduce the elevated platelet count and risk of thrombosis and to ameliorate symptoms—**
Adults: 0.5 mg P.O. q.i.d. or 1 mg P.O. b.i.d. for at least 1 week; then adjust dosage to lowest effective dose needed to maintain platelet count below 600,000/mm³, and ideally to normal range. Don't increase dose by more than 0.5 mg/day in any 1 week; don't exceed 10 mg/day or 2.5 mg in single dose.

ACTION
Reduces platelet production, possibly by decreasing megakaryocyte hypermaturation.

Route	Onset	Peak	Duration
P.O.	Immediate	1 hr	48 hr

ADVERSE REACTIONS
CNS: amnesia, *asthenia,* confusion, ***CVA,*** depression, *dizziness, headache,* syncope, insomnia, migraine, nervousness, pain, paresthesia, malaise, somnolence.
CV: ***arrhythmias,*** angina, chest pain, CV disease, ***heart failure, hemorrhage,*** hypertension, *palpitations,* orthostatic hypotension, vasodilatation, tachycardia, *edema.*
EENT: abnormal vision, amblyopia, diplopia, epistaxis, rhinitis, sinusitis, tinnitus, visual field abnormality.
GI: *abdominal pain,* aphthous stomatitis, constipation, *diarrhea,* dyspepsia, anorexia, eructation, *flatulence,* GI distress, ***GI hemorrhage,*** gastritis, melena, *nausea,* vomiting.
GU: dysuria, hematuria.
Hematologic: anemia, ecchymosis, lymphadenoma, ***thrombocytopenia.***
Metabolic: dehydration.
Musculoskeletal: arthralgia, back pain, leg cramps, myalgia, neck pain.
Respiratory: asthma, bronchitis, *dyspnea,* pneumonia, respiratory disease.
Skin: alopecia, photosensitivity reaction, pruritus, rash, skin disease, urticaria.
Other: chills, fever, flulike symptoms.

INTERACTIONS
Drug-drug. *Sucralfate:* May interfere with anagrelide absorption. Monitor patient closely.
Drug-food. *Any food:* May decrease bioavailability. Advise patient to take drug 1 hour before or 2 hours after meals.

EFFECTS ON LAB TEST RESULTS
• May decrease hemoglobin and platelet count.

CONTRAINDICATIONS
No known contraindications.

NURSING CONSIDERATIONS
• Use with caution in patients with CV disease because drug may cause vasodilation, tachycardia, palpitations, and heart failure.
• Use with caution in patients with creatinine level of 2 mg/dl or more and in those with liver function test values exceeding 1.5 times upper limit of normal.
• During first 2 weeks of treatment, monitor blood counts and liver and renal function test results.
• Platelet counts should be performed every other day during the first week of therapy, then every week thereafter until a maintenance dose is achieved.
• Because it isn't known if drug appears in breast milk, use caution when giving drug to breast-feeding women.

PATIENT TEACHING
• Instruct patient to report increased bleeding, bruising, or cardiac symptoms.
• Instruct woman of childbearing age to use contraception during therapy.

aprotinin
Trasylol

Pregnancy risk category B

AVAILABLE FORMS
Injection: 10,000 kallikrein inactivator units/ml (1.4 mg/ml) in 100-ml and 200-ml vials

INDICATIONS & DOSAGES
➤ **To reduce blood loss or the need for transfusion in patients undergoing coronary artery bypass grafts—**
Adults: Initially 10,000 units (1 ml) I.V. test dose at least 10 minutes before loading dose. If no allergic reaction is evident, anesthesia may be induced while loading dose of 2 million units is given I.V. slowly over 20 to 30 minutes. When loading dose is complete, sternotomy may be performed. Before bypass is initiated, cardiopulmonary bypass circuit is primed with 2 million units of drug by replacing an aliquot of priming fluid with drug. A continuous infusion at 500,000 units/hour is then given I.V. until patient leaves operating room. This is known as regimen A. Or second regimen, known as regimen B, may be given, which is half the dosage of regimen A (except for test dose).

I.V. ADMINISTRATION
● Drug is incompatible with amino acids, corticosteroids, fat emulsions, heparin, and tetracyclines. Don't add other drugs to I.V. container and use separate I.V. line.
● Be prepared to give test dose. Test dose is particularly important in patients who have previously received drug because they have a higher risk of anaphylaxis. In such patients, pretreat with an antihistamine.
● Give all doses through a central line.

ACTION
A naturally occurring protease inhibitor that acts as a systemic hemostatic, decreasing bleeding and turnover of coagulation factors. Inhibits fibrinolysis by affecting kallikrein and plasmin, prevents triggering of the contact phase of the coagulation pathway, and increases the resistance of platelets to damage from mechanical injury and high plasmin levels that occur during cardiopulmonary bypass.

Route	Onset	Peak	Duration
I.V.	Unknown	Unknown	Unknown

ADVERSE REACTIONS
CV: *cardiac arrest, heart failure, ventricular tachycardia, MI, heart block, atrial fibrillation, atrial flutter,* hypotension, supraventricular tachycardia.
GU: *nephrotoxicity, renal failure.*
Metabolic: acidosis, hypervolemia, hypokalemia, hyperglycemia.
Respiratory: pneumonia, respiratory disorder, apnea, asthma, dyspnea.
Other: hypersensitivity reactions, *anaphylaxis,* fever, *shock, sepsis.*

INTERACTIONS
Drug-drug. *Captopril:* Decreased hypotensive effects. Monitor patient closely.
Fibrinolytic drugs: Inhibited fibrinolytic effects. Avoid using together.
Heparin: Prolonged activated clotting time. Monitor clotting time and PTT.

EFFECTS ON LAB TEST RESULTS
● May increase AST, ALT, creatinine, and glucose levels. May decrease potassium levels.
● May alter liver function test values.

CONTRAINDICATIONS
Contraindicated in patients hypersensitive to beef because drug is prepared from bovine lung.

NURSING CONSIDERATIONS
● *Alert:* Use drug cautiously and monitor patient closely for hypersensitivity reaction. Patient may experience anaphylaxis after full therapeutic dose even if they remain asymptomatic after test dose. If symptoms of hypersensitivity occur (skin eruptions, itching, dyspnea, nausea, tachycardia), discontinue infusion immediately, notify prescriber, and provide supportive treatment.
● Obtain history of possible allergies. Patients with history of allergies to drugs or other substances may be at higher risk for developing an allergic reaction to aprotinin.
● To avoid hypotension, make sure patient is supine when loading dose is given. Monitor blood pressure.
● Monitor laboratory studies, including liver function tests.
● Monitor patient for increased creatinine levels and other signs of nephrotoxicity. If nephrotoxicity occurs, it's usually mild and reversible.
● Store drug between 36° and 77° F (2° and 25° C). Protect drug from freezing.

PATIENT TEACHING
● Explain use and administration of drug to patient and family.
● Reassure patient and family that patient will be monitored continuously throughout drug administration.

✳ *NEW DRUG*

balsalazide disodium
COLAZAL

Pregnancy risk category B

AVAILABLE FORMS
Capsules: 750 mg

INDICATIONS & DOSAGES
➤ **Ulcerative colitis—**
Adults: 2.25 g P.O. (three 750-mg capsules) t.i.d., for a total of 6.75 g/day, for 8 weeks.

ACTION

Balsalazide is first converted to mesalamine in the colon, and then converted to 5-aminosalicylic acid. The mechanism of action is unknown, but it appears to be topical. It may decrease inflammation by blocking production of arachidonic acid metabolites in the colon.

Route	Onset	Peak	Duration
P.O.	Unknown	Unknown	Unknown

ADVERSE REACTIONS

CNS: dizziness, fatigue, headache, insomnia.
EENT: pharyngitis, rhinitis, sinusitis.
GI: abdominal pain, anorexia, constipation, cramps, diarrhea, dyspepsia, flatulence, frequent stools, nausea, rectal bleeding, vomiting, dry mouth.
GU: urinary tract infection.
Musculoskeletal: arthralgia, back pain, myalgia.
Respiratory: cough, respiratory infection.
Other: fever, flulike syndrome, pain.

INTERACTIONS

Drug-drug. *Oral antibiotics:* May interfere with release of mesalamine in the colon. Monitor patient for effect.

EFFECTS ON LAB TEST RESULTS

None reported.

CONTRAINDICATIONS

Contraindicated in patients hypersensitive to salicylates or to any component of balsalazide disodium or balsalazide metabolites.

NURSING CONSIDERATIONS

• Use cautiously in patients with history of renal disease or renal dysfunction.
• Hepatotoxicity, including elevated liver function test values, jaundice, cirrhosis, liver necrosis, and liver failure, has occurred with other products containing or metabolized to mesalamine. Although no signs of hepatotoxicity have been reported with balsalazide disodium, monitor patient closely for evidence of hepatic dysfunction.
• Patients with pyloric stenosis may have prolonged retention of drug.

• It isn't known if balsalazide appears in breast milk; use caution when giving drug to a breast-feeding patient.
• Safety and effectiveness beyond 12 weeks haven't been established.
• Safety and effectiveness in pediatric patients haven't been established.

PATIENT TEACHING

• Advise patient not to take drug if he's allergic to aspirin.
• Instruct patient to swallow capsules whole.
• Advise patient to report adverse reactions promptly.

---

becaplermin
Regranex Gel

Pregnancy risk category C

AVAILABLE FORMS

Gel: 100 mcg/g in tubes of 2 g, 7.5 g, 15 g

INDICATIONS & DOSAGES

➤ **Diabetic neuropathic ulcers of the leg that extend into the subcutaneous tissue or beyond and have adequate blood supply—**
Adults: Apply daily in 1/16-inch even thickness to entire surface of wound. The following table shows the length of gel to apply in inches (or centimeters) based on tube size and wound size.

Tube size	Inches	Centimeters
2 g	Ulcer length × ulcer width × 1.3	(Ulcer length × ulcer width) ÷ 2
7.5, 15 g	Ulcer length × ulcer width × 0.6	(Ulcer length × ulcer width) ÷ 4

ACTION

Thought to promote chemotactic recruitment and proliferation of cells involved in wound repair and formation of new granulation tissue.

Route	Onset	Peak	Duration
Topical	Unknown	Unknown	Unknown

ADVERSE REACTIONS

Musculoskeletal: osteomyelitis.
Skin: erythematous rash.
Other: cellulitis, infection.

Reactions may be *common*, uncommon, *life-threatening*, or **COMMON AND LIFE-THREATENING**.

INTERACTIONS
None significant.

EFFECTS ON LAB TEST RESULTS
None reported.

CONTRAINDICATIONS
Contraindicated in patients hypersensitive to drug or its components (such as parabens or m-cresol) and in those with known neoplasms at application site.

NURSING CONSIDERATIONS
● Use cautiously in breast-feeding women.
● **Alert:** Don't use drug in wounds that close by primary intention.
● Drug facilitates complete healing of diabetic ulcers when used as an adjunct to good ulcer care practices, which include initial sharp debridement, infection control, and pressure relief.
● Treatment efficacy hasn't been evaluated for diabetic neuropathic ulcers that don't extend through the dermis into subcutaneous tissue or for ischemic diabetic ulcers.
● To apply drug, calculate length of gel by measuring ulcer's greatest length and width, and use dosage formula. Squeeze calculated length of gel to apply onto clean measuring surface such as waxed paper. Use cotton swab or other application aid to transfer and spread drug over entire ulcer area in a 1/16-inch thick continuous layer. Place a saline-moistened dressing over site and leave in place for about 12 hours. After 12 hours, remove dressing and rinse away residual gel with normal saline solution or water, and apply a fresh moist dressing, without becaplermin, for rest of day.
● Monitor wound size and healing; recalculate amount of drug to be applied at least once weekly. If ulcer doesn't decrease in size by about one-third after 10 weeks, or if complete healing hasn't occurred within 20 weeks, treatment should be reassessed.
● Watch for application site reactions. Sensitization, or irritation caused by parabens or m-cresol, should be considered.
● Drug is for external use only.
● Safety and effectiveness of drug in children younger than age 16 haven't been established.

PATIENT TEACHING
● Instruct patient to wash hands thoroughly before applying gel.
● Advise patient not to touch tip of tube against ulcer or any other surfaces.
● Instruct patient on proper procedure for wound care, including applying gel and changing dressings.
● Stress need to keep area covered with a wet dressing at all times.
● Instruct patient to recap tube tightly after each use.
● Tell patient to store drug in refrigerator (36° to 46° F [2° to 8° C]).
● Instruct patient not to use drug after expiration date.

capsaicin
Capsin◇, Dolorac◇, No Pain-HP◇, Pain Doctor◇, Pain-X◇, Zostrix◇, Zostrix-HP◇

Pregnancy risk category NR

AVAILABLE FORMS
Cream: 0.025% (Zostrix), 0.075% (Zostrix HP), 0.25% (Dolorac)
Gel: 0.025%, 0.05%
Lotion: 0.025%, 0.075%
Roll-on: 0.075%

INDICATIONS & DOSAGES
➤ **Temporary relief from pain after herpes zoster infections; neuralgias, such as postoperative pain and painful diabetic neuropathy; pain from osteoarthritis or rheumatoid arthritis—**
Adults and children older than age 2: Apply to affected areas not more than q.i.d.
➤ **Temporary relief from arthritis pain (Dolorac)—**
Adults and children age 12 and older: Apply thin film to affected area b.i.d.

ACTION
Unknown. May increase release of substance P, a principal neurotransmitter for pain, from peripheral type C sensory fibers to central neurons.

Route	Onset	Peak	Duration
Topical	Unknown	Unknown	Unknown

ADVERSE REACTIONS
Respiratory: cough, irritation.
Skin: redness, *stinging or burning on application.*

INTERACTIONS
None significant.

EFFECTS ON LAB TEST RESULTS
None reported.

CONTRAINDICATIONS
Contraindicated in patients hypersensitive to drug.

NURSING CONSIDERATIONS
• Drug is for external use only.

PATIENT TEACHING
• Warn patient to avoid getting drug in eyes or on broken skin.
• Advise patient not to bandage area tightly after applying drug.
• Tell patient to wash hands after applying drug. However, tell patient to wait approximately 30 minutes to wash hands if using for arthritis of the hands.
• Inform patient that transient burning or stinging is usually evident at initial therapy but decreases with cautious use. This effect persists in patients who use drug less often than t.i.d.
• Tell patient who is taking capsaicin to contact prescriber if symptoms persist beyond 2 to 4 weeks or resolve and shortly reappear.

---

clomiphene citrate
Clomid, Milophene, Serophene

Pregnancy risk category X

AVAILABLE FORMS
Tablets: 50 mg

INDICATIONS & DOSAGES
➤ **To induce ovulation—**
Adults: 50 mg P.O. daily for 5 days starting on day 5 of menstrual cycle (first day of menstrual flow is day 1) if bleeding occurs, or at any time if patient hasn't had recent uterine bleeding. If ovulation doesn't occur, may increase dose to 100 mg P.O. daily for 5 days as soon as 30 days after

previous course. Repeated until conception occurs or until three courses of therapy are completed.

ACTION
Unknown. Appears to stimulate release of follicle-stimulating hormone, luteinizing hormone, and pituitary gonadotropins, resulting in maturation of the ovarian follicle, ovulation, and development of the corpus luteum.

Route	Onset	Peak	Duration
P.O.	Unknown	Unknown	Unknown

ADVERSE REACTIONS
CNS: headache, restlessness, insomnia, dizziness, light-headedness, depression, fatigue.
EENT: blurred vision, diplopia, scotoma, photophobia.
GI: nausea, vomiting, bloating, distention.
GU: urinary frequency and polyuria, abnormal uterine bleeding, *ovarian enlargement,* cyst formation that regresses spontaneously when drug is stopped.
Metabolic: weight gain.
Skin: reversible alopecia, urticaria, rash, dermatitis.
Other: *hot flashes, breast discomfort.*

INTERACTIONS
None significant.

EFFECTS ON LAB TEST RESULTS
None reported.

CONTRAINDICATIONS
Contraindicated during pregnancy and in patients with undiagnosed abnormal genital bleeding, ovarian cyst not related to polycystic ovarian syndrome, hepatic disease or dysfunction, uncontrolled thyroid or adrenal dysfunction, or presence of organic intracranial lesion (such as a pituitary tumor). Also contraindicated in patients with liver disease.

NURSING CONSIDERATIONS
• Monitor patient closely because of potentially serious adverse reactions.
• Long-term cyclic therapy isn't recommended.

• **Alert:** Don't confuse clomiphene with clomipramine or clonidine.

PATIENT TEACHING
• Tell patient that risk of multiple births exists, which increases with higher doses.
• Teach patient to take and chart basal body temperature to ascertain if ovulation has occurred.
• Reassure patient that ovulation typically occurs after first course of therapy. If pregnancy doesn't occur, therapy may be repeated twice.
• Advise patient to stop drug and contact prescriber immediately if pregnancy is suspected because drug may have teratogenic effect.
• **Alert:** Advise patient to stop drug and contact prescriber immediately if abdominal symptoms or pain occur; these symptoms may indicate ovarian enlargement or ovarian cyst. Also tell patient to immediately notify prescriber if signs and symptoms of impending visual toxicity occur, such as blurred vision, diplopia, scotoma, or photophobia.
• Warn patient to avoid hazardous activities, such as driving or operating machinery, until CNS effects are known. Drug may cause dizziness or visual disturbances.

✷ NEW DRUG

eflornithine hydrochloride
Vaniqa

Pregnancy risk category C

AVAILABLE FORMS
Cream: 13.9%, 30-g tube (single or double)

INDICATIONS & DOSAGES
➤ **Reduction of unwanted facial hair in women—**
Adults and children older than age 12:
Apply a thin layer to affected areas of the face and adjacent areas under chin; rub in thoroughly b.i.d., at least 8 hours apart. Don't wash area for at least 4 hours after application.

ACTION
Thought to irreversibly inhibit skin enzyme ornithine decarboxylase activity.

This inhibits cell division and synthesis, thereby slowing the rate of hair growth.

Route	Onset	Peak	Duration
Topical	Unknown	8 hr	Unknown

ADVERSE REACTIONS
CNS: headache, dizziness, asthenia, vertigo.
GI: dyspepsia, anorexia, nausea.
Skin: *acne, pseudofolliculitis barbae,* stinging or burning sensation, dry skin, pruritus, erythema, skin irritation, rash, alopecia, folliculitis, ingrown hair, facial edema.

INTERACTIONS
No known interactions.

EFFECTS ON LAB TEST RESULTS
None reported.

CONTRAINDICATIONS
Contraindicated in patients hypersensitive to drug or its components.

NURSING CONSIDERATIONS
• Application of the cream should be limited to the face and adjacent involved areas under the chin.
• Drug shouldn't cause contact sensitization, phototoxicity, or photosensitization reactions.
• If no improvement is seen after 6 months, treatment should be stopped. Hair will return to normal about 8 weeks after stopping treatment.
• It's unknown if drug appears in breast milk. Use cautiously in breast-feeding women.
• Store drug at 59° to 86° F (15° to 30° C).

PATIENT TEACHING
• Tell patient that product is for external use only and to avoid getting into eyes, nose, or mouth. If drug gets into eyes, tell patient to rinse thoroughly with water and to contact her prescriber.
• Tell patient to apply a thin layer to affected areas of the face and adjacent involved areas under the chin and to rub thoroughly. Tell her not to wash treatment areas for at least 4 hours after application.
• Instruct patient to use product exactly as prescribed.

---

*Liquid contains alcohol.   **May contain tartrazine.   †Canada   ‡Australia   §U.K.   ◇OTC

• Explain to patient that drug works by inhibiting an enzyme in the hair follicle of the skin responsible for hair growth, resulting in slowing of the hair growth rate. Instruct patient to continue current hair removal techniques of tweezing and plucking because drug won't permanently remove hair. Wait at least 5 minutes after hair removal to apply cream.

• Warn patient that results aren't immediate and may vary. Improvement may occur as early as 4 to 8 weeks but may take longer.

• Instruct patient that she may use cosmetics or sunblocks after applying drug but that she should wait a few minutes to allow the cream to be absorbed.

• If adverse effects become bothersome, instruct patient to limit use to once a day. If adverse effects persist or if condition worsens, tell patient to stop drug and to consult prescriber.

---

etanercept
Enbrel

Pregnancy risk category B

AVAILABLE FORMS
Injection: 25-mg single-use vial

INDICATIONS & DOSAGES
➤ **Reduction in signs and symptoms of moderately to severely active rheumatoid arthritis in patients who demonstrate inadequate response to one or more disease-modifying antirheumatic drugs with methotrexate and who don't respond adequately to methotrexate alone**—
Adults: 25 mg S.C. twice weekly, 72 to 96 hours apart.
➤ **Reduction in signs and symptoms of moderately to severely active polyarticular-course juvenile rheumatoid arthritis in patients who have had an inadequate response to one or more disease-modifying antirheumatic drugs**—
Children ages 4 to 17: 0.4 kg/kg (up to maximum of 25 mg per dose) S.C. twice weekly, 72 to 96 hours apart.
✽ *NEW INDICATION:* **Reducing signs and symptoms and delaying structural dam-**
age in patients with moderately to severely active rheumatoid arthritis—
Adults: 25 mg S.C. twice weekly, 72 to 96 hours apart.

ACTION
Binds specifically to tumor necrosis factor (TNF) and blocks its action with cell surface TNF receptors, reducing inflammatory and immune responses found in rheumatoid arthritis.

Route	Onset	Peak	Duration
S.C.	Unknown	72 hr.	Unknown

ADVERSE REACTIONS
CNS: asthenia, *headache,* dizziness.
EENT: *rhinitis,* pharyngitis, sinusitis.
GI: abdominal pain, dyspepsia.
Respiratory: *upper respiratory tract infections,* cough, respiratory disorder.
Skin: *injection site reaction,* rash.
Other: *infections,* malignancies.

INTERACTIONS
None significant.

EFFECTS ON LAB TEST RESULTS
None reported.

CONTRAINDICATIONS
Contraindicated in patients hypersensitive to drug or its components and in those with sepsis.

NURSING CONSIDERATIONS
• Use caution when using in rheumatoid arthritis patients with pre-existing or recent onset of demyelinating disorders, including multiple sclerosis, myelitis, and optic neuritis.
• *Alert:* Anti-TNF therapies, including etanercept, may affect defenses against infection. Notify prescriber and discontinue therapy if serious infection occurs.
• *Alert:* Drug is for S.C. injection only.
• *Alert:* Don't give live vaccines concurrently during therapy.
• Patients with juvenile rheumatoid arthritis should, if possible, be brought up-to-date with all immunizations in compliance with current immunization guidelines before initiating treatment.
• Reconstitute aseptically with 1 ml of supplied sterile bacteriostatic water for in-

---

jection, USP (0.9% benzyl alcohol). Don't filter reconstituted solution during preparation or administration. Inject diluent slowly into vial. Minimize foaming by gently swirling during dissolution rather than shaking. Dissolution takes less than 5 minutes.

• Visually inspect solution for particulates and discoloration before use. Reconstituted solution should be clear and colorless. Don't use solution if it's discolored or cloudy, or if it contains particulate matter.

• Don't add other drugs or diluents to reconstituted solution.

• Use reconstituted solution as soon as possible; may be refrigerated in vial for up to 6 hours at 36° to 46° F (2° to 8° C).

• Injection sites should be at least 1 inch apart; areas where skin is tender, bruised, red, or hard should never be used. Recommended sites include the thigh, abdomen, and upper arm. Rotate sites regularly.

• Patient may develop positive antinuclear antibody or positive anti-double-stranded DNA antibodies measured by radioimmunoassay and *Crithidia luciliae* assay.

• Drug isn't recommended for use in children younger than age 4.

• Needle cover of diluent syringe contains dry natural rubber (latex) and shouldn't be handled by persons sensitive to latex.

PATIENT TEACHING
• If patient will be giving drug, advise him about mixing and injection techniques, including rotation of injection sites.

• Instruct patient to use puncture-resistant container for disposal of needles and syringes.

• Tell patient that injection site reactions generally occur within first month of therapy and decrease thereafter.

• Inform patient of importance of avoiding live vaccine administration during therapy.

• Stress importance of alerting prescriber or other health care providers of etanercept use.

• Instruct patient to promptly report signs and symptoms of infection to prescriber.

• Advise breast-feeding woman to discontinue breast-feeding during therapy.

finasteride
Propecia, Proscar

Pregnancy risk category X

AVAILABLE FORMS
Tablets: 1 mg, 5 mg

INDICATIONS & DOSAGES
Propecia
➤ **Male pattern hair loss (androgenetic alopecia) in men only—**
Adults: 1 mg P.O. daily.
Proscar
➤ **Symptomatic BPH to improve symptoms and reduce risk of acute urine retention and need for surgery, including transurethral resection of prostate and prostatectomy—**
Adults: 5 mg P.O. daily.

ACTION
Competitively inhibits corticosteroid 5 alpha-reductase, an enzyme responsible for formation of potent androgen 5 alpha-dihydrotestosterone (DHT) from testosterone. Because DHT influences development of the prostate gland, decreasing levels of this hormone in adult men should relieve the symptoms related to BPH. In male pattern balding, the balding scalp contains miniaturized hair follicles and increased amounts of DHT. Finasteride decreases scalp and DHT levels in such cases.

Route	Onset	Peak	Duration
P.O.	Unknown	1-2 hr	24 hr

ADVERSE REACTIONS
GU: impotence, decreased volume of ejaculate.
Other: decreased libido.

INTERACTIONS
None significant.

EFFECTS ON LAB TEST RESULTS
None reported.

CONTRAINDICATIONS
Contraindicated in patients hypersensitive to drug. Although drug isn't used in women or children, manufacturer indicates pregnancy as a contraindication.

NURSING CONSIDERATIONS

• Before therapy, patient should be evaluated for conditions that mimic BPH, including hypotonic bladder; prostate cancer, infection, or stricture; or relevant neurologic conditions.

• Carefully monitor patients who have a large residual urine volume or severely diminished urine flow; these patients may not be candidates for drug therapy.

• Carefully evaluate sustained increases in prostate-specific antigen levels, which could indicate noncompliance with therapy.

• Although drug's elimination rate is decreased in elderly patients, dosage adjustments aren't needed.

• Because it's impossible to identify which patients will respond to finasteride, minimum of 6 months of therapy may be needed for treatment of BPH.

• Long-term effects on complications of BPH, including acute urinary obstruction and risk of surgery, are unknown.

PATIENT TEACHING

• Warn woman who is or may become pregnant not to handle crushed tablets because of risk of adverse effects on male fetus.

• Inform patient that 3 months or more of daily use is generally needed to see benefits when drug is used to treat hair loss.

• Tell patient to anticipate baseline and periodic digital rectal examinations.

• Reassure patient that drug may decrease volume of ejaculate but doesn't appear to impair normal sexual function. Impotence and decreased libido have occurred in less than 4% of patients.

✳ *NEW DRUG*

imatinib mesylate
Gleevec

Pregnancy risk category D

AVAILABLE FORMS
Capsules: 100 mg

INDICATIONS AND DOSAGES
➤ **Chronic myeloid leukemia (CML) in blast crisis, in accelerated phase, or in chronic phase after failure of interferon-alpha therapy—**

Adults: Chronic-phase CML: 400 mg P.O. daily as single dose with a meal and large glass of water. *Accelerated-phase CML or blast crisis:* 600 mg P.O. daily as single dose with a meal and large glass of water. Continue treatment as long as patient continues to benefit. May increase daily dose to 600 mg P.O. in chronic phase or to 800 mg P.O. (400 mg P.O. b.i.d.) in accelerated phase or blast crisis.

➤ **Kit (CD117)–positive unresectable or metastatic malignant GI stromal tumors (GIST)—**

Adults: 400 or 600 mg P.O. daily.

Adjust-a-dose: For severe nonhematologic adverse reactions (severe hepatotoxicity or severe fluid retention), withhold drug until event has resolved; resume treatment as appropriate based on initial severity of event. For elevations in bilirubin level more than three times the institutional upper limit of normal (IULN) or liver transaminase levels more than five times IULN, withhold drug until bilirubin level returns to less than 1.5 IULN and transaminase levels to less than 2.5 IULN. May then resume drug at reduced daily dose (400 mg to 300 mg or 600 mg to 400 mg).

For hematologic adverse reactions, see the table on page 1255.

ACTION

Drug inhibits Bcr-Abl tyrosine kinase, which is the abnormal tyrosine kinase created by the Philadelphia chromosome abnormality in CML; in vivo, it inhibits tumor growth of Bcr-Abl transfected murine myeloid cells as well as Bcr-Abl positive leukemia lines derived from CML patients in blast crisis.

Route	Onset	Peak	Duration
P.O.	Unknown	2-4 hr	Unknown

ADVERSE REACTIONS

CNS: *headache,* CEREBRAL HEMORRHAGE, *fatigue, weakness.*
CV: *edema.*
EENT: nasopharyngitis, *epistaxis.*
GI: *anorexia, nausea, diarrhea, abdominal pain, constipation, vomiting, dyspepsia,* GI HEMORRHAGE.

Reactions may be *common*, uncommon, ***life-threatening***, or COMMON AND LIFE-THREATENING.

Dosage Adjustments for Hematologic Adverse Reactions

Indication	Laboratory values	Treatment guidelines
Chronic-phase chronic myeloid leukemia or GI stromal tumors (starting dose 400 mg)	Absolute neutrophil count (ANC) < 1 $\times$ 10^9/L or platelets < 50 $\times$ 10^9/L, or both.	1. Stop Gleevec until ANC $\geq$ 1.5 $\times$ 10^9/L and platelets $\geq$ 75 $\times$ 10^9/L. 2. Resume treatment at 400 mg. 3. If recurrence of ANC < 1 $\times$ 10^9/L, platelets < 50 $\times$ 10^9/L, or both, repeat step 1 and resume Gleevec at reduced dose of 300 mg.
Accelerated phase chronic myeloid leukemia and blast crisis or GI stromal tumors (starting dose 600 mg)	ANC < 0.5 $\times$ 10^9/L occurring after at least 1 month of treatment or platelets < 10 $\times$ 10^9/L, or both.	1. Check if cytopenia is related to leukemia via marrow aspirate or biopsy. 2. If cytopenia is unrelated to leukemia, reduce dose of Gleevec to 400 mg. 3. If cytopenia persists 2 weeks, reduce further to 300 mg. 4. If cytopenia persists 4 weeks and is still unrelated to leukemia, stop Gleevec until ANC $\geq$ 1 $\times$ 10^9/L and platelets $\geq$ 20 $\times$ 10^9/L and then resume treatment at 300 mg.

Hematologic: HEMORRHAGE, NEUTRO-
PENIA, THROMBOCYTOPENIA, *anemia.*
Metabolic: *hypokalemia,* weight increase.
Musculoskeletal: *myalgia, muscle
cramps, musculoskeletal pain, arthralgia.*
Respiratory: *cough, dyspnea, pneumonia.*
Skin: *rash,* pruritus, *petechiae.*
Other: *pyrexia, night sweats.*

INTERACTIONS
Drug-drug. *CYP3A4 inhibitors (clarithromycin, erythromycin, itraconazole, ketoconazole):* Decreased metabolism and increased imatinib levels. Monitor patient
for toxicity.
*CYP3A4 inducers (carbamazepine, dexam-
ethasone, phenobarbital, phenytoin, rifampin):* Increased metabolism and decreased
imatinib levels. Use together cautiously.
*Dihydropyridine–calcium channel block-
ers, certain HMG-CoA reductase inhibitors, cyclosporine, pimozide, triazolo-
benzodiazepines:* Increased levels of these
drugs. Monitor patient for toxicity and obtain drug levels, if appropriate.
Warfarin: Altered metabolism of warfarin.
Avoid using together; use standard heparin
or a low molecular weight heparin.
Drug-herb. *St. John's wort:* May decrease
imatinib effects. Discourage use together.

EFFECTS ON LAB TEST RESULTS
• May increase creatinine, bilirubin, alka-
line phosphatase, AST, and ALT levels.
May decrease potassium levels.
• May decrease hemoglobin and neu-
trophil and platelet counts.

CONTRAINDICATIONS
Contraindicated in patients hypersensitive
to drug or its components.

NURSING CONSIDERATIONS
• Use cautiously in patients with hepatic
impairment.
• Monitor weight daily. Evaluate and treat
unexpected rapid weight gain.
• Monitor patients closely for fluid retention, which can be severe.
• Monitor CBC weekly for first month,
then decrease to biweekly for second
month, and periodically thereafter.
• Because GI irritation is common, patients should take drug with food.
• Monitor liver function tests carefully because hepatotoxicity (occasionally severe)
may occur; decrease dosage as needed.
• Although there are no data on long-term
safety of this drug, monitor renal and liver
toxicity and immunosuppression carefully.
• Elderly patients may have an increased
incidence of edema when taking this drug.
• Consider dosage increases only if there
are no severe adverse reactions or severe
non–leukemia-related neutropenia or
thrombocytopenia in the following circumstances: disease progression (at any
time), failure to achieve a satisfactory
hematologic response after at least 3
months of treatment, or loss of a previously achieved hematologic response.

PATIENT TEACHING
• Tell patient to take drug with food and a
large glass of water.

• Advise patient to report adverse effects, such as fluid retention, to prescriber.
• Advise patient to obtain periodic liver and kidney function tests and blood work to determine blood counts.

---

imiquimod
Aldara

Pregnancy risk category B

AVAILABLE FORMS
Cream: 5% in single-use packets containing 250 mg

INDICATIONS & DOSAGES
➤ **External genital and perianal warts—**
Adults: Apply thin layer to affected area three times weekly before normal sleeping hours and leave on skin for 6 to 10 hours. Continue treatment until there is total clearance of the genital or perianal warts or for maximum of 16 weeks.

ACTION
Exact mechanism unknown. An immune response modifier; has no direct antiviral activity.

Route	Onset	Peak	Duration
Topical	Unknown	Unknown	Unknown

ADVERSE REACTIONS
CNS: headache.
Musculoskeletal: myalgia.
Skin: local itching, burning, pain, soreness, erythema, ulceration, edema, erosion, induration, flaking, excoriation.
Other: flulike symptoms, *fungal infection.*

INTERACTIONS
None significant.

EFFECTS ON LAB TEST RESULTS
None reported.

CONTRAINDICATIONS
No known contraindications.

NURSING CONSIDERATIONS
• Safety of drug in breast-feeding women is unknown.

• Safety and efficacy of drug in patients younger than age 18 haven't been established.
• Drug isn't recommended for treatment of urethral, intravaginal, cervical, rectal, or intra-anal human papilloma viral disease.
• Don't use until genital or perianal tissue is healed from previous drug or surgical treatment.
• Patient usually experiences local skin reactions at site of application or surrounding areas. Use nonocclusive dressings, such as cotton gauze, or cotton undergarments in management of skin reactions. Patient's discomfort or severity of the local skin reaction may require a rest period of several days. Resume treatment once reaction subsides.
• Drug isn't a cure; new warts may develop during therapy.

PATIENT TEACHING
• Advise patient that effect of cream on transmission of genital or perianal warts is unknown. New warts may develop during therapy; drug isn't a cure.
• Tell patient to use cream only as directed and to avoid contact with eyes.
• Tell patient to wash hands before and after applying cream.
• Advise patient to apply cream in thin layer over affected area and rub in until cream isn't visible. Advise patient to avoid excessive use of cream. Tell patient not to occlude area after applying cream and to wash with mild soap and water 6 to 10 hours following application of cream.
• Advise patient that mild local skin reactions, such as erythema, erosion, excoriation, flaking, and edema at site of application or surrounding areas, are common. Tell patient that most skin reactions are mild to moderate. Advise him to report severe skin reactions promptly.
• Instruct uncircumcised man being treated for warts under the foreskin to retract foreskin and clean area daily.
• Advise patient that drug can weaken condoms and vaginal diaphragms and that use together isn't recommended.
• Advise patient to avoid sexual contact while cream is on the skin.
• Tell patient to store drug at temperatures below 86° F (30° C) and to avoid freezing.

Reactions may be *common*, uncommon, **life-threatening**, or COMMON AND LIFE-THREATENING.

infliximab
Remicade

Pregnancy risk category B

AVAILABLE FORMS
Injection: 100-mg vial

INDICATIONS & DOSAGES
➤ **Reduction of signs and symptoms in patients with moderately to severely active Crohn's disease with inadequate response to conventional therapy**—
Adults: 5 mg/kg single I.V. infusion over not less than 2 hours.
➤ **Reduction in number of draining enterocutaneous fistulas in patients with fistulizing Crohn's disease**—
Adults: 5 mg/kg I.V. infused over not less than 2 hours. Additional doses of 5 mg/kg should be given at 2 and 6 weeks after initial infusion.
➤ **Reduction in signs and symptoms of rheumatoid arthritis in patients who have had inadequate response to methotrexate alone**—
Adults: 3 mg/kg I.V. infusion over 2 hours or more, followed by additional 3-mg/kg doses at 2 and 6 weeks after first infusion; then every 8 weeks thereafter. Give with methotrexate. If response is inadequate, dose may be increased to maximum of 10 mg/kg or infusions may be given every 4 weeks.

I.V. ADMINISTRATION
• Vials don't contain antibacterial preservatives; use reconstituted drug immediately. Reconstitute with 10 ml sterile water for injection, using syringe with 21G or smaller needle. Don't shake; gently swirl to dissolve powder. Solution should be colorless to light yellow and opalescent, and may develop a few translucent particles. Don't use if other particles or discoloration exists.
• Dilute total volume of reconstituted drug to 250 ml with normal saline solution for injection. Infusion concentration range is 0.4 to 4 mg/ml. Infusion should begin within 3 hours of preparation and must be given over not less than 2 hours.
• Don't infuse drug in same I.V. line with other drugs.

ACTION
A monoclonal antibody that binds to human tumor necrosis factor (TNF)-alpha to neutralize its activity and inhibit its binding with receptors, thereby reducing the infiltration of inflammatory cells and TNF-alpha production in inflamed areas of the intestine.

Route	Onset	Peak	Duration
I.V.	Unknown	Unknown	Unknown

ADVERSE REACTIONS
CNS: *headache, fatigue,* dizziness, malaise, insomnia.
CV: hypertension, hypotension, tachycardia, chest pain, flushing.
EENT: pharyngitis, rhinitis, sinusitis, conjunctivitis.
GI: *nausea, abdominal pain,* vomiting, constipation, dyspepsia, flatulence, intestinal obstruction, oral pain, ulcerative stomatitis.
GU: dysuria, increased urinary frequency.
Hematologic: anemia, hematoma.
Musculoskeletal: myalgia, arthralgia, arthritis, back pain.
Respiratory: *upper respiratory tract infections,* bronchitis, coughing, dyspnea, respiratory tract allergic reaction.
Skin: rash, pruritus, candidiasis, acne, alopecia, eczema, erythema, erythematous rash, maculopapular rash, papular rash, dry skin, increased sweating, urticaria.
Other: toothache, flu syndrome, ecchymosis, *fever,* chills, pain, peripheral edema, hot flashes, abscess.

INTERACTIONS
Drug-drug. *Vaccines:* Infliximab may affect normal immune response. Don't use together with live-virus vaccines.

EFFECTS ON LAB TEST RESULTS
• May increase liver enzyme levels.
• May decrease hemoglobin.

CONTRAINDICATIONS
Contraindicated in patients hypersensitive to murine proteins or other components of drug. Patients with congestive heart failure should not begin using this drug; clinical trials showed that the heart patients on Remicade got much sicker than those patients who were not using the drug.

---

*Liquid contains alcohol.   **May contain tartrazine.   †Canada   ‡Australia   §U.K.   ◊OTC

NURSING CONSIDERATIONS
• Use cautiously in elderly patients and in patients with active infection or history of chronic or recurrent infections. In patients who have resided in regions where histoplasmosis is endemic, the benefits and risks of infliximab therapy should be carefully considered before initiation of therapy.

• *Alert:* Watch for infusion-related reactions, including fever, chills, pruritus, urticaria, dyspnea, hypotension, hypertension, and chest pain, during administration and for 2 hours following completion. If an infusion-related reaction occurs, discontinue drug, notify prescriber, and be prepared to give acetaminophen, antihistamines, corticosteroids, and epinephrine.

• Watch for development of lymphomas and infection. Patients with chronic Crohn's disease and long-term exposure to immunosuppressants are more likely to develop lymphomas and infections.

• Drug may affect normal immune responses. Patient may develop autoimmune antibodies and lupuslike syndrome; in these cases, drug should be discontinued. Symptoms can be expected to resolve.

• Some patients test positive for antinuclear antibodies.

• Tuberculosis (frequently disseminated or extrapulmonary at clinical presentation), invasive fungal infections, and other opportunistic infections have been observed in patients receiving infliximab. Some of these infections have been fatal.

• Patients should be evaluated for latent tuberculosis infection with a tuberculin skin test. Treatment of latent tuberculosis infection should be initiated prior to therapy with infliximab.

PATIENT TEACHING
• Tell patient about infusion-reaction symptoms and instruct him to report them.

• Inform patient of adverse effects that may occur after infusion, and instruct him to report them promptly.

• Inform breast-feeding woman to stop breast-feeding during therapy.

• Instruct patient to inform prescriber of drug use before receiving vaccines.

isotretinoin
Accutane, Roaccutane‡

Pregnancy risk category X

AVAILABLE FORMS
Capsules: 10 mg, 20 mg, 40 mg

INDICATIONS & DOSAGES
➤ **Severe recalcitrant nodular acne unresponsive to conventional therapy**—
Adults and adolescents: 0.5 to 2 mg/kg P.O. daily in two divided doses with food for 15 to 20 weeks.

ACTION
Unknown. Thought to normalize keratinization, reversibly decrease size of sebaceous glands, and alter composition of sebum to a less viscous form that is less likely to cause follicular plugging.

Route	Onset	Peak	Duration
P.O.	Unknown	3 hr	Unknown

ADVERSE REACTIONS
CNS: headache, fatigue, *pseudotumor cerebri.*
EENT: *conjunctivitis,* corneal deposits, dry eyes, visual disturbances, *epistaxis, drying of mucous membranes, dry nose.*
GI: nonspecific GI symptoms, *nausea, vomiting,* anorexia, *abdominal pain, dry mouth,* gum bleeding and inflammation.
Hematologic: anemia, elevated platelet count, *increased erythrocyte sedimentation rate.*
Metabolic: *hypertriglyceridemia,* hyperglycemia, altered uric acid levels.
Musculoskeletal: *musculoskeletal pain.*
Skin: *cheilosis, rash, dry skin, facial skin desquamation,* peeling of palms and toes, *petechiae, nail brittleness,* thinning of hair, skin infection, photosensitivity reaction, *cheilitis, pruritus, fragility.*

INTERACTIONS
Drug-drug. *Carbamazepine:* Decreased carbamazepine levels. Monitor levels.
Tetracyclines: Increased risk of pseudotumor cerebri. Avoid using together.
Vitamin A, products containing vitamin A: Increased toxic effects of isotretinoin.

Reactions may be *common,* uncommon, *life-threatening,* or COMMON AND LIFE-THREATENING.

Avoid using together without informing prescriber.

Drug-food. *Any food:* Increased absorption of drug. Advise patient to take drug with milk, a meal, or shortly after a meal.

Drug-lifestyle. *Alcohol use:* Increased risk of hypertriglyceridemia. Discourage use together.

Sun exposure: Increased photosensitivity reaction. Advise patient to avoid excessive sunlight exposure.

EFFECTS ON LAB TEST RESULTS
● May increase AST, ALT, alkaline phosphatase, triglyceride, glucose, and uric acid levels.
● May increase platelet count and erythrocyte sedimentation rate.

CONTRAINDICATIONS
Contraindicated in patients hypersensitive to parabens (which are used as preservatives), vitamin A, or other retinoids. Also contraindicated in woman of childbearing age unless patient has had a negative serum pregnancy test within 2 weeks before beginning therapy, will begin drug therapy on second or third day of next menstrual period, and will comply with stringent contraceptive measures for 1 month before therapy, during therapy, and for at least 1 month after therapy.

NURSING CONSIDERATIONS
● Before use, have patient read patient information and sign accompanying consent form.
● Patient must have negative results from two urine or serum pregnancy tests, one of which is performed in the office when the patient is qualified for therapy, the second of which is performed on the second day of the next normal menstrual period or 11 days or more after the last unprotected act of sexual intercourse, whichever is later.
● Monitor baseline lipid studies and liver function tests before therapy and at regular intervals.
● Monitor glucose level regularly and CK levels in patients who participate in vigorous physical activity.
● Most adverse reactions appear to be dose-related, occurring at doses exceeding 1 mg/kg daily. Reactions are generally reversible when therapy is discontinued or dosage is reduced.
● *Alert:* Patient who experiences headache, nausea and vomiting, or visual disturbances should be screened for papilledema. Signs and symptoms of pseudotumor cerebri require immediate discontinuation of drug and prompt neurologic intervention.
● *Alert:* Severe fetal abnormalities may occur if drug is used during pregnancy.
● The FDA and drug manufacturer designed a program, System to Manage Accutane Related Teratogenicity (S.M.A.R.T.), to encourage the safe and appropriate use of drug, which can cause birth defects and fetal death if taken by a pregnant woman.
● If patient becomes pregnant during treatment, prescribers are encouraged to call Roche Medical Services at 1-800-526-6367 or FDA MedWatch at 1-800-FDA-1088.
● Anticipate a second course of therapy, if needed, not to start for at least 8 weeks after completion of first course because improvement may continue after withdrawal of drug.

PATIENT TEACHING
● Advise patient to take drug with or shortly after meals to facilitate absorption.
● Tell patient to immediately report visual disturbances and bone, muscle, or joint pain.
● Warn patient that contact lenses may feel uncomfortable during therapy.
● Warn patient against using abrasives, medicated soaps and cleansers, acne preparations containing peeling drugs, and topical alcohol products (including cosmetics, aftershave, cologne) because these products cause cumulative irritation or excessive drying of skin.
● Tell patient to avoid prolonged sun exposure and to use sunblock. Drug may have additive effect if used with other drugs that cause photosensitivity reaction.
● Advise patient of childbearing age to use two reliable forms of contraception simultaneously, unless abstinence is chosen method of birth control, for 1 month before, during, and 1 month after treatment.

---

*Liquid contains alcohol.   **May contain tartrazine.   †Canada   ‡Australia   §U.K.   ◊OTC

• Manufacturer will supply urine pregnancy tests for female patients for initial, second, and monthly testing during therapy.

• Advise patient not to donate blood during or for 30 days after therapy; severe fetal abnormalities may occur if a pregnant woman receives blood containing isotretinoin.

• Warn patient that transient exacerbations may occur during therapy.

---

leflunomide
Arava

Pregnancy risk category X

AVAILABLE FORMS
Tablets: 10 mg, 20 mg, 100 mg

INDICATIONS & DOSAGES
➤ **Active rheumatoid arthritis to reduce signs and symptoms and to retard structural damage as evidenced by X-ray erosions and joint space narrowing—**
Adults: 100 mg P.O. q 24 hours for 3 days; then 20 mg (maximum daily dose) P.O. q 24 hours. Dose may be decreased to 10 mg daily if higher dose isn't well-tolerated.

ACTION
An immunomodulatory drug that inhibits dihydroorotate dehydrogenase, an enzyme involved in pyrimidine synthesis, and has antiproliferative activity and anti-inflammatory effects.

Route	Onset	Peak	Duration
P.O.	Unknown	6-12 hr	Unknown

ADVERSE REACTIONS
CNS: asthenia, dizziness, headache, paresthesia, malaise, migraine, sleep disorder, vertigo, neuritis, anxiety, depression, insomnia, neuralgia.
CV: angina pectoris, *hypertension,* chest pain, palpitations, tachycardia, vasculitis, vasodilation, varicose veins, peripheral edema.
EENT: pharyngitis, rhinitis, sinusitis, epistaxis, blurred vision, cataracts, conjunctivitis, eye disorder.
GI: mouth ulcer, oral candidiasis, gingivitis, enlarged salivary glands, stomatitis, dry mouth, taste perversion, anorexia, *di-*

arrhea, dyspepsia, gastroenteritis, nausea, abdominal pain, vomiting, cholelithiasis, colitis, constipation, esophagitis, flatulence, gastritis, melena.
GU: urinary tract infection, albuminuria, cystitis, dysuria, hematuria, menstrual disorder, pelvic pain, vaginal candidiasis, prostate disorder, urinary frequency.
Hematologic: anemia.
Metabolic: diabetes mellitus, hyperglycemia, hyperthyroidism, hypokalemia, hyperlipidemia, weight loss.
Musculoskeletal: arthrosis, back pain, bursitis, muscle cramps, myalgia, bone necrosis, bone pain, arthralgia, leg cramps, joint disorder, neck pain, synovitis, tendon rupture, tenosynovitis.
Respiratory: bronchitis, increased cough, pneumonia, *respiratory infection,* asthma, dyspnea, lung disorder.
Skin: *alopecia,* eczema, pruritus, *rash,* dry skin, acne, contact dermatitis, fungal dermatitis, hair discoloration, hematoma, nail disorder, skin nodule, subcutaneous nodule, maculopapular rash, skin disorder, skin discoloration, skin ulcer.
Other: tooth disorder, fever, allergic reaction, flu syndrome, injury or accident, pain, abscess, cyst, hernia, increased sweating, ecchymoses, herpes simplex, herpes zoster.

INTERACTIONS
Drug-drug. *Charcoal, cholestyramine:* Decreased plasma levels of leflunomide. Sometimes used for this effect in overdose.
Methotrexate, other hepatotoxic drugs: Increased risk of hepatotoxicity. Monitor liver enzymes.
NSAIDs (diclofenac, ibuprofen): Increased levels of NSAIDs. Clinical significance is unknown.
Rifampin: Increased active leflunomide metabolite level. Use together cautiously.
Tolbutamide: Increased tolbutamide levels. Clinical significance is unknown.

EFFECTS ON LAB TEST RESULTS
• May increase AST, ALT, glucose, lipid, and CK levels. May decrease potassium levels.

CONTRAINDICATIONS
Contraindicated in patients hypersensitive to drug or its components and in women

who are or may become pregnant or who are breast-feeding. Drug isn't recommended for patients with hepatic insufficiency, hepatitis B or C, severe immunodeficiency, bone marrow dysplasia, or severe uncontrolled infections. Drug isn't recommended for use in patients younger than age 18 and in men attempting to father a child.

NURSING CONSIDERATIONS
• Use cautiously in patients with renal insufficiency.
• Vaccination with live vaccines isn't recommended. The long half-life of drug should be considered when contemplating administration of a live vaccine after stopping drug treatment.
• *Alert:* Drug can cause fetal harm when given to pregnant women; women planning pregnancy should discontinue drug therapy and consult prescriber. Men planning to father a child should discontinue drug therapy and follow recommended leflunomide removal protocol (cholestyramine 8 g, P.O. t.i.d. for 11 days). In addition to cholestyramine, verify drug levels are less than 0.02 mg/L by two separate tests at least 14 days apart. If level is greater than 0.02 mg/L, consider additional cholestyramine treatment.
• Risk of malignancy, particularly lymphoproliferative disorders, is increased with use of some immunosuppressants, including leflunomide.
• Monitor liver enzyme levels (ALT and AST) before starting therapy and monthly thereafter until stable. Frequency can then be decreased based on clinical situation.

PATIENT TEACHING
• Explain need and frequency of required blood tests and monitoring.
• Instruct patient to use birth control during course of treatment and until it has been determined that drug is no longer active.
• Warn patient to immediately notify prescriber if signs or symptoms of pregnancy occur (such as late menses or breast tenderness).
• Advise breast-feeding woman to discontinue breast-feeding during therapy.
• Inform patient that aspirin, other NSAIDs, and low-dose corticosteroids may be continued during treatment. However, use of drug with antimalarials, intramuscular or oral gold, penicillamine, azathioprine, or methotrexate hasn't been adequately studied.

---

levocarnitine (L-carnitine)
Carnitor

Pregnancy risk category B

AVAILABLE FORMS
Capsules: 250 mg ◊
Injection: 1 g/5 ml
Oral liquid: 100 mg/ml
Tablets: 330 mg

INDICATIONS & DOSAGES
➤ **Primary and secondary systemic carnitine deficiency**—
Adults: 990 mg P.O. b.i.d. or t.i.d. Or, 10 to 30 ml (1 to 3 g) of oral liquid daily.
Children: 50 to 100 mg/kg/day P.O. in divided doses.

All doses depend on clinical response. Higher doses may be given. However, for children, maximum dose is 3 g/day.
➤ **Immediate and long-term treatment of secondary carnitine deficiency**—
Adults: 50 mg/kg I.V. slowly over 2 to 3 minutes q 3 to 4 hours.

I.V. ADMINISTRATION
• A loading dose frequently is given to patients with severe metabolic crisis, followed by an equivalent dose over next 24 hours.
• Drug is compatible and stable when mixed in solutions of normal saline solution or lactated Ringer's solution in concentrations ranging from 250 mg/500 ml to 4,200 mg/500 ml.
• Store mixed infusions at room temperature (77° F [25° C]) for up to 24 hours in polyvinyl chloride plastic bags.
• Don't refrigerate solution.

ACTION
Facilitates transport of long-chain fatty acids into cellular mitochondria. The fatty acids are then used to produce energy.

Route	Onset	Peak	Duration
I.V., P.O.	Unknown	Unknown	Unknown

---

*Liquid contains alcohol.   **May contain tartrazine.   †Canada   ‡Australia   §U.K.   ◊OTC

ADVERSE REACTIONS
GI: *nausea, vomiting, cramps, diarrhea.*
Other: *body odor.*

INTERACTIONS
Drug-drug. *D,L-carnitine:* Inhibition of levocarnitine and possible deficiency. Avoid using together.
Valproic acid: Increased requirement for carnitine. Adjust dosage.
Drug-food. *Any food:* Decreased GI upset. Advise patient to dissolve drug in drink or liquid food, or take with meals.

EFFECTS ON LAB TEST RESULTS
None reported.

CONTRAINDICATIONS
No known contraindications.

NURSING CONSIDERATIONS
• Don't use oral formulations in patients with end-stage renal disease, those on dialysis, and those with severely compromised renal function. Only the I.V. formulation has been approved for this population because the major metabolites formed during oral administration of high doses for long periods cannot be efficiently removed by the kidneys and will accumulate.
• Give enteral liquid alone or dissolved in drinks or liquid food.
• Use entire or partial contents of containers of liquid immediately after opening; discard any unused contents.
• Monitor patient's tolerance during first week of therapy and after increasing dosage.
• Monitor blood chemistry results and plasma carnitine levels periodically, as well as vital signs and patient's overall clinical condition.

PATIENT TEACHING
• Tell patient to consume oral liquid slowly to minimize GI distress. If GI intolerance persists, dosage may have to be reduced.
• Caution patient not to share drug with others. Some people have used it to improve athletic performance.
• Warn patient about possible body odor.
• Space doses evenly every 3 to 4 hours and give drug with or after meals, if possible.

• Tell patient to store drug at room temperature.

---

mesalamine
Asacol, Mesasal, Pentasa, Rowasa, Salofalk

Pregnancy risk category B

AVAILABLE FORMS
Capsules (controlled-release): 250 mg
Rectal suspension: 4 g/60 ml
Suppositories: 500 mg
Tablets (delayed-release): 400 mg

INDICATIONS & DOSAGES
➤ **Active mild to moderate distal ulcerative colitis, proctitis, or proctosigmoiditis—**
Adults: 800 mg P.O. (tablets) t.i.d. for total dose of 2.4 g/day for 6 weeks; or 1 g P.O. (capsules) q.i.d. for total dose of 4 g up to 8 weeks; or 500 mg P.R. (suppository) b.i.d. or 4 g as retention enema once daily (preferably h.s.). Rectal dosage form should be retained overnight (for about 8 hours). Usual course of therapy for rectal form is 3 to 6 weeks.

ACTION
Unknown. An active metabolite of sulfasalazine; probably acts topically by inhibiting prostaglandin production in the colon.

Route	Onset	Peak	Duration
P.O., P.R.	Unknown	3-12 hr	Unknown

ADVERSE REACTIONS
CNS: headache, dizziness, fatigue, malaise, asthenia, chills.
CV: chest pain.
GI: abdominal pain, cramps, discomfort, flatulence, diarrhea, rectal pain, bloating, nausea, *pancolitis,* vomiting, constipation, eructation.
GU: interstitial nephritis, nephropathy, ***nephrotoxicity.***
Musculoskeletal: arthralgia, myalgia, back pain, hypertonia.
Respiratory: wheezing.
Skin: itching, rash, urticaria, hair loss.
Other: fever.

Reactions may be *common,* uncommon, *life-threatening,* or COMMON AND LIFE-THREATENING.

INTERACTIONS

Drug-drug. *Lactulose:* May impair release of delayed or extended-release products. Monitor patient closely.
Omeprazole: Increased absorption of mesalamine. Monitor patient closely.

EFFECTS ON LAB TEST RESULTS

• May increase BUN, creatinine, AST, ALT, alkaline phosphatase, LDH, amylase, and lipase levels.

CONTRAINDICATIONS

Contraindicated in patients allergic to mesalamine, any salicylates, or any component of the preparation; also contraindicated in children.

NURSING CONSIDERATIONS

• Use cautiously in patients with renal impairment. Problems haven't been documented, but nephrotoxic potential from absorbed mesalamine exists.
• Shake suspension well before each use and remove sheath before inserting into rectum.
• Intact or partially intact tablets may be seen in the stool. Notify prescriber if this occurs repeatedly.
• Monitor periodic renal function studies in patients on long-term therapy.
• Because the mesalamine rectal suspension contains potassium metabisulfite, it may cause hypersensitivity reactions in patients sensitive to sulfites.
• *Alert:* Don't confuse Asacol with Os-Cal.

PATIENT TEACHING

• Instruct patient to carefully follow instructions supplied with drug and to swallow tablets whole; do not crush or chew.
• Advise patient to discontinue drug if fever or rash occurs. Patient intolerant of sulfasalazine may also be hypersensitive to mesalamine.
• Tell patient to remove foil wrapper from suppositories before inserting into rectum.
• Teach patient about proper use of retention enema.
• Tell patient that enema solution may stain bedsheets and clothing. Protective underpads and linens should be used.

mesna
Mesnex, Uromitexan§

Pregnancy risk category B

AVAILABLE FORMS

Injection: 100 mg/ml

INDICATIONS & DOSAGES

➤ **Prophylaxis of hemorrhagic cystitis in patients receiving ifosfamide—**
Adults: Dosage varies with amount of ifosfamide given; calculated as 20% of ifosfamide dose at time of ifosfamide administration. Usual dose is 240 mg/m^2 as an I.V. bolus with administration of ifosfamide; repeated at 4 and 8 hours after administration of ifosfamide.

I.V. ADMINISTRATION

• Prepare I.V. solution by diluting commercially available ampules with D_5W, dextrose 5% and normal saline solution for injection, normal saline solution for injection, or lactated Ringer's solution to obtain final solution of 20 mg/ml.
• Although diluted solutions are stable for 24 hours at room temperature, it's recommended that they be refrigerated and used within 6 hours. After opening ampule, discard any unused drug.
• Mesna and ifosfamide are compatible in same I.V. infusion.
• *Alert:* Mesna I.V. is incompatible with cisplatin; don't mix them.

ACTION

Prevents ifosfamide-induced hemorrhagic cystitis by reacting with urotoxic ifosfamide metabolites.

Route	Onset	Peak	Duration
I.V.	Unknown	Unknown	Unknown

ADVERSE REACTIONS

CNS: headache, fatigue.
CV: *hypotension.*
GI: *soft stools,* nausea, vomiting, diarrhea, *dysgeusia.*
Musculoskeletal: *limb pain.*
Other: allergy.

INTERACTIONS

None significant.

EFFECTS ON LAB TEST RESULTS
None reported.

CONTRAINDICATIONS
Contraindicated in patients hypersensitive to mesna or compounds containing thiol.

NURSING CONSIDERATIONS
• Mesna isn't effective in preventing hematuria from other causes (such as thrombocytopenia).
• Because mesna is used with ifosfamide and other chemotherapeutic drugs, it's difficult to determine adverse reactions attributable solely to mesna.
• The total daily dose of mesna is 60% of the ifosfamide dose.
• Although formulated to prevent hemorrhagic cystitis from ifosfamide, drug won't protect against other toxicities from drug therapy.
• Monitor urine samples for hematuria daily. Monitor BUN and creatinine levels and intake and output.
• Drug contains benzyl alcohol, which has been linked to fatal gasping syndrome in premature infants.

PATIENT TEACHING
• Explain to patient and family or other caregiver the need for drug and how it's given.
• Instruct patient to report persistent or severe adverse reactions.
• Advise patient to promptly report blood in urine.

---

minoxidil (topical)
Rogaine

Pregnancy risk category C

AVAILABLE FORMS
Topical solution: 2%

INDICATIONS & DOSAGES
➤ **Androgenetic alopecia—**
Adults: 1 ml of 2% solution applied to affected area b.i.d. Maximum daily dose is 2 ml.

ACTION
Unknown. Stimulates hair growth, possibly by dilating arterial microcapillaries around hair follicles.

Route	Onset	Peak	Duration
Topical	Unknown	Unknown	Unknown

ADVERSE REACTIONS
CNS: headache, dizziness, faintness, light-headedness.
CV: edema, chest pain, hypertension, hypotension, palpitations, increased or decreased pulse rate.
EENT: sinusitis.
GI: diarrhea, nausea, vomiting.
GU: urinary tract infection, renal calculi, urethritis.
Metabolic: weight gain.
Musculoskeletal: back pain, tendinitis.
Respiratory: bronchitis, upper respiratory infection.
Skin: *irritant dermatitis,* allergic contact dermatitis, eczema, hypertrichosis, *local erythema, pruritus, dry skin or scalp, flaking,* alopecia, exacerbation of hair loss.

INTERACTIONS
Drug-drug. *Petroleum jelly, topical corticosteroids, topical retinoids, other drugs that may increase skin absorption:* Increased risk of systemic effects of minoxidil. Don't apply minoxidil with other drugs.

EFFECTS ON LAB TEST RESULTS
None reported.

CONTRAINDICATIONS
Contraindicated in patients hypersensitive to drug or components of solution.

NURSING CONSIDERATIONS
• Use cautiously in patients older than age 50 and in those with cardiac, renal, or hepatic disease.
• Patients need to have normal, healthy scalps before beginning therapy because absorption of drug through irritated skin may cause adverse systemic effects.
• Treatment is most likely to succeed in patients with balding area smaller than 4 inches (10 cm) that developed within past 10 years.

PATIENT TEACHING

• Teach patient how to apply topical minoxidil. Hair and scalp should be thoroughly dry before application, and drug shouldn't be applied to other body areas. Tell patient not to use drug on irritated or sunburned scalp or with other drugs on scalp. Tell him to thoroughly wash hands after application.

• Warn patient to avoid inhaling any spray or mist from drug and to avoid spraying around eyes because solution contains alcohol and may be irritating.

• Inform patient that more frequent applications or using more than 2 ml/day won't increase hair growth, but instead may increase adverse reactions. Don't attempt to double doses for missed applications.

• Teach patient to monitor pulse rate and body weight.

• Advise patient of need for medical follow-ups, beginning 1 month after therapy starts and every 6 months thereafter.

• Advise patient that therapy will be prolonged and will continue for at least 4 months before clinical effects appear and that drug must be used daily for optimal results. About 40% of patients will see moderate to dense hair growth.

• Tell patient that discontinuing drug may result in loss of new hair growth. New hair growth is usually fine and may be colorless, but will resemble existing hair after continued treatment.

---

nimodipine
Nimotop

Pregnancy risk category C

AVAILABLE FORMS
Capsules: 30 mg

INDICATIONS & DOSAGES
➤ **Improvement of neurologic deficits after subarachnoid hemorrhage from ruptured congenital aneurysms—**
Adults: 60 mg P.O. q 4 hours for 21 days. Begin therapy within 96 hours after subarachnoid hemorrhage.
Adjust-a-dose: For patients with hepatic failure, 30 mg P.O. q 4 hours for 21 days.

ACTION
Inhibits calcium ion influx across cardiac and smooth-muscle cells, decreasing myocardial contractility and oxygen demand, and dilates coronary and cerebral arteries and arterioles.

Route	Onset	Peak	Duration
P.O.	Unknown	1 hr	Unknown

ADVERSE REACTIONS
CNS: headache, psychic disturbances.
CV: decreased blood pressure, flushing, edema, tachycardia.
GI: nausea, diarrhea, abdominal discomfort.
Musculoskeletal: muscle cramps.
Respiratory: dyspnea, wheezing.
Skin: dermatitis, rash.

INTERACTIONS
Drug-drug. *Antihypertensives:* May increase hypotensive effect. Monitor patient closely.
Calcium channel blockers: May increase CV effects. Monitor patient closely.
Cimetidine: Increased nimodipine bioavailability. Monitor patient closely.

EFFECTS ON LAB TEST RESULTS
None reported.

CONTRAINDICATIONS
No known contraindications.

NURSING CONSIDERATIONS
• Use cautiously in patients with hepatic failure.
• Reserve drug for patients who are in good neurologic condition (for example, Hunt and Hess grades I to III).
• Monitor blood pressure and heart rate in all patients, especially at start of therapy.
• If capsule can't be swallowed, make a hole in each end of capsule with an 18G needle, and extract contents into syringe.
• Empty syringe into patient's nasogastric tube. Flush tube with 30 ml of normal saline solution.
• *Alert:* If using a needle to extract contents of capsule, make sure that drug isn't then given I.V. instead of P.O. Label the syringe, "for oral use only" before withdrawing the contents of the capsule.

PATIENT TEACHING
● Explain use of drug, and review administration schedule with patient and family. Stress importance of compliance for maximum drug effectiveness.
● Instruct patient to report persistent or severe adverse reactions promptly.
● Tell patient not to eat grapefruit or drink grapefruit juice while taking this drug.

olsalazine sodium
Dipentum

Pregnancy risk category C

AVAILABLE FORMS
Capsules: 250 mg

INDICATIONS & DOSAGES
➤ **Maintenance of remission of ulcerative colitis in patients intolerant of sulfasalazine—**
Adults: 500 mg P.O. b.i.d. with meals.

ACTION
Unknown. After oral administration, converts to 5-aminosalicylic acid (5-ASA or mesalamine) in the colon, where it has local anti-inflammatory effect.

Route	Onset	Peak	Duration
P.O.	Unknown	1 hr	Unknown

ADVERSE REACTIONS
CNS: headache, depression, vertigo, dizziness, fatigue.
GI: *diarrhea,* nausea, *abdominal pain,* dyspepsia, bloating, anorexia.
Musculoskeletal: arthralgia.
Skin: rash, itching.

INTERACTIONS
Drug-drug. *Anticoagulants, coumarin derivatives:* Prolonged PT or INR. Monitor bleeding studies.
Drug-food. *Any food:* Decreased GI irritation. Advise patient to take drug with food.

EFFECTS ON LAB TEST RESULTS
None reported.

CONTRAINDICATIONS
Contraindicated in patients hypersensitive to salicylates.

NURSING CONSIDERATIONS
● Use cautiously in patients with renal disease. Although problems haven't been reported, possibility of renal tubular damage from absorbed drug or its metabolites must be considered.
● Regularly monitor BUN and creatinine levels and urinalysis in patients with renal disease.
● Some patients have reported diarrhea during therapy. Although diarrhea appears to be dose-related, it's difficult to distinguish from worsening of disease symptoms.
● Similar drugs have caused exacerbation of disease.
● *Alert:* Don't confuse olsalazine with olanzapine.

PATIENT TEACHING
● Teach patient to take drug in evenly divided doses and with food to minimize adverse GI reactions.
● Instruct patient to report persistent or severe adverse reactions promptly.

orlistat
Xenical

Pregnancy risk category B

AVAILABLE FORMS
Capsules: 120 mg

INDICATIONS & DOSAGES
➤ **Management of obesity, including weight loss and weight maintenance with a reduced-calorie diet; reduction of risk of weight gain after previous weight loss—**
Adults: 120 mg P.O. t.i.d. with each main meal containing fat; during or up to 1 hour after meals.

ACTION
A reversible inhibitor of lipases that forms bond with active site of gastric and pancreatic lipases, inactivating them. Thus, enzymes can't hydrolyze dietary fat, in the form of triglycerides, into absorbable free

fatty acids and monoglycerides. The undigested triglycerides aren't absorbed, resulting in caloric deficit.

Route	Onset	Peak	Duration
P.O.	Unknown	Unknown	Unknown

ADVERSE REACTIONS

CNS: *headache,* dizziness, fatigue, sleep disorder, anxiety, depression.
CV: pedal edema.
EENT: otitis.
GI: *oily spotting, flatus with discharge, fecal urgency, fatty or oily stool, oily evacuation, increased defecation, abdominal pain,* fecal incontinence, nausea, infectious diarrhea, rectal pain, vomiting.
GU: menstrual irregularity, vaginitis, urinary tract infection.
Musculoskeletal: *back pain, leg pain,* arthritis, myalgia, joint disorder, tendonitis.
Respiratory: *influenza, upper respiratory tract infection,* lower respiratory tract infection.
Skin: rash, dry skin.
Other: tooth and gingival disorders.

INTERACTIONS

Drug-drug. *Cyclosporine:* Potential alterations of cyclosporine absorption with variations in dietary intake. Monitor patient's cyclosporine levels if used together.
Fat-soluble vitamins (such as vitamins A and E and beta-carotene): Decreased absorption of vitamins. Separate administration times by 2 hours.
Pravastatin: Slightly increased pravastatin levels and additive lipid-lowering effects of drug. Monitor patient.
Warfarin: May change coagulation values. Monitor INR.

EFFECTS ON LAB TEST RESULTS
None reported.

CONTRAINDICATIONS
Contraindicated in patients hypersensitive to drug or its components and in those with chronic malabsorption syndrome or cholestasis. Exclude organic causes of obesity such as hypothyroidism before starting drug therapy.

NURSING CONSIDERATIONS
● Use cautiously in patients with history of hyperoxaluria or calcium oxalate nephrolithiasis or risk of anorexia nervosa or bulimia.
● Use cautiously in patients receiving cyclosporine therapy because of potential changes in cyclosporine absorption related to variations in dietary intake.
● Drug is recommended for use in patients with an initial body mass index of 30 kg/m^2 or more, or 27 kg/m^2 or more and other risk factors (such as hypertension, diabetes, or dyslipidemia).
● Advise patient to adhere to dietary guidelines. GI effects may increase when patient takes drug with high-fat foods, specifically when more than 30% of total daily calories come from fat.
● Drug reduces absorption of some fat-soluble vitamins and beta-carotene. To ensure adequate nutrition, advise patient to take daily multivitamin supplements that contain fat-soluble vitamins during therapy.
● In diabetic patients, because improved metabolic control may accompany weight loss, dosage of oral antidiabetic or insulin may need to be reduced.
● As with other weight-loss drugs, potential for misuse in certain patients exists (such as those with anorexia nervosa or bulimia).
● *Alert:* Don't confuse Xenical with Xeloda.

PATIENT TEACHING
● Advise patient to follow a nutritionally balanced, reduced-calorie diet that derives only 30% of its calories from fat. Daily intake of fat, carbohydrate, and protein should be distributed over three main meals. If a meal is occasionally missed or contains no fat, tell patient that dose of drug can be omitted.
● To ensure adequate nutrition, advise patient to take daily multivitamin supplements that contain fat-soluble vitamins at least 2 hours before or after administration of drug, such as at bedtime.
● Tell patient with diabetes that weight loss may improve his glycemic control, so dosage of his oral antidiabetic (such as sulfonylureas or metformin) or insulin may need to be reduced during drug therapy.

• Tell woman of childbearing age to inform prescriber if pregnancy or breast-feeding is planned during therapy.

---

pilocarpine hydrochloride
Salagen

Pregnancy risk category C

AVAILABLE FORMS
Tablets: 5 mg

INDICATIONS & DOSAGES
➤ **Xerostomia from salivary gland hypofunction caused by radiotherapy for cancer of head and neck—**
Adults: 5 mg P.O. t.i.d.; may be increased to 10 mg P.O. t.i.d., p.r.n.
➤ **Symptoms of dry mouth in patients with Sjögren's syndrome—**
Adults: 5 mg P.O. q.i.d.

ACTION
A cholinergic parasympathomimetic that increases secretion of salivary glands, eliminating dryness.

Route	Onset	Peak	Duration
P.O.	20 min	1 hr	3-5 hr

ADVERSE REACTIONS
CNS: *dizziness, headache,* tremor, *asthenia.*
CV: hypertension, tachycardia, *flushing,* edema.
EENT: *rhinitis,* lacrimation, amblyopia, pharyngitis, voice alteration, conjunctivitis, epistaxis, *sinusitis, abnormal vision.*
GI: *nausea,* dyspepsia, diarrhea, abdominal pain, vomiting, dysphagia, taste perversion.
GU: *urinary frequency.*
Musculoskeletal: myalgia.
Skin: rash, pruritus, *sweating.*
Other: *chills.*

INTERACTIONS
Drug-drug. *Beta-adrenergic antagonists:* May increase risk of conduction disturbances. Use together cautiously.
Drugs with anticholinergic effects: May antagonize anticholinergic effects. Use together cautiously.

Drugs with parasympathomimetic effects: May result in additive pharmacologic effects. Monitor patient closely.
Drug-food. *High-fat meals:* Reduced drug absorption. Discourage patient from eating high-fat meals.

EFFECTS ON LAB TEST RESULTS
None reported.

CONTRAINDICATIONS
Contraindicated in patients hypersensitive to pilocarpine, in those with uncontrolled asthma, and in those for whom miosis is undesirable, as in acute iritis or narrow-angle glaucoma.

NURSING CONSIDERATIONS
• Use cautiously in patients with CV disease, controlled asthma, chronic bronchitis, COPD, cholelithiasis, biliary tract disease, nephrolithiasis, or cognitive or psychiatric disturbances.
• Don't use drug in breast-feeding women.
• Safety and efficacy of drug in children haven't been established.
• Examine patient's fundus carefully before beginning therapy because retinal detachment has been reported in patients with retinal disease.
• Monitor patient for signs and symptoms of toxicity: headache, visual disturbance, lacrimation, sweating, respiratory distress, GI spasm, nausea, vomiting, diarrhea, AV block, tachycardia, bradycardia, hypotension, hypertension, shock, mental confusion, arrhythmia, and tremors. Immediately notify prescriber of suspected toxicity.

PATIENT TEACHING
• Warn patient that driving ability may be impaired, especially at night, by drug-induced visual disturbances.
• Advise patient to drink plenty of fluids to prevent dehydration.
• Inform elderly patient with Sjögren's syndrome that he may be especially prone to urinary frequency, diarrhea, and dizziness.
• Advise patient not to take drug with a high-fat meal.

---

raloxifene hydrochloride
Evista

Pregnancy risk category X

AVAILABLE FORMS
Tablets: 60 mg

INDICATIONS & DOSAGES
➤ **Prevention of osteoporosis in post-menopausal women—**
Adults: 60 mg P.O. once daily.
➤ **Treatment of osteoporosis in post-menopausal women—**
Adults: 60 mg P.O. daily.

ACTION
A selective estrogen receptor modulator that reduces resorption of bone and decreases overall bone turnover. These effects on bone are manifested as reductions in serum and urine levels of bone turnover markers and increases in bone mineral density.

Route	Onset	Peak	Duration
P.O.	Unknown	Unknown	24 hr

ADVERSE REACTIONS
CNS: depression, insomnia, migraine.
CV: chest pain.
EENT: *sinusitis,* pharyngitis, laryngitis.
GI: nausea, dyspepsia, vomiting, flatulence, GI disorder, gastroenteritis, abdominal pain.
GU: vaginitis, urinary tract infection, cystitis, leukorrhea, endometrial disorder, vaginal bleeding.
Metabolic: weight gain.
Musculoskeletal: *arthralgia,* myalgia, arthritis, leg cramps.
Respiratory: increased cough, pneumonia.
Skin: rash, sweating.
Other: breast pain, *infection, flu syndrome, hot flashes,* peripheral edema, fever.

INTERACTIONS
Drug-drug. *Cholestyramine:* Causes significant reduction in absorption of raloxifene. Avoid using together.
Highly protein-bound drugs (such as clofibrate, diazepam, diazoxide, ibuprofen, in-domethacin, naproxen): May interfere with binding sites. Use together cautiously.
Warfarin: May cause a decrease in PT. Monitor PT and INR closely.

EFFECTS ON LAB TEST RESULTS
● May increase calcium, inorganic phosphate, total protein, albumin, hormone-binding globulin, and apolipoprotein A levels. May decrease total and LDL cholesterol levels and apolipoprotein B levels.

CONTRAINDICATIONS
Contraindicated in women hypersensitive to drug or its components; in those with past or current venous thromboembolic events, including deep vein thrombosis, pulmonary embolism, and retinal vein thrombosis; in women who are pregnant, planning to get pregnant, or breast-feeding; and in children.

NURSING CONSIDERATIONS
● Use cautiously in patients with severe hepatic impairment.
● Watch for signs of blood clots. Greatest risk of thromboembolic events occurs during first 4 months of treatment.
● Discontinue drug at least 72 hours before prolonged immobilization and resume only after patient is fully mobilized.
● Report unexplained uterine bleeding because endometrial proliferation hasn't been linked with drug use.
● Watch for breast abnormalities that occur during treatment. Drug hasn't been linked to breast enlargement, breast pain, or an increased risk of breast cancer.
● Safety and efficacy of drug haven't been evaluated in men.
● Effect on bone mineral density beyond 2 years of drug treatment isn't known.
● Use with hormone replacement therapy or systemic estrogen hasn't been evaluated and isn't recommended.

PATIENT TEACHING
● Advise patient to avoid long periods of restricted movement (such as during traveling) because of increased risk of venous thromboembolic events.
● Inform patient that hot flashes or flushing may occur and that drug doesn't aid in reducing them.

- Instruct patient to practice other bone loss–prevention measures, including taking supplemental calcium and vitamin D if dietary intake is inadequate, performing weight-bearing exercises, and discontinuing alcohol consumption and smoking.
- Tell patient that drug may be taken without regard to food.
- Advise patient to report unexplained uterine bleeding or breast abnormalities during therapy.
- Explain adverse reactions and instruct patient to read patient package insert before starting therapy and to reread it each time prescription is renewed.

---

riluzole
Rilutek

Pregnancy risk category C

AVAILABLE FORMS
Tablets: 50 mg

INDICATIONS & DOSAGES
➤ **Amyotrophic lateral sclerosis—**
Adults: 50 mg P.O. q 12 hours, taken on empty stomach.

ACTION
May protect motor neurons from excitotoxic effects of glutamate by inhibiting glutamate release, inactivating some sodium channels, and interfering with transmitter binding.

Route	Onset	Peak	Duration
P.O.	Unknown	Unknown	Unknown

ADVERSE REACTIONS
CNS: headache, aggravation reaction, *asthenia,* hypertonia, depression, dizziness, insomnia, malaise, somnolence, vertigo, circumoral paresthesia.
CV: hypertension, tachycardia, palpitations, orthostatic hypotension.
EENT: rhinitis, sinusitis.
GI: abdominal pain, *nausea,* vomiting, dyspepsia, anorexia, diarrhea, flatulence, stomatitis, tooth disorder, dry mouth, oral candidiasis.
GU: urinary tract infection, dysuria.
Metabolic: weight loss.
Musculoskeletal: back pain, arthralgia.

Respiratory: *decreased lung function,* increased cough.
Skin: pruritus, eczema, alopecia, exfoliative dermatitis.
Other: phlebitis, peripheral edema.

INTERACTIONS
Drug-drug. *Allopurinol, methyldopa, sulfasalazine:* Increased risk of hepatotoxicity. Monitor patient closely.
Inducers of CYP1A2 (omeprazole, rifampin): May increase riluzole elimination. Monitor patient closely.
Potential inhibitors of CYP1A2 (amitriptyline, caffeine, phenacetin, quinolones, theophylline): May decrease riluzole elimination. Monitor closely.
Drug-food. *Any food:* Decreased bioavailability. Advise patient to take 1 hour before or 2 hours after meals.
Charbroiled foods: May increase elimination of drug. Discourage use together.
Drug-lifestyle. *Alcohol use:* May increase risk of hepatotoxicity. Discourage excessive use.
Smoking: May increase riluzole elimination. Discourage patient from smoking.

EFFECTS ON LAB TEST RESULTS
- May increase AST, ALT, bilirubin, and GGT levels.

CONTRAINDICATIONS
Contraindicated in patients with history of severe hypersensitivity to drug or its components.

NURSING CONSIDERATIONS
- Use cautiously in patients with hepatic or renal dysfunction, in elderly patients, and in women and Japanese patients (who may have lower metabolic capacity to eliminate drug than men and Caucasian patients, respectively).
- Elevations in baseline liver function studies (especially bilirubin) preclude drug use. Perform liver function studies periodically during therapy. In many patients, drug may increase aminotransferase level; if level exceeds five times upper limit of normal or if clinical jaundice develops, notify prescriber.
- Give drug at least 1 hour before or 2 hours after meals to avoid decreased bioavailability.

PATIENT TEACHING

• Tell patient to take drug at same time each day. If a dose is missed, tell him to take next tablet when planned.
• Instruct patient to take drug on an empty stomach to facilitate full dose absorption.
• Instruct patient to report fever to prescriber, who may order a WBC count.
• Warn patient to avoid hazardous activities until CNS effects of drug are known and to limit alcohol use during therapy.
• Tell patient to store drug at room temperature, protect from bright light, and keep out of children's reach.

✴ NEW DRUG

risedronate sodium
Actonel

Pregnancy risk category C

AVAILABLE FORMS
Tablets: 5 mg, 30 mg

INDICATIONS & DOSAGES
➤ **Prevention and treatment of postmenopausal osteoporosis—**
Adults: 5 mg P.O. daily.
➤ **Glucocorticoid-induced osteoporosis in patients who are either starting or continuing glucocorticoid therapy at 7.5 mg or more of prednisone or equivalent daily—**
Adults: 5 mg P.O. daily.
➤ **Paget's disease—**
Adults: 30 mg P.O. daily for 2 months. If relapse occurs or alkaline phosphatase level doesn't normalize, may retreat with same dose and duration 2 months or more after completing first treatment.
Adjust-a-dose: Drug isn't recommended for patients with creatinine clearance below 30 ml/minute.

ACTION
Risedronate reverses the loss of bone mineral density in postmenopausal women, a central factor in the progression of osteoporosis. It does so by reducing bone turnover and bone resorption at remodeling sites by inhibiting osteoclasts. In patients with Paget's disease, drug causes bone turnover to return to normal, as evidenced by reduced levels of alkaline phosphatase (a marker of bone formation) and urinary hydroxyproline/creatinine and deoxypyridinoline/creatinine (markers of bone resorption).

Route	Onset	Peak	Duration
P.O.	1 hr	Unknown	Unknown

ADVERSE REACTIONS
CNS: asthenia, *headache,* depression, dizziness, insomnia, anxiety, neuralgia, vertigo, paresthesia.
CV: *hypertension,* CV disorder, angina pectoris, chest pain, peripheral edema.
EENT: pharyngitis, rhinitis, sinusitis, cataract, conjunctivitis, otitis media, amblyopia, tinnitus.
GI: *nausea, diarrhea, abdominal pain,* flatulence, gastritis, rectal disorder, constipation.
GU: *urinary tract infection,* cystitis.
Hematologic: ecchymosis, anemia.
Musculoskeletal: *arthralgia,* neck pain, *back pain,* myalgia, bone pain, leg cramps, bursitis, tendon disorder.
Respiratory: dyspnea, pneumonia, bronchitis.
Skin: *rash,* pruritus, skin carcinoma.
Other: *infection,* tooth disorder, *pain.*

INTERACTIONS
Drug-drug. *Calcium supplements, antacids that contain calcium, magnesium, or aluminum:* Interference with risedronate absorption. Advise patient to separate administration times.
Drug-food. *Any food:* Interference with risedronate absorption. Advise patient to take drug at least 30 minutes before first food or drink of the day (other than water).

EFFECTS ON LAB TEST RESULTS
• May decrease calcium and phosphorus levels.

CONTRAINDICATIONS
Contraindicated in patients who are hypersensitive to any component of the product, or are hypocalcemic or unable to stand or sit upright for 30 minutes after administration. Drug isn't recommended for patients with severe renal impairment (creatinine clearance below 30 ml/minute).

NURSING CONSIDERATIONS

• Use cautiously in patients with upper GI disorders such as dysphagia, esophagitis, and esophageal or gastric ulcers.

• Risk factors for the development of osteoporosis include family history, previous fracture, smoking, a decrease in bone mineral density below the premenopausal mean, a thin body frame, white or Asian race, and early menopause.

• *Alert:* Follow dosing instructions carefully because benefits of the drug may be compromised by failure to take it according to instructions. Give drug at least 30 minutes before patient's first food or drink of the day (other than water).

• Give drug with sufficient (6 to 8 ounces) plain water to facilitate delivery to the stomach. Don't allow patient to lie down for 30 minutes after taking drug.

• Weight-bearing exercise should be considered along with cessation of smoking and alcohol consumption, as appropriate.

• *Alert:* Bisphosphonates have been linked to such GI disorders as dysphagia, esophagitis, and esophageal or gastric ulcers. Monitor patient for symptoms of esophageal disease (such as dysphagia, retrosternal pain, or severe persistent or worsening heartburn).

• Patients should receive supplemental calcium and vitamin D if dietary intake is inadequate. However, because calcium supplements and calcium-, aluminum-, and magnesium-containing medications may interfere with risedronate absorption, the dosing times should be separated.

• Store drug at 68° to 77° F (20° to 25° C).

• Bisphosphonates can interfere with bone-imaging agents.

PATIENT TEACHING

• Explain that risedronate is used to replace bone lost as a result of certain disease processes.

• Caution patient about the importance of adhering to special dosing instructions.

• Tell patient to take drug at least 30 minutes before the first food or drink of the day other than water. Urge patient to take the drug with a full glass of water (6 to 8 ounces) while sitting or standing. Warn against lying down for 30 minutes after taking risedronate.

• Advise patient not to chew or suck the tablet because doing so could cause mouth irritation.

• Advise patient to contact prescriber immediately if he develops symptoms of esophageal disease (such as difficulty or pain when swallowing, retrosternal pain, or severe heartburn).

• Advise patient to take calcium and vitamin D if dietary intake is inadequate, but to take them at a different time than risedronate.

• Advise patient to stop smoking and drinking alcohol, as appropriate. Also, advise patient to perform weight-bearing exercise.

• Tell patient to store drug in a cool, dry place, at room temperature, and away from children.

• Urge patient to read the Patient Information Guide before starting therapy.

sevelamer hydrochloride
Renagel

Pregnancy risk category C

AVAILABLE FORMS
Capsules: 403 mg
Tablets (film-coated): 400 mg, 800 mg

INDICATIONS & DOSAGES
➤ **Reduction of phosphorus in patients with end-stage renal disease—**
Adults: Initially, 2 to 4 capsules P.O. t.i.d. with meals, depending on severity of hyperphosphatemia. Gradually adjust dosage based on phosphorus level with goal of lowering phosphorus to 6 mg/dl or less. If phosphorus level is 9 mg/dl or more, 4 capsules P.O. t.i.d. with meals; if phosphorus level is between 7.5 and 9 mg/dl, 3 capsules P.O. t.i.d. with meals; if phosphorus level is between 6 and 7.5 mg/dl, 2 capsules P.O. t.i.d. with meals.
Adults not taking a phosphate binder: Initially, 800 to 1,600 mg (one to two 800-mg tablets, two to four 400-mg tablets, or two to four capsules) with each meal, based on phosphorus level. If phosphorus level is greater than 6 and less than 7.5 mg/dl, start with one 800-mg tablet t.i.d., with meals, or two 400-mg tablets or capsules (800 mg) t.i.d., with meals. If

phosphorus level is greater than or equal to 7.5 or less than 9 mg/dl, start with two 800-mg tablets (1,600 mg) t.i.d., with meals, or three 400-mg tablets or capsule (1,200 mg) t.i.d., with meals. If phosphorus is greater than or equal to 9 mg/dl, start with two 800-mg tablets (1,600 mg) t.i.d., with meals, or four 400-mg tablets or capsules (1,600 mg) t.i.d., with meals.
Adults switching from calcium acetate: If taking one 667-mg calcium acetate tablet per meal, start with one 800-mg tablet sevelamer per meal or two 400-mg tablets or capsules sevelamer per meal. If taking two 667-mg calcium acetate tablets per meal, start with two 800-mg tablets of sevelamer per meal or three 400-mg tablets or capsules sevelamer per meal. If taking three 667-mg calcium acetate tablets per meal, start with three 800-mg tablets sevelamer per meal or five 400-mg tablets or capsules sevelamer per meal.
Adjust-a-dose: If phosphorus level is greater than 6 mg/dl, increase 1 tablet or capsule sevelamer per meal at 2-week intervals. If phosphorus level is 3.5 to 6 mg/dl, maintain current sevelamer dose. If phosphorus level is less than 3.5 mg/dl, give 1 tablet or capsule sevelamer per meal.

ACTION
A phosphate binder that inhibits intestinal phosphate absorption and decreases phosphorus levels.

Route	Onset	Peak	Duration
P.O.	Unknown	Unknown	Unknown

ADVERSE REACTIONS
CNS: *headache, pain.*
CV: hypertension, *hypotension, **thrombosis.***
GI: *vomiting,* nausea, constipation, *diarrhea,* flatulence, *dyspepsia.*
Respiratory: increased cough.
Other: *infection.*

INTERACTIONS
None significant.

EFFECTS ON LAB TEST RESULTS
None reported.

CONTRAINDICATIONS
Contraindicated in patients hypersensitive to drug or its components and in those with hypophosphatemia or bowel obstruction.

NURSING CONSIDERATIONS
• Use cautiously in patients with dysphagia, swallowing disorders, severe GI motility disorders, or major GI tract surgery.
• Monitor calcium, bicarbonate, and chloride levels.
• Watch for symptoms of thrombosis (numbness or tingling of limbs, chest pain, shortness of breath), and notify prescriber if they occur.
• Although no known drug interactions have been studied, drug may bind to other drugs and decrease their bioavailability. Give other drugs 1 hour before or 3 hours after sevelamer. Take special precautions when antiarrhythmics or anticonvulsants are taken with sevelamer.
• Don't crush or break capsules, and give only with meals.

PATIENT TEACHING
• Instruct patient to take with meals and adhere to prescribed diet.
• Inform patient that tablets and capsules must be taken whole because contents expand in water; caution him not to open or chew capsules.
• Tell patient to take other drugs as directed, but they must be taken either 1 hour before or 3 hours after sevelamer.
• Inform patient about common adverse reactions and instruct him to report them immediately. Teach patient signs and symptoms of thrombosis (numbness, tingling limbs, chest pain, changes in level of consciousness).

---

sildenafil citrate
Viagra

Pregnancy risk category B

AVAILABLE FORMS
Tablets: 25 mg, 50 mg, 100 mg

INDICATIONS & DOSAGES
➤ **Erectile dysfunction—**
Adults younger than age 65: 50 mg P.O., p.r.n., about 1 hour before sexual activity.

Dosage range is 25 to 100 mg based on effectiveness and toleration. Maximum is one dose daily.

Elderly patients (age 65 and older):
25 mg P.O., p.r.n., about 1 hour before sexual activity. Dosage may be adjusted based on patient response. Maximum is one dose daily.

Adjust-a-dose: For adults with hepatic or severe renal impairment, 25 mg P.O. about 1 hour before sexual activity. Dosage may be adjusted based on patient response. Maximum is one dose daily.

ACTION
Has no direct relaxant effect on isolated human corpus cavernosum, but increases effect of nitric oxide by inhibiting phosphodiesterase type 5 (PDE_5), which is responsible for degradation of cyclic guanosine monophosphate (cGMP) in the corpus cavernosum. When sexual stimulation causes local release of nitric oxide, inhibition of PDE_5 by sildenafil causes increased levels of cGMP in the corpus cavernosum, resulting in smooth-muscle relaxation and inflow of blood to the corpus cavernosum.

Route	Onset	Peak	Duration
P.O.	Unknown	0.5-2 hr	4 hr

ADVERSE REACTIONS
CNS: anxiety, *headache,* dizziness, *seizures,* somnolence, vertigo.
CV: *MI, sudden cardiac death, ventricular arrhythmias, cerebrovascular hemorrhage, transient ischemic attack,* hypertension, flushing.
EENT: diplopia, temporary vision loss, decreased vision, ocular redness or bloodshot appearance, increased intraocular pressure, retinal vascular disease, retinal bleeding, vitreous detachment or traction, paramacular edema, photophobia, color-tinged vision, blurred vision, ocular burning, swelling, pressure, nasal congestion.
GI: *dyspepsia,* diarrhea.
GU: hematuria, prolonged erection, priapism, urinary tract infection.
Musculoskeletal: arthralgia, back pain.
Respiratory: respiratory tract infection.
Skin: rash.
Other: flu syndrome.

INTERACTIONS
Drug-drug. *Beta blockers, loop and potassium-sparing diuretics:* Increased blood levels of major metabolite of sildenafil, N-desmethyl sildenafil. Clinical significance of these interactions isn't known. Monitor patient.
CYP3A4 inducers, rifampin: Reduced sildenafil plasma levels. Monitor effect.
Hepatic isoenzyme inhibitors (such as cimetidine, erythromycin, itraconazole, ketoconazole): May reduce clearance of sildenafil. Avoid using together.
Protease inhibitors, delavirdine: Increased sildenafil plasma concentrations may cause an increase in sildenafil-associated adverse events, including hypotension, visual changes, and priapism. The patient shouldn't exceed 25 mg of sildenafil in a 48-hour period.
Nitrates: Sildenafil increases hypotensive effects. Avoid using together.
Drug-food. *High-fat meal:* Reduced rate of absorption and decreased peak levels. Advise patient to separate administration time from meals.

EFFECTS ON LAB TEST RESULTS
None reported.

CONTRAINDICATIONS
Contraindicated in patients hypersensitive to drug or its components. Concomitant use of organic nitrates at any frequency and in any form is also contraindicated.

NURSING CONSIDERATIONS
• Use cautiously in patients age 65 and older; in patients with hepatic or severe renal impairment, retinitis pigmentosa, bleeding disorders, or active peptic ulcer disease; in those who have suffered an MI, CVA, or life-threatening arrhythmia within last 6 months; in those with history of cardiac failure, coronary artery disease, uncontrolled high or low blood pressure, or anatomic deformation of the penis (such as angulation, cavernosal fibrosis, or Peyronie's disease); and in those with conditions that may predispose them to priapism (such as sickle cell anemia, multiple myeloma, leukemia).
• **Alert:** Drug increases risk of cardiac events. Systemic vasodilatory properties of drug cause transient decreases in supine

---

Reactions may be *common,* uncommon, *life-threatening,* or **COMMON AND LIFE-THREATENING.**

blood pressure and cardiac output (about 2 hours after ingestion). With the potential cardiac risk of sexual activity, drug increases risk for patients with underlying CV disease.

● *Alert:* Serious CV events, including MI, sudden cardiac death, ventricular arrhythmias, cerebrovascular hemorrhage, transient ischemic attack, and hypertension have been reported in temporal association with drug use. Most, but not all, of these incidents involved CV risk factors. Many events occurred during or shortly after sexual activity; a few occurred shortly after drug use without sexual activity; and others occurred hours to days after drug use and sexual activity.

● There is no indication for use of drug in newborns, children, or women.

PATIENT TEACHING

● Advise patient that drug shouldn't be used with nitrates under any circumstances.

● Advise patient of potential cardiac risk of sexual activity, especially in presence of CV risk factors. Instruct patient to notify prescriber of such symptoms as angina pectoris, dizziness, or nausea on initiation of sexual activity and tell him to refrain from further activity.

● Warn patient that erections lasting longer than 4 hours and priapism (painful erections lasting longer than 6 hours) can occur and should be reported immediately. Penile tissue damage and permanent loss of potency may result if priapism isn't treated immediately.

● Inform patient that drug doesn't offer protection against sexually transmitted diseases; protective measures such as condoms should be used.

● Tell patient receiving HIV medications that there is an increased risk of sildenafil-associated adverse events including hypotension, visual changes, and priapism, and that he should promptly report any symptoms to his prescriber. Tell him not to exceed 25 mg of sildenafil in 48 hours.

● Instruct patient to take drug 30 minutes to 4 hours before sexual activity; maximum benefit can be expected less than 2 hours after ingestion.

● Advise patient that drug is most rapidly absorbed if taken on an empty stomach.

● Inform patient that impairment of color discrimination (blue, green) may occur and to avoid hazardous activities that rely on color discrimination.

● Instruct patient to notify prescriber of visual changes.

● Advise patient that drug is effective only in presence of sexual stimulation.

● Caution patient to take drug only as prescribed.

---

sulfasalazine (salazosulfapyridine, sulphasalazine)
Azulfidine, Azulfidine EN-tabs, PMS-Sulfasalazine E.C.†, Salazopyrin†‡, Salazopyrin EN-Tabs†‡

Pregnancy risk category B

AVAILABLE FORMS
Tablets: 500 mg with or without enteric coating

INDICATIONS & DOSAGES
➤ **Mild to moderate ulcerative colitis, adjunctive therapy in severe ulcerative colitis, Crohn's disease—**
Adults: Initially, 3 to 4 g P.O. daily in evenly divided doses; usual maintenance dose is 2 g P.O. daily in divided doses q 6 hours. Dosage may be started with 1 to 2 g, with gradual increase in dosage to minimize adverse effects.
Children older than age 2: Initially, 40 to 60 mg/kg P.O. daily, divided into three to six doses; then 30 mg/kg daily in four doses. Dosage may be started at lower dose if GI intolerance occurs.
➤ **Rheumatoid arthritis in patients who have responded inadequately to salicylates or NSAIDs—**
Adults: 2 g P.O. daily in evenly divided doses. Dosage may be started at 0.5 to 1 g daily to reduce possible GI intolerance.
✳ *NEW INDICATION:* **Polyarticular-course juvenile rheumatoid arthritis in patients who have responded inadequately to salicylates or other nonsteroidal anti-inflammatories—**
Children age 6 and older: 50 mg/kg P.O. daily in two divided doses. Maximum dose is 2 g daily. To reduce possible GI in-

---

tolerance, start with one-quarter to one-third of planned maintenance dose and increase weekly until reaching maintenance dose at 1 month.

ACTION
Unknown.

Route	Onset	Peak	Duration
P.O.	Unknown	3-12 hr	Unknown

ADVERSE REACTIONS
CNS: headache, depression, *seizures,* hallucinations.
GI: *nausea, vomiting, diarrhea,* abdominal pain, anorexia, stomatitis.
GU: *toxic nephrosis with oliguria and anuria,* crystalluria, hematuria, oligospermia, infertility.
Hematologic: *agranulocytosis,* aplastic anemia, megaloblastic anemia, ***thrombocytopenia, leukopenia,*** hemolytic anemia.
Hepatic: jaundice, ***hepatotoxicity.***
Skin: ***erythema multiforme, Stevens-Johnson syndrome,*** *generalized skin eruption,* epidermal necrolysis, exfoliative dermatitis, photosensitivity reaction, urticaria, pruritus.
Other: hypersensitivity reactions, *serum sickness, drug fever,* ***anaphylaxis.***

INTERACTIONS
Drug-drug. *Antibiotics:* May alter action of sulfasalazine by altering internal flora. Monitor patient closely.
Digoxin: May reduce absorption of digoxin. Monitor patient closely.
Folic acid: May decrease absorption. No intervention needed.
Iron: Decreased blood levels of sulfasalazine caused by iron chelation. Monitor patient closely.
Oral anticoagulants: Increased anticoagulant effect. Watch for bleeding.
Oral antidiabetics: Increased hypoglycemic effect. Monitor blood glucose levels.
Oral contraceptives: Decreased contraceptive effectiveness and increased risk of breakthrough bleeding. Suggest nonhormonal form of contraception.

EFFECTS ON LAB TEST RESULTS
• May increase AST and ALT levels.
• May decrease hemoglobin and granulocyte, platelet, and WBC counts.

CONTRAINDICATIONS
Contraindicated in patients hypersensitive to drug or its metabolites, in those with porphyria or intestinal and urinary obstruction, and in children younger than age 2.

NURSING CONSIDERATIONS
• Use cautiously and in reduced doses in patients with impaired hepatic or renal function, severe allergy, bronchial asthma, or G6PD deficiency.
• Although therapeutic response in rheumatoid arthritis has been noted as soon as 4 weeks after starting therapy, it may take 12 weeks of therapy before some patients show benefit.
• Drug colors alkaline urine orange-yellow.
• Give drug with food to decrease GI irritation.
• ***Alert:*** Discontinue drug immediately and notify prescriber if patient shows signs and symptoms of hypersensitivity.
• ***Alert:*** Don't confuse sulfasalazine with sulfisoxazole, salsalate, or sulfadiazine.

PATIENT TEACHING
• Instruct patient to take drug after food intake and to space doses evenly.
• Instruct patient to drink plenty of water.
• Warn patient to avoid ultraviolet light.
• Advise patient that drug may produce an orange-yellow discoloration of skin and urine and may cause contact lenses to turn yellow.
• Instruct patient to notify prescriber immediately if discoloration of skin or urine occurs.
• Advise patient to make sure fluid intake is adequate and to swallow tablets intact; do not crush or chew.

tacrolimus (FK506)
Prograf

Pregnancy risk category C

AVAILABLE FORMS
Capsules: 1 mg, 5 mg
Injection: 5 mg/ml

INDICATIONS AND DOSAGES
➤ **Prevention of liver organ rejection—**
Adults: Initially, 0.05 to 0.1 mg/kg daily as a continuous I.V. infusion given no sooner than 6 hours after transplantation. Maintain I.V. route only until patient can tolerate oral administration (usually within 2 to 3 days); then give 0.15 to 0.3 mg/kg P.O. daily in two divided doses q 12 hours, beginning 8 to 12 hours after stopping infusion. May use oral dosing originally, if tolerated. Give doses at lower end of range, if possible.
Children: 0.1 mg/kg I.V. daily or 0.3 mg/kg P.O. daily given no sooner than 6 hours after transplantation. Maintain I.V. route only until patient can tolerate oral administration (usually within 2 to 3 days); then give 0.3 mg/kg P.O. daily in two divided doses q 12 hours, beginning 8 to 12 hours after stopping infusion.

I.V. ADMINISTRATION
● Because of risk of anaphylaxis, reserve injection for patients unable to take capsules.
● Dilute I.V. form with normal saline solution injection or D₅W injection to a level between 0.004 and 0.02 mg/ml before use.
● Store diluted infusion solution in glass or polyethylene container and discard after 24 hours. Don't store in polyvinyl chloride container because of decreased stability and potential for extraction of phthalates.
● Continuously observe patient receiving drug I.V. for at least 30 minutes after start of infusion and frequently thereafter. Stop infusion if signs or symptoms of anaphylaxis occur. Have an aqueous solution of epinephrine 1:1,000 and a source of oxygen available at patient's bedside.

ACTION
Exact mechanism unknown. Inhibits T-lymphocyte activation. Drug may bind to an intracellular protein, FKBP-12. A complex of tacrolimus-FKBP-12, calcium, calmodulin, and calcineurin then forms, inhibiting the phosphatase activity of calcineurin. This effect may prevent the generation of nuclear factor of activated T cells, a nuclear component thought to initiate gene transcription for the formation of lymphocyte activation and, therefore, to cause immunosuppression.

Route	Onset	Peak	Duration
I.V.	Rapid	1-2 hr	Unknown
P.O.	Unknown	1⅓-3½ hr	Unknown

ADVERSE REACTIONS
CNS: *headache, tremor, insomnia, paresthesia, asthenia.*
CV: *hypertension, peripheral edema.*
GI: *diarrhea, nausea, constipation, anorexia, vomiting, abdominal pain.*
GU: *urinary tract infection, oliguria.*
Hematologic: *anemia, leukocytosis,* THROMBOCYTOPENIA.
Metabolic: *hyperkalemia, hypokalemia, hyperglycemia, hypomagnesemia.*
Musculoskeletal: *back pain.*
Respiratory: *pleural effusion, atelectasis, dyspnea.*
Skin: *pruritus, rash.*
Other: *pain, fever, ascites,* **anaphylaxis.**

INTERACTIONS
Drug-drug. *Antifungals, bromocriptine, calcium channel blockers, cimetidine, clarithromycin, danazol, diltiazem, erythromycin, methylprednisolone, metoclopramide:* May interfere with tacrolimus metabolism. Reduce tacrolimus dosage if needed.
Carbamazepine, phenobarbital, phenytoin, rifamycins: Decreased tacrolimus levels. Increase tacrolimus dosage.
Immunosuppressants (except adrenal corticosteroids): Increased susceptibility to infection. Avoid using together.
Live-virus vaccines: Active infection. Avoid using together.
Nephrotoxic drugs (aminoglycosides, amphotericin B, cisplatin, cyclosporine): Increased risk of nephrotoxicity. Avoid use of tacrolimus and cyclosporine; stop one drug at least 24 hours before starting other. With elevated tacrolimus or cyclosporine levels, further dosing with other drug is usually delayed.
Drug-food. *Any food:* Inhibited drug absorption. Advise patient to take drug on empty stomach.
Grapefruit juice: Increased blood levels of drug in liver transplant patients. Advise these patients to avoid grapefruit juice during therapy.

---

*Liquid contains alcohol.   **May contain tartrazine.   †Canada   ‡Australia   §U.K.   ◇OTC

EFFECTS ON LAB TEST RESULTS
• May increase glucose, creatinine, and BUN levels. May decrease magnesium levels. May increase or decrease potassium levels.
• May increase WBC count and liver function test values. May decrease hemoglobin and platelet count.

CONTRAINDICATIONS
Contraindicated in patients hypersensitive to drug. I.V. form is contraindicated in those hypersensitive to castor oil derivatives.

NURSING CONSIDERATIONS
• Use cautiously in patients with impaired renal or hepatic function.
• Give adult patients doses at lower end of dosing range. Adjust dosage based on assessment of rejection and tolerance. Lower doses may be sufficient as maintenance therapy. Tacrolimus should be used with adrenal corticosteroids in early posttransplant period.
• Drug is being investigated for use in kidney, bone marrow, cardiac, pancreas, pancreatic island cell, and small bowel transplantation. It also may be used to treat autoimmune disease and severe recalcitrant psoriasis.
• Tacrolimus therapy is usually delayed 48 hours or longer in patients with postoperative oliguria.
• Because of risk of hyperkalemia (mild to severe hyperkalemia has been noted in 10% to 44% of liver transplant recipients given tacrolimus), monitor potassium levels and don't use potassium-sparing diuretics.
• *Alert:* Patients receiving drug are at increased risk for developing lymphomas and other malignancies, particularly of skin. Risk appears to be related to intensity and duration of immunosuppression rather than to use of any specific drug.
• A lymphoproliferative disorder related to Epstein-Barr virus (EBV) may occur in immunosuppressed organ transplant recipients. Lymphoproliferative disorder occurs most often in young children who are at risk for primary EBV infection while immunosuppressed or who are switched to tacrolimus after long-term immunosuppressive therapy.

• Antihypertensive therapy may be needed to control blood pressure elevations linked to drug use. Likewise, therapy may be needed to control glucose elevations linked to drug use.
• Black renal transplant patients may need higher doses to maintain comparable whole-blood trough drug levels.
• Closely monitor patient with impaired renal function; dosage may need to be reduced. In patients with persistent elevations of creatinine level who are unresponsive to dosage adjustments, consider changing to another immunosuppressive therapy.
• Closely monitor patient experiencing posttransplant hepatic impairment because of increased risk of renal insufficiency related to high whole-blood levels of tacrolimus. Dosage adjustments may be needed.
• Drug appears in breast milk. Avoid use in breast-feeding women.
• Children without renal or hepatic dysfunction have needed and tolerated higher doses than adults to achieve similar blood levels. Children should receive high end of recommended adult I.V. and oral dosing ranges (0.1 mg/kg I.V. daily and 0.3 mg/kg P.O. daily). Dosage adjustments may be needed.

PATIENT TEACHING
• Tell patient to take capsules on empty stomach because food impairs drug absorption.
• Inform patient of need for repeated laboratory tests during therapy to watch for adverse reactions and monitor drug effectiveness.
• Advise woman of childbearing age to tell prescriber if she becomes pregnant or plans to become pregnant.

☀ *NEW DRUG*

---

tacrolimus (topical)
Protopic

Pregnancy risk category C

AVAILABLE FORMS
Ointment: 0.03%, 0.1%

INDICATION & DOSAGES
➤ **Moderate to severe atopic dermatitis in patients unresponsive to other thera-**

Reactions may be *common*, uncommon, *life-threatening*, or COMMON AND LIFE-THREATENING.

pies or unable to use other therapies because of potential risks—
Adults: Thin layer of 0.03% or 0.1% strength applied to affected areas twice daily and rubbed in completely. Continued for 1 week after affected area clears.
Children age 2 and older: Thin layer of 0.03% strength applied to affected areas twice daily and rubbed in completely. Continue for 1 week after affected area clears.

ACTION
Unknown. Believed to act as an immune system modulator in the skin by inhibiting T-lymphocyte activation, which causes immunosuppression. Drug also inhibits the release of mediators from mast cells and basophils in skin.

Route	Onset	Peak	Duration
Topical	Unknown	Unknown	Unknown

ADVERSE REACTIONS
CNS: *headache,* hyperesthesia, asthenia, insomnia.
CV: peripheral edema.
EENT: *otitis media, pharyngitis,* rhinitis, sinusitis, conjunctivitis.
GI: diarrhea, vomiting, nausea, abdominal pain, gastroenteritis, dyspepsia.
GU: dysmenorrhea.
Musculoskeletal: back pain, myalgia.
Respiratory: *increased cough, asthma,* pneumonia, bronchitis.
Skin: *skin burning, pruritis, skin erythema, skin infection, herpes simplex,* eczema herpeticum, pustular rash, *folliculitis,* urticaria, maculopapular rash, rash, fungal dermatitis, acne, sunburn, tingling, benign skin neoplasm, skin disorder, vesiculobullous rash, dry skin, varicella zoster, herpes zoster, eczema, exfoliative dermatitis, contact dermatitis.
Other: *flulike symptoms, accidental injury, infection, lack of drug effect,* face edema, alcohol intolerance, periodontal abscess, cyst, *allergic reaction, fever,* pain, lymphadenopathy.

INTERACTIONS
Drug-drug. *Calcium channel blockers, cimetidine, CYP3A4 inhibitors (erythromycin, itraconazole, ketoconazole, flu-*

conazole): May interfere with effects of tacrolimus. Use together cautiously.
Drug-lifestyle. *Sun exposure:* Risk of phototoxicity. Advise patient to avoid excessive sunlight or artificial ultraviolet light exposure.

EFFECTS ON LAB TEST RESULTS
None reported.

CONTRAINDICATIONS
Contraindicated in patients hypersensitive to tacrolimus. Don't use in patients with Netherton's syndrome or generalized erythroderma.

NURSING CONSIDERATIONS
● Drug is used only for short-term or intermittent long-term therapy.
● In patients with clinically infected atopic dermatitis, clear infections at treatment site before using drug.
● Don't use occlusive dressings over drug application.
● Use of this drug may increase the risk of varicella zoster, herpes simplex virus, and eczema herpeticum.
● Evaluate all cases of lymphadenopathy to determine its etiology. If a clear etiology is unknown or acute mononucleosis is diagnosed, consider stopping drug.
● Monitor all cases of lymphadenopathy until resolution.
● Local adverse effects are most common during the first few days of treatment.
● Use only the 0.03% ointment on children ages 2 to 15.

PATIENT TEACHING
● Tell patient to wash hands before and after applying drug and to avoid applying drug to wet skin.
● Urge patient not to use bandages or other occlusive dressings.
● Tell patient not to bathe, shower, or swim immediately after application because doing so could wash the ointment off.
● Advise patient to avoid or minimize exposure to natural or artificial sunlight.
● Caution patient not to use drug for any disorder other than that for which it was prescribed.
● Encourage patient to report adverse reactions.

• Tell patient to store the ointment at room temperature.

---

tamsulosin hydrochloride
Flomax

Pregnancy risk category B

AVAILABLE FORMS
Capsules: 0.4 mg

INDICATIONS & DOSAGES
➤ **BPH—**
Adults: 0.4 mg P.O. once daily, given 30 minutes after same meal each day. If no response after 2 to 4 weeks, dose may be increased to 0.8 mg P.O. once daily.

ACTION
Selectively blocks alpha receptors in the prostate, leading to relaxation of smooth muscles in the bladder neck and prostate, improving urine flow and reduction in symptoms of BPH.

Route	Onset	Peak	Duration
P.O.	Unknown	4-5 hr	9-15 hr

ADVERSE REACTIONS
CNS: asthenia, *dizziness, headache,* insomnia, somnolence, syncope, vertigo.
CV: chest pain, orthostatic hypotension.
EENT: amblyopia, pharyngitis, *rhinitis,* sinusitis.
GI: diarrhea, nausea.
GU: abnormal ejaculation.
Musculoskeletal: back pain.
Respiratory: increased cough.
Other: decreased libido, *infection,* tooth disorder.

INTERACTIONS
Drug-drug. *Alpha-adrenergic blockers:* May interact with tamsulosin. Avoid using together.
Cimetidine: Decreased clearance of tamsulosin. Use together cautiously.

EFFECTS ON LAB TEST RESULTS
None reported.

CONTRAINDICATIONS
Contraindicated in patients hypersensitive to drug or its components.

NURSING CONSIDERATIONS
• Monitor patient for decreases in blood pressure.
• Symptoms of BPH and carcinoma of the prostate are similar; rule out carcinoma before starting therapy.
• If treatment is interrupted for several days or more, restart therapy at 1 capsule daily.
• *Alert:* Don't confuse Flomax with Fosamax or Volmax.

PATIENT TEACHING
• Instruct patient not to crush, chew, or open capsules.
• Tell patient to rise slowly from chair or bed during initiation of therapy and to avoid situations in which injury could occur as a result of syncope. Advise him that drug may cause sudden drop in blood pressure, especially after first dose or when changing doses.
• Instruct patient not to drive or perform hazardous tasks for 12 hours following initial dose or changes in dose until response can be monitored.
• Tell patient to take drug about 30 minutes after same meal each day.

---

thalidomide
Thalomid

Pregnancy risk category X

AVAILABLE FORMS
Capsules: 50 mg

INDICATIONS & DOSAGES
➤ **Immediate treatment of cutaneous effects of moderate to severe erythema nodosum leprosum (ENL)—**
Adults: 100 to 300 mg P.O. once daily with water, preferably at h.s. and at least 1 hour after the evening meal.
   Note: If patient weighs less than 50 kg (111 lb), start dosing at lower end of range.
➤ **Prevention and suppression of cutaneous effects of ENL recurrence—**
Adults: Up to 400 mg P.O. daily h.s. or in divided doses, with water, at least 1 hour after meals.

Reactions may be *common*, uncommon, *life-threatening*, or COMMON AND LIFE-THREATENING.

ACTION

Exact mechanism unknown. An immuno-modulatory drug.

Route	Onset	Peak	Duration
P.O.	Unknown	3-6 hr	Unknown

ADVERSE REACTIONS

CNS: *asthenia, drowsiness, somnolence, dizziness,* peripheral neuropathy, *headache,* agitation, insomnia, malaise, nervousness, *paresthesia,* tremor, vertigo.
CV: orthostatic hypotension, **bradycardia,** peripheral edema.
EENT: pharyngitis, sinusitis.
GI: dry mouth, oral candidiasis, abdominal pain, anorexia, constipation, *diarrhea,* flatulence, *nausea.*
GU: albuminuria, *hematuria,* impotence.
Hematologic: neutropenia, increased HIV viral load, anemia, *lymphadenopathy,* LEUKOPENIA.
Musculoskeletal: back pain, neck pain or rigidity.
Skin: acne, fungal dermatitis, nail disorder, pruritus, *rash, maculopapular rash, sweating,* photosensitivity reaction.
Other: human teratogenicity, hypersensitivity reactions, facial edema, fever, chills, accidental injury, infection, pain.

INTERACTIONS

Drug-drug. *Barbiturates, chlorpromazine, reserpine:* Increased sedative activity. Use cautiously together.
Drugs linked to peripheral neuropathy: Increased risk of peripheral neuropathy. Use cautiously together.
Drugs with the potential to reduce efficacy of hormonal contraception (carbamazepine, griseofulvin, HIV-protease inhibitors, phenytoin, rifabutin, rifampin): May cause thalidomide-induced teratogenicity if pregnancy occurs. Patient must be advised to use two other highly effective methods of contraception.
Drug-food. *Any food:* Decreased absorption of drug. Advise patient to take 1 hour after meals.
Drug-lifestyle. *Alcohol use:* Increased sedation. Discourage use together.

EFFECTS ON LAB TEST RESULTS

● May increase AST, ALT, LDH, and lipid levels.

● May decrease hemoglobin and neutrophil and WBC counts.

CONTRAINDICATIONS

Contraindicated in patients hypersensitive to drug or its components; in pregnant women; and in those capable of becoming pregnant except when alternative therapies are inappropriate and patient meets all conditions listed in the System for Thalidomide Education and Prescribing Safety (S.T.E.P.S.) program.

NURSING CONSIDERATIONS

● **Alert:** Give drug only in compliance with all terms outlined in the S.T.E.P.S. program; drug may be prescribed and dispensed only by prescribers and pharmacists registered with the S.T.E.P.S. program.
● All sexually mature patients (men and women) capable of reproduction must meet rigid S.T.E.P.S. program requirements, including ability to understand and carry out instructions, ability and willingness to comply with mandatory contraceptive measures (use of at least two highly effective means of contraception), and written acknowledgment of understanding of all warnings concerning hazards of fetal exposure to drug and risk of contraception failure.
● Sexually mature women who haven't undergone a hysterectomy or who haven't been postmenopausal for at least 24 consecutive months (that is, who have had menses at some time in preceding 24 consecutive months) are considered to be women of childbearing potential even with history of infertility.
● Perform mandatory pregnancy test within 24 hours before starting drug therapy in women of childbearing potential, then weekly during first month of therapy, then monthly for women with regular menstrual cycles. If menstrual cycles are irregular, pregnancy testing continues every 2 weeks during therapy. Retesting is performed if menstrual changes occur, including missed menses.
● Immediately report suspected fetal exposure to FDA via Medwatch, at 1-800-FDA-1088, and to manufacturer.
● Corticosteroids may be given together in patients with moderate to severe neuritis

linked with severe ENL reaction. Corticosteroids can be tapered and discontinued when neuritis improves.

• Patient with history of requiring prolonged treatment to prevent recurrence of cutaneous ENL or who experiences flare during tapering, should use minimum effective dose. Tapering should be attempted every 3 to 6 months at dose reduction rate of 50 mg every 2 to 4 weeks.

• Perform WBC count and differential before initiating therapy and periodically thereafter. Patients with an absolute neutrophil count falling below 750/mm³ during treatment should be reevaluated.

• Monitor patient for signs and symptoms of neuropathy at least once monthly during first 3 months of therapy, then periodically. Notify prescriber immediately if such symptoms as numbness, tingling, or pain in hands or feet occur.

PATIENT TEACHING

• Warn patient of dangers of fetal exposure to any amount of thalidomide. Make sure patient understands and follows the S.T.E.P.S. program.

• Stress that blood and sperm donations are prohibited during therapy.

• Explain that at least two highly reliable means of contraception must be used simultaneously and continuously from at least 1 month before initiation to 1 month after completion of therapy.

• Instruct patient to report signs or symptoms of pregnancy immediately without regard to chances of pregnancy.

• Inform woman of childbearing potential of mandatory pregnancy testing schedule.

• Inform patient that if pregnancy occurs, drug must be discontinued immediately.

• Caution patient that it isn't known whether drug is present in ejaculate of men receiving thalidomide, and that men receiving drug must always use a latex condom when engaging in sexual activity with women of childbearing potential.

• Advise patient to read package insert carefully.

• Instruct woman taking drugs (such as carbamazepine, griseofulvin, HIV-protease inhibitors, phenytoin, rifabutin, rifampin) that reduce the effect of hormonal contraceptive drugs to use two other effective means of contraception.

• Tell breast-feeding woman to discontinue breast-feeding during therapy.

• Stress importance of storing drug at room temperature, protected from light, and out of reach of children or others who may mistakenly take drug.

• Instruct patient to take drug only as prescribed.

• Caution patient against sharing drug with others, including those who also have a thalidomide prescription.

• Warn patient of potential for dizziness and orthostatic hypotension; instruct him to change position slowly when rising.

• Inform patient that drug frequently causes drowsiness and somnolence. Advise patient to avoid hazardous activities and alcohol or other drugs that might cause drowsiness.

• Tell patient to take drug at bedtime with glass of water, at least 1 hour after the evening meal.

• Teach patient signs and symptoms of peripheral neuropathy and to report their occurrence immediately.

• Tell patient to notify prescriber if hypersensitivity reactions, such as erythematous macular rash, fever, tachycardia, and hypotension, or other adverse reactions occur.

• Advise patient to use sunscreen because drug may cause photosensitivity reaction.

---

tolterodine tartrate
Detrol, Detrol LA

Pregnancy risk category C

AVAILABLE FORMS
Capsules (extended-release): 4 mg
Tablets: 1 mg, 2 mg

INDICATIONS & DOSAGES
➤ **Overactive bladder in patients with symptoms of urinary frequency, urgency, or urge incontinence—**
Adults: 2 mg P.O. b.i.d. Dose may be lowered to 1 mg P.O. b.i.d. based on patient response and tolerance.
Adjust-a-dose: For adults with significantly reduced hepatic function or in those who are currently taking drug that inhibits cytochrome P-450 3A4 isoenzyme system, 1 mg P.O. b.i.d.

ACTION
A competitive muscarinic receptor antagonist. Both urinary bladder contraction and salivation are mediated via cholinergic muscarinic receptors.

Route	Onset	Peak	Duration
P.O.	Unknown	1-2 hr	Unknown

ADVERSE REACTIONS
CNS: *dry mouth,* fatigue, paresthesia, vertigo, dizziness, *headache,* nervousness, somnolence.
CV: hypertension, chest pain.
EENT: abnormal vision, xerophthalmia, pharyngitis, rhinitis, sinusitis.
GI: abdominal pain, constipation, diarrhea, dyspepsia, flatulence, nausea, vomiting.
GU: dysuria, micturition frequency, urine retention, urinary tract infection.
Metabolic: weight gain.
Musculoskeletal: arthralgia, back pain.
Respiratory: bronchitis, coughing, upper respiratory tract infection.
Skin: pruritus, rash, erythema, dry skin.
Other: flu syndrome, falls, fungal infection, infection.

INTERACTIONS
Drug-drug. *Antifungal drugs (itraconazole, ketoconazole, miconazole), cytochrome P-450 3A4 inhibitors (such as macrolide antibiotics [clarithromycin, erythromycin]):* Effects haven't been studied. However, tolterodine doses above 1 mg b.i.d. shouldn't be given together.
Fluoxetine: Increased tolterodine levels. Avoid using together.

EFFECTS ON LAB TEST RESULTS
None reported.

CONTRAINDICATIONS
Contraindicated in patients hypersensitive to drug or its components and in those with uncontrolled narrow-angle glaucoma or urine or gastric retention.

NURSING CONSIDERATIONS
● Use with caution in patients with significant bladder outflow obstruction, GI obstructive disorders (such as pyloric stenosis), controlled narrow-angle glaucoma, and hepatic or renal impairment.

● Assess baseline bladder function and monitor therapeutic effects.
● Safety and effectiveness of drug in children haven't been established.

PATIENT TEACHING
● Tell patient that sugarless gum, hard candy, or saliva substitute may help relieve dry mouth.
● Advise patient to avoid driving or other potentially hazardous activities until visual effects of drug are known.
● Advise breast-feeding woman to discontinue breast-feeding during therapy.
● Instruct patient to immediately report signs of infection, urine retention, or GI problems.

---

tretinoin (retinoic acid, vitamin A acid)
Avita, Renova, Retin-A, StieVA-A†

Pregnancy risk category C

AVAILABLE FORMS
Cream: 0.02%, 0.025%, 0.05%, 0.1%
Gel: 0.01%, 0.025%
Solution: 0.05%

INDICATIONS & DOSAGES
➤ **Acne vulgaris—**
Adults and children: Clean affected area and lightly apply once daily h.s.
➤ **Adjunctive for use in the mitigation of fine facial wrinkles in patients who use comprehensive skin care and sunlight avoidance programs—**
Adults: Apply a small, pearl-sized amount (¼ inch or 5 mm in diameter) to cover affected area lightly, once daily in the evening.

ADVERSE REACTIONS
Skin: *feeling of warmth, slight stinging, local erythema, peeling,* chapping, swelling, blistering, crusting, temporary hyperpigmentation or hypopigmentation.

ACTION
Inhibits comedones by increasing epidermal cell mitosis and turnover.

Route	Onset	Peak	Duration
Topical	Unknown	Unknown	Unknown

INTERACTIONS

Drug-drug. *Topical drugs containing benzoyl peroxide, resorcinol, salicylic acid, or sulfur:* Increased risk of skin irritation. Avoid using together.

Topical minoxidil or photosensitizing drugs: Increased risk of skin irritation. Avoid using together.

Drug-lifestyle. *Abrasive cleansers, medicated cosmetics, skin preparations containing alcohol:* Increased risk of skin irritation. Discourage use together.

Sun exposure: Increased photosensitivity reaction. Advise patient to avoid excessive sunlight exposure.

EFFECTS ON LAB TEST RESULTS

None reported.

CONTRAINDICATIONS

Contraindicated in patients hypersensitive to drug or its components. Contraindicated in patients with sunburn.

NURSING CONSIDERATIONS

• Use cautiously in patients with eczema.
• Initially, drug may be applied every 2 to 3 days using a lower concentration to reduce irritation.
• Relapses generally occur within 3 to 6 weeks after therapy is stopped.
• **Alert:** Don't confuse tretinoin with trientine.

PATIENT TEACHING

• Instruct patient to clean area thoroughly before application and to avoid getting drug in eyes, mouth, or mucous membranes.
• Tell patient to wash face with mild soap no more than b.i.d. or t.i.d. Warn patient against using strong or medicated cosmetics, soaps, or other skin cleansers. Also advise him to avoid topical products containing alcohol, astringents, spices, and lime because they may interfere with drug's actions.
• Tell patient using drug for palliation of fine wrinkles to wait 20 minutes after washing face to apply drug, and to avoid washing face or applying another skin product or cosmetic for 1 hour after application.
• Tell patient that normal use of cosmetics is allowed.

• Advise patient not to discontinue drug if transient exacerbation of inflammatory lesions occurs. If severe local irritation develops, advise patient to discontinue drug temporarily and notify prescriber. Dosage will be readjusted when application is resumed. Some redness and scaling are normal reactions.
• Warn patient that he may experience increased sensitivity to wind or cold temperatures.
• Instruct patient to minimize exposure to sunlight or ultraviolet rays during treatment. If he becomes sunburned, he should delay therapy until sunburn subsides. Tell patient who can't avoid exposure to sunlight to use SPF-15 sunblock and to wear protective clothing.
• Warn patient that he may have a temporary increase in lesions, which will improve in 2 to 3 weeks.

Herbal medicines

Herb names	Reported uses	Nursing considerations	Patient teaching
ALOE Aloe Gel, Aloe Latex, Aloe Vera, Cape	Aloe latex is used orally as a cathartic. It's used to treat constipation; to provide evacuation relief for patient with anal fissures, hemorrhoids, or recent anorectal surgery; and to prepare a patient for diagnostic testing of the GI tract. Aloe gel is used to treat minor burns and skin irritation and to aid in wound healing. It may also be effective as an antibacterial.	• Find out why patient is using the herb. • Aloe's laxative effects are apparent within 10 hours of taking it. • Monitor patient for signs of dehydration. Geriatric patients are particularly at risk. • Monitor electrolyte levels, especially potassium, after long-term use. • If patient is using aloe topically, monitor wound for healing.	• Advise patient to consult his health care provider before using an herbal preparation because a treatment with proven efficacy may be available. • Advise patient that when he fills a prescription, he should tell pharmacist of any herb or dietary supplement he's taking. • Caution patient that if he delays seeking medical diagnosis and treatment, his condition could worsen. • If patient is taking digoxin or another drug to control his heart rate, a diuretic, or a corticosteroid, warn him not to take aloe without consulting his health care provider. • Advise patient to reduce dose if cramping occurs after a single dose and not to take aloe for longer than 1 to 2 weeks at a time without consulting his health care provider. • Advise patient to notify his health care provider immediately if he experiences feelings of dehydration, weakness, or confusion, especially if he has been using aloe for a prolonged period.
ANGELICA Nature's Answer, Angelica Root Liquid	Angelica seed is used as a diuretic and diaphoretic. It's also used to treat conditions of the kidneys and the urinary, GI, and respiratory tracts as well as rheumatic and neuralgic symptoms.	• Find out why patient is using the herb. • Monitor patient for persistent diarrhea, which may be a sign of something more serious. • Monitor patient for dermatologic reactions. • Photodermatosis is possible after contact with the plant juice or plant extract.	• Advise patient to consult his health care provider before using an herbal preparation because a treatment with proven efficacy may be available. • Advise patient that when he fills a prescription, he should tell pharmacist of any herb or dietary supplement he's taking. • Caution patient not to delay seeking medical treatment for symptoms that may be related to a serious medical condition. • Advise patient not to take angelica if pregnant or if taking a gastric acid blocker or anticoagulant. • Advise patient to notify his health care provider if he develops a rash.
BITTER MELON BitterMelon, Bitter Melon Juice, Bitter Melon Power,	Used to treat diabetes symptoms. May help treat GI disorders.	• Find out why patient is using the herb. • The juice of bitter melon has a bitter taste. • Bitter melon should be taken only in small doses, for no longer than 4 weeks.	• Advise patient to consult his health care provider before using an herbal preparation because a treatment with proven efficacy may be available. *(continued)*

Adapted from *Nursing Herbal Medicine Handbook*. Springhouse Corporation, Springhouse, Pa.

Herb names	Reported uses	Nursing considerations	Patient teaching
BITTER MELON *(continued)* Bitter Melon Tincture		• The hypoglycemic effects of bitter melon are dose related, so dosage should be adjusted gradually. • **ALERT:** Bitter melon seeds contain vicine, which may cause an acute condition characterized by headache, fever, abdominal pain, and coma.	• Advise patient that when he fills a prescription, he should tell pharmacist of any herb or dietary supplement he's taking.
CAPSICUM *Topical capsaicin products:* Capsin (0.025% or 0.075% lotion), Capzasin-P (0.025% cream), Dolorac (0.025% cream in emollient base), No Pain-HP (0.075% roll-on), Pain Doctor (0.025% cream with methylsalicylate and menthol), Pain-X (0.05% gel), R-Gel (0.025% gel), Zostrix (0.025% cream in emollient base), Zostrix-HP (0.075% cream in emollient base) *Oral capsaicin products:* Cayenne Pepper Capsules and Alcoholic Extract	The FDA has approved topical capsaicin for temporary relief of pain from rheumatoid arthritis, osteoarthritis, postherpetic neuralgia (shingles), and diabetic neuropathy. It's being tested for treatment of psoriasis, intractable pruritus, vitiligo, phantom limb pain, mastectomy pain, Guillain-Barré syndrome, neurogenic bladder, vulvar vestibulitis, apocrine chromhidrosis, and reflex sympathetic dystrophy. It's also used in personal defense sprays. Oral capsicum is used for various GI complaints, including dyspepsia, flatulence, ulcers, and stomach cramps. It's used to treat hypertension and improve circulation. It's also used in some weight-loss and metabolic-enhancement products.	• Find out why patient is using the herb. • Alcoholic extract may be unsuitable for children, alcoholic patients, patients with liver disease, and those taking disulfiram or metronidazole. • Topical product shouldn't be used on broken or irritated skin or covered with a tight bandage. • Adverse skin reactions to topically applied capsaicin are treated by washing the area thoroughly with soap and water. Soaking the area in vegetable oil after washing provides a slower onset but longer duration of relief than cold water. Vinegar water irrigation is moderately successful. Rubbing alcohol may also help. • EMLA, an emulsion of lidocaine and prilocaine, provides pain relief in about 1 hour to skin that has been severely irritated by capsaicin. • **ALERT:** Advise patient to avoid taking capsicum orally for longer than 2 days and then to avoid using again for 2 weeks.	• Advise patient to consult his health care provider before using an herbal preparation because a treatment with proven efficacy may be available. • Advise patient that when he fills a prescription, he should tell pharmacist of any herb or dietary supplement he's taking. • If patient is pregnant or breast-feeding or is planning pregnancy, advise her not to use this herb. • If patient is applying capsicum topically, inform him that it may take 1 to 2 weeks for him to experience maximum pain control. • If patient is using capsicum topically, instruct him to wash his hands before and immediately after applying it and to avoid contact with eyes. Advise contact lens wearer to wash his hands and to use gloves or an applicator if handling his lenses after applying capsicum. • If patient is using capsicum topically, advise him not to use topical capsicum on broken or irritated skin and instruct him not to tightly bandage any area to which he has applied it. • Inform patient not to delay treatment for an illness that doesn't resolve after taking capsicum. If he's applying it topically, advise him to promptly contact his health care provider if his condition worsens or if symptoms persist for 2 to 4 weeks. • Tell patient to store capsicum in a tightly sealed container, away from light.
CHAMOMILE Azulon, Chamomile Flowers, Chamomile	Used orally to treat diarrhea, anxiety, restlessness, stomatitis, hemorrhagic cysti-	• Find out why patient is using the herb. • **ALERT:** People sensitive to ragweed and chrysanthemums or other Compositae	• Advise patient to consult his health care provider before using an herbal preparation because a treatment with proven efficacy may be available.

Adapted from *Nursing Herbal Medicine Handbook*. Springhouse Corporation, Springhouse, Pa.

Herb names	Reported uses	Nursing considerations	Patient teaching
CHAMOMILE *(continued)* Tea, Kid Chamomile, Standardized Chamomile Extract, Wild Chamomile	tis, flatulence and motion sickness.　Used topically to stimulate skin metabolism, reduce inflammation, encourage the healing of wounds, and treat cutaneous burns. Also used for its antibacterial and antiviral effects. Teas are mainly used for sedation or relaxation.	family members (arnica, yarrow, feverfew, tansy, artemisia) may be more susceptible to contact allergies and anaphylaxis. Patients with hay fever or bronchial asthma caused by pollens are more susceptible to anaphylactic reactions.	● Advise patient that when he fills a prescription, he should tell pharmacist of any herb or dietary supplement he's taking. ● If patient is pregnant or is planning pregnancy, advise her not to use chamomile. ● If patient is taking an anticoagulant, advise him not to use chamomile because of possible enhanced anticoagulant effects. ● Advise patient that chamomile may enhance an allergic reaction or make existing symptoms worse in susceptible patients. ● Instruct parent not to give chamomile to any child before checking with a knowledgeable practitioner.
CRANBERRY Cran-Actin, Cranberry-Plus, Emergen-C Cranberry, Ultra Cranberry	Used to prevent urinary tract infections, particularly in women prone to recurrent infection. Also used to prevent kidney stones and to treat asthma, fever, and active urinary tract infection (UTI).	● Find out why patient is using the herb. ● Tinctures may contain up to 45% alcohol. ● Contrary to early investigations focusing on cranberry's ability to acidify the urine, its ability to prevent bacteria from adhering to the bladder wall seems to be more important in preventing UTIs. ● Only the unsweetened, unprocessed form of cranberry juice is effective in preventing bacteria from adhering to the bladder wall. ● Cranberry is safe for use in pregnant and breast-feeding patients. ● When consumed regularly, cranberry may be effective in reducing the frequency of bacteriuria with pyuria in women with recurrent UTIs.	● Advise patient to consult his health care provider before using an herbal preparation because a treatment with proven efficacy may be available. ● Advise patient that when he fills a prescription, he should tell pharmacist of any herb or dietary supplement he's taking. ● Advise patient that an appropriate antibiotic is usually needed to treat an active UTI. ● If patient is using cranberry to prevent a UTI, advise him to notify his health care provider if signs or symptoms of a UTI appear. ● If patient has diabetes, inform him that cranberry juice contains sugar but that sugar-free cranberry supplements and juices are available.
ECHINACEA Coneflower Extract, EchinaCare Liquid, Echinacea, Echinacea Angustifolia Herb, Echinacea Extract, Echinacea Fresh Freeze	Used to stimulate the immune system and treat acute and chronic upper respiratory tract infections and urinary tract infections. Used also to heal wounds, including abscesses, burns, eczema, and skin ulcers. Used as an	● Find out why patient is using the herb. ● Daily dose depends on the preparation and potency but shouldn't exceed 8 weeks. Consult specific manufacturer's instructions for parenteral administration, if applicable. ● Echinacea is considered supportive treatment for infection; it shouldn't be used	● Advise patient to consult his health care provider before using an herbal preparation because a treatment with proven efficacy may be available. ● Advise patient that when he fills a prescription, he should tell pharmacist of any herb or dietary supplement he's taking. ● Advise patient not to delay seeking appropriate medical evaluation for a prolonged illness. *(continued)*

Adapted from *Nursing Herbal Medicine Handbook*. Springhouse Corporation, Springhouse, Pa.

Herb names	Reported uses	Nursing considerations	Patient teaching
ECHINACEA (continued) Dried, Echinacea Glycerite, Echinacea Herbal Comfort, Echinacea Red Root Supreme, Echinacea Root Complex, Echinacea Root Extract, Echinacea Xtra, Echina Fresh, Echinagel, EchinaGuard Liquid, EchinaGuard Pro, Echinex, Enhanced Echinacea, Standardized Echinacea Extract	adjunct to a conventional antineoplastic and to provide prophylaxis against upper respiratory tract infections and the common cold.	in place of antibiotic therapy. • Some active components may be water-insoluble. • Echinacea is usally taken at the first sign of illness and continued for up to 14 days. Regular prophylactic use isn't recommended. • Herbalists recommend using liquid preparations because it's believed that echinacea functions in the mouth and should have direct contact with the lymph tissues at the back of the throat. • Some tinctures contain between 15% and 90% alcohol, which may be unsuitable for children and adolescents, alcoholics, and patients with hepatic disease.	• Advise patient that prolonged use may result in overstimulation of the immune system and possible immune suppression. Echinacea shouldn't be used longer than 14 days for supportive treatment of infection. • The herb should be stored away from direct light. • Warn patients to keep all herbal products away from children and pets.
EPHEDRA Available as combination products, including Chromemate, Escalation, Excel, Herbal Ecstasy, Herbal Fen-Phen, Herbalife, Metabolife, Power Trim, Up Your Gas	Used to treat respiratory tract diseases with mild bronchospasm. Allopathic practitioners have used it since the 1930s to treat asthma, but the herb has become less popular as more specific beta agonists have become available. Also used as a CV stimulant. Pseudoephedrine remains a common ingredient in many OTC cough and cold preparations. Ephedrine is used to treat various other conditions, including chills, coughs, colds, flu, fever, headaches, edema, and nasal congestion; it's	• Find out why patient is using the herb. • Compounds containing ephedra have been linked to several deaths and more than 800 adverse effects, many of which appear to be dose related. • Monitor patient's pulse and blood pressure. • Ephedra shouldn't be used for more than 7 consecutive days because of the risk of anaphylaxis and dependence. • Patients with eating disorders may abuse this herb. • ALERT: Pills containing ephedra have been combined with other stimulants like caffeine and sold as "natural" stimulants in weight loss products. Deaths from overstimulation have been reported. • ALERT: Dosages high enough to produce psychoactive or hallucinogenic effects are toxic to the heart and shouldn't be used.	• Advise patient to consult his health care provider before using an herbal preparation because a treatment with proven efficacy may be available. • Advise patient that when he fills a prescription, he should tell pharmacist of any herb or dietary supplement he's taking. • Advise patient not to use this herb in place of getting the proper medical evaluation for a prolonged illness. • Advise patient with thyroid disease, hypertension, CV disease, or diabetes to avoid using ephedra. • Recommend standard pharmaceutical formulations of ephedrine or pseudoephedrine for those with a valid need for these compounds because preparations may differ in ephedrine alkaloid content by 130%. • Advise patient not to use ephedra-containing products for longer than 7 consecutive days. • Advise patient not to use ephedra at dosages that are purported to produce psychoactive or hallucino-

Adapted from *Nursing Herbal Medicine Handbook*. Springhouse Corporation, Springhouse, Pa.

Herb names	Reported uses	Nursing considerations	Patient teaching
EPHEDRA *(continued)*	also used as an appetite suppressant. The alkaloid-free North American species is used to treat venereal disease.	• Signs and symptoms of toxic reaction include diaphoresis, dilated pupils, muscle spasms, fever, and cardiac and respiratory failure. • If overdose occurs, perform gastric lavage and administer activated charcoal. Treat spasms with diazepam, replace electrolytes with I.V. fluids, and prevent acidosis with sodium bicarbonate infusions.	genic effects because such dosages are toxic to the heart. • Advise patient to watch for adverse reactions, particularly chest pain, shortness of breath, palpitations, dizziness, and fainting. • Instruct patient to store ephedra away from direct light. • Warn patients to keep all herbal products away from children and pets.
FEVERFEW Feverfew, Feverfew Extract, Feverfew Extract Complex, Feverfew Leaf, Feverfew Leaf and Flower, Feverfew LF and FL-GBE, Feverfew Power, Fresh Freeze-Dried Feverfew, Migracare Feverfew Extract, Migracin, MigraSpray, MygraFew, Partenelle, Tanacet	Used most commonly to prevent or treat migraine headaches and to treat rheumatoid arthritis. Used to treat asthma, psoriasis, menstrual cramps, digestion problems, and intestinal parasites; to debride wounds; and to promote menstrual flow. Also used as a mouthwash after tooth extraction, a tranquilizer, and abortifacient, and an external antiseptic and insecticide.	• Find out why patient is using the herb. • If patient is taking an anticoagulant, monitor appropriate coagulation values, such as INR, PTT, and PT. Also, observe patient for abnormal bleeding. • Rash or contact dermatitis may indicate sensitivity to feverfew. Patient should discontinue use immediately. • Abruptly stopping the herb may cause "postfeverfew syndrome," involving tension headaches, insomnia, joint stiffness and pain, and lethargy.	• Advise patient to consult his health care provider before using an herbal preparation because a treatment with proven efficacy may be available. • Advise patient that when he fills a prescription, he should tell pharmacist of any herb or dietary supplement he's taking. • If patient is pregnant, planning to become pregnant, or breast-feeding, advise her not to use feverfew. • Educate patient about the potential risk of abnormal bleeding when combining herb with an anticoagulant, such as warfarin or heparin, or an antiplatelet, such as aspirin or another NSAID. • Caution patient that a rash or abnormal skin alteration may indicate an allergy to feverfew. Instruct patient to stop taking the herb if a rash appears.
FLAX Dakota Flax Gold, Fax Seed Oil, Flax Seed Whole	Used internally to treat diarrhea, constipation, diverticulitis, irritable bowel, colons damaged by laxative abuse, gastritis, enteritis, and bladder inflammation. Used externally to remove foreign objects from the eye. Also used as a poultice for skin inflammation.	• Find out why patient is using the herb. • When flax is used internally, it should be taken with more than 5 oz of liquid per tablespoon of flaxseed. • Cyanogenic glycosides may release cyanide; however, the body only metabolizes these to a certain extent. At therapeutic doses, flax doesn't elevate cyanide ion level. • Although flax may decrease a patient's cholesterol level or increase bleeding time, it isn't necessary to monitor cholesterol level or platelet aggregation.	• Advise patient to consult his health care provider before using an herbal preparation because a treatment with proven efficacy may be available. • Advise patient that when he fills a prescription, he should tell pharmacist of any herb or dietary supplement he's taking. • Warn patient not to treat chronic constipation or other GI disturbances or ophthalmic injury with flax before seeking appropriate medical evaluation because doing so may delay diagnosis of a potentially serious medical condition. • If patient is pregnant, plans to become pregnant, or is breast-feeding, advise her not to use flax. *(continued)*

Adapted from *Nursing Herbal Medicine Handbook*. Springhouse Corporation, Springhouse, Pa.

Herb names	Reported uses	Nursing considerations	Patient teaching
FLAX *(continued)*			• Instruct patient to drink plenty of water when taking flaxseed. • Instruct patient not to take any drug for at least 2 hours after taking flax.
GARLIC Garlicin, Garlic Powermax, Garlinase 4,000, Garli-Pure, Garlique, Garlitrin 4,000, Kwai, Kyolic Liquid, Wellness Garlicell	Used most commonly to decrease total cholesterol and triglyceride levels and increase HDL cholesterol level. Also used to help prevent atherosclerosis because of its effect on blood pressure and platelet aggregation. Used to decrease the risk of cancer, especially cancer of the GI tract. Used to decrease the risk of stroke and heart attack and to treat coughs, colds, fevers, and sore throats. Used orally and topically to fight infection through its antibacterial and antifungal effects.	• Find out why patient is using the herb. • Garlic isn't recommended for patients with diabetes, insomnia, pemphigus, organ transplants, or rheumatoid arthritis, or for post-surgical patients. • Consuming excessive amounts of raw garlic increases the risk of adverse reactions. • Monitor patient for signs and symptoms of bleeding. • Garlic may lower glucose level. If patient is taking an antihyperglycemic, watch for signs and symptoms of hypoglycemia and monitor his glucose level. • **ALERT:** Advise parents not to use garlic oil to treat inner ear infection in children.	• Advise patient to consult his health care provider before using an herbal preparation because a treatment with proven efficacy may be available. • Advise patient that when he fills a prescription, he should tell the pharmacist of any herb or dietary supplement he's taking. • Advise patient not to delay seeking appropriate medical evaluation because doing so may delay diagnosis of a potentially serious medical condition. • Advise patient to consume garlic in moderation, to minimize the risk of adverse reactions. • Discourage heavy use of garlic before surgery. • If patient is using garlic to lower his cholesterol levels, advise him to notify his health care provider and to have his cholesterol levels monitored. • Advise patient that using garlic with anticoagulants may increase the risk of bleeding. • If patient is using garlic as a topical antiseptic, avoid prolonged exposure to the skin because burns can occur.
GINGER Alcohol-Free Ginger Root, Caffeine Free Ginger Root, Ginger Aid Tea, Ginger Kid, GingerMax, Ginger Powder, Ginger Root, Quanterra Stomach Comfort, Travellers, Travel Sickness, Zintona	Used most commonly as an antiemetic in those with motion sickness, morning sickness, and generalized nausea. Used to treat colic, flatulence, and indigestion. Used to treat hypercholesterolemia, burns, ulcers, depression, impotence, and liver toxicity. Used as an anti-inflammatory for those with arthritis and as an antispasmodic. Also used for its anti-	• Find out why patient is using the herb. • Adverse reactions are uncommon. • Monitor patient for signs and symptoms of bleeding. If patient is taking an anticoagulant, monitor PTT, PT, and INR carefully. • Use in pregnant patients is questionable, although small amounts used in cooking are safe. It's unknown if ginger appears in breast milk. • Ginger may interfere with the intended therapeutic effect of conventional drugs. • If overdose occurs, monitor patient for arrhythmias and CNS depression.	• Advise patient to consult his health care provider before using an herbal preparation because a treatment with proven efficacy may be available. • Advise patient that when he fills a prescription, he should tell the pharmacist of any herb or dietary supplement he's taking. • If patient is pregnant, advise her to consult a knowledgeable practitioner before using ginger medicinally. • Educate patients to look for signs and symptoms of bleeding, such as nosebleeds or excessive bruising. • Warn patient to keep all herbal products away from children and pets.

Adapted from *Nursing Herbal Medicine Handbook*. Springhouse Corporation, Springhouse, Pa.

Herb names	Reported uses	Nursing considerations	Patient teaching
GINGER *(continued)*	tumorigenic activity in patients with cancer.		
GINKGO Bioginkgo, Gincosan, Ginkgo Go!, Ginkgo Liquid Extract Herb, Ginkgo Nut, Ginkgo Power, Ginkgo Capsules, Ginkgo, Quanterra Mental Sharpness	Primarily used to manage cerebral insufficiency, dementia, and circulatory disorders such as intermittent claudication. Also used to treat headaches, asthma, colitis, impotence, depression, altitude sickness, tinnitus, cochlear deafness, vertigo, premenstrual syndrome, macular degeneration, diabetic retinopathy, and allergies. Used as an adjunctive treatment for pancreatic cancer and schizophrenia. Also used in addition to physical therapy for Fontaine stage IIb peripheral arterial disease to decrease pain during ambulation with a minimum of 6 weeks of treatment. In Germany, standardized ginkgo extract must contain 22% to 27% ginkgo flavonoids and 5% to 7% terpenoids.	• Find out why the patient is using the herb. • Ginkgo extracts are considered standardized if they contain 24% ginkgo flavonoid glycosides and 6% terpene lactones. • Treatment should continue for at least 6 to 8 weeks, but therapy beyond 3 months isn't recommended. • **ALERT:** Seizures have been reported in children after ingestion of more than 50 seeds. • Patients must be monitored for possible adverse reaction such as GI problems, headaches, dizziness, allergic reactions, and serious bleeding. • Toxicity may cause atonia and adynamia.	• Advise patient to consult his health care provider before using an herbal preparation because a treatment with proven efficacy may be available. • Advise patient that when he fills a prescription, he should tell the pharmacist of any herb or dietary supplement he's taking. • If patient is taking the herb for motion sickness, advise him to begin taking it 1 to 2 days before taking the trip and to continue taking it for the duration of his trip. • Inform patient that the therapeutic and toxic components of ginkgo can vary significantly from product to product. Advise him to obtain his ginkgo from a reliable source. • Warn patient to keep all herbal products away from children and pets. • Advise patient to discontinue use at least 2 weeks before surgery.
GINSENG, ASIAN American Ginseng, American Ginseng Root, Centrum Ginseng, Chikusetsu Ginseng, Manchurian, Ginseng Natural, Ginseng Power Max	Used to manage fatigue and lack of concentration and to treat atherosclerosis, bleeding disorders, colitis, diabetes, depression, and cancer. Also used to help recover health and strength after sickness or weakness.	• Find out why patient is using the herb. • The German Commission E doesn't recommend using ginseng for longer than 3 months. • Ginseng is believed by some to strengthen the body and increase resistance to disease. • **ALERT:** Reports have circulated of a severe reaction known as the ginseng	• Advise patient to consult his health care provider before using an herbal preparation because a treatment with proven efficacy may be available. • Advise patient that when he fills a prescription, he should tell the pharmacist of any herb or dietary supplement he's taking. • Inform patient that the therapeutic and toxic components of ginseng can vary significantly from

(continued)

Herb names	Reported uses	Nursing considerations	Patient teaching
GINSENG, ASIAN *(continued)* 004X G-Sana, Ginseng Up, Gin Zip, Herbal Sure Chinese Red Ginseng, Herbal Sure Korean Ginseng, Himalayan Ginseng, Korean Ginseng, Korean Ginseng Root, Forean White Ginseng, Lynae Ginse-Cool, Manchurian Ginseng, Natural Ginseng, Power Herb Korean Ginseng, Premium Blend Korean Ginseng Extract, Sanchi Ginseng, The Ginseng Solution, Time Release Korean Ginseng Power, Zhuzishen		abuse syndrome in patients taking large doses—more than 3 g per day for up to 2 years. Patients experiencing this syndrome report a feeling of increased motor and cognitive activity combined with significant diarrhea, nervousness, insomnia, hypertension, edema, and skin eruptions.	product to product. Advise him to obtain his ginseng from a reliable source.
GREEN TEA Chinese Green Tea Bags, Green Tea, Green Tea Extract, Green Tea Power, Green Tea Power Caffeine Free, Standardized Green Tea Extract	Used to prevent cancer, hyperlipidemia, atherosclerosis, dental caries, and headaches, and to treat wounds, skin disorders, stomach disorders, and infectious diarrhea. Also used as a CNS stimulant, a mild diuretic, and antibacterial and, topically, as an astringent.	• Find out why patient is using the herb. • Dosage varies with the form of the herb. • Look for products standardized to 80% polyphenol and 55% epigallocatechin gallate. • Daily consumption should be limited to fewer than 5 cups, or the equivalent of 300 mg of caffeine, per day to avoid the adverse effects of caffeine. • Prolonged high caffeine intake may cause restlessness, irritability, insomnia, palpitations, vertigo, headache, and adverse GI effects. Monitor patient's intake. • The adverse GI effects of chlorogenic acid and tannin can be avoided if	• Advise patient to consult his health care provider before using an herbal preparation because a treatment with proven efficacy may be available. • Advise patient that when he fills a prescription, he should tell the pharmacist of any herb or dietary supplement he's taking. • Instruct patient not to consume more than 5 cups a day, or 300 mg of caffeine, to avoid or minimize adverse effects. • Advise patient that heavy consumption may be associated with esophageal cancer secondary to the tannin content in the mixture. • Tell patient that the first signs of toxic reaction are vomiting and abdominal spasm.

Adapted from *Nursing Herbal Medicine Handbook*. Springhouse Corporation, Springhouse, Pa.

Herb names	Reported uses	Nursing considerations	Patient teaching
GREEN TEA *(continued)*		milk is added to the tea mixture. • The tannin content in tea increases the longer it's left to brew; this increases the antidiarrheal properties of the tea. • In children, administering green tea with iron supplements or multivitamins with iron prevents the absorption of iron. • The first signs of a toxic reaction are vomiting and abdominal spasm.	
HAWTHORNE Hawthorne Berry, Hawthorne Extract, Hawthorne Formula, Hawthorne Power	Used to regulate blood pressure and heart rate and to treat atherosclerosis. Used as a cardiotonic and as a sedative for sleep. Used in mild cardiac insufficiency, heart conditions not requiring digoxin, mild stable forms of angina pectoris, and mild forms of bradycardia and palpitations.	• Find out why patient is using the herb. • High doses may cause hypotension and sedation. Monitor patient for CNS adverse effects, and monitor blood pressure. • Hawthorne may interfere with digoxin's effects or serum monitoring. • If patient has heart failure, he should only use hawthorne under close medical supervision and in combination with other standard treatments, only as directed. • Observe patient closely for adverse reactions, especially adverse CNS reactions.	• Advise patient not to delay seeking appropriate medical evaluation because doing so may delay diagnosis of a potentially serious medical condition. • Advise patient to consult his health care provider before using an herbal preparation because a treatment with proven efficacy may be available. • Advise patient that when he fills a prescription, he should tell the pharmacist of any herb or dietary supplement he's taking. • Advise patient to avoid use because of toxic adverse effects and narrow therapeutic index. • Warn patient to keep all herbal products away from children and pets.
HORSE CHESTNUT Horse Chestnut (some products that contain varying amounts of horse chestnut include: Arthro-Therapy, Cell-U-Var Cream, Varicare, Varicosin, and VenoCare Ultra-Joint Response, Venastat)	Used to treat chronic venous insufficiency, varicose veins, leg pain, tiredness, tension, and leg swelling and edema. Extract is used as a conjunctive treatment for lymphedema, hemorrhoids, and enlarged prostate. Horse chestnut has been used as an analgesic, anticoagulant, antipyretic, astringent, expectorant, and tonic. It has also been used to treat skin ulcers,	• Find out why patient is using the herb. • The nuts, seeds, twigs, sprouts, and leaves of horse chestnut are poisonous. Standardized formulations remove most of the toxins and standardize the amount of aescin. • **ALERT:** High doses and nonstandardized forms can be lethal. • Signs and symptoms of toxicity include loss of coordination, salivation, hemolysis, headache, dilated pupils, muscle twitching, seizures, vomiting, diarrhea, depression, paralysis, respiratory and cardiac failure, and death.	• Advise patient to consult his health care provider before using an herbal preparation because a treatment with proven efficacy may be available. • Advise patient that when he fills a prescription, he should tell the pharmacist of any herb or dietary supplement he's taking. • Inform patient that the FDA classifies horse chestnut as an unsafe herb and that deaths have occurred. • Advise patient to use only a standardized extract containing 16% to 21% aescin, at recommended doses, and to discontinue use if he experiences sign of toxic reaction. • Tell patient that this is only symptomatic treatment of chronic venous insufficiency and not a cure. *(continued)*

Adapted from *Nursing Herbal Medicine Handbook*. Springhouse Corporation, Springhouse, Pa.

Herb names	Reported uses	Nursing considerations	Patient teaching
HORSE CHESTNUT *(continued)*	phlebitis, leg cramps, cough, and diarrhea.	● Monitor patient for signs of toxicity and discontinue horse chestnut immediately if any occur. ● Monitor glucose level in patients taking antidiabetics for hypoglycemia.	● Advise patient not to confuse horse chestnut with sweet chestnut, used as a food. ● Advise patient to keep the herb away from children. Consumption of amounts of leaves, twigs, and seeds equaling 1% of a child's weight may be lethal.
KAVA Contained in a variety of products including, but not limited to, the following: Alcohol-Free Fava-Kava, Kavacin, Kava Kava Plus, Kava Kava Root, Fava Tone, St. John's Plus Kava Kava, and Standardized Kava Extract.	Used to treat nervous anxiety, stress, and restlessness. It's used orally to produce sedation, to promote wound healing, and to treat headaches, seizure disorders, the common cold, respiratory tract infection, tuberculosis, and rheumatism. It's also used to treat urogenital infections, including chronic cystitis, venereal disease, uterine inflammation, menstrual problems, and vaginal prolapse. Some herbal practitioners consider kava an aphrodisiac. Kava juice is used to treat skin diseases, including leprosy. It's also used as a poultice for intestinal problems, otitis, and abscesses.	● Find out why patient is using the herb. ● Patient shouldn't use kava with conventional sedative-hypnotics, anxiolytics, MAO inhibitors, other psychopharmacologic drugs, levodopa, or antiplatelet drugs without first consulting a health care provider. ● Adverse effects of kava are mild at suggested dosages. They may occur at start of therapy but are transient. ● Oral use is probably safe for 3 months or less; use for longer than 3 months may be habit forming. ● Kava can cause drowsiness and may impair motor reflexes. ● Patients should avoid taking herb with alcohol because of increased risk of CNS depression and liver damage. ● Periodic monitoring of liver function tests and CBC may be needed. ● Heavy kava users are more likely to complain of poor health: 20% are underweight with reduced levels of albumin, total protein, bilirubin, urea, platelets, and lymphocytes; increased HDL cholesterol and RBCs; hematuria; puffy faces; scaly rashes; and some evidence of pulmonary hypertension. These symptoms resolve several weeks after the herb is stopped. Toxic doses can cause progressive ataxia, muscle weakness, and ascending paralysis, all of which resolve when herb is stopped. Extreme use (more than 300 g	● Advise patient to consult his health care provider before using an herbal preparation because a treatment with proven efficacy may be available. ● Advise patient that when he fills a prescription, he should tell the pharmacist of any herb or dietary supplement he's taking. ● Encourage patients to seek medical diagnosis before taking kava. ● Advise patient that usual doses can affect motor function; caution him against performing hazardous activities. ● Tell patient oral use is probably safe for 3 months or less, but use for longer than 3 months may be habit forming. ● Warn patient to avoid taking herb with alcohol because of increased risk of CNS depression and liver damage.

Adapted from *Nursing Herbal Medicine Handbook*. Springhouse Corporation, Springhouse, Pa.

Herb names	Reported uses	Nursing considerations	Patient teaching
KAVA *(continued)*		per week) may increase gammaglutamyltransferase levels.	
MELATONIN Circadian (controlled-release, not available in U.S.), Mela-T, Melatonex	Used for treating insomnia, jet lag, shift-work disorder, blind entrainment (a condition in which blind people develop insomnia or daytime sleepiness because they feel no circadian rhythm), immune system enhancement, tinnitus, depression, and benzodiazepine withdrawal in geriatric patients with insomnia. Also, used as a cancer therapy adjuvant, antiaging product, contraceptive, and a prophylactic therapy for cluster headaches. Topically, it's used for skin protection against ultraviolet light.	● Find out why patient is using herb. ● Monitor patient for excessive daytime drowsiness. ● May increase human growth hormone levels.	● Advise patient to consult his health care provider before using an herbal preparation or supplement because a treatment with proven efficacy may be available. ● Advise patient that when he fills a prescription, he should tell the pharmacist of any herb or dietary supplement he's taking. ● Warn patient to avoid hazardous activities until full extent of CNS depressant effect is known. ● If patient wishes to conceive, tell her that melatonin may have a contraceptive effect. However, herb shouldn't be used as birth control. ● Although no chemical interactions have been reported in clinical studies, tell patient that melatonin may interfere with therapeutic effects of conventional drugs. ● Warn patient about possible additive effects if taken with alcohol. ● Advise patient to use only the synthetic form (not the animal-derived product) because of concerns about contamination and viral transmission. ● Advise patient not to use melatonin for prolonged periods because safety data aren't available.
MILK THISTLE Liver Formula with Milk Thistle, Milk Thistle Extract, Milk Thistle Phytosome, Milk Thistle Plus, Milk Thistle Power, Milk Thistle Super Complex, Silybin Phytosome, Silymarin Milk Thistle, Simply Milk Thistle, Thisilyn	Used for dyspepsia, liver damage from chemicals, Amanita mushroom poisoning, supportive therapy for inflammatory liver disease and cirrhosis, loss of appetite, and gallbladder and spleen disorders. It's also used as a liver protectant.	● Find out why patient is using herb. ● Mild allergic reactions may occur, especially in people allergic to members of the Astertaceae family, including ragweed, chrysanthemums, marigolds, and daisies. ● Don't confuse milk thistle seeds or fruit with other parts of the plant or with blessed thistle (Cnictus benedictus). ● Silymarin has poor water solubility; therefore, efficacy when prepared as a tea is questionable.	● Advise patient to consult his health care provider before using an herbal preparation because a treatment with proven efficacy may be available. ● Advise patient that when he fills a prescription, he should tell the pharmacist of any herb or dietary supplement he's taking. ● Although no chemical interactions have been reported in clinical studies, advise patient that herb may interfere with therapeutic effect of conventional drugs. ● Warn patient not to take this herb while pregnant or breast-feeding. ● Tell patient to stay alert for possible allergic reactions, especially if allergic to ragweed, chrysanthemums, marigolds, or daisies.

(continued)

Adapted from *Nursing Herbal Medicine Handbook*. Springhouse Corporation, Springhouse, Pa.

Herb names	Reported uses	Nursing considerations	Patient teaching
MILK THISTLE *(continued)*			• Warn patient not to take herb for liver inflammation or cirrhosis before seeking appropriate medical evaluation because doing so may delay diagnosis of a potentially serious medical condition. • Warn patient to keep all herbal products away from children and pets.
NETTLE Freeze-Dried Nettle Capsules, Fresh Nettle Leaf, Nettle Blend, Nettle Leaf, Nettle Leaf Tea, Nettle Organic Tea, Nettle Root, Nettle Seed	Used to treat allergic rhinitis, osteoarthritis, rheumatoid arthritis, kidney stones, asthma, and BPH. Also used as a diuretic, an expectorant, a general health tonic, a blood builder and purifier, a pain reliever and anti-inflammatory, and a lung tonic for ex-smokers. Also used for eczema, hives, bursitis, tendinitis, laryngitis, sciatica, and premenstrual syndrome. Nettle is being investigated for treatment of hay fever and irrigation of the urinary tract.	• Find out why patient is using the herb. • Nettle is reported to be an abortifacient and may affect the menstrual cycle. • Allergic adverse effects from internal use are rare.	• Advise patient to consult his health care provider before using an herbal preparation because a treatment with proven efficacy may be available. • Advise patient that when he fills a prescription, he should tell the pharmacist of any herb or dietary supplement he's taking. • Recommend caution if patient takes an antihypertensive or antidiabetic. • Warn patient that external adverse effects result from skin contact and include burning and stinging that may persist for 12 hours or longer. • Inform patient that capsules and extracts should be stored at room temperature, away from heat and direct light. • Instruct women taking herb to notify health care provider about planned, suspected, or known pregnancy. • Advise patient not to breast-feed while taking this herb.
PASSION FLOWER Passion Flower, Alcohol Free Passion Flower Liquid	Used as a sedative, a hypnotic, an analgesic, and an antispasmodic for treating muscle spasms caused by indigestion, menstrual cramping, pain, or migraines. Also used for neuralgia, generalized seizures, hysteria, nervous agitation, and insomnia. Crushed leaves and flowers are used topically for cuts and bruises.	• Find out why patient is using the herb. • Monitor patient for possible adverse CNS effects. • No adverse effects have been observed with recommended doses. • A disulfiram-like reaction may produce nausea, vomiting, flushing, headache, hypotension, tachycardia, ventricular arrhythmias, and shock leading to death. • Patients with liver disease or alcoholism shouldn't use herbal products that contain alcohol.	• Advise patient to consult his health care provider before using an herbal preparation because a treatment with proven efficacy may be available. • Advise patient that when he fills a prescription, he should tell the pharmacist of any herb or dietary supplement he's taking. • Because sedation is possible, caution patient to avoid hazardous activities. • Warn patient not to take herb for chronic pain or insomnia before seeking medical attention because doing so may delay diagnosis of a potentially serious medical condition. • Caution pregnant patients to avoid this herb. • Advise patient to consult his health care provider before using

Herb names	Reported uses	Nursing considerations	Patient teaching
SAW PALMETTO Centrum Saw Palmetto, Herbal Sure Saw Palmetto, Permixon, PlusStrogen, Premium Blend Saw Palmetto, Pro-active Saw Palmetto, Propalmex, Quanterra Prostate, Saw Palmetto Power, Standardized Saw Palmetto ExtractCap, Super Saw Palmetto	Used to treat symptoms of BPH and coughs and congestion from colds, bronchitis, or asthma. Also used as a mild diuretic, urinary antiseptic, and astringent.	• Find out why patient is using the herb. • Herb should be used cautiously for conditions other than BPH because data about its effectiveness in other conditions are lacking. • Obtain a baseline prostate-specific antigen (PSA) test before patient starts taking herb because it may cause a false-negative PSA result. • Saw palmetto may not alter prostate size. • Laboratory values didn't change significantly in clinical trials using dosages of 160 mg to 320 mg daily.	an herbal preparation because a treatment with proven efficacy may be available. • Advise patient that when he fills a prescription, he should tell the pharmacist of any herb or dietary supplement he's taking. • Warn patient not to take herb for bladder or prostate problems before seeking medical attention because doing so could delay diagnosis of a potentially serious medical condition. • Tell patient to take herb with food to minimize GI effects. • Caution patient to promptly notify health care provider about new or worsened adverse effects. • Warn women to avoid herb if planning pregnancy, if pregnant, or if breast-feeding.
ST. JOHN'S WORT Alterra, Hypercalm, Kira, Quanterra Emotional Balance, St. John's Wort Extracts, Tension Tamer, various combination products	Used orally for mild to moderate depression, anxiety, psychovegetative disorders, sciatica, and viral infections, including herpes simplex virus types 1 and 2, hepatitis C, influenza virus, murine cytomegalovirus, and poliovirus. St. John's wort has also been used to treat bronchitis, asthma, gallbladder disease, nocturnal enuresis, gout, and rheumatism, although it hasn't proven effective in these cases.	• Find out why patient is using the herb. • St. John's wort has been effective in treating mild to moderate depression. • Recommended duration of therapy for depression is 4 to 6 weeks; if no improvement occurs, a different therapy should be considered. • Monitor patient for response to herbal therapy, as evidenced by improved mood and lessened depression. • By using standardized extracts, patient can better control the dosage. Clinical studies have used formulations of standardized 0.3% hypericin as well as hyperforin-stabilized version of the extract. • St. John's wort interacts with many other products; they must be considered before patient takes it with other prescription or OTC products. • Serotonin syndrome may cause dizziness, nausea, vomiting, headache, epigastric pain, anxiety, confusion, restlessness, and irritability.	• Advise patient to consult his health care provider before using an herbal preparation because a treatment with proven efficacy may be available. • Advise patient that when he fills a prescription, he should tell the pharmacist of any herb or dietary supplement he's taking. • Instruct patient to consult a health care provider for a thorough medical evaluation before using St. John's wort. • Encourage patient to discuss depression and to seek regular psychiatric help, as indicated. • If patient takes St. John's wort for mild to moderate depression, explain that several weeks may pass before effects occur. Tell patient that a new therapy may be needed if no improvement occurs in 4 to 6 weeks. • Inform patient that St. John's wort interacts with many other prescription and OTC products and may reduce their effectiveness. • Tell patient that St. John's wort may cause increased sensitivity to direct sunlight. Recommend protective clothing, sunscreen, and limited sun exposure. • Inform patient that a sufficient wash-out period is needed after *(continued)*

Adapted from *Nursing Herbal Medicine Handbook*. Springhouse Corporation, Springhouse, Pa.

Herb names	Reported uses	Nursing considerations	Patient teaching
ST. JOHN'S WORT *(continued)*		● Because St. John's wort decreases the effect of certain prescription drugs, watch for signs of drug toxicity if patient stops using the herb. Drug dosage may need to be reduced. ● St. John's wort has mutagenic effects on sperm cells and oocytes and adverse effects on reproductive cells; therefore, it shouldn't be used by pregnant patients or those planning pregnancy (including men). ● Topically, the volatile plant oil is an irritant. Monitor affected site for adverse effects and improvement. ● Monitor patient for sedative effects and GI complaints.	stopping an antidepressant before switching to St. John's wort. ● Tell patient to report adverse effects to a health care provider. ● Warn patient to keep all herbal products away from children and pets.
TEA TREE OIL Tea Tree Oil, Tea Tree Oil Lotion, Tea Tree Soap	Used topically for contusions, inflammation, myalgia, burns, hemorrhoids, and vitiligo. In traditional Chinese medicine, tea tree oil has been used as a gargle for tonsillitis and as a lotion for dermatoses.	● Find out why patient is using the herb. ● Because of systemic toxicity, tea tree oil shouldn't be used internally. ● Essential oil should be used externally only after being diluted, especially by people with sensitive skin. ● Tea tree oil may cause burns or itching in tender areas and shouldn't be used around nose, eyes, and mouth. ● Diluted essential oil, even as low as 0.25% or 0.5%, is active against microbes. ● Vaginal douches using concentrations as strong as 40% require extreme caution and supervision by a health care provider. ● Pure (100%) essential tea tree oil is rarely used and only with close supervision by a health care provider. ● Other related Melaleuca species are also known as tea trees, such as *M. cajeputi, M. dissitifolia,* and *M. linariiflora* but tea tree oil can be obtained only from *M. alternifolia.*	● Advise patient to consult his health care provider before using an herbal preparation because a treatment with proven efficacy may be available. ● Advise patient that when he fills a prescription, he should tell the pharmacist of any herb or dietary supplement he's taking. ● Tell patient to use very dilute tea tree oil (0.25% to 0.5%) as topical anti-infective. ● Explain that a few drops are sufficient in mouthwash, shampoo, or sitz bath. ● Caution patient not to apply oil to wounds or to skin that's dry or cracked. ● If patient will be using the douche form of this product, stress the need for medical supervision. ● Warn patient to keep all herbal products away from children and pets.

Adapted from *Nursing Herbal Medicine Handbook*. Springhouse Corporation, Springhouse, Pa.

Most common drug errors

Listed below are 25 of the most common drug errors and steps you can take to prevent them.

Drug orders

Prescribing and filling drug orders must be done carefully to avoid potential problems.

Pharmacy computer systems

Error: The Institute for Safe Medication Practices (ISMP) performed a field test on 307 pharmacy computer systems; only four detected all unsafe orders. Many didn't detect potentially lethal orders, including doses that exceeded safe limits, drug ingredient duplications, and orders to administer oral solutions I.V.

Best practice or prevention: Don't rely on the pharmacy computer system to detect all unsafe orders. Before administering a drug, understand the correct dosage, indications, and adverse effects; if necessary, refer to a current drug reference.

Drug name confusion

Error: The approval of Lantus (insulin glargine [rDNA origin]) raises concerns that this drug will be confused with Lente insulin. This mix-up could easily happen with either a verbal or written order.

Best practice or prevention: Be aware of the medications your patient takes regularly and question any deviations from his regular routine. And as with any medication, take your time and read the label carefully.

Abbreviations

Error: Abbreviating drug names is risky. A cancer patient with anemia may receive epoetin alfa, commonly abbreviated EPO, to stimulate RBC production. In one case, when a cancer patient was admitted to a hospital, the doctor wrote, "May take own supply of EPO." However, the patient wasn't anemic. Sensing that something wrong, the pharmacist interviewed the patient, who confirmed that he was taking "EPO"—evening primrose oil—to lower his cholesterol level.

Best practice or prevention: Ask all prescribers to spell out drug names.

Unclear orders

Error: A patient was supposed to receive one dose of the antineoplastic lomustine to treat brain cancer. (Lomustine is typically given as a single oral dose once every 6 weeks.) The doctor's order read "Administer h.s." Because this was misinterpreted to mean every night, the patient received nine daily doses, developed severe thrombocytopenia and leukopenia, and died.

Best practice or prevention: If you're unfamiliar with a drug, check a drug reference before administering it. If a prescriber uses "h.s." but doesn't specify the frequency of administration, clarify the order. When documenting orders, note "h.s. nightly" or "h.s. × one dose today."

Misinterpretation of orders

Error: Several reports to the ISMP involved errors related to insulin orders. In one case, an order was written as "add 10U of regular insulin to each TPN bag," and the pharmacist preparing the solution misinterpreted the dose as 100 units. In another case, a pharmacy technician entering orders misinterpreted a sliding scale when the insulin order used "u" for units, an error that could have caused a 10-fold overdose if a nurse hadn't caught it. Yet another report involved a nurse who received a verbal order to resume an insulin drip but wrote "resume heparin drip." Fortunately, the pharmacist caught the error.

Best practice or prevention: Before administering drugs such as insulin or heparin, which are ordered in units, always check the prescriber's written order against the provided dose. Never abbreviate "units." If you must accept a verbal order, have another nurse listen in; then transcribe that order directly onto an order form and repeat it to ensure that you've transcribed it correctly.

Inadvertent overdose

Error: The inadvertent prescribing of harmful acetaminophen doses has become a disturbing trend. To relieve pain, prescribers may write orders for combined acetaminophen and opioid analgesic tablets (Lortab, Tylox, Darvocet-N) without realizing that the total acetaminophen dose could be toxic.

Consider this order: "Tylox, 1 to 2 tablets every 4 hours, as needed, for pain." By taking the higher dose, the patient would receive 1,000 mg of acetaminophen every 4 hours, exceeding the maximum recommended dose of 4 g/day.

Best practice or prevention: To prevent an acetaminophen overdose from combined analgesics, note the amount of acetaminophen in each drug. Beware of substitutions by the pharmacy because the amount of acetaminophen may vary.

Lipid-based drugs
Error: Serious drug errors, some fatal, have occurred because of confusion between certain lipid-based (liposomal) drugs and their conventional counterparts. The drugs involved include:
• lipid-based amphotericin B (Abelcet, Amphotec, AmBisome) and conventional amphotericin B for injection (available generically and as Fungizone)
• the pegylated liposomal form of doxorubicin (Doxil) and its conventional form, doxorubicin hydrochloride (Adriamycin, Rubex)
• a liposomal form of daunorubicin (DaunoXome, daunorubicin citrate liposomal) and conventional daunorubicin hydrochloride (Cerubidine).
Best practice or prevention: Lipid-based products have different dosages than their conventional counterparts. Check the original order and labels carefully to avoid mix-ups.

Drug preparation
When preparing a drug for administration, be alert for potential problems.

Syringe tip caps and children
Error: A syringe tip cap poses a potential choking hazard to a small child: If you forget to remove the cap from an oral syringe before administering a drug, the cap could blow off into the child's mouth when you press the plunger. If a cap from an oral or a hypodermic syringe gets lost

in the linens, the child may find it later and swallow or aspirate it.
Best practice or prevention: Remove and discard the cap in a secure sharps container before administering the drug; don't place it in a trash can where the child may find it later.

Teach parents about the potential danger of syringe tip caps. Tell them to store a capped syringe where children can't reach it and to remove the cap before giving the drug.

Inattentiveness
Error: When a hospital pharmacy received an order for Fludara (fludarabine), a pharmacy technician asked the pharmacist if Navelbine (vinorelbine) was the same as Fludara (both are antineoplastics). The preoccupied pharmacist said "yes." The technician prepared the Navelbine, but labeled it as Fludara. The pharmacist checked the preparation but didn't notice the error, and the patient received the wrong drug.
Best practice or prevention: To prevent errors of this type, the hospital posted tables of antineoplastics and their dosing guidelines in the pharmacy. As an added safeguard, the pharmacy now sends the empty drug vial or box top with the prepared solution for the nurse to double-check before infusing the drug.

Injectable solution color changes
Error: In two cases, alert nurses noticed that antineoplastics prepared in the pharmacy didn't look the way they should.

The first error involved a 6-year-old child who was to receive 12 mg of methotrexate intrathecally. In the pharmacy, a 1-g vial was mistakenly selected instead of a 20-mg vial, and the drug was reconstituted with 10 ml of normal saline. The vial containing 100 mg/ml was incorrectly labeled as containing 2 mg/ml, and 6 ml of the solution was drawn into a syringe. Although the syringe label indicated 12 mg of drug, the syringe actually contained 600 mg of drug.

When the nurse received the syringe and noted that the drug's color didn't appear right, she returned it to the pharmacy for verification. The pharmacist retrieved the vial used to prepare the dose and drew the remaining solution into another syringe. The solutions in both syringes matched, and no one noticed the vial's 1-g label. The pharmacist concluded that a manufacturing change caused the color difference.

The child received the 600-mg dose and experienced seizures 45 minutes later. A pharmacist responding to the emergency detected the error. The child received an antidote and recovered.

A similar case involved a 20-year-old patient with leukemia who received mitomycin instead of mitoxantrone. The nurse had questioned the drug's unusual bluish tint, but the pharmacist assured her that the color difference was due to a change in manufacturer. Fortunately, the patient didn't suffer any harm.

Best practice or prevention: If a familiar drug seems to have an unfamiliar appearance, investigate the cause. If the pharmacist cites a manufacturing change, ask him to double-check whether he has received verification from the manufacturer. Document the appearance discrepancy, your actions, and the pharmacist's response in the patient record.

Dropper confusion

Error: Ordering drugs such as liquid ferrous sulfate by the dropperful is a dangerous practice. One person might correctly consider the dropper full when the liquid meets the upper calibration mark; another might incorrectly fill the entire length of the dropper. Also, parents administering the drug at home may use a different dropper, which could significantly alter the dose given.

Best practice or prevention: Dosing directions for liquid drugs should always be expressed as weight per volume, such as 15 mg/0.6 ml. Verify the correct dose and teach parents to use only the dropper provided. Show them the mark on the dropper that indicates a full dose and ask them to demonstrate the proper technique.

Incorrect allergy history

Error: After a patient was admitted to the hospital, a nurse faxed a list of the patient's allergies to the pharmacy. The pharmacist couldn't read it, so he accessed the files from the patient's previous admission. However, these records didn't reflect an allergy to the anti-infective cefazolin that the patient had recently developed.

A consulting doctor ordered cefazolin, and the pharmacy processed the order. The medication administration record (MAR) generated by the pharmacy's database didn't indicate the allergy, and the nurse didn't know about it either.

The patient received cefazolin and became hypotensive and unresponsive. The nurse immediately notified the doctor and administered the antihistamine diphenhydramine. The patient recovered and was discharged the next day.

Best practice or prevention: Perform a new allergy history with each admission. If the patient's history must be faxed, name the drugs, note how many are included, and follow the facility's faxing safeguards. If the pharmacy also adheres to strict guidelines, the computer-generated MAR should be accurate.

Drug administration

When administering a drug, be careful to avoid the following problems.

Patient misidentification

Error: Two common errors for nurses who are administering drugs are inadvertently failing to check the patient's identification and confusing patients with similar names. Using a tactic that helps prevent wrong-site surgery—involving the patient in the identification process—could also help prevent these drug errors.

Best practice or prevention: Urge the patient to clearly state his full name, even without being asked, at admission and before accepting drugs, procedures, or treatments. Teach him to offer his identification bracelet for inspection when anyone arrives with drugs and to insist on having it replaced if it's removed.

Herbal remedies

Error: Surveys suggest that about one-third of Americans use herbal products as medicine. Some people take them with conventional drugs; others use them as replacements. Herbal products are available without a prescription. Because government quality assurance standards don't apply to herbal products' manufacturing and labeling, their ingredients may be misrepresented or contaminated.

Research on the effects of herbal products is limited. Because these products may contain a mixture of chemicals, their use carries risks.

Best practice or prevention: Ask the patient about his use of alternative therapies, including herbal products, and record your findings in his medical record. Monitor the patient carefully and report unusual events. Ask the patient to keep a diary of all therapies he uses and to take the diary for review each time he visits a health care professional.

Calculation errors

Error: A physician assistant wrote the following order for a woman being admitted to the hospital for neck surgery: "methylprednisolone 10.6 g (30 mg/kg) over 1 hour IVPB before surgery" to minimize inflammation. The patient weighed 154 lb (70 kg), so the dose should have been 2.1 g, and not 10.6 g. However, neither the pharmacist nor the nurse independently checked the calculation, and the patient received an overdose. She developed significant hyperglycemia and hypokalemia but recovered without injury.

Best practice or prevention: Writing the mg/kg or mg/m^2 dose and the calculated dose provides a safeguard against calculation errors. Whenever a prescriber provides the calculation, double-check it and document that the dose was verified.

Eyedrops for two or more

Error: Using one bottle of eyedrops to treat several patients may seem like a good way to prevent waste, control cost, and save time. Some facilities, for example, administer shared drugs to multiple patients undergoing outpatient cataract surgery. But this practice has risks.

Although eyedrops contain preservatives to prevent bacterial growth, contaminants may remain on the bottle top's inner surfaces or outer grooves. The dropper can also become contaminated if it accidentally touches an infected eye. (Cross-infections have been reported.)

Administering the wrong drug or wrong concentration is more likely because patient names don't appear on the containers. A patient may receive the wrong drops because the nurse can't check the bottle label against his patient identification.

Best practice or prevention: Just as sharing any drug is poor practice, eyedrops shouldn't be used for more than one patient. If unit doses aren't available for surgical patients, each patient should fill his prescriptions before admission and bring his drugs with him.

Trouble with liquids

Error: Liquid medications may be more error-prone than solid medications because of the calculations and dosage measurements needed. Here are a few examples: A 5-year-old boy who was receiving imipramine to treat his enuresis was given a 5-fold overdose because of an incorrectly compounded suspension. A prescription of Augmentin was dispensed with the instruction to take 2½ tsp instead of 2½ ml. And a mother who misunderstood the written directions gave her child 7 ml instead of 0.7 ml of a liquid drug.

Best practice or prevention: Don't assume that liquid medications are less likely to cause harm than other forms, including parenteral ones. Pediatric and geriatric patients commonly receive liquid medications and may be especially sensitive to the effects of an inaccurate dose. If a unit-dose form isn't available, calculate carefully, and double-check your math and the drug label.

Celexa, Celebrex, and Cerebyx confusion

Error: An 80-year-old woman mistakenly received 20 mg of Celexa (citalopram), a selective serotonin reuptake inhibitor (SSRI), b.i.d. for 1 month for arthritis pain. She should have received 100 mg of Celebrex (celecoxib), an NSAID. A member of the pharmacy staff had confused the drug names when pulling the product from the shelf. Although the patient wasn't harmed, the potential for harm was great because she was already taking an SSRI.

Best practice or prevention: Help prevent errors related to Celebrex, Celexa, and the anticonvulsant Cerebyx (fosphenytoin) by asking prescribers to use the generic name and by confirming the drug's indication if the order doesn't clearly state it. For verbal orders, repeat the drug name and your understanding of its indication to the prescriber.

Labels and toxicity

Error: A container of 5% acetic acid, used to clean tracheostomy tubing, was left near nebulization equipment in the room of a 10-month-old infant. A respiratory therapist mistook the liquid for normal saline solution and used it to dilute albuterol for the child's nebulizer treatment. During treatment, the child experienced bronchospasm, hypercapnic dyspnea, tachypnea, and tachycardia.

Best practice or prevention: Leaving potentially dangerous chemicals near patients is extremely risky, especially when the container labels don't indicate toxicity. To prevent such problems, read the label on every drug you prepare and never administer anything that isn't labeled.

Dosage equations

Error: A 13-month study at Albany (N.Y.) Medical Center examined 200 prescribing errors arising from the use of dosage equations. Almost 70% involved pediatric patients, for whom dosage equations are commonly used. Mistakes in decimal point placement, mathematical calculation, or expression of the regimen accounted for over 50% of the errors. Examples include prescribing the entire day's drug as a single dose instead of at intervals or using an entire day's dose at each interval. Use of dosage equations invites drug errors.

Best practice or prevention: Alternatives to dosage equations include using pre-established ranges or tables, incorporating a calculator into a computer order entry system, and requiring both the calculated dose and dosage equation on orders to facilitate independent checks.

After calculating drug dosages, always have another nurse calculate them independently to double-check your results. If doubts or questions remain or if the calculations don't match, ask a pharmacist to calculate the dose before administering the drug.

Misread orders

Error: Two reports concerned incorrect dosing of the tricyclic antidepressant nortriptyline (Pamelor, Aventyl, or, in Australia, Allegron) when ordered for neuropathic pain syndromes. The cases involved 10-mg and 20-mg orders that were misread as 100 mg and 200 mg, respectively. One patient who received an incorrect dose required hospitalization; the other developed sedation and orthostatic hypotension after two doses, which led to recognition of the error.

Best practice or prevention: Nortriptyline and other tricyclic antidepressants aren't prescribed as frequently as they once were. To make sure you're familiar with recommended dosages, refer to a drug handbook and then ask a pharmacist, if necessary.

Air bubbles in pump tubing

Error: After starting an I.V. drip to administer insulin, 2 units/hour, to a 9-year-old patient, a nurse noted air bubbles in the tubing and pump chamber. To remove them and promote proper flow, she disconnected the tubing and increased the pump rate to 200 ml/hour. When the bubbles were cleared, she reconnected the tubing and restarted the infusion without resetting the rate. The child received about 50 units of insulin before the error was detected. Fortunately, the child wasn't harmed.

Best practice or prevention: To clear bubbles from I.V. tubing, never increase the pump's flow rate to flush the line. Instead, remove the tubing from the pump, disconnect it from the patient, and use the flow-control clamp to establish gravity flow. When the bubbles have been removed, return the tubing to the pump, restart the infusion, and recheck the flow rate.

Misplaced decimals

Error: A patient in the intensive care unit was to receive the opioid fentanyl, 12.5 to 25 mcg I.V. every 4 to 6 hours, as needed, for pain. Unit stock consisted of 5-ml ampules of fentanyl 0.05 mg/ml, so each ampule contained 0.25 mg (250 mcg). A nurse preparing a dose confused the volume needed when she converted from milligrams to micrograms and administered

5 ml thinking it contained 25 micrograms. The patient suffered respiratory arrest but was resuscitated.

Best practice or prevention: Numerous serious fentanyl errors have been reported, and a misplaced decimal point caused many of them. A safer alternative for intermittent dosing is I.V. morphine. Fentanyl doses are best prepared in the pharmacy rather than in the unit. If a fentanyl dose must be prepared, refer to dosing charts, follow the facility's protocols, and ask another nurse to check your calculations.

Incorrect administration route

Error: A nurse was caring for a patient who had a jejunostomy tube for oral drugs and a central I.V. line for hyperalimentation and I.V. drugs. At the bedside was a stock bottle of digoxin elixir. After checking the concentration, the nurse used a syringe to withdraw 2.5 ml of elixir for a 0.125-mg dose. She then mistakenly administered the elixir through the central line rather than the jejunostomy tube.

Using an incorrect route put the patient at risk for overdose and secondary infection from unsterile I.V. administration. Fortunately, he was receiving antibiotics for a preexisting infection and suffered no adverse reactions.

Best practice or prevention: This case emphasizes the need to ensure that the right route is being used to administer any drug. When the patient has multiple lines, label the distal end of each line. Using a parenteral syringe to prepare oral liquid drugs increases the chance for error because the syringe tip fits easily into I.V. ports. To safely administer an oral drug through a feeding tube, use a dose prepared by the pharmacy and a syringe with the appropriate tip.

Stress

Error: A nurse-anesthetist administered the sedative midazolam (Versed) to the wrong patient. When she discovered the error, she grabbed what she thought was a vial of the antidote flumazenil (Romazicon), withdrew 2.5 ml, and administered it. When the patient didn't respond, she realized she'd grabbed a vial of ondansetron (Zofran), an antiemetic, instead. Another

practitioner assisted with proper I.V. administration of flumazenil, and the patient recovered without harm.

Best practice or prevention: Committing a serious error can cause enormous stress and cloud your judgment. If you're involved in a drug error, ask another professional to administer the antidote.

Infusion rates

Epinephrine infusion rates
Mix 1 mg in 250 ml (4 mcg/ml).

Dose (mcg/min)	Infusion rate (ml/hr)
1	15
2	30
3	45
4	60
5	75
6	90
7	105
8	120
9	135
10	150
15	225
20	300
25	375
30	450
35	525
40	600

Isoproterenol infusion rates
Mix 1 mg in 250 ml (4 mcg/ml).

Dose (mcg/min)	Infusion rate (ml/hr)
0.5	8
1	15
2	30
3	45
4	60
5	75
6	90
7	105
8	120
9	135
10	150
15	225
20	300
25	375
30	450

Nitroglycerin infusion rates
Determine the infusion rate in ml/hr using the ordered dose and the concentration of the drug solution.

Dose (mcg/min)	25 mg/250 ml (100 mcg/ml)	50 mg/250 ml (200 mcg/ml)	100 mg/250 ml (400 mcg/ml)
5	3	2	1
10	6	3	2
20	12	6	3
30	18	9	5
40	24	12	6
50	30	15	8
60	36	18	9
70	42	21	10
80	48	24	12
90	54	27	14
100	60	30	15
150	90	45	23
200	120	60	30

(continued)

Dobutamine infusion rates

Mix 250 mg in 250 ml of D_5W (1,000 mcg/ml). Determine the infusion rate in ml/hr using the ordered dose and the patient's weight in pounds or kilograms.

Dose (mcg/kg/min)	lb 88 kg 40	99 45	110 50	121 55	132 60	143 65	154 70	165 75	176 80	187 85	198 90	209 95	220 100	231 105	242 110
2.5	6	7	8	8	9	10	11	11	12	13	14	14	15	16	17
5	12	14	15	17	18	20	21	23	24	26	27	29	30	32	33
7.5	18	20	23	25	27	29	32	34	36	38	41	43	45	47	50
10	24	27	30	33	36	39	42	45	48	51	54	57	60	63	66
12.5	30	34	38	41	45	49	53	56	60	64	68	71	75	79	83
15	36	41	45	50	54	59	63	68	72	77	81	86	90	95	99
20	48	54	60	66	72	78	84	90	96	102	108	114	120	126	132
25	60	68	75	83	90	98	105	113	120	128	135	143	150	158	165
30	72	81	90	99	108	117	126	135	144	153	162	171	180	189	198
35	84	95	105	116	126	137	147	158	168	179	189	200	210	221	231
40	96	108	120	132	144	156	168	180	192	204	216	228	240	252	264

Dopamine infusion rates

Mix 400 mg in 250 ml of D_5W (1,600 mcg/ml). Determine the infusion rate in ml/hr using the ordered dose and the patient's weight in pounds or kilograms.

Dose (mcg/kg/min)	lb 88 kg 40	99 45	110 50	121 55	132 60	143 65	154 70	165 75	176 80	187 85	198 90	209 95	220 100	231 105
2.5	4	4	5	5	6	6	7	7	8	8	8	9	9	10
5	8	8	9	10	11	12	13	14	15	16	17	18	19	20
7.5	11	13	14	15	17	18	20	21	23	24	25	27	28	30
10	15	17	19	21	23	24	26	28	30	32	34	36	38	39
12.5	19	21	23	26	28	30	33	35	38	40	42	45	47	49
15	23	25	28	31	34	37	39	42	45	48	51	53	56	59
20	30	34	38	41	45	49	53	56	60	64	68	71	75	79
25	38	42	47	52	56	61	66	70	75	80	84	89	94	98
30	45	51	56	62	67	73	79	84	90	96	101	107	113	118
35	53	59	66	72	79	85	92	98	105	112	118	125	131	138
40	60	68	75	83	90	98	105	113	120	128	135	143	150	158
45	68	76	84	93	101	110	118	127	135	143	152	160	169	177
50	75	84	94	103	113	122	131	141	150	159	169	178	188	197

Nitroprusside infusion rates

Mix 50 mg in 250 ml of D_5W (200 mcg/ml). Determine the infusion rate in ml/hr using the ordered dose and the patient's weight in pounds or kilograms.

Dose (mcg/kg/min)	lb 88	99	110	121	132	143	154	165	176	187	198	209	220	231	242
	kg 40	45	50	55	60	65	70	75	80	85	90	95	100	105	110
0.3	4	4	5	5	5	6	6	7	7	8	8	9	9	9	10
0.5	6	7	8	8	9	10	11	11	12	13	14	14	15	16	17
1	12	14	15	17	18	20	21	23	24	26	27	29	30	32	33
1.5	18	20	23	25	27	29	32	34	36	38	41	43	45	47	50
2	24	27	30	33	36	39	42	45	48	51	54	57	60	63	66
3	36	41	45	50	54	59	63	68	72	77	81	86	90	95	99
4	48	54	60	66	72	78	84	90	96	102	108	114	120	126	132
5	60	68	75	83	90	98	105	113	120	128	135	143	150	158	165
6	72	81	90	99	108	117	126	135	144	153	162	171	180	189	198
7	84	95	105	116	126	137	147	158	168	179	189	200	210	221	231
8	96	108	120	132	144	156	168	180	192	204	216	228	240	252	264
9	108	122	135	149	162	176	189	203	216	230	243	257	270	284	297
10	120	135	150	165	180	195	210	225	240	255	270	285	300	315	330

Therapeutic drug monitoring guidelines

Drug	Laboratory test monitored	Therapeutic ranges of test

aminoglycoside antibiotics (amikacin, gentamicin, tobramycin)	Amikacin peak
	  trough
	Gentamicin/tobramycin
	  peak
	  trough
	Creatinine
		20 to 25 mcg/ml
		5 to 10 mcg/ml
		
		4 to 8 mcg/ml
		1 to 2 mcg/ml
		0.6 to 1.3 mg/dl

amphotericin B	Creatinine BUN Electrolytes (especially potassium and magnesium) Liver function CBC with differential and platelets	0.6 to 1.3 mg/dl 5 to 20 mg/dl Potassium: 3.5 to 5 mEq/L Magnesium: 1.5 to 2.5 mEq/L Sodium: 135 to 145 mEq/L Chloride: 98 to 106 mEq/L * *****
antibiotics	WBC with differential Cultures and sensitivities	*****
biguanides (metformin)	Creatinine Fasting glucose Glycosylated hemoglobin CBC	0.6 to 1.3 mg/dl 70 to 110 mg/dl 5.5% to 8.5% of total hemoglobin *****
clozapine	WBC with differential	*****
digoxin	Digoxin Electrolytes (especially potassium, magnesium, and calcium) Creatinine	0.8 to 2 ng/ml Potassium: 3.5 to 5 mEq/L Magnesium: 1.7 to 2.1 mEq/L Sodium: 135 to 145 mEq/L Chloride: 98 to 106 mEq/L Calcium: 8.6 to 10 mg/dl 0.6 to 1.3 mg/dl
diuretics	Electrolytes Creatinine BUN Uric acid Fasting glucose	Potassium: 3.5 to 5 mEq/L Magnesium: 1.7 to 2.1 mEq/L Sodium: 135 to 145 mEq/L Chloride: 98 to 106 mEq/L Calcium: 8.6 to 10 mg/dl 0.6 to 1.3 mg/dl 5 to 20 mg/dl 2 to 7 mg/dl 70 to 110 mg/dl
erythropoietin	Hematocrit	Women: 36% to 48% Men: 42% to 52%
ethosuximide	Ethosuximide	40 to 100 mcg/ml

Note: ***** For those areas marked with asterisks, the following values can be used:

Hemoglobin: Women: 12 to 16 g/dl
  Men: 14 to 18 g/dl
Hematocrit: Women: 37% to 48%
  Men: 42% to 52%
RBCs: 4 to 5.5 x 10^6/mm^3
WBCs: 5 to 10 x 10^3/mm^3

Differential: Neutrophils: 45% to 74%
  Bands: 0% to 8%
  Lymphocytes: 16% to 45%
  Monocytes: 4% to 10%
  Eosinophils: 0% to 7%
  Basophils: 0% to 2%

Monitoring guidelines

Wait until the administration of the third dose to check drug levels. Obtain blood for peak level 30 minutes after I.V. infusion or 60 minutes after I.M. administration. For trough levels, draw blood just before next dose. Dosage may need to be adjusted accordingly. Recheck after three doses. Monitor creatinine and BUN levels and urine output for signs of decreasing renal function.

Monitor creatinine, BUN, and electrolyte levels at least weekly during therapy. Also, regularly monitor blood counts and liver function test results during therapy.

Specimen cultures and sensitivities will determine the cause of the infection and the best treatment. Monitor WBC with differential weekly during therapy.

Check renal function and hematologic parameters before initiating therapy and at least annually thereafter. If the patient has impaired renal function, don't use metformin because it may cause lactic acidosis. Monitor response to therapy by periodically evaluating fasting glucose and glycosylated hemoglobin levels. A patient's home monitoring of glucose levels helps monitor compliance and response.

Obtain WBC with differential before initiating therapy, weekly during therapy, and 4 weeks after discontinuing the drug.

Check digoxin levels at least 12 hours, but preferably 24 hours, after the last dose is administered. To monitor maintenance therapy, check drug levels at least 1 to 2 weeks after therapy is initiated or changed. Make any adjustments in therapy based on entire clinical picture, not solely on drug levels. Also, check electrolyte levels and renal function periodically during therapy.

To monitor fluid and electrolyte balance, perform baseline and periodic determinations of electrolyte, calcium, BUN, uric acid, and glucose levels.

After therapy is initiated or changed, monitor the hematocrit twice weekly for 2 to 6 weeks until stabilized in the target range and a maintenance dose determined. Monitor hematocrit regularly thereafter.

Check drug level 8 to 10 days after therapy is initiated or changed.

(continued)

* For those areas marked with one asterisk, the following values can be used:

ALT: 7 to 56 U/L
AST: 5 to 40 U/L
Alkaline phosphatase: 17 to 142 U/L
LDH: 60 to 220 U/L
GGT: < 40 U/L
Total bilirubin: 0.2 to 1 mg/dl

Drug	Laboratory test monitored	Therapeutic ranges of test
gemfibrozil	Lipids	Total cholesterol: < 200 mg/dl LDL: < 130 mg/dl HDL: Women: 40 to 75 mg/dl Men: 37 to 70 mg/dl Triglycerides: 10 to 160 mg/dl
heparin	Activated partial thromboplastin time (aPTT)	1.5 to 2 times control
HMG-CoA reductase inhibitors (fluvastatin, lovastatin, pravastatin, simvastatin)	Lipids Liver function	Total cholesterol: < 200 mg/dl LDL: < 130 mg/dl HDL: Women: 40 to 75 mg/dl Men: 37 to 70 mg/dl Triglycerides: 10 to 160 mg/dl *
insulin	Fasting glucose Glycosylated hemoglobin	70 to 110 mg/dl 5.5% to 8.5% of total hemoglobin
lithium	Lithium Creatinine CBC Electrolytes (especially potassium and sodium) Fasting glucose Thyroid function tests	0.5 to 1.4 mEq/L 0.6 to 1.3 mg/dl ***** Potassium: 3.5 to 5 mEq/L Magnesium: 1.7 to 2.1 mEq/L Sodium: 135 to 145 mEq/L Chloride: 98 to 106 mEq/L 70 to 110 mg/dl TSH: 0.2 to 5.4 microU/ml T_3: 80 to 200 ng/dl T_4: 5.4 to 11.5 mcg/dl
methotrexate	Methotrexate CBC with differential Platelet count Liver function Creatinine	Normal elimination: < 10 micromol 24 hours postdose < 1 micromol 48 hours postdose < 0.2 micromol 72 hours postdose ***** 150 to 450 × 10³/mm³ * 0.6 to 1.3 mg/dl
phenytoin	Phenytoin CBC	10 to 20 mcg/ml *****
potassium chloride	Potassium	3.5 to 5 mEq/L
procainamide	Procainamide N-acetylprocainamide CBC	4 to 8 mcg/ml (procainamide) 5 to 30 mcg/ml (combined procainamide and NAPA) *****

Note: ***** For those areas marked with asterisks, the following values can be used:

Hemoglobin: Women: 12 to 16 g/dl
  Men: 14 to 18 g/dl
Hematocrit: Women: 37% to 48%
  Men: 42% to 52%
RBCs: 4 to 5.5 x 10⁶/mm³
WBCs: 5 to 10 x 10³/mm³

Differential: Neutrophils: 45% to 74%
  Bands: 0% to 8%
  Lymphocytes: 16% to 45%
  Monocytes: 4% to 10%
  Eosinophils: 0% to 7%
  Basophils: 0% to 2%

Monitoring guidelines

Therapy is usually withdrawn after 3 months if response is inadequate. Patient must be fasting to measure triglyceride levels.

When drug is given by continuous I.V. infusion, check aPTT every 4 hours in the early stages of therapy. When drug is given by deep S.C. injection, check aPTT 4 to 6 hours after injection.

Perform liver function tests at baseline, 6 to 12 weeks after therapy is initiated or changed, and periodically thereafter. If adequate response isn't achieved within 6 weeks, consider changing the therapy.

Monitor response to therapy by evaluating glucose and glycosylated hemoglobin levels. Glycosylated hemoglobin level is a good measure of long-term control. A patient's home monitoring of glucose levels helps measure compliance and response.

Checking lithium levels is crucial to the safe use of the drug. Obtain lithium levels immediately before next dose. Monitor levels twice weekly until stable. Once at steady state, levels should be checked weekly; when the patient is on the appropriate maintenance dose, levels should be checked every 2 to 3 months. Monitor creatinine, electrolyte, and fasting glucose levels; CBC; and thyroid function test results before therapy is initiated and periodically during therapy.

Monitor methotrexate levels according to dosing protocol. Monitor CBC with differential, platelet count, and liver and renal function test results more frequently when therapy is initiated or changed and when methotrexate levels may be elevated, such as when the patient is dehydrated.

Monitor phenytoin levels immediately before next dose and 2 to 4 weeks after therapy is initiated or changed. Obtain a CBC at baseline and monthly early in therapy. Watch for toxic effects at therapeutic levels. Adjust the measured level for hypoalbuminemia or renal impairment, which can increase free drug levels.

Check level weekly after oral replacement therapy is initiated until stable and every 3 to 6 months thereafter.

Measure procainamide levels 6 to 12 hours after a continuous infusion is started or immediately before the next oral dose. Combined (procainamide and NAPA) levels can be used as an index of toxicity when renal impairment exists. Obtain CBC periodically during longer-term therapy.

(continued)

---

* For those areas marked with one asterisk, the following values can be used:

ALT: 7 to 56 U/L
AST: 5 to 40 U/L
Alkaline phosphatase: 17 to 142 U/L
LDH: 60 to 220 U/L
GGT: < 40 U/L
Total bilirubin: 0.2 to 1 mg/dl

Drug	Laboratory test monitored	Therapeutic ranges of test
quinidine	Quinidine CBC Liver function Creatinine Electrolytes (especially potassium)	2 to 6 mcg/ml ***** * 0.6 to 1.3 mg/dl Potassium: 3.5 to 5 mEq/L Magnesium: 1.7 to 2.1 mEq/L Sodium: 135 to 145 mEq/L Chloride: 98 to 106 mEq/L
sulfonylureas	Fasting glucose Glycosylated hemoglobin	70 to 110 mg/dl 5.5% to 8.5% of total hemoglobin
theophylline	Theophylline	10 to 20 mcg/ml
thyroid hormone	Thyroid function tests	TSH: 0.2 to 5.4 microU/ml T_3: 80 to 200 ng/dl T_4: 5.4 to 11.5 mcg/dl
vancomycin	Vancomycin Creatinine	20 to 35 mcg/ml (peak) 5 to 10 mcg/ml (trough) 0.6 to 1.3 mg/dl
warfarin	INR	For an acute MI, atrial fibrillation, treatment of pulmonary embolism, prevention of systemic embolism, tissue heart valves, valvular heart disease, or prophylaxis or treatment of venous thrombosis: 2 to 3 For mechanical prosthetic valves or recurrent systemic embolism: 2.5 to 3.5

Note: ***** For those areas marked with asterisks, the following values can be used:

Hemoglobin: Women: 12 to 16 g/dl
   Men: 14 to 18 g/dl
Hematocrit: Women: 37% to 48%
   Men: 42% to 52%
RBCs: 4 to 5.5 x 10⁶/mm³
WBCs: 5 to 10 x 10³/mm³

Differential: Neutrophils: 45% to 74%
   Bands: 0% to 8%
   Lymphocytes: 16% to 45%
   Monocytes: 4% to 10%
   Eosinophils: 0% to 7%
   Basophils: 0% to 2%

Monitoring guidelines

Obtain levels immediately before next oral dose and 30 to 35 hours after therapy is initiated or changed. Periodically obtain blood counts, liver and kidney function test results, and electrolyte levels.

Monitor response to therapy by periodically evaluating fasting glucose and glycosylated hemoglobin levels. Patient should monitor glucose levels at home to help measure compliance and response.

Obtain theophylline levels immediately before next dose of sustained-release oral product and at least 2 days after therapy is initiated or changed.

Monitor thyroid function test results every 2 to 3 weeks until appropriate maintenance dose is determined.

Vancomycin levels may be checked with the third dose administered, at the earliest. Draw peak levels ½ hour after the I.V. infusion is completed. Draw trough levels immediately before the next dose is administered. Renal function can be used to adjust dosing and intervals.

Check INR daily, beginning 3 days after therapy is initiated. Continue checking it until therapeutic goal is achieved, and monitor it periodically thereafter. Also, check levels 7 days after any change in warfarin dose or concomitant, potentially interacting therapy.

---

* For those areas marked with one asterisk, the following values can be used:

ALT: 7 to 56 U/L
AST: 5 to 40 U/L
Alkaline phosphatase: 17 to 142 U/L
LDH: 60 to 220 U/L
GGT: < 40 U/L
Total bilirubin: 0.2 to 1 mg/dl

Selected local and topical anesthetics

Drug, indications, dosage	Adverse reactions

Local

bupivacaine hydrochloride
(Marcaine, Sensorcaine)
Dosages given are for the drug without epinephrine and for adults.
Volume listed below refers to the total volume of anesthetic given,
sometimes in incremental doses of 2 to 6 ml.
Epidural block—
0.25% solution: 10 to 20 ml (25 to 50 mg)
0.5% solution: 10 to 20 ml (50 to 100 mg)
0.75% solution: 10 to 20 ml (75 to 150 mg), single-dose only
Caudal block—
0.25% solution: 15 to 30 ml (37.5 to 75 mg)
0.5% solution: 15 to 30 ml (75 to 150 mg)
Spinal block—
0.75% solution (in dextrose 8.25%): 0.8 to 1.6 ml (6 to 12 mg)
Peripheral nerve block—
0.25% solution: 5 ml (12.5 mg)
0.5% solution: 5 ml (25 mg)

CNS: anxiety, nervousness, *seizures* followed by drowsiness.
CV: *arrhythmias, bradycardia, cardiac arrest,* hypotension, myocardial depression.
EENT: blurred vision, tinnitus.
GI: nausea, vomiting.
Respiratory: *respiratory arrest.*
Skin: dermatologic reactions, *status asthmaticus.*
Other: *anaphylactoid reactions, anaphylaxis,* edema.

---

chloroprocaine hydrochloride
(Nesacaine, Nesacaine-MPF)
Dosages given are for the drug without epinephrine and for adults.
Volume listed below refers to the total volume of anesthetic given,
sometimes in incremental doses of 2 to 6 ml.
Infiltration and nerve block—
1% solution: 3 to 20 ml (30 to 200 mg)
2% solution: 2 to 40 ml (40 to 800 mg)
Caudal and epidural block—
2% to 3% solution: 15 to 25 ml (300 to 750 mg)
May be repeated with smaller doses q 40 to 50 minutes. Dose and interval may be increased when combined with epinephrine. Maximum adult dose is 800 mg; when combined with epinephrine, maximum dose is 1 g.

CNS: anxiety, nervousness, *seizures* followed by drowsiness.
CV: *arrhythmias, bradycardia, cardiac arrest,* hypotension, myocardial depression.
EENT: blurred vision, tinnitus.
GI: nausea, vomiting.
Respiratory: *respiratory arrest, status asthmaticus.*
Skin: dermatologic reactions.
Other: *anaphylactoid reactions, anaphylaxis,* edema.

---

etidocaine hydrochloride
(Duranest, Duranest MPF)
Dosages given are for the drug without epinephrine and for adults.
Dose limit is 4 mg/kg or 300 mg per injection. When combined with
epinephrine, dose limit is 5.5 mg/kg or 400 mg per injection. May be
repeated q 2 to 3 hours.
Peripheral nerve block—
1% solution: 5 to 40 ml (50 to 400 mg)
Central neural block (lower limbs, cesarean section, lumbar, epidural)—
1% solution: 10 to 30 ml (100 to 300 mg)
Transvaginal block—
1% solution: 5 to 20 ml (50 to 200 mg)
Caudal block—
1% solution: 10 to 30 ml (100 to 300 mg)

CNS: anxiety, apprehension, nervousness, *seizures* followed by drowsiness.
CV: *arrhythmias, bradycardia, cardiac arrest,* hypotension, myocardial depression.
EENT: blurred vision, tinnitus.
GI: nausea, vomiting.
Respiratory: *respiratory arrest, status asthmaticus.*
Skin: dermatologic reactions.
Other: *anaphylactoid reactions, anaphylaxis,* edema.

Reactions may be *common*, uncommon, *life-threatening*, or COMMON AND LIFE-THREATENING.

Interactions	Nursing considerations

Beta blockers: enhanced sympathomimetic effects when used with bupivacaine and epinephrine. Use with caution.
Butyrophenones, phenothiazines: may reduce or reverse pressor effect of epinephrine. Monitor patient.
Chloroprocaine: may lessen bupivacaine's action. Don't use together.
CNS depressants: may cause additive CNS effects. Reduce dosage of CNS depressants.
Cyclic antidepressants, MAO inhibitors: severe, sustained hypertension when used with bupivacaine and epinephrine. Use with extreme caution.
Enflurane, halothane, isoflurane, related drugs: arrhythmias when used with bupivacaine and epinephrine. Use with extreme caution.

• Contraindicated in children under 12 years, for spinal or topical anesthesia or paracervical block, and in patients with known history of hypersensitivity reactions to local anesthetics of the amide type.
• Some solutions contain sulfites and should be avoided in patients with sulfite hypersensitivity.
• Should not be used for I.V. regional anesthesia (Bier block, Bier's local anesthesia).
• Don't use 0.75% solution for obstetric surgery; lower concentrations are effective and less hazardous.
• Use cautiously in debilitated, elderly, or acutely ill patients and in patients with severe hepatic disease or drug allergies.
• Use solutions with epinephrine cautiously in patients with CV disorders and in body areas with limited blood supply (ears, nose, fingers, toes).
• Keep resuscitation equipment and drugs available.
• Don't use solution with preservatives for caudal or epidural block.
• Discard partially used vials without preservatives.
• Check solution for particles.
• Protect solutions containing epinephrine from light.

Bupivacaine: chloroprocaine may lessen bupivacaine's action. Monitor for effect.
CNS depressants: may cause additive CNS effects. Reduce dosage of CNS depressants.
Sulfonamides: chloroprocaine inhibits the action of sulfonamides. Don't use in conditions in which a sulfonamide drug is required.

• Contraindicated in patients with hypersensitivity to procaine, tetracaine, or other PABA derivatives and for spinal or topical anesthesia. Epidural and caudal blocks are contraindicated in patients with CNS disease.
• Use cautiously in debilitated, elderly, or acutely ill patients; in children; and in patients with drug allergies, paracervical block, or CV disease.
• Keep resuscitation equipment and drugs available.
• Don't use solution with preservatives for caudal or epidural block.
• Don't use discolored solution.
• Check solution for particles.
• Discard partially used vials without preservatives.

CNS depressants: may cause additive CNS effects. Reduce dosage of CNS depressants.
Cyclic antidepressants, MAO inhibitors, phenothiazines: severe, sustained hypertension or hypotension with etidocaine and epinephrine. Use with extreme caution.
Enflurane, halothane, isoflurane, related drugs: arrhythmias when used with etidocaine and epinephrine. Use with extreme caution.

• Contraindicated in patients with inflammation or infection in puncture region, septicemia, severe hypertension, spinal deformities, or neurologic disorders; in children under 14 years; and for spinal anesthesia.
• Contraindicated in patients with known history of hypersensitivity to local anesthetics of the amide type.
• Some solutions contain sulfites and should be avoided in patients with sulfite hypersensitivity.
• Use cautiously in debilitated, elderly, or acutely ill patients; in patients with severe shock, heart block, general drug allergies, or hepatic and renal disease; and as epidural block in obstetric patients.
• Use solutions with epinephrine cautiously in patients with CV disease and in body areas with limited blood supply (ears, nose, fingers, toes).
• Don't use solution with preservatives for caudal or epidural block; check solution for particles.
• Keep resuscitation equipment and drugs available.

(continued)

Drug, indications, dosage	Adverse reactions

Local

lidocaine hydrochloride
[lignocaine hydrochloride]
(Dilocaine, Lidoject-1, Lidoject-2, Nervocaine, Octocaine, Xylocaine)
Dosages given are for drug without epinephrine and for adults.
Volume listed below refers to total volume of anesthetic given, sometimes in incremental doses of 2 to 6 ml.
For anesthesia other than spinal—
Maximum single dose is 4.5 mg/kg or 300 mg. With epinephrine,
maximum dose is 7 mg/kg or 500 mg.
Caudal (obstetric) or epidural (thoracic) block—
1% solution: 20 to 30 ml (200 to 300 mg)
Epidural (lumbar anesthesia) block—
1% solution: 25 to 30 ml (250 to 300 mg)
1.5% solution: 15 to 20 ml (225 to 300 mg)
2% solution: 10 to 15 ml (200 to 300 mg)
Spinal surgical anesthesia—
5% (with 7.5% dextrose): 1.5 to 2 ml (75 to 100 mg)
Caudal (surgery) block—
1.5% solution: 15 to 20 ml (225 to 300 mg)

CNS: anxiety, nervousness,
seizures followed by drowsiness.
CV: *arrhythmias, bradycardia,
cardiac arrest,* myocardial depression, hypotension.
EENT: blurred vision, tinnitus.
GI: nausea, vomiting.
Respiratory: *respiratory arrest,
status asthmaticus.*
Skin: dermatologic reactions.
Other: *anaphylactoid reactions,
anaphylaxis,* edema.

procaine hydrochloride
(Novocain)
Spinal anesthesia—
Adults: initial dose should not exceed 1 g. Before using, dilute 10%
solution with normal saline solution injection, sterile distilled water, or
CSF. For hyperbaric technique, use dextrose solution.
Perineum: 0.5 ml of 10% solution (50 mg) and 0.5 ml diluent injected
at the L4 interspace
Perineum and lower extremities: 1 ml of 10% solution (100 mg) and
1 ml diluent injected at the L3 or L4 interspace
Up to costal margin: 2 ml of 10% solution (200 mg) and 1 ml diluent
injected at the L2, L3, or L4 interspace
Peripheral nerve block—
1% solution: 100 ml (1 g)
2% solution: 50 ml (1 g)
Infiltration—
350 to 600 mg in 0.25% to 0.5% solution. Maximum initial dose is 1 g.

CNS: anxiety, nervousness,
seizures followed by drowsiness.
CV: *arrhythmias, bradycardia,
cardiac arrest,* hypotension,
myocardial depression.
EENT: blurred vision, tinnitus.
GI: nausea, vomiting.
Respiratory: *respiratory arrest,
status asthmaticus.*
Skin: dermatologic reactions.
Other: *anaphylactoid reactions,
anaphylaxis,* edema.

ropivacaine hydrochloride
(Naropin)
Avoid rapid injection of large volume of local anesthetic and use incremental doses. Use smallest dose and concentration required to produce desired result.
Lumbar epidural block in surgery—
0.5% solution: 15 to 30 ml (75 to 150 mg)
0.75% solution: 15 to 25 ml (119 to 188 mg)
1.0% solution: 15 to 20 ml (150 to 200 mg)
Lumbar epidural block for cesarean section—
0.5% solution: 20 to 30 ml (100 to 150 mg)
*Thoracic epidural administration to establish block for postoperative
pain relief—*
0.5% solution: 5 to 15 ml (25 to 75 mg)
Major nerve block (brachial plexus)—
0.5 % solution: 35 to 50 ml (175 to 250 mg)
Field block (minor nerve blocks and infiltration)—
0.5% solution: 1 to 10 ml (5 to 200 mg)
Lumbar epidural block in labor—
Initially, 0.2% solution: 10 to 20 ml (20 to 40 mg); then 6 to 14 ml/
hour (12 to 28 mg/hour) as continuous infusion or 10 to 15 ml/hour
(20 to 30 mg/hour) as incremental "top-up" injections

CNS: anxiety, dizziness, headache, hypoesthesia, pain, paresthesia.
CV: *bradycardia,* chest pain, hypotension, hypertension, tachycardia.
GI: nausea, vomiting.
GU: oliguria, urine retention.
Hematologic: anemia.
Skin: pruritus.
Other: back pain, fever, chills,
postoperative complications, rigors.
*Neonatal—*vomiting, jaundice,
tachypnea, respiratory distress.
*Fetal— **bradycardia,*** fever,
tachycardia, distress.

Reactions may be *common*, uncommon, *life-threatening*, or COMMON AND LIFE-THREATENING.

Interactions	Nursing considerations
Beta blockers: enhanced sympathomimetic effects. Don't use with lidocaine and epinephrine. *Butyrophenones, phenothiazines:* may reduce or reverse the pressor effect of epinephrine. Monitor patient. *CNS depressants:* may cause additive CNS effects. Reduce dosage of CNS depressants. *Cyclic antidepressants, MAO inhibitors:* severe, sustained hypertension when used with lidocaine and epinephrine. Use with extreme caution. *Enflurane, halothane, isoflurane, related drugs:* arrhythmias when used with lidocaine and epinephrine. Use with extreme caution.	• Contraindicated in patients with inflammation or infection in puncture region, septicemia, severe hypertension, spinal deformities, and neurologic disorders. • Also contraindicated in patients with known history of hypersensitivity to local anesthetics of the amide type. • Use cautiously in debilitated, elderly, or acutely ill patients; in patients with severe shock, heart block, or general drug allergies; in obstetric patients; and for paracervical block. • Dose and interval are increased with epinephrine. • Use solutions with epinephrine cautiously in patients with CV disorders and in body areas with limited blood supply (ears, nose, fingers, toes). • Don't use solution with preservatives for spinal, epidural, or caudal block. • Keep resuscitation equipment and drugs available. • Discard partially used vials without preservatives. • Check solution for particles. • Some solutions contain sulfites; they shouldn't be given to patients hypersensitivie to sulfites.
CNS depressants: may cause additive CNS effects. Reduce dosage of CNS depressants. *Echothiophate iodide:* reduced hydrolysis of procaine. Use together cautiously. *Succinylcholine:* prolonged neuromuscular blockade. Use cautiously together. *Sulfonamides:* procaine inhibits the action of sulfonamides. Don't use in conditions in which a sulfonamide drug is required.	• Contraindicated in patients with traumatized urethras and in those with hypersensitivity to chloroprocaine, tetracaine, or other PABA derivatives. • Also contraindicated in obstetric patients with cephalopelvic disproportion, placenta previa, abruptio placentae, floating fetal head, and intrauterine manipulation. • Use cautiously in hyperexcitable patients; in those with CNS disease, infection at puncture site, shock, profound anemia, cachexia, sepsis, hypertension, hypotension, GI hemorrhage, bowel perforation or strangulation, peritonitis, cardiac decompensation, massive pleural effusion, or increased intra-abdominal pressure; and in obstetric patients. • Keep resuscitation equipment and drugs available. • Use preservative-free solution for epidural block. • Discard partially used vials without preservatives.
Amide-type anesthetics: additive effects if given with ropivacaine. Use with caution. *CNS depressants:* may cause additive CNS effects. Reduce dosage of CNS depressants. *Fluvoxamine, imipramine, theophylline, verapamil:* may interact with ropivacaine. Use with caution.	• Contraindicated in patients with known hypersensitivity to drug or local anesthetics of amide type. • Use cautiously (especially when giving repeat doses) in debilitated, elderly, acutely ill, or breast-feeding patients and in patients with hypotension, hypovolemia, impaired CV function, heart block, or hepatic disease. • Don't inject drug rapidly. • Aspiration for blood should be done before all doses to avoid intravascular or subarachnoid injection. • Drug should be used only by personnel familiar with use of drug. Have emergency equipment and personnel available. • Don't use in emergency situations. • Drug should not be used for the production of obstetric paracervical block anesthesia, retrobulbar block, or spinal anesthesia (subarachnoid block). • Should not be used for I.V. regional anesthesia (Bier block). • Use an adequate test dose (3 to 5 ml of short-acting local anesthetic solution containing epinephrine) before induction of complete block.

(continued)

Drug, indications, dosage	Adverse reactions

Local

ropivacaine hydrochloride *(continued)*
Lumbar epidural block in postoperative pain management—
0.2% solution: 6 to 10 ml/hour (12 to 20 mg/hour) as continuous infusion
Thoracic epidural block in postoperative pain management—
0.2% solution: 4 to 8 ml/hour (8 to 16 mg/hour) as continuous infusion
Infiltration (minor nerve block) in postoperative pain management—
0.2% solution: 1 to 100 ml (2 to 200 mg)
0.5% solution: 1 to 40 ml (5 to 200 mg)

---

tetracaine hydrochloride
(Pontocaine)
Dosage for adults varies according to extent of block.
Low spinal (saddle) block in vaginal delivery—
2 to 5 mg as hyperbaric solution (in 10% dextrose)
Perineum and lower extremities: 5 to 10 mg
Up to costal margin: 15 to 20 mg

CNS: anxiety, nervousness, *seizures* followed by drowsiness.
CV: *arrhythmias, bradycardia, cardiac arrest,* hypotension, myocardial depression.
EENT: blurred vision, tinnitus.
GI: nausea, vomiting.
Respiratory: *respiratory arrest, status asthmaticus.*
Skin: dermatologic reactions.
Other: *anaphylactoid reactions, anaphylaxis,* edema.

Topical

proparacaine hydrochloride
(AK-Taine, Alcaine, Ophthaine, Ophthetic)
Anesthesia for tonometry, gonioscopy—
Adults and children: 1 or 2 drops of 0.5% solution instilled in eye just before procedure.
Anesthesia for cataract extraction, glaucoma surgery—
Adults and children: 1 or 2 drops of 0.5% solution instilled in eye q 5 to 10 minutes for five to seven doses.
Removal of foreign bodies or sutures—
Adults and children: 1 or 2 drops 2 to 3 minutes before procedure or q 5 to 10 minutes for one to three doses.

EENT: conjunctival redness, transient eye pain.
Other: hypersensitivity reactions.

---

tetracaine
(Pontocaine Solution)
tetracaine hydrochloride
(Pontocaine)
Anesthesia for tonometry, gonioscopy; removal of corneal foreign bodies, suture removal from cornea; other diagnostic and minor surgical procedures—
Adults and children: 1 to 2 drops of 0.5% in eye just before procedure.

EENT: transient stinging in eye 30 seconds after initial instillation, epithelial damage in excessive or long-term use.
Other: sensitization with repeated use (allergic skin rash, urticaria).

Reactions may be *common,* uncommon, *life-threatening,* or **COMMON AND LIFE-THREATENING.**

Interactions	Nursing considerations
	• Restlessness, anxiety, incoherent speech, light-headedness, numbness and tingling of mouth and lips, metallic taste, tinnitus, dizziness, blurred vision, tremors, twitching, depression, or drowsiness may be early warning signs or symptoms of CNS toxicity. • Don't use in ophthalmic surgery.
CNS depressants: may cause additive CNS effects. Reduce dosage of CNS depressants. *Sulfonamides:* tetracaine inhibits the action of sulfonamides. Don't use in conditions in which a sulfonamide drug is required.	• Safety and efficacy in children haven't been established. • Contraindicated in patients with infection at injection site, CNS disease, or hypersensitivity to procaine or related agents. • Saddle block is contraindicated in patients with cephalopelvic disproportion, placenta previa, abruptio placentae, intrauterine manipulation, and floating fetal head. • Use cautiously in patients with shock, profound anemia, cachexia, hypertension, hypotension, peritonitis, cardiac decompensation, massive pleural effusion, increased intracranial pressure, and infection. Beware of possible sulfite sensitivity. • Keep resuscitation equipment and drugs available. • When CSF is added to powdered drug or solution during spinal anesthesia, solution may be cloudy. Don't use discolored or crystallized solutions. • Protect from light; store in refrigerator.
None significant.	• Contraindicated in patients with hypersensitivity to ester-type local anesthetics, PABA or its derivatives, or to other ingredients in these preparations. • Use cautiously in patients with cardiac disease and hyperthyroidism. • Not for long-term use; may delay wound healing. • Warn patients not to rub or touch eye while cornea is anesthetized. • Warn patients with corneal abrasion that pain is relieved only temporarily. • Check solution for particles. • Don't use discolored solution. • Store in tightly closed container. Refrigerate opened containers.
Cholinesterase inhibitors: prolonged ocular anesthesia and increased risk of toxicity. Use with caution. *Sulfonamides:* interference with sulfonamide antibacterial activity. Wait 30 minutes after anesthesia before instilling sulfonamide.	• Contraindicated in patients with hypersensitivity to drug or similar drugs (such as ester-type local anesthetics), PABA or its derivatives, or other ingredients in these preparations. • Drug doesn't dilate pupils, paralyze accommodation, or increase intraocular pressure. • Don't use discolored, cloudy, or crystallized solution. Keep container tightly closed and refrigerated. • Warn patient not to touch eye while cornea is anesthetized. • Avoid long-term use.

Diagnostic skin tests

Drug, indications, dosage

coccidioidin
BioCox, Spherulin

Suspected coccidioidomycosis—
Adults and children: 0.1 ml of 1:100 dilution I.D. into flexor surface of forearm. In patients who don't react to this form, repeat test using 1:10 dilution. Use 1:1,000 or 1:10,000 dilution if erythema nodosum is evident.

histoplasmin
Histolyn-CYL, Histoplasmin Diluted

To differentiate histoplasmosis from coccidioidomycosis, tuberculosis, sarcoidosis, and other mycotic or bacterial infections—
Adults and children: 0.1 ml I.D. into flexor surface of forearm.

mumps skin test antigen
MSTA

Detection of delayed hypersensitivity to mumps antigens and assessment of cell-mediated immunity—
Adults: 0.1 ml I.D. into flexor surface of forearm.

tuberculin purified protein derivative (Mantoux, PPD, TST)
Aplisol, PPD-Stabilized Solution (Mantoux test), Selavo-PPD Solution, Tubersol

Diagnosis of tuberculosis—
Adults and children: Initially, 1 tuberculin unit (TU; for patients suspected of being highly sensitized) or 5 TU (for patients not expected to be highly sensitized) I.D. into flexor surface of forearm. If patient has a negative reaction, retest with 250 TU.

tuberculosis multiple-puncture tests
Aplitest (dried purified protein derivative [PPD]), Mono-Vacc Test (liquid Old Tuberculin [OT]), Tine Test (dried OT, dried PPD)

Screening for tuberculosis—
Adults and children: Clean skin thoroughly with alcohol and let dry; make skin taut on flexor surface of forearm and press points firmly into selected site. Hold device at injection site for about 3 seconds to ensure deposition of dried tuberculin B in tissue lymph.

Adverse reactions	Nursing considerations
Other: hypersensitivity reactions (vesiculation, ulceration, necrosis), ***anaphylaxis,*** Arthus reaction.	● Pregnancy risk category C. ● Contraindicated in patients hypersensitive to thimerosal or erythema nodosum. ● Read test at 24 and 48 hours. ● A positive result consists of a 5-mm area of induration. Erythema without induration is a negative result.
Skin: urticaria, ulceration, vesiculation, or necrosis in highly sensitive patients. **Other:** ***angioedema, anaphylaxis.***	● Pregnancy risk category C. ● Contraindicated in patients with a history of positive reaction to this test. ● Read test in 48 to 72 hours. ● For cell-mediated immunity with other antigens, reaction should be examined in 24 to 48 hours.
Other: hypersensitivity reactions (vesiculation, ulceration), ***anaphylaxis,*** Arthus reaction.	● Pregnancy risk category C. ● Contraindicated in patients hypersensitive to eggs, egg products, or thimerosal. ● Read test at 48 and 72 hours. ● A 5-mm or larger area of induration, with or without erythema, is a positive result. ● Safety and effiicacy in children haven't been established.
CNS: pain. **Skin:** pruritus, vesiculation. **Other:** hypersensitivity reactions, ***anaphylaxis,*** Arthus reaction, ulceration, necrosis.	● Pregnancy risk category C. ● Contraindicated in patients with a history of positive reaction to tuberculin tests; severe reactions may occur. ● Read test in 48 to 72 hours. If repeat test using 250 TU shows no response, patient is nonreactive. ● A patient who doesn't show a positive reaction to 1 TU or 5 TU on the fiirst test may be retested wit 5 TU. If second test reaction is negative, patient may be tested with 250 TU. Perform any repeat testing on the other forearm. Don't use 250 TU for the initial injection.
Other: hypersensitivity reactions (vesiculation, ulceration, necrosis), ***anaphylaxis.***	● Pregnancy risk category C. ● Contraindicated in patients with a history of positive reaction to tuberculin tests. ● Read test in 48 to 72 hours. Verify questionable or positive reactions with the Mantoux test. ● Because the dose of tuberculin in the multiple-puncture devices can't be precisely controlled, these devices shouldn't be used for periodic checks in patients who are likely to be exposed to clinical tuberculosis.

Reactions may be *common*, uncommon, *life-threatening*, or COMMON AND LIFE-THREATENING.

Selected drugs used for conscious sedation

Defined as the induction of a minimally depressed level of consciousness (LOC), conscious sedation is used during certain short medical procedures to relieve pain and anxiety, produce a hypnotic state, cause short-term amnesia, or achieve a combination of these effects. Over the last decade, conscious sedation has gained widespread popularity and is now performed in gastroenterology, radiology, pulmonology, and cardiac catheterization suites as well as in critical care settings.

Required safeguards

Conscious sedation must occur in a controlled environment with emergency resuscitative equipment readily available. During the procedure, the patient must be able to maintain a patent airway independently and respond appropriately to physical or verbal commands. To avoid deep sedation and cardiopulmonary depression, the sedative dose is titrated to decrease the patient's LOC only to the point of slurred speech and nystagmus.

Drug options

Drugs used for conscious sedation include analgesics, hypnotics, and amnestic drugs. Nurses who administer them must demonstrate understanding of their pharmacology, familiarity with facility policy, and knowledge of and clinical competency in preprocedure patient assessment, procedural monitoring (including ECG, blood pressure, pulse oximetry, and LOC), airway management, postprocedure monitoring, and discharge criteria.

This table gives general dosing guidelines and key nursing considerations for the drugs most commonly used to produce conscious sedation in adults. Administered alone or in combination, these drugs produce varying levels of sedation and commonly have potent synergistic effects.

Drug	Dosage	Key considerations
diazepam (Valium) Drug is a benzodiazepine with anxiolytic, amnestic, anticonvulsant, skeletal muscle relaxant, and sedative-hypnotic properties.	*Adults:* up to 10 mg I.V. given slowly immediately before the procedure is usually adequate. If opiates aren't given concomitantly, up to 20 mg I.V. may be required. Or, 5 to 10 mg I.M. given 30 minutes before the procedure.	• Individualize doses and titrate to achieve desired effect. • Drug is a potent respiratory depressant, particularly when given with opioids. • Hypotension and bradycardia may occur in patients premedicated with a narcotic. • For I.V. administration, give directly into a large vein at no more than 5 mg/minute. • For pharmacologic reversal of sedative effects, administer flumazenil (Romazicon). Individualize dosage; generally, 0.2 mg I.V. over 15 seconds. May repeat p.r.n. Don't exceed 3 mg in any 1-hour period.
fentanyl citrate (Sublimaze) Drug is an opioid agonist that's 100 times more potent than morphine sulfate. Its analgesic activity of 100 mcg is equivalent to 10 mg morphine or 75 mg meperidine.	*Adults:* 0.5 to 1 mcg/kg I.V. titrated in 25-mcg increments over several minutes. *Elderly or debilitated patients with renal or hepatic disease:* individualize and reduce dosage.	• Watch for bradycardia, hypotension, apnea, respiratory depression, and chest wall rigidity. • Drug may cause nausea and vomiting. • Contraindicated in patients with elevated intracranial pressure or head trauma. • If overdose occurs, maintain patent airway and provide respiratory and CV support.

Drug	Dosage	Key considerations
fentanyl citrate (Sublimaze) *(continued)*		• Use naloxone (Narcan), to reverse respiratory and CV depressant effects. Low doses (1 to 4 mcg/kg) have been used to reverse respiratory depression caused by conscious sedation procedures. Patient may need additional doses (0.1 to 0.2 mg) based on total dosage and time elapsed since last narcotic dose.
lorazepam (Ativan) Drug is a benzodiazepine with sedative-hypnotic and anxiolytic properties.	*Adults:* 2 mg I.V. 15 to 20 minutes before the procedure. For greater amnestic effect, give up to 4 mg I.V. *Elderly patients:* use reduced dosage and wait several minutes to evaluate pharmacologic effect before administering additional sedative doses. Don't exceed 2 mg I.V. total for patients older than age 50.	• Individualize doses and titrate to achieve desired effect. • Before I.V. administration, dilute drug with an equal volume of compatible solution and inject directly into the vein or into the tubing of an existing I.V. infusion at a rate not exceeding 2 mg/minute. • Have emergency resuscitation equipment available when administering drug I.V. • For pharmacologic reversal of sedative effects, administer flumazenil (Romazicon). Individualize dosage; generally, 0.2 mg I.V. over 15 seconds. May repeat p.r.n. Don't exceed 3 mg in any 1-hour period.
midazolam (Versed) Drug is an ultrashort-acting, water-soluble benzodiazepine with amnestic, anxiolytic, sedative, muscle relaxant, and anticonvulsant properties.	*Healthy adults:* 0.5 mg I.V. over a 2-minute period. For the initial dose, don't exceed 2.5 mg. Some patients may respond to as little as 0.5 to 1 mg. *Adults age 60 and older or debilitated patients with decreased pulmonary reserve:* incremental 0.25- to 0.5-mg doses administered over a 2-minute period. Wait several minutes to evaluate pharmacologic effect before administering additional sedative doses.	• Individualize doses and titrate to achieve desired effect. • Bolus administration isn't recommended for conscious sedation procedures. • Drug is potent respiratory depressant, particularly when given with opioids. • Hypotension and bradycardia may occur in patients premedicated with a narcotic. • Excessive doses or development of hypoxia may lead to agitation, involuntary movement, hyperactivity, and combativeness. • For pharmacologic reversal of sedative effects, administer flumazenil (Romazicon). Reversal dosage is individualized; generally, 0.2 mg is given I.V. over 15 seconds. May repeat dose to achieve desired effect; however, don't exceed 3 mg in any 1-hour period.
meperidine (Demerol) Drug is an opioid analgesic that's also used as an adjunct to anesthesia.	*Adults:* 50 to 100 mg I.M. or S.C. 30 to 90 minutes before anesthesia.	• Watch for bradycardia, hypotension, respiratory depression, and apnea. • Drug may cause nausea and vomiting. • If I.V. administration is necessary, decrease dosage and administer commercially available injections slowly, preferably as a diluted solution. • Use naloxone (Narcan) to reverse respiratory and CV depressant effects.

Normal laboratory test values

Hematology

Activated partial thromboplastin time
  25 to 36 seconds
Hematocrit
  Men: 42% to 54%
  Women: 38% to 46%
Hemoglobin, total
  Men: 14 to 18 g/dl
  Women: 12 to 16 g/dl
Platelet count
  140,000 to 400,000/mm³
Prothrombin time
  10 to 14 seconds; INR for patients on
  warfarin therapy, 2 to 3 (those with
  pediatric heart valve, 2.5 to 3.5)
Red blood cell (RBC) count
  Men: 4.5 to 6.2 million/mm³ venous
  blood
  Women: 4.2 to 5.4 million/mm³ venous
  blood
RBC indices
  MCH: 26 to 32 fl
  MCHC: 30 to 36 g/dl
  MCV: 84 to 99 fl
Reticulocyte count
  0.5% to 2% of total RBC count
White blood cell (WBC) count
  4,100 to 10,900/mm³
WBC differential, blood
  Basophils: 0.3% to 2%
  Eosinophils: 0.3% to 7%
  Lymphocytes: 16.2% to 43%
  Monocytes: 0.6% to 9.6%
  Neutrophils: 47.6% to 76.8%

Blood chemistry

Alanine aminotransferase
  Men: 10 to 35 units/L
  Women: 9 to 24 units/L
Alkaline phosphatase
  Men ≥ age 19: 98 to 251 units/L
  Women ages 24 to 65: 81 to 282 units/L
  Women ≥ age 65: 119 to 309 units/L
Amylase
  Age ≥ 18: 35 to 115 units/L
Arterial blood gases
  HCO_3^-: 22 to 26 mEq/L
  Pao_2: 75 to 100 mm Hg
  $Paco_2$: 35 to 45 mm Hg
  pH: 7.35 to 7.45
  SaO_2: 94% to 100%

Aspartate aminotransferase
  Men: 8 to 20 units/L
  Women: 5 to 40 units/L
Bilirubin
  Adults: direct, < 0.5 mg/dl;
  indirect, 1.1 mg/dl
BUN
  8 to 20 mg/dl
Calcium
  Men ≥ age 22, women ≥ age 19: 8.9 to
  10.1 mg/dl
Carbon dioxide, total, blood
  22 to 34 mEq/L
Chloride
  100 to 108 mEq/L
Creatine kinase (CK)
  CK-BB: None
  CK-MB: 0 to 7 units/L
  CK-MM: 5 to 70 units/L
  Total: Men ≥ age 18, 52 to 336 units/L;
  women ≥ age 18, 38 to 176 units/L
Creatine
  Men: 0.2 to 0.6 mg/dl
  Women: 0.6 to 1 mg/dl
Creatinine
  Men: 0.8 to 1.2 mg/dl
  Women: 0.6 to 0.9 mg/dl
Glucose, fasting, plasma
  70 to 100 mg/dl
Lactate dehydrogenase (LDH)
  Total: 48 to 115 IU/L
  LDH_1: 14% to 26%
  LDH_2: 29% to 39%
  LDH_3: 20% to 26%
  LDH_4: 8% to 16%
  LDH_5: 6% to 16%
Magnesium
  1.5 to 2.5 mEq/L
  Atomic absorption: 1.7 to 2.1 mg/dl
Phosphates
  1.8 to 2.6 mEq/L
  Atomic absorption: 2.5 to 4.5 mg/dl
Potassium
  3.8 to 5.5 mEq/L
Protein, total
  26.6 to 7.9 g/dl
  Albumin fraction: 3.3 to 4.5 g/dl
Sodium
  135 to 145 mEq/L
Uric acid
  Men: 4.3 to 8 mg/dl
  Women: 2.3 to 6 mg/dl

Table of equivalents

Metric system equivalents

Metric weight

1 kilogram (kg or Kg)	=	1,000 grams (g or gm)
1 gram	=	1,000 milligrams (mg)
1 milligram	=	1,000 micrograms (µg or mcg)
0.6 g	=	600 mg
0.3 g	=	300 mg
0.1 g	=	100 mg
0.06 g	=	60 mg
0.03 g	=	30 mg
0.015 g	=	15 mg
0.001 g	=	1 mg

Metric volume

1 liter (l or L)	=	1,000 milliliters (ml)*
1 milliliter	=	1,000 microliters (µl)

Household		Metric
1 teaspoon (tsp)	=	5 ml
1 tablespoon (T or tbs)	=	15 ml
2 tablespoons	=	30 ml
8 ounces	=	240 ml
1 pint (pt)	=	473 ml
1 quart (qt)	=	946 ml
1 gallon (gal)	=	3,785 ml

Temperature conversions

CELSIUS DEGREES	FAHRENHEIT DEGREES	CELSIUS DEGREES	FAHRENHEIT DEGREES	CELSIUS DEGREES	FAHRENHEIT DEGREES
41.1	106.0	38.1	100.6	35.1	95.2
41.0	105.8	38.0	100.4	35.0	95.0
40.9	105.6	37.9	100.2	34.9	94.8
40.8	105.4	37.8	100.0	34.8	94.6
40.7	105.2	37.7	99.8	34.7	94.4
40.6	105.0	37.6	99.6	34.6	94.2
40.4	104.8	37.4	99.4	34.4	94.0
40.3	104.6	37.3	99.2	34.3	93.8
40.2	104.4	37.2	99.0	34.2	93.6
40.1	104.2	37.1	98.8	34.1	93.4
40.0	104.0	37.0	98.6	34.0	93.2
39.9	103.8	36.9	98.4	33.9	93.0
39.8	103.6	36.8	98.2	33.8	92.8
39.7	103.4	36.7	98.0	33.7	92.6
39.6	103.2	36.5	97.8	33.6	92.4
39.4	103.0	36.4	97.6	33.4	92.2
39.3	102.8	36.3	97.4	33.3	92.0
39.2	102.6	36.2	97.2	33.2	91.8
39.1	102.4	36.1	97.0	33.1	91.6
39.0	102.2	36.0	96.8	33.0	91.4
38.9	102.0	35.9	96.6	32.9	91.2
38.8	101.8	35.8	96.4	32.8	91.0
38.7	101.6	35.7	96.2	32.7	90.8
38.6	101.4	35.6	96.0	32.6	90.6
38.4	101.2	35.4	95.8	32.4	90.4
38.3	101.0	35.3	95.6	32.3	90.2
38.2	100.8	35.2	95.4	32.2	90.0

Weight conversions

1 oz = 30 g	1 lb = 453.6 g	2.2 lb = 1 kg

---

*1 ml = 1 cubic centimeter (cc); however, ml is the preferred measurement term.

Dialyzable drugs

The amount of a drug removed by dialysis differs among patients and depends on several factors, including the patient's condition, the drug's properties, length of dialysis and dialysate used, rate of blood flow or dwell time, and purpose of dialysis. This table indicates the effect of hemodialysis on selected drugs.

Drug	Level reduced by hemodialysis	Drug	Level reduced by hemodialysis
acetaminophen	Yes (may not influence toxicity)	ceftizoxime	Yes
		ceftriaxone	No
acyclovir	Yes	cefuroxime	Yes
allopurinol	Yes	cephalexin	Yes
alprazolam	No	cephalothin	Yes
amikacin	Yes	cephradine	Yes
amiodarone	No	chloral hydrate	Yes
amitriptyline	No	chlorambucil	No
amoxicillin	Yes	chloramphenicol	Yes (very small amount)
amoxicillin/clavulanate potassium	Yes		
		chlordiazepoxide	No
amphotericin B	No	chloroquine	No
ampicillin	Yes	chlorpheniramine	No
ampicillin/clavulanate potassium	Yes	chlorpromazine	No
		chlorthalidone	No
aspirin	Yes	cimetidine	Yes
atenolol	Yes	ciprofloxacin	Yes (only by 20%)
azathioprine	Yes	cisplatin	No
aztreonam	Yes	clindamycin	No
captopril	Yes	clofibrate	No
carbamazepine	No	clonazepam	No
carbenicillin	Yes	clonidine	No
carmustine	No	clorazepate	No
cefaclor	Yes	cloxacillin	No
cefadroxil	Yes	codeine	No
cefamandole	Yes	colchicine	No
cefazolin	Yes	cortisone	No
cefepima	Yes	co-trimoxazole	Yes
cefonicid	Yes (only by 20%)	cyclophosphamide	Yes
cefoperazone	Yes	diazepam	No
cefotaxime	Yes	diazoxide	No
cefotetan	Yes (only by 20%)	diclofenac	No
cefoxitin	Yes	dicloxacillin	No
ceftazidime	Yes	digoxin	No

Drug	Level reduced by hemodialysis	Drug	Level reduced by hemodialysis
diltiazem	No	indapamide	No
diphenhydramine	No	indomethacin	No
dipyridamole	No	insulin	No
disopyramide	Yes	irbesartan	No
doxazosin	No	iron dextran	No
doxepin	No	isoniazid	Yes
doxorubicin	No	isosorbide	No
doxycycline	No	isradipine	No
enalapril	Yes	kanamycin	Yes
erythromycin	Yes (only by 20%)	ketoconazole	No
ethacrynic acid	No	ketoprofen	Yes
ethambutol	Yes (only by 20%)	labetalol	No
ethchlorvynol	Yes	levofloxacin	No
ethosuximide	Yes	lidocaine	No
famotidine	No	lithium	Yes
fenoprofen	No	lomefloxacin	No
flecainide	No	lomustine	No
fluconazole	Yes	loracarbet	Yes
flucytosine	Yes	loratadine	No
fluorouracil	Yes	lorazepam	No
fluoxetine	No	mechlorethamine	No
flurazepam	No	mefenamic acid	No
fosinopril	No	meperidine	No
furosemide	No	mercaptopurine	Yes
gabapentin	Yes	methadone	No
ganciclovir	Yes	methicillin	No
gemfibrozil	No	methotrexate	Yes
gentamicin	Yes	methyldopa	Yes
glipizide	No	methylprednisolone	No
glutethimide	Yes	metoclopramide	No
glyburide	No	metolazone	No
guanfacine	No	metoprolol	No
haloperidol	No	metronidazole	Yes
heparin	No	mexiletine	Yes
hydralazine	No	mezlocillin	Yes
hydrochlorothiazide	No	miconazole	No
hydroxyzine	No	midazolam	No
ibuprofen	No	minocycline	No
imipenem/cilastatin	Yes	minoxidil	Yes
imipramine	No		*(continued)*

Drug	Level reduced by hemodialysis	Drug	Level reduced by hemodialysis
misoprostol	No	ranitidine	Yes
morphine	No	rifampin	No
nabumetone	No	rofecoxib	No
nadolol	Yes	sertraline	No
nafcillin	No	sotalol	Yes
naproxen	No	stavudine	Yes
nelfinavir	Yes	streptomycin	Yes
netilmicin	Yes	sucralfate	No
nifedipine	No	sulbactam	Yes
nimodipine	No	sulfamethoxazole	Yes
nitrofurantoin	Yes	sulindac	No
nitroglycerin	No	temazepam	No
nitroprusside	Yes	theophylline	Yes
nizatidine	No	ticarcillin	Yes
norfloxacin	No	timolol	No
nortriptyline	No	tobramycin	Yes
ofloxacin	Yes	tocainide	Yes
olanzapine	No	tolbutamide	No
omeprazole	No	topirimate	Yes
oxacillin	No	trazodone	No
oxazepam	No	triazolam	No
paroxetine	No	trimethoprim	Yes
penicillin G	Yes	valcyclovir	Yes
pentamidine	No	valproic acid	No
pentazocine	Yes	valsartan	No
phenobarbital	Yes	vancomycin	No
phenylbutazone	No	verapamil	No
phenytoin	No	warfarin	No
piperacillin	Yes		
piroxicam	No		
prazosin	No		
prednisone	No		
primidone	Yes		
procainamide	Yes		
promethazine	No		
propoxyphene	No		
propranolol	No		
protriptyline	No		
quinidine	Yes		

Estimating surface area in children

Pediatric drug dosages should be calculated on the basis of body surface area or body weight. If your pediatric patient is average size, find his weight and corresponding surface area in the box. Otherwise, to use the nomogram, lay a straightedge on the correct height and weight points for your patient, and find the point where it intersects on the surface area scale. *Note:* In premature or full-term newborns, base drug dosages on body weight rather than on body surface area.

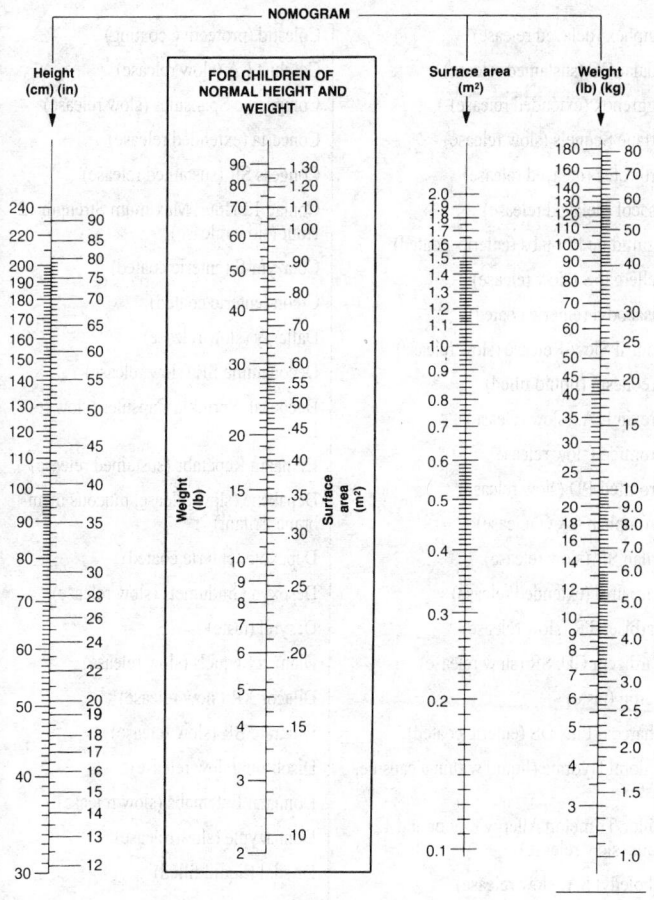

Drugs that shouldn't be crushed

Many drug forms, such as slow-release, enteric-coated, encapsulated beads, wax-matrix, sublingual, and buccal forms, are made to release their active ingredients over a certain period of time or at preset points after administration. The disruptions caused by crushing these drug forms can dramatically affect the absorption rate and increase the risk of adverse reactions.

Other reasons not to crush these drug forms include such considerations as taste, tissue irritation, and unusual formulation—for example, a capsule within a capsule, a liquid within a capsule, or a multiple-compressed tablet. Avoid crushing the following drugs, listed by brand name, for the reasons noted beside them.

Aciphex (delayed release)

Adalat CC (sustained release)

Aggrenox (extended release)

Artane Sequels (slow release)

Arthrotec (delayed release)

Asacol (delayed release)

Azulfidine EN-tabs (enteric coated)

Bellergal-S (slow release)

Bisacodyl (enteric coated)

Bontril Slow-Release (slow release)

Breonesin (liquid filled)

Brexin L.A. (slow release)

Bromfed (slow release)

Bromfed-PD (slow release)

Bromphen (slow release)

Calan SR (slow release)

Carbatrol (extended release)

Carbiset-TR (slow release)

Cardizem CD, SR (slow release)

Ceftin (taste)

Charcoal Plus DS (enteric coated)

Chloral Hydrate (liquid within a capsule, taste)

Chlor-Trimeton Allergy 8-hour and 12-hour (slow release)

Choledyl SA (slow release)

Cipro (taste)

Colace (liquid within a capsule, taste)

Colazal

Colestid (protective coating)

Comhist LA (slow release)

Compazine Spansules (slow release)

Concerta (extended release)

Congess SR (sustained release)

Contac 12 Hour, Maximum Strength 12 Hour (slow release)

Cotazym-S (enteric coated)

Creon (enteric coated)

Dallergy (slow release)

Deconamine SR (slow release)

Deconsal, Sprinkle Capsules (slow release)

Demazin Repetabs (sustained release)

Depakene (slow release, mucous membrane irritant)

Depakote (enteric coated)

Desoxyn Gradumets (slow release)

Desyrel (taste)

Diamox Sequels (slow release)

Dilacor XR (slow release)

Dilatrate-SR (slow release)

Disobrom (slow release)

Donnatal Extentabs (slow release)

Donnazyme (slow release)

Drisdol (liquid filled)

Drixoral (slow release)

Drixoral Sinus (slow release)

Drize (slow release)

Dulcolax (enteric coated)

Ecotrin (enteric coated)

Ecotrin Maximum Strength (enteric coated)

E.E.S. 400 Filmtab (enteric coated)

Effexor XR (extended release)

E-Mycin (enteric coated)

Endafed (slow release)

Entex LA (slow release)

Equanil (taste)

Eryc (enteric coated)

Ery-Tab (enteric coated)

Erythrocin Stearate (enteric coated)

Erythromycin Base (enteric coated)

Eskalith CR (slow release)

Fedahist Gyrocaps, Timecaps (slow release)

Feldene (mucous membrane irritant)

Feocyte (slow release)

Feosol (enteric coated)

Feratab (enteric coated)

Fergon (slow release)

Fero-Grad-500 (slow release)

Ferro-Sequel (slow release)

Feverall Children's Capsules, Sprinkle (taste)

Fumatinic (slow release)

Geocillin (taste)

Gris-PEG (crushing may cause precipitation of larger particles)

Guaifed (slow release)

Guaifed-PD (slow release)

Humibid Sprinkle, DM, DM Sprinkle, LA (slow release)

Hydergine LC (liquid within a capsule)

Hytakerol (liquid filled)

Iberet (slow release)

Iberet-500 (slow release)

ICAPS Plus (slow release)

ICAPS Time Release (slow release)

Ilotycin (enteric coated)

Inderal LA (slow release)

Inderide LA (slow release)

Indocin SR (slow release)

Ionamin (slow release)

Isoptin SR (slow release)

Isordil Sublingual (sublingual)

Isordil Tembids (slow release)

Isosorbide Dinitrate Sublingual (sublingual)

Isuprel Glossets (sublingual)

Kaon-Cl (slow release)

K-Dur (slow release)

Klor-Con (slow release)

Klotrix (slow release)

K-Tab (slow release)

Levsinex Timecaps (slow release)

Lithobid (slow release)

Mestinon Timespans (slow release)

Methylin ER (extended release)

Micro-K (slow release)

Micro-K Extencaps (slow release)

Motrin (taste)

MS Contin (slow release)

Nexium (sustained release)

Nitro-Bid (slow release)

Nitroglyn (slow release)

Nitrong (sublingual)

Nitrostat (sublingual)

Nolamine (slow release)

Norflex (slow release)

Norpace CR (slow release)

Novafed A (slow release)

Oramorph SR (slow release)

Ornade Spansules (slow release)

Pancrease (enteric coated)	Slow-Mag (slow release)
Pancrease MT (enteric coated)	Sorbitrate SA (slow release)
PCE (slow release)	Sparine (taste)
Pentasa (controlled release)	Sudafed 12 Hour (slow release)
Perdiem (wax coated)	Sustaire (slow release)
Phazyme (slow release)	Tamine S.R. (slow release)
Phazyme 95 (slow release)	Tavist-D (multiple compressed tablet)
Phenergan (taste)	Tegretol-XR (extended release)
Phyllocontin (slow release)	Teldrin (slow release)
Plendil (slow release)	Teldrin Spansules (slow release)
Polaramine Repetabs (slow release)	Ten-K (slow release)
Prelu-2 (slow release)	Tenuate Dospan (slow release)
Prevacid (delayed release)	Tessalon Perles (slow release)
Prilosec (slow release)	Theobid Duracaps (slow release)
Pro-Banthine (taste)	Theochron (slow release)
Procainamide HCl SR (slow release)	Theoclear LA (slow release)
Procardia (delayed absorption)	Theo-Dur (slow release)
Procardia XL (slow release)	Theolair-SR (slow release)
Pronestyl-SR (slow release)	Theo-Sav (slow release)
Protonix (delayed release)	Theospan-SR (slow release)
Proventil Repetabs (slow release)	Theo-24 (slow release)
Prozac (slow release)	Theovent (slow release)
Quibron-T/SR (slow release)	Theo-X (slow release)
Quinaglute Dura-Tabs (slow release)	Thorazine Spansules (slow release)
Quinidex Extentabs (slow release)	Tiazac (extended release)
Respaire SR (slow release)	Topamax (bitter taste)
Respbid (slow release)	Toprol XL (slow release)
Ritalin-SR (slow release)	T-Phyl (slow release)
Rondec-TR (slow release)	Tranxene-SD (slow release)
Ru-Tuss (slow release)	Trental (slow release)
Ru-Tuss DE, II (slow release)	Triaminic (slow release)
Sinemet CR (slow release)	Triaminic TR (slow release)
Slo-bid Gyrocaps (slow release)	Triaminic-12 (slow release)
Slo-Niacin (slow release)	Trilafon Repetabs (slow release)
Slo-Phyllin GG, Gyrocaps (slow release)	Trinalin Repetabs (slow release)
Slow FE (slow release)	Triptone Caplets (slow release)
Slow-K (slow release)	Tuss-LA (slow release)

Tuss-Ornade Spansules (slow release)

Tylenol Extended Relief (slow release)

ULR-LA (slow release)

Uniphyl (slow release)

Verelan (slow release)

Voltaren (enteric coated)

Voltaren-XR (enteric coated)

Wellbutrin SR (sustained release)

Wygesic (taste)

ZORprin (slow release)

Zyban (slow release)

Zymase (enteric coated)

English-Spanish drug phrase translator

Medication history

Do you take any medications?
- Prescription?
- Over-the-counter?
- Other?

¿Toma Ud. medicamentos?
- ¿De receta?
- ¿Sin necesidad de receta?
- ¿Otro?

Which prescription medications do you take routinely?
- How often do you take them?
  - Once daily?
  - Twice daily?
  - Three times daily?
  - Four times daily?
  - More often?

¿Qué medicamentos de receta toma Ud. por rutina?
- ¿Con qué frecuencia los toma?
  - ¿Una vez al día?
  - ¿Dos veces al día?
  - ¿Tres veces al día?
  - ¿Cuátro veces al día?
  - ¿Con más frecuencia?

Which over-the-counter medications do you take routinely?
- How often do you take them?
- Once daily?
- Twice daily?
- Three times daily?
- Four times daily?
- More often?

¿Qué medicamentos que no necesitan receta toma Ud. por rutina?
- ¿Con que frecuencia los toma?
- ¿Una vez al día?
- ¿Dos veces al día?
- ¿Tres veces al día?
- ¿Cuatro veces al día?
- ¿Con más frecuencia?

Which medications do you take periodically?

¿Qué medicamentos toma Ud. periódicamente?

Why do you take these medications?

¿Por qué toma Ud. estos medicamentos?

What is the dosage for each medication?

¿Cuál es la dosis para cada uno de los medicamentos?

How does each medication make you feel?

¿Cómo le hace sentirse cada medicamento?

Are you allergic to any medications?

¿Está Ud. alérgico(a) a algúnos medicamentos?

- Which medications?
- What happens when you have an allergic reaction?

- ¿A qué medicamentos?
- ¿Qué pasa cuando Ud. tiene una reacción alérgica?

Medication teaching

PURPOSE OF THE MEDICATION
This medication will:
- elevate your blood pressure.
- improve circulation to your _____.

- lower your blood pressure.
- lower your blood sugar.

Este medicamento hará que:
- su presión sanguínea suba.
- la circulación por (la región del cuerpo) mejore.
- su presión sanguínea baje.
- el nivel de azucar en la sangre baje.

– make your heart rhythm more even.
– raise your blood sugar.
– reduce or prevent the formation of blood clots.
– remove fluid from your body.
– remove fluid from your feet, ankles, or legs.
– remove fluid from your lungs so that they work better.
– remove fluid from your pancreas so that it works better.

– el ritmo del corazón sea más uniforme.
– su nivel de azucar en la sangre suba.
– se reduzca o evite la formación de coágulos de sangre.
– se le quite fluido en el cuerpo.
– se le quite fluido de los pies, tobillos o piernas.
– se le quite fluido de los pulmones para que funcionen mejor.
– se le quite fluido de la páncreas para que funcione mejor.

This medication will help your body to:

– kill the bacteria in your _____.

– slow down your heart rate.
– soften your bowel movements.
– speed up your heart rate.
– use insulin more efficiently.

Este medicamento le ayudará a su cuerpo a:

– destruir la bacteria de la (región infectada).
– reducir el latir del corazón.
– ablandar sus evacuaciones.
– acelerar el latir del corazón.
– usar la insulina más eficazmente.

This medication will help you to:

– breathe better.
– fight infections.
– relax.
– sleep.
– think more clearly.

Este medicamento le ayudará a Ud. a:

– respirar con mayor facilidad.
– luchar contra infecciones.
– relajarse.
– dormir.
– pensar con mayor claridad.

This medication will relieve or reduce:

– the acid production in your stomach.
– anxiety.
– bladder spasms.
– burning in your stomach or chest.
– burning when you urinate.
– diarrhea.
– muscle cramps.
– nausea.
– pain in your _____.

Este medicamento le aliviará o disminuirá:

– la producción de acido en el estómago.
– la angustia.
– espasmos en la vejiga.
– sensación ardiente en el estómago o tórax.
– sensación ardiente al orinar.
– diarrea.
– espasmos en los músculos.
– nausea.
– dolor en la (el) _____.

This medication will help your body to produce more or less:

– antibodies.
– clotting factors.
– insulin.
– platelets.
– red blood cells.
– white blood cells.

Este medicamento le ayudará a su cuerpo a producir más o menos:

– anticuerpos.
– factores o agentes coagulantes.
– insulina.
– plaquetas.
– células rojas de sangre.
– células blancas de sangre.

This medication or treatment will destroy:

– antibodies.
– bacteria.
– cancer cells.
– clotting factors.
– platelets.

Este medicamento o tratamiento destruirá:

– anticuerpos.
– bacteria.
– células cancerosas.
– factores o agentes coagulantes.
– plaquetas.

– red blood cells.

– white blood cells.

– células rojas de sangre.

– células blancas de sangre.

MEDICATION ADMINISTRATION

I would like to give you:

– an injection.

– an I.V. medication.

– a liquid medication.

– a medicated cream or powder.

– a medication through your epidural
  catheter.

– a medication through your rectum.

– a medication through your _____ tube.

– a medication under your tongue.

– some pill(s).

– a suppository.

Quisiera darle a Ud. un(a):

– inyección.

– medicamento por vía intravenosa.

– medicamento en forma líquida.

– medicamento en pomada o polvo.

– medicamento por el catéter epidural.

– medicamento por el recto.

– medicamento por su _____ tubo.

– medicamento debajo de la lengua.

– píldoras.

– supositorio.

This is how you take this medication.

Así se toma este medicamento.

If you can't swallow this pill, I can crush
it and mix it in some food or liquid
such as:

– applesauce.

– pudding.

– yogurt.

Si Ud. no se puede tragar esta píldora,
puedo aplastarla y mezclarla en un ali-
mento/líquido, tal como:

– puré de manzana.

– pudín.

– yogur.

If you can't swallow this pill, I can get it
in another form.

Si Ud. no puede tragarse esta píldora,
puede obtenerla en otra forma.

If you can't swallow a pill, you can crush
it and mix it in soft food.

Si Ud. no se puede tragar la píldora, la
puede moler y mezclarla en un alimento
blando.

I need to mix this medication in juice or
water.

Tengo que mezclar este medicamento en
jugo (zumo) o agua.

I need to give you this injection in your:

– abdomen.

– buttocks.

– hip.

– outer arm.

– thigh.

Tengo que ponerle esta inyección:

– en el abdomen.

– en las nalgas.

– en la cadera.

– en el brazo.

– en el muslo.

I need to give you this medication I.V.

Tengo que darle este medicamento por
vía intravenosa (I.V.).

Place it under your tongue.

Póngaselo debajo de la lengua.

You should feel some burning when it is
under your tongue.

Ud. debiera sentir un ardor cuando se lo
pone debajo de la lengua.

This indicates that it is working.

Esto indica que está tomando efecto.

Some medications are coated with a special substance to protect your stomach
from getting upset.

Algunos medicamentos están cubiertos
con una sustancia especial para prote-
gerle contra un trastorno estomacal.

Do not chew:
- enteric-coated pills.
- long-acting pills.
- capsules.
- sublingual medication.

No masque Ud.:
- píldoras con recubrimientoentérico.
- píldoras de efecto prolongado.
- cápsulas.
- medicamentos sublinguales.

Ask your doctor or pharmacist whether you can:
- mix your medication with food or fluids.
- take your medication with or without food.

Pregúntele Ud. a su doctor o farmacéutico si debiera:
- mezclar su medicamento con un alimento o con líquidos.
- tomar su medicamento con o sin alimento.

You need to take your medication:
- after meals.
- before meals.
- on an empty stomach.
- with meals or food.

Ud. tiene que tomarse el medicamento:
- después de las comidas.
- antes de las comidas.
- con el estómago vacío.
- con las comidas o con un alimento.

SKIPPING DOSES
If you skip or miss a dose:
- Take it as soon as you remember it.
- Wait until the next dose.
- Call the doctor if you are not sure.
- Do not take an extra dose.

Si Ud. omite o se salta una dosis:
- Tómesela encuanto se acuerde.
- Espérese hasta la siguiente dosis.
- Llame al doctor si Ud. no está seguro(a).
- No se tome una dosis extra.

ADVERSE EFFECTS
Some common adverse effects of _____ are:
- constipation
- diarrhea
- difficulty sleeping
- dry mouth
- fatigue
- headache
- itching
- light-headedness
- nausea
- poor appetite
- rash
- upset stomach
- weight loss or gain
- frequent urination.

Unos efectos adversos comunes a _____ son:
- estreñimiento
- diarrea
- dificultad en dormir
- boca seca
- fatiga
- dolor de cabeza
- comezón (picazón)
- mareo
- nausea
- poco apetito
- erupción
- trastorno estomacal
- perdida o aumento de peso
- orinar con frecuencia.

These adverse effects:
- will go away after your body gets used to the medication.
- may persist as long as you take the medication.

Estos efectos adversos:
- desaparecerán una vez que su cuerpo se acostumbre al medicamento.
- puede continuar mientras Ud. tome el medicamento.

If they bother you, speak to your doctor about changing your medication.

Si le molestan a Ud., hable con su doctor acerca de que le cambie el medicamento.

If you have an adverse reaction to your medication, call your doctor right away.

Si Ud. tiene una reacción adversa a su medicamento, llame a su doctor inmediatamente.

OTHER CONCERNS
Tell your doctor if you are pregnant or breast-feeding.

Dígale a su doctor si Ud. está ebarazada o si cría a los pechos.

While you are taking this medication, ask your doctor if:
– you can safely take other over-the-counter medications.
– you can drink alcoholic beverages.
– your medications interact with each other.

Mientras Ud. tome este medicamento, pregúntele a su doctor si:
– puede tomar otros medicamentos que no necesitan receta.
– puede tomar bebidas alcohólicas.
– sus medicamentos interaccionan uno con el otro.

STORING MEDICATION
You should keep your medication:
– in a cool, dry place.
– in the refrigerator.
– at room temperature.
– out of direct sunlight.
– away from heat.
– away from children.

Ud. debiera guardar sus medicamentos:
– en un lugar fresco, seco.
– en el refrigerador.
– al tiempo.
– fuera de la luz de sol.
– lejos de la calefacción.
– lejos del alcance de los niños.

Do not keep your medication:
– in a warm place or near heat.

– in the sun.
– in your pocket.
– in the bathroom medicine cabinet.

No guarde Ud. su medicamento:
– en un lugar caliente ni cerca de la calefacción.
– en el sol.
– en su bolsillo.
– en el botiquín del baño.

TEACHING A PATIENT TO GIVE A SUBCUTANEOUS INJECTION
To give yourself an injection, follow these steps:
– Draw up the medication.
– Replace the cap carefully.
– Decide where you are going to give the injection.
– Clean the skin area with alcohol.
– Gently pinch up a little skin over the area.
– Using a dartlike motion, stab the needle into your skin.
– Gently pull back on the plunger to see if there is any blood in the syringe.
– Steadily push the medication into your skin.
– Pull the needle out.
– Apply gentle pressure with the alcohol wipe.
– Dispose of the needle in a proper receptacle.

Así es como uno se pone una inyección a sí mismo(a):
– Saque el medicamento.
– Coloque de nuevo la tapa con cuidado.
– Decida Ud. donde va a ponerse la inyección.
– Limpie el área de la piel con alcohol.
– Suavemente pellizque un poco de piel sobre el área.
– Con un movimiento rápido, penetre la aguja en su piel.
– Con cuidado retire el émbolo para ver si hay sangre en la jeringa.
– Constantemente empuje el medicamento dentro de su piel.
– Saque la aguja.
– Ejerza presión suavemente con un limpión de alcohol.
– Deshagase de la aguja en un recipiente apropiado.

INSULIN PREPARATION AND ADMINISTRATION

The doctor has ordered insulin for you.

El doctor ha recetado insulina para Ud.

To draw up insulin, follow these steps:

Para extraer la insulina siga las siguientes pasos:

– Wipe the rubber top of the insulin bottle with alcohol.
– Remove the needle cap.
– Pull out the plunger until the end of the plunger in the barrel aligns with the number of units of insulin that you need.

– Push the needle through the rubber top of the insulin bottle.
– Inject the air into the bottle.
– Without removing the needle from the bottle, turn it upside down.
– Withdraw the plunger until the end of the plunger aligns with the number of units you need.
– Gently pull the needle out of the bottle.

– Limpie la tapa de hule (goma) de la botella de la insulina con alcohol.
– Quítele el capuchón a la aguja.
– Saque el émbolo hasta el otro extremo del émbolo en la cuba esté al nivel de la dosis de insulina (número de unidades) que Ud. necesita.
– Empuje la aguja por la tapa de hule (goma) de la botella de insulina.
– Inyecte el aire dentro de la botella.
– Sin sacar la aguja de la botella, póngala al revés.
– Retire el émbolo hasta que llegue la insulina al número de unidades que Ud. necesita.
– Retire Ud. la aguja de la botella suavemente.

To mix insulin, follow these steps:

Para mezclar la insulina siga los siguientes pasos:

– Wipe the rubber tops of the insulin bottles with alcohol.
– Gently roll the cloudy insulin between your palms.
– Remove the needle cap.
– Pull out the plunger until the end of the plunger in the barrel aligns with the number of units of NPH or Lente insulin that you need.

– Push the needle through the rubber top of the cloudy insulin bottle.
– Inject the air into the bottle.
– Remove the needle.
– Pull out the plunger until the end of the plunger in the barrel aligns with the number of units of clear regular insulin that you need.

– Limpie la tapa de hule (goma) de las botellas de insulina con alcohol.
– Suavemente mueva la insulina turbia entre las palmas de la mano.
– Retire el capuchón de la aguja.
– Saque el émbolo hasta que el otro extremo del émbolo en el barril esté al nivel con la dosis de insulina turbia (NPH o insulina Lente) (número de unidades) que Ud. necesita.
– Empuje la aguja por la tapa de goma (hule) de la botella de insulina turbia.
– Inyecte el aire dentro de la botella.
– Saque la aguja.
– Retire el émbolo hasta que el otro extremo del émbolo en el barril esté al nivel con la dosis de insulina clara (regular) (número de unidades) que Ud. necesita.

– Push the needle through the rubber top of the clear insulin bottle.
– Inject the air into the bottle.
– Without removing the needle, turn the bottle upside down.
– Withdraw the plunger until it aligns with the number of units of clear regular insulin that you need.
– Gently pull the needle out of the bottle.

– Empuje Ud. la aguja por la tapa de goma de la botella de insulna clara.
– Inyecte el aire dentro de la botella.
– Sin sacar la aguja, vuelva la botella al revés.
– Retire el émbolo hasta que llegue a la dosis de insulina (regular) clara (número de unidades) que Ud. necesita.
– Suavemente saque Ud. la aguja de la botella.

– Push the needle into the cloudy (NPH or Lente) insulin without injecting it into the bottle.

– Empuje la aguja en la insulina turbia (NPH o insulina Lente) sin inyectarla dentro de la botella.

– Withdraw the plunger until you reach your total dosage of insulin in units (regular combined with NPH or Lente).

– Retire el émbolo hasta que llegue a su dosis total de insulina en unidades (regular y NPH/Lente conbinadas).

– We will practice again.

– Practicaremos juntos(as) otra vez.

Home care phrases

Wash your hands before touching medications.

Lávese Ud. las manos antes de tocar los medicamentos.

Check the medication bottle for name, dose, and frequency (how often it's supposed to be taken).

En el envase del medicamento verifique Ud. el nombre, la dosis y la frecuencia (con que frequencia se debe tomar).

Check the expiration date on all medications.

Verifique Ud. la fecha en la que el medicamento expira.

Store medications according to pharmacy instructions.

Guarde Ud. los medicamentos según las instrucciones de la farmacia.

Under adequate lighting, read medication labels carefully before taking doses.

Bajo luz adecuada, lea Ud. la etiqueta del medicamento con mucho cuidado antes de tomar las dosis.

Don't crush medication without first asking the doctor or pharmacist.

No machaque Ud. el medicamento sin antes preguntárselo al doctor o al farmacéutico.

Contact your doctor if a new or unexpected symptom or another problem appears.

Póngase Ud. en contacto con su doctor si un síntoma nuevo o inesperado u otros problemas aparecen.

Do not stop taking medication unless instructed by your doctor.

No deje Ud. de tomar el medicamento sólo que se lo ordene su doctor.

Discard outdated medications.

Deshágase Ud. de medicamentos caducos.

Never take someone else's medications.

Nunca tome Ud. los medicamentos de otra persona.

Keep a record of your current medications.

Apunte Ud. (tome nota de) sus medicamentos actuales.

General drug therapy phrases

DRUG CLASSES

Analgesic	Analgésico
Anesthetic	Anestético
Antacid	Antiácido
Antianginal agent	Agente antianginal
Antianxiety agent	Agente ansiolítico
Antiarrhythmic agent	Agente antiarrítmico
Antibiotic	Antibiótico
Anticancer agent	Agente anticarcinógeno

English	Spanish
Anticoagulant	Anticoagulante
Anticonvulsant	Anticonvulsivante
Antidepressant	Antidepresivo
Antidiarrheal	Antidiarreico
Antifungal agent	Agente antifúngico
Antigout agent	Agente antigota
Antihistamine	Antihistamínico
Antihyperlipemic agent	Agente hiperlipémico
Antihypertensive agent	Agente antihipertenso
Anti-inflammatory agent	Agente antiinflamatorio
Antimalarial agent	Agente antimalárico
Antiparkinsonian agent	Agente antiparkinsoniano
Antipsychotic agent	Agente antipsicótico
Antipyretic	Antipirético
Antiseptic	Antiséptico
Antispasmodic	Antiespasmódico
Antithyroid agent	Agente antitiroideo
Antituberculosis agent	Agente antituberculoso
Antitussive agent	Agente antitusígeno
Antiviral agent	Agente antiviral
Appetite stimulant	Estimulante para el apetito
Appetite suppressant	Supresor de apetito
Bronchodilator	Broncodilatador
Decongestant	Descongestivo
Digestant	Digestivo (agente que estimula la digestión)
Diuretic	Diurético
Emetic	Emético
Fertility agent	Agente para la fertilidad
Hypnotic	Hipnótico
Insulin	Insulina
Laxative	Laxante
Muscle relaxant	Relajante de músculos
Oral contraceptive	Anticonceptivo oral
Oral hypoglycemic agent	Agente hipoglucémico oral
Sedative	Sedante
Steroid	Esteroide
Thyroid hormone	Hormona de la glándula tiroides
Vaccine	Vacuna
Vasodilator	Vasodilatador
Vitamin	Vitamina

ROUTES

Intradermal	Intradérmica
Intramuscular	Intramuscular
Intravenous	Intravenosa
Oral	Oral
Rectal	Rectal
Subcutaneous	Subcutánea
Topical	Tópica
Vaginal	Vaginal

PREPARATIONS

Capsule	Cápsula
Cream	Pomada
Drops	Gotas
Elixir	Elixir
Injection	Inyección
Inhaler	Inhalador
Lotion	Loción
Lozenge	Pastilla
Powder	Polvo
Spray	Atomizador
Suppository	Supositorio
Suspension	Suspensión
Syrup	Jarabe
Tablet	Tableta

FREQUENCY

Once daily	Una vez al día
Twice daily	Dos veces al día
Three times daily	Tres veces al día
Four times daily	Cuatro veces al día
In the morning	Por la mañana
With meals	Con las comidas
Before meals	Antes de las comidas
After meals	Después de las comidas
Before bedtime	Antes de acostarse
When you have_____	Cuando Ud. tome_____
Only when you need it	Sólo cuando lo necesite
Every four hours	Cada cuatro horas
Every six hours	Cada seis horas
Every eight hours	Cada ocho horas

Acknowledgments

We would like to thank the following companies for granting us permission to include their drugs in the full-color photoguide. We would also like to thank Facts and Comparisons for the use of their resources.

Abbott Laboratories
Biaxin®, Biaxin® XL, Depakote®, Depakote® Sprinkle, E-Mycin®, Ery-Tab®, Hytrin®, Isoptin® SR, Synthroid®, Vicodin®, Vicodin ES®

AstraZeneca LP
Elavil®, Nolvadex®, Prilosec®, Tenormin®, Toprol-XL®, Zestril®

Aventis Pharmaceuticals
Allegra®, Carafate®, DiaBeta®, Lasix®, Trental®

Bayer Corporation
Cipro®

Biovail Corporation
Cardizem®, Cardizem® CD, Cardizem® SR

Bristol-Myers Squibb Company
BuSpar®, Capoten®, Cefzil®, Coumadin®, Desyrel®, Glucophage®, Glucophage® XR, Monopril®, Pravachol®, Serzone®

Forest Pharmaceuticals, Inc.
Celexa®, Levothroid®

Geneva Pharmaceuticals
Trimox®, Pen VK

GlaxoSmithKline
Amoxil®, Amoxil® Chewable, Augmentin®, Augmentin® Chewable, Avandia®, Ceftin®, Compazine®, Coreg®, Imitrex®, Lanoxicaps®, Lanoxin®, Paxil®, Relafen®, Tagamet®, Wellbutrin®, Wellbutrin SR®, Wellcovorin®, Zantac®, Zovirax®, Zyban®

Janssen Pharmaceutica, Inc.
Risperdal®

King Pharmaceuticals, Inc.
Altace®, Levoxyl®

Eli Lilly and Company
Evista®, Prozac®, Sarafem®

Mallinckrodt, Inc.
Pamelor®, Restoril®

McNeil-PPC, Inc.
Concerta®, Motrin®

Merck & Co., Inc.
Cozaar®, Fosamax®, HydroDIURIL®, Mevacor®, Pepcid®, Prinivil®, Singulair®, Vasotec®, Vioxx®, Zocor®

Novartis Pharma Corporation
Gleevec®, Lescol®, Lotensin®, Ritalin®, Ritalin SR®

Ortho-McNeil Pharmaceutical
Levaquin®, Tylenol® with Codeine, Ultracet®

Parke-Davis
Accupril®, Dilantin® Infatabs®, Dilantin® Kapseals®, Lipitor®, Lopid®, Neurontin®, Nitrostat®

Pfizer, Inc.
Cardura®, Celebrex®, Diflucan®, Glucotrol®, Glucotrol XL®, Norvasc®, Procardia®, Procardia XL®, Viagra®, Zithromax®, Zoloft®, Zyrtec®

Pharmacia Corporation
Ambien®, Calan®, Daypro®, Deltasone®, Demulen®, Detrol®, Medrol®, Micronase®, Provera®, Xanax®

Proctor and Gamble Pharmaceuticals, Inc.
Actonel®, Macrobid®

Purdue Pharma L.P.
OxyContin®

Roche Laboratories, Inc.
Bumex®, Klonopin®, Naprosyn®,
Ticlid®, Valium®

Sanofi-Synthelabo, Inc.
Demerol®

**Schering Corporation and Key
Pharmaceuticals, Inc.**
Claritin®, Claritin® Reditabs®, K-Dur®

Schwarz Pharma
Verelan®

Tap Pharmaceuticals, Inc.
Prevacid®

UCB Pharmaceuticals, Inc.
Lortab®

Wallace Laboratories
Soma®

Warner Chilcott Laboratories, Inc.
Eryc®, Estrace®

Women First HealthCare, Inc.
Bactrim DS®

Wyeth-Ayerst Laboratories
Effexor®, Effexor® XR, Inderal®,
Inderal® LA, Phenergan®, Premarin®,
Sonata®

Index

---

t refers to a table; **boldface** refers to full-color photographs.

t refers to a table; **boldface** refers to full-color photographs.

t refers to a table; **boldface** refers to full-color photographs.

t refers to a table; **boldface** refers to full-color photographs.

t refers to a table; **boldface** refers to full-color photographs.

t refers to a table; **boldface** refers to full-color photographs.

Lymphoma *(continued)*
cyclophosphamide for, 908
doxorubicin for, 939
interferon alfa-2b, recombinant, for, 1073
methotrexate for, 929
thiotepa for, 917
vinblastine for, 998
vincristine for, 999-1000
Lymphosarcoma
bleomycin for, 933
chlorambucil for, 905
mechlorethamine for, 913
methotrexate for, 929
vinblastine for, 998
Lysodren, 982

M

Maalox Antacid Caplets, 652
Maalox Antacid Plus Anti-Gas Extra Strength, 650
Maalox Anti-Diarrheal Caplets, 663
Maalox Plus, 650
Maalox Tablets, 650
Maalox Therapeutic Concentrate Suspension, 650
Macrobid, 203, 212, **C20**
Macrocytic anemia, folic acid for, 1178
Macrodantin, 212
Macrodex, 847
Macrolide anti-infectives, 196-202
Macroprolactinoma, bromocriptine for, 510
Madopar‡, 509
Madopar HBS‡, 509
Madopar Q‡, 509
magaldrate, 653-654
Magnaprin, 341
Magnaprin Arthritis Strength, 341
magnesium chloride, 850-851
magnesium citrate, 671-672
magnesium hydroxide, 671-672
Magnesium intoxication, calcium salts for, 845
magnesium oxide, 654-655
magnesium sulfate, 417-418, 671-672, 850-851
Magnesium supplementation, magnesium salts for, 850
Mag-Ox 400, 654
Malaria
atovaquone and proguanil for, 39
chloroquine for, 41
doxycycline for, 125
hydroxychloroquine for, 42
mefloquine for, 43
primaquine for, 44-45
pyrimethamine for, 45-46

Malaria *(continued)*
quinidine for, 242
sulfadiazine for, 133
tetracycline for, 128
Malarone, 39
Malarone Pediatric, 39
Male pattern hair loss
finasteride for, 1253
minoxidil for, 1264
Malignant effusions
bleomycin for, 933
mechlorethamine for, 913
thiotepa for, 917
Malignant hyperthermic crisis, dantrolene for, 575
Mallamint, 844
Malogen†, 727
manganese, 1193-1194
manganese chloride, 1193-1194
Manganese deficiency, manganese for, 1194
manganese sulfate, 1193-1194
Mania
chlorpromazine for, 472
divalproex sodium for, 428
lithium for, 530
mannitol, 835-837
Mantoux test, 1320-1321t
Maox, 654
Marax, 604
Marax-DF Syrup, 604
Marcaine, 1314t
Marinol, 680
Marvelon§, 749
Mastocytosis
cimetidine for, 690
cromolyn sodium for, 639
Matulane, 990
Mavik, 309
Maxair, 622
Maxair Autohaler, 622
Maxalt, 538
Maxalt-MLT, 538
Maxenal†, 566
Maxeran†, 683
Maxidex, 1094
Maxiflor, 1164
Maxipime, 99
Maxitrol Ointment/Ophthalmic Suspension, 1084
Maxivate, 1160
Maxolon‡, 683
Maxzide, 266, 823
Maxzide-25mg, 823
MCT, 1200
measles, mumps, and rubella virus vaccine, live, 1031-1033
measles and rubella virus vaccine, live attenuated, 1033
Measles exposure, immune globulin for, 1056

Measles immunization
measles, mumps, and rubella virus vaccine, live, for, 1032
measles and rubella virus vaccine, live attenuated, for, 1033
measles virus vaccine, live attenuated, for, 1034
measles virus vaccine, live attenuated, 1034-1035
mebendazole, 19
Mechanical ventilation, facilitating
atracurium for, 579
cisatracurium for, 581
mivacurium for, 584
pancuronium for, 585
rocuronium for, 587
succinylcholine for, 588
tubocurarine for, 590
vecuronium for, 591
mechlorethamine hydrochloride, 913-914
meclizine hydrochloride, 682-683
meclozine hydrochloride, 682-683
Medigesic, 341
Medihaler-Iso, 616
Medipren, 355
medium-chain triglycerides, 1200
Medralone-40, 712
Medralone-80, 712
Medrol, 712, **C19**
Medrone§, 712
medroxyprogesterone acetate, 754-755
medroxyprogesterone acetate and estradiol cipionate, 756-757
mefloquine hydrochloride, 43-44
Mefoxin, 109
Megace, 959
Megace OS†, 959
Megacillin†, 81
Megaloblastic anemia
folic acid for, 1178
leucovorin for, 1179
megestrol acetate, 959
Megostat‡, 959
Meibomianitis, gentamicin for, 1088
Melanoma
dacarbazine for, 973
hydroxyurea for, 927
interferon alfa-2b, recombinant, for, 1072-1073
melatonin, 1295t
Melipramine‡, 443
Mellaril, 490
Mellaril Concentrate, 490

---

t refers to a table; **boldface** refers to full-color photographs.

t refers to a table; **boldface** refers to full-color photographs.

---

t refers to a table; **boldface** refers to full-color photographs.

---

t refers to a table; **boldface** refers to full-color photographs.

Visit NDHnow.com

The Web site of *Nursing2003 Drug Handbook* gives you:
- updates on recently approved drugs, new indications, and new warnings
- patient-teaching aids on new drugs, administration techniques, and supportive measures
- news summaries on recent drug developments
- clinical pearls of wisdom
- links to pharmaceutical companies, government agencies, and nursing organizations
- continuing education tests for *Nursing2003 Drug Handbook* and *Nursing Herbal Medicine Handbook*
- career opportunities
- a nursing bookstore.

About NDH2003*Plus!*

NDH2003*Plus!* mini-CD lets you:
- take 10 continuing education tests (and earn up to 40 contact hours)
- customize and print patient-teaching instructions for 200 of the most commonly prescribed drugs, in regular or large print
- view and print monographs on the same 200 common drugs
- learn about potentially dangerous drug interactions
- link directly to **NDHnow.com** for drug updates and important drug news.

Windows system requirements
- Windows 95 or higher
- Pentium 166 or higher
- 64 MB RAM
- 40 MB free hard-disk space

- SVGA monitor with high color (16-bit). Display area must be set to 800 x 600, and display font size must be set to "Small fonts."
- CD-ROM drive and mouse

CAUTION: Don't try to use this mini-CD in a floppy disk drive, Zip drive, certain slot drives, or a car stereo. Don't insert the mini-CD into a CD-ROM drive that requires the mini-CD to be in a vertical position. Placing the CD into such a drive may result in jamming.

Before installing this program, make sure your monitor is set up to display high color (16-bit), your display area is set to 800 x 600, and your display font size is set to "Small fonts." If it isn't, consult your user's manual for instructions about changing the display settings.

To install on Windows 95 or higher:
- Place the mini-CD on the inner ring of the CD-ROM drive tray. Close the tray.
- In a few moments, the CD should automatically start. Once it starts, click the "Install NDH2003*Plus!*" button to install on your computer.

- Click "Start" and select "Run" if the CD doesn't start automatically.
- Type **d:\setup** (where **d** is the letter of your CD-ROM drive), and click *OK*. Follow on-screen instructions for installing the CD.